THE TORONTO NOTES 2009

A comprehensive medical reference and review for the
Medical Council of Canada Qualifying Exam – Part 1 and the
United States Medical Licensing Exam – Step 2

25th Edition

Editors-in-Chief:
Sagar Dugani and Danica Lam

*Life so short, the art so long,
opportunity fleeting, experiment treacherous,
judgement difficult.*

– Hippocrates

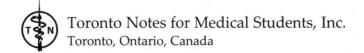
Toronto Notes for Medical Students, Inc.
Toronto, Ontario, Canada

Twenty-fifth Edition

Cover design and photography: Dennis Wei & Jennifer Belanger
Illustrations: Biomedical Communications, University of Toronto
Clipart images: Copyright TASK FORCE ImageGALLERY, © NVTech Inc., Type & Graphics Inc.

Notice:
THIS PUBLICATION HAS NOT BEEN AUTHORED, REVIEWED OR OTHERWISE SUPPORTED BY THE MEDICAL COUNCIL OF CANADA NOR DOES IT RECEIVE ENDORSEMENT BY THE MEDICAL COUNCIL AS REVIEW MATERIAL FOR THE MCCQE. THIS PUBLICATION HAS NOT BEEN AUTHORED, REVIEWED OR OTHERWISE SUPPORTED BY THE NATIONAL BOARD OF MEDICAL EXAMINERS U.S.A. NOR DOES IT RECEIVE ENDORSEMENT BY THE NATIONAL BOARD AS REVIEW MATERIAL FOR THE USMLE.

The editors of this edition have taken every effort to ensure that the information contained herein is accurate and conforms to the standards accepted at the time of publication. However, due to the constantly changing nature of the medical sciences and the possibility of human error, the reader is encouraged to exercise individual clinical judgement and consult with other sources of information that may become available with continuing research. The authors, editors, and publisher are not responsible for errors or omissions or for any consequences from application of the information in this textbook, atlas, or software and make no warranty, expressed or implied, with respect to the currency, completeness, or accuracy of the contents of the publication. In particular, the reader is advised to check the manufacturer's insert of all pharmacologic products before administration.

Canadian Cataloguing in Publication Data

The National Library of Canada has catalogued this publication as follows:

Main entry under title:

The Toronto Notes 2009: Comprehensive Medical Reference
Annual.
Imprint varies.
ISB 978-0-9809397-0-5 (25th ed.)

1. Medicine   2. University of Toronto   3. MCCQE
R735.A1M33   610   C99-091498-6

To the contributors of past, present and future editions

— who invest of themselves for the benefit

of our future doctors and their patients.

And

To the families, friends and loved ones

of those who participated in the Toronto Notes 2009 production —

your support and understanding were much needed, appreciated and

invaluable in the success of this project. Thank You!

The Toronto Notes is dedicated to helping fund many charitable endeavours and medical student initiatives at the University of Toronto's Faculty of Medicine. Some of the programs that current and past Toronto Notes funding has supported include:

Community Affairs Projects
- Saturday Program for Inner City High School and Gr. 8 students
- St. Felix Mentorship Program for Inner City children
- Parkdale Mentorship Program for Gr.10 – 12 students
- Woodgreen Centre
- Let's Talk Science
- Growing up Healthy

Medical School Clubs
- Books with Wings
- Women in Medicine
- UTIHP (University of Toronto International Health Program)
- Complementary and Alternative Medicine
- Peer Support for Students
- History of Medicine Society
- Yearbook

Annual Faculty Showcase Events
- Daffydil, in support of the Canadian Cancer Society
- Earthtones Benefit Concert
- Clerkship Luncheon

Graduating Class
- Bruce Tovee Lecture Series
- Convocation and Ceremonies
- Scholarships and Bursaries to aid medical students with increasing burden of debt

---

NOTE:

Many of you have wondered about the *Toronto Notes* logo, which is based on the rod of Asclepius, an ancient Greek god. The rod of Asclepius consists of a single serpent entwined around a staff. This icon symbolizes both rebirth, by way of a snake shedding its skin, and also authority, by way of the staff.

In ancient Greek mythology, Asclepius was a son of Apollo and a skilled practitioner of medicine who learned the medical arts from the centaur Chiron. Asclepius' healing abilities were so great that he was said to be able to bring back people from the dead. These abilities displeased the gods, who punished Asclepius by placing him in the sky as the constellation Orphiuchus.

The rod of Asclepius is at times confused with the caduceus or wand of Hermes, a staff entwined with two serpents and often depicted with wings. The caduceus is often used as a symbol of medicine or medical professionals, but there is little historical basis for this symbolism.

As you may have guessed, our logo uses a caduceus that is modified to also resemble the CN Tower--our way of recognizing the university and community in which we have been privileged to learn the art and science of medicine.

Thomas O'Brien, HBSc
M.D. Program, University of Toronto

Preface – From the Editors

Dear Reader:

Toronto Notes started out as an informal compilation of notes that the University of Toronto graduating medical school class developed to help each other study for the MCCQE I. Twenty-five years later, it has turned into a package that includes a 1350-page textbook, a pocket clinical handbook, and digital resources that range from an online version of the text to PDA software to interactive learning tools. *Toronto Notes* is now sold throughout the world, and almost all Canadian medical students use *Toronto Notes* throughout their training.

The chapters in the main text cover 29 specialties and topics relevant to the medical trainee, serving as a comprehensive clinical reference that also prepares readers for the MCCQE I and USMLE II exams. The cumulative work of 25 years ensures that each new edition builds upon previous versions, and this 25th edition is no exception. Our staff of more than 120 has worked tirelessly to ensure that we are providing you with up-to-date and accurate information, including the latest practice guidelines, EBM recommendations, clinical pearls, and other helpful learning aids. This edition also boasts 40 new illustrations.

The pocket clinical handbook has also been revamped this year, making it the only bedside resource geared specifically to senior medical students. The new edition has 150 additional pages of ward-ready information. It has been reorganized into a clinically relevant format—with an emphasis on tables, charts, and algorithms—that will put the information you need right at your fingertips.

This year, many of the digital components in the *Toronto Notes* package are also new or improved. These include a much improved website interface with better search capabilities; an expanded PDA edition; new online learning tools: angiography videos and a heart sounds tutorial; a redesigned diagnostic medical imaging learning tool; and a summary question bank that is now entirely online and interactive.

As a customer of *Toronto Notes*, you may be interested to know that our sales revenue goes to support dozens of worthy causes. These include medical student-run community projects for underprivileged children and isolated seniors, charitable fundraising concerts, international health initiatives, and grants and bursaries. None of this would be possible without your support.

Thanks are due as well to everyone who has contributed to this 2009 edition of *Toronto Notes*. In particular, we would like to thank: the editorial board (Billie Au, Sami Chadi, Justine Chan, Deepti Damaraju, Behzad Hassani, Angela Ho, Biniam Kidane, Lesley Mok, Emily Partridge, David Orlov, Elliott Owen, Terence Tang, Erik Venos, Patrick Wong, and Pei Pei Zheng); Elliott Owen for producing so many of our new flowcharts and other such figures; the more than 60 faculty editors who gave so generously of their time and expertise; the Biomedical Communications students who contributed to the illustrations and cover, and in particular Caitlin LaFlamme and Tess Peters; our Production Managers, Karen Jang and Jonathan So; our class presidents, Nam Le and Amol Verma;

and the rest of our classmates who contributed to *Toronto Notes* (more than 100 of them).

We are also grateful for our continuing partnership with our publisher, Type & Graphics. Our professional relationship with them spans many years now, and their dedication and commitment to this project year after year is invaluable. The same goes for our partnership with the University of Toronto Bookstore, which has always supported *Toronto Notes*. We are grateful to the Medical Education Centres at St. Michael's Hospital, Toronto General Hospital, Women's College Hospital, Toronto Western Hospital and Sunnybrook Hospital, and The Office of Health Professions Student Affairs (Faculty of Medicine, University of Toronto) for their support.

Without all of these people, this 25th edition of the *Toronto Notes* would not be in your hands.

We hope that *Toronto Notes 2009* will prove to be a helpful resource to you, regardless of the stage of training in which you find yourselves, and as always, we thank you for your support of our publication.

Sagar Dugani, BSc, MSc   Danica Lam, BASc

Editors-in-chief, *Toronto Notes 2009*
M.D. Program, University of Toronto

Student Contributors

Editors-in-Chief
Sagar Dugani
Danica Lam

Production Managers
Karen Jang
Jon So

Website Editors
Terence Tang
Patrick Wong

Atlas Editors
Lesley Mok
Terence Tang

PDA Program
David Orlov
Trevor MacPhail - programmer

Handbook Editors
Behzad Hassani
Pei Pei Zheng

Associate Editors - Medicine
Deepti Damaraju
Elliott Owen

Associate Editors – Surgery
Sami Chadi
Biniam Kidane

Associate Editors – Primary & Core
Justine Chan
Angela Ho

EBM Editor – Medicine
Erik Venos

EBM Editor – Surgery
Emily Partridge

EBM Editor – Primary & Core
Billie Au

Chapter Editors - Medicine
Tamer Abdelshaheed
Adil Bhatti
Kristen Brown
Jack Brzezinski
Warren Cheung
Ana Florescu
Tom Havey
Andrea Herschorn
Tasha Jeyanathan
Cecilia Kim
Alexandra Kuritzky
Janice Kwan
Alex Mansfield
Neesha Merchant
Michael Mohareb
Emily Ow
Nic Petrescu
Morgan Rosenberg
Suraj Sharma
Rachel Sheps
Anjali Shroff
Taryn Simms
Amol Verma
Laura Waltman
Adina Weinerman
Jonathan Wong
Kit Man Wong
Hannah Wu
Ivan Ying

Chapter Editors – Surgery
CB Allard
Heather Baltzer
Winston Bharat
Ashton Connor
Khaled Hasan
Amir Khoshbin
John Kim
Timothy Leroux
Michelle Lin
Rubini Pathy
Theresa Pazionis
Adrian Sacher
Sharmi Shafi
Nashwah Taha
David Walmsley
Melinda Wu

Chapter Editors – Primary & Core
Larbi Benhabib
Priscilla Che
Sivan Durbin
Malcolm Gooi
Kate Hanneman
Thien Huynh
Karen Jang
Annie Keeler
Katie Ker
Julia Kfouri
Ekta Khemani
Goldie Kurtz
Jennifer Lam
Carrie Lynde
Anna MacDonald
Kelsey Mills
Nayha Mody
Laurel Murphy
Eddie Ng
Thomas O'Brien
Silvia Odorcic
Natasha Pinto
Indra Rasaratnam
Shail Rawal
Fereshte Samji
Kasy Soare
Shanna Spring
Shauna Tsuchiya
Jen Vergel De Dios
Melissa Vyvey
Andrew Willmore

Copy Editors
Sacha Bhinder
Natasha Bollegala
Jenn Boyd
Roderick Cheung
Melissa de Souza
Aruna Dhara
Renu Gupta
Dan Hesse
Thomas Irvine
Danielle Kain
Adam Kaufman
Meghan Kelly
Chana Korenblum
Joe Koval
Joe Krakowski
Tran Le
Micheal McInnis
Erynn Shaw
Laura Sovran
Linda Sun
Evan Taerk
Joanna Tang
Astra Teo
Kate Thompson
Priya Vasa
Keith Wong
Kristin Wynne
Gina Yip

Biomedical Communications

Production Editors
Caitlin S. LaFlamme
Tess N. Peters

Illustrators
Heather K. Ambraska
Jennifer M. Belanger
Steven Bernstein
Janet S.M. Chan

Erin M. Duff
Takami Iijima
Simon P. Ip
Caitlin S. LaFlamme
Michael Marcynuk

Anas Nader
Caitlin C. O'Connell
Susan N. Park
Tess N. Peters
Dennis Wei

Faculty of Medicine Contributors, University of Toronto

Ruby Alvi, MD, CCFP, MHSc
Assistant Professor, Department of Family and
Community Medicine
University of Toronto

Anne M.R. Agur, BSc (OT), MSc, PhD
Professor
Division of Anatomy, Department of Surgery
University of Toronto

Hosanna Au, MD, FRCPC
Assistant Professor, Department of Pediatrics
University of Toronto
Pediatrician, Division of Pediatric Medicine
The Hospital for Sick Children

Dr. Glen Bandiera, MD, MEd
Department of Emergency Services
St. Michael's Hospital

Stacey Bernstein, MD, FRCPC
Assistant Professor, Department of Pediatrics
University of Toronto
Director, Undergraduate Medical Education

Dr. David Black, MD
Clinical Fellow
Division of Gastroenterology
Sunnybrook Health Sciences Centre

Luigi Casella, MD, FRCPC
Associate Professor of Medicine
University of Toronto
Honorary Consultant, St. Michael's Hospital
Division of Cardiology

Alice Y.Y. Cheng, MD, FRCPC
Assistant Professor (Adjunct)
Department of Medicine
Endocrinology and Metabolism
St. Michael's Hospital and Credit Valley
Hospital

Chi-Ming Chow, MDCM, MSc, FRCPC,
FACC, FASE
Assistant Professor of Medicine
University of Toronto
Staff Cardiologist
St. Michael's Hospital

TaeBong Chung, MD, FRCPC
Assistant Professor
Department of Medical Imaging
Staff, Department of Medical Imaging
Mount Sinai Hospital

Jack Colman MD, FRCPC
Associate Professor of Medicine
University of Toronto
Staff Cardiologist, Congenital Cardiac Centre
Peter Munk Cardiac Centre/UHN and
Mount Sinai Hospital

Isabella Devito, MD, FRCPC
Assistant Professor
Department of Anesthesia
Staff, Department of Anesthesia
and Pain Management
University Health Network
and Mount Sinai Hospital

Dr. Alexandra Easson, FACS, FRCSC, MD,
MSc
Division of Surgery, Princess Margaret
Hospital

Walid A. Farhat, MD
Associate Professor, Department of Surgery
Pediatric Urologist
The Hospital for Sick Children
University of Toronto

Dr. Darlene Fenech, MD, MSc, FRCSC
Division of General Surgery
Sunnybrook Health Sciences Centre

Peter Ferguson, MD, MSc, FRCSC
Assistant Professor, Department of Surgery
Division of Orthopaedic Surgery
Mount Sinai Hospital
Department of Surgical Oncology
Princess Margaret Hospital

Arnis Freiberg, MD, FRCS[C], FACS
Professor (Emeritus), Department of Surgery
Staff, Department of Surgery
University Health Network

William Geerts, MD, FRCPC
Professor, Department of Medicine
Thromboembolism Program
Sunnybrook Health Sciences Centre

Richard Glazier, MD, MPH, CCFP, FCFP
Associate Professor, Department of Family &
Community Medicine
Public Health Sciences
Senior Scientist, Institute for Clinical
Evaluative Sciences
Staff Scientist, Centre for Research on Inner
City Health, St. Michael's Hospital

Dr. Wayne Gold, MD, FRCPC
Department of Medicine
Toronto General Hospital

Barry J. Goldlist, MD, FRCPC, FACP, AGSF
Professor, and Director
Division of Geriatric Medicine
University of Toronto
Staff, Department of Medicine
University Health Network

John T. Granton, MD, FRCPC
Associate Professor
Department of Medicine
Divisions of Respirology and
Interdepartmental Division of Critical Care
Program Director, Critical Care Medicine
University Health Network

Philip C. Hébert, MA, PhD, MD, FCFPC
Associate Professor, Department of Family
and Community Medicine
Ethics Consultant, Clinical Ethics Centre
Sunnybrook Health Sciences Centre
Joint Centre for Bioethics

Sender Herschorn, MD, FRCSC
Professor and Chair, Division of Urology
Staff, Sunnybrook Health Sciences Centre
and Women's College Hospital

Jonathan C. Irish, MD, MSc, FRCSC, FACS
Professor, Department of Otolaryngology
Chief, Department of Surgical Oncology
Staff, Department of Otolaryngology/Head
and Neck Surgery
University Health Network
and Mount Sinai Hospital

Nasir Jaffer, MD, FRCPC
Associate Professor
Department of Medical Imaging
Staff, Department of Medical Imaging
Mount Sinai Hospital and
University Health Network

Cheryl Jaigobin, MD, FRCPC, MSc
Assistant Professor, Department of Medicine
Staff, Department of Medicine
Division of Neurology
University Health Network

Dana Jerome, MD, MEd, FRCPC
Assistant Professor
University of Toronto
Staff, Department of Medicine
Division of Rheumatology
Women's College Hospital

Ian Johnson, MD, FRCPC
Associate Professor
Department of Public Health Sciences
University of Toronto

Dr. David Juurlink, MD, PhD, FRCPC
Assistant Professor of Medicine, Pediatrics,
and Health Policy, Management, and
Evaluation, Attending Physician, Division
of General Internal Medicine,
Head, Division of Clinical Pharmacology
and Toxicology,
Sunnybrook Health Sciences Centre

Gabor Kandel, MD, FRCPC
Associate Professor
Department of Medicine
Staff, Department of Medicine
St. Michael's Hospital

Jay S. Keystone, MD, MSc (CTM), FRCPC
Tropical Disease Unit
Toronto General Hospital
Professor of Medicine, University of
Toronto

Sari L. Kives, MD, FRCSC
Assistant Professor
Department of Obstetrics and Gynecology
St. Michael's Hospital
Hospital for Sick Children
ine Contributors, University of Toronto

Dr. William Kraemer, MD, FRCSC
Program Director, Orthopaedic Surgery
The Banting Institue, University of Toronto

Abhaya V. Kulkarni, MD, PhD, FRCSC
Neurosurgeon and Scientist-Track
Investigator
Division of Neurosurgery
Hospital for Sick Children

Wai-Ching Lam, MD, FRCSC
Associate Professor,
Department of Ophthalmology and Vision
Science, University of Toronto

Liesly Lee, MSc, MD, FRCPC
Assistant Professor of Medicine
(Neurology)
Neurology Education Site Director
Sunnybrook Health Sciences Centre
University of Toronto

Jodi Lofchy, MD, FRCPC
Director, Psychiatry Emergency Services
University Health Network
Director, Undergraduate Education
Department of Psychiatry
Associate Professor, University of Toronto

Ryan Mai, MD
Department of Anesthesia
St. Michael's Hospital

Nancy H McKee, MD, FRCS(c), FACS
Professor, Department of Surgery
Plastic & Reconstructive Surgery
Staff, Mount Sinai Hospital

Heather McDonald-Blumer, MD, FRCPR
Program Director, Division of
Rheumatology, University of Toronto
Assistant Director & Staff Rheumatologist
The Rebecca MacDonald Centre for
Arthritis & Autoimmune Disease
Mount Sinai Hospital

Anne McLeod, MD, FRCPC
Assistant Professor
Department of Medicine
Staff, Department of Medicine
University Health Network

Filomena Meffe, MD, FRCSC, MSc
Director, Undergraduate Medical
Education, Department of Obstetrics and
Gynecology
Faculty of Medicine, University of Toronto
Staff, Department of Obstetrics and
Gynecology
St. Michael's Hospital

Azadeh Moaveni, MD, CCFP
Undergraduate Hospital Program Director
Toronto Western Hospital
Lecturer, Department of Family and
Community Medicine, University of Toronto

Dr. Markku Nousiainen, MD, MSc, FRCSC
Holland Orthopaedic & Arthritic Centre
Sunnybrook Health Sciences Centre

Dr. Allan Okrainec, MD, FRCSC
Division of General Surgery
Toronto Western Hospital

Blake C. Papsin, MD, MSc, FRCSC, FACS,
FAAP
Cochlear Americas Chair in Auditory
Development
Associate Professor, Department of
Otolaryngology/Head and Neck Surgery
Staff Otolaryngologist, The Hospital for Sick
Children

Ramesh Prasad, MBBS, MSc, FRCPC,
FACP
Assistant Professor
Department of Medicine
Staff, Department of Medicine
St. Michael's Hospital

James T. Rutka, MD, PhD, FRCSC, FACS,
FAAP
Chairman, Division of Neurosurgery
The University of Toronto

Dr. Fred Saibil, MD, FRCPC
Associate Scientist
Head, Division of Gastroenterology
Sunnybrook Health Sciences Centre

Rayfel Schneider, MBBCh, FRCPC
Associate Chair (Education)
Department of Pediatrics, University of
Toronto
Staff, Division of Rheumatology
The Hospital for Sick Children

Martin Schreiber, MD, FRCPC
Associate Professor
Department of Medicine
Staff, Department of Medicine
St. Michael's Hospital

Neil H. Shear, MD, FRCPC, FACP
Professor
Departments of Medicine, Pharmacology &
Pediatrics
Departmental Division Director for
Dermatology
University of Toronto
and Chief at Sunnybrook Health Sciences
Centre

Margaret Thompson, MD, FRCPC
Assistant Professor
Department of Medicine
Medical Director – Ontario Regional Poison
Information Centre
Staff, Department of Emergency Medicine
St. Michael's Hospital

Jeffrey Tyberg, MD, FRCPC, FACEP
Assistant Professor
Department of Medicine
Division of Emergency Medicine
Chief, Department of Emergency Services
Sunnybrook Health Sciences Centre

Taufik A Valiante, MD PhD FRCS
Assistant Professor, Department of Surgery
Division of Neurosurgery
Co-Director, Epilepsy Program
University Health Network

Herbert P. von Schroeder, MD, MSc, FRCSC
Associate Professor
Department of Surgery
Staff, Divisions of Orthopaedic and Plastic Surgery
University Health Network

Sharon Walmsley, MD, FRCPC
Associate Professor
Department of Medicine
Staff, Department of Medicine
University Health Network

Dr. Michael Weinstein, MD, FRCPC, FAAP
Director, Inpatient Paediatric Medicine
The Hospital for Sick Children

Michael Wiley, BSc, MSc, PhD
Professor and Division Chair
Division of Anatomy,Department of Surgery
University of Toronto

Anna Woo, MD SM, FRCPC, FACC
Staff Cardiologist
Assistant Professor
Division of Cardiology
Toronto General Hospital
University of Toronto

Louis Wu, MD, FRCPC
Assistant Professor
Department of Medical Imaging
Staff, Department of Medical Imaging
St. Michael's Hospital

Jae Yang, MD, FRCPC
Assistant Professor
Department of Medicine
Staff, Department of Medicine
St. Michael's Hospital

Feedback and Errata

We are constantly trying to improve the Toronto Notes and welcome your feedback. If you have found an error in this edition please do not hesitate to contact us. As well, we look forward to receiving any comments regarding any component of the Toronto Notes package and website.

Please send your feedback to: feedback@torontonotes.ca

Alternatively, send mail to: Toronto Notes for Medical Students
Editors-in-chief
c/o The Medical Society
1 King's College Circle
Room 2171A
Toronto, Ontario
M5S 1A8
Canada

email: chiefeditors@torontonotes.ca
Tel: 1-416-946-3047
Fax: 1-416-978-8730

For more information on the Toronto Notes, visit our website: www.torontonotes.ca

Table of Contents

How to Use This Book

This book has been designed to remain as one book or to be taken apart into smaller booklets. Identify the beginning and end of a particular section; then carefully bend the pages along the perforated line next to the spine of the book. Then tear the pages out along the perforation.

The layout of *Toronto Notes 2009* allows easy identification of important information. These items are indicated by icons interspersed throughout the text:

Icon	Significance
	The 'key' icon, found next to headings in the text, identifies key objectives and causal conditions as defined by the Medical Council of Canada or the National Board of Medical Examiners USA. If it appears beside a 'black-bar' title, all subsequent subheadings should be considered key topics.
	The 'pearl' icon, found in the sidebar, identifies concise, important information which will aid in the diagnosis and/or management of conditions discussed in the accompanying text.
	The 'light bulb' icon indicates helpful mnemonic devices and other memory aids.
	The 'flags' icon indicates information or findings that require urgent management or specialist referral.
	The 'camera' icon indicates topics that correspond with images found in the Colour Photo Atlas available on online.
	The 'X-ray' icon indicates topics that correspond to information or images contained within the Radiology Atlas located online.
	The 'PDA' icon indicates topics that corresponds with entries found in the PDA Program – *"Clinical Information Set"*. The program can be downloaded from the website.
	The 'computer' icon indicates topics that correspond with electronic resources such as Functional Neuroanatomy™ or ECG Made Simple™ located online.

Chapter Divisions

To aid in studying and finding relevant material quickly, each chapter is organized in the following general framework:

Basic Anatomy/Physiology Review
- features the high-yield, salient background information students are often assumed to have remembered from their early medical school education

Common Differential Diagnoses
- aims to outline a clinically useful framework to tackle the common presentations and problems faced in the area of expertise

Diagnoses
- the bulk of the book
- etiology, epidemiology, pathophysiology, clinical features, investigations, management, complications, and prognosis

Common Medications
- a quick reference section for review of medications commonly prescribed

Ethical, Legal and Organizational Aspects of Medicine

Goldie Kurtz and Natasha Pinto, chapter editors
Justine Chan and Angela Ho, associate editors
Billie Au, EBM editor
Dr. Philip Hébert, staff editor

Further information on these topics can be found in the *Objectives of the Considerations of the Legal, Ethical and Organizational Aspects of the Practice of Medicine (CLEO)* – which can be downloaded free of charge from the *Medical Council of Canada* website at http://www.mcc.ca/pdf/cleo.pdf

Organization of Health Care in Canada

- one federal, three territorial, and ten provincial systems with uniform federal guidelines
- federal system provides care to Aboriginal groups, the RCMP, the armed forces
- financed by both the public (70%) and private (30%) sectors
- each provincial plan must cover all medically necessary health services delivered in hospitals and by physicians; can choose to cover additional services such as home care and prescription drugs
- non-insured health services and fees are either covered by private insurance or by the individual
- workers' compensation funds cover treatments for work-related injuries and diseases

The current legal foundation of the Canadian health system is based on three statutes:
- *Constitution Act* (1867) - deals primarily with the jurisdictional power between federal and provincial governments
- *Canada Health Act* (1984) - outlines the national terms and conditions
- *Canada Health and Social Transfer Act* (1996) - sets the conditions for fiscal transfers from the federal government to the provinces and territories

Source: Public Health and Preventive Medicine in Canada, Shah, C.P. 5th edition (2003).

History

1867	*British North America Act* (now *Constitution Act*) establishes Canada as a confederacy
	▪ government has only minimal role in health care at this time
	▪ "establishment, maintenance, and management of hospitals" under provincial jurisdiction
1947	Saskatchewan introduces universal hospital insurance
	▪ based on taxes and premiums
	▪ other provinces follow
1957	Federal government passes *Hospital Insurance and Diagnostic Services Act*
	▪ provinces with universal hospital insurance to receive federal funds
	▪ federal government pays for approximately 50% of insured services
1962	Saskatchewan implements universal medical care insurance
	▪ physician services included
1965	*Royal Commission on Health Services (Hall Commission)* recommends federal leadership and financial support with provincial government operation
1966	*Medical Care Act* passed by federal government
	▪ federal government contribution maintained at 50% on average, with poorer provinces receiving more funds
	▪ medical insurance must be:

       ◆ **Comprehensive**   ◆ **Portable**

       ◆ **Universal**   ◆ **Publicly administered**

1977	*Established Programs Financing Act* passed by federal government
	▪ federal government gives "tax points" to provinces by reducing federal taxes and allowing provinces to collect more
	▪ funding no longer tied to direct services → federal influence wanes
	▪ provinces bear greater costs and impose restrictions on physicians
	▪ physicians respond with "extra-billing": patients pay a supplementary fee
1984	*Canada Health Act* passed by federal government
	▪ replaced *Medical Care Act* and *Hospital Insurance and Diagnostic Services Act*
	▪ extra-billing banned by new fifth criterion: **Accessibility**
1996	*Canada Health and Social Transfer Act* passed by federal government
	▪ federal government gives provinces a single grant for health care, social programs, and post-secondary education; division of resources at provinces' discretion
1999	*Social Union Framework Agreement* signed by the Prime Minister and all Premiers and territorial leaders except Quebec
	▪ federal and provincial/territorial governments vow to concentrate their efforts to modernize Canadian social policy
2001	*Kirby* and *Romanow Commissions* appointed
	Kirby Commission (final report, October 2002)
	▪ one-member committee of the Senate: examined history of health care system in Canada, pressures and constraints of current health care system, role of federal government, and health care systems in foreign jurisdictions
	(http://www.parl.gc.ca/37/2/parlbus/commbus/senate/Com-e/soci-e/rep-e/repoct02vol6part8-e.htm#APPENDIX%20A)
	Romanow Commission (final report, November 2002)
	▪ one-member royal commission (former Saskatchewan Premier Roy Romanow) appointed by the Prime Minister to inquire into and undertake dialogue with Canadians on the future of Canada's public health care system
	(http://www.hc-sc.gc.ca/hcs-sss/alt_formats/hpb-dgps/pdf/hhr/ romanow-eng.pdf)

2003   *First Ministers' Accord on Health Care Renewal* signed
- First Ministers agree on an action plan to improve access to quality care for all Canadians and to prepare an annual public report on primary and home care
- 1st Health Council (composed of government and expert/public representatives) appointed to improve accountability in the Canadian health care system

2004   *First Ministers' Meeting on the Future of Health Care* produces a 10-year plan
- priorities of the plan are reductions in waiting times, development of a national pharmacare plan, and primary care reform

2005   *Chaoulli v. Quebec (Attorney General)*, Supreme Court of Canada Decision
- ruled that banning private insurance is unconstitutional under the Quebec Charter of Rights, given that patients do not have access to those services under the public system in a timely way

Key Principles of the *Canada Health Act*

1. Public Administration	-	provincial health care programs must be administered by public authorities
2. Comprehensiveness	-	provincial health care programs must cover all necessary diagnostic, physician, and hospital services
3. Universality	-	all eligible residents must be entitled to health care services
4. Portability	-	emergency health services must be available to Canadians who are outside their home province; the home province must pay at the host-province rate within Canada and at the home-province rate outside of Canada
5. Accessibility	-	user fees, charges, or other obstructions to insured health care services are not permitted

> The federal government can reduce its contributions to provinces that violate the key principles of the *Canada Health Act*.

Health Care Expenditure and Delivery in Canada

- projected total health care expenditure in 2006 was $148 billion, 10.0% of the GDP, approx. $3678 USD per capita; this includes out-of-pocket, government-funded and third-party expenditures (*Canadian Institute of Health Information*)
- the 2006 Canadian health care expenditure increased 5.8% over 2005 spending, (*Canadian Institute of Health Information*)
- the 2006 Canadian health care expenditure as a percentage of GDP ranked eighth out of 30 Organization for Economic Cooperation and Development (OECD) member nations
- 70.4% of health care spending came from public sector sources in 2006, as compared to 45.8% in the U.S.
- in 2006 there were 2.1 physicians per 1000 population, ranking 26th out of OECD member countries

Source: OECD Health Data 2008: How Does Canada Compare. Copyright OECD (2008).

> **A systematic review and meta-analysis of studies comparing mortality rates of private for-profit and private not-for-profit hospitals**
> *CMAJ 2002;166(11):1399-406.*
> Compiled data from 15 U.S. observational studies involving 38 million patients from 1983-1996. Concluded that US private for-profit hospitals are associated with an increased risk of death (RR = 1.020; 95% Confidence Interval (CI) 1.003-1.038; p = 0.02).
> They estimate that switching Canadian hospitals to private for-profit institutions could lead to approximately 2200 extra deaths a year.

Delivery of Health Care

- hospital services in Canada are publicly funded but delivered through private, not-for-profit institutions owned and operated by communities, religious organizations and regional health authorities
- this differs from other countries such as the United States (a mix of public and private funding, as well as private-for-profit and private not-for-profit delivery) and the United Kingdom (primarily public funding and delivery)
- in Canada there have been recent calls for increased private sector involvement in health care via private-for-profit facilities (Lewis *et al*, 2001)
- however, there is good evidence for a negative impact of investor-owned-for-profit delivery on health outcomes such as morbidity and mortality, and on the cost of health care (see sidebar)

> **Payments for care at private for-profit and private not-for-profit hospitals: a systematic review and meta-analysis**
> *CMAJ 2004;170(12):1817-24.*
> Meta-analysis of 8 U.S. observational studies involving more than 350 000 patients. Concluded that care provided by private for-profit hospitals was more expensive (Relative payments for care=1.19; 95% CI=1.07-1.33; p=0.001). If half of Canadian hospitals were converted to private for-profit institutions, an extra $3.6 billion would be paid annually.

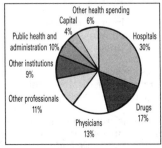

Figure 1. Health expenditure in Canada, 2005
Source: Canadian Institute of Health Information.

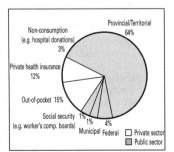

Figure 2. Canadian health care dollars by source of funds, 2005
Source: Canadian Institute of Health Information.

Role of the Provincial Licensing Authorities

Some details in the *Role of the Provincial Licensing Authorities* section are specific to Ontario; general principles apply throughout Canada.

- the medical profession in Canada self-regulates under the authority of provincial legislation; Canada is the only country in the world where the medical profession still regulates itself
- physicians in each province are self-regulated by a licensing authority (e.g. the College of Physicians & Surgeons of Ontario (CPSO)); membership is **mandatory** to practice in that province
- system of self-regulation is based on the premise that the licensing authority must act first and foremost in the interest of the public
- Licensing Authority functions:
  - issuing nontransferable licenses → allows doctors to practice in that province
  - maintaining ethical, legal and competency standards and developing policies to guide doctors
  - investigating complaints against doctors
  - disciplining doctors guilty of professional misconduct or incompetence (in most Canadian jurisdictions there is zero tolerance for sexual misconduct by physicians, resulting in harsh penalties including permanent suspension from the profession)
- role of the CPSO outlined in the *Regulated Health Professions Act of Ontario* (1991)
  - CPSO consists of:
    - ◆ a governing College Council composed of 16 peer-elected physicians, 3 medical faculty-appointed physicians, and 13-15 non-physicians appointed by provincial government
    - ◆ the following committees: Executive, Registration, Complaints, Discipline, Quality Assurance, Fitness to Practice, and Education

Distinction Between Licensure and Certification

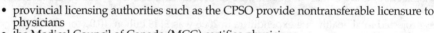

Certification by the LMCC plus either the RCPSC or CFPC is a minimum requirement for licensure by most provincial licensing authorities.

- provincial licensing authorities such as the CPSO provide nontransferable licensure to physicians
- the Medical Council of Canada (MCC) certifies physicians
  - certification is known as the Licentiate of the MCC (LMCC)
  - LMCC is acquired by passing the MCC Qualifying Examination Parts I and II
- the Royal College of Physicians and Surgeons of Canada (RCPSC) certifies specialists who complete an accredited residency program and pass the appropriate specialty exam
  - voluntary membership of RCPSC is designated FRCPC or FRCSC (Fellow of the Royal College of Physicians/Surgeons of Canada)
- the College of Family Physicians of Canada (CFPC) certifies family physicians who complete an accredited residency program and pass the Certification Examination in Family Medicine
- the RCPSC and CFPC are responsible for monitoring ongoing continuing medical education (CME) and professional development

Role of Professional Associations

- provincial medical associations (e.g. the British Columbia Medical Association) represent the economic and professional interests of doctors
  - membership is voluntary, although fee payment is mandatory in some provinces
- the Canadian Medical Association (CMA) is a national association that provides leadership to doctors and advocates for access to high quality health care in Canada
  - membership is voluntary and requires provincial medical association membership
- the CMA represents physicians' concerns at the national level, while the provincial medical associations negotiate fee and benefit schedules with provincial governments
- medical residents
  - represented nationally by the Canadian Association of Interns and Residents
  - represented provincially by Provincial Housestaff Organizations, which uphold the economic and professional interests of residents
- medical students
  - represented at their universities by student societies
  - these bodies collectively form the Canadian Federation of Medical Students
  - francophone medical schools participate in the Federation of Quebec Medical Student Societies
- the Canadian Medical Protective Association (CMPA), a physician-run organization, is a voluntary insurance association that protects the integrity of member physicians by providing legal defense against allegations of malpractice or negligence and by providing risk management and educational programs and general advice

The U.S. Health Care System

- the United States health care system is market-based
- it is funded and delivered by a mixture of the public, private, and voluntary sectors; private-for-profit is the prevailing method of delivery
- public funding is derived from taxes raised at both the federal and state government levels

Health Care Expenditure and Delivery in the U.S.

- health care spending in the U.S. represents a large economic sector:
  - health care comprises over 15% of the gross domestic product (GDP) (highest in the OECD), amounting to $6714 USD per capita in 2006
  - one advantage is the widespread availability of technology – the U.S. has 4 times as many MRI machines per capita than Canada (*OECD Health Data 2008*)
- the U.S. scores poorly on some indicators of population health, with a life expectancy below the OECD average and infant mortality above the OECD average. Several factors have been put forth to account for this discrepancy:
  - poor health of large uninsured population
  - high cost of health care administration in the U.S.
  - the provision of inefficient high-cost, high-intensity care
    - the higher-spending regions in the U.S. do not provide any better quality of care, access to care, health outcomes or satisfaction with care when compared to the lower-spending regions (Fisher *et al*, 2003)
- the U.S. has the highest level of obesity of all OECD nations at 34.3%; this has major implications for future health care spending
Source: OECD Health Data 2008: How Does the United States Compare. Copyright OECD (2008).

> **Cost of Health Care Administration in the United States and Canada**
> *N Engl J Med* 2003; 349:768-75.
> Administrative costs were estimated from data on insurance overhead, employers' costs to manage benefits, and the administrative costs of hospitals, practitioners' offices, nursing homes, and home care. In 1999, the cost of U.S. health administration was $1,059 per capita, more than three times greater than the cost in Canada ($307 per capita).

Access to Health Services in the U.S.

- 70% of Americans under the age of 65 have private health insurance, either employer-sponsored or individually purchased, and a further 12% receive health care through public health insurance; 18%, mainly the poor, have no health insurance (CDC National Centre for Health Statistics)
- access to publicly funded health services occurs primarily through two programs, Medicare and Medicaid (see Table 1), which were created by the 1965 *Social Security Act*
- other federal government-funded health programs include the Military Health Services System, the Veterans Affairs Health Services System, the Indian Health Service, and the Prison Health Service

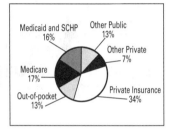

Figure 3. USA health care dollars by source of funds, 2004
Source: Centers for Medicare & Medicaid Services, Office of the Actuary, National Health Statistics Group

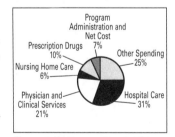

Figure 4. Health expenditure in USA, 2004
Source: Centers for Medicare & Medicaid Services, Office of the Actuary, National Health Statistics Group

Table 1. Medicare and Medicaid program information

	Medicare	Medicaid
Eligibility	People over the age of 65 People with end stage renal disease People of any age meeting the Medicare definition of disability	People who receive funds through social assistance programs Pregnant women People with developmental disabilities Low-income children through the 1997 State Children's Health Insurance Program
Coverage	Basic "Part A" providing inpatient hospital care, home care, limited skilled nursing facility care, and hospice care. Supplemental "Part B" covers outpatient physician and clinic services, and requires payment of a further monthly fee. "Part C" is called Medicare+Choice and offers access to managed care programs for a further fee. In 2006, Medicare recipients can subscribe to a "Part D" prescription drug benefit with payment of a monthly fee.	Basic coverage involves inpatient and outpatient hospital care, laboratory and x-ray services, skilled nursing care, home care, physician services, dental services, and family planning. Financing for Medicaid is provided jointly by the federal and state governments, and program details vary greatly between states. A further 30 optional services are provided depending on the state program.
Co-payment	There is a deductible payable for each benefit period including Part D. Low-income Medicare recipients avoid the deductible and monthly fee. To help pay for out-of-pocket expenditures, and to cover many of the services not insured by Medicare, the majority of Medicare beneficiaries buy supplemental private health insurance called Medisup.	States may impose deductibles, coinsurance, or co-payments on some Medicaid recipients for certain services. Emergency services and family planning services are exempt from such co-payments. Certain Medicaid recipients are excluded from this cost sharing including pregnant women and children under age 18. **Medicaid is not health insurance**– coverage is unreliable as improvement in an individual's financial status can lead to a loss of Medicaid eligibility.

Source: Centers for Medicare and Medicaid Services; http://www.cms.hhs.gov

The Uninsured in the U.S.

- in a 17-year prospective study, adults who lacked health insurance at the outset had a 25% greater mortality than those with private health insurance (Franks *et al*, 1993)
- the uninsured receive fewer diagnostic and treatment services for trauma or myocardial infarction, are less likely to access cancer screening, and the care they receive for chronic conditions such as diabetes often does not meet professional standards (reviewed in *Care Without Coverage: Too Little, Too Late*, Institute of Medicine, 2002)

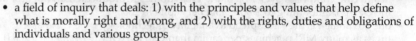

Ethics

- a field of inquiry that deals: 1) with the principles and values that help define what is morally right and wrong, and 2) with the rights, duties and obligations of individuals and various groups
- there are two broad approaches to ethics – **consequentialism** and **deontology**
  - consequentialism distinguishes right from wrong according to an action's outcomes (e.g. the right thing to do is minimize suffering) while deontology is rule or duty-based (e.g. it is always wrong to punish the innocent)
  - there is no one agreed upon ethical theory but most contemporary writers combine both approaches
  - the most widely used approach is **'principlism'** championed by Beauchamp and Childress

The Four Principles Approach to Medical Ethics ('principlism')

1. Respect for Autonomy
  - recognizes an individual's right and ability to decide for themself according to their personal beliefs and values
  - respecting, reflecting, and promoting an individual patient's personal values in decision making to empower him or her
  - patients' decisions may sometimes be different from the recommendation of the physician
  - patients are not expected to act in ways considered reasonable by others, as long as they do not harm others (this principle is not applicable to newborn children or situations where informed consent and choice are not possible or may not be appropriate)
  - autonomy also requires showing fidelity to incapable patients' prior capable views if known, and treating them with inherent worth and dignity

2. Beneficence
  - acting in the patient's 'best interests', where these represent the patient's values, beliefs, and preferences, so far as these are known
  - the aim is to minimize harmful outcomes and maximize beneficial ones
  - physicians recommend treatment based on evidence and professional experience to patients and help them weigh the risks and benefits of various options
  - autonomy should be integrated with the physician's conception of a competent patient's best interests
  - paramount in situations where consent/choice is not possible or may not be appropriate

3. Non-Maleficence
  - obligation to avoid causing harm; *primum non nocere* ("First, do no harm")
  - patients should not be 'worse off' on account of medical care
  - efforts should be made to reduce error and adverse events and ensure patient safety
  - a limit condition of the Beneficence principle

4. Justice
  - fair distribution of benefits and harms within a community, regardless of geography or privilege
  - scarce resources are distributed based on the needs of patients and the benefit they would receive from obtaining a specific resource (e.g. organs for transplantation are fairly distributed if they go to those who are the most unwell, who are the most likely to survive the longest with the transplant, and who have waited the longest to receive a transplant)
  - concept of fairness: Is the patient receiving what he or she deserves? How do treatment decisions impact on others?
  - respects rules of fair play and basic human rights, such as freedom from persecution and the right to have one's interests considered and respected

Four Ethical Principles
1. Autonomy
2. Beneficence
3. Non-maleficence
4. Justice

Autonomy vs. Competence
Autonomy: the right that patients have to make decisions according to their beliefs and preferences
Competence: the ability or capacity to make *specific* decisions for one's self

Adverse Event (AE)
An unintended injury or complication resulting in disability, death or prolonged hospital stay that arises from health care management.

The Canadian Adverse Events Study: the incidence of adverse events among hospital patients in Canada
CMAJ 2004;170(11):1678-86.
Study: Review of random sample of charts in four randomly selected Canadian hospitals for the fiscal year 2000
Patients: 4174 patient charts sampled, 3745 eligible charts (>18 years of age; nonpsychiatric, nonobstetric, minimum 24 hour admission)
Results: AE rate was 7.5% per 100 hospital admissions (95% CI 5.7-9.3). Highly preventable AEs occurred in 36.9% of patients with AEs (95% CI 32.0-41.8%) and death occurred in 20.8% (95% CI 78%-33.8%). An estimated 1521 additional hospital days were associated with AEs. Patients with AEs were significantly older than those without (mean age [and standard deviation] 64.9 [16.7] v. 62.0 [18.4] years; p=0.016). Men & women experienced equal rates of AEs.
Conclusions: The overall incidence rate of AEs of 7.5% suggests that, of the almost 2.5 million annual hospital admissions in Canada similar to the type studied, about 185 000 are associated with an AE and close to 70 000 of these are potentially preventable.

CMA Code of Ethics

- the CMA has developed and approved a **Code of Ethics** that acts as a common ethical framework for Canadian physicians. It was last revised in 2004:
  - sources include the Hippocratic Oath, developments in human rights, recent bioethical discussion
  - may set out different standards of behaviour than does the law
  - prepared by physicians for physicians
  - based on the fundamental ethical principles of medicine
  - statements are general in nature
  - applies to physicians, residents and medical students
- **CMA policy statements** exist to address specific ethical issues not mentioned by the code such as abortion, transplantation, and euthanasia

> The CMA Code of Ethics is a quasi-legal standard for physicians. If the law sets a minimal moral standard for doctors, the Code ratchets up these standards.

Confidentiality

- a full and open exchange of information between patient and physician is central to a therapeutic relationship
- privacy is a **right** of patients (which they may forego), while confidentiality is a **duty** of doctors (which they must respect barring patient consent or the requirements of the law)
- confidentiality is thus important in creating a trusting doctor-patient relationship which allows patients to disclose personal information
- if inappropiately breached by a doctor, he or she can be sanctioned by the court or by their regulatory authority (see *Confidentiality and Reporting Requirements*, ELOAM18)
- based on the ethical principal of patient *autonomy*
  - patients have the right to control their own information
  - patients have the right to expect information concerning them will receive proper protection from unauthorized access by others (see *Privacy*, ELOAM19)
- **confidentiality may be ethically and legally breached in certain circumstances,** for example, the right to confidentiality can be overridden by the threat of harm to others (see *Confidentiality and Reporting Requirements*, ELOAM18)
- unlike the solicitor-client privilege, there is no 'physician-patient privilege' by which a physician, even a psychiatrist, can promise the patient 'absolute confidentiality'
- physicians should seek advice from their local health authority or the CMPA before disclosing HIV status of a patient to someone else
  - many jurisdictions make mandatory not only the reporting of serious communicable diseases like AIDS, but also the reporting of those who harbour the agent of the communicable disease, such as HIV
  - physicians failing to abide by such regulations could be subject to professional or civil actions

> **CMA Code of Ethics**
> "Disclose your patients' personal health information to third parties only with their consent, or as provided for by law, such as when the maintenance of confidentiality would result in a significant risk of substantial harm to others or, in the case of incompetent patients, to the patients themselves. In such cases take all reasonable steps to inform the patients that the usual requirements for confidentiality will be breached."

> **Reasons to Breach Confidentiality**
> - Child abuse
> - Fitness to drive
> - Communicable disease
> - Coroner report
> - Duty to inform/warn

Consent

- the autonomous authorization of a medical intervention by a patient
- applies to both the acceptance and the refusal of treatment

Elements of Ethically Valid Consent (also see *Consent under the Law*, ELOAM16)
- Voluntary – right of the patient to come to a decision freely, without physical force or threats, including psychological coercion or manipulation of salient information
- Capable – ability of the patient to understand the relevant information and appreciate the consequences of their decision
- Informed – disclosure of what a 'reasonable person' in the patient's situation would need to know to make an informed choice

Ethical Principles: Underlying Consent
- usually the principle of respect for patient autonomy overrides the principle of beneficence
- where a patient cannot make an autonomous decision, it is the duty of the substitute decision maker (or the physician in an emergency) to act on the patient's known prior wishes or, failing that, to act in the patient's best interests
- there is a duty to discover, if possible, what the patient would have wanted when capable
- central to determining best interests is understanding the patient's values, beliefs and cultural/religious background as these will affect treatments the patient would find beneficial or harmful

> **CPSO Policy**
> **Consent**
> Obtaining valid consent before carrying out medical, therapeutic and diagnostic procedures has long been recognized as an elementary step in fulfilling the doctor's obligations to the patient.

Obtaining Consent
- a signed consent form only documents the consent – it does not replace the process for obtaining valid consent (see Figure 5)
- consent is not a contract to accept treatment – consent can be withdrawn at any point
- consent is not required in certain situations (see *Consent under the Law, ELOAM16*)

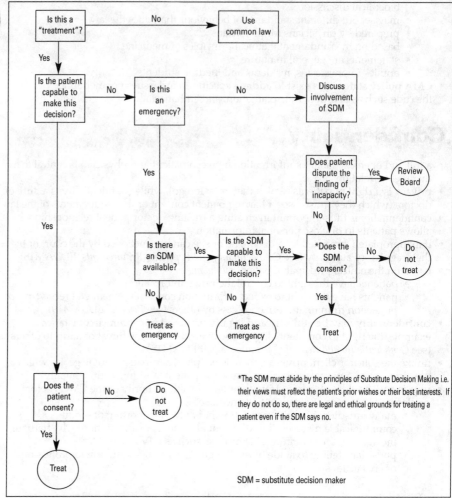

Figure 5. Consent Flowchart
Adapted by P. Hébert from Sunnybrook Health Sciences Centre Consent Guidelines.

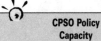

Assessing Capacity

- capacity is the ability to:
  - understand information relevant to a treatment decision
  - appreciate the reasonably foreseeable consequences of a decision or lack of a decision
- **capacity is specific** for each decision (e.g. a person may be capable to consent to having a chest x-ray, but not for a bronchoscopy)
- most Canadian jurisdictions distinguish capacity to make health care decisions from capacity to make financial decisions. A patient may be deemed capable of one but not the other
- **capacity can change over time** (e.g. temporary incapacity secondary to delirium)
- clinical capacity assessment may include:
  - specific capacity assessment, that is, capacity specific to the decision at hand
    1. effective disclosure of information and evaluation of patient's reason for decision
    2. for the ***understanding*** required to accept or refuse a medical treatment, one must understand
       - one's condition,
       - the nature of the proposed treatment,
       - alternatives to the treatment,
       - the consequences of accepting and rejecting the treatment, and
       - the risks and benefits of the various options (test: can the patient recite back what you have disclosed to them?)
    3. for the ***appreciation*** needed for decision making capacity, a person must:

- acknowledge the condition that affects himself or herself,
- be able to assess how the various options would affect him or her,
- be able to reach a decision and adhere to it, and make a choice, not based primarily upon delusional belief (test: are their beliefs responsive to evidence?)
  - general impressions
  - input from psychiatrists, neurologists, etc.
- employ "Aid to Capacity Evaluation" (see Table 2)
- a decision of incapacity may warrant further assessment – psychiatry, legal review boards, such as the courts or, in Ontario, the Consent and Capacity Review Board
- judicial review is open to patients as, if found incapable, they lose certain decision-making rights
- see *Consent Under the Law*, ELOAM16

Table 2. Aid to Capacity Evaluation

Ability to understand the medical problem

Ability to understand the proposed treatment

Ability to understand the alternatives (if any) to the proposed treatment

Ability to understand the option of refusing treatment or of it being withheld or withdrawn

Ability to appreciate the reasonably foreseeable consequences of accepting the proposed treatment

Ability to appreciate the reasonably foreseeable consequences of refusing the proposed treatment

Ability to make a decision that is not substantially based on delusions or depression

Adapted from Etchells et al. (1996).

- ethical principles underlying capacity
  - patient autonomy and respect for persons
  - physician beneficence requires that incapable persons be protected from making harmful decisions
  - even patients found incapable to make a specific decision should still be involved in that decision as much as possible (seek assent and cooperation and explore reasons for dissent)
  - people should be allowed to make their own informed decisions, or to appoint their own substitute decision maker
  - agreement or disagreement does not equal capacity
- age of consent for medical treatment in Canada
  - some provinces have a specific age of consent (PEI, NB, QC, SK, BC), but despite these regulations, common law and case law do deem underage legal minors capable, allowing them the right to make their own choice
  - Ontario has no legislation establishing an age of consent to treatment

Truth Telling

Ethical Basis
- helps to promote and maintain a trusting physician-patient relationship
- patients have a right to be told important information that physicians have regarding their care
- enables patients to make informed decisions about health care and about their lives
  - allows patients to seek medical attention when they should and organize their affairs as they choose

Legal Basis
- required for valid patient consent (see *Consent under the Law*, ELOAM16)
  - goal is to disclose information that a reasonable person in the patient's position would need in order to make an informed decision ("standard of disclosure")
- withholding information can be a breach of fiduciary duty and duty of care
- obtaining consent on the basis of misleading information can be seen as negligent

> **CPSO Policy**
> **Truth Telling**
> Physicians should provide patients with whatever information that will, from the patient's perspective, have a bearing on medical decision-making and communicate that information in a way that is comprehensible to the patient.

Evidence about Truth Telling
- most patients want to know what is wrong with them
- although many patients want to protect family members from bad news, they themselves would want to be informed in the same situation
- truth telling improves compliance and health outcomes
- informed patients are more satisfied with their care when compared to the less well informed
- negative consequences of truth telling can include decreased emotional well-being and suicidal thoughts

Reviewed in Hebert et al., 1997.

Difficulties in Truth Telling
- **Medical error**
  - many jurisdictions and professional associations expect and require physicians to disclose medical error; any event that harms or threatens to harm patients must be disclosed to the patient or the patient's family and reported to the appropriate health authorities

- physicians should disclose to patients the occurrence of adverse events or errors caused by medical management but should not suggest that they resulted from negligence because (a) negligence is a legal determination and (b) error is not equal to negligence; (see *Negligence and Liability*, ELOAM19)
- disclosure allows the injured patient to seek appropriate corrective treatment promptly
- physicians should avoid simple attributions as to cause and sole responsibility of others or oneself
- physicians should offer apologies or empathic expressions of regret ("I wish things had turned out differently"); these can increase trust and are not admissions of guilt or liability

- **Breaking bad news**
  - disclosure of difficult news is important and should be approached with care
  - adequate support should be provided along with the disclosure of difficult news
  - SPIKES protocol was developed to facilitate "breaking bad news" (see sidebar)

Arguments against Truth Telling
- may go against certain cultural norms and expectations
- may lead to patient harm and increased anxiety
- some patients prefer to waive the right to be informed
- medical uncertainty may result in the disclosure of uncertain or inaccurate information

Exceptions to Truth Telling
- waiving the right to know: patient capably decides to decline information
- physicians should explore this desire to determine if it is authentic
- patients should be explicitly offered the opportunity to be told important information or for substitute decision maker/family to be informed
- a patient may waive their right to know the truth about their situation when:
  - disclosure would in itself cause physical or mental harm to the patient
  - a strong cultural component exists that must be respected and acknowledged
  - the patient is incapacitated
  - he or she is in a medical emergency
  - the more weighty the consequences for the patient from non-disclosure, the more carefully one must consider the right to ignorance; arguably, such a patient could be considered as incapacitated and a substitute decision maker may need to be found to whom disclosure can be made
- the doctrine of therapeutic privilege is no longer acceptable in Canadian courts
  - this principle refers to the withholding of information by the clinician in the belief that disclosure of this information would lead to the harm or suffering of the patient
  - clinicians should **avoid** invoking therapeutic privilege and allow patients to make decisions since the burden of proof to justify nondisclosure will be the physician's

Resource Allocation

- resource allocation is the distribution of goods and services to programs and people
- the physician's primary duty is towards his or her individual patients
- physicians have the duty to inform patients about therapeutic options even if they are not available
- ethics relate to **justice**: physicians must make health care resources available to patients in a manner which is fair and equitable, without bias or discrimination
  - need and benefit are considered morally relevant criteria for resource allocation
  - gender, sexual orientation, religion, level of education or age alone are morally irrelevant criteria
- ethical **dilemmas** that arise when deciding how best to allocate resources
  - fair chances versus best outcome – favouring best outcome versus giving all patients fair access to limited resources (e.g. transplant list prioritization)
  - priorities problem – how much priority should treating the sickest patients receive?
  - aggregation problem – modest benefits to many versus significant benefits to few
  - democracy problem – when to rely on a fair democratic process as the only way to arrive at a decision
- guidelines for appropriately allocating resources
  - the physician's primary obligation is to protect and promote the welfare and best interests of his or her patients
  - choose interventions known to be beneficial on the basis of evidence of effectiveness
  - seek the tests or treatments that will accomplish the diagnostic or therapeutic goal for the least cost
  - advocate for one's own patients but avoid manipulating the system to gain unfair advantage for them
  - resolve conflicting claims for scarce resources justly, on the basis of morally relevant criteria such as need and benefit, using fair and publicly defensible procedures
  - inform patients of the impact of cost constraints on care, but do so in a sensitive way
  - seek resolution of unacceptable shortages at the level of hospital management or government

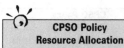

SPIKES Protocol to Break Bad News

S **setting** and listening skills

P patient's **perception** of condition and seriousness

I **invitation** from patient to give information

K **knowledge** – giving medical facts

E **explore** emotions and empathize

S **strategy** and **summary**

WF Baile and R Buckman, 2000.

CPSO Policy Resource Allocation
Physicians should "recognize [their] responsibility to promote fair access to health care resources" and should "use health care resources prudently."

Research Ethics

- involves the systematic analysis of ethical dilemmas arising during research involving human subjects to ensure the following:
    - that study participants are protected
    - that clinical research is conducted to serve the interests of the participants and/or society as a whole
- major ethical dilemmas arise when a physician's obligation to the patient comes into conflict with other obligations and incentives
- any exceptions to disclosure for therapeutic consent do not apply in an experimental situation

Table 3. Ethical Principles for Research Involving Human Subjects (laid out in the *Declaration of Helsinki*, the *Belmont Report*, etc.) Include:

Patient's participation in research should not put him/her at a known or probable disadvantage with respect to medical care

Participant's voluntary and informed choice is usually required
- Consent may not be required in special circumstances: chart reviews without patient contact; emergency situations for which there is no accepted or helpful standard of care and the proposed intervention is not likely to cause more harm than such patients already face

Access to the treatment that is considered standard
- Placebo-controlled trials are generally acceptable where patients still receive the standard of care and are informed about the placebo arm and what that entails

Must employ a scientifically valid design to answer the research question
- Scientific rigour ensured via peer review, expert opinion

Must demonstrate sufficient value to justify the risk posed to participants

Must be conducted honestly (i.e. carried out as stated in the approved protocol)

Findings must be reported promptly and accurately, without exaggeration, to allow practicing clinicians to draw reasonable conclusions

Patients must not be enticed into risky research by the lure of money and investigators must not trade the interests of patients for disproportionate recompense by a sponsor; both participants and investigators are due, however, fair recompense for their time and efforts

Any significant interventional trial ought to have a data safety monitoring board that is independent of the sponsor and can ensure safety of the ongoing trial

> **Guiding Principles for Research Ethics:**
> 1) *Respect for persons* (i.e. informed consent)
> 2) *Beneficence* (i.e. balancing benefits and harms)
> 3) *Justice* (i.e. avoiding exploitation or unjustified exclusion)

> **Informed Consent for Research**
> - the nature of informed consent differs in the contexts of research and clinical practice in that the potential research subject must be informed about:
>   - the purpose of the study
>   - its source of funding
>   - the nature and relative probability of harms and benefits
>   - the nature of the physician's participation including any compensation
> - proposals for research must be submitted to a research ethics board to be scientifically and ethically evaluated and approved

Physician-Industry Relations

- health care delivery in Canada involves collaboration between physicians and the pharmaceutical and health supply industries in the areas of research, education, and clinical evaluation packages (product samples)
- physicians have a responsibility to ensure that their participation in such collaborative efforts is in keeping with their duties to their patients and society
- gifts or free products from the pharmaceutical industry are inappropriate
    - sponsorship for travel and fees for conference attendance may be accepted only where the physician is a conference presenter and not just in attendance
    - physicians receiving such sponsorship must disclose this at presentations or in written articles
- CMA and CPSO guidelines for ethically appropriate physician-industry relations
    - the primary goal should be the advancement of the health of Canadians
    - relationships should be guided by the CMA Code of Ethics
    - the physician's primary obligation is to the patient
    - physicians should avoid any self-interest in their prescribing and referral practices
    - physicians should always maintain professional autonomy, independence and commitment to the scientific method
- physicians are able to set limits on their practice in terms of who they will see; such limits must be free of discriminatory bias

Doctor-Patient Relationship

CMA definition of the doctor-patient relationship:
- the fundamental basis of the therapeutic relationship
- a partnership based on the physician providing expert opinion, information, options and interventions that allow the patient to make informed choices about their health care
- within this relationship, the doctor and patient share the goals of positive health outcomes, good communication, honesty, flexibility, sensitivity, informed consent and, above all, respect

- this relationship has the potential to be unequal due to a power difference
  - patients are ill and lack medical knowledge
  - physicians possess medical knowledge and skills and have their patients' trust
- due to the nature of the doctor-patient relationship, the physician will:
  - place the best interests of the patient first
  - establish a relationship of trust between physician and patient
  - follow through on undertakings made to the patient in good faith
- the physician will accept or refuse patients requesting care:
  - without consideration of race, gender, age, sexual orientation, financial means, religion or nationality
  - without arbitrary exclusion of any particular group of patients, such as those known to be difficult or afflicted with serious disease
  - except in emergency situations, in which case care must be rendered
- once having accepted a patient into care, the physician may terminate the relationship providing:
  - it is not an emergency
  - care has been transferred
  - adequate notice has been given to allow the patient to make alternative arrangements
  - they have other options to find 'medically necessary care'
- the physician will not exploit the doctor-patient relationship for personal advantage – financial, academic or otherwise
- the physician will disclose limitations to the patient where personal beliefs or inclinations limit the treatment the physician is able to offer
- the physician will maintain and respect professional boundaries at all times
  - including physical, emotional, and sexual boundaries
  - regarding treatment of themselves, their families, or friends

> **CPSO Policy**
> **Treating Self and Family Members**
> Physicians will not diagnose or treat themselves or family members except for minor conditions or in emergencies and then only if no other physician is readily available.

> **CPSO Policy**
> **Ending the Physician-Patient Relationship**
> Discontinuing services that are needed is an act of professional misconduct unless done by patient request, alternative services are arranged, or adequate notice has been given.

Personal and Professional Conduct

CANMEDS Competencies
- a framework of professional competencies established by the Medical Council of Canada (MCC) as objectives for the Medical Council of Canada Qualifying Exam (MCCQE)
- further information on MCC objectives can be found at: www.mcc.ca

1. Communicator; Culturally Aware:
- display sensitivity to people of all ages, races, cultures, religions, sexual orientations and genders
- accept or refuse patients without consideration of age, race, culture, religion, sexual orientation and gender
- understand the variation in values and morals and their impact on approaches to care and decision-making
- elicit patients' beliefs, concerns and expectations about their illness
- conduct patient-centered interviews, ensure patient comprehension

2. Collaborator:
- respect all members of the health care team
- identify the roles and competencies of each member, and delegate tasks appropriately
- consult other physicians and health care professionals effectively and appropriately
- consult with patients and families regarding continuing care plans
- be able to outline co-ordination of services (Public Health, Home Care, Social Services, Workers' Compensation, Children's Aid Society, etc.)

3. Health Advocate:
- identify determinants of health:
  - biological (genes, impact of lifestyle)
  - physical (food, shelter, working conditions)
  - social (education, employment, culture, access to care)
- influence public health and health policy in order to protect, maintain and promote the health of individuals and the community

4. Manager:
- describe different remuneration models: fee-for-service, salary, capitation
- meet regulatory requirements in an office practice (medical record-keeping, narcotic control, infection control, etc.)
- be prudent in utilization of finite health care resources, based on anticipated cost-benefit balance
- regulate work schedule such that time is available for continuing education

5. Professional:
- maintain standards of excellence in clinical care and ethical conduct
- exhibit appropriate personal and interpersonal behaviour
- enhance clinical competence through lifelong learning
- accept responsibility for personal actions

- do not exploit the physician-patient relationship for personal advantage (financial, academic, etc.)

6. Scholar:
- commitment to critical appraisal, constructive skepticism
- participate in the learning of peers and others (students, health care professionals, patients)

Areas of Controversy

Euthanasia and Physician-Assisted Suicide
- **euthanasia**: a deliberate act undertaken by one person with the intention of ending the life of another person to relieve that person's suffering where the act is the cause of death
- **physician-assisted suicide**: the act of intentionally killing oneself with the assistance of a physician who deliberately provides the knowledge and/or the means
- ethical issues and arguments:
  - right to make autonomous choices about the time and manner of own death
  - belief that there is no ethical difference between the acts of euthanasia/assisted suicide and foregoing life-sustaining treatments
  - belief that these acts benefit terminally ill patients by relieving suffering
  - patient autonomy has limits
  - death should be the consequence of the morally justified withdrawal of life-sustaining treatments only in cases where there is a fatal underlying condition, and it is the condition (not the withdrawal of treatment) that causes death
- **law**: both euthanasia and physician-assisted suicide are punishable offences under the Criminal Code of Canada
- euthanasia and assisted suicide is distinguished from palliative care because in the latter, the death of the patient is not intended, drugs are used in response to symptoms, and the escalation of drugs is done in proportion to the patient's symptoms

> **Dealing with Controversial & Ethical Issues in Practice**
> - discuss in a non-judgmental manner
> - ensure patients have full access to relevant and necessary information
> - identify if certain options lie outside of your moral boundaries and refer to another physician if appropriate
> - consult with appropriate ethics committees or boards
> - protect freedom of moral choice for students or trainees
> Source: MCC-CLEO Objectives, 1998.

> **Euthanasia: Ethically Appropriate Actions**
> - respect competent decisions to forgo treatment
> - provide appropriate palliative measures
> - decline requests for euthanasia and assisted suicide

Maternal-Fetal Conflict of Rights
- conflict between maternal autonomy and the best interests of the fetus
- ethical issues and arguments:
  - principle of reproductive freedom
    - women have the right to make their own reproductive choices
  - coercion of a woman to accept efforts to promote fetal well-being is an unacceptable infringement of her personal autonomy
- law – upholds a woman's right to life, liberty, and security of person and does not recognize fetal rights
  - if a woman is competent and refuses medical advice, her decision must be respected even if the fetus will suffer as a result
  - the fetus does not have legal rights until it is born alive and with complete delivery from the body of the woman
- *Royal Commission on New Reproductive Technologies* recommendations:
  - medical treatment must never be imposed upon a competent pregnant woman against her wishes
  - no law should be used to confine a pregnant woman in the interest of her fetus
  - the conduct of a pregnant woman in relation to her fetus should not be criminalized
  - child welfare should never be used to control a woman's behaviour during pregnancy
  - civil liability should never be imposed upon a woman for harm done to her fetus during pregnancy
- ethically appropriate actions:
  - a woman is permitted to refuse HIV testing during pregnancy, even if this results in vertical transmission to fetus
  - a woman is permitted to refuse Caesarean section in labour that is not progressing, despite evidence of fetal distress

Advanced Reproductive Technologies (ART)
- types of ART:
  - **non-coital insemination**: intrauterine or intravaginal insemination from either a donor or a woman's partner
  - **hormonal ovarian stimulation**: increases the number of mature oocytes
  - *in vitro* **fertilization**: hormonal ovarian stimulation is used to mature multiple ova which are retrieved and fertilized in the laboratory
- ethical issues and arguments:
  - donor anonymity versus child-centred reproduction (knowledge about genetic medical history)
  - preimplantation genetic testing for diagnosis before pregnancy
  - lack of sufficient data regarding efficacy and complications to provide the full disclosure needed for truly informed consent
  - use of new techniques without patients appreciating their experimental nature

> **Advanced Reproductive Technologies: Ethically Appropriate Actions**
> - educate patients and address contributors to infertility (e.g. stress, alcohol, medications, etc.)
> - investigate and treat underlying health problems causing infertility
> - wait at least one year before initiating treatment with ART (exceptions - advanced age or specific indicators of infertility)
> - educate and prepare patients for potential negative outcomes of ART

- embryo status - the Supreme Court of Canada maintains that fetuses are "unique" but not persons under law; this view would likely apply to embryos as well
- access to ART
  - private versus public funding
  - social factors limiting access to ART (e.g. same-sex couples)
- commercialization of reproduction; reimbursement of gamete donors is currently illegal in Canada

Fetal Tissue

The CMA remains neutral on the issue of embryonic stem cell research.

- pluripotent stem cells have been derived from human embryonic and fetal tissue
- potential uses of stem cells in research:
  - studying human development and factors that direct cell specialization
  - evaluating drugs for efficacy and safety in human models
  - cell therapy: using stem cells grown *in vitro* to repair or replace degenerated/destroyed/malignant tissues (e.g. Parkinson's disease)
  - genetic treatment aimed at altering germ cells is prohibited in Canada and elsewhere
  - genetic treatment aimed at altering somatic cells (i.e. myocardial or immunological cells is acceptable and ongoing)
- ethical issues and arguments:
  - the opinions on embryo status range from full moral status → special moral status → collection of cells
- *Tri-Council Policy Statement: Ethical Conduct for Research Involving Humans* (Government of Canada, 2003)
  - embryo research is permitted up to 14 days post-fertilization
  - embryos created for reproductive purposes that are no longer required may be used
  - gamete providers must give free and informed consent for research use
  - no commercial transactions in the creation and use of the embryos is permitted
  - creation of embryos solely for research purposes is prohibited
  - human cloning is strictly prohibited
- risks of coercion must be minimized:
  - may not pressure fertility treatment team to generate more embryos than necessary
  - only discuss option of using fetal tissue for research after free and informed choice to have a therapeutic abortion has been made
  - physicians responsible for fertility treatment may not be part of a stem cell research team

Abortion

- abortion: the active termination of a pregnancy before fetal viability
  - fetal viability: fetus >500 g weight, or >23-24 weeks gestational age
  - in the case of multiple pregnancy, selective termination of the nonviable or less viable fetus is allowed
- ethical and legal issues and arguments:
  - according to common law, the rights of a fetus are not equal to those of a human being
  - who should have input into the abortion decision (e.g. male partners, patient's guardians)
    - no law currently regulates abortion in Canada – it is a woman's medical decision to be made in consultation with whom she wishes; no mandatory role for spouse/family
- CMA policy on induced abortion:
  - induced abortion should not be used as an alternative to contraception
  - counselling on contraception must be readily available
  - full and immediate counselling services must be provided in the event of unwanted pregnancy
  - there should be no delay in the provision of abortion services
  - no patient should be compelled to have a pregnancy terminated
  - physicians should not be compelled to participate in abortion – if morally opposed, the physician should inform the patient so she may consult another physician
  - no discrimination should be directed towards either physicians who do not perform or assist at induced abortions or physicians who do
  - induced abortion should be uniformly available to all women in Canada and health care insurance should cover all the costs

Genetic Testing

- uses:
  - confirm a clinical diagnosis
  - detect genetic predisposition to a disease
    - allows preventative steps to be taken and helps patient prepare for the future

- give parents the option to terminate a pregnancy or begin early treatment
- ethical dilemmas arise because of the nature of genetic information:
  - it has individual and familial implications
  - it pertains to future disease
  - it often identifies disorders for which there are no effective treatments or preventative steps
- ethical issues and arguments:
  - obtaining informed consent is difficult due to the complexity of genetic information
  - doctor's duty to maintain confidentiality versus duty to warn family members
  - risk of social discrimination (e.g. insurance) and psychological harm
- law:
  - no current specific legislation exists
  - testing requires informed consent
  - no standard of care exists for clinical genetics but physicians are legally obligated to inform patients that prenatal testing exists and is available
  - breach of confidentiality – duty to warn family members
    - ◆ only acceptable if can likely prevent serious harm, such as if treatment or prevention is available (e.g. familial adenomatous polyposis)

N.B.: Canadian law applicable to medical
Genetic Testing: Ethically Appropriate
Actions
- thorough discussion and realistic planning with patient before testing is done
- genetic counselling for delivery of complex information, supportive discussion

CMA Policies on Controversial Issues
- euthanasia and assisted suicide: Canadian physicians should not participate in euthanasia and assisted suicide
- maternal-fetal conflict of rights: a physician must respect the right of a competent pregnant patient to accept or reject any medical care recommended
- assisted reproduction: assisted human reproduction has the potential for both benefit and harm, and therefore needs to be regulated
- use of fetal tissue: the CMA remains neutral on the issue of embryonic stem cell research

Legal Matters

The Doctor-Patient Relationship under the Law

- the laws which regulate the doctor-patient relationship function to protect patients
- these laws are derived from three sources: 1. **the common law** (or, in Quebec, the *Civil Code of Quebec*), 2. **statutes**, and 3. **the Constitution**
- **the common law** is the body of legal rules and principles, derived from judges' decisions, that forms the basis of the Anglo-Canadian legal system. Areas of common law include:
  - *tort law* allows patients to recover damages for wrongful acts committed against them. The most important torts in medical relationships are 1. *negligence* (see *Negligence and Liability*, ELOAM19) and 2. *battery* (the application of force to a person's body without their consent)
  - the doctor-patient relationship constitutes a *contract*. This gives rise to various *contractual rights and obligations* that, if breached, may result in the award of damages
  - a doctor also has a *fiduciary duty* to their patient – that is, an obligation to act in the patient's best interests
- **statutes** are laws passed by provincial legislatures and the federal parliament, for example:
  - in Ontario, the *Health Care Consent Act* (HCCA) regulates consent to treatment (see *Consent under the Law*, ELOAM16)
  - the *Personal Health Information Protection Act* regulates the collection, use and disclosure of health records (see *Privacy of Medical Records*, ELOAM19)
  - the *Criminal Code* and the *Controlled Drugs and Substances Act* regulate the use of many medications
- **the Constitution** is the supreme law of Canada: all other laws must be consistent with it or they are of no force and effect
  - the *Canadian Charter of Rights and Freedoms* guarantees individuals the rights (among others) of life, liberty, security of the person, and equality under the law
  - these rights are subject only to such reasonable limits prescribed by law as can be demonstrably justified in a free and democratic society

N.B.: Canadian law applicable to medical practice varies between jurisdictions and also changes over time.

- Criminal law is nationwide but non-criminal (civil) law varies between provinces.

- This section is meant to serve only as a guide; students and physicians should ensure that their practices conform to local and current laws.

Consent under the Law

- consent of the patient must be obtained before any medical intervention is provided
- consent can be oral or written, although written is usually preferred
- consent can be either expressed or implied; an example of implied consent is a patient holding out their arm for an immunization
- consent is an ongoing process; consent may be withdrawn or changed after it is given
- *Health Care Consent Act* covers consent to treatment, admission to a facility, and personal assistance services (e.g. home care)

Exceptions to Consent
1. Emergencies
- treatment can be provided without consent where a patient is experiencing severe suffering, OR where a delay in treatment would lead to serious harm or death AND consent cannot be obtained from the patient or their substitute decision maker
- emergency treatment should not violate a prior capable expressed wish of the patient (e.g. a signed Jehovah's Witness card)

2. Legislation
- Mental Health legislation allows for:
  - the detention of patients without their consent (see *Consent*, ELOAM7)
  - psychiatric outpatients to be compelled to adhere to a care plan (see <u>Psychiatry</u>)
- Public Health legislation allows medical officers of health to detain, examine, and treat patients without their consent (e.g. a patient with TB refusing to take medication) for the purpose of preventing transmission of communicable diseases (see <u>Population and Community Health</u>)

3. Special Situations
- public health emergencies such as an epidemic or communicable disease treatment
- warrant for information by police

Four basic requirements of valid consent
1. Voluntary
- consent must be given free of coercion or pressure
- the physician must not deliberately mislead the patient about the proposed treatment

2. Capable
- the patient must be able to understand the nature and effect of the proposed treatment

3. Specific
- the consent provided is specific to the particular procedure being proposed and to the particular provider who will carry out the procedure (i.e. the patient must be informed if students will be involved in providing the treatment)

4. Informed
- sufficient information must be provided to allow the patient to make choices in accordance with their wishes. This information should include:
  - the nature of the treatment or investigation proposed and its expected effects
  - all significant risks and special or unusual risks
  - alternative treatments or investigations, and their anticipated effects and significant risks
  - the consequences of declining treatment
  - common risks that are common sense need not to be disclosed (i.e. bruising after venipuncture)
- the **reasonable person test** – the physician must provide all the information that would be needed "by a reasonable person in the patient's position" to be able to make the treatment decision
  - disclose common adverse events (>1 in 200 chance of occurrence) and serious risks such as death, even if remote
- it is the physician's responsibility to make reasonable attempts to ensure that the patient understands the information
- physicians cannot withhold information about a therapeutic option based on personal conscience (e.g. not discussing the option of emergency contraception with a rape victim)

Consequences of failure to obtain valid consent
- treatment without consent is battery, even if the treatment is life-saving
- treatment of a patient on the basis of poorly informed consent may constitute negligence
- the onus of proof that valid consent was not obtained rests with the plaintiff (usually, the patient)

Capacity and Substitute Decision Makers (see *Assessing Capacity*, ELOAM8)
- capable patients are entitled to make their own decisions
- capacity assessments should be conducted by MD and, if possible, in collaboration with other health care professionals (e.g. another physician, a psychiatrist, a mental health nurse)

"Every patient has a right to bodily integrity. This encompasses the right to determine what medical procedures will be accepted and the extent to which they will be accepted. Everyone has the right to decide what is to be done to one's own body. This includes the right to be free from medical treatment to which the individual does not consent."

Ciarlariello v. Schacter, [1993] Supreme Court of Canada decision

---

Major Exceptions to Consent
- Emergencies
- Communicable diseases
- Mental Health legislation

The Supreme Court of Canada expects physicians to disclose the risks that a "reasonable" person would want to know. In practice, this means disclosing minor risks that are common as well as serious risks that happen infrequently.

Consent:
Treatment without consent = battery, including if NO consent or if WRONG procedure

Treatment with poor or invalid consent = negligence

- capable patients can refuse treatment even if it leads to serious harm or death and this does not indicate a lack of capacity

Substitute Decision Makers (SDMs)
- principles a SDM must follow when giving informed consent:
  - act in accordance with wishes previously expressed by the patient, while capable
  - if wishes unknown, SDM must act in the patient's best interest, taking the following into account:
    1. values and beliefs held by the patient while capable
    2. whether well-being is likely to improve with vs. without treatment
    3. whether the benefit expected by the treatment outweighs the risk of harm
    4. whether a less intrusive treatment would be as beneficial as the one proposed
  - the final decision of the SDM should be made in consultation with the MD
- most provinces have legislated hierarchies for SDMs; the hierarchy in Ontario is:
  1. patient's legally appointed guardian
  2. patient's appointed attorney for personal care, if a power of attorney confers authority for treatment consent (see *Power of Attorney*, ELOAM18)
  3. representative appointed by the Consent and Capacity Board
  4. spouse or partner
  5. child (age 16 or older) or parent (unless the parent has only a right of access)
  6. parent with only a right of access
  7. brother or sister
  8. other relative(s)
  9. public guardian and trustee

If the MD feels the SDM is not acting in the patient's best interest, the MD can apply to Consent and Capacity Board for another SDM.

Treatment of the Incapable Patient
- obtain informed consent from SDM
- an incapable patient can only be detained against his/her will to receive treatment if he/she meets criteria for certification under the *Mental Health Act* (see <u>Psychiatry</u>). In such a situation:
  - document assessment in chart
  - notify patient of assessment using appropriate Mental Health Form(s) (Form 42)
  - notify Rights Advisor

Treatment of the Incapable Patient in an Emergency Situation
- emergency treatment may be administered without consent if the physician believes the incapable patient is:
  - experiencing extreme suffering
  - at risk of sustaining serious bodily harm if treatment is not administered promptly
- MD must document reasons for incapacity and why situation is emergent
- if a SDM is not available, MD can treat without consent until the SDM is available or the situation is no longer emergent

Administration of treatment for an incapable patient in an Emergency Situation is applicable if the patient is:
1. experiencing extreme suffering
2. at risk of sustaining serious bodily harm if treatment is not administered promptly

Pediatric Aspects of Capacity Covered by the *HCCA*
- no age of consent – consent depends on one's decision-making ability (capacity)
- this causes a dilemma with patients who are infants or children; adolescents are usually treated as adults
- it is assumed that infants and children lack mature decision-making capacity for consent but they should still be involved (e.g. be provided the information appropriate to their comprehension level)
- preferably, assent should be gained from patient, if not capable of giving consent
- most likely SDM in hierarchy is a parent or legal guardian
- in the event that the physician believes the SDM is not acting in the child's best interest, an appeal must be made to the local child welfare authorities
- parents have access to medical record
- should open parental chart to record specific parental information
- maintain chart for 10 years after child's 18th birthday

In the pediatric population there is no age of consent.

Other Types of Capacity Not Covered by the *HCCA*
- testamentary (ability to make a will)
- fitness (ability to stand trial)
- financial (ability to manage property – Form 21 of the *Mental Health Act*)
- personal (ability to care for oneself on a daily basis)

Criteria for Financial Competence
- covered by the *Mental Health Act and Substitute Decision Act*
- patient must:
  - appreciate importance of financial capability and reason for exam
  - have realistic appreciation of own strengths/weaknesses in managing finances
  - understand nature and extent of assets, liabilities, income, and expenses
  - have recently demonstrated ability to make reasonable financial decisions and be expected to do so in future

- have appropriately used available resources, and indicate willingness to do so in future
- if MD determines the patient is incapable of managing property, a Form 21 is completed and the Public Guardian and Trustee becomes the temporary guardian until a substitute can be found; those eligible as substitute guardians are the patient's spouse/partner, relative, or attorney
- Form 21 can only be filled out if the patient is an inpatient of a psychiatric facility
- Form 24 to be filled out in order to continue financial incapacity upon discharge from hospital

Instructional Advance Directives
- allow patients to exert control over their care once they are no longer capable
- in an advanced directive, the patient sets out their decisions about future health care, including who they want to make their treatment decisions and what types of interventions they would want
- the advanced directive takes effect once the patient is incapable with respect to treatment decisions
- in Ontario, a person can appoint a "power of attorney for personal care" to carry out his/her advance directives
- patients should be encouraged to review these documents with their family and their physicians, and to reevaluate it often as their illness progresses to ensure it is current with their wishes

Power of Attorney

Legal Terms and Definitions

Power of Attorney for Personal Care
- a legal document in which one person gives another person the authority to make personal care decisions (health care, nutrition, shelter, clothing, hygiene, safety) on their behalf if they become mentally incapable

Guardian of the Person
- someone who is appointed by the Court to make decisions on behalf of an incapable person in some or all areas of personal care, in the absence of a power of attorney for personal care

Continuing Power of Attorney for Property
- a legal document in which a person gives someone else the legal authority to make decisions about their finances if they become unable to make those decisions themselves

Guardian of Property
- someone who is appointed by the Public Guardian and Trustee or the Courts to look after an incapable person's property or finances

Public Guardian and Trustee
- acts as a substitute decision maker of last resort on behalf of those mentally incapable people who have no one who is willing or able to act on their behalf

Confidentiality and Reporting Requirements

- physicians have a legal duty to maintain the confidentiality of their patients' medical information
- this legal duty is imposed by both provincial health information legislation and by various precedent-setting cases in the common law
- the right to confidentiality is not absolute
- disclosure of health information can take place: 1) with the patient's consent, and 2) without the patient's consent in certain circumstances defined by statutory and common law

The legal aspects of confidentiality can be complex; advice should always be sought from provincial licensing authorities and/or legal counsel when in doubt.

Statutory Reporting Obligations
- specific instances where legislation has defined that the public interest overrides the patient right to confidentiality; these requirements vary by province, but may include:
    1. suspected child abuse or neglect: reported to local child welfare authorities (e.g. Children's Aid Society)
    2. fitness to drive a vehicle or fly an airplane if a pilot: reported to provincial Ministry of Transportation (see Geriatric Medicine)
    3. communicable diseases: reported to local public health authority (see Population and Community Health)

4. improper conduct of other physicians or health professionals: report to college or regulatory body of the health professional (sexual impropriety by physicians is required reporting in some provinces)
5. vital statistics must be reported and reporting may vary by province (in Ontario, births are required to be reported within 30 days to Office of Registrar General or local municipality; death certificates must be completed by a physician and then forwarded to municipal authorities)
6. reporting to coroners (see *Physician Responsibilities Regarding Death*, ELOAM20)
- physicians who fail to report in these situations are subject to prosecution and penalty, and may be liable if a third party has been harmed

Duty to Inform/Warn
- the physician has a duty to inform the police or a potential victim (in appropriate circumstances) if a patient expresses a serious intention to inflict harm
- first established by a Supreme Court of California decision in 1976; not yet tested in Canadian courts
- is obliged by the CMA Code of Ethics and is allowed for by some provincial health information laws
- applies in a situation where:
    1. there is a clear risk to an identifiable person or group of persons;
    2. there is a risk of serious bodily harm or death; and
    3. the danger is imminent
- see sidebar for additional guidelines

Disclosure for Legal Proceedings
- disclosure of health records can be compelled by a court order, warrant or subpoena

Privacy of Medical Records

- privacy is a right underpinning health care in Canada
- privacy of health information is protected by professional codes of ethics, provincial and federal legislation, the *Canadian Charter of Rights and Freedoms*, and the fiduciary duty
- the federal government created the *Personal Information Protection and Electronic Documents Act* (PIPEDA) which established principles for the collection, use, and disclosure of information that is part of commercial activity (e.g. physician practices, pharmacies, private labs)
- PIPEDA has been superseded by provincial legislation in many provinces, including the *Ontario Personal Health Information Protection Act (PHIPA)*

Duties of physicians with regards to the privacy of health information
- inform patients of your information-handling practices through various means (i.e. the posting of notices, brochures and pamphlets, and/or through normal discussions between a patient and a health care provider)
- obtain the patient's express consent to disclose information to third parties
    - under Ontario privacy legislation, you do not need to get the patient's express consent to share information between health care team members involved in the "circle of care." However, the patient may withdraw consent for this sharing of information
- provide a patient with access to their own medical records
    - there are limited reasons why: a patient may not be able to access their medical information, including when there is a potential for harm either to the patient or to a third party
- provide secure storage of information and implement measures to limit access to patient records
- ensure proper destruction of information that is no longer necessary

Negligence and Liability

- **negligence** is the breach of a legal duty of care which results in damage
- negligence is a legal finding, not a medical one
- physicians may be found negligent when all the following four conditions are met:
    1. the physician owed a **legal duty of care to the patient** (the existence of a doctor-patient relationship generally suffices)
    2. the **duty of care was breached** (e.g. by failure to provide the **standard of care**)
    3. the patient was **injured or harmed**
    4. the harm or injury was caused by the breach of the duty of care
- the **standard of care** is one that would reasonably be expected under similar circumstances of an ordinary, prudent physician of the same training, experience, and specialization
- errors of judgement are not necessarily negligent

- making the wrong diagnosis is not negligent if a reasonable doctor might have made the same mistake in the same circumstances (i.e. misdiagnosing appendicitis as pelvic inflammatory disease)
  - failure to reconsider the diagnosis if the patient does not respond to treatment may be negligent
- physicians can also be held liable for the negligent actions of their employees or other individuals they are supervising

Physician Competence and Conduct

Provincial legislation deems sexual abuse of a patient as professional misconduct.

Source: Regulated Health Professions Act, 1991, section 4.

- the competence and conduct of physicians is legally regulated in certain respects to protect patients and society
- physicians are legally required to maintain a license with the appropriate authority
- physicians must ensure that patients have access to continuous on-call coverage and are never abandoned
- sexual conduct with patients, even when consented to by the patient, is a serious matter that can lead to criminal, civil, and disciplinary action
  - sexual conduct includes intercourse, undue touching, inappropriate reference to sexual matters, sexual jokes, and physician presence when capable patients undress or dress themselves
  - physicians may have a personal relationship with a patient providing a year has passed since the last therapeutic contact
  - physicians are prohibited from personal relationships with patients for whom they saw for psychotherapy
  - in Ontario, physicians must report to appropriate authorities any colleagues of whom they have information regarding sexual impropriety
- physicians must maintain adequate records for each patient, including:
  - showing that care has been continuous and comprehensive
  - minimal standards for record keeping include: diagnosis, differential diagnosis, appropriate tests and referrals, coherent patient record (full standards available on CPSO website, www.cpso.on.ca)
  - keeping records for 10 years in most jurisdictions
  - although the medical record is the property of the physician or an institution, the patient or the patient's delegate must be allowed full access to information in the medical record upon (usually written) request
- in the hospital environment, physicians must ensure their own competence, respect hospital by-laws and regulations, practice only within the limits of granted privileges, cooperate with other hospital personnel, and maintain adequate hospital records

CMA Code of Ethics
Report any unprofessional conduct by colleagues to the appropriate authority.

Physician Responsibilities Regarding Death

- physicians are required by law to complete a medical certificate of death unless the coroner needs notification (see below); failure to report death is a criminal offence

Role of the Coroner

Notify Coroner if Death Occurs due to:
- Violence, negligence, misconduct
- Pregnancy
- Sudden or unexpected causes
- Disease **NOT** treated
- Cause **other** than disease
- Suspicious circumstances

- *Coroner's Act* (specific to Ontario, similar in other provinces) requires physicians to notify a coroner or police officer if death occurs:
  - due to violence, negligence, misconduct, misadventure, or malpractice
  - during pregnancy or is attributable to pregnancy
  - suddenly and unexpectedly
  - from disease which was not treated by a legally qualified medical practitioner
  - from any cause other than disease
  - under suspicious circumstances
- coroner investigates these deaths, as well as deaths that occur in psychiatric institutions, jails, foster homes, nursing homes, hospitals to which a person was transferred from a facility, institution or home, etc.
- in consultation with forensic pathologists and other specialists, the coroner establishes:
  - the identity of the deceased
  - where and when the death occurred
  - the medical cause of death
  - the means of death
    - natural
    - accidental
    - suicide
    - homicide
    - undetermined
- coroners do not make decisions regarding criminality or legal responsibility

Anesthesia and Perioperative Medicine

Khaled Hasan and John Kim, chapter editors
Sami Chadi and Biniam Kidane, associate editors
Emily Partridge, EBM editor
Dr. Isabella Devito and Dr. Ryan Mai, staff editors

Basic Anatomy Review

- normal airway begins at nares
- resistance to airflow through nasal passages accounts for approximately 2/3 of total airway resistance
- pharyngeal airway extends from posterior aspect of nose to cricoid cartilage
- the larynx consists of muscles, ligaments and a collection of cartilages (thyroid, cricoid, arytenoids, corniculates, and epiglottis)
- the curved MacIntosh blade is placed in the valleculae – depressions on either side of the glossoepiglottic fold
- the glottic opening (triangular space formed between the true vocal cords) is the narrowest segment of the laryngeal opening in adults
- when intubating, the glottic opening is used as the space through which one visualizes proper placement of the endotracheal tube (ETT)
- the trachea begins at the level of the thyroid cartilage (opposite C6)
- the trachea bifurcates into the right and left main bronchi at the level of T5

Pre-Operative Assessment

- the purpose of the pre-operative assessment is to identify the patient's medical and surgical problems; to allow for the arrangement of further investigations, consultations and treatments for patients whose conditions are not optimized; and to plan anesthetic techniques

History & Physical

History
- indication for surgery
- surgical/anesthetic Hx: previous anesthetics/complications, previous intubations, medications, drug allergies
- PMH
  - CNS: seizures, stroke, raised intracranial pressure (ICP), spinal disease
  - CVS: coronary artery disease (CAD), myocardial infarction (MI), congestive heart failure (CHF), hypertension (HTN), valvular disease, dysrhythmias, peripheral vascular disease (PVD), conditions requiring endocarditis prophylaxis, exercise tolerance, CCS class, NYHA class
  - respiratory: smoking, asthma, chronic obstructive pulmonary disease (COPD), recent upper respiratory tract infection (URTI), sleep apnea
  - GI: gastroesophageal reflux disease (GERD), liver disease
  - renal: insufficiency, dialysis
  - hematologic: anemia, coagulopathies, blood dyscrasias
  - MSK: conditions associated with difficult intubations – arthritis, rheumatoid arthritis (RA), cervical tumours, cervical infections/abscess, trauma to cervical spine, Down syndrome, scleroderma, obesity, conditions affecting neuromuscular junction (e.g. myasthenia gravis)
  - endocrine: diabetes, thyroid, adrenal disorders
  - other: morbid obesity, pregnancy, ethanol/other drug use
- FHx: malignant hyperthermia, atypical cholinesterase (pseudocholinesterase), other abnormal drug reactions

Physical Examination
- oropharynx and airway assessment to determine the likelihood of difficult intubation
- ability to assume "sniffing position" - assesses likeliness of difficult intubation - upper cervical spine extension, lower cervical spine flexion
- no single test is specific or sensitive – all aid in determining the ease of intubation
  - Mallampati Classification (see Figure 1)
  - Wilson Risk Sum (score that factors in patient's weight, head and neck movement, jaw movement, receding mandible, and buck teeth)
  - thyromental distance (the distance of the lower mandible in the midline from the mentum to the thyroid notch)
    - this measurement is performed with the adult patient's neck fully extended
    - <3 finger breadths, or <6 cm in adults is associated with difficult intubation
  - mouth opening (<2 finger breadths associated with difficult intubation, few studies have been performed to assess its predictive value)
  - tongue size

Lee's Cardiac Risk Scoring System for Patients Undergoing Non-Cardiac Surgery

Risk Factors (CCDrsH)
Coronary artery disease
Congestive heart failure
Diabetes Mellitus: Type I or II
Renal insufficiency: Creatinine ≥175
Stroke, history of cerebral vascular disease
High risk surgery: Intraabdominal, thoracic or vascular

Risk Factors	Adverse Cardiac Event
0-1	≤1%
2	4-6%
≥3	9-11%

Patients with higher risks based on the Lee risk scoring system can be subjected to the following for possible risk reduction:
1. Perioperative beta-blockers
2. Regional anesthesia
3. Cardiac investigation/intervention if appropriate

Lee TH, Marcantonio ER, Mangione CM et al. Derivation and prospective validation of a simple index for prediction of cardiac risk of major noncardiac surgery. Circulation 1999; 100: 1043-9.
Goldman L, Caldera DL, Nussbaum SR et al. Multifactorial index of cardiac risk in noncardiac surgical procedures. N Eng J Med 1977; 297: 845-50.
Detsky AS, Abrams B, McLaughlin JR et al. Predicting cardiac complications in patients undergoing noncardiac surgery. J Gen Intern Med 1986; 1: 211-9.
Mangano DT, Layug EL, Wallace A, Tateo I. Effect of atenolol on mortality and cardiac morbidity after noncardiac surgery. N Engl J Med 1996; 335:1713-20.

- dentition, dental appliances/prosthetic caps – must inform patients of the rare possibility of damage
- nasal passage patency (if planning nasotracheal intubation)
- bony landmarks and suitability of anatomy for regional anesthesia if relevant
- focused physical exam on CNS, CVS, and respiratory (includes airway) systems
- general assessment of nutrition, hydration, and mental status
- pre-existing motor and sensory deficits
- sites for IV, central venous pressure (CVP) and pulmonary artery (PA) catheters

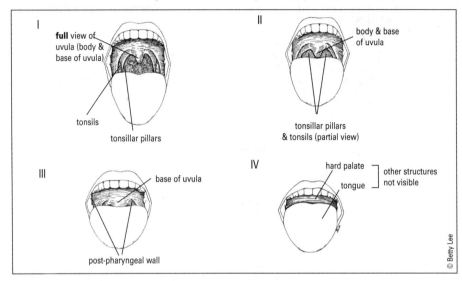

Figure 1. Mallampati Classification of Upper Airway Visualization

Pre-Operative Airway Assessment: Wilson Risk Sum

Risk Factor	Level	Score
Weight	<90 kg	0
	90-110 kg	1
	>110 kg	2
Head and Neck Movements	Above 90°	0
	90° +/- 10°	1
	Below 90°	2
Jaw Movement	IG <5 cm or Sublux >0 cm	0
	IG <5 cm or Sublux = 0 cm	1
	IG <5 cm or Sublux <0 cm	2
Receding Mandible	Normal	0
	Moderate	1
	Severe	2
Buck Teeth	Normal	0
	Moderate	1
	Severe	2

IG = inter-incisor gap i.e. mouth opening
A score of 2 or more is a difficult intubation

Pre-Operative Investigations

Table 1. Suggested Indications for Specific Investigations in the Pre-Operative Period

Test	Indications
CBC	major surgery requiring group and screen or cross and match chronic cardiovascular, pulmonary, renal, or hepatic disease malignancy known or suspected anemia, bleeding diathesis or myelosuppression patient less than 1 year of age
Sickle cell screen	genetically predisposed patient (hemoglobin electrophoresis if screen is positive)
INR, aPTT	anticoagulant therapy, bleeding diathesis, liver disease
Electrolytes and Creatinine	hypertension, renal disease, diabetes, pituitary or adrenal disease, digoxin or diuretic therapy; or other drug therapies affecting electrolytes, age >50
Fasting glucose level	diabetes (should be repeated on day of surgery)
Pregnancy (β-HCG)	women who may be pregnant
ECG	heart disease, hypertension, diabetes, other risk factors for cardiac disease (may include age), subarachnoid hemorrhage, CVA, head trauma, age (male >40 y.o., female >50 y.o.)
Chest radiograph	cardiac or pulmonary disease, malignancy, age >60

Guidelines to the Practice of Anesthesia, Revised 2006. Supplement to the Canadian Journal of Anesthesia, Vol 53(12), Dec. 2006.
Reproduced with permission ©Canadian Anesthesiologists' Society.

Impact of Anesthesia Management Characteristics on Severe Morbidity and Mortality
Anesthesiology 2005; 102(2):257-258.

Study: Case-control study of patients undergoing anesthesia
Patients: 803 cases and 883 controls were analyzed among a cohort of 869,483 patients undergoing anesthesia between 1995-1997. Cases were defined as patients who either remained comatose or died within 24 hours of receiving anesthesia. Controls were defined as patients who neither remained comatose nor died within 24 hours of receiving anesthesia.
Intervention: General, regional, or combined anesthesia to patients undergoing a surgical procedure.
Main Outcome: coma or death within 24 hours of receiving anesthesia
Results: The incidence of 24-hour postoperative death was 8.8 per 10,000 anesthetics (95% CI, 8.2–9.5) and the incidence of coma was 0.5 (95% CI, 0.3-0.6). Anesthesia management risk factors that were associated with a decreased risk of morbidity and mortality were: equipment check with protocol and documentation, directly available anesthesiologist with no change during anesthesia, 2 persons present at emergence of anesthesia, reversal of muscle relaxation, and postoperative pain medication.

Fasting Guidelines

Fasting Guidelines Prior to Surgery (Canadian Anesthesiologists' Society)
- **8 hours** after a meal that includes meat, fried or fatty foods
- **6 hours** after a light meal (such as toast, crackers and clear fluid) or after ingestion of infant formula or nonhuman milk
- **4 hours** after ingestion of breast milk or jello
- **2 hours** after clear fluids (water, black coffee, tea, carbonated beverages, juice without pulp)

Effects of extended-release metoprolol succinate in patients undergoing non-cardiac surgery (POISE trial): a randomized controlled trial
POISE study group. 2008 The Lancet 371(9627):1839-47

Background: Non-cardiac surgery is associated with substantial risk of cardiac side effects, and patients with identified cardiac risk factors may benefit from prophylactic/preventative treatment. This study was designed to investigate the effects of perioperative beta blockers in patients with diagnosed atherosclerotic disease or patients with defined cardiovascular risk factors undergoing non-cardiac surgical procedures.
Methods: 8351 patients were randomly assigned to receive extended-release metoprolol succinate (n=4174) or placebo (n=4177). Study treatment was started 2-4 h before surgery and continued for 30 days. Study endpoints included cardiovascular death, non-fatal myocardial infarction, and non-fatal cardiac arrest.
Results: Metoprolol was associated with a significant reduction in MI events (176 [4.2%] vs 239 [5.7%] patients; hazard ratio 0.73, 95% confidence interval 0.60-0.89; p=0.0017). However, metoprolol was associated with increased rates of death (129 [3.1%] vs 97 [2.3%] patients; HR 1.33, CI 1.03-1.74; p=0.0317) and stroke (41 [1.0%] vs 19 [0.5%] patients; 2.17, 1.26-3.74; p=0.0053).
Conclusions: This study highlights the potential risk associated with perioperative beta blockers in patients with increased risk for cardiac side effects undergoing non-cardiac surgery. Further studies are needed to determine the potential risks and benefits associated with this regimen in the perioperative setting.

Effect of Atenolol on Mortality and Cardiovascular Morbidity After Noncardiac Surgery
NEJM 1996;335:1713-1720.

Study: Randomized, double-blind, placebo-controlled trial.
Patients: 200 patients with, or at risk for, coronary artery disease (CAD) who were scheduled for elective noncardiac surgery requiring general anesthesia were enrolled.
Intervention: 101 patients were randomized to the placebo group and 99 were randomized to receive atenolol intravenously before and immediately after the surgery, followed by oral administration daily while in hospital. Patients were followed for 2 years.
Results: Overall mortality after hospital discharge was significantly reduced in the atenolol group compared to the placebo group at 6 months post-discharge (0% vs. 8%, p<0.001); 1 year (3% vs. 14%, p=0.005); and 2 years post-discharge (10% vs. 21%, p=0.019). Cardiovascular complications were also reduced in the atenolol group compared to the placebo group with a higher event-free survival rate during the 2-year period (83% vs. 68%, p=0.008).
Conclusions: Treatment with atenolol during hospitalization in patients with or at risk for CAD undergoing elective noncardiac surgery can reduce mortality and the incidence of cardiovascular complications for as long as 2 years after surgery.

The Effect of Bisoprolol on Perioperative Mortality and Myocardial Infarction in High-Risk Patients Undergoing Vascular Surgery
NEJM 1999;341:1789-1794.

Study: Prospective, randomized, multi-centre trial.
Patients: 112 patients undergoing elective major vascular surgery who were considered high-risk for death from cardiac causes or nonfatal myocardial infarction were enrolled and followed for 30 days post-operatively. High-risk patients were identified as having specific clinical cardiac risk factors and positive results on dobutamine echocardiography.
Intervention: The 112 patients were randomized with 53 patients assigned to receive standard perioperative care and 59 patients assigned to receive standard perioperative care plus bisoprolol. Bisoprolol was administered daily (orally, or intravenously when necessary) from a minimum of 1 week pre-operatively to 30 days post-operatively.
Results: Death from cardiac causes was reduced in the bisoprolol group vs. the standard care group (3.4% vs. 17%, p=0.02) and nonfatal myocardial infarction occurrence was also lower in the bisoprolol group (0% vs. 17%, p<0.001).
Conclusions: Treatment with bisoprolol can reduce the perioperative incidence of cardiac-related death and nonfatal myocardial infarction in high-risk patients undergoing major vascular surgery.

American Society of Anesthesiology (ASA) Classification

- common classification of physical status at time of surgery
- a gross predictor of overall outcome, NOT used as stratification for anesthetic risk (mortality rates)
  - **ASA 1:** a healthy, fit patient
  - **ASA 2:** a patient with mild systemic disease, e.g. controlled Type 2 diabetes, controlled essential HTN, obesity, smoker
  - **ASA 3:** a patient with severe systemic disease that limits activity, e.g. angina, prior MI, COPD, DM, obesity
  - **ASA 4:** a patient with incapacitating disease that is a constant threat to life, e.g. CHF, renal failure, acute respiratory failure
  - **ASA 5:** a moribund patient not expected to survive 24 hours with/without surgery, e.g. ruptured abdominal aortic aneurysm (AAA), head trauma with increased ICP
- for emergency operations, add the letter **E** after classification

Myocardial Infarction

- ACC/AHA Guidelines (2002) recommends postponing elective surgery 4-6 weeks following an MI
- this period carries increased risk of reinfarction/death
- reinfarction risk is classically quoted as:
  - <3 months after MI – 37% patients may reinfarct
  - 3-6 months after MI – 15%
  - >6 months after MI – risk remains constant at 5%
- reinfarction carries a 50% mortality rate
- if operative procedure is essential and cannot be delayed, invasive monitoring and post-operative intensive care unit (ICU) monitoring reduce the risk to 6%, 2% and 1% respectively for the above time periods
- mortality with peri-operative MI is 20-50%
- perioperative beta-blockade is recommended to reduce post-operative adverse cardiac events
- treatment of patients at risk for CAD with atenolol while in hospital reduces mortality and cardiovascular complications (Mangano, et al. NEJM 1996; 335:1713-1720)
- in high-risk patients, perioperative MI and mortality of vascular surgery is reduced by bisoprolol (Poldermans, et al. NEJM. 1999; 341:1789-1794)

Pre-Operative Optimization

Medications

- pay particular attention to cardiac and respiratory meds, narcotics and drugs with many side effects and interactions
- **pre-operative medications to start:**
  - prophylaxis
    - risk of GE reflux – sodium citrate 30 cc PO 30 minutes to 1 hour pre-op
    - risk of infective endocarditis – antibiotics
    - risk of adrenal suppression – steroid coverage
    - risk of DVT – heparin SC
- optimization of co-existing disease → bronchodilators (COPD, asthma), nitroglycerin and beta-blockers (CAD risk factors)
- **pre-operative medications to stop:**
  - oral hypoglycemics – stop on morning of surgery
  - antidepressants (tricyclics, MAOI's) – stop on morning of surgery
- **pre-operative medication to adjust:**
  - insulin, prednisone, coumadin, bronchodilators

Hypertension

- assess for absence/presence of end-organ damage and treat accordingly
- target dBP <110 mmHg
- target sBP <180 mmHg
- mild to moderate HTN is not an independent risk factor for perioperative cardiovascular complication (Lette et al. Ann Surg 1992; 216:192 -204)

Endocrine Disorders

- adrenocortical insufficiency; e.g. Addison's, exogenous steroid use
  - steroid coverage suggested if steroid use of >1 week in past 6 months
- diabetes mellitus
  - hypoglycemia
    - caused by drugs and surgical stresses and masked by anesthesia
    - prevent with dextrose/insulin infusion and blood glucose monitoring
  - end organ damage – be wary of damage to CVS, renal and nervous systems
- pheochromocytoma
  - adrenergic crisis with surgical manipulation → prone to large swings in blood pressure (BP) and heart rate (HR)
  - prevention with alpha and beta adrenergic blockade pre-op
- hyperthyroidism
  - can experience sudden release of thyroid hormone (thyroid storm)
  - treatment: β-blockers + pre-op prophylaxis

Respiratory Diseases

- asthma
  - bronchospasm from intubation, delivery of gaseous anesthetics
  - prevent with inhaled salbutamol immediately pre-op
  - avoid non-selective β-blockers, caution with $β_2$ specific
  - deep breathing/incentive spirometry if >1 pulmonary risk factor
- smokers
  - abstain at least 8 weeks pre-op
  - if unable, abstaining even 24 hours pre-op has shown benefit

Aspiration

- risk of aspiration in GE sphincter incompetence, GERD, hernia
- avoid inhibiting airway reflexes, reduce gastric volume and acidity
- employ rapid sequence induction and always use cuffed ETT
- increased risk with laryngeal mask (instead of ETT)

Monitoring

Canadian Guidelines to the Practice of Anesthesia and Patient Monitoring
- an anesthetist present – "the only indispensable monitor"
- a completed pre-anesthetic checklist – including ASA class, NPO policy, Hx, investigations
- a perioperative anesthetic record – HR and BP q5min, dose and route of drugs and fluids
- continuous monitoring: clinical and quantitative measurement of
  a) oxygenation b) ventilation c) circulation d) temperature

Routine Monitors for All Cases
- BP cuff, telemetry, pulse oximeter (O_2 saturation), stethoscope, temperature probe, gas analyzer, capnometer (end tidal carbon dioxide to indicate adequacy of ventilation)

Elements to Monitor
- anesthetic depth
  - inadequate
    - blink reflex present, HTN, tachycardia
  - excessive
    - hypotension, bradycardia
- oxygenation
  - pulse oximetry, inspired oxygen concentration
- ventilation
  - verification of correctly positioned ETT, chest excursions, breath sounds, end tidal carbon dioxide analysis
- circulation
  - pulse, heart sounds, BP, telemetry, oximetry, central venous pressure, pulmonary capillary wedge pressure
- temperature
  - temperature probe

Cardioselective Beta-Blockers for Reversible Airway Disease
Salpeter S et al. *Cochrane Database of Systematic Reviews 2003*; Issue 3

Purpose: To assess the effect of cardioselective beta-blockers in patients with asthma or COPD. These drugs, while having been shown to be of benefit in patients with HTN, CHF, and CAD, have traditionally been considered contraindicated in patients with reversible airway disease.
Study: Systematic review of randomized, blinded, placebo-controlled trials of single dose or continued treatment of the effects of cardioselective beta-blockers in patients with reversible airway disease.
Patients: 29 trials.
Main Outcomes: Pulmonary function tests.
Results: Single dose cardioselective beta-blockers produced a 7.46% reduction in FEV1 but with a 4.63% increase in FEV1 with beta 2-agonist, compared to placebo. Treatment lasting 3 to 28 days produced no change in FEV1, symptoms, or inhaler use, whilst maintaining an 8.74% response to beta 2-agonist. There was no significant change in FEV1 treatment effect for those patients with COPD.
Conclusion: Cardioselective beta-blockers given in mild to moderate reversible airway disease or COPD do not produce adverse respiratory effects in the short term. Given their demonstrated benefit in conditions such as CHF, cardiac arrhythmias and HTN, these agents should not be withheld from such patients. Long-term safety still needs to be established.

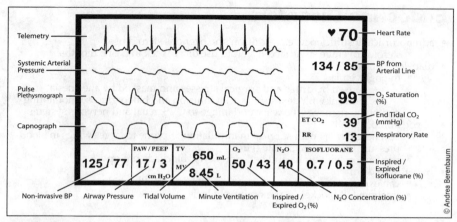

Figure 2. Typical Anesthesia Monitor

Induction Agents

Intravenous and Volatile Inhalational Agents

The role of intraoperative management is to achieve anesthesia, analgesia, amnesia, areflexia, and autonomic stability. Induction may be achieved with intravenous agents, volatile agents or both. The IV induction agents include a selection of non-opioid drugs used to provide amnesia and blunt reflexes. These are initially used to draw the patient into the maintenance phase of general anesthesia (GA) rapidly, smoothly and with little adverse effects. This can be carried out by propofol, sodium thiopental or ketamine. Propofol and ketamine can also be used for the maintenance phase of GA. Intravenous induction agents are relatively simple in their administration and are described in Table 7. General concepts of volatile agents are discussed below with their specific properties explained in Table 9.

MAC (minimum alveolar concentration)
- definition: the alveolar concentration of an agent at one atmosphere (atm) of pressure that will prevent movement in 50% of patients in response to a surgical stimulus (e.g. abdominal incision)
- often 1.2-1.3 times MAC will ablate response in the general population
- potency of inhalational agents is compared using MAC
- MAC values are roughly additive when mixing N_2O with another volatile agent (i.e. 0.5 MAC of a potent agent + 0.5 MAC of N_2O = 1 MAC of potent agent; however, this only applies to movement, not other effects such as blood pressure changes and does not hold over the entire N_2O dose range)
- MAC-intubation – the MAC of anesthetic that will inhibit movement and coughing during endotracheal intubation, generally 1.3 MAC
- MAC-block adrenergic response (MAC-BAR) – the MAC necessary to blunt the sympathetic response to noxious stimuli, generally 1.5 MAC
- MAC-awake – the MAC of a given volatile anesthetic at which a patient will open his eyes to command, usually 0.3-0.4 of the usual MAC value

Conditions which require ↑ MAC
- hyperthermia, chronic EtOH/drug abuse, acute amphetamine use, hyperthyroidism, ↑ Na, increased neurotransmitter levels (MAOI use, cocaine, levodopa, ephedrine)

Conditions which require ↓ MAC
- ↑ age, hypothermia, ↓↓ BP, other anesthetics (e.g. benzodiazepines, opioids), acute EtOH/drug use, pregnancy, hypothyroidism, certain psychiatric drugs (clonidine, reserpine)

Conditions that do not alter MAC
- gender, duration of anesthesia, CO_2 tension (21-95 mmHg), metabolic acid-base status, hypertension

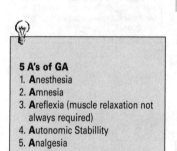

5 A's of GA
1. **A**nesthesia
2. **A**mnesia
3. **A**reflexia (muscle relaxation not always required)
4. **A**utonomic Stabillity
5. **A**nalgesia

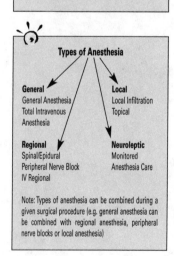

Types of Anesthesia

General   **Local**
General Anesthesia   Local Infiltration
Total Intravenous   Topical
Anesthesia

Regional   **Neuroleptic**
Spinal/Epidural   Monitored
Peripheral Nerve Block   Anesthesia Care
IV Regional

Note: Types of anesthesia can be combined during a given surgical procedure (e.g. general anesthesia can be combined with regional anesthesia, peripheral nerve blocks or local anesthesia)

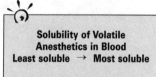

Solubility of Volatile Anesthetics in Blood
Least soluble → Most soluble

Nitrous oxide < desflurane < sevoflurane < isoflurane < halothane

Muscle Relaxants and Reversing Agents

- note: specific muscle relaxants are described in Tables 10 and 11

Anatomy and Physiology of Neuromuscular Junction (NMJ)
- pre-junctional motor nerve endings containing acetylcholine (ACh) vesicles
- synaptic cleft filled with extracellular fluid
- postsynaptic skeletal muscle membrane contains nicotinic cholinergic receptors
- action potential arrives at the nerve → release of ACh into the cleft → ACh binds to nicotinic cholinergic receptors → change in membrane permeability to ions, membrane potential → action potential spreads across the surface of the muscle → muscle contraction → ACh rapidly diffuses away from muscles and is hydrolyzed by acetylcholinesterase → return of normal ionic gradients → NMJ and muscle return to non-depolarized state
- refer to Neurology for NMJ diagram

Muscle Relaxants
- muscle relaxation produces the following desired effects:
  - facilitates intubation
  - assists with mechanical ventilation
  - prevents muscle stretch reflex and decreases muscle tone
  - allows access to the surgical field (intracavitary surgery)
- never use without adequate preparation and equipment to maintain airway and ventilation
- interrupts transmission at the NMJ
- provides skeletal muscle paralysis, including the diaphragm, but spares involuntary muscles such as the heart and smooth muscle
- actions potentiated by all potent inhalational agents
- nerve stimulator used intraoperatively to assess level of nerve block

Reversing Agents for Non-Depolarizing Relaxants
(e.g. neostigmine, pyridostigmine, edrophonium)
- reversal agents are **acetylcholinesterase inhibitors**
  - inhibits enzymatic degradation of ACh; increases amount of ACh at nicotinic and muscarinic receptors, displacing non-depolarizing muscle relaxant
  - muscarinic effects of reversing agents result in unwanted bradycardia, salivation, increased bowel peristalsis
- anticholinergic agents, atropine or glycopyrrolate, are simultaneously administered to minimize muscarinic effect
- degree of muscular blockade assessed with nerve stimulator commonly applied to ulnar or facial nerve
  - no twitch response seen with complete neuromuscular blockade

Plasma Cholinesterase Deficiency
- inherited condition leading to a marked reduction in the hydrolysis of succinylcholine
- patients with abnormal cholinesterase activity are otherwise healthy and can only be identified by a specific blood test
- most severe form has a frequency of 1:3200
- patients experience a prolonged neuromuscular block that can be increased from several minutes to several hours following a normal intubating dose of succinylcholine
- management includes controlled ventilation, reassurance and sedation during the prolonged neuromuscular block, sending blood samples to confirm the diagnosis and identify the genotype and advising family members to be tested

Airway Management

- multiple options for airway management including endotracheal intubation, laryngeal mask airway (LMA) and bag and mask ventilation (see Table 2)
- an LMA consists of a wide-bore PVC tube with a distal inflatable laryngeal cuff. When in place, the laryngeal cuff rests in the patient's pharynx, just above the vocal cords at the junction of the larynx and esophagus
- LMA contraindicated for patients with high risk of aspiration

Tracheal Intubation

Equipment for Intubation
- oxygen source and self-inflating bag
- face mask (appropriate size and one size larger and smaller)
- oropharyngeal and nasopharyngeal airways
- endotracheal tubes (appropriate size and one size smaller)

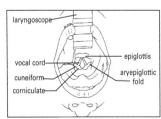

Figure 3. Landmarks for Intubation

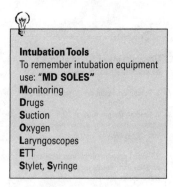

Intubation Tools
To remember intubation equipment
use: **"MD SOLES"**
Monitoring
Drugs
Suction
Oxygen
Laryngoscopes
ETT
Stylet, **S**yringe

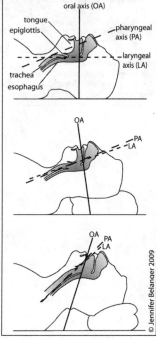

Figure 4. Anatomic Considerations in Laryngoscopy

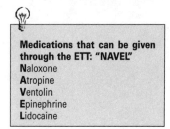

Medications that can be given through the ETT: "NAVEL"
Naloxone
Atropine
Ventolin
Epinephrine
Lidocaine

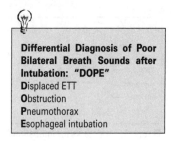

Differential Diagnosis of Poor Bilateral Breath Sounds after Intubation: "DOPE"
Displaced ETT
Obstruction
Pneumothorax
Esophageal intubation

- tracheal stylet
- syringe for tube cuff inflation
- suction
- laryngoscopes

Preparing for Intubation
- failed attempts at intubation can make further attempts difficult due to tissue trauma
- plan, prepare and assess for potential difficulties (see *Pre-operative Assessment*)
- ensure equipment is available and working (e.g. test ETT cuff, check laryngoscope light, machine check)
- pre-oxygenate/denitrogenate: patient breathes 100% O_2 for 3-5 min or for 4 vital capacity breaths
- may need to suction mouth and pharynx first

Proper Positioning for Intubation
- **"sniffing position"**: **flexion** of lower C-spine (C5,6) i.e. bow head forward, and **extension** of upper C-spine at atlanto (C1)-occipital joint, i.e. nose in the air
- aligns the three axes of mouth, pharynx, and larynx to allow visualization from the oral cavity to the glottis (see Figure 6)
- contraindicated in known/suspected C-spine fracture
- caution in rheumatoid arthritis

Proper Distance of Tube Insertion
- a malpositioned endotracheal tube (ETT) is a potential hazard for intubated patient
- if the ETT is inserted too deeply, it may result in right endobronchial intubation which is associated with left-sided atelectasis and right-sided tension pneumothorax
- too shallow a placement may lead to accidental extubation, vocal cord trauma and laryngeal paralysis as a result of pressure injury by the cuff of the ETT
- the tip of ETT should be located at the midpoint of the trachea at least 2 cm above the carina and the proximal end of the cuff should be placed at least 2 cm below the vocal cords
- approximately 20-23 cm mark at the right corner of the mouth for men and 19-21 cm for women

Confirmation of Tracheal Placement of ETT
- direct
  - visualization of ETT passing through cords
  - bronchoscopic visualization of ETT in trachea
- indirect
  - end-tidal CO_2 ($ETCO_2$) in exhaled gas measured by capnograph
  - auscultate for equal breath sounds bilaterally and absent breath sounds over epigastrium
  - chest movement and no abdominal distention
  - feel the normal compliance of lungs when ventilating patient
  - condensation of water vapour in ETT visible during exhalation
  - refilling of reservoir bag during exhalation
  - AP or lateral CXR: ETT tip at midpoint of thoracic inlet and carina (lateral CXR more sensitive and specific)

Table 2. Methods of Supporting the Airway

	Bag and Mask ± oral airway	Laryngeal Mask Airway (LMA)	Endotracheal Tube (ETT)
Advantages/Indications	- basic - non-invasive - readily available	- easy to insert - less airway trauma/irritation than ETT - less chance of laryngospasm - frees up hands (vs. face mask)	"the **5 P's**" - ensures airway **P**atency - **P**rotects against aspiration - allows **P**ositive pressure ventilation - allows suctioning to prevent **P**ulmonary toilet - a route for **P**harmacological administration
Disadvantages/ Contraindications	- risk of aspiration if ↓ LOC - cannot ensure airway patency - inability to deliver precise tidal volume - operator fatigue	- risk of gastric aspiration - PPV>20 cm H_2O needed - limited TMJ mobility - C-spine or laryngeal cartilage fracture - oropharyngeal, retropharyngeal pathology or foreign body	- insertion can be difficult - muscle relaxant usually needed - laryngospasm may occur on extubation or on failed intubation - sympathetic stress due to intubation

Other Info	- facilitate airway patency with jaw thrust and chin lift	- does NOT protect against laryngospasm or gastric aspiration
		- primarily used in spontaneously ventilating patient
		- Sizing (approx):
		  Male: 4.0-5.0
		  Female: 3.0-4.0
			- necessary for rapid sequence induction
			- auscultate to avoid endobronchial intubation
			- Sizing (approx):
			  Male: 8.0–9.0 mm
			  Female: 7.0–8.0 mm
			  Pediatric: (age/4) + 4 mm

- esophageal intubation suspected when
  - end-tidal CO_2 zero or near zero on capnograph
  - abnormal sounds during assisted ventilation
  - impairment of chest excursion
  - hypoxia/cyanosis
  - presence of gastric contents in ETT
  - distention of stomach/epigastrium with ventilation

Complications During Laryngoscopy and Intubation
- mechanical
  - dental damage (e.g. chipped teeth)
  - laceration (lips, gums, tongue, pharynx, esophagus)
  - laryngeal trauma
  - esophageal or endobronchial intubation
  - accidental extubation
  - insufficient cuff inflation or cuff laceration: allows leaking and aspiration
- systemic
  - laryngospasm
  - bronchospasm

Rapid Sequence Induction (RSI)

- indicated when patient has "full stomach" i.e. predisposed to regurgitation/aspiration
  - ↓ level of consciousness (LOC)
  - trauma
  - meal within 6 hours
  - sphincter incompetence suspected (GERD, hiatus hernia, nasogastric (NG) tube)
  - ↑ abdominal pressure (pregnancy, obesity, bowel obstruction, acute abdomen)
- preoxygenate/denitrogenate: patient breathes 100% O_2 for 3-5 minutes or for 4 vital capacity breaths prior to induction of anesthesia (do NOT bag ventilate)
- assistant performs "Sellick's" maneuver: pressure on cricoid cartilage to compress esophagus between cartilage and C6 to prevent reflux/aspiration
- administration of induction agent immediately followed by fast acting muscle relaxant
- intubate shortly after administration of muscle relaxant (approximately 45-60 seconds)
- must use cuffed ETT to prevent aspiration of gastric contents
- inflate cuff, verify correct placement of ETT, release cricoid cartilage pressure
- ventilation when ETT in place and cuff inflated

Difficult Airway

- difficulties with bag and mask ventilation, supraglottic airway, endotracheal intubation, infraglottic airway or surgical airway
- algorithms exist for difficult airways (e.g. Anesthesiology 2003; 98:3273, Anaesthesia 2004; 59:675)
- pre-op assessment (history of previous difficult airway, airway examination) and pre-oxygenation are important preventative measures
- if difficult airway expected, consider:
  - awake intubation
  - intubating with bronchoscope, trachlight (lighted stylet), fibre-optic laryngoscope, glidescope, etc.
- if intubation unsuccessful after induction
  1. ventilate with 100% O_2 via bag and mask
  2. CALL FOR HELP
  3. consider returning to spontaneous ventilation and/or waking patient
- if bag and mask ventilation inadequate:
  1. attempt ventilation with oral airway
  2. CALL FOR HELP
  3. consider/attempt LMA
  4. emergency non-invasive airway ventilation (e.g. rigid bronchoscope, jet ventilation, combitube, etc.)
  5. emergency invasive airway access (i.e. cricothyrotomy or tracheostomy)

Predicting Difficult Intubation in Apparently Normal Patients
Anesthesiology 2005; 103:429–37

Purpose: To assess widely available bedside tests and widely used laryngoscopic techniques in the prediction of difficult intubations.
Study: Meta-analysis
Selection Criteria: Prospective studies where at least one bedside diagnostic test was used, which also reported absolute numbers of true-positive, false-negative, true-negative, and false-negative results or derivable from published data, and use of a standard laryngoscope. Exclusion criteria included any study with insufficient data, with patients whose airway was anatomically abnormal, or with complex or not commonly used scoring systems. Also excluded were retrospective studies, studies requiring impractical and costly diagnostic tests that are not yet widely accepted such as radiologic examinations, and studies involving a special laryngoscope or technique.
Patients: 35 studies encompassing 50,760 patients were included
Definitions: Difficult intubation was defined usually as Cormack–Lehane grade of 3 or greater, but some authors reported the requirement of a special technique, multiple unsuccessful attempts, or a combination of these as the accepted standard for difficult intubation.
Results: The overall incidence of difficult intubation was 5.8% (95% CI, 4.5–7.5%) for the overall patient population, 6.2% (95% CI, 4.6–8.3%) for normal patients excluding obstetric and obese patients, 3.1% (95% CI, 1.7–5.5%) for obstetric patients, and 15.8% (95% CI, 14.3–17.5%) for obese patients.
Mallampati score: SN: 49% SP:86% PLR:3.7 NLR:0.5, Thyromental distance: SN:20% SP:94% PLR:3.4 NLR:0.8 Sternomental distance: SN:62% SP:82% PLR:5.7 NLR:0.5, Mouth opening: SN:22% SP:97% PLR: 4.0 NLR:0.8 ,Wilson risk-sum: SN:46% SP:89% PLR:5.8 NLR:0.6, Combination Mallampati and thyromental distance: SN:36% SP:87% PLR:9.9 NLR:0.6
Conclusions: A combination of the Mallampati test and thyromental distance is the most accurate at predicting difficult intubation. The positive likelihood ratio (9.9) is supportive of the test as a good predictor of difficult intubation.
PLR: Positive likelihood ratio; NLR: Negative likelihood ratio; SN: Sensitivity; SP: Specificity

Intraoperative Management

Oxygenation

- in general the goal of oxygen therapy is to maintain oxygen saturation greater than 90%
- below an SaO_2 of 90%, a small $\downarrow$ in saturation corresponds to a large drop in P_aO_2
- in intubated patients oxygen is delivered via the endotracheal tube
- in patients who are not intubated there are many oxygen delivery systems available; the choice depends on the amount of oxygen required (FiO_2) and the degree to which precise control of delivery is needed
- cyanosis can be detected at $SaO_2 = 80\%$, frank cyanosis at $SaO_2 = 67\%$

Low Flow Systems

- acceptable if tidal volume 300-700 ml, respiratory rate (RR) <25, consistent ventilation pattern
- provide O_2 at flows between 0-8 L/min
- dilution of oxygen with room air results in a decrease in the inspired oxygen concentration
- an increase in minute ventilation (tidal volume x RR) results in a decrease in the inspired oxygen concentration
- **nasal canula**
  - well tolerated if flow rates <5-6 L/min, at high flows drying of nasal mucosa occurs
  - the nasopharynx acts as an anatomic reservoir that collects O_2
  - the delivered oxygen concentration (FiO_2) can be estimated by adding 4% for every additional litre of O_2 delivered (e.g. normal tidal volume and RR, flow rate 1-6 L/min, $FiO_2 = 24$-44%)

Reservoir Systems

- use a volume reservoir to accumulate oxygen during exhalation increasing the amount of oxygen available for the next breath
- **simple face mask (Hudson face mask)**
  - covers patient's nose and mouth and provides an additional reservoir beyond nasopharynx
  - fed by small bore O_2 tubing at a rate of at least 6 L/min to ensure that exhaled CO_2 is flushed through the exhalation ports and not rebreathed
  - FiO_2 of 55% can be achieved at O_2 flow rates of 10 L/min
- **non-rebreather mask**
  - reservoir bag and a series of one-way valves direct gas flow from the bag on inhalation and allow release of expired gases on exhalation
  - O_2 flow rates of 10-15 L/min are needed to maintain the reservoir bag inflation and should deliver FiO_2 greater than 80%

High Flow Systems

- generates flows of up to 50-60 L/min
- meets/exceeds patient's inspiratory flow requirement
- delivers consistent and predictable concentration of O_2
- **Venturi mask**
  - delivers specific percentages of oxygen by varying the size of air entrapment
  - port determines the oxygen concentration (e.g. can vary to achieve 24%, 28%, 35%, 50%)
  - enables control of gas humidity
- **Puritan mask**
  - delivers the highest level of humidified oxygen

Ventilation

- muscle relaxant given for intubation and surgical access also affects muscles of respiration
- in these patients minute ventilation is maintained with positive pressure ventilation
- if no muscle relaxant is given patients may have sufficient spontaneous respirations to maintain ventilation, or assisted/controlled ventilation can be used
- mechanical ventilation has many other indications in and out of the operating room (OR) including:
  - apnea
  - hypoventilation (many causes)

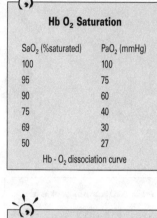

Hb O_2 Saturation

SaO_2 (%saturated)	PaO_2 (mmHg)
100	100
95	75
90	60
75	40
69	30
50	27

Hb - O_2 dissociation curve

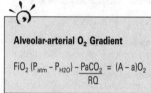

Alveolar-arterial O_2 Gradient

$$FiO_2 (P_{atm} - P_{H2O}) - \frac{PaCO_2}{RQ} = (A - a)O_2$$

Arterial O_2 Content

$$CaO_2 = (SaO_2)(Hb)(1.34) + (PaO_2)(0.003)$$

CaO_2 = arterial O_2 content

SaO_2 = % hemoglobin saturation

PaO_2 = arterial O_2 pressure

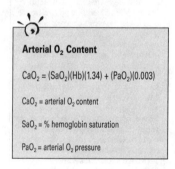

Suspect difficult ventilation with: "BONES"
Beard
Obesity/**O**bstetrics
No teeth
Elderly
Sleep apnea

- intraoperative position limiting respiratory excursion (e.g. prone, Trendelenburg)
- required hyperventilation (to lower intracranial pressure)
- deliver positive end expiratory pressure (PEEP)
- increased intrathoracic pressure (e.g. laparoscopic procedure)
- complications of mechanical ventilation include:
  - $\downarrow CO_2$ due to hyperventilation
  - $\downarrow$ BP due to $\downarrow$ venous return from $\uparrow$ intrathoracic pressure
  - alkalemia with aggressive correction of chronic hypercarbia
  - nosocomial pneumonia/bronchitis
- see Respirology for ventilatory modes

Causes of Intraoperative Hypocapnea
- hyperventilation
- inadequate sampling volume
- incorrect placement of sampling catheter
- hypothermia
- incipient pulmonary edema
- air embolism
- decreased blood flow to lungs

Causes of Intraoperative Hypercapnea
- hypoventilation
- low bicarbonate
- anesthetic breathing circuit error
  - inadequate fresh gas flow
  - rebreathing, faulty circuit absorber valves
  - exhausted soda lime
- hyperthermia
- improved blood flow to lungs after resuscitation or hypotension
- water in capnography device

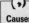

Causes of Intraoperative Hypoxia

Inadequate oxygen supply: i.e. breathing system disconnection, obstructed or malpositioned ETT, leaks in the anesthetic machine, loss of main oxygen supply

Hypoventilation

Ventilation-perfusion inequalities: i.e. atelectasis, pneumonia, pulmonary edema, pneumothorax

Reduction in oxygen carrying capacity: i.e. anemia, carbon monoxide poisoning, methemoglobinemia, hemoglobinopathy

Leftward shift of the hemoglobin-oxygen saturation curve: i.e. hypothermia, decreased 2,3-DPG, alkalosis, hypocarbia, carbon monoxide poisoning

Right-to-Left cardiac shunt

Temperature

Hypothermia
- intraoperative temperature losses are common
- OR environment (cold room, IV fluids, instruments) and open wound increase heat loss
- prevent with inflated warming blanket and warmed IV fluids (if giving platelet transfusion put through a line that does not go through warmer, warmer distorts viability of platelets)

Hyperthermia
- drugs (e.g. atropine)
- blood transfusion reaction
- infection/sepsis
- medical disorder (e.g. thyrotoxicosis)
- malignant hyperthermia (see *Uncommon Complications* section for presentation and management)
- over-zealous warming efforts

Mild Hypothermia (32°-35°C) Impact on Outcomes

Reduces resistance to wound infections by impairing immune function
Increases the period of hospitalization by delaying healing
Reduces platelet function and impairs activation of coagulation cascade increasing blood loss and transfusion requirements
Triples the incidence of V-tach and morbid cardiac events
Decreases the metabolism of anesthetic agents prolonging post-op recovery

Heart Rate

Intraoperative Tachycardia
- confirm it is sinus tachycardia vs. other rhythms (e.g. atrial fibrillation/flutter, paroxysmal atrial tachycardia, accessory pathway syndromes, ventricular tachycardia)
- sinus tachycardia is often due to increased sympathetic tone
- shock/hypovolemia/blood loss
- anxiety/pain/light anesthesia
- full bladder
- anemia
- febrile illness/sepsis
- drugs (e.g. atropine, cocaine, dopamine, epinephrine, ephedrine, isoflurane, isoproterenol, pancuronium)
- Addisonian crisis, hypoglycemia, transfusion reaction, malignant hyperthermia

Intraoperative Bradycardia
- **must** rule out hypoxemia
- increased parasympathetic tone vs. decreased sympathetic tone
- decreased cardiac conduction (see Cardiology and CV Surgery)

Intraoperative Management

- baroreceptor reflex due to increased intracranial pressure or increased blood pressure
- vagal reflex (occulocardiac reflex, carotid sinus reflex, airway manipulation)
- drugs (e.g. succinylcholine, opioids, edrophonium, neostigmine, halothane, digoxin, β-blockers)
- high spinal/epidural anesthesia

Blood Pressure

Causes of Intraoperative Hypotension/Shock (sBP<90 mmHg or MAP <60)

Intraoperative Shock
"SHOCKED"
Sepsis or **S**pinal shock
Hypovolemic/**H**emorrhagic
Obstructive
Cardiogenic
anaphylacti**K**
Extra/other
Drugs

a) hypovolemic/hemorrhagic shock
- most common form of shock, due to blood loss or dehydration
- class 1 hemorrhage (0-15%) of blood volume or <3% total body water (TBW)
  - decreased peripheral perfusion only of organs able to withstand prolonged ischemia (skin, fat, muscle, bone)
  - patient feels cold, postural hypotension and tachycardia, cool, pale, moist skin, low JVP, decreased CVP, increased peripheral vascular resistance, concentrated urine
  - treatment: rapidly infuse 1-2 L of balanced salt solutions (BSS), then maintenance fluids
- class 2 hemorrhage (15-30%) of blood volume or approximately 6% of TBW
  - decreased perfusion of organs able to tolerate only brief periods of ischemia
  - thirst, supine hypotension and tachycardia, oliguria or anuria
  - treatment: rapidly infuse 2 L of BSS then re-evaluate continued needs
- class 3 hemorrhage (30-40%)
  - decreased perfusion of organs tolerable to ischemia and mildly decreased perfusion to heart and brain
  - marked tachypnea, tachycardia, decreased sBP, oliguria, confusion
- class 4 hemorrhage (>40%) of blood volume or approximately 9% of TBW
  - decreased perfusion of heart and brain
  - agitation, confusion, obtundation, supine hypotension and tachycardia, rapid deep breathing, anuria
  - treatment: rapidly infuse 2 L of BSS
  - replace blood losses with BSS (1:3) or PRBCs, colloid (1:1)
  - maintain urine output >0.5 mL/kg/hr

b) obstructive shock
- cardiac compressive shock
- ↑ JVP, distended neck veins, ↑ systemic vascular resistance, insufficient cardiac output (CO)
- occurs with tension pneumothorax, cardiac tamponade, pulmonary embolism, pulmonary HTN, aortic and mitral stenosis

c) cardiogenic shock
- myocardial dysfunction may be due to: dysrhythmias, MI, cardiomyopathy, acute valvular dysfunction
- ↑ JVP, distended neck veins, ↑ systemic vascular resistance, ↓ CO

d) septic shock
- bacterial, viral, fungal
- endotoxins/mediators cause pooling of blood in veins and capillaries
- associated with contamination of open wounds, intestinal injury or penetrating trauma
- clinical features: fever, ↓ JVP, wide pulse pressure, ↑ cardiac output, ↑ HR, ↓ systemic vascular resistance
- initial treatment: antibiotics, volume expansion

e) spinal/neurogenic shock
- decreased sympathetic tone
- hypotension without tachycardia or peripheral vasoconstriction (warm skin)

f) anaphylactic shock
- type I hypersensitivity
- acute/subacute generalized allergic reaction due to an inappropriate or excessive immune response
  - treatment
    - moderate reaction: generalized urticaria, angioedema, wheezing, tachycardia, NO hypotension
      - epinephrine (1:1,000) 0.3-0.5 mg SC = 0.3-0.5 mL
      - antihistamines: diphenhydramine (Benadryl™) 25-50 mg IM
      - salbutamol (Ventolin™) 1 cc via nebulizer
    - severe reaction/evolution: severe wheezing, laryngeal/pulmonary edema, shock

－　must ensure airway and IV access
－　epinephrine 0.1-0.3 mL (0.1-0.3 mg) of 1:1000 solution IV (or via ETT if no IV access) to start, repeat as needed
－　epinephrine infusion may be given at 0.05-0.2 μg/kg/min
－　antihistamines: Benadryl™ 50 mg IV (~1 mg/kg)
－　steroids: hydrocortisone (Solucortef™) 100 mg IV (~1.5 mg/kg) or methylprednisolone (Solumedrol™) 1 mg/kg IV q6h x 24h
－　large volumes of crystalloid may be required

g) drugs
  ▪ vasodilators, high spinal anesthetic interfering with sympathetic outflow
h) other
  ▪ transfusion reaction, Addisonian crisis, thyrotoxicosis, hypothyroid

Causes of Intraoperative Hypertension

- pain, anxiety due to inadequate anesthesia
- pre-existing essential hypertension, coarctation, pre-eclampsia, etc.
- hypoxemia/hypercarbia
- hypervolemia
- drugs (e.g. ephedrine, epinephrine, cocaine, phenylephrine, ketamine)
- allergic/anaphylactic reaction

Fluid Balance

- TOTAL REQUIREMENT = MAINTENANCE + DEFICIT+ ONGOING LOSS
- in surgical settings this formula must take into account many factors including pre-operative fasting/decreased fluid intake, increased losses during or before surgery, fluid shifting during surgery and fluids given with blood products and medications

What Is The Maintenance?

- average healthy adult requires approximately 2,500 mL water/day
  ▪ 200 mL/day GI losses
  ▪ 800 mL/day insensible losses (respiration, perspiration)
  ▪ 1,500 mL/day urine (beware of renal failure)
- increased requirements with fever, sweating, GI losses (vomiting, diarrhea, NG suction), adrenal insufficiency, hyperventilation, and polyuric renal disease
- decreased requirements with anuria/oliguria, SIADH, highly humidified atmospheres, and CHF
- **4/2/1 rule** to calculate maintenance requirements
  ▪ 4 mL/kg/hour first 10 kg
  ▪ 2 mL/kg/hour second 10 kg
  ▪ 1 mL/kg/hour for remaining weight >20 kg
- maintenance electrolytes
  ▪ Na: 3 mEq/kg/day
  ▪ K: 1 mEq/kg/day
- e.g. 50 kg patient maintenance requirements
  ▪ fluid = 40 + 20 + 30 = 90 mL/hour = 2,160 mL/day
  ▪ Na = 150 mEq/day (therefore 66 mEq/L)
  ▪ K = 50 mEq/day (therefore 22 mEq/L)
- above patient's requirements roughly met with 2/3 D5W, 1/3 NS
  ▪ e.g. 2/3 + 1/3 @ 100 mL/hour with 20 mEq KCl per litre

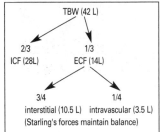

Figure 5. Total Body Water Division in a 70 kg Adult

What Is The Deficit?

- patients should be adequately hydrated prior to anesthesia
- TBW = 60% total body weight (e.g. for a 70 kg adult TBW = 70 x 0.6 = 42 L)
- total Na content determines ECF volume, [Na] determines ICF volume
- hypovolemia due to volume contraction
  ▪ extra-renal Na loss
    ◆ GI: vomiting, NG suction, drainage, fistulae, diarrhea
    ◆ skin/resp: insensible losses (fever), sweating, burns
    ◆ vascular: hemorrhage
  ▪ renal Na and H_2O loss
    ◆ diuretics
    ◆ osmotic diuresis
    ◆ hypoaldosteronism
    ◆ salt-wasting nephropathies
  ▪ renal H_2O loss
    ◆ diabetes insipidus (central or nephrogenic)

- hypovolemia with normal or expanded ECF volume
  - decreased cardiac output
  - redistribution
    - hypoalbuminemia: cirrhosis, nephrotic syndrome
    - capillary leaking: acute pancreatitis, rhabdomyolysis, ischemic bowel
- replace water and electrolytes as determined by patient's needs
- with chronic hyponatremia correction must be done gradually over >48 hours to avoid CNS central pontine myelinolysis

Table 3. Signs and Symptoms of Dehydration

Percentage of Body Water Loss	Severity	Signs and Symptoms
3%	Mild	Decreased skin turgor, sunken eyes, dry mucous membranes, dry tongue, reduced sweating
6%	Moderate	Oliguria, orthostatic hypotension, tachycardia, low volume pulse, cool peripheries, reduced filling of peripheral veins and CVP, hemoconcentration, apathy
9%	Severe	Profound oliguria or anuria and compromised CNS function with or without altered sensorium

What Are the Ongoing Losses?
- tubes
  - Foley catheter, NG, surgical drains
- third spacing (other than ECF, ICF)
  - pleura, GI, retroperitoneal, peritoneal
  - evaporation via exposed viscera, burns
- blood loss
- ongoing loss due to type of surgery
  - minor surgery   4 cc/kg/hr
  - internal surgery   6 cc/kg/hr
  - major surgery   8 cc/kg/hr

IV Fluid Solutions

- replacement fluids include crystalloid and colloid solutions
- improves perfusion but NOT O_2 carrying capacity of blood

Crystalloid Infusion
- salt-containing solutions that distribute within ECF
- maintain euvolemia in patient with blood loss: 3 mL crystalloid infusion per 1 mL of blood loss for volume replacement (i.e. **3:1** replacement)
- if large volumes to be given, use balanced fluid such as Ringer's lactate or Plasmalyte™ as too much normal saline (NS) may lead to hyperchloremic metabolic acidosis

Table 4. IV Fluid Solutions

		ECF	Ringer's Lactate	0.9 NS	0.45 NS	D5W	2/3 + 1/3	Plasmalyte
mEq/L	Na	142	130	154	77	–	51	140
	K	4	4	–	–	–	–	5
	Ca	4	3	–	–	–	–	–
	Mg	3	–	–	–	–	–	3
	Cl	103	109	154	77	–	51	98
	HCO$_3$	27	28*	–	–	–	–	27
mOsm/L		280-310	273	308	407	253	269	294

* converted from lactate

Colloid Infusion (also see *Blood Products*, A15)
- collected from donor blood (fresh frozen plasma, albumin, RBCs) or synthetics (e.g. starch products)
- distributes within intravascular volume
- **1:1** ratio (infusion:blood loss) only in terms of replacing volume

Initial Distribution of IV Fluids
- H_2O follows ions/molecules to their respective compartments

Blood Products

- see <u>Hematology</u>

Red Blood Cells (RBCs) (U = unit)
- 1 U RBCs = approx. 300 mL
- 1 U RBCs increases Hb by approx. 10 g/L in a 70 kg patient
- RBCs may be diluted with colloid/crystalloid to decrease viscosity
- decision to transfuse based on initial blood volume, premorbid Hb level, present volume status, expected further blood loss, patient health status
- MASSIVE transfusion = >1 x blood volume/24 hours

Autologous RBCs
- replacement of blood volume with one's own RBCs
- marked decrease in complications (infectious, febrile, etc.)
- alternative to homologous transfusion in elective procedures, but only if adequate Hb and no infection
- pre-op phlebotomy with hemodilution prior to elective surgery (up to 4 U collected >2 days before surgery)
- intraoperative salvage and filtration (cell saver)

Non-RBC Products
- fresh frozen plasma (FFP)
  - contains all plasma clotting factors and fibrinogen close to normal plasma levels
  - to prevent/treat bleeding due to coagulation factor depletion/deficiencies, liver failure, massive transfusions
  - for liver failure, factor deficiencies, massive transfusions
- cryoprecipitate
  - contains Factors VIII and XIII, vWF, fibrinogen
- platelets
  - used in thrombocytopenia, massive transfusions, impaired platelet function
- albumin
  - selective intravascular volume expander
- erythropoietin
  - can be used preoperatively to stimulate erythropoiesis
- Pentaspan™
  - colloid, do not give >2 L/70 kg/24 hours

Transfusion Reactions

Immunosuppression
- some studies show associations between perioperative transfusion and post-operative infection, earlier cancer recurrence, and poorer outcome

Nonimmune
- infectious risks: HIV, hepatitis B/C, Epstein-Barr virus (EBV), cytomegalovirus (CMV), brucellosis, malaria, salmonellosis, measles, syphilis
- hypervolemia
- electrolyte changes: increased K in stored blood
- coagulopathy
- hypothermia
- citrate toxicity
- hypocalcemia

Calculating Acceptable Blood Losses (ABL)
- blood volume
  - term infant   80 mL/kg
  - adult male   70 mL/kg
  - adult female   60 mL/kg
- calculate estimated blood volume (EBV) (e.g. in a 70 kg male, approx. 70 mL/kg)
  - EBV = 70 kg x 70 mL/kg = 4900 mL
- decide on a transfusion trigger, i.e. the Hb level at which you would begin transfusion, (e.g. 70 g/L for a person with Hb(i) = 150 g/L)
  - Hb(f) = 70 g/L
- calculate

$$ABL = \frac{Hb(i) - Hb(f)}{Hb(i)} \times EBV$$

$$= \frac{150 - 70}{150} \times 4900 = 2613 \text{ mL}$$

- therefore in order to keep the Hb level above 70 g/L, RBCs would have to be given after approximately 2.6 L of blood has been lost

A Multicenter, Randomized, Controlled Clinical Trial of Transfusion Requirements in Critical Care.
NEJM 1999; 340: 409-417

Purpose: To determine whether a restrictive strategy of RBC transfusion and a liberal strategy produced equivalent results in critically ill patients.
Study: Randomized controlled trial with 60 day follow-up.
Patients: 838 critically ill patients with euvolemia after initial treatment who had Hb concentrations of less than 90 g/L within 72 hours after admission to the ICU. Mean age 57.5 years, 62.5% male.
Intervention: Patients were randomly assigned to either a restrictive strategy of transfusion, in which RBC were transfused if the Hb dropped <70g/L and Hb concentrations were maintained between 70-90 g/L, or to a liberal strategy, in which transfusions were given when the Hb dropped <100 g/L and Hb concentrations were maintained between 100-120 g/L.
Main Outcomes: All cause mortality rates at 30 and 60 days, mortality rates during the stay in ICU and hospitalization, survival times during the first 30 days, and rates of organ failure and dysfunction.
Results: Overall, 30-day mortality was similar in the two groups. However, the rates were significantly lower with the restrictive transfusion strategy among patients who were less acutely ill (8.7% vs. 16.1%) and who were less than 55 years of age (5.7% vs. 13%), but not among patients with clinically significant cardiac disease.
The mortality rate during hospitalization was significantly lower in the restrictive-strategy group (22.2% vs. 28.1%).
Conclusions: A restrictive strategy of RBC transfusion is at least as effective as, and possibly superior to, a liberal transfusion strategy in critically ill patients, with the possible exception of patients with acute MI and unstable angina.

Table 5. Immune Transfusion Reactions

Reaction	Cause	Presentation	Management
Non-hemolytic: Febrile	- alloantibodies to WBC, platelet, or other donor plasma antigens	- mild fever <38°C with or without rigors; may be >38°C with restlessness and shivering - nausea, facial flushing, headache, myalgias, hypotension, chest and back pain - occurs quickly; near completion of transfusion or within 2 hours	- rule out fever due to hemolytic reaction or bacterial contamination - mild <38°C: decrease infusion rate and give antipyretics - severe: stop transfusion, give antipyretics, antihistamines, and symptomatic treatment
Non-hemolytic: Allergic	- mild allergic reaction due to IgE alloantibodies to substances in donor plasma - mast cells activated with histamine release - usually occurs in pre-exposed (e.g. multiple transfusions, multiparous)	- often have history of similar reactions - abrupt onset pruritic erythema/urticaria on arms and trunk, occasionally with fever - less common: involvement of face, larynx and bronchioles	- mild: slow transfusion rate, IV antihistamines - moderate to severe: stop transfusion, IV antihistamines, subcutaneous epinephrine, hydrocortisone, IV fluids, bronchodilators - prophylactic: antihistamines 15-60 minutes prior to transfusion, washed or deglycerolized frozen RBC
Non-hemolytic: Anaphylactoid	- in IgA deficient patients with anti-IgA antibodies receiving IgA-containing blood - immune complexes activate mast cells, basophils, eosinophils, and complement system = severe symptoms after transfusion of RBC, plasma, platelets, or other components with IgA	- rare, potentially lethal - apprehension, urticarial eruptions, dyspnea, hypotension, laryngeal and airway edema, wheezing, chest pain, shock, sudden death	- circulatory support with fluids, catecholamines (epinephrine), bronchodilators - respiratory assistance as indicated - evaluate for IgA deficiency and anti-IgA antibodies - future transfusions must be free of IgA: washed/deglycerolized RBCs free of IgA, blood from IgA deficient donor
Transfusion Related Acute Lung Injury (TRALI)	- form of noncardiogenic pulmonary edema - immunologic cause; not due to fluid overload or cardiac failure	- occurs 2-4 hours post transfusion - respiratory distress: mild dyspnea to severe hypoxia - chest x-ray: consistent with acute pulmonary edema, but pulmonary artery and wedge pressures are not elevated	- usually resolves within 48 hrs with O_2, mechanical ventilation, supportive treatment
Hemolytic Acute (intravascular hemolysis)	- caused by donor incompatibility with recipient's blood - often due to clerical error - antibody coated RBC is destroyed by activation of complement system - ABO incompatibility common cause, other RBC Ag-Ab systems can be involved	- fever, chills, chest or back pain, hypotension, tachycardia, nausea, flushing, dyspnea, wheezing, hypoxemia, hemoglobinuria, diffuse bleeding due to DIC, acute renal failure	- stop transfusion - notify blood bank, confirm or rule out diagnosis – clerical check, direct Coombs', repeat grouping, Rh screen and crossmatch, serum haptoglobin - manage hypotension with fluids, inotropes, other blood products - maintain urine output with crystalloids, furosemide, dopamine, alkalinize urine - component treatment if DIC, repeat grouping, Rh screen and crossmatch, serum haptoglobin - manage hypotension with fluids, inotropes, other blood product - component treatment
Hemolytic Delayed (extravascular hemolysis)	- caused by donor incompatibility with recipient's blood - generally mild, caused by antibodies to Rh system, Kell, Duffy, or Kidd antigens - the level of antibody at the time of transfusion is too low to be detected or to cause hemolysis, later the level of antibody is increased due to secondary stimulus	- occurs in recipients sensitized to RBC antigens by previous blood transfusion or pregnancy - anemia, mild jaundice, fever 1 to 21 days post transfusion	- supportive - direct Coombs and reexamination of pretransfusion specimens from the patient and donor for diagnosis

Extubation

- performed by trained, experienced personnel because reintubation may be required
- laryngospasm more likely in semiconscious patient; must ensure level of consciousness is adequate
- general guidelines
  - ensure patient has normal neuromuscular function and hemodynamic status
  - ensure patient is breathing spontaneously with adequate rate and tidal volume
  - allow ventilation (spontaneous or controlled) with 100% O_2 for 3-5 minutes
  - suction secretions from pharynx
  - deflate cuff, remove ETT on inspiration (vocal cords abducted)
  - ensure patient breathing adequately after extubation
  - ensure face mask for O_2 delivery available
  - proper positioning of patient during transfer to recovery room (e.g. lateral decubitus, head elevated)

Complications of Extubation
- early
  - aspiration
  - laryngospasm
- late
  - transient vocal cord incompetence
  - edema (glottic, subglottic)
  - pharyngitis, tracheitis

Post-Operative Care

- pain management should be continuous from OR to post-anesthetic unit to hospital ward and home
- pain service may assist with management of post-operative inpatients

Post-Operative Nausea and Vomiting
- more likely to occur if young age, female gender, eye/middle ear/gynecological surgery, obese, history of post-anesthetic nausea/vomiting
- some anesthetic agents tend to cause more nausea post-operatively than others (e.g. opioids, nitrous oxide)
- hypotension and bradycardia must be ruled out
- pain/surgical manipulation also cause nausea
- often treated with dimenhydrinate (Gravol™), metoclopramide (Maxeran™) (not with bowel obstruction), prochlorperazine (Stemetil™), ondansetron (Zofran™), granisetron

Risk Factors for Postoperative Nausea and Vomiting (PONV):
1. young age
2. female
3. history of PONV
4. non-smoker
5. type of surgery: ophtho, ENT, abdo/pelvic, plastics
6. type of anesthetic: N_2O, opioids, volatile agents

Post-Operative Confusion and Agitation
- ABCs first! – confusion or agitation can be caused by airway obstruction, hypercapnea, hypoxemia
- neurologic status (Glasgow Coma Scale, pupils), residual paralysis from anesthetic
- pain, distended bowel/bladder
- fear/anxiety/separation from caregivers/language barriers
- metabolic disturbance (hypoglycemia, hypercalcemia, hyponatremia – especially post-TURP)
- intracranial cause (stroke, raised intracranial pressure)
- drug effect (ketamine, anticholinergics)
- elderly patients are more susceptible to post-operative delirium

Pain Service

Definitions
- nociception: detection, transduction and transmission of noxious stimuli
- pain: perception of nociception which occurs in the brain

Acute Pain
- pain of short duration (<6 weeks) usually associated with surgery, trauma or acute illness, often associated with inflammation
- usually limited to the area of damage/trauma and resolves spontaneously with healing

Acute Pain Mechanism
- tissue damage by thermal, mechanical or chemical forces results in activation of free nerve endings called nociceptors (pain receptors)
- sensory pathways transmit information from peripheral pain receptors to CNS
- 1st order afferent neuron synapses with 2nd order afferent neuron in the dorsal horn of spinal cord → 2nd order synapses with 3rd order in the thalamus → 3rd order sends axonal projections into the sensory cortex
- substance P is a key neurotransmitter involved in the propagation of nociceptive signals across the synapses between 1st and 2nd order sensory neurons
- sensory pathways can be modulated by the higher centres in the CNS to limit the amount of afferent nociceptive stimulation which can be perceived as pain
- the most important site of modulation is the synapse between 1st and 2nd order sensory neurons in the outer layers of the dorsal horn where efferent modulatory neurons descend from the brainstem
- modulatory neurons release neurotransmitter substances (endorphins, enkaphlins, norepinephrine, serotonin, GABA) which dampen the nociceptive transmission by impairing the release of substance P or by making the post-synaptic membrane more difficult to depolarize

Pharmacological Management of Acute Pain
- ask the patient to rate the pain to determine whether it is mild, moderate or severe
- **analgesic ladder**:
  - mild pain – acetaminophen, non-steroidal anti-inflammatories (NSAIDs)
  - moderate – codeine, oxycodone
  - severe – oxycodone, morphine, hydromorphone, fentanyl
- **acetaminophen**
  - 1st line for mild acute pain
  - analgesic and antipyretic but no anti-inflammatory properties
  - adjunct to opioid analgesia in moderate and severe pain
  - be cautious of liver toxicity
  - limited by analgesic ceiling – above certain dose there is no analgesic effect
- **NSAIDs**
  - mild to moderate acute pain
  - analgesic and anti-inflammatory properties → good for management of acute pain due to tissue damage and inflammation
  - significant inter-individual variation in efficacy and side effect profile
  - limited by analgesic ceiling
- **opioids**
  - produces analgesia by acting at several levels of the nervous system:
    - dampens nociceptive transmission between 1st and 2nd order sensory neurons in the dorsal horn by binding to pre-synaptic, post-synaptic and interneuron opioid receptors
    - activates descending modulatory pathways resulting in the release of inhibitory neurotransmitters (i.e. noradrenaline, serotonin, GABA)
    - inhibits the inflammatory response in the periphery and decreases hyperalgesia
    - affects mood and anxiety and alleviates the affective component of perceived pain
  - key advantage of opioids is that, unlike acetaminophen and NSAIDs, they have no maximum dose and can be titrated to manage even severe forms of pain (i.e. no analgesic ceiling)
  - respiratory drive depression can occur with opioids
  - see Clinical Pharmacology for opioid analgesic equivalencies
- oral opioid analgesics
  - codeine, oxycodone, morphine, hydromorphone
  - mild and moderate acute pain
  - side effects such as respiratory depression, constipation and abdominal pain limit dosage titration

Analgesia Ladder

Mild pain
Acetaminophen
NSAIDS

Moderate pain
Codeine
Oxycodone

Severe pain
Oxycodone
Morphine
Hydromorphone
Fentanyl

Use NSAIDs with Caution in Patients with:
1. asthma
2. coagulopathy
3. GI ulcers
4. renal insufficiency
5. pregnancy, 3rd trimester

Common side effects of opioids
1. Nausea & vomiting
2. Constipation
3. Sedation
4. Pruritis
5. Abdominal pain
6. Urinary retention
7. Respiratory depression

- may be prescribed alone but most commonly prescribed in combination with NSAIDs or acetaminophen
- parenteral opioids
  - morphine, hydromorphone, meperidine, fentanyl
  - severe acute pain
- other methods of opioid administration
  - intrathecal administration (spinal block)
    - superior analgesia with much smaller doses of opioids
    - higher concentration of narcotics in the brainstem may lead to respiratory depression, sedation, nausea and vomiting, pruritus
  - continuous infusion into epidural space
    - opioids can be administered over a period of several days

- **Patient Controlled Analgesia (PCA)**
  - involves the use of computerized pumps that can deliver a constant infusion as well as bolus breakthrough doses of parenterally administered opioid analgesics limited by lockout intervals
  - most commonly used agents for PCA are morphine and hydromorphone
  - refer to Table 8 for suggested infusion rate, PCA dose, and lockout intervals

Opioid Antagonists (naloxone, naltrexone)
- opioid toxicity manifests primarily at CNS – manage ABCs
- opioid antagonists competitively inhibit opioid receptors, predominantly mu receptors
- naloxone is short acting ($t_{1/2} = 1$ hr); effects of narcotic may return when naloxone wears off, therefore the patient must be observed closely following its administration
- naltrexone is longer acting ($t_{1/2} = 10$ hrs); less likely to see return of narcotic effects
- relative overdose of naloxone may cause nausea, agitation, sweating, tachycardia, hypertension, re-emergence of pain, pulmonary edema, seizures (essentially opioid withdrawal)

PCA Parameters
1. loading dose
2. bolus dose
3. lockout interval
4. continuous infusion (optional)
5. max. 4 hr limit (optional)

Advantages of PCA
Better pain control
Fewer side effects
Accomodates patient variability
Accomodates changes in opioid requirements

Regional Anesthesia

Definition of Regional Anesthesia

- local anesthetic agent (LA) applied around a peripheral nerve at any point along the length of the nerve (from spinal cord up to, but not including, the nerve endings) for the purposes of reducing or preventing impulse transmission
- no CNS depression (unless overdose of local anesthetic); patient conscious
- regional anesthetic techniques categorized as follows:
  - epidural and spinal anesthesia
  - peripheral nerve blockades
  - IV regional anesthesia

Preparation for Regional Anesthesia

Patient Preparation
- thorough pre-operative evaluation and assessment of patient
- technique explained to patient
- IV sedation may be indicated before block
- monitoring should be as extensive as for general anesthesia

Relative Indications for Regional Anesthesia
- avoids some of the dangers of general anesthesia (e.g. known difficult intubation, severe respiratory failure, etc.)
- patient specifically requests regional anesthesia
- high quality post-operative pain relief
- general anesthesia not available/contraindicated
- titration of LA dosage for differential blockade, e.g. can block pain but preserve motor function

Contraindications to Peripheral Nerve Blockade
- allergy to local anesthetic
- patient refusal, lack of cooperation
- lack of resuscitation equipment
- lack of IV access
- certain types of pre-existing neurological dysfunction (eg. ALS, MS)
- local infection at block site

Contraindications to Spinal/Epidural Anesthesia
- absolute contraindications include:
  - lack of proper equipment or properly trained personnel
  - lack of IV access
  - allergy to LA
  - infection at puncture site or underlying tissues
  - uncorrected hypovolemia
  - coagulation abnormalities
  - raised ICP
  - sepsis/bacteremia
  - hemodynamic instability/uncorrected hypovolemia
- relative contraindications include:
  - bacteremia
  - pre-existing neurological disease
  - aortic/mitral valve stenosis (i.e. fixed CO states)
  - previous spinal surgery, other back problems
  - severe/unstable psychiatric disease or emotional instability

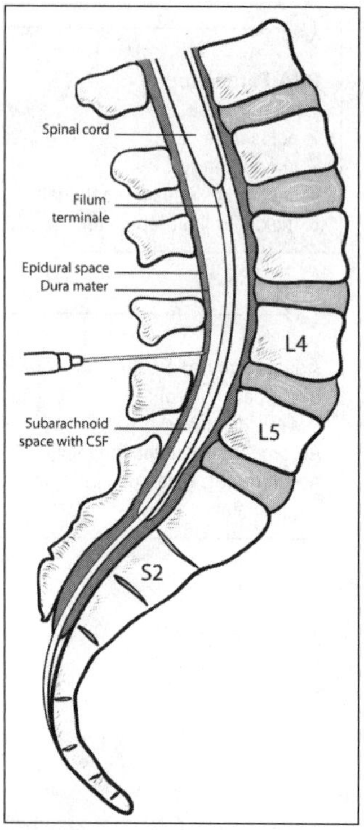

Complications of Regional Anesthesia
- failure of technique
- systemic drug toxicity due to overdose or intravascular injection
- peripheral neuropathy due to intraneural injection
- pain or hematoma at injection site
- infection
- sympathetic blockade with hypotension and bradycardia (occurs early, followed by sensory then motor blockade)

Epidural and Spinal Anesthesia

Anatomy of Spinal/Epidural Area
- spinal cord extends to L2, dural sac to S2 in adults
- nerve roots (cauda equina) from L2 to S2
- needle inserted below L2 should not encounter cord, thus L3-L4, L4-L5 interspace commonly used
- structures penetrated
  - skin, subcutaneous fat
  - supraspinous ligament
  - interspinous ligament
  - ligamentum flavum (last layer before epidural space)
  - dura + arachnoid for spinal anesthesia

Figure 6. Landmarks for Placement of Epidural/Spinals

The figure on the left shows a lateral view of the lumbar spine with labels:
- Spinal cord
- Filum terminale
- Epidural space
- Dura mater
- Subarachnoid space with CSF
- L4
- L5
- S2

Landmarking epidural/spinal anesthesia

Spinous processes should be maximally flexed

L4 spinous process is found between iliac crests

Common sites of insertion are L3-L4 and L4-L5

Classic Presentation of Dural Puncture Headache
1. onset 6 hrs - 3 days after dural puncture
2. postural component (worse sitting)
3. occipital or frontal localization
4. ± tinnitus, diplopia

Table 6. Epidural versus Spinal Anesthesia

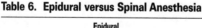

	Epidural	Spinal
onset	• significant blockade requires 10-15 minutes • slower onset of side effects	• rapid blockade (onset in 2-5 minutes)
effectiveness	• effectiveness of blockade can be variable	• very effective blockade
deposition site	• LA deposited in epidural space (potential space between ligamentum flavum and dura) • initial blockade is at the spinal roots followed by some degree of spinal cord anesthesia as LA diffuses into the subarachnoid space through the dura	• LA injected into subarachnoid space in the dural sac surrounding the spinal cord and nerve roots
difficulty	• technically more difficult; greater failure rate	• easier to perform
patient positioning	• position of patient not as important; specific gravity not an issue	• hyperbaric LA solution – position of patient important
specific gravity/spread	• solutions injected here spread throughout the potential space; specific gravity of solution does not affect spread	• LA solution may be made hyperbaric (of greater specific gravity than the cerebrospinal fluid by mixing with 10% dextrose, thus increasing spread of LA to the dependent (low) areas of the subarachnoid space)
dosage	• larger volume/dose of LA (usually > toxic IV dose)	• smaller dose of LA required (usually < toxic IV dose)
continuous infusion	• use of catheter allows for continuous infusion or repeat injections	• none

Table 6. Epidural versus Spinal Anesthesia (continued)

	Epidural	Spinal
complications	• failure of technique • hypotension • bradycardia if cardiac sympathetics blocked (only if ~T2-4 block) • epidural or subarachnoid hematoma • accidental subarachnoid injection can produce spinal anesthesia (and any of the above complications) • systemic toxicity of LA (accidental intravenous) • catheter complications (shearing, kinking, vascular or subarachnoid placement) • infection • dural puncture	• failure of technique • hypotension • bradycardia if cardiac sympathetics blocked (only if ~T2-4 block), i.e. "high spinal" • epidural or subarachnoid hematoma • post-spinal headache (CSF leak) • persistent paresthesias (usually transient) • spinal cord trauma, infection
combined spinal-epidural	• combines the benefits of rapid, reliable, intense blockade of spinal anesthesia together with the flexibility of an epidural catheter	

Peripheral Nerve Blocks

- relatively safe – avoid intraneural injection and neurotoxic agents
- provides good operating conditions
- e.g. brachial plexus block, femoral nerve block, digital ring block, etc.

Local Anesthesia

Local Infiltration, Hematoma Blocks

- note: local anesthetics are described in Table 13

Local Infiltration
- injection of tissue with local anesthetic agent (LA), producing a lack of sensation in the infiltrated area due to LA acting on nerve endings
- one of the simplest and safest techniques of providing anesthesia
- suitable for small incisions, suturing, excising small lesions
- can use fairly large volumes of dilute LA to infiltrate a large area
- low concentrations of epinephrine (1:100,000-1:200,000) cause vasoconstriction thus reducing bleeding and prolonging the effects of LA by reducing systemic absorption

Fracture Hematoma Block
- special type of local infiltration for pain control during manipulation of certain fractures
- hematoma created by fracture is infiltrated with LA to anesthetize surrounding tissues
- sensory blockade may be only partial
- no muscle relaxation

Topical Anesthetics

- various preparations of local anesthetics available for topical use, may be a mixture of agents, e.g. EMLA cream is a combination of 2.5% lidocaine and prilocaine
- must be able to penetrate the skin or mucous membrane

Local Anesthetic Agents

Definition and Mode of Action
- LA are drugs that block the generation and propagation of impulses in excitable tissues: nerves, skeletal muscle, cardiac muscle, brain
- LA substances bind to a Na channel receptor on the cytosolic side of the Na channel (i.e. must be lipid soluble), inhibiting Na flux and thus blocking impulse conduction
- different types of nerve fibres undergo blockade at different rates

Reduction of Postoperative Mortality and Morbidity with Epidural or Spinal Anaesthesia: Results from Overview of Randomised Trials
BMJ 2000; 321:1-12

Purpose: To obtain reliable estimates of the effects of neuraxial blockade with epidural or spinal anesthesia on postoperative morbidity and mortality.
Study: Systematic review of all trials with randomization to intraoperative neuraxial blockade versus not.
Patients: 141 trials including 9559 patients.
Main Outcomes: All cause mortality, MI, PE, DVT, transfusion requirements, pneumonia, other infections, respiratory depression, and renal failure.
Results: Overall mortality was reduced by about a third in patients allocated to neuraxial blockade. Neuraxial blockade reduced the odds of PE by 55%, DVT by 44%, transfusion requirements by 50%, pneumonia by 39%, and respiratory depression by 59%. There were also reductions in MI and renal failure. The proportional reductions in mortality did not clearly differ by surgical group, type of blockade (epidural or spinal), or in those trials in which neuraxial blockade was combined with general anesthesia compared with trials in which neuraxial blockade was used alone.
Conclusions: Neuraxial blockade reduces postoperative mortality and other serious complications.

Where Not to Use Local Anesthetic Agent (LA) with Epinephrine
Nose, **H**ose (penis), **F**ingers, and **T**oes

Absorption, Distribution, Metabolism
- LA readily crosses the blood-brain barrier (BBB) once absorbed into the bloodstream
- **ester-type** LA (procaine, tetracaine) broken down by plasma and hepatic esterases; metabolites excreted via kidneys
- **amide-type** LA (lidocaine, bupivicaine) broken down by hepatic mixed function oxidases (P450 system); metabolites excreted via kidney

Selection of LA
- choice of LA depends on
    - onset of action: influenced by pKa (the lower the pKa, the higher the concentration of the base form of the LA and the faster the onset of action)
    - duration of desired effects: influenced by protein binding (long duration of action when the protein binding of LA is strong)
    - potency: influenced by lipid solubility (agents with high lipid solubility will penetrate the nerve membrane more easily)
    - unique needs (e.g. sensory blockade with relative preservation of motor function by bupivicaine at low doses)
    - potential for toxicity

Systemic Toxicity
- occurs by accidental intravascular injection, LA overdose, or unexpectedly rapid absorption
- systemic toxicity manifests itself mainly at CNS and CVS
- CNS effects first appear to be excitatory due to initial block of inhibitory fibres; then subsequent block of excitatory fibres
- CNS effects (in approximate order of appearance)
    - numbness of tongue, perioral tingling, metallic taste
    - disorientation, drowsiness
    - tinnitus
    - visual disturbances
    - muscle twitching, tremors
    - unconsciousness
    - convulsions, seizures
    - generalized CNS depression, coma, respiratory arrest
- CVS effects
    - vasodilation, hypotension
    - decreased myocardial contractility
    - dose-dependent delay in cardiac impulse transmission
        - prolonged PR, QRS intervals
        - sinus bradycardia
    - CVS collapse
- treatment of systemic toxicity
    - early recognition of signs
    - 100% O_2, manage ABCs
    - diazepam or sodium thiopental may be used to increase seizure threshold
    - if the seizures are not controlled by diazepam or thiopental, consider using succinylcholine (stops muscular manifestations of seizures, facilitates intubation)

Obstetrical Anesthesia

- adequate anesthesia requires a clear understanding of maternal and fetal physiology

Physiologic Changes in Pregnancy
1. **airway**
    - upper airway becomes edematous and friable
    - ↓FRC and ↑O_2 consumption → desaturation
2. **cardiovascular system**
    - ↑blood volume > ↑RBC mass → mild anemia
    - ↓SVR proportionally greater than ↑CO → ↓BP
    - prone to ↓BP due to aortocaval compression
3. **central nervous system**
    - ↓MAC due to hormonal effects
    - ↑block height due to engorged epidural veins
4. **gastrointestinal system**
    - delayed gastric emptying
    - ↑volume and acidity of gastric fluid
    - ↓LES tone
    - ↑abdominal pressure
    - combined this leads to an ↑risk of aspiration

The Effect of Epidural Analgesia on Labour, Maternal, and Neonatal Outcomes: A Systematic Review
Am J Obstet Gynecol 2002; 186:S69-77

Study: Meta-analysis of 14 studies with sample size of 4324 women
Selection Criteria: Randomized controlled trials and prospective cohort (PC) studies between 1980-2001 in which epidural analgesia was compared to parenteral opioid administration during labour
Types of Participants: Healthy women with uneventful pregnancies.
Intervention: Participants were randomized to either epidural analgesia or parenteral opioid administration during labour for labour pain relief.
Outcomes and Results: Maternal – there were no differences between the 2 groups in first-stage labour length, incidence of Caesarean delivery, incidence of instrumented vaginal delivery for dystocia, nausea, or mid-to-low back pain post-partum. However, second-stage labour length was longer (mean=15 min) and there were greater reports of fever and hypotension in the epidural group. Also, lower pain scores and greater satisfaction with analgesia were reported among the epidural group. There was no difference in lactation success at 6 weeks and urinary incontinence was more frequent in the epidural group immediately post-partum, but not at 3 months or 1 year (evidence from PC studies only). Neonatal – there were no differences between the 2 groups for incidence of fetal heart rate abnormalities, intrapartum meconium, poor 5-min Apgar score, or low umbilical artery pH. However, the incidence of poor 1-min Apgar scores and need for neonatal naloxone were higher in the parenteral opioid group.
Conclusions: Epidural analgesia is a safe intrapartum method for labour pain relief and women should not avoid epidural analgesia for fear of neonatal harm, Caesarean delivery, breastfeeding difficulties, long-term back pain or long-term urinary incontinence.

Options for Analgesia during Labour

1) **psychoprophylaxis** – Lamaze method
   - patterns of breathing and focused attention on fixed object
2) **systemic medication**
   - easy to administer, but risk of maternal or neonatal depression
   - common drugs: opioids (morphine, meperidine)
3) **inhalational analgesia**
   - easy to administer, makes uterine contractions more tolerable, but does not relieve pain completely
   - 50% nitrous oxide
4) **regional anesthesia**
   - provides excellent analgesia with minimal depressant effects
   - hypotension is the most common complication
   - maternal BP monitored q2-5 min for 15-20 min after initiation and regularly thereafter
   - techniques used: epidural, combined spinal epidural, pudendal blocks, spinal, paracervical, lumbar sympathetic blocks

Options for Caesarean Section

1) **regional**: spinal or epidural
2) **general**: used when contraindications or time precludes regional blockade
   - potential complications of anesthesia in Caesarean Section:
     - pulmonary aspiration under general anesthesia: due to increased gastroesophageal reflux
     - hypotension and/or fetal distress: caused by occlusion of the inferior vena cava/aorta by the gravid uterus (**aortocaval compression**); corrected by turning patient in the left lateral decubitus (LLD) position or using left uterine displacement (LUD)
     - unintentional total spinal anesthesia
     - LA induced seizures: intravascular injection of LA
     - postdural puncture headache
     - nerve injury (rare)

Nociceptive Pathways in Labour and Delivery
- Labour
  - cervical dilation and effacement
  - visceral nerve fibres entering the spinal cord at T10-L1
- Delivery
  - distention of lower vagina and perineum
  - somatic nociceptive impulses via the pudendal nerve entering the spinal cord at S2-S4

Correcting Aortocaval Compression

Turn patient to left lateral decubitus position

Left uterine displacement by placing wedge under right hip

Pediatric Anesthesia

Respiratory System

- in comparison to adults, **anatomical differences** in infants include:
  - large head, short trachea/neck, large tongue, adenoids and tonsils
  - narrow nasal passages (obligate nasal breathers until 5 months)
  - narrowest part of airway at the level of the cricoid vs. glottis in adults
  - epiglottis is longer, U shaped and angled at 45 degrees, carina is wider and is at the level of T2 (T4 in adults)
- **physiologic differences** include:
  - faster RR, immature respiratory centres which are depressed by hypoxia/hypercapnea (airway closure occurs in the neonate at the end of expiration)
  - less oxygen reserve during apnea – decreased total lung volume, vital and functional reserve capacity together with higher metabolic needs
  - greater V/Q mismatch – lower lung compliance due to immature alveoli (mature at 8 years)
  - greater work of breathing – greater chest wall compliance, weaker intercostals/diaphragm and higher resistance to airflow
- a pediatric breathing unit is required for all children <20 kg

Cardiovascular System

- blood volume at birth is approximately 80 mL/kg; transfusion should be started if >10% of blood volume lost
- children have a high pulse rate and a low BP
- CO is increased by increasing HR, not stroke volume because of low heart wall compliance; therefore, bradycardia → severe compromise in CO

Temperature Regulation

- vulnerable to hypothermia
- minimize heat loss by use of warming blankets, covering the infant head, humidification of inspired gases and warming of infused solutions

Central Nervous System

- the MAC of halothane is increased from the adult (i.e. 0.75% adult, 0.87% neonates, 1.2% infant)

To increase alveolar minute ventilation in neonates, increase respiratory rate not tidal volume.

Neonate   30-40 bpm

$$1\text{-}13 \text{ yrs} \quad \frac{(24 - [\text{age}/2])}{\text{min}}$$

Poiseuille's Law

$$\text{flow} = \frac{(\Delta\text{pressure}) \, (\pi) \, (\text{radius})^4}{(8) \, (\text{viscosity})(\text{length})}$$

ETT Sizing in Pediatrics
Diameter of tracheal tube in children (mm) after 1 year = [age/4] + 4
Length of tracheal tube (cm) = (age/2) + 12

A Comparison of Three Methods for Estimating Appropriate Tracheal Tube Depth in Children
Paediatr Anaesth 2005; 15(10):846-851.

Study: Prospective, randomized controlled trial
Patients: 60 infants and children (age range 3 months – 7 years) scheduled for fluoroscopic procedures requiring general anesthesia and intubation with an endotracheal tube (ETT).
Intervention: Patients were randomly assigned to one of three methods of endotracheal intubation: 1) 'mainstem' method – deliberate endobronchial (mainstem) intubation with subsequent withdrawal of the ETT to 2cm above the carina. 2) 'marker' method – alignment of a double-black line marker on the tip of the ETT with the vocal cords. 3) 'formula' method – placement of the ETT to a depth calculated using the formula: ETT depth (cm) = 3 x ETT size (mmID).
Main outcome: "Appropriate" ETT placement, defined as placement with position of the ETT tip between the sternoclavicular junction and 0.5 cm above the carina as determined by fluoroscopy.
Results: The mainstem method was associated with the highest rate of appropriate ETT placement (73%) compared to the marker method (53%, p=0.03, RR=1.56) and the formula method (42%, p=0.006, RR=2.016). There was no difference between the marker and formula methods (p=0.2, RR=1.27), but there was a higher success of ETT placement with the marker method compared to the formula method for patients aged 3-12 months (p=0.0056, RR=4.0).
Conclusions: Deliberate intubation of the mainstem bronchus with subsequent withdrawal of the ETT tip to above the carina most reliably resulted in appropriate depth of the ETT in infants and children.

- the neuromuscular junction is immature for the first 4 weeks of life and thus there is an increased sensitivity to non-depolarizing relaxants
- parasympathetics mature at birth, sympathetics mature at 4-6 months → autonomic imbalance
- infant brain is 12% of body weight and receives 34% of CO (adult: 2% body weight and 14% CO)

Glucose Maintenance
- infants less than 1 year can become seriously hypoglycemic during preoperative fasting and postoperatively if feeding is not recommenced as soon as possible
- after 1 year children are able to maintain normal glucose homeostasis in excess of 8 hours

Pharmacology
- higher dose requirements because of higher TBW (75% vs. 60% in adults) and greater volume of distribution
- barbiturates/opioids more potent due to greater permeability of BBB
- muscle relaxants
    - non-depolarizing
        - immature NMJ, variable response
    - depolarizing
        - must be pretreated with atropine or may get profound bradycardia, sinus node arrest due to PNS > SNS (also dries oral secretions)
        - more susceptible to arrhythmias, hyperkalemia, rhabdomyolysis, myoglobinemia, masseter spasm, and malignant hyperthermia

Uncommon Complications

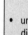

Malignant Hyperthermia (MH)

- hypermetabolic disorder of skeletal muscle
- due to an uncontrolled increase in intracellular Ca (because of an anomaly of the ryanodine receptor which regulates the Ca channel in the sarcoplasmic reticulum of skeletal muscle)
- autosomal dominant (AD) inheritance
- incidence of 1-5:100,000, may be associated with skeletal muscle abnormalities such as dystrophy or myopathy
- anesthetic drugs triggering MH crises
    - volatile anesthetics: enflurane, halothane, isoflurane, desflurane and sevoflurane (any drug ending in "-ane")
    - depolarizing relaxants: succinylcholine (SCh), decamethonium

Clinical Picture
- onset: immediate or hours after contact with trigger agent
- hypermetabolism
    - increased oxygen consumption
    - increased end-tidal CO_2 on capnograph
    - tachycardia/dysrhythmia
    - tachypnea/cyanosis
    - increased temperature – late sign
    - hypertension
    - diaphoresis
- muscle symptoms
    - trismus (masseter spasm) common but not specific for MH (occurs in 1% of children given SCh with halothane anesthesia)
    - tender, swollen muscles
    - trunk or total body rigidity

Complications
- death
- coma
- disseminated intravascular coagulation (DIC)
- muscle necrosis/weakness
- myoglobinuric renal failure/hepatic dysfunction
- electrolyte abnormalities (e.g. hyperkalemia) and secondary arrhythmias
- ARDS
- pulmonary edema

Signs of Malignant HT
- unexplained rise in end-tidal carbon dioxide
- increase in minute ventilation
- tachycardia
- hyperthermia (late sign)
- rigidity

Complications of MH
- death
- coma
- disseminated intravascular coagulation (DIC)
- muscle necrosis/weakness
- myoglobinuric renal failure/hepatic dysfunction
- electrolyte abnormalities (e.g. hyperkalemia) and secondary arrhythmias
- ARDS
- pulmonary edema

Prevention
- suspect MH in patients with a family history of problems/death with anesthetic
- dantrolene prophylaxis no longer routine
- avoid all trigger medications (use regional if possible) and use "clean" equipment
- central body temp and end-tidal CO_2 monitoring

Malignant Hyperthermia Management
1) notify surgeon, discontinue volatile agents and succinylcholine, hyperventilate with 100% oxygen at flows of 10 L/min or more. Halt the procedure as soon as possible
2) Dantrolene 2.5 mg/kg rapidly IV, through large-bore IV if possible
   - repeat until there is control of signs of MH. Sometimes up to 30 mg/kg is necessary
3) Bicarbonate 1-2 mEq/kg if blood gas values are not available for metabolic acidosis
4) cool the patient with core temp >39C
   - lavage open body cavities, stomach, bladder, rectum, apply ice to surface, infuse cold saline IV
   - stop cooling if temp <38C and is falling to prevent drift to <36C
5) dysrhythmias usually respond to treatment of acidosis and hyperkalemia
   - use standard drug therapy except Ca channel blockers as they may cause hyperkalemia and cardiac arrest in presence of dantrolene
6) hyperkalemia
   - treat with hyperventilation, bicarbonate, glucose/insulin, calcium
   - bicarb 1-2 mEq/kg IV, calcium chloride 10 mg/kg or calcium gluconate 10-50 mg/kg for life-threatening hyperkalemia and check glucose levels hourly
7) follow $ETCO_2$, electrolytes, blood gases, CK, core temperature, urine output and colour with Foley catheter, coagulation studies
   - if CK and/or potassium rises more than transiently or urine output falls to less than 0.5 ml/kg/hr, induce diuresis to >1 ml/kg/hr urine to avoid myoglobinuria-induced renal failure

> **Basic principles of MH Management**
> - call for help
> - turn off potential triggering agents
> - notify operating personnel
> - administer dantrolene 2.5mg/kg q5minutes
> - cool patient to 38°C
> - monitor and correct blood gases, electrolytes, and glucose

Common Medications

Table 7. Intravenous Induction Agents

	propofol (Diprivan™)	thiopental (Pentothal™, sodium thiopental, sodium thiopentone)	ketamine (Ketalar™, Ketaject™)	Benzodiazepines (midazolam (Versed™), diazepam (Valium™), lorazepam (Ativan™))
class	• alkylphenol - hypnotic	• ultra-short acting thiobarbiturate-hypnotic	• phencyclidine (PCP) derivative – dissociative	
action	• inhibitory at GABA synapse • ↓cerebral metabolic rate + blood flow, ↓ICP, ↓SVR, ↓BP, and ↓SV	• ↓time Cl channels open • facilitating GABA and supressing glutamic acid • ↓cerebral metabolism + ↓blood flow, CPP, ↓CO, ↓BP, ↓reflex tachycardia, ↓respiration	• may act on NMDA, opiate and other receptors • ↑HR, ↑BP, ↑SVR, ↑coronary flow, ↑myocardial O_2 uptake, CNS + respiratory depression, bronchial smooth muscle relaxation	• causes ↑glycine inhibitory neurotransmitter, facilitates GABA • produces antianxiety and skeletal muscle relaxant effects • minimal cardiac depression
indications	• induction • maintenance • total intravenous anesthesia (TIVA)	• popular for induction • control of convulsive states	• major trauma, hypovolemia, severe asthma because sympathomimetic	• used for sedation, amnesia and anxiolysis
caution	• allergy (egg, soy) • pts who cannot tolerate sudden ↓BP (i.e. fixed cardiac output or shock)	• allergy to barbiturates • uncontrolled hypotension, shock, cardiac failure • porphyria, liver disease, status asthmaticus, myxedema	• ketamine allergy • TCA medication (interaction causes HTN and dysrrhythmias) • history of psychosis • pt cannot tolerate HTN (i.e. CHF, ↑ICP, aneurysm)	• marked respiratory depression
dosing	• IV induction: 2.5-3.0 mg/kg (less with opioids or premeds) TIVA • unconscious <1 min • lasts 4-6 min • $t_{1/2}$=0.9 hrs • ↓post-op sedation, recovery time, N/V	• IV induction: 3-5 mg/kg TIVA • unconscious about 30s • lasts 5 min • accumulation with repeat dosing-not for maintenance • $t_{1/2}$=5-12 hrs • post-op sedation lasts hours	• IV induction 1-2 mg/kg • dissociation in 15s, analgesia, amnesia and unconsciousness in 45-60s • unconscious for 10-15 min, analgesia for 40min, amnesia for 1-2 hrs • $t_{1/2}$ = ~3 hrs	• onset less than 5 minutes if given IV • duration of action long but variable/somewhat unpredictable
special considerations	• 20-30% ↓BP due to vasodilation • reduce burning at IV site by mixing with lidocaine	• combining with rocuronium causes precipitate to form	• high incidence of emergence reactions (vivid dreaming, out-of-body sensation, illusions) • pretreat with glycopyrrolate to ↓ saliva	• antagonist: flumazenil (Anexate™) competitive inhibitor, 0.2 mg IV over 15 s; • repeat with 0.1 mg/min (max of 2 mg) , $t_{1/2}$ of 60 minutes • midazolam also has amnestic (antegrade) effects +↓risk of thrombophlebitis

Table 8. Opioids

Agent	Infusion rate	PCA dose	PCA lockout interval	
morphine	0.3 - 0.9 mg/h	0.2 - 0.3 mg	30 minutes	
fentanyl	25 - 50 ug/h	20 - 30 ug	15 minutes	
hydromorphone	0.1 - 0.2 mg/h	0.15 ug	30 minutes	

Agent	Moderate Dose	Onset	Duration	Special Considerations
morphine	0.2-0.3 mg/kg	Moderate	Moderate	Histamine release leading to decrease in BP
meperidine (Demerol™)	2-3 mg/kg	Moderate	Moderate	Anticholinergic, hallucinations, less pupillary constriction than morphine, metabolite build up may cause seizures
codeine	0.5-1 mg/kg	Moderate	Moderate	Primarily postoperative use, not for IV use
hydromorphone (Dilaudid™)	30-80 µg/kg	Moderate	Moderate	
fentanyl	3-10 µg/kg	Rapid	Short	Transient muscle rigidity in very high doses
remifentanil	0.5-1.5 µg/kg	Rapid	Ultra short	Only use during induction and maintenance of anesthesia

Table 9. Volatile Inhalational Agents

	sevoflurane	desflurane	isoflurane	enflurane	halothane	nitrous oxide (N_2O)*
MAC(% gas in O_2)	2.0	6.0	1.2	1.7	0.8	104
CNS	↑ ICP	↑ ICP	↓ cerebral metabolic rate ↑ ICP	EEG seizure-like activity, ↑ ICP	↑ ICP and CBF	
Resp	Respiratory depression (↓↓TV, ↑ RR), ↓ response to respiratory CO_2 reflexes, bronchodilation					
CVS	Less ↓ of contractility, Stable HR	Tachycardia with rapid ↑ in concentration	↓ BP and CO ↑ HR, theoretical chance of coronary steal**	Stable HR ↓ contractility	↓ BP, CO, HR and conduction. Sensitizes myocardium to epinephrine induced arrhythmias	Can cause ↓ HR in pediatric cases Myocardial depression in those with existing heart disease
MSK	Muscle relaxation, potentiation of other muscle relaxants, uterine relaxation					

*Properties and Adverse Effects of N_2O
Due to its high MAC, nitrous oxide is combined with other anesthetic gases to attain surgical anesthesia. A MAC of 104% is possible in a pressurized chamber only.
Second Gas Effect: *see Determinants of Speed of Onset of Volatile Anesthetics, A7.*
Expansion of closed spaces: closed spaces such as a pneumothorax, the middle ear, bowel lumen and ETT cuff will markedly enlarge if N_2O is administered.
Diffusion hypoxia: During anesthesia, the washout of N_2O from body stores into alveoli can dilute the alveolar $[O_2]$, creating a hypoxic mixture if the original $[O_2]$ is low.
**Coronary Steal: N_2O causes small vessel dilation which may compromise blood flow to poorly perfused areas of heart.

Table 10. Depolarizing Muscle Relaxants (Non-competitive): succinylcholine (SCh)

Mechanism of Action	mimics ACh and binds to ACh receptors causing prolonged depolarization, initial fasciculation may be seen, followed by temporary paralysis secondary to blocked ACh receptors by SCh
Intubating Dose	1-2 mg/kg
Onset	**30-60 seconds – RAPID (fastest of all muscle relaxants)**
Duration	**5-10 minutes – SHORT (no reversing agent for SCh)**
Metabolism	SCh is hydrolyzed by **plasma cholinesterase** (pseudocholinesterase), found only in plasma and not at the NMJ
Indications	- assist intubation - ↑ risk of aspiration (need rapid paralysis and airway control) - short procedures e.g. full stomach, DM, hiatal hernia, obesity, pregnancy, trauma - ECT - laryngospasm

Side Effects	1. **SCh also stimulates muscarinic cholinergic autonomic receptors (in addition to nicotinic receptors)**
	     - may cause bradycardia, dysrhythmias, sinus arrest, increased secretions of salivary glands (especially in children)
	2. **hyperkalemia**
	     - disruption of motor nerve activity causes proliferation of extrajunctional (outside NMJ) cholinergic receptors
	     - depolarization of an increased number of receptors by SCh may lead to massive release of potassium out of muscle cells
	     - pts at risk: - 3rd degree burns 24 hrs-6 mths after injury
	                - traumatic paralysis or neuromuscular diseases (e.g. muscular dystrophy)
	                - severe intra-abdo infections
	                - severe closed head injury
	                - upper motor neuron lesions
	3. can trigger **malignant hyperthermia**
	4. increase ICP/intraocular pressure (IOP)/intragastric pressure (no increased risk of aspiration if competent lower esophageal sphincter)
	5. **fasciculations, post-op myalgia** – may be minimized if small dose of non-depolarizing agent given before SCh administration

Contraindications **Absolute**	known hypersensitivity or allergy, positive history of malignant hyperthermia, myotonia (m. congenita, m. dystrophica, paramyotonia congenital), high risk for hyperkalemic response
Relative	known history of plasma cholinesterase deficiency, myasthenia gravis, myasthenic syndrome, familial periodic paralysis, open eye injury

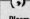

Plasma Cholinesterase
Plasma cholinesterase is produced by the liver and metabolizes SCh, ester local anesthetics, and mivacurium. A prolonged duration of blockade by SCh occurs with:
(a) **decreased quantity** of plasma cholinesterase, e.g. liver disease, pregnancy, malignancy, malnutrition, collagen vascular disease, hypothyroidism
(b) **abnormal quality** of plasma cholinesterase, i.e. normal levels but impaired activity of enzymes, genetically inherited

Table 11. Non-depolarizing Muscle Relaxants (Competitive)

Mechanism of Action	competitive blockade of postsynaptic ACh receptors preventing depolarization					
Classification	**Short**	**Intermediate**			**Long**	
	mivacuronium	rocuronium	vecuronium	cisatracurium	pancuronium	doxacurium
Intubating Dose (mg/kg)	0.2	0.6	0.1	0.1	0.1	0.05
Onset (min)	2-3	1.5	2-3	3	3-5	5-7
Duration (min)	15-25	30-45	45-60	40-60	90-120	90-120
Metabolism	plasma cholinesterase	liver (major) renal (minor)	liver	Hofmann elimination	renal (major) liver (minor)	renal
Indications	Assist intubation, assist mechanical ventilation in some ICU patients, reduce fasciculations and post-op myalgias secondary to SCh					
Side Effects						
Histamine release	Yes	No	No	No	No	Yes
Other					tachycardia	
Considerations	↑ duration of action in renal or liver failure	quick onset of rocuronium allows its use in rapid sequence induction cisatracurium is good for patients with renal or hepatic insufficiency			pancuronium if ↑ HR & BP desired doxacurium if cardiovascular stability needed	

Table 12. Reversal Agents for Non-Depolarizing Relaxants

- Reversal agents are acetylcholinesterase inhibitors
- Atropine and glycopyrrolate are anticholinergic agents administered during the administration of reversal agents to minimize muscarinic effects

Cholinesterase Inhibitor	Neostigmine	Pyridostigmine	Edrophonium
Onset & Duration	Intermediate	Longest	Shortest
Mechanism of action	Inhibits enzymatic degredation of ACh, increases ACh at nicotinic and muscarinic receptors, displacing non-depolarizing muscle relaxants Muscarinic effects of reversing agents include unwanted bradycardia, salivation and increased bowel peristalsis		
Dose	0.04-0.08 mg/kg	0.1-0.4mg/kg	0.5-1mg/kg
Recommended Anticholinergic	Glycopyrrolate	Glycopyrrolate	Atropine
Dose of Anticholinergic per mg of Cholinesterase Inhibitor	0.2mg	0.05mg	0.014mg

Table 13. Local Anesthetic Agents

	Max. dose	Max. dose with epinephrine	Potency	Duration
chlorprocaine	11 mg/kg	14 mg/kg	low	15-30 min
lidocaine	5 mg/kg	7 mg/kg	medium	1-2 hours
bupivicaine	2.5 mg/kg	3 mg/kg	high	3-8 hours

Notes

C

Cardiology and Cardiovascular Surg

Michael Mohareb, Suraj Sharma and Kit Man Wong, chapter editors
Deepti Damaraju and Elliott Owen, associate editors
Erik Venos, EBM editor
Dr. Luigi Casella, Dr. Chi-Ming Chow, Dr. Jack Colman and Dr. Anna Woo, staff editors

Basic Anatomy Review

Coronary Circulation

- arterial supply to the heart is from the right and left coronary arteries, arising from the root of the aorta (see Figures 1 and 2)
  - right coronary artery (RCA)
    - acute marginal branches
    - atrioventricular (AV) nodal artery
    - posterior interventricular artery (PIV) = posterior descending artery (PD)
  - left main coronary artery (LCA): two major branches
    - left anterior descending artery (LAD)
      - septal branches
      - diagonal branches
    - left circumflex artery (LCx)
      - obtuse marginal branches
- dominance of circulation
  - right-dominant circulation: PIV and at least one posterolateral branch arise from RCA (80%)
  - left-dominant circulation: PIV and at least one posterolateral branch arise from LCx (15%)
  - balanced circulation: dual supply of posteroinferior LV from RCA and LCx (5%)
- the sinoatrial (SA) node is supplied by the SA nodal artery, which may arise from the RCA (60%) or LCA (40%)
- most venous blood from the heart drains into the RA through the coronary sinus, although a small amount drains through thebesian veins into all four chambers, contributing to the physiologic R-L shunt

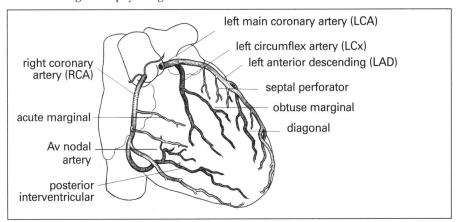

Figure 1. Anatomy of the Coronary Arteries (right anterior oblique projection)

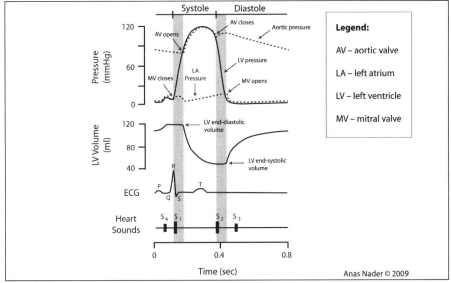

Figure 2. Cardiac Cycle

Cardiac Anatomy

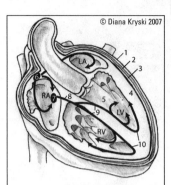

1. parietal pericardium   6. sinoatrial node
2. pericardial cavity   7. atrioventricular node
3. visceral pericardium   8. bundle of His
4. myocardium   9. R, L bundle branches
5. endocardium   10. Purkinje fibres

Figure 3. Conduction and Layers

- layers of the heart
    - endocardium
    - myocardium
    - pericardium
        - visceral pericardium
        - pericardial space
        - parietal pericardium
- valves
    - tricuspid valve (TV): separates RA and RV
    - pulmonic valve (PV): separates RV and PA
    - mitral valve (MV): separates LA and LV
        - the mitral valve has 2 cusps; all others have 3
    - aortic valve (AV): separates LV and ascending aorta
- conduction system
    - in the normal heart, rhythm is controlled by the SA node near the junction of the SVC and RA
    - impulses from the SA node travel through the atria → AV node → bundle of His
    - bundle of His splits into left and right bundle branches (LBB and RBB)
    - left bundle branch splits into anterior and posterior fascicles
    - RBB and fascicles of LBB give off Purkinje fibres which conduct impulses to ventricular myocardium

Differential Diagnoses of Common Presentations

Cardiac Murmur
- valvular heart disease
- atrial/ventricular septal defect
- patent ductus arteriosus
- arteriovenous fistula
- functional murmur

Claudication
- Vascular
    - atherosclerotic disease
    - vasculitis (e.g. Buerger's disease, Takayasu's disease)
    - diabetic neuropathy
    - venous disease (e.g. DVT, varicose veins)
    - popliteal entrapment syndrome
- Neurologic
    - neurospinal disease (e.g. spinal stenosis)
    - reflex sympathetic dystrophy
- MSK
    - osteoarthritis
    - rhematoid arthritis/connective tissue disease
    - remote trauma

Syncope
- Hypovolemia
    - blood loss
    - decreased fluid intake
    - increased fluid losses
    - third spacing
- Cardiac
    - Structural or obstructive causes
        - myocardial disease (e.g. acute coronary syndrome)
        - aortic stenosis
        - hypertrophic obstructive cardiomyopathy (HOCM)
        - cardiac tamponade/constrictive pericarditis
    - Arrhythmias
        - Bradyarrythmias
            - sick sinus syndrome
            - sinus node ischemia
            - AV block
            - pacemaker dysfunction
        - Tachyarrhythmias
            - SVT
            - ventricular fibrillation
            - Torsade de Pointes
- Respiratory
    - massive PE
    - pulmonary hypertension
    - hypoxia
    - hypercapnia
- Neurologic
    - stroke/TIA (esp. vertebrobasilar insufficiency)
    - migraine
    - seizure
    - vasovagal
- Metabolic
    - anemia
    - hypoglycemia
- Drugs
    - antihypertensives
    - antiarrhythmics
    - beta blockers, CCBs
- Psychiatric
    - panic attack

Local Edema
- inflammation/infection
- venous or lymphatic obstruction
    - thrombophlebitis
    - chronic lymphangitis
    - resection of regional lymph nodes
    - filariasis

Generalized Edema
- Increased hydrostatic pressure
    - Increased fluid retention
        - Cardiac causes e.g. CHF
        - Hepatic causes e.g. cirrhosis
        - Renal causes e.g. acute and chronic renal failure
    - Vasodilators (especially CCBs)
    - Refeeding edema
- Decreased oncotic pressure
    - Hypoalbuminemia
- Hormonal
    - hypothyroidism
    - exogenous steroids
    - pregnancy
    - estrogens

Chest Pain
*can be fatal acutely
- pulmonary
    - pneumonia
    - pulmonary embolism (PE)*
    - pneumothorax/hemothorax*
    - empyema
    - pulmonary neoplasm

- bronchiectasis
- TB
- cardiac
  - MI/angina*
  - myocarditis
  - pericarditis/Dressler's syndrome*
  - cardiac tamponade*
- gastrointestinal
  - esophageal: spasm, GERD, esophagitis, ulceration, achalasia, neoplasm
  - PUD
  - gastritis
  - pancreatitis
  - biliary colic
- mediastinal
  - lymphoma
  - thymoma
- vascular
  - dissecting aortic aneurysm
- surface structures
  - costochondritis
  - rib fracture
  - skin (bruising, shingles)
  - breast

Palpitations
- Cardiac
  - arrhythmias (PAB, PVB, SVT, VT)
  - mitral valve prolapse
  - valvular heart disease
  - hypertrophic cardiomyopathy
- Endocrine
  - thyrotoxicosis
  - pheochromocytoma
  - hypoglycemia
- Systemic
  - fever
  - anemia
- Drugs
  - tobacco, caffeine, alcohol, epinephrine, ephedrine, aminophylline, atropine
- Psychiatric
  - panic attack

ST Segment Changes
- ST Elevation
  - acute ST-elevation myocardial infarction (STEMI)
  - ventricular aneurysm
  - left bundle branch block (LBBB)
  - acute pericarditis (diffuse ST changes)

- ischemia with reciprocal changes
- post myocardial infarction (MI)
- vasospastic (Prinzmetal's) angina
- hypothermia (Osborne waves)
- early repolarization (normal variant correlate with old ECGs)
- ST depression
  - acute non-ST elevation myocardial infarction (NSTEMI) or ischemia
  - LVH or RVH with strain
  - post MI
  - STEMI with reciprocal changes
  - digitalis effect ("scooping")
  - left or right bundle branch block
  - Wolff-Parkinson-White syndrome (WPW)

Dyspnea
- cardiovascular
  - acute MI
  - CHF/LV failure
  - aortic stenosis
  - mitral stenosis
  - elevated pulmonary venous pressure
- respiratory
  - airway disease
    - asthma
    - COPD exacerbation
    - upper airway obstruction (anaphylaxis, foreign body, mucus plugging)
  - parenchymal lung disease
    - ARDS
    - pneumonia
    - interstitial lung disease
  - pulmonary vascular disease
    - PE
    - pulmonary HTN
    - pulmonary vasculitis
  - pleural disease
    - pneumothorax
    - pleural effusion
- neuromuscular and chest wall disorders
  - C-spine injury
  - polymyositis, myasthenia gravis, Guillain-Barré syndrome
  - kyphoscoliosis
- anxiety/psychosomatic
- severe anemia

Cardiac Diagnostic Tests

Electrocardiography (ECG)

ECG Basics

- the electrocardiogram (ECG) is a graphic representation of the electrical activity of the heart recorded from the surface of the body
- on the ECG graph
  - the horizontal axis represents time
    1 mm (1 small square) = 40 msec
    5 mm (1 large square) = 200 msec (at paper speed 25 mm/sec)
  - the vertical axis represents voltage
    1 mm (1 small square) = 0.1 mV
    10 mm (2 large squares) = 1 mV (at standard gain setting)
- leads
  - standard 12-lead ECG
    - limb leads: I, II, III, aVL, aVR, aVF
    - precordial leads: V1-V6
  - additional leads
    - right-sided leads: V3R-V6R (useful in RV infarction and dextrocardia)

Overview of diagnostic tests
- Cardiac biomarkers (Tn, CK-MB) – in symptomatic state
- ECG – at rest, with stress, or in symptomatic state
- Echocardiography – at rest, or with stress
- Nuclear imaging – with stress
- Angiography (cardiac catheterization)
- CTA
- MRA/MRI

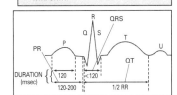

Figure 4. ECG Waveforms and Normal Values

Approach to ECGs

Rate Calculation
• Examples
• Practice

Approach to ECGs Summary
• Rate
• Rhythm
• Axis
• Conduction
• Chamber enlargement/ hypertrophy
• Ischemia/infarction
• Miscellaneous

Axis
• Definition
• Calculation method
• Examples
• Practice

LAD	RAD
Left Ant. Hemiblock	RVH
Inferior MI	Left Post.
WPW	Hemiblock
RV Pacing	PE
Normal Variant	COPD
	Lateral MI
	WPW
	Dextrocardia

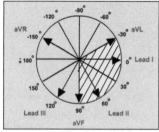

Figure 5. QRS Axis on Frontal Plane

Intraventricular conduction abnormalities
• Examples

Rate
• normal = 60-100 bpm
• regular rhythm
  ▪ to calculate the rate, divide 300 by number of large squares between 2 QRS complexes (there are 300 large squares in 1 minute: 300 X 200 msec = 60 sec), or divide 1500 by the number of small squares between 2 QRS complexes
  ▪ or remember 300-150-100-75-60-50-43 (rate falls in this sequence with the number of additional large squares between QRS)
• irregular rhythm
  ▪ rate = 6 x number of R-R intervals in 10 seconds (the "rhythm strips" are 10 second recordings)

Rhythm
• regular = R-R interval is the same across the tracing
• irregular = R-R interval varies across the tracing
  ▪ regularly-irregular = repeating pattern of varying R-R intervals
  ▪ irregularly irregular = R-R intervals vary erratically
• normal sinus rhythm (NSR)
  ▪ P wave precedes each QRS; QRS follows each P wave
  ▪ P wave axis is normal (positive in leads I, aVF)
  ▪ Rate between 60-100 bpm

Axis
• mean axis indicates the direction of the mean vector
• can be determined for any waveform (P, QRS, T)
• the standard ECG reported QRS axis usually refers to the mean axis of the frontal plane. It indicates the mean direction of ventricular depolarization forces
• QRS axis in the horizontal plane is not routinely calculated. It is directed posteriorly and to the left
  ▪ the transition from negative to positive is usually in lead V3
• QRS axis in the frontal plane (see Figure 6)
  ▪ normal axis: -30° to 90° (i.e., positive QRS in leads I and II)
  ▪ left axis deviation (LAD): axis <-30°
  ▪ right axis deviation (RAD): axis >90°

Intraventricular Conduction Abnormalities

Right Bundle Branch Block (RBBB)	Left Bundle Branch Block (LBBB)
Complete RBBB • QRS duration >120 msec • positive QRS in lead V1 (rSR' or occasionally broad R wave) • broad S waves in leads I, V5-6 (>40 msec) • usually secondary T wave inversion in leads V1-2	**Complete LBBB** • QRS duration >120 msec • in leads I, aVL and usually V5 and V6, a broad notched or slurred R wave • deep broad S waves in leads V1-2 • secondary ST-T changes (-ve in leads with broad R waves, +ve in V1-2) are usually present • LBBB usually masks ECG signs of myocardial infarction
Incomplete RBBB • QRS duration >90 and <120 msec • in lead V1 rsR', or rsr', with r' >30 msec	**Incomplete LBBB** • In V1 and V6: R not preceded by q, but followed by negative T wave • rS or QS in V1 +/- V2 • QRS duration 0.10 to 120 msec

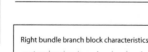
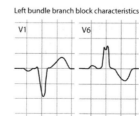
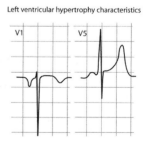

Right bundle branch block characteristics   Left bundle branch block characteristics   Left ventricular hypertrophy characteristics

Figure 6. RBBB, LBBB and Left Ventricular Hypertrophy Characteristics

Left Anterior Fascicular Block (LAFB) (Left Anterior Hemiblock)	• left axis deviation (-30° to -90°)
	  ▪ i.e. small q and prominent R in leads I and aVL
	  ▪ i.e. small r and prominent S in leads II, III, and aVF

Left Posterior Fascicular Block (LPFB) (Left Posterior Hemiblock)	• right axis deviation (110° to 180°)
	  ▪ i.e. small r and prominent S in leads I and aVL
	  ▪ i.e. small q and prominent R in leads II, III, and aVF

Bifascicular Block	• RBBB pattern • the first 60 msec (1.5 small squares) of the QRS shows the pattern of LAFB or LPFB • bifascicular block refers to impaired conduction in two of the three fascicles, most commonly a RBBB and left anterior hemiblock; the appearance on an ECG meets the criteria for both types of blocks

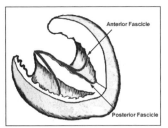

Figure 7. Ventricular Conduction System

Nonspecific Intraventricular block
• QRS duration >120 msec
• absence of criteria for LBBB or RBBB

Hypertrophy and Chamber Enlargement

• left ventricular hypertrophy (LVH)
  ▪ S in V1 + R in V5 or V6 >35 mm above age 40, (>40 mm for age 31-40, >45 mm for age 21-30)
  ▪ R in aVL >11 mm
  ▪ R in I + S in III >25 mm
  ▪ additional criteria:
    ♦ LV strain pattern (ST depression and T wave inversion in leads I, aVL, V4-V6)
    ♦ left atrial enlargement
• right ventricular hypertrophy (RVH)
  ▪ right axis deviation
  ▪ R/S ratio >1 or qR in lead V1
  ▪ RV strain pattern: ST segment depression and T wave inversion in leads V1-2
• left atrial enlargement (LAE)
  ▪ negative component of P wave in lead V1 ≥1 mm wide and ≥1 mm deep
  ▪ additional criterion
    ♦ P wave >120 msec, notched in lead II ("P mitrale")
• right atrial enlargement (RAE):
  ▪ P wave >2.5 mm in height in leads II, III, or aVF ("P pulmonale")

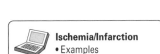

Hypertrophy and Chamber Enlargement
• Examples

Ischemia/Infarction

• look for the anatomic distribution of the following ECG abnormalities (see Table 1)
• ischemia
  ▪ ST segment depression
  ▪ T wave inversion
• injury
  ▪ transmural (involving the epicardium) - ST elevation in the leads facing the area injured/infarcted; transient ST elevation may occur in patients with coronary artery spasm (e.g. Prinzmetal angina)
  ▪ subendocardial – marked ST depression in the leads facing the affected area; it may be accompanied by enzyme changes and other signs of myocardial infarction

Ischemia/Infarction
• Examples

Significant ECG changes
• look for ST changes starting at 80 msec from J point
• J point = the junction between the QRS complex and the ST segment
• ST elevation: at least 1mm in 2 adjacent limb leads, or at least 1-2mm in adjacent precordial leads
• ST depression: downsloping or horizontal
• Q wave: pathological if QRS ≥1 small square (≥40 msec) or >25% height of R

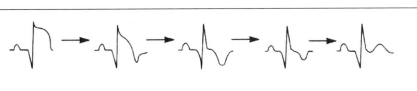

Acute days (avg. 3-5 hours) ST segment elevation	**Recent** weeks-months T wave inversion	**Old** months-years (avg. > 6 months) Significant Qs

Figure 8. ECG changes with infarction

- evolving infarction
  - "typical" sequential changes of evolving myocardial infarction
    - 1st - hyperacute T waves (tall, symmetric T waves) in the leads facing the infarcted area, with or without ST elevation
    - 2nd - ST elevation (injury pattern) in the leads facing the infarcted area
      - usually in the first hours post infarct
      - in acute posterior infarction, there is ST depression in V1-V3 (reciprocal to ST elevation in the posterior leads, that are not recorded in the standard 12-lead ECG)
    - 3rd - significant Q waves (hours to days post-infarct)
    - 4th - inverted T waves (one day to weeks after infarction)
    - this classical sequence, however, does not always occur, e.g.
      - Q waves of infarction may appear in the very early stages, with or without ST changes
      - Non-Q wave infarction: there may be only ST or T changes, despite clinical evidence of infarction
- completed infarction
  - abnormal Q waves (note that wide Q waves may be found in III and aVL in normal individuals)
    - duration >40 msec (>30 msec in aVF for inferior infarction)
    - Q/QRS voltage ratio is >25%
  - abnormal R waves (R/S ratio >1, duration >40 msec) in V1 and more frequently in V2 are found in posterior infarction (usually in association with signs of inferior and/or lateral infarction)

Table 1. Areas of Infarction/Ischemia (right dominant anatomy)

Vessel Usually Involved	Infarct Area	Leads
left anterior descending (LAD)	anteroseptal	V1, V2
	anterior	V3, V4
	anterolateral	I, aVL, V3-V6
	extensive anterior	I, aVL, V1-V6
right coronary artery (RCA)	inferior	II, III, aVF
	right ventricle	V3R & V4R (right sided chest leads)
	posterior MI (assoc. with inf. MI)	V1 and V2 (prominent R waves)
circumflex	lateral	I, aVL, V5-6
	isolated posterior MI	V1 and V2 (prominent R waves)

Miscellaneous ECG Changes

Electrolyte Disturbances
- hyperkalemia (see Figure 9)
  - mild to moderate (K 5-7 mmol/L): tall peaked T waves
  - severe (K >7 mmol/L): progressive changes: P waves flatten and disappear; QRS widens and may show bizarre patterns, axis shifts left or right; ST shift with tall T waves

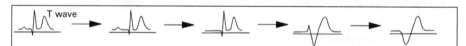

Figure 9. Hyperkalemia

- hypokalemia (see Figure 10)
  - ST segment depression, prolonged QT interval, low T waves, prominent U waves (U>T)

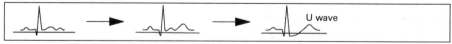

Figure 10. Hypokalemia

- hypercalcemia: shortened QT interval
- hypocalcemia: prolonged QT interval

Hypothermia
- sinus bradycardia
- when severe, prolonged QRS and QT intervals
- atrial fibrillation with slow ventricular response and other atrial/ventricular dysrhythmias
- Osborne J waves: "hump-like" waves at the junction of the J point and the ST segment

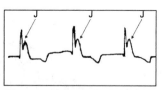

Figure 11. Osborne J Waves of a hypothermic patient

Pericarditis
- early – diffuse ST segment elevation ± PR segment depression, upright T waves
- later – isoelectric ST segment, flat or inverted T waves
- tachycardia

Low Voltage
- definition: total QRS height in precordial leads <10 mm and limb leads <5 mm
- differential diagnosis
  - myocardial disease
    - ischemia
      - infiltrative or dilated cardiomyopathy, myocarditis
  - pericardial effusion
  - thick chest wall/barrel chest: COPD, obesity
  - generalized edema
  - hypothyroidism/myxedema
  - inappropriate voltage standardization

Drug Effects
- digitalis
  - therapeutic levels may be associated with "dig effect" (see Figure 12):
    - ST downsloping or "scooping"
    - T wave depression or inversion
    - QT shortening ± U waves
    - slowing of ventricular rate in atrial fibrillation
  - toxic levels associated with:
    - arrhythmias: paroxysmal atrial tachycardia (PAT) with conduction blocks; severe bradycardia in atrial fibrillation, accelerated junctional rhythms, PVCs, ventricular tachycardia
    - "regularization" of ventricular rate in atrial fibrillation due to a junctional rhythm and AV dissociation
- amiodarone, quinidine, phenothiazines, tricyclic antidepressants, antipsychotics, some antihistamines, some antibiotics: prolonged QT interval, U waves

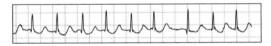

Figure 12. Atrial fibrillation, ST change due to digitalis ("digitalis effect")

Pulmonary Disorders
- cor pulmonale (often secondary to COPD)
  - low voltage, RAD, poor R wave progression
  - RAE and RVH with strain
  - multifocal atrial tachycardia (MAT)
- massive pulmonary embolism (PE)
  - sinus tachycardia and atrial fibrillation/atrial flutter are the most common arrhythmias
  - RAD, RVH with strain – most specific sign is $S_1Q_3T_3$ (S in I, Q and inverted T wave in III)

Other Cardiac Diagnostic Tests

Cardiac Biomarkers

- provide diagnostic & prognostic information and identify increased risk of mortality in acute coronary syndromes

Table 2. Cardiac Enzymes

Enzyme	Peak	Duration Elevated	DDx of Elevation
Troponin I, Troponin T	1-2 days	Up to 2 weeks	MI, CHF, AF, acute pulmonary embolism, myocarditis, chronic renal insufficiency, sepsis, hypovolemia
CK-MB	1 day	3 days	myocardial infarction, myocarditis, pericarditis, muscular dystrophy, cardiac defibrillation, etc.

- check troponin I at presentation and 8h later ± creatine kinase-MB (CK-MB) (depends on local laboratory protocol)
- new CK-MB elevation can be used to diagnose reinfarction, troponin cannot

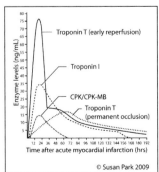

Figure 13. Cardiac Enzymes

- other biomarkers of cardiac disease:
  - AST and LDH also increased in myocardial infarction (low specificity)
  - BNP and NT-proBNP – secreted by ventricles in response to increased end-diastolic pressure and volume
    - DDx: CHF, AF, PE, COPD exacerbation, pulmonary hypertension

Use of B-Type Natriuretic Peptide in the Evaluation and Management of Acute Dyspnea (BASEL)
N Engl J Med 2004;350;647-54
Study: Prospective, randomized controlled trial.
Patients: 452 patients (mean age 71 yrs. 58% male) with acute dyspnea; Patients with severe renal disease or cardiogenic shock were excluded.
Intervention: Patients were randomized to assessment including measurement of B-type natriuretic peptide or standard assessment.
Primary Outcome: Time to discharge and total cost of treatment.
Results: Median time to discharge was significantly shorter in the intervention group when compared with the control group (8.0 vs. 11.0 days, p=0.001). Total cost was also significantly lower in the intervention group ($5410 vs. $7264, p=0.006). In addition, the measurement of B-type natriuretic peptide significantly reduced the need for admission to hospital and intensive care. The 30-day mortality rates were similar (10% vs. 12%, p=0.45).
Conclusions: In patients with acute dyspnea, measurement of B-type natriuretic peptide improves clinical outcomes (need for hospitalization or intensive care) and reduces time to discharge and total cost of treatment.

Ambulatory ECG

- indications for outpatient management: palpitations, syncope, antiarrhythmic drug monitoring, and arrhythmia surveillance in patients with documented or potentially abnormal rhythms, surveillance of non-sustained arrhythmias that can lead to prophylactic intervention
- available technologies:
  - Holter monitor
    - battery operated, continually records up to 3 leads for 24-48 hrs
    - symptoms recorded by patient on Holter clock for correlation with ECG findings
  - continuous loop recorder (diagnostic yield 66-83%)
    - worn continuously and can record data before and after patient activation for symptomatic episodes
  - external and implantable devices
    - external devices can be transtelephonically downloaded
    - implantable loop recorder (ILR) – implanted subcutaneously to the right or left of the sternum; triggered by placing an activator over it; anterograde and retrograde recording time is programmable; cannot be transtelephonically downloaded; left in place for 14 to 18 months

Echocardiography

Transthoracic Echocardiography (TTE)
- ultrasound beams are directed across the chest wall to obtain images of the heart
- indications: evaluation of left ventricular ejection fraction (LVEF), wall motion abnormalities, myocardial ischemia and complications of MI, chamber sizes, wall thickness, valve morphology, proximal great vessels, pericardial effusion, unexplained hypotension, murmurs, syncope
- may use with Doppler, which can help to quantify degree of valvular stenosis or regurgitation

Transoesophageal Echocardiography (TEE)
- ultrasound probe inserted into the esophagus to allow for better resolution of the heart and its structures
- better visualization of posterior structures, such as left atrium, mitral and aortic valves
- invasive procedure, used to complement transthoracic echocardiography
- indications: intracardiac thrombi, tumours, valvular vegetations (infective endocarditis), aortic dissection, aortic atheromas, prosthetic valve function, shunts, technically inadequate transthoracic studies
- may use with Doppler, which can help to quantify degree of valvular stenosis or regurgitation

Stress Echocardiography
- echocardiography in combination with either physiologic (exercise treadmill or bike testing) or pharmacologic (dobutamine infusion) stress
- validated in demonstrating myocardial ischemia
- provides information on the global left ventricular response to exercise
- regional wall motion is analyzed at rest and with stress

Contrast Echocardiography
- contrast agents injected into the bloodstream to improve imaging of the heart
- conventional agent: agitated saline (contains microbubbles of air)
- allows visualization of right heart and intracardiac shunts, most commonly patent foramen ovale (PFO)
- newer contrast agents are capable of crossing the pulmonary bed and achieving left heart opacification following intravenous injection

Exercise Testing

- exercise testing is a cardiovascular stress test using treadmill or bicycle exercise with electrocardiographic and blood pressure monitoring
- ACC/AHA 2003 guidelines for use:
  - patients with intermediate (10-90%) pretest probability of CAD based on age, gender and symptoms
  - complete RBBB
  - ST depression <1mm at rest
- **note**: less useful in cases of marked resting ST-T abnormalities, LBBB, digoxin use, WPW, LVH with strain pattern, less accurate in women
- **exercise test results stratify patients into risk groups**
  - low risk patients can be treated medically without invasive testing
  - intermediate risk patients may need additional testing in the form of exercise imaging studies or cardiac catheterization
  - high risk patients should be referred for cardiac catheterization

Most commonly used treadmill protocols:
- The Bruce Protocol
- For older individuals or those with limited exercise capacity: either The Modified Bruce or The Modified Naughton Protocol

Contraindications to Exercise Testing

Absolute	Relative
• acute myocardial infarction (within two days)	• left main coronary stenosis
• uncontrolled cardiac arrhythmias causing symptoms or hemodynamic compromise	• hemodynamically significant aortic stenosis
• symptomatic severe aortic stenosis	• high-degree atrioventricular block
• acute aortic dissection	• electrolyte abnormalities
• acute myocarditis or pericarditis	• tachyarrhythmias or bradyarrhythmias
• acute pulmonary embolus or pulmonary infarction	• hypertrophic cardiomyopathy and other forms of outflow tract obstruction
• unstable angina not previously stabilized by medical therapy	• severe arterial hypertension
• uncontrolled symptomatic heart failure	• mental or physical impairment leading to inability to exercise adequately

Duke Treadmill Score
Weighted index combining:
1) treadmill exercise time using standard Bruce protocol
2) maximum net ST segment deviation (depression or elevation)
3) exercise-induced angina.
Provides diagnostic and prognostic information (such as 1 year mortality) for the evaluation of patients with suspected coronary heart disease.

Prognostic Markers

- maximum exercise capacity, markers related to exercise-induced ischemia (exercise-induced ST-segment depression, exercise-induced ST segment elevation (in leads without pathological Q waves and not in aVR), exercise-induced angina, and inadequate blood pressure response in post infarct patients
- the most commonly used ECG criteria for a positive exercise test: ≥1 mm of horizontal or downsloping ST-segment depression or elevation (at least 60 to 80 msec after the end of the QRS complex)

Absolute Indications for Terminating Exercise Stress Test

- drop in systolic blood pressure of >10 mm Hg from baseline despite an increase in workload, when accompanied by other evidence of ischemia
- moderate to severe angina
- ST elevation (>1 mm) in leads without diagnostic Q-waves (other than V1 or aVR)
- increasing nervous system symptoms (e.g. ataxia, dizziness, or near syncope)
- signs of poor perfusion (cyanosis or pallor)
- technical difficulties in monitoring ECG or systolic blood pressure
- subject's desire to stop
- sustained ventricular tachycardia

Most important prognostic factors in exercise testing
- ST depression
- ST elevation
- inadequate blood pressure compensation

Nuclear Cardiology

- myocardial perfusion imaging (MPI) with gated single photon emission computed tomography (SPECT)
- role in evaluating myocardial viability, detecting ischemia, and simultaneously assessing perfusion and left ventricular function by ECG gated SPECT
- stress
  - exercise
    - treadmill test (unless contraindicated)
  - vasodilator stress with intravenous drugs
    - dipyridamole (Persantine™), adenosine
      - act to increase coronary flow
- images of the heart obtained during stress and at rest 3-4h later
  - fixed defect – impaired perfusion at rest and during stress (infarcted)
  - reversible defect – impaired perfusion only during stress (ischemic)

Patients with normal perfusion studies at peak stress have a <1%/year incidence of death after nonfatal MI and are thus often spared further invasive evaluation for assessment of their symptoms.

Higher sensitivity and specificity compared to standard exercise ECG testing when used to diagnose CAD.

The degree of severity shown on the scan reveals the likelihood of further cardiac event rates independent of the patient's history, examination, resting ECG, and stress ECG result.

ACC/AHA 2003 Guidelines for Use
Stable angina, baseline ECG abnormalities, post-revascularization assessment, heart failure, patients unable to exercise, preoperative risk assessment for patients undergoing noncardiac surgery.

Tracers
- thallium-201 (^{201}Tl, a K analogue)
- technetium-99 (^{99}Tc)-labelled tracer (sestamibi/Cardiolite™ or hexamibi/Myoview™)

Summary of Stress Testing
- Exercise ECG
    - initial evaluation in patients without hard-to-interpret ECGs who are able to exercise
- Exercise Stress Echo
    - when ECG is uninterpretable
    - intermediate pre-test probability with normal/equivocal exercise ECG
    - post-ACS when used to decide on potential efficacy of revascularization
- Dobutamine Stress Echo
    - in patients unable to exercise and same indications as exercise echo
- Exercise Myocardial Perfusion Imaging (MPI)
    - when ECG is uninterpretable
    - intermediate pre-test probability with normal/equivocal exercise ECG
    - in patients with previous imaging whose symptoms have changed
- Dipyridamole/Adenosine MPI
    - to diagnose CAD in possible ACS patients with non-diagnostic ECG and negative serum biomarkers
    - when ECG is uninterpretable due to LBBB or V-paced rhythm
    - in patients unable to exercise and same indications as exercise MPI

Table 3. Sensitivity and Specificity of Various Stress Testing

Testing Modality	Sensitivity	Specificity
Exercise ECG	68	77
Planar Thallium MPI (exercise or pharmacologic stress)	79	73
Thallium SPECT MPI (exercise or pharmacologic stress)	88	77
Stress Echocardiography	76	88
PET scanning	91	82

Sensitivity and specificity of various stress testing modalities in the detection of coronary artery lesions. If positive, findings were confirmed with angiography. Derived from the meta-analysis by Garber AM and Solomon NA. Cost-effectiveness of alternative test strategies for the diagnosis of coronary artery disease. Ann Intern Med 1999; 130(9):719-28.

Cardiac Catheterization and Angiography

- invasive: catheters are introduced percutaneously into arterial and venous circulation under conscious sedation and contrast is injected
- arterial access most commonly through the femoral artery; radial approach gaining favour especially for obese and outpatients
- venous access through the femoral vein or internal jugular vein
- same day procedure as outpatient:
    - indications for prehospitalization: anticoagulation therapy, renal failure, diabetes, contrast allergy
- catheterization permits direct measurement of intracardiac pressures, transvalvular and mean peak pressure gradients, valve areas, cardiac output, shunt data, oxygen saturations, and visualization of coronary arteries, cardiac chambers and great vessels

Right Heart Catheterization (Swan-Ganz catheter)
- right atrial, right ventricular, pulmonary artery pressures are recorded
- pulmonary capillary wedge pressure
    - obtained by advancing the catheter to wedge into the distal pulmonary artery
        - records pressures measured from the pulmonary venous system
        - in the absence of pulmonary venous disease, will reflect left atrial pressure

Left Heart Catheterization
- systolic and end-diastolic pressure tracings recorded; left ventricular size, wall motion and ejection fraction can be assessed by injecting contrast into the left ventricle (left ventriculography)
- cardiac output (measured by the Fick oxygen method or the indicator dilution method)

Coronary Angiography (see Figure 14)
- coronary vasculature accessed via the coronary ostium

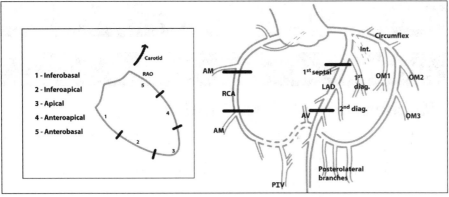

Figure 14. Coronary Angiogram Schematic (RCA = right coronary artery, AM = acute marginal, LAD = left anterior descending, OM = obtuse marginal)

Coronary Angiography
Gold standard for localizing and quantifying CAD.

Prognosticators
- angiographic variables may provide valuable information regarding lesion severity, complexity, location and prognosis

Diagnostic Catheterization
- outcomes related to complications for diagnostic catheterization should be <1%
- procedure related complications: vascular injury, renal failure, stroke, MI
  - mortality rate 0.1-0.2%
- inadequate diagnostic procedures should occur in far fewer than 1% of cases
- provocative pharmacological agents can be used to unmask pathology
  - fluid loading may unmask latent pericardial constriction
  - afterload reduction or inotropic stimulation may be used to increase the outflow tract gradient in hypertrophic cardiomyopathy
  - coronary vasoreactive agents (e.g. methylergonovine, acetylcholine)
  - a variety of pulmonary vasoreactive agents in primary pulmonary hypertension (e.g. oxygen, calcium channel blockers, adenosine, nitric oxide, or prostacyclin)

Hemodynamically significant stenosis is defined as 70% or more narrowing of the luminal diameter.

Contrast-Enhanced CT Coronary Angiography

- fast ECG-synchronized multi-slice CT image acquisition in the heart has enabled non invasive imaging of the coronary arterial tree

Magnetic Resonance Imaging (MRI)

- offers high spatial resolution, eliminates the need for iodinated contrast, and does not involve exposure to ionizing radiation
- particular value in assessment of congenital cardiac anomalies, abnormalities of the aorta, and assessment of viable myocardium

CARDIAC DISEASE

Arrhythmias

Mechanisms of Arrhythmias

- automaticity is the property of the myocardial cell to generate an action potential. It is influenced by:
  - neurohormonal factors (sympathetic and parasympathetic)
  - abnormal metabolic conditions (e.g. hypoxia, acidosis, hypothermia)
  - electrolyte abnormalities
  - drugs (e.g. digitalis)
  - local ischemia/infarction
  - other cardiac pathology

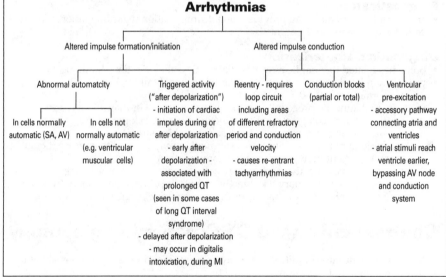

Figure 15. Mechanism of Arrhythmias

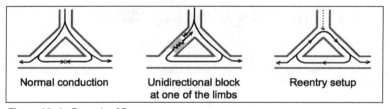

Figure 16. An Example of Reentry

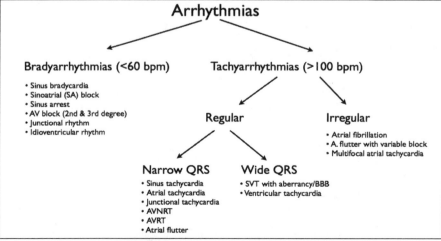

Figure 17. Clinical Approach to Arrhythmias

Bradyarrhythmias and AV Conduction Blocks

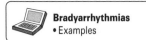

Bradyarrhythmias
• Examples

Sinus Bradycardia
- P axis normal (P waves positive in I and aVF)
- rate <60/min
- marked sinus bradycardia (<50/min) may be seen in normal adults, particularly athletes, and in elderly individuals
- caused by
    - increased vagal tone or vagal stimulation
    - vomiting
    - episodes of myocardial ischemia or infarction (inferior MI)
    - sick sinus node
    - increased intracranial pressure
    - hypothyroidism
    - hypothermia
    - drugs (beta-blockers, calcium blockers, etc.)
- treatment: if symptomatic, atropine during acute episodes; atrial pacing for sick sinus node syndrome; if drug-induced, reduction or withdrawal of drugs

Sinus Arrhythmia (SA)
- normal P waves, with variation of the P-P interval
- "respiratory SA" is normal: rate increases with inspiration, slows with expiration
- "non-respiratory SA" is seen more often in the elderly, and when marked it may be due to sinus node dysfunction. Usually it does not require treatment

Sinus Pause/Sinus Arrest
- sinus pause: a temporary pause (>2 sec) without P wave
- the P-P prolongation is not phasic or gradual (unlike sinus arrhythmia) and is not a multiple of the normal P-P interval (unlike sino-atrial block)
- sinus arrest is prolonged or permanent
- escape beats or rhythm may occur:
    - atrial escape: P waves with abnormal morphology
    - junctional escape: P waves not seen, or follow the QRS (retrograde P), rate 40-60 bpm
    - ventricular escape: no P wave; wide, abnormal QRS; slow rate (20-40 bpm)

Sick Sinus Syndrome (SSS)
- characterized by sinus node dysfunction (marked bradycardia, sinus pause/arrest, sinoatrial block)
- frequently associated with episodes of atrial tachyarrhythmias
- when symptomatic, electronic pacemaker is indicated

AV Conduction Blocks

1st Degree AV Block
- prolonged PR interval (>200 msec)
- frequently found among otherwise healthy adults
- no treatment required

2nd Degree AV Block
- some of the atrial impulses are not conducted to the ventricles
- can describe block by ratio of P waves to # of QRS (e.g. 2:1, 3:1, 4:1 increases in severity)
- second degree AV block is further subdivided into:
    - Type I (Mobitz I) 2nd Degree AV Block
        - a gradual prolongation of the PR interval precedes the failure of conduction of a P wave (Wenckebach phenomenon)
        - AV block is usually in AV node
        - frequently benign

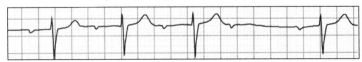

Figure 18. Second Degree AV Block with Wenckebach Phenomenon (Mobitz I) (Lead V_1)

- Type II (Mobitz II) 2nd Degree AV Block
    - the PR interval is constant; there is an abrupt failure of conduction of a P wave
    - AV block is usually distal to the AV node
    - increased risk of high grade or 3rd degree AV block

Type II (Mobitz II)
2° AV block is an indication for permanent pacing.

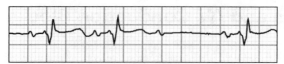

Figure 19. Second Degree AV Block Mobitz II (Lead V$_1$)

2:1 AV block
- often not possible to determine whether the block is type I or type II
- prolonged or repeated recordings may clarify the diagnosis

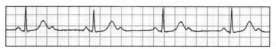

Figure 20. 2:1 AV Block (Lead II)

High Grade 2nd Degree AV Block
- 2 or more consecutive P waves that are not conducted
- usually without progressive prolongation of PR intervals (type II pattern)
- more likely to progress to 3rd degree AV block

3rd Degree AV Block
- complete failure of conduction of the supraventricular impulses to the ventricles
- ventricular depolarization initiated by an escape pacemaker distal to the block
- QRS can be narrow or wide (junctional vs. ventricular escape rhythm)
- PP and RR intervals are constant, variable PR intervals
- no relationship between P waves and QRS complexes (P waves "marching through")
- mangement (see *Electrical Pacing*)

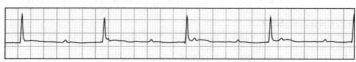

Figure 21. Third degree AV Block (Complete Heart Block) (Lead II)

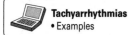
Tachyarrhythmias
- Examples

Supraventricular Tachyarrhythmias and Pre-excitation Syndromes

Presentation
- symptoms, when present, include: palpitations, dizziness, dyspnea, chest discomfort, presyncope/syncope
- may precipitate congestive heart failure (CHF), hypotension, or ischemia in patients with underlying disease
- untreated tachycardias can cause cardiomyopathy (rare)
- includes supraventricular and ventricular rhythms

Supraventricular Tachyarrhythmias (SVT)
- the term is used to designate any of the tachyarrhythmias that originate in the atria or AV junction, when a more specific diagnosis of its mechanism and site of origin cannot be made
- characterized by narrow QRS, unless there is pre-existing BBB or aberrant ventricular conduction (abnormal conduction due to a change in cycle length)

Sinus Tachycardia
- sinus rhythm with rate >100 bpm
- occurs in normal subjects with increased sympathetic tone (exercise, emotions, pain), alcohol use, caffeinated beverages, drugs (e.g. beta-adrenergic agonists, anticholinergic drugs, etc.)
- etiology: fever, hypotension, hypovolemia, anemia, thyrotoxicosis, heart failure, MI, shock, pulmonary embolism, etc.
- treatment: treat underlying disease; consider β-blocker if symptomatic, rate modifying CCB if β-blockers contraindicated

Premature Beats
- premature atrial contraction (PAC)
  - ectopic supraventricular beat originating in the atria
  - P wave morphology of the PAC usually differs from that of a normal sinus beat
- junctional premature beat
  - ectopic supraventricular beat that originates in the vicinity of the AV node
  - P wave is usually not seen or retrograde P wave may follow closely the QRS complex
- treatment usually not required

Atrial Flutter
- rapid, regular atrial depolarization from a re-entry circuit within the atrium
- atrial rate 250-350 bpm, usually 300 bpm
- AV block usually occurs. It may be fixed (2:1, 3:1, 4:1, etc.) or variable
- etiology: CAD, thyrotoxicosis, MV disease, cardiac surgery, COPD, pulmonary embolism, pericarditis
- ECG: sawtooth flutter waves in inferior leads (II, III, aVF); narrow QRS (unless aberrancy)
- in atrial flutter with 2:1 block, carotid sinus massage (first check for bruits), Valsalva maneuver or adenosine may decrease AV conduction and bring out flutter waves
- treatment:
  - acute: if unstable (e.g. hypotension, CHF, angina): electrical cardioversion
  - if stable:
    - (1) rate control: β-blocker, diltiazem, verapamil, or digitalis
    - (2) chemical cardioversion: sotalol, amiodarone, type I antiarrhythmics OR electrical cardioversion
  - anticoagulation guidelines same as for patients with AFib (see *AFib*)
  - long-term: antiarrhythmics, catheter ablation

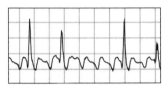

Figure 22. Atrial Flutter with Variable Block

Multifocal Atrial Tachycardia (MAT)
- irregular rhythm caused by presence of 3 or more atrial foci (may mimic AFib)
- atrial rate 100-200 bpm; at least 3 distinct P wave morphologies and PR intervals vary, some P waves may not be conducted
- occurs more commonly in patients with COPD, and hypoxemia; less commonly in patients with hypokalemia, hypomagnesemia, sepsis, theophylline or digitalis toxicity
- treatment: treat the underlying cause; CCBs may be used (e.g. diltiazem, verapamil), β-blockers may be contraindicated because of severe pulmonary disease
- no role for electrical cardioversion, antiarryhthmics or ablation

Atrial Fibrillation (AFib)
- most common sustained arrhythmia; incidence increases with age (8% of population over 80)
- rapid, disorganized and asynchronous activity of atria due to simultaneous discharge and reentry at multiple atrial foci
- cardiac function is affected (loss of atrial contraction, irregular and rapid ventricular response, decreased cardiac output and coronary flow)
- symptoms: palpitation, fatigue, when acute and with rapid ventricular response may cause syncope and precipitate or worsen heart failure
- may be asymptomatic
- associated with thromboembolic events
- etiology: HTN, CAD, valvular disease, pericarditis, cardiomyopathy, myocarditis, ASD, following surgery, PE, COPD, thyrotoxicosis, SSS (Sick Sinus Syndrome), alcohol ("holiday heart")
- may present in young subjects without demonstrable disease ("lone AFib") and in the elderly without underlying heart disease
- ECG findings: no organized P waves, chaotic baseline with fibrillatory waves, irregularly irregular ventricular response, narrow QRS (unless aberrancy or previous BBB)
- atrial rate 400-600/min; ventricular rate depends on AV node conduction, typically 100-180 bpm when untreated
- wide QRS complexes due to aberrancy may occur following a long-short cycle sequence ("Ashman phenomenon")
- loss of atrial contraction - no "a" wave seen in JVP, no S4

Atrial Fibrillation – AFFIRM trial
NEJM 2002; 347:1825-33.
Study: Randomized, multicenter trial with mean follow-up of 3.5 years.
Patients: 4060 patients (mean age 70 yrs, 61% male, 89% white) with atrial fibrillation and a high risk of stroke or death, in whom anticoagulant therapy was not contraindicated.
Intervention: Rate control (using β-blockers, verapamil, diltiazem, or digoxin alone or in combination) vs. rhythm control (using an antiarrhythmic drug chosen by the treating physician).
Main outcome: Overall mortality.
Results: There was no difference in mortality between the two groups. There were more hospitalizations and adverse drug effects in the rhythm-control group.
Conclusion: Rate-control was as effective as rhythm-control in atrial fibrillation, and may be better tolerated. Anticoagulation should be continued.
See also AF-CHF trial: NEJM 2008; 358: 2667-2677.

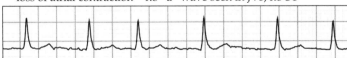

Figure 23. Atrial Fibrillation

Table 4. CHADS2 Risk Prediction for Non-Valvular AFib
(JAMA 2001; 285(22):2864-70)

Risk Factor	Points
Congestive Heart Failure	1
Hypertension	1
Age>75	1
Diabetes	1
Stroke/TIA (prior)	2

CHADS Score	Stroke Risk (%/Yr)	Anticoagulation Recommendation
0-1	1.9-2.8 (low)	aspirin 81-325 mg
2-3	4.0-5.9 (mod)	coumadin (INR 2-3)
4-6	8.5-18.2 (high)	coumadin (INR 2-3)

Oral anticoagulants versus antiplatelet therapy for preventing stroke in patients with non-valvular atrial fibrillation and no history of stroke or transient ischemic attacks.
Cochrane Database Syst Rev. 2007;(3):CD006186.
Purpose: To characterize the relative effect of long-term oral anticoagulant treatment compared with antiplatelet therapy on major vascular events in patients with non-valvular AF and no history of stroke or transient ischemic attack (TIA).
Study Selection: All unconfounded, randomized trials in which long-term (more than four weeks) adjusted-dose oral anticoagulant treatment was compared with antiplatelet therapy in patients with chronic non-valvular AF.
Results: Eight randomized trials, including 9,598 patients, tested adjusted-dose warfarin versus aspirin (in dosages ranging from 75 to 325 mg/day) in AF patients without prior stroke or TIA. The mean overall follow-up was 1.9 years per participant.

Measure	OR (95% CI)
All stroke	0.68 (0.54 to 0.85)
Ischemic stroke	0.53 (0.41 to 0.68)
Systemic emboli	0.48 (0.25 to 0.90)
Disabling or fatal strokes	0.69 (0.47 to 1.01)
Myocardial infarction	0.69 (0.47 to 1.01)
Vascular death	0.93 (0.75 to 1.15)
All cause mortality	0.99 (0.83 to 1.18)
Intracranial hemorrhage	1.98 (1.20 to 3.28)

Conclusions: Adjusted-dose warfarin and related oral anticoagulants reduce stroke, disabling stroke and other major vascular events by about one third in those with non-valvular AF, when compared with antiplatelet therapy.

Management (adapted from ACC/AHA/ESC guidelines 2006)

Major objectives:
1) to control rate: beta-blockers, diltiazem, verapamil (in patients with heart failure: digoxin, amiodarone)
2) to prevent thromboembolism
   - assess stroke risk: determine CHADS2 score in patients with nonvalvular AFib (see sidebar)
   - if no risk factors, ASA 81-325 mg daily
   - 1 moderate risk factor, ASA or warfarin (INR 2.0-3.0, target 2.5)
   - >1 moderate risk factor or any high risk factor (prior stroke, TIA or embolism, mitral stenosis, prosthetic valve), warfarin
3) to restore sinus rhythm *if feasible*

Other objectives:
- to prevent and manage myocardial and hemodynamic consequences of AFib
- to identify and treat causes of AFib and associated conditions
- to improve and maintain quality of life

Newly Discovered AFib
- if the episode is self limited and not associated with severe symptoms, no need for antiarrhythmic drugs. Anticoagulants beneficial if risk for stroke is high
- if AFib persists, 2 options:
  - a) rate control and anticoagulants
  - b) cardioversion; if AFib >48 hrs, anticoagulate for 3 weeks prior and 4 weeks after cardioversion. Long term anticoagulation as indicated by stroke risk stratification (CHADS2 score)

Recurrent AFib/Permanent AFib
- if episodes are brief or minimally symptomatic, antiarrhythmic drug may be avoided; rate control and antithrombotic therapy are appropriate
- if symptoms are bothersome or episodes are prolonged, antiarrhythmic drugs (flecainide, propafenone or sotalol for patients with no or minimal heart disease; amiodarone for patients with LV dysfunction; beta-blockers, amiodarone and sotalol for CAD patients)
- patients who have undergone at least one attempt to restore sinus rhythm may remain in AFib after recurrence: permanent AFib may be accepted (with rate control and antithrombotics as indicated by CHADS2 score)

AV Nodal Re-Entrant Tachycardia (AVNRT)
- sudden onset and offset
- fast regular rhythm; rate 150-250 bpm
- usually initiated by a supraventricular or ventricular premature beat
- AVNRT accounts for 60-70% of all paroxysmal SVTs
- retrograde P waves may be seen but are usually lost in the QRS complex
- treatment
  - acute: Valsalva or carotid massage (check first for bruits), adenosine is first choice if unresponsive to vagal maneuvers; if no response, try metoprolol, digitalis, diltiazem; electrical cardioversion if patient hemodynamically unstable (hypotension, angina, or CHF)
  - long-term: 1st line: β-blocker, diltiazem, digitalis, 2nd: anti-arrhythmic drugs (flecainide, propafenone), 3rd: catheter ablation

The carotid massage is actually not a massage, but rather constant pressure directed posteriorly against the carotid artery for 5-10 seconds.

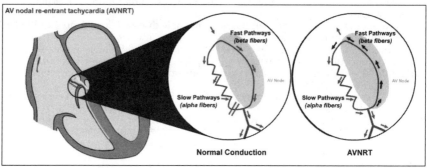

Figure 24. Pathways for AVNRT (see ECG Made Simple online for details)

Pre-excitation Syndromes

Wolff-Parkinson-White (WPW) Syndrome
- congenital defect, present in 1.5-2/1000 of the general population
- accessory bypass pathway (Kent bundle) connects atria and ventricle
- activation through bypass pathway reaches the ventricle earlier than through the AV node and the normal conduction system
- typical ECG pattern is due to the stimulation of the ventricle through the bypass tract
- early activation, slow conduction in the ventricular myocardium produce the "delta wave" (initial slurred upstroke of QRS complex)
- followed by the stimulus going through the AV node and the normal conduction system, generating a "fusion complex"
- ECG features:
  - PR interval <120 msec.
  - "delta wave"(the leads showing the delta wave vary with the site of the bypass)
  - wide QRS complex due to the premature activation
  - secondary ST segment and T wave changes
  - tachyarrythmias may occur, most often AVRT and AFib

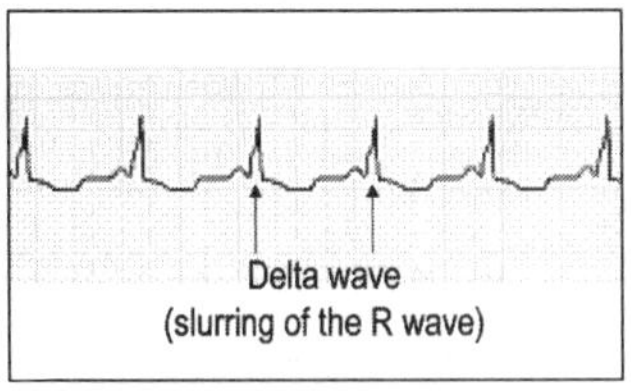

Atrial Fibrillation in WPW Patients
- as most atrial stimuli are conducted through the bypass tract, the ventricular rate is very rapid (>200/min) and the QRS complex very wide
- treatment: electrical cardioversion, IV procainamide or IV amiodarone
- do not use drugs that slow AV node conduction (digitalis, beta blockers) as they may increase conduction through the bypass tract and precipitate VFib
- long term: ablation of bypass tract when possible

AV Re-Entrant Tachycardia (AVRT)
- re-entrant loop via accessory pathway and normal conduction system
- initiated by a premature atrial or ventricular complex
- orthodromic AVRT: stimulus from a premature complex travels up the bypass tract (V to A) and down the AV node (A to V). Narrow QRS complex (no delta wave because stimulus travels through normal conduction system)
- antidromic AVRT: more rarely stimulus goes up the AV node (V to A) and down the bypass tract (A to V). Wide and abnormal QRS as ventricular activation is only via the bypass tract.
- treatment:
  - acute: similar to AVNRT except avoid long-acting AV nodal blockers, e.g. digitalis & verapamil
  - long-term: for recurrent arrhythmias, ablation of the bypass tract is recommended. Drugs such as flecainide and procainamide can be used

![Delta wave ECG](Figure 25)

Figure 25. Delta wave of WPW syndrome

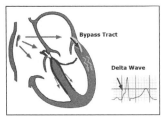

Figure 26. WPW: bypass tract and delta wave

Ventricular Tachyarrhythmias

Premature Ventricular Contraction (PVC) or Ventricular Premature Beat (VPB)
- QRS width >120 msec, no preceding P wave, bizarre QRS morphology
- origin: LBBB pattern = RV site; RBBB pattern = LV site
- PVCs may be benign but are usually significant in the following situations:
  - consecutive (≥3 = VT) or multiform (varied origin)
  - PVC falling on the T wave of the previous beat ("R on T phenomenon"): may precipitate ventricular tachycardia or VFib

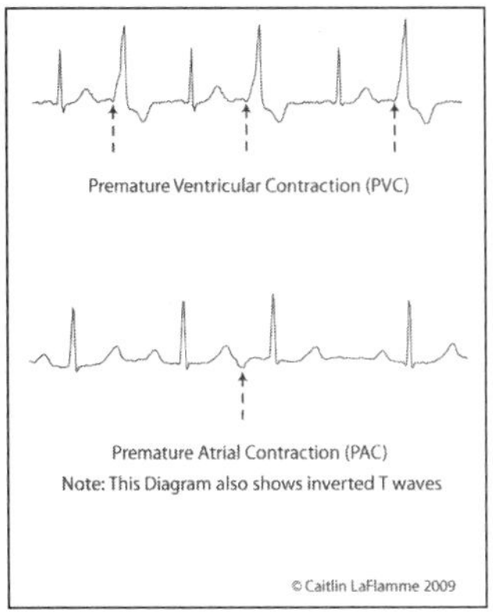

Accelerated Idioventricular Rhythm
- ectopic ventricular rhythm
- rate 50-100 bpm
- more frequently occurs in the presence of sinus bradycardia, and is easily overdriven by a faster supraventricular rhythm
- frequently occurs in patients with acute myocardial infarction or other types of heart disease (cardiomyopathy, hypertensive, valvular) but it does not affect prognosis and does not usually require treatment

Ventricular Tachycardia (VT)
- 3 or more consecutive ectopic ventricular complexes
  - rate >100 bpm (usually 140-200)
  - "sustained VT" if it lasts longer than 30 sec.
  - ECG characteristics : wide regular QRS tachycardia (QRS usually >140 msec); AV dissociation; bizarre QRS pattern. Also favour Dx of VT: left axis or right axis deviation; nonspecific intraventricular block pattern; monophasic or biphasic QRS in V1 with RBBB; QRS concordance in V1-V6
  - occasionally during VT supraventricular impulses may be conducted to the ventricles generating QRS complexes with normal or aberrant supraventricular morphology ("ventricular capture") or summation pattern ("fusion complexes")

Premature Ventricular Contraction (PVC)

Premature Atrial Contraction (PAC)
Note: This Diagram also shows inverted T waves

© Caitlin LaFlamme 2009

Figure 27. PVC and VPB

Table 5. Wide Complex Tachycardia: Clues for Differentiating VT vs. SVT with Aberrancy*	
Clinical Clues	
Presenting symptoms	not helpful
History of CAD and previous MI	VT
Physical Exam	
Cannon "a" waves	VT
Variable S1	VT
Carotid sinus massage/ adenosine terminates arrhythmia	SVT**
ECG Clues	
AV dissociation	VT
Capture or fusion	VT
QRS width >140 msec	VT
Extreme axis deviation	
(left or right superior axis)	VT
Positive QRS concordance	
(R wave across chest leads)	VT
Negative QRS concordance	
(S wave across chest leads)	may suggest VT
Axis shift during arrhythmia	VT (polymorphic)

* if patient >65 and previous MI or structural heart disease, then chance of VT >95%
** May terminate VT in some patients with no structural heart disease

Arrhythmias that may present as a wide QRS tachycardia
- ventricular tachycardia
- SVT with aberrant conduction (rate related)
- SVT with preexisting BBB or nonspecific intraventricular conduction defect
- AV conduction through a bypass tract in WPW patients during an atrial tachyarrhythmia (e.g. atrial flutter, atrial tachycardia)
- antidromic AVRT in WPW patients (see Pre-excitation Syndromes)

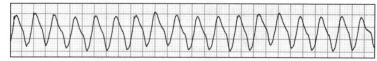

Figure 28. Ventricular Tachycardia

- treatment:
  - sustained VT (longer than 30 seconds) is an emergency, requiring immediate treatment
  - hemodynamic compromise – electrical cardioversion
  - no hemodynamic compromise – electrical cardioversion, lidocaine, amiodarone, type Ia agents (procainamide, quinidine)

Torsade de Pointes
- polymorphic VT – "twisting of the points"
- looks like usual VT except that QRS complexes "rotate around the baseline" changing their axis and amplitude
- ventricular rate greater than 100, usually 150-300
- etiology: patients with prolonged QT intervals are predisposed
  - congenital long QT syndromes
  - drugs – e.g. Class IA (quinidine), Class III (sotalol), phenothiazines (TCAs), erythromycin, quinolones, antihistamines
  - electrolyte disturbances – hypokalemia, hypomagnesemia
  - nutritional deficiencies causing above electrolyte abnormalities
- treatment: IV magnesium, temporary pacing, isoproterenol and correct underlying cause of prolonged QT, electrical cardioversion if hemodynamic compromise

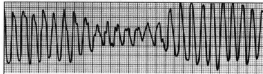

Figure 29. Torsades de Pointes

Ventricular Fibrillation (VFib)
- chaotic ventricular arrythmia, with very rapid irregular ventricular fibrillatory waves of varying morphology
- terminal event, unless advanced cardiac life-support (ACLS) procedures are promptly initiated to maintain ventilation and cardiac output, and electrical defibrillation is carried out
- most frequent cause of sudden death
- refer to ACLS algorithm for complete therapeutic guidelines

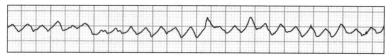

Figure 30. Ventricular Fibrillation

Electrophysiology (EPS) Studies

- invasive test used to better characterize arrhythmias
- mostly viewed as supplemental to ECG recordings which are commonly sufficient for diagnosis and management
- provide useful information when ECG data are nondiagnostic or unobtainable
- bradyarrhythmias: sinus node dysfunction, atrioventricular (AV) block, and intraventricular conduction delay
- tachyarrhythmias: mainly used to map tachyarrythmias for possible ablation or to assess inducibility of ventricular tachycardia

Electrical Pacing

- the decision to implant a pacemaker usually is based on symptoms of a bradyarrhythmia or tachyarrhythmia in the setting of heart disease

Pacemaker Indications
- SA node dysfunction (most common): symptomatic bradycardia +/- hemodynamic instability)
    - common manifestations include: syncope, near syncope, transient lightheadedness, or severe fatigue
- SA node dysfunction is commonly caused by one or more of the following: intrinsic disease within the sinus node (e.g. idiopathic degeneration, fibrosis, ischemia, or surgical trauma), abnormalities in autonomic nervous system function, and drug effects
- AV nodal - infranodal block: Mobitz II, complete heart block

Pacing Techniques
- temporary: transvenous (jugular, subclavian, femoral) or external pacing
- permanent: transvenous into RA, apex of RV or both
    - can sense and pace atrium, ventricle or both
    - new generation = rate responsive, able to respond to physiologic demand
    - biventricular
- nomenclature e.g. "VVIR"
    1. chamber paced (atrium, ventricle, dual)
    2. chamber sensitive (atrium, ventricle, dual)
    3. response to sensing (inhibit, trigger, dual (I&T))
    4. programmability (e.g. rate responsive)
    5. arrhythmia control (pace, shock, dual, none)

Implantable Cardioverter Defibrillators (ICDs)

- sudden cardiac death (SCD) usually results from ventricular fibrillation (VFib), sometimes preceded by monomorphic or polymorphic ventricular tachycardia (VT)
- ICDs detect ventricular tachyarrhythmias and are highly effective in terminating VT/VFib and in aborting SCD
- several studies demonstrate mortality benefit vs. antiarrhythmics in 2° prevention (AVID, CASH, CIDS)
- benefit for 1° prevention of SCD in patients with ischemic & non-ischemic cardiomyopathy, depressed left ventricular ejection fraction (LVEF), prolonged QRS (MADIT-I, MADIT-II, MUSTT, SCD-HeFT studies)
- very expensive: ongoing trials to determine cost effectiveness of 1° prevention and define benefit in various subgroups
- see *Heart Failure* for current treatment recommendations

Catheter Ablation

Techniques
- radiofrequency (RF) energy: a low-voltage high-frequency form of electrical energy (similar to cautery). RF energy produces small, homogeneous, necrotic lesions approximately 5-7 mm in diameter and 3-5 mm in depth

Indications
- paroxysmal SVT
    - AVNRT: accounts for more than half of all cases
    - an extra pathway lies in or near the AV node, which creates a reentry circuit
- accessory pathway (orthodromic reciprocating tachycardia): 30% of SVT
    - reentrant rhythm, with an accessory AV connection as the retrograde limb
    - cured by targeting the accessory pathway
- atrial flutter: flutter focus in RA
- atrial fibrillation: potential role for pulmonary vein ablation
- ventricular tachycardia: commonly arises from the right ventricular outflow tract and less commonly originates in the inferoseptal left ventricle near the apex (note: majority of cases of VT are due to scarring from previous MI and cannot be ablated)

Major Complications
- approximately 1% of patients
- death: 0.1-0.2%
- cardiac: high grade AV block requiring permanent pacemaker, tamponade, pericarditis
- vascular: hematoma, vascular injury, thromboembolism, TIA/stroke
- pulmonary: pulmonary embolism

Systematic review: implantable cardioverter defibrillators for adults with left ventricular systolic dysfunction.
Ann Intern Med. 2007;147:251-62.
Purpose: To summarize the evidence on the benefits and harms of implantable cardioverter defibrillators (ICDs) in adult patients with LV systolic dysfunction.
Study Selection: Twelve randomized, controlled trials (RCTs) (8,516 patients) that reported on mortality, and 76 observational studies (96,951 patients) that examined safety or effectiveness.
Results: In adult patients with LV systolic dysfunction, 86% of whom had New York Heart Association class II or III symptoms, ICDs reduced all-cause mortality by 20% in the RCTs and by 46% in the observational studies. Death associated with implantation of ICDs occurred during 1.2% of procedures. The frequency of post-implantation complications per 100 patient-years included 1.4 device malfunctions, 1.5 lead problems, and 0.6 site infection. Rates of inappropriate discharges per 100 patient-years ranged from 19.1 in RCTs to 4.9 in observational studies.
Conclusions: Implantable cardioverter defibrillators are efficacious in reducing mortality in adult patients with LV systolic dysfunction, and this benefit extends to non-trial populations. Improved risk stratification tools to identify patients who are most likely to benefit from ICD are needed.

Ischemic Heart Disease (IHD)

Epidemiology
- commonest cause of cardiovascular morbidity and mortality
- atherosclerosis and thrombosis are by far the most important pathogenetic mechanisms
- male:female ratio = 2:1 with all age groups included (Framingham study), 8:1 for age <40, 1:1 for age >70
- peak incidence of symptomatic IHD is age 50-60 (men) and 60-70 (women)
- for primary prevention of ischemic heart disease, please see Family Medicine
- risk factors as per Table 6

Table 6. Risk Factors For Atherosclerotic Heart Disease

Major Risk Factors	Minor Risk Factors
smoking	male, postmenopausal female
diabetes mellitus (DM)	obesity
hypertension (HTN)	sedentary lifestyle
family history (FHx) of MI	hyperhomocysteinemia
first degree male relative <55 or	
first degree female relative <60	
hyperlipidemia	

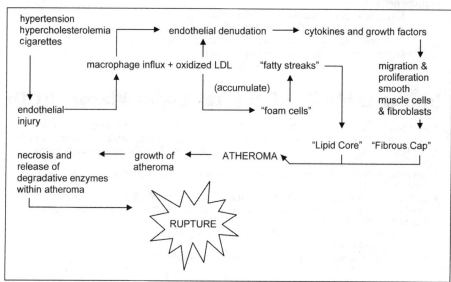

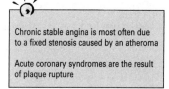

Chronic stable angina is most often due to a fixed stenosis caused by an atheroma

Acute coronary syndromes are the result of plaque rupture

Figure 31. Pathophysiology of Atherosclerosis (Jon Kenny ©2006)

Chronic Stable Angina

Definition
- symptom complex resulting from an imbalance between oxygen supply and demand in the myocardium
- factors influencing supply:
  - luminal diameter (most important factor)
  - duration of diastole
  - hemoglobin
  - SaO_2
- factors influencing demand
  - heart rate
  - contractility
  - wall stress

Etiology and Pathophysiology
- decreased myocardial oxygen supply
  - atherosclerosis, vasospasm
  - tachycardia (↓ duration of diastole)
  - anemia
  - hypoxemia
  - congenital anomalies

- increased myocardial oxygen demand
  - tachycardia
  - hyperthyroidism ($\uparrow$ contractility, $\uparrow$ HR)
  - myocardial hypertrophy, aortic stenosis ($\uparrow$ wall tension)

Signs and Symptoms
- typical: retrosternal chest pain, tightness or discomfort radiating to left ($\pm$ right) shoulder/arm/neck/jaw, associated with diaphoresis, nausea, anxiety
- predictably precipitated by the "3 E's": Exertion, Emotion and Eating
- brief duration, lasting <10-15 minutes and typically relieved by rest and nitrates
- Levine's sign: clutching fist over sternum when describing chest pain
- anginal equivalents: dyspnea, acute left ventricular failure, flash pulmonary edema

Clinical Assessment (ACC 2002 Guidelines)
- history, physical and directed risk factor assessment
- labs: Hb, fasting glucose, fasting lipid profile
- ECG (at rest and during episode of chest pain if possible)
- CXR (suspected heart failure, valvular disease, pericardial disease, aortic dissection/aneurysm, or signs or symptoms of pulmonary disease)
- stress testing (see *Cardiac Diagnostic Tests*, C5) or angiography
- echocardiography:
  - to assess systolic murmur suggestive of aortic stenosis (AS), mitral regurgitation (MR) and/or hypertrophic cardiomyopathy (HCM)
  - to assess LV function in patients with Hx of prior MI, pathological Q waves, signs or symptoms of congestive heart failure (CHF)

Differential Diagnosis
- cardiovascular
  - aortic dissection
  - pericarditis
- respiratory (e.g. PE, pneumothorax, pneumonia)
- gastrointestinal (e.g. peptic ulcer disease, gastroesophageal reflux disease, esophagitis, esophageal spasm, esophageal rupture)
- musculoskeletal (e.g. rib fracture, costochondritis, muscle spasm)
- neurological (e.g. herpes zoster)
- psychiatric (e.g. anxiety)

Treatment (ACC 2002 Guidelines)
- goals of treatment: reduce myocardial oxygen demand and/or increase oxygen supply
- **CONSERVATIVE**
  - lifestyle modification, treatment of risk factors, enrollment in an exercise program
- **MEDICATION**
  - enteric coated ASA (ECASA), clopidogrel when ASA absolutely contraindicated
  - β-blockers (first line therapy – decrease overall mortality)
    - increase coronary perfusion and decrease demand (HR, contractility) and BP (afterload)
    - cardioselective agents are preferred (e.g. metoprolol, atenolol) to avoid peripheral effects (inhibition of vasodilation and bronchodilation via β2 receptors)
    - avoid intrinsic sympathomimetics (e.g. acebutolol) which increase demand
  - nitrates – used for symptomatic control, no clear impact on survival
    - decrease preload (venous dilatation) and afterload (arteriolar dilatation), and increase coronary perfusion
    - maintain daily nitrate-free intervals to prevent nitrate tolerance (tachyphylaxis)
  - statins (see <u>Endocrinology</u>, <u>Family Medicine</u> for target lipid guidelines)
  - calcium channel blockers (CCBs) (second line or combination)
    - increase coronary perfusion and decrease demand (HR, contractility) and BP (afterload)
    - caution: verapamil/diltiazem combined with β-blockers may cause symptomatic sinus bradycardia or AV block
  - ACE inhibitors (ACEIs)
    - not used to treat angina – however, angina patients tend to have risk factors for cardiovascular disease which do warrant use of an ACEI (e.g. hypertension, diabetes, proteinuric renal disease, previous MI with LV dysfunction)
    - class IIa evidence of benefit in all patients at high risk for cardiovascular disease
    - class I evidence in patients with concomitant DM, renal dysfunction or LV systolic dysfunction

    ◆ growing evidence for angiotensin II receptor blockers (ARBs) when ACEIs
      are contraindicated
    ◆ ACEIs do not treat symptoms of angina
• **INVASIVE**
    ▪ revascularization (see *Coronary Revascularization* and *COURAGE trial*)

VARIANT ANGINA (Prinzmetal's Angina)
• myocardial ischemia secondary to coronary artery vasospasm, with or without
  atherosclerosis
• uncommonly associated with infarction or LV dysfunction
• typically occurs between midnight and 8 AM, unrelated to exercise, relieved by nitrates
• typically ST elevation on ECG
• diagnose by provocative testing with ergot vasoconstrictors (rarely done)
• treat with nitrates and CCBs

SYNDROME X
• typical symptoms of angina but normal angiogram
• may show definite signs of ischemia with exercise testing
• thought to be due to inadequate vasodilator reserve of coronary resistance vessels
• better prognosis than overt epicardial atherosclerosis

Acute Coronary Syndromes (ACS)

Definition
• coronary atherosclerosis with superimposed thrombus on ruptured plaque
• other causes of unstable angina:
    ▪ coronary thromboembolism (e.g. infective endocarditis, intracavity thrombus,
      paradoxical embolism) or cholesterol embolism
    ▪ severe coronary vasospasm
    ▪ coronary dissection
    ▪ increased demand can also contribute (e.g. tachycardia, anemia)

Spectrum of ACS
• unstable angina (UA)/non-ST elevation myocardial infarction (NSTEMI)
• ST elevation myocardial infarction (STEMI)
• sudden cardiac death

Investigations
• history and physical
    ▪ note that up to 30% of MIs are unrecognized or "silent" due to atypical
      symptoms – most common in DM, elderly, post-heart transplant (because of
      denervation)
• ECG, CXR
• labs
    ▪ serum cardiac biomarkers for myocardial damage (see *Cardiac Biomarkers*
      section)
    ▪ CBC, INR/aPTT, electrolytes and magnesium, creatinine, urea, glucose, serum
      lipids
    ▪ draw serum lipids within 24-48 hours because values are unreliable from 2 to 48
      days post-MI

Unstable Angina (UA)/Non ST Elevation MI (NSTEMI)

Definition
• syndrome of acute plaque rupture and thrombosis with incomplete or transient vessel
  occlusion
• unstable angina is clinically defined by any of the following:
    ▪ accelerating pattern of pain: ↑ frequency, ↑ duration, with ↓ exertion,
      ↓ response to treatment
    ▪ angina at rest
    ▪ new onset angina
    ▪ angina post-MI or post-procedure (e.g. percutaneous coronary intervention
      [PCI], coronary artery bypass grafting [CABG])
• NSTEMI is clinically defined by the presence of 2 of 3 criteria:
    ▪ symptoms of angina/ischemia
    ▪ rise and fall of serum markers of myocardial necrosis
    ▪ evolution of ischemic ECG changes (without ST elevation or new LBBB)
• acute phase of UA/NSTEMI:
    ▪ risk of progression to MI or the development of recurrent MI or death is highest
      in the early period
    ▪ at 1 to 3 months after the acute phase, most patients resume a clinical course
      similar to that in patients with chronic stable coronary disease
• majority of NSTEMIs do not result in the development of Q waves

---

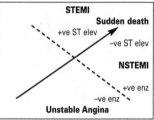

Recommendations for Coronary Angiography (ACC/AHA 2002 Recommendations)
• disabling (CCS classes III and IV) chronic stable angina despite medical therapy
• high-risk criteria on clinical assessment or non-invasive testing
• sudden cardiac death, serious ventricular arrhythmia, or CHF
• uncertain diagnosis or prognosis after non-invasive testing
• inability to undergo non-invasive testing

STEMI
Sudden death
+ve ST elev
–ve ST elev
NSTEMI
+ve enz
–ve enz
Unstable Angina

Figure 32. ACS Specturm
(Courtesy of Dr. M. Husain)

The most compelling features that increase the likelihood of MI are ST-segment elevation, new Q-wave, chest pain radiating to both the right and left arm simultaneously, presence of an S3 and hypotension.

The most compelling features that decrease the likelihood of MI are normal ECG report, pleuritic chest pain, pain reproduced on palpation, sharp or stabbing chest pain, and positional chest pain.
(Is This Patient Having a Myocardial Infarction? JAMA 1998; 280: 1256-63.)

Management of NSTEMI (ACC/AHA 2007)

General measures
- ABCs: assess and correct hemodynamic status first
- bed rest, cardiac monitoring, oxygen
- nitroglycerin SL followed by IV
- morphine IV

Anti-platelet and anticoagulation therapy
- ASA (162-325 mg chewed)
- clopidogrel 300 mg loading dose then 75 mg OD if ASA contraindicated and in addition to ASA for some
- subcutaneous low molecular weight heparin (LMWH) or IV unfractionated heparin UH (LMWH is preferable to UH except in renal failure or if CABG is planned within 24h)
- if PCI is planned: clopidogrel 300 mg loading dose and IV GP IIb/IIIa inhibitor

- β-blockers (first dose IV) followed by oral administration
  - non-dihydropyridine CCB in absence of severe LV dysfunction in patients with continuing or frequently recurring ischemia when β-blockers are contraindicated (evidence suggests that CCBs do not prevent MI or decrease mortality)

Conservative vs. invasive strategies (FRISC II, TACTICS-TIMI 18, RITA 3, ICTUS)
- early coronary angiography ± revascularization if possible is recommended in UA/NSTEMI with any of the following high-risk indicators (class I):
  - recurrent angina/ischemia at rest despite intensive anti-ischemic therapy
  - CHF or LV dysfunction
  - hemodynamic instability
  - high TIMI risk score (3 or higher)
  - sustained VT
  - dynamic ECG changes
  - high-risk findings on non-invasive stress testing
  - PCI within the previous 6 months
  - repeated presentations for ACS despite Tx and without evidence of ongoing ischemia or high risk features (class IIa)
- **note: thrombolysis is NOT indicated for UA/NSTEMI**

Post-discharge therapy
- **CONSERVATIVE**
  - education, risk factor modification
- **MEDICATION**
  - drugs required in hospital to control ischemia should be continued after discharge in patients who do not undergo revascularization
  - ECASA 81-162mg OD
  - clopidogrel 75mg OD (at least 1 month, some suggest 9-12 months)
  - ± warfarin x 3 months if high risk (large anterior MI, LV thrombus, LVEF <30%, history of VTE, chronic AFib)
  - β-blocker (e.g. metoprolol 25-50 mg bid or atendol 50-100 mg OD)
  - statin early, intensive, irrespective of cholesterol level (e.g. atorvastatin 80 mg OD)
  - ACEI (and/or ARB)
  - for patients with LV dysfunction or CHF
  - for all ACS patients with diabetes (class I)
  - for all post-ACS patients (class IIa)
  - nitrates for symptomatic relief of ongoing angina if necessary
  - ± aldosterone antagonist (if on ACEI and LVEF < 40% and CHF or DM)
  - CCB (NOT recommended as first-line treatment, consider as alternative to β-blocker)
- **INVASIVE**
  - risk stratification as per Figure 34
- Predischarge:
  - stress ECG (if not fully revascularized)
  - echo

ST Elevation Myocardial Infarction (STEMI)

Definition
- syndrome of acute plaque rupture and thrombosis with total coronary occlusion resulting in myocardial necrosis
- STEMI is clinically defined by new ischemic ECG changes plus one or both of ischemic symptoms and elevated cardiac enzymes
  - ECG criteria (see *Electrocardiography*):
    - ST elevation in 2 contiguous leads (≥1 mm in limb leads or ≥2 mm in precordial leads) or new LBBB

Management of UA/NSTEMI
Acute
1. General Measures
2. Antiplatelet and Anticoagulation
3. β-blocker
4. Decide Conservative vs. Invasive

Further Therapy
- conservative
- medication
- invasive (consider if still high risk)

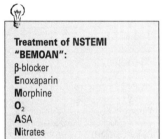

Treatment of NSTEMI "BEMOAN":
β-blocker
Enoxaparin
Morphine
O$_2$
ASA
Nitrates

TIMI Risk Score for UA/NSTEMI

Characteristics	Points
Historical	
Age ≥65 yrs	1
≥3 risk factors for CAD	1
Known CAD (stenosis ≥50%)	1
Aspirin use in past 7 days	1
Presentation	
Recent (≤24 hr) severe angina	1
ST-segment deviation ≥0.5 mm	1
↑ cardiac markers	1
Risk Score = Total Points	(0-7)

CAD = coronary artery disease
NSTEMI = non ST-segment elevation myocardial infarction
TIMI = thrombolysis in myocardial infarction
UA = unstable angina
JAMA 2000;284:835-842.

Management of STEMI (ACC/AHA 2007)

Acute Management
- note: after the diagnosis of STEMI is made, do not wait for results of further investigations before implementing reperfusion therapy
- goal: thrombolysis (EMS-to-needle) within 30 minutes or PCI (EMS-to-balloon) within 90 minutes depending on capabilities of hospital

General Measures
- ABCs: assess and correct hemodynamic status first
- bedrest, telemetry, oxygen
- nitroglycerin sublingual or IV
- morphine IV

Anti-platelet and Anticoagulation Therapy
- ASA 162-325 mg chewed
- if PCI is planned: clopidogrel 300 mg loading dose then 75 mg OD, IV GP IIb/IIIa inhibitor
- anticoagulation options depend on reperfusion strategy:
  - primary PCI: UH during procedure; bivalirudin possible alternative
  - thrombolysis: LMWH (enoxaparin) until D/C from hospital; can use UH as alternative because of possible rescue PCI
  - no reperfusion: LMWH (enoxaparin) until discharge from hospital
- continue LMWH or UH followed by oral anticoagulation at discharge if at high risk for thromboembolic event (large anterior MI, AFib, severe LV dysfunction, CHF, previous DVT or PE, or Echo evidence of mural thrombus)

- β-blocker (first dose IV) followed by oral administration
  - if bradycardia is present, consider administering atropine (COMMIT/CCS2 trial: ↑mortality in patients with hemodynamic compromise with early beta-blockers given IV)

Reperfusion Options
- if skilled PCI practitioners are available, early PCI (≤12 hrs after symptom onset and <90 mins after presentation) has been shown to improve mortality versus thrombolysis, with fewer intracranial hemorrhages and recurrent MIs (ACC/AHA Class I recommendations)
- thrombolysis preferred if the patient presents ≤12 hrs of symptom onset, and <30 min after presentation to hospital; has contraindications to PCI or PCI cannot be administered within 90 mins by a skilled practitioner (ACC/AHA 2004 Guidelines)
- categorization of PCI in management of STEMI:
  - primary: PCI without prior administration of thrombolytic therapy – data suggest that when available and performed in experienced centres, primary PCI is the method of choice to establish reperfusion (JAMA 2004;291:736-39)
  - rescue: PCI following failed thrombolytic therapy (diagnosed clinically when, upon completion of thrombolytic infusion, ST segment elevation fails to resolve below half its initial magnitude and patient still having chest pain)

Table 7. Contraindications and Cautions for Thrombolysis in STEMI

Absolute	Relative
Prior intracranial hemorrhage	Chronic, severe, poorly controlled hypertension
Known structural cerebral vascular lesion	Uncontrolled hypertension (sBP>180, dBP>110)
Known malignant IC neoplasm	Current anticoagulation
Significant closed-head or facial trauma (≤3 months)	Noncompressible vascular punctures
Ischemic stroke (≤3 months)	Ischemic stroke (≥3 months)
Active bleeding	Recent internal bleeding (≤2-4 weeks)
Suspected aortic dissection	Prolonged CPR or major surgery (≤3 weeks)
	Pregnancy
	Active peptic ulcer

Long Term Management/Secondary Prevention
- **CONSERVATIVE**
  - education, risk factor modification
- **MEDICATION**
  - drugs required in hospital to control ischemia should be continued after discharge in patients who do not undergo revascularization
  - ECASA 81-162 mg OD
  - clopidogrel 75 mg OD (for up to 12 mos depending on stent placement, some say longer)
  - ± warfarin x 3 months if high risk (large anterior MI, LV thrombus, LVEF <30%, history of VTE, chronic AFib)
  - β-blockers (e.g. metoprolol 25-50 mg bid or atendol 50-100 mg OD)
  - statin early, intensive, irrespective of cholesterol level (e.g. atorvastatin 80 mg OD)
  - ACEI (prevent adverse ventricular remodeling)

Management of STEMI
Acute
1. General Measures
2. Decide on Reperfusion
   - primary PCI
   - thrombolysis
   - no reperfusion
3. Antiplatelet/Anticoagulation
4. β-blocker

Further Therapy
   - conservative
   - medication
   - invasive (consider if still high risk)

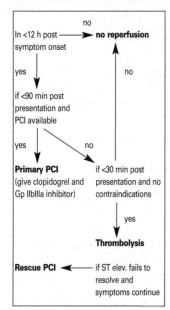

Figure 33. Reperfusion Strategy

Enoxaparin versus unfractionated heparin with fibrinolysis for ST-elevation myocardial infarction
N Engl J Med 2006;354:1477-88
Study: Prospective, randomized, controlled multicentre trial.
Patients: 20,479 patients (median age 60 yrs. 77% male) with STEMI who were scheduled to undergo fibrinolysis.
Intervention: Patients were randomized to receive either enoxaparin or weight based unfractionated heparin in addition to thrombolysis and standard therapies.
Primary Outcome: Death or recurrent nonfatal MI 30 days post-event.
Results: The composite primary outcome occurred less often in the enoxaparin group compared with those who received unfractionated heparin (9.9% vs. 12.0%, p<0.001, NNT=47). Taken separately, there was a trend toward reduced mortality (6.9% vs. 7.5%, p=0.11) and a significant reduction in nonfatal reinfarction (3.0% vs. 4.5%, p<0.001) in the enoxaparin group. The risk of major bleeding was significantly increased in the enoxaparin group (2.1% vs. 1.4%, p<0.001, NNH=142).
Conclusion: In patients with STEMI receiving thrombolysis, enoxaparin is superior to unfractionated heparin in preventing recurrent nonfatal MI and may lead to a small reduction in mortality.

- ◆ recommended for asymptomatic patients, even if LVEF >40% (HOPE trial)
- ◆ recommended for symptomatic CHF, reduced LVEF (<40%), anterior MI (ACC/AHA 2004 Guidelines)
- ◆ use ARBs in patients who are intolerant of ACEIs
  - ▪ nitrates (alleviate ischemia but do not improve outcome; use caution in right-sided MI patients who are pre-load dependent)
  - ▪ ± aldosterone antagonists
    - ◆ if on ACEI and β-blockers and LVEF <40% and CHF or DM
    - ◆ EPHESUS trial showed significant mortality benefit of eplerenone by 30 days
- • CCB (NOT recommended as first-line treatment, consider as alternative to β-blockers)
- • **INVASIVE**
  - ▪ risk stratification as per Figure 34
- • Predischarge:
  - ▪ stress ECG (if not fully revascularized)
  - ▪ echo

Prognosis

- • 5-15% of hospitalized patients will die
  - ▪ risk factors
    - ◆ infarct size/severity
    - ◆ age
    - ◆ co-morbid conditions
    - ◆ development of heart failure or hypotension
- • post-discharge mortality rates
  - ▪ 6-8% within first year, half of these within first 3 months
  - ▪ 4% per year following first year
  - ▪ risk factors
    - ◆ LV dysfunction
    - ◆ residual myocardial ischemia
    - ◆ ventricular arrhythmias
    - ◆ history of prior MI
- • complications as per Table 8

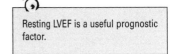

Resting LVEF is a useful prognostic factor.

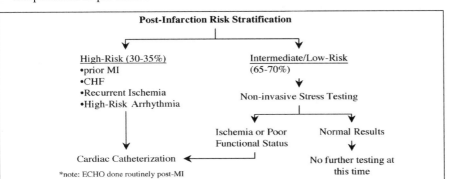

Figure 34. Post-Infarction Risk Stratification

Table 8. Complications of Myocardial Infarction

Complication	Etiology	Presentation	Therapy
Arrhythmia			
1. tachycardia	sinus, AFib, VT, VFib	first 48 hrs	see *Arrhythmias*, C14
2. bradycardia	sinus, AV block	first 48 hrs	
Myocardial Rupture			
1. LV free wall	transmural infarction	1-7 days	surgery
2. papillary muscle (→MR)	inferior infarction	1-7 days	surgery
3. ventricular septum (→VSD)	septal infarction	1-7 days	surgery
Shock/CHF	infarction or aneurysm	within 48 hours	inotropes, intra-aortic balloon pump
Post-infarct Angina	persistent coronary stenosis multivessel disease	anytime	aggressive medical therapy PCI or CABG
Recurrent MI	reocclusion	anytime	see above
Thromboembolism	mural/apical thrombus DVT	7-10 days, up to 6 months	anticoagulation
Pericarditis (Dressler's syndrome)	inflammatory autoimmune	1-7 days 2-8 weeks	ASA

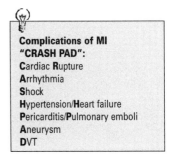

Complications of MI "CRASH PAD":
Cardiac **R**upture
Arrhythmia
Shock
Hypertension/**H**eart failure
Pericarditis/**P**ulmonary emboli
Aneurysm
DVT

Treatment Algorithm for Chest Pain

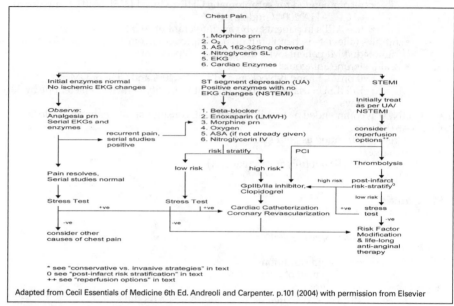

Figure 35. Treatment Algorithm for Chest Pain

Sudden Cardiac Death

Definition
- unanticipated, non-traumatic cardiac death in stable patient, within 1 hour of symptom onset; ventricular fibrillation is most common cause

Etiology
- primary cardiac pathology
  - ischemia/MI
  - LV dysfunction
  - severe ventricular hypertrophy
    - hypertrophic cardiomyopathy (HCM)
    - AS
  - long QT syndrome
  - congenital heart disease

Management
- acute – resuscitate with prompt CPR and defibrillation
- investigate underlying cause (cardiac catheterization, electrophysiologic studies)
- treat underlying cause
- anti-arrhythmic drug therapy: amiodarone, β-blockers
- ICD

Coronary Revascularization

Percutaneous Coronary Intervention (PCI)

- interventional technique aimed at relieving significant coronary stenosis
- main techniques: balloon angioplasty, stenting
- less common techniques: rotational/directional/extraction atherectomy

Indications
- medically refractory angina
- NSTEMI/UA with high TIMI risk score is within 90 min of presentation
- primary/rescue PCI for STEMI

Balloon Angioplasty and Intracoronary Stenting
- coronary lesions dilated with balloon inflation
- majority of patients receive intracoronary stent(s) to reduce recurrence (restenosis) of lesion(s)

- primary success is >90%
- major complication is restenosis, felt to be due to elastic recoil and neointimal hyperplasia (occurs in 20%)
- recent development: drug-eluting stents (DES)
  - coated with antiproliferative drugs (sirolimus, paclitaxel)
  - aim to prevent neointimal hyperplasia and restenosis
  - problem of late stent thrombosis with DES

Adjunctive Therapies
- ASA and heparin decrease post-procedural complications
- further reduction in ischemic complications has now been demonstrated using GpIIb/IIIa inhibitors in coronary angiography and stenting (abciximab, eptifibatide, tirofiban)
- following stent implantation, patients treated with ASA and clopidogrel
  - dual antiplatelet therapy (ASA and clopidogrel) needed at least 12 months after DES

Procedural Complications
- mortality and emergency bypass rates <1%
- nonfatal MI: approximately 2-3%

Coronary Artery Bypass Graft (CABG) Surgery

- the objective of CABG is complete revascularization of the myocardium; goals include relieving symptoms (angina, heart failure) and thus improving quality of life, and/or prolonging life

Indications

- Class I: there is evidence and/or general agreement that a given procedure or treatment is useful and effective:
  - CABG
    - significant left main artery disease
    - triple vessel disease, survival benefit greatest in patients with abnormal LV function (EF <50%)
    - two-vessel disease with significant proximal left anterior descending (LAD) disease and with abnormal LV function (EF <50%) or demonstrable ischemia on noninvasive testing
    - one or two vessel disease without significant LAD disease who have survived sudden cardiac death or sustained VT
  - CABG or PCI
    - patients with one or two vessel disease without significant LAD disease but with a large area of viable myocardium and high risk criteria on noninvasive testing
    - recurrent stenosis associated with a large area of viable myocardium or high risk criteria on noninvasive testing
- Class IIa: weight of evidence/opinion is in favour of usefulness/efficacy
  - CABG or PCI
    - one vessel disease with significant proximal LAD
    - repeat CABG for multiple saphenous vein graft stenosis, with high risk criteria on noninvasive testing, especially when LAD graft at risk. PCI may be appropriate for focal lesions, or multiple lesions in poor surgical candidates
    - one or two vessel disease without significant proximal LAD disease but with a moderate area of viable ischemia on noninvasive testing

Operative Issues
- isolated proximal disease in large coronary arteries (>1.0-1.5 mm) is ideal for bypass surgery; small, diffusely diseased coronary arteries are not suitable for bypass surgery
- arteries with severe stenoses (>50% diameter reduction) are bypassed, except those of small calibre (<1 mm in diameter)

Choice of Resvascularization Procedure

Advantages of PCI over CABG
- Less invasive technique
- Less periprocedural morbidity and mortality
- Shorter periprocedural hospitalization

Advantages of CABG over PCI
- Greater ability to achieve complete revascularization
- Less need for repeated revascularization procedures

Indications for PCI over CABG
- Single or double-vessel disease
- Inability to tolerate surgery

Indications for CABG over PCI
- Triple-vessel or left main disease
- Diabetes mellitus
- Plaque morphology unfavourable for PCI

Table 9. Risk Factors for CABG Mortality and Morbidity

Risk Factors for CABG Mortality (decreasing order of significance)	Risk Factors for CABG postop morbidity or length of stay (decreasing order of significance)
• urgency of surgery (emergent or urgent)	• reoperation
• reoperation	• emergent procedure
• older age	• preoperative intra-aortic balloon pump (IABP)
• poor left ventricular function (see below)	• congestive heart failure
• female gender	• CABG + valve surgery
• left main disease	• older age
• others include catastrophic conditions (cardiogenic shock,	• renal dysfunction
ventricular septal rupture, ongoing CPR), dialysis-dependent	• COPD
renal failure, end-stage COPD, diabetes, cerebrovascular disease,	• diabetes
and peripheral vascular disease	• cerebrovascular disease

- left ventricular function is an important determinant of outcome of all heart diseases
- patients with severe LV dysfunction usually have poor prognosis, but surgery can sometimes dramatically improve LV function
- assess viability of non-functioning myocardial segments using thallium myocardial imaging, PET scanning or MRI

Conduits for CABG

- saphenous vein grafts (SVG)
  - at 10 years, 50% occluded, 25% stenotic, 25% angiographically normal
- left internal thoracic/mammary artery (LITA/LIMA)
  - LIMA to LAD is the most preferred option; excellent long term patency (90-95% at 15 years), improved event-free survival (angina, MI), decreased late cardiac events; no increase in operative risk
- right internal thoracic/mammary artery (RITA/RIMA)
  - used in bilateral ITA grafting; pedicled RIMA patency comparable to LIMA (free RIMA patency less)
  - patients receiving bilateral ITAs have less risk of recurrent angina, late myocardial infarction, angioplasty, reoperation and death; however, higher rates of sternal infection, dehiscence and mediastinitis especially in elderly, obese or diabetic patients
- radial artery (free graft)
  - approximately 85-90% patency at 5 years
  - prone to severe vasospasm postoperatively due to muscular wall; patients often placed on CCB (e.g. nifedipine XL 20 mg OD) postoperatively
- right gastroepiploic artery
  - good long term patency (80-90% at 5 years)
  - primarily used as an in situ graft to bypass the RCA
  - use limited because of the fragile quality of the artery, other technical issues, increased operative time (laparotomy incision) and incisional discomfort with associated ileus
- for younger patients (<60 years of age), complete arterial revascularization is preferred due to longer term graft patency
- redo bypass grafting
  - operative mortality 2-3 times higher than first operation
  - 10% perioperative MI rate
  - reoperation undertaken only in symptomatic patients who have failed medical therapy and in whom angiography has documented progression of the disease
  - increased risk with redo-sternotomy secondary to adhesions which may result in laceration to aorta, RV, IMA and other bypass grafts

Off-Pump Coronary Artery Bypass (OPCAB) Surgery

- despite the success of CABG with cardiopulmonary bypass (CPB), the deleterious effects of CPB include:
  - stroke and neurocognitive defects (microembolization of gaseous and particulate matter)
  - immunosuppression
  - systemic inflammatory response leading to:
    - myocardial dysfunction
    - renal dysfunction
    - neurological injury
    - respiratory dysfunction
    - coagulopathies

Procedure
- OPCAB avoids the use of CPB by allowing surgeons to operate on a beating heart
  - stabilization devices allow local cardiac wall motion fixation around the distal anastomotic site (e.g. Genzyme Immobilizer™) while positioning devices allow the surgeon to lift the beating heart to access the lateral and posterior vessels (Medtronic Octopus and Starfish system™)
  - procedure is safe and well tolerated by most patients; however, OPCAB surgery remains technically more demanding and has a steeper learning curve

Indications
- use in poor candidates for CPB who have: calcified aorta, poor LVEF, severe peripheral vascular disease (PVD), severe COPD, CRF, coagulopathy, transfusion issues (i.e. Jehovah's Witness), good target vessels, anterior/lateral wall revascularization, target revascularization in older, sicker patients
- **absolute contraindications** include: hemodynamic instability, poor quality target vessels including intramyocardial vessels, diffusely diseased vessels and calcified coronary vessels
- **relative contraindications** include: cardiomegaly/CHF, critical left main disease, small distal targets, recent or current acute MI, cardiogenic shock, LVEF <35%

Outcomes
- OPCAB decreases in-hospital morbidity (decreased incidence of chest infection, inotropic requirement, supraventricular arrhythmia), blood product transfusion, ICU stay, length of hospitalization, and decreased CK-MB and troponin I levels
- no significant difference in terms of survival at 2 years, frequency of cardiac events (MI, PCI, CHF, recurrent angina, redo CABG) or medication usage when compared to on-pump CABG

Cardiac Transplantation

- for end-stage heart disease; majority due to ischemic cardiomyopathy (60%) or idiopathic cardiomyopathy (20%), and minority due to valvular or congenital problems
- worldwide 1-year survival is 79%, 5-year survival about 60%, annual mortality rate of 4%
- donor hearts are considered from patients up to age 50-55
- matching is according to blood type, body size and weight (should be within 25%), and HLA tissue matching (if time allows)

Indications for Surgery
- severe cardiac disability despite maximal medical therapy (recurrent hospitalizations for CHF, NYHA III or IV, peak metabolic oxygen consumption <15 ml/kg/min)
- symptomatic cardiac ischemia refractory to conventional treatment (unstable angina not amenable to CABG or angioplasty with LVEF <30%; recurrent, symptomatic ventricular arrhythmias)
- exclusion of all surgical alternatives to cardiac transplantation (revascularization for significant reversible ischemia, valve replacement for critical aortic valve disease, valve replacement or repair for severe MR)

Prerequisites
- emotionally stable with social support
- medically compliant and motivated
- contraindications: incurable malignancy, major systemic illness, irreversible major organ disease (e.g. renal, hepatic), active systemic infection (e.g. Hep C, HIV), obesity, irreversible pulmonary hypertension (pulmonary vascular resistance [PVR] >6 Wood units), severe COPD (FEV_1 <1 L), or active drug addiction or alcoholism
- typically age <70 years

Complications
- rejection
  - common, however less than 5% have serious hemodynamic compromise
  - no noninvasive tests to detect rejection, and the gold standard remains endomyocardial biopsies
  - risk of acute rejection is greatest during the first 3 months after transplant
- infection
  - leading cause of morbidity and mortality after cardiac transplantation
  - risk peaks early during the first few months after transplantation and then declines to a low persistent rate

---

EuroSCORE risk prediction algorithm for cardiac surgical mortality
S.A.M. Nashef et. al. Eur J Cardiothorac Surg 1999; 16:9

Predictor/Definition	Risk points*
Age/Peer 5 years or part thereof over 60 years	1
Sex/Female	1
Chronic pulmonary disease/Long-term use of bronchodilators or steroids for lung disease	1
Extracardiac arteriopathy/Any one or more of the following: claudication carotid occlusion or >50 percent stenosis previous or planned intervention on the abdominal aorta, limb arteries or carotids	2
Neurological dysfunction/Disease severely affecting ambulation or day-to-day functioning	2
Previous cardiac surgery Requiring opening of the pericardium	3
Serum creatinine/>200 micromol/L (2.3 mg/dL) preoperatively	2
Active endocarditis/Patient still under antibiotic treatment for endocarditis at the time of surgery Any one or more of the following ventricular tachycardia or fibrillation or aborted sudden death, preoperative cardiac massage	3
Critical preoperative state/ preoperative ventilation before arrival in the anesthetic room, preoperative inotropic support, intraaortic balloon counterpulsation preoperative acute renal failure (anuria or oliguria <10 mL/hour)	3
Unstable angina Rest angina requiring IV nitrates until arrival in the anesthetic room	2
LV dysfunction/Moderate or LV ejection fraction 30 to 50 percent	1
Poor or LV ejection fraction <30 percent	3
Recent myocardial infarct/<90 days	2
Pulmonary hypertension/Systolic pulmonary artery pressure >60 mmHg	2
Emergency operation/Carried out on referral before the beginning of the next working day	2
Other than isolated CABG/Major cardiac procedure other than or in addition to CABG	2
Surgery on thoracic aorta/For disorder of ascending, arch or descending aorta	3
Postinfarct septal rupture	4

- low risk 0-2 points (estimated mortality 1.3%)
- medium risk 3-5 points (estimated mortality 2.9%)
- high risk >6 points (estimated mortality 10.9 to 11.5%)

- allograft coronary artery disease
    - approximately 50% develop graft CAD within 5 years of transplantation
    - the most common cause of late death following transplantation
- malignancy
    - develop in 15% of cardiac transplant recipients
    - second most common cause of late death following transplantation
    - cutaneous neoplams most common, followed by non-Hodgkin's lymphoma and lung cancer
- immunosuppressive medication side effects

Ventricular Assist Devices (VADs)

- works to unload the ventricle while maintaining its output; also results in decreased myocardial oxygen consumption, permitting recovery of the myocardium that is not irreversibly injured
- can support the left (LVAD), right (RVAD) or both ventricles (BiVAD)
- indications
    - bridge to transplantation
    - postoperative mechanical support when unable to separate from cardiopulmonary bypass despite inotropic and IABP support
    - postoperative cardiogenic shock
- long-term implantation is being studied for its effectiveness in transplant and non-transplantable patients

Heart Failure

Congestive Heart Failure (CHF)

Definitions
- forward heart failure – heart unable to maintain adequate cardiac output to meet demands and/or able to do so only by elevating filling pressure
- backward heart failure – heart unable to accommodate venous return resulting in vascular congestion (systemic or pulmonary)
    - e.g.: pulmonary edema – severe pulmonary congestion $2°$ to backwards left-heart failure
- heart failure can involve left side of heart (left heart failure), right side (right heart failure) or both (biventricular failure) (See Table 10)
- components of ineffective ventricular filling (diastolic dysfunction) and/or emptying (systolic dysfunction)
- most cases associated with poor cardiac output (low-output heart failure); however, some not due to intrinsic cardiac disease but instead due to increased demand (high-out put heart failure)

Pathophysiology
- primary insults (myocyte loss, overload) → pump dysfunction, which leads to:
    - remodeling (dilatation, hypertrophy)
    - neurohumoral activation → necrosis and apoptosis
- both pathways result in further damage (restarting the cycle), and edema, tachycardia, vasoconstriction, congestion
- compensatory response to myocardial stress (perpetuate disease process)
    - increased end-systolic ventricular pressure (pressure overload) e.g. HTN, aortic stenosis → hypertrophy
    - increased end-diastolic ventricular volume (volume overload) e.g. aortic regurgitation → cardiac dilatation
- systemic response to ineffective circulating volume
    - activation of sympathetic nervous and renin-angiotensin-aldosterone systems result in
        - salt and water retention with intravascular expansion
        - increased heart rate and myocardial contractility
        - increased afterload

Dichotomies of Heart Failure:
Forward vs. Backward
Left-sided vs. Right-sided
Systolic dysfunction vs.
    Diastolic dysfunction
Low output vs. High output

Systolic Dysfunction (impaired ventricular ejection)
- impaired myocardial contractile function → decreased ejection fraction (LVEF) and stroke volume (SV) → decreased cardiac output (CO)
- findings: apex beat displaced, S3, ↑ heart size on CXR, ↓ LVEF, LV dilatation

- causes:
  - ischemic
  - non-ischemic
    - hypertension
    - diabetes mellitus
    - alcohol (and other toxins)
    - myocarditis
    - dilated cardiomyopathy

Diastolic Dysfunction (impaired ventricular filling)
- at least 1/3 of all HF patients have normal systolic function (i.e. normal ejection fraction)
- increased LV filling pressures produce venous congestion upstream (i.e. pulmonary and systemic venous congestion)
- findings: HTN, apex beat sustained, S4, normal-sized heart on CXR, LVH on ECG/echo, normal LVEF
- causes of decreased compliance:
  - transiently by ischemia (relaxation of myocardium is active and requires ATP)
  - permanently
    - severe hypertrophy (HTN, AS, HCM)
    - restrictive cardiomyopathy (RCM)
    - MI

High-Output Heart Failure
- caused by demand for increased cardiac output
- often exacerbates existing heart failure or decompensates a patient with other cardiac pathology, but is infrequently a primary cause of heart failure
- differential diagnosis: anemia, thiamine deficiency (beriberi), hyperthyroidism, A-V fistula or L-R shunting, Paget's disease of bone, renal disease, hepatic disease

Etiologies of Primary Insults
- consider predisposing, precipitating and perpetuating factors
- see sidebar for top five etiologies
- less common causes of CHF
  - toxic e.g. anthracyclines, radiation, uremia, catecholamines
  - infectious e.g. Chagas' disease (very common cause in South America), Coxsackie virus, HIV
  - endocrine e.g. hyperthyroidism, DM, acromegaly
  - infiltrative e.g. sarcoidosis, amyloidosis, hemochromatosis
  - genetic e.g. HCM, Friedreich's Ataxia, muscular dystrophy
  - congenital heart disease
  - metabolic e.g. thiamine deficiency, selenium deficiency
  - peripartum

Precipitants of Symptomatic Exacerbations
- consider natural progression of disease vs. new precipitant, and search for reversible cause
- see differential diagnosis ("HEART FAILED")
- differential can also be organized as follows:
  - new cardiac insult/disease: MI, arrythmia, valvular disease
  - new demand on CV system: hypertension, anemia, thyrotoxicosis, infection etc.
  - failure to take medications as prescribed

Table 10. Signs and Symptoms of L vs. R Heart Failure

	Left Failure	Right Failure
Low cardiac output (forward)	fatigue	(Right heart failure can mimic most of the symptoms of forward left heart failure if decreased RV output leads to LV underfilling)
	syncope	
	systemic hypotension	
	cool extremities	
	slow capillary refill	
	peripheral cyanosis	
	pulsus alternans	
	mitral regurgitation	tricuspid regurgitation
	S3	S3 (right-sided)
Venous congestion (backward)	dyspnea, orthopnea, PND	peripheral edema
	cough	elevated JVP with AJR and Kussmaul's sign
	crackles	hepatomegaly
		pulsatile liver

Sidebars:

> Use ejection fraction to grade LV dysfunction:
> Grade I (EF >60%) (Normal)
> Grade II (EF = 40-59%),
> Grade III (EF = 21-39%)
> Grade IV (EF ≤20%)

> **What are the five most common causes of CHF?**
> 1. coronary artery disease (60-70%)
> 2. HTN
> 3. idiopathic (often in the form of dilated cardiomyopathy)
> 4. valvular (e.g. AS, AR and MR)
> 5. alcohol (may cause dilated cardiomyopathy)

> **Precipitants of Heart Failure "HEART FAILED":**
> **H**TN (common)
> **E**ndocarditis/environment (e.g. heat wave)
> **A**nemia
> **R**heumatic heart disease and other valvular disease
> **T**hyrotoxicosis
> **F**ailure to take meds (very common)
> **A**rrhythmia (common)
> **I**nfection/ischemia/infarction (common)
> **L**ung problems (PE, pneumonia, COPD)
> **E**ndocrine (pheochromocytoma, hyperaldosteronism)
> **D**ietary indiscretions (common)

> The most common cause of right heart failure is left heart failure

> New York Heart Association (NYHA) Functional Classification of Heart Failure
> - Class I: ordinary physical activity does not cause symptoms of HF
> - Class II: comfortable at rest, ordinary physical activity results in symptoms
> - Class III: marked limitation of ordinary activity; less than ordinary physical activity results in symptoms
> - Class IV: inability to carry out any physical activity without discomfort; symptoms may be present at rest

Investigations
- identify and assess precipitating factors and treatable causes of CHF
- blood work – CBC, electrolytes, BUN, creatinine ± TSH, ferritin, B-natriuretic peptide (BNP)
- ECG (look for chamber enlargement, arrhythmia, ischemia/infarction)
- CXR – see Diagnostic Medical Imaging
- echocardiography – LVEF, cardiac dimensions, flow or wall motion abnormalities, valvular disease, pericardial effusion
- radionuclide angiography (MUGA) – LVEF
- myocardial perfusion scintigraphy (thallium or sestamibi SPECT)

TREATMENT

Acute Management of Pulmonary Edema ("LMNOP")
- treat acute precipitating factors (e.g. ischemia, arrhythmias)
- **L** - Lasix™ (furosemide) dose varies from 40-500 mg IV
- **M** - morphine 2-4 mg IV – decreases anxiety, venodilation (decreases preload)
- **N** - nitroglycerin (topical/IV)
- **O** - oxygen
- **P** - positive airway pressure (CPAP or BiPAP) – decreases preload and need for ventilation
- **P** - position – sit patient up with legs hanging down unless patient is hypotensive
- other vasodilators/inotropes as necessary in ICU setting
  - nitroprusside (IV)
  - hydralazine (PO)
  - sympathomimetics
    - dopamine
      - low dose causes selective renal vasodilation (high potency D_1 agonist)
      - medium dose provides inotropic support (medium potency β_1 agonist)
      - high dose increases systemic vascular resistance (SVR) (low potency α_1 agonist), which in most cases is undesirable
    - dobutamine – selective inotrope ($\beta 1$ agonist) and arterial vasodilator (α_1 antagonist)
    - phosphodiesterase inhibitors (milrinone)
      - inotropic effect and vascular smooth muscle relaxation (decreased SVR), similar to dobutamine
      - adverse effect on survival when used as long-term oral agent
- consider PA catheter to monitor pulmonary capillary wedge pressure (PCWP) if patient is unstable or a cardiac etiology is uncertain (PCWP >18 indicates likely cardiac etiology)
- mechanical ventilation as needed
- rarely used but potentially life-saving measures:
  - intra-aortic balloon pump (IABP)
  - L or R ventricular assist device (LVAD/RVAD)
  - cardiac transplant

Long Term Management of Heart Failure (ACC/AHA 2005 Guidelines)

Conservative Measures
- symptomatic measures
  - oxygen in hospital, bedrest, elevation of head of bed
- lifestyle measures (grade B evidence)
  - diet, exercise, DM control, smoking cessation, ↓ alcohol consumption, patient education, sodium and fluid restriction
- multidisciplinary heart failure clinics (grade B evidence)
  - for management of individuals at higher risk, or with recent hospitalization

Pharmacological Therapy
- vasodilators
  - ACEIs: standard of care – slow progression and improve survival (CONSENSUS, SOLVD, SAVE trials)
    - all symptomatic patients functional class II-IV (grade A)
    - all asymptomatic patients with LVEF <40% (grade A)
    - post-MI (see IHD section)
    - target dose as used in mortality trials, or maximum tolerated dose
  - angiotensin II receptor blockers (ELITE-II, CHARM, Val-HeFT trials)
    - second line to ACEI if not tolerated (grade B), or as adjunct to ACEI if β-blockers not tolerated (grade A)
  - hydralazine and nitrates (Ve-HeFT-I trial)

"The best findings for detecting increased filling pressure are jugular venous distension and radiographic redistribution."

"The best findings for detecting systolic dysfunction are an abnormal apical impulse, radiographic cardiomegaly, Q-waves or LBBB on an electrocardiogram."

"Diastolic dysfunction is difficult to diagnose but is associated with elevated blood pressure during heart failure."

(Can the Clinical Examination Diagnose Left-Sided Heart Failure in Adults? JAMA 1997; 277:1712-99)

Acute Treatment of Pulmonary Edema
Lasix™
Morphine
Nitroglycerin
Oxygen
Positive airway pressure and **P**osition upright

- ◆ second line to ACEI, decrease in mortality not as great as with ACEI (Ve-HeFT-II trial)
- β-blockers: standard of care – slow progression and improve survival (metoprolol: MERIT; carvedilol: US-CARVEDILOL, COPERNICUS trials)
  - ▪ class I-III with LVEF <40% (grade A)
  - ▪ stable class IV patients (grade A)
  - ▪ **note: should be used cautiously, titrate slowly because may initially worsen CHF; not routinely used in acute CHF**
- aldosterone antagonists: mortality benefit in severe CHF (spironolactone: RALES; eplerenone: EPHESUS trial)
  - ▪ spironolactone for class IIIb and IV CHF already on ACEI and loop diuretic (grade A)
  - ▪ eplerenone may be considered if intolerable endocrine side effects
  - ▪ note: potential for life threatening hyperkalemia
    - ◆ monitor K after initiation and avoid if Cr >220 μmol/L or K >5.2 mmol/L
- diuretics: symptom control, management of fluid overload
  - ▪ furosemide (40-500 mg OD) for potent diuresis
  - ▪ metolazone may be used with furosemide to increase diuresis
  - ▪ furosemide, metalozone, and thiazides oppose the hyperkalemia induced by β-blockers, ACEIs, ARBs, and aldosterone antagonists
- inotropes: digoxin improves symptoms and decreases hospitalizations, no effect on mortality (DIG trial)
  - ▪ indications: patient in sinus rhythm and symptomatic on ACEI (grade A), or CHF and atrial fibrillation (grade B)
  - ▪ patients on digitalis glycosides may worsen if these are withdrawn
- anti-arrhythmic drugs: for use in CHF with arrhythmia
  - ▪ can use amiodarone, β-blocker, or digitalis (grade B)
- anticoagulants: warfarin for prevention of thromboembolic events
  - ▪ prior thromboembolic event or atrial fibrillation (grade B)
  - ▪ possible benefit in other patients with LVEF <30% or LV thrombus (controversial)
- CCBs (equivocal effect on survival) – not currently recommended
- selected drugs contraindicated in CHF:
  - ▪ NSAIDs, class I/III antiarrhythmic agents, metformin, thiazolidinediones, cGMP phosphodiesterase inhibitors (sildenafil, vardenafil, tadalafil) with borderline low blood pressure

> **Chronic Treament of CHF**
>
> ACE inhibitors*
> Beta blockers*
> ± Aldosterone antagonists* (if severe CHF)
> Diuretic
> ± Inotrope
> ± Antiarrythmic
> ± Anticoagulant
>
> * = Mortality Benefit

Procedural Interventions
- resynchronization therapy: symptomatic improvement with biventricular pacemaker (MIRACLE trial)
  - ▪ consider if QRS >130 ms, LVEF <35%, and severe symptoms despite optimal therapy (grade B)
  - ▪ greatest benefit likely with marked LV enlargement, MR, QRS >150 ms, high diuretic requirement
- ICD: mortality benefit in 1° and 2° prevention of Sudden Cardiac Death (MADIT-I, MUSTT, MADIT-II trials)
  - ▪ prior MI, optimal medical therapy, LVEF <30%, clinically stable (grade B)
  - ▪ prior MI, NSVT, LVEF 30-40%, EPS inducible VT (grade B)
- LVAD/RVAD (see *Ventricular Assist Devices*, C32)
- cardiac transplantation (see *Cardiac Transplantation*, C31)
- valve repair if patient is a good surgical candidate and has significant valve disease contributing to CHF (see *Valvular Heart Disease*, C39)

Sleep-Disordered Breathing

- 45-55% of patients with CHF have sleep disturbances, including Cheyne-Stokes breathing and sleep apnea (central or obstructive)
- associated with a worse prognosis and greater LV dysfunction
- nasal continuous positive airway pressure (CPAP) is effective in treating Cheyne-Stokes respiration/sleep apnea with improvement in cardiac function and symptoms

Myocardial Disease

Definition of Cardiomyopathy (CMP):
- intrinsic or primary myocardial disease not 2° to congenital, hypertensive, coronary, valvular, or pericardial disease
- usually classified as dilated, hypertrophic or restrictive cardiomyopathy (functional classification)
- LV dysfunction 2° to MI often termed "ischemic cardiomyopathy", but this is not a true cardiomyopathy (i.e. primary myocardial disorder) since the primary pathology is CAD

Dilated Cardiomyopathy (DCM)

Definition
- dilation and impaired systolic function of one or both ventricles

Etiology
- idiopathic (presumed viral or genetic) ~50% of DCM
- alcohol
- familial
- uncontrolled tachycardia
- collagen vascular disease: SLE, PAN, dermatomyositis, progressive systemic sclerosis
- infectious: viral (Coxsackie B, HIV), Chagas disease, Lyme disease, Rickettsial diseases, acute rheumatic fever
- neuromuscular disease: Duchenne muscular dystrophy, myotonic dystrophy, Friedreich's ataxia
- metabolic: uremia, nutritional deficiency (thiamine, selenium, carnitine)
- endocrine: hyper/hypothyroidism, DM, pheochromocytoma
- peripartum
- toxic: cocaine, heroin, glue sniffing, organic solvents
- drugs: chemotherapies (anthracycline, cyclophosphamide), anti-retrovirals, chloroquine, clozapine
- radiation induced

Signs and Symptoms
- may present as
    - CHF
    - systemic or pulmonary emboli
    - arrhythmias
    - sudden death (major cause of mortality due to fatal arrhythmia)

Investigations
- ECG – variable ST-T wave abnormalities, poor R wave progression, conduction defects (e.g. BBB), arrhythmias (non-sustained VT)
- CXR – global cardiomegaly (globular heart), signs of CHF
- echo – 4-chamber enlargement, global hypokinesis, depressed LVEF, MR and TR, mural thrombi
- endomyocardial biopsy – not routine, used to rule out a treatable cause
- angiography – in selected patients to exclude ischemic HD

Management
- treat underlying disease: e.g. abstinence from EtOH
- treat CHF: see *Heart Failure*, C32
- thromboembolism prophylaxis: anticoagulation with warfarin
    - indicated for: AFib, history of thromboembolism or documented thrombus
    - LVEF <30% (controversial)
- treat symptomatic or serious arrhythmias
- immunize against influenza and *S. pneumoniae*
- consider surgical options (eg. LVAD, transplant, volume reduction surgery) in appropriate candidates with severe, refractory disease

Prognosis
- depends on etiology
    - better with reversible underlying cause, worst with infiltrative diseases, HIV, drug-induced
- cause of death usually CHF or sudden death 2° to ventricular arrhythmias
- systemic emboli are significant source of morbidity

Myocarditis

Definition
- inflammatory process involving the myocardium ranging from acute to chronic; an important cause of dilated cardiomyopathy

Etiology
- idiopathic
- infectious
  - viral (most common): Coxsackie B, echovirus, poliovirus, HIV, mumps
  - bacterial: *S. aureus, C. perfringens, C. diphtheriae, Mycoplasma, Rickettsia*
  - fungi
  - spirochetal (Lyme disease – *Borrelia burgdorferi*)
  - Chagas disease (*Trypanosoma cruzi*), toxoplasmosis
- toxic: catecholamines, chemotherapy, cocaine
- hypersensitivity, eosinophilic: drugs (antibiotics, diuretics, lithium, clozapine), insect/snake bites
- systemic diseases: collagen vascular diseases (SLE, RA, others), sarcoidosis, autoimmune
- other: giant cell myocarditis, acute rheumatic fever

Signs and Symptoms
- constitutional illness
- acute CHF
- chest pain – due to pericarditis or cardiac ischemia
- arrhythmias
- systemic or pulmonary emboli
- sudden death

Investigations
- ECG – non-specific ST-T changes ± conduction defects
- bloodwork
  - increased CK, troponin, LDH, and AST with acute myocardial necrosis ± increased WBC, ESR, ANA, rheumatoid factor, complement levels
  - blood culture, viral titres and cold agglutinins for *Mycoplasma*
- CXR – enlarged cardiac silhouette
- echo – dilated, hypokinetic chambers, segmental wall motion abnormalities
- myocardial biopsy (in limited cases)

Management
- supportive care
- restrict physical activity
- treat CHF
- treat arrhythmias
- anticoagulation
- treat underlying cause if possible

Prognosis
- usually self-limited and often unrecognized, many recover
- sudden death in young adults
- may progress to dilated cardiomyopathy
- few may have recurrent or chronic myocarditis

Table 11. Summary Table for CHF and Myocardial Disease

Congestive Heart Failure & Myocardial Disease				
Systolic Heart Failure		**Diastolic Heart Failure**		
Dilated Cardiomyopathy	**Secondary Causes**	**Hypertrophic Cardiomyopathy**	**Restrictive Cardiomyopathy**	**Secondary Causes**
Idiopathic, infectious (e.g. myocarditis), Alcohol, Familial, Collagen vascular disease, etc.	Coronary artery disease, MI, Diabetes, Valvular (e.g. AR, MR)	Genetic disorder affecting cardiac sarcomeres (most common cause of sudden cardiac death in young athletes)	Amyloidosis, Sarcoidosis, Scleroderma, Hemochromatosis, Fabry's, Pompe's Disease, Loeffler's, etc.	Hypertension, Diabetes, Valvular (e.g. AS), Post-MI, Transiently by ischemia, etc.

Hypertrophic Cardiomyopathy (HCM)

Definition
- defined as unexplained ventricular hypertrophy (not due to systemic HTN or AS)
  - most causes involve asymmetric pattern of hypertrophy (septal hypertrophy most common)

Etiology and Pathophysiology
- histopathologic features are myocyte disarray, hypertrophy, and interstitial fibrosis
- cause is felt to be a genetic defect involving one of the cardiac sarcomeric proteins (>200 mutations associated with AD inheritance, incomplete penetrance)
- prevalence of 1/500 - 1/1000 in general population

Hemodynamic Classification
- hypertrophic obstructive cardiomyopathy (HOCM): dynamic LV outflow tract (LVOT) obstruction, either resting or provocable
- non-obstructive hypertrophic cardiomyopathy: no LVOT obstruction
- many patients have diastolic dysfunction (impaired filling, decreased ventricular compliance)

Signs and Symptoms (of HOCM)
- clinical manifestations: asymptomatic (common therefore screening important), SOBOE, angina, presyncope/syncope (due to LV outflow obstruction or arrhythmia), CHF, arrhythmias, SCD
- pulses: rapid upstroke, bifid carotid pulse (in HOCM)
- precordial palpation: PMI localized, sustained, double impulse, 'triple ripple' (triple apical impulse in HOCM), LV lift
- precordial auscultation: normal or paradoxically split S2, S4, harsh systolic diamond-shaped murmur at LLSB or apex, enhanced by squat to standing or Valsalva (murmur secondary to LVOT obstruction as compared to aortic stenosis); often with pansystolic murmur due to mitral regurgitation

Investigations
- ECG – LVH, high voltages across precordium, prominent Q waves or tall R wave in V1, P wave abnormalities
- echo – asymmetric septal hypertrophy (less commonly apical), systolic anterior movement of mitral valve and MR
- cardiac catheterization (usually performed only when patient being considered for invasive therapy)

Management
- avoid factors which increase obstruction, including volume depletion and strenuous exertion
- treatment of HOCM
  - medical agents: β-blockers, disopyramide, verapamil (only in patients with no resting/provocable obstruction)
- patients with drug-refractory symptoms:
  - surgical myectomy
  - septal ethanol ablation
  - dual-chamber pacing
- treatment of ventricular arrhythmias – amiodarone or ICD
- first-degree relatives of patients with HCM should be screened annually during adolescence (physical, ECG, 2D echo), then serially every 5 years

Prognosis
- potential complications: AFib, VT, CHF, sudden death (most common cause of SCD in young athletes)
- major risk factors for sudden death
  - history of survived cardiac arrest/sustained VT
  - family history of multiple premature sudden deaths
  - other factors associated with increased risk of sudden cardiac death:
    - syncope
    - non-sustained VT on ambulatory monitoring
    - marked ventricular hypertrophy (max wall thickness ≥30 mm)

Restrictive Cardiomyopathy (RCM)

Definition
- restricted ventricular filling in a non-dilated, non-hypertrophied ventricle 2° to myocardial abnormality (stiffening, fibrosis and/or decreased compliance)

Etiology
- infiltrative: amyloidosis, sarcoidosis
- non-infiltrative: scleroderma, idiopathic myocardial fibrosis
- storage diseases: hemochromatosis, Fabry's disease, glycogen storage diseases
- endomyocardial:
    - endomyocardial fibrosis, Loeffler's endocarditis or eosinophilic endomyocardial disease
    - radiation heart disease
    - carcinoid syndrome (may have associated TV or PV dysfunction)

Clinical Manifestations
- CHF (usually with preserved LV systolic function), arrhythmias
- elevated JVP with prominent x and y descents, Kussmaul's sign
- S4

Investigations
- ECG – low voltage, non-specific, diffuse ST-T wave changes ± nonischemic Q waves
- CXR – mild cardiac enlargement
- echo
- cardiac catheterization – ↑ end-diastolic ventricular pressures
- endomyocardial biopsy – to determine etiology (especially for infiltrative RCM)

Management
- exclude constrictive pericarditis
- treat underlying disease
- supportive care and treatment for CHF, arrhythmias
- heart transplant – might be considered for CHF refractory to medical therapy

Prognosis
- depends on etiology

Valvular Heart Disease

Infective Endocarditis (IE)

- see Infectious Diseases

- AHA 2007 guidelines recommend IE prophylaxis
    - only for patients with prosthetic valve material, past history of IE, certain types of congenital heart disease or cardiact transplant recipients who develop valvulopathy only for the following procedures
        - dental
        - respiratory tract
        - procedures on infected skin/skin structures/MSK structures
        - *not GI/GU procedures specifically*

Rheumatic Fever

- see Pediatrics

Prognosis
- acute complications: myocarditis (DCM/CHF), conduction abnormalities (sinus tachycardia, AFib), valvulitis (acute MR), pericarditis (not usually constrictive pericarditis)
- chronic complications: rheumatic valvular heart disease – fibrous thickening, adhesion, calcification of valve leaflets resulting in stenosis/regurgitation, increased risk of IE ± thromboembolism
- onset of symptoms usually after 10-20 year latency from acute carditis of rheumatic fever
- mitral valve most commonly affected

Choice of Valve Prosthesis

Table 12. Mechanical Valve vs. Bioprosthetic Valve

Mechanical Valve	Bioprosthetic Valve
• Good durability	• Limited long-term durability (mitral<aortic)
• Less preferred in small aortic root (stenotic)	• Good flow in small aortic root sizes
• Increased risk of thromboembolism (1-3%/year): long-term anticoagulation with warfarin	• Decreased risk of thromboembolism: long-term anticoagulation not needed for aortic valves
• Target INR aortic valves: 2.0-3.0 mitral valves: 2.3-3.5	• Some recommendation for limited anticoagulation for mitral valves
• Increased risk of hemorrhage: 1-2%/year	• Decreased risk of hemorrhage

Summary of Valvular Diseases

Table 13. Valvular Heart Disease

A bedside clinical prediction rule for detecting moderate or severe aortic stenosis
Type: Blinded cross sectional study
Who: 124 patients of an ambulatory cardiology clinic. Patients were examined for: 1) murmur over the right clavicle; 2) murmur loudest at second right intercostal space 3) reduced intensity of S2; 4) reduced volume of the carotid pulse 5) delayed carotid upstroke.
Methods: Patients were examined by blinded investigators, and the clinical examination findings were compared to findings on subsequent echocardiography. Moderate to severe aortic stenosis was defined as a valve area < 1.2 cm² or a peak intensity gradient of > 25 mmHg.
Results: Absence of a murmur over the right clavicle ruled out aortic stenosis while presence of ≥3 of the 4 associated symptoms ruled in aortic stenosis (LR=40).
Conclusions: Bedside techniques can accurately rule in and rule out moderate to severe aortic stenosis.
Etchells E, Glenns V, Shadowitz S, Bell C, Siu S. *J Gen Intern Med.* 1998 Oct;13(10):699-704. Department of Medicine, Toronto Hospital, Ont, Canada.

AS

Anas Nader ©2009

Etiology
Congenital (bicuspid, unicuspid valve), calcification (wear and tear), rheumatic disease
AVA: N=3-4 cm²
severe AS=<1.0 cm²
critical AS <0.5 cm²

Pathophysiology
Outflow obstruction —> increased EDP —> concentric LVH —> LV failure —> CHF, subendocardial ischemia

Symptoms
Exertional angina, syncope, dyspnea, PND, orthopnea, peripheral edema

Physical Exam
Narrow pulse pressure, brachial-radial delay, pulsus parvus et tardus, sustained PMI
Auscultation: crescendo-decrescendo SEM radiating to R clavicle & carotid, musical quality at apex (Gallavardin phenomenon), S4, soft S2 w/paradoxical splitting, S3 (late)

Investigations
ECG: LVH & strain, LBBB, LAE, AFib
CXR: post-stenotic aortic root dilatation, calcified valve, LVH, LAE, CHF
ECHO: reduced valve area, pressure gradient, LVH, reduced LV function

Treatment
Asymptomatic: serial echos, avoid exertion
Symptomatic: avoid nitrates/arterial dilators & ACEIs in severe AS
Surgery if: symptomatic or LV dysfunction

Surgical Options
Valve replacement : aortic rheumatic valve disease & trileaflet valve
–pregnancy
–balloon valvuloplasty (in young)

AR

Anas Nader ©2009

Etiology
Supravalvular: aortic root disease (Marfan's, atherosclerosis & dissecting aneurysm, connective tissue disease)
Valvular: congenital (bicuspid AV, large VSD), IE
Acute Onset: IE, aortic dissection, trauma, failed prosthetic valve

Pathophysiology
Volume overload —> LV dilatation —> increased SV, high sBP & low dBP —> increased wall tension —> pressure overload —> LVH (low dBP —> decreased coronary perfusion)

Symptoms
Usually only becomes symptomatic late in disease when LV failure develops
Dyspnea, orthopnea, PND, syncope, angina

Physical Exam
Waterhammer pulse, bisferiens pulse, femoral-brachial sBP > 20 (Hill's test: wide pulse pressure), hyperdynamic apex, displaced PMI, heaving apex
Auscultation: early decrescendo diastolic murmur at LLSB (cusp) or RLSB (aortic root), best heard sitting, leaning forward, on full expiration, soft S1, absent S2, S3 (late)

Investigations
ECG: LVH, LAE
CXR: LVH, LAE, aortic root dilatation
echo/TTE: quantify AR, leaflet or aortic root anomalies
Cath: if >40 yrs and surgical candidate to assess for ischemic heart disease
Exercise testing: hypotension with exercise

Treatment
Asymptomatic: serial echos, afterload reduction (ACEIs if normal LV function)
Symptomatic: avoid exertion, treat CHF
Surgery if: NYHA class III-IV CHF, LVEF < 50% with/without symptoms, increasing LV size

Surgical Options
Valve replacement:–most patients
Valve repair: limited role, repair of valves to improve coaptation
Aortic root replace (Bentall proced.): when ascending aortic aneurysm present, valved conduit used

MS

Anas Nader ©2009

Etiology
Rheumatic disease most common cause; congenital (rare)
Severe MS is MVA <1.2 cm²

Pathophysiology
MS —> fixed CO & LAE —> increased LA pressure —> pulmonary vascular resistance and CHF; worst with AFib (no atrial kick), tachycardia (decreased atrial emptying time) & pregnancy (increased preload)

Symptoms
SOBOE, orthopnea, fatigue, palpitations, peripheral edema, malar flush, pinched and blue facies (severe MS)

Physical Exam
AFib, no "a" wave on JVP, left parasternal lift, palpable diastolic thrill at apex
Auscultation: mid-diastolic rumble at apex, best with bell in LLD position following exertion, loud S1, OS following loud P2 (heard best during expiration), long murmur & short A2-OS interval correlate with worse MS

MR

Anas Nader ©2009

Etiology
Mitral valve prolapse
Congenital cleft leaflets, LV dilatation/aneurysm (CHF, DCM, myocarditis), IE abscess, Marfan's syndrome, HOCM, acute MI, myxoma, MV annulus calcification, chordae/papillary muscle trauma/ischemia/rupture, rheumatic disease

Pathophysiology
Reduced CO —> increased LV & LA pressure —> LV & LA dilatation —> CHF & pulmonary HTN

Symptoms
Dyspnea, PND, orthopnea, palpitations, peripheral edema

Physical Exam
Displaced, hyperdynamic apex, left parasternal lift, apical thrill
Auscultation: holosystolic murmur at apex, radiating to axilla +/- mid-diastolic rumble, loud S2 (if pulmonary HTN), S3

Table 13. Valvular Heart Disease (continued)

MS (continued)

Investigations
ECG: NSR/AFib, LAE (P mitrale), RVH, RAD
CXR: LAE, CHF, MV calcification
echo/TTE: valvular anomalies
Cath: concurrent CAD if >40 yrs (male) or >50 yrs (female)

Treatment
Avoid exertion, fever (increased LA pressure), treat AFib and CHF, increase diastolic filling time (β-blockers, digitalis)
Surgery if: NYHA class III-IV CHF and failure of medical therapy (usually MVA <1.2 cm²)

Surgical Options
Percutaneous balloon valvuloplasty: young rheumatic pts & good leaflet morphology, asymptom pts with mod-sev MS, new-onset AFib, pulmon HTN
Contraindication: Left atrial thrombus, mod-sev MR
Open Mitral Commissurotomy: If mild calcif +leaflet/chordal thickening
–restenosis in 50% pts in 8yrs
Valve replacement: mod-sev calcif & sev scarred leaflets

TS

Etiology
Rheumatic disease, congenital, carcinoid, fibroelastosis; usually accompanied by MS

S_1 S_2 os S_1

Anas Nader ©2009

Pathophysiology
Increased RA pressure —> right heart failure —> decreased CO and fixed on exertion

Symptoms
Peripheral edema, fatigue, palpitations

Physical Exam
Prominent "a" waves in JVP, +ve abdominojugular reflex, Kussmaul's sign, diastolic rumble 4th left intercostals space

Investigations
ECG: RAE
CXR: dilatation of RA without pulmonary artery enlargement
Echo: diagnostic

Treatment
Preload reduction (diuretics)
Surgery if: usually only if other surgery needed (e.g. MVR)

Surgical Options
Commissurotomy
Valve Replace:
–if severely diseased valve
–bioprosthesis preferred

PS

Etiology
Usually congenital, rheumatic disease (rare), carcinoid

click

S_1 S_2 S_1

Anas Nader ©2009

Pathophysiology
Increased RV pressure —> RV hypertrophy —> right heart failure

Symptoms
Chest pain, syncope, fatigue, peripheral edema

Physical Exam
Systolic murmur at 2nd LICS accentuated by inspiration, pulmonary ejection click, right-sided S4

Investigations
ECG: RVH
CXR: prominent pulmonary arteries enlarged RV
echo: diagnostic

Treatment
Balloon valvuloplasty if severe symptoms

Surgical Options
Percutaneous or open balloon valvuloplasty

MR (continued)

Investigations
ECG: LAE, left atrial delay (bifid P waves), +/- LVH
CXR: LVH, LAE, pulmonary venous HTN
echo: severity of MR, LV function, leaflets
Swan-Ganz: prominent LA "v" wave

Treatment
Asymptomatic: serial echos
Symptomatic: decrease preload (diuretics), decrease afterload (ACEIs) for severe MR & poor surgical candidate; stabilize acute MR with vasodilators b/f surgery
Surgery if: acute MR with CHF, papillary muscle rupture, NYHA class III-IV CHF, AFib, LVEF <60%, increasing LV size, earlier surgery if valve repairable

Surgical Options
Valve repair:– >75% of pts with MR & myxomatous MV disease (MVP)
–annuloplasty rings, leaflet repair, chordae transfers/shorten/replacement
Valve replacement: failure of repair, heavily calcified annulus
Advantage of Repair:low rate of endocarditis, no anticoagulation, less chance of re-operation

TR

Etiology
RV dilatation, IE (IV drug use), rheumatic disease, congenital (Ebstein anomaly), carcinoid

S_1 S_2 S_1

Anas Nader ©2009

Pathophysiology
RV dilatation —> TR —> further RV dilatation —> right heart failure

Symptoms
Peripheral edema, fatigue, palpitations

Physical Exam
"cv" waves in JVP, +ve abdominojugular reflux, Kussmaul's sign, holosystolic murmur at LLSB accentuated by inspiration, left parasternal lift

Investigations
ECG: RAE, RVH, AFib
CXR: RAE, RV enlargement
echo: diagnostic

Treatment
Preload reduction (diuretics)
Surgery if: usually only if other surgery needed (e.g. MVR)

Surgical Options
Annuloplasty, i.e. repair (rarely replacement)

PR

Etiology
Pulmonary HTN, IE, rheumatic disease, tetrology of Fallot, post-repair

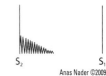

S_1 S_2 S_1

Anas Nader ©2009

Pathophysiology
Increased RV volume —> increased wall tension —> RV hypertrophy —> right heart failure

Symptoms
Chest pain, syncope, fatigue, peripheral edema

Physical Exam
Early diastolic murmur at LLSB, Graham Steell (diastolic) murmur 2nd and 3rd LICS increasing with inspiration

Investigations
ECG: RVH
CXR: prominent pulmonary arteries if pulmonary HTN; enlarged RV
echo: diagnositc

Treatment
Rarely requires treatment; valve replacement if severe

Surgical Options
Pulmonary valve replacement

Table 13. Valvular Heart Disease (continued)

Mitral Valve Prolapse

Etiology
Myxomatous degeneration of chordae; thick, bulky leaflets that crowd orifice; Marfan's syndrome; pectus excavatum, straight back syndrome, other MSK abnormalities; <3% of population, F=M

Pathophysiology
MV displaced into LA during systole; no causal mechanisms found for symptoms

Symptoms
Prolonged, stabbing chest pain, dyspnea, anxiety/panic, palpitations, fatigue, presyncope

Physical Exam
Auscultation: mid-systolic click (billowing of mitral leaflet into LA; tensing of redundant valve tissue); mid to late systolic murmur at apex, accentuated by Valsalva or squat-to-stand maneuvers

Investigations
ECG: non-specific ST-T wave changes, PSVT, ventricular ectopy
Echo: systolic displacement of thickened MV leaflets into LA

Treatment
Asymptomatic: no treatment; reassurance
Symptomatic: ß-blockers and avoidance of stimulants (caffeine) for significant palpitations, anticoagulation if systemic emboli

Surgical Options
None unless symptomatic and significant MR

Pericardial Disease

Acute Pericarditis

Etiology of Pericarditis/Pericardial Effusion
- idiopathic is most common: usually presumed to be viral
- infectious
  - viral: Coxsackie virus A, B (most common), echovirus
  - bacterial: *S. pneumoniae, S. aureus*
  - TB
  - fungal: histoplasmosis, blastomycosis
- post-MI: acute (direct extension of myocardial inflammation, 1-7 days), Dressler's syndrome (autoimmune, 2-8 weeks)
- post-cardiac surgery (e.g. CABG), other trauma
- metabolic: uremia (common), hypothyroidism
- neoplasm: Hodgkin's, breast, lung, renal cell carcinoma, melanoma
- collagen vascular disease: SLE, polyarteritis, RA, scleroderma
- vascular: dissecting aneurysm
- other: drugs (e.g. hydralazine), radiation, infiltrative disease (sarcoid)

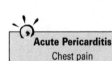

Acute Pericarditis
Chest pain
Friction rub
ECG changes

Signs and Symptoms
- diagnostic triad: chest pain, friction rub, and ECG changes
- pleuritic chest pain – alleviated by sitting up and leaning forward
- pericardial friction rub – may be uni-, bi- or triphasic
- ± fever, malaise

Investigations
- ECG – initially diffuse elevated ST segments ± depressed PR segment, the elevation in the ST segment is concave upwards → 2-5 days later ST isoelectric with T wave flattening and inversion
- CXR – normal heart size, pulmonary infiltrates
- Echo – assess pericardial effusion

Treatment
- treat the underlying disease
- anti-inflammatory agents (high dose NSAIDs/ASA, steroids if severe or recurrent); analgesics

Prognosis
- complications: recurrence, atrial arrhythmia, pericardial effusion, tamponade, constrictive pericarditis (uncommon)

Pericardial Effusion

Etiology
- transudative (serous)
  - CHF, hypoalbuminemia/hypoproteinemia, hypothyroidism
- exudative (serosanguinous or bloody)
  - causes similar to the causes of acute pericarditis
  - may develop acute effusion secondary to hemopericardium (trauma, post MI myocardial rupture, aortic dissection)
- physiological consequences depend on type and volume of effusion, rate of effusion development, and underlying cardiac disease

Signs and Symptoms
- may be asymptomatic or similar to acute pericarditis
- dyspnea, cough
- extra-cardiac (esophageal/recurrent laryngeal nerve/tracheo-bronchial/phrenic nerve irritation)
- JVP increased with dominant "x" descent
- arterial pulse normal to decreased volume, decreased pulse pressure
- auscultation: distant heart sounds ± rub

Investigations
- ECG – low voltage, flat T waves
- CXR – cardiomegaly, rounded cardiac contour
- Echo (procedure of choice) – fluid in pericardial sac
- pericardiocentesis – definitive method of determining transudate vs exudate, identify infectious agents, neoplastic involvement

Treatment
- mild: frequent observation with serial echocardiograms, treat the cause, anti-inflammatory agents for inflammation
- severe: may develop cardiac tamponade

Cardiac Tamponade

Etiology
- major complication of rapidly accumulating pericardial effusion; cardiac tamponade is a clinical diagnosis
- any cause of pericarditis but especially trauma, malignancy, uremia, idiopathic, proximal aortic dissection with rupture

Pathophysiology
- high intra-pericardial pressure → decreased venous return → decreased diastolic ventricular filling → decreased CO → hypotension & venous congestion

Signs and Symptoms
- tachypnea, dyspnea, shock
- pulsus paradoxus (inspiratory fall in systolic BP >10 mmHg during quiet breathing)
- JVP "x" descent only, absent "y" descent
- hepatic congestion/peripheral edema

Investigations
- ECG – electrical alternans (pathognomonic variation in R wave amplitude), low voltage
- Echo – pericardial effusion, compression of cardiac chambers (RA and RV) in diastole
- cardiac catheterization

Treatment
- pericardiocentesis – echo or ECG-guided
- pericardiotomy
- avoid diuretics and vasodilators (these decrease venous return to already under-filled RV → decrease LV preload → decrease CO)
- fluid administration may temporarily increase CO
- treat underlying cause

Classic quartet of tamponade: hypotension, increased JVP, tachycardia, pulsus paradoxus.

Beck's triad: hypotension, increased JVP, muffled heart sounds.

Constrictive Pericarditis

Etiology
- chronic pericarditis resulting in fibrosed, thickened, adherent, and/or calcified pericardium
- any cause of acute pericarditis may result in chronic pericarditis
- major causes are post-viral, TB, radiation, uremia, post-cardiac surgery, idiopathic

Signs and Symptoms
- dyspnea, fatigue, palpitations
- abdominal pain
- may mimic CHF (especially right-sided HF)
  - ascites, hepatosplenomegaly, edema
- increased JVP, Kussmaul's sign (paradoxical increase in JVP with inspiration), Friedreich's sign (prominent "y" descent)
- BP usually normal
- precordial examination: ± pericardial knock (early diastolic sound)
- see Table 14 for differentiation from cardiac tamponade

Investigations
- ECG – non-specific: low voltage, flat T wave, ± AFib
- CXR – pericardial calcification, effusions
- Echo/CT/MRI – pericardial thickening
- cardiac catheterization

Treatment
- medical: diuretics, salt restriction
- surgical: pericardiectomy (if refractory to medical therapy)

Table 14. Differentiation of Constrictive Pericarditis vs. Cardiac Tamponade

Characteristic	Constrictive Pericarditis	Tamponade
JVP	"y" > "x"	"x" > "y"
Kussmaul's sign	present	absent
pulsus paradoxus	uncommon	always
pericardial knock	present	absent
hypotension	variable	severe

Congenital Cardiac Disease

- see Pediatrics. Note: more adults than children now live with congenital heart defects

VASCULAR DISEASE

Peripheral Arterial Disease

Acute Arterial Occlusion/Insufficiency

Definition
- acute occlusion/rupture of a peripheral artery
- urgent management required: >6 hours results in irreversible ischemia and myonecrosis
- lower extremity > upper extremity; femoropopliteal > aortoiliac

Etiology
- embolus
  - cardiac embolus (80-90%): history of MI <3 months, valvular disease, AFib, cardiomyopathy, endocarditis, atrial myxoma
  - arterial embolus: proximal arterial aneurysm, atheroembolism

- venous embolus (intracardiac shunt); may have Hx of OCP use
- Hx of TIAs/strokes
- thrombus
  - atherosclerotic, congenital anomaly, infection, hematological disorders and stasis
- trauma
  - arterial catheterization, intra-arterial drug injection induced, aortic dissection, severe venous thrombophlebitis, prolonged immobilization
- idiopathic

Clinical Features
- general
  - pain in lower extremity progressing within hours to a feeling of cold, numbness, loss of function and sensation
  - symptoms (6 **P**'s) – all may not be present
    - Pain: absent in 20% of cases due to prompt onset of anesthesia and paralysis
    - Pallor: within a few hours becomes mottled cyanosis
    - Paresthesia: light touch (small fibres) lost first then sensory modalities (large fibres)
    - Paralysis/Power loss: most important, heralds impending gangrene
    - Polar (cold)
    - Pulselessness: not reliable
- embolus vs. thrombus – dramatically different treatment
- see Table 15

Table 15. Differentiation of arterial embolism and thrombosis

Presentation	Embolus	Thrombus
Onset	Acute	Progressive, acute-on-chronic
Loss of function/sensation	Prominent	Less profound
Hx of claudication	No	Yes
Atrophic changes	No	Yes
Contralateral limb pulses	Yes	Decreased or absent

Investigations
- CXR, ECG, arteriography

Treatment
- immediate heparinization with 5000 IU bolus and continuous infusion to maintain PTT >60 seconds
- absent power and sensation – emergent revascularization
- present power and sensation – work-up (including angiogram)
- definitive treatment
  - embolus: embolectomy
  - thrombus: thrombectomy ± graft, ± bypass
  - irreversible ischemia: amputation
- identify and treat underlying cause
- continue heparin post-op, start warfarin post-op day 1 for 3 months

Complications
- compartment syndrome with prolonged ischemia; requires fasciotomy
- renal failure and multi-organ failure due to toxic metabolites from ischemic muscle

Prognosis
- 12-15% mortality rate
- 5-40% morbidity rate (amputation)

Chronic Arterial Occlusion/Insufficiency

Etiology
- predominantly due to atherosclerosis: primarily lower extremities with symptoms related to the location of obstruction

Risk Factors
- major: smoking, DM, hyperhomocysteinemia
- minor: HTN, hyperlipidemia, family history, obesity, sedentary lifestyle, male gender

Clinical Features
- claudication:
  1. pain with exertion: usually in calves or any exercising group

Signs of peripheral vascular insufficiency "SICVD":
Symmetry of leg musculature
Integrity of skin
Colour of toe nails
Varicose veins
Distribution of hair

2. relieved by short rest: 2 to 5 minutes, and no postural changes necessary
3. reproducible: same distance to elicit pain, same location of pain, same amount of rest to relieve pain
- pulses may be absent at some locations, bruits may be present
- signs of poor perfusion: hair loss, hypertrophic nails, atrophic muscle, skin ulcerations and infections, slow capillary refill, prolonged pallor with elevation and rubor on dependency, venous troughing (collapse of superficial veins of foot)
- other manifestations of atherosclerosis: CVD, CAD, impotence, splanchnic ischemia

Differential Diagnosis
- osteoarthritis (OA): worse at night and varies day-to-day
- neurogenic claudication: due to spinal stenosis or radiculopathy; pain very similar but relieved by longer rest and postural changes
- varicose veins: localized pain, typically less severe, after exercise and never at rest; related to the presence and site of varices
- inflammatory processes: Buerger's disease, Takayasu's arteritis
- other: popliteal entrapment (e.g. tumour, Baker's cyst), radiation injury, remote trauma

Investigations
- non-invasive
  - ankle-brachial index (ABI) (grade IA recommendation): measure brachial and ankle pressures bilaterally (use highest value) generally, ABI <0.90 abnormal, rest pain appears at <0.3 (see Table 16)

Table 16. Ankle-Brachial indices and degrees of ischemia

ABI recording	Degree of Ischemia
>0.95	normal/no ischemia
0.85 – 0.94	mild
0.50 – 0.84	moderate
0.26 – 0.49	severe
<0.25	consider limb salvage
>1.2	suspect wall calcification (most common in diabetics)

  - CTA and MRA – excellent correlation with arteriography, where available, can replace it for intervention planning (IA recommendation)
  - Doppler segmental pressures and pulse volume recordings, transcutaneous oxygen studies (photoplethysmography) treadmill exercise claudication test and real-time duplex scanning considered by vascular specialist (Grade 3C)
- invasive
  - arteriography (gold standard): defines site and size of occlusion, and collateral flow status, operative planning tool

Treatment (ACC/AHA 2005) (see Figure 36)
- conservative
  - risk factor modification (smoking cessation improves prognosis, treatment of HTN, hyperlipidemia and/or DM)
  - exercise program – develops collateral circulation, improves exercise tolerance
  - foot care (especially DM)
- pharmacotherapy:
  - anti-platelet agents (ECASA, clopidogrel or ticlopidine)
  - cilostazol (cAMP-phosphodiesterase inhibitor with anti-platelet and vasodilatory effects, now available in Canada)
  - pain relief: opiate analgesia (morphine sulphate), supplemented by NSAIDs; if opiate analgesia inadequate, possibility of lumbar sympathectomy
- surgical/interventional
  - indications: claudication interfering with lifestyle, rest pain, pre-gangrene/gangrene
  - surgical options: endovascular (stenting/angioplasty) or arterial bypass grafts
  - bypass graft sites: aortofemoral, axillofemoral, femoropopliteal, distal arterial
  - graft choices: in situ graft – reversed vein graft, synthetic – polytetrafluoroethylene graft (Gor-Tex™) or Dacron®
  - amputation: if not suitable for revascularization and persistent serious infections and/or gangrene

Prognosis
- conservative therapy: 60-80% improve, 20-30% stay the same, 5-10% deteriorate, 5% will require intervention within 5 years, <4% will require amputation

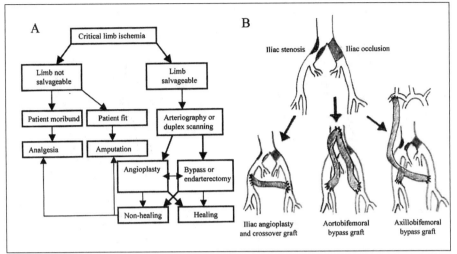

Figure 36. Treatment options for critical limb ischemia. (A) Algorithm for the treatment of critical limb ischemia. (B) Surgical treatment options for the treatment of aortoiliac disease.
Modified from Beard JD. Chronic lower limb ischemia. BMJ. 2000;320:854-857.

Hypertension

- see Family Medicine

Pulmonary Hypertension

- see Respirology

Carotid Artery Disease

- see Neurosurgery

Aortic Disease

Aortic Dissection

Definition
- tear in aortic intima allowing blood to dissect into the media; acute <2 weeks, chronic >2 weeks

Classification (see Figure 37)
- DeBakey
  - Type I – involves ascending and descending aorta
  - Type II – ascending aorta only (stops at the innominate artery)
  - Type IIIA – descending thoracic aorta only (distal to left subclavian artery and proximal to diaphragm)
  - Type IIIB – Type IIIA plus abdominal aorta
- Stanford
  - Type A – involves ascending aorta and aortic arch; requires emergency surgery
  - Type B – only involves aorta distal to subclavian artery; emergency surgery only if complications of dissection (requires long-term follow-up to assess aneurysm size)

Etiology
- most common: damage to aortic media (smooth muscle and elastic tissue), leading to degenerative/cystic changes due to hypertension
- other: cystic medial necrosis, atherosclerosis, connective tissue disease (Marfan's, Ehlers-Danlos), congenital conditions (coarctation of aorta, bicuspid aortic valves, patent ductus arteriosus), infection, trauma, arteritis (Takayasu's)

Epidemiology
- incidence of 5.2 in 1 000 000
- male:female = 3.2:1.0

- small increased incidence in African-Canadians (related to higher incidence of hypertension)
- lowest incidence in Asians

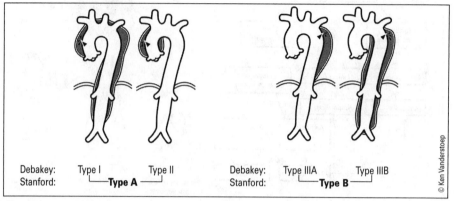

Figure 37. Classification of Aortic Dissection

Clinical Features
- sudden onset tearing chest pain that radiates to back with:
  - hypertension (75-85% of patients)
  - asymmetric BPs and pulses between arms
  - ischemic syndromes due to occlusion of aortic branches: coronary (MI), carotids (ischemic stroke, Horner's syndrome), splanchnic (ischemic gut)
  - "unseating" of aortic valve cusps (new diastolic murmur in 20-30%)
  - rupture into pleura (dyspnea, hemoptysis) or peritoneum (hypotension, shock) or pericardium (cardiac tamponade)
  - renal insufficiency
  - lower limb ischemia (cold legs)

Investigations
- CXR:
  - pleural cap (pleural effusion in lung apices)
  - widened mediastinum
  - left pleural effusion with extravasation of blood
- TEE: can visualize aortic valve and thoracic aorta but not abdominal aorta
- ECG: LVH (90%), ± MI, pericarditis, heart block
- CT, aortography, MR – definitive imaging studies
- bloodwork: LDH (r/o ischemic gut), amylase (r/o pancreatitis), troponin (r/o MI)

Treatment
- pharmacologic
  - sodium nitroprusside and β-blocker to lower BP and decrease cardiac contractility
- surgical
  - resection of intimal tear, reconstitution of flow through true lumen, replacement of the affected aorta with prosthetic graft, correction of any predisposing factors (e.g. bicuspid aortic valve, PDA, etc)
  - post-operative complications: renal failure, intestinal ischemia, stroke, paraplegia, persistent leg ischemia, death
  - Type A: requires emergent surgery with cardiopulmonary bypass, may require hypothermic circulation for transverse arch dissections, valve replacement and coronary re-implantation for aortic root involvement, initial mortality rate without surgery is 1-2% per hour for first 48 hours
  - Type B: initially managed medically – 10-20% require urgent operation for complications (expansion, rupture, compromise of branch arteries, refractory HTN, or ongoing pain)

Aortic Aneurysm

Definition of Aneurysm
- localized dilatation of an artery that is beyond its normal diameter (1.5x diameter)
  - true aneurysm: involving all vessel wall layers (intima, media and adventitia)
  - false aneurysm: disruption of the aortic wall or the anastomotic site between vessel and graft with containment of blood by fibrous capsule made of surrounding tissue
- aneurysms can rupture, thrombose, embolize or erode and fistulize

Classification
- thoracic (TAA): ascending, transverse arch, descending
- thoracoabdominal
- abdominal (AAA): 90-98% are infrarenal

> **ACC/AHA 2005** Guidelines define an AAA when minimum AP diameter of abdominal aorta ≥3.0 cm

Etiology
- degenerative
- atherosclerotic
- traumatic
- mycotic (Salmonella, Staphylococcus, usually suprarenal)
- connective tissue disorder (Marfan syndrome, Ehlers-Danlos)
- vasculitis
- ascending thoracic are associated with bicuspid aortic valve

> **Classic Triad of Ruptured AAA**
> - pain
> - hypotension
> - pulsatile abdominal mass

Epidemiology
- incidence 4.7 to 31.9 per 100 000 for AAA and 5.9 per 100 000 for TAA
- high risk groups:
  - 65 years and older
  - male:female = 3.8:1
  - peripheral vascular disease, CAD, CVD
  - family history of AAA

Clinical Features
- common presentation: due to acute expansion or disruption of wall
  - syncope, pain (chest, abdominal, flank, back)
  - hypotension
  - palpable mass above the umbilicus, pulsatile abdominal mass in two directions
  - airway or esophageal obstruction, hoarseness (left recurrent laryngeal nerve paralysis), hemoptysis, or hematemesis
  - distal pulses may be intact
- 75% asymptomatic (discovered incidentally)
- uncommon presentation
  - partial bowel obstruction
  - ureteric obstruction and hydronephrosis
  - GI bleed (duodenal mucosal hemorrhage, aortoduodenal fistula)
  - aortocaval fistula
  - distal embolization (blue toe)
- associated diseases
  - hypertension, PVD, CAD, COPD, renal insufficiency

> **ACC/AHA 2005** Guidelines suggest
> 1. men ≥60 yrs with AAA in first-degree relative should have U/S screening for AAA
> 2. men 60-75 yrs who have ever smoked should have one-time U/S screening for AAA

Investigations
- abdominal U/S (100% sensitive, up to ± 0.6 cm accuracy in size determination)
- CT (accurate visualization, size determination)
- MRI (accurate visualization, limited access)
- aortogram (not for diagnosis because false negative normal lumen size due to thrombus formation; indicated for associated renovascular HTN, peri-renal AAA, visceral angina, iliac disease)
- Doppler/duplex (r/o vascular tree aneurysms elsewhere)

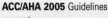

Treatment

Conservative
- cardiovascular risk factor reduction: smoking cessation, HTN control, DM and hyperlipidemia control
- regular exercise
- watchful waiting, U/S q 6 months to 3 yrs depending on size and location

> **Management of Ruptured AAA**
> - no imaging
> - straight to OR (confirm diagnosis by laparotomy)
> - crossmatch 10 units PRBCs
> - start IV if possible

Surgical
- when risk of rupture greater than or equal to risk of surgery
- risk of rupture depends on:
  - size
  - rate of enlargement >0.4 cm/yr
  - symptoms, comorbidities (HTN, COPD, dissection), smoking
- elective AAA repair mortality: 2-5%, elective TAA repair mortality <10% (highest with proximal aortic and thoracoabdominal repairs)
- consider revascularization for patients with CAD before elective repair of aneurysm
- indications:
  - general: ruptured, symptomatic, mycotic, associated with acute Type A dissection or complicated Type B dissection or when risk of rupture is greater than risk of surgery (size >5.5 cm or >2x normal lumen size)
  - ascending thoracic aortic aneurysms
    - symptomatic, enlarging, diameter >5.5 cm or >2x normal lumen size, >4.5 cm & aortic regurgitation (annuloaortic ectasia); ≥5 cm in Marfan syndrome

Risk of AAA Rupture	
Size	1-year rupture risk
<4 cm	0%
4-4.99 cm	1%
5-5.99 cm	11%
6-6.99 cm	25%

> **Repair of asymptomatic AAA is generally not justified for:**
> Males <5.0 cm
> Females <4.5 cm

- contraindications: life expectancy <1 year, terminal disease (e.g. cancer), significant co-morbidities (recent MI, unstable angina), decreased mental acuity, advanced age
- surgical options:
  - open surgery (laparotomy) with graft replacement (see Figure 38)
    - possible complications
      - early: renal failure, spinal cord injury (paraparesis or paraplegia), impotence, arterial thrombosis, anastomotic rupture or bleeding, peripheral emboli
      - late: graft infection/thrombosis, aortoenteric fistula, anastomotic (pseudo) aneurysm
  - endoluminal graft placement under image guidance
    - newer procedure; high success rates in patients with suitable anatomy and experienced centres
    - advantages: decreased morbidity and mortality, procedure time, need for transfusion, ICU admissions, length of hospitalization, and recovery time
    - disadvantages: endoleak rates as high as 20-30%, device failure increasing as longer follow-up periods are achieved, re-intervention rates 10-30%, cost-effectiveness is an issue (devices are very expensive)
    - complications
      - early: immediate conversion to open repair, groin hematoma, arterial thrombosis, iliac artery rupture, and thromboemboli
      - late: endoleak, severe graft kinking, migration, thrombosis, rupture of aneurysm

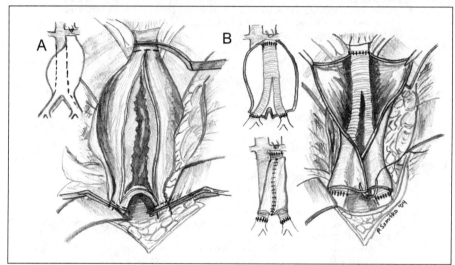

Figure 38. Replacement of an infrarenal abdominal aortic aneurysm with a synthetic bifurcation graft. (A) Arterial clamps are placed at the proximal end of the aneurysm (below the left renal vein) and the common iliac arteries. (B) The aneurysmal segment is replaced with a synthetic bifurcation graft and the outer wall of the aorta is closed over the graft.

Peripheral Venous Disease

Deep Venous Thromboembolism

- see Hematology

Superficial Thrombophlebitis

Definition
- erythema, induration, and tenderness along the superficial vein; usually spontaneous but can follow venous cannulation

Etiology
- infectious: suppurative phlebitis (complication of intravenous cannulation; associated with fever, chills)
- trauma

- inflammatory: varicose veins, migratory superficial thrombophlebitis, Buerger's disease, SLE
- hematologic: polycythemia, thrombocytosis
- neoplastic: occult malignancy (especially pancreatic)
- idiopathic

Clinical Features
- most common in greater saphenous vein and its tributaries
- pain and cord-like swelling along course of involved vein
- areas of induration, erythema and tenderness correspond to dilated and often thrombosed superficial veins
- complications:
  - simultaneous DVT (up to 20% of cases), pulmonary embolus (rare unless DVT)
  - recurrent superficial thrombophlebitis

Migratory superficial thrombophlebitis is often a sign of underlying malignancy ("Trousseau's disease").

Investigations
- non-invasive tests (e.g. Doppler ultrasonography) to exclude associated DVT

Treatment
- conservative
  - bedrest and elevation of limb
  - moist heat, compression bandages, mild analgesic, anti-inflammatory and anti-platelet (e.g. ASA), ambulation
- surgical excision of involved vein
  - indication: failure of conservative measures (symptoms that persist over 2 weeks)
  - suppurative thrombophlebitis: broad-spectrum IV antibiotics and excision

Varicose Veins

Definition
- distention of tortuous superficial veins resulting from incompetent valves in the deep, superficial, or perforator systems
- distribution: greater saphenous vein and tributaries (most common), esophagus, anorectum, scrotum

Etiology
- primary
  - main factor: inherited structural weakness of valves
  - contributing factors: increasing age, female gender, OCP use, occupations requiring long hours of standing, pregnancy, obesity
- secondary
  - malignant pelvic tumours with venous compression
  - congenital anomalies – arteriovenous fistulae

Epidemiology
- most common form of venous disorder of lower extremity
- 10-20% of population

Clinical Features
- diffuse aching, fullness/tightness, nocturnal cramping
- aggravated by prolonged standing (end of day), premenstrual
- visible long, dilated and tortuous superficial veins along thigh and leg
- ulceration, hyperpigmentation, and induration (secondary varicosities)
- associated esophageal varices (GI bleed), hemorrhoids, varicocele
- Brodie-Trendelenberg test (valvular competence test)
  - with patient supine, raise leg and compress saphenous vein at thigh; have patient stand; if veins fill quickly from top down then incompetent valves; use multiple tourniquets to localize incompetent veins

Complications
- recurrent superficial thrombophlebitis
- hemorrhage: external or subcutaneous
- ulceration, eczema, lipodermatosclerosis, and hyperpigmentation

Treatment
- largely a cosmetic problem
- conservative: elevation of leg and/or elastic stockings
- surgical: high ligation and stripping of the long saphenous vein and its tributaries, sclerotherapy, endovenous laser therapy (EVLT)

Prognosis
- natural history benign, slow with predictable complications
- almost 100% symptomatic relief with treatment if varicosities are primary
- good cosmetic results with treatment
- significant post-operative recurrence, especially with sclerosing agent injection

Chronic Venous Insufficiency

Definition
- chronic elevation of deep venous pressure and blood pooling in lower extremities

Etiology
- calf muscle pump dysfunction and valvular incompetence (valvular reflux) due to phlebitis, varicosities, or DVT
- venous obstruction
- AV fistulas, venous malformations

Clinical Features
- pain (most common), ankle and calf edema – relieved by foot elevation
- pruritis, brownish hyperpigmentation (hemosiderin deposits)
- stasis dermatitis
- ulceration: shallow, above medial malleolus, weeping (wet), painless, irregular outline
- signs of DVT/varicose veins/thrombophlebitis

Investigations
- ambulatory venous pressure measurement (gold standard)
- Doppler U/S (most commonly used)
- photoplethysmography

Treatment
- conservative
  - elastic compression stockings, leg elevation, avoid prolonged sitting/standing
  - ulcers: zinc-oxide wraps, split-thickness skin grafts, antibiotics, debridement
- surgical
  - if conservative measures fail, or if recurrent/large ulcers
  - surgical ligation of perforators in region of ulcer, greater saphenous vein stripping
  - venous bypass if short segment obstruction

Lymphedema

Definition
- obstruction of lymphatic drainage resulting in edema with high protein content

Etiology
- primary: Milroy's syndrome
- secondary:
  - infection: filariasis (#1 cause worldwide), post-operative
  - malignant infiltration: axillary, groin or intrapelvic
  - radiation/surgery (axillary, groin LN removal): #1 cause in North America

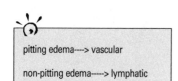

pitting edema----> vascular

non-pitting edema-----> lymphatic

Clinical Features
- classically non-pitting edema
- impaired limb mobility; discomfort/pain; psychological distress

Treatment
- avoid limb injury (can precipitate or worsen lymphedema)
- skin hygiene
  - daily skin care with moisturizers
  - topical treatment of fungal infection; systemic treatment of bacterial infection
- external support
  - intensive: compression bandages
  - maintenance: lymphedema sleeve
- exercise
  - gentle daily exercise of affected limb, gradually increasing ROM
  - must wear a sleeve/bandages when doing exercises
- massage and manual lymph drainage therapy

Prognosis
- if left untreated, becomes resistant to treatment due to subcutaneous fibrosis
- cellulitis causes rapid increase in swelling: can lead to sepsis and death

Common Medications

Table 18. Commonly Used Cardiac Therapeutics

Drug class	Examples	Mechanism of action	Indications	Side effects	Contraindications
ANGIOTENSIN CONVERTING ENZYME INHIBITORS (ACEIs)	enalapril (Vasotec™), perindopril (Coversyl™), ramipril (Altace™), lisinopril	Inhibit ACE-mediated conversion of angiotensin I to angiotensin II (AT II), causing peripheral vasodilation and decreased aldosterone synthesis	HTN, CAD, CHF, post-MI, DM	Dry cough, 10% hypotension, fatigue, hyperkalemia, renal insufficiency, angioedema	Bilateral renal artery stenosis, pregnancy, caution in decreased GFR
ANGIOTENSIN II RECEPTOR BLOCKERS (ARBs)	candesartan, irbesartan, valsartan	Block AT II receptors, causing similar effects to ACEIs	Same as ACEIs, although evidence is generally less for ARBs. Often used when ACEIs are not tolerated.	Similar to ACEIs, but do not cause dry cough	Same as ACEIs
β-BLOCKERS β₁ antagonists β₁,β₂ antagonists α₁,β₁,β₂ antagonists β₁ antagonists with ISA	atenolol, metoprolol, bisoprolol propranolol labetalol, carvedilol acebutalol	Block β-adrenergic receptors, decreasing HR, BP, contractility, and myocardial oxygen demand, slow conduction through the AV node	HTN, CAD, acute MI, post-MI, CHF, (start low and go slow) AFib, SVT	Hypotension, fatigue, light-headedness, depression, bradycardia, hyperkalemia, bronchospasm, impotence, depression of counterregulatory response to hypoglycemia, exacerbation of Raynaud's phenomenon and claudication	Sinus bradycardia, 2nd or 3rd degree heart block, hypotension, WPW. Caution in asthma, claudication, Raynaud's phenomenon, and decompensated CHF
CALCIUM CHANNEL BLOCKERS (CCBs) Benzothiazepines Phenylalkylamines (non-dihydropyridines)	diltiazem verapamil	Block smooth muscle and myocardial calcium channels causing effects similar to β-blockers Also vasodilate	HTN, CAD, SVT, diastolic dysfunction	Hypotension, bradycardia, edema Negative inotrope	Sinus bradycardia, 2nd or 3rd degree heart block, hypotension, WPW, CHF
Dihydropyridines	amlodipine (Norvasc™), nifedipine (Adalat™), felodipine (Plendil™)	Block smooth muscle calcium channels causing peripheral vasodilation	HTN	Hypotension, edema, flushing, headache, light-headedness	Severe aortic stenosis and liver failure
DIURETICS Thiazides	hydrochlorthiazide, chlorthalidone, metolazone	Reduce Na reabsorption in the DCT	HTN (drugs of choice for uncomplicated HTN)	Hypotension, hypokalemia, polyuria	Sulfa allergy, pregnancy
Loop diuretics	furosemide (Lasix™)	Blocks Na/K ATPase in the loop of Henle	CHF, pulmonary or peripheral edema	Hypovolemia, hypokalemic metabolic alkalosis	Hypovolemia, hypokalemia
Aldosterone receptor antagonists	spironolactone, eplerenone	Antagonize aldosterone receptors	HTN, CHF, hypokalemia	Edema, hyperkalemia, gynecomastia	Renal insufficiency, hyperkalemia, pregnancy

Table 18. Commonly Used Cardiac Therapeutics (continued)

Drug class	Examples	Mechanism of action	Indications	Side effects	Contraindications
INOTROPES	Digoxin (Lanoxin™)	Inhibit Na/K-ATPase, leading to increased intracellular Na and Ca concentration and increased myocardial contractility. Also slows conduction through the AV node	CHF; AFib	AV block, tachyarrhythmias, bradyarrhythmias, blurred or yellow vision (van Gogh syndrome), anorexia, nausea and vomiting	2nd or 3rd degree AV block, hypokalemia, WPW
ANTICOAGULANTS					
Coumarins	warfarin (Coumadin™)	Antagonizes vitamin K, leading to decreased synthesis of clotting factors II, VII, IX, and X	Atrial fibrillation, LV dysfunction, prosthetic valves	Bleeding (by far the most important side effect), paradoxical thrombosis, skin necrosis	Recent surgery or bleeding, bleeding diathesis, pregnancy
Heparins	unfractionated heparin low molecular weight heparins (LMWHs): dalteparin, enoxaparin, tinzaparin	Antithrombin III agonist, leading to decreased clotting factor activity	Acute MI; when immediate anticoagulant effect needed	Bleeding, osteoporosis, heparin-induced thrombocytopenia (less in LMWHs)	Recent surgery or bleeding, bleeding diathesis, thrombocytopenia, renal insufficiency (for LMWHs)
ANTIPLATELETS					
Salicylates	ASA (Aspirin™)	Irreversibly acetylates platelet COX-1, preventing thromboxane A2-mediated platelet aggregation	CAD, acute MI, post-MI, post-PCI and CABG	Bleeding, GI upset, gastrointestinal ulceration, impaired renal perfusion	Active bleeding or peptic ulcer disease (PUD)
Thienopyridines	clopidogrel (Plavix™) ticlopidine (Ticlid™)	Block platelet ADP receptors	Acute MI, post-MI, post-PCI and CABG	Bleeding, thrombotic thrombocytopenic purpura, neutropenia (ticlopidine)	Active bleeding or PUD
Gp IIbIIIa inhibitors	eptifibatide, tirofiban, abciximab	Block binding of fibrinogen to Gp IIbIIIa	Acute MI, particularly if PCI is planned	Bleeding	Recent surgery or bleeding, bleeding diathesis
THROMBOLYTICS	alteplase, reteplase, tenecteplase, streptokinase	Convert circulating plasminogen to plasmin, which lyses cross-linked fibrin	Acute STEMI	Bleeding	See Table 7, C26
NITRATES	nitroglycerin	Relax vascular smooth muscle, producing venous and arteriolar dilation	CAD, MI, CHF (isosorbide dinitrate plus hydralazine)	Headache, dizziness, weakness, postural hypotension	Concurrent use of cGMP phosphodiesterase inhibitors, angle closure glaucoma, increased ICP
LIPID LOWERING AGENTS					
Statins	atorvastatin (Lipitor™), pravastatin (Pravachol™), rosuvastatin (Crestor™), simvastatin (Zocor™), lovastatin (Mevacor™)	Inhibit hydroxymethylglutaryl CoA reductase, which catalyzes the rate-limiting step in cholesterol synthesis	Dyslipidemia (1° prevention of CAD), CAD, post-MI	Myalgia, rhabdomyolysis, abdominal pain	Liver or muscle disease

Antiarrhythmics

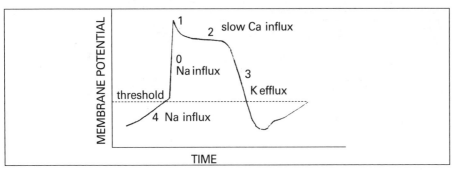

Figure 39. Representative Action Potential

Table 19. Antiarrhythmic* drugs (Vaughn-Williams Classification)

Class	Agent	Indications	Side Effects	Mechanism of Action
Ia	quinidine procainamide disopyramide	SVT, VT	Torsades de Pointes (all Ia), diarrhea lupus-like syndrome anti-cholinergic effects	• moderate Na channel blockade • slows phase 0 upstroke • prolongs repolarization, slowing conduction
Ib	lidocaine mexiletine	VT	confusion, stupor, seizures GI upset, tremor	• mild Na channel blockade • shortens phase 3 repolarization
Ic	propafenone flecainide encainide	SVT, VT AFib	exacerbation of VT (all Ic) negative inotropy (all Ic) bradycardia and heart block (all Ic)	• marked Na channel blockade • markedly slows phase 0 upstroke
II	propranolol metoprolol etc.	SVT, AFib	bronchospasm, negative inotropy, bradycardia, AV block, impotence, fatigue	• β-blocker • decreases phase 4 depolarization
III	amiodarone** sotalol	SVT, VT AFib SVT, VT, AFib	photosensitivity, pulmonary toxicity, hepatotoxicity, thyroid disease, ↑INR Torsades de Pointes, bradycardia, heart block and β-blocker side effects	• blocks K channel • prolongs phase 3 repolarization, which prolongs effective refractory period
IV	verapamil diltiazem	SVT AFib	bradycardia, AV block hypotension	• CCB • slows phase 4 spontaneous depolarization, slowing AV node conduction

*All antiarrhythmics have potential to be proarrhythmic   **amiodarone has class I, II, III, and IV properties

Table 20. Actions of Alpha and Beta Adrenergic Receptors

Adapted from the Family Practice Notebook (http://www.fpnotebook.com/NEU194.htm)

Target System	Alpha Receptors		Beta Receptors	
	Alpha 1	Alpha 2	β1	β2
Cardiovascular	• constriction of vascular smooth muscle • constriction of skin, skeletal muscle and splanchnic vessels		• ↑ myocardial contractility • accelerate SA node	• ↓ vascular smooth muscle tone
	• ↑ myocardial contractility • ↓ heart rate	• peripherally act to modulate vessel tone • vasoconstrict and dilate; oppose Alpha 1 vasoconstrictor activity	• accelerate ectopic pacemakers	
Respiratory				• bronchodilation
Dermal	• pilomotor smooth muscle contraction • apocrine constriction			
Ocular	• radial muscle contraction		• ciliary muscle relaxation	
Gastrointestinal	• inhibition of myenteric plexus • anal sphincter contraction			
Genitourinary	• pregnant uterine contraction • penile and seminal vesicle ejaculation		• stimulation of renal renin release	• bladder wall relaxation • uterine relaxation
	• urinary bladder contraction	• smooth muscle wall relaxation		
Metabolic	• stimulate gluconeogenesis and glycogenolysis at the liver	• fat cell lipolysis	• fat cell lipolysis	• gluconeogenesis • glycogenolysis

Table 21. Commonly Used Drugs that Act on Alpha and Beta Adrenergic Receptors

Adapted from the Family Practice Notebook (http://www.fpnotebook.com/NEU194.htm)

Mechanism of Action	Alpha Receptors			Beta Receptors		
	α1	α1 and α2	α2	β1	β1 and β2	β2
Agonist		Epinephrine			Isoproterenol	
		Norepinephrine			Epinephrine	
	Phenylephrine		Clonidine	Norepinephrine		Albuterol
	Methoxamine			Dobutamine		Terbutaline
Antagonist		Phentolamine			Propranolol	
					Timolol	
	Prazosin		Yohimbine		Nadolol	
	Phenoxybenzamine				Pindolol	
				Metoprolol	Carvedilol	Butoxamine
				Acebutolol		
				Alprenolol		
				Atenolol		
				Esmolol		

Landmark Cardiac Trials

Table 22. Congestive Heart Failure

Trial	Reference	Results
VeHEFT-1	*NEJM* 1986; 341:1547-52.	Hydralazine & isorbide dinitrate decreased mortality in patients with CHF.
SOLVD	*NEJM* 1991; 325:293-302.	Addition of enalapril to conventional therapy significantly reduced mortality and hospitalizations for CHF in patients with chronic CHF and decreased ejection fractions.
VeHEFT-2	*NEJM* 1991; 325:303-10.	Enalapril decreased mortality compared to hydralazine & isorbide dinitrate in patients with CHF.
US-CARVEDILOL	*NEJM* 1996; 334:1349-55.	When added to digoxin, diuretics, and an ACE inhibitor, carvedilol reduced the risk of cardiovascular related death and hospitalization in patients with CHF.
PRAISE	*NEJM* 1996; 335:1107-14.	Amlodipine had no significant mortality benefit over placebo in CHF, but may decrease mortality in patients with non-ischemic dilated cardiomyopathy.
DIG	*NEJM* 1997; 336:525-33.	Digoxin decreased rate of hospitalization, improved symptoms and exercise capacity, but had no mortality benefit in patients with CHF.
ELITE I	*Lancet* 1997; 349:747-52.	Compared to captopril, losartan was associated with lower all-cause mortality in CHF patients over 65.
MERIT	*Lancet* 1999; 353:2001-7.	Metoprolol added to ACE inhibitors and diuretics significantly reduced morbidity and mortality in NYHA class II-IV CHF.
RALES	*NEJM* 1999; 341:709-17.	Spironolactone in addition to standard treatment significantly reduced mortality in patients with NYHA class III-IV CHF.
ELITE II	*Lancet* 2000; 355:1582-7.	In elderly CHF patients, losartan was not superior to captopril in improving all-cause mortality, but was significantly better tolerated.
COMET	*Lancet* 2003; 362: 7-13.	Compared with metoprolol, carvedilol was associated with a reduction in all cause mortality.
COPERNICUS	*NEJM* 2001; 344:1651-58.	Carvedilol in addition to standard treatment significantly reduced the risk of death or hospitalization in patients with severe CHF.
EPHESUS	*NEJM* 2003; 348:1309-21.	In addition to standard therapy, eplerenone (a selective aldosterone blocker) reduced morbidity and mortality in patients with post-acute MI heart failure. The risk of hyperkalemia was increased.
BNP	*NEJM* 2002; 347:161-167	BNP was more accurate than clinical evaluation in identifying heart failure as cause of dyspnea
PRIDE	*Am J Cardiol* 2005; 95:948-54	NTproBNP level lower than 300 pg/mLl was optimal for ruling out heart failure, with a negative predictive value of 99% regardless of age
AF-CHF	*NEJM* 2008;358:2667-2677	In patients with atrial fibrillation and CHF, rhythm control does not reduce cardiovascular mortality compared to rate control

Table 23. Ischemic Heart Disease

Trial	Reference	Results
ESSENCE	*NEJM* 1997; 337:447-52.	Compared to unfractionated heparin, enoxaparin significantly reduced the risk of death, MI, or recurrent angina in patients with unstable angina or non-Q-wave MI.
PURSUIT	*NEJM* 1998; 339:436-443.	In patients with ACS who did not have persistent ST-elevation, eptifibatide (Gp IIb/IIIa inhibitor) in addition to standard therapy significantly reduced the risk of death or non-fatal MI at 4, 7, and 30 days. The risk of bleeding was increased.
BARI	*NEJM* 1996; 335:217-25.	Patients with multivessel disease treated with CABG or PTCA had similar 5-year mortality rates. Those treated with PTCA were more likely to require subsequent revascularization. CABG conferred a survival benefit in diabetics.
HOPE	*NEJM* 2000; 342:145-53.	In patients without LV dysfunction who had CAD, Hx of CVD, PVD, or DM + 1 other CVD risk factor, ramipril significantly reduced the risks of death, MI and stroke.
CURE	*NEJM* 2001; 345:494-502.	Clopidogrel plus aspirin significantly reduced the risk of CVD death, non-fatal MI, or stroke, in patients with mild MI or unstable angina, compared to aspirin alone. The risk of major bleeding was increased.
COMMIT/CCS2	*J Am Coll Cardiol* 2005; 45(suppl13):1213-1613.	No mortality benefit for early IV administration of β-blockers in STEMI, if also undergoing vascularization. Increased mortality in patients with hemodynamic compromise.
COURAGE	*NEJM* 2007; 356(15):1503-1516	PCI offers limited benefits beyond optimal medical therapy in patients with stable CAD

Notes

Clinical Pharmacology

Ekta Khemani and Laurel Murphy, chapter editors
Justine Chan and Angela Ho, associate editors
Billie Au, EBM editor
Dr. David Juurlink, staff editor

General Principles

Drug Nomenclature

- chemical name: describes the chemical structure; the same in all countries (e.g. N(4-hydroxyphenyl) acetamide is acetaminophen)
- drug company code: a number; usually for drugs that are not yet marketed
- non-proprietary (generic) name: shortened form of chemical name; listed in pharmacopoeia (e.g. acetaminophen)
- proprietary (trade) name: the brand name or registered trademark (e.g. Tylenol™)
- street name: slang term used for a drug of abuse

Phases of Clinical Testing

- phase I
  - first administration to healthy human volunteers, following animal studies; to determine pharmacokinetics and pharmacodynamics
- phase II
  - first administration to patients, small studies; to determine therapeutic efficacy, dose range, pharmacokinetics, pharmacodynamics
- phase III
  - double blind, large sample; to compare a new drug to placebo or standard of care, safety and efficacy
- phase IV
  - post-marketing surveillance, wide distribution; to determine rare adverse reactions, effects of long-term use, determine ideal dosing

> At the time of drug launch, only phase I, II, III data available, therefore true effectiveness and safety may be unknown.

Drug Administration and Site of Action

- choice of route of administration depends on:
  - properties of the drug
  - local and systemic effects (limiting action or adverse events)
  - desired onset and/or duration of action
  - patient characteristics

Common Latin Abbreviations

q	each, every
od/bid/tid/qid	once/twice/three times/four times a day
qhs	at bedtime
ac/pc/cc	before/after/with meals
prn	as necessary
gtt	drops
ung	ointment
ud	as directed
od/os/ou	right/left/each eye
ad/as/au	right/left/each ear

Table 1. Routes of Drug Administration

Route	Advantage	Disadvantage
Oral (PO)	Convenient, easy to administer Large surface area for absorption Inexpensive relative to parenteral administration	Drug metabolism by gastrointestinal secretions Incomplete absorption Hepatic first-pass effect Potential GI irritation
Buccal Sublingual (SL)	Rapid onset of action No hepatic first-pass effect	Must be lipid soluble Must be non-irritating Short duration of action
Rectal (PR)	Almost no hepatic first-pass effect Convenient if patient is NPO, vomiting or unconscious	Inconvenient Irritation at site of application Erratic absorption
Intravenous (IV)	Direct to systemic circulation No hepatic first-pass effect Slow infusion or rapid onset of action Easy to titrate dose	Requires IV access, aseptic technique Hard to remove once administered Vascular injury, extravasation Expensive Risk of infection, bleeding
Intra-arterial	Direct to specific organs (heart, brain) No hepatic first-pass effect	Risk of infection, bleeding, vascular complications
Intramuscular (IM)	Depot storage if oil-based = slow release of drug Aqueous solution = rapid onset of action	Pain at site of injection
Subcutaneous (SC)	Non-irritating drugs, small volumes Constant, even absorption Alternative to IV	Pain at site of injection Smaller volumes than IM May have tissue damage from multiple injections

Table 1. Routes of Drug Administration (continued)

Route	Advantage	Disadvantage
Intrathecal	Direct into cerebrospinal fluid (CSF) Bypass blood-brain barrier (BBB) and blood-CSF barrier	Infection Possibility of brain herniation and coning
Inhalation	Immediate action in lungs Rapid delivery to blood Local or systemic action No hepatic first-pass effect	Must be a gas, vapour or aerosol
Topical	Easy to administer Localized Limited systemic absorption	Effects are mainly limited to site of application
Transdermal	Drug absorption through intact skin Rapid onset of action No hepatic first-pass effect	Irritation at site of application Delayed onset of action Hydrophilic drugs are not easily absorbed
Others: Intraperitoneal, Intra-articular	Local effect	Risk of infection

Overview of Drug Disposition

Pharmacology = Pharmacokinetics
- the study of "what the body does to a drug"; movement of a drug in the body
- subdivided into ADME: absorption, distribution, metabolism and elimination

\+ Pharmacodynamics
- the study of "what a drug does to the body"; the interaction of a drug with its receptor and the resultant effect
- includes dose-response relationship, drug-receptor binding

Pharmacokinetics (ADME)

- definition: the relationship between drug administration, the time-course of distribution, and the concentration achieved in the body
    - the manner in which the body handles a drug
- examines the rate and extent at which drug concentrations change in the body by observing:
    - input processes
        - absorption
    - output processes responsible for drug delivery and removal from the body
        - distribution, metabolism (biotransformation), elimination

Absorption

- definition: movement of the drug from the site of administration into the plasma
- important for the main routes of administration, except IV

Mechanisms of Drug Absorption
- most drugs are absorbed into the systemic circulation via passive diffusion
- other mechanisms: active transport, facilitated diffusion, pinocytosis/phagocytosis

Factors Affecting the Rate and Extent of Drug Absorption
- partition coefficient of the drug ($P_{oil/water}$), i.e. the relative solubility of a drug in oil (lipid) vs. water
    - drugs with high lipid solubility can rapidly diffuse across cell membranes (e.g. anesthetics are very lipid soluble and therefore have a rapid onset of action)
- local blood flow at the site of administration (e.g. sublingual vessels provide significant blood flow and therefore rapid absorption)
- molecular size
    - drugs with a small molecular weight (MW) absorb faster than drugs with high MW

Partition Coefficient (P)
- the ratio of a drug's solubility in lipid as compared to water
- more relevant when thought of in terms of a drug's solubility in membrane as compared to extracellular fluid
- a large P means that a drug is highly soluble in lipid and will thus cross membranes easily, i.e. highly absorbed

Drug Ionization and the Henderson-Hasselbach Equation

Ionization reaction for a weak acid:
$HA \rightleftharpoons A^- + H^+$; $pK_a = pH + \log [HA/A^-]$
(Henderson-Hasselbach equation)
  For a weak acid of $pK_a = 4.4$,
  at a gastric pH of 1.4,
  non-ionized:ionized $= HA:A^- = 1: 0.001$

Therefore, drug is mainly non-ionized and diffuses across membrane

Ionization reaction for a weak base:
$BH^+ \rightleftharpoons B + H^+$; $pKa = pH + \log [BH^+/B]$

The amount of drug that reaches the systemic circulation (bioavailability) is highly dependent on absorption and the first-pass effect. Properties of the drug, route of administration and patient factors should be considered to ensure clinical effectiveness.

- pH and drug ionization
  - drugs are usually weak acids (e.g. acetylsalicylic acid) or weak bases (e.g. ketoconazole); therefore, they have an ionized and non-ionized form
  - pH and pK_a determine the ratio of ionized:non-ionized forms (Henderson-Hasselbach equation)
  - non-ionized forms cross cell membranes much faster than ionized forms
- total surface area for absorption
  - the small intestine has villi, which increase the surface area for absorption, making it the primary site of absorption for most oral drugs

Bioavailability (F)
- definition: the fraction of drug that reaches the systemic circulation in an unchanged state following administration
- factors affecting bioavailability:
  - drug absorption
  - metabolism in the gut wall
  - hepatic first-pass effect
- IV and intra-arterial dose have 100% bioavailability (F = 1)
- drugs with a low bioavailability may be ineffective orally (e.g. penicillin G is destroyed by gastric enzymes and needs to be administered IV)

Hepatic First-Pass Effect
- definition: the metabolism of a drug by the liver following absorption, but before it reaches systemic circulation
- occurs with PO administration of a drug: GI tract (absorption) → portal vein → liver (first-pass metabolism) → systemic circulation; significant first-pass effect can drastically reduce a drug's bioavailability
- occurs to much lesser extent with PR administration, because drug absorbed in colon bypasses the portal system: colon (absorption) → internal pudendal veins → IVC → systemic circulation
- drugs with a high hepatic first-pass effect include:
  - levodopa, morphine, propranolol, lidocaine, organic nitrates
- drugs with low hepatic extraction (little or no first pass effect) include:
  - diazepam, digoxin, phenytoin, warfarin

Efflux Pump
- p-glycoprotein (pgp) is a protein in the GI tract and renal epithelium that acts as an efflux pump involved in the transport of drugs out of cells
- pgp blocks intestinal absorption of certain hydrophobic drugs
- some drugs (eg. macrolide antibiotics) inhibit pgp and can increase absorption of drugs that are substrates for pgp proteins
- some tumours also overexpress pgps leading to multi-drug resistance to chemotherapeutic agents

Distribution

- definition: process by which drugs move between different body compartments and to the site of action
- major body fluid compartments: plasma, interstitial fluid, intracellular fluid, transcellular fluid (e.g. CSF, peritoneal, pleural)
- tissue compartments: fat, brain

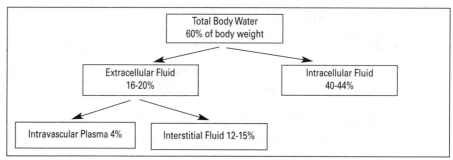

Figure 1. Distribution of Total Body Water (TBW)

Factors Affecting the Rate and Extent of Drug Distribution

- physicochemical properties of the drug (e.g. partition coefficient)
- pH of fluid
- plasma protein binding
- binding within compartments
- cardiac output
- regional blood flow
- percentage body fat

Volume of Distribution (V_d)

- actual V_d: the anatomic volume of body fluid into which a drug will distribute
- maximum "actual V_d" = total body water (40L for average adult)
- apparent V_d: the theoretical volume of body fluid into which a drug will distribute
    - a calculated value that does not correspond to an anatomical space
    - the value takes into account drug distribution into tissues and protein binding
    - this value is used in dosing patients
- for example, amiodarone distributes into total body water (TBW = actual V_d = 40 L), but it also distributes to and concentrates in fat tissues; this gives an apparent V_d of 400 L, i.e. to achieve a given plasma concentration of amiodarone, we dose as if the drug distributes into 400 L of body fluid

Principles of Protein Binding

- drug molecules in the blood exist in two forms:
    1) bound to plasma proteins
        - acidic drugs bind to albumin
        - basic drugs bind to α_1-acid glycoprotein
    2) free
        - only free drug can leave the circulation, distribute into tissues and exert an effect
        - free drug is subject to metabolism and elimination
- within the plasma, the fraction of free drug is in equilibrium with the fraction of bound drug, i.e. as free drug leaves the circulation, more drug unbinds to equilibrate with the portion that is left
- the fraction of drug that is bound is determined by:
    - drug concentration
    - drug affinity for protein binding site
    - number of binding sites/protein concentration
- saturation of binding sites may result in a large increase in free drug concentration, potentially leading to toxicity
- in hypoalbuminemia (liver failure or nephrotic syndrome), the dose of highly binding drugs must be lowered to avoid toxicity
- multiple drugs and endogenous substances can compete for the same protein binding sites, leading to increased free drug concentration and increased effect/toxicity
    - e.g. ASA displaces acidic drugs that are highly protein bound such as phenytoin, therefore increasing the risk of toxicity; sulfonamide displaces bilirubin from protein binding sites: this can lead to jaundice and kernicterus in neonates
- in general, only drugs that are highly protein bound (>90%) are involved in drug interactions due to competitive binding

Depots

- a body compartment (i.e. a type of tissue) where drug molecules tend to be stored
- fat is a depot for very lipid soluble drugs (e.g. diazepam)
- some oil-based medications are injected IM for slow release (e.g. depot medroxyprogesterone)

Barriers (relative)

- body structures that limit or prevent diffusion of drug molecules
    - placenta
    - blood brain barrier (BBB) – barrier composed of tight junctions (between capillary endothelial cells) and astrocytes
    - need to consider dosing route if drugs are meant to cross these barriers

Special consideration must be given in dosing patients in hypoalbuminemic states to prevent drug toxicity. Highly protein-bound drugs will exert a greater effect in these patients than in healthy individuals because of higher levels of free drug.

Examples of highly protein-binding drugs: warfarin, digoxin, diazepam, furosemide, amitriptyline

Main Factors Governing Penetration of BBB
1. Small molecular size (<500 Daltons)
2. High lipid solubility
3. Active transport mechanisms

Common Drugs that Cross BBB
- general anesthetics
- alcohol
- nicotine
- caffeine
- l-dopa
- narcotics
- psychotropic medications

Metabolism (Biotransformation)

- definition: chemical transformation of a drug *in vivo*
- main site of biotransformation in the body: liver
- other sites: GI tract, lung, plasma, kidney
- goal is to make compounds more hydrophilic to enhance renal elimination
- as a result of the process of biotransformation
    - a pro-drug may be activated to an active drug (e.g. nitroglycerin to nitric oxide)
    - a drug may be changed to another active metabolite (e.g. codeine to morphine)
    - a drug may be changed to a toxic metabolite (e.g. halogenated alkenes to toxins)
    - a drug may be inactivated (e.g. procaine to PABA)

Drug Metabolizing Pathways
- phase I (P450) reactions
    - introduce or unmask polar chemical groups on a parent compound in order to increase water solubility (e.g. oxidation-reduction, hydrolysis, hydroxylation reactions)
    - mediated by cytochrome P450 enzymes found in the endoplasmic reticulum or cell cytoplasm
    - product of the reaction can be excreted or undergo phase II reactions
- phase II (conjugation) reactions
    - conjugation with polar endogenous substrates (e.g. glucuronidation, glutathione conjugation, sulfation)
    - increases water solubility and renal elimination

Factors Affecting Drug Biotransformation
- genetic polymorphism of metabolizing enzymes
    - individuals may metabolize drugs faster or slower depending on their genotype
    - this may lead to toxicity or ineffectiveness of a drug at a normal dose
    - genetic diversity in CYP2D6 results in phenotypes that correspond to poor, intermediate, extensive, and ultrarapid metabolizers of drugs using this enzyme pathway (e.g. isoniazid is metabolized by N-acetylation; patients with the "slow acetylator" phenotype are predisposed to peripheral neuropathy from isoniazid toxicity)
- enzyme inhibition due to competition from other drugs and micronutrients
    - inhibition of CYP3A4 is particularly important as it leads to an increased concentration of the substrate drug
    - erythromycin, ketoconazole, indinavir and grapefruit juice inhibit CYP3A4 and predispose a patient to drug toxicity from other medications metabolized by this pathway
    - other enzyme inhibitors: valproic acid, ciprofloxacin
- enzyme induction
    - certain medications enhance gene transcription leading to an increase in the activity of a metabolizing enzyme
    - a single drug may stimulate multiple P450 isoenzymes simultaneously
    - by inducing the P450 enzyme system, a drug may induce its own metabolism (e.g. carbamazepine) and/or induce other drugs' metabolism (e.g. phenobarbital can induce the metabolism of oral contraceptives and bilirubin)
    - other potent enzyme inducers: phenytoin, dexamethasone
- liver dysfunction caused by disease
    - hepatitis, alcoholic liver disease, biliary cirrhosis, and hepatocellular carcinoma may decrease drug metabolism; however, the reduction in metabolism may not be clinically significant due to the liver's reserve
- renal disease
- age
    - neonates and the elderly have reduced biotransformation capacity, therefore doses must be adjusted accordingly
- nutrition
    - insufficient protein and fatty acid intake decrease P450 biotransformation
    - vitamin and mineral deficiencies may also impact metabolizing enzymes
- alcohol
    - acute alcohol ingestion inhibits P450 2E1
    - chronic alcohol consumption can induce the P450 2E1 enzyme and increase the generation of the toxic metabolite and cause hepatocellular damage
- smoking
    - cigarette smoke induces CYP1A2 thereby increasing the metabolism of some drugs (e.g. smokers may require higher doses of theophylline because it is metabolized by CYP1A2)

Cytochrome P450 System
The P450 enzymes are a superfamily of heme proteins that are grouped into families and subfamilies according to their amino acid sequence. These proteins are responsible for the metabolism of drugs, chemicals and other substances.

Nomenclature: CYP3A4
"CYP" = cytochrome P450 protein

1st Arabic # = family
letter = subfamily
2nd Arabic # = isoform

The CYP1, CYP2, and CYP3 families metabolize most drugs in humans. The most important isoforms are CYP3A4 and CYP2D6; therefore, anticipate drug interactions if prescribing drugs using these enzymes.

Some Common Examples of P450 Inhibitors and Inducers

P450 inhibitors "MINCE"
Metronidazole
Isoniazid, **I**ndinavir
Naringin or bergamottin (bioflavenoid in grapefruit)
Ciprofloxacin, **C**imetidine
Erythromycin (macrolides)

P450 inducers
phenytoin
phenobarbital
rifampin
smoking

The very young and the very old are very sensitive to the actions of drugs.

Elimination

- definition: removal of drug from the body

Routes of Drug Elimination
- kidneys
    - main organ of drug excretion
    - two mechanisms for renal elimination:
        1) glomerular filtration
            - a passive process
            - only the free drug fraction can be filtered
            - rate of drug filtration depends on the GFR, degree of protein binding of the drug, and the size of drug
        2) tubular secretion:
            - an active process that is saturable
            - both the protein-bound fraction, and the free drug can be secreted
            - two distinct transport mechanisms for weak acids and weak bases
                i)   acids: penicillin, salicylic acid, probenecid, chlorothiazide
                ii) bases: quinine, quaternary ammonium compounds (e.g. choline)
            - drugs may competitively block each other's secretion if both use the same secretion system (e.g. probenecid was historically used to reduce the excretion of penicillin and increase its levels)
    - tubular reabsorption: drugs can be passively reabsorbed back to the systemic circulation, countering elimination mechanisms
    - elimination rate depends on renal function, which decreases with age and is affected by many disease states; renal function is assessed clinically using serum creatinine (Cr) levels
    - thus, in those with renal impairment, dosage adjustments may be required for medications affected by renal elimination
    - the Cockcroft-Gault equation can estimate creatinine clearance (CrCl) in adults 20 years of age and older:
        - for males, $\text{CrCl (mL/min)} = \dfrac{[(140 - \text{age in yrs}) \times \text{Weight (kg)}] \times 1.2}{\text{SCr } (\mu\text{mol/L})}$
        - for females, above equation x 0.85
- stool
    - some drugs and metabolites are actively excreted in the bile (e.g. corticosteroids) or directly into the intestinal tract from systemic circulation
    - enterohepatic circulation
        - counteracts stool elimination
        - some glucuronic acid conjugates are excreted in the bile and hydrolyzed in the intestines by bacteria; this results in the release of the drug in its original form and allows for systemic reabsorption
        - can substantially prolong the duration of drug in the body
- lungs
    - elimination of anesthetic gases and vapours by exhalation
- sweat, saliva, tears
    - saliva concentrations of some drugs parallel their plasma concentration (e.g. rifampin)

Avoid toxicity from drug or metabolite accumulation by adjusting a drug's dosage according to the elimination characteristics of the patient (e.g. in renal impairment).

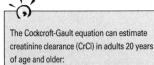

The Cockcroft-Gault equation can estimate creatinine clearance (CrCl) in adults 20 years of age and older:

for males
CrCl (mL/min) =
[(140 – age in yrs) x Weight (kg)] x 1.2
SCr (μmol/L)

for females, multiply above equation x 0.85

It takes 5 half-lives to reach steady state with repeated dosing or to eliminate a drug once dosing is stopped.

Pharmacokinetics Calculations

- definition: the quantitative description of the rates of the various steps of drug disposition, i.e. how drugs move through the body
- the pharmacokinetic principles of ADME (absorption, distribution, metabolism and elimination) can be graphically represented on the concentration vs. time graph (see Figure 2)

Time-Course of Drug Action
- many kinetic parameters are measured using IV dosing, thus there is no absorption phase and distribution for most drugs is rapid
    - therefore, elimination is the main process measured
- the concentration axis is converted to a $\log_{10}$ concentration to allow for easier mathematical calculations (see Figure 3)

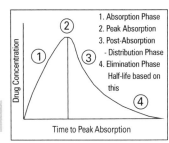

Figure 2. Time Course of Drug Action

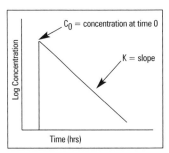

Figure 3. Log Concentration vs. Time Graph (IV bolus dose)

Half-Life ($t_{1/2}$)

- definition: the time it takes for the blood level of a drug to fall to one-half (50%) during elimination
- for most drugs, half-life correlates with the elimination phase
- in general, it takes five half-lives to either reach steady state (with repeated dosing) or for drug elimination (once dosing is stopped)

# of Half Lives	1	2	3	3.3
Concentration	50%	75%	87.5%	90%

Steady State

- the concentration at which the same amount of drug entering the system is eliminated from the system
- time is important for therapeutic monitoring since drug levels are reliable only when the drug has reached this steady state (see Figure 4)
- special situations
    - drugs with a long half-life and the clinical need to rapidly increase the blood concentration may be addressed by giving a loading dose (e.g. phenytoin)
    - drugs with a very short half-life and the need for a long term effect; multiple, frequently repeated doses are too inconvenient, so use a continuous infusion (e.g. nitroprusside, insulin, heparin)

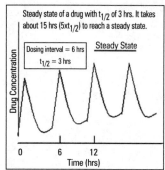

Figure 4. Steady State of a Drug

Steady state of a drug with $t_{1/2}$ of 3 hrs. It takes about 15 hrs ($5 \times t_{1/2}$) to reach a steady state.

Dosing interval = 6 hrs
$t_{1/2}$ = 3 hrs

Clearance

- a quantitative measurement of the rate of removal of a substance from the body
- clearance = volume of body fluid from which a substance is removed per unit of time
- consider:
    - clearance from a specific part of the body
    - total body clearance

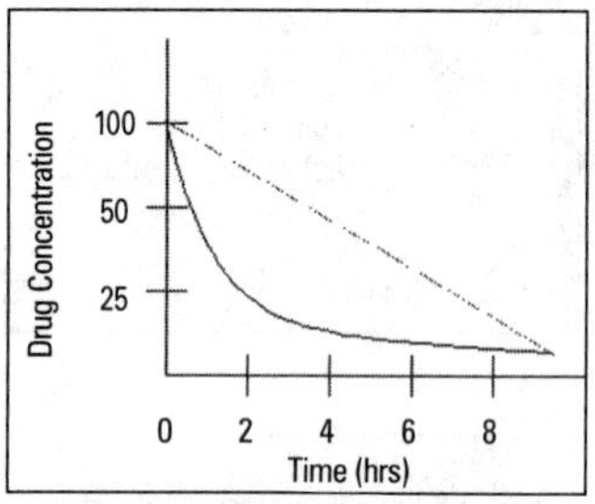

Elimination Kinetics

- first-order kinetics (the most common type)
    - a constant fraction of drug is eliminated per unit time
    - the amount of drug eliminated is based on the concentration of drug present
    - this relationship is linear and predictable (see Figure 5)
- zero-order kinetics (less common, associated with toxicities)
    - non-linear kinetics
    - the rate of elimination of the drug is constant regardless of the drug concentration
    - clearance slows as drug concentration rises
    - some drugs can follow first-order kinetics until elimination is saturated (usually at large doses) at which point the clearance decreases
    - some drugs follow zero-order kinetics at therapeutic levels (e.g. phenytoin)

Figure 5. First and Zero Order Kinetics. In first order kinetics (solid line), a constant fraction of the drug is eliminated per unit time; in zero order kinetics (dashed line), a constant amount of the drug is eliminated per unit time.

Principles of Pharmacokinetics

- volume of distribution (V_d) : relates the amount of drug in the body to the plasma concentration. The volume of distribution of plasma-protein bound drugs can be altered by liver and kidney disease

  Vd = amount of drug in tbe body / plasma drug concentration

- clearance (CL): relates the rate of elimination to the plasma concentration

  CL = rate of elimination of drug / plasma drug concentration

- half-life ($t_{1/2}$) = 0.7 x Vd / CL

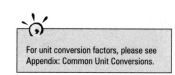

For unit conversion factors, please see Appendix: Common Unit Conversions.

Loading vs Maintenance Dosing

Loading Dose	Maintenance Dose
Use when you need an IMMEDIATE effect	Consider either: after a loading dose OR beginning with maintenance doses
Often Parenteral medication	Steady-state levels achieved after around 5 half lives
Rational: Give large dose of medication to "fill up" the volume of distribution	Can be given as either a continuous infusion (relatively rare, short half-life drug) OR (much more commonly) as intermittent doses

Pharmacodynamics

Dose-Response Relationship

- efficacy and potency are two important pharmacodynamic characteristics of a drug
- the principles of efficacy and potency can be quantified using dose-response curves
- with gradual dose-response relationships, the response of the drug reflects the number of receptors that are effectively occupied

Efficacy
- a measure of the ability of a drug to elicit an effect at its receptor
- independent of concentration
- measured as E_{max} = the maximal **response** that a drug can elicit (see Figure 6)
- e.g. if Drug A causes a greater maximum intensity of response than Drug B (regardless of dose), then Drug A is more efficacious than Drug B
- reflects drug response under ideal circumstances (e.g. controlled clinical trial)

Potency
- a measure of the effect produced by a certain concentration of a drug
- measured as ED_{50} (or EC_{50}) = the effective **concentration** of a drug needed to produce 50% of the maximal possible effect (see Figure 6)
- one may compare the ED_{50} of two or more drugs that have parallel log dose-response curves
- the drug that reaches its ED_{50} at the lower dose is the more potent
- if the potency of a drug is low, this may be overcome by increasing the dose of the drug (e.g. 30 mg vs. 15 mg); this is not problematic provided that the higher dose not cause adverse side effects

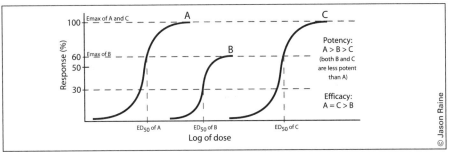

Figure 6. Log Dose-Response Curve Illustrating Efficacy and Potency

Effects of Drugs on Receptors

- drugs that act on specific receptors can be broadly classified as agonists or antagonists (see Figure 7)

Agonists
- drugs that bind to endogenous ligands and exert an effect
- have two main properties:
  - affinity: the ability of the agonist to bind to the receptor (e.g. the β2-agonist salbutamol binds to β2-receptors)
  - efficacy: the ability to cause a response via the receptor interaction (e.g. binding of salbutamol to β2-receptors results in activation of smooth muscle relaxation)
- full agonists: can elicit a maximal effect at a receptor
- partial agonists: can only elicit a partial effect, no matter how high the concentration, i.e. they have reduced efficacy as compared to full agonists

Antagonists
- drugs that have affinity (can bind to a receptor), but no efficacy
- these are drugs that block the action of an agonist or of an endogenous ligand

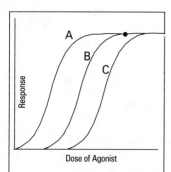

A → C increasing dose of competitive antagonist.

At each dose of antagonist, increasing the concentration of agonist can overcome the inhibition

Figure 8. The Log Dose-Response Curve for Competitive Reversible Antagonism

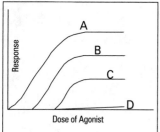

A → D increasing dose of irreversible antagonist.

With one dose of antagonist, increasing dose of agonist does not completely overcome antagonism, as seen in B. Eventually with high enough antagonist concentrations, no amount of agonist can elicit a response, as seen in D.

Figure 9. The Log Dose-Response Curve for Non-Competitive Irreversible Antagonism

- chemical antagonism
    - direct chemical interaction between agonist and antagonist prevents agonist binding to receptor (e.g. chelating agents for removal of heavy metals)
- functional antagonism
    - interaction of two agonists that act at different receptors independent of each other but have opposite physiological effects
        - e.g. acetylcholine at the muscarinic receptor decreases HR, constricts pupil, stimulates intestinal motility; whereas epinephrine at the adrenergic receptor increases HR, dilates pupil, decreases intestinal motility
- reversible competitive antagonism (most common in clinical practice) (see Figure 8)
    - antagonist binds to the same receptor as the agonist, thus displacing it
    - the antagonist binds reversibly
    - increasing the concentration of agonist can overcome the antagonism through competition
- irreversible antagonism
    - competitive (see Figure 9)
        - irreversible binding of the antagonist to the same receptor as the agonist
        - blocks the agonist from binding
        - e.g. acetylsalicylic acid is a competitive irreversible antagonist of cyclooxygenase
    - non-competitive (see Figure 9)
        - binding of antagonist to an alternate site, separate from but usually near to the agonist receptor
        - binding of antagonist produces allosteric effects which change the ability of the agonist to bind
        - e.g. organophosphates are non-competitive irreversible antagonists of acetylcholinesterase

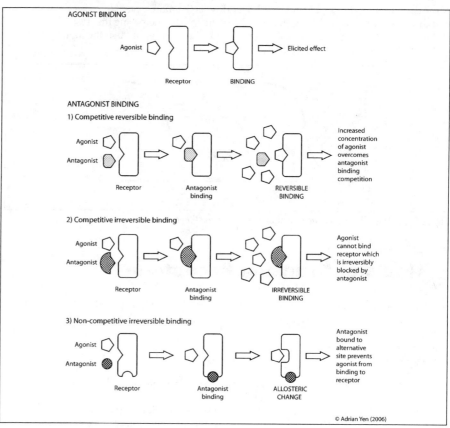

Figure 7. Mechanism of Agonists and Antagonists

Effectiveness and Safety

- the two most clinically relevant properties of any drug are effectiveness and safety
- effectiveness
  - ED_{50} (Effective Dose - 50%): the dose of a drug needed to cause a therapeutic effect in 50% of a test population of subjects
- safety
  - LD_{50} (Lethal Dose - 50%): the dose of a drug needed to cause death in 50% of a test population of subjects (usually rodents)
  - TD_{50} (Toxic Dose - 50%): the dose needed to cause a harmful effect in 50% of a test population of subjects

Therapeutic Index (TI)

- defined as TD_{50}/ED_{50} (see Figure 10)
- reflects the "margin of safety" for a drug – the likelihood of a high dose causing serious toxicity or death
- the larger the TI, the safer a drug (e.g. amoxicillin has a wide TI, therefore therapeutic monitoring is not needed, whereas warfarin has a narrow TI and must have accurate therapeutic monitoring)
- factors can change the ED_{50}, LD_{50} or TD_{50}:
  - presence of interacting drugs
  - changes in drug absorption, distribution, metabolism, elimination

Drugs with a narrow TI have a high likelihood of causing toxicity and need therapeutic monitoring.

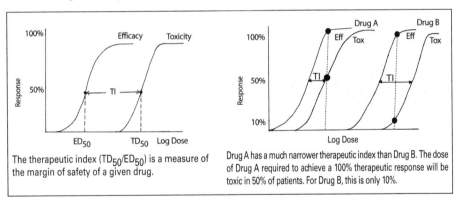

The therapeutic index (TD_{50}/ED_{50}) is a measure of the margin of safety of a given drug.

Drug A has a much narrower therapeutic index than Drug B. The dose of Drug A required to achieve a 100% therapeutic response will be toxic in 50% of patients. For Drug B, this is only 10%.

Figure 10. ED_{50}, TD_{50}, and the Therapeutic Index (TI)

Therapeutic Drug Monitoring (TDM)

- definition: using serum drug concentration data to optimize drug therapy (e.g. dose adjustment, monitor compliance)
- TDM is often used for drugs that have:
  - narrow therapeutic index (TI)
  - unpredictable dose-response relationship
  - significant consequences associated with therapeutic failure or toxicity
  - wide interpatient pharmacokinetic variability
- serum drug samples are usually taken when the drug has reached steady state (e.g. trough level – the lowest level before the next dose), therefore sampling times are generally before the next dose
- examples of drugs whose levels need to be monitored: warfarin (via INR monitoring rather than serum levels), digoxin (if patient is symptomatic), lithium, heparin, carbamazepine, phenytoin, theophylline

Adverse Drug Reactions (ADRs)

- in Canada, an estimated 1.6% of patients admitted to hospitals experience a serious adverse drug reaction
- classification of adverse drug reactions
  - type A: predictable, dose-related
  - type B: unpredictable, not dose-related

In Canada, an estimated 1.6% of patients admitted to hospitals experience a serious adverse drug reaction.

Type A

- side effects: excessive but characteristic pharmacological effect from usual dose of a drug (e.g. β-blockers causing bradycardia)
- overdose/toxicity: exaggerated but characteristic pharmacological effect from supratherapeutic dose
- teratogen: drug may produce developmental defects in fetus
- characteristics:
  - account for more than 80% of all ADRs
  - extension of pharmacological effect
  - dose-related and generally not severe
  - usually do not require discontinuation
  - dose reduction or titration may help minimize effect

Type B

Sulfa-containing Medications
- sulfamethoxazole
- thiazide diuretics
- sulfasalazine
- sulfonylureas

- idiosyncratic: uncharacteristic response to drug, unrelated to pharmacology (e.g. sulfa-containing medications)
- pseudoallergenic: mimics immune-mediated reaction
- allergic/immune-mediated: does not occur on first exposure (up to 7 d), immediate with subsequent exposure, may occur with low dose, resolves within 3-4 days of discontinuation
- characteristics:
  - usually more severe
  - usually require discontinuation
  - not dose-related

Approach to Suspected ADRs

- history and physical examination: signs and symptoms of the reaction (e.g. rash, fever, hepatitis, anaphylaxis, etc.), timing, risk factors, medication history, dechallenge (response when drug is removed) and rechallenge (response when drug is given again)
- check with literature, Health Canada and FDA; contact the pharmaceutical company
- differentiate between drug therapy vs. disease pathophysiology
- treatment: stop the drug, supportive care, symptomatic relief
- Canadian Adverse Drug Reaction Monitoring Program:
  http://www.hc-sc.gc.ca/dhp-mps/medeff/report-declaration/index_e.html
- should report all suspected ADRs which are: 1) unexpected; 2) serious; or 3) reactions to recently marketed drugs (on the market < 5 years) regardless of nature or severity

Table 2. Sample of Clinically Relevant Adverse Drug Reactions and Interactions

Drug(s)	Adverse Drug Reaction	Comments
Beta blockers	Bradycardia	Dose dependent
Vancomycin	Red Man Syndrome	Pruritic erythematous rash on upper body Related to rapid infusion of first dose Not considered "allergy"
ACEI	Cough	Switch ACEI to ARB
Sulfa drugs	Stevens-Johnson Syndrome Toxic Epidermal Necrolysis	Life threatening
Penicillin	Rash	Many children with EBV infection will develop a rash when given amoxicillin ; this is NOT a true penicillin allergy
Warfarin with acetaminophen or amiodarone	Increased INR	Many other drugs interact with warfarin
Aminoglycosides	Ototoxicity and nephrotoxicity	Dose dependent
Acetaminophen Valproic acid Chinese herbs	Hepatotoxicity	Many other drugs are hepatotoxic (e.g. statins, OCPs, isoniazid)

Variability in Drug Response

- each person is unique in their dosing requirements
- recommended patient dosing is based on clinical research and represents mean values for a select population
    - the majority of patients will experience the desired therapeutic effect of a drug with minimal ADRs on the recommended dose, but not all patients will achieve this effect
    - dosing may need to be adjusted, or the medication may need to be changed altogether
- the causes of individual variability in drug response are many, but can be broadly divided into problems with intake, pharmacokinetics, and pharmacodynamics
- a variety of factors may increase or decrease a patient's response to a medication at a given dose
- more than one factor may be affecting a patient; be open minded and flexible when prescribing and dosing medication
- some possible causes of variable responses to a drug:
    - intake
        - compliance
            - if a patient is non-compliant, consider why and try to find a solution
            - e.g. dosing schedule is too hard to follow; medication is non-palatable; medication is too expensive
    - pharmacokinetics
        - absorption
            - is the patient not absorbing due to vomiting, diarrhea or steatorrhea?
            - is the hepatic first pass effect too high due to enzyme induction, or too low because of liver disease?
            - is change in absorption due to drug interactions (e.g. calcium carbonate chelates iron)
        - distribution
            - does the patient have a very high or low percentage body fat?
            - is the BBB intact or disrupted?
        - metabolism
            - is the patient elderly or a neonate?
            - does the patient have a certain genetic polymorphism? – patient may lack enzymes to metabolize drugs (e.g. acetylcholinesterase deficiency, CYP polymorphism)
            - does the patient have liver dysfunction?

- is metabolism increased due to enzyme induction or decreased due to enzyme inhibition?
  ◆ elimination
    - is there kidney or liver dysfunction?
    - is there obstruction of the bile elimination pathway?
- pharmacodynamics
  ◆ is the variability due to genetic variability in drug response? (e.g. malignant hyperthermia due to specific anesthetic agents)
  ◆ is the variability due to drug interactions? (e.g. polypharmacy) does this person have a disease process that affects drug pharmacodynamics?
  ◆ is this person tolerant to the medication?

Autonomic Pharmacology

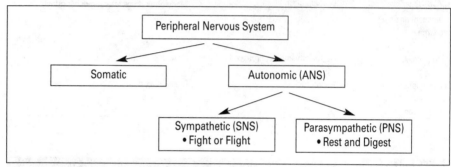

Figure 11. Subdivisions of the Peripheral Nervous System

- most organs are innervated by both sympathetic and parasympathetic nerves; these have opposing effects (see Figure 12)
- sympathetic and parasympathetic efferent fibers originate bilaterally in lateral horn of the spinal cord
- almost all autonomic nervous system (ANS) efferent tracts are divided into preganglionic and postganglionic nerves:

$$\text{preganglionic nerves} \xrightarrow{\text{ACh}} \text{ganglionic synapse} \xrightarrow{\text{ACh or NE}} \text{postganglionic nerve} \rightarrow \text{synapse on target organ}$$

- sympathetic preganglionic fibers originate in the spinal cord at spinal levels T1-L3, and terminate in one of two ganglia:
    1) paravertebral ganglia, i.e. the sympathetic trunk, that lie in a chain close to the vertebral column
    2) pre-vertebral ganglia, i.e. celiac and mesenteric ganglia, that lie within the abdomen
- parasympathetic preganglionic fibers originate in the spinal cord in the lower brainstem and in the sacral spinal cord at levels S2-S4; they terminate in the ganglionic cells located near or within the target organ
- both sympathetic and parasympathetic pre-ganglionic nerves release acetylcholine (ACh)
- post-ganglionic sympathetic nerves release norepinephrine (NE), while post-ganglionic parasympathetic nerves release ACh
- the exceptions are post-ganglionic sympathetics to sweat glands, and a few skeletal muscles and some blood vessels, which also release ACh

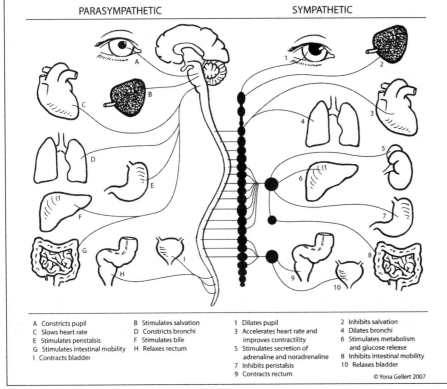

Figure 12. Autonomic Nervous System

Parasympathetic Nervous System (PNS)

- acetylcholine (ACh) is the neurotransmitter of the parasympathetic nervous system
- ACh receptors include:
    - nicotinic (pre-ganglionic) receptors located in the autonomic ganglia, and nicotinic (post-ganglionic) receptors in the adrenal medulla and neuromuscular junction (NMJ)
    - muscarinic (only post-ganglionic) receptors
        - M_1 located in the CNS
        - M_2 receptors located on smooth muscle, cardiac muscle and glandular epithelium
- acetylcholine action is terminated by metabolism in the synaptic cleft by acetylcholinesterase and in the plasma by pseudocholinesterase
    - e.g. acetylcholinesterase inhibitors are used to increase ACh levels in conditions such as myasthenia gravis and Alzheimer's Disease

Sympathetic Nervous System (SNS)

- norepinephrine is the major neurotransmitter of the SNS
- receptors include:
    - β_1 predominately in cardiac tissue
    - β_2 predominately in smooth muscle and glands
    - α_1 predominately on post-synaptic receptors in smooth muscles and glands
    - α_2 predominately on pre-synaptic terminals, where they feed back to inhibit sympathetic nervous system response; also exist as post-synaptic terminals in the brain, uterus and vascular smooth muscle
- norepinephrine action is terminated by reuptake by the presynaptic membrane, diffusion from the synaptic cleft and degradation by monoamine oxidase (MAO) and catechol-O-methyl transferase (COMT)

Table 3. Direct Effects of Autonomic Innervation on the Cardiorespiratory System

| Organ | Sympathetic Nervous System | | Parasympathetic Nervous System | |
	Receptor	Action	Receptor	Action
Heart				
1. Sinoatrial Node	β_1	increased HR	M	decreased HR
2. Atrioventricular Node	β_1	increased conduction	M	decreased conduction
3. Atria	β_1	increased contractility	M	decreased contractility
4. Ventricles	β_1	increased contractility	M	decreased contractility
Blood Vessels				
1. Skin, Splanchnic	α_1, α_2	constriction	M	dilatation
2. Skeletal Muscle	α_1	constriction	M	dilatation
	β_2	dilatation	M	dilatation
3. Coronary	α_1, α_2	constriction	M	dilatation
	β_2	dilatation	M	dilatation
Lungs				
1. Bronchiolar Smooth Muscle	β_2	relaxation	M	contraction
2. Bronchiolar Glands	α_1, β_2	increased secretion	M	stimulation

Opioid Analgesic Equivalencies

Table 4. Opioid Equivalent Doses

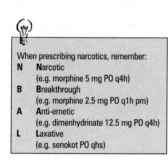

When prescribing narcotics, remember:
N **N**arcotic
     (e.g. morphine 5 mg PO q4h)
B **B**reakthrough
     (e.g. morphine 2.5 mg PO q1h prn)
A **A**nti-emetic
     (e.g. dimenhydrinate 12.5 mg PO q4h)
L **L**axative
     (e.g. senokot PO qhs)

Generic Name	Proprietary Name	Route Oral (mg)	Route IV (mg)	Comments
Morphine	MSIR™ ("immediate release") (PO); MS Contin™, M-Eslon™ (controlled release PO); various names for IV form	30-60	10	- Parenteral 10 mg morphine is usual standard for comparison - Morphine PO:IV = 60:10 for opioid naïve patient, 30:10 for others - Do not crush, break, or chew oral controlled release morphine
Codeine	Tylenol #1,#2,#3 Codeine Contin™, generics	200	120	- Metabolized to morphine (~7- 10% of Caucasians are non-metabolizers, due to CYP2D6 polymorphisms) - Limited by potential toxicities of the acetaminophen with which it is often combined - No additional benefit at doses >~200 mg
Oxycodone	OxyContin™ Oxy IR™, Endocodone™ Percocet™, Percodan™ (combination with ASA or acetaminophen)	30	15	- Often formulated in combination with acetaminophen/aspirin - Use caution if administrating additional acetaminophen or aspirin
Hydrocodone	Vicodin™, Lortab™	20	Not Available	- Limited by potential toxicities of the acetaminophen or ibuprofen with which it is combined - Quick onset of action and thus highly addictive
Hydromorphone	Dilaudid™	7.5	1.5	- PO especially useful for initial dose titration and prn supplementation - IV form often used subcutaneously
Meperidine	Demerol™	300	75	- Not a 1st line opioid. May cause seizures due to the accumulation of normeperidine, its breakdown product - It should not be used longer than 48 h nor more than 600 mg/24 h - Contraindicated with MAOIs - Rarely used anymore

Table 4. Opioid Equivalent Doses (continued)

Generic Name	Proprietary Name	Route Oral (mg)	IV (mg)	Comments
Fentanyl	Sublimaze™	Not Available	0.1	- Minimal experience outside the hospital setting
Fentanyl (transdermal)	Duragesic™	Transdermal 50 μg/h patch = Morphine 100 mg PO/24 h = 16 mg PO q4h = 1.4 mg/h IV		- Usually for stable pain, especially in patients with GI dysfunction
Methadone	Dolophine™	20	10	- Long, variable half-life, which may complicate titration
Levorphanol	Levodromoran™	4	2	- Long half-life with relatively short dosing interval

- when converting from one opioid to another, use 50-75% of the equivalent dose to allow for incomplete cross-tolerance
- rapid titration and prn use may be required to ensure effective analgesia for the first 24 hours
- dose equivalencies provided in the above table are approximate; individual patients vary
- the opioids often used to manage mild to moderate pain include codeine, hydrocodone, and oxycodone
- moderate to severe pain is often managed using morphine, hydromorphone, oxycodone, fentanyl, methadone, or levorphanol
- note that usual starting therapeutic doses are lower than those listed above

Table 5. Common Drug Endings

Ending	Category	Example
-afil	Erectile dysfunction	sildenafil
-ane	Inhaled general anesthetic	halothane
-azepam	Benzodiazepine	lorazepam
-azole	Antifungal	ketoconazole
-olol	β-Blocker	propanolol
-pril	ACE inhibitor	captopril
-terol	β2 agonist	albuterol
-tidine	H2 agonist	cimetidne
-tropin	Pituitary hormone	somatotropin
-zosin	α1 antagonist	prazosin

Notes

Carrie Lynde and Shanna Spring, chapter editors
Justine Chan and Angela Ho, associate editors
Billie Au, EBM editor
Dr. Neil H. Shear, staff editor

Introduction to the Skin

Skin Anatomy

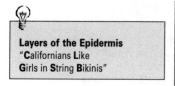

Layers of the Epidermis
"**C**alifornians **L**ike
Girls in **S**tring **B**ikinis"

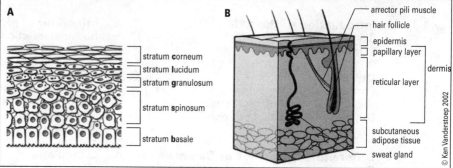

Figure 1. A cross-section of the various layers of skin. Epidermal layer is detailed in A.

Skin
- divided anatomically into epidermis, dermis, and subcutaneous tissue
- **epidermis**
  - avascular → receives its nutrition from the dermal capillaries
  - derived from keratinocytes with the youngest presenting at the 'base' (see layers Figure 1A)
  - cells progress from stratum basale to stratum corneum in about four weeks
    - stratum basale (germinativum): mitotic figures that give rise to keratinocytes
    - stratum spinosum (prickle cells): junctions in this layer (tonofilaments) give the epidermis its strength
    - stratum granulosum: flat cells containing basophilic granules which characterize skin
    - stratum lucidum: comprised of transparent layers of packed dead cells
    - stratum corneum: flat scales of the resistant protein keratin
    - other epidermal cells include melanocytes, Langerhans cells, and white blood cells
- **dermis** – comprised of connective tissue divided into two regions:
  - papillary: contains numerous capillaries that supply nutrients to the dermis and epidermis
  - reticular: provides a strong structure for skin; consists of collagen bundles woven together along with elastic fibres, fibroblasts, and macrophages
- **subcutaneous tissue** (subdermal)
  - consists primarily of lipid in fat cells

Skin Appendages
- epidermal in origin; can extend into the dermis
- include hair, nails, and cutaneous glands (sebaceous glands, apocrine and eccrine sweat glands)

Cutaneous Glands
- **sebaceous gland** – part of pilosebaceous unit, produces sebum which is secreted into the hair follicle via the sebaceous duct, where it covers the skin surface (protective function). Sebum has some antifungal properties
  - found over entire skin surface except palms and soles
- **apocrine sweat gland** – apocrine duct empties into hair follicle above sebaceous gland
  - found in axillae and perineum
  - main function is to produce scent
- **eccrine sweat gland** – not part of pilosebaceous unit
  - found over entire skin surface except lips, nail beds and glans penis
  - important in temperature regulation via secretion of sweat to cool skin surface

Skin Function

- protection
  - with continuous recycling and avascularity, the skin is a barrier to numerous insults:
    - UV radiation, mechanical/chemical insults, pathogens, and dehydration
- thermal regulation
  - insulation to maintain body temperature in cool environments
    - via hair and subcutaneous adipose tissue
  - dissipation of heat in warm environments
    - via increased activity of sweat glands and increased blood flow within the vascular network of the dermis
- sensation
  - largest sensory organ of the body with touch, pain, and temperature sensation
- metabolic function
  - vitamin D synthesis
  - energy storage (mainly in the form of triglycerides)

Definitions

Primary Morphological Lesions

Definition

- an initial lesion that has not been altered by trauma or manipulation, and has not regressed

Table 1. Types of Lesions

Profile	<1 cm Diameter	≥1 cm Diameter
Flat Lesion	Macule (e.g. freckle)	Patch (e.g. vitiligo)
Raised Superficial Lesion	Papule (e.g. wart)	Plaque (e.g. psoriasis)
Palpable Deep (dermal or subcutaneous)	Nodule (e.g. dermatofibroma)	Tumour (e.g. lipoma)
Elevated Fluid-filled Lesions	Vesicle (e.g. herpes simplex virus (HSV))	Bulla (e.g. bullous pemphigoid)

- **cyst**: a nodule containing semi-solid or fluid material
- **pustule**: an elevated lesion containing purulent fluid (white, grey, yellow, green)
- **erosion**: a disruption of the skin involving the epidermis alone, heals without scarring
- **ulcer**: a disruption of the skin that extends into the dermis or deeper; heals with scarring
- **indurated**: descriptive term for a lesion that is hard or firm
- **scar**: replacement fibrosis of dermis and subcutaneous tissue (hypertrophic or atrophic)
- **wheal**: a special form of papule or plaque that is blanchable and transient, formed by edema in the dermis (e.g. urticaria)

Describe a lesion with SCALDA
S ize
C olour (e.g. hyperpigmented, hypopigmented, erythematous)
A rrangement (e.g. solitary, linear, reticulated, grouped, herpetiform)
L esion morphology (see Table 1)
D istribution (e.g. dermatomal, intertriginous, symmetrical/asymmetrical, follicular)
A lways check hair, nails, mucous membranes and intertriginous areas

Secondary Morphological Lesions

Definition

- develop during the evolutionary process of skin disease, or are created by manipulation or complication of primary lesion (e.g. rubbing, scratching, infection)
- **crust**: dried fluid (serum, blood, or purulent exudate) originating from a lesion (e.g. impetigo)
- **scale**: excess keratin (e.g. seborrheic dermatitis)
- **fissure**: a linear slit-like cleavage of the skin
- **excoriation**: a scratch mark
- **lichenification**: thickening of the skin and accentuation of normal skin markings (e.g. chronic atopic dermatitis)
- **xerosis**: pathologic dryness of skin (xeroderma), conjunctiva (xerophthalmia), or mucous membranes
- **atrophy**: histological decrease in size and number of cells or tissues resulting in thinning or depression of the skin

Other Morphological Lesions

- **comedones**: collection of sebum and keratin
    - open comedo (blackhead)
    - closed comedo (whitehead)
- **purpura**: extravasation of blood into dermis resulting in hemorrhagic lesions; non-blanchable
    - **petechiae**: small pinpoint purpura
    - **ecchymoses**: large flat purpura, "bruise"
- **telangiectasia**: dilated superficial blood vessels; blanchable

Patterns and Distribution

- **acral**: relating to the hands and feet (e.g. hand, foot and mouth disease)
- **annular lesions**: ring shaped e.g. granuloma annulare
- **follicular lesions**: involving hair follicles (e.g. folliculitis)
- **guttate lesions**: "drop-like" lesions found on the skin (e.g. guttate psoriasis)
- **Koebner phenomenon**: isomorphic response, appearance of lesions at an injury site (e.g. molluscum, lichen planus, psoriasis, warts)
- **morbilliform**: macules and papules (e.g. measles)
- **reticular lesions**: lesions following a net-like pattern (e.g. livedo reticularis)
- **satellite lesions**: lesions scattered outside of primary lesion (e.g. candida diaper dermatitis)
- **serpignous lesions**: lesions following a snake-like pattern (e.g. cutaneous larva migrans)
- **target (iris) lesions**: concentric ring lesions (like a dartboard, e.g. erythema multiforme)
- **other descriptive terms**: discrete, clustered, linear, confluent, dermatitic

Differential Diagnoses of Common Presentations

Table 2. Differential Diagnosis of Common Presenting Problems

Lesion	Infectious	Inflammatory	Drug/Toxin	Miscellaneous
Discrete Red Papule	Folliculitis Furuncle Scabies	Acne vulgaris Lichen planus Rosacea, Psoriasis Urticaria	Bites/stings	Vascular: hemangioma, pyogenic granuloma Other: dermatofibroma, milaria rubra
Red Scales	Pityriasis rosea Secondary syphilis Tinea	Dermatitis (atopic, contact, nummular, seborrheic) Discoid lupus, Lichen planus, Psoriasis	Gold	Neoplastic: mycosis fungoides
Brown Macule		Post-inflammatory hyper pigmentation	UV Radiation: actinic/solar lentigo, freckle (ephelide)	Congenital: café-au-lait spots, congenital nevus, epidermal/junctional nevus Neoplasia: lentigo maligna, malignant melanoma, pigmented BCC Melasma/chloasma ("mask of pregancy")
Vesicle	Cat-Scratch disease Impetigo Viral: HSV, zoster, varicella, molluscum, coxsackie, scabies	Acute contact dermatitis Dyshidrotic eczema		Other: dermatits herpetiformis, porphyria cutanea tarda
Bullae	Bullous impetigo	Acute dermatitis EM/SJS/TEN Lupus erythematosus	Fixed drug eruption	Autoimmune: bullous pemphigoid, pemphigus vulgaris Other: dermatitis herpetiformis, porphyria cutanea tarda
Pustule	Candida Dermatophyte Impetigo Sepsis Varicella	Acne vulgaris Rosacea Dyshidrotic eczema Pustular folliculitis Pustular psoriasis	Acute generalized exanthematous pustulosis (usually secondary to drug reaction)	Other: hidradenitis suppurativa
Oral Ulcer	Aspergillosis CMV Coxsackie Cryptococcosis HSV/HZ HIV, TB, Syphilis	Allergic stomatitis EM/SJS/TEN Lichen planus Seronegatives, SLE Recurrent aphthous stomatitis	Chemotherapy Radiation therapy	Autoimmune: pemphigus vulgaris Congenital: XXY Hematologic: sickle cell disease Neoplasia: BCC, SCC
Skin Ulcer	Plague Syphilis TB Tularemia	RA, SLE, vasculitis Ulcerative colitis (pyoderma gangrenosum)		Autoimmune: necrobiosis lipoidica diabeticorum (e.g. DM) Congenital: XXY Hematologic: sickle cell disease Neoplasia: SCC Vascular: arterial, neurotropic, pressure, venous, aphthous, leukoplakia, traumatic

Common Skin Lesions

Cysts

Table 3. Cysts

	Epidermal Cyst (Sebaceous cyst)	Pilar (Trichelemmal) Cyst	Dermoid Cyst	Ganglion Cyst	Milium (milia pl)
Definition	Keratin-containing cyst lined by epidermis	Thick walled cyst lined with stratified squamous epithelium and filled with dense keratin	Rare, congenital hamartomas Thick walled cyst filled with dense keratin	Cystic lesion that originates from joint or tendon sheath, called a mucous cyst when found on fingertip	small epidermoid cyst
Epidemiology	Most common cutaneous cyst Youth – mid age	2nd most common cutaneous cyst F>M	Rare	Older age	Any age, 40-50% of infants
Etiology/ Pathophysiology	Epithelial cells displaced into dermis, becomes filled with keratin and lipid-rich debris; May be post-traumatic	Idiopathic Post-trauma	Arise from inclusion of epidermis along embryonal cleft closure lines	Associated with osteoarthritis	Primarily arise from pluripotential cells in epidermal or adnexal epithelium; Secondarily from blistering, ulceration, trauma, topical corticosteroid atrophy, or cosmetic procedures
Signs & Symptoms	Round, yellow/flesh-coloured, slow growing, mobile, firm, fluctuant, nodule or tumour	Often presents with multiple, hard, varying sized nodules under the scalp, **lacks central punctum**	Most commonly found at lateral third of eyebrow or midline under nose	Usually solitary, rubbery, translucent; a clear gelatinous viscous fluid may be extruded	1-2 mm superficial, white to yellow subepidermal papules occuring on eyelids, cheeks, and forehead at sites of trauma and within pilosebaceous follicles
Clinical Course	Central punctum may rupture (foul, cheesy odour, creamy colour) and produce inflammatory reaction; Increase in size and number over time, especially in pregnancy	Rupture causes pain and inflammation	If nasal midline, risk of extention into CNS	Stable	In newborns spontaneously resolves in first 4 weeks of life
Treatment	Excise completely before it becomes infected	Excision	Excision	Drainage ± steroid injection if painful Compression daily for 6 weeks Excision if bothersome	Incision and expression of contents Laser ablation and electrodesiccation Multiple facial milia responds to topical retinoid therapy

Fibrous Lesions

DERMATOFIBROMA

Definition/Pathophysiology
- button-like benign dermal tumour due to fibroblast proliferation in dermis

Etiology
- unknown; often associated with history of minor trauma (e.g. shaving) or insect bites

Epidemiology
- adults, F>M

Differential Diagnosis
- blue nevus, dermatofibrosarcoma protruberans, Kaposi's sarcoma, malignant melanoma

Signs and Symptoms
- firm, red-brown, solitary, well-demarcated dermal papules or nodules with central dimpling and hyperpigmentation
- majority are asymptomatic but pruritus and tenderness are common
- site: legs > arms > trunk
- Fitzpatrick's sign: pressure causes skin retraction (dimple)

Treatment
- no treatment usually needed (excise if bothersome or diagnosis uncertain)
- cryotherapy if certain of diagnosis

SKIN TAGS (PAPILLOMA, ACHROCORDON, FIBROEPITHELIAL POLYP)

Definition
- benign outgrowth of skin

Epidemiology
- middle-aged and elderly, F>M, obese

Signs and Symptoms
- small, soft, skin-coloured or tan, pedunculated papule or papilloma, 1-10 mm
- sites: neck, axillae, and trunk

Treatment
- clipping, cautery

Hyperkeratotic Lesions

SEBORRHEIC KERATOSIS

Definition
- benign neoplasm of epidermal cells

Epidemiology
- unusual <30 years old
- autosomal dominant inheritance

Differential Diagnosis
- malignant melanoma (lentigo maligna, nodular melanoma), melanocytic nevi, pigmented BCC, solar lentigo, spreading pigmented actinic keratosis

Signs and Symptoms (usually asymptomatic)
- round/oval, well-demarcated, discrete waxy papule/plaque, ± pigment, warty surface, "stuck on" appearance
- sites: face, trunk, upper extremities (may occur at any site except palms or soles)
- colour varies (white to pink to jet black)
- surface crumbles when picked

Clinical Course
- over time, increase in pigmentation, "stuck on" plaque appears warty

Investigations
- biopsy only if diagnosis uncertain

Treatment
- none required, but often sought for cosmetic or physical ("in the way") reasons
- liquid nitrogen
- curettage

ACTINIC KERATOSIS (SOLAR KERATOSIS)

Definition
- common, persistent, keratotic lesions with malignant potential

Pathophysiology
- UV radiation damage to keratinocytes from repeated sun exposure (especially UVB)
- pleomorphic keratinocytes, parakeratosis, and atypical keratinocytes

Epidemiology
- common with increasing age, M>F
- skin phototypes I-III (see Table 22)
- melanin is protective

Differential Diagnosis
- Bowen's disease, chronic cutaneous lupus erythematosus, superficial basal cell carcinoma

Signs and Symptoms
- discrete yellow-brown, scaly, adherent patches on a background of sun damaged skin
- sandpaper-like, gritty sensation felt on stroking these lesions
- <1 cm, round/oval
- sites: areas of sun exposure – face, ears, scalp if bald, neck, sun exposed limbs

Types of Actinic Keratoses (AKs)
- erythematous
  - typical AK lesion
- hypertrophic
  - thicker, rough papule/plaque
- cutaneous horn
  - firm hyperkeratotic outgrowth
- actinic cheilitis
  - confluent AKs on the lip
- pigmented
  - flat, tan-brown, scaly plaque
- spreading pigmented
- proliferative
- conjunctival
  - type of pinguecula or pterygium

Clinical Course
- may transform into SCC (1-10%)

Investigations
- biopsy lesions that are refractory to treatment

Treatment
- 5-FU (fluorouracil) cream applied over 2-3 weeks, Aldara™ (imiquimod) cream applied over 8-10 weeks
- liquid nitrogen

KERATOACANTHOMA

Definition
- epithelial neoplasm with atypical keratinocytes in epidermis
- considered a clinically distinct variant of a well-differentiated SCC capable of spontaneous regression

Epidemiology
- >50 years, rare under 20 years
- skin phototypes I-III (see Table 22)

Etiology
- associated with human papilloma virus (HPV)
- associated with UV radiation and chemical carcinogens (tar, mineral oil)

Differential Diagnosis
- treat as SCC until proven otherwise

Signs and Symptoms
- erythematous, skin-coloured, firm, dome-shaped nodule with central keratin-filled crater, smooth surface (resembles an erupting volcano)
- lesion is quite tender during the proliferative phase
- sites: sun-exposed skin

Clinical Course
- rapidly grows to ~2.5 cm in 6 weeks, with keratotic plug in centre of nodule by 6 weeks
- attains full size in <4 months, may spontaneously regress in <10 months
- disfiguring scar after regression
- rarely, keratoacanthomas show intravascular and perineural invasion, and lymph node metatasis

Treatment
- surgical excision is advisable given lack of features predicting prognosis
- curettage and electrocautery
- if on lip treat as SCC

Vascular Lesions

HEMANGIOMAS

Definition
- benign proliferation of vessels in the dermis
- red or blue nodules that blanch with pressure
- includes vascular malformations and vascular lesions

A) VASCULAR MALFORMATIONS

1. NEVUS FLAMMEUS (PORT-WINE STAIN)

Definition
- vascular malformation of dermal capillaries that follow a dermatomal distribution

Etiology
- congenital
- associated with Sturge Weber syndrome (V1, V2 distribution)

Epidemiology
- 0.3% incidence

Signs and Symptoms
- follows dermatomal distribution, rarely crosses midline
- red to blue macule present at birth
- most common site: nape of neck

Clinical Course
- papules/nodules may develop in adulthood, no involution

Treatment
- laser or camouflage (i.e. make-up)

2. SALMON PATCH (NEVUS SIMPLEX)

Definition
- pink-red irregular patches resulting from dilation of dermal capillaries
- midline macule on glabella known as "Angel Kiss," on nuchal region known as "Stork Bites"

Epidemiology
- 1/3 newborns

Clinical Course
- majority regress spontaneously

Treatment
- no treatment required

B) VASCULAR LESIONS

1. CAVERNOUS HEMANGIOMA
(CAPILLARY/VENOUS/LYMPHATIC MALFORMATIONS)

Definition
- deeply situated proliferation of thick-walled blood vessels, venous malformation without endothelial proliferation

Signs and Symptoms
- soft, compressible, bluish, subcutaneous mass that feels like a bag of worms when palpated
- site: anywhere (distribution may indicate underlying cranial abnormality)

Clinical Course
- can ulcerate
- tend to persist, generally do not involute

Treatment
- surgical removal

2. CAPILLARY/INFANTILE HEMANGIOMA (STRAWBERRY NEVUS)

Definition
- benign vascular proliferation of endothelial lining

Epidemiology
- congenital (usually occur within 1st month of life)

Signs and Symptoms
- red/blue nodules

Clinical Course
- appears by age 9 months, increases in size over months, then regresses
- 50% of lesions resolve by 5 years old
- Kasabach-Merritt syndrome (consumptive thrombocytopenia if hemangioma enlarges rapidly)
- can be part of PHACES syndrome

Treatment
- may consider excision if not gone by school age
- systemic corticosteroids and INF-α may be indicated for rapidly growing lesions

Treatment of Hemangiomas of Infancy
Natural history for most is spontaneous resolution, however, 10% require treatment due to functional impairment (visual compromise, airway obstruction, high output cardiac failure) or cosmetic disfigurement. Oral corticosteroids are the first-line therapy.

Hemangiomas: Considerations for Evaluation, Referral +/or Treatment
- Life threatening
- Function Threatening
- Large facial
- Beard distribution
- Ulcerating
- Lumbosacral
- Multiple

3. SPIDER ANGIOMA (SPIDER TELANGIECTASIA)

Definition
• central arteriole with slender branches resembling legs of a spider

Epidemiology
• associated with hyperestrogenic state (e.g. in hepatocellular disease, pregnancy, oral contraceptive pill (OCP))

Differential Diagnosis
• ataxia telangiectasia, hereditary hemorrhagic telangiectasia, telangiectasia in systemic scleroderma

Signs and Symptoms
• faintly pulsatile, blanchable, red macule
• sites: face, forearms, and hands

Treatment
• electro or laser surgery

A spider angioma will blanch when the tip of a paperclip is applied to the centre of the lesion.

4. CHERRY ANGIOMA (CAMPBELL DEMORGAN SPOT)

Definition
• benign vascular neoplasm

Epidemiology
• >30 years old

Signs and Symptoms
• bright red to deep maroon, dome-shaped vascular papules, 1-5 mm
• site: trunk
• less friable compared to pyogenic granulomas

Clinical Course
• increase in number over time

Treatment
• no treatment usually needed
• laser or electrocautery for small lesions
• excisions of large lesions if necessary

5. PYOGENIC GRANULOMA

Definition
• rapidly developing hemangioma

Epidemiology
• <30 years old

Pathophysiology
• proliferation of capillaries with erosion of epidermis and neutrophilia

Differential Diagnosis
• glomus tumour, nodular malignant melanoma, SCC, nodular BCC

Signs and Symptoms
• bright red, dome-shaped sessile or pedunculated nodule
• sites: fingers, lips, mouth, trunk, toes

Clinical Course
• lesions bleed frequently and persist for months

Treatment
• surgical excision with histologic examination
• electrocautery
• laser
• cryotherapy

Pyogenic Granuloma is a misnomer: it is neither pyogenic nor granulomatous.

Pigmented Lesions

SEBORRHEIC KERATOSIS (see *Hyperkeratotic Lesions*, D6)

MELANOCYTIC NEVI (MOLES) (see Table 5)
- be suspicious of new pigmented lesions in individuals over age 40
- average number of moles per person: 18-40

HYPERPIGMENTED MACULES
- purpura (e.g. solar, ASA, anti-coagulants, steroids, hemosiderin stain)
- post-inflammatory
- melasma
- melanoma
- fixed drug eruption

Table 4. Pigmented Lesions

	Solar Lentigo (Aging spots, Liver Spots)	Dermal Melanocytosis (Slate grey nevus of childhood, "Mongolian Spot")	Freckles (Ephelides)	Becker's Nevus
Definition	Benign melanocytic proliferation in an area of previous sun damage	Congenital hyperpigmented macule	Commonly acquired hyperpigmented macules secondary to sun exposure	Asymptomatic pigmented hamartoma
Pathophysiology	Increased number of melanocytes in dermal-epidermal junction due to chronic sun exposure	Ectopic melanocytes in dermis	Increased melanin within basal layer keratinocytes	Increased melanin in basal cells
Epidemiology	Most common in Caucasians >40 years old Skin phototype I-III	99% occurs in Asian and Aboriginal infants	Skin phototypes I and II (most common in blonde and red haired individuals)	M>F Often becomes noticeable at puberty
Differential Diagnosis	Lentigo maligna, seborrheic keratosis, pigmented solar keratosis	Ecchymosis	Junctional nevi Juvenile lentigines	Congenital melanocytic nevus
Signs and Symptoms	Well demarcated brown/black irregular macules Sites: sun-exposed skin, especially dorsum of hands and feet	Grey-blue macule Commonly on lumbosacral area; usually a single lesion	Usually <5 mm Sharply demarcated light brown-ginger macules Lesions multiply & grow darker with sun exposure	Light brown macule/patch with a papular verrucous surface & sharply demarcated borders Sites: trunk and shoulders Hair growth follows onset of pigmentation and is localized to areas of pigmentation
Clinical Course and Treatment	Laser therapy, shave excisions, cryotherapy	Usually fades in early childhood but may persist into adullthood	Do not require treatment and usually fade in the winter. Broad-spectrum sunscreens may prevent the appearance of new freckles	Benign lesion extends for 1-2 years and then remains stable, rarely fading Cosmetic management as desired (usually too large to remove)

Miscellaneous Lesions

KELOID

Definition
- excessive proliferation of collagen following trauma to skin; tissue extends beyond boundaries of scar

Epidemiology
- predilection for darker skin
- M=F

Signs and Symptoms
- skin-coloured or red-bluish papules/ nodules; firm and small with claw-like extensions
- differentiate from a hypertrophic scar, which is confined to injured skin
- may continue to expand in size for years
- can be pruritic and painful
- sites: earlobes, shoulders, sternum, scapular area

Treatment
- intralesional corticosteroid injections
- cryotherapy
- silicone compression

Table 5. Melanocytic Nevi Classification

Type	Age of Onset	Description	Histology	Treatment
Congenital Nevus	• birth	• sharply demarcated pigmented brown plaque with regular/ irregular contours ± coarse hairs • >1.5 cm • rule out leptomeningeal involvement if on head/neck	• nevomelanocytes in epidermis (clusters) and dermis (strands)	• surgical excision if suspicious, due to increased risk of developing melanoma
Acquired Melanocytic Nevus	• early childhood to age 40 • involute by age 60	• benign neoplasm of pigment-forming nevus cell • well circumscribed, round, uniformly pigmented macules/papules • <1.5 cm • can be classified according to site of nevus cells (see below)		• excisional biopsy required if on scalp, soles, mucous membranes, anogenital area, or if variegated colours, irregular borders, pruritic, bleeding, exposed to trauma
Junctional Nevus	• childhood • majority progress to compound nevus	• flat, irregularly bordered, uniformly tan-dark brown, sharply demarcated smooth macule	• melanocytes at dermal-epidermal junction above basement membrane	• same as above
Compound Nevus	• any age	• domed, regularly bordered, smooth, round, tan-dark brown papule • face, trunk, extremities, scalp • NOT found on palms or soles	• melanocytes at dermal-epidermal junction; migration into dermis	• same as above
Dermal Nevus	• adults	• soft, dome-shaped, skin-coloured to tan/brown papules or nodules, often with telangiectasia • sites: face, neck	• melanocytes exclusively in dermis	• same as above
Dysplastic Nevus (Clark's Melanocytic Nevus)	• childhood	• variegated macule/papule with irregular indistinct borders and focal elevation • >6 mm • risk factors: positive family history 100% lifetime risk of malignant melanoma with 2 blood relatives with melanoma (0.8% risk for general population)	• hyperplasia and proliferation of melanocytes in the basal cell layer	• follow q2-6 months with colour photographs • excisional biopsy if lesion changing or highly atypical
Halo Nevus	• first 3 decades	• brown oval/round papules surrounded by hypomelanosis • same sites as neocellular nevus (NCN) • spontaneous involution with regression of centrally located pigmented nevus	• dermal or compound neocellular nevus (NCN) surrounded by hypomelanosis, lymphocytes, histiocytes	• none required • excision if colour variegated or irregular borders • associated with vitiligo, metastatic melanoma
Blue Nevus	• childhood and late adolescence	• uniformly blue to blue-black macule/papule with smooth border • < 6 mm	• pigmented melanocytes and melanophages in dermis	• remove if suddenly appears or has changed

Acneiform Eruptions

Acne Vulgaris/Common Acne

Definition and Clinical Features
- a common inflammatory pilosebaceous disease categorized with respect to severity
    - Type I – **comedonal**, sparse, no scarring
    - Type II – comedonal, **papular**, moderate ± little scarring
    - Type III – comedonal, papular, and **pustular**, with scarring
    - Type IV – **nodulocystic** acne, risk of severe scarring
- predilection sites: face, neck, upper chest, and back
- epidemiology
    - common during the teen years
    - severe disease affects males 10x more frequently than females
    - incidence decreases in adulthood

Pathogenesis
- increased sebum production
- sebum is comedogenic, an irritant, and is converted to free fatty acids (FFA) by microbial lipases made by anaerobic diphtheroid *Propionibacterium acnes*
- free fatty acids + bacteria → inflammation + delayed hypersensitivity reaction → hyperkeratinization of follicle lining with resultant plugging → inflammatory papules and comedones

Exacerbating Factors
- menstruation/hormonal factors (androgens increase sebum production)
- OCP: specifically those containing progestins with significant androgenic effects (norethindrone acetate, levo/norgestrel)
- topical acnegenic agents
    - steroids, tars, ointments, oily cosmetics, etc.
- systemic medications: lithium, phenytoin, steroids, halogens (chloracne), androgens, iodides, bromides, danazol
- NB: foods are not a major aggravating factor

Differential Diagnosis
- folliculitis, keratosis pilaris (upper arms, face, thighs), perioral dermatitis, rosacea

Table 6. Acne Treatments and Mechanisms of Action

MILD ACNE
Topical Therapies

Drug name	Mechanism of Action	Notes
clindamycin phosphate (e.g. Dalacin T™)	Lincosamide antibiotic; inhibits protein synthesis	Generally regarded as unsafe in lactation
erythromycin	Macrolide antibiotic; inhibits protein synthesis	Local skin reactions include burning, peeling, dryness, pruritus, erythema
benzoyl peroxide	Protein oxidant with bactericidal effect	Dry skin, contact dermatitis. Apply to the point of dryness and erythema, but not discomfort
BenzaClin™ gel	1% clindamycin and 5% benzoyl peroxide	See above
erythromycin + benzoyl peroxide (Benzamycin™)	3% erythromycin and 5% benzoyl peroxide	See above
adapalene (e.g. Differin™)	Comedolytic	Less irritating than tretinoin. No interaction with sun, expensive
tretinoin (e.g. Retin-A™)	Comedolytic	Sun sensitivity and irritation

Table 6. Acne Treatments and Mechanisms of Action (continued)

MODERATE ACNE

After topical treatments have failed, add oral antibiotics, such as tetracycline (500 mg PO daily to bid), erythromycin (500 mg PO bid).
Antibiotics require 3-6 months of use before assessing efficacy. May also consider hormonal therapy, including antiandrogens.

Drug name	Mechanism of Action	Notes
tetracycline	Systemic antibiotic	Use caution with regard to drug interactions: do not use with isotretinoin Not to be used as the sole treatment or first line treatment
cyproterone acetate-ethinyl estradiol (Diane-35™)	cyproterone: potent anti-androgenic, progestogenic and antigonadatrophic activity ethinyl estradiol: increases level of sex hormone binding globulin (SHBG), reducing circulating plasma levels of androgens	After 35 years of age, estrogen/progesterone should only be considered in exceptional circumstances, carefully weighing the risk/benefit ratio with physician guidance Also used for other androgen-dependent symptoms, including seborrhea, alopecia, and mild hirsutism.

SEVERE ACNE

Consider systemic retinoids after above treatments have failed

Drug name	Mechanism of Action	Notes
isotretinoin (Accutane Roche™, Clarus™)	Retinoid that inhibits sebaceous gland function and keratinization	Teratogenic: contraindicated during pregnancy Baseline lipid profile, hepatic enzymes and beta-hCG before treatment May transiently exacerbate acne. Drug may be discontinued at 16-20 weeks when nodule count has dropped by >70%. A second course may be initiated after 2 months prn. Refractory cases may require 3 of more courses of isotretinoin. Highly unsafe in pregnancy; generally regarded as unsafe in lactation. Reliable contraception is necessary. May cause depression. Signed informed consent is needed when prescribing

Isotretinoin & Lipids
Case reports indicate isotretinoin-induced hypertriglyceridemia can be successfully controlled with concurrent hypolipidemic therapy.

Perioral Dermatitis

Definition
- distinctive pattern of discrete erythematous micropapules that often become confluent, forming inflammatory plaques on perioral and periorbital skin

Epidemiology
- 15-40 years old
- predominantly females

Signs and Symptoms
- initial lesions usually in nasolabial folds
- symmetry common
- rim of sparing around vermilion border of lips

Exacerbating Factors
- inappropriate use of potent topical corticosteroids

Treatment
- topical: metronidazole 0.75% gel or 0.75-1% cream to area bid
- systemic: tetracycline

Rosacea

Definition
- chronic acneiform, inflammatory skin disease

Pathophysiology
- unknown

Epidemiology
- although found in all skin types, although highest prevalence in fair skinned people (10% prevalence in Sweden)
- 30-50 years old
- F>M

Signs and Symptoms
- typically affecting the convexities of the central face, especially forehead, nose, cheeks and chin
- may also affect the scalp, neck, and the upper part of body
- differentiated from acne by the absence of comedones

Guidelines for the Diagnosis of Rosacea

Presence of one or more of the following primary features:
- Flushing (transient erythema)
- Nontransient erythema
- Papules and pustules
- Telangiectasia

May include one or more of the following secondary features:
- Burning or stinging
- Plaque
- Dry appearance
- Edema
- Ocular manifestations
- Peripheral location
- Phymatous changes

Subtypes and Variants of Rosacea and Their Characteristics

SUBTYPE

Erythromatotelangiectatic
Flushing, persistent central facial erythema ± telangiectasia

Papulopustular
Persistent central facial erythema
Transient, central facial papules or pustules or both

Phymatous
Thickening skin, irregular surface nodularities and enlargement
Nose, chin, forehead, cheeks or ears

Ocular
Foreign body sensation in the eye, burning or stinging, dryness, itching, ocular photosensitivity, blurred vision, telangiectasia of the sclera or other parts of the eye, or periorbital edema

VARIANT

Granulomatous
Noninflammatory, hard, brown, yellow, or red cutaneous papules or nodules of uniform size

- dome-shaped red papules with or without pustules that often occur in crops
- pustulation and papulation may develop contributing to a florid and ruddy complexion
- non-transient erythema is the commonest sign of rosacea
- in longstanding rosacea, signs of thickening, induration, lymphedema in the skin may become apparent
- phyma: a distinct swelling caused by lymphedema and hypertrophy of subcutaneous tissue, and particularly affects the nose (rhinophyma)
- ocular changes are common in rosacea: conjunctivitis, keratitis, iritis

Exacerbating Factors
- heat, cold, wind, sun, stress, drinking hot liquids, alcohol, caffeine, spices (triggers of vasodilatation)

Clinical Course
- characterized by remissions and exacerbations
- all forms of rosacea can progress from mild to moderate to severe
- unclear whether a patient can change from one subtype to another
- flushing (transient erythema) with a burning sensation is common initially
- early diagnosis and prompt treatment are recommended to prevent worsening

Treatment
- avoid topical corticosteroids
- cosmetic camouflage
- telangiectasia: treated by physical measures; vessels can be ablated using electrical hyfrecators, vascular lasers, and intense pulsed light therapies
- phymas: treated by physical ablation or removal; paring, electrosurgery, cryotherapy, laser therapy (CO_2, Argon, Nd:YAG)

Table 7. Specific Rosacea Treatments

1st Line	2nd Line	3rd Line
Oral tetracyclines (250-500 mg PO bid)	Topical clindamycin	Oral retinoids
Topical metronidazole	Topical erythromycin 2% solution	Topical sulfur
Oral erythromycin (250-500 mg PO bid)	Topical benzoyl peroxide	
	Oral metronidazole	
	Ampicillin	

Dermatitis (Eczema)

Definition
- inflammation of the skin

Signs and Symptoms
- symptoms include pruritus and pain
- acute dermatitis: papules, vesicles
- subacute dermatitis: scaling, crusting
- chronic dermatitis: results from scratching, lichenification, xerosis and fissuring

Asteatotic Dermatitis

Definition and Clinical Features
- diffuse, mild pruritic dermatitis secondary to dry skin
- very common in elderly, especially in the winter (a.k.a. "winter itch") but starts in the fall

Treatment
- skin rehydration with moisturizing routine
- ± mild corticosteroid creams

Atopic Dermatitis (Eczema)

Definition
- subacute and chronic eczematous reaction associated with Type I (IgE-mediated) hypersensitivity reaction (release of histamine) and Th2 cellular response producing prolonged severe pruritus

Etiology
- associated with personal or family history of atopy (asthma, hay fever, anaphylaxis, eosinophilia)
- polygenic inheritance: one parent >60% chance for child; two parents >80% chance for child
- frequently affects infants, children, and young adults
- females only slightly more at risk than males (1.3:1 over the age of 2 years)
- almost 15% of children in developed countries under the age of 5 are affected; half of these cases are diagnosed by 1 year of age
- half of all patients with AD are over 18 years of age
- the earlier the onset, the more severe and persistent the disease
- long-term condition with 1/3 of patients continuing to show signs of AD into adulthood
- childhood onset and hereditary forms are associated with a defect in the protein filaggrin

Signs and Symptoms
- inflammation, lichenification, excoriations are secondary to relentless scratching
- atopic palms: prominent palmar creases
- associated with
  - keratosis pilaris (hyperkeratosis of hair follicles, "chicken skin")
  - xerosis
  - occupational hand dryness
- patients usually suffer from three flares per year

Distribution
- infant (onset at 2-6 months old): face, scalp, extensor surfaces
- childhood (>18 months): flexural surfaces
- adult: hands, feet, flexures, neck, eyelids, forehead, face, wrists

Investigations
- no prerequisite investigations to diagnose atopic dermatitis
- may consider: skin biopsy, immunoglobulin serum levels (often elevated serum IgE level), patch testing, and skin prick tests to look for contact or environmental allergies

Treatment
- majority of cases are mild and easily managed
- goal: reduce signs and symptoms, prevent or reduce recurrences, and provide long-term management to prevent progression from early disease to full AD flare
- treatment maximized (i.e. less flare-ups, modified course of disease) if diagnosis made early and treatment plan individualized
  - individualized based on age, severity, sites and extent of involvement, presence of infection, previous responses to therapy
- reassure patients that although there is no absolute cure, the disease can be controlled
- avoid triggers of AD: irritants (detergents and solvents, certain clothing, water hardness), inappropriate bathing habits (long hot showers), microbes (*S. aureus*), stress, sweating, contact allergens, and environmental aeroallergens (dust mites)
- enhance barrier function of the skin
  - simplest and most important aspect of controlling AD
  - involves regular application of moisturizers +/- diluted corticosteroid wet-wrap dressings
    - emollients hydrate the skin and reduce pruritus
  - twice daily application is recommended even in absence of symptoms, especially after bathing or swimming
    - bathing promotes hydration when followed by the application of moisturizers to the skin
- consider psychological support for some patients

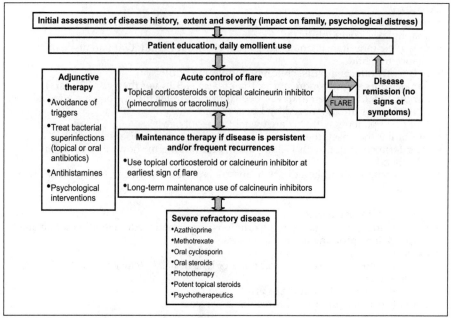

Figure 2. Atopic dermatitis treatment algorithm

Adapted from: Ellis C, et al. ICCAD II Faculty. International Consensus Conference on Atopic Dermatitis II (ICCAD II): clinical update and current treatment strategies. *Br J Dermatol.* 2003; 148 (Suppl 63):3-10.

- **anti-inflammatory therapies**
    a) topical corticosteroids:
    - effective, rapid symptomatic relief for acute flares
    - different formulations and potencies suitable for nearly any area of skin
    - best applied immediately after bathing
    - control inflammation with a potent topical steroid; prescribe a milder one following resolution of acute flare
    - systemic immunosuppression may be needed in severe cases
    - flares may respond to systemic anti-staphylococcal therapy
    - side effects:
        - skin atrophy, purpura, striae, steroid acne, perioral dermatitis, and glaucoma when used around the eyes

    b) topical immunomodulators:
    - long-term management
    - calcineurin inhibitors such as pimecrolimus (Elidel™) and tacrolimus (Protopic™)
        - block calcineurin and inhibit inflammatory cytokine transcription in activated T-cells and other inflammatory cells
    - significant adverse events may include skin burning and transient irritation
    - advantages of long-term management of AD over long-term corticosteroid use
        - rapid, sustained effect in controlling pruritus
        - produce no skin atrophy
        - safe for the face and neck
        - no significant systemic toxicities associated with their use

Prognosis
- 50% clear by age 13, few persist >30 years of age

Complications
- infections are common: diagnose early and treat appropriately (i.e. antibiotic, antifungal, antiviral therapy); infections must be resolved before applying anti-inflammatory treatments
    - topical mupirocin or fusidic acid is often sufficient
    - oral antibiotics (i.e. cloxacillin, cephalexin) for widespread *S. aureus* infections

Contact Dermatitis

Definition
- cutaneous inflammation from the interaction between external agent(s) and the skin

Table 8. Contact Dermatitis

	Irritant Contact Dermatitis	Allergic Contact Dermatitis
Mechanism of reaction	toxic injury to skin; non-immune mechanism	cell-mediated delayed (Type IV) hypersensitivity reaction
Type of reaction	erythema, dryness, fine scale, burning acute: quick reaction, sharp margins (e.g. from acid/ alkali exposure) cumulative insult: slow to appear, poorly defined margins (e.g. from soap), more common	erythema with a papulovesicular eruption swelling, pruritus
Frequency of contact dermatitis	majority; will occur in anyone given sufficient concentration of irritants	minority; patient acquires susceptibility to allergen that persists indefinately
Area of involvement	palmar surface of hand usually involved	dorsum of hand usually involved; often discrete area of skin involvement
Examples	soaps, weak alkali, detergents, organic solvents, alcohol, oils	many allergens are irritants, so may coincide with irritant dermatitis See sidebar for most common examples
Treatment	Avoidance of irritants Compresses Barrier moisturizers Topical/ oral steroids	Patch testing to determine specific allergen Avoid allergen and its cross-reactants Wet compresses soaked in Burow's solution (drying agent) Steroid cream (hydrocortisone 1%, betamethasone valerate 0.05% or 0.1% cream; bid) Systemic steroids prn (prednisone 1mg/kg, taper over 2 weeks)

Dyshidrotic Dermatitis

Definition
- "tapioca pudding" papulovesicular dermatitis of hands and feet, followed by painful crackling/fissuring

Pathophysiology
- NOT caused by hyperhidrosis (excessive sweating)
- emotional stress may precipitate the dermatitis

Signs and Symptoms
- acute vesicular lesions that coalesce into plaques, which dry and develop scaling
- acute stage often very pruritic
- secondary infection common
- lesions heal with desquamation and may lead to chronic lichenification
- sites: palms and soles ± dorsal surfaces of hands and feet

Treatment
- topical
  - high potency corticosteroid with saran wrap occlusion to increase penetration
- intralesional triamcinolone
- systemic
  - prednisone in severe cases
  - antibiotics for secondary *S. aureus* infection

Nummular Dermatitis

Definition and Clinical Features
- annular, coin-shaped, pruritic, erythematous plaques
- dry, scaly, lichenified
- often associated with atopy and dyshidrotic dermatitis
- secondary bacterial infection common

Treatment
- moisturization
- potent corticosteroid ointment e.g. Cyclocort™ ointment bid

---

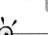

Top Ten Allergens as Identified by The North American Contact Dermatitis Group

Test Substance	Allergic reactions (%)	
Nickel Sulfate	14.2	found in some jewelry, buckles
Neomycin sulfate	13.1	most commonly used topical antibiotic
Balsam of Peru	11.8	fragrance material
Fragrance mix	11.7	a mix of eight different fragrance components which was developed to allow for allergen testing in cosmetics
Thimerosal	10.9	a common preservative that is used in vaccines, contact lens solution, cosmetics
Sodium gold	9.5	used in jewellery, dentistry, thiosulfate electronics
Formaldehyde	9.3	a colourless gas found in many workplaces, cosmetics, medications, textiles, resins, plastic bottles
Quaternium-15	9.0	a component in many shampoos, moisturizers, conditioners and soaps
Cobalt chloride	9.0	a hard metal found in cosmetics, jewellery, buttons, tools
Bacitracin	8.7	a topical antibiotic

Lichen Simplex Chronicus

Definition and Clinical Features
- chronic dermatitis resulting from continued rubbing/scratching of skin
- may develop secondarily to another pruritic skin disease
- lichenified (thickened) skin

Treatment
- treat pruritus to break the itch-scratch cycle
  - antihistamines, topical antipruritics
- topical corticosteroids (extremely potent)

Seborrheic Dermatitis

Definition
- greasy, erythematous, yellow, non-pruritic scaling papules and plaques; occurs in areas rich in sebaceous glands

Etiology
- possible etiologic association with *Pityrosporum ovale* (yeast)

Epidemiology
- common in infants and at puberty
- increased incidence in immunocompromised patients e.g. HIV
- in adults, can cause dandruff (pityriasis sicca)

Signs and Symptoms
- infants – one cause of "cradle cap"
- children – may be generalized with flexural and scalp involvement
- adults – diffuse in areas of scalp margin with yellow to white flakes, pruritus, and underlying erythema
- sites: scalp, eyebrows, eyelashes, beard, face, trunk, body folds, genitalia
- face: eyebrows, sides of nose, posterior ears, glabella
- chest: over sternum

Treatment
- face: Nizoral™ cream OD + mild steroid cream OD or bid
- scalp: salicylic acid in olive oil or Derma-Smoothe FS™ lotion (peanut oil, mineral oil, fluocinolone acetonide 0.01%) to remove dense scales, 2% ketoconazole shampoo (Nizoral™), ciclopirox (Stieprox™) shampoo, selenium sulfide (e.g. Selsun™) or zinc pyrithione (e.g. Head and Shoulders™) shampoo, steroid lotion (e.g. betamethasone valerate 0.1% lotion bid)

Stasis Dermatitis

Definition and Clinical Features
- persistent skin inflammation of the lower legs with brown pigmentation, erythema, xerosis, and scaling
- associated with venous insufficiency

Treatment
- support stockings
- rest and elevate legs
- moisturizer to treat xerosis
- mild topical corticosteroids to control inflammation

Complications
- ulceration (common in medial malleolus), secondary bacterial infections

Papulosquamous Diseases

Lichen Planus

Definition
- acute or chronic inflammation of mucous membranes or skin characterized by violaceous papules, especially on flexural surfaces

Epidemiology
- association with hepatitis C
- may be triggered by severe emotional stress

Signs and Symptoms
- small, polygonal, flat-topped, shiny, violet papules; resolves with hyperpigmented macules
- Wickham's striae: greyish lines over surface; pathognomonic
- sites: wrists, ankles, mucous membranes in 60% (mouth, vulva, glans), nails, scalp
- mucous membrane lesions: lacy, whitish reticular network, milky-white plaques/papules; increased risk of SCC in erosions and ulcers
- nails: longitudinal ridging; dystrophic
- scalp: scarring alopecia
- spontaneously resolves in weeks or lasts for years (mouth and shin lesions)
- Koebner phenomenon: develops in areas of trauma

Treatment
- topical corticosteroids with occlusion or intradermal steroid injections
- short courses of oral prednisone (rarely)
- photochemotherapy for generalized or resistant cases
- oral retinoids for erosive lichen planus in mouth

> **The 6 P's of Lichen Planus**
> **P**urple, **P**ruritic, **P**olygonal, **P**eripheral, **P**apules, **P**enis (i.e. mucosa)

Pityriasis Rosea

Definition and Clinical Features
- acute, self-limiting, erythematous eruption characterized by red, oval plaques/patches with central scales that do not extend to edge of lesion
- sites: trunk, proximal aspects of arms and legs
- long axis of lesions follows parallel to ribs producing "Christmas tree" pattern on back
- varied degree of pruritus
- most start with a "herald" patch which precedes other lesions by 1-2 weeks

Etiology
- suspected human herpes virus 7

Treatment
- no treatment needed; clears spontaneously in 6-12 weeks, reassurance
- topical corticosteroids when post-inflammatory pigmentation is a concern

> Secondary syphilis can present with a non-pruritic papulosquamous eruption but usually ALSO has palmar lesions.

Psoriasis

Classification
- plaque psoriasis
- guttate psoriasis
- erythrodermic psoriasis
- pustular psoriasis
- psoriatic arthritis

Differential Diagnosis
- atopic dermatitis, mycosis fungoides (cutaneous T-cell lymphoma), seborrheic dermatitis, tinea

PLAQUE PSORIASIS

Definition
- a common chronic and recurrent disease characterized by well-circumscribed erythematous papules/plaques with silvery-white scales, mostly at sites of repeated trauma

Pathophysiology
- decreased epidermal transit time from basal to horny layers
- shortened cell cycle of psoriatic and normal skin → excess keratinization with scales

Epidemiology
- multifactorial inheritance

> **PSORIASIS: Pathophysiology**
> **P**ink papules/**P**laques/**P**inpoint bleeding (Auspitz sign)/**P**hysical injury (Koebner phenomenon)
> **S**ilver scale/**S**harp margins
> **O**nycholysis/**O**il spots
> **R**ete **R**idges with **R**egular elongation
> **I**tching
> **A**rthritis/**A**bscess (Monro)/**A**utoimmune
> **S**tratum corneum with nuclei
> **I**mmunologic
> **S**tratum granulosum absent

> **Woronoff's Ring**
> Woronoff's ring: blanched halo that surrounds psoriatic lesions after topical or phototherapy treatments.

Psoriasis Treatment Approach

1st line
Topical corticosteroids (moderate to very potent)
Topical Vitamin D analogues
Topical Retinoid
Coal Tar Therapy
Anthralin (dithranol)
Topical Salicylic Acid

2nd line
Phototherapy
PUVA, UVB, Narrowband UVB
Cyclosporin
Methotrexate
Acitretin

3rd line
Biological therapies (alefacept, etanercept, infliximab, etc.)

Calcipotriol is a vitamin D derivative
Dovobet™ = calcipotriene combined with betamethasone dipro-portionate and is considered to be the most potent topical psoriatic therapy.

Signs and Symptoms
- worse in winter (lack of sun and humidity)
- Koebner phenomenon (isomorphic response): induction of new lesion by injury
- Auspitz' sign: bleeds from minute points when scale is removed
- sites: scalp, extensor surfaces of elbows and knees, trunk, nails, pressure areas
- usually non-pruritic
- exacerbating factors: drugs (lithium, ethanol, chloroquine, β-blockers), sunlight, stress, obesity

Treatment
- preventative measures: avoid sunburns, avoid drugs that exacerbate the condition (β-blockers, lithium, corticosteroid rebound phenomenon, interferon, etc.)
- first-line treatment mainly involves topical treatments, usually prescribed if less than 5-10% of the body surfaces are involved. If the affected area is >10%, use topical medications as adjuncts to phototherapy or systemic drugs
- systemic treatments should be considered if:
  - psoriatic lesions cover >10% of the body surface area
  - unsuccessful topical therapies
  - disease is causing psychological distress

Table 9. Topical Treatment of Psoriasis

Treatment	Mechanism	Comments
lubricants	Reduce fissure formation	Petrolatum is effective
salicylic acid 1-12%	Remove scales	
tar (LCD: Liquor carbonis detergens) 20% coal tar solution	Inhibits DNA synthesis, increases cell turnover	Poor long term compliance
calcipotriene (Dovonex™, Dovobet™)	Binds to skin 1,25-dihydroxyvitamin D3 to inhibit keratinocyte proliferation	Not to be used on face or skin folds
corticosteroid ointment	Reduce scaling and thickness	Use appropriate potency steroid in different areas for degree of psoriasis
tazarotene (Tazarac™) (gel/cream)	Retinoid derivative	Use on nails
UVB	UVB 290-320 nm or 311 nm Narrow Band UVB (NBUVC)	Use with topicals

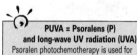

PUVA = Psoralens (P) and long-wave UV radiation (UVA)
Psoralen photochemotherapy is used for treatment of psoriasis as well as a number of other dermatologic disorders. Psoralens, which are linear furocoumarins found in plants and made synthetically, are applied topically via solutions/creams/baths or given orally followed by UVA exposure at a wavelength of 350-360 nm. The therapeutic effect of PUVA in psoriasis is due to the conjunction of psoralens with epidermal DNA which inhibits DNA replication and causes cell cycle arrest.

Table 10. Systemic Treatment of Psoriasis

Treatment	Adverse Effects
methotrexate	Bone marrow toxicity, hepatic cirrhosis
psoralens and long wave ultraviolet radiation (PUVA)	Pruritus, burning, cataracts, skin cancer
acitretin	Alopecia, cheilitis, teratogenicity, epistaxis, xerosis, hypertriglyeridemia
cyclosporine	Renal toxicity, hypertension, immunosuppression
"Narrow band" UVB (311-312 nm)	Well tolerated

Case reports indicate that patients inadequately controlled or intolerant to etanercept may benefit from switching to efalizumab.

Mechanism of Biologicals
"-mab" = monoclonal antibody
"-rcept" = receptor

Table 11. "Biologicals" approved in Canada

Treatment	Route	Dosing Schedule	Effectiveness	Action
alefacept (Amevive™)	IM	weekly	+	T-cell
efalizumab (Raptiva™)	SC	weekly	++	T-cell
etanercept (Enbrel™)*	SC	twice weekly initially	+++	TNF
adalimumab (Humira™)*	SC	once every 2 weeks	++++	TNF
infliximab (Remicade™)*	IV	~every 2 months	+++++	TNF

*Can also be used to treat Psoriatic Arthritis

GUTTATE PSORIASIS ("DROP-LIKE")

Definition and Clinical Features
- discrete, scattered salmon-pink scaling papules
- sites: generalized, sparing palms and soles
- often antecedent streptococcal pharyngitis

Treatment
- UVB phototherapy, sunlight, lubricants
- penicillin V or erythromycin if Group A β-hemolytic *Streptococcus* on throat culture

ERYTHRODERMIC PSORIASIS

Definition and Clinical Features
- generalized erythema with fine desquamative scale on surface
- associated symptoms: arthralgia, severe pruritus
- may present in patient with previous mild plaque psoriasis
- aggravating factors: lithium, β-blockers, NSAIDs, antimalarials, phototoxic reaction, infection

Treatment
- hospitalization, bedrest, IV fluids, sun avoidance, monitor fluid and electrolytes
- treat underlying aggravating condition
- methotrexate, UV, oral retinoids, biologicals

PUSTULAR PSORIASIS

Definition and Clinical Features
- sudden onset of erythematous macules and papules which evolve rapidly into pustules, very painful
- can be generalized or localized to palms/soles
- patient usually has history of psoriasis; may occur with sudden withdrawal from steroid therapy

Treatment
- methotrexate, oral retinoids, biologicals

PSORIATIC ARTHRITIS
- 5 categories
  - asymmetric oligoarthropathy
  - distal interphalangeal (DIP) joint involvement (predominant)
  - rheumatoid pattern – symmetric polyarthropathy
  - psoriatic arthritis mutilans (most severe form)
  - predominant spondylitis or sacroiliitis
  - see <u>Rheumatology</u>

Vesiculobullous Diseases

Bullous Pemphigoid

Definition
- chronic autoimmune bullous eruption characterized by pruritic, tense, subepidermal bullae on an erythematous or normal skin base

Pathophysiology
- IgG produced against dermal-epidermal basement membrane leads to subepidermal bullae

Epidemiology
- 60-80 years old
- associated with malignancy (rarely)

Pemphigu<u>s</u> Vulgaris vs.
Bullous Pemphigoi<u>d</u>
S = **S**uperficial
D = **D**eeper at the junction

Signs and Symptoms
- sites: flexor aspect of forearms, axillae, medial thighs, groin, abdomen, mouth (33%)

Investigations
- immunofluorescence shows deposition of IgG and C3 at basement membrane
- anti-basement membrane antibody (IgG) (pemphigoid antibody detectable in serum)

Prognosis
- generalized bullous eruption heals without scarring
- can be fatal

Treatment
- prednisone ± steroid-sparing agents (e.g. azathioprine)
- topical potent steroids (clobetasol) may be as effective as systemic steroids
- tetracycline ± nicotinamide is effective for some cases
- dapsone for milder cases

Pemphigus Vulgaris

Definition
- autoimmune blistering disease characterized by flaccid, non-pruritic epidermal bullae/vesicles on an erythematous or normal skin base

Pathophysiology
- IgG produced against epidermal desmoglein 3 leads to intraepidermal bullae

Epidemiology
- 40-60 years old, higher prevalence in Jewish, Mediterranean, Asian populations
- associated with thymoma, myasthenia gravis, malignancy, and use of D-penicillamine

Signs and Symptoms
- may present with erosions and secondary bacterial infection
- sites: mouth (90%), scalp, face, chest, axillae, groin, umbilicus
- Nikolsky's sign: sliding or rubbing pressure on skin → separation of epidermis
- Asboe-Hanson sign: pressure applied to bulla causes it ot extend laterally

Investigations
- immunofluorescence: shows IgG and C3 deposition intraepidermally
- circulating serum anti-desmoglein IgG antibodies

Prognosis and Clinical Course
- begins with mouth lesions, followed by skin lesions
- first localized (6-12 months) then generalized
- lesions heal with hyperpigmentation but no scar
- may be fatal unless treated with immunosuppressive agents

Treatment
- prednisone 2.0-3.0 mg/kg until no new blisters, then 1.0-1.5 mg/kg until clear, then taper
- steroid-sparing agents – azathioprine, methotrexate, gold, cyclophosphamide, cyclosporine, intravenous immunoglobulin (IVIG), mycophenolate mofetil
- plasmapheresis for acutely high antibody levels

Pemphigus Foliaceus
An autoimmune intraepidermal blistering disease that is more superficial than pemphigus vulgaris due to antibodies against desmoglein 1, an intracellular adhesion molecule. Appears as crusted patches and erosions which can initially be managed with topical steroids if localized. Active widespread disease is treated like pemphigus vulgaris.

Dermatitis Herpetiformis

Definition
- intensely pruritic grouped papules/vesicles/urticarial wheals on an erythematous base
- almost always excoriated, rarely seen as blisters

Etiology
- 90% have HLA B8, DR3, DQWZ
- 90% associated with gluten-sensitive enteropathy (celiac) (80% are asymptomatic)
- 30% have thyroid disease; some have intestinal lymphoma or iron/folate deficiency

Epidemiology
- 20-60 years old, M:F = 2:1

Signs and Symptoms
- sites: extensor surfaces of elbows/knees, sacrum, buttocks, scalp
- lesions grouped, bilaterally symmetrical
- pruritus, burning, stinging

Treatment
- dapsone for pruritus
- gluten-free diet

Table 12. Summary of Vesiculobullous Diseases

	Pemphigus Vulgaris	Bullous Pemphigoid	Dermatitis Herpetiformis
Antibody	IgG	IgG	IgA
Site	Intercellular space	Basement membrane	Dermal
Infiltrate	Eosinophils and neutrophils	Eosinophils	Neutrophils
Treatment	High dose steroids Immunosuppressive agent (e.g. Imuran, mycophenolic acid)	Tetracyclin Clobetasol cream	Gluten-free diet Dapsone
Association	Malignancy with paraneoplastic pemphigus	Malignancy (rarely)	Gluten enteropathy Thyroid disease Intestinal lymphoma

Porphyria Cutanea Tarda

Definition
- autosomal dominant or sporadic skin disorder associated with the presence of excess heme, characterized by tense vesicles/bullae in photoexposed areas subjected to trauma

Etiology
- associated with alcohol abuse, DM, drugs (estrogen therapy, NSAID), HIV, hepatitis C, increased iron indices

Epidemiology
- 30-40 years old, M>F

Signs and Symptoms
- facial hypertrichosis, brown hypermelanosis vesicles, and bullae in photodistribution (dorsum of hands and feet)
- sites: light-exposed areas subjected to trauma, dorsum of hands and feet, nose, and upper trunk

Investigations
- urine + 5% HCl shows orange-red fluorescence under Wood's lamp (UV rays)
- 24-hour urine for uroporphyrins (elevated)
- stool contains elevated coproporphyrins
- immunofluorescence shows IgE at dermal-epidermal junctions

Treatment
- discontinue aggravating substances (alcohol, estrogen therapy)
- phlebotomy to decrease body iron load
- low dose hydroxychloroquine if phlebotomy contraindicated

Drug Eruptions

Erythema Multiforme (EM), Stevens-Johnson Syndrome (SJS), Toxic Epidermal Necrolysis (TEN)

- disorders with varying presence of characteristic skin lesions, blistering and mucous membrane involvement
- note that EM is considered to be distinct from the SJS - TEN spectrum

> Erythema multiforme is a clinical diagnosis. Resonable evidence exists for the following as precipitating factors:
> - HSV (Predominant precipitating factor)
> - Histoplasma capsulatum
> - Orf virus

Table 13. Comparison of Erythema Multiforme, Stevens-Johnson Syndrome, Toxic Epidermal Necrolysis

	Erythema Multiforme (EM)	Stevens-Johnson Syndrome (SJS)	Toxic Epidermal Necrolysis (TEN)
Lesion	• macules/papules with central vesicles • classic bull's-eye pattern of concentric light and dark rings (target lesions) • bilateral and symmetric • all lesions appear within 72 hours • no edema • lesion "fixed" for at least 7 days	• EM with more mucous membrane involvement • "Atypical lesions" – red circular patch with dark purple centre • "sicker" (high fever) • sheet-like epidermal detachment in <10% (Nikolsky sign)	• severe mucous membrane involvement, and blistering • "atypical lesions" – 50% have no target lesions • diffuse erythema then necrosis and sheet-like epidermal detachment in >30%
Sites	• dorsa of hands and forearms • mucous membrane involvement (lips, tongue, buccal mucosa) is possible • extremities with face > trunk • involvement of palms and soles	• generalized with prominent face and trunk involvement • palms and soles may be spared	• generalized • nails may also shed
Other Complications	• burning and stinging • recurrences • secondary bacterial infection	• scarring, contractures, eruptive nevomelanocytic nevi, corneal scarring, blindness, phimosis and vaginal synechiae	• tubular necrosis and acute renal failure, epithelial erosions of trachea
Constitutional symptoms	• weakness, malaise	• prodrome 1-14 days prior to eruption with fever and flu-like illness	• high fever >38°C
Etiology	• infection – HSV, or *Histoplasma capsulatum*	• 15% are drug-related (NSAIDs, anticonvulsants, sulfonamides, penicillins) • occurs up to 1-3 weeks after drug exposure with more rapid onset upon rechallenge	• 50% are definitely drug related • <5% are due to viral infection, immunization
Differential diagnosis	• giant urticaria, granuloma annulare, mycosis fungoides, vasculitis	• scarlet fever, phototoxic, eruption, GVHD, SSSS, exfoliative dermatitis, Kawasaki disease, paraneoplastic pemphigus	• scarlet fever, phototoxic eruption, GVHD, SSSS, exfoliative dermatitis
Course and Prognosis	• lesions last 2 weeks and heal without complications	• 4-6 week course • 5% mortality	• 30% mortality due to fluid loss, regrowth of epidermis by 3 weeks, secondary infection
Treatment	• symptomatic treatment (oral antihistamines, oral antacids) • corticosteroids in severely ill (controversial) • prophylactic oral acyclovir for 6-12 months for herpes simplex virus (HSV)-associated EM with frequent recurrences	• prolonged hospitalization • withdraw suspect drug • intravenous fluids • corticosteroids – controversial • infection prophylaxis • consider IVIG	• as for Stevens-Johnson syndrome • admit to burn unit • debride frankly necrotic tissue • consider IVIG

SSSS = Staphylococcal Scalded Skin Syndrome   GVHD = Graft Versus Host Disease

Drug Hypersensitivity Syndrome

- initial **fever**, followed by symmetrical bright red **exanthematous eruption** that may lead to **internal organ involvement** (hepatitis, arthralgia, nephritis, pneumonitis, lymphadenopathy, and/or hematologic abnormalities)
- classically occurs approximately 10 days after first exposure to the drug
- siblings at risk
- sulfonamides and anticonvulsants (phenytoin, phenobarbital, carbamazepine, lamotrigine) most common
- 10% mortality if undiagnosed and untreated

Exanthematous Eruptions (Maculopapular Eruptions/Morbilliform)

- symmetrical, widespread, erythematous patches or plaques with or without scales
- the "classic" and most common adverse drug reaction
- often starts on trunk or areas of sun exposure
- may progress to generalized exfoliative dermatitis especially if the drug is continued
- associated with penicillin > sulfonamides > phenytoin
- see *Pediatric Exanthems* section, D44

Fixed Drug Eruption

- sharply demarcated erythematous oval patches on the skin or mucous membranes
  - sites: face, mucosa, genitalia
  - reoccurs in same location upon subsequent exposure to the drug (fixed location)
- most common causes: antimicrobials (tetracycline, sulfonamides), anti-inflammatories, psychoactive agents (barbiturates), phenolphthalein

Photosensitivity Eruptions

- phototoxic reaction: "an exaggerated sunburn" confined to sun-exposed areas
- photoallergic reaction: an eczematous eruption that may spread to areas not exposed to light
- chlorpromazine, doxycycline, thiazide diuretics, procainamide

Serum Sickness-Like Reaction

- a symmetric drug eruption resulting in fever, arthralgia, lymphadenopathy, and skin rash
- usually appears 5-10 days after drug
- skin manifestations: usually urticaria; can be morbilliform
- cefaclor most common in kids; buproprion (Zyban™) in adults

Angioedema

- deeper swelling of the skin involving subcutaneous tissues often with swelling of the eyes, lips, and tongue
- may or may not accompany urticaria
- can have hereditary or acquired forms; acquired form occurs with urticaria
- hereditary angioedema – does not occur with urticaria
  - onset in childhood; 80% have positive family history
  - recurrent attacks; 25% die from laryngeal edema
  - triggers: minor trauma, emotional upset, temperature changes
- treatment: prophylaxis with danazol or stanozolol
  - epinephrine pen to temporize until patient reaches hospital in acute attack

> **Wheal**
> - typically erythematous flat-topped, palpable lesions varying in size with circumscribed dermal edema
> - associated with mast cell release of histamine
> - may be pruritic
> - individual lesion lasts <24 hrs

Urticaria

(also known as "Hives"; see Table 14 for classification)
- transient, red, pruritic well-demarcated wheals
- second most common type of drug reaction, though can be due to many other things
- due to release of histamine from mast cells in dermis
- each lesion lasts less than 24 hours, though condition may be chronic
- can also result after physical contact with allergen

> **Urticaria**
> The name urticaria dates back to the 18th century where contact with nettles (*Urtica dioica*) was believed to cause swelling and burning of skin.

Table 14. Classification of Urticaria

Type	Approach to Diagnosis

Acute Urticaria
>2/3 of cases
Attacks lasts <6 weeks
Individual lesion <24 hrs
	Drugs
	    especially aspirin, NSAIDs
	Foods
	    nuts, shellfish, eggs, fruit
	Idiopathic
	Infection
	Insect stings
	Percutanous absorption
	    cosmetics, work exposures
	Stress
	Systemic diseases
	    systemic lupus erythematosis (SLE), endocrinopathy, neoplasm

Chronic Urticaria
<1/3 of cases
Attacks last >6 weeks
Individual lesion lasts <24 hrs
	IgE-dependent: trigger associated
	    Idiopathic (90% of chronic urticaria patients)
	    Drugs (antibiotics, hormones, local anesthetics)
	    Physical contact (animal saliva, plant resins, latex, metals, lotions, soap)
	    Insect stings (bees, wasps, hornets)
	    Aeroallergens
	    Foods and additives
	    Parasitic infections
	Direct mast cell release
	    Opiates, muscle relaxants, radio-contrast agents
	Complement-mediated
	    Serum sickness, transfusion reactions
	    Infections, viral/bacterial (>80% of urticaria in pediatric patients)
	    Urticarial vasculitis
	Arachidonic acid metabolism
	    ASA, NSAIDs
	Physical
	    Dermatographism (friction, rubbing skin), cold (ice cube, cold water), cholinergic (hot shower, exercise), solar, pressure (shoulder strap, buttocks), aquagenic (exposure to water), adrenergic (stress), heat
	Other
	    Mastocytosis, urticaria pigmentosa

Vasculitic Urticaria
Lesions last >24 hrs
Painful, non-pruritic
Requires biopsy
	Idiopathic
	Infections
	    Hepatitis
	Autoimmune diseases
	    SLE
	Drug hypersensitivity
	    cimetidine and diltiazem

Mastocytosis (Urticaria Pigmentosa)
Rare disease due to excessive infiltration of the skin by mast cells. It manifests as many reddish-brown elevated plaques and macules. Applying pressure to a lesion produces a wheal surrounded by intense erythema (Darier's sign), due to mast cell degranulation. This occurs within minutes.

Infections

Bacterial Infections

- often involve the epidermis, dermis, hair follicles or periungual region
- may also be systemic

Superficial Skin (Epidermal)

Table 15. Comparison of Impetigo Vulgaris and Bullous Impetigo

	Impetigo Vulgaris	Bullous Impetigo
Definition and Clinical Features	• acute purulent infection which appears vesicular and progresses to golden yellow "honey-crusted" lesions surrounded by erythema • sites: commonly involves the face, arms, legs and buttocks	• scattered, thin-walled bullae containing clear yellow or slightly turbid fluid with no surrounding erythema • sites: trunk, intertriginous areas, face
Etiology	• agent: Group A β-hemolytic *Streptococcus* (GAS), *S. aureus*, or both	• *S. aureus* group II elaborating exfoliating toxin
Epidemiology	• preschool and young adults living in crowded conditions, poor hygiene, neglected minor trauma	• neonates and older children, can be epidemic
Differential Diagnosis	• infected eczema, HSV, varicella virus	• bullous drug eruption, pemphigus vulgaris, bullous insect bites, thermal burns
Investigations	• Gram stain and culture of blister fluid or biopsy	• Gram stain and culture of blister fluid or biopsy
Treatment	• remove crusts, use saline compresses and topical antiseptic soaks bid • topical antibacterials such as 2% mupirocin or fusidic acid tid, continued for 7-10 days after resolution • systemic antibiotics such as cloxacillin or cephalexin for 7-10 days	• cloxacillin for 7-10 days • topical antibacterials such as fusidic acid or mupirocin, continued for 7-10 days after oral antibiotic is stopped • complication: high levels of toxin in immunocompromised or young children may lead to generalized skin peeling or SSSS

Deeper Skin (Dermal)

Table 16. Comparison of Erysipelas and Cellulitis

	Erysipelas	Cellulitis
Lesion	• upper dermis • may be confluent, erythematous, raised, warm plaque • very painful (once called St. Anthony's fire)	• lower dermis/subcutaneous fat • unilateral erythematous flat lesion, often with vesicles poorly demarcated, not uniformly raised • tender
Distribution	• face and legs	• commonly legs
Etiology	• GAS	• GAS, *S. aureus* (large sized wounds), *H. influenzae* (periorbital), *Pasteurella multocida* (dog/cat bite)
Systemic Symptoms	• fever, chills, headache, weakness (more serious)	• fever, leukocytosis, lymphadenopathy (less common)
Complications	• scarlet fever, streptococcal gangrene, fat necrosis, coagulopathy • spreads through lymphatics	• less likely
Treatment	• first line: penicillin, cloxacillin or cefazolin • second line: clindamycin or cephalexin • if allergic to penicillin use erythromycin	• first line: cloxacillin or cefazolin/cephalexin • second line: erythromycin or clindamycin • children: cefuroxime • diabetes mellitus (DM) (foot infections): trimethoprim-sulfamethoxazole (TMP/SMX) and metronidazole

• clinical diagnosis therefore rarely do skin/blood culture.
• if suspect necrotizing fasciitis, do immediate biopsy and frozen section histopathology.
• differential diagnosis: deep vein thrombosis (DVT) (less red, less hot, smoother), superficial phlebitis, contact dermatitis, photosensivity reaction, stasis dermatitis, panniculitis, vasculitis

Common Hair Follicle Infections

Table 17. Comparison of Superficial Folliculitis, Furuncles and Carbuncles

	Superficial Folliculitis	Furuncles (Boils)	Carbuncles
Definition	• superficial infection of the hair follicle • pseudofolliculitis: inflammation of follicle due to friction, irritation, or occlusion	• red, hot, tender, inflammatory nodules involving subcutaneous tissue that arises from a hair follicle • sites: hair-bearing skin (thigh, neck, face, axillae, perineum, buttocks)	• deep-seated abscess formed by multiple coalescing furuncles
Etiology	• normal non-pathogenic bacteria (*Staphylococcus* - most common; *Pseudomonas* - hot tub) • *Pityrosporum*	• *S. aureus*	• *S. aureus*
Signs and Symptoms	• acute lesion consists of a dome-shaped pustule at the mouth of hair follicle • pustule ruptures to form a small crust • sites: primarily scalp, shoulders, anterior chest, upper back, other hair-bearing areas	• develops as a red, tender nodule with central yellowish point, which forms over summit and ruptures	• usually in areas of thicker skin • occasionally ulcerates • lesions drain through multiple openings to the surface • systemic symptoms may be associated
Treatment	• antiseptic (Hibitane™) • topical antibacterial (fusidic acid, mupirocin, or erythromycin) • oral cloxacillin for 7-10 days	• incise and drain large carbuncles to relieve pressure and pain • if afebrile: hot wet packs, topical antibiotic • if febrile/cellulitis: culture blood and aspirate pustules (Gram stain and C&S) • cloxacillin for 1-2 weeks (especially for lesions near external auditory canal/ nose, with surrounding cellulitis, and not responsive to topical therapy)	• same as for furuncles

Sexually Transmitted Infections

SYPHILIS

Definition and Clinical Features
• sexually transmitted infection caused by *Treponema pallidum* characterized initially by a painless ulcer (chancre)
• transmitted sexually, congenitally, or rarely, by transfusion
• following inoculation, becomes a systemic infection with secondary and tertiary stages

Table 18. Stages of Syphilis

	Primary Syphilis	Secondary Syphilis	Tertiary Syphilis
Clinical Features	• single red, indurated, PAINLESS chancre, that develops into painless ulcer with raised border and scanty serous exudate • chancre develops at site of inoculation after 3 weeks of incubation and heals in 4-6 weeks; chancres may also develop on lips or anus • regional non-tender lymphadenopathy appears <1 week after onset of chancre • DDx: chancroid (painful), HSV (multiple lesions)	• 2-6 months after primary infection (patient may not recall presence of primary chancre) • associated with generalized lymphadenopathy, splenomegaly, headache, chills, fever, arthralgias, myalgias, malaise, photophobia • lesions heal in 1-5 weeks and may recur for 1 year • three types of lesions: 1) macules and papules, flat top, scaling, non-pruritic, sharply defined, circular/annular rash DDx: pityriasis rosea, tinea corporis, drug eruptions, lichen planus 2) condyloma lata: wart-like moist papules around genital/perianal region 3) mucous patches: macerated patches mainly found in oral mucosa	• extremely rare • 3-7 years after secondary • main skin lesion: 'Gumma' – a granulomatous non-tender nodule
Investigations and Diagnosis	• cannot be based on clinical presentation alone • VDRL negative – repeat weekly for 1 month • fluorescent treponemal antibody-absorption (FTA-ABS) test has greater sensitivity and may detect disease earlier in course • darkfield examination – spirochete in chancre fluid or lymph node aspirate	• VDRL positive • FTA-ABS +ve; –ve after 1yr following appearance of chancre • darkfield +ve in all secondary syphilis except macular exanthem	• as in primary syphilis, VDRL can be falsely negative
Treatment	• penicillin G, 2.4 million units IM, single dose	• as for primary syphilis	• treatment: penicillin G, 2.4 million units IM weekly

Natural History of Untreated Syphilis
• Inoculation
• Primary syphilis (10-90 d after infection)
• Secondary syphilis (simultaneous to primary syphilis or up to 6 mo after healing of primary lesion)
• Latent syphilis
• Tertiary syphilis (2-20 y)

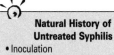

Latent Syphilis
The period between healing of clinical lesions and appearance of late manifesations. 70% of untreated patients will remain in this stage for the rest of their lives and are immune to new primary infection.

GONOCOCCEMIA

Definition
• disseminated gonococcal infection

Etiology
• *Neisseria gonorrheae*

Signs and Symptoms
• hemorrhagic, tender, pustules on a purpuric/petechial background
• sites: distal aspects of extremities
• associated with fever, arthritis, urethritis, proctitis, pharyngitis and tenosynovitis
• conjunctivitis if infected via birth canal

Treatment
• notify Public Health authorities
• screen for other sexually transmitted infections (STIs)
• cefixime 400 mg PO (drug of choice) or ceftriaxone 125 mg IM

Dermatophytoses

Definition
• infection of skin, hair and nails caused by dermatophytes (fungi that live within the epidermal keratin and do not penetrate deeper structures)

Etiology and Pathophysiology
• *Trichophyton, Microsporum, Epidermophyton* species (*Pityrosporum* is a superficial yeast)
• digestion of keratin by dermatophytes results in scaly skin, broken hairs, crumbling nails

Investigations
- skin scrapings, hair, and nail clippings analyzed with potassium hydroxide (KOH) prep → look for hyphae and mycelia

Treatment
- topicals as first line agents for tinea corporis/cruris and tinea pedis (interdigital type) e.g. clotrimazole or terbinafine cream applied OD or bid, until one week after complete resolution of lesions
- oral therapy is indicated for onychomycosis or tinea capitis [e.g. terbinafine (Lamisil™ – liver toxicity, CYP 2D6 inhibitor) or itraconazole (Sporanox™ – heart failure reported, CYP 3A4 inhibitor)]

Table 19. Different Manifestations of Dermatophyte Infection

	Definition and Clinical Features	Differential Diagnosis	Investigations	Treatment
Tinea Capitis	• superficial fungal infection of scalp, eyelashes, and eyebrows involving hair shafts and follicles • round, scaly patches of alopecia, possibly with broken off hairs, pruritic • a kerion (boggy, elevated, purulent inflamed nodule/plaque) may form secondary to infected by bacteria and result in scarring • affects children (mainly black), immunocompromised adults • very contagious and may be transmitted from barber, hats, theatre seats, pets • may have occipital lymphadenopathy	• alopecia areata, psoriasis, seborrheic dermatitis, trichotillomania	• Wood's light examination of hair: green fluorescence only for *Microsporum* infection • culture of scales/hair shaft • microscopic examination of a KOH preparation of scales or hair shafts	• griseofulvin x 8 weeks or terbinafine (Lamisil™) x 2-4 weeks • NB- oral agents are required to penetrate the hair root • adjunctive antifungal shampoos or lotions may be helpful • e.g. slenium sulfide, ketoconazole, ciclopirox
Tinea Corporis (Ringworm)	• pruritic, scaly, round/oval plaque with active erythematous margin and central clearing • site: trunk, limbs, face	• granuloma annulare, pityriasis rosea, psoriasis, seborrheic dermatitis	• microscopic examinations of KOH prep of scales scraped from active margin shows hyphae • scales can be cultured	• topicals – 1% clotrimazole or 2% miconazole bid for 2-4 weeks
Tinea Cruris ("Jock Itch")	• scaly patch/plaque with a well-defined, curved border and central clearing on medial thigh • does not involve scrotum • pruritic, erythematous, dry/macerated	• candidiasis (involvement of scrotum and has satellite lesions), contact dermatitis, erythrasma	• same as for tinea corporis	• topicals – 1% clotrimazole or 2% miconazole bid for 2-4 weeks
Tinea Pedis (Athlete's Foot)	• pruritic scaling and/or maceration of the web spaces and powdery scaling of soles • acute infection: interdigital (esp. 4th web space) red/white scales, vesicles, bullae, often with maceration • may present as flare-up of chronic tinea pedis • frequently become secondarily infected by bacteria • chronic: non-pruritic, pink, scaling keratosis on soles and sides of feet • predisposing factors: heat, humidity, occlusive footwear	• atopic dermatitis, contact dermatitis, dyshidrotic dermatitis, erythrasma, intertrigo (interdigital), psoriasis	• same as for tinea corporis	• topicals – 1% clotrimazole or 2% miconazole bid for 2-4 weeks

Table 19. Different Manifestations of Dermatophyte Infection (continued)

	Definition and Clinical Features	Differential Diagnosis	Investigations	Treatment
Tinea Manuum	• acute: blisters at edge of red areas on hands • chronic: single dry scaly patch • primary fungal infection of the hand is rare; usually associated with tinea pedis	• atopic dermatitis, contact dermatitis, granuloma annulare, psoriasis	• same as for tinea corporis	• topicals – 1% clotrimazole or 2% miconazole bid for 2-4 weeks
Tinea Unguium (Onychomycosis)	• crumbling, distally dystrophic nails; yellowish, opaque with subungual hyperkeratotic debris • toenail infections usually precede fingernail infections • T. rubrum (90% of all toenail infections)	• Psoriasis, lichen planus, contact dermatitis, traumatic onychodystrophies, bacterial infections	• KOH prep of scales from subungual scraping shows hyphae on microscopic exam • subungual scraping or nail clippings may be cultured on Sabouraud's agar	• terbinafine (Lamisil™) (6 weeks for fingernails, 12 weeks for toenails) • itraconazole (Sporanox™) 7 days on, 3 weeks off (2 pulses for fingernails, 3 pulses for toenails) • topical- ciclopirox (Penlac™); nail laquer

Viral Infections

HERPES SIMPLEX

Signs and Symptoms
- herpetiform (i.e. grouped) umbilicated vesicles on an erythematous base
- caused by HSV
- vesicles located on skin or mucous membranes
- transmitted via contact with erupted vesicles or via asymptomatic viral shedding
- primary
  - children and young adults
  - usually asymptomatic; may have high fever, regional lymphadenopathy, malaise
- followed by antibody formation and latency of virus in nerve root ganglion
- secondary
  - recurrent form seen in adults; much more common than primary
  - prodrome: tingling, pruritus, pain
  - triggers for recurrence: fever, sunburn, physical trauma, menstruation, emotional stress, upper respiratory tract infection (URTI)

Classification
- 2 biologically and immunologically different subtypes: HSV-1 and HSV-2

HSV-1
- most commonly "cold sores" (grouped vesicles which quickly burst and commonly occur at the muco-cutaneous junction)
- recurrent on face, lips but NOT on mucous membranes (unlike aphthous ulcers)

Treatment
- treat during prodrome to prevent vesicle formation
- topical antiviral (Zovirax™) cream, apply 5-6x/day, 4-7 days for facial/genital lesions
- oral antivirals are far more effective and have an easier dosing schedule

HSV-2
- sexually transmitted; incubation 2-20 days
- gingivostomatitis (entire buccal mucosa involved with erythema and edema of gingiva)
- vulvovaginitis (edematous, erythematous, extremely tender, profuse vaginal discharge)
- urethritis (watery discharge in males)
- recurrent on vulva, vagina, penis, lasting 5-7 days
- diagnosis
  - negative darkfield, negative serology for syphilis, negative bacterial cultures
  - Tzanck smear with Giemsa stain shows multinucleated giant epithelial cells
  - tissue culture and electron microscopy of vesicular fluid
  - skin biopsy
  - antibody titres increase one week after primary infection only (no increase with recurrent lesions)

Both HSV-1 and HSV-2 can occur on face or genitalia.

Differential Diagnosis of Genital Ulcerations
- *Candida balanitis*, chancroid, multiple syphilitic chancres

Treatment of HSV-2
* rupture vesicle with sterile needle
* wet dressing with aluminum subacetate solution, Burow's compression, or betadine solution
* acyclovir 400 mg po bid: 10 days for 1st episode
* famciclovir and valacyclovir may be substituted and have better enteric absorption
* in case of herpes genitalis, look for and treat any other sexually-transmitted infections

Complications
* dendritic corneal ulcer
* EM
* herpes simplex encephalitis
* HSV infection on atopic dermatitis causing Kaposi's varicelliform eruption (eczema herpeticum)

HERPES ZOSTER (SHINGLES)

Definition
* dermatomal infection caused by varicella zoster in a person who has already had the primary infection (chicken pox)

Risk Factors
* immunosuppression, old age, occasionally associated with hematologic malignancy

Signs and Symptoms
* unilateral dermatomal eruption occurring 3-5 days after pain and paresthesia of that dermatome
* vesicles, bullae, and pustules on an erythematous, edematous base
* lesions may become eroded/ulcerated and last days-weeks
* pain is pre-herpetic, synchronous with rash, or post-herpetic
* severe post-herpetic neuralgia often occurs in elderly
* involvement of tip of nose suggests eye involvement

Distribution
* thoracic (50%), trigeminal (10-20%), cervical (10-20%); disseminated in HIV patients

Differential Diagnosis
* before thoracic skin lesions occur, must consider other causes of chest pain, contact dermatitis, localized bacterial infection, zosteriform herpes simplex virus (more pathogenic for the eyes than varicella zoster)

Treatment
* compress with normal saline, Burow's, or betadine solution
* analgesics (NSAIDs, amitriptyline)
* for patients over 50 years old, with severe acute pain or ophthalmic involvement: famciclovir or valacyclovir for 7 days or acyclovir for 7 days if immunocompromised; must initiate within 72 hours to be of benefit
* gabapentin 300-600 mg PO tid
* early and sufficient treatment helps reduce the incidence of post-herpetic neuralgia

MOLLUSCUM CONTAGIOSUM

Definition and Clinical Features
* discrete dome-shaped and umbilicated pearly, white papules caused by DNA pox virus (molluscum contagiosum virus (MCV))
* sites: eyelids, beard (likely spread by shaving), neck, axillae, trunk, perineum, buttocks

Epidemiology
* common in children and AIDS patients
* transmission: direct contact, auto-inoculation, sexual

Treatment
* topical cantharidin (a keratolytic)
* liquid nitrogen cryotherapy
* curettage
* Aldara™ (immune system modulation) (iniquimod)

Herpes Zoster typically involves a single dermatome; lesions rarely cross the midline.

WARTS (HUMAN PAPILLOMA VIRUS (HPV) INFECTIONS)

Table 20. Different Manifestations of HPV Infection

	Definition and Clinical Features	Differential Diagnosis
Verruca Vulgaris (Common Warts)	• hyperkeratotic, elevated discrete epithelial growths with papillated surface caused by HPV – at least 80 types are known • located at trauma sites: fingers, hands, knees of children and teens • paring of surface reveals punctate, red-brown specks (dilated capillaries)	• molluscum contagiosum, seborrheic keratosis
Verruca Plantaris (Plantar Warts) and Verruca Palmaris (Palmar Warts)	• hyperkeratotic, shiny, sharply marginated growths • commonly caused by HPV 1, 2, 4, 10 • located at pressure sites: heads of metatarsal, heels, toes • paring of surface reveals red-brown specks (capillaries), interruption of epidermal ridges	• need to scrape ("pare") lesions to differentiate wart from callus and corn
Verruca Planae (Flat Warts)	• multiple discrete, skin coloured, flat topped papules grouped or in linear configuration • common in children • commonly HPV 3, 10 • sites: face, dorsa of hands, shins, knees	• syringoma, seborrheic keratosis, molluscum contagiosum, lichen planus
Condyloma Acuminata (Genital Warts)	• skin-coloured pinhead papules to soft cauliflower like masses in clusters on genitalia and perianal areas • commonly HPV 6 and 11 • HPV 16, 18, 31, 33 cause cervical dysplasia, squamous cell cancer and invasive cancer • often occurs in young adults, infants, children • can be asymptomatic, lasting months to years • highly contagious, transmitted sexually and non-sexually (e.g. Koebner phenomenon via scratching, shaving), and can spread without clinically apparent lesions • Investigations: acetowhitening (subclinical lesions seen with 5% acetic acid x 5 minutes and hand lens) • Complications: fairy-ring warts (satellite warts at periphery of treated area of original warts)	• condyloma lata (secondary syphilitic lesion, darkfield strongly +ve), molluscum contagiosum

Wart vs. Corn vs. Callous
Distinguishing features of Corns, Callouses, and Warts

Corns (underlying bony protuberance)
Paring reveals a whitish yellow central translucent keratinous core

Callouses
Paring reveals layers of yellowish keratin with no thrombosed capillaries or interruption of epidermal ridges

Verruca vulgaris (Warts)
Paring reveals multiple bleeding points and thrombosed capillaries

Treatment for skin warts
First Line Therapies
salicylic acid preparations (patches, solutions, creams, ointments)
silver nitrate stick
topical cantharone
glutaraldehyde
occlusive methods (duct tape)

Second Line Therapies
liquid nitrogen cryotherapy
topical imiquimod

Third Line Therapies
curettage
cautery
surgery
laser
oral cimetidine (particularly children)
topical 5-fluorouracil
topical tretinoin (flat warts)
localized heat therapy
intralesional bleomycin (plantar warts)

Treatment for Anogenital warts
First line therapies
imiquimod 5% cream
podophyllotoxin (solution, cream, or gel)
podophyllin resin
cryotherapy

Second line therapies
trichloroacetic acid
topical 5-fluorouracil
electrodessication (ED)
surgical excision
(with cold steel or scissors)
CO_2 laser

Table 21. Treatment of Warts

Treatment	Type of Wart	Notes
Destructive		
liquid nitrogen/electrodesiccation	All	dyschromia, pain, 10-30 seconds
surgery	Resistant	scar, recurrence
laser	Resistant	CO_2 and Nd:Yag lasers
Caustic Acids		
cantharidin (topical)	Small, common	keratolytic irritation, blisters, hyperpigmentation
mono-di-and tri-chloracetic acid	Common	irritation, blisters, scar
Chemotherapeutic Agents		
podophyllotoxin*	Genital	erythema, erosions, ulcers, pain
bleomycin (intralesional)*	Common	pain, nail loss/dystrophy, Raynaud's phenomenon
Hypersensitivity Agents		
dinitrochlorobenzene (DNCB)	Common, plantar	causes an allergic/hypersensitivity reaction
Immune Response Modifiers		
5% imiquimod cream (Aldara™)*	Genital	erythema, burning, erosion
Miscellaneous		
no treatment	Common	65-90% resolve spontaneously over several years
salicylic acid 40% minimum	Common, plantar	over the counter (OTC), use with occulsion
tretinoin (topical)*	Flat	irritation
cimetidine (oral)*	Resistant	best in children
canthrone plus	Common, plantar	cantharidin + podophyllin + salicylic acid
duct tape		
± occlusion/callous scraping/paring		

* = Avoid in pregnancy

Yeast Infections

CANDIDIASIS

Candidal paronychia
- painful red swellings of periungual skin mucous membranes
- glossitis (thrush), balanitis, vulvovaginitis

Candidal intertrigo
- macerated/eroded erythematous patches that may be covered with papules and pustules, located in intertriginous areas often under breast, groin, or interdigitally
- peripheral "satellite" pustules
- predisposing factors – obesity, diabetes, systemic antibiotics, immunosuppression, malignancy
- intertrigo starts as non-infectious maceration from heat, moisture and friction; evidence that it has been infected by Candida is a pustular border
- treatment: keep area dry, miconazole cream bid until rash clears

PITYRIASIS (TINEA) VERSICOLOUR

Definition
- chronic asymptomatic superficial fungal infection with brown/white scaling macules

Etiology and Pathophysiology
- *Pityrosporum ovale (Malassezia furfur)*
- microbe produces carboxylic acid → inflammatory reaction inhibiting melanin synthesis yielding variable pigmentation
- affinity for sebaceous glands; require fatty acids to survive

Epidemiology
- *Pityrosporum ovale* also associated with folliculitis and seborrheic dermatitis
- predisposing factors: summer, tropical climates, Cushing's syndrome, prolonged corticosteroid use

Signs and Symptoms
- affected skin darker than surrounding skin in winter, lighter in summer (does not tan)
- sites: upper trunk most common

Investigations
- KOH prep of scales for hyphae and spores

Oral Terbinafine (Lamisil™) is not effective because it is not secreted by sebaceous glands.

Treatment
- scrub off scales with soap and water
- selenium sulfide body lotion
- ketoconazole cream or PO daily for 10 days if more extensive

Parasitic Infections

SCABIES

Definition
- a transmissible parasitic skin infection due to *Sarcoptes scabiei*, a mite, characterized by superficial burrows, intense pruritus (especially nocturnal), and secondary infection

Epidemiology/Pathogenesis
- risk factors: sexual promiscuity, crowding, poverty, nosocomial
- immunocompromised: "Crusted (Norwegian) Scabies"; all over body, millions of mites
- scabies mite remains alive 2-3 days on clothing/sheets
- incubation = 1 month, then pruritus begins
- re-infection followed by hypersensitivity in 24 hours

Differential Diagnosis
- asteatotic eczema, dermatitis herpetiformis (vesicles, urticaria, eosinophilia, no burrows), lichen simplex chronicus (neurodermatitis)

Signs and Symptoms
- primary lesion: superficial linear burrows
- secondary lesions: small urticarial crusted papules, eczematous plaques, excoriations
- sites: axillae, groin, buttocks, hands/feet (especially web spaces), sparing of head and neck (except in infants)

Investigations
- microscopic examination of root and content of burrow with KOH for mite, eggs, feces

Treatment
- bathe, then apply permethrin 5% cream (i.e. Nix™) or permethrin 1% (Kwellada P™) from neck down to soles of feet (must be left on for 8-14 hours and may require second treatment 7 days after first treatment)
- change underwear and linens; wash with detergent in hot water cycle then machine dry
- ± antihistamine
- treat family and contacts
- pruritus may persist for 2-3 weeks due to prolonged hypersensitivity reaction

LICE (PEDICULOSIS)

Definition and Clinical Features
- intensely pruritic red excoriations, morbilliform rash, caused by louse (a parasite)
- scalp lice: nits (i.e. louse eggs) on hairs
  - red excoriated skin with secondary bacterial infection, lymphadenopathy
- pubic lice: nits on hairs
  - excoriations
- body lice: nits and lice in seams of clothing
  - excoriations and secondary infection mainly on shoulders, belt-line and buttocks

Differential Diagnosis
- bacterial infection of scalp, seborrheic dermatitis

Treatment
- permethrin 1% (Nix™ cream rinse) (ovicidal) or permethrin 1% (RC & Cor™, Kwellada-P™ shampoo)
- comb hair with fine-toothed comb using dilute vinegar solution to remove nits
- repeat in 7 days
- bedding, clothing and towels should be changed and washed with detergent in hot water cycle then machine dried

Leukoplakia

Definition
- white plaque or patch that is not characterized pathologically or clinically as any other disease
- seen as a precancerous or premalignant condition
- oral form is strongly associated with tobacco use and alcohol consumption

Epidemiology
- 1-5% prevalence in adult population after 30 years of age; peak at age 50
- M>F, fair-skinned
- most common oral mucosal premalignant lesion

Differential Diagnosis
- lichen planus, oral hairy leukoplakia

Signs and Symptoms
- sharply demarcated borders, homogeneous or speckled white plaque
- most often found on floor of mouth, soft palate, and ventral and lateral surfaces of the tongue

Investigations
- biopsy is mandatory because it is a premalignant lesion

Treatment
- low risk sites (buccal/labial mucosal or hard palate): eliminate carcinogenic habits, follow-up
- moderate/dysplastic lesions: excision, cryotherapy

Pre-Malignant Skin Conditions

- **nevus sebaceous:** salmon-coloured waxy plaques on scalp; usually solitary, hairless, 10% become basal cell carcinomas (BCC)
- **actinic keratosis:** See D6; 1-10% become squamous cell carcinoma (SCC)
- **dysplastic nevi:** See Table 5
- **giant, congenital hairy nevi:** 10% malignant melanoma
- **lentigo maligna** may transform into malignant melanoma (MM)

Work-up of Nonmelanoma Skin Cancers (NMSC)
- **History**: duration, growth rate, family/personal hx of skin cancer, prior therapy to the particular lesion
- **Physical**: determine exact location, size, whether circumscribed, tethering to deep structures, full skin exam, lymph node exam (basosquamous/SCCs)
- **Biopsy**: if shallow lesion/shallow therapy considered, do shave biopsy; otherwise punch biopsy

Malignant Skin Tumours

Table 22. Skin Phototypes (Fitzpatrick)

Phototypes	Colour of Skin	Skin's Response to Sun Exposure (without SPF protection)
Sun Exposure		
I	White	Always burns, never tans
II	White	Always burns, little tan
III	White	Slight burn, slow tan
IV	Pale brown	Slight burn, faster tan
V	Brown	Rarely burns, dark tan
VI	Dark brown/black	Never burns, dark tan

Basal Cell Carcinoma

Definition
- malignant proliferation of basal cells of the epidermis (primarily tangential growth)
- subtypes: noduloulcerative, pigmented, superficial, sclerosing

Epidemiology
- 75% of all malignant skin tumours >40 years, increased prevalence in the elderly
- M>F, skin phototypes I and II, chronic cumulative sun exposure
- usually due to UV light, therefore >80% on face
- may also be caused by scar formation, radiation, trauma, arsenic exposure or genetic predisposition (Gorlin syndrome)

Margins
- **smaller lesions**: electrodesiccation and curettage with 2-3 mm margin of normal skin
- **deep infiltrative lesions**: surgical excision with 3-5 mm margins beyond visible and palpable tumour border; may require skin graft or flap

Differential Diagnosis
- intradermal melanocytic nevus, nodular malignant melanoma (biopsy), sebaceous hyperplasia, SCC

Signs and Symptoms
- noduloulcerative (typical)
  - skin-coloured papule/nodule with rolled, translucent ("pearly") telangiectatic border and depressed/eroded/ulcerated centre
- pigmented variant
  - flecks of pigment in translucent lesion with surface telangiectasia
  - may mimic malignant melanoma
- superficial variant
  - scaly plaque with fine telangiectasia at margin
- sclerosing variant
  - flesh/yellowish-coloured, shiny papule/plaque with indistinct borders

Treatment
- electrodesiccation and curettage
- surgical excision ± microscopically controlled surgery (Mohs surgery - unique minimally invasive stepwise excision)
- radiotherapy (less traumatic, useful in areas difficulty to reconstruct; requires skilled physician because of many complications)
- cryotherapy
- life-long follow-up
- 95% cure rate if lesion is less than 2 cm in diameter
- slow growing lesion, locally invasive and rarely metastatic (<0.1%)
- imiquimod 5% cream (Aldara™) can be used for primary superficial lesions if surgical management is inappropriate

Cutaneous T-Cell Lymphoma

Definition
- T-cell lymphoma, first manifested in skin

Epidemiology
- >50 years old, M:F 2:1

Differential Diagnosis
- nummular dermatitis, psoriasis

Signs and Symptoms
- two major forms:
  - **Mycosis Fungoides** (limited superficial type)
    - characterized by erythematous patches/plaques/nodules/tumours which may be pruritic, poikiloderma ("cigarette-paper skin"; atrophy, telangiectasia and pigment changes)
    - leonine facies (caused by extensive infiltration)
    - mildly symptomatic, usually excellent prognosis
  - **Sezary Syndrome** (widespread systemic type)
    - rare variant characterized by universal erythroderma ("redman syndrome"), lymphadenopathy, WBC >20 x 10^9 cells per litre with Sezary cells
    - hair loss, pruritus
    - fatigue, fever, often fatal

Investigations
- skin biopsy (histology, lymphocyte antigen "cell" markers, TcR gene arrangement)
- blood smear looking for Sezary cells or flow cytometry (e.g. CD4: CD8 >10 is Sezary)
- imaging (for systemic involvement)

Treatment
- **Mycosis Fungoides**
  - topical steroids and/or PUVA, narrow band (311-313 mm), UVB (NBUVB)
- **Sezary Syndrome**
  - oral retinoids and interferon, extra-corporeal photophoresis
  - may need radiotherapy → total skin electron beam radiation
  - may maintain on UV therapy

Malignant Melanoma

Definition
- malignant neoplasm of pigment forming cells (melanocytes and nevus cells)
- several different subtypes based on pathology (see below)

Epidemiology
- incidence 1:100
- risk factors: numerous moles, fair skin, red hair, positive personal/family history, large congenital nevi, familial dysplastic nevus syndrome (100%)
- most common sites: back (M), calves (F)
- worse prognosis if: male, on scalp, hands, feet, late lesion, no pre-existing nevus present

Signs and Symptoms
- malignant characteristics of a mole: see mnemonic "**ABCDE**"
- sites: skin, mucous membranes, eyes, CNS

Prognostic Indicators
- ulceration or microulceration upstages risk
- number of nodes more important than size of nodes
- sentinel node status is single most important prognostic factor for recurrence and survival

Lentigo maligna
- malignant melanoma in situ (normal and malignant melanocytes confined to the epidermis)
- 2-6 cm, tan/brown/black uniformly flat macule or patch with irregular borders
- lesion grows radially and produces complex colours
- sites: face, sun exposed areas
- 1/3 evolve into lentigo maligna melanoma

Lentigo maligna melanoma (15% of all melanomas)
- malignant melanocytes invading into the dermis
- flat, brown, stain-like lesion that gradually enlarges with loss of skin surface markings
- with time, colour changes from uniform brown to dark brown with black and blue hues
- found on all skin surfaces, especially those often exposed to sun
- not associated with preexisting acquired nevi

Superficial spreading melanoma (60-70% of all melanomas)
- atypical melanocytes initially spread laterally in the epidermis then invade the dermis
- irregular, indurated, enlarging plaques with red/white/blue discolouration, focal papules and nodules
- ulcerate and bleed with growth

Nodular melanoma (30% of all melanomas)
- atypical melanocytes that initially grow vertically with little lateral spread
- uniformly ulcerated, blue-black, and sharply delineated plaque or nodule
- rapidly fatal

Acrolentiginous melanoma (5% of all melanomas)
- ill-defined dark brown, blue-black macule
- palmar, plantar, subungual skin
- melanomas on mucous membranes have poor prognosis

Treatment
- excisional biopsy preferable, otherwise incisional biopsy
- remove full depth of dermis and extend beyond edges of lesion only after histologic diagnosis
  - beware of lesions that regress – tumour is usually deeper than anticipated
- lymph node dissection shows survival advantage if nodes uninvolved
- chemotherapy (cis-platinum, BCG), high dose interferon α for stage II (regional) and stage III (distant) disease
- radiotherapy is curative for uveal melanomas, palliative for bone and brain metastases

American Joint Committee on Cancer Staging System
Based on Breslow's Thickness of Invasion
- T1   <1.0 mm
- T2   1.01-2.0 mm
- T3   2.01-4.0 mm
- T4   >4.0 mm
- a = no ulceration; b = ulceration

- Stage I   T1a - T2a   5-year survival 90%
- Stage II   T2b - T4b   5-year survival 70%
- Stage III   any nodes   5-year survival 45%
- Stage IV   any mets   5-year survival 10%

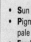

Does this Patient have a Mole or Melanoma?
JAMA 1998; 279(9): 696-701.

ABCDE checklist:
A - **A**symmetry
B - **B**order (irregular)
C - **C**olour (varied)
D - **D**iameter (increasing or >6 mm)
E - **E**nlargement, elevation, evolution

Sensitivity 92% (CI 82-96%)
Specificity 100% (CI 54-100%)

**Risk Factors for Melanoma
(no SPF is a SIN)**
- **S**un exposure
- **P**igment traits (blue eyes, fair/red hair, pale complexion)
- **F**reckling

- **S**kin reaction to sunlight (increased incidence of sunburn)
- **I**mmunosuppressive states (e.g. renal transplantation)
- **N**evi (dysplastic nevi; increased number of benign melanocytic nevi)

Node dissection for lesions >10 mm
- assess sentinel nodes
  - if macroscopically or microscopically positive, a lymph node dissection should be preformed prior to wide excision of the primary melanoma to ensure accurate lymphatic mapping

Squamous Cell Carcinoma

Definition
- a malignant neoplasm of keratinocytes (primarily vertical growth)

Epidemiology
- primarily on sun-exposed skin in the elderly, M>F, skin phototypes I and II, chronic sun exposure, second most common type
- predisposing factors include UV radiation, ionizing radiation therapy/exposure, immunosuppression, PUVA, atrophic skin lesions, chemical carcinogens such as arsenic, tar and nitrogen mustards
- organ transplant recipients
  - SCC is most common cutaneous malignancy
  - increased mortality

Differential Diagnosis
- BCC, Bowen's disease, melanoma, nummular eczema, psoriasis

Signs and Symptoms
- indurated erythematous nodule/plaque with surface scale/crust, and eventual ulceration
- more rapid enlargement than BCC
- sites: face, ears, scalp, forearms, dorsum of hands

Treatment
- surgical excision with primary closure, skin flaps or grafting
- lifelong follow-up (more aggressive treatment than BCC)

Prognosis
- prognostic factors include: immediate treatment, negative margins, and small lesions
- SCCs that arise from actinic keratosis metastasize less frequently (~1%) than other SCCs (e.g. arising de novo in old burns) (2-5% of cases)
- overall control is 75% over 5 years, 5-10% metastasize

BOWEN'S DISEASE (SQUAMOUS CELL CARCINOMA IN SITU)

Definition
- erythematous plaque with a sharply demarcated red and scaly border

Signs and Symptoms
- often 1-3 cm in diameter and found on the skin and mucous membranes
- evolves to SCC in 10-20% of cutaneous lesions and >20% of mucosal lesions

Treatment
- biopsy required for diagnosis
- as for BCC
- topical 5-fluorouracil (Efudex™) or imiquimod (Aldara™) used if extensive and as a tool to identify margins of poorly defined tumours

Heritable Disorders

Ichthyosis Vulgaris

Definition
- a generalized disorder of hyperkeratosis leading to dry skin, associated with atopy and keratosis pilaris

Epidemiology
- 1:300 incidence
- autosomal dominant inheritance
- associated with atopic dermatitis

Signs and Symptoms
- "fish-scale" appearance especially on extremities with sparing of flexural creases, palms and soles, scaling without inflammation

Treatment
- immersion in bath and oils
- emollient or humectant creams, and creams or oils containing urea

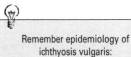
Remember epidemiology of ichthyosis vulgaris:
2 A.D.
atopic **d**ermatitis and
autosomal **d**ominant

Neurofibromatosis (Type I; von Recklinghausen's Disease)

Definition
- autosomal dominant disorder with excessive and abnormal proliferation of neural crest elements

Epidemiology
- autosomal dominant inheritance
- incidence 1:3,000

Signs and Symptoms
- diagnostic criteria include 2 or more of:
  1) more than 6 café-au-lait spots >1.5 cm in an adult,
     and more than 5 café-au-lait spots >0.5 cm in a child under age 5
  2) axillary or inguinal freckling
  3) iris hamartomas (Lisch nodules)
  4) optic gliomas
  5) neurofibromas, and others
  6) distinctive bony lesion
  7) first degree relative with neurofibromatosis type 1
- associated with pheochromocytoma, astrocytoma, bilateral acoustic neuromas, bone cysts, scoliosis, precocious puberty, developmental delay, and renal artery stenosis

Treatment
- follow closely for malignancy, transformation of neurofibroma to neurofibrosarcoma
- excise suspicious or painful lesions
- see Pediatrics

Vitiligo

Definition
- primary pigmentary disorder characterized by hypopigmentation and depigmentation

Epidemiology
- 1% incidence, polygenic
- 30% with positive family history
- associated with other autoimmune disease especially thyroid disease, DM, Addison's disease, pernicious anemia
- may be precipitated by trauma (Koebner phenomenon)

Signs and Symptoms
- acquired destruction of melanocytes characterized by sharply marginated white patches
- sites: extensor surfaces and periorificial areas (mouth, eyes, anus, genitalia)
- associated with streaks of depigmented hair, chorioretinitis

Investigations
- rule out other autoimmune diseases: autoimmune thyroiditis, pernicious anemia, Addison's disease, Type I DM
- Wood's lamp to detect lesions

Treatment
- sun avoidance and protection
- topical immunomodulator (i.e. tacrolimus, pimecrolimus) or a topical steroid for 6-12 months prior to attempting phototherapy
- camouflage preparations
- PUVA
- "bleaching" normal pigmented areas (total white colour) if widespread loss of pigmentation

Skin Manifestations of Systemic Disease

Skin Manifestations of Internal Conditions

Table 23. Skin Manifestations of Internal Conditions

Disease	Related Dermatoses
AUTOIMMUNE DISORDERS	
Buerger's disease	Superficial migratory thrombophlebitis, pallor, cyanosis, gangrene, ulcerations
Cutaneous lupus erythematosus	Sharply marginated annular or psoriaform bright red plaques with scales, telangiectasia, marked scarring, diffuse non-scarring alopecia
Dermatomyositis	Periorbital and perioral violaceous erythema, heliotrope with edema, Gottron's papules (violaceous flat-topped papules with atrophy), periungual erythema, telangiectasia, calcinosis cutis
Polyarteritis nodosa	Polyarteritic nodules, stellate purpura, erythema, gangrene, splinter hemorrhages, livedo reticularis
Rheumatic fever	Petechiae, urticaria, erythema nodosum, erythema multiforme, rheumatic nodules
Scleroderma	Raynaud's, nonpitting edema, waxy/shiny/tense atrophic skin (morphea), ulcers, cutaneous calcification, periungual telangiectasia, acrosclerosis
Systemic lupus erythematosus	Malar erythema, discoid rash (erythematous papules or plaques with keratotic scale, follicular plugging, atrophic scarring on face, hands, and arms), hemorrhagic bullae, palpable purpura, urticarial purpura, patchy/diffuse alopecia, mucosal ulcers, photosensitivity
Ulcerative colitis (UC)	Pyoderma gangrenosum
ENDOCRINE DISORDERS	
Addison's disease	Generalized hyperpigmentation or limited to skin folds, buccal mucosa and scars
Cushing's syndrome	Moon facies, purple striae, acne, hyperpigmentation, hirsutism, atrophic skin with telangiectasia
Diabetes mellitus	Infections (boils, carbuncles, candidiasis, *S. aureus*, dermatophytoses, tinea pedis and cruris, infectious eczematoid dermatitis), pruritus, eruptive xanthomas, necrobiosis lipoidica diabeticorum, granuloma annulare, diabetic foot, diabetic bullae, acanthosis nigricans, calciphylaxis
Hyperthyroid	Moist, warm skin, seborrhea, acne, nail atrophy, hyperpigmentation, toxic alopecia, pretibial myxedema, acropachy, onycholysis
Hypothyroid	Cool, dry, scaly, thickened, hyperpigmented skin; toxic alopecia with dry, coarse hair, brittle nails, myxedema, loss of lateral 1/3 eyebrows
HIV	
Infections	Viral (HSV, HZV, HPV, cytomegalovirus, molluscum contagiosum, oral hairy leukoplakia), bacterial (impetigo, acneiform folliculitis, dental caries, cellulitis, bacillary epithelioid angiomatosis, syphilis), other (candidiasis)
Inflammatory dermatoses	Seborrhea, psoriasis, pityriasis rosea, vasculitis
Malignancies	Kaposi's sarcoma, lymphoma, BCC, SCC, malignant melanoma
MALIGNANCY	
Adenocarcinoma	
Gastrointestinal (GI)	Peutz-Jeghers: pigmented macules on lips/oral mucosa
Cervix/anus/rectum	Paget's Disease: eroding scaling plaques of perineum
Carcinoma	
Breast	Paget's Disease: eczematous and crusting lesions of breast
GI	Palmoplantar keratoderma: thickened skin of palms/soles
Thyroid	Sipple's Syndrome: multiple mucosal neuromas
Breast/GU/lung/ovary	Dermatomyositis: heliotrope erythema of eyelids and purplish plaques over knuckles
Lymphoma/Leukemia	
Hodgkin's	Ataxia Telangiectasia: telangiectasia on pinna, bulbar conjunctiva
Acute Leukemia	Ichthyosis: generalized scaling especially on extremities
	Bloom's Syndrome: butterfly erythema on face, associated with short stature
Multiple Myeloma	Amyloidosis: large, smooth tongue with waxy papules on eyelids, nasolabial folds and lips, as well as facial petechiae
OTHERS	
Liver disease	Pruritus, hyperpigmentation, spider nevi, palmar erythema, white nails, porphyria cutanea tarda, xanthomas, hair loss
Renal disease	Pruritus, pigmentation, half and half nails
Pruritic urticaria papules and plaques of pregnancy	Erythematous papules or urticarial plaques in distribution of striae distensae: buttocks, thighs, upper inner arms and lower backs
Cryoglobulinemia	Palpable purpura in cold-exposed areas, Raynaud's, cold urticaria, acral hemorrhagic necrosis, bleeding disorders, related to hepatitis C infection

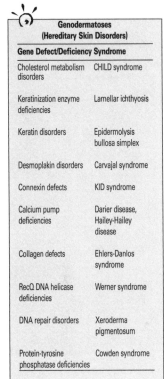

Genodermatoses (Hereditary Skin Disorders)	
Gene Defect/Deficiency	**Syndrome**
Cholesterol metabolism disorders	CHILD syndrome
Keratinization enzyme deficiencies	Lamellar ichthyosis
Keratin disorders	Epidermolysis bullosa simplex
Desmoplakin disorders	Carvajal syndrome
Connexin defects	KID syndrome
Calcium pump deficiencies	Darier disease, Hailey-Hailey disease
Collagen defects	Ehlers-Danlos syndrome
RecQ DNA helicase deficiencies	Werner syndrome
DNA repair disorders	Xeroderma pigmentosum
Protein-tyrosine phosphatase deficiencies	Cowden syndrome

Raynaud's Phenomenon DDx COLD HAND:
Cryoglobulins/ **C**ryofibrinogens
Obstruction/ **O**ccupational
Lupus erythematosus, other connective tissue disease
Diabetes mellitus/ **D**rugs
Hematologic problems (polycythemia, leukemia, etc)
Arterial problems (atherosclerosis)
Neurologic problems (vascular tone)
Disease of unknown origin (idiopathic)

Acanthosis Nigricans
An asymptomatic dark thickened velvety hyperpigmentation of flexural skin most commonly around the neck. Associated with diabetes, obesity and other endocrine disorders and malignancy. It is a cutaneous marker of tissue insulin resistance.

Nails and Disorders of the Nail Apparatus

Table 24. Nail Changes in Systemic and Dermatological Conditions

Nail Abnormality	Definition/Etiology	Associated Disease
NAIL CHANGES		
Clubbing	Proximal nail plate has greater than 180 degree angle to nail fold, watch-glass nails, bulbous digits	Cyanotic heart disease, bacterial endocarditis, pulmonary disorders, GI disorders, etc.
Koilonychia	Spoon shaped nails	Iron deficiency, malnutrition, diabetes
Onycholysis	Separation of nail plate from nail bed	Psoriasis, dermatophytes, thyroid disease
Onychogryphosis	Hypertrophy of the nail plate and subungal hyperkeratosis	Poor circulation, chronic inflammation, tinea
Onychohemia	Subungual hematoma	Trauma to nail bed
Onychomycosis	Fungal infection of nail (e.g. dermatophyte, yeast, mould)	HIV, diabetes, peripheral arterial disease
Onychocryptosis (Ingrown toenail)	Often hallux with congenital malalignment, painful inflammation, granulation tissue	Tight fitting shoes, excessive nail clipping
SURFACE CHANGES		
Wedge Shaped	Distal margin has v-shaped indentation	Darier's disease (Follicular Dyskeratosis)
Pterygium inversus unguium	Distal nail plate does not separate from underlying nail bed	Scleroderma
Pitting	Punctate depressions that migrate distally with growth	Psoriasis, alopecia areata, eczema
Transverse ridging	Transverse depressions often more in central portion of nail plate	Serious acute illness slows nail growth (Beau's lines), eczema, chronic paronychia, trauma
Transverse white lines	Bands of white discolouration	Poisons, hypoalbuminemia (Muherke's lines)
COLOUR CHANGES		
Yellow		Tinea, jaundice, tetracycline, pityriasis rubra pilaris, yellow nail syndrome
Green		*Pseudomonas*
Black		Melanoma, hematoma
Brown		Nicotine use, psoriasis, poisons
Splinter Hemorrhages	Extravasation of blood from longitudinal vessels of nail bed Blood attaches to overlying nail plate and moves distally as it grows	Trauma, bacterial endocarditis, blood dyscrasias, psoriasis
Oil spots	Brown-yellow discolouration	Psoriasis
LOCAL CHANGES		
Herpetic whitlow	HSV infection of distal phalanx	Genital herpes infection
Paronychia	Local inflammation of the nail fold around the nail bed	Acute: painful infection Chronic: constant wetting (e.g. dishwashing, thumbsucking)
Nail fold telangiectasias	Cuticular hemorrhages, roughness, capillary changes	Scleroderma, SLE

Alopecia (Hair Loss)

Hair Growth

- hair grows in a cyclic pattern that is defined in three stages:
  - growth stage = anagen phase
  - degenerative stage = catagen phase
  - resting stage = telogen phase
- total duration of the growth phase reflects the type and location of hair
  - eyebrow, eyelash, and axillary hairs have a short anagen phase in relation to the telogen phase
- growth of the hair follicles is also based on the hormonal response to testosterone and dihydrotestosterone (DHT)
  - this response is genetically controlled

Non-Scarring (Non-Cicatricial) Alopecia

PHYSIOLOGICAL

Definition
- male-pattern alopecia (androgenic alopecia)

Pathophysiology
- action of testosterone on hair follicles

Epidemiology
- early 20's-30's (female androgenic alopecia is diffuse and occurs in 40's and 50's)

Signs and Symptoms
- fronto-temporal areas progressing to vertex, entire scalp may be bald

Treatment
- minoxidil (Rogaine™) lotion to reduce rate of loss/partial restoration
- spironolactone in women (anti-androgenic effects), cyproterone acetate (Diane-35™)
- finasteride (Propecia™) (5-α-reductase inhibitor) 1 mg/d in men
- hair transplant

PHYSICAL
- trichotillomania: impulse-control disorder characterized by compulsive hair pulling with irregular patches of hair loss, and with remaining hairs broken at varying lengths
- traumatic (e.g. tight "corn-row" braiding of hair)

TELOGEN EFFLUVIUM

Definition
- uniform decrease in hair density secondary to an increased number of hairs in telogen phase (resting phase)
- 5% of hair normally in resting phase, about to shed (telogen)

Precipitating Factors
- post-partum, high fever, oral contraceptives, malnutrition, severe physical/mental stress, Fe deficiency

Clinical Course
- 2-4 month latent period after stimulus
- regrowth occurs within few months but may not be complete

ANAGEN EFFLUVIUM

Definition
- hair loss due to insult to hair follicle impairing its mitotic activity (growing phase)

Precipitating Factors
- chemotherapeutic agents (most common), other meds (bismuth, levodopa, colchicine, cyclosporine), exposure to chemicals (thallium, boron, arsenic)
- dose-dependent effect

Clinical Course
- 7-14 days after single pulse of chemotherapy; most clinically apparent after 1-2 months
- reversible effect; follicles resume normal mitotic activity few weeks after agent stopped

Hair Loss: "TOP HAT"
T telogen effluvium, tinea capitis
O out of Fe, Zn
P physical – trichotillomania, "corn-row" braiding
H hormonal – hypothyroidism, androgenic
A autoimmune – SLE, alopecia areata
T toxins – heavy metals, anticoagulants, chemotherapy, Vit. A, SSRIs

Non-scarring alopecia vs. Scarring alopecia

Non-scarring (non-cicatricial) alopecia
Autoimmune
　alopecia areata
Endocrine
　hypothyroidism
　androgens
Micronutrient deficiencies
　iron
　zinc
Toxins
　heavy metals
　anticoagulants
　chemotherapy
　Vitamin A
Trauma to the hair follicle
　trichotillomania
　'corn-row' braiding
Other
　severe illness
　childbirth

Scarring (cicatricial) alopecia
Developmental/Hereditary Disorders
　Aplasia cutis congenita
　Epidermal nevi
　Romberg's syndrome
　Generalized follicular hamartoma
Primary causes
　Group 1: Lymphocytic
　　Lupus erythematosus
　　Lichen planopilaris
　　Classic Pseudopelade
　Group 2: Neutrophilic
　　Folliculitis decalvans
　Group 3: Mixed
　　Acne keloidalis nuchae
Secondary causes
　Infectious agents
　　Bacterial (i.e. post-cellulitis)
　　Fungal (i.e. tinea capitis)
　Neoplasms (i.e. BCC, SCC, lymphomas, and metastatic tumours)
　Physical agents
　　Mechanical trauma
　　Burns
　　Radiotherapy
　　Caustic chemicals

ALOPECIA AREATA

Definition
- autoimmune disorder characterized by patches of complete hair loss (loss of telogen hairs) localized to scalp, eyebrows, beard, eyelashes
- alopecia totalis – loss of all scalp hair and eyebrows
- alopecia universalis – loss of all body hair

Signs and Symptoms
- associated with dystrophic nail changes - fine stippling
- "exclamation mark" pattern (hairs fractured and have tapered shafts, i.e. looks like "!")
- may be associated with pernicious anemia, vitiligo, thyroid disease, Addison's disease

Treatment
- generally unsatisfactory
- intralesional triamcinolone acetonide (corticosteroids) can be used for isolated patches
- wigs
- UV or PUVA therapy
- immunomodulatory (diphencyprone)

Prognosis
- spontaneous regrowth may occur within months of first attack (worse prognosis if young at age of onset and extensive loss)
- frequent recurrence often precipitated by emotional distress

METABOLIC ALOPECIA

Etiology
- drugs: chemotherapy, danazol, vitamin A, retinoids, anticoagulants, thallium, antithyroid drugs, OCPs, allopurinol, propanoid, salicylates, gentamicin, levodopa
- toxins: heavy metals
- endocrine: hypothyroidism

Scarring (Cicatricial) Alopecia

Definition
- irreversible loss of hair follicles with fibrosis

Scarring alopecia: absent hair follicles on exam → biopsy required
Non-scarring alopecia: intact hair follicles on exam → biopsy not required

Etiology
- physical: radiation, burns
- infections: fungal, bacterial, TB, leprosy, viral (herpes zoster)
- inflammatory
  - lichen planus (lichen planopilaris)
  - collagen-vascular
  - discoid lupus erythematosus (treatment with topical/intralesional steroid or antimalarial); note that SLE can cause an alopecia unrelated to discoid lupus lesions which are non-scarring
  - scleroderma: "coup de sabre" with involvement of centre of scalp

Investigations
- biopsy from active border

Pediatric Exanthems

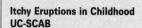

Definition
- exanthem: an eruption on the skin occuring as a symptom of a systemic disease typically with a fever
- enanthem: an eruption on a mucous membrane occuring in the context of an exanthem

Itchy Eruptions in Childhood
UC-SCAB

Urticaria
Contact dermatitis
Scabies
Chicken pox
Atopic dermatitis
Bites

Table 25. Common Pediatric Exanthems

Exanthem	Etiology	Clinical Description	Important Complications	Management
Chicken pox	Human herpes virus (HHV) 3 Incubation 10-21d, communicable 1-2d pre-rash to 5d post-rash	Diffuse vesicular pustular eruption beginning on thorax spreading to extremities New lesions every 2-3d Enanthems	Necrotizing fasciitis, encephalitis, cerebellar ataxia, disseminated intravascular coagulation (DIC), hepatitis	Supportive therapy, Acyclovir if severe, Varicella Zoster Immunoglobulin (within 96 hrs of contact), Varicella vaccine

Table 25. Common Pediatric Exanthems (continued)

Exanthem	Etiology	Clinical Description	Important Complications	Management
Enteroviral	Enteroviruses Most common exanthem in summer and fall	Polymorphous rash (macules, papules, vesicles, petechiae, urticaria)	None	Supportive care for majority Serious cases (immunosuppressed) can be treated with pleconaril
Erythema Infectiosum	Parvovirus B19 Incubation 4-14d Peaks in winter and spring	Slapped cheeks (red, flushed cheeks) then 1-4 days later lacy/reticular maculo-papular rash of trunk/extremities	STAR complex (Sore Throat, Arthritis, Rash) Fetal infection (anemia, fetal hydrops or death) aplastic crisis in sickle cell patients	No treatment: children often feel well NSAIDs for symptomatic arthropathy
Gianotti-Crosti Syndrome	Epstein-Barr virus most common, hepatitis B, coxsackie, parvovirus Spring and early summer	Symmetric papular eruption of face, buttocks, and extremities	None	Supportive treatment
Hand, foot and mouth disease	Coxsackie A and B viruses Highly contagious virus	Vesicular eruption of palms and soles with an erosive stomatitis	Pulmonary neurological death	Supportive treatment
Kawasaki disease	No proven viral etiology, but infectious etiology suggested Superantigen toxin-mediated bacterial process proposed Late winter to early spring	Fever ≥5 days and 4/5: unilateral lymphadenopathy; puffy/red palms and soles; red, cracked lips/strawberry tongue; skin rash; non-purulent bilateral conjunctivitis	Most common cause of vasculitis and acquired heart disease in children CNS, GI tract, kidney, eyes	Aspirin, intravenous immune globulin, baseline echo and repeat in 6 weeks
Measles	Paramyxovirus Incubation 10-14d, communicable 4d before and after rash	Erythematous macular eruption beginning on head and spreading downwards, desquamates, no palm or sole involvement Enanthem: Koplik spots (grey/white papules on buccal mucosa)	Otitis media, pneumonia, encephalitis, SJS, glomerular nephritis, myocarditis/pericarditis	Vitamin A, immunoglobulin, measles/mumps/rubella (MMR) vaccine
Roseola	HHV 6, HHV 7 Incubation 9-10d	Pink macules and papules on trunk, neck, proximal extremities, and occasionally face Eruption after high fever ends	Neurological involvement Viral reactivation in immunosuppressed patients	Supportive treatment Antipyretics during the febrile period
Rubella	RNA virus of the Togaviridae family Incubation 16-18d	1-5 days following mild prodrome (fever, headache, respiratory symptoms), a pink maculo-papular rash erupts on face spreading in a cephalocaudal direction Occipital and retroauricular nodes	STAR complex Congenital rubella (cataract, glaucoma, thrombocytopenia, hepatitis, deafness, congenital heart disease)	Supportive treatment MMR vaccine Serologic testing in rubella-exposed pregnant women
Scarlet Fever	Group A β-hemolytic *streptococci* toxin types A,B, and C Late fall, winter, and early spring	Generalized rash, red papules, "sand-paper" texture, desquamation, flexural accentuation, enanthem (strawberry tongue, petechiae on palate) Pastia's lines – linear petechial streaks in axillary, inguinal, and antecubital areas	Mastoiditis, otitis, sinusitis, pneumonia, meningitis, myocarditis, arthritis, hepatitis, rheumatic fever, and glomerulonephritis	10-14 day course of penicillin

Partially adapted from: Pope E. *Pediatric Exanthems*. Lecture presentation to 2006/2007 University of Toronto Year 3 Medical Students

Erythema Nodosum

Definition
- acute or chronic inflammation of subcutaneous fat (panniculitis)

Etiology
- infections: GAS, primary tuberculosis (TB), histoplasmosis, *Yersinia*
- drugs: sulfonamides, oral contraceptives (also pregnancy), analgesics, trans-retinoic acid
- inflammation: sarcoidosis, Crohn's > Ulcerative Colitis
- malignancy: acute leukemia, Hodgkin's lymphoma
- 40% are idiopathic

Epidemiology
- 15-30 years old, F:M = 3:1
- lesions last for days and spontaneously resolve in 6 weeks

N – **NO** cause (idiopathic)
O in 40%
Drugs (sulfonamides, OCP, etc.)
Other infections (GAS+)
Sarcoidosis
Ulcerative colitis & Crohn's
Malignancy (leukemia, Hodgkin's lymphoma)

Signs and Symptoms
- round, red, tender, poorly demarcated nodules
- sites: asymmetrically arranged on lower legs, knees, arms
- associated with arthralgia, fever, malaise

Investigations
- chest x-ray (to rule out chest infection and sarcoidosis)
- throat culture, antistreptolysin O (ASO) titre, purified protein derivative (PPD) skin test

Treatment
- symptomatic: bed rest, compressive bandages, wet dressings
- NSAIDs
- treat underlying cause

Pruritus

Definition
- a sensation provoking a desire to scratch

Etiology
- dermatologic – generalized
  - asteatotic dermatitis ("winter itch")
  - pruritus of senescent skin (may not have dry skin, any time of year)
  - infestations: scabies, lice
  - drug eruptions: ASA, antidepressants, opiates
  - psychogenic states
- dermatologic – local
  - atopic and contact dermatitis, lichen planus, urticaria, insect bites, dermatitis herpetiformis
  - infection: varicella, candidiasis
  - lichen simplex chronicus
  - prurigo nodularis
- systemic disease – usually generalized
  - hepatic: obstructive biliary disease, cholestatic liver disease of pregnancy
  - renal: chronic renal failure, uremia secondary to hemodialysis
  - hematologic: Hodgkin's lymphoma, multiple myeloma, leukemia, polycythemia vera, hemochromatosis, Fe deficiency anemia, cutaneous T-cell lymphoma
  - neoplastic: lung, breast, gastric (internal solid tumours)
  - endocrine: carcinoid, DM, hypothyroid/thyrotoxicosis
  - infectious: HIV, trichinosis, echinococcosis, hepatitic C
  - psychiatric: depression, psychosis
  - neurologic: post-herpetic neuralgia, multiple sclerosis

Treatment
- treat underlying cause
- cool water compresses to relieve pruritus
- topical corticosteroid and antipruritics (e.g. menthol, camphor, phenol, mirtazapine, capsaicin)
- systemic antihistamines: H1 blockers are most effective, most useful for urticaria
- phototherapy with UVB or PUVA

Wounds and Ulcers

Key to a wound that does not heal ...
- Relentless debridement of biofilm and antimicrobials
- Biopsy any wound without signs of healing after 3 months to rule out cancer!

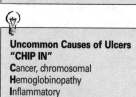

Uncommon Causes of Ulcers "CHIP IN"
Cancer, chromosomal
Hemoglobinopathy
Inflammatory
Pyoderma gangrenosum
Infections
Necrobiosis lipoidica diabeticorum

Table 26. Different Types of Ulcers and Treatment

Ulcer Type	Symptoms and Signs	Treatment
Arterial	Wound at tips of toes, cold feet with claudication, gangrene, distal hyperemia, decreased pedal pulses	1. Doppler study 2. If ankle:brachial ratio <0.4, consider amputation 3. If gangrenous, paint with betadine 4. Otherwise, dressings to promote moist interactive wound healing
Venous	Wound at malleolus, stasis change, edema, previous venous injury	1. Local wound dressing: moist interactive healing 2. Compression: preferably four layers 3. After wound heals, support stockings for life
Neurotropic and Diabetic	Wound at pressure point or secondary to unknown trauma, common at base of 1st metatarsal phalangeal (MTP)	1. Pressure downloading by using proper shoes/seats 2. Promote moist interactive wound healing 3. Appropriate broad-spectrum antibiotic coverage
Vasculitic	Livedo reticularis, petechiae, extreme tenderness, delayed healing	1. Biopsy to determine vasculitis 2. Serum screening for vasculitis 3. Treat vasculitis 4. Local moist interactive wound healing

Common Medications

Topical Steroids

Table 27. Potency Ranking of Topical Steroids

Relative Potency	Relative Strength	Generic Names	Trade Names	Usage
Weak	x1	hydrocortisone 1%	Emo Cort™	Intertriginous areas, children, face, thin skin
Moderate	x3	hydrocortisone 2% 17-valerate - 0.2% desonide mometasone furorate	Westcort™ Tridesilon™ Elocom™	Arm, leg, trunk
Potent	x6	betamethasone - 0.1% 17-valerate - 0.1% amcinonide	Betnovate™ Celestoderm - V™ Cyclocort™	Body
Very Potent	x9	betamethasone dipropionate - 0.05% fluocinonide - 0.05%	Diprosone™ Lidex, Topsyn gel™	Palms and soles
Extremely Potent	x12	clobetasol propionate (most potent) betamethasone dipropionate ointment halobetasol propionate	Dermovate™ Diprolene™ Ultravate™	Palms and soles

Body site: Relative Percutaneous Absorption

forearm	1.0
plantar foot	0.14
palm	0.83
back	1.7
scalp	3.7
forehead	6.0
cheeks	13.0
scrotum	42.0

•calculation of strength of steroid compared to hydrocortisone on forearm: relative strength of steroid x relative percutaneous absorption

Side effects of Topical Steroids
1) Local: atrophy
           perioral dermatitis
           steroid acne
           rosacea
           contact dermatitis
           tachyphylaxis (tolerance)
2) Systemic: suppression of HPA axis

Sunscreens and Preventative Therapy

Sunburn
- erythema 2-6 hours post UV exposure often associated with edema, pain and blistering with subsequent desquamation of the dermis, and hyperpigmentation
- chronic UVB exposure leads to photoaging, immunosuppression, photocarcinogenesis
- prevention: avoid peak UVR (10 am to 4 pm), wear appropriate clothing, wide-brimmed hat, sunglasses, and broad-spectrum sunscreen
- clothing with UV protection expressed as UV protection factor (UPV) is analogous to SPF of sunscreen

Sunscreens
- sun protection factor (SPF): under ideal conditions, an SPF of 10 means that a person who normally burns in 20 minutes will burn in 200 minutes following the application of the sunscreen, regardless of how often the sunscreen is applied
- topical chemical: absorbs UV light
  - requires application at least 15-60 minutes prior to exposure, should be reapplied every 2 hours (more often if sweating, swimming)
  - UVB absorbers: PABA, salicylates, cinnamates, benzylidene camphor derivatives
  - UVA absorbers: benzophenones, anthranilates, dibenzoylmethanes, benzylidene camphor derivatives
- topical physical: reflects and scatters UV light
  - titanium dioxide, zinc oxide, kaolin, talc, ferric chloride and melanin, all are effective against the UVA and UVB spectrum
  - less risk of sensitization than chemical sunscreens and waterproof, but may cause folliculitis or miliaria
- some sunscreen ingredients may cause contact or photocontact allergic reactions, but are uncommon

Treatment
- sunburn: if significant blistering present, consider treatment in hospital; otherwise, symptomatic treatment
- antioxidants, both oral and topical are being studied for their abilities to protect the skin; topical agents are limited by their ability to penetrate the skin

Sunburn therapy
- symptomatic therapy
  - cool, wet compresses and baths
  - moisturizers for dryness and peeling
  - oral anti-inflammatory: 400 mg ibuprofen q6h to relieve pain, minimize erythema, and edema
  - topical corticosteroids: soothes and decreases erythema, especially with immediate application
  - does not reduce damage
  - oral steroids and antihistamines have no role

UV RADIATION
- UVA (320-400 nm)
  - penetrates skin more effectively than UVB or UVC
  - responsible for tanning, burning, wrinkling and premature skin aging
  - penetrates clouds, glass and is reflected off water, snow and cement
- UVB (290-320 nm)
  - absorbed by the outer dermis
  - is mainly responsible for burning and premature skin aging
  - primarily responsible for BCC, SCC
  - does not penetrate glass and is substantially absorbed by ozone
- UVC (200-290 nm)
  - is filtered by ozone layer

UVA- Aging
UVB- Burning
SPF = burn time with cream/burn time without cream

Sun Protection: "Seek, Slip, Slap, Slop."
Seek Shade, **Slip** on a shirt, **Slap** on a hat, **Slop** on sunscreen.

Dermatological Therapies

Table 28. Oral therapies that are important in dermatology

Drug Name	Dosing Schedule	Indications	Comments
acitretin (Soriatane™)	25-50 mg PO OD; maximum 75 mg/d	Severe psoriasis Other disorders of hyperkeratinization (ichthyosis, Darier's disease)	Monitoring strategies: Monitor lipids, LFTs at baseline and q1-2wk until stable Contraindications: Women of childbearing potential unless strict contraceptive requirements are met Drug interactions: Other systemic retinoids, methotrexate, tetracyclines, certain contraceptives May be combined with PUVA phototherapy (known as re-PUVA)
antivirals	famcyclovir (Famvir™) 250 mg PO tid x 7-10 days (for 1st episode of genital herpes) 125 mg PO bid x 5d (for recurrent genital herpes) valacyclovir (Valtrex™) 1000 mg PO bid x 7-10 d (for 1st episode of genital herpes) 500 mg PO bid x 5 d (for recurrent genital herpes)	Chickenpox Herpes zoster Genital Herpes Acute and prophylactic to reduce transmission in infected patients Herpes labialis	Side effects: Headache, nausea, diarrhea, abdominal pain Reduce dose if impaired renal function Side effects: Dizziness, depression, abdominal pain Reduce dose if impaired renal function Drug interactions: cimetidine
cyclosporin (Neoral™)	2.5-4 mg/kg/d PO div bid Max 4 mg/kg/d. Supplied in capsules After 4 weeks may increase by 0.5 mg/kg/d q2wks Concomitant dose of magnesium may protect the kidneys	Psoriasis May also be effective in: Lichen Planus Dermatitis herpetiformis Erythema multiforme Recalcitrant urticaria Recalcitrant atopic dermatitis	Blood pressure, renal function Contraindications: Abnormal renal function, uncontrolled hypertension, malignancy (except non-melanoma skin cancer), uncontrolled infection, immunodeficiency (excluding autoimmune disease), hypersensitivity to drug Long term effects preclude use of cyclosporin for >2 years; discontinue earlier if possible May consider rotating therapy with other drugs to minimize adverse effects of each drug
dapsone	50-100-150 mg PO OD tapering to 25-50 mg PO OD to as low as 50 mg 2x/wk	Pemphigus vulgaris Dermatitis herpetiformis	Monitoring strategies: Obtain thio purine methyl transferase and G6PD levels before initiating; in the initial two weeks obtain methemoglobin levels and follow the blood counts carefully for the first few months Side effects: Neuropathy Hemolysis (Vitamin C and E supplementation can help prevent this) Drug interactions: Substrate of CYP2C8/9 (minor), 2C19 (minor), 2E1 (minor), 3A4 (major) Often a dramatic response within hours
isotretinoin (Accutane Roche™)	0.5-1 mg/kg/day given OD, to achieve a total dose of 120 mg/kg (i.e.16-20 weeks)	Severe nodular and/or inflammatory acne Acne conglobata Recalcitrant acne	Contraindications: Teratogenic – in females, reliable contraception is necessary Generally regarded as unsafe in lactation Side effects: Night blindness, decreased tolerance to contact lenses. May transiently exacerbate acne Monitoring strategies: Baseline lipid profile and hepatic enzymes before treatment, beta-HCG Drug interactions: Do not use at the same time as tetracycline or minocycline – both cause pseudotumour cerebri Discontinue vitamin A supplements Drug may be discontinued at 16-20 weeks when nodule count has dropped by >70%. A second course may be initiated after 2 months prn Refractory cases may require ≥3 courses
itraconazole (Sporanox™)	100-400 mg PO OD, depending on infection treated. Supply: 100 mg tablet TCo, TCr: 200 mg PO OD x 7 days, TP: 100 mg PO OD x 28 days; or, 200 mg PO bid x 7 days, TV: 200 mg PO OD x 7 days. Toenails with or without fingernail involvement: 200 mg PO bid x 7 days once per month, repeated 3x. Fingernail involvement only: 200 mg bid PO x 7 days once per month, repeated 2x	Tinea capitis Onychomycosis May also be used in: Tinea corporis Tinea cruris Tinea pedis Pityriasis versicolor If extensive or recalcitrant	Side effects: Serious hepatotoxicity Contraindications: CHF Drug Interactions: Inhibits CYP 3A4. Increases concentration of some drugs metabolized by this enzyme Give capsules with food, capsules must be swallowed whole

Table 28. Oral therapies that are important in dermatology (continued)

Drug Name	Dosing Schedule	Indications	Comments
ivermectin (Mectizan™, Stromectol™)	200-250 µg/kg PO qwkly x 2. Take once as directed; repeat one week later	Onchocerciasis (USA only) **Not licensed for use in Canada** Also effective for: Scabies	No significant serious side effects Efficacious
methotrexate (Trexall™)	10-25 mg qwk, PO, IM, or IV Max: 30 mg/wk To minimize side effects, consider folic acid supplementation: 1 mg to 5 mg six days/week	Psoriasis Atopic dermatitis Cutaneous T-cell lymphoma Lymphomatoid papulosis May also be effective in: Cutaneous Sarcoidosis	Monitoring strategies: Baseline renal, liver, and hematological studies Contraindications: Pregnancy, lactation, alcohol abuse, liver dysfunction, immunodeficiency syndrome, blood dyscrasias hypersensitivity to drug Restricted to severe, recalcitrant or disabling psoriasis not adequately responsive to other forms of therapy Especially efficacious in nail psoriasis Consider combining with cyclosporine to allow lower doses of both drugs
minocycline (Minocin™)	50-100 mg PO bid. Taper to 50 mg PO OD as acne lessens.	Acne vulgaris Rosacea	Contraindications: Caution if impaired renal or liver function Drug interactions: Do not use with isotretinoin (Accutane™) Side effects: Extensive; affects multiple organ systems including CNS, teeth, eyes, bones, renal, and skin (photosensitivity, and blue pigmentation) Not be used as the sole treatment, or the first treatment Alternative to tetracycline
terbinafine (Lamisil™)	250 mg PO OD x 2 weeks Fingernails x 6 wks Toenails x 12 wks Confirm diagnosis prior to treatment	Tinea capitis Onychomycosis May also be used in: Tinea corporis Tinea cruris Tinea pedis If extensive or recalcitrant	Contraindications: Pregnancy, chronic or active liver disease Drug interactions: Potent inhibitor of CYP 2D6; use with caution when also taking β-blockers, certain anti-arrhythmic agents, MAOI type B, and/or antipsychotics Drug concentrates rapidly in skin, hair and nails at levels associated with fungicidal activity
tetracycline	250-500 mg PO daily (acne) Taken 1 hour before or 2 hours after a meal	Acne vulgaris Rosacea Bullous pemphigoid	Contraindications: Severe renal or hepatic dysfunction Pregnancy/lactation

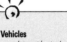

Vehicles
- ointment (water in oil): hydrate, greasy
- cream (oil in water): hydrate, variable
- lotion (oil in water): drying, cosmesis
- solutions (water, alcohol, propylene glycol)
- gel (solution that melts on contact with skin): drying

Table 29. Topical therapies that are important in dermatology

Drug Name	Dosing Schedule	Indications	Comments
calcipotriol (Dovonex™)	0.005% cream, ointment, scalp solution, apply bid. For maintenance therapy apply OD	Psoriasis	Burning, itching, skin irritation, worsening of psoriasis Avoid face, mucous membranes, eyes; wash hands after application Maximum weekly dosage of cream by age: 2-5 years – 25 g/wk 6-10 years – 50 g/wk 11-14 years – 75 g/wk >14, adults – 100g/wk
imiquimod (Aldara™)	5% cream applied 3x/wk Apply at bedtime, leave on 6-10 hours, then wash off with mild soap and water. Max. duration 16 weeks	Genital Warts Cutaneous warts Actinic keratosis Superficial basal cell carcinoma	Avoid natural/artificial sun exposure Local skin and application site reactions; Erythema, ulceration, edema, flu-like symptoms Works best for warts on mucosal surfaces May induce inflammation and erosion
permethrin (Kwellada™ P Lotion and Nix™ dermal cream)	5% cream, applied once overnight to all skin areas from neck down	Scabies (Kwellada-P lotion, Nix™ Dermal Creme) Pediculosis (Kwellada-P Crème Rinse™, Nix Crème Rinse™)	Do not use in children <2 yrs old Hypersensitivity to drug, or known sensitivity to chrysanthemums Local reactions only (resolve rapidly); including burning, pruritis Low toxicity, excellent results Consider 2nd application after 7 days
pimecrolimus (Elidel™)	1.0% cream bid Use for as long as lesions persist and d/c upon resolution of symptoms	Atopic dermatitis (mild to moderate)	Burning Lacks adverse effects of steroids May be used on all skin surfaces including head, neck, and intertriginous areas Expensive
tacrolimus topical (Protopic™)	0.03% (children) or 0.1% (adults) ointment bid Continue for duration of disease PLUS x 1 week after clearing.	Atopic dermatitis (mild to moderate)	Burning Lacks adverse effects of steroids May be used on all skin surfaces including head, neck, and intertriginous areas Expensive

Notes

DM | Diagnostic Medical Imaging

Thien Huynh and Edmund Ng, chapter editors
Justine Chan and Angela Ho, associate editors
Billie Au, EBM editor
Dr. TaeBong Chung, Dr. Nasir Jaffer and Dr. Louis Wu, staff editors

Please see the Essentials of Medical Imaging software for illustrations of the content in this chapter

Imaging Modalities

X-Ray Imaging

- x-rays, or Roentgen rays, are a form of electromagnetic energy of short wavelength
- as x-ray photons traverse matter, they can be absorbed (process known as "attenuation") and/or scattered
- the density of a structure determines its ability to attenuate or "weaken" the x-ray beam (air < fat < water < bone < metal)
- structures that have high attenuation, e.g. bone, appear white on the resulting images
- two broad categories of x-ray based imaging are plain films and computed tomography (CT)

Plain Films
- images are produced by passing x-rays through the patient
- exiting x-rays interact with a detection device to produce a 2-dimensional projection image
- structures closer to the film appear sharper and less magnified
- **contraindications**: pregnancy (relative)
- **advantages**: inexpensive, non-invasive, readily available
- **disadvantages**: radiation exposure, generally poor at distinguishing soft tissues

Computed Tomography (CT)
- x-ray beam opposite a detector moves in a continuous 360° arc as patient is advanced through the imaging system with subsequent computer assisted reconstruction of anatomical structures in the axial plane
- attenuation is quantified in Hounsfield units: +1000 (bone) > +40 (muscle and soft tissue) > 0 (water) > –120 (fat) > –1000 (air)
- by adjusting the "window width" (range of Hounsfield units displayed) and "window level" (midpoint value of the window width), can maximally visualize certain anatomical structures (e.g. CT chest can be viewed using "lung", "soft tissue" and "bone" settings)
- **contraindications**: pregnancy (relative), contraindications to contrast agents
- **advantages**: spiral CT has fast data acquisition, CT angiography less invasive than conventional angiography, delineates surrounding soft tissues, excellent at delineating bones, excellent at identifying lung nodules/liver metastases, may be used to guide biopsies, helical CT may allow 3D reconstruction
- **disadvantages**: high radiation exposure, IV contrast injection, anxiety of patient when going through scanner, relatively high cost, limited availability compared to plain films

Ultrasound (U/S)

- high frequency sound waves are transmitted from a transducer and passed through tissues; reflections of the sound waves are picked up by the transducer and transformed into images
- reflection occurs when the sound waves pass through tissue interfaces of different acoustic densities such that part of the wave energy is reflected as an "echo"
- structures are described based on their echogenicity; hyperechoic structures appear bright whereas hypoechoic structures appear dark on brightness-modulated images
- higher ultrasound frequencies result in greater resolution but greater attenuation (i.e. deeper structures more difficult to visualize)
- **artifacts:** acoustic shadowing refers to the loss of information below an interface (e.g. gallstone) that strongly reflects sound waves; enhancement refers to the increase in reflection amplitude from structures that lie below a structure (e.g. cyst) that weakly attenuates ultrasound
- **Doppler**: determines the velocity of blood flowing past the transducer based on the Doppler effect
- **Duplex scan**: Doppler + visual images
- **advantages**: relatively low cost, non-invasive, no radiation, real time imaging, may be used for guided biopsies, many different imaging planes (axial, sagittal), determines cystic versus solid
- **disadvantages**: highly operator-dependent, air in bowel may prevent imaging of midline structures in the abdomen, may be limited by patient habitus

Typical Effective Doses from Diagnostic Medical Exposures

Diagnostic Procedure	Equivalent Number of Chest x-rays	Approximate Equivalent Period of Natural Background Radiation (~2.2 mSv/year)
X-ray examinations:		
Limbs and joints	<0.5	<1.5 days
Chest (single PA film)	1	3 days
Skull	3.5	11 days
Thoracic spine	35	4 months
Lumbar spine	65	7 months
Hip	15	7 weeks
Pelvis	35	4 months
Abdomen	50	6 months
IVU	125	14 months
Barium swallow	75	8 months
Barium follow through	150	16 months
Barium enema	350	3.2 years
CT head	115	1 year
CT chest	400	3.6 years
CT abdomen or pelvis	500	4.5 years
Radionuclide studies:		
Lung ventilation (Xe-133)	15	7 weeks
Lung perfusion (Tc-99m)	50	6 months
Kidney (Tc-99m)	50	6 months
Thyroid (Tc-99m)	50	6 months
Bone (Tc-99m)	200	1.8 years
Dynamic cardiac (Tc-99m)	300	2.7 years
PET head (F-18 FDG)	250	2.3 years

Source: European Commission, Radiation Protection Report 118, "Referral guidelines for imaging." Directorate-General for the Environment of the European Commission, 2000.

Magnetic Resonance Imaging (MRI)

- non-invasive technique that does not use ionizing radiation
- able to produce images in virtually any plane
- patient is placed in a magnetic field; protons (H+) align themselves along the plane of magnetization due to intrinsic polarity. A pulsed radiofrequency beam is subsequently turned on which deflects all the protons off their aligned axes due to absorption of energy from the radiofrequency beam. When the radiofrequency beam is turned off, the protons return to their pre-excitation axis, giving off the energy they absorbed. It is this energy that is measured with a detector and interpreted by a computer to generate MR images
- the MR image reflects the signal intensity as picked up by the receiver. This signal intensity is dependent on:
  - (1) hydrogen density: tissues with low hydrogen density (cortical bone, lung) generate little to no MR signal and appear black. Tissues with high hydrogen density (water) appear white on MRI
  - (2) magnetic relaxation times (T1 and T2): reflect quantitative alterations in MR signal strength due to intrinsic properties of the tissue and its surrounding chemical and physical environment (see Table 1)

Table 1. MR Signal Intensities

Tissue or Body Fluid	T1 - weighted	T2 -weighted
Gas	Nil	Nil
Mineral-rich tissue (e.g. cortical bone, calculi)	Nil	Nil
Collagenous tissue (e.g. ligaments, tendons, scars) Hemosiderin	Low	Low
Fat	High	Medium to high
Protein-containing fluid (e.g. abscess, complex cyst) Synovium Nucleus pulposus	Medium	High

High bound-water tissues:
   Muscle, hyaline cartilage
   Liver, pancreas, adrenal
	Low	Low to medium

High free-water tissues:
   CSF, urine, bile, edema
   Simple cysts
   GU organs, including kidney
   Thyroid
	Low	High

Hemorrhage: Hyperacute (<24 hours); hyperacute venous hemorrhage is slightly less bright than arterial on T2 due to deoxyhemoglobin	Low	Low
Acute (1–6 days) reflects deoxyhemoglobin	Low	High

Chronic (>7 days) reflects methemoglobin
       • intracellular
       • extracellular
	High
	High
		Low
		High

Neuropathology:
   Ischemia
   Edema
   Demyelination
   Most malignant tumours
	Low	High

Meningioma	Medium / Isointense	Medium / Isointense

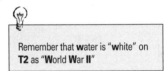

Remember that **w**ater is "**w**hite" on **T2** as "**W**orld **W**ar **II**"

Positron Emission Tomography Scans (PET)

- non-invasive technique that involves exposure to ionizing radiation (~7mSv)
- nuclear medicine imaging technique that produces images of functional processes in the body
- positron-producing radioisotope, such as 18-fluorodeoxyglucose (18-FDG) is chemically incorporated into a metabolically active molecule (glucose), injected into subject, travels to target organ, accumulates in tissues of interest, and radioactive substance begins to decay, sending off gamma rays which are detected by PET scanner
- **advantages**: oncologic early staging (breast, lung, brain), shows metabolism and function of tissues (not only anatomic), follow progression of cancer treatments, early signs of CAD
- **disadvantage**: cost, ionizing radiation, lack of anatomic reference (unless used with CT/MRI)
- **contraindications**: pregnancy

Contrast Enhancement

Contrast Agents in X-Ray Imaging
- contrast media are used to examine structures that do not have inherent contrast differences relative to their surroundings
- contrast can be administered by mouth (anterograde), rectum (retrograde) or intravenous injection prior to x-ray imaging
- contrast agents used include barium sulphate (GI studies), iodine (intravenous pyelogram (IVP), endoscopic retrograde cholangio-pancreatography (ERCP), hysterosalpingography) and gas (air or CO_2 used in GI double contrast exams)

Table 2. Types of Contrast Routes

	Advantages	Disadvantages	Contraindications
Suppository (Barium Enema)	delineates intraluminal anatomy, may demonstrate patency, lumen integrity, or large filling defects; under fluoroscopy, may also give information on function of an organ	risk of contrast reaction; may cause renal failure in dehydrated patients with diabetes, myeloma patients, or patients with pre-existing renal disease	previous adverse reaction to contrast, renal failure, multiple myeloma, dehydration, diabetes, severe heart failure; barium enema is also contraindicated in toxic megacolon, acute colitis, and suspected perforation (use Hypaque™)
IV Contrast	same as above	same as above	previous adverse reaction to contrast, renal failure, multiple myeloma, dehydration, diabetes, severe heart failure

Contrast Agents in MR Imaging
- gadolinium-chelates used to highlight the blood vessels or highly vascular structures (e.g. tumours)

Contrast Reactions
- contrast agents generally safe drugs; adverse reactions exist but they are uncommon
  - anaphylactoid reaction
  - contrast induced nephropathy
- treatment: diphenhydramine ± IV epinephrine

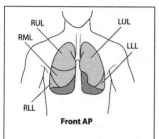

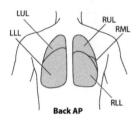

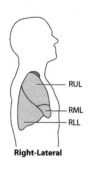

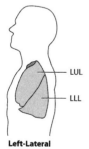

Legend:
RUL: Right Upper Lobe
RML: Right Middle Lobe
RLL: Right Lower Lobe
LUL: Left Upper Lobe
LLL: Left Lower Lobe

Anas Nader © 2009

Figure 1. Lobes

Chest Imaging

Modalities

Chest X-ray
- chest x-ray should be the initial imaging study in all patients with suspected thoracic disease
- standard views: erect posterior to anterior (PA) and left lateral (minimize distortion of heart size by positioning heart closer to film)
- supplemental films may include oblique, lordotic, and (left or right) lateral decubitus views
- patient condition may require AP rather than PA, and supine rather than erect (i.e. bedridden)
- always attempt to obtain a previous study for comparison

Computed Tomography (CT) Scan
- indications for CT in thoracic disease:
  - evaluation of abnormality detected on chest x-ray
  - staging lung malignancies, metastatic disease
  - differentiation of empyema from lung abscess
  - detection of pulmonary embolism (PE protocol)
  - detection and evaluation of aortic dissection
  - determine biopsy approach and may be used to guide biopsy
- high-resolution CT takes fine-cut images of limited areas of the lung. Indications:
  - evaluation of a diffusely abnormal chest x-ray
  - baseline investigation for patients with diffuse lung disease
  - lung disease in a patient with normal CXR and abnormal pulmonary function tests
  - characterization of a solitary pulmonary nodule
  - hemoptysis

Thoracic Ultrasound
- pleural effusions may be identified and tapped, pleural lesions identified and biopsied
- anterior mediastinal masses may be identified and biopsied
- "real-time" imaging can evaluate diaphragmatic excursion

Other Modalities in Chest Imaging
- MRI: brachial plexus, pancoast tumour, cardiac
- nuclear medicine: V/Q scan, bone scan

Approach to the Chest X-Ray (CXR)

Basics
- Identification: date of exam, patient name, sex, age, indications for the study
- Markers: R and/or L
- Position: medial ends of clavicles should be equidistant from spinous process at midline
- Quality: degree of penetration (e.g. thoracic disc spaces should be just visible through heart), lack of motion artifact
- Respiration: right hemidiaphragm at 6th anterior interspace or 10th rib posteriorly on good inspiration; poor inspiration results in poor aeration, vascular crowding, compression and widening of central shadow

Approach
- Soft tissues: neck, axillae, pectoral muscles, breasts/nipples, chest wall
  - nipple markers can help identify nipples (which may mimic lung nodules)
  - look for the amount of soft tissue present and presence of any soft tissue masses
  - look for the presence of air in the soft tissues
- Abdomen (see *Gastrointestinal Tract*, DM10): look for free air under the diaphragm
- Bones: C-spine, T-spine, shoulder girdle, ribs, sternum (seen best on lateral film)
- Central shadow: trachea, heart, great vessels, mediastinum, spine; look for mediastinal or tracheal shift
- Hila: pulmonary vessels, mainstem and segmental bronchi, lymph nodes
- Lungs: lung parenchyma, pleura, diaphragm; lungs on lateral film should become darker when going inferiorly
- Absent structures: review the above, noting ribs, breasts, lung lobes

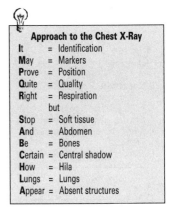

Approach to the Chest X-Ray		
It	=	Identification
May	=	Markers
Prove	=	Position
Quite	=	Quality
Right	=	Respiration
		but
Stop	=	Soft tissue
And	=	Abdomen
Be	=	Bones
Certain	=	Central shadow
How	=	Hila
Lungs	=	Lungs
Appear	=	Absent structures

The Portable CXR
- an x-ray where equipment is brought to the bedridden patient (e.g. in ER, ICU, or general ward)
- resulting radiographs may not be as high in quality as stationary CXR
- generally poor inspiration (vascular crowding and accentuation of normal structures) – shot in AP (apparent increased heart size)
- good for following a patient's progress (e.g. tracking an effusion, pulmonary edema, or line placement)

Common CXR Signs

Kerley B Lines
- thickened connective tissue planes that occur most commonly in pulmonary edema and lymphangitic carcinomatosis
- horizontal, <2 cm long and 1 mm thick, at periphery of lung, reach lung edge

Air Bronchograms
- normally bronchiole walls are not visible because they are filled with air and are surrounded by air
- when surrounding alveoli are filled with fluid, dark, branching markings are visible (air bronchograms)

Silhouette Sign
- in normal CXR, diaphragm and mediastinum are visible because of difference in radiodensity between lung and these structures; i.e. there is an "interface" between the tissues
- "silhouette sign" refers to loss of normally appearing interfaces, implying opacification due to consolidation (most common), atelectasis, mass, etc. in adjacent lung
- silhouetting of different structures is associated with disease in specific parts of the lung (Table 3). Note that pleural or mediastinal disease can also produce the silhouette sign

Table 3. Localization Using the Silhouette Sign

Interface Lost	Location of Lung Pathology
Superior vena cava / right superior mediastinum	Right upper lobe
Right heart border	Right middle lobe
Right hemidiaphragm	Right lower lobe
Aortic knob / left superior mediastinum	Left upper lobe
Left heart border	Lingula
Left hemidiaphragm	Left lower lobe

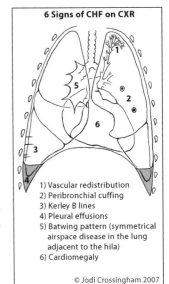

6 Signs of CHF on CXR
1) Vascular redistribution
2) Peribronchial cuffing
3) Kerley B lines
4) Pleural effusions
5) Batwing pattern (symmetrical airspace disease in the lung adjacent to the hila)
6) Cardiomegaly

© Jodi Crossingham 2007

Figure 2. 6 Signs of CHF on CXR

Snowball Sign
- if the mass looks like a snowball just before impact, it is localized in the lungs
- if the mass looks like a flattened snowball after impact, it is localized in the surrounding structures (i.e. chest wall, pleura, or mediastinum)

Common CXR Abnormalities

LUNG

Air Space Disease

DDx of airspace disease
- pus (e.g. pneumonia)
- fluid (e.g. pulmonary edema)
- blood (e.g. pulmonary hemorrhage)
- cells (e.g. bronchioalveolar carcinoma; lymphoma)
- protein (e.g. alveolar proteinosis)

- air space disease refers to a pathological process primarily in the alveoli; it is synonymous with consolidation
  - cardinal features of airspace disease:
    - air bronchogram:
      - lucent branching bronchi visible through opacification
    - airspace nodules:
      - fluffy, patchy, poorly marginated appearance with later tendency to coalesce
      - may take on lobar or segmental distribution

Interstitial Disease

DDx of interstitial disease
- pulmonary edema
- collagen disease (e.g. fibrosis)
- sarcoidosis
- pneumoconiosis
- metastatic disease (e.g. lymphangitic permeation)
- inflammatory conditions (e.g. early viral pneumonia, interstitial pneumonia)

- pathological process involving the interlobular connective tissue (i.e. "scaffolding of the lung")
  - cardinal features of interstitial disease:
    - linear densities: Kerley B lines (see *Common CXR Signs*, DM5)
    - reticular pattern: thin, well-defined linear densities, often in net-like or "honeycomb" arrangement
    - nodular pattern: multiple, discrete, nodular densities, <5 mm diameter
    - reticulonodular: combination of reticular and nodular patterns
- both air space and interstitial disease may occur simultaneously (e.g. pulmonary edema)

Pulmonary Edema

DDx of pulmonary edema
- cardiogenic
- renal failure, volume overload
- non-cardiogenic (e.g. acute respiratory distress syndrome (ARDS))

- look for vascular redistribution/enlargement, pleural effusion, cardiomegaly (may be present in cardiogenic edema and fluid overloaded states)
- edema fluid initially collects in interstitium:
  - loss of definition of pulmonary vasculature
  - peribronchial cuffing
  - Kerley B lines
  - reticulonodular pattern
  - thickening of interlobar fissures
- as pulmonary edema progresses, fluid begins to collect in alveoli causing diffuse air space disease often in a "bat wing" or "butterfly" pattern in perihilar regions with tendency to spare the outermost lung fields

Atelectasis
- loss of lung volume, ranging from subsegmental collapse to collapse of an entire lung
- 5 causes of atelectasis:
  1. **obstructive**: most common and most important type; collapse of alveoli develops within a few hours of airway obstruction as air distal to obstruction is reabsorbed
     - obstructive atelectasis may occur secondary to neoplasm, foreign body, inflammation or mucus plug (seen in cystic fibrosis)
  2. **compressive**: physical compression due to adjacent tumour, bulla, effusion, enlarged heart
  3. **traction (cicatrization)**: due to scarring, which distorts alveoli and contracts the lung
  4. **adhesive**: due to lack of surfactant ($\downarrow$ surfactant = $\downarrow$ lung distensibility); can be congenital (i.e. hyaline membrane disease)
  5. **passive (relaxation)**: a result of air or fluid in the pleural space (i.e. pleural effusion, pneumothorax)
- direct signs of atelectasis:
  - displacement or deviation of a fissure (most important)
  - increased opacity
  - crowding of vessels
  - silhouette sign
- indirect signs of atelectasis (secondary to volume loss):
  - hilar shift toward collapse (most important)
  - mediastinal shift toward collapse (except in tension pneumothorax)
  - diaphragm elevation
  - compensatory hyperinflation in other areas
- in the absence of a known etiology, persisting atelectasis must be investigated to rule out a bronchogenic carcinoma

Pulmonary Nodule (see Table 4)

- differential diagnosis:
  - malignancy (primary or metastatic)
  - benign neoplasm: hamartoma, bronchial adenoma
  - granuloma
  - simulated: nipple, bone lesion, skin lesion, foreign body, artifact
  - less common causes include abscess, hematoma, infarct, loculated pleural effusion, organized pneumonia, sarcoidosis, cystic disease, vascular lesions

> **DDx for cavitating lung nodule**
> **C**ancer
> **A**utoimmune
> **V**ascular
> **I**nfection
> **T**rauma
> **Y**outh (Congenital)

Table 4. Characteristics of Benign & Malignant Pulmonary Nodules

	Malignant	Benign
Margin	ill-defined/spiculated ("corona radiata")	well-defined
Contour	lobulated	smooth
Calcification	eccentric or stippled	diffuse, central, popcorn, concentric
Doubling Time	20-460 days	<20 days or >460 days
Other Features	cavitation, collapse, adenopathy, pleural effusion, lytic bone lesions, smoking history	

- doubling time: time required for a lesion to double in volume; this corresponds to a 1.26x increase in diameter
- 2-year follow-up is recommended; if no change, then >99% chance benign
- CT scan excellent for determining the pattern of calcification and presence of fat (as in hamartoma)
- clinical information and CT appearance determine level of suspicion of malignancy
- if high probability, invasive testing is indicated
- if low probability, repeat CXR or CT in 1-3 months and then every 6 months for 2 years
- invasive tests include fine needle aspiration under CT or fluoroscopic guidance. This is more sensitive (>90% for malignancy) than transbronchial biopsy for peripheral lesion, but carries increased morbidity
- generally transbronchial biopsy is better for central lesions; transthoracic better for peripheral lesions

PLEURA

Pleural Effusion

- in an uncomplicated effusion fluid is higher laterally than medially, forming a meniscus with the pleura; a horizontal fluid level is seen only in a hydropneumothorax (both fluid and air within pleural cavity)
- pooling of fluid occurs first in the posterior recess, then spreads laterally and anteriorly; therefore, the lateral film is most sensitive for pleural effusion (min 75cc of fluid accumulation on lateral film compared to 200cc of fluid on PA to first detect pleural effusion)
- lateral decubitus film with effusion in dependent position will show layering unless effusion is loculated
- supine film with effusion will show diffuse haziness
- effusion may exert mass effect, shift trachea and mediastinum to opposite side or cause atelectasis of adjacent lung
- ultrasound is superior to plain film for detection of small effusions and may also aid in thoracentesis

> **Elevated Hemidiaphragm**
> suggests:
> - intra-abdominal process
> - pregnancy
> - diaphragmatic paralysis
> - atelectasis
> - lung resection
> - pneumonectomy
>
> Pleural effusion also may result in **apparent elevation**.
>
> **Depressed Hemidiaphragm**
> suggests:
> - asthma
> - COPD
> - large pleural effusion
> - tumour

Pneumothorax

- upright chest film allows visualization of visceral pleura as curvilinear line paralleling chest wall, separating partially collapsed lung from pleural air
- more obvious on expiratory (increased contrast between lung and air) or lateral decubitus film (air collects superiorly)
- more difficult to detect on supine film; look for the "deep (costophrenic) sulcus" sign, "double diaphragm" sign (dome and anterior portions of diaphragm outlined by lung and pleural air, respectively), hyperlucent hemithorax, sharpening of adjacent mediastinal structures
- mediastinal shift may occur if air is under tension ("tension pneumothorax")

Asbestos

- asbestos exposure may cause various pleural abnormalities including benign plaques (most common) that may calcify, diffuse pleural fibrosis, effusion, and malignant mesothelioma

MEDIASTINUM (see online imaging)

Mediastinal Mass

- according to Felson's, the mediastinum is divided into three compartments; this provides the approach to the differential diagnosis of a mediastinal mass
- anterior (anterior line formed by anterior trachea and posterior border of heart and great vessels)
  - 4 T's: thyroid, thymic neoplasm (e.g. thymoma), teratoma, and "terrible" lymphoma
  - thymic or pericardial cyst, epicardial fat pad
  - foramen of Morgagni hernia
- middle (extending behind anterior mediastinum to a line 1 cm posterior to the anterior border of the thoracic vertebral bodies)
  - esophageal carcinoma, esophageal duplication cyst
  - metastatic disease
  - lymphadenopathy (all causes)
  - hiatus hernia
  - bronchogenic cyst
- posterior (posterior to the line described above)
  - neurogenic tumour (e.g. neurofibroma, schwannoma)
  - multiple myeloma
  - pheochromocytoma
  - neurenteric cyst, thoracic duct cyst
  - lateral meningocele
  - Bochdalek hernia
  - extramedullary hematopoiesis
- in addition, any compartment may give rise to lymphoma, lung cancer, aortic aneurysm or other vascular abnormality, abscess, and hematoma

Enlarged Cardiovascular Shadow

- heart borders
  - on PA view, right heart border is formed by right atrium; left heart border is formed by left atrium and left ventricle
  - on lateral view, anterior heart border is formed by right ventricle; posterior border is formed by left atrium (superior to left ventricle) and left ventricle
- cardiothoracic ratio = greatest transverse dimension of the central shadow relative to the greatest transverse dimension of the thoracic cavity
  - in an adult, good quality erect PA chest film, cardiothoracic ratio of >0.5 is abnormal; DDx of ratio >0.5:
    - cardiomegaly (myocardial dilatation or hypertrophy)
    - pericardial effusion
    - poor inspiratory effort/low lung volumes
    - pectus excavatum
  - ratio <0.5 does not exclude enlargement (e.g. cardiomegaly + concomitant hyperinflation)
- pericardial effusion
  - globular heart
  - loss of indentations on left mediastinal border
  - peri- and epicardial fat pad separation on lateral film ("sandwich sign")
- right atrial (RA) enlargement
  - increase in curvature of right heart border
  - enlargement of superior vena cava (SVC)
- left atrial (LA) enlargement
  - straightening of left heart border
  - increased opacity of lower right side of cardiovascular shadow (double heart border)
  - elevation of left main bronchus (specifically, the upper lobe bronchus on the lateral film), distance between left main bronchus and "double" heart border >7 cm, splayed carina (late sign)
- right ventricular (RV) enlargement
  - elevation of cardiac apex from diaphragm
  - anterior enlargement leading to loss of retrosternal air space on lateral
  - increased contact of RV against sternum
- left ventricular (LV) enlargement
  - displacement of cardiac apex inferiorly and posteriorly
  - "boot-shaped" heart
  - Rigler's sign: on lateral film, from junction of inferior vena cava (IVC) and heart at level of the left hemidiaphragm, measure 1.8 cm posteriorly then 1.8 cm superiorly → if cardiac shadow extends beyond this point, then LV enlargement is suggested [Note: not to be confused with Rigler's sign in the abdomen]

DDx Anterior Mediastinal Mass:
4 Ts
Thyroid
Thymus
Teratoma
"Terrible" lymphoma

DDx of ↑ Cardiothoracic Ratio
- cardiomegaly (myocardial dilatation or hypertrophy)
- pericardial effusion
- poor inspiratory effort/low lung volumes
- pectus excavatum

Tubes, Lines, and Catheters

- provides information about patient health status
- ensure appropriate placement and assess potential complications of lines and tubes
- avoid mistaking a line/tube for pathology (e.g. oxygen rebreather mask for pneumothoraces)

Central Venous Catheter
- primarily used to administer fluids, medications, and vascular access for hemodialysis – also monitor central venous pressure
- if monitoring pressure – catheter tip must be proximal to venous valves
- tip must be located distal to (above) right atrium as this prevents catheter from producing arrhythmias or perforating wall of atrium
- tip of well positioned central venous catheter projects over silhouette of SVC in a zone demarcated superiorly by the anterior first rib end and clavicle and inferiorly by top of RA
- course should parallel course of superior vena cava – if appears to bend as it approaches wall of SVC – or perpendicular – possibility of catheter damaging and ultimately perforating wall of SVC
- **complications**: pneumothorax, bleeding (mediastinal, pleural), air embolism

Endotracheal Tube
- frontal chest film: tube projects over trachea and shallow oblique or lateral chest radiograph will help determine in 3 dimension
- look for progressive gaseous distention of stomach while lung volumes remain low
- 4 cm above tracheal carina – avoids selective intubation of right/left mainstem bronchus as patient moves, low enough so it doesn't rub against vocal chords
- tube should not be inflated to point that continuously and completely occludes tracheal lumen – pressure induced necrosis of tracheal mucosa and predispose to rupture or eventual stenosis
- maximum inflation diameter <3.0 cm – ensure diameter of balloon is less than tracheal diameter above and below balloon
- **complications**: aspiration (pharenchymal opacities), pharyngeal perforation (subcutaneous emphysema, pneumomediastinum, mediastinitis)

Nasogastric Tube
- tip and sideport of NG tube should be positioned distal to esophagogastric junction and proximal to gastric pylorus
- radiographic confirmation of tube is mandatory because clinical techniques for assessing tip position may be unreliable
- **complications**: aspiration (parenchymal opacities), intracranial perforation (trauma patients), pneumothorax

Swan-Ganz catheter
- monitor pulmonary capillary wedge pressure (usually a resasonable approximation of left atrial end-diastolic pressure) and to measure cardiac output in patients suspected of having left ventricular dysfunction
- tip of Swan-Ganz catheter should be positioned within right or left main pulmonary arteries or in one of their large, lobar branches
- if tip is located more distally, increased risk of prolonged pulmonary artery occlusion resulting in pulmonary infarction or, rarely, pulmonary artery rupture
- **complications**: pneumothorax, bleeding (mediastinal, pleural), air embolism

Chest Tube
- ideally placed to evacuate gas or fluid from pleural space
- gas tend to collect in most nondependent portion of pleural space, while fluid lies in most dependent part
- chest tube to evacuate fluid usually in dorsal and caudad portion of pleural space – for pneumothoraces: ventral and cephalad portions of pleural space
- tube may lie in fissure as long as clinically performing function
- **complications**: lung perforation (mediastinal opacities)

Gastrointestinal (GI) Tract

Modalities

Abdominal X-Ray (AXR)

- acute abdomen: bowel perforation, toxic megacolon, bowel ischemia, small bowel obstruction (SBO), large bowel obstruction (LBO)
- chronic symptoms: constipation, calcifications (gallstones, renal stones, urinary bladder stones, etc.)
- AXR – 3 most common views: supine, upright and left lateral decubitus (LLD)

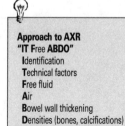

3 Views of Abdomen
- CXR
- Supine AXR
- Erect/Upright AXR

Table 5. Differentiating Small and Large Bowel

Property	Small Bowel	Large Bowel
Mucosal Folds	uninterrupted valvulae conniventes (or plicae circularis)	interrupted haustra extend only partway across lumen
Location	central	peripheral (picture frame)
Maximum diameter	3 cm	6 cm (9 cm at cecum)
Maximum fold thickness	3 mm	5 mm
Other	rarely contains solid fecal material	commonly contains solid fecal material

- bilateral flank fat stripes adjacent to ascending and descending colon
- abdomen divided into 2 cavities:
    - peritoneal cavity - lined by peritoneum that wraps around most of the bowel, the spleen and most of the liver; forms a recess lateral to both the ascending and descending colon (paracolic gutters)
    - retroperitoneal cavity - contains duodenum (2nd, 3rd, and 4th parts), ascending and descending colon and the rectum, pancreas, kidneys, adrenal glands, ureters, bladder, psoas muscles, and the abdominal aorta; the contour of several of these organs can often be seen on radiographs

Abdominal CT

- plain CT: renal colic, hemorrhage
- contrast CT:
    - portal venous phase: majority of cases
    - biphasic (arterial and portal venous phases): liver, pancreas, bile duct tumours
    - oral: barium or water soluble (water soluble if suspected perforation) given in most cases to demarcate GI tract
    - rectal: given for investigation of colonic lesions
    - IV: given immediately before or during CT to allow identification of arteries and veins
    - caution: contrast allergy (give pre-medication = steroids and antihistamine)
    - contraindication: impaired renal function

Approach to Abdominal X-Ray (AXR)

- **Mnemonic: "IT Free ABDO"**
- **I = identification:** date, name, age of patient, type of study
- **T = technical factors:** good coverage, appropriate penetration, identify view
- **Free = free fluid**
    - assess distance between lateral fat stripes and adjacent colon for evidence of free peritoneal fluid in the paracolic gutters
    - pooling of the bowel to the centre of the supine film
    - ascites (free fluid in the peritoneal cavity) and blood (hemoperitoneum) are the same density on the radiograph, therefore, cannot be differentiated
    - large amounts of fluid → diffuse increased opacification on supine film; bowel floats to centre of anterior abdominal wall
- **A = Air**

Approach to AXR
"IT Free ABDO"
Identification
Technical factors
Free fluid
Air
Bowel wall thickening
Densities (bones, calcifications)
Organs

Table 6. Abnormal Air on Abdominal X-Ray

Air	Appearance	Common Etiologies
Extraluminal		
intraperitoneal (pneumoperitoneum)	upright film: air under diaphragm LLD film: air between liver and abdominal wall supine film: gas outlines of structures not normally seen: • inner & outer bowel wall (Rigler's sign) • falciform ligament • peritoneal cavity ("football" sign)	perforated viscus postoperative (up to 10 days to be resorbed)
retroperitoneal	gas outlining retroperitoneal structures allowing increased visualization: • psoas shadows • renal shadows	perforation of retroperitoneal segments of bowel: duodenal ulcer, post-colonoscopy
Intramural (pneumatosis intestinalis)	lucent air streaks in bowel wall, 2 types: 1. linear 2. rounded (cystoides type)	linear: ischemia, necrotizing enterocolitis rounded/cystoides: • primary (idiopathic) • secondary to COPD
Intraluminal	dilated loops of bowel, air-fluid levels	adynamic (paralytic) ileus, mechanical bowel obstruction (see Table 8)
Loculated	mottled, localized in abnormal position without normal bowel features	abscess (evaluate with CT)
Biliary	air centrally over liver cholangitis, emphysematous cholecystitis	sphincterotomy, gallstone ileus, erosive peptic ulcer
Portal venous	air peripherally over liver in branching pattern	bowel ischemia/infarction

What's in the Retroperitoneum?
1) Duodenum (2nd, 3rd, 4th part)
2) Ascending, descending colon
3) Rectum
4) Kidneys, ureters, bladder, adrenals
5) Psoas, quadratus lumborum
6) Aorta, inferior vena cava

Table 7. Adynamic Ileus vs. Mechanical Obstruction

Feature	Adynamic Ileus	Mechanical Obstruction
Calibre of bowel loops	normal or dilated	usually dilated
Air-Fluid levels (erect and LLD films only)	same level in a single loop	multiple air fluid levels giving "step ladder" appearance, dynamic (indicating peristalsis present) "string of pearls" (row of small gas accumulations in the dilated valvulae conniventes)
Other	air throughout GI tract generalized or localized • in a localized ileus (e.g. pancreatitis, appendicitis): dilated loop "sentinel loop" remains in the same location on serial films, usually adjacent to the area of inflammation	dilated bowel up to the point of obstruction (i.e. transition point) no air distal to obstructed segment "hairpin" (180°) turns in bowel ileocecal valve (ICV) function in large bowel obstruction: • competent ICV: bowel distention from site of obstruction to valve; cecal distention >10 cm represents increased risk for perforation • incompetent ICV: small and large bowel distended; radiographic appearance more similar to paralytic ileus

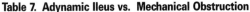

- volvulus ("twisting of the bowel upon itself") – from most to least common:
    - sigmoid: "coffee bean" sign (massively dilated sigmoid projects to right or mid-upper abdomen) with proximal large bowel dilation; see Table 6
    - cecal: massively dilated bowel loop projecting to left or mid-upper abdomen with small bowel dilation
    - gastric: rare
    - small bowel: "corkscrew sign" (rarely diagnosed on plain films, seen best on CT)
- toxic megacolon
    - manifestation of fulminant colitis
    - extreme dilatation of colon (>6.5 cm) with mucosal changes including foci of edema, ulceration and pseudopolyps, loss of normal haustral pattern
- **B = bowel wall thickening**
    - increased soft-tissue density in bowel wall, thumb-like indentations in bowel wall "thumb-printing", or a picket-fence appearance of the valvulae conniventes ("stacked coin" appearance)
    - encountered in IBD, infection, ischemia, hypoproteinemic states, and submucosal hemorrhage

- D = densities
  - bones – look for gross abnormalities of lower ribs, vertebral column and bony pelvis
  - abnormal calcifications – approach by location
    - RUQ: renal stone, adrenal calcification, gallstone, porcelain gallbladder
    - RLQ: ureteral stone, appendicolith, gallstone ileus
    - LUQ: renal stone, adrenal calcification, tail of pancreas
    - LLQ: ureteral stone
    - central: aorta/aortic aneurysm, pancreas, lymph nodes
    - pelvis: phleboliths (calcified veins), uterine fibroids, bladder stones
- O = organs
  - kidney, liver, gallbladder, spleen, pancreas, urinary bladder, psoas shadow
  - outlines can occasionally be identified because they are surrounded by more lucent fat, but all are best visualized with other imaging modalities (CT, MRI)

Approach to Abdominal Computed Tomography (CT)

A Comparison of Colonoscopy and Double-Contrast Barium Enema for Surveillance after Polypectomy
NEMJ 2006 June 15; 342:1766-1772

Study: Randomized, blinded clinical trial.
Patients: Part of National Polyp Study. Total of 580 patients with previous polypectomy.
Intervention: Patients received a total of 862 paired colonoscopy and double-contrast barium enema (DCBE) studies. Endoscopist was blinded to DCBE results (performed prior to colonoscopy).
Main outcomes: For either modality, detection of polyps, size of polyps detected.
Results: Positive colonoscopy studies, 242. Positive barium enema studies, 222 (26%), of which 94 were coincident with colonoscopy findings. Detection rate for DCBE (39%) was significantly related to polyp size. For polyps sized 0.5 cm or less on colonoscopy, 32% of DCBE studies were positive. For polyps sized 0.6 to 1.0 cm, 53% of polyps were detected with DCBE. In the 139 paired examinations with positive DCBE results and negative colonoscopy results, 19 polyps of which 12 were adenomas were detected on colonoscopic re-examination.
Conclusion: Colonoscopy is a more effective method of surveillance than DCBE. No endpoints vis-à-vis patient outcome were examined in this study.

1. look through all images in Gestalt fashion to identify any obvious abnormalities
2. look at each organ/structure individually, from top to bottom evaluating size and shape of each area of increased or decreased density
3. evaluate the following:
   - visible lung (bases), liver, gallbladder, spleen, pancreas
   - adrenals, kidneys, ureters, and bladder
   - stomach, duodenum, small bowel mesentery, and colon/appendix
   - retroperitoneum: aorta, vena cava, and mesenteric vessels; look for adenopathy in vicinity of vessels
   - peritoneal cavity for fluid or masses
   - vertebrae, spinal cord and bony pelvis
   - abdominal wall and adjacent soft tissue

CT and Bowel Obstruction
- cause of bowel obstruction rarely found on plain films – CT is best choice for imaging

CT Colonography (virtual colonoscopy)
- emerging imaging technique for evaluation of intraluminal colonic masses (i.e. polyps, tumours)
- CT scan of the abdomen after the instillation of air into a prepped colon
- computer rendering of 2-dimensional CT images into a 3-dimensional intraluminal view of the colon in order to look for polyps
- lesions seen on 3D rendering correlated with 2D axial images
- indications: surveillance in low-risk patients, incomplete colonoscopy, staging of identified colonic lesions

Contrast Studies

Table 8. Types of Contrast Studies

Study	Description	Indications	Assessment	Diseases
Cine Esophagogram	- contrast agent swallowed - recorded for later playback and analysis		cervical esophagus	aspiration, webs, Zenker's diverticulum, cricopharyngeal bar, laryngeal tumour
Barium Swallow	- contrast agent swallowed under fluoroscopy, selective images captured	dysphagia, r/o GERD, post esophageal surgery	thoracic esophagus	achalasia, hiatus hernia, esophagitis, cancer, esophageal tear: 1) Mallory Weiss tear (mucosal) 2) Submucosal tear (submucosal) 3) Boerhaave's tear (transmural)
Upper GI Series	- double contrast study - (1) barium to coat mucosa, then (2) gas pills for distention - patient NPO after midnight	dyspepsia, investigate possible UGI bleed, weight loss/anemia, post gastric surgery	thoracic esophagus, stomach, duodenum	ulcers, neoplasms, filling defects
Barium Enema	- colon filled retrograde with barium and air or CO_2 - bowel prep the night before procedure	altered bowel habits, suspected LGI bleed, weight loss, anemia, r/o large bowel obstruction, suspected perforation, check surgical anastamosis, history of polyps	large bowel rectum may be obscured by tube - therefore must do sigmoidoscopy to exclude rectal lesions	diverticulosis, neoplasms, IBD, intussusception (can be reduced with barium or air enema), volvulus
Hypaque Enema	- water soluble contrast with or without bowel prep	post operatively to assess anastomoses for leak/obstruction, perforation	large bowel	perforation, obstruction
Small Bowel Follow Through	- single contrast images following UGI series	GI bleed with nondiagnostic upper GI series/barium enema, weight loss/anemia, diarrhea, IBD, malabsorption, abdominal pain, post small bowel surgery	entire small bowel	neoplasms, IBD, malabsorption, infection
Small Bowel Enema (enteroclysis)	duodenal intubation 1) barium/methyl cellulose infusion and fluoroscopic evaluation 2) CT enteroclysis with water infusion	IBD, malabsorption, weight loss/anemia, Meckel's diverticulum	entire small bowel	as above

Specific Visceral Organ Imaging

Liver
- U/S: assessment of cysts, abscesses, tumours, biliary tree
- differentiation of benign hemangiomas from primary liver tumours and metastases as well as cirrhosis and portal hypertension
  - CT ± IV contrast
  - MRI ± IV contrast
- Findings:
  - altered liver size, contour, density
  - fatty infiltration: liver appears less dense than spleen (reverse true if healthy) on CT scan
  - advanced cirrhosis: liver small and irregular (fibrous scarring, segmental atrophy, regenerating nodules)
  - varices (caput medusa, esophageal varices, porto-systemic shunts, dilated splenic vein)
  - splenomegaly and ascites
- investigation of liver masses
  - require contrast to visualize certain hepatic masses
  - hepatic blood supply: 20% hepatic artery, 80% portal vein
  - 3 phases of enhancement following IV contrast bolus:
    - arterial phase (20-30 sec)
      - early and late arterial phase possible on MDCT
      - late arterial phase best for discriminating hypervascular HCC
    - portal venous phase (60-70 sec)
      - provides maximum enhancement of hepatic tissue
      - most tumours supplied by hepatic artery and relatively hypovascular, therefore, appear as low-attenuation masses in portal
    - equilibrium phase (120 - 180 sec)

Revised Estimates of Diagnostic Test Sensitivity and Specificity in Suspected Biliary Tract Disease
Archives of Internal Medicine. 154(22): 2573-81, 1994 Nov 28
Purpose: To assess the sensitivity and specificity of tests used to diagnose cholelithiasis and acute cholecystitis, including ultrasonography, oral cholecystography, radionucleotide scanning with Technetium, MRI, CT.
Study Characteristics: Meta-analysis of 30 studies evaluating the use of different imaging modalities in the diagnosis of biliary tract disease.
Participants: No limits.
Main Outcomes: Sensitivity and specificity of the different imaging modalities, using the gold standard of surgery, autopsy, or 3 month clinical follow-up for cholelithiasis. For acute cholecystitis, pathologic findings, confirmation of an alternate disease, or clinical resolution during hospitalization for cholecystitis were uses as the standard.
Results: For evaluating cholelithiasis, U/S had the best unadjusted sensitivity (0.97; 95% CI, 0.95 to 0.99) and specificity (0.95, 95% CI, 0.88 to 1.00) and adjusted (for verification bias) sensitivity (0.84, 95% CI 0.76 to 0.92) and specificity (0.99; 95% CI, 0.097 to 1.00). For evaluating acute cholecystitis, radionucleotide scanning has the best sensitivity (0.97; 95% CI, 0.96 to 0.98) and specificity (0.90; 95% CI, 0.86 to 0.95).
Conclusions: U/S is the test of choice for diagnosing cholelithiasis and radionucleotide scanning is the superior test for diagnosing acute cholecystitis.

Table 9. Imaging of Liver Masses

Mass	U/S	CT
Metastases	Multiple masses of variable echotexture	Usually low attenuation on contrast enhanced scan
HCC	Single/multiple masses, or diffuse infiltration	Small: hypervascular enhances in arterial phase Large: low-attenuation
Simple cyst	Well-defined, anechoic, acoustic enhancement	Well-defined, low attenuation, homogenous
Abscess	Poorly defined, irregular margin, hypoechoic contents	Low-attenuation lesion with an irregular enhancing wall
Hydatid cyst	Simple/multiloculated cyst	Low-attenuation simple or multiloculated cyst; calcification
Hemangioma	Homogenous hyperechoic mass	Peripheral globular enhancement in arterial phase scans; central-filling and persistent enhancement on delayed scans
Focal nodular hyperplasia	Well-defined mass, central scar seen in 50%	Equal attenuation to liver in portal venous phase, enhancement in arterial phase
Hepatic adenoma	Most common in young women taking oral contraceptives. Well-defined mass with hyperechoic areas due to hemorrhage	Well-defined margin with heterogeneous texture due to hemorrhage or fat

Spleen
- U/S, CT, and/or nuclear medicine scan
- primary lymphoma > splenic metastases
- CT for splenic trauma (hemorrhage)

Biliary Tree
- U/S
  - bile ducts usually visualized only if dilated, secondary to obstruction (e.g. choledocholithiasis, benign stricture, mass)
- CT
  - dilated intrahepatic ductules seen as branching, tubular structures following pathway of portal venous system
- ERCP, MRCP, PTC: further evaluation of obstruction

Pancreas
- tumours
  - U/S: mass is more echogenic than normal pancreatic tissue
  - CT: preferred modality for diagnosis/staging
- ductal dilation secondary to stone/tumour
  - MRCP: imaging of ductal system using MRI cholangiography
  - ERCP: assessment of pancreatic and bile ducts via Ampulla of Vater; therapeutic potential (stent placement, stone retrieval); complication = acute pancreatitis occurs in 5% of diagnostic procedures and 10% of therapeutic procedures
- pancreatitis and/or its complications: pseudocyst, abscess, necrosis, splenic artery aneurysm (see *"itis" Imaging* below)

"itis" Imaging

Acute Cholecystitis
- U/S very accurate – thick wall, pericholecystic fluid, gallstones, dilated gallbladder, positive sonographic Murphy's sign
- nuclear medicine (HIDA scan) may be helpful in equivocal cases, but is not often used; it has equivalent sensitivity and specificity to ultrasound

Acute Appendicitis
- U/S very useful – thick-walled appendix, appendicolith, dilated fluid-filled appendix
- U/S may also demonstrate other causes of RLQ pain (e.g. ovarian abscess, IBD, ectopic pregnancy)
- CT: enlargement of appendix (>6 mm in outer diameter), enhancement of appendiceal wall, adjacent inflammatory stranding, appendicolith
- CT: done to facilitate percutaneous abscess drainage

Computed Tomography and Ultrasonography to Detect Acute Appendicitis in Adults and Adolescents
Annals of Internal Medicine. 141(7): 537-546, 2004 Oct 5
Purpose: To review the diagnostic accuracy of CT and ultrasonography in the diagnosis of acute appendicitis.
Study Characteristics: Meta-analysis of 22 prospective studies evaluating the use of CT or ultrasonography, followed by surgical or clinical follow-up in patients with suspected appendicitis.
Participants: Age 14 and older with a clinical suspicion of appendicitis.
Main Outcomes: Sensitivity and specificity using surgery or clinical follow-up as the gold standard.
Results: CT (12 studies) had an overall sensitivity of 0.94 (95% CI, 0.91 to 0.95) and a specificity of 0.95 (95% CI, 0.93 to 0.96). Ultrasonography (14 studies) had an overall sensitivity of 0.86 (95% CI, 0.83 to 0.88) and a specificity of 0.81 (95% CI, 0.78 to 0.84).
Conclusions: CT is more accurate for diagnosing appendicitis in adults and adolescents, although verification bias and inappropriate blinding of reference standards were noted in the included studies.

Acute Diverticulitis
- most common site is rectosigmoid (diverticula are outpouchings of colon wall)
- CT is imaging modality of choice, although U/S is sometimes used
  - oral and rectal contrast given before CT to opacify bowel
  - cardinal signs: thickened wall, mesenteric infiltration, gas-filled diverticula, abscess
  - CT can be used for percutaneous abscess drainage before or in lieu of surgical intervention
  - sometimes difficult to distinguish from perforated cancer (therefore, send abscess fluid for cytology and follow up with colonoscopy)
  - if chronic, may see fistula (most common to bladder) or sinus tract (linear or branching structures)

Acute Pancreatitis
- clinical/biochemical diagnosis
- imaging used to support diagnosis and evaluate for complications (diagnosis cannot be excluded by imaging alone)
- U/S good for screening and follow up (although useless if ileus present as gas obscures pancreas)
    - hypoechoic enlarged pancreas
- CT is useful in advanced stages of pancreatitis and in assessing for complications and is increasingly becoming the 1st line imaging test
    - enlarged pancreas, edema, stranding changes in surrounding fat with indistinct fat planes, mesenteric and Gerota's fascia thickening, pseudocyst in lesser sac, abscess (gas or thick-walled fluid collection), pancreatic necrosis (low attenuation gas-containing non-enhancing pancreatic tissue), hemorrhage
    - CT-guided needle aspiration and/or drainage done for abscess drainage when clinically indicated
    - pseudocyst may be followed by CT and drained if symptomatic

Angiography of GI Tract

- GI tract arterial blood supply:
    - celiac artery : hepatic, splenic, gastroduodenal, left/right gastric
    - superior mesenteric artery (SMA): jejunal, ileal, ileo-colic, right colic, middle colic
    - inferior mesenteric artery (IMA): left colic, superior rectal
- imaging of GI tract vessels:
    - conventional angiogram: invasive (puncture femoral artery), catheter used
        - aortography: catheter injection into abdominal aorta
        - selective arteriography of individual vessels
    - CT angiogram: IV contrast (no catheterization required), computer generated images

Genitourinary (GU) System

Modalities

CT Urography
- historically, intravenous urography (IVU) provided anatomical and functional information about the urogenital system; this has largely been replaced by CT urography
- excretory-phase CT is new imaging technique of choice exclusively to assess the renal collecting systems. It has a high sensitivity (95%) in detecting upper urinary tract uroepithelial malignancies, and is also useful for detecting renal calculi
- indications include hematuria (with negative cystoscopy and U/S studies ruling out parenchymal causes), unexplained hydronephrosis on U/S, evaluation of the renal collecting system post-trauma (e.g. post pelvic surgery)
- CT features of various renal lesions are as follows:
    - renal cysts: fluid filled lesions with smooth, well-defined borders, low density, no enhancement with contrast (smooth walled, bright lesions on non-contrast CT may suggest hyperdense cysts consisting of debris from proteinaceous material or previous hemorrhage into a benign cyst)
    - complex renal cysts: thick walled, may contain calcifications, some may be septated, walls may enhance with contrast
    - renal cell carcinoma: less-defined borders, same density as kidney, enhancement with contrast (characterizing vascularity) ± areas of necrosis
    - angiomyolipoma (a benign renal neoplasm composed of fat, vascular, and smooth muscle elements): fat density seen on non-contrast CT, some enhancement with contrast (less intense than renal cell carcinoma)

U/S
- initial study for evaluation of kidney size and nature of renal masses (solid vs cystic renal masses vs complicated cysts)
- technique of choice for screening patients with suspected hydronephrosis (no intravenous contrast injection, no radiation to patient , and can be used in patients in renal failure)
- solid renal masses: echogenic (bright on U/S)
- cystic renal masses: smooth well-defined walls with anechoic interior (dark on U/S)
- complicated cysts: internal echoes within a thickened, irregular-walled cyst

- transrectal U/S (TRUS) useful to evaluate prostate gland and guide biopsies
- Doppler U/S to assess renal vasculature

Retrograde Pyelography
- used to visualize the urinary collecting system via a cystoscope, ureteral catheterization, and retrograde injection of contrast medium
- ordered when the intrarenal collecting system and ureters can't be opacified using intravenous techniques (patient with impaired renal function, high grade obstruction)
- only yields information about the collecting systems (renal pelvis and associated structures); no information regarding the parenchyma of the kidney

Voiding Cystourethrogram (VCUG)
- bladder filled with contrast to the point where voiding is triggered
- real-time images via fluoroscopy (continuous x-ray imaging) to visualize bladder
- contractility and evidence of vesicoureteric reflux
- indications: children with recurrent UTIs, hydronephrosis, hydroureter, suspected lower urinary tract obstruction or vesicoureteral reflux

Retrograde Urethrogram
- used mainly to study strictures or trauma to the male urethra

MRI
- strengths: high spatial and tissue resolution, lack of exposure to ionizing radiation and nephrotoxic contrast agents
- indicated over CT for depiction of renal masses in patients with previous nephron sparing surgery, patients requiring serial follow-ups (no radiation dosage), patients with reduced renal function and patients with solitary kidneys

Renal Scan
- 2 radionuclide tests for kidney – renogram and morphological scan
- renogram
  - to assess renal function and collecting system
  - useful in evaluation of renal failure, workup of urinary tract obstruction and hypertension, investigation of renal transplant
  - intravenous injection of a radionuclide, technetium-99m pentetate (Tc99m-DTPA) or iodine-labelled hippurate, and imaged at 1-second intervals with a gamma camera over 30 minutes to assess perfusion. Delayed static images over the next 30 minutes can be used to assess renal function and the collecting system
- morphological
  - to assess renal anatomy
  - study done with Tc99m-DMSA and Tc99m-glucoheptonate
  - useful in investigation of renal mass and cortical scars

Neuroradiology

Modalities

- CT is modality of choice for most neuropathology; even under circumstances when MRI is preferred, CT is frequently the initial study because of its speed, availability and lower cost
- CT is preferred for:
  - acute head trauma: CT is best for visualizing "bone and blood." MRI is used in this setting only when CT fails to detect an abnormality in the presence of strong clinical suspicion
  - acute stroke
  - suspected subarachnoid or intracranial hemorrhage
  - meningitis: rule out mass lesion (e.g. abscess) prior to lumbar puncture
  - tinnitus and vertigo: CT and MRI are used in combination to detect bony abnormalities and CN VIII tumours, respectively

Skull Films
- rarely performed; CT is modality of choice
- indications include:
  - facial fracture
  - sinus disease
  - penetrating trauma

Approach to interpretation of skull films
- bony vault
- sella turcica
- facial bones
- basal foramina
- sinuses
- calcifications
- soft tissues

- destructive bony lesions (e.g. metastases)
- metabolic disease
- skull anomalies
- post-operative changes
- generally not indicated for non-penetrating head trauma
- standard views (each designed to demonstrate a particular area of the skull)
  - PA (frontal bones, frontal/ethmoid sinuses, nasal cavity, superior orbital rims, and mandible)
  - Lateral (frontal, parietal, temporal, and occipital bones, mastoid region, sella turcica, orbital roofs, and lateral aspects of facial bones)
  - Towne's view/occipital; "half-axial" (occipital bone, mastoid and middle ear regions, foramen magnum, and zygomatic arches)
  - Base view (basal structures of skull, including major foramina)
  - Water's view/occipitomental (facial bones and sinuses)
  - panoramic view (mandible)

CT

- excellent study for evaluation of bony abnormalities
- often done first without and then with intravenous contrast to show vascular structures or anomalies
- vascular structures and areas of blood-brain barrier impairment are opaque (white/show enhancement) with contrast injection
  - when in doubt, look for circle of Willis or confluence of sinuses to determine presence of contrast enhancement
- posterior fossa obscured by bone
- rule out skull fracture, epidural hematoma (lenticular shape), subdural hematoma (crescentic shape), subarachnoid hemorrhage, space occupying lesion, hydrocephalus, and cerebral edema

Myelography

- introduction of water-soluble, low-osmotic-contrast media into subarachnoid space using lumbar puncture followed by x-ray or CT scan
- excellent study for disc herniations, traumatic nerve root avulsions
- use has decreased due to MRI

MRI (see Table 1)

- shows brain anatomy in fine detail
- clearly distinguishes white from grey matter (especially T1-weighted series)
- multiplanar reconstruction helpful in pre-op assessment

Cerebral Angiography

- evaluation of vascular lesions such as atherosclerotic disease, aneurysms, vascular malformations
- digital subtraction angiography (DSA) commonly used to create images of vessels

Nuclear Medicine

- SPECT using HMPAO (technetium-99m labelled derivative of propylamine oxane) imaging assesses cerebral blood flow by diffusing rapidly across the blood brain barrier and becoming trapped within cells
- PET imaging assesses cerebral metabolic activity

Selected Pathology

- see Neurosurgery for intracranial mass lesions
- see Neurosurgery and Plastic Surgery for head trauma
- see Emergency Medicine for vertebral trauma

Cerebrovascular Disease (see Neurology and Neurosurgery)

- carotid artery disease
  - evaluate with Duplex Doppler U/S
  - MR angiography or CT angiography if carotid angioplasty or endarterectomy is under consideration (conventional angiography reserved for inadequate MRA or CTA)
- infarction
  - early changes
    - CT
      - usually normal within 6 hours of infarction
      - edema (loss of grey-white matter differentiation – "insular ribbon" sign, effacement of sulci, mass effect)

Attenuation:
bone (= bright) > grey matter > white matter ("fatty" myelin) > CSF > air (= dark)

Approach to head CT
- soft tissues
- bone
- sinuses
- sulci
- cortical parenchyma
- ventricular system
- cisterns (supracellar, ambient, prepontine, cisterna magna)
- symmetry
- midline structures (fornix, pineal gland, falx shift)

DDx for ring enhancing lesion on CT with contrast: "MAGICAL DR"
*Metastases
*Abscess
*Glioblastoma
(high grade astrocytoma)
Infarct
Contusion
AIDS
Lymphoma
Demyelination
Resolving hematoma
[* by far the 3 most common Dx's]

Transient ischemic attacks are not associated with radiological findings.

Early Signs of Brain Infarction at CT: Observer Reliability and Outcome after Thrombolytic Treatment – Systematic Review
Radiology 2005; 235:444–453

Study: Systematic review of 15 studies between 1990-2003 that investigated inter-observer agreement of early CT signs of acute ischemic stroke, and prognostic value of early CT signs in patient outcome. There was a median of 30 CTs and 6 raters per study.
Patients: 3468 adult patients who underwent CT within 6 hours of stroke
Main Outcome: Degree of inter-observer agreement between stroke signs on CT, and risk of death or dependency (using validated stroke scales) based on CT signs using after 1-3 months.
Results: Prevalence of all early infarction signs was 61%±21, and interobserver agreement was 0.14-0.78 (k statistic) for any early infarct sign. Average sensitivity of detecting early ischemic stroke was 66% (range 20%-87%) and average specificity was 87% (range 56%-100%). Experience improved detection, but knowledge of patient history did not. An increased risk of poor outcome (death or dependency) was associated with any early infarction sign, with an odds ratio of 3.11 (95%CI 2.77-3.49).

DDx suspected MS lesion
Vasculopathy: ischemia, vasculitis, hypertension, migraine
Demyelinating disease: MS, progressive multifocal leukoencephalpathy, age-related
Inflammatory process: sarcoid, lyme

– within 24 hours, development of low-density, wedge-shaped area of infarction extending to periphery (orrelating to vascular territory distal to affected artery)
– refer to **Functional Neuroanatomy software**
– in case of ischemic stroke, may see hyperattenuating (bright) artery (hyperdense MCA sign) – intravascular thrombus or embolus
– in case of hemorrhagic stroke or transformation (common in basal ganglia and cortex), may see bright acute blood surrounded by edema
   ◆ MRI
– edema with high signal on T2-weighted images and FLAIR (fluid-attenuated inversion – recovery) image (loss of grey-white matter differentiation, effacement of sulci, mass effect)
– diffusion-weighted image (DWI) shows acute high signal changes demonstrating restricted movement of water (indicative of cytotoxic edema)
– apparent diffusion coefficient (ADC) image shows low signal intensity in acute ischemia (nadir 3-5 days, returns to baseline 1-4 weeks)
   ▪ subacute changes (CT and MRI)
      ◆ edema and mass effect more prominent
      ◆ gyral enhancement with contrast indicative of blood-brain barrier breakdown
   ▪ chronic changes (CT and MRI)
      ◆ encephalomalacia (parenchymal volume loss) with dilatation of adjacent ventricles

Multiple Sclerosis (MS)
- acute phase: plaques undergo inflammatory reaction with edema, cellular infiltration and spectrum of demyelination
- chronic phase: astrocytic hypoplasia, resolution of cellular inflammation and loss of myelin
- MRI is the most sensitive diagnostic test (>90%), but not specific
   ▪ ischemic demyelination can produce similar features
   ▪ confluent multiple sclerosis lesions can be mistaken for a neoplamnm
   ▪ specificity greatly improved if periventricular plaques are accompanied by lesions in the cerebellum, cerebral peduncles, corpus callosum and spinal cord
- T2-weighted MRI shows multiple hyperintense round or ovoid white matter plaques from myelin breakdown in periventricular or subcortical distribution ("Dawson's finger")
- T1-weighted MRI shows iso- or low intensity regions ("black-holes")
- most common locations include periventricular white matter (>80%), corpus callosum (particularly at callosal-septal interface, 50-80%), visual pathways (optic neuritis), posterior fossa, and brainstem
- FLAIR imaging superior for supratentorial white matter lesions; may not detect posterior fossa, brainstem and spinal lesions
- enhancement lasts 2-8 weeks but may persists 6+ months; clinical suspicion for neoplasm required if nodule/plaque enhances for 3+ months
- lesions tend to be confluent and >6 mm in diameter
- new lesions with active demyelination may enhance with gadolinium contrast, ranging from nodular enhancement to ring or arc shape; older, less active lesions do not enhance

Degenerative Spinal Abnormalities (see Neurosurgery and Orthopaedics)
- spondylosis
   ▪ mild: slight disc space narrowing and spur formation
   ▪ severe (spondylosis deformans): marked disc space narrowing, facet joint narrowing, spur formation; may result in stenosis of the intervertebral foramina or vertebral canal
   ▪ if symptomatic, evaluate with CT, MRI, and/or myelography
- herniated disc
   ▪ if symptomatic, evaluate with CT, MRI, and/or myelography

Musculoskeletal System (MSK)

- see Orthopaedics

Modalities

Plain Film/X-Ray
- initial study used in most evaluations of bone
- minimum of two films at right angles to each other (usually AP and lateral) to rule out a fracture
- image proximal and distal joints (particularly important where there are paired bones e.g. radius/ulna)
- not very effective in evaluating soft tissue injury
- fast, inexpensive, readily available

CT
- evaluation of bone cortex and type of cortical expansion
- for comminuted fractures and complex structures (skull, spine, acetabulum, calcaneus, sacrum)
- IV contrast may be used to determine lesion vascularity
- evaluation of soft tissue calcification/ossification

MRI
- excellent for visualization of bone marrow and surrounding soft tissues (ligaments, tendons, joint capsules, menisci, cartilage)
- can visualize vascular structures without need for contrast

Ultrasound
- diagnose tendon and ligament injury (e.g. rotator cuff injury)
- determine if lesions are cystic or solid
- guided biopsy of soft tissue lesions
- Doppler – determines vascularity of structures

Nuclear Medicine (Skeletal Scintigraphy)
- determine the location and extent of bony lesions
- radioisotopes localize to areas of increased bone turnover or calcification – growth plate in children, tumours, infections, fractures, metabolic bone disease (e.g. Paget's), sites of reactive bone formation in arthritis, and periostitis
- very sensitive, not specific (trauma, infection, inflammation look the same)

> **P**lain **F**ilm **F**irst for **F**ractures
> **C**T for **C**ortex
> **M**RI for **M**arrow

> **Approach to Fractures**
> 1) Look for fracture lines (abnormal black lines)
> 2) Look for discontinuation/disruption of cortex border
> 3) Look for joint space narrowing/widening
> 4) Look for soft tissue involvement (swelling, calcification)

Approach to Interpretation of Bone X-Rays

- identification – name, age of patient, type of study, region of investigation
- soft tissues – swelling, calcification/ossification
- joints – alignment, joint space, presence of effusion, osteophytes, erosions, bone density, overall pattern and symmetry of affected joint
- bone – periosteum, cortex, medulla, trabeculae, density, articular ends, bone destruction, bone production, appearance of the edges or borders of any lesions (see Figure 3)

Trauma

Fracture/Dislocation
- description of fractures
  - patient (name, age, sex)
  - views (e.g. AP and lateral of right wrist)
  - site of fracture
    - bone (e.g. tibia, scaphoid, etc.)
    - region of bone (e.g. proximal, distal, metaphyseal, epiphyseal, diaphyseal)
    - intra-articular vs. extra-articular
  - pattern of fracture line
    - simple: a single break divides bone in two pieces
    - comminuted: bone broken into more than two pieces
  - displacement (described with reference to distal fragment)
  - soft tissue involvement
    - calcification, gas, foreign bodies
    - open (compound) vs. closed
    - type of fracture
      - stress: fracture due to repetitive small trauma
      - pathologic: fracture in area of bone weakened by disease
- for specific fracture descriptions and characteristics of fractures, see Orthopaedics

> **Types of Fractures**
> - transverse
> - oblique
> - spiral
> - avulsion
> - impacted

> **Types of Displacements**
> - translation
> - angulation
> - rotation
> - impaction
> - dislocation

Arthritis

- see Rheumatology

Bone Tumour

Approach
- metastatic tumours to bone are much more common than primary bone tumours, particularly if age >40 years
    - diagnosis usually requires a biopsy if primary not located
    - few benign tumours/lesions have potential for malignant transformation
    - CT is the best way to identify the extent of a bone lesion in the cortex, or extent of cortical involvement
    - MRI is good for tissue delineation and preoperative assessment of surrounding soft tissues, and medullary/marrow involvement
    - plain film is less sensitive than other modalities

Considerations
- age – most common tumours by age group:
    - <1 year of age: metastatic neuroblastoma
    - 1-20 years of age: Ewing's tumour in tubular bones
    - 10-30 years of age: osteosarcoma and Ewing's tumour in flat bones
    - >40 years of age: metastases, multiple myeloma and chondrosarcoma
- single or multiple lesions: multiple lesions are more suggestive of malignant process or metabolic disease
- cortical thickening: new bone formation, suggestive of osteomyelitis, malignancy, or pathological fractures

Characteristics of Tumours
- see Figure 3 and Table 10
    - margins/zones of transition
        - transition area from normal bone to area of lesion, reflects aggressiveness of the lesion
        - well-defined lesion with narrow zone of transition (i.e. sharp cut-off between normal and abnormal) suggest a non-aggressive process
        - sclerosed borders are suggestive of a non-aggressive process
        - an ill-defined lesion with a permeative pattern is suggestive of malignancy
    - expansile
        - intact, ballooned cortex is more likely benign
        - destruction of cortex is more likely malignant
    - periosteal reaction
        - mature well-formed solid periosteal reaction: most likely a non-aggressive process
    - soft tissue
        - soft tissue mass: matrix tumour, osseous, cartilage

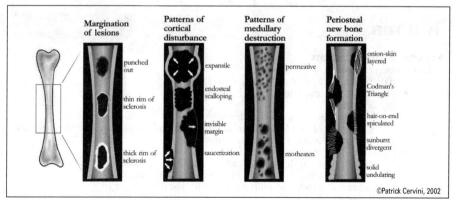

Figure 3. Radiographic Appearance of Bone Remodelling and Destruction Processes

Table 10. Characteristics of Benign and Malignant Bone Lesions

Benign	Malignant
single lesion	multiple lesions (metastatic/multiple myeloma) (some syndromes have multiple benign lesions)
no bone pain	bone pain
sharp area of delineation	poor delineation of lesion – wide zone of transition
overlying cortex intact	loss of overlying cortex/bony destruction
no or simple periosteal reaction	periosteal reaction – aggressive
sclerotic margins with sharp zone of transition	wide zone of transition
no soft tissue mass	soft tissue mass

Note: for specific bone tumours see Orthopaedics

Metastatic Bone Tumours
- all malignancies have potential to metastasize to bone
- metastases are 20-30x more common than primary bone tumours
- when a primary malignancy is first detected, a bone scan is often part of the initial work-up
- may present with pathological fractures or pain
- biopsy or determination of primary is the only way to confirm the diagnosis
- metastasis can cause a lytic (decreased density) or a sclerotic (increased density) reaction when seeding to bone

Table 11. Characteristic Bone Metastases of Common Cancers

Lytic	Sclerotic	Expansile	Peripheral
breast	prostate	thyroid	lung
lung	breast	renal	kidney
thyroid	treated tumours		melanoma
kidney			
multiple myeloma			

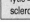

lytic = decreased density
sclerotic = increased density

Most Common Metastatic Bone Tumours
(in order of frequency)
"**Be** **L**ike **P**eople **T**hat **K**now"
Breast
Lung
Prostate
Thyroid
Kidney

Infection

Osteomyelitis
- Tc99m, followed by indium-111 labelled white cell scan or gallium radioisotope scan is the best modality to establish the presence of bone infection
- plain film
  - visible 8-10 days after process has begun
  - osteomyelitic changes on plain film
    - soft tissue swelling that is deep and extends from the bone with loss of tissue planes (because fat becomes edematous)
    - local simple periosteal reaction over the area of bone
    - pockets of air (from anaerobes) may be seen in the tissue planes
    - metaphysis over the area of infection may appear mottled and nonhomogeneous with a classic "moth-eaten" appearance

Bone Abscess
- classical appearance known as Brodie's abscess on plain film
  - overlying cortex has periosteal new bone formation
  - sharply outlined radiolucent area with variable thickness in zone of transition
  - variable thickness periosteal sclerosis
  - sequestrum: a piece of dead bone within a Brodie's abscess
  - a sinus tract or cloaca may communicate between the abscess through the cortex to the surface of the bone

Metabolic Bone Disease

Osteoporosis
- with increasing age, hormonal changes lead to bone resorption exceeding bone formation
- reduction in amount of normal bone; fewer and thinner trabeculae; diffuse process; affecting all bones
- Dual X-ray Absorptiometry (DEXA) – gold standard for measuring bone mineral density (BMD)

Diagnostic sensitivity of DEXA highest when BMD measured at lumbar spine and proximal femur.

- T-Score: the number of standard deviations from the young adult mean
  - used to diagnosis osteoporosis and is a measure of current fracture risk
  - most clinically valuable
  - $-2.5 < t < -1$ = osteopenia
  - $t < -2.5$ = osteoporosis
- Z-score: the number of standard deviations from the age-matched mean
- appearance on plain film:
  - increase in bone lucency
  - compression of vertebral bodies
  - biconcave vertebral bodies ("codfish" vertebrae)
  - long bones have appearance of thinned cortex and increased medullary cavity
  - look for complications of osteoporosis (e.g. insufficiency fractures: hip, vertebrae, sacrum, pubic rami, calcaneus most common)

Osteoporosis
Reduced amount of bone

OsteoM**alacia**
Normal amount of bone, but reduced **M**ineralization of normal osteoid

Osteomalacia/Rickets
- reduction in bone density due to unmineralized osteoid
- initial radiological appearance of both osteoporosis and osteomalacia is osteopenia (coarse and poorly defined bone texture)
- seams of unmineralized osteoid
- "fuzzy", ill-defined trabeculae
- softening and arching of long bones
- Looser's zones (pseudofracture)
  - characteristic radiological feature
  - fissures or clefts at right angles to and extending through cortex of long bones
  - DDx: osteomalacia, chronic renal disease, fibrous dysplasia, hyperthyroidism, Paget's, osteodystrophy, x-linked hypophosphatemia

Hyperparathyroidism
- most common cause is renal osteodystrophy (also caused by malignancy)
- skeletal manifestations of chronic renal insufficiency
  - chondrocalcinosis
  - intra-articular deposits of calcium
  - calcifications of the soft tissues (including arteries and peri-articular soft tissue)
  - resorption of bone typically in hands (subperiosteal and at tufts), SI joints (subchondral), skull ("salt and pepper" appearance), osteoclastomas (brown tumours)
  - "rugger jersey spine": band-like osteosclerosis at superior/inferior margins of vertebral bodies

Paget's Disease
- abnormal remodelling of bone – especially skull, spine, pelvis
- may involve single or multiple bones
- 3 phases: 1st lytic, 2nd mixed (lytic/sclerotic), 3rd sclerotic
- features:
  - coarsening of the trabeculae with bone expansion
  - bone softening/bowing
  - bone scan will reveal high activity, especially at bone ends
  - thickened cortex
- complications:
  - pathological fractures
  - cardiac failure
  - early OA
  - nerve entrapment in base of skull
  - malignant degeneration

Nuclear Medicine

Thyroid

Radioactive Iodine Uptake (see Endocrinology)
- an index of thyroid function (trapping and organification of iodine)
- radioactive I-131 or I-123 PO in fasting patient
  - measured as a percentage of administered iodide taken up by thyroid
- increased RAIU: toxic multinodular goiter, toxic adenoma, Graves' (although may be normal)
- decreased RAIU: subacute thyroiditis, late Hashimoto's disease, hormone suppression
- falsely decreased in patient with recent radiographic contrast studies, high dietary iodine (i.e. seaweed)

Thyroid Imaging (Scintiscan)
- Tc99m pertechnetate IV or radioactive iodine
- provides functional anatomic detail

- hot (hyperfunctioning) lesions
    - adenoma, toxic multinodular goiter
    - usually benign, cancer very unlikely (less than 1%)
- cold (hypofunctioning) lesions
    - cancer must be considered until biopsy negative even though only 6-10% are cancerous
- cool lesions
    - cancer must be considered as a cool lesion may represent cold nodules superimposed on normal tissue
    - if cyst suspected, correlate with U/S
- serum thyroglobulin to detect recurrent thyroid cancer post treatment.

Radioiodine Ablation
- I-131 for Graves, multinodular goiter, thyroid cancer

Respiratory

V/Q Scan
- examine areas of lung in which ventilation and perfusion do not match
- ventilation scan
    - patient breathes radioactive gas through a closed system, filling alveoli proportional to ventilation
    - ventilation scan defects indicate: airway obstruction, chronic lung disease, bronchospasm, tumour mass obstruction
- perfusion scan
    - radiotracer injected IV → trapped in pulmonary capillaries (1 in 1500 arterioles occluded) according to blood flow
    - gives a map of pulmonary circulation
    - relatively contraindicated in severe pulmonary HTN and right-to-left shunt
- PE areas of lung are well ventilated but not perfused (unmatched defect)
- PE is wedge-shaped, extend to periphery, usually bilateral and multiple
- reported as high probability, intermediate, low or normal
- V/Q scans for PE have been largely replaced by spiral CT scan with contrast (see <u>Respirology</u>)

V/Q Scan
For PE investigation: normal scan makes PE unlikely.
Probablity of PE: High 80-100%, intermediate 20-80%, low <20%.

Ventilation scan defects indicate:
airway obstruction, chronic lung disease, bronchospasm, tumour mass obstruction.

Perfusion scan defects indicate:
reduced blood flow due to PE, COPD, asthma, bronchogenic carcinoma, inflammatory lung diseases (pneumonia, sarcoidosis), mediastinitis, mucus plug, vasculitis.

Cardiac

Myocardial Perfusion Scanning
- for investigation of angina, atypical chest pain, coronary artery disease (CAD), post bypass follow-up
- thallium-201 (a radioactive analogue of potassium) or Tc99m MIBI
- injected at peak exercise (physical stress) or after persantine challenge (vasodilator) and again later at rest
- persistent defect (at rest and stress) suggests infarction; reversible defect (only during stress) suggests ischemia
- used to discriminate between reversible (ischemia) vs. irreversible (infarction) changes when other investigations are equivocal
- see <u>Cardiology</u>

Active uptake of radiolabel by myocardium proportional to regional blood flow.

Persistent defect (at rest and stress) suggests infarction; reversible defect (only during stress) suggests ischemia.

Radionuclide Ventriculography
- Tc99m attached to red blood cells
- first pass through right ventricle (RV) → pulmonary circulation → left ventricle (LV) provides information about RV function
- cardiac MUGA scan (MUltiple GAted acquisition scan) sums multiple cardiac cycles
    - evaluation of LV function
    - images are obtained by gating (synchronizing) the count acquisitions to the ECG signal
    - MUGA scan can be used to study the function of the heart at a particular stage of contraction
- provides information on ejection fraction (normal = 55-65%), ventricular volume, and wall motion

MUGA scan can be used to study the function of the heart at a particular stage of contraction. Superior to ECHO only in its reproducibility in EF measurement (precise).

Pyrophosphate Scintigraphy
- technetium pyrophosphate concentrates in bone and necrotic tissue
- used to detect infarcted tissue 1-5 days post-MI when ECG and enzyme results are equivocal or unreliable
- sensitivity and specificity about 90% in transmural infarct

Technetium pyrophosphate concentrates in bone and necrotic tissue.

Bone

Bone Scan
- isotopes
  - technetium Tc99m:
    - triphasic bone scan: perfusion → blood pool → delayed bone images
    - uptake can distinguish bone vs. soft tissue infection and septic arthritis vs. osteomyelitis vs. peripheral cellulitis
    - acute osteomyelitis: increased activity in blood pool and delayed bone images, usually does not cross joint
    - septic arthritis & cellulitis: increased activity in blood pool and normal or slightly increased activity in delayed images, may cross joint
  - indium-111 WBC: tracks the active migration of the WBC – more specific for infection
  - gallium-67 citrate: may see uptake in some tumours, also more specific for infection
- radioactive tracer binds to hydroxyapatite of bone matrix
- increased binding when increased blood supply to bone and/or high bone turnover (active osteoblasts)
- positive bone scan
  - bone metastases from breast, prostate, lung, thyroid
  - primary bone tumour
  - arthritis
  - fracture
  - infection
  - anemia
  - Paget's disease
- multiple myeloma: typically normal or cold (false negative); need a skeletal survey
- superscan: good visualization of bone, but not kidneys, due to diffuse metastases

Indications for a Bone Scan
- bone pain of unknown origin
- AVN
- suspected malignancy
- staging malignancy (cancer of breast, prostate, kidney, thyroid or lung)
- follow up after treatment
- detection and follow up of primary bone disease
- assessment of skeletal trauma
- detection of soft tissue calcification
- renal failure

Abdomen

Liver/Spleen Scans
- IV injection of technetium-labelled sulphur colloid (usually technetium) that is phagocytosed by reticuloendothelial (Kupffer's) cells of liver and spleen
- "cold spots": lesions displacing the normal reticuloendothelial system (RES) (tumour, abscess, cyst, hemangioma, infarct)
- diffuse patchy reduction in uptake: diffuse parenchymal disease (e.g. cirrhosis)

HIDA (Hepatobiliary IminoDiacetic Acid) Scan
- IV injection of radiotracer (HIDA) which is bound to protein, taken up, and excreted by hepatocytes into biliary system
- can be performed in non-fasting state but prefer NPO after midnight
- gallbladder visualized when cystic duct is patent, usually seen by 30 min to 1 hour
- if gallbladder is not visualized, suspect obstructed cystic duct (acute or chronic cholecystitis)
- acute cholecystitis: no visualization of gallbladder at 4-hour or after administration of morphine at 1-hour
- chronic cholecystitis: no visualization of gallbladder at 1-hour but seen at 4-hour or after morphine administration
- differential diagnosis of obstructed cystic duct: acute cholecystitis, decreased hepatobiliary function (commonly due to alcoholism), bile duct obstruction, parenteral nutrition, fasting less than 4 hours or more than 24 hours
- filling of gallbladder rules out cholecystitis (<1% probability)
- assess bile leaks post-operatively

RBC Scan
- IV injection of radiotracer with sequential images of the abdomen (Tc99m labelled RBC)
- GI bleed
  - if bleeding acutely at <0.5 mL/min, the focus of activity in the images generally indicates the site of the acute bleed, look for a change in shape and location on sequential image
  - if bleeding acutely at >0.5 mL/min, use angiography (more specific)
  - RBC scan is more sensitive for lower GI bleed
- liver lesion evaluation
  - hemangioma has characteristic appearance, cold early, fills in later

Renal Scan
- see *Genitourinary System*, DM15

Inflammation and Infection

- use gallium-67 citrate, or indium-111 or Tc99m labelled WBCs
- gallium accumulates in skeleton, lacrimal glands, nasopharynx, normal liver, spleen, bone marrow, sites of inflammation, some neoplasms (lymphomas)
- labelled WBCs accumulate in normal spleen, liver, bone marrow, sites of inflammation and infection (abscess, sarcoid, osteomyelitis)

Brain

- SPECT Tc99m-HMPAO imaging assesses cerebral blood flow, taken up in cortical and subcortical grey matter; used for CVA, vasculitis, dementia
- PET imaging assesses metabolic activity by using 18-FDG
- CSF imaging, intrathecal administration of 111-In DTPA to evaluate CSF leak or to differentiate normal pressure hydrocephalus from other causes of hydrocephalus

Interventional Radiology

Vascular Procedures

Angiography
- injection of contrast material through a catheter placed directly into an artery (or vein) to delineate vascular anatomy
- catheter can be placed into a large vessel (e.g. aorta, vena cava) for a "flush" or selectively placed into a branch vessel for more detailed examination of smaller vessels and specific organs
- more recently, non-invasive evaluation of vascular structures is being performed (colour Doppler U/S, CT angiography (CTA) and MR angiography (MRA))
- **indications**: aneurysm, peripheral ischemia, coronary, carotid and cerebral vascular disease, PE, trauma, bleeding, vascular malformations
- significant complications occur in <5% of patients
- **complications**: puncture site hematoma, infection, pseudoaneurysm, AV fistula, dissection, thrombosis, embolic occlusion of a distal vessel
- see *Neuroradiology*, DM16 and *Angiography of GI tract*, DM15

Contraindications to Intravascular Contrast Media
- anaphylactoid reaction
- renal failure
- multiple myeloma
- dehydration
- diabetes
- severe heart failure

Percutaneous Transluminal Angioplasty (PTA)
- introduction and inflation of a balloon into a stenosed vessel to restore distal blood supply
- common alternative to surgical bypass grafting with five year patency rates similar to surgery, depending on site
- renal, iliac, femoral, mesenteric, subclavian and carotid artery stenoses are amenable to treatment
- vascular stents may help improve long term results by keeping the vessel wall patent after PTA
- covered stents (a.k.a. stent grafts) may provide an alternative treatment for aneurysms and AV fistulas
- **complications**: similar to angiography, but includes vessel rupture

Thrombolytic Therapy
- infusion of a fibrinolytic agent (urokinase, streptokinase, TNK, tPA – used most commonly) via a catheter inserted directly into a thrombus
- can restore blood flow in a vessel obstructed with a thrombus or embolus
- **indications**: treatment of ischemic limb (most common indication), early treatment of MI or stroke to reduce organ damage, treatment of venous thrombosis (DVT of leg or PE)
- **complications**: bleeding, stroke, distal embolus, reperfusion injury with myoglobinuria and renal failure if advanced ischemia present

Advanced ischemia patients should receive surgery rather than thrombolysis.

Embolization
- injection of occluding material into vessels
- permanent agents: coils, balloons, glue
- temporary: gel foam, autologous blood clots
- **indications**: management of hemorrhage (epistaxis, trauma, GI bleed), treatment of AVM, pre-operative treatment of vascular tumours (bone metastases, renal cell carcinoma), varicocele embolization for infertility, symptomatic uterine fibroids
- **complications**:
  - post embolization syndrome (pain, fever, leukocytosis)
  - unintentional embolization of a non-target organ with resultant ischemia

Inferior Vena Cava Filter
- insertion of metallic "umbrellas" to mechanically trap emboli preventing a PE
- inserted via femoral vein, jugular vein, or antecubital vein
- placed infrarenally to avoid renal vein thrombosis
- **indications**: contraindication to anticoagulation, failure of adequate anticoagulation (i.e. recurrent PE despite therapeutic anticoagulant levels), complication of anticoagulation

Central Venous Access
- variety of devices available
  - peripherally inserted central catheter (PICC), external tunnelled catheter (Hickmann), subcutaneous port (Portacath™)
- **indications**: chemotherapy, TPN, long-term antibiotics, administration of fluids and blood products, blood sampling
- **complications**: venous thrombosis, infection, pneumothorax

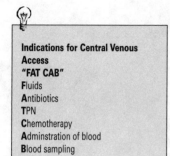

Indications for Central Venous Access
"FAT CAB"
Fluids
Antibiotics
TPN
Chemotherapy
Adminstration of blood
Blood sampling

Nonvascular Interventions

Percutaneous Biopsy
- replaces an open surgical procedure
- many sites are amenable to biopsy using U/S, fluoroscopy or CT guidance
- complications:
  - false negative biopsies due to sampling error or tissue necrosis
  - pneumothorax in 30% of lung biopsies, chest tube required in approximately 5%
  - pancreatic biopsies are associated with risk of inducing pancreatitis
  - transjugular liver biopsies can be performed to minimize bleeding complications in patients with uncorrectable coagulopathies or ascites

ERCP is the primary modality for distal common bile duct obstructions.

Abscess Drainage
- placement of a drainage catheter into an infected fluid collection
- administer broad spectrum IV antibiotics prior to procedure
- routes: percutaneous (most common), transvaginal, transrectal
- complications:
  - bacteremia with sepsis
  - hemorrhage, injury to intervening structures (e.g. bowel)

Percutaneous Biliary Drainage (PBD)/Cholecystostomy
- placement of drainage catheter ± metallic stent into obstructed biliary system (PBD) or gallbladder (cholecystostomy) for relief of jaundice or infection
- percutaneous access can be used to crush or remove stones
- indications:
  - cholecystostomy: acute acalculous cholescytitis
  - percutaneous biliary drainage: biliary obstruction secondary to stone or tumour
- complications:
  - acute: sepsis, hemorrhage
  - long-term: tumour overgrowth and stent occlusion

Percutaneous Nephrostomy
- placement of catheter into renal collecting system
- **indications**: hydronephrosis (urinary obstruction as a result of a stone or tumour)
- **complications**: hematuria, pseudoaneurysm, AV fistulas

Gastrostomy/Gastrojejunostomy
- percutaneous placement of catheter directly into either stomach (gastrostomy) or through stomach into small bowel (gastrojejunostomy)
- indications:
  - feeding: inability to eat (most commonly CNS lesion, e.g. stroke) or esophageal obstruction
  - decompression: gastric outlet obstruction
- **complications**: gastroesophageal reflux with aspiration, peritonitis, hemorrhage, bowel injury

Radiofrequency (RF) Ablation
- U/S or CT guided probe is inserted into tumour, RF energy delivered through probe causes heat deposition and tissue destruction
- **indications:** most commonly used for hepatic tumours (hepatocellular carcinoma and metastases)
- **complications:** destruction of neighbouring tissues and structures

ER Emergency Medicine

Anna MacDonald and Andrew Willmore, chapter editors
Justine Chan and Angela Ho, associate editors
Billie Au, EBM editor
Dr. Glen Bandiera, Dr. Margaret Thompson and Dr. Jeffrey Tyberg, staff editors

Initial Patient Assessment and Management

1. Rapid Primary Survey (RPS)

- Airway maintenance with cervical spine (C-spine) control
- Breathing and ventilation
- Circulation (pulses, hemorrhage control)
- Disability (neurological status)
- Exposure (complete) and Environment (temperature control, provider safety)
- restart sequence from beginning if patient deteriorates

IMPORTANT: always watch for signs of shock while doing primary survey (see Table 1)

A. AIRWAY

- first priority is to secure airway
- assume a cervical injury in every trauma patient and immobilize with collar
- assess ability to breathe and speak
- signs of obstruction
  - agitation, confusion, "universal choking sign"
  - respiratory distress
  - failure to speak, dysphonia
  - cyanosis
  - stridor (noisy breathing)
- think about ability to maintain patency in future
- can change rapidly, therefore reassess frequently

Airway Management

- goals
  - permit adequate oxygenation and ventilation
  - facilitate ongoing patient management
  - give drugs via endotracheal tube (ETT) if IV not available
- N.B. start with basic management techniques before progressing to advanced (see below)

1. Basic Airway Management

- don't forget to protect the C-spine
- head-tilt or jaw thrust (if C-spine injury suspected) to open the airway
- sweep and suction to clear mouth of foreign material

2. Definitive Airway Management

- ETT intubation with inline stabilization of spine (see Figure 1)
  - orotracheal ± Rapid Sequence Intubation (RSI)
  - nasotracheal - may be better tolerated in conscious patient
    - relatively contraindicated with basal skull fracture
- does not provide 100% protection against aspiration
- indications for intubation
  - unable to protect airway (e.g. Glasgow Coma Scale (GCS) ≤8; airway trauma)
  - inadequate oxygenation with spontaneous respiration (O_2 saturation <90% with 100% O_2 or rising pCO_2)
  - profound shock
  - anticipate in trauma, overdose, congestive heart failure (CHF), asthma, chronic obstructive pulmonary disease (COPD) and smoke inhalation injury
  - anticipated transfer of critically ill patients
- rescue airway devices (used to obtain/maintain airway if intubation not possible)
  - laryngeal mask airway
  - intubate LMA
  - combination esophageal/tracheal devices
- surgical airway (if unable to intubate using oral/nasal route and unable to ventilate)
  - cricothyroidotomy

3. Rescue or Temporising Measures

- nasopharyngeal airway
- oropharyngeal airway (not if gag present)
- "rescue" airway devices (e.g. laryngeal mask airway (LMA); combitube)
- transtracheal jet ventilation through cricothyroid membrane
  - used as last resort to ventilate

Approach to the Critically Ill Patient
1. Rapid Primary Survey (RPS)
2. Resuscitation (often concurrent with RPS)
3. Detailed Secondary Survey
4. Definitive Care

Noisy breathing is obstructed breathing until proven otherwise.

If IV access is not available, the following drugs can be given down an ETT ("**NAVEL**"):
Naloxone (**N**arcan)
Atropine
Ventolin (Salbutamol)
Epinephrine
Lidocaine

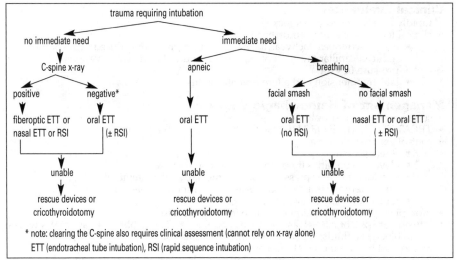

Figure 1. Approach to Endotracheal Intubation in an Injured Patient

B. BREATHING

- LOOK   mental status (anxiety, agitation, decreased LOC), colour, chest movement (bilateral or asymmetrical), respiratory rate/effort, nasal flaring
- LISTEN   sounds of obstruction (e.g. stridor), breath sounds, symmetry of air entry, air escaping
- FEEL   flow of air, tracheal shift, chest wall for crepitus, flail segments, sucking chest wounds, subcutaneous emphysema

Breathing Assessment

- measurement of respiratory function: rate, pulse oximetry, arterial blood gas (ABG), A-a gradient

Management of Breathing

- treatment modalities:
  - nasal prongs → simple face mask → oxygen reservoir → CPAP/BiPAP
  - Venturi mask: used to precisely control O_2 delivery
  - Bag-Valve mask and CPAP to supplement ventilation

C. CIRCULATION

Definition of Shock

- inadequate organ and tissue perfusion with oxygenated blood (brain, kidney, extremities)
- not a level of blood pressure

Shock in a trauma patient is hemorrhagic until proven otherwise.

Causes of Shock (SHOCKE)
S - **S**pinal/neurogenic, **S**eptic
H - **H**emorrhagic
O - **O**bstructive (e.g. tension pneumothorax, cardiac tamponade, pulmonary embolism)
C - **C**ardiogenic (e.g. blunt myocardial injury, arrhythmia, MI)
K - anaphylacti**K**
E - **E**ndocrine (e.g. Addison's, myxedema\ coma)

Table 1. Estimation of Degree of Hemorrhagic Shock

Class	I	II	III	IV
Blood Loss	<750 cc	750-1500 cc	1500-2000 cc	>2000 cc
(% of blood volume)	(<15%)	(15-30%)	(30-40%)	(>40%)
Pulse	<100	>100	>120	>140
Blood pressure	Normal	Normal	Decreased	Decreased
Respiratory rate	20	30	35	>45
Capillary refill	Normal	Decreased	Decreased	Decreased
Urinary output	30 cc/hr	20 cc/hr	10 cc/hr	None
Fluid replacement	Crystalloid	Crystalloid	Crystalloid + blood	Crystalloid + blood

Table 2. Major Types of Shock

Hypovolemic	Cardiogenic	Distributive	Obstructive
- Hemorrhage (External and Internal)	- Myocardial Ischemia	- Septic	- Cardiac tamponade
- Severe burns	- Arrhythmias	- Anaphylactic	- Tension pneumothorax
- High output fistulas	- Congestive Heart Failure	- Neurogenic	- Pulmonary embolism
	- Cardiomyopathies	(Spinal cord injury)	- Aortic stenosis
	- Cardiac valve problems		- Constrictive pericarditis

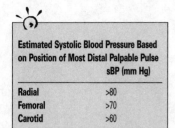

Estimated Systolic Blood Pressure Based on Position of Most Distal Palpable Pulse
                 sBP (mm Hg)

Radial	>80
Femoral	>70
Carotid	>60

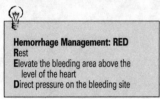

Hemorrhage Management: RED
Rest
Elevate the bleeding area above the level of the heart
Direct pressure on the bleeding site

Since only 30% of infused isotonic crystalloids remains in intravascular space, you must give 3x estimated blood loss.

Clinical Evaluation
- rapidly assess for cause of shock
- clinical features of acute hemorrhage
  - early: tachypnea, tachycardia, narrow pulse pressure, reduced urine output, reduced capillary refill, cool extremities and reduced central venous pressure (CVP)
  - late: hypotension and altered mental status

Management of Hemorrhagic Shock
- secure airway and supply O_2
- TREAT THE CAUSE OF THE SHOCK
- control external bleeding
  - direct pressure
  - elevate extremities if no obvious unstable fracture
  - consider vascular pressure points (brachial, axillary, femoral)
  - do not remove impaled objects as they tamponade bleeding
  - tourniquet only as last resort
- prompt surgical consultation for active internal bleeding
- infusion of 1-2 L of NS/RL as rapidly as possible → 2 large bore (14 gauge) IVs wide open
- warm blood/IV fluids, especially for massive transfusions
- replace lost blood volume at ratio of 3:1 with crystalloid
- if inadequate response, consider ongoing blood loss (e.g. chest, abdomen, pelvis, extremities) → operative intervention required
- indications for blood transfusion
  - severe hypotension on arrival
  - shock persists following crystalloid infusion
  - rapid bleeding
- transfusion options with packed red blood cells (PRBCs)
  - cross matched if possible
  - type-specific (provided by most blood banks within 10 minutes)
    - preferred to O-negative uncross-matched blood if both available
  - O-negative (children and women of child-bearing age)
  - O-positive if no time for crossmatch (males/postmenopausal women)
  - anticipate complications with massive transfusions
  - consider replacement of other blood products (plalelets, FFP) after 2u PRBCs
- transfusion with fresh frozen plasma (FFP)
  - used for clinical evidence of impaired hemostasis
  - ongoing hemorrhage, PT >1.5x normal range

D. DISABILITY
- assess level of consciousness by AVPU method (see sidebar) or GCS

Glasgow Coma Scale (GCS)
- for use in trauma patients with decreased LOC; good indicator of severity of injury and neurosurgical prognosis
- often used for metabolic coma, but less meaningful
- most useful if repeated and used for monitoring of trend
  - change in GCS with time is more relevant than the absolute number
  - patient with deteriorating GCS needs immediate attention
  - prognosis based on best post-resuscitation GCS

The "**AVPU**" method of assessing level of consciousness:
A – **A**lert
V – responds to **V**erbal stimuli
P – responds to **P**ainful stimuli
U – **U**nresponsive

Table 3. Glasgow Coma Scale

Eyes Open		Best Verbal Response		Best Motor Response	
Spontaneously	4	Answers questions appropriately	5	Obeys commands	6
To voice	3	Confused, disoriented	4	Localizes to pain	5
To pain	2	Inappropriate words	3	Withdraws from pain	4
No response	1	Incomprehensible sounds	2	Decorticate (flexion)	3
		No verbal response	1	Decerebrate (extension)	2
				No response	1

- best reported as a 3 part score: Eyes + Verbal + Motor = Total
- provides indication of degree of injury
  - 13-15 = mild injury
  - 9-12 = moderate injury
  - ≤8 = severe injury
- if patient intubated, GCS score reported out of 10 + T (T= tubed, i.e. no verbal component)

E. EXPOSURE/ENVIRONMENT
- undress patient completely; logroll to examine back
- essential to assess entire body for possible injury

- keep patient warm with a blanket ± radiant heaters; avoid hypothermia
- warm IV fluids/blood
- keep providers safe (contamination, combative patient)

Unproven or Harmful Treatments for Hemorrhage Shock
- Trendelenberg position
- steroids (used only in spinal cord injury)
- MAST garments
- vasopressors

2. Resuscitation

- done simultaneously with primary survey
- attend to ABCs
- manage life-threatening problems as they are identified
- vital signs q5-15 minutes
- ECG, BP and O_2 monitors
- Foley catheter and nasogastric (NG) tube if indicated
- tests and investigations: CBC, electrolytes, BUN, Cr, glucose, amylase, INR/PTT, β-hCG, toxicology screen, cross & type

3. Detailed Secondary Survey

- done after rapid primary survey problems have been addressed
- identifies major injuries or areas of concern
- full physical exam and X-rays (C-spine, chest, pelvis - required in blunt trauma, consider T-spine and L-spine)
- CT may replace screening spine xrays

HISTORY
- "SAMPLE": **S**igns and **S**ymptoms, **A**llergies, **M**edications, **P**ast medical history, **L**ast meal, **E**vents related to injury

PHYSICAL EXAMINATION

Head and Neck
- pupils
  - assess equality, size, symmetry, reactivity to light
    - inequality suggests local eye problem or lateralizing CNS lesion
- reactivity/level of consciousness (LOC)
  - reactive pupils + decreased LOC → metabolic or structural cause
  - non-reactive pupils + decreased LOC → structural cause (especially if asymmetric)
- extraocular movements and nystagmus
- fundoscopy (papilledema, hemorrhages)
- palpation of facial bones, scalp
- tympanic membranes, fluid in ear canal, hemotympanum, Battle's sign (mastoid bruising), neck tenderness
- relative afferent pupillary defect (swinging light test) - optic nerve damage

Foley contraindications
- blood at urethral meatus
- scrotal hematoma
- high-riding prostate on DRE

NG tube contraindications
- significant mid-face trauma
- basal skull fracture

Chest
- inspect for flail segment, contusion
- palpate for subcutaneous emphysema
- auscultate lung fields

Abdomen
- assess for peritonitis, abdominal distention, and evidence of intra-abdominal bleeding
- FAST (Focused Abdominal Sonogram in Trauma), diagnostic peritoneal lavage (DPL) or CT
- rectal exam for gastrointestinal (GI) bleed, high riding prostate and anal tone (best to do during the log roll)
- bimanual exam in females as appropriate

Musculoskeletal (MSK)
- examine all extremities for swelling, deformity, contusion, tenderness
- log roll and palpate thoracic and lumbar spines
- palpate iliac crests and pubic symphysis, pelvic stability (lateral, AP, vertical)

Neurological
- GCS
- alterations of rate and rhythm of breathing are signs of structural or metabolic abnormalities
  - progressive deterioration of breathing pattern implies a failing CNS
- full cranial nerve exam
- assessment of spinal cord integrity
  - conscious patient: assess distal sensation and motor ability
  - unconscious patient: response to painful or noxious stimulus applied to extremities

Signs of increased intracranial pressure (ICP)
- deteriorating LOC (hallmark of increasing ICP)
- deteriorating respiratory pattern
- Cushing reflex (high BP, low heart rate, irregular respirations)
- lateralizing CNS signs (e.g. cranial nerve palsies, hemiparesis)
- seizures
- papilledema (occurs late)
- N/V and H/A

4. Definitive Care

- continue therapy
- continue patient evaluations and special investigations
- specialty consultations including OR as needed
- disposition: home, admission, or transfer to another setting (e.g. OR, ICU)

Ethical Considerations

Consent to Treatment: Adults

- emergency rule: consent not needed when patient is at imminent risk from a serious injury (e.g. severe suffering, loss of limb, vital organ or life) AND obtaining consent is either: a) not possible (e.g. patient is comatose); OR b) would increase risk to the patient (e.g. time delay)
  - the emergency rule assumes that most people would want to be saved in an emergency
- any capable and informed patient can refuse any treatment or part of treatment, even if it is life-saving
  - consider: is the patient truly capable? Does pain, stress, or psychological distress impair their judgment?
- exceptions to the Emergency Rule: treatment cannot be initiated if:
  1. a competent patient has previously refused the same or similar treatment and there is no evidence to suggest the patient's wishes have changed
  2. an advance directive is available – e.g. do not resuscitate (DNR) order
- refusal of help in a suicide situation is not an exception; care must be given
- if in doubt, initiate treatment, care can be withdrawn if appropriate at a later time or if wishes clarified by family

Consent to Treatment: Children

- treat immediately if patient is at imminent risk
- parents/guardians have right to make treatment decisions
- if parents refuse treatment that is life-saving or will potentially alter the child's quality of life, Children's Aid Society (CAS) must be contacted – consent of CAS is needed to treat

Other Issues of Consent

- need consent for HIV testing of patient and for administration of blood products

Duty to Report

- law may vary depending on province and/or state
  - gunshot wounds, potential drunken drivers, suspected child abuse, various communicable diseases
  - medical unsuitability to drive

Traumatology

Epidemiology

- statistics
  - leading cause of death in patients <45 yrs
  - 4th highest cause of death in North America
  - causes more deaths in children/adolescents than all diseases combined
- trimodal distribution of death
  - minutes: lethal injuries, death usually at the scene
  - death within 4-6 hours – "golden hour" (but decreased mortality with trauma care)
  - days-weeks: death from multiple organ dysfunction, sepsis, etc.
- injuries generally fall into two categories
  - blunt (most common): motor vehicle collision (MVC), pedestrian-automobile impact, motorcycle collision, fall, assault, sports, etc.
  - penetrating (increasing in incidence): gunshot wound, stabbing, impalement
- high risk injuries:
  - MVC at high speed, resulting in ejection from vehicle
  - motorcycle collisions
  - vehicle vs. pedestrian crashes
  - fall from height >12 ft (3.6 m)

Jehovah's Witnesses
- capable adults have the right to refuse medical treatment
- may refuse whole blood, PRBCs, platelets, plasma and WBCs even if life-saving
- should be questioned directly about the use of albumin, immunoglobulins, hemophilic preparations
- do not allow for autologous transfusion unless there is uninterrupted extra corporeal circulation
- usually ask for the highest possible quality of care without the use of the above interventions (e.g. crystalloids for volume expansion, attempts at bloodless surgery)
- patient will generally sign hospital forms releasing medical staff from liability
- most legal cases involve children of Jehovah's Witnesses; if life-saving treatment is refused CAS is contacted

Considerations for Traumatic Injury

- important to know the mechanism of injury in order to anticipate traumatic injuries
- always look for an underlying cause (alcohol, medications, illicit substances, seizure, suicide attempt, medical problem)
- always inquire about head injury, loss of consciousness, amnesia, vomiting, headache and seizure activity

Motor Vehicle Collision (MVC)
- vehicle(s) involved: weight, size, speed, amount of damage
- type of crash (to assess location of possible injuries)
  - lateral/T-bone or head-on: head, cervical spine, thoracic, abdominal, pelvic and lower extremity
  - rear-end: hyper-extension of cervical spine (whiplash injury to neck)
  - roll over: energy dissipated, less likely severe injury if victim restrained by seatbelt, however still significant potential morbidity
- location of patient in vehicle
- use and type of seatbelt
  - lap belt: spine and abdominal injury
  - shoulder belt: look for major vessel injury
- ejection of patient from vehicle/entrapment of patient under vehicle
- airbag deployment
- use of helmet in motorcycle or bicycle collisions

Pedestrian-Automobile Impact
- high morbidity and mortality
- vehicle speed is an important factor
- site of impact on car
  - children tend to be run over
  - adults tend to be struck in lower legs, impact again on car (truncal injury) and thrown to the ground (head injury)

Vehicle vs. Pedestrian Crash
In adults look for triad of injuries:
1. tibia-fibula or femur fracture
2. truncal injury
3. craniofacial injury

Falls
- 1 storey = 12 feet (3.6 m)
- distance of fall: 50% mortality at 4 stories and 95% mortality at 7 stories
- position in which patient landed and type of surface
- assess for shock, lower extremity, spine and pelvic fractures

Gunshot Wounds (GSW)
- type of gun
  - handgun injuries: medium or high velocity, extent of injury may be limited to a small area
  - hunting and rifle injuries: high velocity, widespread injury
  - shotgun: widespread tissue destruction
- type of ammunition (e.g. hollow point bullets)
- range of shot
  - close range: massive tissue destruction, deposition of wadding into wound
- characterize route of entry and site of exit wound (if any)
- GSW with hypotension: immediate transport to OR
  - hypotension indicates severe blood loss (>2 L blood loss in 70 kg patient is required to produce hypotension)

Stab Wounds
- route/direction of entry, length of blade
- type of penetration (stab, slash, impalement)
- victim recollection and witness reports are often inaccurate and may not correlate with depth/severity of wound
- if blade in-situ, DO NOT REMOVE – it may be tamponading bleeding vessel (to be removed in OR)

Always completely expose and count the number of wounds

Head Trauma

- see Neurosurgery
- 60% of trauma admissions have head injuries
- 60% of MVC-related deaths are due to head injury

Specific Injuries
- fractures (diagnosed by CT of head, often not visible on x-ray)
  A) skull fractures:
    - vault fractures:
      - linear, non-depressed
        - most common
        - typically occur over temporal bone, in area of middle meningeal artery (commonest cause of epidural hematoma)
      - depressed
        - open (associated overlying scalp laceration, torn dura) vs. closed
    - basal skull
      - typically occur through floor of anterior cranial fossa (longitudinal more common than transverse)
      - clinical diagnosis superior (Battle's sign, raccoon eyes, CSF otorrhea/rhinorrhea, hemotympanum)
  B) facial fractures (see Plastic Surgery)
- neuronal injury
  A) diffuse:
    - concussion
      - mild: temporary disturbance of neurological function, complete recovery
      - classical: temporary, reversible neurological disturbance, with temporary (<6 hrs) LOC, complete recovery
    - diffuse axonal injury
      - mild: coma 6-24 hrs, possibly lasting deficit
      - moderate: coma >24hrs, little or no signs of brainstem dysfunction
      - severe: coma >24hrs, frequent signs of brainstem dysfunction
  B) focal injuries
      - contusions
      - intracranial hemorrhage (epidural, subdural, intracerebral)

ASSESSMENT OF BRAIN INJURY

History
- pre-hospital status
- mechanism of injury

Physical Examination
- assume C-spine injury until ruled out
- vital signs
    - shock (not due to isolated brain injury, except in infants)
    - Cushing's response to increasing ICP (bradycardia, hypertension, irregular respirations)
- severity of injury determined by:
  1) level of consciousness
    - Glasgow Coma Scale (GCS): GCS ≤8 intubate, any change in score of 3 or more = serious injury
  2) pupils: size, anisocoria >1 mm (in patient with altered LOC), response to light
  3) lateralizing signs (motor/sensory), may become more subtle with increasing severity of injury
- re-assess frequently

Investigations
- labs: CBC, electrolytes, coags, glucose, tox screen
- CT scan
- skull X-rays - little value in the management of blunt head injury in adults
    - for diagnosis of calvarium fractures (not brain injury)
    - may help localize foreign body after penetrating head injury
- C-spine imaging, often with CT neck and head CT

Management
- general
    - ABCs
    - treat other injuries, must treat hypotension, hypoxia (both contribute significantly to mortality)

Signs of basal skull fracture
- Battle's sign (bruised mastoid process)
- Hemotympanum
- Raccoon eyes (periorbital bruising)

Warning signs of severe head injury:
- GCS <8
- deteriorating GCS
- unequal pupils
- lateralizing signs

N.B. alteration of consciousness is a hallmark of brain injury

---

Canadian CT Head Rule

CT Head is only required for patients with minor head injuries with any one of the following:

High risk (for neurological intervention)
- GCS score <15 at 2 h after injury
- Suspected open or depressed skull fracture
- Any sign of basal skull fracture (hemotympanum, "raccoon" eyes, cerebrospinal fluid otorrhea/rhinorrhoea, Battle's sign)
- Vomiting ≥2 episodes
- Age ≥65 years

Medium risk (for brain injury on CT)
- Amnesia before impact >30 min
- Dangerous mechanism (pedestrian struck by motor vehicle, occupant ejected from motor vehicle, fall from height >3 feet or five stairs)

Minor head injury is defined as witnessed loss of consciousness, definite amnesia, or witnessed disorientation in a patient with a GCS score of 13-15.

The Lancet. May 5, 2001. 357: 9266; 1391-1396.

Treatment of Increased ICP
- Elevate head of bed
- Mannitol
- Hyperventilate
- Paralyzing agents

- early neurosurgical consultation for acute and subsequent patient management
- medical
  - seizure treatment/prophylaxis
    - benzodiazepines, phenytoin, phenobarbital
    - steroids are of no proven value
  - treat suspected raised ICP → consider the following:
    - raise head of stretcher 20° if patient hemodynamically stable
    - intubate and hyperventilate (100% O_2) to a pCO_2 of 30-35 mmHg
    - mannitol 1g/kg infused as rapidly as possible (reserved for head-injured patients with signs of increased ICP)
    - consider paralysing meds if agitated/high airway pressures
    - maintenance of cerebral perfusion pressure is critical
- surgical

Disposition
- neurosurgical ICU admission for severe head injuries (HI)
- in hemodynamically unstable patient with other injuries, prioritize most life-threatening injuries and try to maintain cerebral perfusion
- for minor head injury not requiring admission, provide 24-hour HI protocol to competent caregiver, follow-up with neurology as even seemingly minor HI may cause lasting deficits

Spine and Spinal Cord Trauma

- assume cord injury with significant falls (>12 ft), deceleration injuries, blunt trauma to head, neck or back
- spinal immobilization (cervical collar, spine board during patient transport only) must be maintained until spinal injury has been ruled out (see Figure 2)
- vertebral injuries may be present without spinal cord injury; normal neurologic exam does not exclude spinal injury
- spine may be unstable despite normal C-spine X-ray (SCIWARA = spinal cord injury without radiologic abnormality)
- injuries can include: complete/incomplete transection, cord edema, spinal shock

History
- mechanism of injury, previous deficits, SAMPLE
- neck pain, paralysis/weakness, parasthesia

Physical Exam
- ABCs
- abdo: ecchymosis, tenderness
- neuro: complete exam, including mental status
- spine: maintain neutral position, palpate C-spine for tenderness, step-off; log-roll, then palpate thoracic and lumbar spine; assess rectal tone
- extremities: check cap refill, suspect thoracolumbar injury with calcaneal fractures

Investigations
- labs: CBC, electrolytes, creatinine, glucose, coags, cross and type, tox screen
- imaging:
  - full C-spine X-ray series for trauma (AP, lateral, odontoid)
- thoracolumbar X-rays
  - AP and lateral views
  - indicated in:
    - patients with C-spine injury
    - unconscious patients (with appropriate mechanism of injury)
    - patients with symptoms or neurological findings
    - patients with deformities that are palpable when patient log-rolled
    - patients with back pain
    - patients with suggestive injuries, e.g. bilateral calcaneal fractures
- consider CT (for subtle bony injuries), MRI (for soft tissue injuries) if appropriate

Collar everyone with at least one of the following criteria:
- midline tenderness
- neurological symptoms or signs
- significant distracting injuries
- head injury
- intoxication
- dangerous mechanism
- history of LOC

If a fracture is found, be suspicious, look for another fracture.

Note: Patients with penetrating trauma (especially gunshot and knife wounds) can also have spinal cord injury.

Of the investigations, the lateral C-spine X-ray is the single most important film. 95% of radiologically visible abnormalities are found on this film.

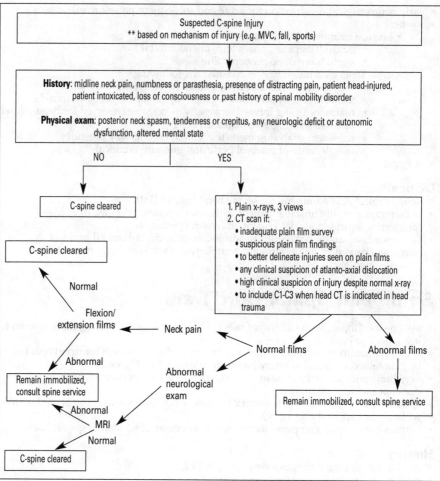

Figure 2. Approach to clearing the C-spine

Management of Cord Injury
- immobilize
- evaluate ABCs
- treat shock (maintain sBP >100 mmHg)
- insert NG and Foley catheter
- high dose steroids: methylprednisolone 30 mg/kg bolus, then 5.4 mg/kg/hr drip, start within 6-8 hrs of injury (controversial and recently has less support)
- complete imaging of spine
- spine consult
- continually reassess high cord injuries as edema can travel up cord
- if cervical cord lesion, watch for respiratory insufficiency
    - low cervical transection (C5-T1) produces abdominal breathing (phrenic innervation of diaphragm still intact)
    - high cervical cord injury (above C4) may require intubation and ventilation
- beware hypotension (neurogenic shock)
    - treatment: warm blanket, Trendelenberg position (occasionally), volume infusion, consider vasopressors

APPROACH TO C-SPINE X-RAYS
- 3-view C-spine series is the screening modality of choice in low-risk patients, CT in high-risk
    - lateral C1-T1 ± swimmer's view (see Figure 3 and Table 4 for interpretation)
        - lateral view is BEST, identifies 90-95% of radiologically apparent injuries

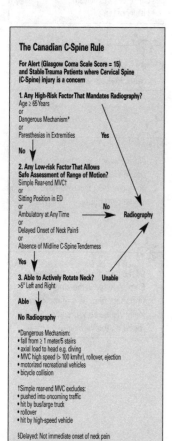

The Canadian C-Spine Rule

For Alert (Glasgow Coma Scale Score = 15) and Stable Trauma Patients where Cervical Spine (C-Spine) injury is a concern

1. Any High-Risk Factor That Mandates Radiography?
Age ≥ 65 Years
or
Dangerous Mechanism*
or
Paresthesias in Extremities   **Yes**

No ↓

2. Any Low-risk Factor That Allows Safe Assessment of Range of Motion?
Simple Rear-end MVC†
or
Sitting Position in ED
or
Ambulatory at Any Time   **No** → **Radiography**
or
Delayed Onset of Neck Pain§
or
Absence of Midline C-Spine Tenderness

Yes ↓

3. Able to Actively Rotate Neck?   Unable
>5° Left and Right

Able ↓

No Radiography

*Dangerous Mechanism:
- fall from ≥ 1 meter/5 stairs
- axial load to head e.g. diving
- MVC high speed (> 100 km/hr), rollover, ejection
- motorized recreational vehicles
- bicycle collision

†Simple rear-end MVC excludes:
- pushed into oncoming traffic
- hit by bus/large truck
- rollover
- hit by high-speed vehicle

§Delayed: Not immediate onset of neck pain

JAMA. Oct 17, 2001. 286;(15); 1841-1848.

Table 4. Interpretation of Lateral View: The ABCS

A - Adequacy and Alignment
- **must see C1 to C7-T1 junction**; if not, downward traction of shoulders, swimmer's view, bilateral supine obliques, or CT scan needed
- lines of contour (in children <8 years of age: can see physiologic subluxation of C2 on C3, and C3 on C4, but the spinolaminal line is maintained)
- fanning of spinous processes - suggests posterior ligamentous disruption
- widening of facet joints
- check atlanto-occipital joint:
  - line extending inferiorly from clivus should transect odontoid
  - atlanto-axial articulation - widening of predental space (normal: <3 mm in adults, <5 mm in children) indicates injury of C1 or C2

B - Bones
- height, width and shape of each vertebral body
- pedicles, facets, and laminae should appear as one - doubling suggests rotation

C - Cartilage
- intervertebral disc spaces – wedging anteriorly or posteriorly suggests vertebral compression

S - Soft Tissues
- widening of retropharyngeal (normal: <7 mm at C1-4, may be wide in children <2 yrs on expiration) or retrotracheal spaces (normal: <22 mm at C6-T1, <14 mm in children <5 yrs)

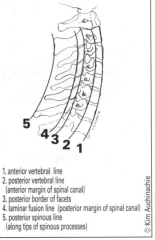

1. anterior vertebral line
2. posterior vertebral line (anterior margin of spinal canal)
3. posterior border of facets
4. laminar fusion line (posterior margin of spinal canal)
5. posterior spinous line (along tips of spinous processes)

© Kim Auchinachie

Figure 3. Lines of Contour on a Lateral C-Spine X-Ray

- odontoid view (open mouth or oblique submental view) (see Figure 4)
  - examine the dens for fractures
    - beware of artifact (horizontal or vertical) caused by the radiological shadow of the teeth overlying the dens
    - if unable to rule out fracture, repeat view or consider CT or plain film tomography
  - examine lateral aspects of C1 and spacing relative to C2
- AP view
  - alignment of spinous processes in the midline
  - spacing of spinous processes should be equal
  - check vertebral bodies

Supine Oblique Views
- rarely used
- detects some injuries not visible on the usual 3 views but CT is best
- better visualization of posterior element fractures (lamina, pedicle, facet joint)
- can be used to visualize the C7-T1 junction

Sequelae of C-spine Fractures
- decreased descending sympathetic tone (neurogenic/spinal shock) responsible for most sequelae
- cardiac
  - no autoregulation, falling BP, decreasing HR, vasodilation
  - management: give IV fluids ± vasopressors
- respiratory
  - no cough reflex (risk of aspiration pneumonia)
  - no intercostal muscles ± diaphragm
  - management: intubate and maintain vital capacity
- gastrointestinal
  - ileus, vasodilation, bile and pancreatic secretion continues (>1L/day), risk of aspiration, GI stress ulcers
  - management: NG tube may be required for suctioning, feeding, etc.
- renal
  - hypoperfusion → give IV fluids
  - kidney still producing urine (bladder can rupture if patient not urinating)
  - management: Foley catheter may be required (measure urine output)
- skin
  - vasodilation, heat loss, no thermoregulation, atrophy (risk of skin ulcers)
- muscle
  - flaccidity, atrophy, decreased venous return
- penis
  - priapism

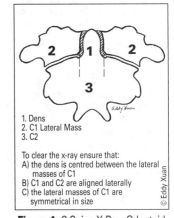

1. Dens
2. C1 Lateral Mass
3. C2

To clear the x-ray ensure that:
A) the dens is centred between the lateral masses of C1
B) C1 and C2 are aligned laterally
C) the lateral masses of C1 are symmetrical in size

© Eddy Xuan

Figure 4. C-Spine X-Ray: Odontoid View

Prevertebral soft tissue swelling is only 49% sensitive for injury.

20% of C-spine fractures are accompanied by other spinal fractures, so ensure thoracic and lumbar spine x-rays are normal before proceeding to OR.

Chest Trauma

* two types:
  * A. found and managed in 1° survey
  * B. found and managed in 2° survey

A. LIFE-THREATENING CHEST INJURIES FOUND IN 1° SURVEY

* see Table 5

Trauma to the chest accounts for, or contributes to 50% of trauma deaths.

80% of all chest injuries can be managed non-surgically with simple measures such as intubation, chest tubes, and pain control.

3 way seal for open pneumothorax (i.e. sucking chest wound)
Allows air to escape during the expiratory phase (so that you don't get a tension pneumothorax) but seals itself to allow adequate breaths during the inspiratory phase.

DDx of Life Threatening Chest Injuries (HOT and FAT CHEST):
Hemothorax
Open pneumothorax
Tension pneumothorax

Flail chest
Airway obstruction
Tamponade

Contusion: pulmonary, myocardial
Hernia: traumatic, diaphragmatic
ESophageal perforation
Tracheobronchial disruption/
Traumatic injury

Table 5. Life-Threatening Chest Injuries Found in 1° Survey

Physical Exam	Investigations	Management
Airway Obstruction	• anxiety, stridor, hoarseness, altered mental status • apnea, cyanosis	• do not wait for ABG to intubate	• definitive airway management • intubate early • remove FB if visible with laryngoscope prior to intubation
Tension Pneumothorax • clinical diagnosis • one-way valve causing accumulation of air in pleural space	• respiratory distress, tachycardia, distended neck veins, cyanosis, asymmetry of chest wall motion • tracheal deviation away from pneumothorax • percussion hyperresonance • unilateral absence of breath sounds	• non-radiographic diagnosis	• needle thoracostomy – large bore needle, 2nd ICS mid clavicular line, followed by chest tube in 5th ICS, anterior axillary line
Open Pneumothorax • air entering chest from wound rather than trachea	• gunshot or other wound (hole >2/3 tracheal diameter) ± exit wound • unequal breath sounds	• ABG: decreased pO_2	• air-tight dressing sealed on 3 sides • chest tube • surgery

Massive Hemothorax
• >1500 cc blood loss in chest cavity
	• pallor, flat neck veins, shock
	• unilateral dullness
	• absent breath sounds, hypotension
		• usually only able to do supine CXR – entire lung appears radioopaque as blood spreads out over posterior thoracic cavity	• restore blood volume
			• chest tube
			• thoracotomy if:
			  • >1500 cc total blood loss
			  • ≥200 cc/hr continued drainage

Flail Chest • free-floating segment of chest wall due to >2 rib fractures, each at 2 sites • underlying lung contusion (cause of morbidity and mortality)	• paradoxical movement of flail segment • palpable crepitus of ribs • decreased air entry on affected side	• ABG: decreased pO_2, increased pCO_2 • CXR: rib fractures, lung contusion	• O_2 + fluid therapy + pain control • judicious fluid therapy in absence of systemic hypotension • positive pressure ventilation • ± intubation and ventilation
Cardiac Tamponade • clinical diagnosis • pericardial fluid accumulation impairing ventricular function	• penetrating wound (usually) • Beck's triad: hypotension, distended neck veins, muffled heart sounds • tachycardia, tachypnea • pulsus paradoxus • Kussmaul's sign	• echocardiogram • bedside ultrasound (FAST)	• IV fluids • pericardiocentesis • open thoracotomy

B. POTENTIALLY LIFE-THREATENING CHEST INJURIES FOUND IN 2° SURVEY

- need to have high index of suspicion, usually dependent on mechanism of injury
- see Table 6

Table 6. Potentially Life-Threatening Chest Injuries Found in 2° Survey

Physical Exam	Investigations	Management
Pulmonary Contusion	• blunt trauma to chest • interstitial edema impairs compliance and gas exchange	• CXR: areas of opacification of lung within 6 hours of trauma • air bronchograms	• maintain adequate ventilation • monitor with ABG, pulse oximeter and ECG • chest physiotherapy • positive pressure ventilation if severe
Ruptured Diaphragm	• blunt trauma to chest or abdomen (e.g. high lap belt in MVC)	• CXR: abnormality of diaphragm/lower lung fields/NG tube placement • CT scan and endoscopy - sometimes helpful for diagnosis • thoracoscopy/laparoscopy definitive	• laparotomy for diaphragm repair and because of associated intra-abdominal injuries
Esophageal Injury	• usually penetrating trauma (pain out of proportion to degree of injury)	• CXR: mediastinal air (not always) • esophagram (Gastrograffin) • flexible esophagoscopy	• early repair (within 24 hrs.) improves outcome but all require repair
Aortic Tear • 90% tear at subclavian (near ligamentum arteriosum), most die at scene • salvageable if diagnosis made rapidly	• sudden high speed deceleration (e.g. MVC, fall, airplane crash), complaints of chest pain, dyspnea, hoarseness frequently absent) • decreased femoral pulses, differential arm BP (arch tear)	• CXR, CT scan, transesophageal echo (TEE), aortography (gold standard) • see sidebar for CXR features	• thoracotomy (may treat other severe injuries first)
Blunt Myocardial Injury (Rare)	• blunt trauma to chest (usually in setting of multi-system trauma and therefore difficult to diagnose) • physical examination: overlying injury, i.e. fractures, chest wall contusion	• ECG: arrhythmias, ST changes • patients with a normal ECG and normal hemodynamics never get dysrhythmias	• O₂ • antiarrhythmic agents • analgesia

Ruptured diaphragm is more often diagnosed on the left side, as liver conceals right side defect.

X-ray features of **A**ortic tear (**ABC WHITE**):
- depressed left mainstem **B**ronchus
- pleural **C**ap
- **Wi**de mediastinum (most consistent)
- **H**emothorax
- **I**ndistinct aortic knuckle
- **T**racheal deviation to right side
- **E**sophagus (NG tube) deviated to right

C. OTHER POTENTIALLY LIFE-THREATENING INJURIES RELATED TO THE CHEST

1. Penetrating Neck Trauma
- includes all penetrating trauma to the three zones of the neck (Figure 5)
- management: injuries deep to platysma require further evaluation by angiography, contrast CT or surgery
- do not explore penetrating neck wounds except in the OR

2. Airway Injuries
- always maintain a high index of suspicion
- larynx
  - history: strangulation, clothes line, direct blow, blunt trauma, any penetrating injury involving platysma
  - triad: hoarseness, subcutaneous emphysema, palpable fracture crepitus
  - other symptoms: hemoptysis, dyspnea, dysphonia
  - investigations: CXR, CT scan, arteriography (if penetrating)
  - management
    - airway – manage early because of edema
    - C-spine may also be injured, consider mechanism of injury
    - surgical – tracheotomy vs. repair
- trachea/bronchus
  - frequently missed
  - history: deceleration, penetration, increased intra-thoracic pressure; complaints of dyspnea, hemoptysis
  - examination: subcutaneous air, Hamman's sign (crunching sound synchronous with heart beat)
  - CXR: mediastinal air, persistent pneumothorax
  - persistent air leak after chest tube inserted for pneumothorax
  - management: surgical repair if >1/3 circumference

If penetrating neck trauma present, DON'T:
- clamp structures (can damage nerves)
- probe
- insert NG tube (leads to bleeding)
- remove weapon/impaled object

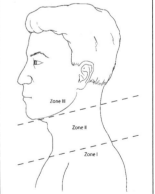

© Adrian Yen (2006)

Zone III: superior aspect of neck
Zone II: midportion of neck (cricoid to the angle of mandible)
Zone I: base of neck (thoracic inlet to cricoid cartilage)

Figure 5. Zones of the Neck in Trauma

Abdominal Trauma

- two mechanisms:
    - blunt trauma: usually causes solid organ injury (spleen injury is most common)
    - penetrating trauma: usually causes hollow organ injury or liver injury (most common)

BLUNT TRAUMA
- results in two types of hemorrhage
    - intra-abdominal bleed
    - retroperitoneal bleed
- adopt high clinical suspicion of bleeding in multi-system trauma

History
- mechanism of injury, SAMPLE history

Physical Exam
- often unreliable in multi-system trauma
    - slow blood loss not immediately apparent
    - other injuries may mask symptoms
    - serial examinations are required
- abdomen:
    - inspect: contusions, abrasions, seatbelt sign, distention
    - auscultate: bruits, bowel sounds
    - palpate: tenderness, rebound tenderness, rigidity, guarding
    - DRE: rectal tone, blood, bone fragments, prostate location
    - placement of NG, foley catheter should be considered part of the abdo exam
- other systems to assess: CVS, respiratory (possibility of diaphragm rupture), pelvis, back, neuro as it pertains to abdo sensation, GU

Investigations
- labs: CBC, electrolytes, coags, cross & type, glucose, creatinine, CK, lipase, amylase, liver enzymes, ABG, blood EtOH, β-hCG, U/A, tox screen
- imaging: see Table 7

Table 7.   Imaging in Abdominal Trauma

Imaging	Strengths	Limitations
X-Ray	Chest (looking for free air under diaphragm, diaphragmatic hernia, air fluid levels), pelvis, cervical, thoracic, lumbar spines	No soft tissue
CT scan	Most specific test	Radiation exposure 20x more than xray Cannot use if hemodynamic instability
Diagnostic Peritoneal Lavage (DPL)	Most sensitive test Tests for intra-peritoneal bleed	Cannot test for retroperitoneal bleed or diaphragmatic rupture Cannot distinguish lethal from trivial bleed Results can take up to 1 hr
Ultrasound: FAST (Focused Abdominal Sonogram for Trauma)	Identifies presence/absence of free fluid in peritoneal cavity RAPID exam: less than 5 minutes Can also examine pericardium and pleural cavities	NOT used to identify specific organ injuries If patient has ascites, FAST will be falsely positive

- imaging must be done if:
    - equivocal abdominal examination, suspected intra-abdominal injury or distracting injuries
    - multiple trauma patient resulting in unreliable physical exam (altered sensorium, i.e. secondary to drugs, alcohol, head trauma, or distracting injury; spinal cord injury resulting in abdominal anesthesia)
    - unexplained shock/hypotension
    - multiple trauma patients who must undergo general anesthesia for orthopaedic, neurosurgical, or other injuries
    - fractures of lower ribs, pelvis, spine

Management
- general: ABCs, fluid resuscitation and stabilization
- surgical: watchful wait vs. laparotomy
- solid organ injuries: decision based on hemodynamic stability, not the specific injuries
- hemodynamically unstable or persistently high transfusion requirements → laparotomy
- hollow organ injuries: laparotomy
- even if low suspicion of injury: admit and observe for 24 hours

PENETRATING TRAUMA
- high risk of gastrointestinal perforation and sepsis
- history: size of blade, calibre/distance from gun, route of entry

---

Seatbelt injuries may cause
- retroperitoneal duodenal trauma
- intraperitoneal bowel transection
- mesenteric injury
- L-spine injury

Indications for Foley & NG tube in abdo trauma
Foley catheter: unconscious or multiply injured patient who cannot void spontaneously. **Contraindications**: blood at the meatus, an ecchymotic scrotum, or a "high-riding" prostate on DRE (retrograde cystourethrogram is indicated to rule out a urethral tear or ruptured bladder) **NG tube**: used to decompress the stomach and proximal small bowel **Contraindications**: facial fractures or basal skull fractures suspected.

Criteria for Positive Lavage
- >10 cc gross blood
- bile, bacteria, foreign material
- RBC count >100,000 x 10⁶/L
- WBC >500 x 10⁶/L, amylase >175 IU

Laparotomy is mandatory if penetrating trauma and:
- shock
- peritonitis
- evisceration
- free air in abdomen
- blood in NG tube, Foley catheter, or on rectal exam

- local wound exploration (not reliable) with the following exceptions:
  - thoracoabdominal region (may cause pneumothorax)
  - back or flanks (muscles too thick)

Management
- general: ABCs, fluid resuscitation and stabilization
- gunshot wounds → always require laparotomy
- stab wounds → "rule of thirds" (see sidebar)

"Rule of Thirds" for stab wounds:
- 1/3 do not penetrate peritoneal cavity
- 1/3 penetrate but are harmless
- 1/3 cause injury requiring surgery

Genitourinary Tract Injuries

- see Urology

Etiology
- blunt trauma – often associated with pelvic fractures
  - renal contusions (minor injury – parenchymal ecchymoses with intact renal capsule)
  - renal parenchymal tears/laceration: non-communicating (hematoma) vs. communicating (urine extravasation, hematuria)
  - extraperitoneal rupture of bladder from pelvic fracture fragments
  - intraperitoneal rupture of bladder from trauma and full bladder
  - anterior (bulbous) urethral damage with pelvic fractures
  - ureter: rare, at uretero-pelvic junction
- penetrating trauma
  - damage to: kidney, bladder, ureter (rare)
- acceleration/deceleration injury
  - renal pedicle injury – high mortality rate (laceration and thrombosis of renal artery, renal vein, and their branches)
- iatrogenic
  - ureter (from instrumentation)

Gross hematuria suggests bladder injury.

History
- mechanism of injury
- hematuria (microscopic or gross), blood on underwear
- dysuria, urinary retention
- history of hypotension

Physical Examination
- abdominal pain, flank pain, costovertebral angle (CVA) tenderness, upper quadrant mass, perineal lacerations
- DRE: sphincter tone, position of prostate, presence of blood
- scrotum: ecchymoses, lacerations, testicular disruption, hematomas
- bimanual exam, speculum exam
- extraperitoneal bladder rupture: pelvic instability, suprapubic tenderness from mass of urine or extravasated blood
- intraperitoneal bladder rupture: acute abdomen (not in first hour or two)

In the case of gross hematuria, the GU system is investigated from distal to proximal (i.e. urethrogram, cystogram, etc.)

Investigations
- plain film: look for fractures (lower rib, lower thoracic, upper lumbar vertebrae, pelvis)
- renal: CT scan (best, if hemodynamically stable), intravenous pyelogram (IVP) during laparotomy, renal arteriography (if renal artery injury suspected)
- ureter: retrograde ureterogram
- bladder: urinalysis, CT scan, urethrogram, ± retrograde cystoscopy, ± cystogram (distended bladder + post-void)
- urethra: retrograde urethrography

Management
- urology consult
- renal
  - minor injuries – conservative management
    - bedrest, hydration, analgesia, antibiotics
  - major injuries – admit
    - conservative management with frequent reassessments, serial urinalysis, ± reimaging
    - surgical repair (exploration, nephrectomy) (e.g. hemodynamically unstable or continuing to bleed >48h, major urine extravasation, renal pedicle injury, all penetrating wounds and major lacerations, infections, renal artery thrombosis)
- ureter
  - uretero-uretostomy
- bladder
  - extraperitoneal: minor rupture: Foley drainage x 10-14 days
    major rupture: surgical repair
  - intraperitoneal: drain abdomen and surgical repair
- urethra
  - anterior: conservative, if cannot void → Foley or suprapubic cystostomy and antibiotics
  - posterior: suprapubic cystostomy (avoid catheterization) ± surgical repair

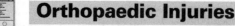

Orthopaedic Injuries

* see <u>Orthopaedics</u> (*Shoulder, Knee, Wrist, Ankle*)

Goals of ED Treatment
* identify injuries accurately and address potentially life/limb threatening problems appropriately
* reduce and immobilize fractures (cast/splint) as appropriate
* provide adequate pain relief
* arrange proper follow-up if necessary

History
* use SAMPLE
* mechanism of injury may be very important

Physical Examination
* **Look** (inspection): "**SEADS**" **S**welling, **E**rythema, **A**trophy, **D**eformity, **S**kin changes (e.g. bruises)
* **Feel** (palpation): all joints/bones – local tenderness, swelling, warmth, crepitus, joint effusions, subtle deformity
* **Move**: joints affected plus above and below injury – active ROM preferred to passive
* **Neurovascular status**: distal to injury (BEFORE and AFTER reduction)

LIFE AND LIMB THREATENING INJURIES
* threat to life is usually due to blood loss (e.g. up to 3 L in pelvic fractures, 1.5 L per long bone fracture)
* threat to limb is usually due to interruption of blood supply to distal part of limb or to susceptible part of bone

Table 8. Life and Limb Threatening Orthopedic Injuries

Life Threatening Injuries	Limb Threatening Injuries
• Major pelvic fractures	• Fracture/dislocation of ankle (talar AVN)
• Traumatic amputations	• Crush injuries
• Massive long bone injuries (beware fat emboli)	• Compartment syndrome
• Vascular injury proximal to knee/elbow	• Open fractures
	• Dislocations of knee/hip
	• Fractures above knee/elbow

Open Fractures
* communication between fracture site and external surface of skin – risk of osteomyelitis
* remove gross debris, irrigate, cover with sterile dressing – formal irrigation and debridement often done in the OR
* control bleeding with pressure (no clamping)
* splint
* antibiotics (1st generation cephalosporin and aminoglycoside) and tetanus prophylaxis
* must secure definitive surgical care within 6-8 hours

Vascular Injuries
* realign limb/apply longitudinal traction and reassess pulses (e.g. Doppler probe)
* surgical consult

Compartment Syndrome
* increased interstitial pressure in an anatomical "compartment" (forearm, calf) with little room for expansion, resulting in ↓perfusion and potential muscle/nerve necrosis
* **excessive** pain which is worse with passive stretching and refractory to analgesia is the hallmark sign early on; also look for "the 6 Ps" (see sidebar)
* requires prompt decompression - remove constrictive casts, dressings; fasciotomy may be needed emergently

UPPER EXTREMITY INJURIES
* anterior shoulder dislocation
    * axillary nerve (lateral aspect of shoulder) and musculocutaneous nerve (extensor aspect of forearm) at risk
    * seen on lateral view: humeral head anterior to glenoid
        * reduce (traction, scapular manipulation), immobilize in internal rotation, re-X-ray, out-patient appointment with ortho
        * with forceful injury, look for fracture
* Colles' fracture (Figure 6)
    * distal radius fracture with dorsal displacement
    * from **f**all **o**n an **o**utstretched **h**and (FOOSH)
    * AP film: shortening, radial deviation, radial displacement
    * lateral film: dorsal displacement, volar angulation

Description of Fractures ("SOLARTAT")
Site
Open vs. closed
Length
Articular
Rotation
Translation
Alignment/angulation
Type (i.e. Salter-Harris, etc.)

Reasons for Emergent Orthopaedic Consultation
- compartment syndrome
- irreducible dislocation
- circulatory compromise
- open fracture
- injury requiring surgical repair

When dealing with an open fracture, remember "STAND"
Splint
Tetanus prophylaxis
Antibiotic
Neurovascular status (before and after)
Dressings (to cover wound)

Vascular injury/compartment syndrome is suggested by "The **6 Ps**":
Pulse discrepancies
Pallor
Paresthesia/hypoesthesia
Paralysis
Pain (especially when refractory to usual analgesics)
Polar (cold)

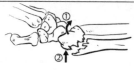

lateral view

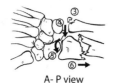

A- P view

1. dorsal tilt
2. dorsal displacement
3. ulnar styloid fracture
4. radial displacement
5. radial tilt
6. shortening

© Willa Bradshaw 2005

Figure 6. Colles' fracture

- reduce, immobilize with splint, out-patient with ortho or immediate ortho referral if complicated fracture
- if involvement of articular surface, emergent ortho referral
- scaphoid fracture
  - tenderness in anatomical snuff box, pain on scaphoid tubercle, pain on axial loading of thumb
  - negative X-ray: thumb spica splint, re-X-ray in 1 week ± bone scan
  - positive X-ray: thumb spica splint x 6-8 weeks
  - risk of avascular necrosis (AVN) of scaphoid if not immobilized
  - outpatient ortho appointment

LOWER EXTREMITY INJURIES

- ankle and foot fractures
  - see Ottawa Ankle and Foot rules (Figure 8)
- knee injuries
  - see Ottawa Knee rules (Figure 9)
- avulsion of the base of 5th metatarsal
  - occurs with inversion injury
  - supportive tensor or below knee walking cast for 3 weeks
- calcaneal fracture
  - associated with fall from height
  - associated injuries may involve ankles, knees, hips, pelvis, lumbar spine

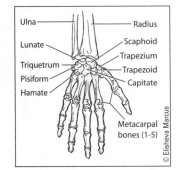

Figure 7. Carpal Bones

Reasons for Splinting
- reduces pain
- reduces further damage to vessels and nerves
- reduces risk of inadvertently converting a closed fracture into an open fracture
- facilitates patient transport

An ankle radiographic series is required only if there is any pain in malleolar zone and any of these findings:
1. bone tenderness at A
or
2. bone tenderness at B
or
3. inability to bear weight both immediately and in emergency department

A foot radiographic series is required only if there is any pain in midfoot zone and any of these findings:
1. bone tenderness at C
or
2. bone tenderness at D
or
3. inability to bear weight both immediately and in emergency department

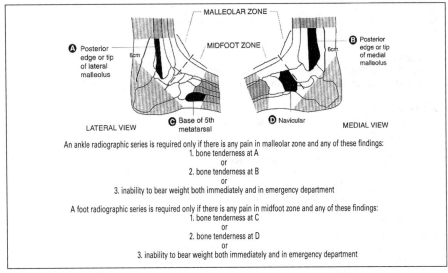

Figure 8. Ottawa Ankle Rules
Reprinted with permission from Stiell et. al. (1994) *JAMA* 271(11):827-832, copyright © (1994), American Medical Association.

A knee x-ray examination is required only for acute injury patients with one or more of:
- age 55 years or older
- tenderness at head of fibula
- isolated tenderness of patella*
- inability to flex to 90°
- inability to bear weight both immediately and in the emergency department (four steps)**

*no bony tenderness of knee other than patella
**unable to transfer weight twice onto each lower limb regardless of limping

Figure 9. Ottawa Knee Rules
Reprinted with permission from: Stiell et. al. (1997) *JAMA* 278(23):611-5, copyright © (1997), American Medical Association.

Wound Management

Goals of ED Treatment
- identify injuries and stop any active bleeding – direct pressure
- manage pain
- wound examination and exploration (history and physical)
- cleansing ± antibiotic and tetanus prophylaxis
- repair and dressing

Tetanus Prophylaxis
- both tetanus toxoid (Td) and immunoglobulin (TIG) are safe (and indicated) in pregnancy

Table 9. Guidelines for Tetanus Prophylaxis for Wounds

Immunization History	Non Tetanus Prone Wounds		Tetanus Prone Wounds[1]	
	Td[2]	TIG[3]	Td	TIG
Uncertain or <3 doses	Yes	No	Yes	Yes
3 or more, none for >10 years	Yes	No	Yes	No
3 or more, >5 but <10 years ago	No	No	Yes	No
3 or more, <4 years ago	No	No	Yes	No

[1] wounds >6 hours old, >1 cm deep, puncture wounds, avulsions, wounds resulting from missiles, crush wounds, burns, frostbite, wounds contaminated with dirt, feces, soil, or saliva
[2] 0.5 mL IM tetanus and diphtheria toxoids (Td), adsorbed   [3] tetanus immune globulin (TIG), 250 units deep IM
Source: MMWR 2001; 50(20); 418, 427. MMWR 1991; 40(RR12); 1-52.

Bruises
- tender swelling (hematoma) following blunt trauma
- is patient on anticoagulants? do they have a coagulopathy (e.g. liver disease)?

Abrasions
- partial to full thickness break in skin
- management
  - clean thoroughly, ± local anesthetic, with brush to prevent foreign body impregnation (tattooing)
  - antiseptic ointment (Polysporin™ or Vaseline™) for 7 days for facial and complex abrasions
  - tetanus prophylaxis – see Table 9

Lacerations
- see Plastic Surgery
- consider every structure deep to a laceration injured until proven otherwise
- in hand injury patient, include following in history: handedness, occupation, mechanism of injury, previous history of injury
- physical exam
  - think about underlying anatomy
  - examine tendon function actively against resistance and neurovascular status distally
  - clean and explore under local anesthetic; look for partial tendon injuries
  - x-ray wounds if a foreign body is suspected (e.g. shattered glass) and not found when exploring wound (remember: not all foreign bodies are radiopaque), or if suspect intra-articular involvement
- management
  - disinfect skin/use sterile techniques
  - irrigate copiously with normal saline
  - analgesia ± anesthesia
- maximum dose of lidocaine:
  - 7 mg/kg with epinephrine
  - 5 mg/kg without epinephrine
- in children, topical anesthetics such as LET (lidocaine, epinephrine and tetracaine) and in selected cases a short-acting benzodiazepine (midazolam or other agents) for sedation and amnesia are useful
- secure hemostasis
- evacuate hematomas, debride non-viable tissue, remove hair and remove foreign bodies
- ± prophylactic antibiotics
- suture unless delayed presentation, a puncture wound, or mammalian bite
- take into account patient and wound factors when considering suturing
- advise patient when to have sutures removed

Acute treatment of contusions (**RICE**):
Rest
Ice
Compression
Elevation

Suture To	Close with nylon or other nonabsorbable suture	Approx. Duration (days)
Face	6-0	5
Not Joint	4-0	7
Joint	3-0	10
Scalp	4-0	7
Mucous Membrane	absorbable (vicryl)	N/A

N.B. Patients on steroid therapy may need sutures in for longer periods of time

---

Alternatives to Sutures
- tissue glue
- Steristrips™
- staples

Where **not** to use local anesthetic with epinephrine:
Ears, **N**ose, **F**ingers, **T**oes and **H**ose (**P**enis)

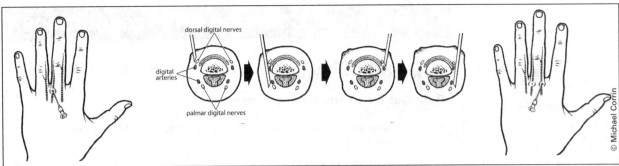

Figure 10. Digital Block – Local Anesthesia of Digits

Cellulitis
- see Plastic Surgery
- localized infection of the dermis
- bacterial (*S. aureus*, GAS, *H. influenzae*, rarely pseudomonas, MRSA) infection of skin and subcutaneous tissues
- look for "rubor, calor, dolor, tumor" (erythema, warmth, pain, swelling)
- have high index of suspicion in patients who are immunocompromised (e.g. HIV, DM), vasculopaths, IV drug users
- treat with immobilization and elevation of infected area, antibiotics, analgesics, and close follow-up
- antibiotics for common cellulitis: cefazolin IV then cephalexin PO (alt: clindamycin PO, vancomycin IV then linezolid PO); consider MRSA

Differential Diagnosis of cellulitis
Necrotizing Fasciitis
Gas gangrene
Cutaneous anthrax
Vaccinia vaccination
Insect bite (hypersensitivity)
Acute gout
DVT
Fixed drug reaction
Kawasaki's
Pyoderma gangrenosum

Abscess
- may be associated with a retained foreign body
- look for warm, swollen, painful, erythematous fluctuant masses
- ensure absence of systemic symptoms and presence of subcutaneous air in simple abscesses
- anesthetize locally
- treat with incision and drainage ± antibiotics – apply warm compress, give analgesics

Which Abscesses Need Antibiotics?
- evidence of systemic illness (e.g. cellulitis)
- immunocompromised patient
- patient at risk for endocarditis

Trauma in Pregnancy

- Priorities: Airway, Breathing, Circulation

Early wound irrigation and debridement are the most important factors in decreasing infection.

Hemodynamic Considerations
- near term, inferior vena caval compression in the supine position can decrease cardiac output by 30-40%
  - use left lateral decubitus (LLD) positioning or hip bolster to alleviate compression and increase blood return
- BP drops 5-15 mmHg systolic in 2nd trimester, increases to normal by term
- HR increases 15-20 beats per minute by 3rd trimester

Blood Considerations
- physiologic macrocytic anemia of pregnancy (Hb 100-120)
- WBC increases to high of 20,000

The best treatment for the fetus is the effective treatment of the mother.

Shock
- pregnant patients may lose 35% of blood volume without typical signs of shock (i.e. tachycardia, hypotension)
- the fetus may be in "shock" due to contraction of the uteroplacental circulation
- fetal HR changes are an indication of maternal circulatory compromise

Management Differences
- place bolster under right hip to stop inferior vena cava compression
- fetal monitoring (continuous tocographic monitoring if possible viable fetus i.e. >20 weeks)
- early obstetrical consult
- do not avoid necessary x-rays, but shield as much as posssible
- consider need for RhoGAM if mother Rh–

Approach to Common ER Presentations

Abdominal Pain

Rule Out Life-Threatening Causes
- CVS: MI, aortic dissection, ruptured AAA (tearing pain)
- GI : perforated viscus, hepatic/splenic injury, ischemic bowel (diffuse pain)
- GU: ectopic pregnancy

Additional Differential Diagnosis
- GI: appendicitis, diverticulitis, bowel obstruction, hepatitis, cholecystitis, pancreatitis
- urinary: cystitis, pyelonephritis, ureteral calculi
- genital
    - female: pelvic inflammatory disease (PID), endometriosis, salpingitis/tubo-ovarian abscess, ovarian torsion/cyst
    - male: testicular torsion, epididymitis
- other: diabetic ketoacidosis (DKA), Herpes Zoster Virus (HZV), intra-abdominal abscess, pneumonia, lead poisoning, porphyria, sickle cell crisis

History and Physical Examination
- determine onset, course, location and character of pain: PQRST
- associated GU, GI, respiratory, CV symptoms
- abdominal trauma/surgeries
- general appearance, vitals
- respiratory, CVS
- back: CVA tenderness, ecchymoses
- extremities: differential pulses, psoas/obturator sign
- abdomen, including DRE, pelvic exam (females), genital exam (males)

Investigations
- do not delay consultation if patient unstable
- CBC, electrolytes, glucose, LFTs, amylase, BUN/creat, U/A, + others if indicated: β-hCG, lactate, ECG
- AXR: look for calcifications, free air, gas pattern, air fluid levels
- CXR upright: look for pneumoperitoneum (free air under diaphragm)
- U/S: biliary tract, ectopic pregnancy, AAA, free fluid
- CT: trauma, AAA, pancreatitis, nephro/urolithiasis, appendicitis

Management
- NPO, IV, NG tube, analgesics
    - growing evidence that small amounts of narcotic analgesics improve diagnostic accuracy of physical exam of surgical abdomen
- consult as necessary: general surgery, vascular, gynecology, etc.

Disposition
- Admission: in addition to a surgical abdomen, admission is sometimes required for workup of abnormal findings on investigation, IV antibiotics, pain control, etc.
- Discharge: patients with a negative lab and imaging workup who improve clinically during their stay can be discharged. Instruct the patient to return if severe pain, fever, or persistent vomiting develop. Follow up with FP in 24-48 hours

Acute Pelvic Pain

Etiology
- gynecological
    - 2nd most common gynecological complaint after vaginal bleeding
    - ruptured ovarian cysts – most common cause of pelvic pain, follicular cyst most common type
    - ovarian torsion – rare, 50% will have ovarian tumour
    - leiomyomas (uterine fibroids) – especially with torsion of a pedunculated fibroid or in pregnant patient (degeneration)
    - ectopic pregnancy – ruptured/expanding/leaking
    - spontaneous abortion – threatened or incomplete
    - infection – PID, endometritis, tubo-ovarian abscess
    - dysmenorrhea and endometriosis – rarely cause new onset acute pelvic pain

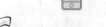

Red Flags
- extremes of age
- unstable vital signs
- fever
- signs/symptoms of shock
- rapid onset severe pain

Abdominal Assessment (DR. GERM):
Assess in all 4 quadrants for
Distention
Rigidity
Guarding
Eviceration/**E**cchymosis
Rebound tenderness
Masses

Unstable patients should not be sent for imaging.

All women of childbearing age assumed to be pregnant until proven otherwise.

- non-gynecological
  - GI – appendicitis, constipation, bowel obstruction, gastroenteritis, diverticulitis, IBD, IBS
  - GU – cystitis, pyelonephritis, ureteral stone
  - other – porphyria, abdominal angina, aneurysm, hernia, zoster

History and Physical Exam
- determine onset, course, location and character of the pain
- associated symptoms: vaginal bleeding, bowel or bladder symptoms, radiation
- vitals
- gynecological exam
- abdominal exam

Investigations
- β–hCG for all women of childbearing age
- CBC and differential, PTT, INR
- pelvic and abdominal US – evaluate adnexa, look for free fluid in the pelvis or masses, evaluate thickness of endometrium
- doppler flow studies for ovarian torsion

Management
- general: analgesia, determine if admission and consults needed
  - gynecology consult if history and physical suggestive of serious cause
  - other consults as indicated – general surgery, urology, etc.
- specific:
  - ovarian cysts
    - unruptured or ruptured and hemodynamically stable – analgesia and follow-up
    - ruptured with significant hemoperitoneum – may require surgery
  - ovarian torsion – surgical detorsion or removal of ovary
  - uncomplicated leiomyomas, endometriosis and secondary dysmenorrhea can usually be treated on an outpatient basis, discharge with gynecology follow-up
  - PID: requires broad spectrum antibiotics

Disposition
- patients requiring IV therapy or surgery should be admitted
- patients to be discharged should be given clear instructions for appropriate follow up

Altered Level of Consciousness (LOC)

Definitions
- altered mental status – collective, non-specific term referring to change in cognitive function, behaviour, or attentiveness
- delirium – acute, transient, fluctuating, potentially reversible organic brain disorder presenting as altered LOC or attentiveness
- dementia – insidious, progressive, organic brain disorder with change in memory, judgment, personality and cortical function
- lethargy – state of decreased awareness and alertness (patient may appear wakeful)
- stupor – unresponsiveness from which the patient can be aroused
- coma – a sleep-like state, non arousable to consciousness
- use the GCS to evaluate LOC (see *Initial Patient Assessment and Management*, ER4)

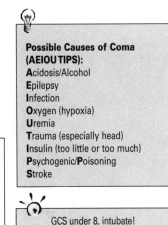

Possible Causes of Coma (AEIOU TIPS):
Acidosis/Alcohol
Epilepsy
Infection
Oxygen (hypoxia)
Uremia
Trauma (especially head)
Insulin (too little or too much)
Psychogenic/**P**oisoning
Stroke

GCS under 8, intubate!

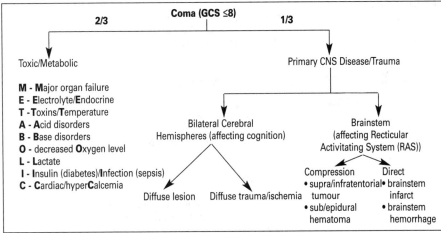

Figure 11. Etiology of Coma

MANAGEMENT OF ALTERED LOC

History
- obtained from family, friends, police, paramedics, old chart, etc.
- onset and progression
  - abrupt onset suggests CNS hemorrhage/ischemia or cardiac cause
  - progression over hours to days suggests progressive CNS lesion or toxic/metabolic cause
- preceding events
  - it is essential to determine patient's baseline LOC preceding deterioration
  - antecedent trauma, seizure activity, fever
- past medical history (e.g. similar episode, depression)

Physical Examination
- vitals including temperature, cardiac, chest, respiratory, abdominal exam, and the "five Ns" (see sidebar)
- complete neuro exam in particularly examination of the eyes

Investigations
- rapid blood sugar, CBC, electrolytes, Cr, BUN, LFTs, glucose, serum osmolality, ABGs, coags, troponins, U/A
- ECG, CXR, Head CT
- drug levels of specific toxins if indicated

Diagnosis
- administer appropriate universal antidotes (see sidebar)
  - thiamine 100 mg IV if history of EtOH or patient looks malnourished
  - one ampule D50W IV if low blood sugar on finger-stick
  - naloxone 0.4-2 mg IV or IM if opiate overdose suspected
- distinguish between structural and toxic-metabolic coma
  - structural coma
    - pupils, extraocular movements and motor findings are asymmetric or absent
  - toxic-metabolic coma
    - dysfunction at lower levels of the brainstem (e.g. caloric unresponsiveness)
    - respiratory depression in association with an intact upper brainstem (e.g. equal and reactive pupils; see exceptions in Table 10)
    - extraocular movements and motor findings are symmetric or absent

Table 10. Toxic - Metabolic Causes of Fixed Pupils

Dilated	Dilated to Normal	Constricted
• anoxia	• hypothermia	• cholinergic agents (e.g. organophosphates)
• anticholinergic agents (e.g. atropine, TCAs)	• barbiturates	• opiates (e.g. heroin), except meperidine
• methanol (rare)		

- essential to re-examine frequently – status can change rapidly
- diagnosis may become apparent only with the passage of time
  - delayed deficit after head trauma suggestive of epidural hematoma (characteristic "lucid interval")

Disposition
- readily reversible alteration of LOC: discharge if adequate follow-up care available
- ongoing decreased LOC: admit to service based on tentative diagnosis
- transfer patient if appropriate level of care not available

Chest Pain

Rule Out Life-Threatening Causes
- CVS: acute coronary syndrome/acute MI, pericarditis/cardiac tamponade, aortic dissection
- respiratory: pulmonary embolism (PE)/tension pneumothorax
- GI: esophageal rupture/pneumomediastinum

Additional Differential Diagnosis
- cardiac: stable angina
- respiratory: pneumonia, spontaneous pneumothorax (young, thin, tall)
- GI: peptic ulcer disease (PUD), pancreatitis, cholecystitis, esophagitis, reflux
- MSK: rib fractures, costochondritis, zoster, etc.
- psychogenic/anxiety (diagnosis of exclusion)

Initial Resuscitation and Management
- O_2, IV, cardiac monitoring, CXR (portable if unstable), ECG

History
- must evaluate cardiac risk factors (DM, HTN, hyperlipidemia, smoking, 1st degree relative with CAD <50 yo)
- classic presentations (but presentation seldom classic)
  - aortic dissection: sudden severe tearing pain, often radiating to back
  - pulmonary embolism: pleuritic chest pain (75%), dyspnea, anxiety, tachycardia
  - pericarditis: anterior precordial pain, pleuritic, relieved by sitting up and leaning forward
  - acute coronary syndrome (ACS): retrosternal squeezing/pressure pain, radiation to arm/neck, dyspnea, nausea/vomiting, syncope
  - esophageal: frequent heartburn, acid reflux, dysphagia, relief with antacids
- ACS more likely to be atypical in females, diabetics, and >80 years

Physical Examamination
- vitals
  - BP in BOTH arms: >20 mmHg difference suggests thoracic aortic dissection
- palpate chest wall for tender points, but be aware that 25% of patients with acute MI have chest wall tenderness
  - consider a diagnosis of MSK disease only if more serious causes excluded and palpation fully reproduces pain and symptoms
- cardiac exam, respiratory exam, peripheral vascular exam

Investigations
- CBC, electrolytes
- serial cardiac enzymes
  - normal CK does NOT rule out MI
  - troponin I more sensitive (but positive later than CK-MB; can have false positives in renal failure, must follow for 8 hrs post onset of symptoms)
- ECG
  - always compare with previous
  - PE and acute MI may have normal ECG in up to 50% of cases
  - consider 15-lead ECG if hypotensive or if ECG shows inferior MI or AV node involvement
- CXR
  - always compare with previous
  - PE
    - 50% completely normal
    - atelectasis, elevated hemidiaphragm, pleural effusion
  - aortic dissection
    - mediastinal widening, bulging aortic arch, separation of intima calcification from edge of aortic shadow, depressed left main bronchus
    - change from previous CXR is the most accurate finding
    - CXR is normal in 20% of thoracic dissections
  - pneumothorax
    - may need inspiration and expiration views
- ABGs – normal in 20% of patients with PE; not sensitive enough to rule out PE
- D-dimer, V/Q scan or helical CT, venous leg Doppler, if PE suspected (see Wells' Score)
- negative D-dimer rules out PE in low probability patients
- patients with intermediate or high probability Wells' score require imaging

Disposition
- patients at risk of developing dysrhythmias should be admitted to a monitored bed
- consult cardiology for patients with ACS. Obtain a cardiothoracic surgery consultation for patients with valvular lesions by echocardiogram, esophageal rupture, or aortic dissection
- discharge is appropriate for patients with a low probability of life-threatening illness due to resolving symptoms and negative workup. Instruct the patient to return if they develop SOB or increased chest pain. Patient should follow up with family physician

ACUTE MYOCARDIAL INFARCTION
- see Cardiology

Management
- immediate stabilization
  - oxygen 4L/min
  - IV access
  - cardiac monitors
  - "STAT" ECG
  - cardiac enzymes (CK, Troponins)

Signs and Symptoms of MI (PULSE):
Persistent chest pain
Upset stomach
Lightheadedness
Shortness of breath
Excessive sweating

Signs of PE on CXR
Westermark's sign: abrupt tapering of a vessel on chest film.
Hampton's hump: a wedge-shaped infiltrate that abuts the pleura.

Wells' Score for PE
Previous Hx of DVT/emboli +1.5
HR >100: +1.5
Recent immobility or Sx: +1.5
Clinical signs of DVT: +3
Alternate Dx less likely than PE: +3
Hemoptysis: +1
Cancer: +1

Low probability = 0-2
Intermediate probability = 2-6
High probability = >6

Every Acute MI patient in the ER must be greeted by BMONA right away:
β-Blockade
Morphine
Oxygen
Nitroglycerin
ASA

Addition of Clopidogrel to Aspirin and Fibrinolytic Therapy for Myocardial Infarction with ST-Segment Elevation
NEJM. 352(12): 1179-1191, 2005 Mar
Purpose: To assess the benefit of adding clopidogrel to aspirin and fibrinolytic therapy in ST-elevation MI.
Study Characteristics: Double-blind, RCT, following intention-to-treat analysis, with 3491 patients and clinical follow-up at 30 days.
Participants: Individuals presenting within 12 hours of onset of ST-elevation MI (mean age 57, 80.3% male, 50.3% smokers, 9.1% previous MI). Those presenting after 12 hours, age >75, or with previous CABG were excluded.
Intervention: Clopidogrel (300 mg loading dose followed by 75 mg od until day of angiogram) or placebo, in addition to aspirin, a fibrinolytic agent, and heparin when appropriate.
Primary Outcome: Composite of occluded infarct-related artery on angiography (Thrombosis in Myocardial Infarction flow grade 0 or 1), or death or recurrent MI prior to angiography.
Results: Rates of primary end point were 21.7% in the placebo group and 15.0% in the clopidogrel group (95% CI, 24-47%). Among the individual components of the primary end point, clopidogrel had a significant effect on the rate of an occluded infarct-related artery and the rate of recurrent MI, but no effect on the rate of death from any cause. At 30 days clinical follow-up, there was no difference in rate of death from cardiovascular causes, a significant reduction in the odds of recurrent MI, and a non-significant reduction in recurrent ischemia with need for urgent revascularization. The rates of major bleeding and intracranial hemorrhage were similar between the two groups.
Conclusion: Addition of clopidogrel improves the patency rate of infarct-related arteries and reduces ischemic complications, both of which are associated with improved long-term survival after MI. The trial was not powered to detect a survival benefit and none was seen.

- ASA 160-325mg chewed
- nitroglycerin 0.3 mg SL q5min x 3 (IV for CHF, HTN, unresolved pain)
- morphine 2-5 mg IV q5-30min if unresponsive to NTG
- metoprolol 5 mg slow IV q5min x 3 if no contraindication (beware in inferior wall AMI)
- thrombolytics or primary percutaneous coronary intervention (PCI)
  - agents include t-PA, r-PA, Streptokinase, and TNK
  - evaluate indications and contraindications prior to use
- enoxaparin (Low Molecular Weight Heparin) 1 mg/kg SC bid (30mg IV STAT post TNK infusion)
- other – antiarrythmics, cardioversion, defibrillation, transthoracic pacing, angioplasty
- cardiology consult

Headache

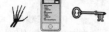

- see Neurology

Etiology
- **the common**
  - common migraine (no aura)/classic migraine (involves aura)
    - gradual onset, unilateral/bilateral, throbbing
    - nausea/vomiting, photo/phonophobia
    - treatment: analgesics, neuroleptics, vasoactive meds
  - tension/muscular headache
    - never during sleep, gradual over 24 hours
    - posterior/occipital
    - increased with stressors
    - treatment: modify stressor, local measures, NSAIDs
- **the deadly**
  - subarachnoid hemorrhage (SAH) – see Neurosurgery
    - sudden onset, increased with exertion
    - "worst" headache, nausea and vomiting, meningeal signs
    - diagnosis: CT, LP (5-10% of patients with SAH have negative initial CT)
      - sensitivity of CT decreases with time and is much less sensitive by 48-72 hr
    - management: urgent neurosurgery consult
  - increased ICP
    - worst in morning, supine, or bending down
    - physical exam: neurological deficits, cranial nerve palsies, papilledema
    - diagnosis: CT scan
    - management: consult neurosurgery
  - meningitis (see Infectious Diseases)
    - fever, nausea/vomiting, meningeal signs, purpuric rash
    - altered level of consciousness
    - perform CT to rule out SAH then do LP for diagnosis
    - treatment: early empiric antibiotics (depending on age group), steroid therapy
  - temporal arteritis (not immediately deadly but causes great morbidity) (see Ophthalmology)
    - one-sided scalp tenderness, jaw claudication, visual disturbances
    - labs: elevated ESR
    - temporal artery biopsy is gold standard for diagnosis
    - treatment: high-dose steroids immediately if TA suspected

Disposition
- admit if underlying diagnosis is critical or emergent, if there are abnormal neurological findings, if patient is elderly or immunocompromised (don't manifest symptoms as well), or if pain is refractory to oral medications
- most patients can be discharged with appropriate analgesia and follow up with their family physician. Instruct patients to return for fever, vomiting, neurologic changes, or increasing pain

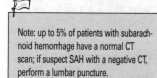
Note: up to 5% of patients with subarachnoid hemorrhage have a normal CT scan; if suspect SAH with a negative CT, perform a lumbar puncture.

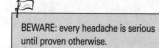
BEWARE: every headache is serious until proven otherwise.

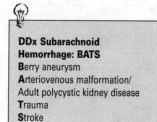
DDx Subarachnoid Hemorrhage: BATS
Berry aneurysm
Arteriovenous malformation/ Adult polycystic kidney disease
Trauma
Stroke

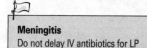
Meningitis
Do not delay IV antibiotics for LP

Seizures

- see Neurology

Definition
- paroxysmal alteration of behaviour and/or EEG changes resulting from abnormal, excessive activity of neurons

Categories
- generalized seizure (consciousness always lost): tonic/clonic, absence, myoclonic, atonic
- partial seizure (focal): simple partial, complex partial
- causes: trauma, intracranial hemorrhage, structural abnormality, infection, toxins/drugs, metabolic disturbance (hypo/hyperglycemia, hypo/hypernatremia, hypocalcemia, hypomagnesemia); primary seizure disorder
- differential diagnosis: syncope, pseudoseizures, migraines, movement disorder, narcolepsy/cataplexy, myoclonus

History
- from patient and bystander: flaccid and unconscious, often with deep rapid breathing
- preceding aura, rapid onset, loss of bladder/bowel control, tongue-biting

Physical Examination
- injuries to head and spine, bony prominences (e.g. elbows), tongue laceration, aspiration, urinary incontinence

Investigations
- known seizure disorder: anticonvulsant levels
- Accucheck
- first time seizure: CBC, serum glucose, electrolytes, BUN, creatinine, Ca, Mg; consider prolactin, β-hCG, tox screen
- initial: CT; X-ray suspected extremily injuries. Definitive: MRI, EEG

Table 11. Management of Status Epilepticus

Time (min)	Steps
0-5	Give oxygen; ensure adequate ventilation Monitor: vital signs, electrocardiography, oximetry Establish IV access; obtain blood samples for glucose level, CBC, lytes, toxins, and anticonvulsant levels
6-9	Give glucose (preceded by thiamine in adults)
10-20	Intravenously administer either 0.1 mg/kg of lorazepam at 2 mg/min or 0.2 mg/kg of diazepam at 5 mg/min. Diazepam can be repeated if seizures do not stop after 5 min; if diazepam is used to stop the status, then phenytoin should be administered promptly to prevent the recurrence of status
21-60	If status persists, administer 15-20 mg/kg of phenytoin intravenously no faster than 50 mg/min in adults and 1 mg/kg/min in children
>60	If status does not stop after 20 mg/kg of phenytoin, give additional doses of 5 mg/kg to a maximal dose of 30 mg/kg. If status persists, then give 20 mg/kg of phenobarbital IV at 100 mg/min. When phenobarbital is given after a benzodiazepine, ventilatory assistance is usually required If status persists, then give general anaesthesia (e.g., pentobarbital). Vasopressors or fluid volume are usually necessary. Electroencephalogram should be monitored. Neuromuscular blockade may be needed.

Source: Cecil's Essentials of Medicine, 7th edition, Table 125-7. Used with permission.

Disposition
- the decision to admit or discharge should be based on the underlying disease process identified. If a patient has returned to baseline function and is neurologically intact, then discharge with outpatient follow up is often an option
- first-time seizure patients being discharged should be referred to a neurologist for follow up. Admitted patients should generally have a neurology consult
- patient should not drive until medically cleared (local regulations vary)
  - complete notification form to appropriate authority re: ability to drive

Syncope

- definition: sudden, transient loss of consciousness and postural tone with spontaneous recovery
- usually caused by generalized cerebral hypoperfusion

Causes of Syncope by System (HEAD, HEART, VeSSELS):
Hypoxia/**H**ypoglycemia
Epilepsy
Anxiety
Dysfunctional brainstem

Heart attack
Embolism (PE)
Aortic obstruction
Rhythm disturbance
Tachycardia

Vasovagal
Situational
Subclavian steal
ENT (glossopharyngeal neuralgia)
Low systemic vascular resistance
Sensitive carotid **S**inus

Etiology
- cardiogenic: arrhythmia, outflow obstruction (e.g. PE, tamponade, tension pneumo, pulmonary HTN), MI, valvular disease
- non-cardiogenic: peripheral vascular (hypovolemia), vaso-vagal, cerebrovascular disorders, CNS, metabolic disturbances

History
- gather details from witnesses
- distinguish between syncope and seizure (see <u>Neurology</u>)
  - signs and symptoms during presyncope, syncope and postsyncope
  - past medical history, drugs

Physical Examination
- postural BP and HR
- cardiovascular, respiratory and neuro exam

Investigations
- ECG (tachycardia, bradycardia, blocks, WPW, long QT interval), bedside glucose
- as indicated: CBC, electrolytes, BUN, creatinine, ABGs, Troponin, Mg, Ca, β-hCG (tailor to clinical presentation and patient's premorbid condition)
- consider drug screen

Management
- ABCs, IV, O_2, monitor
- examine for signs of trauma caused by syncopal episode
- cardiogenic syncope: admit to medicine/cardiology
- non-cardiogenic syncope: discharge with follow-up as indicated by cause

Disposition
- decision to admit is based on etiology (e.g. cardiac or neurologic)
- most patients will be discharged
- on discharge, instruct patient to follow up with family physician. Educate re: avoiding orthostatic or situational syncope. Patients with recurrent syncope should avoid high risk activities (e.g. driving)

Sexual Assault

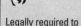
Legally required to report sexual assault if victim is <16 years of age.

Epidemiology
- 1 in 4 women and 1 in 10 men will be sexually assaulted in their lifetime
- it is estimated that only 7% of rapes are reported

General Approach
- ABCs, treat acute, serious injuries
- ensure patient is not left alone and provide ongoing emotional support
- set aside adequate time for exam (usually 1.5 hours)
- obtain consent for medical exam and treatment, collection of evidence, disclosure to police (notify police as soon as consent obtained)
- Sexual Assault Kit (document injuries, collect evidence) if <72hrs since assault
- label samples immediately and pass directly to police
- offer community crisis resources (e.g. shelter, hotline)
- do not report unless victim requests (legally required if <16 years old)

History
- ensure privacy for the patient -- others should be asked to leave
- who? how many? when? where did penetration occur? what happened? any weapons or physical assault?
- post-assault activities (urination, defecation, change of clothes, shower, douche, etc.)
- gynecologic history
  - gravity, parity, last menstrual period
  - contraception
  - last voluntary intercourse (sperm motile 6-12 hours in vagina, 5 days in cervix)
- don't forget the general medical history - acute injury/illness, chronic diseases, psychiatric history, medications, allergies, etc.

Physical Examination
- evidence collection is always secondary to treatment of serious injuries
- never re-traumatize a patient with the examination
- general examination
  - mental status
  - sexual maturity
  - patient should remove clothes and place in paper bag
  - document abrasions, bruises, lacerations, torn frenulum/broken teeth (indicates oral penetration)
- pelvic exam and specimen collection
  - ideally before urination or defecation
  - examine for seminal stains, hymen, signs of trauma
  - collect moistened swabs of dried seminal stains
  - pubic hair combings and cuttings
  - speculum exam
    - lubricate with water only
    - vaginal lacerations, foreign bodies
    - Pap smear
    - oral/cervical/rectal culture for gonorrhea and chlamydia
    - posterior fornix secretions if present or aspiration of saline irrigation
    - immediate wet smear for motile sperm
    - air-dried slides for immotile sperm, acid phosphatase, ABO group
- others
  - fingernail scrapings
  - saliva sample from victim

Investigations
- VDRL - repeat in 3 months if negative
- serum β-hCG
- blood for ABO group, Rh type, baseline serology (e.g. hepatitis, HIV)

Management
- involve local/regional sexual assault team
- medical
  - suture lacerations
  - tetanus prophylaxis
  - gynecology consult for foreign body, complex lacerations
  - assumed positive for gonorrhea and chlamydia
    - management: azithromycin 1 g PO x 1 dose
      (alt: doxycycline 100 mg PO bid x 7 days)
      and cefixime 400 mg PO x 1 dose
  - may start prophylaxis for hepatitis B and HIV
  - pre and post counselling for HIV testing
  - pregnancy prophylaxis offered
    - levonorgestrel 0.75 mg STAT, repeat in 12 hours (Plan B™)
- psychological
  - high incidence of psychological sequelae
  - have victim change and shower after exam completed

Risk of Sexually Transmitted Disease After Sexual Assault
Gonorrhea: 6-18%
Chlamydia: 4-17%
Syphilis: 0.5-3%
HIV: <1%

Disposition
- discharge if injuries/social situation permit
- follow-up with MD in rape crisis centre within 24 hours
- best if patient does not leave ED alone

DOMESTIC VIOLENCE
- women are usually the victims, but male victimisation also occurs
- identify the problem (need high index of suspicion)
  - suggestive injuries (bruises, sprains, abrasions, occasionally fractures, burns or other injuries; often do not match up with history provided)
  - somatic symptoms (chronic and vague complaints)
  - psychosocial symptoms (your 'gut feeling' e.g. overbearing partner that won't leave patient's side)
- if disclosed, be supportive and assess danger
- how to secretly get patient alone to question re: abuse? Order an x-ray

How do you get a patient who is accompanied by her partner alone without arousing suspicion?
Order an x-ray

Management
- treat injuries
- ask about sexual assault and children at home
- document findings
- plan safety
- follow-up: family doctor/social worker

Medical Emergencies

Anaphylaxis and Allergic Reactions

Etiology
- exaggerated immune response classically IgE mediated, sensitization then re-exposure
- anaphylaxis: a severe hypersensitivity reaction affecting multiple systems
- urticaria: a hypersensitivity reaction causing an itchy skin eruption
- angioedema: swelling that occurs in the tissue just below the surface of the skin, most often around the lips and eyes
- anaphylactoid reaction: non-IgE mediated, may occur with first exposure (e.g. radiocontrast dyes); presentation and treatment same as for anaphylaxis

> **Most common triggers for anaphylaxis**
> - penicillin
> - stings
> - nuts
> - shellfish

History and Physical Examination
- general – marked anxiety, apprehension, tremor, cold sensation
- skin – generalized urticaria, edema, erythema, pruritus
- respiratory – nasal congestion, sneezing, coryza, cough, hoarseness, sensation of throat tightness, dyspnea, stridor, wheeze
- eyes – itch, tearing, conjunctival injection
- cardiovascular – hypotension, tachycardia, weakness, dizziness, syncope, chest pain, arrhythmia, MI
- GI – abdominal pain, nausea, vomiting, diarrhea

Management
- remove causative agent; secure ABCs
- epinephrine:
    - on scene – epi-pen (injectable epinephrine) if available
    - moderate signs and symptoms (minimal airway edema, mild bronchospasm, cutaneous reactions)
        - adult: 0.3-0.5 mL of 1:1000 solution IM epinephrine
        - child: 0.01 mL/kg/dose up to 0.4 mL/dose 1:1000 epinephrine
    - severe signs and symptoms (laryngeal edema, severe bronchospasm and shock)
        - epinephrine via IV or ETT starting at 1 ml of 1:10,000 (0.1 mg) in adults; 0.01 mL/kg in children
        - cardiac monitoring, ECG
- diphenhydramine (Benadryl™) 50 mg IM or IV q4-6h
- methylprednisolone 50-100 mg IV dose depending on severity
- salbutamol (Ventolin™) via nebulizer if bronchospasm present
- glucagon (for those on β-blockers with resistant hypotension) 5-15 μg q1min IV

Disposition
- monitor for min 4-6 hours in ED
- can have second phase reaction up to 48 hours later, patient may need to be supervised
- 3 day course of:
    - H1 antagonist (Certrizine 10 mg PO od)
    - H2 antagonist (ranitidine 150 mg PO od)
    - corticosteroid (prednisone 50 mg PO od)

Asthma

> Beware of the silent asthmatic! This is a medical emergency and may require emergency intubation.

- see Respirology
- chronic inflammatory airway disease with episodes of bronchospasm and inflammation resulting in airflow obstruction

Investigations
- O₂ sat
- peak flow meter
- ± ABG
- CXR if diagnosis in doubt or concerns of pneumonia, pneumothorax, etc.

Table 12. Asthma Assessment and Management

Classification	History and Physical Examination	Management

Respiratory arrest imminent	• exhausted, confused, diaphoretic, cyanotic
	• silent chest, ineffective respiratory effort
	• decreased HR
	• O_2 sat <90% despite supplemental O_2
		• 100% O_2, cardiac monitor, IV access
		• intubate
		• β-agonist: MDI 4–8 puffs
		  OR nebulizer 5 mg continually
		• anticholinergics: MDI 4–8 puffs q20 min x 3
		  OR nebulizer 0.5 mg q20 min x 3
		• IV steroids: methylprednisolone 125 mg,
		  hydrocortisone 500 mg

Severe Asthma	• agitated, diaphoretic, laboured respirations • difficulty speaking in full sentences • no relief from β-agonist • O_2 sat <90%, FEV_1 <50%	• anticipate need for intubation • similar to above management (β-agonist may be less frequent; q15-20 min)
Moderate Asthma	• SOB at rest, cough, congestion, chest tightness • nocturnal symptoms • inadequate relief from β-agonist • FEV_1 50-80%	• O_2 to achieve O2-sat >90% • β-agonist – puffer or neb q1h • steroids: prednisone 40-60 mg PO • anticholinergics
Mild Asthma	• exertional SOB/cough with some nocturnal symptoms • good response to β-agonist • FEV_1 >80%	• β-agonist • monitor FEV_1 • consider steroids (nebulized or PO)

> **Treatment of Asthma**
> **ASTHMA**
> **A**drenergics (beta-agonists)
> **ST**eroids
> **H**ydration
> **M**ask (O2)
> **A**ntibiotics (if cuncurrent infection)

Disposition
• β-agonist MDI regular use (2-4 puffs q2-4h) until symptoms controlled then prm
• prednisone 30-60 mg/day for 7-14 days with no taper
• inhaled steroid
• F/U with primary care physician

Cardiac Dysrhythmias

• see <u>Cardiology</u>

Bradyarrhythmias and AV conduction blocks
• AV conduction blocks
  ■ 1st degree - prolonged PR interval (>200 msec), no treatment required
  ■ 2nd degree
    ♦ Mobitz I - gradual prolongation of PR then dropped QRS, usually benign
    ♦ Mobitz II - PR constant with dropped QRS, can progress to 3rd degree
      AV block
  ■ 3rd degree - P unrelated to QRS, PP and RR intervals constant
    ♦ atropine and transcutaneous pacemaker (TCP)
    ♦ if TCP fails consider dopamine, epinephrine IV
  ■ longterm treatment for Mobitz II and 3rd degree block - internal pacemaker
• sinus bradycardia (rate <60 bpm)
  ■ can be normal
  ■ causes: vomiting, myocardial infarction/ischemia, increase ICP, sick sinus node,
    hypothyroidism, drugs (e.g. β-blockers, CCBs)
  ■ treat if symptomatic (hypotension, chest pain)
    ♦ acute: atropine +/- transcutaneous pacing
    ♦ sick sinus: transcutaneous pacing
    ♦ drug induced: discontinue/reduce offending drug

Supraventricular Tachyarrhythmias (narrow QRS)
• sinus tachycardia
  ■ causes: increased sympathetic tone, drugs, fever, hypotension, anemia,
    thyrotoxicosis, MI, PE, etc.
  ■ treat underlying cause, consider β-blocker if symptomatic
• regular rhythm
  ■ vagal maneuvres, adenosine 6 mg IV push, if no conversion give 12 mg, can
    repeat 12 mg dose once
  ■ rhythm converts: probable re-entry tachycardia
    ♦ monitor for recurrence
    ♦ treat recurrence with adenosine or longer acting (diltiazem, β-blockers)
  ■ rhythm does not convert: atrial flutter, ectopic atrial tachycardia, junctional
    tachycardia
    ♦ rate control (diltiazem, β-blockers) and consult cardiology

> If the patient with tachyarrhythmia is unstable, perform immediate cardioversion.

> **Clinical features of instability:**
> • hypotension (sBP < 90)
> • CHF or pulmonary edema
> • chest pain
> • altered LOC (may indicate shock)

- irregular rhythm
  - probable atrial fibrillation, atrial flutter or multifocal atrial tachycardia
  - rate control (diltiazem, ⊟blockers)

Atrial Fibrillation

If patient has Wolff-Parkinson-White and is in A Fib use amiodarone or procainamide. Avoid AV nodal blocking agents (adenosine, digoxin, diltiazem, verapamil) as this can increase conduction through bypass tract.

- etiology: HTN, CAD, thyrotoxicosis, EtOH (holiday heart), valvular disease, pericarditis, cardiomyopathy
- treatment principles: stroke prevention, treat symptoms, identify / treat underlying cause
- decreases cardiac output by 20-30%
- acute management
  - if symptomatic or first presentation - cardiovert
    - electrical cardioversion: synchronized DC cardioversion
    - chemical cardioversion: amiodarone, procainamide, flecainide, propafenone (if decreased IV function use amiodarone)
  - if onset of A fib is >24-48 hrs: anticoagulate 3 wks prior to cardioversion or do transesophageal echo to rule out clot
- long term management: rate control (maybe rhythm control), consider anticoagulation

Ventricular Tachyarrhythmias (wide QRS)

- ventricular tachycardia (VT)
  - definition: 3 or more consecutive ventricular beats at >100 bpm
  - etiology: CAD with MI is most common cause
  - treatment: sustained VT (>30 seconds) is an emergency
    - hemodynamic compromise: DC cardioversion
    - no hemodynamic compromise: DC cardioversion, lidocaine, amiodarone, procainamide
- ventricular fibrillation - call a code, follow ACLS for pulseless arrest
- torsades de pointes
  - looks like VT but QRS 'rotates around baseline' with changing axis and amplitude
  - etiology: prolonged QT due to drugs (quinidine, TCAs, erythromycin, quinolones, etc.), electrolyte imbalance (hypokalemia, hypomagnesemia), congenital
  - treatment:
    - IV Mg, temporary pacing, isoproterenol
    - correct cause of prolonged QT
    - DC cardioversion if hemodynamic compromise

Chronic Obstructive Pulmonary Disease (COPD)

- see Respirology

History and Physical Examination
- worsening dyspnea or tachypnea
- acute change in frequency, quantity and colour of sputum production
- trigger: pneumonia, urinary tract infection, PE, CHF, drugs

Investigations
- CBC, electrolytes, ABG, CXR, ECG, PFTs

Management
- keep O_2 sat 88-92% (BEWARE OF CO_2 RETAINERS, but do not withhold O_2 if hypoxic)
- ipratriopium is bronchodilator of choice, add salbutamol
- steroids: prednisone 40 mg PO (tapered over 3 weeks)
- antibiotics: TMP-SMX, cephalosporins, quinolones (if signs of infection)
- ventilation (chance of ventilator dependency)
- lower threshold to admit if co-morbid illness

Disposition
- can use up to 4-6 puffs qid of ipratropium and salbutamol for exacerbations
- continue antibiotics if started and give tapering steroids

Congestive Heart Failure

- see Cardiology

Etiology
- decreased myocardial contractility: ischemia, infarction, cardiomyopathy, myocarditis
- pressure overload states: hypertension, valvular abnormalities, congenital heart disease
- restricted cardiac output: myocardial infiltrative disease, cardiac tamponade
- volume overload

Causes of Exacerbation or Precipitants
- cardiac: acute myocardial infarction or ischemia, cardiac tachyarrhythmias (e.g, atrial fibrillation), uncontrolled hypertension
- medications: non-compliance with or change in cardiac medications, NSAIDS, steroids
- dietary: increased sodium intake
- increased cardiac output demand – infection, anemia, hyperthyroidism, pregnancy
- other: pulmonary embolus, physical overexertion, renal failure

History/Presentation
- left-sided heart failure
  - dyspnea, decreased exercise tolerance, paroxysmal nocturnal dyspnea, orthopnea, nocturia, fatigue, possibly altered mental status
  - in severe cases pulmonary edema: severe respiratory distress, pink frothy or white sputum, rales, S3 or S4
- right-sided heart failure
  - dependant edema, jugular venous elevation, hepatic enlargement, ascites
- patients often present with a combination of right-sided and left-sided symptoms

Physical Examination
- vitals: tachypnea, tachycardia, hypo- or hypertension, hypoxia
- respiratory: crackles, wheezes
- cardiac: laterally displaced apex, S3 or S4, jugular venous distention, hepato-jugular reflex
- abdominal: hepatomegaly, ascites
- peripheral vascular: peripheral or sacral edema, weak peripheral pulses, pulsus alternans (alternating weak and strong pulse), cool extremities

Investigations
- labs: CBC, electrolytes, AST, ALT, bilirubin, creatinine, BUN, cardiac enzymes
- chest X-ray
- ECG: look for MI, ischemia
  - in CHF: LVH, atrial enlargement, conduction abnormalities
- ABG: if severe or refractory to treatment
  - hypoxemia, hypercapnia and acidosis are signs of severe CHF
- echocardiogram: not usually used in emergency evaluation, previous results may aid in diagnosis

Management (acute)
- ABC, may require intubation if severe hypoxia
- sit upright, cardiac monitoring and continuous pulse oximetry
- IV TKVO only, Foley catheter (to follow effectiveness of diuresis)
- 100% O$_2$ by mask
  - if poor response may require CPAP, BiPAP, or intubation
- drugs:
  - 0.3 mg nitro SL q5min PRN ± topical nitro patch (0.2-0.8 mg/hr)
  - if not responding or ischemia: 10-200 μg/min IV, titrate
  - diuretic if volume overloaded (e.g. furosemide 40-80 mg IV)
  - morphine 1-2 mg IV prn
    - if hypotensive may require dobutamine (2.5 μg/kg/min IV) or dopamine (5-10 μg/kg/min IV), titrate up to sBP 90-100
  - ASA 160 mg chew and swallow
- treat precipitating factor (e.g. treat pneumonia)
- cardiology or medicine consult

Causes of CHF Exacerbation (FAILURE):
Forgot medication
Arrhythmia/anemia
Ischemia/infarction/infection
Lifestyle (i.e. too much salt)
Upregulation of cardiac output (pregnancy, hyperthyroidism)
Renal failure
Embolism (pulmonary)

Hospital management required if:
- acute MI
- pulmonary edema or severe respiratory distress
- severe complicating medical illness (e.g. pneumonia)
- anasarca
- symptomatic hypotension or syncope
- refractory to outpatient therapy
- thromboembolic complications requiring interventions
- clinically significant arrhythmias
- inadequate social support for safe outpatient management
- persistant hypoxia requiring supplemental oxygen

CHF on CXR
Grade 1: pulmonary vascular redistribution
Grade 2: perihilar infiltrates
Grade 2: interstitial edema, Kerley B lines
Grade 4: alveolar edema, bilateral infiltrates
may also see cardiomegaly, pleural effusions

Acute Treatment of CHF (LMNOP):
Lasix (furosemide)
Morphine
Nitroglycerine
Oxygen
Position (sit upright)

Diabetic Emergencies

- see Endocrinology

Diabetic Ketoacidosis (DKA)

- severe insulin deficiency resulting in dehydration and electrolyte abnormalities
- history and physical examination – often young, type 1 DM, may be first presentation of undiagnosed DM (may occur in small percentage of type 2 patients)
    - early symptoms:
        - polyuria, polydipsia, malaise
    - late signs and symptoms:
        - anorexia, nausea, vomiting, dyspnea (often due to acidosis), fatigue
        - abdominal pain
        - drowsiness, stupor, coma
        - Kussmaul's respiration
        - fruity acetone breath
- investigations
    - CBC, glucose, electrolytes, BUN/creatinine, Ca, Mg, phosphate
    - urine glucose and ketones
    - ABG
    - ECG (MI possible precipitant; electrolyte disturbances may predispose to arrhythmia)
- management
    - rehydration
        - bolus of NS, then high rate NS infusion (but beware of overhydration and cerebral edema, especially in pediatric patients)
    - insulin
        - initial bolus of 5-10 U short-acting/regular insulin (or 0.2 U/kg) IV in adults
        - followed by continuous infusion at 5-10 U (or 0.1 U/kg) per hour
        - some advocate for no bolus and use infusion only
        - add D5W when blood glucose <15 mM
    - potassium
        - essential to avoid hypokalemia: replace KCl (20 mEq/L if adequate renal function and initial K <5.5 mmol/L)
        - use cardiac monitoring if potassium levels normal or low
    - bicarbonate is not given unless patient is at risk of death or shock

Hyperosmolar Hyperglycemic State (HHS)

- state of extreme hyperglycemia (due to relative insulin deficiency, increased counter-regulatory hormones, gluconeogenesis) and dehydration (due to osmotic diuresis) in type 2 DM, high mortality
- history and physical examination
    - mental disturbances, coma, delirium, seizures
    - polyuria
    - nausea, vomiting
- investigations
    - CBC, electrolytes, creatinine, BUN, glucose, Mg, phosphate, urine glucose and ketones
    - ABG
    - ECG
- management
    - rehydration with NS (total water deficit estimated at average 100 cc/kg body weight)
    - O_2 and cardiac monitoring, frequent electrolytes and glucose monitoring
    - insulin as required
    - identify and treat cause

Hypoglycemia

- very common ED presentation
- management focus:
    1. treatment of hypoglycemia
    2. investigation of cause (most often due to exogenous insulin, EtOH, sulfonylureas)
- history and physical examination
    - last meal, known diabetes, prior similar episodes, drug therapy
    - liver / renal / endocrine / neoplastic disease
    - depression, EtOH or drug use
- management:
    - IV access and rapid BG
    - D50W 50 mL IV push, glucose PO if mental status permits
        - if IV access not possible, glucagon 1-2 mg IM, repeat x 1 in 10-20 min.
    - O_2, cardiac, frequent BG monitoring
    - thiamine 100 mg IM
    - full meal as soon as mental status permits
    - if episode due to long acting insulin, sulfonylureas, watch for prolonged hypoglycemia due to long $t_{1/2}$
    - search for cause

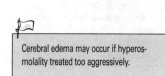

Precipitating Factors in DKA (the 5 Is):
Infection
Ischemia
Infarction
Intoxication
Insulin missed

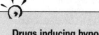

4 criteria for DKA Dx: hyperglycemia, metabolic acidosis, hyperketonemia, ketonuria.

Cerebral edema may occur if hyperosmolality treated too aggressively.

Drugs inducing hypoglycemia

Insulin	Sulfa abx
Sulfonylureas	Cotrimazole
Ethanol	Ampicillin
Salicylates	Tetracycline
Acetaminophen	Amphetamines,
NSAIDS	cocaine
β-adrenergic agonists	Pyridoxine
Lithium	ACE-I
Calcium	Theophylline
MAOI	Quinine
Coumadin	

DVT and Pulmonary Embolism

- see Respirology

Risk Factors
- Virchow's triad
  - alterations in blood flow
  - injury to endothelium
  - hypercoagulable state (including pregnancy, use of OCP, malignancy)
- most significant risk factors
  - major surgery or trauma
  - permanent immobilization
  - malignancy, other hypercoagulable state
  - prior venous thromboembolism

History/Presentation
- DVT: calf pain, leg swelling/erythema/edema
- PE: dyspnea, pleuritic chest pain, tachypnea, hemoptysis, cyanosis, low O2 sat
- presence of risk factors
- clinical signs/symptoms are unreliable for diagnosis and exclusion of DVT/PE so investigation often needed (see Figures 12 and 13)

Investigations
- ECG and CXR are useful to look for other causes (e.g. ACS, pneumonia)
- D-dimer is only useful if it is negative in low risk patients
- Duplex scan has high Sn and Sp for proximal clot but only 73% Sn for DVT
- CT angiography has high Sn and Sp for PE
- V/Q scan useful when CT angio not available
- pulmonary angiography is the gold standard but is more invasive

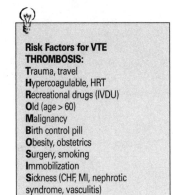

Risk Factors for VTE THROMBOSIS:
Trauma, travel
Hypercoagulable, HRT
Recreational drugs (IVDU)
Old (age > 60)
Malignancy
Birth control pill
Obesity, obstetrics
Surgery, smoking
Immobilization
Sickness (CHF, MI, nephrotic syndrome, vasculitis)

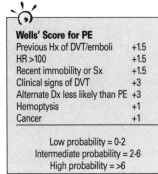

Wells' Score for PE
Previous Hx of DVT/emboli	+1.5
HR >100	+1.5
Recent immobility or Sx	+1.5
Clinical signs of DVT	+3
Alternate Dx less likely than PE	+3
Hemoptysis	+1
Cancer	+1

Low probability = 0-2
Intermediate probability = 2-6
High probability = >6

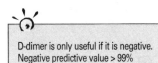

D-dimer is only useful if it is negative. Negative predictive value > 99%

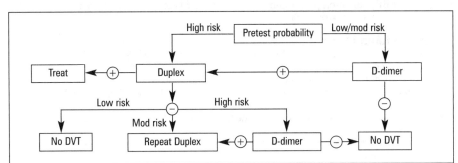

Figure 12. Approach to Suspected DVT

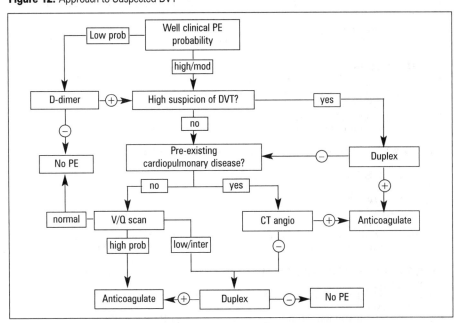

Figure 13. Approach to Suspected PE

Management of DVT/PE
- LMWH unless patient also has renal failure
  - dalteparin 200 IU/kg SC q24h or enoxaparin 1.5 mg/kg SC q24h
- warfarin started at same time as LMWH
- LMWH discontinued when INR has been therapeutic (2-3) for 2 consecutive days
- early ambulation with analgesia is safe if appropriately anticoagulated
- IVC filter or surgical thrombectomy considered if anticoagulation is contraindicated
- consider thrombolysis if extensive DVT or PE causing hemodynamic compromise

Disposition
- often can be treated as outpatient
- admit if hemodynamically unstable, require supplemental O2, major comorbidities, lack of sufficient social supports, unable to ambulate, need invasive therapy
- long term anticoagulation
  - if reversible risk factor: 3-6 months of warfarin
  - idiopathic VTE: may need longer term warfarin (5 yrs or more)

Hypertensive Emergencies

Hypertensive Emergency (Hypertensive Crisis)
- definition: acute elevation of BP associated with end-organ damage (CNS, eyes, heart, or kidneys)
- immediate goal of IV therapy is to reduce the dBP by 10-15% (to approx. 110 mmHg) in 30-60 min (5-10 min for aortic dissection)
- treatment may be initiated in the ED followed by prompt admission to ICU for continuous BP monitoring
- BP should NOT be lowered rapidly in patients with major cerebrovascular event
  - BP lowering attempted if dBP >120 to 130 mmHg; aim to reduce dBP by 20% in the first 24h
  - ↑BP is an attempt to maintain cerebral perfusion pressure; decreasing BP too fast may extend or worsen stroke

Hypertensive Urgency
- definition: severely elevated blood pressure (usually dBP >115) with no evidence of end-organ damage
- most commonly due to non-compliance with medications
- treatment: gradually reduce pressure over 24-48 hours to a level appropriate for the patient
- goal is to differentiate hypertensive emergencies from hypertensive urgencies

History and Physical Examination
- prior hypertensive crises
- antihypertensive medications prescribed and BP control
- MAOIs, substance use, use of stimulants or withdrawal from sedatives including EtOH
- blood pressure measurement in all limbs
- fundoscopic exam (hemorrhages, papilledema, etc.)

Investigations
- CBC, electrolytes, BUN, creatinine, urinalysis
- peripheral blood smear – to detect microangiopathic hemolytic anemia
- CXR – if SOB or chest pain
- ECG, troponins, CK if chest pain
- CT head – if neurological findings or severe headache

Treatment of Hypertensive Emergencies (see Table 13)

HYPERTENSIVE EMERGENCIES

Hypertensive Encephalopathy
- pathophysiology: cerebral hyperperfusion due to blood pressure in excess of the capacity for cerebral autoregulation
- signs and symptoms: headache, nausea, vomiting, mental status changes (lethargy to coma), fundoscopic changes, over hours can lead to coma and death

Pregnancy Induced Hypertension (PIH)
- see Obstetrics
- watch for HTN, seizures, proteinuria, thrombocytopenia, increased AST, clonus, and hyperreflexia
- initial treatment = magnesium sulfate IV; often lowers BP sufficiently without other agents, check reflexes when on drip

Evidence of end-organ damage
CNS: headache, focal neurological signs, seizures
CVS: angina, CHF, back pain (aortic dissection)
Renal: hematuria oliguria
Eyes: papilledema, retinal hemorrhages

With CNS manifestations of severe hypertension, it is often difficult to differentiate causal relationships (i.e. hypertension could be secondary to primary cerebral event [Cushing effect]).

Cardiovascular Emergencies
- left ventricular failure (LVF)
  - pathophysiology: decreased LV function due to increased afterload, increased oxygen demand and decreased coronary blood flow
  - signs and symptoms: chest pain, SOB
  - avoid diazoxide, hydralazine, minoxidil as these drugs increase oxygen demand
- thoracic aortic dissection (see Cardiology)

Hypertensive Renal Emergencies
- renal failure can be either the cause or effect of a hypertensive emergency
- hypertension associated with deteriorating renal function is considered an emergency
- diagnosis: proteinuria, RBCs and RBC casts in urine, elevated BUN and creatinine
- treatment: IV calcium channel blockers, ± emergent ultrafiltration

Catecholamine-Induced Hypertensive Emergencies
- etiology
  - discontinuation of short-acting sympathetic blocker (e.g. clonidine, propranolol)
  - pheochromocytoma
  - sympathomimetic drugs (cocaine, amphetamines, phencyclidine)
  - MAOI with sympathomimetics or tyramine-containing foods (cheese, red wine)
- treatment: re-administer sympathetic blocker if due to withdrawal (e.g. clonidine, propranolol)

Catecholamine Induced Hypertensive Emergencies
Avoid use of non-selective β-blockers as they inhibit β-mediated vasodilation and leave α-adrenergic vasoconstriction unopposed.

Most commonly used agents are labetalol and nitroprusside.

Table 13. Most commonly used agents for the treatment of hypertensive crisis

Drug	Dosage*	Onset of Action	Duration of Action	Adverse Effects	Special Indications
VASODILATORS					
• Sodium Nitroprusside (vascular smooth muscle dilator) 1st line	0.25–10 μg/kg/min	Immediate	3-5 min	N/V, muscle twitching, sweating, cyanide intoxication, coronary steal syndrome	Most hypertensive emergencies (esp CHF, aortic dissection) Use in combination with β–blockers (i.e. esmolol) in aortic dissection Caution with high ICP and azotemia
• Nicardipine (CCB)	2 mg IV bolus, then 4 mg/kg/hr IV	15-30 min	40 min	Tachycardia, headache, flushing, local phlebitis	Most hypertensive emergencies (i.e. encephalopathy, RF, eclampsia, sympathetic crisis) Caution with acute CHF
• Fenoldopam Mesylate (dopamine receptor antagonist)	0.05-0.1 μmg/kg/min IV	<5 min	8-10 min	Tachycardia, headache, nausea, flushing (i.e. acute RF)	Most hypertensive emergencies Caution with glaucoma
• Enalapril (ACEI)	0.625 – 1.25 mg IV q6h	15-30 min	12-24 hr in high renin states not seen in studies	Theoretical fall in pressure Avoid in acute MI, pregnancy, acute RF	Acute LV failure
• Nitroglycerin	5-20 μg/min IV	1-2 min	3-5 min	Hypotension, bradycardia, headache, lightheadedness, dizziness	MI/ Pulmonary edema
• Hydralazine	5-10 mg IV/IM q20min (max 20 mg)	5-20 min	2-6 hrs	Dizziness, drowsiness, headache, tachycardia, Na retention	Eclampsia
ADRENERGIC INHIBITORS					
• Labetalol	20 mg IV bolus q10 min or 0.5-2 mg/min	5-10 min	3-6 hr burning in throat, dizziness, nausea, heart block, orthostatic hypotension	Vomiting, scalp tingling, Avoid in acute CHF, HB > 1st degree	Most hypertensive emergencies (esp. eclampsia)
• Esmolol	250-500 ug/kg/min for 1 min, then 50 ug/kg/min for 4 min; repeat	1-2 min	10-20 min bronchospasm	Hypotension, nausea, SVT dysrythmias, perioperative HTN Avoid in acute CHF, HB > 1st degree	Aortic dissection, acute MI
• Phentolamine	5-15 mg q5-15 min	1-2 min	3-10 min	Tachycardia, headache, flushing	Catecholamine excess (ie. pheo)

*Hypotension may occur with all of these agents

Differentiation of UMN Disease versus LMN Disease

Category	UMN Disease	LMN Disease
Muscular deficit	Muscle groups	Individual muscles
Reflexes	Increased	Decreased/ absent
Tone	Increased	Decreased
Fasciculations	Absent	Present
Atrophy	Absent/ minimal	Present

Thrombolysis for Acute Ischemic Stroke
Cochrane Database of Systematic Reviews 2005; Issue 3
Purpose: To review the efficacy and safety of thrombolysis in acute ischemic stroke.
Study Characteristics: Systematic review of 18 RCTs (16 double-blind) with 5727 patients.
Participants: Patients with acute ischemic stroke confirmed by CT.
Intervention: Any thrombolytic agent, any dose, intravenously or intra-arterial.
Primary Outcomes: Early outcomes (7 to 10 days) include deaths from all causes or symptomatic intracranial hemorrhages. Late outcomes (3 and 6 months) include deaths from all causes, or poor functional outcome at follow-up (death or dependency) as measured by Rankin or Barthel scores.
Results: Thrombolytic therapy is associated with an excess of early deaths (OR 1.81; 95% CI, 1.46-2.24) and symptomatic intracranial hemorrhage (OR 3.37; 95% CI, 2.68-4.22). Use of a thrombolytic agent within three hours of stroke is effective in reducing death or dependency at 3 to 6 months (OR 0.66, 95% CI 0.53 to 0.83) without a statistically significant increase in deaths (OR 1.13, 95% CI 0.86 to 1.48). When given within six hours, thrombolytic therapy significantly reduced the proportion of patients dead or dependent at three to six months (OR 0.84, 95% CI 0.75 to 0.95), but also significantly increased the odds of death (OR 1.33, 95% CI 1.15 to 1.53). Non-random comparisons of rt-PA suggest it may be associated with slightly less hazard and more benefit than other thrombolytics.
Conclusions: Thrombolytic therapy increases immediate hazard in patients, but when used within three hours of ischemic stroke decreases death or dependency without significant increase in mortality.

Stroke

- see Neurology
- can be ischemic (80% of all strokes) or hemorrhagic

History
- consider acute stroke if acute neurological deficit (focal or global) or altered LOC
- more likely to be hemorrhagic if: nausea, vomiting, headache, change in LOC, seizure
- common symptoms of stroke: abrupt onset of hemiparesis/monoparesis, visual loss/ field deficits, diplopia, dysarthria, ataxia, vertigo, aphasia, sudden decrease in LOC
- determine time of symptom onset for consideration of thrombolytic therapy
- DDx includes hypoglycemia, Todds paralysis, peripheral nerve injury, Bell's palsy, tumour

Physical Examination
- vitals
- if decreased LOC: assess for ability to protect airway
- rule out trauma, infection, meningeal irritation
- search for cardiovascular causes of stroke
  - ocular fundi (retinopathy, emboli, hemorrhage)
  - CVS (murmurs, gallops)
  - PVS (auscultate for carotid bruits)
- neuro:
  - mental status, LOC, cranial nerves, motor function, sensory function, cerebellar function, gait, deep tendon reflexes
  - confirm presence of stroke syndrome, and distinguish from stroke mimics (seizure, systemic infection, brain tumour, positional vertigo, Bell's palsy)
  - establish neurological baseline should patient improve/deteriorate

Table 14. Stroke Syndromes

Region of Stroke	Stroke Syndrome
Anterior Cerebral Artery	• Primarily frontal lobe function affected • Altered mental status, impaired judgement, contralateral lower extremity weakness and hypoesthesia, gait apraxia
Middle Cerebral Artery	• Contralateral hemiparesis (arm & face weakness > leg weakness) and hypoesthesia, ipsilateral hemianopsia, gaze preference to side of lesion • ± agnosia, receptive/expressive aphasia
Posterior Cerebral Artery	• Affects vision and thought • Homonymous hemianopsia, cortical blindness, visual agnosia, altered mental status, impaired memory
Vertebrobasilar Artery	• Wide variety of CN, cerebellar and brainstem deficits: vertigo, nystagmus, diplopia, visual field deficits, dysphagia, dysarthria, facial hypoesthesia, syncope, ataxia • Loss of pain and temperature sensation ipsilateral face and contralateral body

Investigations
- CBC, electrolytes, blood glucose, coagulation studies, ± cardiac biomarkers, ± toxicology screen
- CT scan, non-contrast: look for hemorrhage, ischemia
- ECG: rule out atrial fibrillation, acute MI as source of emboli

Management
- ABC's with RSI if GCS ≤8/rapidly decreasing GCS/inadequate airway protection reflexes
- IV ± cardiac monitoring
  - judge fluid rate carefully to avoid overhydration (cerebral edema) as well as underhydration (underperfusion of the ischemic penumbra)
- BP control: only treat severe hypertension (sBP >200, dBP >100, mean arterial BP >140) or hypertension associated with hemorrhagic stroke transformation, cardiac ischemia, aortic dissection, or renal damage; use IV nitroprusside or labetalol
- cerebral edema control: hyperventilation, mannitol to decrease ICP if necessary
- consult neurosurgery, neurology as indicated

Medications
- acute ischemic stroke: thrombolytics (rt-PA, e.g. alteplase) if within 3 hours of symptom onset with no evidence of hemorrhage on CT scan
- antiplatelet agents: prevent recurrent stroke or stroke after TIAs, e.g. aspirin (1st-line); clopidogrel, ticlopidine (2nd-line)

Gynecology/Urology Emergencies

Vaginal Bleed

- see <u>Gynecology</u> and <u>Obstetrics</u>

Etiology
- pregnant patient
  - 1st/2nd trimester pregnancy: ectopic pregnancy, abortion (threatened, incomplete, complete, missed, inevitable, septic), molar pregnancy
  - 2nd/3rd trimester pregnancy: placenta previa, placental abruption, premature rupture of membranes, preterm labour
  - either: trauma, bleeding cervical polyp
- postpartum
  - postpartum hemorrhage, uterine inversion, retained placental tissue, endometritis
- non-pregnant patients
  - dysfunctional uterine bleeding, uterine fibroids , pelvic tumors, trauma, endometriosis, PID, exogenous hormones

Vaginal bleeding can be life threatening! Always start with ABC's and ensure your patient is stable.

History
- last menstrual period, sexual activity, contraception, history of PID
- pregnancy details
- determine amount of blood
- urinary, GI symptoms

Physical Examination
- look for signs of hypovolemia
- pelvic examination – NOT if suspected placenta previa (ultrasound first)
- speculum exam
  - if pregnant use sterile speculum
- bimanual examination
  - sterile gloves if pregnant
  - if patient is near term with possible rupture of membranes and without other indications defer bimanual examination (infection risk)

Investigations
- β-hCG test for all patients with child-bearing potential
- CBC, blood and Rh type, quantitative β-hCG, PTT, INR
- type and cross if significant blood loss
- 1st/2nd trimester/non-pregnant:
  - ultrasound (U/S) – intrauterine pregnancy, ectopic pregnancy, traumatic injury, foreign body
  - must correlate U/S findings with β-hCG if U/S is non-diagnostic
- 2nd/3rd trimester pregnancy:
  - U/S if no fetal heart tones, no documented intrauterine pregnancy or unknown lie of placenta
  - DIC panel if placental abruption – platelets, PTT, INR, fibrinogen
- postpartum:
  - U/S for retained products
  - β-hCG if concerned about retained tissue

Need β-hCG ≥1200 to see interuterine changes on transvaginal U/S

Management
- ABCs
- pulse oximeter and cardiac monitors if unstable
- Rh immune globulin for vaginal bleeding in pregnancy and Rh-negative mother
- 1st/2nd trimester pregnancy:
  - ectopic pregnancy: definitive treatment with surgery or methotrexate
  - intrauterine pregnancy, no concerns of coexistent ectopic: discharge patient with obstetrics follow up
  - U/S indeterminate or β-hCG > 1000-2000 IU for further work-up and/or gynecology consult
  - abortions: if complete, discharge if stable, for all others get gynecology consult
- 2nd/3rd trimester pregnancy:
  - placenta previa or placental abruption: obstetrics consult for possible admission
- postpartum:
  - uterine inversion: replace uterus immediately, may require operative management
  - postpartum hemorrhage: extraction of placenta if retained, hysterectomy if uncontrolled bleeding

Vaginal bleeding (and its underlying causes) can be a very emotionally taxing presentation for patients.
Ensure appropriate support is provided.

- retained tissue: D&C
- endometritis: IV antibiotics
- non-pregnant
  - dysfunctional uterine bleeding
    - <35-40 years of age: Provera™ 10 mg PO x 10 days, warn patient of a withdrawal bleed, discharge if stable
    - if unstable, admit for IV hormonal therapy, possible D&C
    - >35-40 years of age: uterine sampling necessary prior to initiation of hormonal treatment to rule out endometrial cancer, U/S for any masses felt on exam
  - structural abnormalities: fibroids or uterine tumors may require excision for diagnosis/treatment, U/S for workup of other pelvic masses, Pap smear/biopsy for cervical lesions

Disposition
- the decision to admit or discharge should be based on the stability of the patient, as well as the nature of the underlying cause. Consult gynecology for admitted patients
- if patient can be safely discharged, ensure follow up with family physician or gynecologist (if available). Instruct patient to return to emerg for increased bleeding, presyncope, etc.

Pregnant Patient in the ER

Table 15. Complications of Pregnancy

Trimester	Fetal	Maternal
First 1-14 wk	Pregnancy failure • Spontaneous abortion • Fetal demise • Gestational trophoblastic disease	Ectopic pregnancy Anemia Hyperemesis gravidarum UTI/ pyelonephritis
Second 15-27 wk	Disorders of fetal growth • IUGR • oligo/polyhydramnios	Gestational diabetes mellitus Rh incompatibility UTI/ pyelonephritis
Third 28-40 wk	Vasa previa	Preterm labor/ PPROM Preeclampsia/eclampsia Placenta previa Placental abruption Uterine rupture DVT

Nephrolithiasis (Renal Colic)

Epidemiology and Risk Factors
- 10% of population (twice as common in males)
- recurrence 50% at 5 yrs
- peak incidence 30-50 years of age

Clinical Features
- urinary obstruction —> upstream distention of ureter or collecting system —> severe colicky pain
- writhing, never comfortable, nausea, vomiting, hematuria (90% microscopic), diaphoresis, tachycardia, tachypnea
- occasionally gross symptoms of trigonal irritation (frequency, urgency)
- fever, chills, rigors in secondary pyelonephritis

Differential Diagnosis of Renal Colic
- acute ureteral obstruction (other causes)
  - UPJ obstruction
  - sloughed papillae
  - clot colic from gross hematuria
  - extrinsic (e.g. tumour)
- acute abdomen – biliary, bowel, pancreas, AAA
- gynecological – ectopic pregnancy, torsion/rupture of ovarian cyst
- pyelonephritis (fever, chills, pyuria)
- radiculitis (L1) – herpes zoster, nerve root compression

Investigations
- screening labs
  - CBC → elevated WBC in presence of fever suggests infection
  - electrolytes, Cr, BUN → to assess renal function
  - urinalysis: R&M (WBCs, RBCs, crystals), C&S
- imaging
  - non-contrast spiral CT is the study of choice
  - abdominal ultrasound may demonstrate stone or hydronephrosis
  - intravenous pyelogram (not used very much anymore)
- strain all urine → stone analysis

Management
- analgesics, antiemetics, IV fluids
- urology consult is indicated, especially if stone >5mm, or if patient has signs of obstruction or infection
- α–blocker helpful to increase stone passage in select cases

Disposition
- see admission criteria (sidebar)
- most patients can be discharged. Ensure patient is stable, has adequate analgesia, and is able to tolerate oral meds. Follow up with family doctor in 24-48 hours

Indinavir stones are the only stones that are radiolucent on spiral CT as well as on plain film.

Indications for Admission to Hospital
- intractable pain
- fever (suggests infection)
- single kidney with ureteral obstruction
- bilateral obstructing stones
- intractable vomiting
- comprised renal function

Ophthalmology Emergencies

Ophthalmologic Foreign Body and Corneal Abrasion

- see also Ophthalmology

History
- patient may complain of pain, tearing, itching, redness, photophobia, foreign body sensation
- elicit history of potential trauma to eye
- mechanism of foreign body insertion – if high velocity injury suspected (welding, metal grinding, metal striking metal), must obtain orbital x-rays or ultrasound to exclude presence of intraocular metallic foreign body

Physical Examination
- visual acuity with best corrected vision
- pupils, extraocular movement, external ocular structures
- fundoscopy
- tonometry – measurement of intraocular pressure (with Tonopen) – normal pressure: 10-20 mmHg
- slit lamp exam
  - start with unaffected eye
  - systematic examination of anterior segment structures and vitreous
  - proparacaine anaesthetic drops may ease examination
  - look for rust ring with metallic foreign body, corneal edema, anterior chamber cells/flare
  - may use fluoroscein dye which stains de-epithelialized cornea green when viewing with cobalt blue filter

Management
- copious irrigation with saline for any foreign body
- remove foreign body under slit lamp exam with cotton swab or sterile needle
- antibiotic drops qid until healed
- patching may not improve healing or comfort – do not patch contact lens wearers
- limit use of topical anesthetic to examination only
- consider tetanus prophylaxis
- ophtho consult if globe penetration suspected

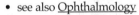

ALWAYS assess visual acuity in both eyes when a patient presents to the ER with an ophthalmologic complaint.

Contraindications to pupil dilation:
- shallow anterior chamber
- iris-supported lens implant
- potential neurological abnormality requiring pupillary evaluation
- caution with CV disease – mydriatics can cause tachycardia

Initial Management of Opthalmologic Emergencies
- see Ophthalmology
- ruptured globe - stabilize any foreign body, shield eye with no pressure, elevate head of bed to 30º, tetanus prophylaxis, IV antibiotics, NPO, analgesic, antiemetic, sedation PRN
- retinal artery occlusion - globe massage, paper bag breathing, carbogen inhalation (95% oxygen, 5% carbon dioxide)
- chemical burn - immediate copious irrigation, may consider topical anaesthetic drops to facilitate irrigation
- acute angle-closure glaucoma - IV or PO acetazolamide, topical pilocarpine and timolol

Disposition
- most patients can be discharged with outpatient opthamology follow up
- admit patients requiring emergent opthalmologic procedures or IV antibiotics

Otolaryngolgy Emergencies

Acute Otitis Externa (OE)

Etiology
- bacteria (~90% of OE): *P. aeruginosa, P. vulgaris, E. coli, S. aureus*
- fungus: *Candida albicans, Aspergillus niger*
- risk factors: swimming, Q-tips, hearing aids, headphones, etc.

Clinical Features
- pain, otorrhea, conductive hearing loss, post auricular lymphadenopathy
- complicated otitis externa: pinna and or periauricular soft tissue inflamed

Treatment
- clean ear under magnification with irrigation, suction, dry swabbing, and C&S
- bacterial etiology
    - antipseudomonal drops + steroid – e.g. Cipro HC™
    - do not use aminoglycoside if the tympanic membrane is ruptured
    - consider using a pope wick if external canal edematous
    - systemic antibiotics if either cervical lymphadenopathy or cellulitis
- fungal etiology – requires repeated debridement and antifungals
- ± analgesics

Disposition
- most patients can be discharged – follow up with family physician if symptoms do not resolve with antibiotic drops

Acute Sinusitis

- see Otolaryngology

Etiology
- acute bacterial infection of the paranasal sinuses
- maxillary sinus most commonly affected
- organisms
    - Bacterial: S. pneumo (35%), H. flu (35%), *M. catarrhalis*
    - Viral: rhinovirus, influenza, parainfluenza

Investigations
- not usually necessary (diagnosis is clinical)
- 4-view radiographic exam (used infrequently): look for air fluid level, opacification of sinus, mucosal thickening
- CT not cost effective for routine diagnosis

Otitis externa has two forms: a benign infection of the outer canal that could occur in anybody and a potentially lethal disease which usually occurs in elderly, immunosuppressed or diabetic patients.

Pulling on the pinna is extremely painful in otitis externa, but is usually tolerated in otitis media.

Table 16. Clinical Diagnosis of Sinusitis = 2 major symptoms or 1 major and 2 minor symptoms

Major Symptoms	Minor Symptoms
Facial pain/pressure	Headache
Facial fullness	Halitosis
Nasal obstruction	Fatigue
Purulent nasal discharge	Dental pain
Postnasal drip	Cough
Hyposmia	Ear pain/pressure
Fever	

Treatment
- antibiotics: amoxicillin 500 mg tid x 10 days
- adjunctive therapy: decongestants, saline irrigation
- do not use antihistamines (may interfere with mucous clearance)

Disposition
- discharge
- follow up with family doctor after antibiotic regime

Epistaxis

- see Otolaryngology
- 90% of nosebleeds stem from the anterior nasal septum (at Kiesselbach's plexus located in Little's area)
- can be life-threatening!

Etiology
- most commonly caused by trauma (digital, blunt, foreign bodies), but can also be caused by barometric changes, nasal dryness, chemicals (cocaine, Otrivin™), or systemic disease (coagulopathies, hypertension, etc.)

Investigations
- CBC, PT/PTT (if indicated)
- x-ray, CT as needed

Treatment
- aim is to localize bleeding and achieve hemostasis
- first-aid: ABC's, lean forward, pinch soft part of nose for 20 minutes
- assess blood loss: vitals, IV normal saline, cross match 2 units packed RBC if significant
- determine site of bleeding: use topical anaesthetic/vasoconstrictor to facilitate. Use nasal speculum and good lighting
- attempt to control the bleeding:
  - first line: Otrivin™ or cocaine
  - second line: cauterize with silver nitrate (one side of septum only!)
  - if these fail, or if bleeding is posterior → nasal packing
  - if packing fails, consult ENT

Disposition
- most patients can be discharged. Ensure vitals are stable, bleeding is controlled, and patient has appropriate follow-up
- educate patients about prevention (e.g. humidifiers, saline spray, topical ointments, avoiding irritants, managing hypertension, etc.)
- admission may be required for severe cases. Consult ENT

Thrombocytopenic patients – use resorbable packs to avoid risk of re-bleeding caused by pulling out the removable pack.

Environmental Injuries

Heat Exhaustion and Heat Stroke

Heat Exhaustion
- clinical features relate to loss of circulating volume caused by exposure to heat stress
- "water depletion": heat exhaustion (HE) occurs if lost fluid not adequately replaced
- "salt depletion": HE occurs when losses replaced with hypotonic fluid

> Heat exhaustion (HE) may closely resemble heat stroke. HE may eventually progress to heat stroke. Therefore if diagnosis is uncertain treat as heat stroke.

Heat Stroke
- life-threatening emergency resulting from failure of normal compensatory heat-shedding mechanisms
- divided into classical and exertional subtypes (see Table 17)

Table 17. Heat Exhaustion vs. Heat Stroke

	Heat Exhaustion	Classical Heat Stroke	Exertional Heat Stroke
Clinical Features	• non-specific malaise, headache, fatigue • body temp <40.5°C (usually normal) • no coma or seizures • dehydration (↑ HR, orthostatic hypotension)	• occurs in setting of high ambient temperatures (e.g. heat wave, poor ventilation) • often patients are older, poor, and sedentary or immobile • dry, hot skin • temp usually >40.5°C • altered mental status, seizures, delirium, coma • may have elevated AST, ALT	• occurs with high endogenous heat production (e.g. exercise) and overwhelmed homeostatic mechanisms • patients often younger, more active • skin often diaphoretic • other symptoms as for classical HS, but may also have DIC, acute renal failure, rhabdomyolysis, marked lactic acidosis
Treatment	• rest in a cool environment • normal saline IV if orthostatic hypotension; otherwise replace losses slowly PO	• cool down body temperature with water mist (e.g. spray bottle) and standing fans • ice water immersion also effective; monitor body temp closely to avoid hypothermic overshoot • secure airway because of risk of seizures and aspiration • give fluid resuscitation if still hypotensive after above therapy • avoid α-agonists (epinephrine, etc.) peripheral vasoconstriction and antipyretics (ASA, etc.)	

- if patient does not respond relatively quickly to cooling treatments, consider other possible etiologies of hyperpyrexia (e.g. meningitis, thyroid storm, anticholinergic poisoning, delirium tremens, other infections, etc.)

Hypothermia and Cold Injuries

- predisposing factors: extremes of age, lack of housing, drug overdose, EtOH ingestion, trauma (incapacitating), cold water immersion, outdoor sports
- treatment based on: (a) re-warming and (b) supporting cardiorespiratory function
- complications: coagulopathy, acidosis, ventricular arrhythmias (Vfib), asystole, volume/electrolyte depletion
- labs: CBC, electrolytes, ABG, serum glucose, creatinine/BUN, Mg, Ca, amylase, coags
- imaging: CXR (aspiration pneumonia, pulmonary edema are common)
- monitors: ECG, rectal thermistor, Foley catheter, NG tube, monitor metabolic status frequently

Table 18. Classification of Hypothermia

Class	Temp	Symptoms/Signs
Mild	32-34.9°C	Tachypnea, tachycardia, ataxia, dysarthria, shivering
Moderate	28-31.9°C	Loss of shivering, arrythmias, Osborne (J) waves on ECG, decreased LOC, combative behaviour, muscle rigidity, dilated pupils
Severe	<28°C	Coma, hypotension, acidemia, ventricular fibrillation, asystole, flaccidity, apnea

Re-warming Options
- gentle fluid and electrolyte replacement in all (due to cold diuresis)
- Passive External Re-warming (PER):
  - suitable for most stable patients with core temperature >32.2°C
  - involves covering patient with insulating blanket; body generates heat and re-warms through metabolic process, shivering
- Active External Re-warming (AER)
  - involves use of warming blankets
  - beware "afterdrop" phenomenon (warming of extremities causes vasodilation and movement of cool pooled blood from extremities to core, resulting in a drop in core temperature → cardiac arrest)
  - safer when done in conjunction with active core re-warming (below)
- Active Core Re-warming (ACR)

- generally for patients with core temperature <32.2°C, and/or with cardiovascular instability
- avoids "afterdrop" seen with AER alone
- re-warm core by using:
  - warmed humidified oxygen, IV fluids
  - peritoneal dialysis with warm fluids
  - gastric/colonic/pleural irrigation with warm fluids
  - external circulation (cardiopulmonary bypass machine) is most effective, fastest

Cardiac Arrest in the Hypothermic Patient
- do all procedures gently or may precipitate ventricular fibrillation (VF)
- check pulse and rhythm for at least 1 minute; may have profound bradycardia
- if any pulse at all (even very slow) do NOT do CPR
- if in VF try to defibrillate up to max 3 shocks if T_c <30°C
- intubate gently if required, ventilate with warmed, humidified O_2
- medications (vasopressors, antiarrhythmics) may not be effective at low temperatures
  - controversial; may try one dose
- focus of treatment is re-warming!

FROSTBITE

Classification
- ice crystals form between cells
- classified according to depth – similar to burns (1st to 3rd degree)
- **1st degree**
  - symptoms: initial paresthesia, pruritus
  - signs: erythema, edema, hyperemia, no blisters
- **2nd degree**
  - symptoms: numbness
  - signs: blistering (clear), erythema, edema
- **3rd degree**
  - symptoms: pain, burning, throbbing (on thawing); may be painless if severe
  - signs: hemorrhagic blisters, skin necrosis, edema, no movement

Management
- treat for hypothermia: O_2, IV fluids, maintenance of body warmth
- remove wet and constrictive clothing
- immerse in 40-42°C agitated water for 10-30 minutes (very painful; administer adequate analgesia)
- clean injured area, leave injured region open to air
- consider aspiration/debridement of blisters (controversial)
- debride skin gently with daily whirlpool immersion (topical ointments not required)
- tetanus prophylaxis
- consider penicillin G as frost bite injury at high risk of infection
- surgical intervention may be required to release restrictive eschars
- never allow a thawed area to re-chill/freeze

Burns

- see Plastic Surgery

Management
- remove noxious agent/stop burning process
- establish airway if needed (indicated with burns >40% BSA or smoke inhalation injury)
- resuscitation for 2nd and 3rd degree burns
  - Parkland Formula: Ringer's lactate 4 cc/kg/%BSA burned; give 1/2 in first 8 hours, 1/2 in next 16 hours
  - urine output is best measure of resuscitation, should be 40-50 cc/hr or 0.5 cc/kg/hr; avoid diuretics
- pain relief - continuous morphine infusion at 2 mg/hr with breakthrough bolus
- burn wound care – prevent infection, clean with mild soap and water, sterile dressings
- escharotomy or fasciotomy for circumferential burns (chest, extremities)
- topical antibiotics, systemic antibiotics infrequently indicated
- tetanus prophylaxis

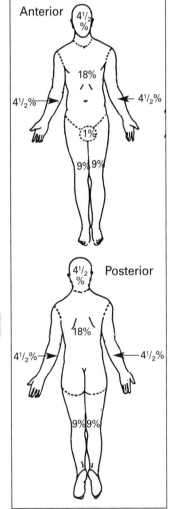

Figure 14. Rule of 9's for Total Body Surface Area (BSA)

Use palm of the patient's hand to estimate 1% of BSA affected.

High Risk Factors for Infection:
- puncture wounds
- crush injuries
- wounds greater than 12 hours old
- hand or foot wounds, wounds near joints
- immunocompromised patient
- patient age greater than 50 years
- prosthetic joints or valves
  (risk of endocarditis)

Physical Examination
- burn size:
  - rule of nines (see Figure 14); does not include superficial
- burn depth:
  - superficial: epidermis only (e.g. sunburn)
  - partial thickness: into superficial dermis deep or hair follicles, sweat glands
  - full thickness: all layers of the skin
  - deep: to fat, muscle, even bone

Disposition
- admit if:
  - 2nd degree burns to >10% BSA; any significant 3rd degree burns
  - 2nd degree on face, hands, feet, perineum or across major joints
  - electrical, chemical burns and inhalation injury
  - burn victims with underlying medical problems or immunosuppressed patients

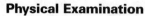

Inhalation Injury

Intubate early if you suspect inhalation injury.

Biological Weapons
Microbes (anthrax, Q fever, viruses), bacterial toxins (ricin, botulinum), mycotoxins and others are usually spread by droplets (aerosols).

Diluted household bleach (1:19 with water) is good for most biohazard materials for decontamination.

Use contact isolation protocols, and treat for the specific agent.

Etiology
- carbon monoxide (CO) poisoning (see *Toxicology* section, ER46)
- direct thermal injury – limited to upper airway
- smoke causes bronchospasm and edema from particulate matter and toxic inhalants (tissue asphyxiates, pulmonary irritants, systemic toxins)

History and Physical
- risk factors: closed space fires, period of unconsciousness, noxious chemicals involved
- cherry red skin/blood (usually a post-mortem finding)
- singed nasal hairs, soot on oral/nasal membranes, sooty sputum
- hoarseness, stridor, dyspnea
- decreased LOC, confusion
- PO_2 normal but O_2 sat low suggests CO poisoning

Investigations
- true O_2 sat must be measured (not pulse oximeter nor PO_2 from ABG)
- measure carboxyhemoglobin levels
- ABG
- CXR ± bronchoscopy

Management
- CO poisoning: 100% O_2 ± hyperbaric O_2 (controversial)
- direct thermal injury: humidified oxygen, early intubation, pulmonary toilet, bronchodilators

Bites

High risk criteria for infection
Wound factors:
- puncture wounds
- crush injuries
- wounds > 12 hrs old
- hand or foot wounds
- wounds near joints

Patient factors:
- immunocompromised
- age > 50 years
- prosthetic joints or valves

Mammalian Bites
- see Plastic Surgery
- history
  - time and circumstances of bite, symptoms, allergies, tetanus immunization status, comorbid conditions, rabies risks, HIV/hepatitis risk (human bite)
  - high morbidity associated with clenched fist injuries (CFIs), "fight bites"
- physical examination
  - assess type of wound: abrasion, laceration, puncture, crush injury
  - assess for direct tissue damage: skin, bone, tendon, neurovascular status
- investigations
  - if bony injury or infection suspected check for fracture and gas in tissue with X-rays
  - ALWAYS get skull films in children with scalp bite wounds, ± CT to rule out cranial perforation
- initial management
  - wound cleansing and copious irrigation as soon as possible
  - irrigate/debride puncture wounds if feasible, but not if sealed or very small openings; avoid hydrodissection along tissue planes
  - debridement is important in crush injuries to reduce infection and optimize cosmetic and functional repair
  - culture wound if signs of infection (erythema, necrosis or pus); obtain anaerobic cultures if wound foul smelling, necrotizing, or abscess; notify lab that sample is from bite wound

- prophylactic antibiotics
  - types of infections resulting from bites: cellulitis, lymphangitis, abscesses, tenosynovitis, osteomyelitis, septic arthritis, sepsis, endocarditis, meningitis
  - a 3-5 day course of antibiotics is recommended for all bite wounds to the hand and should be considered in other bites if any high-risk factors present (efficacy not proven)
  - dog and cat bites (pathogens: *Pasteurella multocida, S. aureus, S. viridans*)
    - 80% of cat bites, 5% of dog bites become infected
    - 1st line: amoxicillin + clavulinic acid
  - human bites (pathogens: *Eikenella corrodens, S. aureus, S. viridans*, oral anaerobes)
    - 1st line: amoxicillin + clavulinic acid
  - rabies (see <u>Infectious Diseases</u>)
    - reservoirs: warm-blooded animals except rodents, lagomorphs (e.g. rabbits)
    - post-exposure vaccine is effective; treatment depends on local prevalence (contact public health)
  - suturing
    - vascular structures (i.e. face and scalp) are less likely to get infected, therefore consider suturing
    - avascular structures (i.e. pretibial regions, hands and feet) by secondary intention
- tetanus immunization if ≥10 yrs or incomplete primary series

> **Consider admission if:**
> - moderate to severe infections
> - infections in immunocompromised patients
> - not responding to oral Rx
> - penetrating injuries to tendons, joints, CNS
> - open fractures

Snake Bites

- history, physical exam, investigations and initial management similar to mammalian bites
- additional management issues
  - snake bites are rarely fatal but proper precautions must be taken
  - supportive management, observe for compartment syndrome, analgesia, tetanus prophylaxis
  - contact regional Poison Control Centre for consultation
  - constriction band should be placed proximal to bite
  - observe for signs and symptoms of envenomation 15min-2hrs after bite (pain, sweating, edema, chills, weakness, numbness, tingling, HR changes, faintness, ecchymosis, N/V); if no envenomation then remove band and monitor closely for 24 hrs
  - if envenomation present, administer antivenom

Insect Bites

- Bee Stings
  - 5 types of reactions to stings (local, large local, systemic, toxic, unusual)
  - history and physical exam key to diagnosis; no lab test will confirm
  - investigations: CBC, electrolytes, BUN, creatinine, glucose, ABGs, ECG
  - ABC management, epinephrine 0.1 mg IV over 5 minutes if shock, antihistamines, cimetidine 300 mg IV/IM/PO, steroids, β-agonists for SOB/wheezing 3 mg in 5 mL NS via nebulizer, local site management
- West Nile Virus (see <u>Infectious Diseases</u>)
  - severity: asymptomatic 80%, flu-like symptoms 20%, encephalitis <1%
  - clues: aseptic meningitis/encephalitis in late summer in prevalent area
  - incubation 3-14 days, symptoms last 3-6 days
  - general symptoms: fever, malaise, anorexia, headache, altered mental status, motor weakness, ataxia, extrapyramidal signs, GI signs, myalgias, lymphadenopathy, rash, myocarditis, optic neuritis
  - diagnosis: CSF and serum for serology
  - investigations: CBC, electrolytes, CSF, CT/MRI
  - management: ABCs, IV fluids for dehydration, antibiotics if signs of meningitis (based on CSF analysis), analgesia, antipyretics, interferon-alpha 2b, ribavirin

Near Drowning

- most common in children <4 yrs and teenagers
- causes lung damage, hypoxemia and may lead to hypoxic encephalopathy
- must also assess for shock, C-spine injuries, hypothermia, SCUBA-related injuries (barotrauma, air emboli, lung re-expansion injury)
- complications: volume shifts, electrolyte abnormalities, hemolysis, rhabdomyolysis, ATN, DIC

Physical Examination
- ABC's, vitals – watch closely for hypotension
- lungs: rales (ARDS, pulmonary edema), decreased breath sounds (pneumothorax)
- CVS: murmurs, arrhythmias, JVP (CHF, pneumothorax)
- H&N: assess for C-spine injuries
- neuro: GCS or AVPU, pupils, focal deficits

Investigations
- labs: CBC, electrolytes, ABGs, Cr, BUN, urinalysis
- imaging: CXR (pulmonary edema, pneumothorax)
- ECG

Management
- ABCs, treat for trauma, shock, hypothermia
- cardiac and O_2 sat monitor, IV access
- intensive respiratory care:
  - ventilatory assistance if decreased respirations, pCO_2 >50 mmHg, or pO_2 <60 mmHg on max O_2
  - may require intubation for airway protection, ventilation, pulmonary toilet
  - high flow O_2/CPAP/BiPAP may be adequate but some may need mechanical ventilation with PEEP
- arrhythmias: usually respond to corrections of hypoxemia, hypothermia, acidosis
- vomiting: very common, insert NG suction to avoid aspiration
- convulsions: usually respond to O_2; if not, diazepam 5-10 mg IV slowly
- bronchospasm: bronchodilators
- bacterial pneumonia: not necessary to prophylax with antibiotics unless contaminated water or hot-tub (*Pseudomonas*)
- must observe for 24 hours as non-cardiogenic pulmonary edema may develop late

Disposition
- not significant submersion - discharge after short observation
- significant submersion (even if asymptomatic) - long period of observation (24 hrs) as pulmonary edema may appear late
- CNS symptoms or hypoxemia - admit
- severe hypoxemia, decreased LOC - ICU

Toxicology

Alcohol Related Emergencies

- see Psychiatry

Acute Intoxication
- slurred speech, CNS depression, disinhibition, lack of coordination
- nystagmus, diplopia, dysarthria, ataxia → may progress to coma
- frank hypotension (peripheral vasodilation)
- if obtunded rule out:
  - head trauma/intracranial hemorrhage
  - associated depressant, street drugs, toxic alcohols
    - synergistic → respiratory/cardiac depression
  - hypoglycemia (screen with bedside glucometer)
  - hepatic encephalopathy
    - precipitating factors: GI bleed, infection, sedation, electrolyte abnormalities, protein meal
  - Wernicke's encephalopathy ("WACO")
  - post-ictal state, basilar stroke

Withdrawal
- beware withdrawal signs – see Table 19
- treatment
  - diazepam 10-20 mg IV or PO OR lorazepam 2-4 mg IV or PO q1hr until calm
  - may use CIWA protocol and give benzodiazepines as above when CIWA >= 10
  - thiamine 100 mg IM then 50-100 mg/day and fluid resus with D5NS
  - magnesium sulfate 4 g IV over 1-2 h (if hypomagnesemic)
  - admit patients with delerium tremens (DT)

EtOH levels correlate poorly with intoxication.

EtOH intoxication may invalidate informed consent.

Wernicke's encephalopathy (**WACO**):
Ataxia
Coma
Ocular findings: nystagmus, CN VI paresis

Table 19. Alcohol Withdrawal Signs

Time since last drink	Syndrome	Description
6-8 hr	mild withdrawal	• generalized tremor, anxiety, agitation, but no delirium • autonomic hyperactivity (sinus tachycardia), insomnia, nausea, vomiting
1-2 days	alcoholic hallucinations	• visual (most common), auditory and tactile hallucinations • vitals often normal
8 hr-2 days	withdrawal seizures	• typically brief generalized tonic-clonic seizures • may have several within a few hours
3-5 days	delirium tremens (DT)	• 5% of untreated withdrawal patients • severely confused state, fluctuating levels of consciousness • agitation, insomnia, hallucinations/delusions, tremor • tachycardia, hyperpyrexia, diaphoresis • high mortality rate

CIWA Withdrawal Symptoms
Nausea and vomiting
Tremor
Paroxysmal sweats
Anxiety
Agitation
Visual/tactile/auditory disturbances
Headache
Disorientation

10 symptoms each scored out of 7 except orientation is out of 4.

Seizures
- associated with ingestion and withdrawal
- withdrawal seizures
  - occur 8-48 hrs after last drink (typically brief generalized tonic-clonic seizures)
  - if >48 hrs, think of DT (see Table 19)
- prophylaxis: diazepam 20 mg PO q1h x 3 minimum
- CT head if focal seizures have occurred

Cardiovascular Complications
- hypertension (HTN)
- cardiomyopathy: SOB, edema
- arrhythmias ("holiday heart")
  - atrial fibrillation (most common), atrial flutter, PVC, PAC, SVT, VT (especially torsade if hypomagnesemic/hypokalemic)

Metabolic Abnormalities
- alcoholic ketoacidosis
  - history of chronic alcohol intake with abrupt decrease/cessation
  - malnourished, abdominal pain with nausea and vomiting
  - anion gap (AG) metabolic acidosis, urine ketones, low glucose and normal osmolality
  - treatment: dextrose, thiamine (50-100 mg prior to dextrose), volume repletion (with NS)
  - generally resolves in 12-24 hr
- other alcohols (see also *Toxicology*)
  - ethylene glycol → CNS, CVS, renal findings
  - methanol
    - early: lethargy, confusion
    - late: headache, visual changes, N/V, abdominal pain, tachypnea
  - both produce severe metabolic acidosis with AG and osmolar gap
  - EtOH co-ingestion is protective
  - treatment
    - fomepizole 15 mg/kg IV bolus or
    - IV 10% EtOH bolus and drip to achieve blood level of 20 mmol/L
    - alcohol loading may be done PO
    - urgent hemodialysis required
- other abnormalities associated with alcohol: hypomagnesemia, hypophosphatemia, hypocalcemia, hypoglycemia, hypokalemia

Common Deficiencies
- thiamine
- niacin
- folate
- glycogen
- magnesium
- potassium

Gastrointestinal Abnormalities
- gastritis
  - common cause of abdominal pain and GI bleed in chronic alcohol users
- pancreatitis
  - serum amylase very unreliable in patients with chronic pancreatitis, may need serum lipase
  - hemorrhagic form (15%) associated with increased mortality
  - fluid resuscitation very important
- hepatitis
  - AST/ALT ratio >2 suggests alcohol as the cause as well as elevated GGT with acute ingestion
- peritonitis/spontaneous bacterial peritonitis
  - occasionally accompanies cirrhosis
  - leukocytosis, fever, generalized abdominal pain/tenderness
  - paracentesis for diagnosis (common pathogens: *E. coli, Klebsiella,* Strep)
- GI bleeds
  - most commonly gastritis or ulcers, even if patient known to have varices
  - consider Mallory-Weiss tear secondary to retching
  - often complicated by underlying coagulopathies
  - minor – treat with antacids
  - severe or recurrent – endoscopy

Miscellaneous Problems
- rhabdomyolysis
  - presents as acute weakness associated with muscle tenderness
  - usually occurs after prolonged immobilization
  - increased creatinine kinase (CK), hyperkalemia
  - myoglobinuria – may lead to acute renal failure
  - treatment: IV fluids, forced diuresis (mannitol 20% 15 mg/kg IV over 30 min)
- increased infections – due to impaired host defences, compromised immunity, poor living conditions

Disposition
- before patient leaves ED ensure
  - stable vital signs
  - can walk unassisted
  - fully oriented
- offer social services to find shelter or detox program
- ensure patient can obtain any medications prescribed and can complete any necessary follow-up

Approach to the Overdose Patient/Toxic Exposure

History
- who? age, weight, underlying medical problems, medications
- what? substance and how much
- when? time since exposure determines prognosis and need for decontamination, symptoms since
- how? route
- why? intention, suicidality

Physical Examination
- focus on: ABCs, LOC/GCS, vitals, pupils

Principles of Toxicology
- 5 principles to consider with all ingestions
  i. resuscitation (ABCs)
  ii. screening (toxidrome? clinical clues?)
  iii. decrease absorption of drug
  iv. increase elimination of drug
  v. antidote available?

Suspect overdose when:
- altered level of consciousness/coma
- young patient with life-threatening arrhythmia
- trauma patient
- bizarre or puzzling clinical presentation

ABCs of Toxicology

- basic axiom of care is symptomatic and supportive treatment
- address underlying problem only once patient is stable
  - **A** Airway (consider stabilizing the C-spine)
  - **B** Breathing
  - **C** Circulation
  - **D1** Drugs
    - ACLS as necessary to resuscitate the patient
    - universal antidotes
  - **D2** Draw bloods
  - **D3** Decontamination (decrease absorption)
  - **E** Expose (look for specific toxidromes)/Examine the Patient
  - **F** Full vitals, ECG monitor, Foley, X-rays, etc.
  - **G** Give specific antidotes, treatments
  - Go back and reassess
  - Call Poison information
  - Obtain corroborative history from family, bystanders

D1 – Universal Antidotes

- treatments that will not harm patients and may be essential

Oxygen
- do not deprive a hypoxic patient of oxygen no matter what the antecedent medical history (i.e. even COPD with CO_2 retention)
- if depression of hypoxic drive, intubate and ventilate
- exception: paraquat or diquat (herbicides) inhalation or ingestion (oxygen radicals increase morbidity)

Glucose
- give to any patient presenting with altered LOC
- measure blood glucose prior to glucose administration if possible
- adults: 0.5-1.0 g/kg (1-2 mL/kg) IV of D50W
- children: 0.25 g/kg (2-4 mL/kg) IV of D25W

Thiamine (Vitamin B₁)
- 100 mg IV/IM to all patients with IV/PO glucose
- a necessary cofactor for glucose metabolism, but do not delay glucose if thiamine unavailable
- to prevent Wernicke-Korsakoff syndrome
- must assume all undifferentiated comatose patients are at risk

Populations at risk for thiamine deficiency:
- alcoholics
- anorectics
- hyperemesis of pregnancy
- malnutrition states

Naloxone
- antidote for opioids: administration is both diagnostic and therapeutic (1 min onset of action)
- used for the undifferentiated comatose patient if narcotics are suspected etiology
- loading dose
  - adults
    - 2 mg initial bolus IV/IM/SL/SC or via ETT (ETT dose = 2-2.5x IV dose)
    - if no response after 2-3 minutes, increase dose by 2 mg increments until a response or to max 10 mg
    - known chronic user, suspicious history, or evidence of track marks, give 0.01 mg/kg
  - child
    - 0.01 mg/kg initial bolus IV/IO/ETT
    - 0.1 mg/kg if no response and narcotic still suspected to max of 10 mg
- maintenance dose
  - may be required because half-life of naloxone much shorter than many narcotics
    - hourly infusion rate at 2/3 of initial dose that produced patient arousal

Administration of naloxone can cause opiate withdrawal in chronic users

D2 - Draw Bloods

- essential bloods (see Table 21 for interpretation)
  - CBC, electrolytes, BUN/creat, glucose, INR/PTT, osmolality
  - ABGs, measure O_2 sat
  - acetylsalicylic acid (ASA), acetaminophen, EtOH levels
- potentially useful bloods
  - drug levels – NOT serum drug screen
  - Ca, Mg, PO_4
  - protein, albumin, lactate, ketones, liver enzymes, CK - depending on drug and clinical presentation

Serum Drug Levels
- treat the patient, not the drug level
- negative tox screen does not rule out a toxic ingestion - signifies only that the specific drugs tested were not detectable in the specimen
- specific drugs available on general screen vary by institution; check before ordering
- urine screens also available (qualitative only)

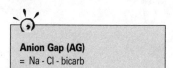

Plasma Osmolar Gap (POG)
= (2 Na + glucose + urea) - plasma osmolarity

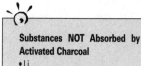

Anion Gap (AG)
= Na - Cl - bicarb

Table 20. Toxic Gaps (see Nephrology)

Metabolic Acidosis

Increased AG: "MUDPILES CAT" (* = toxic)
  Methanol*
  Uremia
  Diabetic ketoacidosis/Starvation ketoacidosis
  Phenformin*/Paraldehyde*
  Isoniazid, iron, ibuprofen
  Lactate (anything that causes seizures or shock)
  Ethylene glycol*
  Salicylates*
  Cyanide, carbon monoxide*
  Alcoholic Ketoacidosis
  Toluene, theophylline*

Decreased AG
• error
• electrolyte imbalance (increased $Na^+/K^+/Mg^{2+}$)
• hypoalbuminemia (50% fall in albumin
  ~5.5 mmol/L decrease in the AG)
• Li, Br elevation
• paraproteins (multiple myeloma)

Normal AG
• high K: pyelonephritis, obstructive nephropathy, renal tubular acidosis (RTA), IV, TPN
• low K: small bowel losses, acetazolamide, RTA I, II

Increased POG: "MAE DIE" (if it ends in "-ol", it will likely ↑ the POG)
  Methanol
  Acetone
  Ethanol
  Diuretics (glycerol, mannitol, sorbitol)
  Isopropanol
  Ethylene Glycol
  Note: normal osmolar gap does not rule out toxic alcohol; only an elevated gap is helpful

Increased O$_2$ saturation gap
• carboxyhemoglobin
• methemoglobin
• sulfmethemoglobin

Table 21. Use of the Clinical Laboratory in the Initial Diagnosis of Poisoning

Test	Finding	Selected Causes
ABG	• hypoventilation (↑ pCO$_2$) • hyperventilation (↓ pCO$_2$)	• CNS depressants (opioids, sedative-hypnotic agents, phenothiazines, EtOH) • salicylates, CO, other asphyxiants
Electrolytes	• ↑ anion-gap metabolic acidosis • hyperkalemia • hypokalemia	• **"MUDPILES CAT"**: see "Metabolic Acidosis" above • digitalis glycosides, fluoride, potassium • theophylline, caffeine, β-adrenergic agents, soluble barium salts, diuretics
Glucose	• hypoglycemia	• oral hypoglycemia agents, insulin, EtOH, ASA
Osmolality and Osmolar Gap	• elevated osmolar gap	• **"MAE DIE"**; see "Toxic Gaps" above
ECG	• wide QRS complex • prolonged QT interval • atrioventricular block	• TCAs, quinidine, other class Ia and Ic antiarrhythmic agents • quinidine and related antiarrhythmics, terfenadine, astemizole • Ca^{2+} antagonists, digitalis glycosides, phenylpropanolamine
Abdominal X-Ray	• radiopaque pills or objects	• **"CHIPES"**: **C**alcium, **C**hloral hydrate, **C**Cl$_4$, **H**eavy metals, **I**ron, **P**otassium, **E**nteric coated **S**alicylates, and some foreign bodies
Serum Acetaminophen	• elevated level (>140 mg/L or 1000 µmol/L 4 hours after ingestion)	• may be only sign of acetaminophen poisoning

D3 – Decontamination and Enhanced Elimination

Ocular Decontamination
• saline irrigation to neutralize pH; alkali exposure requires ophthalmology consult

Dermal Decontamination (wear protective gear)
• remove clothing, brush off toxic agents, irrigate all external surfaces

Gastrointestinal Decontamination
• single dose activated charcoal (SDAC)
  ▪ adsorption of drug/toxin to AC prevents availability
  ▪ contraindications: caustics, SBO, perforation
  ▪ dose: 10 g/g drug ingested or 1g/kg body weight
  ▪ odourless, tasteless, prepared as slurry with H$_2$O
• whole bowel irrigation
  ▪ 500 mL (child) to 2000 mL (adult) of balanced electrolyte solution/hour by mouth until clear effluent per rectum (polyethylene glycol solution)
  ▪ indications
    ♦ awake, alert patient who can be nursed upright
    ♦ delayed release product
    ♦ drug/toxin not bound to charcoal
    ♦ drug packages (if any evidence of breakage → emergency surgery)
    ♦ recent toxin ingestion

Substances NOT Absorbed by Activated Charcoal
• Li
• Fe
• Alcohols
• Lead
• Caustics

- contraindications
    - ◆ evidence of ileus, perforation, or obstruction
- surgical removal in extreme cases
    - indicated for drugs that are toxic, form concretions, or cannot be removed by conventional means
- no evidence for the use of cathartics (or ipecac)

EXTRA-CORPOREAL DRUG REMOVAL (ECDR)

Urine Alkalinization
- may be used for: ASA, methotrexate, phenobarb, chlorpropamide
- weakly acidic substances can be trapped in alkali urine (pH >7.5) to increase elimination

Multidose Activated Charcoal (MDAC)
- may be used for: carbamazepine, phenobarb, quinine, theophylline
- for toxins which undergo enterohepatic recirculation
- removes drug that has already been absorbed by drawing them back into GI tract
- various regimens: 12.5 g (1/4 bottle) PO q1h or 25 g (1/2 bottle) PO q2h until non-toxic

Hemodialysis
- indications/criteria for hemodialysis
    - toxins that have high water solubility, low protein binding, low molecular weight, adequate concentration gradient, small volume of distribution (Vd) or rapid plasma equilibration
    - removal of toxin will cause clinical improvement
    - advantage is shown over other modes of therapy
    - predicted that drug or metabolite will have toxic effects
    - impairment of normal routes of elimination (cardiac, renal, or hepatic)
    - clinical deterioration despite maximal medical support
- useful for the following toxin blood levels:
    - methanol
    - ethylene glycol
    - salicylates
    - lithium
    - phenobarbital: 430-650 mmol/L
    - chloral hydrate ($\rightarrow$ trichloroethanol): >200 mg/kg
- others include theophylline, carbamazepine, valproate, methotrexate

E - Examine the Patient

- vital signs (including temperature), skin (needle tracks, colour), mucous membranes, pupils, odours and CNS
- head-to-toe survey including:
    - C-spine
    - signs of trauma, seizures (incontinence, "tongue biting", etc.), infection (meningismus), chronic alcohol/drug abuse (track marks, nasal septum erosion)
- mental status

Table 22. Specific Toxidromes

Toxidrome	Overdose Signs and Symptoms		Examples of Drugs
Anticholinergics	Hyperthermia	"Hot as a hare"	Antidepressants (e.g. TCAs)
	Dilated pupils	"Blind as a bat"	Cyclobenzaprine (Flexeril™)
	Dry skin	"Dry as a bone"	Carbamazepine
	Vasodilation	"Red as a beet"	Antihistamines (e.g. diphenhydramine)
	Agitation/hallucinations	"Mad as a hatter"	Antiparkinsonians
	Ileus	"The bowel and bladder lose	Antipsychotics
	Urinary retention	their tone and the heart	Antispasmotics
	Tachycardia	goes on alone"	Belladonna alkaloids (e.g. atropine)
Cholinergics	"DUMBELS"		Natural plants
	Diaphoresis, Diarrhea, Decreased blood pressure		mushrooms, trumpet flower
	Urination		Anticholinesterases
	Miosis		physostigmine
	Bronchospasm, Bronchorrhea, Bradycardia		insecticides (organophosphate, carbamates)
	Emesis, Excitation of skeletal muscle		nerve gases
	Lacrimation		
	Salivation, Seizures		

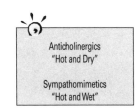

Anticholinergics
"Hot and Dry"

Sympathomimetics
"Hot and Wet"

Table 22. Specific Toxidromes (continued)

Toxidrome	Overdose Signs and Symptoms	Examples of Drugs
Extrapyramidal	Dysphonia, dysphagia Rigidity and tremor Motor restlessness, crawling sensation (akathisia) Constant movements (dyskinesia) Dystonia (muscle spasms, laryngospasm, trismus, oculogyric crisis, torticollis)	Major tranquilizers Antipsychotics
Hemoglobin Derangements	Increased respiratory rate Decreased level of consciousness Seizures Cyanosis unresponsive to O_2 Lactic acidosis	Carbon monoxide poisoning (carboxyhemoglobin) Drug ingestion (methemoglobin, sulfmethemoglobin)
Narcotics, Sedatives/ Hypnotics, EtOH	Hypothermia Hypotension Respiratory depression Dilated or constricted pupils (pinpoint in opiate OD) CNS depression	EtOH Benzodiazepines Opiates (morphine, heroin, etc.) Barbiturates GHB
Sympathomimetics	Increased temperature CNS excitation (including seizures) Tachycardia, hypertension Nausea and vomiting Diaphoresis Dilated pupils	Caffeine Amphetamines Cocaine, LSD, PCP Ephedrine & other decongestants Thyroid hormone Sedatives, EtOH withdrawal
Serotonin Syndrome	Mental status changes, autonomic hyperactivity, neuromuscular abnormalities, hyperthermia, diarrhea, HTN	MAOI, TCA, SSRI, opiate analgesics, Cough medicine, weight reduction medications

Note: ASA poisoning and hypoglycemia mimic sympathomimetic toxidrome

G – Give Specific Antidotes and Treatments

Table 23. Protocol for Warfarin Overdose

INR	Management
<5.0*	Cessation of warfarin administration, observation, serial INR/PT
5.1–9.0*	If no risk factors for bleeding, hold warfarin x 1-2 days and reduce maintenance dose OR Vitamin K 1-2 mg PO if patient at increased risk of bleeding or fresh frozen plasma (FFP) if active bleed
9.1–20.0*	Hold warfarin, Vitamin K 2-4 mg PO, serial INR/PT, additional Vitamin K if necessary or FFP if active bleed
>20.0 or	FFP 10-15 mL/kg, Vitamin K 10 mg IV over 10 min, increase Vitamin K dosing (q4h) if needed

Urine Alkalinization Treatment for ASA Overdose

- urine pH >7.5
- fluid resuscitate first, then 3 amps $NaHCO_3$/litre of DSW @ 1.5 x maintenance
- add 20-40 mEq KCl/litre if patient is able to urinate

**Table 24. Specific Antidotes and Treatments –
call local poison information centre for specific doses and treatment recommendations**

Toxin	Treatment	Considerations
Acetaminophen	Decontaminate (charcoal) N-acetylcysteine	Often clinically silent; evidence of liver/renal damage delayed >24 hrs Toxic dose >200 mg/kg (>7.5g adult) Monitor drug level immediately and @ 4 hrs post-ingestion; also liver Enzymes, INR, PTT, BUN, Cr Hypoglycemia, metabolic acidosis, encephalopathy → poor prognosis
ASA	Decontaminate (activated charcoal) Alkalinize urine (see Table 23); want urine pH >7.5	Monitor serum pH and drug levels closely Monitor K+ level; may require supplement for urine alkalinization Hemodialysis may be needed if intractable metabolic acidosis, very high levels, or end-organ damage (i.e. unable to diurese)
Anticholinergics	Decontaminate (activated charcoal) Supportive care	Special antidotes available. Consult PIC
Benzodiazepines	Decontaminate (activated charcoal) Supportive care	
β-blockers	Decontaminate (charcoal). Consider glucagon or high dose insulin euglycemia therapy (HDIE)	Consult PIC

**Table 24. Specific Antidotes and Treatments –
call local poison information centre for specific doses and treatment recommendations
(continued)**

Toxin	Treatment	Considerations
Calcium Channel Blockers	CaCl 1-4 g of 10% sol'n IV if hypotensive Atropine or isoproterenol if severe Other: high-dose insulin, also known as HDIE (high dose insulin euglycemia) inotropes or aggressive supportive therapy	Order ECG, lytes (especially Ca, Mg, Na, K), glucagon may help (2-5 mg)
Cyanide	Cyanide antidote kit or hydroxycobalamin	
Digoxin	Decontaminate (charcoal) Digoxin-specific Ab fragments 10-20 vials IV if acute; 3-6 if chronic 1 vial (40 mg) neutralizes 0.5 mg of toxin	Use for life-threatening arrhythmias unresponsive to conventional therapy, 6 hr serum digoxin >19 nmol/L, initial K+ >5 mM, ingestion >10 mg (adult) / >4 mg (child) Common arrhythmias include V-fib, V-tach, and conduction blocks
Acute Dystonic Rxn	Benztropine: 1-2 mg IM/IV then 2 mg PO x 3 days OR Diphenhydramine 1-2 mg/kg IV, then 25 mg PO qid x 3 days	Benztropine (Cogentin™) has euphoric effect and potential for abuse
Heparin	Protamine sulfate 25-50 mg IV	
Insulin/ oral hypoglycemic	Glucose IV/PO/NG tube Glucagon: 1-2 mg IM (if no access to glucose)	Glyburide carries highest risk of hypoglycemia among oral agents; Consider octreotide for oral hypoglycemics (50-100 ug SC q6h) in these cases; consult local PIC
Ethanol	Thiamine 100 mg IM/IV Manage airway and circulatory support	Hypoglycemia very common in children Mouthwash = 70% EtOH; perfumes and colognes = 40-60% EtOH Order serum EtOH level and glucose level; treat glucose level appropriately
Ethylene glycol/ Methanol	Ethanol (10%) 10 ml/kg over 30 min, then 1.5 ml/h or fomepizole (4-methylpyrazole) 15 mg/kg IV load Over 30 min, then 10 mg/kg q12h	CBC, lytes, glucose, ethanol level Consider hemodialysis
CO Poisoning	See ER40	
Opioids	See ER47	
TCAs	Aggressive supportive care NaHCO$_3$ bolus for wide QRS/seizures	Flumazenil antidote contraindicated in combined TCA/benzodiazepine overdose Also consider cardiac and Hypotension support, gastric decontamination, seizure control Intralipid therapy (consult local PIC)
MDMA	Decontaminate (charcoal), supportive care	Monitor CK; treat rhabdomyolysis with high flow fluids
Cocaine	Decontaminate (charcoal) if oral Aggressive supportive care	β-blockers are contraindicated in acute cocaine toxicity

Disposition from the Emergency Department

- methanol, ethylene glycol
  - delayed onset, admit and watch clinical and biochemical markers
- TCAs
  - prolonged/delayed cardiotoxicity warrants admission to monitored (ICU) bed
  - if asymptomatic and no clinical signs of intoxication: 6 hour ED observation adequate with proper decontamination
  - sinus tachycardia alone (most common finding) with history of OD warrants observation in ED
- hydrocarbons/smoke inhalation
  - pneumonitis may lag 6-8 hours
  - consider observation for repeated clinical and radiographic examination
- ASA, acetaminophen
  - if borderline level, get second level 2-4 hours after first
- oral hypoglycemics
  - admit all patients for minimum 24 hours if hypoglycemic
  - observe asymptomatic patient for at least 8 hours

Psychiatric Consultation
- once patient medically cleared, arrange psychiatric intervention if required
- beware - suicidal ideation may not be expressed

Psychiatric Emergencies

Approach to Common Psychiatric Presentations

- see Psychiatry
- before seeing patient, ensure your own safety; have security/police available if necessary

History

- safety
    - assess suicidality: suicidal ideation, intent, plan, lethal means, past attempts, future planning
    - assess homicidality: access to weapons, intended victim, history of violence
    - command hallucinations
- mood symptoms
- psychotic symptoms: delusions, hallucinations, disorganized speech, disorganized or catatonic behavior, negative symptoms (affective flattening, alogia, avolition)
- substance use history: most recent use, amount, previous withdrawal reactions
- past psychiatric history, medications, compliance with medications
- medical history: obtain collateral if available

Physical

- complete physical exam focusing on: vitals, neurological exam, signs of head trauma, signs of drug toxicity, signs of metabolic disorder
- mental status exam: general appearance, speech, mood and affect, thought content and form, perceptions, cognition including MMSE, judgment, insight, reliability

Investigations

- investigations vary with: patient's age, established psychiatric diagnosis vs. first presentation, history and physical suggestive of organic cause
- as indicated: blood glucose, urine and serum toxicology screen, pregnancy test, electrolytes, TSH, AST/ALT, bilirubin, serum creatinine, BUN, osmolality
- blood levels of psychiatric medications
- CT head if suspect neurological etiology
- LP if indicated

Acute Psychosis

Differential Diagnosis

- primary psychotic disorder (e.g. schizophrenia)
- secondary to medical condition (e.g. delerium)
- drugs: substance intoxication or withdrawal, medications (e.g. steroids, anticholinergics)
- infectious (CNS)
- metabolic (hypoglycemic, hepatic, renal, thyroid)
- structural (hemorrhage, neoplasm)

Management

- violence prevention
    - remain calm, empathetic and reassuring
    - ensure safety of staff and patients, have extra staff and/or security on hand
    - patients demonstrating escalating agitation or overt violent behavior may require physical restraint and/or chemical tranquilization (see *Violent Patient*)
- treat agitation: whenever possible, offer medication to patients as opposed to administering with force (helps calm and engage patient)
    - benzodiazepines – lorazepam 2 mg PO or IM
    - antipsychotics – olanzapine 5 mg PO, haloperidol 5 mg PO/IM
- treat underlying medical condition
- psychiatry or Crisis Intervention Team consult

Key functions of emergency psychiatric assessment:
1. Is the patient medically stable?
2. Rule out medical cause
3. Is psychiatric consult needed?
4. Are there safety issues (SI, HI)?
5. Is patient certifiable?

Features that suggest organic etiology:

A   age >40 years old
B   babbling (incoherent speech or speech difficulties)
C   concerning vital signs
D   disorientation
E   emotional lability
F   fluctuating course
G   global impairment of cognitive function
H   headaches
I   immodesty
J   just started (sudden onset)
K
L   loss of consciousness
M   movement abnormalities (tremor, ataxia, psychomotor retardation)
N   neurological findings (focal)
O   other abnormalities on physical exam
P   perceptions (visual hallucinations)

Suicidal Patient

Epidemiology
- attempted suicide F>M, completed suicide M>F
- second leading cause of death in people <24 yo

Management
- ensure patient safety: close observation, remove potentially dangerous objects from person and room
- assess thoughts (ideation), means, action (preparatory, practice attempts), previous attempts
- admit if there is evidence of intent and organized plan, access to lethal means, psychiatric disorder, intoxication (suicidal ideation may resolve with few days of abstinence)
- patient may require certification if unwilling to stay voluntarily
- do not start long-term medications in the emergency department
- psychiatry or crisis team consult

High risk patients
"SAD PERSONS"
Sex = male
Age >45 years old
Depression
Previous attempts
Ethanol use
Rational thinking lost
Suicide in family
Organized plan
No spouse, no support system
Serious illness

Hospitalize if total number of risk factors ≥7, consider hospitalization if 5-6 risk factor

Violent Patient

Differential Diagnosis
- rule out lethal organic cause (see *Acute Psychosis* section, ER54)
- leading organic causes are EtOH, drugs, and head injuries

Prevention
- be aware and look for prodromal signs of violence: anxiety, restlessness, defensiveness, verbal attacks
- try to de-escalate the situation: address the patient's anger, empathize

Restraints
- pharmacological
  - often necessary – may mask clinical findings and impair exam
  - haloperidol 5-10 mg IM (be prepared for dystonic reactions, especially with multiple doses of neuroleptics over a short period) + lorazepam 2 mg IM/IV
  - look for signs of anticholinergic OD first (see *Toxicology* section, ER52)
- physical
  - present option to patient in firm but non-hostile manner
  - sufficient people to carry it out safely (trained security, show of force)
  - restrain supine or on side; preferably 4-point restraints, never less than 2-points (opposite arm and leg)
  - suction and airway support available in case of vomiting
- once restrained, search person/clothing for drugs and weapons

Common Pediatric ER Presentations

Modified Coma Score

Table 25. Modified GCS

Modified GCS for infants

Eye opening	Verbal Response	Motor Response
4 – spontaneously	5 – coos, babbles	6 – normal, spontaneous movement
3 – to speech	4 – irritable cry	5 – withdraws to touch
2 – to pain	3 – cries to pain	4 – withdraws to pain
1 – no response	2 – moans to pain	3 – decorticate flexion
	1 – no response	2 – decerebrate extension
		1 – no response

Modified GCS for Children <4 yr

Eye opening	Verbal Response	Motor Response
4 – spontaneously	5 – oriented, social, speaks, interacts	6 – normal, spontaneous movement
3 – to speech	4 – confused speech, disoriented, consolable	5 – localizes pain
2 – to pain	3 – inappropriate words, not consolable/aware	4 – withdraws to pain
1 – no response	2 – incomprehensible, agitated, restless, not aware	3 – decorticate flexion
	1 – no response	2 – decerebrate extension
		1 – no response

Any infant <1 year of age with a large, boggy scalp hematoma requires skull x-rays ± CT.

Respiratory Distress

- see Pediatrics

History and Physical Examination
- infants not able to feed, older children not able to speak in full sentences
- anxious, irritable, lethargic – may indicate hypoxia
- tachypnea >60, retractions
- pulsus paradoxus
- wheezing, grunting, vomiting

Table 26. Stridorous Upper Airway Diseases: Diagnosis

Feature	Croup	Bacterial Tracheitis	Epiglottitis[1]
Age range (yrs)	0.5-4	5-10	2-8
Prodrome	Days	Hrs to days	Minutes to hrs
Temperature	Low grade	High	High
Radiography	Steeple sign	Exudates in trachea	Thumb sign
Etiology	Parainfluenza	*S. aureus*/GAS	H flu type b
Barky Cough	Yes	Yes	No
Drooling	Yes	No	Yes
Appear Toxic	No	Yes	Yes
Intubation? ICU?	No	Yes	Yes
Antibiotics	No	Yes	Yes
NOTE:			No oral exam

[1]rare now with Hib vaccine in common use

- **management of croup**
  - humidified O_2
  - racemic epinephrine q1h x 3 doses, observe for 'rebound effects'
  - dexamethasone x 1 dose
  - consider bacterial tracheitis/epiglottitis if unresponsive to croup therapy
- **management of bacterial tracheitis**
  - start croup therapy
  - usually require intubation, ENT consult, ICU
  - start abx (e.g. cloxacillin), pending C&S
- **management of epiglottitis**
  - 4 D's: drooling, dyspnea, dysphagia, dysphonia + tripod sitting
  - do NOT EXAMINE OROPHARYNX or AGITATE patient
  - immediate anaesthesia, ENT call - intubate
  - then IV fluids, Abx, blood cultures
- **management of asthma**
  - supplemental O_2 if sats <90% or PaO_2 <60%
  - bronchodilator therapy: salbutamol (Ventolin™) 0.15 mg/kg by masks q20 min x 3
  - add 250-500 μg ipratropium (Atrovent™) to first 3 doses salbutamol
  - give corticosteroid therapy as soon as possible after arrival (prednisolone 2 mg/kg, dexamethasone 0.3 mg/kg)
  - $MgSO_4$ if critically ill, not responding to inhaled bronchodilators, steroids; give IV bolus, then infusion
  - IV β_2-agonists if critically ill and not responding to above

Febrile Infant and Febrile Seizures

FEBRILE INFANT
- see Pediatrics
- for fever >38°C without obvious focus:
  - <28 days
    - admit
    - full septic work up (CBC & diff, blood C&S, urine C&S, CSF, CXR if indicated)
    - treat empirically with broad spectrum IV antibiotics
  - 28-90 days
    - as above unless infant meets Rochester criteria (see below)
  - >90 days
    - toxic: admit, treat, full septic workup
    - non-toxic and no focus: investigate as indicated by history and physical

Rochester Criteria for Febrile Infants age 28-90 days old:
- non toxic - looking
- previously well (>37 weeks GA, home with mother, no hyperbilirubinemia, no prior antibiotics or hospitalizations, no chronic/underlying illness)
- no skin, soft tissue, bone, joint, or ear infection on physical exam
- WBC 5000-15,000; bands <1500; urine <10 WBC/HPF, stool <5 WBC/HPF

FEBRILE SEIZURES
- see Pediatrics

Etiology
- children aged 6 months to 5 years with fever or history of recent fever
- simple vs complex febrile seizures

Table 27. Simple vs Complex Febrile Seizures

Characteristic	Simple	Complex
Duration	<15 min	>15 min
Type of seizure	Generalized	Focal features
Frequency	1 in 24 hours	>1 in 24 hours

- normal neurological exam afterward
- no evidence of intracranial infection or history of previous non-febrile seizures
- often positive family history of febrile seizures
- relatively well looking after seizure

Investigations and Management
- if it is a febrile seizure: treat fever and look for source of fever
- if not a febrile seizure: treat seizure and look for source of seizure
  - note: may also have fever but may not meet criteria for febrile seizure

Abdominal Pain

- see Pediatrics

History
- nature of pain, associated fever, timing, quality, pattern of pain
- associated GI, GU symptoms
- anorexia, decreased fluid intake

Physical Exammination
- HEENT, respiratory, abdominal exam including DRE, testicular/genital exam

Table 28. Differential Diagnosis of Abdominal Pain in Infants/Children/Adolescents

Medical	Surgical
Colic	Malrotation with volvulus
UTI	Hirschprung's
Constipation	Necrotizing enterocolitis
Gastroenteritis	Incarcerated hernia
Sepsis	Intussusception
HSP (Henoch Schonlein purpura)	Duodenal atresia
Inflammatory Bowel Disease	Appendicitis
HUS (Hemolytic Uremic Syndrome)	Cholecystitis
Pneumonia	Pancreatitis
Strep Throat	Testicular torsion
SCD crisis	Ectopic pregnancy
DKA	Trauma
Functional	Pyloric stenosis

*remember to keep an index of suspicion for child abuse

Rashes

- see Pediatrics and Dermatology

Measles
- maculopapular rash starting at hairline, spreading to face/trunk preceded by 3 C's (cough, coryza, conjunctivitis)
- complications: pneumonia, OM, encephalitis
- management: Vit A if hospitalized and/or immuncompromised; respiratory isolation, treat contacts with immune globulin

Erythema Infectiosum
- caused by Parvovirus B19 ('fifth disease')
- 'slapped cheeks', maculopapular lacy-like rash on trunk/limbs
- complications: STAR (sore throat, arthritis, rash), aplastic crisis
- management: supportive, respiratory isolation x 7d

VZV/Chicken Pox
- itchy, vesicular, maculo-papular rash at multiple stages
- complications: impetigo, necrotizing fasciitis, acute encephalitis, acute cerebellar ataxia, hepatitis, DIC
- management: symptomatic, acyclovir only for complicated cases, respiratory + contact isolation
- prevention: VZIG within 96 hrs of exposure, Varicella vaccine (Varivax ™)
- uncomplicated cases can be discharged. Educate parents to follow isolation precautions (don't go back to school until all lesions have fully crusted over)

Kawasaki Disease
- leading cause of acquired cardiac disease in children; can cause coronary artery aneurysms
- fever >5 d plus 4 of 5 of the following:
  - unilateral lymphadenopathy
  - bilateral, non-purulent conjunctivitis
  - cracked lips, strawberry tongue
  - rash
  - puffy, red palms and soles
- management:
  - admit
  - acute phase: IVIG 2g/kg and ASA 100 mg/kg/day until fever resolves
  - subacute: ASA 3-5 mg/kg/day until platelets normalize, or indefinitely in case of cardiac disease
  - ECG and echocardiography with echocardiography follow-up at 2, 6, 12 months

Common Infections

- see Pediatrics

Table 29. Antibiotic Treatment of Pediatric Bacterial Infections

Infection	Pathogens	Treatment
Meningitis Sepsis		
Neonatal	GBS, *E.coli*, *Listeria*, *S. aureus*, Gram negative bacilli	• ampicillin + aminoglycoside (gentamicin) or • ampicillin + cefotaxime ± cloxacillin if risk of *S. aureus*
1-3 months	same pathogens as above and below	• ampicillin + cefotaxime ± cloxacillin if risk of *S. aureus*
>3 mos	*S. pneumococcus*, *H. influenzae* type b (>5 yrs), meningococcus	• cefuroxime • ceftriaxone or cefotaxime, if risk of meningitis • vancomycin, if penicillin/cephalosporin- resistant pneumococci
Otitis Media		
1st line	*S. pneumoniae*, *H. influenzae* type b, *M. Catarrhalis*	• amoxicillin
2nd line		• high dose amoxicillin or clavulin
Treatment Failure		• high dose clavulin or cefuroxime or ceftriaxone
Strep Pharyngitis		
	group A β-hemolytic *Streptococcus*	• penicillin/amoxicillin or erythromycin (pencillin allergy)
UTI		
	E. Coli, *Proteus*, *H. Influenzae*, *Pseudomonas*, *S. saprophyticus*, *Enterococcus*, GBS	• amoxicillin/ampicillin or • trimethoprim-sulfamethoxazole
Pneumonia		
1-3 mos	viral, *S. pneumoniae*, *C. trachomatis*, *B. pertussis*, *S. aureus*, *H. influenzae*	• cefuroxime ± macrolide (erythromycin) or • ampicillin ± macrolide
3 mos-5yrs	viral, *S. pneumoniae*, *S. aureus*, *H. influenzae*, *Mycoplasma pneumoniae*	• ampicillin/amoxicillin or cefuroxime
>5 years	as above	• ampicillin/amoxicillin + macrolide or cefuroxime + macrolide

Child Abuse and Neglect

- see <u>Pediatrics</u>
- obligation to report **any** suspected/known case of child abuse or neglect to CAS yourself (**do not delegate**)
- document injuries
- consider skeletal survey X-rays, ophtho consult, CT head
- injury patterns associated with child abuse:
  - **head injuries**: torn frenulum, dental injuries, bilateral black eyes, traumatic hair loss, diffuse severe CNS injury, retinal hemorrhage
  - **Shaken Baby Syndrome**: diffuse brain injury, subdural/subarachnoid hemorrhage, retinal hemorrhage, minimal/no evidence of external trauma, associated bony fractures
  - **skin injuries**: bites, bruises/burns in shape of an object, glove/stocking distribution of burns, bruises of various ages, bruises in protected areas
  - **bone injuries**: rib fractures without major trauma, femur fractures age <1 year of age, spiral fractures of long bones in non-ambulatory children, metaphyseal fractures in infants, multiple fractures of various ages, complex/multiple skull fractures
  - **genitourinary/gastrointestinal injuries**: chronic abdominal/perineal pain, injury to genitals/rectum, STI/pregnancy, recurrent vomiting or diarrhea

Presentation of Neglect
- Failure to thrive, developmental delay
- Inadequate or dirty clothing, poor hygiene
- Child exhibits poor attachment to parents, no stranger anxiety

Procedural Sedation

- procedural sedation: the technique of sedative or dissociative agent administration with or without analgesics to induce a state that allows a patient to tolerate an unpleasant or painful procedure while maintaining all protective cardiorespiratory functions (i.e. a depressed level of consciousness without loss of a patient's protective airway reflexes)
  - must weigh degree of pain and expected relief versus risk/complications of sedation and procedure

Requirements for Safe Procedural Sedation in the Emergency Department
- airway suitable for safe intubation and ventilation
- appropriate equipment/personnel available
- intact and functioning cardiorespiratory and neurological system
- ideally, NPO for minimum 4-6 hours
- anesthetic history and drug allergies, include manifestations
- appropriate IV access, monitoring (oxygen saturation, BP, HR, etc.)
- informed consent obtained

Common Procedural Sedation Medications (titrate to effect)
- see *Commonly Used Medications* section, ER60

Commonly Used Medications

Drug	Dosing Schedule	Indications	Comments
fentanyl	0.5-1.0 µg/kg IV	Procedural sedation	Very short acting narcotic (complication=apnea)
midazolam	50 µg/kg IV	Procedural sedation	Short acting benzodiazepine (complication=apnea when used with narcotic) fentanyl and midazolam often used together for procedural sedation
propofol	0.25-0.5 mg/kg IV	Procedural sedation	Short acting Anesthetic/sedative (complication=apnea, decreased BP)
flumazenil	0.3 mg IV bolus q5min x 3doses	Reversal of procedural sedation	Benzodiazepine antagonist NB don't use in chronic benzo
lidocaine with epi	max 7 mg/kg SC	Local anesthetic	Not to be used in fingers, nose, toes, penis, ears
lidocaine w/o epi	max 5 mg/kg SC	Local anesthetic	
Polysporin®	apply to affected area bid-tid	Superficial infections	
morphine (MS Contin)	15-30 mg PO q8-12h 0.1-0.2 mg/kg max 15 mg IV q4h	Mild to moderate acute/chronic pain Prescribed in combination with NSAIDs or acetaminophen	GI and constipation side effects DO NOT CRUSH, CUT or CHEW
Percocet 10/325®	1-2 tabs PO q6h pm	Moderate pain control	Oxycodone + acetaminophen Max 4 g acetaminophen OD
acetaminophen	325-650 mg PO q4-6h pm	Pain control	Max 4 g OD
Tylenol #3®	1-2 tabs q4-6h prn	Pain control	Max 4 g acetaminophen OD
Ibuprofen	200-800 mg PO tid prn max 1200 mg/d	Mild to moderate acute pain Analgesia and anti-inflammatory properties	
thiamine	Wernicke's encephalopathy: 100 mg IV/IM initially then 50-100 mg IM/IV OD/PO x 3d	To treat/prevent Wernicke's encephalopathy	Caution use in pregnancy
diazepam	anxiety: 2-10 mg PO tid/qid alcohol withdrawal: 10-20 mg PO/IV q1h titrated to signs/symptoms	Anxiety Alcohol withdrawal	
lorazepam	anxiety: 0.5-2 mg PO/IM/IV q6-8h status epilepticus; 4 mg IV repeat up to q5min	Anxiety Status epilepticus	
phenytoin	status epilepticus: Load 20 mg/kg IV @ less then 50 mg/min then 5-10 mg/kg IV @ less then 50 mg/min	Status epilepticus Continuous ECG, BP monitoring recommended	Begin maintenance dose 12hr after loading dose
epinephrine	anaphalaxis: 0.1-0.5 mg IM; can repeat q10-15min	Anaphalaxis	Max 1 mg/dose
salbutamol	2 puffs inhaled q4-6h (4yrs) max 12 puffs/day	Asthma	Caution with cardiac abnormalities
Ipratropium bromide	2-3 puffs tid-qid, max 12 puffs/day	Asthma	Contraindicated with peanut/soy allergy Caution with narrow-angle glaucoma
nitroglycerin	acute angina: 0.3-0.6 mg SL q5min, OR 5 µg/min IV increasing by 5-20 µg/min q3-5min	Angina Acute MI	Not to be used with other anti-hypertensives
ASA	325-650 mg PO q4h max 4g/day stroke/MI risk: 81-325 mg PO OD	Pain control Cardiac prevention	
β-blockers (metoprolol)	5 mg slow IV q5min x 3 if no contraindications	Acute MI	
enoxaparin	1 mg/kg SC BID	Acute MI	
insulin R	bolus 5-10 U (0.2 U/kg) then 5-10 U (0.1 U/kg) per hour	Hyperglycemia	Monitor blood glucose levels Consider K replacement also measure blood glucose levels before administration
glucose	0.5-1.0 g/kg (1-2 ml/kg) IV of D50W	Hypoglycemia/DKA	
furosemide (Lasix™)	CHF: 40-80 mg IV HTN: 10-40 mg PO BID	CHF HTN	Monitor for electrolyte imbalances
haloperidol	2.5-5.0 mg PO/IM initial effective dose 6-20 mg/day	Psychosis	Monitor with Parkinsons; results in CNS depression
naloxone	0.5-2 mg or 0.01-0.02 mg/kg initial bolus IV/IM/SL/SC or via ETT (2-2.5x IV dose), increase dose by 2 mg until response/max 10 mg	Comatose patient Opioid overdose Reversal in procedural sedation	
charcoal	30-100 g PO in 250 ml H_2O	Poisoning/overdose	

Endocrinology

Tasha Jeyanathan, Emily Ow and Hannah Wu, chapter editors
Deepti Damaraju and Elliott Owen, associate editors
Erik Venos, EBM editor
Dr. Alice Cheng, staff editor

Basic Anatomy Review

Major Endocrine Organs

ADH and oxytocin are synthesized by the hypothalamus. They are transported via neurons to the posterior pituitary and are subsequently secreted into the systemic circulation from this location.

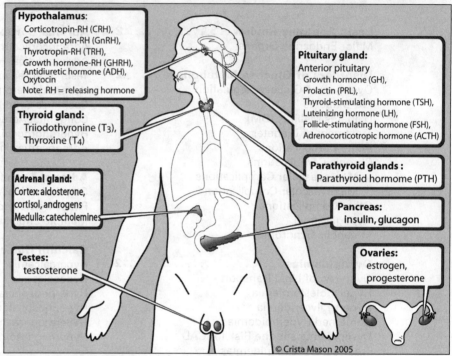

Figure 1. Endocrine System

Disorders of Glucose Metabolism

Overview of Glucose Regulation

DPP-IV inhibitors are newer antihyperglycemic agents that inhibit the degradation of endogenous incretin hormones like GLP-1.
They stimulate insulin secretion and inhibit glucagon release from the pancreas.
DPP-IV inhibitors also delay gastric emptying.

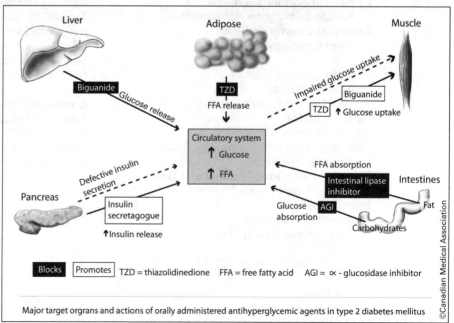

Major target organs and actions of orally administered antihyperglycemic agents in type 2 diabetes mellitus

Figure 2. Antihyperglycemic Agents

Pre-Diabetes

- 1-5% per year go on to develop diabetes mellitus
- 50-80% revert to normal glucose tolerance
- weight loss may improve glucose tolerance
- increased risk of developing macrovascular complications
- lifestyle modifications ↓ progression to DM by 51%

Diagnostic Criteria
- impaired fasting glucose (IFG): fasting blood glucose (FBG) 6.1-6.9 mmol/L (110-125 mg/dL)
- impaired glucose tolerance (IGT): 2h 75 g oral glucose tolerance test (OGTT) 7.8-11.0 mmol/L (140-200 mg/dL)

Diabetes Mellitus (DM)

Definition
- syndrome of disordered metabolism and inappropriate hyperglycemia secondary to an absolute/relative deficiency of insulin, or a reduction in biological effectiveness of insulin, or both

Diagnostic Criteria
- any one of the following are considered diagnostic of diabetes:
  - presence of classic symptoms of DM (polyuria, polydipsia, polyphagia, weight loss, blurry vision, nocturia, ketonuria) PLUS random blood glucose (BG) ≥11.1 mmol/L (200 mg/dL)
  - FBG ≥7.0 mmol/L (126 mg/dL)
  - 2h 75 g OGTT ≥11.1 mmol/L (200 mg/dL)

Etiology and Pathophysiology

Table 1. Etiologic Classification of Diabetes Mellitus

I.	Type 1 diabetes (immune-mediated β cell destruction, usually leading to absolute insulin deficiency)
II.	Type 2 diabetes (ranges from predominantly insulin resistance with relative insulin deficiency to a predominantly insulin secretory defect with insulin resistance 2° to β cell dysfunction)
III.	Other specific causes of diabetes:
	a. Genetic defects of β cell function (e.g. MODY - Maturity-Onset Diabetes of the Young) or insulin action
	b. Diseases of the exocrine pancreas:
	• pancreatitis, pancreatectomy, neoplasia, cystic fibrosis, hemochromatosis ("bronze diabetes")
	c. Endocrinopathies:
	• acromegaly, Cushing's syndrome, glucagonoma, pheochromocytoma, hyperthyroidism
	d. Drug-induced:
	• Glucocorticoids, thyroid hormone, β–adrenergic agonists, thiazides, phenytoin, clozapine
	e. Infections:
	• congenital rubella, CMV, coxsackie
	f. Genetic syndromes associated with diabetes:
	• Down's syndrome, Klinefelter's syndrome, Turner's syndrome
IV.	Gestational Diabetes Mellitus

Intensive insulin therapy for Type 1 DM – DCCT
NEJM 1993;329 (14):977-86
Study: Randomized controlled trial (mean follow-up 6.5 years).
Patients: 1441 patients with Type 1 DM (mean age 27 y; 53% men; 96% white), stratified according to retinopathy and nephropathy at baseline (mild vs. none). Exclusions included hypertension, hypercholesterolemia, severe complications of DM, and severe medical conditions.
Intervention: Conventional therapy (1-2 insulin injections per day, daily self-monitoring of blood glucose) vs. Intensive therapy (3+ insulin injections per day, self-monitoring of blood glucose 4+ times per day, with dosage adjusted to meet targets).
Main outcomes: retinopathy (fundus photographs), nephropathy (urinary albumin excretion >40 mg/24hr), neuropathy (abnormal neuro exam).
Results: Patients in the intensive therapy group had lower mean HbA1C levels (p<0.001).

Complication	RRR % (95%CI)
Retinopathy	63 (52-71)
Nephropathy	39 (21-52)
Neuropathy	60 (38-74)

Conclusion: Intensive blood glucose control delayed the onset and reduced the progression of microvascular complications in Type 1 DM.

Blood glucose control in Type 2 DM – UKPDS 33
Lancet 1998;352:837-53
Study: Randomized controlled trial (mean follow-up 10 years).
Patients: 3867 patients with newly diagnosed Type 2 DM (mean age 53 y, 61% men, 81% white, mean fasting plasma glucose (FPG) 6.1-15.0 mmol/L). Exclusions included severe cardiovascular disease, renal disease, retinopathy, and others.
Intervention: Intensive treatment with a sulfonylurea or insulin (target FPG <6 mmol/L) vs. conventional treatment with diet alone (target FPG <15 mmol/L without hyperglycemic symptoms).
Main outcomes: Diabetes-related endpoints (MI, angina, heart failure, stroke, renal failure, amputation, retinopathy, blindness, death from hyperglycemia or hypoglycemia), diabetes-related death, and all-cause mortality.
Results: Patients allocated to intensive treatment had lower median HbA1C levels (p<0.001).

Outcome	RRR % (p value)
Diabetes-related endpoint	12 (0.029)
Diabetes-related death	10 (0.34)
All-cause mortality	6 (0.44)

Patients allocated to intensive therapy had more hypoglycemic episodes and greater weight gain.
Conclusion: Intensive blood glucose control reduces microvascular, but not macrovascular complications in Type 2 DM.

Dietary advice for treatment of Type 2 DM in adults
Cochrane Database Syst Rev. 2007;(3):CD004097.
Purpose: To assess the effects of type and frequency of different types of dietary advice for adults with Type 2 DM.
Study Selection: Randomised controlled trials, of six months or longer, in which dietary advice was the main intervention.
Results: Thirty-six articles reporting a total of eighteen trials following 1467 participants were included. The review assessed low-fat/high-carbohydrate diets, high-fat/low-carbohydrate diets, low-calorie (1000 kcal per day) and very-low-calorie (500 kcal per day) diets and modified fat diets. The results suggest that adoption of regular exercise is a good way to promote better glycemic control in type 2 diabetic patients, however all of these studies were at high risk of bias.
Conclusions: There are no high quality data on the efficacy of the dietary treatment of Type 2 DM, however the data available indicate that the adoption of exercise appears to improve HbA1C at six and twelve months in people with Type 2 DM.

Table 2. Comparison of Type 1 and Type 2 Diabetes Mellitus

	Type 1	Type 2
Onset	• usually <30 years of age	• usually >40 years of age • increasing incidence in pediatric population secondary to obesity
Epidemiology	• more common in Caucasians • rare in Asians, Hispanics, Aboriginals, and Blacks • accounts for 5-10% of all DM	• more common in Blacks, Hispanics, Aboriginals, Asians • accounts for >90% of all DM
Etiology	• autoimmune	• complex & multifactorial
Genetics	• MZ twin concordance is 30-40% • associated with HLA class II DR3 and DR4, with either being present in up to 95% of Type 1 DM • certain DQ alleles also confer a risk	• greater heritability than Type 1 DM • MZ twin concordance is 70-90% • polygenic • non-HLA associated
Pathophysiology	• synergistic effects of genetic, immune, and environmental factors that result in β cell destruction resulting in impaired insulin secretion • autoimmune process is believed to be triggered by environmental factors (?viruses, bovine milk protein, nitrosurea compounds) • pancreatic cells are infiltrated with lymphocytes resulting in islet cell destruction • 80% of β cell mass is destroyed before features of diabetes present	• impaired insulin secretion, peripheral insulin resistance (likely due to receptor and post receptor abnormality), and excess hepatic glucose production
Natural history	• after initial presentation, honeymoon period often occurs where glycemic control can be achieved with little or no insulin treatment as residual cells are still able to produce insulin • as those cells are destroyed, there is complete insulin deficiency	• early on, glucose tolerance remains normal despite insulin resistance as β cells compensate with increased insulin production • as insulin resistance & compensatory hyperinsulinism continue, the β cells are unable to maintain the hyperinsulinemic state which results in glucose intolerance and diabetes
Circulating autoantibodies	• islet cell Ab present in up to 60-85% • most common islet cell Ab is against glutamic acid decarboxylase (GAD) • up to 60% have Ab against insulin	• <10%
Risk Factors	• personal history of other autoimmune diseases including Graves', myasthenia gravis, autoimmune thyroid disease, and pernicious anemia	• age ≥40 y • fatty liver • abdominal obesity/overweight • hyperuricemia • first-degree relative with DM • race/ethnicity (Black, Aboriginal, Hispanic, Asian-American, Pacific Islander) • history of IGT or IFG • HTN • dyslipidemia • PCOS • GDM • schizophrenia
Body Habitus	• normal to wasted	• typically overweight with increased central obesity
Treatment	• insulin	• lifestyle modifications • oral antihyperglycemic agents • insulin therapy
Acute Complication	• diabetic ketoacidosis	• hyperosmolar nonketotic hyperglycemic state
Screening	• subclinical prodrome can be detected in first and second-degree relatives of those with Type 1 DM by the presence of pancreatic islet autoantibodies	• screen individuals with risk factors (see above)

Treatment of Diabetes

Diet
- daily carbohydrate intake 50-55% of energy, protein 15-20% of energy and fat <30% of energy
- intake of both saturated and polyunsaturated fats <10% of total calories each
- limit sodium, alcohol and caffeine
- Type 1: carbohydrate counting is used to titrate insulin regimen
- Type 2: weight reduction

Lifestyle
- regular physical exercise can improve insulin sensitivity, and lower lipid concentrations and blood pressure
- smoking cessation

Medical Treatment – Oral Antihyperglycemic Agents (Type 2 DM)
- initiate oral antihyperglycemic therapy within 2-3 months if lifestyle management does not result in glycemic control
- initiate immediately if HbA1C >9.0%
- see *Common Medications* for details on oral antihyperglycemic agents

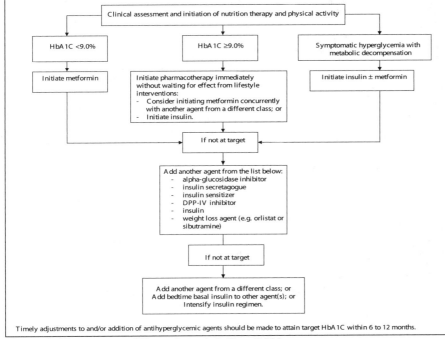

Figure 3. Management of Hyperglycemia in Type 2 DM
(adapted from *Can J Diabetes*. 2008; 32(suppl1):S56)

Insulin (see Figure 4)
- used for Type 1 DM, may be used in Type 2 DM at any point in treatment
- doses adjusted based on individual patient needs to meet target glycemic control
- administration: subcutaneous injections, continuous subcutaneous insulin infusion pump, IV infusion (regular insulin only)
- preparations given as bolus: rapid-acting analogue, short-acting
- preparations given as basal: intermediate, long-acting analogues
- insulin mixtures (%R and %NPH): 10/90, 20/80, 30/70, 40/60, 50/50
- premixed analogues: Humalog Mix 25®, Novomix 30®
- estimated total daily insulin requirement: 0.5-0.7 units/kg

Dosing Schedule
1. Oral agent + basal insulin (NPH, detemir, glargine) (Type 2 only)
    - starting with 10 units qhs, titrate up until FBG <7.0 mmol/L

2. Twice daily injection with insulin mixture
    - insulin mixture used depends on the distribution of carbohydrates in meals but usually start with 30/70
    - estimate total daily insulin requirement then split dose into 2/3 in AM and 1/3 before supper
    - AM bolus targets pre-lunch BG and AM basal targets pre-supper BG
    - PM bolus targets bedtime BG and PM basal targets FBG

Effects of intensive glucose lowering in Type 2 DM. The ADVANCE trial.
N Engl J Med. 2008;358:2545-59.
Study: Multicentre, randomized, controlled trial.
Patients: Patients with Type 2 DM, a glycated hemoglobin level of at least 7.5%, and who had either established cardiovascular disease or additional cardiovascular risk factors. Patients who were morbidly obese, had a recent hypoglycemic event, or who had pre-existing kidney disease were excluded.
Intervention: Patients (n=10,251, mean age 62.2 years, median glycated hemoglobin 8.1%) were randomized to receive comprehensive intensive therapy targeting a glycated hemoglobin level of less than 6.0% or to receive standard therapy targeting a level of 7.0 to 7.9%.
Outcomes: The primary outcome was the first occurrence of nonfatal myocardial infarction or nonfatal stroke or death from cardiovascular causes. Death from any cause was one of several prespecified secondary outcomes
Results: The planned average follow-up was 5.6 years, although the finding of higher mortality in the intensive-therapy group led to a discontinuation of intensive therapy after a mean of 3.5 years. At 1 year, stable median glycated hemoglobin levels of 6.4% and 7.5% were achieved in the intensive-therapy group and the standard-therapy group, respectively. During follow-up, the primary outcome occurred in 352 patients in the intensive-therapy group, as compared with 371 in the standard-therapy group (hazard ratio, 0.90; 95% confidence interval [CI], 0.78 to 1.04; P=0.16). At the same time, 257 patients in the intensive-therapy group died, as compared with 203 patients in the standard-therapy group (hazard ratio, 1.22; 95% CI, 1.01 to 1.46; P=0.04). Hypoglycemia requiring assistance and weight gain of more than 10 kg were more frequent in the intensive-therapy group (P<0.001).
Conclusions: As compared with standard therapy, the use of intensive therapy to target normal glycated hemoglobin levels for 3.5 years increased mortality and did not significantly reduce major cardiovascular events. This harm may be due either to the approach used for rapidly lowering glycated hemoglobin levels or to the levels that were achieved.

Canadian Diabetes Guidelines 2008

	Target	Optimal
HbA1C	<0.07	<0.06
Fasting plasma glucose	4-7mmol/L	4-6mmol/L
2h post prandial glucose	5-10mmol/L	5-8mmol/L
Lipids	as per high or moderate risk group	
Blood pressure	<130/80	

Intensive blood glucose control and vascular outcomes in patients with Type 2 DM. The ACCORD trial.
N Engl J Med. 2008;358:2560-72.
Study: Multicentre, randomized, controlled trial.
Patients: Patients (n= 11,140) with a diagnosis of Type 2 DM at 30 years of age or older, an age of at least 55 years at the time of study entry, and a history of major macrovascular or microvascular disease or at least one other risk factor for vascular disease.
Intervention: A strategy of intensive blood glucose control (target HbA1C value, 6.5%) or a strategy of standard glucose control (with target HbA1C levels defined on the basis of local guidelines). Patients who were randomly assigned to undergo intensive glucose control were given gliclazide (modified release, 30 to 120 mg daily) and were required to discontinue any other sulfonylurea.
Outcomes: Primary study outcomes were a composite of macrovascular events and a composite of microvascular events, considered both jointly and separately. Macrovascular events were defined as death from cardiovascular causes, nonfatal myocardial infarction, or nonfatal stroke. Microvascular events were defined as new or worsening nephropathy or retinopathy.
Results: The median duration of follow-up was 5.0 years. Intensive blood glucose control reduced the incidence of major microvascular events (9.4% vs. 10.9%; hazard ratio, 0.86; 95% CI, 0.77 to 0.97; P=0.01), primarily because of a reduction in the incidence of nephropathy (4.1% vs. 5.2%; hazard ratio, 0.79; 95% CI, 0.66 to 0.93; P=0.006), with no significant effect on retinopathy (P=0.50). There were no significant effects of the type of glucose control on major macrovascular events (hazard ratio with intensive control, 0.94; 95% CI, 0.84 to 1.06; P=0.32), death from cardiovascular causes (hazard ratio with intensive control, 0.88; 95% CI, 0.74 to 1.04; P=0.12), or death from any cause (hazard ratio with intensive control, 0.93; 95% CI, 0.83 to 1.06; P=0.28). Severe hypoglycemia, although uncommon, was more common in the intensive-control group (2.7%, vs. 1.5% in the standard-control group; hazard ratio, 1.86; 95% CI, 1.42 to 2.40; P<0.001).
Conclusions: A strategy of intensive glucose control, involving gliclazide (modified release) and other drugs as required, that lowered the HbA1C value to 6.5% reduced the incidence of major microvascular events due to a reduced incidence of nephropathy. There was no significant reduction in major macrovascular events, death from cardiovascular causes, or death from any cause. Hypoglycemia was more common in the intensive control group.

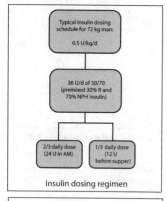

Insulin dosing regimen

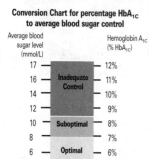

Conversion Chart for percentage HbA₁c to average blood sugar control

Conversion chart adapted from Nathan DM et al. The clinical information value of a glycosylated hemoglobin assay. *NEJM* 1984;310:341-6.

- disadvantages: requires rigid meal timing and carbohydrate content; limited ability to respond to increased or decreased BG

3. MDI (multiple daily injections of insulin)
   - estimate total daily insulin requirement then take 20% of this daily dose before breakfast, lunch, and dinner using regular, aspart or lispro (total 60%)
   - the remaining 40% is given as NPH, glargine or detemir at bedtime
   - advantages: flexible meal timing and carbohydrate content; ability to respond to increased or decreased BG, or planned exercise
   - disadvantages: multiple injections, requires motivation

Table 3. Kinetics of Different Insulin Preparations

Insulin	Brand Names	Insulin type	Onset (h)	Peak (h)	Duration of action (h)
Bolus					
Aspart	Novorapid®	Rapid	5-10 min	30-40 min	2-3
Lispro	Humalog®				
Regular (R), Toronto	Humulin R® Novolin Toronto®	Short	1/2 - 1	1-3	5-7
Basal					
NPH/(N)	Humulin N® Novolin NPH®	Intermediate	2-4	6-10	14-18
Ultralente (U)	Humulin U® Novolin Ultralente®	Long	4-5	---	18-28
Detemir	Levemir®	Long	2-4	--	16-20
Glargine	Lantus®	Long	2-4	--	18-20

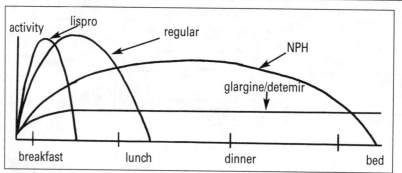

Figure 4. Duration of Activity of Different Insulins

Glucose Monitoring
- frequent self-monitoring and recording of BG is now standard management
- HbA1C reflects glycemic control over 3 months and is a measure of patient's long-term diabetes control
- HbA1C ≥10% indicates poor control
- American Diabetes Association (ADA) suggests HbA1C <7.0%, American Association of Clinical Endocrinologists (AACE) <6.5%
- Canadian Diabetes Association (CDA) guidelines: target <7.0%
- there may be harm associated with strategy to target HbA1C <6.0% in certain patients with Type 2 DM (see EBM box re: ACCORD trial)

Variable Insulin Dose Schedule ("Sliding/Supplemental/Correction Scale")
- patient takes usual doses of basal insulin but varies doses of bolus insulin based on BG reading at time of dose
- use baseline bolus insulin dose when within BG target range; add or subtract units when above or below target
- commonly used in hospital or in perioperative management of diabetes
- allows acute corrections but poor control overall → reactive correction after the period of hypo or hyperglycemia rather than anticipating the BG level

Insulin Pump Therapy
- external battery-operated pump continuously delivers basal dose of lispro or aspart through small subcutaneous catheter
- at meals, patient programs pump to deliver extra insulin bolus
- basal dose may be increased or decreased based on activity, sleep, etc.
- advantages: flexibility in meals and activity
- disadvantages: very expensive, increased risk of DKA if pump inadvertently disconnected, frequent BG testing required

Acute Complications

Table 4. Acute Complications of Diabetes Mellitus: Hyperglycemic Comatose States

	Diabetic Ketoacidosis (DKA)	Hyperglycemic Hyperosmolar Nonketotic State (HONK)
Pathophysiology	• usually occurs in Type 1 DM • insulin deficiency with ↑ counterregulatory hormones (glucagon, cortisol, catecholamines, GH) • can occur with insulin lack (noncompliance, poor dosage, 1st presentation) or increased stress (surgery, infection, exercise) • unrestricted hepatic glucose production → hyperglycemia → osmotic diuresis → dehydration and electrolyte disturbance → ↓ Na (pseudohyponatremia) • fat mobilization → ↑ FFA → ketoacids → metabolic acidosis • severe hyperglycemia exceeds the renal threshold for glucose and ketone reabsorption → glucosuria and ketonuria • total body K depletion but serum K may be normal or elevated 2° to shift from ICF to ECF due to insulin lack, ↑ plasma osmolality • total body PO₄ depletion	• occurs in Type 2 DM • often precipitated by sepsis, stroke, MI, CHF, renal failure, trauma, drugs (glucocorticoids, immunosuppressants, phenytoin, diuretics), dialysis, recent surgery, burns • partial or relative insulin deficiency decreases glucose utilization in muscle, fat, and liver while inducing hyperglucagonemia and hepatic glucose production • presence of a small amount of insulin prevents the development of ketosis by inhibiting lipolysis • characterized by hyperglycemia, hyperosmolality, and dehydration without ketosis • more severe dehydration compared to DKA secondary to more gradual onset and ↑ duration of metabolic decompensation plus the impaired fluid intake which is common in bedridden or elderly • volume contraction → renal insufficiency → ↑ hyperglycemia, ↑ osmolality → shift of fluid from neurons to ECF → mental obtundation and coma
Clinical Features	• polyuria, polydipsia, polyphagia with marked fatigue, nausea, vomiting • dehydration (orthostatic changes) • LOC may be ↓ with high serum osmolality (osm >330 mmol/L) • abdominal pain • fruity smelling breath • Kussmaul's respiration	• onset is insidious → preceded by weakness, polyuria, polydipsia • history of decreased fluid intake • history of ingesting large amounts of glucose containing fluids • dehydration (orthostatic changes) • ↓ LOC → lethargy, confusion, comatose • Kussmaul's respiration is absent unless the underlying precipitant has also caused a metabolic acidosis
Serum	• ↑ BG (11-55 mmol/L, 198-990 mg/dL), ↓ Na (spurious 2° to hyperglycemia → for every ↑ in BG by 10 mmol/L (180 mg/dL) there is a ↓ in Na by 3 mmol/L) • normal or ↑ K, ↓ HCO₃, ↑ BUN, ↑ Cr, ketonemia, ↓ PO₄ • ↑ osmolality	• ↑ BG (44.4-133.2 mmol/L, 800-2400 mg/dL) • in mild dehydration, may have hyponatremia (spurious 2° to hyperglycemia → for every ↑ in BG by 10 mmol/L (180 mg/dL) there is a ↓ in Na by 3 mmol/L) ▪ if dehydration progresses, may get hypernatremia • ketosis usually absent or mild if starvation occurs • ↑ osmolality
ABG	• metabolic acidosis with ↑ AG plus possible 2° respiratory alkalosis • if severe vomiting/dehydration there may be a metabolic alkalosis	• metabolic acidosis absent unless underlying precipitant leads to acidosis (e.g. lactic acidosis in MI)
Urine	• +ve for glucose and ketones	• -ve for ketones unless there is starvation ketosis • glycosuria

Treatment	• immediate resuscitation and emergency measures if patient is stuporous or comatose
	• monitor degree of ketoacidosis with AG not BG or serum ketone level
	• rehydration:
	  - 1L/h NS in first 2 hrs
	  - after 1st 2 L, 300-400 ml/h 0.45% NS
	  - once BG reaches 13.9 mmol/L (250 mg/dL) then switch to D5W to maintain BG in the range of 13.9-16.6 mmol/L (250-300 mg/dL)
	• insulin therapy:
	  - critical to resolve acidosis, not hyperglycemia
	  - use only regular insulin (R)
	  - initially load 0.15 U/ kg body weight insulin R bolus
	  - maintenance 0.1 U/kg/h insulin R infusion
	  - check serum glucose hourly
	• K replacement:
	  - as acidosis is corrected, hypokalemia may develop
	  - when K 3.5-5.5 mmol/L add KCL 30-40mEq/L IV fluid to keep K in the range of 3.5-5 mEq/L
	• HCO₃:
	  - if pH <7.0 or if hypotension, arrhythmia, or coma is present with a pH of < 7.1 give HCO₃ in 0.45% NS
	  - do not give if pH >7.1 (risk of metabolic alkalosis!)
	  - can give in case of life-threatening hyperkalemia
	• ± mannitol (for cerebral edema)
		• same resuscitation and emergency measures as DKA
		• rehydration:
		  - IV fluids: 1 L/h NS initially
		  - evaluate corrected serum Na
		  - if serum Na high or normal, switch to 0.45% NS (4-14 ml/kg/h)
		  - if serum Na low, maintain NS (4-14 ml/kg/h)
		  - when serum BG reaches 13.9 mmol/L (250 mg/dL) switch to D5W
		• K replacement:
		  - less severe K depletion compared to DKA
		  - if serum K<3.3 mmol/L, hold insulin and give 40 mEq K replacement
		  - if K is 3.3-5.4, give KCl 20-30 mEq/L IV fluid
		  - if serum K ≥5.5 mmol/L, check K every 2 h
		• search for precipitating event
		• insulin therapy:
		  - use only regular insulin (R)
		  - initially load 0.15 U/ kg body weight insulin R bolus
		  - maintenance 0.1 U/kg/h insulin R infusion or IM
		  - check serum glucose hourly
		  - in general lower insulin requirement compared to DKA

Prognosis	• 2-5% mortality in developed countries • serious morbidity from sepsis, respiratory complications, thromboembolic complications, and cerebral edema	• overall mortality approaches 50% primarily because of the older patient population and underlying etiology

The 6 I's Precipitating DKA:
Infection
Ischemia or Infarction
Iatrogenic (glucocorticoids)
Intoxication
Insulin missed
Intra-abdominal process
(e.g. pancreatitis, cholecystitis)

Average fluid loss runs at 3-6 L in DKA, and 8-10 L in HONK.

Effect of a multifactorial intervention on mortality in Type 2 DM. The Steno-2 Study
N Engl J Med. 2008;358:580-91.
Study: Single centre, randomized, controlled trial.
Patients: Patients (n=160) with Type 2 DM and persistent microalbuminuria
Intervention: Random assignment to receive either conventional multifactorial treatment or intensified, target-driven therapy involving a combination of medications and focused behaviour modification. Targets included a HbA1C level of <6.5%, a fasting serum total cholesterol level of <4.5 mmol/L, a fasting serum triglyceride level of <1.7 mmol/L, a systolic blood pressure of <130 mm Hg, and a diastolic blood pressure of <80 mm Hg. Patients were treated with blockers of the renin–angiotensin system because of their microalbuminuria, regardless of blood pressure, and received low-dose aspirin as primary prevention.
Outcomes: The primary end point in the follow-up trial was the time to death from any cause. Other endpoints examined death from cardiovascular causes and various cardiovascular events along with diabetic neuropathy, nephropathy, and retinopathy.
Results: Twenty-four patients in the intensive-therapy group died, as compared with 40 in the conventional-therapy group (hazard ratio, 0.54; 95% confidence interval [CI], 0.32 to 0.89; P=0.02). Intensive therapy was associated with a lower risk of death from cardiovascular causes (hazard ratio, 0.43; 95% CI, 0.19 to 0.94; P=0.04) and of cardiovascular events (hazard ratio, 0.41; 95% CI, 0.25 to 0.67; P<0.001). One patient in the intensive-therapy group had progression to end-stage renal disease, as compared with six patients in the conventional-therapy group (P=0.04). Fewer patients in the intensive-therapy group required retinal photocoagulation (relative risk, 0.45; 95% CI, 0.23 to 0.86; P=0.02).
Conclusions: In at-risk patients with Type 2 DM, intensive intervention with multiple drug combinations and behaviour modification had sustained beneficial effects with respect to vascular complications and on rates of death from any cause and from cardiovascular causes.

Chronic Complications

Macrovascular Complications

- increased risk of coronary artery disease (CAD), ischemic stroke, and peripheral vascular disease (PVD) secondary to accelerated atherosclerosis
- coronary artery disease
  - risk of myocardial infarction (MI) is 3-5x higher in diabetics compared to age matched controls
  - CAD is the leading cause of death in Type 2 DM
  - patients with DM are considered as "high risk" under the risk stratification for CAD (see *Dyslipidemias*, E12)
- ischemic stroke
  - risk of stroke is approximately 2.5x higher in diabetics
  - level of glycemia is either a risk factor for stroke or a predictor of a poorer outcome in patients who suffer a stroke
  - HbA1C level is a significant and independent predictor of the risk of stroke
- peripheral vascular disease
  - manifested by intermittent claudication in lower extremities, intestinal angina, foot ulceration
  - risk of gangrene in the feet is 30x higher in diabetics compared to age matched controls
  - risk of lower extremity amputation is 15x higher in diabetics
- treatment
  - tight blood pressure control (<130/80 mmHg)
  - tight glycemic control
  - tight low density lipoprotein (LDL) cholesterol control (LDL <2.0 mmol/L)
  - low-dose ASA in patients with CVD or increased likelihood of CV events
  - ACE inhibitor or angiotensin receptor blocker (ARB) in high-risk patients
  - smoking cessation

Microvascular Complications

DIABETIC RETINOPATHY (see also Ophthalmology)

Epidemiology
- Type 1 DM – 25% affected at 5 years, 100% at 20 years
- Type 2 DM – 25% affected at Dx, 60% at 20 years
- leading cause of blindness in North America between the ages of 20-74
- most important factor is disease duration

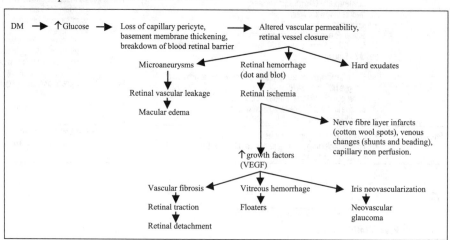

Figure 5. Pathophysiology of Diabetic Retinopathy

Clinical Features
- nonproliferative
  - asymptomatic but with macular involvement may impair vision
  - microaneurysms, hard exudates, dot and blot hemorrhages
- preproliferative
  - 10-40% progress to proliferative within 1 year
  - macular edema, cotton wool spots, venous shunts and beading, intra retinal microvascular abnormalities (IRMA)
- proliferative
  - neovascularization, fibrous scarring, vitreous hemorrhage, retinal detachment
  - great risk for loss of vision secondary to vitreous hemorrhage (floaters) and/or retinal detachment

Treatment and Prevention
- tight glycemic control (delays onset, decreases progression)
- if hypertension is present, treat aggressively
- panretinal laser photocoagulation for treatment of neovascularization
- vitrectomy
- annual follow-up visits with an eye specialist (optometrist or ophthalmologist); examination through dilated pupils whether they are symptomatic or not (immediate referral after diagnosis of Type 2 DM; 5 years after diagnosis of Type 1 DM)
- interval for follow-up should be tailored to severity of retinopathy

DIABETIC NEPHROPATHY (see also Nephrology)

Epidemiology
- diabetes-induced renal failure is the most common cause of renal failure in North America
- 20-40% of persons with Type 1 DM (after 5-10 years) and 4-20% with Type 2 DM have progressive nephropathy

Pathophysiology
- thickening of capillary basement membrane and glomerular mesangium resulting in glomerulosclerosis and renal insufficiency
- diffuse glomerulosclerosis is more common than nodular intercapillary glomerulosclerosis (Kimmelstiel-Wilson lesions)

Screening
- random urine test for albumin to creatinine ratio (ACR) plus urine dipstick test for all Type 2 DM patients at diagnosis, then annually, and for postpubertal Type 1 DM patients with ≥5 years duration of DM

Clinical Features
- initial changes include microalbuminuria, increased GFR (up to 140%), enlarged kidneys
- microalbuminuria: ACR of >2.0 mg/mmol (men) or >2.8 mg/mmol (women)
- macroalbuminuria: ACR of >20.0 mg/mmol (men) or >28.0 mg/mmol (women)
- over 15 years progresses to cause hypertension, persistent proteinuria (macroalbuminuria), nephrotic syndrome, and renal failure
- a high HbA1C is an independent risk factor for progression to microalbuminuria

Treatment and Prevention
- tight glycemic control
- tight blood pressure control <130/80 with angiotensin converting enzyme (ACE) inhibitors or angiotensin receptor blockers (ARBs)
- numerous studies have shown that even in the absence of glycemic control, ACE inhibitors or ARBs reduce the level of albuminuria and reduce the rate of progression of renal disease in normotensive and hypertensive patients with Type 1 or Type 2 DM
- Type 1 DM → if normotensive or hypertensive and patient has microalbuminuria or macroalbuminuria → ACE inhibitors 1st line; ARBs 2nd line
- Type 2 DM → if normotensive or hypertensive and patient has microalbuminuria or macroalbuminuria → ARBs 1st line or ACE inhibitors if creatinine clearance (CrCl) >60 ml/min; ARB if CrCl ≤60 ml/min
- consider use of non-dihydropyridine calcium channel blocker (e.g. diltiazem) in those unable to tolerate both ACE inhibitors and ARBs
- limit use of nephrotoxic drugs and dyes
- protein restriction (controversial)
- renal failure may necessitate hemodialysis and renal transplant

Management of diabetic retinopathy: a systematic review
JAMA. 2007;298:902-16.

Purpose: To review the best evidence for primary and secondary intervention in the management of diabetic retinopathy (DR), including diabetic macular edema.

Study Selection: All English-language randomized controlled trials (RCTs) with more than 12 months of follow-up and meta-analyses were included. Delphi consensus criteria were used to identify well-conducted studies.

Results: Forty-four studies (including 3 meta-analyses) met the inclusion criteria. Tight glycemic and blood pressure control reduces the incidence and progression of DR. Pan-retinal laser photocoagulation reduces the risk of moderate and severe visual loss by 50% in patients with severe nonproliferative and proliferative retinopathy. Focal laser photocoagulation reduces the risk of moderate visual loss by 50% to 70% in eyes with macular edema. Early vitrectomy improves visual recovery in patients with proliferative retinopathy and severe vitreous hemorrhage. Intravitreal injections of steroids may be considered in eyes with persistent loss of vision when conventional treatment has failed. There is insufficient evidence for the efficacy or safety of lipid-lowering therapy, medical interventions, or antivascular endothelial growth factors on the incidence or progression of DR.

Conclusions: Tight glycemic and blood pressure control remains the cornerstone in the primary prevention of DR. Pan-retinal and focal retinal laser photocoagulation reduces the risk of visual loss in patients with severe DR and macular edema, respectively. There is currently insufficient evidence to recommend routine use of other treatments.

DIABETIC NEUROPATHY (see also Neurology)

Epidemiology
- approximately 50% of patients within 10 years of onset of Type 1 DM and Type 2 DM

Pathophysiology
- mechanism poorly understood
- acute cranial nerve palsies and diabetic amyotrophy are thought to be due to ischemic infarction of involved peripheral nerve
- the more common motor and sensory neuropathies are thought to be related to metabolic or osmotic toxicity secondary to increased sorbitol and/or decreased myoinositol (possible mechanisms include accumulation of advanced glycation end (AGE) products, oxidative stress, protein kinase C, nerve growth factor deficiency)
- can have peripheral sensory neuropathy, motor neuropathy, or autonomic neuropathy

Screening
- 128 Hz tuning fork or 10 g monofilament at diagnosis and annually in people with Type 2 DM and after 5 years duration of Type 1 DM

Clinical Features

Effects of treatments for symptoms of painful diabetic neuropathy: systematic review.
BMJ. 2007;335:87
Purpose: To evaluate the effects of treatments for the symptoms of painful diabetic neuropathy.
Study Selection: Randomised controlled trials comparing topically applied and orally administered drugs with a placebo in adults with painful diabetic neuropathy.
Results: 25 included reports compared anticonvulsants (n=1270), antidepressants (94), opioids (329), ion channel blockers (173), N-methyl-D-aspartate antagonist (14), duloxetine (805), capsaicin (277), and isosorbide dinitrate spray (22) with placebo. The odds ratios in terms of 50% pain relief were 5.33 (95% confidence interval 1.77 to 16.02) for traditional anticonvulsants, 3.25 (2.27 to 4.66) for newer generation anticonvulsants, and 22.24 (5.83 to 84.75) for tricyclic antidepressants. The odds ratios in terms of withdrawals related to adverse events were 1.51 (0.33 to 6.96) for traditional anticonvulsants, 2.98 (1.75 to 5.07) for newer generation anticonvulsants, and 2.32 (0.59 to 9.69) for tricyclic antidepressants. Insufficient dichotomous data were available to calculate the odds ratios for ion channel blockers.
Conclusion: Anticonvulsants and antidepressants are still the most commonly used options to manage diabetic neuropathy. Oral tricyclic antidepressants and traditional anticonvulsants are better for short term pain relief than newer generation anticonvulsants. Evidence of the long term effects of oral antidepressants and anticonvulsants is still lacking. Further studies are needed on opioids, N-methyl-D-aspartate antagonists, and ion channel blockers.

Table 5. Clinical Presentation of Diabetic Neuropathies

Peripheral Sensory Neuropathy	Motor Neuropathy	Autonomic Neuropathy
• paresthesias (tingling, itching), neuropathic pain, radicular pain, numbness, decreased tactile sensation • bilateral and symmetric with decreased perception of vibration and pain/temperature; especially true in the lower extremities but may also be present in the hands • decreased ankle reflex • symptoms may first occur in entrapment syndromes e.g. carpal tunnel • neuropathic ulceration of foot	• less common than sensory neuropathy • delayed motor nerve conduction and muscle weakness/atrophy • may involve one nerve trunk (mononeuropathy) or more (mononeuritis multiplex) • some of the motor neuropathies spontaneously resolve after 6-8 wks • reversible CN palsies: III (ptosis/ophthalmoplegia), VI (inability to laterally deviate eye), and VII (Bell's palsy) • diabetic amyotrophy: refers to pain, weakness, and wasting of hip flexors or extensors	• postural hypotension, resting fixed tachycardia, decreased response to Valsalva maneuver • gastroparesis and alternating diarrhea and constipation • urinary retention and erectile dysfunction

Treatment and Management
- tight glycemic control
- for neuropathic pain syndromes: tricyclic antidepressants (e.g. amitriptyline), pregabalin, anti-epileptics (e.g. carbamazepine, gabapentin), and capsaicin
- foot care education
- Jobst fitted stocking and tilting of head of bed may decrease symptoms of orthostatic hypotension
- treat gastroparesis with domperidone and/or metoclopramide (dopamine antagonists), erythromycin (stimulates motilin receptors)
- medical, mechanical and surgical treatment for erectile dysfunction: PDE-5 inhibitors (e.g. sildenafil, tadalafil, vardenafil), intracorporeal injections of vasoactive drugs, vacuum therapy (see Urology)

 ## Other Complications

Dermatologic
- diabetic dermopathy: atrophic brown spots commonly in pretibial region known as "shin spots" secondary to increased glycosylation of tissue proteins or vasculopathy
- eruptive xanthomas secondary to increased triglycerides (TG)
- necrobiosis lipoidica diabeticorum: rare complication characterized by thinning skin over the shins allowing visualization of subcutaneous vessels

Bone and Joint Disease
- juvenile cheiroarthropathy: chronic stiffness of hand secondary to contracture of skin over joints secondary to glycosylated collagen and other connective tissue proteins
- Dupuytren's contracture
- bone demineralization: bone density 10-20% below normal
- frozen shoulder

Cataracts

- subcapsular and senile cataracts secondary to glycosylated lens protein or increased sorbitol causing osmotic change and fibrosis

Infections

- see Infectious Diseases

Hypoglycemia

- characterized by Whipple's Triad:
    1. serum glucose <2.5 mmol/L (45 mg/dL) in males and <2.2 mmol/L (40 mg/dL) in females
    2. neuroglycopenic symptoms or adrenergic symptoms (autonomic response)
    3. relief provided by administration of glucose

Etiology and Pathophysiology

Table 6. Common causes of Hypoglycemia

Fasting		Nonfasting (Reactive)
Hyperinsulinism	**Without hyperinsulinism**	
• exogenous insulin	• severe hepatic dysfunction	• alimentary
• sulfonylurea reaction	• chronic renal insufficiency	• functional
• autoimmune hypoglycemia (autoantibodies to insulin or insulin receptor)	• hypocortisolism	• noninsulinoma pancreatogenous hypoglycemic syndrome
	• alcohol use	• occult diabetes
• pentamidine	• non-pancreatic tumours	• leucine sensitivity
• pancreatic β cell tumour – insulinoma	• inborn error of carbohydrate metabolism, glycogen storage disease, gluconeogenic enzyme deficiency	• hereditary fructose intolerance
		• galactosemia
		• newborn infant of diabetic mother

Clinical Features

- adrenergic symptoms (typically occur first; caused by autonomic nervous system activity)
    - palpitations, sweating, anxiety, tremor, tachycardia, hunger
- neuroglycopenic symptoms (caused by ↓activity of CNS)
    - dizziness, headache, clouding of vision, mental dullness, fatigue, confusion, seizures, coma

Investigations

- electrolytes, BUN/creatinine, LFTs, drugs/toxins

Treatment

- for fasting hypoglycemia, must treat underlying cause
- for reactive hypoglycemia, frequent small feeds
- see Emergency Medicine
- bloodwork to be drawn when patient is hypoglycemic (i.e. during hospitalized 72-hour fast): serum ketones, insulin, proinsulin, C-peptide, cortisol, and GH
- treatment of hypoglycemic episode in the unconscious patient or patient NPO
    - D50W 50 mL (1 ampule) IV or 1 mg glucagon SC (if no IV available)
    - may need ongoing glucose infusion once BG >5mmol/L

Metabolic Syndrome

- defined by having three or more risk factors (see Table 7)
- postulated syndrome related to insulin resistance associated with hyperglycemia, hyperinsulinemia, hypertension, central obesity, and dyslipidemia
- obesity aggravates extent of insulin resistance
- complications include atherosclerosis, CAD, MI, and stroke
- not to be confused with syndrome X related to angina pectoris with normal coronary arteries (Prinzmetal angina)

Treatment of Acute Hypoglycemic Episode (Blood Glucose < 4.0 mmol/L) in the Awake Patient (e.g. able to self-treat)

1) Eat 15 g of carbohydrates (CHO) (e.g. 3 x 5 g glucose tablets; 3 packets sugar dissolved in water; 3/4 cup of juice)
↓
2) Wait 15 minutes
↓
3) Retest Blood Glucose (BG)
↓
4) Repeat steps 1-3 until BG >5 mmol/L
↓
5) Eat next scheduled meal. If next meal is >1 hour away, eat snack including 15 g of CHO and protein

Hypoglycemia Unawareness: (Type 1 DM >>> Type 2 DM) patient remains asymptomatic until severely hypoglycemic levels are reached

Causes:
- ↓glucagon/epinephrine response
- hx of repeated hypoglycemia or low HbA1C
- autonomic dysfunction

Use C-peptide levels to distinguish between exogenous and endogenous source of hyperinsulinemia

decreased = endogenous

decreased or normal = exogenous

Table 7. International Diabetes Federation Worldwide Definition of the Metabolic Syndrome 2005

Note: ethnospecific waist circumference values also available

Risk Factor	Defining level
Abdominal Obesity	
Men	Waist Circumference ≥94 cm (37 inches)
Women	Waist Circumference ≥80 cm (31.5 inches)
Triglyceride level	≥1.7 mmol/L (150.4 mg/dL)
HDL-C level	
Men	<1.0 mmol/L (<40 mg/dL)
Women	<1.3 mmol/L (<50 mg/dL)
Blood pressure	≥130/85 mm Hg
Fasting glucose level	≥5.6 mmol/L (>100 mg/dL)

Dyslipidemias

Definition
- metabolic disorders characterized by elevations of fasting plasma cholesterol, and/or triglycerides (TG), and/or low HDL

Overview of Lipid Transport

- lipoproteins are spherical complexes that consist of a lipid core surrounded by a shell of water-soluble proteins and phospholipids
- lipoproteins transport lipids within the body

Table 8. Lipoproteins

Lipoprotein	Apolipoproteins	Function
Exogenous pathway		
Chylomicron	• B-48, C, E, A-I, A-II, A-IV	• transport dietary TG from gut to adipose tissue and muscle
Endogenous Pathway		
VLDL	• B-100, C, E	• transports hepatic synthesized TG from liver to adipose tissue and muscle
IDL	• B-100, E	• product of hydrolysis of VLDL by lipoprotein lipase resulting in depletion of TG core but enriched in cholesterol esters
LDL	• B-100	• formed by further removal of residual TG from IDL core by hepatic lipase resulting in greater enriched particles with cholesterol esters • transports cholesterol from liver to peripheral tissues
HDL	• A-I, A-II, C, E	• transports cholesterol from peripheral tissues to liver • acts as a reservoir for apolipoproteins

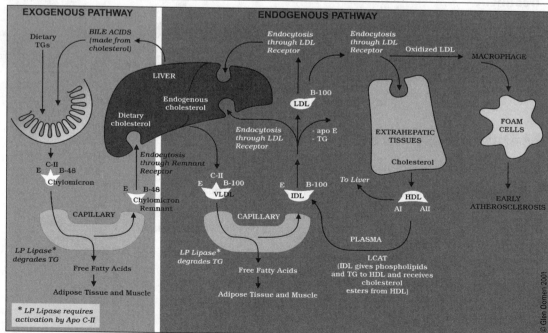

Figure 6. Exogenous and Endogenous Biosynthetic Lipid Pathways

Hypercholesterolemia

PRIMARY HYPERCHOLESTEROLEMIA

Table 9. The Primary Hypercholesterolemias

Hypercholesterolemia	Epidemiology	Etiology/ Pathophysiology	Labs	Clinical Presentation	Treatment
Familial Hypercholesterolemia (Frederickson Type IIa)	heterozygote: 1/500 in US population	• autosomal dominant with high penetrance • deficiency in the normal LDL receptor on cell membranes	• increased total cholesterol (TC) • increased LDL	• tendinous xanthomatosis (achilles, patellar, and extensor tendons of hand) • arcus corneae • xanthelasma • heterozygotes: premature CAD, 50% risk of MI in men by age 30 • homozygotes: manifest CAD and other vascular disease early in childhood and can be fatal (<20 y) if untreated	• heterozygotes: improvement of LDL with dual combination of HMG CoA reductase inhibitors, niacin, or bile acid sequestrants • homozygotes: partial control with portacaval shunt or LDL apheresis in conjunction with niacin; large dose atorvastatin is modestly effective
Polygenic Hypercholesterolemia (Frederickson Type IIa)		• Most common • Few mild inherited defects in cholesterol metabolism	↑TC ↑ LDL	• asymptomatic until vascular disease develops	• HMG CoA reductase inhibtors, bile acid sequestrant, niacin

SECONDARY HYPERCHOLESTEROLEMIA

Etiology
- diet
- anorexia nervosa
- hypothyroidism
- cholestatic liver disease (primary biliary cirrhosis)
- nephrotic disease
- monoclonal gammopathy
- drugs (cyclosporin, diuretics, carbamazepine)

Hypertriglyceridemia

PRIMARY HYPERTRIGLYCERIDEMIA

Table 10. The Primary Hypertriglyceridemias

Hypertriglyceridemia	Etiology/ Pathophysiology	Labs	Clinical Presentation	Treatment
Familial Lipoprotein Lipase deficiency (Frederickson Type I)	• autosomal recessive deficiency in the lipoprotein lipase or its cofactor	↑ chylomicrons, moderate ↑ in VLDL	• hepatosplenomegaly • splenic infarct • anemia, granulocytopenia, thrombocytopenia 2° to hypersplenism • pancreatitis • lipemia retinalis • eruptive xanthomata	• decrease dietary fat intake to <10% of total calories
Familial Hypertriglyceridemia (Frederickson Type IV)	• several genetic defects resulting in ↑ hepatic VLDL synthesis or ↓ removal of VLDL	↑VLDL	• eruptive xanthomata • lipemia retinalis • recurrent epigastric pain • premature CAD • early adulthood develop syndrome of obesity, hypertriglyceridemia, hyperinsulinemia & hyperuricemia	• ↓ dietary fat intake • abstain from EtOH • fibrate or niacin

SECONDARY HYPERTRIGLYCERIDEMIA

Etiology
- obesity / metabolic syndrome
- alcohol
- diabetes mellitus
- drugs (corticosteroids, estrogen, hydrochlorothiazide, retinoic acid, β-blockers without intrinsic sympathomimetic action (ISA), anti-retroviral drugs)
- chronic liver failure
- hepatitis
- hypothyroidism

- polyclonal and monoclonal hypergammaglobulinemia
- glycogen storage disease
- hypopituitarism and acromegaly

Combined Hyperlipidemia

Table 11. Primary Combined Hyperlipidemias

Hyperlipidemia	Epidemiology	Etiology/Pathogenesis	Labs	Clinical Presentation	Treatment
Familial Combined Hyperlipidemia (Frederickson Type IIb)	• most common form of hyperlipidemia	• over-population of VLDL and associated ↑ LDL 2° to excess hepatic synthesis of apolipoprotein B • autosomal dominant	↑LDL ↑VLDL	• xanthelasma • CAD and other vascular disease	• weight reduction • decrease fat, cholesterol, and EtOH in diet • niacin, fibrates • HMG CoA reductase inhibitors
Dysbetalipoproteinemia (Frederickson Type III)		• abnormal apoprotein E	↑IDL ↑VLDL	• tuberous, eruptive, planar xanthomata • IGT • CAD and PVD	• weight reduction • ↓ fat, cholesterol, and EtOH in diet • fibrate, HMG CoA reductase inhibitors, niacin

Dyslipidemia and the Risk for CAD

- ↑ LDL is a major risk factor for atherosclerosis and CAD
- ↑ LDL is associated with ↑ risk of cardiovascular disease and mortality
- ↑ HDL is associated with ↓ cardiovascular disease and mortality
- hypertriglyceridemia is an independent risk factor for CAD in people with DM and in postmenopausal women

Screening
- screening is recommended for:
  - men over 40 years of age
  - women who are postmenopausal or over 50 years of age
  - those with CAD
  - those with family history of hyperlipidemia or premature CAD
  - those with other risk factors (DM, smoking, abdominal obesity, hypertension)
  - those with manifestations of hyperlipidemia (e.g. xanthelasma, xanthoma or arcus corneae)
  - those with evidence of symptomatic or asymptomatic atherosclerosis
- in order to stratify risk for CAD and determine target lipid levels for treatment, establish:
  - presence of CAD, PVD, and cerebrovascular disease
  - risk factors for CAD
  - presence of hyperlipidemia and clinical symptoms (tendon xanthoma, xanthelasma, eruptive xanthoma, lipemia retinalis, arcus corneae)

Table 12. Risk Factors for CAD
(modified from National Cholesterol Education Program)

Positive Risk Factors	Negative Risk Factors	Non-traditional Positive Risk Factors
• age: males >45 years, females >55 years; premature menopause • family history of CAD: MI or sudden death in first-degree male relative <45 or in first-degree female relative <55 • current smoker • hypertension (HTN): BP >140/90 mmHg or currently on antihypertensive medications • ↓HDL cholesterol <0.90 mmol/L (<35 mg/dL) • DM or IGT • hypertriglyceridemia TG >2.3 mmol/L (>205 mg/dL) • abdominal obesity (BMI ≥27; waist hip ratio ≥0.9 in males, ≥0.8 in females)	• high HDL cholesterol	• ↑Apo B (apolipoprotein B) • ↓Apo A-1 (apolipoprotein A-1) • small dense LDL • ↑fibrinogen • ↑PAI-1 • ↑IL-6 (interleukin 6) • ↑TNF (tumour necrosis factor) • ↑CRP (c-reactive protein) • ↓adiponectin • ↑homocysteine

Intensive lipid lowering in CAD: TNT
NEJM 2005;352(14):1425-35
Study: Multicentre, randomized, double-blinded trial with median follow-up of 4.9 years.
Patients: 10,001 patients with CAD and LDL-C <3.4.
Intervention: 80 mg versus 10 mg atorvastatin daily.
Main outcomes: Death from CAD, MI, cardiac arrest, or stroke.
Results: A primary event occurred in 8.7% of the patients receiving intensive therapy, compared to 10.9% of patients receiving standard therapy (RR 0.78, p<0.001). There was no difference in overall mortality. Incidence of persistent transaminase elevations was higher in the intensive therapy group (1.2% versus 0.2%, p<0.001).
Conclusion: Intensive statin therapy is associated with lower rates of CAD events than standard therapy, but also a higher rate of transaminase elevation.

Simvastatin to lower CAD risk –The Heart Protection Study
Lancet 2002;360:7-22
Study: Randomized, double-blind, placebo-controlled trial (median follow-up 5.0 years).
Patients: 20,536 patients with coronary disease, other occlusive arterial disease, or diabetes (aged 40-80 years) who had a total cholesterol level of 3.5mmol/L.
Intervention: Simvastatin 40 mg/day or placebo.
Main Outcomes: Mortality, fatal or non-fatal vascular events.
Results: The use of simvastatin significantly decreased total mortality (12.9 vs. 14.7, p=0.0003) and the first event rate of any cardiovascular event by 25% (p<0.0001).
Conclusion: Treatment with simvastatin improved survival and cardiovascular outcomes in high-risk CAD patients.

Statins and CHD in dyslipidemia – 4S trial
Lancet 1994; 344:1383-89
Study: Randomized, double-blind, placebo-controlled trial (median follow-up 5.4 years).
Patients: 4444 patients with angina or previous MI (52% ≥ 60 yrs; 82% men) with serum cholesterol of 5.5-8.0 mmol/L, triglycerides ≤ 2.5 mmol/L.
Intervention: Simvastatin 20 mg/day or placebo, with dosage titrated to reach target cholesterol level of 3.0-5.2 mmol/L.
Main outcomes: Total mortality, major coronary events.
Results: In the simvastatin group, the mean changes in total, LDL, and HDL cholesterol, and triglycerides, were -25%, -35%, +8%, and -10% respectively, with little change observed in the placebo group. Simvastatin significantly reduced the risks of death (RRR 0.70, p=0.0003), and major coronary events (RRR 0.66, p<0.00001).
Conclusion: Long-term treatment with simvastatin lowered cholesterol and improved survival in CHD patients.

Factors Affecting Risk Assessment

- metabolic syndrome (clustering of cardiovascular risk factors)
- apolipoprotein B (apoB):
  - each atherogenic particle (VLDL, IDL, LDL and lipoprotein(a)) contains one molecule of apoB
  - the serum concentration of apoB reflects the total number of particles and may be useful in assessing cardiovascular risk and adequacy of treatment in high risk patients and those with metabolic syndrome

Table 13. Optimal Target Levels of Apolipoprotein B by Risk Group

	High	Moderate	Low
Target apoB levels (g/L)	<0.85	<1.05	<1.2

- C-reactive protein (CRP) levels:
  - highly sensitive and may be clinically useful in identifying those at a higher risk of cardiovascular disease than predicted by the global risk assessment

Treatment of Dyslipidemias

Approach to Treatment

For clinical guidelines see *Can J Cardiol* 2006; 22(11):913-27.

- estimate 10-year risk of CAD using Framingham model (see Family Medicine)
- establish treatment targets according to level of risk (see Table 14 below)

Table 14. Target LDL by Risk Group

Level of Risk	10-year Risk of CAD	Target LDL (mmol/L)	(mg/dL)	Target TC/HDL
High	≥20%	<2.0	<78	<4
Moderate	10-19%	<3.5	<136.5	<5
Low	<10%	<5.0	<195	<6

Treatment of Hypercholesterolemia

- conservative: 4-6 month trial unless in high risk group in which case medical treatment should start immediately
  - diet
    - ↓ fat: <30% calories
    - ↓ saturated fat: <10% calories
    - ↓ cholesterol: <300 mg/day
    - ↑ fibre: >25-35 g/day
  - ↓ EtOH
  - smoking cessation
  - aerobic exercise: 30-60 minutes/day, 4-7 times/week
  - target body mass index (BMI) <25
- medical
  - HMG-CoA reductase inhibitors, ezetimibe, bile acid sequestrants, niacin (see *Common Medications,* E52 for further details)

Treatment of Hypertriglyceridemia

- conservative: 4-6 month trial
  - diet
    - ↓ fat and simple carbohydrates
    - ↑ omega-3 fatty acids
  - control blood sugars
  - ↓ EtOH
  - smoking cessation
  - aerobic exercise: 30-60 minutes/day, 4-7 times/week
  - target body mass index (BMI) <25
- medical: fibrates, niacin (see *Common Medications,* E53 for further details)
  - indications:
    - failed conservative measures
    - TG >10 mmol/L (885 mg/dL) to prevent pancreatitis
    - combined hyperlipidemia

For Statin Follow-Up
- lipids and liver enzymes every 4-6 months or if patient complains of jaundice, RUQ pain, dark urine
- CK at baseline and if patient complains of myalgia
- d/c statin if CK >10 x upper limit of normal

Simvastatin with or without ezetimibe in familial hypercholesterolemia
N Engl J Med. 2008;358:1431-43.
Study: Double-blind, randomized, 24-month trial.
Patients: Patients with familial hypercholesterolemia (n=720).
Intervention: Daily therapy with 80 mg of simvastatin either with placebo or with 10 mg of ezetimibe
Outcome: The primary outcome measure was the change in the mean carotid-artery intima-media thickness, which was defined as the average of the means of the far-wall intima-media thickness of the right and left common carotid arteries, carotid bulbs, and internal carotid arteries.
Results: The primary outcome, the mean (+/-SE) change in the carotid-artery intima-media thickness, was 0.0058+/-0.0037 mm in the simvastatin-only group and 0.0111+/-0.0038 mm in the simvastatin-plus-ezetimibe (combined-therapy) group (P=0.29). Secondary outcomes (consisting of other variables regarding the intima-media thickness of the carotid and femoral arteries) did not differ significantly between the two groups. At the end of the study, the mean (+/-SD) LDL cholesterol level was 4.98+/-1.56 mmol per liter in the simvastatin group and 3.65+/-1.36 mmol per liter in the combined-therapy group (a between-group difference of 16.5%, P<0.01). The differences between the two groups in reductions in levels of triglycerides and C-reactive protein were 6.6% and 25.7%, respectively, with greater reductions in the combined-therapy group (P<0.01 for both comparisons). Side-effect and safety profiles were similar in the two groups
Conclusions: In patients with familial hypercholesterolemia, combined therapy with ezetimibe and simvastatin did not result in a significant difference in changes in intima-media thickness, as compared with simvastatin alone, despite decreases in levels of LDL cholesterol and C-reactive protein.

Classification of Weight in Adults:

Classification	BMI
Underweight	<18.5
Normal	18.5-24.9
Overweight	25-29.9
Obese	≥30
- Class I	30-34.9
- Class II	35-39.9
- Class III	≥40

Note: Classifications are different for different ethnicities.

Meta-analysis: the effect of dietary counseling for weight loss.
Ann Intern Med. 2007;147:41-50.
Purpose: To perform a meta-analysis of the effect of dietary counseling compared with usual care on body mass index (BMI) over time in adults.
Study Selection: English-language randomized, controlled trials (> or =16 weeks in duration) in overweight adults that reported the effect of dietary counseling on weight. The authors included only weight loss studies with a dietary component.
Results: Random-effects model meta-analyses of 46 trials of dietary counseling revealed a maximum net treatment effect of -1.9 (95% CI, -2.3 to -1.5) BMI units (approximately -6%) at 12 months. Meta-analysis of changes in weight over time (slopes) and meta-regression suggest a change of approximately -0.1 BMI unit per month from 3 to 12 months of active programs and a regain of approximately 0.02 to 0.03 BMI unit per month during subsequent maintenance phases. Different analyses suggested that calorie recommendations, frequency of support meetings, inclusion of exercise, and diabetes may be independent predictors of weight change.
Limitations: The interventions, study samples, and weight changes were heterogeneous. Studies were generally of moderate to poor methodological quality. They had high rates of missing data and failed to explain these losses. The meta-analytic techniques could not fully account for these limitations.
Conclusions: Compared with usual care, dietary counseling interventions produce modest weight losses that diminish over time. In future studies, minimizing loss to follow-up and determining which factors result in more effective weight loss should be emphasized.

Long term pharmacotherapy for obesity and overweight: updated meta-analysis.
BMJ. 2007;335:1194-9.
Purpose: To summarise the long-term efficacy of anti-obesity drugs in reducing weight and improving health status.
Study Selection: Double blind randomised placebo controlled trials of approved anti-obesity drugs used in adults (age over 18) for one year or longer.
Results: Thirty trials of one to four years' duration met the inclusion criteria: 16 orlistat (n=10 631 participants), 10 sibutramine (n=2623), and four rimonabant (n=6365). Of these, 14 trials were new and 16 had previously been identified. Attrition rates averaged 30-40%. Compared with placebo, orlistat reduced weight by 2.9 kg (95% confidence interval 2.5 kg to 3.2 kg), sibutramine by 4.2 kg (3.6 kg to 4.7 kg), and rimonabant by 4.7 kg (4.1 kg to 5.3 kg). Patients receiving active drug treatment were significantly more likely to achieve 5% and 10% weight loss thresholds. Orlistat reduced the incidence of diabetes and improved concentrations of total cholesterol and low density lipoprotein cholesterol, blood pressure, and glycaemic control in patients with diabetes but increased rates of gastrointestinal side effects and slightly lowered concentrations of high density lipoprotein. Sibutramine lowered concentrations of high density lipoprotein cholesterol and triglycerides but raised blood pressure and pulse rate. Rimonabant improved concentrations of high density lipoprotein cholesterol and triglycerides, blood pressure, and glycaemic control in patients with diabetes but increased the risk of mood disorders.
Conclusions: Orlistat, sibutramine, and rimonabant modestly reduce weight, have differing effects on cardiovascular risk profiles, and have specific adverse effects.

Obesity

Definition
- presence of abnormal absolute amount or relative proportion of body fat
- Body Mass Index (BMI)
  - weight/height^2 (kg/m^2 or lbs/inches^2 x 703)
  - BMI >27 leads to increased health risk
- obesity: 20% or greater above ideal body weight (IBW) or BMI >30
- morbid obesity: 170% of IBW or BMI >40

Epidemiology
- 15-25% of North American adults

Etiology and Pathophysiology
- positive energy balance: energy input > energy output
- multifactorial
- increasing age is a risk factor
- genetic variations in energy expenditure
- behaviour/lifestyle - diet and exercise
- secondary causes
  - endocrine: Cushing's syndrome, PCOS, hypothyroidism
  - drugs: antidepressants, antiepileptics, antipsychotics, high dose glucocorticoids
  - hypothalamic injury: trauma, surgical, lesions in ventromedial or paraventricular median nucleus

Treatment
- treatment should be based on medical risk
- comprehensive approach including caloric restriction, increased physical activity and behaviour modification
- diet
  - caloric restriction with a balanced diet with reduced fat, sugar and alcohol
- exercise
- behaviour modification
  - individual or group therapy, self-monitoring, stimulus control, stress management, cognitive change, crisis intervention
- drug therapy
  - pancreatic lipase inhibitor: orlistat (Xenical™)
  - satiety enhancer: sibutramine (Meridia™)
- surgical therapy
  - gastroplasty ("stomach stapling")
  - laparoscopic banding of stomach (effective but costly)
  - liposuction
    - weight loss is regained by fat accumulation at the same site or elsewhere
    - not advocated if patient has significant medical comorbidities
    - does not reduce metabolic risks

Complications
- cardiovascular
  - hypertension, CAD, congestive heart failure (CHF), varicose veins, sudden death from arrhythmia
- respiratory
  - dyspnea, sleep apnea, pulmonary embolus, infections
- gastrointestinal
  - gallbladder disease, gastroesophageal reflux disease (GERD), fatty liver
- musculoskeletal
  - osteoarthritis
- endocrine/metabolic
  - IGT → Type 2 DM, hyperuricemia, hyperlipidemia, PCOS, hirsutism, irregular menses, infertility
- increased risk of neoplastic diseases
  - endometrial, post-menopausal breast, prostate, and colorectal cancers

Pituitary Gland

Pituitary Hormones

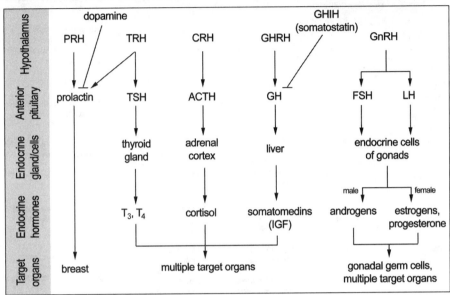

Figure 7. Hypothalamo-pituitary hormonal axes
CRH = corticotrophin-releasing hormone; GnRH = gonadotropin-releasing hormone; GHIH = growth hormone-inhibiting hormone; GHRH = growth hormone-releasing hormone; PRH = prolactin-releasing hormone; TRH = thyrotropin-releasing hormone

Hypothalamic Control of Pituitary
- trophic and inhibitory factors control the release of pituitary hormones
- most hormones are primarily under trophic stimulation except prolactin which is primarily under inhibitory control with dopamine
- transection of the pituitary stalk (i.e. dissociation of hypothalamus and pituitary) leads to pituitary hypersecretion of prolactin and hyposecretion of all remaining hormones

Anterior Pituitary Hormones
- growth hormone (GH), luteinizing hormone (LH), follicle stimulating hormone (FSH), thyroid stimulating hormone (TSH), adrenocorticotropic hormone (ACTH), and prolactin (PRL)

Hypothalamic Hormones
- antidiuretic hormone (ADH) and oxytocin
- peptides synthesized in the supraoptic and paraventricular nuclei of the hypothalamus

Table 15. The Physiology and Action of Pituitary Hormones

Hormone	Inhibitory Stimulus	Secretory Stimulus	Physiology	Function
GH	• glucose challenge • glucocorticoids • hypothyroidism • somatostatin • dopamine agonists • IGF-1 (long-loop)	• insulin induced hypoglycemia • exercise • REM sleep • arginine, clonidine, propranalol, L-dopa • GHRH	• polypeptide • acts indirectly through serum factors synthesized in the liver: IGF (somatomedins) • serum GH undetectable for most of the day and is suppressed after meals that are high in glucose • sustained rise during sleep	• needed for linear growth • IGF stimulates growth of bone and cartilage
PRL	• tonically by dopamine • D$_2$ receptor agonists	• sleep • stress • pregnancy • hypoglycemia • mid-menstrual cycle • breast feeding • TRH • sexual activity • dopamine antagonists • drugs: psychotropics, anti-hypertensives, opiates, high dose estrogen	• polypeptide • episodic secretion	• promotes milk production • inhibits GnRH secretion

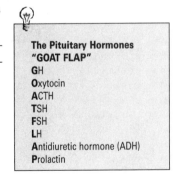

The Pituitary Hormones
"GOAT FLAP"
GH
Oxytocin
ACTH
TSH
FSH
LH
Antidiuretic hormone (ADH)
Prolactin

Table 15. The Physiology and Action of Pituitary Hormones (continued)

Hormone	Inhibitory Stimulus	Secretory Stimulus	Physiology	Function

LH/FSH	• estrogen
	• progesterone
	• testosterone
	• inhibin
	• continuous GnRH infusion
		• pulsatile GnRH	• polypeptide
			• glycoproteins (similar α subunit TSH and hCG)
			• secreted in pulsatile fashion
				• stimulate gonads via cAMP
				• ovary:
				  • LH stimulates theca cells to produce androgens which are subsequently converted to estrogens in granulosa cells
				  • LH induces luteinization in follicles
				  • FSH stimulates growth of granulosa cells in ovarian follicle and controls estrogen formation
				• testes:
				  • LH stimulates testosterone from Leydig cells
				  • FSH stimulates Sertoli cells to produce spermatozoa

ACTH	• dexamethasone • cortisol	• CRH • metyrapone • insulin induced hypoglycemia • fever, pain, stress	• polypeptide • pulsatile and diurnal variation (peaks at 2-4 am; lowest at 6pm-12 am)	• stimulates growth of adrenal cortex and secretion of its hormones
TSH	• circulating thyroid hormones (T_3, T_4) • opiates, dopamine	• TRH • epinephrine • prostaglandins	• glycoprotein	• stimulates growth of thyroid and secretion of T_4 and T_3 via cAMP
ADH	• ↓ serum osmolality	• hypovolemia or ↓ effective circulatory volume • ↑ serum osmolality • stress, pain, fever, paraneoplastic	• octapeptide • osmoreceptors in hypothalamus detect serum osmolality • contracted plasma volume is a more potent stimulus than osmolality	• acts at renal collecting ducts to stimulate insertion of aquaporin channels to increase water reabsorption thereby concentrating urine
Oxytocin	• EtOH	• suckling and distention of female genital tract	• nonapeptide	• causes uterine contraction • physiologic importance is unknown • breast milk secretion

Growth Hormone (GH)

GH DEFICIENCY
• cause of short stature in children (see <u>Pediatrics</u>)
• controversial significance in adults

GH EXCESS

Gigantism
• excess GH secretion before epiphyseal fusion

Acromegaly
• excess GH secretion in adults (after epiphyseal fusion)

Etiology
• pituitary adenoma secreting GH, carcinoid or pancreatic islet tumours secreting ectopic GHRH resulting in excess GH

Pathophysiology
• secretion remains pulsatile, but the nocturnal surge, glucose suppressibility, and hypoglycemic stimulation are lost
• proliferation of bone, cartilage, soft tissues, organomegaly
• insulin resistance and IGT

Clinical Features
• enlargement of hands and feet, coarsening of facial features, thickening of calvarium, prognathism, infraorbital puffiness, thickening of skin, ↑oiliness, sweating, acne, sebaceous cysts, fibromata mollusca, acanthosis nigricans, arthralgia, degenerative osteoarthritis (OA), thyromegaly, renal calculi, hypertension, cardiomyopathy, and DM

Investigations
• glucose suppression test is the most specific test → ↑GH in OGTT
• insulin-like growth factor-1 (IGF-1)

Treatment
• surgery, octreotide (somatostatin analogue), growth hormone receptor antagonist, bromocriptine, radiation

Signs and Symptoms of Acromegaly "ABCDEF"
Arthralgia/**A**rthritis
Blood pressure raised
Carpal tunnel syndrome
Diabetes
Enlarged organs
Field defect (visual)

Prolactin (PRL)

HYPERPROLACTINEMIA

Etiology
- prolactinoma is the most common pituitary adenoma (prolactin secreting tumours may be induced by estrogens and grow during pregnancy)
- pituitary stalk lesions
- primary hypothyroidism ($\uparrow$TRH)
- chronic renal failure resulting in decreased clearance, biliary cirrhosis
- medications with anti-dopaminergic properties are a common cause of high prolactin levels: antipsychotics, antidepressants, antihypertensives, anti-migraine agents (triptans/ergotamines), bowel motility agents (metoclopramide), H_2-blockers (e.g. ranitidine)

Clinical Features
- galactorrhea, infertility, hypogonadism

Investigations
- serum PRL, TSH, liver enzyme tests, creatinine
- MRI

Treatment
- long acting dopamine agonist: bromocriptine, cabergoline or quinagolide (Norprolac™)
- surgery ± radiation (rare)
- these tumours are very slow-growing and sometimes require no treatment
- if medication-induced, consider stopping medication if possible

Luteinizing Hormone (LH) and Follicle Stimulating Hormone (FSH)

HYPOGONADOTROPISM

Clinical Features
- hypogonadism, amenorrhea, erectile dysfunction (ED), loss of body hair, fine skin, testicular atrophy, failure of pubertal development

Treatment
- pergonal, hCG, or GnRH analogue if fertility desired
- symptomatic treatment with estrogen/testosterone

HYPERGONADOTROPISM
- 2° hypersecretion in gonadal failure

Antidiuretic Hormone (ADH)

DIABETES INSIPIDUS (DI)

Definition
- disorder resulting from deficient ADH action resulting in the passage of large volumes of dilute urine

Diagnostic Criteria
- fluid deprivation will differentiate true DI (high urine output persists, urine osmolality < plasma osmolality) from psychogenic DI (psychogenic polydipsia)
- response to exogenous ADH will distinguish central from nephrogenic DI

Etiology and Pathophysiology
- central DI: insufficient ADH due to post-pituitary surgery, tumours, stalk lesion, hydrocephalus, histiocytosis, trauma, familial central DI
- nephrogenic DI: collecting tubules in kidneys resistant to ADH (drugs including lithium, hypercalcemia, hypokalemia, chronic renal disease, hereditary nephrogenic DI)
- psychogenic polydipsia must be ruled out

Clinical Features
- passage of large volumes of dilute urine, polydipsia, dehydration

Treatment
- DDAVP/vasopressin for total DI
- DDAVP, chlorpropamide, clofibrate, or carbamazepine for partial DI
- nephrogenic DI treated with solute restriction and thiazide diuretics

SYNDROME OF INAPPROPRIATE ADH SECRETION (SIADH)

Diagnostic Criteria
- hyponatremia with corresponding plasma hypo-osmolality, urine sodium concentration above 40 mEq/L, urine less than maximally diluted (>100 mosm/kg), euvolemia (edema absent), and absence of adrenal, renal or thyroid insufficiency

> **Diagnosing Subtypes of DI After DDAVP:**
> **C**oncentrated urine = **C**entral
> **N**o effect = **N**ephrogenic

Etiology and Pathophysiology
- malignancy (lung, pancreas, lymphoma)
- CNS disease (inflammatory, hemorrhage, tumour, Guillain-Barré syndrome)
- respiratory disease (TB, pneumonia, empyema)
- drugs (vincristine, chlorpropamide, cyclophosphamide, carbamazepine, nicotine, morphine, DDAVP, oxytocin)
- stress (post-surgical)

Treatment
- treat underlying cause, fluid restriction, and demeclocycline (antibiotic with anti-ADH properties)

Pituitary Pathology

PITUITARY ADENOMA (see also Neurosurgery)

Clinical Features
- related to size and location
  - visual field defects (usually bitemporal hemianopsia), oculomotor palsies, increased ICP (may have headaches)
  - skull radiograph: "double floor" (large sella or erosion), calcification
  - CT and MRI far more sensitive for diagnosis
- related to destruction of gland
  - hypopituitarism
- related to increased hormone secretion
  - PRL (galactorrhea), GH (acromegaly in adults, gigantism in children), ACTH (Cushing's disease = Cushing's syndrome caused by a pituitary tumour), tumours secreting LH, FSH and TSH are rare

EMPTY SELLA SYNDROME
- occurs when subarachnoid space extends into sella turcica, partially filling it with CSF resulting in remodeling and enlargement of sella turcica and flattening of the pituitary gland
- usually eupituitary
- may have headaches
- MRI: herniation of diaphragm sellae and the presence of CSF in the sella turcica
- no treatment necessary

PITUITARY APOPLEXY
- acute hemorrhage/infarction of pituitary tumour
- sudden severe headache, altered level of consciousness
- ocular symptoms: ophthalmoplegia with pituitary tumour likely indicates apoplexy since tumour rarely gets big enough to encroach on cranial nerves
- neurosurgical emergency: acute decompression of pituitary via trans-sphenoidal route

HYPOPITUITARISM

Etiology
- the eight "I"s:
  - Invasive: generally primary tumours
  - Infarction: e.g. Sheehan's syndrome
  - Infiltrative disease: e.g. sarcoidosis, hemochromatosis, histiocytosis
  - Iatrogenic: following surgery or radiation
  - Infectious: e.g. syphilis, TB
  - Injury: severe head trauma
  - Immunologic: autoimmune destruction
  - Idiopathic: familial forms, congenital midline defects

Clinical Features
- typical clinical progression in panhypopituitarism (GH (most common deficiency) → LH/FSH → ACTH → TSH)
- fall in GH is clinically not apparent
- fall in PRL is variable, but may present as decreased lactation
- gonadotropin insufficiency causes erectile dysfunction in men and amenorrhea or infertility in women
- TSH deficiency produces clinical hypothyroidism
- ACTH deficiency leads to adrenal insufficiency

Investigations
- Triple Bolus Test
  - stimulates release of all anterior pituitary hormones in normal individuals
  - rapid sequence IV infusion of insulin, gonadotropin releasing hormone (GnRH) and thyroid releasing hormone (TRH)
  - insulin (usual dose 0.15 units/kg of human regular insulin) → hypoglycemia → increased GH and ACTH
  - GnRH (100 μg IV push) → increased LH and FSH
  - TRH (200 μg IV push over 60 sec) → increased TSH and PRL

Thyroid

Thyroid Hormones

Thyroid Hormone Synthesis
- the synthesis of T_4 (thyroxine) and T_3 (triiodothyronine) by the thyroid gland involves trapping and oxidation of iodide, iodination of thyroglobulin, and release of T_4 and T_3
- free T_4 (0.03%) and free T_3 (0.3%) represent the hormonally active fraction of thyroid hormones
- the remaining fraction is bound to thyroxine binding globulin (TBG) and albumin and is hence biologically inactive
- T_3 is more biologically active (3-8x more potent), but T_4 has longer half-life
- 85% of T_4 is converted to T_3 or reverse T_3 (RT_3) in the periphery by 5' or 5 deiodinase, respectively
- RT_3 is metabolically inactive but produced in times of stress to decrease metabolic activity
- most of the plasma T_3 pool is derived from the peripheral conversion of T_4

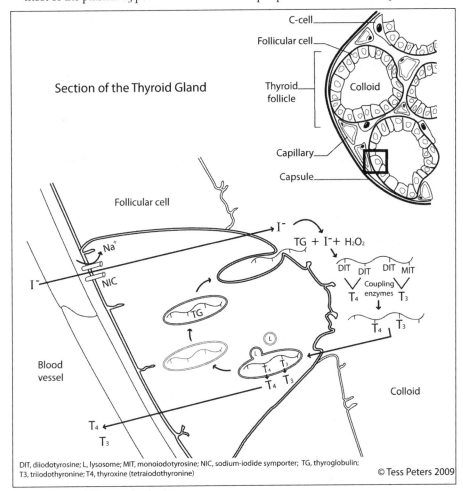

DIT, diiodotyrosine; L, lysosome; MIT, monoiodotyrosine; NIC, sodium-iodide symporter; TG, thyroglobulin; T3, triiodothyronine; T4, thyroxine (tetraiodothyronine)

© Tess Peters 2009

Figure 8. Thyroid Hormone Synthesis

Regulation of Thyroid Function
- extrathyroid
  - stimulation of thyroid by TSH, epinephrine, prostaglandins (cAMP stimulators)
  - T_3 negatively feeds back on anterior pituitary to inhibit TSH and on hypothalamus to inhibit TRH
- intrathyroid (autoregulation)
  - increasing iodide supply inhibits iodide organification, thus decreasing T_3 and T_4 synthesis (Wolff-Chaikoff effect)
  - varying thyroid sensitivity to TSH in response to iodide availability
  - increased ratio of T_3 to T_4 in iodide deficiency
  - increased activity of peripheral 5' deiodinase in hypothyroidism to increase T_3 production despite low T_4 levels

Tests of Thyroid Function and Structure

TSH
- sensitive TSH (sTSH) is the single best test for assessing thyroid function
- hyperthyroidism
  - primary: TSH is low and does not rise in response to TRH because of negative feedback from increased levels of circulating T_3 and T_4
  - secondary: increased TSH which results in increased T_3 and T_4
- hypothyroidism
  - primary: increased TSH (most sensitive test) because of less negative feedback from T_3 and T_4
  - secondary: TSH is low with variable response to TRH depending on the site of the lesion (pituitary or hypothalamic)

Free T_3 and Free T_4
- total T_3 and T_4 levels depend on amount of TBG
- TBG increases with pregnancy, oral contraceptive (OCP) use, acute infectious hepatitis, biliary cirrhosis
- TBG decreases with androgens, glucocorticoids, cirrhosis, hyponatremia, phenytoin, ASA, NSAIDS, nephrotic syndrome, severe systemic illness
- free T_3 and T_4 are independent of TBG and measure biological activity
- standard assessment of thyroid function measures TSH and if necessary free T_4 and free T_3

Thyroid Autoantibodies
- thyroglobulin antibodies (TgAb), thyroid peroxidase (microsomal antibodies), TSH receptor inhibiting antibodies
  - increased in Hashimoto's disease
- thyroid stimulating immunoglobulin (TSI)
  - increased in Graves' disease

Plasma Thyroglobulin
- used to monitor residual thyroid activity post-thyroid ablation, e.g. for thyroid cancer recurrence
- undetectable levels = remission
- normal or elevated levels = probable persistent, recurrent, or metastatic disease

Serum Calcitonin
- not routinely done to investigate most thyroid nodules
- ordered if suspicious of medullary thyroid carcinoma or family history of MEN IIa or IIb syndromes

Thyroid Imaging/Scans
- normal gland size 15-20 g (estimated by palpation)
- thyroid U/S
  - to detect size of gland, solid vs. cystic nodule
- thyroid scan (Technetium-99)
  - differentiates between hot (functioning) and cold (non-functioning) nodules
  - to distinguish between three major types of high-uptake hyperthyroidism
    - Graves' disease (diffuse uptake)
    - toxic multinodular goiter (multiple discrete areas)
    - solid toxic adenoma (single intense area of uptake)
  - test of structure – order if there is a thyroid nodule and patient is hyperthyroid
- radioactive iodine uptake (RAIU)
  - RAIU measures the turnover of iodine by thyroid gland in vivo
  - in areas of low iodine intake and endemic goitre, 24 h RAIU may be as high as 60-90%
  - in areas of high iodine intake, normal 24 h RAIU will be 8-30%
  - RAIU is high in Graves' disease or toxic nodular goitre and low in subacute thyroiditis, active phase of Hashimoto's thyroiditis, and excess iodine intake (e.g. amiodarone)
  - test of function – order if patient is hyperthyroid

Thyroid Biopsy
- fine needle aspiration (FNA) for cytology
  - differentiates between benign and malignant disease

Hyperthyroidism

Definition
- excess production of thyroid hormone
- thyrotoxicosis: denotes clinical, physiological, and biochemical findings in response to elevated thyroid hormone

Epidemiology
- 1% of general population (4-5% of elderly women)
- F:M = 5:1

Etiology and Pathophysiology

Table 16. Differential Diagnosis of Hyperthyroidism

Disorder	TSH	T_4 and T_3	Thyroid Antibodies	RAIU	Other
Graves' disease	↓	↑	TSI	↑	
Toxic Nodular Goitre	↓	↑	—	↑	
Toxic Nodule	↓	↑	—	↑	
Thyroiditis					
• Subacute	↓	↑	Up to 50% of cases	↓	In classical subacute thyroiditis, ESR ↑
• Silent					
• Postpartum					
McCune-Albright syndrome	↓	↑	—	—	At least 2 of polyostotic fibrous dysplasia, café au lait spots, and autonomous endocrine hyperfunction
Jod Basedow	↓	↑	—	↓	iodine induced
Extrathyroidal sources of thyroid hormone:					
• Endogenous: (struma ovariae, ovarian teratoma, metastatic follicular ca)	↓	↑	—	↓	
• Exogenous (drugs)					
Excessive Thyroid stimulation					
• Pituitary thyrotrophoma	↑	↑	—	↑	
• Pituitary thyroid hormone receptor resistance	↑	↑	—	↑	
• ↑ hCG (e.g. pregnancy)	↓	↑	—	↑	

Clinical Features

Table 17. Clinical Features of Hyperthyroidism

General	• fatigue, heat intolerance, irritability, fine tremor
Cardiovascular	• tachycardia, atrial fibrillation, palpitations
	• elderly patients may have only cardiovascular symptoms, commonly new onset atrial fibrillation
GI	• weight loss with ↑ appetite, thirst, increased frequency of bowel movements (hyperdefecation)
Neurology	• proximal muscle weakness, hypokalemic periodic paralysis (common in Orientals)
GU	• scant menses, ↓ fertility
Dermatology	• fine hair, skin moist and warm, vitiligo, soft nails with onycholysis (Plummer's nails), clubbing (acropachy), palmar erythema, pretibial mxyedema
MSK	• ↓ bone mass, proximal muscle weakness
Hematology	• leukopenia, lymphocytosis, splenomegaly, lymphadenopathy (occasionally in Graves' disease)

> **Signs and Symptoms of hyperTHYROIDISM:**
> **T**remor
> **H**eart rate up
> **Y**awning (fatigued)
> **R**estlessness
> **O**ligomenorrhea/amenorrhea
> **I**ntolerance to heat
> **D**iarrhea
> **I**rritability
> **S**weating
> **M**uscle wasting/weight loss

Treatment
- antithyroid drugs (thionamides: propylthiouracil (PTU) or methimazole (MMI))
- β-blockers
- radioactive iodine thyroid ablation
- surgery

Graves' Disease

Definition
- syndrome characterized by hyperthyroidism with any one of the following features including diffuse goiter, ophthalmopathy, dermopathy (need not appear together)

Epidemiology
- most common cause of thyrotoxicosis
- occurs at any age with peak in 3rd and 4th decade
- F > M = 7:1, 1.5-2% of U.S. women
- familial predisposition: 15% of patients have a close family member with Graves' disease and 50% have family members with positive circulating antibodies
- association with HLA B8 and DR3
- may be associated with other autoimmune disorders in family (e.g. pernicious anemia, Hashimoto's disease)

Etiology and Pathophysiology
- autoimmune disorder due to a defect in T-suppressor cells
- B-lymphocytes produce TSI that bind the TSH receptor and stimulate the thyroid
- immune response can be triggered by pregnancy (especially postpartum), iodine excess, lithium therapy, viral or bacterial infections, glucocorticoid withdrawal
- cause of ophthalmopathy uncertain (can occur even when euthyroid)
  - antibodies against extraocular muscle antigens (fibroblasts implicated) with lymphocytic infiltration
  - glycosaminoglycan deposition
- dermopathy may be related to cutaneous glycosaminoglycan deposition

Clinical Features
- diffuse goiter ± bruit
- ophthalmopathy: proptosis, lid lag, lid retraction, diplopia, characteristic stare, conjunctival injection
- dermopathy (rare): pretibial myxedema (thickening of dermis)
- acropachy: clubbing and thickening of distal phalanges

Investigations
- increased free T_4 (and/or increased T_3)
- positive for TSI
- TRH stimulation test (with a flat TSH response) is diagnostic, if sTSH and free T_4 are inconclusive

Treatment
- thionamides
  - propylthiouracil (PTU) or methimazole (MMI)
  - inhibit thyroid hormone synthesis by inhibiting the peroxidase catalyzed reactions, thereby inhibiting organification of iodide, blocking the coupling of iodotyrosines, and inhibiting peripheral deiodination of T_4 to T_3
  - most useful in young patients with small glands and mild disease
  - continue treatment until remission occurs (20-40% of patients achieve spontaneous remission at 6-18 mos of treatment)
  - small goitre and recent onset are good indicators for long-term remission with medical therapy
  - MMI contraindicated in pregnancy
  - major side effects: hepatitis and agranulocytosis
  - minor side effects: rash, fever and arthralgias
  - iodinated contrast agents: sodium ipodate and iapanoic acid can inhibit conversion of T_4 to T_3 and is especially effective in combination with MMI
- symptomatic treatment with β-blockers
- thyroid ablation with radioactive ^{131}I if PTU or MMI trial does not produce disease remission
  - high incidence of hypothyroidism after ^{131}I, requiring lifelong thyroid hormone replacement
  - contraindicated in pregnancy
- subtotal thyroidectomy (indicated rarely for large goitres)
  - risks include hypoparathyroidism and vocal cord palsy
- ophthalmopathy
  - prevent drying
  - high dose prednisone in severe cases
  - orbital radiation, surgical decompression

Prognosis
- course involves remissions and exacerbations unless gland is destroyed by radioactive iodine or surgery
- some patients remain euthyroid after treatment however many develop hypothyroidism
- lifetime follow-up care needed
- risk of relapse is 37%, 21%, 6% in thionamindes, radioiodine ablation, and surgery groups respectively

Radioiodine therapy for Graves' disease and the effect on ophthalmopathy - a systematic review
Clin Endocrinol (Oxf). 2008 Apr 21
Purpose: To assess whether radioiodine therapy (RAI) for Graves' disease GD is associated with increased risk of ophthalmopathy compared with antithyroid drugs (ATDs) or surgery. To assess the efficacy of glucocorticoid prophylaxis in the prevention of occurrence or progression of ophthalmopathy, when used with RAI.
Study Selection: Randomized controlled trials regardless of language or publication status.
Results: RAI was associated with an increased risk of ophthalmopathy compared with ATD (Relative Risk (RR) 4.23, 95% confidence interval (CI): 2.04 to 8.77) but compared with thyroidectomy, there was no statistically significant increased risk (RR 1.59, 95% CI 0.89 to 2.81). The risk of severe GO was also increased with RAI compared with ATD (RR 4.35, 95% CI 1.28 to 14.73). Prednisolone prophylaxis for RAI was highly effective in preventing the progression of GO in patients with pre-existing GO (RR 0.03; 95% CI 0.00 to 0.24). The use of adjunctive ATD with RAI was not associated with any significant benefit on the course of GO.
Conclusions: Radioiodine therapy for Graves' disease is associated with a small but definite increased risk of development or worsening of Graves' ophthalmopathy compared with antithyroid drugs. Steroid prophylaxis is beneficial for patients with pre-existing Graves' ophthalmopathy.

Subacute Thyroiditis (Thyrotoxic Phase)

Definition
- acute inflammatory disorder of the thyroid gland characterized by an initial thyrotoxic state followed by hypothyroidism

Etiology and Pathophysiology
- acute inflammation of the thyroid, probably viral in origin, characterized by giant cells and lymphocytes

- often preceded by upper respiratory tract infection (URTI)
- disruption of thyroid follicles by inflammatory process results in the release of stored hormone

Clinical Features
- initially presents with fever, malaise, and soreness in neck
- thyroid gland enlarges
- two forms
  - painful ("DeQuervain's") thyroid, ears, jaw and occiput
  - painless ("Silent")
- usually transient thyrotoxicosis with a subsequent hypothyroidism phase due to depletion of stored hormone, finally resolving in a euthyroid state over a period of months

Laboratory Investigation
- elevated free T_4, T_3, low TSH, RAIU markedly reduced
- marked elevation of ESR in painful variety only
- as disease progresses, values consistent with hypothyroidism may appear
- rise in RAIU reflects gland recovery

Treatment
- high-dose anti-inflammatories (e.g. ASA) can be used for painful form (increases peripheral T_4 conversion)
- prednisone may be required for severe pain, fever, or malaise
- β-adrenergic blockade is usually effective in reversing most of the hypermetabolic and cardiac symptoms
- if symptomatically hypothyroid may treat short-term with thyroxine

Prognosis
- full recovery in most cases, but permanent hypothyroidism in 10% of painless thyroiditis

Postpartum Thyroiditis

Definition
- painless thyroiditis occurring in the postpartum period

Epidemiology
- occurs in 5-10% of postpartum mothers and is symptomatic in 1/3 of patients

Etiology and Pathophysiology
- autoimmune-mediated

Clinical Features
- thyrotoxicosis 2-3 months postpartum with a subsequent hypothyroid phase at 4-8 months postpartum
- may be mistakenly diagnosed as postpartum depression

Treatment
- same as silent thyroiditis

Prognosis
- most resolve spontaneously without need for supplementation
- may recur with subsequent pregnancies

Toxic Adenoma/Toxic Multinodular Goitre

Etiology and Pathophysiology
- autonomous thyroid hormone production from a functioning adenoma that is hypersecreting T_3 and T_4
- may be singular (toxic adenoma) or multiple (toxic multinodular goitre, aka Plummer's disease)

Clinical Features
- goitre with adenomatous changes
- occurs more frequently in elderly people
- tachycardia, heart failure, arrhythmia, weight loss, nervousness, weakness, tremor, and sweats
- atrial fibrillation is a common presentation in the elderly

Investigations
- low TSH, high T_3 and T_4 (with a larger increase in T_3)
- thyroid scan with increased uptake in nodule(s), and suppression of the remainder of the gland

Treatment
- initiate therapy with PTU or MMI to attain euthyroid state in order to avoid radiation thyroiditis
- then use high dose radioactive iodine to ablate tissue over weeks
- propranolol often necessary for symptomatic treatment prior to definitive therapy
- surgery may be used as 2nd line treatment

Thyrotoxic Crisis/Thyroid Storm

Definition
- acute exacerbation of all of the symptoms of thyrotoxicosis presenting in a life threatening state secondary to uncontrolled hyperthyroidism

Etiology and Pathophysiology
- often precipitated by infection, trauma, or surgery in a hyperthyroid patient

Differential Diagnosis
- sepsis, pheochromocytoma, malignant hyperthermia, drugs

Clinical Features
- hyperthyroidism
- extreme fever (hyperthermia), tachycardia, vomiting, diarrhea, vascular collapse, hepatic failure with jaundice, and confusion
- arrhythmia $\rightarrow$ congestive heart failure, pulmonary edema
- mental status changes ranging from delirium to coma

Laboratory Investigations
- increased free T_3, T_4, undetectable TSH
- ± anemia, leukocytosis, hypercalcemia, elevated LFTs

Treatment
- principles are the same as in hyperthyroidism except use higher doses and frequencies
- initiate prompt therapy; do not wait for confirmation from lab
- propranolol (IV) for tachycardia and to $\downarrow$ peripheral conversion of T_4 to T_3 (watch for CHF)
- supportive: fluid and electrolytes, diuresis, vasopressors, cooling blanket, acetaminophen for pyrexia
- high dose PTU
- iodide (NaI, KI, Lugol's solution) to inhibit release of thyroid hormone
- lithium to inhibit release of thyroid hormone
- dexamethasone to block peripheral conversion, to lower body temperature, and to treat possible underlying autoimmune condition
- if extreme, plasmapheresis or dialysis to remove high circulating thyroid hormone
- treat precipitant

Prognosis
- 50% mortality rate

Hypothyroidism

Definition
- clinical syndrome caused by cellular responses to insufficient thyroid hormone production

Epidemiology
- 2-3% of general population
- F:M = 10:1
- 10-20% of women over age 50 have subclinical hypothyroidism (normal T_4, TSH mildly elevated)

Etiology and Pathophysiology
- primary hypothyroidism (90%)
    - inadequate thyroid hormone production secondary to intrinsic thyroid defect
    - iatrogenic: post-ablative (^{131}I or surgical thyroidectomy)

- autoimmune: Hashimoto's thyroiditis, chronic thyroiditis, idiopathic, burnt out Graves'
  - hypothyroid phase of subacute thyroiditis
  - drugs: goitrogens (iodine), PTU, MMI, lithium
  - infiltrative disease (progressive systemic sclerosis, amyloid)
  - iodine deficiency
  - congenital (1/4000 births)
  - neoplasia
- secondary hypothyroidism: pituitary hypothyroidism
  - insufficiency of pituitary TSH
- tertiary hypothyroidism: hypothalamic hypothyroidism
  - decreased TRH from hypothalamus (rare)
- peripheral tissue resistance to thyroid hormone (Refetoff syndrome)

Table 18. Interpretation of Serum TSH and Free T$_4$ in Hypothyroidism

	Serum TSH	Free T$_4$
Overt Primary Hypothyroidism	↑	↓
Subclinical Primary Hypothyroidism	↑	Normal
Secondary Hypothyroidism	↓ or not appropriately elevated	↓

Clinical Features

Table 19. Clinical Features of Hypothyroidism

General	• fatigue, cold intolerance, slowing of mental and physical performance, hoarseness, macroglossia
CVS	• slow pulse, pericardial effusion, bradycardia, hypertension, worsening CHF + angina, hypercholesterolemia, hyperhomocysteinemia, myxedema heart
GI	• weight gain with poor appetite, constipation
Neurology	• paresthesia, slow speech, muscle cramps, delay in relaxation phase of deep tendon reflexes ("hung reflexes"), Carpal Tunnel syndrome, asymptomatic increase in CK seizures
GU	• menorrhagia, amenorrhea, impotence
Dermatology	• puffiness of face, periorbital edema, cool and pale, dry and rough skin, hair dry and coarse, eyebrows thinned (lateral 1/3), discoloration (carotenemia)
Hematology	• anemia: 10% pernicious due to presence of anti-parietal cell antibodies
Respiratory	• decreased exercise capacity, hypoventilation secondary to weak muscles, decreased pulmonary responses to hypoxia, sleep apnea due to macroglossia

Treatment

- L-thyroxine (dose range: 0.05-0.2 mg PO OD)
- elderly patients and those with CAD: start at 0.025 mg daily and increase gradually (start low, go slow)
- after initiating L-thyroxine, serum T$_4$ & TSH need to be evaluated in 6 weeks; doses adjusted until TSH returns to normal reference range
- once maintenance dose achieved, follow-up with patient annually
- secondary/tertiary hypothyroidism:
  - need to r/o and/or treat adrenal insufficiency
  - monitor via measuring free T$_4$ level NOT ONLY TSH

CONGENITAL HYPOTHYROIDISM

- see Pediatrics

Hashimoto's Thyroiditis

- chronic autoimmune thyroiditis characterized by both cellular and humoral factors in the destruction of thyroid tissue
- two major forms: goitrous and atrophic; two forms share same pathophysiology but differ in the extent of lymphocytic infiltration, fibrosis, and thyroid follicular cell hyperplasia
- goitrous variant usually presents with a rubbery goiter and euthyroidism, then hypothyroidism becomes evident
  - is associated with fibrosis
- atrophic variant patients are hypothyroid from the start
  - is associated with thyroid lymphoma

Thyroid hormone replacement for subclinical hypothyroidism
Cochrane Database Syst Rev. 2007;(3):CD003419
Purpose: To assess the effects of thyroid hormone replacement for subclinical hypothyroidism.
Study Selection: randomised controlled trials comparing thyroid hormone replacement with placebo or no treatment in adults with subclinical hypothyroidism. Minimum duration of follow-up was one month.
Results: We did not identify any trial that assessed (cardiovascular) mortality or morbidity. Seven studies evaluated symptoms, mood and quality of life with no statistically significant improvement. One study showed a statistically significant improvement in cognitive function. Six studies assessed serum lipids, there was a trend for reduction in some parameters following levothyroxine replacement. Some echocardiographic parameters improved after levothyroxine replacement therapy, like myocardial relaxation, as indicated by a significant prolongation of the isovolumic relaxation time as well as diastolic dysfunction. Only four studies reported adverse events with no statistically significant differences between groups.
Conclusions: In current RCTs, levothyroxine replacement therapy for subclinical hypothyroidism did not result in improved survival or decreased cardiovascular morbidity. Data on health-related quality of life and symptoms did not demonstrate significant differences between intervention groups. Some evidence indicates that levothyroxine replacement improves some parameters of lipid profiles and left ventricular function.

Signs and Symptoms of hypothyroidism "HIS FIRM CAP":

Hypoventilation
Intolerance to cold
Slow HR

Fatigue
Impotence
Renal impairment
Menorrhagia/amenorrhea

Constipation
Anemia
Paresthesia

Etiology and Pathophysiology
- defect in clone of T-suppressors leads to cell-mediated destruction of thyroid follicles
- B-lymphocytes produce antibodies against thyroid components including: thyroglobulin, thyroid peroxidase, TSH receptor, Na/I symporter

Risk Factors
- gender: female
- genetic susceptibility: increased frequency in patients with Down's syndrome, Turner's syndrome, certain HLAs, cytotoxic T-lymphocyte-associated protein 4 (CTLA-4)
- family Hx or personal Hx of other autoimmune diseases
- cigarette smoking
- high iodine intake
- stress and infection

Investigations
- high TSH, low T_3, low T_4
- presence of thyroid peroxidase and thyroglobulin antibodies in serum

Treatment
- if hypothyroid, replace with L-thyroxine (analog of T_4)
- if euthyroid, also treat with L-thyroxine if significant anti-thyroid antibody present

Riedel's Struma/Woody Thyroiditis

- rare type of chronic thyroiditis
- fibrotic inflammatory process that extends from the thyroid into surrounding tissues

Clinical Features
- ill-defined, firm mass with "woody" consistency on palpation
- possible compressive symptoms of dysphagia, stridor, hoarseness, pain

Treatment
- surgical wedge resection of the isthmus (to prevent tracheal compression)
- tamoxifen, prednisone

Myxedema Coma

Definition
- severe hypothyroidism complicated by trauma, sepsis, cold exposure, MI, inadvertent administration of hypnotics or narcotics, and other stressful events
- rare but serious mortality of up to 60% despite therapy

Clinical Features
- hypothermia, hyponatremia, hypoglycemia, hypotension, bradycardia, hypoventilation, unresponsiveness

Investigations
- decreased free T_3 and T_4, increased TSH, decreased glucose
- check ACTH and cortisol for evidence of adrenal insufficiency

Treatment
- aggressive treatment required
- ABCs – patient should be in ICU setting
- corticosteroids (due to the possibility of concomitant adrenal insufficiency): hydrocortisone 100 mg q8h
- L-thyroxine 0.2-0.5 mg IV loading dose, then 0.1 mg IV OD until oral therapy tolerated
- supportive measures: mechanical ventilation, fluids, vasopressor drugs, passive rewarming, IV dextrose
- monitor for arrhythmia

Sick Euthyroid Syndrome (SES)

Definition
- denotes the changes in circulating thyroid hormones in patients with serious illness, trauma, or stress
- not due to intrinsic thyroid or pituitary disease.

Pathophysiology
- the abnormalities in SES include alterations in
  - peripheral transport and metabolism of thyroid hormone
  - regulation of TSH secretion
  - thyroid function itself

Labs
- initially decreased free T_3 followed by decreased TSH and finally decreased free T4

Etiology

Table 20. Etiology of SES

Types of SES	Features
normal-T_4 variant	• low free T_3, normal free T_4, normal TSH • proposed mechanism: inhibition of peripheral 5' monodeiodination of T_4 to T_3
low-T_4 variant	• low free T_3, low free T_4, normal or low TSH • low T_4 likely due to inhibited T_4 binding to serum proteins and accelerated metabolic clearance • poorer prognosis

Treatment
• treat the underlying disease; thyroid hormone replacement worsens the outcome

Non-Toxic Goitre

Definition
• generalized enlargement of the thyroid gland in a euthyroid individual that does not result from inflammatory or neoplastic processes

Pathophysiology
• the appearance of a goitre is more likely during adolescence, pregnancy, and lactation because of increased thyroid hormone requirements
  ▪ early stages: goitre is usually diffuse
  ▪ later stages: multinodular non-toxic goitre with nodule, cyst formation and areas of ischemia, hemorrhage, and fibrosis

Etiology
• iodine deficiency or excess
• goitrogens: brassica vegetables (turnip, cassava)
• drugs: iodine, lithium, para-aminosalicylic acid
• any disorder of hormone synthesis with compensatory growth
• peripheral resistance to thyroid hormone

Treatment
• remove goitrogens
• suppression with L-thyroxine (rarely used)
• surgery may be necessary for severe compressive symptoms

Complications
• compression of neck structures causing stridor, dysphagia, pain, and hoarseness
• multinodular goitre may become autonomous leading to toxic multinodular goitre and hyperthyroidism

Thyroid Nodules

Definition
• clearly defined discrete mass, separated from the thyroid parenchyma
• palpable nodules are found in approximately 4% of the population
• M:F = 1:4

Etiology
• benign tumours (e.g. follicular adenoma)
• thyroid malignancy
• hyperplastic area in a multinodular goiter
• cyst: true thyroid cyst, area of cystic degeneration in a multinodular goiter

Investigations
• FNA: for all nodules >1-1.5 cm
• thyroid function tests
• thyroid scan: 15-20% of cold nodules (minimal ^{131}I uptake into nodule) are malignant, very low malignant potential if hot (significant ^{131}I uptake into nodule)

Thyroid Malignancies

• see <u>Otolaryngology</u>

Adrenal Cortex

Adrenocorticotropin Hormone (ACTH)

- a polypeptide secreted in a pulsatile fashion from the anterior pituitary with diurnal variability (peak: 0200-0400; trough: 1800-2400)
- part of a prohormone (pro-opiomelanocorticotropin, POMC) which contains α, β and γ MSH, β-endorphin and lipotropin as well as ACTH
- stimulates growth of adrenal cortex and secretion of its hormones via cAMP
- stimulates release of glucocorticoids, androgens and, to a limited extent, mineralocorticoids
- some melanocyte stimulating activity

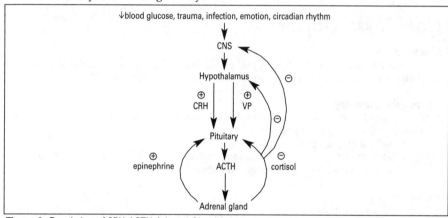

Figure 9. Regulation of CRH-ACTH-Adrenal Gland Axis

Adrenocortical Hormones

- all derived from cholesterol
    - mineralocorticoids (aldosterone) from zona glomerulosa
    - glucocorticoids (cortisol) from zona fasciculata
    - androgens from zona reticularis

Aldosterone
- a mineralcorticoid, which regulates extracellular fluid (ECF) volume through Na retention and K excretion (by stimulation of distal tubule Na/K ATPase)
- regulated by the renin-angiotensin-aldosterone system
- negative feedback to juxtaglomerular apparatus (JGA) by long loop (aldosterone via volume expansion) and short loop (angiotensin II via peripheral vasoconstriction)

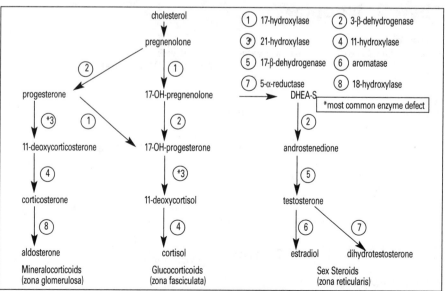

Figure 10. Pathways of Major Steroid Synthesis in the Adrenal Gland and Their Enzymes

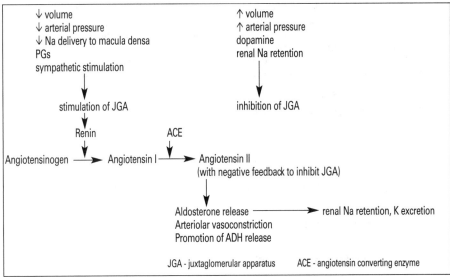

Figure 11. Renin-Angiotensin-Aldosterone Axis, see Nephrology

Cortisol

Table 21. Physiological Effects of Glucocorticoids

Stimulatory Effects	Inhibitory Effects
• stimulate hepatic glucose production (gluconeogenesis) • increase insulin resistance in peripheral tissues • increase protein catabolism • stimulate leukocytosis and lymphopenia	• inhibit bone formation; stimulate bone resorption • inhibit fibroblasts, causing collagen and connective tissue loss • suppress inflammation; impair cell-mediated immunity

Androgens

- sex steroids regulated by ACTH; primarily responsible for adrenarche (growth of axillary and pubic hair)
- principal adrenal androgens are dihydroepiandrosterone (DHEA), androstenedione and 11-hydroxyandrostenedione
- proportion of total androgens (adrenal to gonadal) increases in old age

Tests of Adrenocortical Function

Table 22. Markers of Adrenocortical Function

Plasma cortisol	diurnal variation response to stimulation or suppression more informative
24 hour urinary free cortisol	correlates well with secretory rates good screening test for adrenal hyperfunction
Serum ACTH	high in primary adrenal insufficiency low in secondary adrenal insufficiency
Serum DHEA-S	the main adrenal androgen

Dexamethasone (DXM) Suppression Tests (DST)

- gold standard to determine presence and etiology of hypercortisolism
- principle: DXM suppresses pituitary ACTH, so plasma cortisol should be lowered by negative feedback if HPA axis were normal
- single dose DST: simple and reasonably accurate screening test
    - DXM 1 mg given at 2300h would suppress pituitary ACTH production in healthy individuals, so that the normal 0800h peak of plasma cortisol would fail to develop
    - 95% of Cushing's syndrome patients would fail to suppress
    - <20% false +ve results due to simple obesity, depression, alcohol, other medications
- confirmatory tests
    - low dose DST: 0.5 mg DXM q6h for 48 hours, then 24 hour urinary free cortisol (UFC) twice → normally the UFC level would be reduced to < 54 nmol/day

- high dose DST (8 mg/day): 70-80% of those with adrenal cortex hyperplasia due to hypersecretion of pituitary ACTH would show suppression, whereas adrenal cortisol-producing adenoma/carcinoma and ectopic ACTH would show no changes in UFC levels or serum cortisol
    - however, 30-40% of ectopic ACTH tumours may partially suppress
- plasma ACTH assay supplements DST for differentiation of the various etiologies of Cushing's

Short Cosyntropin Stimulation Test
- for diagnosing adrenal insufficiency, note: dexamethasone treatment does not interfere with this assay
- cosyntropin is an ACTH analogue
- 250 μg cosyntropin IM or IV, measure serum cortisol and ACTH at baseline, and cortisol at 30 and 60 minutes
- physiological response: increase in plasma cortisol level by >250-500 μmol/L or doubling of baseline and an absolute level of >550 μmol/L (rules out primary adrenal insufficiency)
- inappropriate response: inability to stimulate plasma cortisol rise

Hyperaldosteronism

PRIMARY HYPERALDOSTERONISM

Definition
- diastolic hypertension without edema; decreased renin and increased aldosterone secretion both of which are unresponsive to increases in volume

Etiology
- aldosterone-producing adrenal adenoma (Conn's syndrome) (75%)
- adrenal hyperplasia (25%):
  (a) idiopathic
  (b) glucocorticoid-remediable aldosteronism
- adrenal carcinoma (1%)
- adrenal enzyme defect (see Pediatrics)

Clinical Features
- hypertension refractory to standard treatment
- polyuria, polydipsia, nocturia
- fatigue, weakness, paresthesia, headache
- severe cases: tetany, intermittent paralysis

Investigations
- electrolytes: ↓K, ↓Mg, ↑Na
- high 24 hour urinary or plasma aldosterone + low random plasma renin

Treatment
- medical: spironolactone or amiloride; hydrochlorothiazide (HCTZ) or ACE inhibitor might be added for better blood pressure control
- surgical: removal of adenoma

SECONDARY HYPERALDOSTERONISM

Definition
- increase in aldosterone in response to activation of renin-angiotensin system

Etiology and Pathophysiology

Table 23. Etiology and Pathophysiology of Hyperreninism

	Etiology	Pathophysiology
(a) **primary hyperreninism**	• renin-producing tumour	
(b) **secondary hyperreninism**	• renal artery stenosis	• hypoperfusion of kidneys
	• CHF, cirrhosis, nephrosis	• decreased effective circulating volume
	• diuretics/laxative abuse	• JGA hyperplasia
	• Bartter's syndrome	

Cushing's Syndrome

Definition
- results from chronic glucocorticoid excess (endogenous or exogenous sources)

Etiology
- ACTH-dependent (85%): bilateral adrenal hyperplasia and hypersecretion due to:
  - ACTH-secreting pituitary adenoma (Cushing's disease responsible for 80% of ACTH-dependent)
  - ectopic ACTH-secreting tumour (e.g. small cell lung carcinoma, bronchial, carcinoid, pancreatic, adrenal or thyroid tumours)
- ACTH-independent (15%)
  - long-term use of exogenous glucocorticoids
  - primary adrenocortical tumours: adenoma and carcinoma (uncommon)
  - bilateral adrenal nodular hyperplasia

Clinical Features

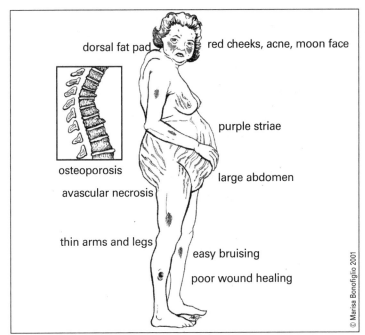

Figure 12. Features of Cushing's Syndrome

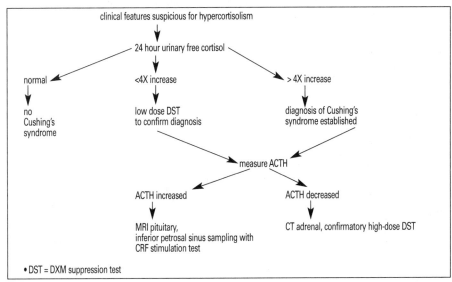

Figure 13. Hypercortisolism: Algorithm for Diagnosis

Treatment
- pituitary
    - transsphenoidal resection, with glucocorticoid supplement peri- and post-operatively
    - irradiation: only 50% effective, with significant risk of hypopituitarism
- adrenal
    - adenoma: unilateral adrenalectomy (curative)
    - carcinoma: palliative (frequent metastases, poor prognosis); adjunctive chemotherapy often not useful
- ectopic ACTH tumour - usually bronchogenic cancer (paraneoplastic syndrome)
    - chemotherapy/radiation for primary tumour
    - agents blocking adrenal steroid synthesis: metyrapone or ketoconazole
    - poor prognosis

Congenital Adrenal Hyperplasia

- see Pediatrics

Hyperandrogenism

Definition
- state of having excessive secretion of androgens

Etiology and Pathophysiology

Table 24. Etiology of Hyperandrogenism

Constitutional/Familial	family history, predisposing ethnic background
Medications androgen-mediated	anabolic steroids, ACTH, androgens, progestational agents
Ovarian	PCOS (see Gynecology, GY24) ovarian hyperthecosis theca cell tumours
Adrenal	congenital hyperplasia (CAH, late-onset CAH) tumours
Pituitary	Cushing's disease - high ACTH

Clinical Features

Hirsutism
- male pattern growth of androgen-dependent terminal body hair in women: back, chest, upper abdomen, face, linea alba

Virilization
- masculinization: hirsutism, temporal balding, clitoral enlargement, deepening of voice, acne
- increase in musculature

Defeminization
- loss of female secondary sex characteristics (i.e. amenorrhea, decreased breast size)

Investigations
- increased testosterone
- increased LH/FSH, seen commonly in PCOS as ratio >2.5
- DHEA-S as measure of adrenal androgen production
- 17-OH progesterone is elevated in CAH due to 21-OH deficiency

Treatment
- discontinue causative medications
- oral contraceptives (e.g. cyproterone acetate – blocks androgen receptor; found in Diane 35™)
- spironolactone - acts as peripheral androgen antagonist
- cosmetic therapy
- low dose glucocorticoid if CAH suspected

Two conditions that do NOT represent true hirsutism
1. androgen-independent hair (e.g. lanugo hair)
2. drug-induced hypertrichosis (e.g.phenytoin,diazoxide, cyclosporine, minoxidil)

Adrenocortical Insufficiency

PRIMARY (ADDISON'S DISEASE)

Etiology

Table 25. Etiology of Primary Adrenocortical Insufficiency

Autoimmune (70-90%) (most common in developed world) (60-75% of pts have antibodies against adrenal enzymes and 3 zones of the cortex)	Isolated adrenal insufficiency Polyglandular autoimmune syndrome type I & II
Infection	TB (7-20%) (most common in developing world) Fungal: histoplasmosis, paracoccidioidomycosis HIV Syphilis African trypanosomiasis
Metastatic Ca	Lung, breast, stomach, colon, lymphoma
Adrenal hemorrhage or infection	Coagulopathy in adults or Waterhouse-Friderichsen syndrome in children (meningococcal or Pseudomonas septicemia), heparin, coumadin
Drugs	Ketoconazole, rifampin, phenytoin, barbituates, megestrol acetate
Others	Adrenoleukodystrophy Congenital adrenal hypoplasia Familial glucocorticoid deficiency or resistance

SECONDARY ADRENOCORTICAL INSUFFICIENCY

- inadequate pituitary ACTH secretion
- multiple etiologies (see *Hypopituitarism*, E20), including withdrawal of exogenous steroids that have suppressed pituitary ACTH production

Clinical Features

Table 26. Clinical Features of Adrenocortical Insufficiency

	Acute Adrenal Crisis	Chronic Addison's	2° Adrenal Insufficiency
Clinical Features	Weight loss Weakness Dehydration Hypotension Vitiligo Hyperpigmentation (buccal mucosa, flexor/palmar creases) Nx/Vx + Hx of wt loss + anorexia Acute abdomen Unexplained hypoglycemia Unexplained fever Other autoimmune endocrine deficiencies (e.g. hypothyroidism, gonadal failure)	Weight loss Weakness Fatigue Hypotension Vitiligo Hyperpigmentation Anorexia GI: Nx/Vx, constipation, abdo pain, diarrhea Salt craving Postural dizziness Myalgia Arthralgia	Many of the signs and symptoms seen in primary adrenal insufficiency are also present here EXCEPT: NO hyperpigmentation GI: less common NO salt craving
Labs	Hyponatremia Hyperkalemia Hypercalcemia Azotemia Eosinophilia Anemia Lymphocytosis Hypoglycemia	Hyponatremia Hyperkalemia Hypercalcemia Azotemia Eosinophilia Anemia Low cortisol unresponsive to exogenous ACTH High ACTH Adrenal antibodies if autoimmune etiology	NO hyperkalemia Hyponatremia often present Low cortisol, low ACTH Hypoglycemia is more common

Treatment

- acute condition - can be life-threatening
    - IV NS or D5W/NS in large volumes (2-3 L)
    - hydrocortisone 100 mg IV q6-8h for 24h, then gradual tapering
    - identify and correct precipitating factors
- maintenance
    - hydrocortisone 15-20 mg PO qam and 5-10 mg qpm
    - Florinef™ (fludrocortisone, synthetic mineralocorticoid) 0.05-0.2 mg PO daily if mineralocorticoid deficient
    - increase dose of steroid 2- to 3- fold for a few days during illness or for surgery
    - medical alert bracelet for patient

ABC of Adrenaline
Adrenaline activates
β-receptors, increasing
Cyclic AMP

Adrenal Medulla

Catecholamine Metabolism

- catecholamines are synthesized from tyrosine in postganglionic sympathetic nerves and chromaffin cells of adrenal medulla
- predominant adrenal catecholamine = epinephrine (adrenaline)
- predominant peripheral catecholamine = norepinephrine (noradrenaline)

Pheochromocytoma

Definition
- rare catecholamine secreting tumour derived from chromaffin cells of the sympathetic system

Epidemiology
- most commonly a single tumour of adrenal medulla
- 10% extra-adrenal (95% of which are intra-abdominal), 10% multiple tumours, 10% malignant, 10% familial
- rare cause of hypertension (<0.2% of all hypertensives)
- curable if recognized and properly treated, but fatal if not

Etiology and Pathophysiology
- most cases sporadic
- familial: associated with multiple endocrine neoplasia II (MEN II) (50%), von Hippel-Lindau (10-20%), paraganglioma (20%), or neurofibromatosis type 1 (NF I) (0.1-5.7%)
- tumours, via unknown mechanism, able to synthesize and release catecholamines
- signs and symptoms caused by hypersecretion of catecholamines

Classic Triad of
PHEochromocytoma
Palpitations
Headache
Episodic sweating

Clinical Features
- 50% suffer from paroxysmal HTN, and the rest have sustained HTN
- classic triad: episodic "pounding" headache, palpitations/tachycardia, diaphoresis
- other symptoms: tremor, anxiety, chest or abdominal pain, nausea/vomiting, visual blurring, wt loss, polyuria, polydipsia
- other signs: orthostatic hypotension, papilledema, increased ESR, hyperglycemia, dilated cardiomyopathy
- symptoms may be triggered by stress, exertion, anesthesia, abdominal pressure, certain foods (especially tyramine containing foods)

Investigations
- urine catecholamines
    - increased catecholamine metabolites (vanillylmandelic acid + metanephrines) and free catecholamines
    - total metanephrines: most sensitive test; >6.5 μmol/day or 1.2 mg/day
- plasma catecholamines
    - >2000 pg/ml (11.8 mmol/L) diagnostic; >950 pg/ml (5.6 mmol/L) suggestive → proceed to clonidine suppression test (rarely done)
    - elevated plasma epinephrine unsuppressed by clonidine (central α-adrenergic) diagnostic
- CT scan
    - if CT is negative, meta-iodo-benzoguanidine (MIBG) scintigraphy, Octreoscan, or MRI might help

Treatment
- adequate pre-operative preparation
- α-blockade for BP control - phenoxybenzamine (14-21 days pre-op), IV phentolamine (peri-operative)
- β-blockade for HR control – propranolol (initiate only after adequate α-blockade)
- metryosine (catecholamine synthesis inhibitor) + phenoxybenzamine or prazosin also used
- volume restoration with vigorous salt-loading
- surgical removal of tumour with careful pre-operative and post-operative ICU monitoring
- rescreen urine one month post-operatively

Multiple Endocrine Neoplasm (MEN)

- neoplastic syndromes involving multiple endocrine glands
- tumours of neuroectodermal origin
- autosomal dominant inheritance with variable penetrance
- genetic screening for RET proto-oncogene on chromosome 10 has long term benefit
  - early cure and prevention of medullary thyroid cancer

Table 27. MEN Classification

Type	Chromosome Implicated	Tissues Involved	Clinical Manifestations
MEN I **Wermer's** **syndrome**	11 (PYGM gene)	• Pituitary	Ant. pituitary adenoma, often non-secreting but may secrete GH and PRL
		• Parathyroid	Primary hyperparathyroidism from hyperplasia
		• Entero-pancreatic endocrine	Pancreatic islet cell tumours Gastrinoma (peptic ulcers) Insulinomas (hypoglycemia) VIPomas (secretory diarrhea)
MEN II **3 distinct syndromes**	10 (RET proto-oncogene) autosomal dominant		
IIa **Sipple's** **syndrome**		• Thyroid • Adrenal medulla • Parathyroid • Skin	Medullary thyroid cancer (MTC) (>90%) Pheochromocytoma (40-50%) 1° parathyroid hyperplasia (10-20%) Cutaneous lichen amyloidosis
Familial **Medullary** **Thyroid Ca.** **(a variant of IIa)**		• Thyroid	Medullary thyroid ca without other clinical manifestations of MEN IIa or IIb
IIb		• Thyroid	Medullary thyroid ca: most common component, more aggressive and earlier onset than MEN IIa
		• Adrenal medulla • Neurons	Pheochromocytoma Mucosal neuroma, intestinal ganglioneuromas
		• MSK	Marfanoid habitus (no aortic abnormalities) Parathyroid hyperplasia-NOT a feature
		• GI	Chronic constipation Megacolon

> **MEN I - Wermer's Syndrome affects the 3 Ps**
> **P**ituitary
> **P**arathyroid
> **P**ancreas

History
- MEN I
  - symptoms of hyperparathyroidism, gastrinoma (abdominal pain, diarrhea, peptic ulcer diseases), and insulinoma
- MEN II
  - family history of MEN syndromes
  - symptoms related to MTC, hyperparathyroidism, or pheochromocytoma
  - scaly skin rash (cutaneous lichen amyloidosis in MEN IIa)

Physical
- clinical picture depends on the endocrine organs involved and the hormones secreted
- MEN I
  - hyperparathyroidism – nephrolithiasis, bone abnormalities, MSK complaints, generalized weakness, and alterations of mental status in severe hypercalcemia
  - gastrinoma – upper abdominal pain due to peptic ulcers and esophagitis
  - glucagonoma – rash, anorexia, anemia, diarrhea, glossitis
  - pituitary tumor – headache, visual-field defects, prolactinoma (erectile dysfunction, decreased libido, amenorrhea, galactorrhea), acromegaly
  - carcinoid syndrome – flushing, diarrhea, bronchospasm

- MEN II – physical signs are very variable and often subtle
  - MTC – neck mass or thyroid nodule; non-tender, anterior neck lymph nodes
  - pheochromocytoma - elevated BP and HR

Investigations
- MEN I
  - laboratory
    - gastrinoma – elevated serum gastrin level (>200 ng/mL) after IV injection of secretin at 2 IU/kg of body weight
    - insulinoma – fasting blood glucose (hypoglycemia)
    - glucagonoma – elevated blood glucose and glucagon levels
    - pituitary tumours – assess GH and prolactin levels
    - hyperparathyroidism – PTH levels; bone density scan (DEXA)
  - imaging
    - MRI for pituitary tumors, gastrinoma, insulinoma
- MEN II
  - laboratory
    - genetic screening for RET mutations in all index patients; if a mutation is identified, screen family members who are at risk
    - calcitonin levels, urine catecholamines, vanillylmandelic acid and metanephrine screen (pheochromocytoma); serum Ca and PTH levels (hyperparathyroidism)
    - pentagastrin +/- Ca stimulation test if calcitonin level is within reference range
  - imaging
    - CT or MRI for imaging of the adrenals
  - metaiodobenzylguanidine (MIBG) scan for pheochromocytoma
  - radionuclide scanning for determining the extent of metastasis
  - octreoscan for examining the spread of MTC
  - FNA (fine-needle aspiration) for thyroid nodules

Treatment
- MEN I
  - surgery is indicated for hyperparathyroidism, insulinoma, glucagonoma, pituitary tumours (transsphenoidal surgery with external radiation when medical treatment fails)
  - PPI for acid hypersecretion in gastrinoma
  - bromocriptine or other dopamine agonists to suppress prolactin secretion
  - somatostatin for symptomatic carcinoid tumors
- MEN II
  - surgery for MEN IIa
  - pre-op treatment:
    - PG inhibitors to alleviate diarrhea associated with thyroid cancer
    - α-blocker for at least 2 weeks for pheochromocytoma
    - hydration for hypercalcemia; if remains severely hypercalcemic, consider calcitonin or bisphosphonates
  - post-op treatment:
    - hormone replacement following total thyroidectomy and bilateral adrenalectomy
    - calcium supplement and/or vitamin D for post-op hypoparathyroidism

Calcium Homeostasis

- normal total serum Ca: 2.25-2.62 mmol/L; 9.0-10.5 mg/dL
- ionic/free Ca levels: 1.15-1.31 mmol/L; 4.6-5.25 mg/dL
- serum Ca is about 50% protein bound (mostly albumin)
- regulated mainly by two factors: parathyroid hormone (PTH) and vitamin D
- actions mainly on three organs: GI tract, bone, and kidney

Parathyroid Hormone (PTH)
- secretion increased by low serum Ca and inhibited by low serum Mg (chronic)
- not influenced directly by PO_4 (except by PO_4 effect on the ionic calcium levels)

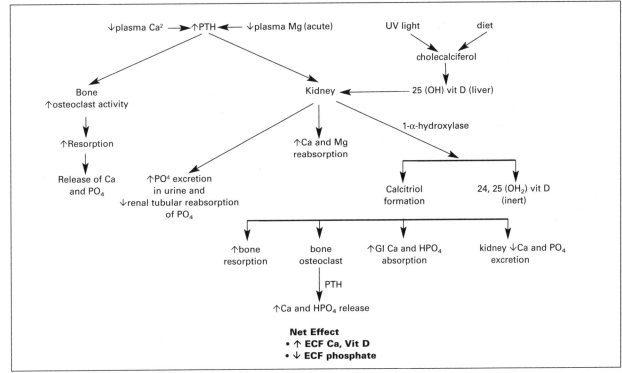

Figure 14. Parathyroid Hormone (PTH) Regulation

Vitamin D
- necessary for Ca and PO_4 absorption from GI tract
- cholecalciferol formed in the skin by the action of UV light

Calcitonin
- polypeptide secreted by thyroid C cells
- secretion enhanced by Ca, GI hormones, pentagastrin
- major actions
  - decreased osteoclastic bone resorption (pharmacological effect)
  - increased renal PO_4 and Na clearance
  - acute net effect: decreased serum Ca when given in pharmacologic doses

Magnesium
- major intracellular divalent cation
- Ca is reabsorbed from the kidney with Mg, and thus Ca balance is difficult to maintain in Mg deficiency

Phosphorus
- intracellular cation
- found in all tissues and necessary for most biochemical processes as well as bone formation

Table 28. Summary of Effects

Hormone	Net Effect
Parathyroid Hormone (PTH)	↑ Ca ↑ Vit D ↓ PO_4
Vitamin D	↑ Ca ↑ PO_4
Calcitonin (in pharmacologic doses)	↓ Ca

Hypercalcemia

Definition

- total corrected serum Ca >2.62 mmol/L (10.5 mg/dL) OR ionized Ca >1.35 mmol/L (5.4 mg/dL)
- corrected Ca (mmol/L) = measured Ca + $\frac{0.25 (40 - \text{albumin})}{10}$

- for every ↓ in albumin by 10, ↑ in Ca by 0.25

benign (less likely malignant):
Ca <2.75 mmol/L (11 mg/dL)

pathologic (more likely malignant):
Ca >3.25 mmol/L (13 mg/dL)

Pseudohypercalcemia: increased protein binding leading to an elevation in serum total Ca without a rise in the ionized/free form, e.g. hyperalbuminemia from severe dehydration.

Watch Out For:
- volume depletion via diuresis
- arrhythmias

High or Normal PTH		
Primary Hyperparathyroidism (major cause of hypercalcemia) • Solitary adenoma 81% • Hyperplasia 15% • Carcinoma 4% • MEN I and IIa	Suspect if: • positive FHx • Hx of MENI/IIa • Hx of childhood H+N radiation • postmenopausal woman • normal physical exam	• Presentation: 50% asymptomatic, renal calculi, neuromuscular disease, decreased bone density and associated consequences • asymptomatic with prolonged hyperparathyroidism • Investigations: serum Ca, PO_4, PTH, diagnostic imaging for renal calculi and osteopenia • Treatment: continued surveillance vs. surgery
Secondary Hyperparathyroidism	Suspect if: • chronic renal failure due to decreased Vit D synthesis	
Tertiary Hyperparathyroidism	Suspect if: • chronic renal failure • renal transplant patient	• Persistent increase in PTH after correction of secondary hyperparathyroidism
Familial hypocalciuric hypercalcemia (FHH) • Autosomal dominant • positive FHx	Suspect if: • asymptomatic patient • hypocalciuric	• Mutation in calcium sensing receptor gene leads to inappropriate secretion of PTH and excessive tubal reabsorption of calcium • DDx of hypocalciuria: FHH, milk alkali syndrome, thiazide, primary hyperparathyroidism if concomitant Vit D deficiency
Drug induced • Lithium		• Increase in set point where PTH secretion will be suppressed
Low PTH		

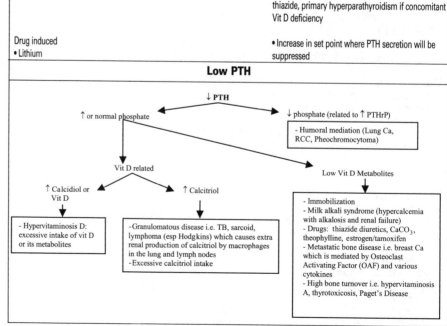

Figure 15. Etiology and Clinical Approach to Hypercalcemia

Clinical Features
- symptoms dependent on the absolute Ca value and the rate of its rise (may be asymptomatic)

Table 29. Symptoms of Hypercalcemia

Cardiovascular	GI	Renal	Rheumatological	MSK	Psychiatric		Neurologic
Hypertension	Constipation	Polyuria	Gout	Weakness	↑alertness ⌐		Hypotonia
Arrhythmia	Anorexia	Polydipsia	Pseudogout	Bone pain (**bones**)	Anxiety		Hyporeflexia
Short QT	Nausea	Nephrogenic DI	Chondrocalcinosis		Depression		Myopathy
Deposition of Ca	Vomiting	Nephrolithiasis (**stones**)			Cognitive	>3 mmol/L	Paresis
on valves,	(**groans**)	Renal failure			dysfunction	(12 mg/dL)	
coronary arteries,	PUD	(irreversible)			Organic brain		
myocardial fibres	pancreatitis				syndromes ⌐		
					Psychosis >4 mmol/L (16 mg/dL)		
					(**moans**)		

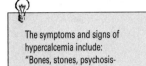

The symptoms and signs of hypercalcemia include: "Bones, stones, psychosis-based moans, and abdominal groans"

Treatment
- treatment depends on the Ca level and the symptoms
- treat acute, symptomatic hypercalcemia aggressively

Table 30. Treatment of Hypercalcemia

Increase urinary Ca excretion	Isotonic saline (4-5 L) ± loop diuretic (i.e. furosemide) but only if hypervolemic
Diminish bone resorption	Bisphosphonates (Tx of choice) • inhibit osteoclast activity • indicated in malignancy-related hypercalcemia IV pamidronate is most commonly used several days (2-4 days) until full effect but effect is long-lasting (2-4 weeks) Calcitonin → additive effect with bisphosphonates • inhibits osteoclastic bone resorption and promotes renal excretion of calcium • acts rapidly but often transient response (↓ by 0.3-0.5 mmol/L (1.2 mg/dL - 2.0 mg/dL) beginning within 4-6 hours) • combination of calcitonin and steroids may prolong reduction in calcium • tachyphylaxis may occur Mithramycin (rarely used) - effective when patient cannot tolerate large fluid load (dangerous - hematotoxic and hepatotoxic)
Decrease GI Ca absorption	Corticosteroids in hypervitaminosis D and hematologic malignancies • anti-tumour effects → ↓ calcitriol production by the activated mononuclear cells in lung and lymph node • slow to act (5-10 days); need high dose
Dialysis	
Chelation	EDTA or IV phosphate (rarely used) Oral phosphate in chronic hypercalcemia

The most common cause of hypercalcemia in hospital inpatients is malignancy-associated hypercalcemia

- Usually occurs in the later stages of disease
- Most commonly seen in renal, breast, ovarian and squamous tumors, as well as lymphoma and multiple myeloma.
- Mechanism: Secretion of parathyroid hormone-related protein (PTHrP) which mimics PTH action by preventing renal calcium excretion and activating osteoclast-induced bone resorpion.

Primary hyperparathyroidism is the most common cause of hypercalcemia in healthy outpatients.

Others
- prostaglandin inhibitors
- surgical treatment if indicated
- avoid immobilization

Hypocalcemia

Definition
• total corrected serum Ca <2.25 mmol/L (9.0 mg/dL)

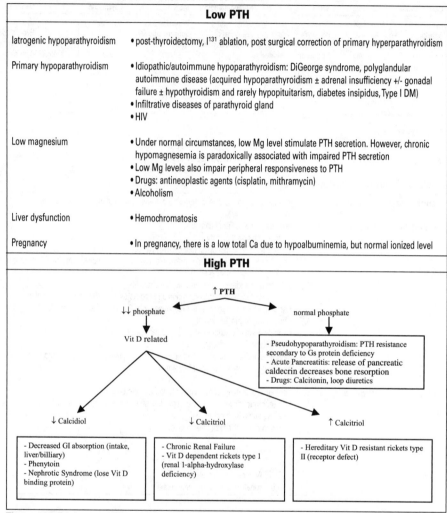

Low PTH	
Iatrogenic hypoparathyroidism	• post-thyroidectomy, I[131] ablation, post surgical correction of primary hyperparathyroidism
Primary hypoparathyroidism	• Idiopathic/autoimmune hypoparathyroidism: DiGeorge syndrome, polyglandular autoimmune disease (acquired hypoparathyroidism ± adrenal insufficiency +/- gonadal failure ± hypothyroidism and rarely hypopituitarism, diabetes insipidus, Type I DM) • Infiltrative diseases of parathyroid gland • HIV
Low magnesium	• Under normal circumstances, low Mg level stimulate PTH secretion. However, chronic hypomagnesemia is paradoxically associated with impaired PTH secretion • Low Mg levels also impair peripheral responsiveness to PTH • Drugs: antineoplastic agents (cisplatin, mithramycin) • Alcoholism
Liver dysfunction	• Hemochromatosis
Pregnancy	• In pregnancy, there is a low total Ca due to hypoalbuminemia, but normal ionized level

Figure 16. Etiology and Clinical Approach to Hypocalcemia

Clinical Features
• most characteristic symptom is tetany

Differential Diagnosis of Tetany
• metabolic alkalosis (with hyperventilation)
• hypokalemia
• hypomagnesemia

Table 31. Clinical Features of Hypocalcemia

Acute Hypocalcemia	Chronic Hypocalcemia
Delirium	CNS: lethargy, seizures, psychosis, basal ganglia calcification, Parkinson's, dystonia, hemiballismus, papilledema, pseudotumour cerebri
Laryngospasm (with stridor)	
Paresthesia	CVS: prolonged QT interval
Hyperreflexia	GI: steatorrhea
Tetany	ENDO: impaired insulin release
Psychiatric Sx: emotional instability, anxiety and depression	SKIN: dry, scaling, alopecia, brittle and transversely fissured nails, moniliasis, abnormal dentition
Chvostek's sign (tap CNVII)	OCULAR: cataracts
Trousseau's sign (carpal spasm)	MSK: generalized muscle weakness and wasting

Signs and Sympotms of Acute Hypocalcemia

• Paresthesias: perioral, hands and feet
• Chvostek's sign: percussion of the facial nerve just anterior to the external auditory meatus elicits unilateral spasm of the orbicularis oculi or orbicularis oris muscle
• Trousseau's sign: inflation of a blood pressure cuff above systolic pressure for 3 minutes elicits carpal spasm and paresthesia

Treatment
- correct underlying disorder
- mild/asymptomatic (ionized Ca >0.8 mmol/L, 3.2 mg/dL)
  - treat by increasing dietary Ca by 1000 mg/day
- acute/symptomatic hypocalcemia (ionized Ca <0.7 mmol/L, 2.8 mg/dL)
  - immediate treatment required
  - IV calcium gluconate 1-2 g in 10-20 mins followed by slow infusion if necessary
- goal is to raise Ca to low normal range (2.0-2.1 mmol/L, 8.0-8.4 mg/dL) to prevent symptoms but allow maximum stimulation of PTH
- if PTH recovery not expected, requires long-term therapy with vitamin D and calcium
- do not correct hypocalcemia if it is suspected to be a transient response

Hyperphosphatemia

- pathophysiology: 2 general mechanisms

Etiology
- **increased intake**
  - GI intake (rectal enema, GI bleeding)
    - IV phosphate load (K-Phos, blood transfusion)
    - endogenous phosphate (tumour lysis syndrome, rhabdomyolysis, hemolysis)
- **reduced renal clearance**
  - ARF/CRF
  - hypoparathyroidism
  - acromegaly
  - tumour calcinosis (ability of kidney to specifically clear phosphate is defective)

Clinical Features
- non-specific

Treatment
- low PO_4 diet, phosphate binders (e.g. $CaCO_3$)

Hypophosphatemia

- pathophysiology: 4 general mechanisms

Etiology
- **inadequate intake**
  - starvation
  - malabsorption (diarrhea, steatorrhea)
  - antacid use
  - alcoholism
- **renal losses**
  - hyperparathyroidism
  - diuretics
  - x-linked or AD hypophosphatemic rickets
  - Fanconi syndrome
- **excessive skeletal mineralization**
  - osteoblastic metastases
  - post parathyroidectomy (referred to as 'hungry bone syndrome')
- **PO_4 shift into ICF**
  - recovery from metabolic acidosis
  - respiratory alkalosis
  - starvation refeeding (stimulated by insulin)

Clinical Features
- non-specific (CHF, coma, hypotension, weakness)

Treatment
- treat underlying cause, supplement with oral PO_4: 2-4 g/d divided bid-qid (start at 1000 mg/d to minimize diarrhea)

Hypermagnesemia

- pathophysiology: 2 general mechanisms

Use of calcium or calcium in combination with vitamin D supplementation to prevent fractures and bone loss in people aged 50 years and older: a meta-analysis
Lancet. 2007;370:657-66.
Purpose: To determine whether supplementation with calcium or calcium in combination with vitamin D reduces fractures of all types and percentage change of bone-mineral density from baseline.
Study Selection: Randomized trials that recruited people aged 50 years or older.
Results: In trials that reported fracture as an outcome (17 trials, n=52 625), treatment was associated with a 12% risk reduction in fractures of all types (risk ratio 0.88, 95% CI 0.83-0.95; p=0.0004). In trials that reported bone-mineral density as an outcome (23 trials, n=41 419), the treatment was associated with a reduced rate of bone loss of 0.54% (0.35-0.73; p<0.0001) at the hip and 1.19% (0.76-1.61%; p<0.0001) in the spine. The fracture risk reduction was significantly greater (24%) in trials in which the compliance rate was high (p<0.0001). The treatment effect was better with calcium doses of 1200 mg or more than with doses less than 1200 mg (0.80 vs 0.94; p=0.006), and with vitamin D doses of 800 IU or more than with doses less than 800 IU (0.84 vs 0.87; p=0.03).
Conclusions: Evidence supports the use of calcium, or calcium in combination with vitamin D supplementation, in the preventive treatment of osteoporosis in people aged 50 years or older. For best therapeutic effect, we recommend minimum doses of 1200 mg of calcium, and 800 IU of vitamin D (for combined calcium plus vitamin D supplementation).

Bisphosphonates in osteoporosis
NEJM 1995;333:1437-43
Study: Randomized, blinded, placebo-controlled trial (3 year follow-up).
Patients: 994 post-menopausal women (mean 64 yrs, 87% white) with low BMD (t≤2.5). Exclusions included hx of glucocorticoid use, other disorders of bone, active PUD, and renal or hepatic insufficiency.
Intervention: alendronate 5 mg, 10 mg, 20 mg, or placebo, each once daily. All received calcium 500 mg/day. In the 3rd year, women in the 20 mg group were blindly switched to 5 mg.
Main outcomes: Change in BMD, new vertebral fractures, and height.
Results: Women in all 3 alendronate groups had significant increases in BMD, while those in the placebo group had significant decreases. Women taking alendronate had fewer new vertebral fractures (RRR 52%, NNT 34, 95% CI 16 to 518), and a lower mean loss of height (p=0.005). There were no significant differences between groups for non-vertebral fractures, adverse effects, or discontinuation rates.
Conclusion: In post-menopausal women with osteoporosis, alendronate increased BMD, and reduced the risk of new vertebral fractures.

Etiology
- Mg-containing antacids given to those with severe renal failure
- IV administration of large doses of $MgSO_4$ (e.g. for pre-eclampsia - see Obstetrics)

Clinical Features
- drowsiness, hyporeflexia, respiratory depression, decreased deep tendon reflexes

Treatment
- stop Mg-containing products

Hypomagnesemia

- pathophysiology: 2 general mechanisms

Etiology
- GI
    - starvation
    - malabsorption
    - vomiting
    - alcoholism
    - acute pancreatitis
- excess renal loss
    - 2° hyperaldosteronism due to cirrhosis and CHF
    - hyperglycemia
    - hypokalemia
    - hypercalcemia
    - diuretics

Clinical Features
- seizures, paresthesia, Chvostek and Trousseau signs

Treatment
- Mg IM/IV (note: cellular uptake of Mg is slow therefore repletion requires sustained correction)
- discontinue diuretics
- in patients requiring diuretics, use a K-sparing diuretic to reduce the amount of magnesuria

Metabolic Bone Disease

Osteoporosis

Definition
- a condition characterized by decreased bone mass and microarchitectural deterioration of bone tissue with a consequent increase in bone fragility and susceptibility to bone fracture

Etiology and Pathophysiology

Primary Osteoporosis

Etiology
- post-menopausal decline in estrogen or increased age

Commonly Seen Fractures
- vertebral, hip, wrist, proximal humerus, pelvis

Secondary Osteoporosis
- gastrointestinal diseases
    - gastrectomy
    - malabsorption
    - chronic liver disease
- bone marrow disorders
    - multiple myeloma
    - lymphoma
    - leukemia
- endocrinopathies
    - Cushing's syndrome
    - hyperparathyroidism
    - hyperthyroidism
    - premature menopause
    - diabetes

- malignancy
  - multiple myeloma
  - breast cancer
  - prostate cancer
- drugs
  - corticosteroid therapy → 2nd most common cause of osteoporosis
    - individuals receiving 7.5 mg of prednisone daily for over 3 mo should be assessed for bone-sparing therapy
    - mechanism: increased resorption + decreased formation
  - phenytoin
  - chronic heparin therapy
  - androgen deprivation therapy
  - aromatase inhibitors
- others
  - rheumatologic disorders
    - rheumatoid arthritis
    - SLE
    - ankylosing spondylitis
  - renal disease
  - poor nutrition
  - immobilization

Risk Factors

Table 32. Risk Factors for Osteoporosis

Major Risk Factors	Minor Risk Factors
• Age >65 years	**Lifestyle/Diet**
• Vertebral compression fracture	• Smoker
• Fragility fracture after age 40	• Excessive alcohol intake
• Family history of osteoporotic fracture (especially maternal hip fracture)	• Excessive caffeine intake
• Propensity to fall (general frailty, poor balance, decreased visual acuity)	• Low dietary calcium intake
• Osteopenia apparent on x-ray film	• Weight <57 kg
	• Weight loss >10% of weight at age 25
Secondary to medical disease	
• Malabsorption syndrome	**Secondary to medical disease**
• Primary hyperparathyroidism	• Rheumatoid Arthritis
	• Past history of clinical hyperthyroidism
Hormonal deficiency	
• Early menopause (before age 45)	**Drugs**
• Hypogonadism	• Chronic anticonvulsant therapy
	• Chronic heparin therapy
Drugs	
• Systemic glucocorticoid therapy of >3 months duration	

Clinical Features
- commonly asymptomatic
- collapsed vertebrae → height loss
- fractures
  - "Fragility fractures": fracture with fall from standing height
  - hip, vertebrae, humerus, and wrist most common
  - Dowager's hump = collapse fracture of vertebral bodies in mid-dorsal region
  - X-ray: vertebral compression and crush fractures, wedge fractures, "codfishing" sign (weakening of subchondral plates and expansion of intervertebral discs)
- pain, especially backache, associated with fractures

Investigations
- usually normal serum Ca, PO_4, alkaline phosphatase
- also measure 25(OH)-vit D, TSH, serum and urine protein electrophoresis, celiac workup and 24 hr urinary Ca excretion to r/o secondary causes
- **Densitometry**
  - dual-energy x-ray absorptiometry (DEXA) – the gold standard in diagnosis of osteoporosis, (quantitative CT, ultrasonography)
  - lumbar spine and femur
  - compared with gender and ethnicity–matched controls
  - bone mineral density 1.5-2.5 SD below mean= osteopenia; >2.5 SD below mean = osteoporosis

Screening: Who should we screen?
- good evidence to recommend screening postmenopausal women to prevent fragility fractures; screening is effective at identifying postmenopausal women at risk and treatment reduces the risk of fractures (grade A recommendation)
- screening for postmenopausal women: age ≥65 years OR previous fragility fracture OR weight <60 kg OR SCORE questionnaire ≥6 OR ORAI score ≥9, if YES should have DEXA performed, if NO should be reassessed in 1-2 years time.
  note: SCORE and ORAI are risk assessment tools for osteoporosis (available online)

Key Risk of Osteoporosis
- age > 65
- low bone mineral density***
- history of fragility fracture >age 40
- family history of osteoporotic fracture
***Those who have suffered a previous osteoporotic fracture should be considered to have osteoporosis even if their BMD is not in the range associated with osteoporosis.

Calcium Content in Common Foods		
	Standard Portion	Calcium (elemental)
Milk and Milk products		
Cheese – Brick, Cheddar, Colby, Edam, Gouda	1.75 oz/50 g	353 mg
Cheese – cottage, creamed, 2%, 1%	1/2 cup/125 mL	87 mg
Cheese – Mozzarella	1.75 oz/50 g	269 mg
Cheese – Swiss, Gruyère	1.75 oz/50 g	493 mg
Ice cream	1/2 cup/125 mL	93 mg
Milk – powder, dry	3 tbsp/45 mL	159 mg
Milk – whole, 2%, 1%, skim	1 glass/250 mL	315 mg
Yogourt	175 g	320 mg
Meat, fish, poultry and alternatives		
Almonds	1/2 cup/125 mL	200 mg
Beans – cooked	1 cup/250 mL	90 mg
Sardines, with bones	8 small	153 mg
Sesame seeds	1/2 cup/125 mL	100 mg
Soybeans – cooked	1 cup/250 mL	175 mg
Tofu – with calcium sulfate	1/2 cup/125 mL	130 mg
Breads and cereals		
Bread – white/wheat	1 slice/30 g	25 mg
Muffin – bran	1/35 g	50 mg
Fruits and vegetables		
Broccoli – raw	1/2 cup/125 mL	38 mg
Figs – dried	10	270 mg
Orange	1 medium/180 g	52 mg
Combination dishes		
Baked beans – canned	1 cup/250 mL	163 mg
Lasagna – homemade	1 cup/250 mL	286 mg
Soup made with milk	1 cup/250 mL	189 mg

Adapted from Health Canada: Canadian Nutrient File, 1991.

Bisphosphonates are considered 1st – line treatment in women with established osteoporosis.

Alendronate for the primary and secondary prevention of osteoporotic fractures in postmenopausal women
Cochrane Database Syst Rev. 2008;(1):CD001155.

Etidronate for the primary and secondary prevention of osteoporotic fractures in postmenopausal women
Cochrane Database Syst Rev. 2008;(1):CD003376.

Risedronate for the primary and secondary prevention of osteoporotic fractures in postmenopausal women
Cochrane Database Syst Rev. 2008;(1):CD004523.

Purpose: To assess the efficacy of three bisphosponates in the primary and secondary prevention of osteoporotic fractures in postmenopausal women.
Study Selection: Women receiving at least one year of bisphosphonates for postmenopausal osteoporosis were compared to those receiving placebo or concurrent calcium/vitamin D or both. The outcome was fracture incidence.
Results: Levels of evidence:
http://www.cochranemsk.org/review/writing/
%RRR and %ARR for 5 year fracture incidence reduction.

	Aledronate (10 mg/d)
1° Prevention - Vertebral	45% RRR, 2% ARR (Gold)
1° Prevention - Hip	Not significant
1° Prevention - Wrist	Not significant
2° Prevention - Vertebral	45% RRR, 6% ARR (Gold)
2° Prevention - Hip	53% RRR, 1% ARR (Gold)
2° Prevention - Wrist	50% RRR, 2% ARR (Gold)
	Etidronate (400 mg/d)
1° Prevention - Vertebral	Not significant
1° Prevention - Hip	Not significant
1° Prevention - Wrist	Not significant
2° Prevention - Vertebral	47% RRR, 5% ARR (Silver)
2° Prevention - Hip	No benefit
2° Prevention - Wrist	No benefit
	Risedronate (5 mg/d)
1° Prevention - Vertebral	Not significant
1° Prevention - Hip	Not significant
1° Prevention - Wrist	Not significant
2° Prevention - Vertebral	39% RRR, 5% ARR (Gold)
2° Prevention - Hip	26% RRR, 1% ARR (Silver)
2° Prevention - Wrist	Not significant

Factors necessary for mineralization
- quantitatively and qualitatively normal osteoid formation
- normal concentration of calcium and phosphate in ECF
- adequate bioactivity of ALP
- normal pH at site of calcification
- absence of inhibitors of calcification

- screening for all men > 65 OR younger men with secondary causes of osteoporosis or other risk factors for fracture

Treatment of osteoporosis in women

Prevention and Lifestyle Modification: All postmenopausal women
- diet: adequate intake of calories, elemental calcium (1000-1500 mg/day), vit D 400-800 IU/day
- exercise: recommended 3x30 min weight-bearing exercises per week
- cessation of smoking, reduce daily caffeine intake
- discontinuation/avoidance of osteoporosis-inducing drugs

Drug Therapy: Postmenopausal women, positive screen for osteoporosis
- bisphosphonates: inhibitors of osteoclast binding; alendronate or risedronate
- selective estrogen-receptor modulator (SERM): agonistic effect on bone but antagonistic effect on uterus and breast; raloxifene prevents osteoporotic fractures (grade A to B recommendation), improves lipid profile, decreases breast cancer risks, but can increase the risk of DVT/PE, stroke mortality, hot flashes and leg cramps

Drug Therapy: Postmenopausal women, positive screen for osteoporosis + fragility fracture
- bisphosphonates (aledronate, risedronate, etidronate, IV pamidronate, IV zoledronic acid) or SERM (raloxifene) or parathyroid hormone (18-24 mos duration)
- if above not tolerated, calcitonin or HRT can be considered
- calcitonin (2nd-line treatment) - osteoclast receptor binding; 200 IU OD administered nasally; calcitriol 0.25 ug bid
- HRT – for most women the risks may outweigh benefits (grade D recommendation), combined estrogen-progestin therapy prevents number of hip, vertebral and total fractures (risks of bone health vs. breast cancer risk/cardiovascular risk)
- combination therapy (synergistic): estrogen + bisphosphonate

Potential New Treatments
- strontium
- growth factors

Treatment of osteoporosis in men
- consider therapy in the following patients:
  - men > 65 with a T-score less than -2.5 (at any measured site)
  - men > 50 with a fragility or vertebral compression fracture and a T-score less than -1.5
  - men of any age receiving glucocorticoid therapy for 3 months or more and a T-score less than -1.5
  - men of any age with hypogonadism and a T-score less than -1.5
- therapy in men should include:
  - diet: 1500 mg Calcium OD (Grade C evidence) and Vitamin D3 > 800 IU OD (Grade A evidence)
  - Bisphosphonate therapy: Alendronate 70mg/wk OR risedronate 35mg/wk OR cyclical etidronate 400mg/d for 14 d per 90-d cycle (Grade A evidence)

Osteomalacia and Ricketts

- ricketts – osteopenia with disordered calcification leading to higher proportion of osteoid (unmineralized) tissue prior to epiphyseal closure (in childhood)
- osteomalacia – osteopenia with disordered calcification leading to higher proportion of osteoid (unmineralized) tissue after epiphyseal closure (in adulthood)

Etiology and Pathophysiology

Vitamin D Deficiency
- leads to secondary hyperparathyroidism and hypophosphatemia
- deficient uptake or absorption
  - nutritional deficiency
  - malabsorption: post-gastrectomy, small bowel disease (e.g. Celiac sprue), pancreatic insufficiency
- defective 25-hydroxylation
  - liver disease
  - anticonvulsant therapy
- loss of vit D binding protein
  - nephrotic syndrome
- defective 1-α-25 hydroxylation
  - hypoparathyroidism
  - renal failure

Mineralization Defect
- abnormal matrix
  - osteogenesis imperfecta
  - fibrogenesis imperfecta
  - axial osteomalacia
- enzyme deficiency
  - hypophosphatasia (inadequate ALP bioactivity)
- presence of calcification inhibitors
  - bisphosphonates, aluminum, high dose fluoride, anticonvulsants

Phosphate Deficiency
- decreased intake
  - antacids
- impaired renal reabsorption
  - primary defect: Wilson's syndrome, Fanconi syndrome, multiple myeloma
  - secondary defect: primary hyperparathyroidism, oncogenic osteomalacia

Table 33. Clinical Presentations of Ricketts and Osteomalacia

Ricketts	Osteomalacia
• skeletal pain and deformities, bowlegs	• not as dramatic
• fracture susceptibililty	• diffuse skeletal pain
• weakness and hypotonia	• bone tenderness
• disturbed growth	• fractures
• ricketic rosary	• gait disturbances (waddling)
(prominent costochondral junctions)	• proximal muscle weakness
• Harrison's groove	• hypotonia
(indentation of lower ribs)	
• hypocalcemia	

Investigations

Table 34. Laboratory Findings in Osteomalacia and Ricketts

Disorder	Serum phosphate	Serum calcium	Serum ALP	Other features
Vit D deficiency	↓	↓ to Normal	↑	↓ calcitriol
Hypophosphatemia	↓	Normal	↓ to Normal	
Proximal RTA	↓	Normal	Normal	Assoc with hyperchloremic metabolic acidosis
Conditions assoc with abnormal matrix formation	Normal	Normal	Normal	

- **radiologic findings**
  - pseudofractures, fissures, narrow radiolucent lines – thought to be healed stress fractures or the result of erosion by arterial pulsation
  - loss of radiologic distinctness of vertebral body trabecula, concavity of the vertebral bodies
  - changes due to secondary hyperparathyroidism: subperiosteal resorption of the phalanges, bone cysts, resorption of the distal ends of long bones
  - others: bowing of tibia, coxa profundus hip deformity
- **bone biopsy**
  - usually not necessary but considered the gold standard for diagnosis

Treatment
- depends on the underlying cause
- vitamin D supplementation
- PO_4 supplements if low serum PO_4 is present
- Ca supplements for isolated calcium deficiency
- HCO_3 if chronic acidosis

Renal Osteodystrophy

- represents a mixture of four types of bone disease
  - low turn-over osteomalacia – from acidosis and retention of toxic metabolites
  - osteoporosis – metabolic acidosis dissolution of bone buffers
  - osteitis fibrosa cystica – from increased PTH
  - osteosclerosis – from increased PTH
- metastatic calcification secondary to hyperphosphatemia may occur

Pathophysiology
- metabolic bone disease secondary to chronic renal failure
- combination of hyperphosphatemia (inhibits $1,25(OH)_2$-vit D synthesis) and loss of renal mass (reduced 1-α-hydroxylase)

Clinical Features
- soft tissue calcifications → necrotic skin lesions if vessels involved
- osteodystrophy → generalized bone pain and fractures
- pruritus
- neuromuscular irritability and tetany may occur
- radiologic features of osteitis fibrosa cystica, osteomalacia, osteosclerosis, osteoporosis

Treatment
- prevention
  - maintenance of normal serum Ca and PO_4 by restricting PO_4 intake to 1 g/day
  - Ca supplements
  - PO_4 binding agents
  - prophylactic use of vitamin D with close monitoring to avoid hypercalcemia and metastatic calcification

Paget's Disease of Bone

Definition
- a metabolic disease characterized by excessive bone destruction and repair

Epidemiology
- a common disease: 5% of the population, 10% of population >80 years old

Etiology
- postulated to be related to a slow progressing viral infection of osteoclasts, possibly paramyxovirus
- strong familial incidence

Pathophysiology
- initiated by increased osteoclastic activity leading to increased bone resorption; osteoblastic activity increases in response to produce new bone that is structurally abnormal and fragile

Differential Diagnosis
- primary bone lesions
  - osteogenic sarcoma
  - multiple myeloma
  - fibrous dysplasia
- secondary bone lesions
  - osteitis fibrosa cystica
  - metastases

Clinical Features
- usually asymptomatic (routine x-ray finding or elevated alkaline phosphatase)
- severe bone pain (e.g. pelvis, femur, tibia) is often the presenting complaint
- skeletal deformities – bowed tibias, kyphosis, frequent fractures
- skull involvement – headaches, increased hat size, deafness
- increased warmth over involved bones due to increased vascularity

Investigations
- laboratory
  - serum alkaline phosphatase is usually very high (unless burnt out)
  - normal or increased serum Ca
  - normal serum PO_4
  - increased urinary hydroxyproline (indicates resorption)
- imaging
  - evaluate the extent of disease with bone scan
  - initial lesion may be destructive and radiolucent
  - involved bones are expanded with cortical thickening and denser than normal
  - multiple fissure fractures in long bones

Complications
- local
  - fractures
  - osteoarthritis
  - cranial nerve compression and palsies, e.g. deafness
  - spinal cord compression
  - osteosarcoma/sarcomatous change
    - 1 to 3%
    - indicated by marked bone pain, new lytic lesions and sudden increased alkaline phosphatase
- systemic
  - hypercalcemia and nephrolithiasis
  - high output congestive heart failure due to increased vascularity

Comparison of a single infusion of zoledronic acid with risedronate for Paget's disease
N Engl J Med. 2005;353:898-908
Study: Two identical, randomized, double-blind, actively controlled trials (combined for analysis)
Patients: 357 men and women who were older than 30 years of age and had radiologically-confirmed Paget's disease of bone. All but 4 patients had alkaline phosphatase levels that were more than twice the upper limit of normal
Intervention: One 15-minute infusion of 5 mg of zoledronic acid with 60 days of oral risedronate (30 mg per day) with follow up at 6 months.
Primary Outcome: Rate of therapeutic response at six months, defined as a normalization of alkaline phosphatase levels or a reduction of at least 75 percent in the total alkaline phosphatase excess.
Results: At six months, 96.0 percent of patients receiving zoledronic acid had a therapeutic response (169 of 176), as compared with 74.3 percent of patients receiving risedronate (127 of 171, P<0.001). Alkaline phosphatase levels normalized in 88.6 percent of patients in the zoledronic acid group and 57.9 percent of patients in the risedronate group (P<0.001). Zoledronic acid was associated with a shorter median time to a first therapeutic response (64 vs. 89 days, P<0.001). Higher response rates in the zoledronic acid group were consistent across all demographic, disease-severity, and treatment-history subgroups and with changes in other bone-turnover markers. The physical-component summary score of the Medical Outcomes Study 36-item Short-Form General Health Survey, a measure of the quality of life, increased significantly from baseline at both three and six months in the zoledronic acid group and differed significantly from those in the risedronate group at three months. Pain scores improved in both groups. During post-trial follow-up (median, 190 days), 21 of 82 patients in the risedronate group had a loss of therapeutic response, as compared with 1 of 113 patients in the zoledronic acid group (P<0.001).
Conclusions: A single infusion of zoledronic acid produces more rapid, more complete, and more sustained responses in Paget's disease than does daily treatment with risedronate.

Treatment
- symptomatic therapy
- treat if ALP >3x normal
- bisphosphonates, e.g. alendronate 40 mg PO OD x 6 mo or risedronate 30 mg PO OD x 3 mo OR zolendronic acid 5 mg IV per year
- calcitonin 50-100 U/day subcutaneous injection
- adequate calcium and vitamin D intake to prevent development of secondary hyperparathyroidism

Male Reproductive Endocrinology

Androgen Regulation

- both positive and negative feedback may occur by androgens directly or after conversion to estrogen
- testosterone (from the Leydig cell) primarily involved in negative feedback on LH, whereas inhibin (from the Sertoli cell) suppresses FSH secretion

Tests of Testicular Function

- testicular size (lower limit = 4 cm x 2.5 cm)
- LH, FSH, testosterone
- human chorionic gonadotropin (hCG) stimulation test
  - assesses ability of Leydig cell to respond to gonadotropin
- semen analysis
  - semen volume, sperm count, morphology and motility
- testicular biopsy
  - indicated in the context of normal FSH and azoospermia/oligospermia

Hypogonadism

- deficiency in gametogenesis or testosterone production

Etiology
- causes include primary (testicular failure) and secondary (hypothalamic-pituitary failure)
- primary hypogonadism is more common than secondary

HYPERGONADOTROPIC HYPOGONADISM (PRIMARY HYPOGONADISM)

Definition
- primary testicular failure; characterized by increased LH and FSH, increased FSH:LH, decreased level of serum testosterone and sperm count

Etiology
- congenital
  - chromosomal defects, i.e. Klinefelter syndrome, Noonan syndrome
  - cryptorchidism
  - male pseudohermaphroditism
  - bilateral anorchia
  - myotonic dystrophy
  - mutation in the FSH or LH receptor gene
  - varicocele
  - disorders of androgen synthesis
- germ cell defects
  - Sertoli cell only syndrome (arrest of sperm development)
  - Leydig cell aplasia/failure
- infection/inflammation
  - orchitis – mumps, tuberculosis, lymphoma, leprosy
  - genital tract infection
- physical factors
  - trauma, heat, irradiation, testicular torsion
- drugs
  - marijuana, alcohol, chemotherapeutic agents, ketoconazole, glucocorticoid
- autoimmune
- chronic systemic disease
  - acquired immunodeficiency syndrome (AIDS)
- idiopathic

> **Two distinct features of primary hypogonadism**
> 1. The decrease in sperm count is affected to a greater extent than the decrease in serum testosterone level
> 2. Likely to be associated with gynecomastia

HYPOGONADOTROPIC HYPOGONADISM (SECONDARY HYPOGONADISM)

Definition
- hypothalamic-pituitary failure; characterized by decreased or normal LH, subnormal level of testosterone and sperm count

Two features of secondary hypogonadism
1. Associated with an equivalent decrease in sperm count and serum testosterone
2. Less likely to be associated with gynecomastia

Etiology
- congenital
  - Kallman's syndrome, Prader-Willi syndrome, abnormal subunit of LH or FSH
- infection
  - tuberculosis, meningitis (rare)
- endocrine
  - Cushing's syndrome
  - hypothyroidism
  - hypopituitarism (pituitary tumours, pituitary apoplexy, hypothalamic lesions)
  - estrogen-secreting tumours (testicular, adrenal)
- drugs
  - alcohol, marijuana, spironolactone, ketoconazole, GnRH agonists, prior androgen use, chronic narcotic administration
- chronic illness
  - cirrhosis, CRF, AIDS
  - sarcoidosis, Langerhans cell histiocytosis, hemochromatosis
- critical illness
  - surgery, MI, head trauma
- idiopathic

Investigations
- laboratory – FSH, LH, prolactin, testosterone, TSH
- semen analysis

Treatment
- medications – testosterone replacement or pulsatile GnRH/hCG
- surgery – only if testicular tissues are not functioning

DEFECTS IN ANDROGEN ACTION

Etiology
- complete androgen insensitivity (testicular feminization)
- incomplete androgen insensitivity
  - 5-α-reductase deficiency
  - mixed gonadal dysgenesis
  - defects in testosterone synthesis
- infertile male syndrome
- undervirilized fertile male syndrome

Clinical Features
- depends on age of onset
- fetal life
  - ambiguous genitalia and male pseudohermaphroditism
- prepubertal
  - poor secondary sexual development, poor muscle development
  - eunuchoid skeletal proportions (upper/lower segment ratio <1; arm span/height ratio >1)
- postpubertal
  - decreased libido, erectile dysfunction, infertility
  - decreased facial and body hair if very significant androgen deficiency (very low levels required to maintain sexual hair)
  - fine wrinkles in the corners of mouth and eyes
  - osteoporosis with longstanding hypogonadism

Treatment
- appropriate gender assignment in the newborn
- hormone replacement or supplementation
- psychological support
- gonadectomy for crytochidism
- reduction mammoplasty for gynecomastia

Infertility

(see Urology)

Erectile Dysfunction

(see Urology)

Gynecomastia

Definition
- True gynecomastia refers to benign proliferation of the glandular component of the male breast, resulting in the formation of a concentric, rubbery, firm mass extending from the nipple(s)
- pseudogynecomastia or lipomastia refers to enlargement of soft adipose tissue, especially seen in obese individuals and does not warrant further evaluation

Etiology

Physiologic
- puberty
- elderly
- neonatal (maternal hormone)

Pathologic
- endocrinopathies – primary hypogonadism, hyperthyroidism, extreme hyperprolactinemia, adrenal disease
- tumours – pituitary, adrenal, testicular, breast
- chronic diseases – liver, renal, malnutrition
- drugs – spironolactone, cimetidine, digoxin, chemotherapy, marijuana
- congenital/genetic – Klinefelter's syndrome
- other – idiopathic, familial

> **Causes of Gynecomastia**
> **DOC TECH:**
> **D**rugs
> **O**ther
> **C**ongenital
> **T**umour
> **E**ndocrine
> **CH**ronic disease

Pathophysiology
- decreased androgen production + increased estrogen production
- increased availability of estrogen precursors for peripheral conversion to estrogen
- androgen receptor blockage + binding of androgen to sex hormone binding globulin (SHBG)

Epidemiology

Table 35. Occurence of Gynecomastia

3 peaks	% affected
infancy	60-90
puberty	4-69
ages 50-80	24-65

History
- recent change in breast characteristics
- history of trauma to testicles
- history of mumps
- alcohol and/or drug use
- family history
- sexual dysfunction

Physical Exam
- signs of feminization
- breast
- GU
- stigmata of liver or thyroid disease

Investigations
- laboratory - serum TSH, PRL, LH, FSH, free testosterone, estradiol, LFTs, βhCG (if βhCG is elevated, need to locate the primary tumour)
- CXR and CT of chest/abdomen/pelvis
- testicular U/S to rule out testicular mass

Treatment
- medical
  - correct the underlying disorder, discontinue responsible drug
  - androgens for hypogonadism
  - anti-estrogens – tamoxifen, clomiphene
- surgical
  - usually required if have macromastia; gynecomastia present for > 1 year; or failed medical treatment and for cosmetic purposes

Common Medications

DIABETES MEDICATIONS

Drug Class	Mechanism of Action	Generic Drug Name	Canada Name	US Name (if different)	Dosing	Indications	Contraindications	Side Effects	Comments
Biguanide	• sensitizes peripheral tissues to insulin → increases glucose uptake • decreases hepatic glucose production	metformin	Glucophage® Glumetza®		500 mg OD titrated to 1000 mg bid maximum	• useful in obese Type 2 DM • improves both fasting and postprandial hyperglycemia • also ↓TG	ABSOLUTE: • moderate to severe liver dysfunction • mild renal dysfunction • cardiac dysfunction	• GI upset (abdo discomfort, bloating, diarrhea) • lactic acidosis • anorexia	↓ HbA1C 1.0-1.5%
Insulin secretagogue	• stimulates insulin release from β cells by causing K channel closure → depolarization → Ca mediated insulin release • use in nonobese Type 2 DM	sulfonylureas: glyburide	Diabeta®, Euglucon®	Micronase® Glynase PreTab®	2.5-5.0 mg/day titrated to >6 mg bid Max: 20 mg/day		ABSOLUTE: • moderate to severe liver dysfunction RELATIVE: • adjust dose in patients with severe kidney dysfunction (and avoid glyburide in these patients) • avoid glyburide in the elderly INTERACTIONS: Do not combine with a non-sulfonylurea or preprandial insulin	• hypoglycemia • weight gain	↓ HbA1C 1.0-1.5%
		gliclazide	Diamicron® Diamicron MR		40-160 mg bid 30-120 mg OD				
		glimepiride	Amaryl™		1-8 mg OD				
		non-sulfonylureas: repaglinide	GlucoNorm®		0.5-4 mg tid	• Short t₁/₂ of 1 hour causes brief but rapid ↑ in insulin, therefore effective for post prandial control	ABSOLUTE: • severe liver dysfunction • severe renal dysfunction INTERACTIONS: Do not combine with a non-sulfonylurea or preprandial insulin	• hypoglycemia • weight gain	↓ HbA1C 1.0-1.5% for repaglinide and 0.5-1.0% for nateglinide
		nateglinide	Starlix®		60-120 mg tid				
Insulin sensitizers (thiazolidinedione)	• sensitizes peripheral tissues to insulin → increases glucose uptake • decreases FFA release from adipose • binds to nuclear receptor	rosiglitazone	Avandia®		2-8 mg OD		ABSOLUTE: • severe liver dysfunction • NYHA >class II CHF INTERACTIONS: Do not combine with insulin	• peripheral edema • pulmonary edema • CHF • anemia • weight gain • fractures	↓ HbA1C 1.0-1.5%
		pioglitazone	Actos™		15-45 mg OD				
α-glucosidase inhibitor	• ↓ carbohydrate GI absorption by inhibiting brush border α-glucosidase	acarbose	Glucobay™		25 mg OD titrated to 100 mg tid	• ↓ postprandial hyperglycemia	ABSOLUTE: • inflammatory bowel disease • severe liver dysfunction	• flatulence • abdominal cramps • diarrhea	↓ HbA1C 0.5-1.0%
Dipeptidyl peptidase-IV (DPP-IV) inhibitor	• inhibits degradation of endogenous antihyperglycemic incretin hormones • incretin hormones stimulate insulin secretion, inhibit glucagon release, and delay gastric emptying	sitagliptin	Januvia™		100 mg OD		ABSOLUTE: • Type 1 DM • DKA RELATIVE: • adjust dose in patients with kidney dysfunction	• nasopharyngitis • URTI • headache	↓ HbA1C 0.5-1.0%

For insulin formulations, please refer to E5-E6

DYSLIPIDEMIA MEDICATIONS

Drug Class	Mechanism of Action	Generic Drug Name	Canada Name	US Name (if different)	Dosing	Indications	Contraindications	Side Effects
HMG CoA reductase inhibitor	• inhibits cholesterol biosynthesis, ↓ LDL synthesis, ↑ LDL clearance, modest ↑ HDL, limited ↓ VLDL	atorvastatin fluvastatin lovastatin pravastatin rosuvastatin simvastatin	Lipitor™ Lescol™ Mevacor™ Pravachol™ Crestor™ Zocor™		10-80 mg/day 20-80 mg/day 20-80 mg/day 10-40 mg/day 10-40 mg/day 10-80 mg/day	• used for ↑TG, ↑ LDL, secondary	• active liver disease • persistent ↑ in AST, ALT	• GI symptoms • rash, pruritus • ↑ liver enzymes • myositis
Fibrates	• ↓ lipolysis in adipose tissue, ↓ VLDL, ↓ TG, modest ↓ LDL, modest ↑ HDL	bezafibrate fenofibrate gemfibrozil	Bezalip™ Lipidil™ Lopid™		400 mg/day 67-200 mg/day 600-1200 mg/day	• used for ↑TG, hyperchylomicronemia	• hepatic disease • renal disease	• GI upset • ↑ risk of gallstone formation
Niacin	• inhibits secretion of hepatic VLDL via lipoprotein lipase (LPL) pathway —> decreased VLDL and LDL decrease; decreased clearance of HDL	nicotinic acid	Niaspan™	Niacor™	1.5-3 g/day	• used for ↑ LDL, ↑VLDL	• hypersensitivity • hepatic dysfunction • active PUD • overt DM • hyperuricemia	• generalized flushing • abnormal liver enzymes • pruritus • IGT • severe hypertension
Bile acid sequestrants	• resins that bind bile acids in intestinal lumen and prevent absorption thereby ↓ LDL	cholestyramine colestipol	Questran™ Prevalite™ Colestid™		2-24 g/day 5-30 g/day	• used for ↑ LDL	• complete biliary obstruction • pregnancy • lactation	• constipation • nausea • flatulence • bloating
Cholesterol absorption inhibitors	• inhibits cholesterol absorption at the small intestine brush border	ezetimibe	Ezetrol™	Zetia™	10 mg/day	• used for ↑ LDL, Apo B	• hypersensitivity • hepatic dysfunction	• fatigue • pharyngitis • sinusitis • abdominal pain • diarrhea • arthralgia

THYROID MEDICATIONS

Drug Class	Mechanism of Action	Generic Drug Name	Canada Name	US Name (if different)	Dosing	Indications	Contraindications	Side Effects
Antithyroid Agent	• decreases thyroid hormone production by inhibiting iodine and peroxidase from interacting with thyroglobulin to form T4 and T3 • also interferes with conversion of T4 to T3	propylthiouracil (PTU)	Propyl-Thyracil™		Start 100 mg PO tid, then adjust accordingly Thyroid storm: start 200-300 PO qid, then adjust accordingly	• hyperthyroidism	• hypersensitivity • relative: renal failure, liver disease	• nausea, vomiting • rash • drug-induced hepatitis • agranulocytosis
		methimazole (MMI)	Tapazole™		Start 5-20 mg PO OD, then adjust accordingly		• pregnancy, lactation	• hepatitis
Thyroid hormone	• synthetic form of thyroxine (T4)	levothyroxine l-thyroxine	Synthroid™ Levothroid™ Unithroid™	Levoxyl™	0.05-2.0 mg/day, in elderly patients start at 0.025 mg/day	• hypothyroidism	• recent MI, thyrotoxicosis	• symptoms of hyperthyroidism • tachycardia • angina • weight loss • hyperthermia • diarrhea • insomnia • tremors • muscle weakness

METABOLIC BONE DISEASE MEDICATIONS

Drug Class	Mechanism of Action	Generic Drug Name	Canada Name	US Name (if different)	Dosing	Indications	Contraindications	Side Effects
Bisphosphonates	• inhibits osteoclast-mediated bone resorption	alendronate	Fosamax®		5 mg OD 10 mg OD or 70 mg once weekly 5-10 mg OD 40 mg OD for 6 months	• prevention of postmenopausal osteoporosis • treatment of osteoporosis • glucocorticoid-induced osteoporosis • Paget's disease	• esophageal stricture or achalasia (oral) • unable to stand or sit upright for >30 min (oral) • hypersensitivity • hypocalcemia • renal insufficiency	• GI • MSK pain • headache • osteonecrosis of the jaw
		risedronate	Actonel®		5 mg OD or 35 mg once weekly 5 mg OD	• treatment and prevention of postmenopausal osteoporosis • treatment and prevention of glucocorticoid-induced osteoporosis • Paget's disease		
		etidronate	Didronel®		30 mg OD for 2 months 400 mg OD x 14 days q 3 months with calcium PO	• osteoporosis • symptomatic Paget's disease • prevention and treatment of heterotopic ossification after total hip replacement or spinal cord injury		
		ibandronate		Boniva®	2.5 mg OD or 150 mg once monthly	• treatment and prevention of postmenopausal osteoporosis (US only)		
		pamidronate	Aredia®		IV	• hypercalcemia of malignancy • Paget's disease • osteolytic bone metastases of breast cancer • osteolytic lesions of multiple myeloma		
		zoledronate	Zometa® Aclasta®		IV	• hypercalcemia of malignancy • treatment and prevention of skeletal complications related to cancer		
Selective Estrogen Receptor Modulators	• decreases resorption of bone through binding to estrogen receptors	raloxifene	Evista®		60 mg OD	• treatment and prevention of postmenopausal osteoporosis (2nd line)	• lactation • pregnancy • active or past history of DVT, PE or retinal vein thrombosis	• hot flashes • leg cramps • increased risk of fatal stroke, venous thromboembolism
Calcitonin	• inhibits osteoclast-mediated bone resorption	salcatonin	Miacalcin®		One spray (200 IU) per day, alternating nostrils	• treatment of postmenopausal osteoporosis, greater than 5 years postmenopause	• clinical allergy to calcitonin-salmon	• rhinitis • epistaxis • sinusitis • nasal dryness
PTH	• stimulates new bone formation by preferential stimulation of osteoblastic activity over osteoclastic activity	teriparatide	Forteo®		20 µg SC OD	• treatment of postmenopausal women with osteoporosis who are at high risk for fracture • treatment of men with primary or hypogonadal osteoporosis who are at high risk for fracture	• Paget's disease • prior external beam or implant radiation therapy involving the skeleton • bone metastases • metabolic bone diseases other than osteoporosis	• orthostatic hypotension • hypercalcemia • dizziness • leg cramps

METABOLIC BONE DISEASE MEDICATIONS (continued)

Drug Class	Mechanism of Action	Generic Drug Name	Canada Name	US Name (if different)	Dosing	Indications	Contraindications	Side Effects
Calcium	• Inhibits PTH secretion				1500 mg/day (including diet) Divide in 3 doses	• osteopenia • osteoporosis • prevention of metabolic bone disease	• caution with renal stones	• vomiting • constipation • dry mouth
Vitamin D	• Regulation of calcium and phosphate homeostasis	cholecalciferol (vitamin D3)			800 IU/day	• osteopenia • osteoporosis • prevention of metabolic bone disease	• caution in patients on digoxin (risk of hypercalcemia may precipitate arrhythmia)	• hypercalcemia • headache • nausea, vomiting • constipation
		ergocalciferol (vitamin D2)	Osteoforte® Deltalin®		50000 IU	• osteoporosis in patients with liver dysfunction, refractory rickets, hypoparathyroidism	• hypercalcemia • malabsorption syndrome • decreased renal function	
		calcitriol (1,25[OH]$_2$-D)	Rocaltrol® Calcijex®		Start 0.25 µg/day Titrate up by 0.25 µg/day at 4-8 week intervals to 0.5-1 µg/day	• hypocalcemia and osteodystrophy in patients with chronic renal failure on dialysis	• hypercalcemia • vitamin D toxicity	
					Start 0.25 µg/day Titrate up by 0.25 µg/day at 2-4 week intervals to 0.5-2 µg/day	• hypoparathyroidism		

Notes

FM | Family Medicine

Larbi Benhabib, Thomas O'Brien and Kasy Soare, chapter editors
Justine Chan and Angela Ho, associate editors
Billie Au, EBM editor
Dr. Ruby Alvi and Dr. Azadeh Moaveni, staff editors

Four Principles of Family Medicine

College of Family Physicians of Canada Guidelines
1. The family physician is a **skilled clinician**
   - skilled in diagnosis and management of diseases common to population served
   - recognizes importance of early diagnosis of serious life threatening illnesses
2. Family medicine is a **community-based discipline**
   - has good knowledge of, and access to, community services
   - responds/adapts to changing needs and changing circumstances
   - collaborates as a team member or a leader
3. The family physician is a **resource to a defined practice population**
   - serves as a health resource
   - promotes self-directed life-long learning
   - advocates for public policy to promote health
4. The **patient-physician relationship is central** to the role of the family physician
   - committed to the person, not just disease
   - promotes continuity of patient care

Patient-Centred Clinical Method

| Patient's Agenda: FIFE |
| Feelings |
| Ideas |
| Function |
| Expectations |

- explore/define patient problems and decide on management together
- consider both agendas
  - doctor's agenda: history, physical, investigation, diagnosis, plan
  - patient's agenda: FIFE (see sidebar), i.e. "How do you feel about...", "What do you think is going on?", "How is this affecting you?", "What would you like to happen today?"
- find common ground in management and follow-up planning

The Periodic Health Examination (PHE)

- Canadian Task Force on Preventive Health Care established in 1976, first published in 1979, last updated in 2005
  - reviews the literature for evidence pertaining to prevention of conditions
  - aids in developing clinical practice guidelines
  - incorporates primary and secondary preventive measures
  - most notable recommendation is the abolition of the annual physical exam; replaced by the periodic health examination (PHE)

Purpose of the PHE

- primary prevention
  - identify risk factors for common diseases
  - counsel patients to promote healthy behaviour
- secondary prevention
  - presymptomatic detection of disease to allow early treatment and prevent disease progression
- update clinical data
- enhance patient-physician relationship

Adult Periodic Health Exam

- male and female evidence-based preventative care checklist forms are available online at www.cfpc.ca under programs > for your practice > clinical tools

Table 1. Periodic Health Exam

	General Population	Special Populations	

Discussion	Dental hygiene (community fluoridation, brushing, flossing) (A)
	Noise control and hearing protection (A)
	Smokers: counsel on smoking cessation, provide
	    nicotine replacement therapy (A)
	    referral to smoking cessation program (B)
	    dietary advice on leafy green vegetables & fruits (B)
	Seat belt use (B)
	Injury prevention (bicycle helmets, smoke detectors) (B)
	Moderate physical activity (B)
	Avoid sun exposure and wear protective clothing (B)
	Problem drinking screening and counselling (B)
	Counselling to protect against STIs (B)
	Nutritional counselling and dietary advice on fat and cholesterol (B)
		Pediatrics: Home visits for high risk families (A)
		    Inquiry into developmental milestones (B)
		Adolescents: Counsel on sexual activity and contraceptive
		    methods (A)
		    Counsel to prevent smoking initiation (B)
		Perimenopausal women:
		    Counsel on osteoporosis
		    Counsel on risks/benefits of hormone replacement therapy (B)
		Adults >65: Follow-up on caregiver concern of cognitive impairment (A)
		    Multidisciplinary post-fall assessment (A)	

Physical	Clinical breast exam (women 50-69) (A)
	Blood pressure measurement (B)
	BMI measurement in obese adults (B)
		Pediatrics: Repeated examinations of hips, eyes and hearing (especially
		    in first year of life) (A)
		    Serial heights, weights and head circumference (B)
		    Visual acuity testing after age 2 (B)
		Adults >65: Visual acuity (Snellen sight chart) (B)
		    Hearing impairment (inquiry, whispered voice test,
		    audioscope) (B)
		First degree relative with melanoma: Full body skin exam (B)	

Tests	Multiphase screening with the Hemoccult test
	    (adults >50 q1-2yrs) (A)
	Sigmoidoscopy (adults >50) (frequency not established) (B)
	Bone mineral density: if at risk (1 major or 2 minor criteria)
	Fasting lipid profile (C):
	    women >50 or post-menopausal; earlier if at risk
	    men >40; earlier if at risk (optimal frequency unknown,
	    at least q5yrs)
	Fasting blood glucose: >40 or sooner if at risk;
	    q3yrs or more frequently if risk factors present
	Syphilis screen if at risk (D)
	Men: PSA testing screening guidelines not established (I)
	Women: Mammography (women 50-69) q1-2yrs (A)
	    Pap smear (women 18-69) (B); annually if 2 or more
	    consecutive negative PAPs q3yrs (more frequently
	    if concerns)
		Pediatrics: Routine hemoglobin for high risk infants (B)
		    Blood lead screening of high risk infants (B)
		Diabetics: Urine dipstick (A)
		    Fundoscopy (B)
		TB high risk groups: Mantoux skin testing (A)
		STI high risk groups: Voluntary HIV antibody screening (A)
		    Gonorrhea screening (A)
		    Chlamydia screening in women (B)
		FAP: Sigmoidoscopy and genetic testing (B)
		HNPCC: Colonoscopy (B)	

Therapy	Folic acid supplementation to women of child-bearing age (A)
	Varicella vaccine for children ages 1-12 and susceptible
	    adolescents/adults (A)
	Rubella vaccine for all non-pregnant women of
	    child-bearing age (B)
	Pharmacologic treatment of hypertension with dBP
	    >90 mmHg (adults 21-64, elderly specific subgroups) (A)
	Tetanus vaccine: routine booster q10yrs if had 1° series (A)
		Pediatrics: Routine immunizations (A)
		    Hepatitis B immunization (A)
		Influenza high risk groups: Outreach strategies for vaccination (A);
		    annual immunization (B), now recommended for all
		TB high risk groups: INH prophylaxis for household contacts/skin test
		    converters (B)
		    INH prophylaxis for high risk sub-groups (B)
		Immunocompetent / ≥65 / COPD: Pneumococcal vaccine (A)	

Reference: Canadian Task Force on Preventative Health Care, 2005. http://www.ctfphc.org

Classification of Recommendations:

A   **good** evidence to recommend the clinical preventative action

B   **fair** evidence to recommend the clinical preventative action

C   existing evidence is **conflicting** and does not allow to make a recommendation for or against use of the clinical preventative action; however, other factors may influence decision-making

D   **fair** evidence to recommend against the clinical preventative action

E   **good** evidence to recommend against the clinical preventative action

I   **insufficient** evidence (in quantity or quality) to make a recommendation; however, other factors may influence decision-making

When ordering fasting bloodwork
- results are valid only if obtained with ≥12 hours of fasting
- remember, "fasting" means no food, no drink, no gum, no medications

Guidelines Advisory Committee (GAC) Recommendations for Breast Cancer Screening
For women aged 40-69 years, there is fair evidence to recommend that routine teaching of breast self-examination (BSE) be excluded from the PHE. Research shows fair evidence of no benefit to BSE and good evidence of harm.

Health Promotion and Counselling

- health promotion is the most effective preventative strategy
- 40-70% of productive life lost annually is preventable
- there are several effective ways to promote healthy behavioural change, such as discussions appropriate to a patient's present stage of change

Motivational Strategies for Behavioural Change

Table 2. Motivational Strategies for Behavioural Change

Patient's Stage of Change	Physician's Aim	Physician's Plan
Pre-contemplation	Encourage patient to consider the possibility of change Assess readiness for change Increase patient's awareness of the problem and its risks	Raise issue in a sensitive manner Offer (not impose) a neutral exchange of information to avoid resistance
Contemplation	Understand patient's ambivalence and encourage change Build confidence and gain commitment to change	Offer opportunity to discuss pros and cons of change, using reflective listening
Preparation	Explore options and choose course most appropriate to patient Identify high-risk situations and develop strategies to prevent relapse Continue to strengthen confidence and commitment	Offer realistic options for change and opportunity to discuss inevitable difficulties
Action	Help patients design ways to reward themselves for success Develop strategies to prevent relapse Support and reinforce convictions towards long-term change	Offer positive reinforcement and explore ways of coping with obstacles Encourage self-rewards to positively reinforce change
Maintenance	Help patient maintain motivation Review identifying high-risk situations and strategies for preventing relapse	Discuss progress and signs of impending relapse
Relapse	Help patient view relapse as a learning experience Provide support appropriate to his or her present level of readiness post-relapse	Offer a non-judgmental discussion about circumstances surrounding relapse and how to avoid relapse in the future Reassess patient's readiness to change

Adapted from Hunt P (2001). Motivating Change. Nursing Standard, 16(2): 45-52, 54-55.

Nutrition

General Population
- Canada's Food Guide appropriate for individuals >2 years old
- counsel on variety, portion size, and plate layout (see Figure 1)

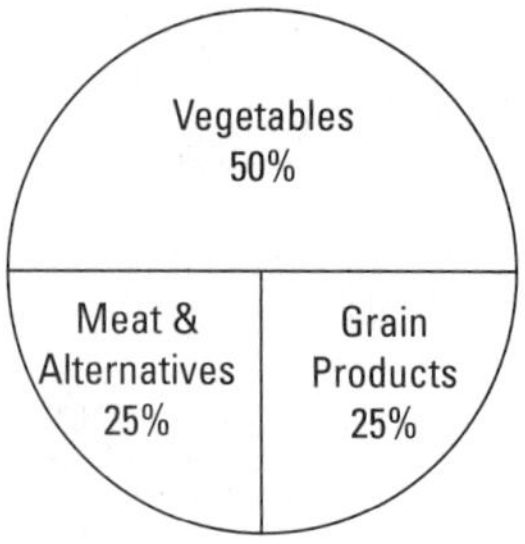

Table 3. Canada's Food Guide 2007 Recommendations for Adults

Food group	Servings/day	Choose more often
Grain products	6-7	Whole grain and enriched grain products
Vegetables and fruit	7-10	Dark green vegetables, orange vegetables and fruit
Milk products	2-3 Children 2-8 years: 2 Youth 9-18 years: 3-4 Pregnant/breastfeeding: 3-4	Lower-fat dairy products
Meat and alternatives	2-3	Lean meat, poultry, fish, peas, beans, lentils

Cardiovascular Disease Prevention

Table 4. Dietary guidelines for reducing risk of cardiovascular disease in general population

Food item	Recommendations	Effects
Fat	Fat intake <30% of total energy Saturated fat <10% of energy Cholesterol <300 mg/d Limit trans fatty acids	Lower LDL
ω-3 fatty acid rich foods	≥2 servings/wk of either fish (especially fatty fish like salmon) or ω-3 rich plant sources (e.g. flaxseed, canola oil, soybean oil, nuts)	Decreased: sudden death, arrhythmia, blood-clotting tendency; Lower TG
Salt	<6 g/d (100 mmol or 2300 mg/d of sodium)	Lower BP
Alcohol	≤2 drinks/d for men ≤1 drink/d for women	Lower BP

References: Canada's Food Guide to Healthy Eating. Health Canada. Last updated 2007.
http://www.hc-sc.gc.ca/fn-an/food-guide-aliment/fg_rainbow-arc_en_cie_ga_e.html
Krauss RM, et al. (2000). AHA Dietary Guidelines. Revision 2000: A statement for healthcare professionals from the nutrition committee of the American Heart Association. *Stroke*, 31: 2751-66.

Vegetables
50%

Meat & Alternatives
25%

Grain Products
25%

Figure 1. Plate Layout

Handy serving size comparisons
- 3oz meat, fish, poultry → palm of hand
- 1 cup dairy (milk/yogurt) → size of fist
- bread/grains → one slice, palm of hand
- ½ cup rice/pasta → one hand cupped
- 1 cup of fruit/vegetables → two cupped hands
- 1oz cheese → full length of thumb
- 1 tsp oil/butter → tip of thumb
- nuts/chips/snacks → palm covered

Table 5. Introduction to Vitamins and Minerals

Vitamin/Mineral	Dietary Source	Signs of Deficiency	Signs of Toxicity
Folate (vit B9)	Green leafy vegetables, organ meats, dried yeast, dried beans, legumes, citrus, fortified grains	Macrocytic anemia, diarrhea, glossitis, lethargy, stomatitis	None known from foods; seizures
Cyanocobalamin (vit B12)	Meats, organ meats, beef, pork, milk, cheese, fish	Megaloblastic anemia, glossitis, leukopenia, weakness, peripheral neuropathy (esp. foot drop)	None known from foods
Ascorbic acid (vit C)	Citrus fruits, tomatoes, potatoes, red berries, peppers	Scurvy, keratosis of hair follicles, impaired wound healing, anemia, depression, lethargy, bleeding	Osmotic diarrhea, N/V, oxalate kidney stones, interference with anticoagulation therapy
Vitamin A	Fish liver oils, egg yolk, dairy products, green leafy or orange/yellow vegetables and fruit	Dermatitis, night blindness, keratomalacia, xeropthalmia	N/V, headache, dizziness, deep bone pain, peeling skin, gingivitis, alopecia, hepatotoxicity
Vitamin D	Fish, fish liver oils, fortified milk, egg yolk, sunlight	Osteomalacia, muscle weakness, bone pain, hypophosphatemia, hypocalcemia	Excess bone & soft tissue calcification, kidney stones, hypercalcemia, anorexia, renal failure
Vitamin E	Polyunsaturated vegetable oils, nuts, eggs, wheat germ, whole grains	Rare hemolysis, anemia, neuronal axonopathy, myopathy	Prolonged clotting time, impaired neutrophil function
Vitamin K	Green leafy vegetables, liver, vegetable oils, intestinal flora	Bleeding, purpura, bruising, prolonged clotting time	Jaundice
Calcium	Dairy products, dark, green & leafy vegetables, fortified soy, fortified orange juice	Tetany, arrhythmias, congestive heart failure, altered nerve conduction, osteomalacia	Metastatic calcification, weakness, renal failure, psychosis
Magnesium	Soy, clams, wheat germ, almonds, dairy products, green leaves, nuts, cereal grains, seafood	Weakness, convulsions, neuromuscular irritability and dysfunction, failure to thrive	Hypotension, cardiac disturbances, respiratory failure
Potassium	Meat, milk, bananas, prunes, raisins, orange, grapefruit, potatoes, legumes	Polyuria, impaired muscle contraction, ECG changes (prolonged QT interval, prominent u-waves), peritoneal distention, dyspnea, paralysis, cardiac disturbances	Mental confusion, hypotension, weakness, ECG changes (flattened P-waves, peaked T-waves), paralysis, cardiac disturbances
Iron	Meat, fish, poultry, organ meats, eggs, prunes, peas, beans, lentils, soy, raisins, fortified grain products	Glossitis, fatigue, tachycardia, microcytic hypochromic anemia, koilonychias, enteropathy	Nutritional hemosiderosis, organ damage

Adapted from Mosby's *Family Practice Sourcebook: An Evidence-Based Approach to Care*, 4th edition, edited by Dr. Michael Evans (pp. 343-345). Copyright © 2006 Elsevier Canada, a division of Reed Elsevier Canada, Ltd. All rights reserved. Reprinted by permission of Elsevier Canada, 2007.

Table 6. Macronutrient distribution ranges

Age (years)	Macronutrient as % of daily calories		
	Protein	Fat	Carbohydrate
1 to 3	5 - 20	30 - 40	45 - 65
4 to 18	10 - 30	25 - 35	45 - 65
19 or older	10 - 35	20 - 35	45 - 65

Adapted from Dietary Reference Intakes Tables, Health Canada.http://www.hc-sc.gc.ca/fn-an/nutrition/reference/table/index_e.html

Obesity

- see Endocrinology
- Body Mass Index (BMI) = weight (kg)/height (m)^2
  = weight (lbs)/height (inch)^2 x 703
- waist circumference (WC)
  - considered newest "vital sign" and should be measured in all adults to assess obesity related health risks
  - specific cutoff points exist for different ethnic backgrounds (as recommended by the 2006 Canadian Clinical Practice Guidelines on obesity)
  - measurement of waist-hip ratio has no advantage over waist circumference alone

Energy Content of Food
- Carbohydrates 4 kcal/g
- Protein 4 kcal/g
- Fat 9 kcal/g
- Ethanol 7 kcal/g

Calculating Total Daily Energy Expenditure (TDEE)
- roughly 35 kcal/kg/day (use ideal wt if obese)
- varies by age, weight, sex, and activity level
- average 2000-2100 kcal/d for women, 2700-2900 kcal/d for men

Canadian Cancer Society (CCS) Recommendations for Vitamin D use
- based on CCS research on Vitamin D and the prevention of colorectal, breast and prostate cancer
- in consultation with their healthcare provider, the Society is recommending that:
  - adults living in Canada should consider taking Vitamin D supplementation of 1,000 international units (IU) a day during the fall and winter
  - adults at higher risk of having lower Vitamin D levels should consider taking Vitamin D supplementation of 1,000 IU/day all year round. This includes people: who are older, with dark skin, who don't go outside often, and who wear clothing that covers most of their skin

Burning Fat
1 pound of human fat results in 3500 kcal of energy when burned through activity.

Losing Weight
• aim for caloric intake 500-1000 kcal/d less than TDEE
• results in 1-2 lb (0.5-1 kg) weight loss per week
• achieved by combination of increased activity and/or decreased caloric intake

Ideal Body Weight
Males: 50 kg + (2.3 kg × # of inches over 5 feet tall)
Females: 45.5 kg + (2.3 kg × # of inches over 5 feet tall)

E.g. for 5'10" male, IBW = 50 kg + 23 kg = 73 kg

Adverse Medical Consequences of Obesity
• type 2 DM   • dyslipidemia
• CAD   • osteoarthritis
• stroke   • sleep apnea
• HTN   • certain cancers
• gallbladder disease   • CHF
• non-alcoholic steatohepatitis   • low back pain
• increased total mortallity
• complications of pregnancy

"The latest evidence on fad diets..."
Comparison of the Atkins, Ornish, Weight Watchers, and Zone diets for weight loss and heart disease risk reduction. JAMA, Jan 2005 vol 293(1): 43-53.
Purpose – To assess the effectiveness and adherence rates of four popular diets for weight loss and reduction of cardiac risk factors.
Study Characteristics – Single center RCT at academic medical center in Boston, MA; 160 participants were randomized to either Atkins (carbohydrate restriction), Zone (macronutrient balanced and low glycemic load), Weight Watchers (low calorie/portion size), or Ornish (fat restriction) diet groups for a period of 18 months.
Participants – Adults aged 22 to 72 years with known HTN, dyslipidemia, or fasting hyperglycemia.
Results – Assuming that participants who discontinued the study remained at baseline, the mean weight loss at 1 year (and self selected dietary adherence rates per self report) were 2.1 kg for Atkins (53% of participants completed, P=0.009), 3.2 kg for the Zone (65% of participants completed, P=0.002), 3.0 kg for Weight Watchers (65% completed, P<0.001), 3.3 kg for Ornish (50% completed, P=0.007). Each diet significantly reduced the LDL/HDL ratio by ~10% (P<0.05), with no significant effects on blood pressure or glucose. Amount of weight loss was associated with adherence level (r = 0.60; P<.001) but not with diet type (r = 0.07; P = 0.40). Weight loss for each diet was significantly associated with reduction in levels of total/HDL cholesterol (r=0.36), C-reactive protein (r=0.37), and insulin (r=0.39), with no significant difference between diets.
Conclusion – Each popular diet was associated with modest weight loss and reduction of several cardiac risk factors. Adherence level, and not diet type, was the most important predictor of weight loss and cardiac risk factor reduction.

Table 7. Classification of Weight by BMI, Waist Circumference, and Associated Disease Risks in Adults

	BMI (kg/m²)	Obesity Class	Men ≤102 cm (40 in) Women ≤88 cm (35 in)	Men > 102 cm (40 in) Women > 88 cm (35 in)
Underweight	< 18.5		-	-
Normal	18.5 - 24.9		-	-
Overweight	25.0 - 29.9		Increased	High
Obesity	30.0 - 34.9	I	High	Very High
	35.0 - 39.9	II	Very High	Very High
Extreme Obesity	40.0 +	III	Extremely High	Extremely High

From: Classification of Overweight and Obesity by BMI, Waist Circumference, and Associated Disease Risks, National Institute of Health, National Heart Lung and Blood Institute, Obesity Education Initiative, http://www.nhlbi.nih.gov/health/public/heart/obesity/lose_wt/bmi_dis.htm

Epidemiology
• in Canada, prevalence of obesity is 23%, and 59% are overweight
• obesity rate in people of aboriginal origin is 1.6 times higher than the national average
• proportion of children aged 6-11 who are overweight has more than doubled in the last 25 years; percentage of overweight adolescents has tripled
• overweight and obesity rates in children are directly proportional to screen time (see *Exercise* section)
• only 10-15% of population consume <30% fat
• obese persons generally consume more energy-dense foods which tend to be highly processed, micronutrient poor, and high in fats, sugars, or starch

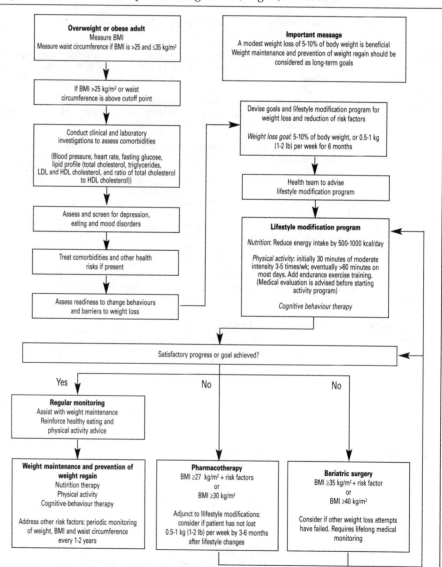

Figure 2. 2006 Canadian clinical practice guidelines on the management and prevention of obesity in adults and children [summary]
Reprinted from, CMAJ 10-Apr-07; 176(8), Page(s) S1-S13 by permission of the publisher. © 2006 Canadian Medical Association

Dyslipidemia

- see Endocrinology
- defined as abnormal elevation of plasma cholesterol or triglyceride levels
- increased risk associated with obesity, DM, EtOH use

Assessment
- measure fasting serum TC, LDL-C, HDL-C, and TG
- often measured in adults over age 20 at least once every 5 years
- screen for secondary causes: hypothyroid, chronic kidney disease, DM, nephrotic syndrome, liver disease
- assess for presence of CAD risk factors
- risk category
  - estimated using the model for 10-year CAD risk developed from the Framingham data
  - gives recommended values for LDL-C and TC:HDL-C ratio (no longer gives target TG levels, keep TG as low as possible)

Table 8. Target Lipid Values for Primary Prevention of CAD in mmol/L (mg/dL)

Risk Category	LDL-C (mmol/L)		Total-C:HDL-C ratio
High (10-yr risk of CAD ≥20%, or history of DM or any atherosclerotic disease)	<2.0 (<100)	and	<4
Moderate (10-yr risk 11-19%)	<3.5 (<130)	and	<5
Low (10-yr risk ≤10%)	<5.0 (<130 with ≥2 risk factors) (<160 with ≤1 risk factors)	and	<6

Reference: McPherson, Ruth et al. (2006). Canadian Cardiovascular Society position statement –Recommendations for the diagnosis and treatment of dyslipidemia and prevention of cardiovascular disease. Can J Cardiol 6;22(11):913-927.

Management
- use level of risk to guide intensity of treatment
- lifestyle modification
  - dietary modification: <7% of calories from saturated fat, increase soluble fibre
  - increased physical activity
  - smoking cessation
  - patient should employ consistent lifestyle modifications for at least 3 months before considering drug therapy
- pharmacologic therapy (lipid-lowering agents)
  - statins (HMG-CoA reductase inhibitor; see Table 8)
    - currently recommended as 1st line mono-therapy following unsuccessful lifestyle modifications
    - risk of myopathy and hepatotoxicity with intensive therapy is rare (0.1% and 1% of patients respectively) but must consider risk-benefit ratio in individual patients – must follow LFTs q6mths
    - see table 8 for common statins
  - other agents: bile acid sequestrants, nicotinic acid, fibrates, psyllium, cholesterol absorption inhibitors (e.g. ezetimibe)
- after initiating drug therapy, lipids should be measured after 6 weeks, and at 3 months
  - if adequate response is achieved, evaluate lipids every 4-6 months
  - monitor ALT, AST, CK at baseline then 6 weeks later for signs of transaminitis or myositis; tolerate rise in CK or creatinine ≤25%; repeat ALT, AST and CK with lipid bloodwork
- isolated hypertriglyceridemia
  - normal HDL-C and TC, elevated TG
  - mild ≥2.0 mmol/L (≥200 mg/dL); marked ≥4.5 mmol/L (≥400 mg/dL)
  - principal therapy is lifestyle modifications
    - weight loss, exercise, avoidance of smoking and alcohol, effective blood glucose control in diabetics, ↑ omega-3 fatty acid intake
  - drug therapy
    - nicotinic acid
    - fibrates
- emerging risk factors (from Framingham group)
  - lipoprotein a
  - metabolic syndrome
  - genetic risk
  - hormone replacement therapy
  - infectious agents

Hyperlipidemia Signs:
1. atheromata – plaques in blood vessel walls
2. xanthoma – plaques or nodules composed of lipid-laden histiocytes in the skin (esp. the eyelids)
3. tendinous xanthoma – lipid deposit in tendon (esp. Achilles)
4. corneal arcus (arcus senilis) – lipid deposit in cornea

LDL cannot be calculated when TG ≥4.5 mmol/L

CLINICAL DEFINITION OF METABOLIC SYNDROME
1) Central obesity
   Men - waist circumference ≥ 94cm
   Women - waist circumference ≥ 80cm
   plus any TWO of the following four factors:

Risk Factor	Defining Level
TG level	≥1.7 mmol/L (150 mg/dL)
HDL-C level:	
Men	<1.0 mmol/L (40 mg/dL)
Women	<1.3 mmol/L (50 mg/dL)
Blood pressure	≥130/85 mmHg
Fasting glucose level	≥ 5.6 mmol/L (100 mg/dL)

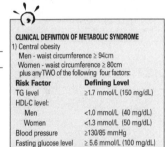

Model for Calculating the 10-year Risk of CAD in a Patient Without Diabetes Mellitus or Clinically Evident Cardiovascular Disease*, Using Framingham Data

STEP 1: DETERMINE RISK POINTS

Risk Factor	Risk Points Men	Women	Risk Factor	Risk Points Men	Women
Age, year					
30-34	-1	-9	55-50	4	7
35-39	0	-4	60-64	5	8
40-44	1	0	65-69	6	8
45-49	2	3	70-74	7	8
50-54	3	6			
Total cholesterol level, mmol/L					
<4.14	-3	-2	6.22-7.24	2	2
4.15-5.17	0	0	≥7.25	3	3
5.18-6.21	1	1			
HDL-C level, mmol					
<0.90	2	5	1.30-1.55	0	0
0.91-1.16	1	2	≥1.56	-2	-3
1.17-1.29	0	1			
Systolic blood pressure, mmHg					
<120	0	-3	140-159	2	2
120-129	0	0	≥160	3	3
130-139	1	1			
Smoker					
No	0	0	Yes	2	2

Record the points	Men	Women
Age	—	—
Total cholesterol	—	—
HDL-C	—	—
Blood pressure	—	—
Smoker	—	—
Add total risk point	—	—

STEP 2: CALCULATE RISK**

Total Risk Points	10-year Risk, % Men	Women	Total Risk Points	10-year Risk, % Men	Women
1	3	2	10	25	10
2	4	3	11	31	11
3	5	3	12	37	13
4	7	4	13	45	15
5	8	4	14	≥53	18
6	10	5	15		20
7	13	6	16		24
8	16	7	17		>27
9	20	8			

*For example, a 55-year-old man who has a total cholesterol level of 5.43 mmol/L, an HDL-C level of 1.23 mmol/L, a systolic blood pressure of 148 mmHg and who smokes would have a total risk score of 9. His 10-year risk for CAD would be 20%, the risk for the average person of his age in the study population is 16%.
**Risk of CAD outcomes including angina pectoris, unstable angina, nonfatal myocardial infarction and coronary death over subsequent 10 years for a Framingham Study participant with that specific risk score.
Reference: Recommendations for the management of dyslipidemia and the prevention of cardiovascular disease: Summary of the 2003 update. Reprinted from CMAJ 28 October 2003; 169(1): 921-924 by permission of the publisher. ©2003 Canadian Medical Association.

Comparative Tolerability of the HMG-CoA Reductase Inhibitors
Drug Safety 2000 Sep;23 (3);197-213
Study: Review
Results: 1. Multiple trials have demonstrated that there is no evidence to support that statin therapy leads to increased incidence of cataract formation. 2. Studies have demonstrated that statin therapy does not lead to statistically significant disturbances in sleep or cognition compared to placebo. 3. Studies demonstrate that the incidence of hepatotoxicity and elevated transaminases depends on statin dose and in general, all statins are similar in their rates of liver toxicity. 4.Statins metabolized solely by CYP3A4 (e.g. Lovastatin, Simvastatin, Atorvastatin, Cerivastatin) are more likely to result in hepatotoxicity or rhabdomyolysis if used in combination with a CYP3A4 inhibiting drug (e.g. Ketoconazole, grapefruit juice, erythromycin).

Table 9. Common Statins (HMG-CoA Reductase Inhibitors) and other lipid lowering agents
see Endocrinology

Drug	Starting Dose	Maximum Dose
Statins		
atorvastatin (Lipitor™)	10 mg PO OD	80 mg PO OD
lovastatin (Mevacor™)	20 mg PO qhs	80 mg PO qhs
pravastatin (Pravachol™)	40 mg PO OD	80 mg PO OD
simvastatin (Zocor™)	20 mg PO qhs	80 mg PO qhs
rosuvastatin (Crestor™)	10 mg PO qhs	40 mg PO qhs
fluvastatin (Lescol™)	20 mg PO qhs	80 mg PO qhs
Resins (bile acid sequestrants)		
cholestyramine (Questran™)	2 g PO OD	24 g PO OD
colestipol (Colestid™)	5 g PO OD	30 g PO OD
Fibrates		
Fenofibrate (Lipidil™)	67-200 mg PO OD	200 mg PO OD
Bezafibrate (Bezalip™)	200 mg PO bid-tid	600 mg PO bid-tid
Gemfibrozil (Lopid™)	600 mg PO bid	1200 mg PO bid
Other		
Ezetimibe (Ezetrol™)	10 mg PO OD	10 mg PO OD
Nicotinic Acid	50-100 mg PO bid-tid 6 g/day	

Exercise

Epidemiology
- 25% of population exercises regularly, 50% occasionally, 25% sedentary
- screen time (time spent watching TV/movies, playing computer games, or surfing the internet) has been increasing steadily in the last several years while amount of time spent being physically active has been decreasing
- excessive screen time can promote overweight and obesity, encourage violent and antisocial behaviours, and foster attention deficit difficulties
- current recommendation from international pediatric societies is that children (>2 years old) should limit their screen time to less than 2 hours/day

Incidence of Hospitalized Rhabdomyolysis in Patients Treated with Lipid-Lowering Drugs
JAMA.2004;292(21):2585-2590
Study: Retrospective cohort study
Patients:252 460 patients treated with lipid-lowering agents
Main outcome: Rabdomyolysis requiring hospitalization
Results: Of 252 460 patients, 24 cases of rhabdomyolysis requiring hospitalization occurred. Incidence rates per 10,000 person-years with 95%CI for each statin menotherapy are:
   Atorvastatin 0.54 (0.22-1.12)
   Cerivastatin 5.34(1.46-13.68)
   Pravastatin 0 (0-1.11)
   Simvastatin 0.49 (0.06-1.76)
   Fenofibrate 0 (0-14.58)
   Gemfibrozil 3.70 (0.76-10.82)
Incidence of rhabdomyolysis increased to 5.98 (95%CI, 0.72-216.0) if atorvastatin, pravastatin or simvastatin was used with a fibrate, and up to 1035 (95%CI, 389-2117) if cerivastatin was combined with a fibrate

Management
- assess current level of fitness, motivation and access to exercise
- encourage warm up and cool down periods to allow transition between rest and activity, and to avoid injuries
- exercise with caution for patients with CAD, diabetes (risk of hypoglycemia), exercise induced asthma
- balanced exercise program incorporating all types of exercise
  1. aerobic (endurance) exercise for 15-60 min 4-7x/wk
     - improves cardiac function, lowers BP, increases HDL, increases insulin sensitivity
     - target HR: 60-80% of maximum HR
     - maximum HR=220–age
  2. weight-bearing (isometric) exercise 10-20 min 2-4x/wk
     - builds muscle strength, improves bone density, improves posture
  3. stretching routine 10-12 min 4-7x/wk
     - prevents cramps, stiffness, injuries, back problems
- other benefits of exercise:
  - increases feeling of well-being and libido
  - improves quality of sleep
  - decreases depression/anxiety
  - weight control
  - improves self-esteem

Use caution when prescribing combined statin and fibrate therapy as there have been recent concerns regarding the safety of certain combinations.

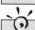

For each 1% reduction in total cholesterol, there is a 2% reduction in risk of CAD.

Smoking Cessation

Epidemiology
- smoking is the single most preventable cause of premature illness and death
- 70% of smokers see a physician each year
- 2006 Canadian data from the Canadian Tobacco Use Monitoring Survey (CTUMS) on population age 15 or older:
  - 19% are current smokers (lowest since 1965)
  - smoke an average of 15.5 cigarettes/day
  - highest prevalence in age group 20-24
  - more teenage boys smoke than teenage girls (16% vs. 14%)
  - in 2006, smoking rate decreased significantly among youth aged 15-19, from 18% down to 15%
  - percentage of ex-smokers growing (27% reported that they had quit)

Physician Advice for Smoking Cessation
Cochrane Database of Systematic Reviews 2004; Issue 4
Reviewers' conclusions: Simple advice has a small effect on cessation rates. Additional manoeuvres appear to have only a small effect, though more intensive interventions are marginally more effective than minimal interventions.

Management

- **general approach**
  - identify tobacco users, elicit smoking habits, previous quit attempts and results
  - every smoker should be offered treatment
  - ≥4 counselling sessions >10 min each with 6-12 month follow-up yield better results
  - 14% abstinent with counselling vs. 10% without counselling (OR 1.55)
  - approach depends on patient's stage of change (see *Motivational Strategies for Behavioural Change* section)
- **willing to quit**
  - follow the 5 As (see sidebar)
  - provision of social support, community resources
  - pregnant patients – advise to quit first without pharmacotherapy; use pharmacotherapy only if benefits > risks; consult Motherisk
  - Nicotine Replacement Therapies (NRT)
    - 19.7% abstinent at 12 months with NRT vs. 11.5% for placebo (OR 1.66)
    - no difference in abstinence for different forms of NRT
    - reduce cravings and withdrawal symptoms and do not contain other harmful substances that are in cigarettes
    - precautions: immediate post-MI, serious/worsening angina, serious arrhythmia
  - Bupropion SR (Zyban™)
    - 21% abstinent at 12 months vs. 8% for placebo (OR 2.73)
  - Varenicline (Champix™)
    - partial nicotine receptor agonist (reduces cravings) and partial (competitive) nicotinic receptor antagonist to reduce the response to smoked nicotine
    - indicated as an alternative to bupropion or NRT

Table 10. Types of Nicotine Replacement Therapy

Type	Dosage	Comment	Side Effects
Nicotine gum (OTC)	2 mg if <25 cig/d 4 mg if >25 cig/d 1 piece q1-2h for 1-3 mos (max. 24 pieces/d)	Chew until "peppery" taste then "park" between gum and cheek to facilitate absorption Continue to chew-park intermittently for 30 min	Mouth soreness Hiccups Dyspepsia Jaw ache Most SE's are transient
Nicotine patch (OTC)	Use for 8 weeks 21 mg/d x 4 weeks 14 mg/d x 2 weeks 7 mg/d x 2 weeks	Start with lower dose if <10 cig/d Change patch q24h and rotate sides	Skin irritation Insomnia Palpitations Anxiety
Nicotine inhaler (OTC)	6-16 cartridges/day for up to 12 weeks	Nicotine inhaled through mouth and absorbed in the mouth and throat, but not in the lungs	Local irritation Coughing
Nicotine nasal spray (Rx)		Not available in Canada	

Table 11. Bupropion as Treatment for Smoking Cessation

Mechanism	Dosage	Prescribing*	Contraindications
Inhibits re-uptake of dopamine and/or norepinephrine **side effects: insomnia, dry mouth	1. 150 mg qAM x 3 days, 2. Then 150 mg bid x 7-12 wks; 3. For maintenance consider 150 mg bid for up to 6 months	1. Decide on a quit date 2. Continue to smoke for first 1-2 wks of treatment and then completely stop (therapeutic levels reached in 1 wk)	Seizure disorder Eating disorder MAOI use in past 14 days Simultaneous use of bupropion (Wellbutrin™) for depression

*may be used in combination with nicotine replacement therapies

Table 12. Varenicline as Treatment for Smoking Cessation

Mechanism	Dosage	Prescribing*	Contraindications
partial nicotinic receptor agonist, and competitive antagonist to exogenous nicotine **side effects: nausea, vomitting, constipation, headache, dream disorder, insomnia	1. 0.5mg qAM x 3 days 2. Then 0.5 mg bid x 4 days 3. Continue 1mg BID x 12 weeks plus +/- additonal 12 weeks as maintenance	Begin treatment 1 week before quit date, then stop smoking as planned	Caution with pre-existing psychiatric condition

*may be used in combination with nicotine replacement therapies

- **unwilling to quit**
  - motivational intervention (5 Rs) – see sidebar
  - risks of smoking:
    - short-term: SOB, asthma exacerbation, impotence, infertility, pregnancy complications, heartburn, URTI
    - long-term: MI, stroke, COPD, lung CA, other cancers
    - environmental: higher risk in spouse/children of lung CA, SIDS, asthma, respiratory infections

Assist patient in developing quit plan "STAR"
Set quit date
Tell family and friends (for support)
Anticipate challenges (e.g. withdrawal)
Remove tobacco products (e.g. ashtrays/lighters)

The 5 As for patients willing to quit:
Ask if patient smokes
Advise patient to quit
Assess willingness to quit
Assist in quit attempt
Arrange follow-up

Nicotine Replacement Therapy for Smoking Cessation
Cochrane Database of Systematic Reviews 2004; Issue 3
Reviewers' conclusions: All of the commercially available forms of NRT (gum, transdermal patch, nasal spray, inhaler and sublingual tablets/lozenges) are effective as part of a strategy to promote smoking cessation. They increase the odds of quitting approximately 1.5 to 2 fold regardless of setting. The effectiveness of NRT appears to be largely independent of the intensity of additional support provided to the smoker. Provision of more intense levels of support, although beneficial in facilitating the likelihood of quitting, is not essential to the success of NRT.

Antidepressants for Smoking Cessation
Hughes JR et al. *Cochrane Database of Systematic Reviews 2006; Issue 3*
Reviewers' conclusions: The antidepressants bupropion and nortriptyline can aid smoking cessation but selective serotonin reuptake inhibitors (e.g. fluoxetine) do not.

The 2-3 Pattern of Smoking Cessation
- onset of withdrawal is 2-3h after last cigarette
- peak withdrawal is at 2-3 days
- expect improvement of withdrawal symptoms at 2-3 weeks
- resolution of withdrawal at 2-3 months
- highest relapse rate within 2-3 months

The 5 Rs for patients unwilling to quit:
Relevance to patient (health concerns, family/social situations)
Risks of smoking
Rewards of quitting
Roadblocks to quitting
Repetition of motivational intervention at each visit

- benefits of smoking cessation:
  - improved health, save money, food tastes better, good example to children
- obstacles:
  - fear of withdrawal, weight gain, failure, lack of support
- repetition:
  - reassure unsuccessful patient that most people try many times before successfully quitting (average number of attempts before success is 7)
- **recent quitter**
  - highest relapse rate within 3 months of quitting
    - minimal practice: congratulate on success, encourage ongoing abstinence, review benefits, problems
    - prescriptive interventions: address problems of weight gain, negative mood, withdrawal, lack of support

Alcohol

- see Psychiatry

Definition
- diagnostic categories occur along a continuum
  - abstinence
  - low-risk drinking
    - ≤2 drinks/day
    - ≤9 drinks/wk for women, ≤14 drinks/wk for men
  - at-risk drinking
    - consumption above low-risk level but no alcohol-related physical or social problems
  - alcohol abuse
    - consumption above low-risk level with one or more of a) alcohol-related physical or social problems b) continued use despite hazardous consequences c) inability to fulfill major life roles d) legal problems associated with use, but no evidence of alcohol dependence
  - alcohol dependence (see Psychiatry)

Epidemiology
- 10-15% of patients in family practice are problem drinkers (see Psychiatry)
- >500,000 Canadians are alcohol-dependent
- 20-50% of hospital admissions, 10% of premature deaths, 30% of suicides, and 50% of fatal traffic accidents in Canada are alcohol-related
- more likely to miss diagnosis in women, elderly, patients with high socioeconomic status

Assessment
- screen for alcohol dependence
  - CAGE questionnaire (see sidebar)
  - if CAGE positive, explore with further questions for alcohol abuse (see Psychiatry)
- assess drinking profile
  - setting, time, place, occasion, with whom
  - impact on: family, work, social
  - quantity-frequency history
    - how many drinks per day?
    - how many days per week?
    - maximum number of drinks on any one day in the past month?
- if identified positive for alcohol problem
  - screen for other drug use
  - identify medical/psychiatric complications
  - ask about drinking and driving
  - ask about past recovery attempts and current readiness for change

Investigations
- GGT and MCV for baseline and follow-up monitoring
- AST, ALT (usually, AST:ALT approaches 2:1 in an alcoholic)
- CBC (anemia, thrombocytopenia), PT (decreased clotting factors production by liver)

Management
- intervention should be consistent with patient's motivation for change (motivational interviewing)
- regular follow-up is crucial
- 10% of patients in alcohol withdrawal will have seizures or delirium tremens
- Alcoholics Anonymous/12-step program

STANDARD DRINK EQUIVALENTS
One standard drink = 14 g of pure alcohol
- beer (5% alcohol) = 12 oz
- wine (12-17%) = 5 oz
- fortified wine = 3 oz
- hard liquor (80 proof) = 1.5 oz

ALCOHOL METABOLIZED PER HOUR
- alcohol metabolism is constant (zero-order kinetics) regardless of blood alcohol level
- average metabolism ranges between 13-25 mg/dL blood per hour or 100-200 mg/kg/hour.
- equivalent to 0.5-1 standard drinks per hour or BAL decrease of 0.01% per hour
- metabolism elevated in chronic alcoholics

CAGE Questionnaire:

C Have you ever felt the need to CUT down on your drinking?

A Have you ever felt ANNOYED at criticism of your drinking?

G Have you ever felt GUILTY about your drinking?

E Have you ever had a drink first thing in the morning to steady your nerves or get rid of a hangover? (EYE OPENER)

≥2 for men or ≥1 for women indicates possibility of problem drinking and need for further assessment (sensitivity 85%, specificity 89%)

Adverse Medical Consequences of Problem Drinking
- GI: gastritis, dyspepsia, pancreatitis, liver disease, bleeds, diarrhea, oral/esophageal cancer
- cardiac: hypertension, alcoholic cardiomyopathy
- neurologic: Wernicke-Korsakoff syndrome, peripheral neuropathy
- hematologic: anemia, coagulopathies
- other: trauma, insomnia, family violence, anxiety/depression, social/family dysfunction, sexual dysfunction, fetal damage

- outpatient/day programs for those with chronic, resistant problems
  - family treatment (Al-Anon, Alateen, screen for spouse/child abuse)
- in-patient program if:
  - dangerous or highly unstable home environment
  - severe medical/psychiatric problem
  - addiction to drug that may require in-patient detoxification
  - refractory to other treatment programs
- pharmacologic
  - diazepam for withdrawal
  - disulfiram (Antabuse™)
    - ◆ blocks conversion of acetaldehyde to acetic acid (which leads to flushing, headache, nausea/vomiting, hypotension if alcohol is ingested)
  - naltrexone
    - ◆ competitive opioid antagonist that reduces cravings and pleasurable effects of drinking
    - ◆ note: prescription opioids become ineffective; may trigger withdrawal in opioid-dependent patients

Prognosis
- relapse is common and should not be viewed as failure
- monitor regularly for signs of relapse
- 25-30% of abusers exhibit spontaneous improvement over 1 year
- 60-70% of individuals with jobs and families have an improved quality of life 1 year post-treatment

Common Presenting Problems

Abdominal Pain

- see Gastroenterology and General Surgery

Epidemiology
- 20% of individuals have experienced abdominal pain within the last 6-12 months
- 90% resolve in 2-3 weeks
- only 10% are referred to specialists
- <10% admitted to hospital

Etiology
- most common diagnosis is "nonspecific abdominal pain", which has no identifiable cause and is usually self-limited
- GI disorders (e.g. PUD, pancreatitis, IBD, appendicitis, gastroenteritis, IBS, diverticular disease, biliary tract disease)
- urinary tract disorders (e.g. UTI, renal calculi)
- gynecological disorders (e.g. PID, ectopic pregnancy, endometriosis)
- cardiovascular disorders (e.g. CAD, AAA, ischemic bowel)
- other: toxic ingestion, foreign body, psychogenic

Pathophysiology
- type of pain
  - somatic pain – sharp, localized pain
  - visceral pain – dull, generalized pain
- location of pain
  - epigastric (foregut) – distal esophagus, stomach, proximal duodenum, biliary tree, pancreas, liver
  - periumbilical (midgut) – distal duodenum to proximal 2/3 of transverse colon
  - hypogastric (hindgut) – distal 1/3 of transverse colon to rectosigmoid region

In patient > 50 years old, keep a high index of suspicion for AAA - its presentation may mimic renal colic or diverticulitis.

Investigations
- guided by findings on history and physical
- bloodwork
  - CBC + differential, electrolytes, BUN, Cr, amylase, lipase, AST, ALT, ALP, bilirubin, glucose, INR/PTT, tox screen, β-hCG
- imaging
  - abdominal x-ray (gas pattern, free air)
  - ultrasound (gallbladder disease, gynecological problems)
  - CT scan
- other tests
  - urinalysis
  - fecal occult blood
  - endoscopy (for peptic ulcers, gastritis, tumours, etc.)
  - *H. pylori* testing (urea breath test, serology)

If pain precedes nausea/vomiting, cause of abdominal pain is more likely to be surgical.

Acne Vulgaris (Common Acne)

- see <u>Dermatology</u>

> **Comedone:** a dilated hair follicle filled with keratin, bacteria and sebum

Definition and Clinical Features
- an inflammatory disease involving the sebaceous glands of the skin; characterized by papules and/or pustules and/or comedones
- may affect face, neck, back, and upper chest
- prevalence: 75% of teenagers and young adults

Pathogenesis
- excess sebum production
  - excellent growth medium for *Propionibacterium acnes*
  - FFA and bacteria cause inflammation, delayed hypersensitivity reaction
- hyperkeratinization of follicle with plugging, resulting in inflammatory papules and comedones
- exacerbating factors
  - oil-based makeup, hair gels and sprays, cooking oils
  - emotional stress, menstruation, hormonal factors
  - systemic medications, including steroids, lithium, phenytoin, androgens
  - OCP containing high progestin doses (e.g. levo/norgestrel)
  - recent studies have shown that intake of dairy and high glycemic index foods may worsen acne by means of IGF-mediated inflammatory pathway

> **CLASSIFICATION OF ACNE VULGARIS**
> **Non-inflammatory Acne**
> - open comedones: black heads
> - closed comedones: white heads
>
> **Inflammatory Acne**
> (in order of lesion formation)
> - papules
> - pustules
> - nodules
> - cysts
> - scars

Management
- general recommendations
  - do not squeeze lesions: may cause inflammation and scarring
  - limit face washing to 2-3 times per day, and avoid abrasive soaps
  - use water-based cosmetics
  - trial of decreased dairy products and high glycemic index foods
- topical therapy (used first, and then in combination with oral therapy if necessary)
  - topical retinoids – tretinoin, adapalene, tazarotene
  - topical antimicrobials – benzoyl peroxide 2.5-10%, clindamycin, erythromycin
  - salicylic acid
- oral therapy
  - oral antibiotics – tetracycline, doxycycline, minocycline
  - hormonal agents (female patients) – estrogen-containing oral contraceptives
  - oral retinoid – isotretinoin (Accutane™)
    - teratogenic and requires monthly bloodwork - used with caution
    - reserved for severe cases of cystic acne (face, neck, back, etc.)
    - reduces sebum production, causes atrophy of sebaceous glands, increases skin cell turnover (comedolytic), and inhibits bacterial growth in skin
    - need baseline CBC, pregnancy test, LFT's, cholesterol and TG prior to initiation of therapy, and repeat tests at 2 weeks and then q 4 weeks
    - women of childbearing age must be using some form of birth control
    - counsel male patients not to share medication with female partners
    - continue use of contraception for at least 1 month after discontinuation

> **A low-glycemic-load diet improves symptoms in acne vulgaris patients: a randomized controlled trial**
> Am J Clin Nutr. 2007;86:107-15
> **Study:** Randomized, observer-blinded, with monthly follow-up x 3 months
> **Patients:** 43 males aged 15-25 years
> **Intervention:** Low glycemic-load diet with 25% of calories from protein and 45% from low glycemic index carbohydrates vs the control diet with carbohydrate dense foods
> **Main outcome:** # acne lesions
> **Results:** Total acne lesions were significantly decreased (p<0.03) in the low glycemic load diet (-23.5±3.9) versus control (-12.0±3.5). The low glycemic load diet also resulted in better insulin sensitivity reduced BMI.

Allergic Rhinitis

Definition
- inflammation of the nasal mucosa that is triggered by an allergic reaction
- classified as seasonal or perennial
  - seasonal:
    - experience symptoms during a specific time of the year
    - usually to outdoor allergens, varies with geographic area
    - common allergens: trees, grass and weed pollens, and airborne moulds
  - perennial:
    - experience symptoms throughout the year with variation in severity
    - common allergens include dust mites, animal dander, and moulds

> **Differential Diagnosis**
> - acute viral infection
> - vasomotor rhinitis
> - deviated septum
> - nasal polyps
> - acute/chronic sinusitis
> - drug-induced rhinitis
> - pregnancy

Etiology
- increased IgE levels to certain allergens → excessive degranulation of mast cells → release of inflammatory mediators (i.e. histamine) and cytokines → local inflammatory reaction

Epidemiology
- affects approximately 40% of children and 20-30% of adults
- prevalence has increased in developed countries, particularly in the past two decades
- associated with asthma, sinusitis and otitis media

Assessment
- identify allergens
- take an environmental/occupational history
- ask about related conditions (e.g. atopic dermatitis, asthma, sinusitis, and family Hx)

Management
- minimize exposure to allergens
  - most important aspect of management, often sufficient (may take months)
- pharmacologic agents
  - oral antihistamines - first line therapy for mild symptoms
    - e.g. cetirizine (Reactine™), fexofenadine (Allegra™), loratadine (Claritin™)
  - intranasal corticosteroids for moderate/severe or persistent symptoms
  - intranasal decongestants (use must be limited to <5 days to avoid rhinitis medicamentosa - see sidebar)
- allergy skin testing
  - for patients with chronic rhinitis
  - symptoms not controlled by allergen avoidance, pharmacological therapy
  - may identify allergens to include in immunotherapy treatment
- immunotherapy (allergy shots)
  - reserved for severe cases unresponsive to pharmacologic agents
  - consists of periodic (usually weekly) subcutaneous injections of custom prepared solutions of one or more antigens to which the patient is allergic

> **Rhinitis medicamentosa -** Rebound nasal congestion. Occurs with prolonged use (>5-7 days) of vasoconstrictive medications. Patient may become dependent, requiring more frequent dosing to achieve the same decongestent effect. See Otolaryngology.

Anxiety

- see Psychiatry

Epidemiology
- 25-30% of patients in primary care settings have psychiatric disorders
- many are undiagnosed or untreated; hence the need for good screening
- high rate of coexistence of anxiety disorders and depression

Screening
- screening questions
  - Do you tend to be an anxious or nervous person?
  - Have you felt unusually worried about things recently?
  - Has this worrying affected your life? How?
- if positive response, follow up with symptom-specific questions (see Figure 3)

Assessment
- associated symptoms
- risk factors
  - family history of anxiety or depression, past history of anxiety, stressful life event, social isolation, gender (women), co-morbid psychiatric diagnosis
- assess substance abuse, co-morbid depression, suicidal ideations/self-harm
- to differentiate anxiety disorders, consider symptoms and their duration (see Figure 3)

Management
- patient education (emphasize commonness, good recovery rate of anxiety conditions)
- lifestyle advice (decrease caffeine and alcohol intake, exercise more, relaxation techniques)
- self-help materials, community resources (support groups)
- cognitive behavioural therapy (cognitive interventions, exposure therapy, etc.)
- pharmacotherapy (start low, go slow)
  - for GAD:
    - 1st line - paroxetine, escitalopram, sertraline, venlafaxine XR
    - 2nd line - lorazepam, diazepam, alprazolam, imipramine, buproprion XL
    - 3rd line - trazodone, mirtazapine, risperidone, adjunctive olanzapine
    - 3rd line therapy may be used as an adjunct or used for those patients who fail 1st and 2nd line therapy alone or combined
    - due to side effects, dependence and withdrawal issues, benzodiazepines are best used on a short-term basis (i.e. 1-2 months)
    - therapy should continue for at least 1 year after relief of symptoms
  - for pharmacotherapy specific to other types of anxiety, see Psychiatry

> **Differential Diagnosis (see Figure 3)**
> - panic disorder
> - GAD
> - PTSD
> - OCD
> - social phobia
> - specific phobia
> - separation anxiety (children)
> - other: GMC, mood disorder, psychotic disorder

> **Rule Out**
> - cardiac (post MI, arrhythmias)
> - endocrine (hyperthyroidism, diabetes, pheochromocytoma)
> - respiratory (asthma, COPD)
> - somatoform disorders
> - psychotic disorders
> - mood disorders (depression, bipolar)
> - personality disorder (OCPD)
> - drugs (amphetamines, thyroid preparations, caffeine, OTC for colds/decongestants, alcohol/benzodiazepine withdrawal)

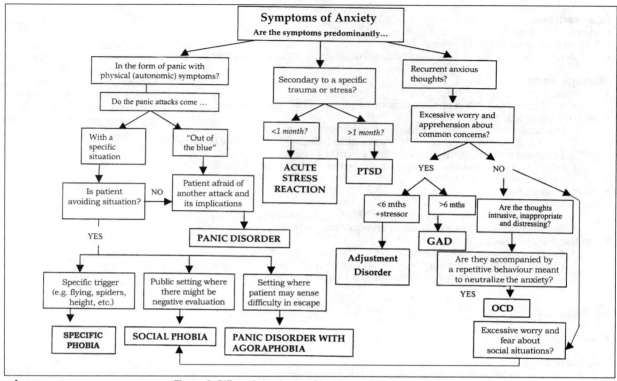

Figure 3. Differentiating Anxiety Disorders
Adapted from: Anxiety Review Panel. Evans M, Bradwejn J, Dunn L (Eds) (2000). Guidelines for the Treatment of Anxiety Disorders in Primary Care. Toronto: Queen's Printer of Ontario, pp. 41.

Asthma/COPD

- see Respirology

Definition
- asthma
  - chronic but reversible airway inflammation characterized by periodic attacks of wheezing, shortness of breath, chest tightness, and coughing
  - airways hyperresponsive to triggers/antigens leading to acute obstructive symptoms by bronchocontriction, mucous plugs and increased inflammation
  - cannot be diagnosed at first presentation
  - called Reactive Airway Disease until recurrent presentations
- chronic obstructive pulmonary disease (COPD)
  - a group of chronic, progressive, expiratory lung diseases characterized by limited airflow with variable degrees of air sac enlargement and lung tissue destruction
  - emphysema and chronic bronchitis are the most common forms of COPD

Table 13. Differentiating COPD from Asthma

	COPD	Asthma
Age of Onset	Usually in 6th decade	Any age (but 50% of cases diagnosed in children <10 yo)
Role of Smoking	Directly related	Known trigger
Reversibility of Airflow Obstruction	Airflow obstruction is chronic and persistent	Airflow obstruction is episodic and usually reversible with therapy
Evolution	Slow, cumulative disabling pattern	Episodic, less than 50% will outgrow
History of Allergy	Infrequent	Over 50% patients
Precipitators	Environmental irritants (air pollution), cigarette smoking, antiprotease deficiency, viral infection, occupational exposure (firefighters, dusty jobs)	Environmental irritants (dust, pollen), furry animals, cold air, exercise, URTIs, cigarette smoke, use of β-blockers/ASA
Symptoms/Signs	Chronic cough, sputum and/or dyspnea	Wheeze (hallmark symptom), dyspnea, chest tightness, cough which is worse in cold, at night, and in early am prolonged expiration

What Colour is Your Inhaler?

Name	Body / Cap Colour
β2-agonists	
Ventolin™	light blue/navy
Serevent™	teal/light teal
Bricanyl™	blue/white
ICS	
Flovent™	orange/peach
Pulmicort™	white/brown
Combined	
Advair™	purple discus
Symbicort™	red/white
Other	
Atrovent™	clear/green
Combivent™	clear/orange
Spiriva™	white/turquoise

Differential Diagnosis of Asthma
- chronic obstructive pulmonary disease
- cystic fibrosis
- vocal cord dysfunction
- congestive heart failure
- mechanical obstruction of airways (e.g. tumours)

When prescribing Ventolin™, watch out for signs of hypokalemia: lethargy, irritability, paresthesias, myalgias, weakness, palpitations, nausea, vomitting, polyuria.

Signs of poorly controlled asthma
- β2 agonist use >4x/wk
- asthma-related absence from work/school
- exercise induced asthma
- night-time symptoms >1x/wk

Table 13. Differentiating COPD from Asthma (continued)

	COPD	Asthma
Diffusion Capacity	Decreased (more so in pure emphysema)	Normal (for pure asthma)
Hypoxemia	Chronic in advanced stages	Not usually present Episodic with severe attacks
Spirometry	May have improvement with bronchodilators but not universally seen	Marked improvement with bronchodilators or steroids
Chest X-ray	Often normal Increased bronchial markings (chronic bronchitis) and chronic hyperinflation (emphysema) often co-exist	Often normal or episodic hyperinflation Hyperinflation during asthma attack
Management	First Line: Ipratropium bromide (Atrovent™) Others: salbutamol (Ventolin™), fluticasone (Flovent™), tiotropium bromide (Spiriva™), oral prednisone, oxygen, salmeterol (Serevent™) at bedtime Get flu shot and Pneumovax™	Combination of reliever medications (SABAs) taken on prn basis and controller medications (see below) taken on a regular basis to achieve control of asthma symptoms (see sidebar) Controller medications Step 1: Low-dose ICS Step 2: Medium/high-dose ICS or low-dose ICS plus either LABA, LT modifier, or long-acting theophylline Step 3: Medium/high-dose ICS plus either LABA, LT modifier, or long-acting theophylline Step 4: As above plus immunotherapy +/- oral glucocorticosteroids

SABA = short-acting β-agonist   LABA = Long-acting β-agonist   ICS = inhaled glucocorticosteroids   LT modifier = leukotriene modifier

Asthma Control Targets
- daytime symptoms <2x per week
- no limitation of activities
- no nocturnal symptoms
- use of reliver medication <2x per week
- normal lung function (PEF, FEV1)
- no exacerbations

Benign Prostatic Hypertrophy (BPH)

- see Urology

Definition
- hyperplasia of the stroma and epithelium in the periurethral transition zone

History
- include current/past health, surgeries, trauma, current and OTC meds - see Table 14

Differential Diagnosis
- prostate cancer
- urethral obstruction
- bladder neck obstruction
- neurogenic bladder
- cystitis
- prostatitis

Table 14. Symptoms of BPH

Obstructive symptoms	Irritative symptoms	Late complications
Hesitancy (difficulty starting urine flow)	Urgency	Hydronephrosis
Diminution in size and force of urinary stream	Frequency	Loss of renal concentrating ability
Stream interruption (double voiding)	Nocturia	Systemic acidosis
Urinary retention (bladder does not feel completely empty)	Urge incontinence	Renal failure
Post-void dribbling	Dysuria	
Overflow incontinence		

Investigations
- physical exam must include DRE for size, symmetry, nodularity, and texture of prostate (prostate is symetrically enlarged, smooth and rubbery in BPH)
- urinalysis for hematuria (common symptom)
- PSA level
  - measured if life expectancy is >10 years, as it will change management (e.g. of voiding symptoms)
  - is considered normal when <4.0 μg/mL; however, must take into account patient's age and rate of PSA increase (PSA velocity)
  - uncertain how to deal with values between 4-10 μg/mL
  - if >10 μg/mL can diagnose prostate pathology
- optional testing includes:
  - Cr, BUN
  - post-void residual volume by ultrasound
  - voiding diary
  - uroflow
  - sexual function questionnaire
- tests NOT recommended as part of routine initial evaluation include:
  - cystourethroscopy
  - cytology
  - prostate ultrasound or biopsy
  - IVP

Management
- referral to urologist if symptoms other than mild
- **watchful waiting with lifestyle modification**
  - for patients with mild symptoms, or moderate/severe symptoms considered by the patient to be non-bothersome
  - lifestyle modification includes:
    - fluid restriction (avoid alcohol and caffeine)
    - avoidance/monitoring of certain medications (e.g. antihistamines, diuretics, antidepressants, decongestants)
    - pelvic floor exercises
    - bladder retraining - organized voiding
- pharmacology - for moderate/severe bothersome symptoms
  - alpha receptor antagonists (e.g. terazosin (Hytrin™), doxazosin (Cardura™), tamsulosin (Flomax™), alfuzosin (Xatral™)) → relaxation of smooth muscle around the prostate and bladder neck
  - 5-α reductase inhibitor (e.g. finasteride (Proscar™))
    - only for patients with demonstrated prostatic enlargement due to BPH
    - inhibits enzyme responsible for conversion of testosterone into DHT thus reducing growth of prostate
  - phytotherapy (e.g. saw palmetto berry extract, *Pygeum africanum*)
    - more studies required before being recommended as standard therapy
    - considered safe for use
- surgery
  - TURP: transurethral resection of the prostate
    - absolute indications - failed medical therapy, intractable urinary retention, benign prostatic obtruction leading to renal insufficiency
    - complications include: impotence, incontinence, ejaculatory difficulties (retrograde ejaculation), decreased libido
  - TUIP: transurethral incision of the prostate - for prostates <30 g
  - other invasive procedures include: TUVP (transurethral electrovaporization of prostate), laser prostatectomy, open prostatectomy
  - minimally invasive surgical therapies (MISTS) include:
    - TUMT: transurethral microwave therapy
    - TUNA: transurethral needle ablation
    - stents - for severe urinary obstruction in non-surgical candidate

Bronchitis (acute)

Definition
- acute infection of the tracheobronchial tree causing inflammation with resultant bronchial edema and mucus formation

Epidemiology
- fifth most common diagnosis in family medicine, most common is URTI

Etiology
- 80% viral: rhinovirus, coronavirus, adenovirus, influenza, parainfluenza, RSV
- 20% bacterial: *M. pneumoniae, C. pneumoniae, S. pneumoniae*

Investigations
- acute bronchitis is typically a clinical diagnosis
- sputum culture/Gram stain is not very informative
- CXR if suspect pneumonia (cough >3 weeks, abnormal vital signs, localized chest findings) or CHF
- pulmonary function tests with methacholine challenge if suspect asthma

Management
- primary prevention
  - frequent hand washing, smoking cessation, avoid irritant exposure
- symptomatic relief: rest, fluids (3-4 L/day when febrile), humidity, analgesics and antitussives as required
- bronchodilators, i.e. albuterol, may offer improvement of symptoms
- current literature does not support routine antibiotic treatment for the management of acute bronchitis because it is most likely to be caused by a viral infection
  - antibiotics may be useful if elderly, comorbidities, pneumonia is suspected, or if the patient is toxic (refer to *Antibiotic Quick Reference Guide*)
  - antibiotics in children show no benefit

Differential Diagnosis
- URTI
- asthma
- acute exacerbation of chronic bronchitis
- sinusitis
- pneumonia
- bronchiolitis
- pertussis
- environmental/occupational exposures
- post-nasal drip
- others: reflux esophagitis, CHF, bronchogenic CA, aspiration syndromes, CF, foreign body

How to tell if viral or bacterial?
Bacterial infections tend to give a higher fever, excessive amounts of purulent sputum production, and may be associated with concomitant COPD.

NB: purulent sputum is not necessarily bacterial.

Chest Pain

- see Cardiology
- see Emergency Medicine

Differential Diagnosis

Table 15. Differential Diagnosis of Chest Pain

Cardiac	Pulmonary	GI	MSK/Neuro	Psychologic
Angina*	Pneumonia	GERD	Costochondritis	Anxiety
MI*	Pneumothorax*	PUD	Intercostal strain	Panic
Pericarditis*	PE*	Perforated viscus*	Arthritis	Depression
Myocarditis	Pulmonary HTN	Esophageal spasm	Rib fractures	
Aortic dissection*	Lung CA	Cholecystitis	Herpes zoster	
Endocarditis		Hepatitis		

*Emergent

Investigations

- ECG, CXR, and others if indicated (cardiac enzymes, D-dimers, LFTs, etc.)
- refer to Emergency Department if suspect serious etiology (e.g. aortic dissection, MI)

Management of Common Causes of Chest Pain

- angina/ischemic heart disease:
    - acute: nitroglycerin (NTG) (wait 5 minutes between sprays and if no effect after 3 sprays call ambulance or go to Emergency Department)
    - long term: See Figure 4
- MI:
    - "MONA" (Morphine, Oxygen, NTG, ASA)
    - ± reperfusion therapy with tPA or streptokinase if within 6 hours (Note: can only use SK once in lifetime)
    - start β-blocker (e.g. metoprolol starting dose 12.5 mg PO OD, increase gradually to 50 mg PO bid)
- endocarditis
    - IV Penicillin G 20 million Units OD or IV ampicillin 12 g OD
- GERD:
    - antacids, H_2 blockers, PPIs
- costochondritis:
    - NSAIDs

Risk Factors for Coronary Artery Disease:

Major
1. Smoking
2. Diabetes
3. Hypertension
4. Hyperlipidemia
5. Family history

Minor
1. Obesity
2. Sedentary lifestyle
3. Age

High-risk symptoms and signs of chest pain include:
- severe pain
- pain for >20 min
- new onset pain at rest
- severe SOB
- loss of consciousness
- hypotension
- tachycardia
- bradycardia
- cyanosis

MI in Eldery Women
Elderly women can often present with dizziness, lightheadedness or weakness, in the absence of chest pain.

Stable Ischemic Heart Disease

↓

life-style modification (address diet, alcohol, smoking, exercise)
manage concomitant disorders (e.g. hypertension, diabetes, hyperthyroidism, anemia)
anti-platelet therapy for *all* patients (aspirin 81 mg po OD unless contraindicated or failed)
β-blocker for *all post-MI* patients or those with heart failure
ACE inhibitor for patients >55 years or with any coincident indication
statin therapy for patients with coronary disease

↓ if symptoms persist

start a β-blocker (if not already using it)/switch to β-1 selective blocker
sublingual nitrate for prophylaxis and acute symptom relief

↓ if symptoms persist

add long-acting (oral or transdermal) nitrate
+/- calcium channel blocker

↓ if symptoms persist

assess suitability for coronary artery revascularization

Figure 4. Treatment Algorithm for Stable Ischemic Heart Disease
References: Ontario Drug Therapy Guidelines for Stable Ischemic Heart Disease in Primary Care (2000). Ontario Program for Optimal Therapeutics. Toronto: Queen's Printer of Ontario, pp. 10.
Guidelines on the management of stable angina pectoris. Recommendations of the Task Force of the European Society of Cardiology; 2006. p63.

Common Cold (Acute Rhinitis)

Definition
- viral upper respiratory tract infection (URTI) with inflammation

Epidemiology
- most common diagnosis in family medicine; peaks in winter months
- incidence: adults = 2-4/year, children = 6-10/year
- organisms
    - mainly rhinoviruses (30-35% of all colds)
    - others: coronavirus, adenovirus, RSV, influenza, parainfluenza, echovirus, coxsackie virus
- incubation: 1-5 days
- transmission: person-person contact via secretions on skin/objects and by aerosol droplets

Risk Factors
- psychological stress, excessive fatigue, allergic nasopharyngeal disorders, smoking, sick contacts

Clinical Features
- symptoms
    - local – nasal congestion, clear to mucopurulent secretions, sneezing, sore throat, conjunctivitis, cough
    - general – malaise, headache, myalgias, mild fever
- signs
    - boggy and erythematous nasal/oropharyngeal mucosa, enlarged lymph nodes
    - normal chest exam
- complications
    - secondary bacterial infection: otitis media, sinusitis, bronchitis, pneumonia
    - asthma/COPD exacerbation

Differential Diagnosis
- allergic rhinitis, pharyngitis, influenza, laryngitis, croup, sinusitis, bacterial infections

Management
- patient education
    - symptoms peak at day 1-3 and usually subside within 1 week
    - cough may persist for days to weeks after other symptoms disappear
    - no antibiotics indicated because of viral etiology
    - secondary bacterial infection can present within 3-10 days after onset of cold symptoms
- prevention
    - frequent hand washing, avoidance of hand to mucous membrane contact, use of surface disinfectant
- symptomatic relief
    - rest, hydration, gargling warm salt water, steam
    - analgesics and antipyretics: acetaminophen, ASA (not in children because risk of Reye's syndrome)
    - cough suppression: dextromethorphan or codeine if necessary
    - zinc gluconate lozenge use is controversial
    - decongestants, antihistamines
- patients with reactive airway disease will require increased use of bronchodilators and inhaled steroids

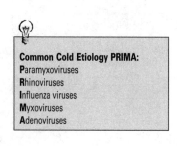

Common Cold Etiology PRIMA:
Paramyxoviruses
Rhinoviruses
Influenza viruses
Myxoviruses
Adenoviruses

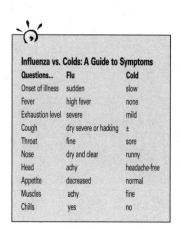

Influenza vs. Colds: A Guide to Symptoms		
Questions...	Flu	Cold
Onset of illness	sudden	slow
Fever	high fever	none
Exhaustion level	severe	mild
Cough	dry severe or hacking	±
Throat	fine	sore
Nose	dry and clear	runny
Head	achy	headache-free
Appetite	decreased	normal
Muscles	achy	fine
Chills	yes	no

Contraception

- see Gynecology

Table 16. Contraception Table

	Advantages	Disadvantages
Combined OCP	99.9% effective with perfect use, 92-97% effective with typical use, cycle control, ↓dysmenorrhea,↓menstrual flow, ↓ovarian cancer, ↓endometrial cancer, ↓ risk of fibroids, ↓ acne, ↓ hirsutism	Irregular bleeding, systemic hormonal side effects (breast tenderness, nausea, mood changes), no STI protection, slightly ↑risk of venous thromboembolism (VTE), MI, and stroke, decreased quantity of breast milk postpartum
Progestin Only Pill (e.g. Micronor®)	99.5% effective with perfect use, ↓ menstrual flow, ↓ cramping , no ↑ risk of VTE, MI or stroke, suitable for postpartum	Irregular bleeding, no STI protection, contraceptive reliability requires regular pill-taking at the same time each day (within 3 hours), no pill free interval
Transdermal Patch (e.g. Evra®)	Easy to use, changed weekly, same advantages of OCP use	Same as OCP, skin irritation
NuvaRing® (inserted by patient)	Easy to use (in for 3 weeks, out for 1), same advantages of OCP, less systemic hormonal side effects	Same as OCP, vaginitis, some women may be uncomfortable with self-insertion
DMPA IM progesterone injection q12 wks (e.g. DepoProvera®)	99% effective against pregnancy, infrequent dosing, ↓ menstrual flow or amenorrhea, ↓ risk of endometrial cancer	Irregular bleeding, delayed return of fertility, no STI protection, systemic hormonal side effects (most common is headache), wt gain, ↓ bone mineral density (check after 5 years)
Male Condom	97% effective against pregnancy and STIs when used properly, when used properly WITH spermicide they are close to 99.9% effective, no Rx required	Allergy to latex, irritation, only effective before the expiry date, must be applied properly, can only be used once, some find them cumbersome
Diaphragm	94% effective with perfect use with spermicide, non-hormonal, female-controlled method of contraception, ↓ risk of cervical cancer	Must be left in 6 hours after intercourse, must be used with spermicide, incomplete STI protection, latex allergy, must be fitted by health care worker, ↑ risk of UTI, risk of toxic shock syndrome
Sponge	One-size-fits-all barrier method, does not require fitting by MD, available in pharmacies, 80-90% effective in nulliparous women	Relatively expensive, only ~60% effective in parous women, incomplete STI protection, risk of toxic shock syndrome
Intrauterine Device (IUD)	99% effective against pregnancy, effective for 5 yrs, no daily regimen required, can be easily removed, ideal in post-partum women	No STI protection, ↑ relative risk of PID in first month, must be inserted by MD, risk of post-insertion vaso-vagal response, risk of uterine rupture is 0.6-1.6 per 1000, 2-10% expulsion rate
Levonorgestrel IUD (e.g. Mirena®)	↓ menstrual flow, less systemic hormonal side effects than OCP	Hormonal side effects (see *combined OCP*), expensive (~$400)
Copper IUD (e.g. Nova T®)	↓ risk of endometrial cancer, less expensive (~$170)	Irregular bleeding or ↑ menstrual flow, 6-20% women discontinue use in first 5 yrs because of pain or ↑ bleeding
Fertility Awareness (e.g. symptothermal method)	↑ awareness of gynecological health, reasonable for couples for whom an accidental pregnancy would be acceptable	High probability of failure if not used consistently and correctly, no STI protection
Lactational amenorrhea	98% effective in breastfeeding women if menses not returned, fully or nearly fully breastfeeding baby and baby is under 6 months old	Increased pregnancy rates if infant receiving supplementary food; breastfeeding must be regular even through the night

Emergency Contraception (EC)
- see Gynecology
- hormonal EC (Yuzpe™ or Plan B™, usually 2 doses taken 12 hrs apart) or post-coital IUD insertion
- hormonal EC is effective if taken within 72 hrs of unprotected intercourse (reduces chance of pregnancy by 75-85%); does not affect an established pregnancy
- post-coital IUDs inserted within 5 days of unprotected intercourse are significantly more effective than hormonal EC (reduces chance of pregnancy by ~99%)
- pregnancy test should be performed if no menstrual bleeding within 21 days of either treatment
- advance provision of hormonal emergency contraception increases the use of emergency contraception without decreasing the use of regular contraception
- pharmacists across Canada can now dispense Plan B™ without a doctor's prescription (as of April 2005)

> **Absolute Contraindications to Combined OCP**
> - known/suspected pregnancy
> - undiagnosed abnormal vaginal bleeding
> - thromboembolic disorders
> - cerebrovascular or coronary artery disease
> - estrogen dependent tumours (breast, uterus)
> - acute liver disease

Differential Diagnosis
- other psychiatric disorders (e.g. anxiety, personality, bipolar, schizoaffective, SAD, substance abuse/withdrawal)
- early dementia
- endocrine (hyper/hypothyroidism, DM)
- liver failure, renal failure
- chronic fatigue syndrome
- vitamin deficiency (pernicious anemia, pellagra)
- medication side effects (β-blockers, benzos)
- infections (mononucleosis)
- menopause
- cancer (50% of patients with tumours, especially of brain, lung and pancreas, develop symptoms of depression before the diagnosis of cancer is made)

Criteria for Depression
M Depressed **M**ood
S Increased/decreased **S**leep
I Decreased **I**nterest
G **G**uilt
E Decreased **E**nergy
C Decreased **C**oncentration
A Increased/decreased **A**ppetite
P **P**sychomotor agitation/retardation
S **S**uicidal ideation

Must Ask About/Rule Out
- bipolar/manic/hypomanic episodes
- psychosis
- anxiety
- bereavement
- substance use/abuse/withdrawal
- suicidal/homicidal ideation

Common Antidepressants and Dosing:

Drug	Starting Dose	Maximum Dose
citalopram (Celexa™)	20 mg PO OD	60 mg PO OD
escitalopram (Cipralex™)	10 mg PO OD	20 mg PO OD
fluoxetine (Prozac™)	20 mg PO q am	80 mg PO OD
paroxetine (Paxil™)	20 mg PO q am	50 mg PO OD
sertraline (Zoloft™)	50 mg PO OD	200 mg PO OD
fluvoxamine (Luvox™)	50 mg PO OD	300 mg PO OD
venlafaxine (Effexor™)	75 mg PO OD	375 mg PO OD
(Effexor XR™)	37.5 mg PO OD	225 mg PO OD
bupropion (Wellbutrin™-immed)	100 mg PO bid	450 mg PO OD
(Sustained release)	100 mg PO qam	400 mg PO OD
amitriptyline (Elavil™)	25 mg PO qhs	300 mg PO OD
mirtazapine (Remeron™)	15 mg PO qhs	45 mg PO OD

Combined pharmacotherapy and psychological treatment for depression: a systematic review
Arch Gen Psychiatry 2004 Jul;61(7):714-9
Study: Systematic review of randomized clinical trials.
Patients: 16 trials comprising 1842 patients.
Intervention: Antidepressant treatment alone vs. combination of psychological intervention and antidepressant therapy.
Main outcomes: Efficacy of and adherence to therapy.
Results: Overall, combined therapy was significantly more effective than antidepressant therapy alone (OR 1.86), however there was no difference in the rate of dropouts and non-responders in either treatment arm. In studies lasting >12 weeks, combined therapy showed a reduction in dropouts compared to non-responders (OR 0.59).

Depression

- see Psychiatry

Etiology
- often presents as non-specific complaints (e.g. chronic fatigue, pain)
- depression is a clinical diagnosis and tests are done in order to rule out other causes of symptoms
- 2/3 of depressed persons may not receive appropriate treatment for their depression
- identification and early treatment improve outcomes

Screening Questions
- Are you depressed? (high specificity and sensitivity)
- Have you lost interest or pleasure in the things you usually like to do (anhedonia)?
- Do you have problems sleeping? (for those not willing to admit depression)

Assessment
- risk factors
- personal or family history of depression
- medications and potential substance abuse problems
- suicidality/homicidality
  - fill out Form 1 (in Ontario): application by physician to hospitalize a patient against his/her will for psychiatric assessment (up to 72 hours)
- functional impairment (e.g. work, relationships)
- at least 5 out of 9 criteria including anhedonia and depressed mood ≥2 weeks for actual diagnosis to be met (refer to criteria sidebar)
- validated depression rating scales: Beck's depression inventory, Zung's self-rating depression scale, Children's depression inventory
- routine medical workup (physical examination, CBC, TSH, electrolytes, urinalysis, glucose etc.)

Treatment
- goal: full remission of symptoms and return to baseline psychosocial function
- phases of treatment
  - acute phase (8-12 weeks): relieve symptoms and improve quality of life
  - maintenance phase (6-12 months after symptom resolution): prevent relapse/recurrence, must stress importance of continuing medication treatment for full duration to patients
- treatment can consist of pharmacotherapy alone or psychotherapy alone
- combination of antidepressant drug therapy and psychotherapy results in synergistic effects (see EBM box)

Common Medications
- SSRIs:
  - paroxetine (Paxil™), fluoxetine (Prozac™), sertraline (Zoloft™), citalopram (Celexa™), fluvoxamine (Luvox™)
  - block serotonin reuptake
  - side effects: sexual dysfunction (impotence, ↓ libido, delayed ejaculation, anorgasmia), headache, GI upset, weight loss, tremors, insomnia, fatigue
  - first-line therapy for teens is fluoxetine; paroxetine is not recommended for teens (controversial)
- SNRIs:
  - venlafaxine (Effexor™)
  - block serotonin and NE reuptake
  - side effects: insomnia, tremors, tachycardia, sweating
- SDRIs:
  - bupropion (Wellbutrin™)
  - block dopamine and NE reuptake
  - side effects: headache, insomnia, nightmares, seizures, less sexual dysfunction than SSRIs
- TCAs:
  - amitriptyline (Elavil™)
  - block serotonin and NE reuptake
  - side effects: sexual dysfunction, weight gain, tremors, tachycardia, sweating
  - note: narrow therapeutic window, lethal in overdose
- Other:
  - mirtazapine (Remeron™)
  - hypericium (St John's Wort)

Prognosis
- up to 40% resolve spontaneously within 6-12 months
- risks of recurrence:
  - 50% after 1 episode
  - 70% after 2 episodes
  - 90% after 3 episodes

Diabetes Mellitus (DM)

- see Endocrinology

Epidemiology
- major health concern, affecting up to 10% of Canadians
- Type 1 Diabetes (DM1): 10-15% of DM, peak incidence age 10-15,
- Type 2 Diabetes (DM2): 85-90% of DM, peak incidence age 50-55, up to 60,000 new cases in Canada per year
- gestational diabetes mellitus (GDM): 2-4% of all pregnancies
- incidence of Type 2 DM is rising dramatically as a result of an aging population, rising rates of obesity, and sedentary lifestyles
- leading cause of new-onset blindness and renal dysfunction
- Canadian adults with diabetes are twice as likely to die prematurely, compared to persons without diabetes

DM RELATED SYMPTOMS
Hyperglycemia: polyphagia, polydipsia, polyuria, weight change, blurry vision, yeast infections
Diabetic ketoacidosis (DKA): fruity breath, anorexia, N/V, fatigue, abdo pain, Kussmaul breathing, dehydration
Hypoglycemia: hunger, anxiety, tremors, palpitations, sweating, headache, fatigue, confusion, seizures, coma

Risk Factors
- Type 1 DM:
    - personal history of autoimmune disease, family history
- Type 2 DM:
    - first degree relative with DM
    - age ≥40 years
    - obesity (especially abdominal), hypertension, hyperlipidemia, coronary artery disease, vascular disease
    - prior GDM, macrosomic baby (>4 kg)
    - PCOS
    - history of IGT or IFG
    - presence of complications associated with diabetes
- both:
    - member of a high risk population (e.g. Aboriginal, Hispanic, Asian or African descent)

DKA can be triggered by infection, ischemia, infarction, intoxication, medication non-compliance

Diagnosis
- persistent hyperglycemia is the hallmark of all forms of diabetes

Table 17. Diagnosis of Insulin Associated Disorders

Condition	Diagnostic Criteria
Diabetes mellitus	One of the following on 2 occasions: Random BG ≥11.1 mmol/L (200 mg/dL) with symptoms of DM (fatigue, polyuria, polydipsia, unexplained weight loss) OR Fasting BG ≥7.0 mmol/L (126 mg/dL) OR BG 2 hours post 75 g OGTT ≥11.1 mmol/L (200 mg/dL) OR HbA1c ≥7% or 0.07
Impaired fasting glucose (IFG)	Fasting BG = 6.1-6.9 mmol/L (110-124 mg/dL)
Impaired glucose tolerance (IGT)	BG 2 hours post 75 g OGTT = 7.8-11.0 mmol/L (141-198 mg/dL)

Screening
- Type 2 DM
    - mass screening for Type 2 DM is not recommended
    - test FBG in everyone ≥40 q3 yrs
    - more frequent and/or earlier testing if:
        - presence of ≥1 risk factor (as previously listed)
- GDM
    - all pregnant women between 24-28 weeks gestation
    - non-fasting 1 hr 50 g OGCT ≥10.3 mmol/L (186 mg/dL) is diagnostic
    - if between 7.8-10.2 mmol/L (141-184 mg/dL) do confirmatory fasting 2 hr 75 g OGTT
    - if develop GDM, have a 50% chance of developing Type 2 DM over 20 years

Goals of Therapy
- general goals of therapy
    - to avoid the acute complications (e.g. ketoacidosis, hyperglycemia, infection)
    - to prevent long-term complications
        - microvascular: nephropathy, retinopathy, neuropathy
        - macrovascular: CAD, CVD, PVD
    - to minimize negative sequelae associated with therapies (e.g. hypoglycemia, weight gain)
- specific goals of therapy
    - fasting or preprandial glucose
        - ideal: 4-6 mmol/L (72-108 mg/dL)
        - recommended: 4-7 mmol/L (72-126 mg/dL)
        - suboptimal (action may be required): 7.1-10.0 mmol/L (128-180 mg/dL)
        - inadequate (action required): >10.0 mmol/L (180 mg/dL)

**Long-term non-pharmacological weight loss inter-
ventions for adults with prediabetes**
Cochrane Database of Systematic Reviews 2006; Issue 3
A meta-analysis, using 9 studies comprising 5168
patients, investigated the effectiveness of diet control,
physical activity, behavioural weight programs and
weight control interventions in adults with prediabetes.
The analysis was limited by heterogeneous patient populations, but when compared with usual care, weight
loss was 2.8 kg and BMI decrease was 1.3 kg/m2 at one
year. Modest but non-significant improvements in
glycemic control, BP and blood lipid concentrations
were noted. Studies with a follow-up of 3-6 years
showed a significant decrease in diabetes onset when
compared with controls.

- 2 hours postprandial glucose
  - ideal: 5-8 mmol/L (90-144 mg/dL)
  - recommended: 5-10 mmol/L (90-180 mg/dL)
- HbA1c
  - ideal: ≤0.06
  - recommended: ≤0.07
  - suboptimal: 0.07-0.084
  - inadequate: >0.084
- blood pressure:
  - adults: <130/80 (DM and HTN guidelines)
- lipids
  - LDL cholesterol <2.0 mmol/L
  - triglyceride <1.5 mmol/L
  - total cholesterol/HDL ratio <4.0

Assessment and Monitoring

Table 18. Assessment and Monitoring

	Initial Assessment	q2-4months	Annually
History	• symptoms of hyperglycemia, ketoacidosis, hypoglycemia • past medical history • functional inquiry • family history • risk factors • medications • sexual function • waist circumference (AC) • lifestyle	• diabetes-directed history • screen for awareness and frequency of hypoglycemia and DKA • glucose monitoring • use of insulin and oral agents	• diabetes-directed history • screen for awareness and frequency of hypoglycemia and DKA • glucose monitoring • use of insulin and oral agents • sexual function • conception counselling • lifestyle counselling • psychosocial issues
Physical	• general: Ht, Wt, BMI, BP • head and neck: fundoscopy oral exam, thyroid exam • cardiovascular exam: signs of CHF pulses, bruits • abdominal exam (e.g. for organomegaly) • hand/foot/skin exam • neurological exam	•Wt, BP, BMI, AC • foot exam for sensation, ulcers, or infection	• complete neuro exam for peripheral neuropathy • remainder of exam as per PHE
Investigations	• FBG, HbA1c, fasting lipids, • urine dip for proteinuria, 24-hr urine collection • ECG	• HbA1c q3 months • FBG as needed	• fasting lipid profile • resting or exercise ECG if age >35 • dipstick analysis for gross proteinuria; if negative: annual microalbuminuria screening with random albumin:creatinine ratio for Type 2 and Type I (5 yrs post puberty) if positive: 24-hr urine for endogenous creatinine clearance rate and microalbuminuria q6-12months
Management	• nutritional and physical education • consider referral to diabetes education program if available • monitoring: methods and frequency • medication counselling: oral hypoglycemics and/or insulin, method of administration, dosage adjustments • ophthalmology consult Type I within 5 yrs Type 2 at diagnosis	• assess progress towards long term complications • adjust treatment plan if necessary	• calibrate home glucose monitor • arrange ophthalmology follow up annually for Type I • q2 years for Type 2 • influenza vaccination annually

**Dietary advice for treatment of Type
2 DM in adults**
*Cochrane Database of Systematic
Reviews* 2007; Issue 3
A meta-analysis, using thirty-six articles
reporting a total of eighteen trials following
1467 participants, showed that there is no
high quality data on the efficacy of dietary
treatment of type 2 diabetes. However the
data available indicates that the adoption
of exercise appears to improve glycosylated hemoglobin at six and twelve months in
people with type 2 diabetes. There is an
urgent need for well-designed studies.

Nonpharmacologic Management
- diet
  - all people with DM should see a registered dietician
  - strive to attain healthy body weight
  - decrease combined saturated fats and trans-fatty acids to <10% of calories
  - avoid simple sugars, encourage complex carbohydrates, choose low-glycemic index foods
- physical activity and exercise
  - encourage 30-45 minutes of moderate exercise 3-5 days/week
  - promotes cardiovascular fitness, increases insulin sensitivity, lowers BP and improves lipid profile
  - if insulin treated, may require alterations of diet, insulin regimen, injection sites and self-monitoring

Self-monitoring of Blood Glucose
- Type 1 DM: 3 or more self tests/day is associated with a 1% reduction in HbA1c
- Type 2 DM: optimum frequency of self tests remains unclear
- if FBG >14 mmol/L, perform ketone testing to rule out DKA
- if bedtime level is <7 mmol/L, have bedtime snack to reduce risk of nocturnal hypoglycemia

Calculate total insulin required:
Type 1: 0.5-0.7 units/kg/day
Type 2: 0.3 units/kg/day

Table 19. Insulin

Type	Onset (minutes)	Peak (hours)	Duration (hours)
Insulin Lispro (Humalog™)	15	1	4
Regular Insulin (Humulin™)	45	4	8
NPH Insulin/Lente	90	8	14
Ultralente Insulin	120	12	24
Glargine (Lantus™)	90	No peak (flat action profile)	21

Oral Hypoglycemics (DM2)
- if glycemic targets not met within 2-4 months of lifestyle management, oral antihyperglycemic agents should be initiated
- if targets not obtained after 2-4 months of single agent use, try combination therapy
- available agents:
  - biguanide: metformin (Glucophage™)
  - thiazolidinedione: troglitazone (Rezulin™), rosiglitazone (Avandia™)
  - alpha glucosidase inhibitor: acarbose (Precose™)
  - nonsulfonylureas: nateglinide (Starlix™), repaglinide (Gluconorm™)
  - sulfonylureas: glyburide (DiaBeta™), glimepiride (Amaryl™), gliclazide (Diamicron™)
  - DPP-4 inhibitor: sitagliptin (Januvia™)

Other Medications Used in DM
- ACE inhibitors used for:
  - all hypertensive DM patients
  - elevated microalbuminuria (30-300 mg albumin in 24 h)
  - overt nephropathy (>300 mg albumin in urine in 24 h)
  - ARBs are second line for these conditions
- ASA
  - recommended for all diabetics, unless contraindicated
- statins
  - as required to attain target lipid profile

Health Canada Recommendations on management of rosiglitazone use in DM2
Rosiglitazone is indicated for:
- use as monotherapy, in patients not controlled by diet and exercise alone
- for patients inadequately controlled on metformin or a sulfonylurea, rosiglitazone should be added to, not substituted for, metformin or the sulfonylurea
- in Canada, rosiglitazone is not approved for use:
  - with insulin therapy
  - with the combination of metformin AND a sulfonylurea
  - in patients with pre-diabetes
- contraindicated in patients with NYHA Class III and IV cardiac status
- should be used with caution in any patient with NYHA Class I and II cardiac status
- patients should be monitored for signs and symptoms of fluid retention, edema, and rapid weight gain
- maximum daily dose used in combination with a sulfonylurea should not exceed 4mg

Metformin Monotherapy for type 2 diabetes mellitus
Cochrane Database of Systematic Reviews 2005; issue 3
A Cochrane Review of 29 trials with 37 arms (5259 participants) compared metformin with sulphonylureas, placebo, diet, thiazolidinediones, insulin, meglitinides, and glucosidase inhibitors. The authors concluded that metformin may prevent some vascular complications and mortality in overweight and obese DM2 patients and as such may be considered first line therapy. There is no evidence that the studied alternative therapies have more benefit for glycaemia control, body weight, or lipids than does metformin.

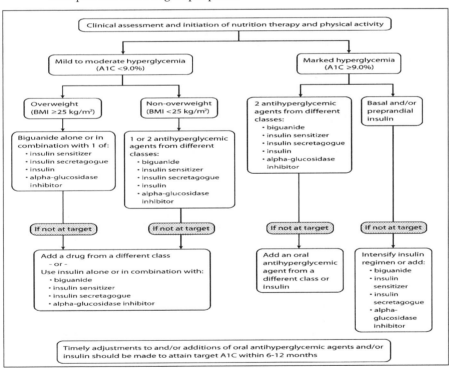

Figure 5. Management of Hyperglycemia in Type 2 Diabetes
Canadian Diabetes Association Clinical Practice Guidelines Expert Committee. Canadian Diabetes Association 2003 Clinical Practice Guidelines for the Prevention and Management of Diabetes in Canada. *Can J Diabetes.* 2003; 27(suppl 2): S39. (used with permission)

Dizziness

- see Otolaryngology

Epidemiology
- 70% see general practitioners initially; only 4% referred to specialists
- frequency proportional to age; commonest complaint of ambulatory patients age >75

Differential Diagnosis

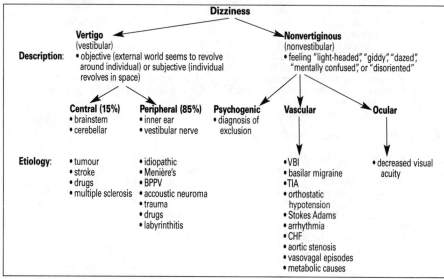

Figure 6. Differential Diagnosis of Dizziness

History
- clarify type of dizziness
  - vertigo, pre-syncope, dysequilibrium, light-headedness
  - ask about onset, precipitating/alleviating factors, preceding infections and activities, associated symptoms, previous experiences of dizziness
- duration (seconds to minutes vs. hours vs. days to weeks vs. persistent)
- exacerbations
  - worse with head movement or eye closure (vestibular)
  - no change with head movement and eye closure (nonvestibular)
  - worse with exercise (cardiac/pulmonary causes)
- associated symptoms
  - neurologic (central)
    - transient diplopia, dysphagia, dysarthria, ataxia (TIA, VBI, migraine)
    - persistent sensory and/or motor deficits (CNS)
  - audiologic (peripheral)
    - hearing loss, tinnitus, otalgia, aural fullness, recruitment
  - others
    - nausea, vomiting (peripheral vestibular disorders)
    - SOB, palpitations (hyperventilation, cardiac problem)
- general medical history
  - history of HTN, diabetes, heart disease, fainting spells, seizures, cerebrovascular disease, migraines
  - ototoxic drugs: aminoglycosides (gentamicin, streptomycin, tobramycin), erythromycin, ASA, antimalarials
  - hypotension (secondary to diuresis): furosemide, caffeine, alcohol

Physical Exam/Investigations
- syncopal
  - cardiac, peripheral vascular, and neurologic exams
  - bloodwork, ECG, 24-hr Holter, treadmill stress test, loop ECG, tilt table testing, carotid and vertebral doppler, EEG
- vertiginous
  - ENT and neurologic exams
  - Dix-Hallpike, consider audiometry and MRI if indicated
- non-syncopal, non-vertiginous
  - cardiac and neurologic exams
  - 3-minute hyperventilation trial, ECG, EEG

Dix-Hallpike Test
- have the patient seated with legs extended and head at 45° rotation
- rapidly shift patient to supine position with head fully supported in slight extension (for 45 seconds)
- observe for rotatory nystagmus and ask about sensation of vertigo

Treatment
- dependent on results of history, physical and investigations
- treatments include education, lifestyle modification, physical maneuvers (e.g. Epley for BPPV), symptomatic management (e.g. antiemetics), pharmacotherapy and surgery
- refer when significant central disease suspected, when vertigo of peripheral origin is persistent (lasting >2-4 weeks), or if atypical presentation

Domestic Violence/Elder Abuse

INTIMATE PARTNER VIOLENCE

Definition
- includes physical, sexual, emotional, psychological and financial abuse (see Emergency Medicine)

Epidemiology
- lifetime prevalence of intimate partner violence against women is between 25% to 30%
- MD recognition rates as low as 5%
- occurs in all socioeconomic, educational and cultural groups with increased incidence in pregnancy, disabled women, and 18-24 age group
- women who experience abuse have increased rates of injury, death and a number of health consequences including 50-70% increase in gynecological, central nervous system, stress-related problems
- 25-50% chance of child abuse or neglect in families where abuse occurs

Presentation
- multiple visits with vague, ill-defined complaints such as:
  - headaches, gastrointestinal symptoms, insomnia, chronic pain, hyperventilation
  - may also present with injuries inconsistent with history

Management
- screen ALL patients
  - always have a high index of suspicion
  - MD often first person to get disclosure
  - health care visits are an important opportunity for physicians to address intimate partner violence (e.g. the Preventative Care Checklist Form includes an inquiry into relationship issue)
  - asking about abuse is the strongest predictor of disclosure
  - several screening tools exist to identify victims of partner violence (see sidebar)
  - make sure to determine the victim's level of immediate and long term danger and ask if there are weapons in the house
- community resources arranged/provided
  - safety planning includes ensuring that there is access to an exit in the home, establishing a safe place to go and having money, clothes, keys, medications, important documents and other emergency items prepared should the patient need to leave quickly
  - shelter or helpline number with legal advocacy and counselling services
  - involve social workers or domestic violence advocates
  - marital counseling not appropriate until woman is safe and violence is under control
- appointment for follow-up to assess whether condition is better or worse
- reassure patient she/he is not to blame and that the assault is a crime
  - goal is to convey the message that "As your doctor, I am concerned for your safety" and "Your partner has a problem that he/she needs help with" and "I want to help you"
  - report suspected or known child abuse (mandatory)
  - spousal abuse is a criminal act, but not reportable without the woman's/man's permission
- exit plans developed to ensure patient safety
  - victim most at risk for homicide when attempting to leave home or following separation
- DOCUMENT all evidence of abuse related visits for medico-legal purposes (see sidebar)

ELDER ABUSE

Definition
- mistreatment of older people by those in a position of trust, power, or responsibilty for their care
- older adults living alone, or with others (e.g. private residences, family, home care or community care, institutions)

Screening Instruments for Domestic Violence

A) WAST-SHORT
1. In general how would you describe your relationship?
   a. lot of tension
   b. some tension
   c. no tension

2. Do you and your partner work out arguments with . . .?
   a. great difficulty
   b. some difficulty
   c. no difficulty

Endorsing either question 1 ("a lot of tension") or question 2 ("great difficulty") makes intimate partner violence exposure likely

B) HITS
How often does your partner:
1. physically **H**urt you?
2. **I**nsult you?
3. **T**hreaten you with harm?
4. **S**cream or curse at you?

Each question on HITS to be answered on a 5 point scale ranging from 1 (= never) to 5 (= frequently)
A total score of 10.5 is significant

How to document abuse
- take photographs (with permission) of known or suspected injuries
- use an injury location chart or "body map" when documenting physical findings
- document any investigations ordered (e.g. X-ray)
- write legibly or use a computer
- set off the patient's own words in quotation marks
- avoid phrases that imply doubt about the patient's reliability (e.g. "patient claims that...")
- record the patient's demeanor (e.g. upset, agitated)
- record the time of day the patient is examined and how much time has elapsed since the abuse occurred

- types of abuse:
  - psychological abuse (e.g. threatening, intimidating, insulting, demeaning, withholding information that may be important to them, ignoring)
  - financial abuse (e.g. stealing, pressuring to sell or share home, misusing power of attorney)
  - physical abuse (e.g. hitting, burning, locking in room, inappropriate use of physical restraints, withholding or misusing medication)
  - sexual abuse
  - neglect

Epidemiology
- 7% of adults in Canada age >65 reported experiences of emotional or financial abuse
- older adults who live with someone are more likely to be abused than those who live alone
- 2/3 of reported abuse cases involved family members, most often adult children followed by spouses
- older females are more likely to be abused than older males
- men are more likely than women to be victimized by an adult child (45% vs 35%)
- women are more likely than men to experience violence at the hands of a spouse (30% vs. 19%) (Statistics Canada, 2004)
- reasons for under-reporting: fear, shame, cognitive impairment, language/cultural barriers, and social and geographic isolation

Risk Factors
- women
- older age (age 80 and older)
- physical and mental frailty

Screening
- the Canadian Task Force determined that there was insufficient evidence to include or exclude case finding for elder abuse as part of the periodic health examination, but recommended that physicians be alert for indicators of abuse and institute measures to prevent further abuse
- general questions such as "Do you feel safe at home?" and move into more specific questions about different kinds of abuse

Presentation
- signs that an older adult is being abused may include:
  - depression, fear, anxiety, passivity, unexplained injuries, dehydration, malnutrition, poor hygiene, rashes, pressure sores, and over-sedation/inappropriate medication use

Management
- gather information from all sources (e.g. family members, health care providers, neighbours)
- perform a thorough physical examination
- ensure immediate safety and devise a plan for follow-up
- additional steps depend on whether the patient accepts intervention and whether they are capable of making decisions about their care
- interventions may include use of protective and legal services, senior resource nurses, elder abuse intervention teams and senior support groups

Dysuria

- see Urology

Definition
- the sensation of pain, burning or discomfort on urination

Epidemiology
- in adulthood, more common in women than men
- approximately 25% of women report one episode of acute dysuria per year
- most common in women 25-54 years of age and in those who are sexually active
- in men, dysuria becomes more prevalent with increasing age

Etiology
- infectious
  - most common cause
  - presents as cystitis, urethritis, pyelonephritis, vaginitis, or prostatitis
- non-infectious
  - hormonal conditions (postmenopausal hypoestrogenism), obstruction (BPH, urethral strictures), neoplasms, allergic reactions, chemicals, foreign bodies, trauma

Does this woman have an acute uncomplicated urinary tract infection?
JAMA. May 2002; 287: 2701-2710
Purpose: To review the accuracy and precision of history taking and physical examination for diagnosing a UTI in a woman.
Study Characteristics: Systematic review of 9 studies looking at the accuracy or precision of history or physical examination in diagnosing uncomplicated UTI.
Participants: Healthy women. Infants, children or adolescents, pregnant women, nursing home patients, and patients with complicated UTI were excluded.
Main Outcomes: Precision and accuracy of history taking and physical exam.
Results: No studies examined precision as an outcome. Four symptoms and one sign significantly increased the probability of UTI: dysuria, frequency, hematuria, back pain, and CVA tenderness. Four symptoms and one sign significantly decreased the probability of UTI: absence of dysuria, absence of back pain, a history of vaginal discharge, a history of vaginal irritation, and vaginal discharge on examination.
Conclusions: Women who present with 1 or more symptoms of a UTI have a probability of infection approaching 50%, effectively ruling in infection. In contrast, for women presenting with 1 or more symptoms of a UTI, the combination of additional historical elements, physical examination, and urinalysis is unable to lower the post-test probability of disease to a level where it can be ruled out and additional testing, such as culture, should be pursued.

Table 20. Etiology, Signs and Symptoms of Dysuria

Infection	Etiology	Signs and Symptoms
UTI/Cystitis	E. coli, S. saprophyticus, Proteus mirabilis, Enterobacter, Klebsiella, Pseudomonas	Internal dysuria throughout micturition, frequency, urgency, incontinence, hematuria, nocturia, back pain, suprapubic discomfort, low grade fever (rare)
Urethritis	C. trachomatis, N. gonorrhea, Trichomonas, Candida, herpes	Initial dysuria, urethral/vaginal discharge, history of STI
Vaginitis	Candida, Gardnerella, Trichomonas, C. trachomatis, atrophic, herpes, lichen sclerosis	External dysuria/pain, vaginal discharge, irritation, dyspareunia, abnormal vaginal bleeding
Prostatitis	E. coli, C. trachomatis, S. saprophyticus, Proteus mirabilis, Enterobacter, Klebisella, Pseudomonas	Dysuria, fever, chills, urgency, frequency, tender prostate
Pyelonephritis	E. coli, S. saprophyticus, Proteus mirabilis, Enterobacter, Klebsiella, Pseudomonas	Internal dysuria, fever, chills, flank pain radiating to groin, CVA tenderness, nausea or vomiting

Investigations
- no investigations necessary when history and physical consistent with uncomplicated UTI – treat empirically (note: urinalysis can be performed when indicated by dipstick or microscopy)
- radiologic studies and other diagnostic tests if atypical presentation
- urinalysis/urine R&M: pyuria, bacteriuria, hematuria
- urine C&S
- if vaginal/urethral discharge present: wet mount, Gram stain, KOH test, vaginal pH, culture for yeast and Trichomonas
- endocervical or urethral swab for N. gonorrheae and C. trachomatis
- renal U/S or voiding cystourethrogram (VCUG) in children with >1 UTI

Management
- see Urology
- UTI/cystitis
  - pregnant women with bacteriuria (2-7%) must be treated even if asymptomatic, due to risk of preterm labour
  - need to follow with monthly urine cultures and retreat if still infected
  - in patients with recurrent UTIs (>3 per year), consider prophylactic antibiotics
  - if complicated UTI, patients require longer courses of broader spectrum antibiotics
- urethritis
  - when swab is positive for chlamydia or gonorrhea must report to Public Health
  - all patients should return 4-7 days after completion of therapy for clinical evaluation

Risk Factors for Complicated Urinary Tract Infection
- male sex
- pregnancy
- recent urinary tract instrumentation
- functional or anatomic abnormality of the urinary tract
- chronic renal disease
- diabetes
- immunosuppression
- indwelling catheter

Prevention of UTIs:
- maintain good hydration (especially with cranberry juice)
- wipe urethra from front to back to avoid contamination of the urethra with feces from the rectum
- avoid feminine hygiene sprays and scented douches
- empty bladder immediately before and after intercourse

Epistaxis

- see Otolaryngology

Table 21. Characteristics of Anterior vs. Posterior Bleeds

	Anterior (90%)	Posterior (10%)
Location/ Origin	Little's Area/ Kiesselbach's Plexus	Woodruff's Plexus/Sphenopalatine Artery
Age	2-10, 50-80	Usually >50
Common Cause	Trauma (digital, fracture, foreign body, Sx), dry air, cool climate, post URTI, nasal dryness, chemical (nasal sprays, cocaine), tumour	Systemic: hepatic disease, primary/secondary bleeding disorder, medications (ASA, NSAIDs, warfarin), HTN, atherosclerosis
Treatment	Conservative: • Position: upright leaning forward with direct digital pressure over ala for >10 min("pinch" up to cartilage) • Humidifier in bedroom, nasal saline sprays, bacitriacin or Vaseline application to Little's area • Silver nitrate • Gelfoam/Hemostat • Nasal packing with Vaseline gauze, nasal catheter or sponge • Cotton soaked in vasoconstrictor (oxymetazoline 0.5%) and topical anesthetic (4% lidocaine) placed in anterior nasal cavity with direct pressure for >10 min • Investigations: CBC, Hct, cross & type, INR, PTT (only if severe), CT/nasopharyngoscopy if suspected tumour	Emergency: ENT/ER consult for posterior packing with an intranasal balloon/Foley catheter Embolization/surgery
Prognosis	Usually stops with >10 min of pressure to nose	Copious bleed. Often swallowed and vomited May lead to hypovolemic shock if not treated promptly

Erectile Dysfunction (ED)

* see Urology

Definition
* consistent or recurrent inability to attain and/or maintain penile erection sufficient for sexual performance of ≥3 months duration

Epiemiology
* ~20% of men aged 40 are affected
* ~50% of men aged 70 are affected

Etiology
* organic: vascular (90%) (arterial insufficiency, atherosclerosis), endocrine (low testosterone), anatomic (structural abnormality e.g. Peyronie's), neurologic (post-op, DM), medications (clonidine, antihypertensives, psychotropics)
* psychogenic (10%)

Major Causes of ED:
Vascular, Neurologic, Endocrine, Diabetes, Drugs, Psychogenic

Table 22. Differentiation Between Organic and Psychogenic Erectile Dysfunction

Characteristic	Organic	Psychogenic
Onset	Gradual	Acute
Circumstances	Global	Situational
Course	Constant	Varying
Non-coital erection	Poor	Rigid
Psychosexual problem	Secondary	Long history
Partner problem	Secondary	At onset
Anxiety and fear	Secondary	Primary

Walsh: Campbell's Urology, 8th ed. Table 46-4.

History
* comprehensive sexual, medical and psychosocial history
* time course
  * last satisfactory erection
  * onset: gradual or sudden
  * attempts at sexual activity
* quantify
  * presence of morning or night time erections
  * stiffness (scale of 1-10)
  * ability to initiate an erection with sexual stimulation
  * ability to maintain erection with sexual stimulation
  * erection stiffness during sex (scale of 1-10)
* qualify
  * partner or situation specific
  * loss of erection before penetration or climax
  * degree of concentration required to maintain an erection
  * percentage of sexual attempts satisfactory to patient and/or his partner
  * ask about significant bends in penis or pain with erection
  * ask about difficulty with specific positions
  * ask about impact on quality of life and relationship

Investigations
* hypothalamic-pituitary-gonadal axis evaluation: testosterone (free + total), prolactin, LH
* risk factor evaluation: fasting glucose, HbA1c, lipid profile
* other: TSH, CBC, urinalysis
* specialized testing:
  * psychological and/or psychiatric consultation
  * in-depth psychosexual and relationship evaluation
  * nocturnal penile tumescence and rigidity (NPTR) assessment
  * vascular diagnostics (e.g. Doppler studies, angiography)

Management

Table 23. Management of Erectile Dysfunction

Nonpharmacologic	Pharmacologic	Surgical
Lifestyle changes (alcohol, smoking, exercise)	Suppository (MUSE: male urethral suppository for erection)	Implants
Relationship/sexual counselling	Oral agents	Vascular repair
Vacuum devices	Injections	Realignment

Modifiable risk factors and erectile dysfunction: can lifestyle changes modify risk?
Urology 2000; 56: 302-306
Study: A prospective cohort study designed to examine whether changes in smoking, heavy alcohol consumption, sedentary lifestyle, and obesity are associated with the risk of ED in men aged 40-70.
Results: Obesity was associated with ED (P=0.006), with baseline obesity conferring higher risk regardless of subsequent weight loss. Level of phyical activity was associated with ED (P=0.01): those initiating physical activity or remaining active had a lower risk of ED, while those who remained sedentary had a higher risk. As compared to their sedentary peers, those who initiated exercise in midlife had a 70% reduced ED rate. Changes in smoking or alcohol intake were not associated with ED (P>0.3).
Conclusion: Although making lifestyle changes in midlife may be too late to reverse the effects of smoking, obesity, and alcohol consumption on ED, initiating physical activity in midlife may in fact reduce ED relative to peers who remain sedentary. Adopting a healthy lifestyle early in life may be the best approach to reducing the risk of developing ED in later years.

- pharmacologic treatment
  - phosphodiesterase type 5 inhibitors (see Table 24)
  - alpha adrenergic blockers (e.g. yohimbine)
  - serotonin antagonist and reuptake inhibitor (e.g. trazodone)
  - testosterone - currently only indicated in patients presenting with hypogonadism and testosterone deficiency (N.B. breast/prostate cancer are absolute contraindications)

Table 24. Phosphodiesterase Type 5 Inhibitors

Examples	Dosing (1 dose/day)	Specifics	Side Effects	Contraindications
sildenafil (Viagra™)	25-100 mg/dose	Take 0.5-4 hr prior to intercourse May last 24 hours	Flushing, headache, indigestion	Not to be used in patients taking nitrates
tadalafil (Cialis™)	5-20 mg/dose	Effects may last 36 hours	as above	as above
vardenafil (Levitra™)	2.5-20 mg/dose	Take 1 hr prior to intercourse	as above	as above

Fatigue

Epidemiology
- 25% of office visits to family physicians
  - peaks in ages 20-40
  - women 3-4x > men
- 50% have associated psychological complaints/problems, especially if <6 month duration

Differential Diagnosis

Table 25. Differential diagnosis of fatigue: PS VINDICATE

P	Psychogenic	Depression, sleep disorder, life stresses, anxiety disorder, chronic fatigue syndrome, fibromyalgia
S	Sedentary	Unhealthy/sedentary lifestyle
V	Vascular	Stroke
I	Infectious	Viral (e.g. mononucleosis, hepatitis), bacterial (e.g. TB), fungal, parasitic, HIV
N	Neoplastic	Any malignancy
	Nutrition	Anemia (Fe deficiency, B_{12} deficiency)
	Neurogenic	Myasthenia gravis, multiple sclerosis, Parkinson's Disease
D	Drugs	β-blockers, antihistamines, anticholinergics, benzodiazepines, antiepileptics, antidepressants
I	Idiopathic	
C	Chronic illnesses	CHF, lung diseases (e.g. COPD, sarcoidosis), renal failure, chronic liver disease
A	Autoimmune	SLE, RA, mixed connective tissue disease, polymyalgia rheumatica
T	Toxin	Substance abuse (e.g. alcohol), heavy metal
E	Endocrine	Hypothyroidism, diabetes, Cushing's syndrome, adrenal insufficiency, pregnancy

Common causes are in bold

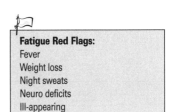

Fatigue Red Flags:
Fever
Weight loss
Night sweats
Neuro deficits
Ill-appearing

Investigations
- psychosocial causes are common, so usually minimal investigation is warranted
- physical causes of fatigue usually have associated symptoms/signs that can be elicited from a focused history and physical examination
- investigations should be guided by findings on history and physical and may include the following:
  - CBC + differential, electrolytes, BUN, Cr, ESR, glucose, TSH, ferritin, B_{12}, total protein, albumin, AST, ALT, ALP, bilirubin, calcium, phosphate, ANA, β-hCG
  - urinalysis, CXR, ECG
  - additional tests: serologies (Lyme disease, hepatitis B and C screen, HIV, ANA) and PPD skin tests

Treatment
- treat the cause
- if etiology undetermined (underlying cause cannot be identified in 1/3 of patients)
  - physician support, REASSURANCE and follow-up, especially with fatigue of psychogenic etiology
  - supportive counselling, behavioural, or group therapy
  - encourage patient to stay physically active to maximize function
  - review all medications, OTC, and herbal remedies, watching for drug-drug interactions and side effects
  - prognosis: after 1 year, 40% are no longer fatigued

Exercise therapy for chronic fatigue
Cochrane Depression, Anxiety, and Neurosis Group.
Cochrane Database of Systematic Reviews 2005;
Issue 3
Purpose: To determine the effectiveness of exercise
therapy for Chronic Fatigue Syndrome (CFS).
Study Characteristics: Systematic review of 5 RCTs
with 336 patients.
Participants: All ages with a clinical diagnosis of CFS.
Interventions: Exercise therapy alone was compared
with treatment as usual (or relaxation and flexibility),
pharmacotherapy (fluoxetine), or exercise therapy
combined with either pharmacotherapy or patient
education.
Main Outcomes: Chalder Fatigue Scale (self-rated
scale of physical and mental fatigue), or any other
fatigue scale.
Results: At 12 weeks, patients undergoing exercise
therapy were less fatigued than controls (SMD -0.77;
95% CI, -1.26 to -0.28). Physical functioning was also
significantly improved, but there were more dropouts
with exercise therapy. Compared with fluoxetine,
patients receiving exercise therapy were less fatigued
(WMD -1.24; 95% CI, -5.31 to 2.83). Patients receiving
combination therapy with exercise therapy and either
fluoxetine or patient education, did better than those on
monotherapy.
Conclusions: Patients may benefit from exercise therapy, and combination therapy with either fluoxetine or
education may offer additional benefit. Further high
quality trials are needed.

CHRONIC FATIGUE SYNDROME (CFS)

Definition (CDC 2006) – must meet both criteria
1. new or definite onset of unexplained, clinically evaluated, persistent or relapsing chronic fatigue, not relieved by rest, which results in occupational, educational, social, or personal dysfunction
2. concurrent presence of at least 4 of the following symptoms for a minimum of 6 months:
   - impairment of short-term memory or concentration, severe enough to cause significant decline in function
   - sore throat
   - tender cervical or axillary lymph nodes
   - muscle pain
   - multi-joint pain with no swelling or redness
   - new headache
   - unrefreshing sleep
   - post-exertion malaise lasting >24 hours
- exclusion criteria: medical conditions that may explain the fatigue, certain psychiatric disorders (depression with psychotic or melancholic features, schizophrenia, eating disorders), substance abuse, severe obesity (BMI >45)

Epidemiology
- F>>M, Caucasians > other groups, majority in their 30s
- CFS found in <5% of patients presenting with fatigue

Etiology
- unknown cause, likely multifactorial
- may include infectious agents, immunological factors, neurohormonal factors, and/or nutritional deficiency

Investigations
- no specific laboratory tests diagnose CFS

Treatment
- promote sleep hygiene
- provide support and reassurance that most patients improve over time
- non-pharmacological
  - regular physical activity
  - optimal diet
  - psychotherapy (e.g. CBT), family therapy, support groups
- pharmacological
  - intended for relief of symptoms (e.g. antidepressants, anxiolytics, NSAIDs, antimicrobials, antiallergy therapy, antihypotensive therapy (increase dietary sodium, fludrocortisone))

Headache

- see Neurology

Primary Headaches

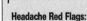

Table 26. Primary Headaches

	Migraine	Tension-type	Cluster	Caffeine withdrawal
Epidemiology	12% of adults F>M 20% with aura 80% without aura	38% of adults, can be episodic or chronic	<0.1% of adults, M>>F	~50% of people drinking ≥2.5cups/d
Duration	5-72 hrs	May occur as isolated incident or daily, duration is variable	<3hrs at same time of day	Begins 12-24hrs after last caffeine intake, can last ~1wk
Pain	Classically unilateral & pulsatile, but 40% are bilateral, moderate-severe intensity, nausea/vomiting, photo/phonophobia	Mild to moderate pain, bilateral, fronto-occipital or generalized pain, band-like pain, +/- contracted neck/scalp muscles, associated with little disability	Sudden, unilateral, severe, usually centered around eye, frequently awakens patient	Severe, throbbing, associated with drowsiness, anxiety, muscle stiffness, nausea, waves of hot or cold sensations

Table 26. Primary Headaches (continued)

	Migraine	Tension-type	Cluster	Caffeine withdrawal
Triggers	Numerous (e.g. food, sleep disturbance, stress, hormonal, fatigue, weather, high altitude) Aggravated by physical activity	Stressful events, NOT aggravated by physical activity	Often alcohol	Caffeine removal
Treatment of acute headache	1st line- acetaminophen, ASA, +/-caffeine 2nd line- NSAIDs 3rd line- 5HT agonists +/- antiemetic	Rest & relaxation NSAIDs	Sumatriptan Dihydroergotamine High-flow O$_2$ Intranasal lidocaine	Caffeine Acetaminophen or ASA +/- caffeine
Prophylactic Therapy	1st line- β-blockers 2nd line-TCAs 3rd line - anticonvulsants	Rest & relaxation, physical activity, biofeedback	Lithium carbonate, prednisone, methysergide	Cut down on caffeine

Secondary Headaches
- caused by underlying organic disease
- account for <10% of all headaches, may be life-threatening
- etiology
  - space-occupying lesion
  - systemic infection (meningitis, encephalitis)
  - stroke
  - subarachnoid hemorrhage
  - systemic disorders (thyroid disease, hypertension, pheochromocytoma, etc)
  - temporal arteritis
  - traumatic head injuries
  - TMJ or C-spine pathology
  - serious ophthalmological and otolaryngological causes of headache
- treatment
  - based on underlying disorder
  - analgesics may provide symptomatic relief

Investigations
- indicated only when red flags are present
- may include:
  - CBC for suspected systemic or intracranial infection
  - ESR for suspected temporal arteritis
  - neuroimaging (CT or MRI) to rule out intracranial pathology
  - CSF analysis for suspected hemorrhage, infection, tumour or disorders related to CSF

Hearing Impairment

- see Otolaryngology

Definition
- hearing impairment: a raised hearing threshold measured as decibels of hearing loss relative to the normal population at specific frequencies
- hearing disability: hearing impairment that interferes with performing daily tasks

Epidemiology
- 90% of age-related hearing loss (presbycusis) is sensorineural
- 10% of the population is hard of hearing or deaf
- hearing loss detectable by audiology is present in greater than 1/3 of people over 65
- associated with significant physical, functional and mental health consequences

Classification
- conductive (sound does not reach cochlea)
- sensorineural (sound is not converted or transmitted via neural signals)
- mixed

Assessment
- detection maneuvers
  - infants
    - universal newborn hearing screening program
  - elderly
    - whispered-voice test
      - whisper six test words 6 inches to 2 feet away from the patient's ear out of the visual field, ask patient to repeat the words (with non-test ear distraction)

Does this patient have hearing impairment?
JAMA 2006;295:416-428
Purpose: To evaluate bedside clinical maneuvers used to evaluate the presence of hearing impairment.
Study: Evidence-based review of studies examining the accuracy or precision of screening questions and tests. 24 studies were included in this analysis.
Conclusions: Elderly patients who admit to having hearing impairment should be offered audiometry, while those who do not should undergo a whispered-voice test. Those who hear the whispered voice require no further testing, while those who do not require audiometry. The Weber and Rinne tests are not useful in screening for hearing impairment.

- tuning fork test
  - Rinne and Weber (not for general screening)
- audioscope
  - delivers pure tone frequencies to obtain thresholds for frequencies of 250-8000 Hz

Management
- counsel about noise control and hearing protection programs (A-grade evidence)
- refer patients with hearing loss for a complete audiological examination
- hearing amplification (e.g. hearing aids), assistive listening devices, and cochlear implants can dramatically improve quality of life

Hypertension

Epidemiology
- 20-25% of Canadian adults have HTN (and up to 50% undiagnosed)
- only 16% have adequate BP control
- approximately 50% of adult Canadians are hypertensive by age 60
- 3rd leading risk factor associated with death
  - risk factor for CAD, CHF, cerebrovascular disease, renal failure, peripheral vascular disease

Symptoms of hypertension are usually NOT PRESENT (This is why it is called the "Silent Killer")

May have occipital headache upon awakening or organ specific complaints if advanced disease.

Definition
- hypertension
  - BP ≥140/90 mmHg
- isolated systolic hypertension
  - sBP ≥140 and dBP <90
  - associated with progressive reduction in vascular compliance
  - usually begins 5th decade; up to 11% of 75 year olds
- accelerated hypertension
  - significant recent increase in BP over previous hypertensive levels associated with evidence of vascular damage on fundoscopy but without papilledema
- malignant hypertension
  - sufficient elevation in BP to cause papilledema and other manifestations of vascular damage (retinal hemorrhages, bulging discs, mental status changes, increasing creatinine)
  - not defined by absolute level of BP, but often requires BP of >200/140
  - develops in about 1% of hypertensive patients
- hypertensive urgency
  - sBP >210 or dBP >120 with minimal or no target-organ damage
- hypertensive emergency
  - high BP + acute target-organ damage (see sidebar)

HYPERTENSIVE EMERGENCIES
1. Accelerated malignant HTN with papilledema
2. Cerebrovascular:
   Hypertensive encephalopathy
   CVA with severe hypertension
   Intracerebral hemorrhage
   SAH
3. Cardiac:
   Acute aortic dissection
   Acute refractory LV failure
   Acute MI with persistent ischemic pain after CABG
4. Renal:
   Acute glomerulonephritis
   Renal crises from collagen vascular diseases
   Severe hypertension following renal transplantation
5. Excessive circulating catecholamines:
   Pheochromocytoma
   Tyramine containing foods or drug interactions with MAOIs
   Sympathomimetic drug use (e.g. cocaine)
   Rebound HTN after cessation of anti-hypertensive drugs (e.g. clonidine)
6. Eclampsia
7. Surgical:
   Severe HTN prior to emergent surgery
   Severe post-op HTN
   Post-op bleeding from vascular suture lines
8. HTN following severe burns
9. Severe epistaxsis

Etiology
- essential (primary) hypertension (>90%)
  - undetermined cause
- secondary hypertension (10%)
- watch for labile, "white coat" hypertension (office-induced elevated BP)

Predisposing Factors
- family history
- obesity (especially abdominal)
- alcohol consumption
- stress
- sedentary lifestyle
- smoking
- male gender
- age >30
- excessive salt intake/fatty diet
- African American ancestry
- dyslipidemia

Table 27. Causes of Secondary Hypertension

Obstructive Sleep Apnea	common cause of 2° HTN
Renal	renovascular HTN renal parenchymal disease, glomerulonephritis, pyelonephritis, polycystic kidney
Endocrine	1° hyperaldosteronism pheochromocytoma Cushing's syndrome hyperthyroidism/hyperparathyroidism hypercalcemia of any cause
Vascular	coarctation of the aorta renal artery stenosis
Drug-induced	estrogens steroids NSAIDs MAOIs lithium decongestants cocaine amphetamines alcohol

Investigations
- for all patients with hypertension (D)
  - CBC, electrolytes, Cr, FBG, Total Chol, HDL, LDL, TG, 12-lead ECG, urinalysis
- for specific patient subgroups (D)
  - DM or renal disease: urinary protein excretion
  - increasing Cr or history of renal disease or proteinuria: renal ultrasound, captopril renal scan (B)
  - if suspected endocrine cause: plasma aldosterone, plasma renin
  - if suspected pheochromocytoma: 24 hr urine for metanephrines and creatinine (C)
  - echocardiogram for left ventricular dysfunction assessment if indicated (C)

Diagnosis
- suspect secondary causes and consider further investigations if:
  - onset of HTN < age 30 or > age 55
  - HTN refractory to treatment (≥3 drugs)
  - accelerated or malignant hypertension
  - suspicious clinical situation
    - paroxysmal headache, palpitations and diaphoresis (pheochromocytoma)
    - renal bruits (renovascular hypertension)
    - hypokalemia and hypernatremia (hyperaldosteronism)
- home or ambulatory BP monitoring can also be used in the diagnosis of HTN (C)
  - consider if patient is:
    - suspected to be nonadherent
    - diabetic, chronic kidney disease
    - masked hypertension
    - suspected of having "white coat" hypertension
    - fluctuating office BP readings
  - BP values should be based on morning (before medications) and evening readings over a 7 day period (C)

Keys to Grade of Recommendations for Hypertension Diagnosis and Treatment
Grade
A   high levels of internal validity and statistical precision
B/C lower levels of internal validity and statistical precision
D   expert opinion

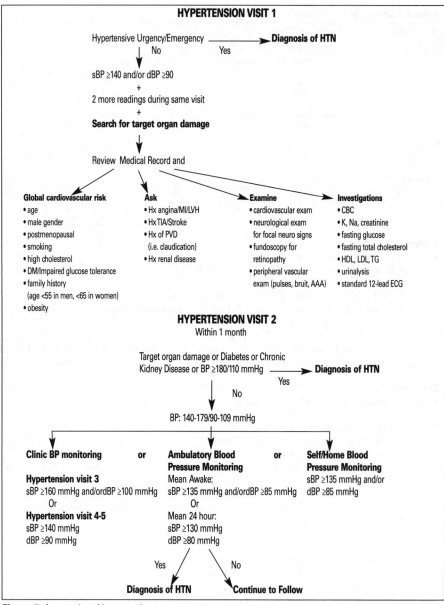

Figure 7. Approach to Hypertension
Adapted from: *The Canadian Journal of Cardiology*, 2006; 22(7):577.

Treatment
- target BP is <140/90 mmHg
  - <130/80 if DM or chronic kidney disease
- **lifestyle modification (in all HTN patients)**
  - may be sole necessary therapy in patients with stage 1 HTN (140-159/90-99)
  - smoking cessation
  - alcohol restriction to low risk drinking guidelines (see *Alcohol* section) (B)
  - weight loss if BMI >25 (at least 4.5 kg) and/or waist circumference is ≥102 cm for men and ≥88 for women (B); BP will decrease by 2/1 mmHg for each 1 kg of wt loss
  - aerobic exercise of moderate intensity 30-60, 4-7x/week (B); higher intensity exercise is no more effective (B)
  - individualized cognitive behavioural intervention if stressed (B)
  - diet
    - follow Canada's Food Guide (see *Nutrition* section) and DASH (reduced cholesterol and saturated fats) (B)
    - salt restriction to target of <100 mmol/day (<2.3 g) of sodium (B)
    - potassium/magnesium/calcium supplementations NOT effective for HTN (B)
- **pharmacological therapy**
  - indications
    - dBP >90 mmHg with target organ damage or independent cardiovascular risk factors (A)

      ◆ dBP >100 mmHg (A) or sBP >160 mmHg (A) without target organ damage or cardiovascular risk factors

Table 28. First-line Monotherapy Agents for Uncomplicated HTN (diastolic ± systolic)

	Mechanism of Action	Example Drugs	Important Notes
Thiazides/ Diuretics	Inhibit Na and Cl resorption at kidneys → increased Na excretion → water loss	Hydrochlorothiazide Furosemide	Monitor serum K because risk of hypokalemia
β-Blocker	Blocks B$_2$ receptors to reduce contractility of cardiac and smooth muscle	"-lols" Atenolol Metoprolol Propanolol	Not recommended as 1st line agents for patients >60 y.o. due to lack of benefit (A)
ACE inhibitor	Inhibits conversion of Angiotensin I to Angiotensin II (a potent vasoconstrictor) → vasodilation	"-prils" Ramipril (Altace™) Enalapril (Vasotec™) Captopril	Should not be used as 1st line agent for those of African American descent If not well tolerated, can prescribe ARBs (A)
Calcium Channel Blocker (CCB)	Inhibits Ca influx into cardiac and smooth muscle → vasodilation and reduced cardiac contractility	Dihydropyridine CCBs Amlodipine (Norvasc™) Nifedipine (Adalat™) Felodipine Non-dihydropyridine CCBs Diltiazem (Cardiazem™) Verapamil	Dihydropyridines act primarily at peripheral vasculature Non-dihydropyridines have both cardiac and vascular effects Short-acting nifedipine should not be used
Angiotasin Receptor Blocker (ARB)	Blocks angiotensin receptors → vasodilation	"-sartans" Losartan (Cozaar™) Irbesartan (Avarpo™) Valsartan (Diovan™)	

Reference: 2008 Canadian Hypertension Education Program Recommendations: The short Clinical Summary - An Annual Update

- if adverse effects, substitute with another drug from above group
- if partial response to standard dose monotherapy, use combination therapy (C)
- caution with combo of non-DHP CCB and β-blocker (D)
- if still not controlled or adverse effects, try other classes of anti-hypertensives (D) (e.g. α-blocker, ARB, centrally acting agents, nondihydropyridine calcium channel blocker (CCB))
- choice of therapy in patients with unique conditions (see Table 29)
- most patients will require combination therapy for optimal control

Follow-Up
- assess and encourage adherence to pharmacological and non-pharmacological therapy at every visit
- lifestyle modification
  - q3-6 months
- pharmacological
  - q1 month until 2 consecutive BP readings under target
  - more often for symptomatic HTN, severe HTN, antihypertensive drug intolerance, target organ damage
  - q3-6 months once at target BP
- referral is indicated for cases of refractory hypertension, suspected secondary cause or worsening renal failure
- hospitalization is indicated for malignant hypertension

Table 29. Pharmacologic treatment of hypertension in patients with unique conditions

Condition or Risk Factor	Recommended Drugs	Alternative Drugs	Not Recommended
Isolated Systolic HTN	Monotherapy with low dose diuretics	Long acting dihydropyridine CCB or ARB	Monotherapy with β-blockers
Ischemic Heart Disease (IHD)	β-blockers, ACE inhibitors	Long-acting CCB ARB (if intolerant to ACEI)	Short-acting CCB
Left Ventricular Hypertrophy	ACEI, ARB, CCB, thiazide diuretics, β-blockers (if <60)		Vasodilators and hydralazine, minoxidil
Cerebrovascular Disease (stroke/TIA)	ACEI/diuretic combination preferred		
Systolic Dysfunction	ACEI, β-blockers (diuretics as additive therapy)	ARB (if intolerant to ACEI) hydralazine + isosorbide dinitrate (if ACEI + ARB contraindicated)	Non-DHP CCB
Dyslipidemias	As for uncomplicated IHD	As for uncomplicated IHD	β-blockers without ISA

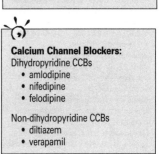

Dieting to reduce body weight for controlling hypertension in adults
Cochrane Database of Systemic Reviews 1998: Issue 4
A systematic review of eighteen trials showed that weight-reducing diets in overweight hypertensive persons can affect modest weight loss in the range of 3-9% of body weight and are probably associated with modest blood pressure decreases of roughly 3 mmHg systolic and diastolic. Weight-reducing diets may decrease dosage requirements of persons taking antihypertensive medications.

Calcium Channel Blockers:
Dihydropyridine CCBs
- amlodipine
- nifedipine
- felodipine

Non-dihydropyridine CCBs
- diltiazem
- verapamil

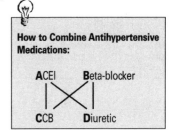

How to Combine Antihypertensive Medications:

ACEI   Beta-blocker

CCB   Diuretic

Table 29. Pharmacologic treatment of hypertension in patients with unique conditions (continued)

Condition or Risk Factor	Recommended Drugs	Alternative Drugs	Not Recommended
Peripheral Vascular Disease		As for uncomplicated IHD	As for uncomplicated IHD
	β-blockers (if severe disease)		
Diabetes Mellitus			
With Nephropathy (urinary albumin ≥30 mg/d)	ACEI or ARB	Add thiazide diuretic, long-acting CCB, or ACEI/ARB combo	If creatinine >150 µmol/L, use loop diuretic instead of thiazide diuretic
Without Nephropathy	1. ACEI or ARB, or 2. thiazide diuretic or DHP CCB	Combo of first-line drugs Cardioselective β-blockers long-acting CCB	If creatinine >150 µmol/L, use loop diuretic instead of thiazide diuretic
Renal Disease	ACEI (thiazide diuretics as additive therapy)	ARB (if intolerant to ACEI) volume overload: loop diuretics instead of thiazide	ACEI/ARB contraindicated in renal artery stenosis
Asthma	K-sparing + thiazide diuretics for patients on salbutamol		β-blockers, unless specific indications like angina or post-MI
Gout			Thiazides, but asymptomatic hyperuricemia is not a contraindication
Smoking	Low dose thiazides ACEI		β-blockers
Pregnancy	Methyldopa Hydralazine	Labetolol Nifedipine	ACEI
Elderly (>60)	As for uncomplicated IHD, except for use of β-blockers		β-blockers not recommended as first-line treatment
Emergency	(BP >169/90) = labetolol, nifedipine		
If >3 cardiovascular RFs or established atherosclerotic disease	Statin, ASA		Caution with use of ASA in patients with uncontrolled BP

ISA = intrinsic sympathomimetic activity, ARB = angiotensin II receptor blockers, ACEI = angiotensin converting enzyme inhibitor
Adapted from: McAlister FA, Zarnke KB, Campbell NRC, et al. (2002). The 2001 Canadian recommendations for the management of hypertension: Part two – Therapy. *Can J Cardiol*, 18(6):625-641. AND The 2006 Canadian Hypertension Education Program Recommendations.

Thiazides as First-Line Antihypertensive Therapy – ALLHAT
JAMA 2002;288:2981-97
Study: Randomized, double-blind, active-controlled clinical trial with mean follow-up of 4.9 years.
Patients: 33,357 participants (mean age 67y, 53% male, 47% white) with stage 1 or 2 hypertension and at least one other CHD risk factor.
Intervention: Participants were randomly assigned to receive chlorthalidone (12.5-25mg/d), amlodipine (2.5-10mg/d), or lisinopril (10-40mg/d). Target BP was <140/90 mmHg, achieved by titrating the assigned study drug, and adding open-label agents when necessary.
Outcomes: The primary outcome was combined fatal CHD or non-fatal MI. Secondary outcomes were all-cause mortality, stroke, combined CHD, and combined CVD.
Results: There were no significant differences in either the primary outcome or all-cause mortality between treatment groups. For amlodipine vs. chlorthalidone, secondary outcomes were similar except for a higher 6-year rate of heart failure with amlodipine (10.2% vs. 7.7%; p<0.001). For lisinopril vs. chlorthalidone, lisinopril had higher 6-year rates of combined CVD (33.3% vs. 30.9%; p<0.001), stroke (6.3% vs. 5.6%; p=0.02) and heart failure (8.7% vs. 7.7%; p<0.001).
Conclusion: Thiazide-type diuretics are superior to CCB and ACEI for preventing one or more major forms of CVD, with similar risks of death and non-fatal MI.

Low Back Pain

- see Orthopaedics

Definition
- acute: <6 weeks
- subacute: 6-12 weeks
- chronic: >12 weeks

Epidemiology
- 5th most common reason for visiting a physician
- lifetime prevalence: 90%
- peak prevalence: age 45-60
- largest WSIB category
- most common cause of chronic disability for persons <45 years old
- 90% resolve in 6 weeks, <5% become chronic

Etiology
- source of pain can be local, radicular, referred, or related to a psychiatric illness
- 98% mechanical cause
  - ligamentous/muscle strain, facet joint degeneration, disc injury, spondylosis, spondylolisthesis, compression fracture, spinal stenosis, pregnancy
  - worse with movement, improved with rest
- 2% non-mechanical cause
  - most concerning when pain is worse at rest and does not change with position
- surgical emergencies
  - cauda equina syndrome: LBP, areflexia, lower extremity weakness, fecal incontinence, urinary retention, saddle anesthesia, decreased anal tone
  - abdominal aortic aneurysm: pulsatile abdominal mass

Red Flags for Back Pain:
B: bowel or bladder dysfunction
A: anesthesia (saddle)
C: constitutional symptoms/malignancy
K: chronic disease
P: paresthesias
A: age >50
I: IV drug use
N: neuromotor deficits

- medical conditions
  - neoplastic (primary, metastatic, multiple myeloma)
  - infectious (osteomyelitis, TB)
  - metabolic (osteoporosis, osteomalacia, Paget's disease)
  - rheumatologic (ankylosing spondylitis, polymyalgia rheumatica)
  - referred pain (perforated ulcer, pancreatitis, pyelonephritis, ectopic pregnancy, herpes zoster), no change with position

Physical Exam
- neurologic exam for L4, L5, S1 helps determine level of spinal involvement (muscle strength, sensation, reflexes), see <u>Neurosurgery</u>
- peripheral pulses
- special tests:
  - straight leg raise (positive if pain at <70 degrees, aggravated by dorsiflexion of ankle), positive test is indicative of sciatica
  - crossed straight leg raise (more specific; raising uninvolved leg elicits pain in leg with sciatica)
  - femoral stretch test (patient prone, knee flexed, examiner extends hip) to diagnose L4 radiculopathy

Investigations
- plain films not recommended in initial evaluation
- indications for lumbar spine x-ray:
  - no improvement after 1 month
  - fever >38°C
  - unexplained weight loss
  - prolonged corticosteroid use
  - significant trauma
  - progressive neuromotor deficit
  - suspicion of ankylosing spondylitis
  - history of cancer (rule out metastases)
  - alcohol/drug abuse (increased risk of osteomyelitis, trauma, fracture)
- CBC, ESR, urinalysis (infection, cancer)
- bone scan (infection, tumour, occult fracture), EMG if indicated
- consider CT or MRI (worsening neurologic deficits, infection, tumour)

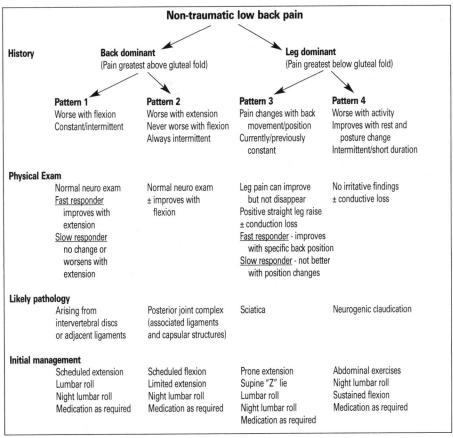

Figure 8. Approach to Nontraumatic Low-Back Pain

Adapted from: American Academy of Orthopaedic Surgeons. Acute Care: Nontraumatic Low Back Pain. *Orthopaedic Knowledge Update: Spine 2* 2001: 153-166

Spinal manipulative therapy for low back pain
Cochrane Database of Systematic Reviews 2004; Issue 3
Last substantive amendment: 17 September 2003.
This systematic review of 39 RCTs compared spinal manipulative therapy with other therapies for low back pain. For acute and chronic low back pain, spinal manipulative therapy was superior only to sham therapy or therapies judged to be ineffective or even harmful. It had no statistical or clinical advantage over analgesics, physical therapy, exercises, back school or physician care.
Conclusions: For acute and chronic low-back pain, there is no evidence that spinal manipulative therapy is superior to other treatments.

Massage for low back pain
Cochrane Database of Systematic Reviews 2004; Issue 3
This systematic review of 8 randomized trials assessed the use of massage therapy for non-specific low back pain as compared to a variety of other treatments.
Conclusions: For some patients with subacute or chronic non-specific low back pain, massage may be beneficial – especially with education and exercises. Some evidence suggests that acupuncture massage may be more effective than classic massage.

Non-steroidal anti-inflammatory drugs for low back pain
Cochrane Database of Systematic Reviews 2004; Issue 3
This systematic review of 51 randomized and double-blind controlled trials assessed the effects of NSAIDs in treating non-specific low back pain and whether one type of NSAID was more effective.
Conclusions: NSAIDs are effective for short-term symptomatic relief in acute low back pain and no specific type of NSAID appears to be better.

Treatment
- reassurance and education if no underlying serious condition
  - 70% improve in 2 weeks, 90% in 6 weeks
- recommend comfort measures
  - limited bed rest (>2-4 days bed rest has potentially debilitating effects and no proven efficacy)
  - staying active (within limits of pain) leads to more rapid recovery and less chronic disability
  - activity modification (temporarily avoid activities that stress spine, e.g. heavy lifting, prolonged unsupported sitting)
  - heat or cold therapies
  - notes for work or WSIB to endorse "modified, appropriate work" vs. time off
  - encourage early return to work or activities
- pharmacological
  - acetaminophen
  - NSAIDs
  - muscle relaxants sometimes helpful but may cause drowsiness and are no better than NSAIDs
  - short term muscle relaxant use <7 days may be helpful
  - NOT narcotics
- physical methods
  - short course of massage may be beneficial
  - NO proven efficacy of spinal traction, TENS, biofeedback, acupuncture, injections (trigger-point, facet joint) or spinal manipulation
- if no improvement after one month of conservative therapy, consider further investigations
- x-rays and appropriate labs in presence of any red flags
- surgical evaluation if:
  - suspected cauda equina syndrome
  - worsening neurologic deficit
  - intractable pain not responding to conservative therapy

Menopause/HRT

- see Gynecology

Epidemiology
- Canadian female life span = 81.2 years
- mean age of menopause = 51.4 years
- a woman will spend over 1/3 of her life in menopause

Clinical Features
- urogenital tract: atrophy, vaginal dryness, incontinence
- blood vessels and heart: vasomotor instability, hot flashes, increased risk of heart disease
- bones: bone loss, fractures, loss of height
- brain: depression, mood swings, memory loss

Management
- encourage physical exercise, smoking cessation, and a balanced diet with adequate intake/supplementation of calcium/vitamin D (1500mg/800IU OD)
- hormone replacement therapy (HRT)
  - routine use of HRT is no longer recommended
  - regimens: cyclic estrogen + progesterone, continuous estrogen + progesterone, estrogen only (no uterus), estrogen ring, estrogen gel
  - helps with symptomatic relief of estrogen deprivation
  - decreases risk of osteoporotic fractures, colorectal cancer
  - increases risk of breast cancer, coronary heart disease, stroke, and pulmonary embolism
  - initiation of HRT requires a thorough discussion of each patient's history, symptoms and risk factors, and of the overall short and long-term benefits and risks
- consider venlafaxine, SSRI, gabapentin to ease with vasomotor instability

Estrogen plus progestin and the risk of coronary heart disease.
N Engl J Med. 2003 Aug 7;349(6):523-34
Study: Randomized controlled trial, after a mean follow-up of 5.2 years. Planned duration was 8.5 years but the data and safety monitoring board recommended terminating the trial because the overall risks exceeded the benefits.
Patients: 16,608 postmenopausal women, age 50 to 79 years at base line.
The intervention was conjugated equine estrogens (0.625 mg per day) plus medroxyprogesterone acetate (2.5 mg per day) or placebo.
Purpose: Final results with regard to estrogen plus progestin and CHD from the Women's Health Initiative (WHI).
Main Outcomes: Nonfatal MI or death due to coronary heart disease.
Results: Combined HRT was associated with a hazard ratio for coronary artery disease of 1.24. The elevation in risk was most apparent at one year (hazard ratio 1.81).
Conclusions: Estrogen plus progestin does not confer cardiac protection and may increase the risk of CHD among generally healthy postmenopausal women, especially during the first year after the initiation of hormone use. This treatment should not be prescribed for the prevention of cardiovascular disease.

Osteoarthritis

* see Rheumatology

Epidemiology
* most common form of arthritis seen in primary care
* prevalence: 10-12%, increases with age
* results in long-term disability in 2-3% of patients with OA
* almost everyone over the age of 65 shows signs of OA on x-ray, but only 33% of these will be symptomatic

Clinical Features
* pain with weight bearing, improved with rest
* morning stiffness or gelling <30 min
* deformity, bony enlargement, crepitus, limitation of movement
* usually affects distal joints of hands, spine, hips, and knees

Investigations
* no laboratory tests for the diagnosis of OA
* radiographic features:
  * joint space narrowing
  * subchondral sclerosis
  * subchondral cyst formation
  * osteophytes

Management
* goals: relieve pain, preserve joint motion and function, prevent further injury
* non-pharmacological
  * patient education, weight loss, exercise (OT/PT), assistive devices (canes, orthotics, raised toilet seats)
* pharmacological
  * keep in mind co-morbid conditions such as HTN, peptic ulcer disease, renal disease
  * medications do not alter natural course of OA
  * 1st line: acetaminophen 325-1000 mg qid prn (OA is not an inflammatory disorder)
  * 2nd line: NSAIDs (COX-2 selective NSAIDs (Celebrex™, Mobicox™) recommended if long-term therapy or if high risk for serious GI problems)
  * combination analgesics (e.g. acetaminophen and codeine)
  * intra-articular corticosteroid injections (not more than 3-4x/yr) may be helpful in acute flares (benefits last 4-6 wks, can be up to 6 mo)
  * intra-articular hyaluronans injections
  * topical NSAID (Pennsaid™)
  * capsaicin cream (Zostrix™)
* surgery
  * consider if persistent significant pain and functional impairment despite optimal pharmacotherapy (e.g. debridement, osteotomy, total joint arthroplasty)

Osteoporosis

* see Endocrinology

Epidemiology
* age related disease characterized by decreased bone mass and increased susceptibility to fractures
* affects 1 in 6 Canadian women over the age of 50

Table 30. Risk Factors for Osteoporosis

Major Risk Factors	Minor Risk Factors
Age >65 years	Rheumatoid arthritis
Vertebral compression fracture	Past history of clinical hyperthyroidism
Fragility fracture after age 40	Chronic anticonvulsant therapy
Family history of osteoporotic fracture (especially maternal hip fracture)	Low dietary calcium intake
Systemic glucocorticoid therapy of >3 months duration	Smoker
Malabsorption syndrome	Excessive alcohol intake
Primary hyperparathyroidism	Excessive caffeine intake
Propensity to fall	Weight <57 kg
Osteopenia apparent on x-ray film	Weight loss >10% of weight at age 25
Hypogonadism	Chronic heparin therapy
Early menopause (before age 45)	

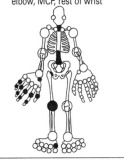

Figure 9. Common sites of involvement in OA

* hand (DIP, PIP, 1st CMC)
* hip
* knee
* 1st MTP
* L-spine (L4-L5, L5-S1)
* C-spine
* uncommon: ankle, shoulder, elbow, MCP, rest of wrist

Vioxx™ is now off the market due to concerns about increasing cardiovascular events.

Glucosamine therapy for treating osteoarthritis
Cochrane Database of Systematic Reviews 2005; Issue 3
Study: To evaluate the effectiveness and toxicity of glucosamine in OA.
Study Characteristics: Meta-analysis of 20 single and double blinded RCTs with 2570 patients. Participants: Age >18 with diagnosis of OA at any site other than the TMJ.
Intervention: Rotta brand and non-Rotta brand glucosamine preparations, administered by any route, and compared against placebo or another treatment.
Main Outcomes: Indicators of response to treatment included changes in pain, function (as assessed using validated questionnaire such as the WOMAC or Lequesne index), global assessment (patient and physician), and radiographically measured structural benefits. Toxicity was also considered.
Results: Analysis of pooled data from all trials showed that glucosamine was more effective than placebo, and was associated with a 28% improvement in pain from baseline (SMD -0.61; 95% CI, -0.95 to -0.28) and an improvement in function using the Lequesne index (SMD -0.51; 95% CI, -0.96 to -0.05); however, the results were not consistently positive. Measurements using the WOMAC scales for pain, function, and stiffness did not reach statistical significance. Subgroup analyses restricted to studies with adequate concealment, or to those in which non-Rotta preparations were used, did not show a benefit of glucosamine for pain and function using the WOMAC index. Two RCTs showed glucosamine slowed radiological progression of OA of the knee (SMD 0.24; 95% CI, 0.04-0.43). The number of patients reporting adverse events was the same for glucosamine as placebo (RR=0.97; 95% CI, 0.88-1.08).
Conclusions: Glucosamine may represent a safe and effective treatment for both symptoms and structural disease in OA. Results are nonetheless heterogeneous and further study is needed to clarify its effectiveness. Differences in the effectiveness of Rotta and non-Rotta preparations, highlight variability between glucosamine preparations, and patients should be made aware of this fact.

Diagnosis
- defined in terms of a bone mineral density (BMD) T-score < –2.5 SD
- osteopenia defined by BMD T-score between –1 S.D. and –2.5 SD
- mass BMD screening is not recommended
- measure BMD in:
  - all patients >65 years of age
  - all patients with one major or two minor risk factors for osteoporosis (see Table 30)
- measure BMD using dual x-ray absorptiometry (DEXA)
- suspect osteoporosis in women with back pain, a decrease in height or thoracic kyphosis

Management
- institute a fall prevention program for those at risk, optimize eyesight
- lifestyle
  - weight bearing exercise, smoking cessation, decrease EtOH intake
- diet
  - for women without documented osteoporosis, calcium and vitamin D supplementation alone prevents osteoporotic fractures (grade B recommendation).
  - calcium (1500 mg/day) and vitamin D (800 IU/day) intake in diet or supplements
- pharmacological
  - for women with osteoporosis, bisphosphonates (e.g. risedronate, alendronate) or Selective Estrogen Receptor Modulators (e.g. raloxifene) prevent osteoporotic fractures (grade A to B recommendation)
  - for women with severe osteoporosis (osteoporosis plus at least 1 fragility fracture), alendronate, risedronate, parathyroid hormone (limited duration), raloxifene, etidronate and oral pamidronate therapy (grade A to B recommendation)
  - if none of these drugs is tolerated, hormone replacement therapy (HRT) or calcitonin can be considered
  - severe esophagitis is the major side effect of bisphosphonate use
- HRT, calcitonin
  - there is fair evidence that combined estrogen–progestin therapy decreases the incidence of total, hip and nonvertebral fractures; however, for most women the risks may outweigh the benefits (grade D recommendation), see Gynecology

Sexually Transmitted Infections (STIs)

- see Gynecology

Definition
- diverse group of infections caused by multiple microbial pathogens
- all can be spread by either secretions or fluids from mucosal surfaces

Etiology
- bacteria: *Chlamydia trachomatis*, *Neisseria gonorrheae*, *Treponema pallidum* (syphilis)
- viruses: HSV, HIV, HPV, hepatitis B, hepatitis C (especially IV drug users)

Epidemiology
- high incidence rates worldwide
- Canadian prevalence rates in clinical practice:
  - common: chlamydia, gonorrhea, PID, genital warts, genital herpes (increasing incidence)
  - less common: hepatitis B, HIV & syphilis (both increasing in incidence), trichomoniasis
  - rare: chancroid, lymphogranuloma venereum, granuloma inguinale
- genital tract infections (NOT sexually transmitted): vulvovaginal candidiasis (VVC), bacterial vaginosis (BV)
- three most common infections associated with vaginal discharge in adult women are BV, VVC, and trichomoniasis

Risk Factors
- sexually active males and females <25 y.o.
- early age of 1st intercourse
- street involved and/or substance use, men who have sex with men
- unprotected sex, previous STI, contact with known case of STI
- new partner in past 2 months, >2 partners in past 12 months

History
- sexual history
    - level of sexual activity and type (oral, anal and/or vaginal intercourse)
    - age of first intercourse, sexual orientation, sexual activity during travel
    - total number of partners in the past year/month/week and duration of involvement with each
- STI history
    - STI awareness, previous STIs and testing, partners with previous STIs
    - contraception history, last Pap test and results
    - local symptoms such as genital burning, itching, discharge, sores, vesicles
    - associated symptoms such as fever, arthralgia, lymphadenopathy
    - partner communication with regards to STIs

Investigations/Screening
- individuals who are symptomatic or asymptomatic and at increased risk should be screened for chlamydia, gonorrhea, HIV, hepatitis B, and syphilis
- Pap test if one not performed in the preceding 12 months

Management
- prevention
    - primary prevention is vastly more effective than treating STIs and their sequelae
    - offer Hep B vaccine if not immune
    - discuss STI risk factors (e.g. decreasing the number of sexual partners)
    - direct advice to ALWAYS use condoms or to abstain from intercourse
    - condoms not 100% effective against HPV, herpes, genital warts
    - consider new HPV vaccine (see Gynecology)
- an STI patient is not considered treated until the management of his/her partner(s) is ensured (contact tracing by Public Health)
- patients should abstain from sexual activity until treatment completion
- STI mandatory reporting: chlamydia, gonorrhea, hepatitis B, HIV, syphilis

> When an STI is detected in a pre-pubertal child, evaluation for sexual abuse is always required.

Table 31. Diagnosis and Treatment of Common STIs

	Symptoms & Signs	Investigations	Treatment	Complications
Gonococcal Urethritis/Cervicitis (Neisseria gonorrheae)	M: burning, irritation, unexplained pyuria, urethral discharge W: mucopurulent endocervical discharge, dysuria, pelvic pain, vaginal bleeding M & W: often asymptomatic, can involve rectal symptoms in cases of unprotected anal sex	M: urine PCR, urethral swabs for stain & culture W: endocervical swab for culture, vaginal swab for wet mount & gram stain	Mandatory reporting to public health Cefixime 400 mg PO, single dose + Non-Gonococcal urethritis/cervicitis Rx* F/U in 2 wks for test of cure if symptoms persist	Arthritis, ↑ risk of acquiring and transmitting HIV M: urethral strictures, epididymitis, infertility W: PID, infertility, ectopic pregnancy, perinatal infection, chronic pelvic pain
Non-Gonococcal Urethritis/Cervicitis (Usually *Chlamydia trachomatis***)	~70% asymptomatic If symptoms appear (usually 2-6 wks after infection) then similar to gonococcal symptoms (see above)	Same as above	Mandatory reporting to public health Azithromycin 1g PO, single dose + Gonococcal urethritis/cervicitis Rx* Same follow up as above	Same as above
Human Papilloma Virus (genital warts)	Most are asymptomatic M: cauliflower lesions (condylomata acuminata) on skin/mucosa of penile/anal area W: cauliflower lesions AND/OR pre-neoplastic/neoplastic lesions on cervix, vagina, or vulva	None needed if simple condylomata Potential biopsy of suspicious lesions W: screening for cervical dysplasia through regular Pap smears	For condylomata: cryotherapy, electrocautery, topical therapy (podophyllotoxin) For cervical dysplasia: colposcopy & possible excision, dependent on grade of lesion	M & W: anal cancer W: cervical/vaginal/vulvar cancer
Genital Herpes (HSV-1 and -2)	1° episode: painful vesicoulcerative genital lesions, +/- tender lymphadenopathy & fever, protracted course Recurrent episodes: less extensive lesions, shorter course, may have "trigger factors"	Swab of vesicular content for culture, type-specific serologic testing for HSV-1 & HSV-2 antibodies	1° episode: Acyclovir 200 mg PO 5x/day for 5-10 days, OR Famciclovir 250 mg PO tid for 5 days, OR Valacyclovir 1000 mg PO bid for 10 days Recurrent Episodes: Valacyclovir 500 mg PO bid OR 1 g qd for 3 days, OR Famciclovir 125 mg PO bid for 5 days, OR Acyclovir 200 mg PO 5 times/day for 5d, or 800 mg PO tid for 2 days	Genital pain, urethritis, aseptic meningitis, cervicitis, ↑ risk of acquiring and transmitting HIV
Infectious Syphillis (Treponema pallidum)	1°: painless sore 2°: rash & flu-like symptoms Latent Phase: asymptomatic 3°: neurologic, cardiovascular, and tissue complications	Specimen collection from 1° & 2° lesions; screen high risk individuals with serologic syphilis testing; universal screening of pregnant women	Mandatory reporting to Public Health Benzathine penicillin G IM (dose depends on stage) Notify partners (last 3-12 mths) Continuous follow-up and testing until patients are seronegative	↑ risk of acquiring and transmitting HIV Chronic neurologic and cardiovascular sequelae

* N.B. if urethritis/cervicitis is suspected, always treat for both gonococcal and non-gonococcal types (i.e. Cefixime AND Azithromycin)
** most common reportable STI in Canada

Sinusitis

- see Otolaryngology

Definition
- inflammation of the mucous membranes of the nasal cavity and paranasal sinuses, fluid within these cavities, and/or the underlying bone

Etiology
- may be divided into
  - acute: <4 weeks
  - recurrent: 4 or more episodes per year, each lasting at least 10 days, with an absence of symptoms in between
  - chronic: ≥12 weeks
- common pathogens: rhinovirus, influenza, parainfluenza, *S. pneumoniae*, *H. influenzae*, *M. catarrhalis*

Risk Factors
- medical conditions: respiratory infections, allergic rhinitis, cystic fibrosis, immunodeficiency
- anatomic: deviated septum, polyps, adenoid hypertrophy, tumour
- irritants: environmental, tobacco smoke, air pollution, chlorine
- iatrogenic: topical decongestant overuse, cocaine, trauma

Investigations
- radiography is warranted only when the diagnosis of sinusitis is in doubt
- all patients with pronounced frontal headaches should have a radiograph performed to rule out frontal sinusitis
- CT scans are not cost-effective and should not be used routinely to diagnose sinusitis

> **Signs of Sinusitis**
> - nasal congestion
> - history of purulent nasal discharge
> - facial pain/facial pressure
> - maxillary toothache
> - poor response to decongestants
> - abnormal transillumination
> - purulent secretions (on physical)

Management
- acute sinusitis
  - 40% of patients will recover spontaneously; however, antimicrobial therapy is beneficial
    - 1st line: amoxicillin x 10 days (TMP-SMX if penicillin allergic)
    - 2nd line: amoxicillin + clavulanate, clarithromycin, ceflacor, cefixime
  - adjunct therapy
    - saline nasal spray, humidification
    - topical or systemic decongestants; for short-term use only
    - nasal corticosteroid spray for chronic sinusitis only
    - antihistamines are contraindicated
  - referral to ENT if:
    - failure of second-line therapy
    - ≥3 episodes per year
    - development of complications (mucocele, orbital extension, meningitis, intracranial abscess, venous sinus thrombosis)

Sleep Disorders

- see Respirology

Definition
- most often characterized by one of three complaints:
  - insomnia
    - difficulty falling asleep, difficulty maintaining sleep, early-morning wakening, non-refreshing sleep
  - parasomnias
    - night terrors, nightmares, restless leg syndrome, somnambulism (performing complex behaviour during sleep with eyes open but without memory of event)
  - excessive daytime sleepiness

Epidemiology
- 1/3 of patients in primary care setting have occasional sleep problems
- 10% have chronic sleep problems
- more common in women and with increasing age

Etiology
- primary sleep disorders
  - primary insomnia, obstructive sleep apnea, restless legs syndrome, narcolepsy, periodic limb movements of sleep
- secondary causes
  - medical (COPD, asthma, CHF, hyperthyroidism, chronic pain, BPH)

- drugs (EtOH, caffeine, nicotine, β-agonists, antidepressants, steroids)
- psychiatric disorders (especially mood and anxiety disorders)
- lifestyle factors (shift work)

Investigations
- complete sleep diary every morning for 1-2 wks
    - record bedtime, sleep latency, total sleep time, awakenings, quality of sleep
- rule out specific medical problems (CBC + differential, TSH)
- sleep study referral if suspect periodic leg movements of sleep or sleep apnea
- night time polysomnogram or daytime multiple sleep latency test

Treatment
- treat and manage any suspected medical or psychiatric cause
- psychologic treatment
    - sleep hygiene
        - avoid caffeine, nicotine, EtOH; exercise regularly; comfortable sleep environment; regular sleep schedule; no napping
    - relaxation therapy (e.g. deep breathing meditation, biofeedback)
    - stimulus control therapy (re-association of bed/bedroom with sleep; re-establishment of a consistent sleep-wake schedule; reduce activities that cue staying awake)
    - sleep restriction therapy: total time in bed should closely match the total sleep time of the patient (improves sleep efficacy)
- pharmacologic treatment
    - short-acting benzodiazepines (e.g. lorazepam, oxazepam, temazepam) should be used <7 consecutive nights to break cycle of chronic insomnia

Specific Problems
- **primary insomnia**
    - majority of cases
    - person reacts to the insomnia with fear or anxiety around bedtime or with a change in sleep hygiene
    - can progress to a chronic disorder (psychophysiological insomnia)

- **snoring**
    - results from soft tissue vibration at the back of the nose and throat due to turbulent airflow through narrowed air passages
    - risk factors: male gender, obesity, alcohol consumption, ingestion of tranquilizers or muscle relaxants, and smoking
    - PE: obesity, nasal polyps, septal deviation, hypertrophy of the nasal turbinates, and enlarged uvula and tonsils
    - investigations (only if severely symptomatic): (1) nocturnal polysomnography and (2) airway assessment (CT/MRI)
    - treatment
        - sleep on side (position therapy), weight loss
        - nasal dilators (noninvasive external dilator made with elastic adhesive backing applied over nasal bridge); tongue-retaining devices; mandibular advancement devices
    - at risk of developing obstructive sleep apnea

- **obstructive sleep apnea (OSA)**
    - apnea resulting from upper airway obstruction due to collapse of the base of the tongue, soft palate with uvula, and epiglottis
    - respiratory effort is present
    - leads to a distinctive snoring, choking, awakening type pattern as body rouses itself to open airway = resuscitative breath
    - apneic episodes can last from 20 sec to 3 min
    - can have 100-600 episodes/night
    - diagnosis based on nocturnal polysomnography: >15 apneic episodes per hour of sleep with arousal recorded
    - consequences:
        - daytime somnolence, nonrestorative sleep
        - poor social and work performance
        - mood changes: anxiety, irritability, depression
        - sexual dysfunction: poor libido, impotence
        - morning headache (due to hypercapnia)
        - HTN (2x ↑ risk), CAD (3x ↑ risk), stroke (4x ↑ risk), arrhythmias
        - pulmonary hypertension, RV dysfunction, cor pulmonale (due to chronic hypoxemia)
        - memory loss, decreased concentration, confusion

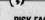

RISK FACTORS
- 2% women, 4% men between ages 30-60
- obesity causing upper airway narrowing: BMI >28 kg/m² present in 60-90% of cases
- children: commonly tonsils, adenoids
- aging which causes decreased muscle tone
- persistent URTIs, allergies, nasal tumours, hypothyroidism (due to macroglossia)
- FHx

- investigations:
  - blood gas not helpful, TSH if clinically indicated
  - evaluate BP, inspect nose, oropharynx (i.e. for enlarged adenoids or tonsils)
  - nocturnal polysomnography (Sleep Lab)
- treatment:
  - modifying factors: avoid sleeping supine, lose weight, avoid EtOH, sedatives, narcotics, inhaled steroids if nasal swelling present
  - primary treatment of OSA is CPAP; maintains patent airway in 95% of OSA cases
  - dental appliances to modify mandibular position
  - surgery: somnoplasty, tonsillectomy & adenoidectomy (in children), uvulopalatopharyngoplasty (UPPP)
  - report patient to Ministry of Transportation if OSA is not controlled by CPAP

- **central sleep apnea**
  - definition:
    - brain fails to send appropriate signals to the breathing muscles to initiate respirations
    - defining feature is absent respiratory effort
    - often secondary to CNS diseases: brainstem infarction, infection, neuromuscular disease
  - investigations: PFTs, nocturnal polysomnography, MRI
  - treatment: CPAP or mechanical ventilation (if brainstem origin)
  - prognosis: poor

Social Phobia

- see Psychiatry

Definition
- a marked and persistent fear of one or more social or performance situations in which the person is exposed to unfamiliar people or to possible scrutiny by others

Epidemiology
- lifetime prevalence rate of up to 16%; F:M = 1.5:1
- often begins in early childhood and adolescence
- can lead to significant psychiatric comorbidity including: depression, other anxiety disorders, alcohol and substance abuse and eating disorders
- is often under-recognized and under-treated by family practitioners

History
- fear of being humiliated or embarassed in one or more social or performance situations
- commonly feared situations include public speaking, eating, drinking, writing in front of others, using public restrooms, speaking on the telephone and social gatherings
- the fear is recognized as excessive or unreasonable
- the avoidance, anticipation and distress of the social situation interferes significantly with social and occupational functioning
- can often present with somatic complaints of insomnia, fatigue, palpitations, chest pain, shortness of breath, dizziness, trembling hands, sweating, blushing and GI complaints

Physical
- presenting with symptoms of hyperhidrosis, tremor, blushing, stuttering, hypertension and tachycardia
- thorough mental status examination

Management
- cognitive behavioural therapy
- exposure therapy, cognitive restructuring and social skills training to decrease anxiety and weaken the tendency to avoid social situations
  - exposure therapy is the most firmly established therapeutic maneuver
- drug therapy
  - effective treatments include SSRIs, MAOIs and anxiolytics; no TCAs
  - SSRIs are becoming the new drugs of choice because of effectiveness and lack of significant negative side effects
  - beta blocker or benzodiazepine in acute social situations

Sore Throat (Pharyngitis)

Definition
- acute pharyngitis is an inflammation of the oropharynx
- may be caused by a wide range of infectious organisms, most of which produce a self-limited infection with no significant sequelae

Etiology
- viral
  - adenovirus, rhinovirus, influenza virus, RSV, EBV, coxsackie virus, herpes simplex virus, CMV, HIV
- bacterial
  - group A β-hemolytic *Streptococcus* (GABHS)
  - other bacterial causes:
    - Group C and G β-hemolytic *Streptococcus*, *Neisseria gonorrheae*, *Chlamydia pneumoniae*, *Mycoplasma pneumoniae*, *Corynebacterium diphtheriae*

Epidemiology
- viral
  - most common cause, occurs year round
- bacterial
  - Group A β-hemolytic *Streptococcus*
    - most common bacterial cause
    - 5-15% of adult cases and up to 50% of all pediatric cases of acute pharyngitis
    - most prevalent between 5-17 years old
    - occurs most often in winter months

Clinical Features
- viral
  - pharyngitis, conjunctivitis, rhinorrhea, hoarseness, cough
  - nonspecific flu-like symptoms such as fever, malaise, and myalgia
  - often mimics bacterial infection
  - coxsackie virus (hand, foot and mouth disease)
    - primarily late summer, early fall
    - sudden onset of fever, pharyngitis, headache, abdominal pain and vomiting
    - appearance of small vesicles that rupture and ulcerate on soft palate, tonsils, pharynx
    - ulcers are pale gray, several mm in diameter, have surrounding erythema, may appear on hands and feet
  - herpes simplex virus
    - like coxsackie virus but ulcers are fewer and larger
  - EBV (infectious mononucleosis)
    - pharyngitis, tonsillar exudate, fever, lymphadenopathy, fatigue, rash
- bacterial
  - symptoms: sore throat, absence of cough, fever, malaise, headache, abdominal pain
  - signs: fever, tonsillar or pharyngeal erythema/exudate, swollen/tender anterior cervical nodes
  - complications
    - rheumatic fever
    - glomerulonephritis
    - suppurative complications (abscess, sinusitis, otitis media, pneumonia, cervical adenitis)
    - meningitis
    - impetigo

Table 32. Sore Throat Score: Approach to diagnosis and management of GABHS

	POINTS
Cough absent?	1
History of fever >38°?	1
Tonsillar exudate?	1
Swollen, tender anterior nodes?	1
Age 3-14 years?	1
Age 15-44 years?	0
Age >45 years?	−1

In communities with moderate levels of strep infection (10-20% of sore throats):

Score	0	1	2	3	4
Chance patient has strep	2-3%	3-7%	8-16%	19-34%	41-61%
Suggested action	NO culture or antibiotic		Culture all, treat only if culture is positive		Culture all, treat with antibiotics on clinical grounds[1]

[1]Clinical grounds include a high fever or other indicators that the patient is clinically unwell and is presenting early in the course of the illness.
Limitations: *This score is not applicable to patients less than 3 years of age.
                  *If an outbreak or epidemic of illness caused by GAS is occuring in any community, the score is invalid and should not be used.
Adapted from: Centor RM et al (1981). *Med Decis Making.* 1: 239-46.
McIssac WI, White D, Tannenbaum D, Low DE (1998). *CMAJ.* 158(1):75-83.

Investigations
- suspected GABHS
  - see Table 32 for approach to diagnosis and management of GABHS
  - gold standard for diagnosis is throat culture
  - rapid test for streptococcal antigen: high specificity (95%), low sensitivity (50-90%)
    - if rapid test positive, treat patient
    - if rapid test negative, take culture and call patient if positive to start antibiotics
- suspected EBV (infectious mononucleosis)
  - peripheral blood smear, heterophile antibody test (i.e. the latex agglutination assay, or "monospot")

Management
- GABHS
  - see Table 32
  - no increased incidence of rheumatic fever with 48-hour delay in treatment
  - incidence of glomerulonephritis is not decreased with antibiotic treatment
  - 10-day antibiotic course
    - adults: penicillin V 300 mg PO tid
    - children: amoxicillin 40 mg/kg/day PO divided q8h
    - erythromycin if penicillin allergic
  - routine follow-up and/or post-treatment throat cultures are not required for most patients
  - follow-up throat culture recommended only for: patients with history of rheumatic fever, patients whose family member has history of acute rheumatic fever, suspected strep carrier
- viral pharyngitis
  - antibiotics NOT indicated
  - symptomatic therapy: acetaminophen/NSAIDs for fever and muscle aches, decongestants
- infectious mononucleosis (EBV)
  - antibiotics NOT indicated; administering ampicillin produces rash
  - self-limiting course; rest during acute phase is beneficial
  - if acute airway obstruction give corticosteroids, consult ENT
  - supportive care, i.e. acetominophen or NSAIDS for fever, sore throat, malaise
  - avoid heavy physical activity and contact sports for at least one month or until splenomegaly resolves because risk of splenic rupture

Complementary and Alternative Medicine (CAM)

Epidemiology
- 50-75% of Canadians report some use of CAM over lifetime, while only half of these will disclose this use to their physician
- use is highest in Western provinces, lowest in Atlantic provinces
- more likely to be used by younger patients, those with higher education and higher income
- examples: chiropractic, acupuncture, massage, naturopathy, homeopathy, traditional Chinese medicine, craniosacral therapy, osteopathy
- most commonly used for: back/neck problems, gynecological problems, anxiety, headaches, digestive problems and chronic fatigue syndromes

Herbal Products
- over 50% of Canadians use natural health products
- most commonly used include echinacea, ginseng, ginkgo, garlic, St John's Wort, and soy
- relatively few herbal products have been shown to be effective in clinical trials
- many patients believe herbal products are inherently safe and are unaware of potential side effects and interactions with conventional medicines
- all natural health products (NHPs) must be regulated under *The Natural Health Products Regulations* as of January 1, 2004, including herbal remedies, homeopathic medicines, vitamins, minerals, traditional medicines, probiotics, amino acids and essential fatty acids (such as omega-3)
- always ask patients whether they are taking any herbal product, herbal supplement or other natural remedy. If yes, explore further, i.e.:
  - Are you taking any prescription or non-prescription medications for the same purpose as the herbal product?
  - Are you allergic to any plant products?
  - Are you pregnant or breast-feeding?
- information resources include National Centre for Complementary and Alternative Medicine (www.nccam.nih.gov), Health Canada website

---

Zinc for the common cold
Cochrane Database of Systematic Reviews 2004;
Issue 3
Last substantive amendment: 15 February 1999.
This systematic review of 7 randomized control trials investigated the effects of zinc lozenges for cold (acute upper respiratory tract infection) symptoms. Two trials suggested the lozenges were effective in reducing severity and duration of symptoms; overall the lozenges did not appear to be effective.
Conclusions: The evidence for zinc lozenges treating the common cold is inconclusive, and there is a potential for side effects.

Echinacea for preventing and treating the common cold
Cochrane Database of Systematic Reviews 2004;
Issue 3
Last substantive amendment: 01 October 1998.
This systematic review of 16 trials assessed the effect of Echinacea in preventing and treating common colds. Trials compared preparations containing Echinacea with placebo, no treatment, or an alternative common cold treatment. Variations in preparations and quality of Echinacea made meta-analysis difficult but in general, results suggested some preparations of Echinacea may be better than placebo.
Conclusions: Most trials of Echinacea show positive data in its ability to prevent and treat the common cold, however there is not enough evidence to recommend a specific Echinacea product or preparation.

St. John's Wort for depression
Cochrane Database of Systematic Reviews 2006;
Issue 3
A meta-analysis of 37 trials, including 26 which compared St. John's Wort with placebo and 14 which compared St. John's Wort with standard antidepressants. The main outcome measure was the ratio of responders to non-responders, and the main outcome measure for adverse effects was the number of patients dropping out due to adverse experiences. Significant heterogeneity was noted among placebo-controlled trials, but trials were statistically homogeneous for trials comparing St. John's Wort with antidepressants. For major depression, compared with placebo, the OR for 6 larger trials was 1.15 and 5 smaller trials, 2.06. Compared with SSRIs and tricyclics, the response rates were 0.98 and 1.03, respectively. Fewer patients on St. John's Wort dropped out due to adverse effects compared to those taking tricyclics (OR 0.25), and a similar but non-significant trend was seen when compared with SSRIs (OR 0.60). Drawing solid conclusions is difficult given the degree of study heterogeneity and number of conflicting studies.

Table 33. Common Herbal Products

Common Name	Reported Uses	Possible Adverse Effects	Possible Drug Interactions
Chamomile	Mild sedative, anxiolytic, GI complaints, common cold	Allergic/contact dermatitis, anaphylaxis	Anxiolytics, sedatives
Echinacea	Common cold, flu, wound treatment, urinary tract infections, cancer	Hypersensitivity, hepatotoxicity with prolonged use, avoid use if immunosuppressed	Potentiates warfarin
Evening primrose	Dysmenorrhea, menopausal sx, inflammation, allergies, eczema, arthritis, MS	Headache, restlessness, nausea, diarrhea, may decrease seizure threshold	Anticoagulants, antiplatelets
Feverfew	Migraine prevention, rheumatoid arthritis, anti-inflammatory	Edginess, upset stomach, skin rash, miscarriage	Anticoagulants, antiplatelets
Flaxseed oil	Laxative, menopausal sx, source of omega-3 fatty acids	Diarrhea	Do not take with other medications as fibre content can bind drugs
Garlic	Elevated lipids, hypertension, hyperglycemia, antimicrobial	GI irritation, contact dermatitis, may increase post-op bleeding	Anticoagulants, potentiates antihypertensives
Ginger	Nausea, motion sickness, dyspepsia, anti-inflammatory	Heartburn, not to be used for morning sickness	None known
Ginkgo biloba	Increases peripheral circulation (AD, dementia, intermittent claudication), premenstrual syndrome, vertigo	Headache, cramping, bleeding, mild digestive problems; reports of intracranial hemorrhage	Anticoagulants, thiazide diuretics, MAO inhibitors
Ginseng	Energy enhancer, decreases stress, adjunct support for chemotherapy/radiation	Hypertension, nervousness, insomnia, breakthrough bleeding, palpitations	Stimulant medications, antihypertensives, hormonal therapies
Glucosamine (Chondroitin)	Osteoarthritis	GI distress, headache, drowsiness, palpitations	Caution if shellfish allergy
Saw palmetto	BPH, adjunct to finasteride	Mild GI distress	α-adrenergics, finasteride
St. John's Wort	Mild to moderate depression	Photosensitivity, increased liver enzymes, drowsiness, dizziness, nausea, headaches	CNS depressants, C/I with indinavir
Valerian root	Sedative, anxiolytic, muscle relaxant, PMS	Drowsiness, headache, digestive problems, paradoxical insomnia	CNS depressants, antihistamines

Reference: Zink T, Chaffin J (1998). Herbal "health" products: What family physicians need to know, *American Family Physician* 58(5):1133-1140.

Primary Care Models

Table 34. Primary Care Models

	Characteristics
Comprehensive care model	• model for physicians in solo practice • regular office hours with limited after-hours availability
Family health group	• group of at least 3 physicians • regular office hours, some after-hours availability as well as on-call to telephone health advisory services
Family health team	• groups of health care professionals (e.g. doctors, nurses, nurse practioners, dieticians, social workers) • wider range of services (e.g. rehabilitation, palliative care) • regular office hours plus increased after-hours availability
Family health network	• group of at least 3 physicians; can utilize nurse practitioners • regular office hours plus telephone health advisory services to provide around the clock primary care coverage
Family health organization	• groups of physicians working in tandem with allied health professionals • provide care via regular office hours, after-hours clinics and around the clock telephone health advisory services

Antibiotic Quick Reference*

CONDITION	MICROORGANISM	ANTIBIOTIC
RESPIRATORY/ENT		
Acute Rhinitis (common cold)	Viral: Rhinovirus, Adeno, RSV, Influenza etc.	None
Pharyngitis (sore throat)	Viral: Adeno, Rhinovirus	None
Strep Pharyngitis	Grp. A β-Hemolytic *Strep* *S. Pneumoniae*	penicillin V 300 PO tid x 10d amoxicillin 40 mg/kg/d PO tid x10d penicillin allergy: erythromycin 400 mg PO OD x 10d
Sinusitis	*S. pneumoniae* *H. influenzae* *M. catarrhalis* Grp A *Strep* Anaerobes *S. Aureus*	1st line: amoxicillin 500 mg PO tid x 7d (If penicillin allergy: TMP/SMX DS 1 tab PO bid) 2nd line: amox/clavulin 500/125 mg PO tid x 7-10d 3rd line: clarithromycin XL 1000 mg PO OD x 14d

Acute Otitis Media	Viral
	S. pneumoniae
	H. influenzae
	M. catarrhalis
		Children under 10:
		    1st line: amoxicillin 40-50 mg/kg/d PO bid/tid x 7d
		    2nd line: ↑ dose to 80-90 mg/kg/d
		    (max dose = 1500 mg/d) x 3d
		    3rd line: cefaclor, cefprozil, macrolides
		Age over 10: amoxicillin 500 mg PO tid x 7-10d
		    penicillin allergy: TMP/SMX or cefuroxime

Otitis Externa	*Pseudomonas* *S. aureus* Fungal	Diabetic: ciprofloxacin 500 mg PO bid x 14d Non-diabetic: 1st line: Buro-sol™ 2-3 drops tid 2nd line: Cortisporin™ otic solution 4 drops tid

Bronchitis	Viral: Rhinovirus, Adenovirus, RSV, Influenza
	S. pneumoniae
	H. influenzae
	M. catarrhalis
		No Abx Rx if viral-related
		1st line: tetracycline 250 mg PO qid or
		    erythromycin 1 g PO bid x 7-10d
		2nd line: doxycycline 100 mg PO bid x 1d
		    then 100 mg PO OD x 10d
		3rd line: clarithromycin 250-500 mg PO bid or
		    azithromycin 500 mg x 1d then 250 mg PO OD x 4d

Community Acquired Pneumonia	Susceptible to β-lactams:
	  S. pneumoniae
	
	  H. influenzae
	  S. aureus
	Not susceptible to β-lactams:
	  Mycoplasma
	  Chlamydia pneumoniae
	  Legionella pneumoniae
		adult dosing (no respiratory comorbidities):
		erythromycin 500 mg PO qid x 10-14d
		clarithromycin 250-500 mg PO bid x 10-14d
		azithromycin 500 mg PO 1st dose then 250 mg PO OD x 4d

Dental Infections/ Periapical and Periodontal Abscesses	Oral Flora	Pen V potassium 500 mg PO qid x 7-10d clindamycin 300 mg PO qid x 7-10d
GASTROENTEROLOGY		

Diarrhea – Enteritis	*Shigella*
	Salmonella
	Campylobacter
	E. coli
	Yersinia
		N.B. In children order a stool C&S prior to antibx to r/o
		    E.coli 0157:H7
		adult: ciprofloxacin 500 mg PO bid ± erythromycin 500 mg PO
		    qid x 7d

Diarrhea – post abx	*C. difficile*	metronidazole 500 mg PO tid x 10-14d

Peptic Ulcer Disease (non-NSAID related)	*H. pylori*	HP-PAC (7 blister card pack):
		    lansoprazole 30 mg PO bid +
		    clarithromycin 500 mg PO bid +
		    amoxicillin 1 g PO bid x 7d
		if penicillin allergy:
		    metronidazole 500 mg PO bid + clarithromycin 250 mg
		    PO bid + omeprazole 20 mg PO bid x 7-14d

CONDITION	MICROORGANISM	ANTIBIOTIC
GENITOURINARY		

UTI/Cystitis	*Klebsiella*
	E. coli
	Enterobacter
	Proteus
	S. saprophyticus
		1st line: TMP/ SMX 1 DS tablet bid x 3d
		2nd line: ciprofloxacin 250 mg PO bid x 3d,
		nitrofurantoin (Macrobid™) 100 mg PO bid x 3d
		pregnancy:
		    amoxicillin 250 -500 mg PO tid x 7d
		    N.B. nitrofurantoin is contraindicated in pregnancy
		    after 38 wks

Vaginal Candidiasis/ Yeast	*Candida*	fluconazole 150 mg PO single dose miconazole 2% vag. cream = Monistat 7™: One applicator (5g) intravag. qhs x 7d
Lice: Head and Pubic (Crabs)	*Pediculosis humanus capitis* *Phthirus pubis*	permethrin cream 5%: apply as liquid on to washed hair for 10min, then rinse. Repeat in 1 wk M: 60 g tube
Gonorrhea/ Chlamydia	*N. gonorrheae* *C. trachomatis*	cefixime 400 mg PO single dose + azithromycin 1 g PO single dose or doxycycline 100 mg PO bid x 7d
Herpes	Herpes simplex virus	acyclovir 400 mg PO tid x 10d valacyclovir 500-1000mg PO bid x 5-7d
Vaginitis	*Gardnerella vaginalis* *Bacteroides* *Mycoplasma hominis*	metronidazole 500 mg PO bid x 7d
DERMATOLOGIC		
Mastitis	*S. aureus*	cloxacillin 500 mg PO qid x 7d cephalexin 500 mg PO qid x 7d
Tinea Cruris/Pedis (Jock Itch/Athlete's Foot)	Trichophyton	clotrimazole 1% cream – apply bid ketoconazole 2% cream – apply bid
Cellulitis (uncomplicated)	β-Hemolytic *Strep sp.* *Staphylococcus*	*1st line:* cephalexin 500 mg PO qid x 10-14d 2nd line: cloxacillin 500 mg PO qid x 10-14d or clindamycin 300 mg PO qid x 10-14d
OPHTHALMOLOGY		
Conjunctivitis (viral)	Adenovirus	none note: very contagious
Conjunctivitis (bacterial)	*S. aureus* *S. pneumoniae* *E. coli*	sulfacetamide: 1-2 gtts q2-6h x 7-10d gentamicin: 1-2 gtts q4h x 7-10d erythromycin ointment: apply to lid margins bid-qid, M: 3.5 g tube
Blepharitis	*S. aureus* *S. epidermidis*	erythromycin ophthalmic ointment: apply to lid margins bid-tid, M: 3.5 g tube

*All doses are adult doses unless otherwise specified
*This chart is not all-encompassing and is non-inclusive of special exceptions (i.e. pregnancy, poor renal clearance etc)

G

Gastroenterology

Tom Havey, Cecilia Kim and Morgan Rosenberg, chapter editors
Deepti Damaraju and Elliott Owen, associate editors
Erik Venos, EBM editor
Dr. Gabor Kandel and Dr. Fred Saibil, staff editors
with contributions from Dr. David Black

Differential Diagnosis of Common Presenting Complaints

Commonly Forgotten Causes of Vomiting
Drugs
Uremia
CNS Disease
Pregnancy

Differential Diagnosis of a Large/Bloated Abdomen (12Fs):
• **F**at
• **F**eces
• **F**etus
• **F**latus
• **F**luid
• **F**atal Growth
• **F**ull stomach
• **F**labby muscles
• **F**aking it/ False pregnancy
• **F**ibroids
• "**F**eels like it" (IBS)
• Combination of **F**actors

Acute Upper Abdominal Pain
Remember to consider "sounds from the attic" (chest) e.g. myocardial infarction, pneumonia, dissecting aneurysm.

Table 1. Differential Diagnosis of Common Presenting Complaints

NAUSEA/ VOMITING	With Abdominal Pain		Without Abdominal Pain/Non-GI	
	Relieved by Vomiting	Not Relieved by Vomiting	Headache/Dizziness	No Other Symptoms
	Gastric outlet obstruction	Gallbladder disease	Cerebral tumour	Drugs
	Small bowel obstruction	Pancreatitis	Migraine	Uremia
		Myocardial infarction	Vestibular	Pregnancy
		Hepatitis	Cerebellar hemorrhage	Metabolic (e.g. hypercalcemia)
				Gastroparesis (e.g. diabetes)
				Ketoacidosis

DYSPHAGIA	Mechanical	Motility	Other	
	Stricture/Esophagitis	Achalasia	Foreign body	
	Cancer	Diffuse esophageal spasm		
	Extrinsic compression	Scleroderma		
	Schatzki ring/esophageal web	Myasthenia gravis		
	Zenker's diverticulum			

ABDOMINAL DISTENTION	Fluid Portal HTN	Normal Portal Pressure	Flatulence	Feces	Other
	Cirrhosis	Cancer esp. ovarian	Irritable bowel syndrome (IBS)	Colonic obstruction	Pregnancy
	Cardiac failure	Pancreatitis		Constipation	Obesity
	Hepatic vein thrombosis	TB	Diet (e.g. lactose intolerance)		Blood

ACUTE ABDOMINAL PAIN	Generalized/ Periumbilical	RUQ	RLQ	LUQ	LLQ
	Gastroenteritis	Hepatitis	Appendicitis	Myocardial infarction (MI)	IBD
	SBO	Biliary colic	IBD	Pancreatitis	Diverticulitis
	Colonic obstruction	Acute cholecystitis	Ureteral stone	Splenic infarction	Sigmoid volvulus
	Mesenteric ischemia	PUD	Salpingitis	Pyelonephritis	Ureteral stone
	Peritonitis	Pyelonephritis	Ruptured corpus uteum cyst		Salpingitis
	Abdominal aortic aneurysm		Ovarian torsion		Ruptured corpus luteum cyst
	Sickle cell crisis		Ruptured ectopic pregnancy		Ruptured ectopic pregnancy
	Perforation				

CHRONIC/RECURRENT ABDOMINAL PAIN	Inflammatory	Neoplastic/Vascular	Toxin	Other	
	PUD	Gastric cancer	Lead poisoning	Mittleschmertz	
	Biliary colic	Recurrent bowel obstruction		Endometriosis (see Gynecology)	
	IBD	Mesenteric ischemia		Porphyria	
	Chronic pancreatitis	Sickle cell anemia		IBS (functional)	
				Radiculopathy	

ACUTE DIARRHEA (see Infectious Diseases)	Invasive	Non-invasive		
	Bacterial	**Bacterial**	**Viral**	
	Salmonella enteritidis	*Staphylococcus aureus*	Rotavirus	
	Shigella	*B. cereus*	Norwalk	
	Salmonella typhi	*C. perfringens*	Cytomegalovirus	
	Campylobacter	*Vibrio cholerae*		
	Yersinia			
	E. coli (EHEC 0157:H7)			
	C. difficile	**Protozoal**	**Drugs**	
	Protozoal	*Giardia lamblia*	Antacids	
	E. histolytica (amebiasis)		Antibiotics	
	Strongyloides		Laxatives (Magnesium)	
			Colchicine	
			Many others	

Table 1. Differential Diagnosis of Common Presenting Complaints (continued)

CHRONIC DIARRHEA	Inflammatory	Secretory	Steatorrhea	Osmotic
	(a) ORGANIC			
	IBD Ischemic	Stimulant laxatives Malignancy Large, rectal villous adenoma Zollinger-Ellison (ZE) Carcinoid Addison's disease VIP secreting tumour of pancreas Diabetes mellitus Cryptosporidiosis	Celiac sprue *Giardia* Chronic pancreatitis	Drugs/Laxatives Lactose intolerance
	(b) FUNCTIONAL IBS Anal sphincter dysfunction			

CONSTIPATION	GI	Systemic	Psych/Social
	IBS Colon cancer Anorectal pathology Mechanical obstruction (e.g. neoplasm)	Electrolytes (K, Ca) Hypothyroidism Scleroderma & other CTD Neurological diseases (e.g. MS, Parkinson's)	Drugs Voluntary retention Lifestyle/Diet Depression Long car trips/Travel/Inactivity

DYSPEPSIA	Common	Uncommon	Rare
	Functional dyspepsia Drug side effect Peptic ulcer GERD	Angina Crohn's disease Cancer Gallstones Aerophagia	*Giardia* Malabsorption (celiac sprue)

UPPER GI BLEED	Common	Uncommon	Rare
	Peptic ulcer disease (PUD) Esophageal varices Mallory-Weiss tears Erosive esophagitis Gastritis	Tumours Arteriovenous malformation Dieulafoy's lesion Gastric antral vascular ectasia (GAVE)	Aorto-enteric fistulas Hemobilia

LOWER GI BLEED	Common	Uncommon	Rare
	Ischemic Colitis Infectious Colitis Diverticulosis Inflammatory Bowel Disease (IBD) Tumours (polyps,cancer) Hemorrhoids	Radiation Colitis Angiodysplasia Post-polypectomy	Intussusception Vasculitides Perforation Stercoral Ulcer Coagulopathies

Esophagus

Basic Anatomy Review

- mucosa: stratified squamous epithelium
- submucosa: connective tissue, lymphocytes, plasma cells, nerve cells
- muscularis propria: inner circular, outer longitudinal muscle
- muscle: upper 1/3 striated muscle, lower 1/3 smooth muscle, separated by transition zone comprised of both
- blood supply:
  - thoracic part: esophageal arteries and terminal branches of bronchial arteries
  - abdominal part: left gastic artery, left phrenic artery
- venous drainage:
  - thoracic part: esophageal veins → azygous system
  - abdominal part: left gastric vein → portal system
- lymphatic drainage: left gastric lymph nodes
- innervation: vagus nerve
- physiologic anatomic compressions (three): aortic arch, left main bronchus, diaphragm
- upper esophageal sphincter (UES)
  - cricopharyngeus + caudal fibers of inferior pharyngeal constrictor muscle
- lower esophageal sphincter (LES)
  - internal muscles: intrinsic muscle of distal esophagus, sling fibers of proximal stomach

- external muscles: crural diaphragm
- normal resting pressure = 15-30 mmHg above intragastric pressure
- relaxes at onset of swallowing
- contraction: cholinergic innervation (via vagus nerve)
- relaxation: non-adrenergic, non-cholinergic input via nitric oxide and VIP
- peristalsis: rhythmic contractions that propel solid contents onward
  - neuronal control via brainstem "swallowing center" (cranial nerve nuclei)
  - primary = induced by swallowing
  - secondary = induced by esophageal distention (e.g. during reflux)
  - tertiary = spontaneous (abnormal) and non-peristaltic

Dysphagia

Definition
- difficulty swallowing, sensation of food "sticking" after swallowing

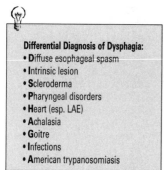

Key Questions in Dysphagia:
- solids, liquids or both
- intermittent, progressive
- heartburn
- change in eating habits/diet

Differential Diagnosis of Dysphagia:
- **D**iffuse esophageal spasm
- **I**ntrinsic lesion
- **S**cleroderma
- **P**haryngeal disorders
- **H**eart (esp. LAE)
- **A**chalasia
- **G**oitre
- **I**nfections
- **A**merican trypanosomiasis

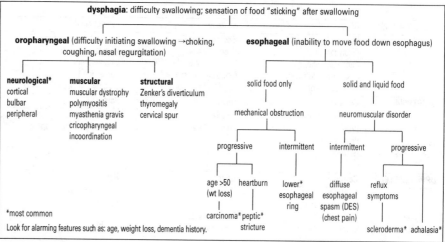

Figure 1. Approach to Dysphagia

Odynophagia

Definition
- pain on swallowing
- causes: usually due to ulceration of esophageal mucosa
  - infection: candida, herpes, CMV (common only in immunosuppressed patients, especially AIDS)
  - inflammation/ulceration (e.g. caustic damage)
  - drugs: tetracyclines (e.g. doxycycline), wax-matrix potassium chloride, quinidine, iron, vitamin C, various antibiotics
  - radiation

Dyspepsia

Definition
- intermittent epigastric discomfort, characteristically develops after eating
- most common cause is functional dyspepsia (i.e. dyspepsia in which all investigations fail to identify an organic cause)
- causes: see Table 1

Gastroesophageal Reflux Disease (GERD)

Definition
- reflux of gastric contents, especially acid, aborally (toward the mouth), rather than distally into duodenum

Etiology
- LES relaxes inappropriately – most common
- low basal LES tone (especially in scleroderma)

- contributing factors include: delayed esophageal clearance, delayed gastric emptying, increased intra-abdominal pressure
- acid hypersecretion (rare) – Zollinger-Ellison syndrome (gastrin-secreting tumour)
- hiatus hernia worsens reflux, does not cause it (see General Surgery)

Epidemiology
- most common condition affecting the esophagus

Clinical Features
- most common symptom is "heartburn" (pyrosis 80% sensitive and specific for reflux) ± bitter regurgitation, water brash; sensation of a lump in the throat; frequent belching

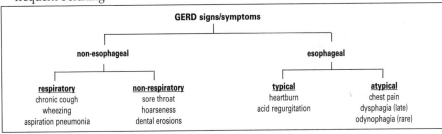

Figure 2. Signs and Symptoms of GERD

Investigations
- usually a clinical diagnosis based on symptom history and relief following a trial of pharmacotherapy (proton pump inhibitor (PPI): symptom relief 80% sensitive for reflux)
- gastroscopy indications:
  - rule out conditions which can mimic reflux (e.g. cancer, peptic ulcer, infective esophagitis)
  - distinguish between esophagitis (indicating aggressive treatment) and non-erosive reflux disease (NERD - goal of treatment is symptom relief)
  - diagnose Barrett's esophagus (requires endoscopic surveillance for cancer)
- esophageal manometry
  - may be done to diagnose abnormal peristalsis and/or decreased LES tone, but cannot detect presence of reflux; must be done before surgery
  - surgical fundoplication more likely to be successful if lower esophageal pressure is diminished; less likely to be successful if abnormal peristalsis
- acid perfusion (Bernstein) test: indicated if reflux known to be present but symptoms are atypical (e.g. chest pain)
  - helps to determine if reflux is cause of symptoms
  - test is done by perfusing esophagus first with isotonic saline then with 0.1 normal HCl; test is positive if symptoms reproduced only by acid perfusion
- barium swallow: to assess presence of strictures
- 24-hour pH monitoring most accurate test but rarely used

Management
- step-down approach: start with proton pump inhibitors (most effective therapy)
- step-up approach: start with diet (more helpful in relieving symptoms), lifestyle changes (elevate head of bed at night, tilt entire body)
- proton pump inhibitors are the mainstay of treatment and are the most effective therapy, usually need to be continued on maintenance therapy
- main approach is three-phase management involving a combination of lifestyle modification (Phase I), pharmacotherapy with H_2 blockers and proton pump inhibitors (PPIs; Phase II), and maintenance therapy or surgery for refractory cases (Phase III)
- on-demand: antacids (MgOH, AlOH) and H_2-RAs can be used for NERD

Complications
- reflux esophagitis: esophageal inflammation from prolonged acid regurgitation; can progress to esophageal peptic stricture, bleeding
- stricture (scarring)
- risk of Barrett's esophagus (columnar metaplasia) and esophageal adenocarcinoma (0.4% risk per year), mandates surveillance gastroscopy

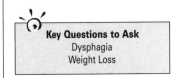

Key Questions to Ask
Dysphagia
Weight Loss

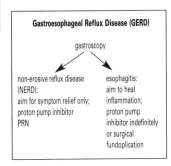

Gastroesophageal Reflux Disease (GERD)

gastroscopy

non-erosive reflux disease (NERD): aim for symptom relief only; proton pump inhibitor PRN

esophagitis: aim to heal inflammation; proton pump inhibitor indefinitely or surgical fundoplication

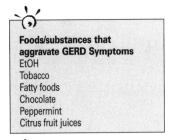

Foods/substances that aggravate GERD Symptoms
EtOH
Tobacco
Fatty foods
Chocolate
Peppermint
Citrus fruit juices

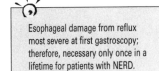

Esophageal damage from reflux most severe at first gastroscopy; therefore, necessary only once in a lifetime for patients with NERD.

Barrett's Esophagus

Definition
- metaplasia of normal squamous epithelium to abnormal columnar epithelium containing foci of intestinal metaplasia and resulting displacement of the squamocolumnar junction proximal to the gastroesophageal junction
- cell of origin unknown

Etiology
- thought to be acquired via long standing GERD and consequent damage to squamous epithelium
- a significant proportion of patients with Barrett's Esophagus (BE) do not report symptoms of GERD (up to 25%)

Epidemiology
- in North America and Western Europe, 0.5-2.0% of adults are thought to have BE
- up to 10% of GERD patients will have already developed BE by the time they seek medical attention
- more common in males, >50 yrs, Caucasians and smokers

Pathophysiology
- endoscopy shows erythematous epithelium in distal esophagus; diagnosis of BE relies on biopsy demonstrating the presence of specialized intestinal epithelium of any length within the esophagus
- persistent presence of BE predisposes to premalignant changes in abnormal columnar epithelium, characterized as low- or high-grade dysplasia
- often occurs in the presence of increased gastric acid secretion

Significance
- BE and dysplastic states lead to increased incidence of esophageal adenocarcinoma; rate of malignant transformation approximately 0.5-1.0% per year for all BE patients prior to dysplasia
- risk of malignant transformation in high-grade dysplasia is significantly higher; studies have reported on a 32-59% transformation rate over 5-8 years of surveillance

Treatment
- acid suppressive therapy with high-dose proton pump inhibitor indefinitely; provides symptom relief but does not accurately correlate to the level of acid suppression achieved
- anti-reflux surgery (fundoplication)
- endoscopic ablation of dysplastic areas
- endoscopic mucosal resection
- endoscopic surveillance every 3 years once diagnosis of BE established; frequency increased to annually once presence of low-grade dysplasia detected on biopsy
- surgical intervention recommended for most patients with high-grade dysplasia

Prognosis
- little evidence to suggest that anti-secretory medications lead to the regression of BE, or prevent progression to dysplasia and/or adenocarcinoma
- vigorous surveillance and endoscopic intervention is thought to reduce the risk of death from adenocarcinoma
- most patients with BE are elderly and die of causes other than esophageal cancer
- validity and significance of the evidence supporting each therapy remains in dispute; large prospective study currently underway to elucidate the natural history of BE and efficacy of acid suppressive therapy in altering/arresting progression to dysplasia or cancer

Esophageal Motor Disorders

Symptoms
- dysphagia with solids and liquids
- chest pain (in some disorders)

Diagnosis
- esophageal motility study (esophageal manometry)

Causes (Table 2)
- idiopathic
- achalasia (painless)
- scleroderma (painless)
- diffuse esophageal spasm (DES) - rare

Table 2. Esophageal Motor Disorders

Disorder	Achalasia	Scleroderma	Diffuse Esophageal Spasm
Definition	• failure of smooth muscle relaxation at lower esophageal sphincter (LES) • progressive loss of peristaltic function	• see Rheumatology • disease of collagen	• normal peristalsis interspersed with frequent, repetitive, spontaneous, high pressure, non-peristaltic waves (tertiary peristalsis)
Etiology	• usually idiopathic • incomplete relaxation of LES with swallowing • high LES resting pressure in most (2° to canceris pseudo-achalasive) • Chagas disease (T. cruzi)	• dysphagia: can be due to reflux or dysmotility, usually both	• unknown
Pathophysiology	• unknown (↑ impaired inhibition related to ↓ NO release)	• blood vessel damage → intramural neuronal dysfunction → distal esophageal muscle weakening → aperistalsis and loss of LES tone → reflux → stricture → dysphagia	• unknown
Diagnosis	• chest x-ray: no air in stomach, with dilated esophagus • barium studies: esophagus terminates in narrowing at the sphincter, giving a "bird's beak" appearance • endoscopy to r/o malignancy • motility study for definitive diagnosis	• ↓pressure in LES • ↓peristalsis in body of esophagus	• barium x-ray: "Corkscrew pattern", tertiary waves
Treatment	• dilatation of LES with balloon, ± GERD prophylaxis, 50% good response, can repeat, risk of perforation (5%) • injection of botulinum toxin into LES (temporary) • surgery (myotomy)	• medical: aggressive GERD therapy (proton pump inhibitors bid) • surgery: anti-reflux surgery (gastroplasty, last resort)	• reassurance • medical: nitrates, calcium channel blockers, anticholinergics have variable benefit • surgical: long esophageal myotomy if unresponsive to above treatment (rarely helpful); balloon dilatation

Endoscopic pneumatic dilation versus botulinum toxin injection in the management of primary achalasia.
Cochrane Database Syst Rev.2006;(4)CD005046.
Purpose: To compare the efficacy and safety of two endoscopic treatments, pneumatic dilation and intrasphincteric botulinum toxin injection, in the treatment of esophageal achalasia
Study Selection: Randomised controlled trials comparing PD to BTX injection in patients with primary achalasia.
Results: Six studies involving 178 participants were included. Two studies were excluded from the meta-analysis of remission rates on the basis of clinical heterogeneity of the initial endoscopic protocols. There was no significant difference in remission between PD or BTX treatment within four weeks of the initial intervention, with a relative risk of remission of 1.15 (95% CI 0.95 to 1.38, P=0.39) for PD compared to BTX. There was also no significant difference in the mean esophageal pressures between the treatment groups; weighted mean difference for PD of -0.77 (95% CT-2.44 to 0.91, P=0.37). Data on remission rates following the initial endoscopic treatment was available for two studies at six months and three studies at 12 months. At six months 22 of 29 PD participants were in remission compared to 11 of 43 BTX participants, relative risk of 2.67 (95% CI 1.58 to 4.52, P=0.0002). No serious adverse outcomes occured in participants receiving BTX, whilst PD was complicated by perforation in three cases.
Conclusion: The results of this meta-analysis would suggest that PD is the more effective endoscopic treatment in the long term (greater than six months) for patients with achalasia.

Esophageal Structural Disorders

Diverticula

Definition
• outpouchings of one or more layers of pharyngeal or esophageal wall

Clinical Features
• commonly associated with motility disorders
• dysphagia, regurgitation, retrosternal pain, intermittent vomiting, may be asymptomatic

Classification
• classified according to location
• pharyngoesophageal (Zenker's) diverticulum
  ▪ most frequent form of esophageal diverticulum
  ▪ posterior pharyngeal outpouching most often on the left side, above cricopharyngeal muscle and below the inferior pharyngeal constrictor muscle
  ▪ symptoms: dysphagia, regurgitation of undigested food, halitosis
  ▪ treatment: myotomy of cricopharyngeal muscle ± excise or suspend sac
• mid-esophageal diverticulum
  ▪ secondary to mediastinal inflammation, motor disorders
  ▪ usually asymptomatic: no treatment required

Benign Stricture

• presents as intermittent or progressive dysphagia in face of reflux symptoms
• diagnose with barium study or endoscopy

Treatment
• endoscopic dilatation and indefinite proton pump inhibitor
• anti-reflux surgery if above unsuccessful

Esophageal Cancer

(see <u>General Surgery</u>)

Webs and Rings

- web = partial occlusion (upper esophagus)
- ring = circumferential narrowing (lower esophagus)

Clinical Features
- asymptomatic with lumen diameter >12 mm, provided peristalsis is normal
- dysphagia with large food boluses
- Plummer-Vinson or Patterson-Kelly syndrome
  - upper esophageal web with iron deficiency, plus cheilosis (dry scaling, and fissuring of the lips) and koilonychia (concave outer nail surface)
  - usually in middle aged females (>40 years)
  - elevated risk of hypopharyngeal carcinoma
- Schatzki's ring
  - mucosal ring at squamo-columnar junction above a hiatus hernia
  - causes intermittent dysphagia for solids
  - treatment involves tearing ring with bougie

Infectious Esophagitis

Definition
- severe mucosal inflammation and ulceration as a result of viral or fungal infection

Risk Factors
- diabetes
- malignancy (chemotherapeutic agents)
- immunocompromised states

Symptoms
- odynophagia, dysphagia
- diagnosis is via endoscopic visualization and biopsy

Treatment
- Candida (most common): nystatin swish and swallow, ketoconazole, fluconazole
- Herpes (second most common): often self-limiting; acyclovir/vancyclovir/famciclovir
- CMV: IV gancyclovir, famciclovir

Stomach and Duodenum

Basic Anatomy Review

Stomach
- chief function is enzymatic digestion of ingested material into chyme, and propulsion of chyme into duodenum; see Table 3 and Figure 3 for a summary of the gastric cell types and their products
- consists of four parts:
  - cardia: adjacent to gastroesophageal junction
  - fundus: superior part, under the left leaf of the diaphragm
  - body: lies between fundus and pylorus
  - pylorus: funnel-shaped, pyloric antrum leads to pyloric canal; distal part is thickened to form the pyloric sphincter which controls discharge of stomach contents into the duodenum
- blood supply: arises from the celiac axis and its branches – left gastric artery, right gastric artery (branch of hepatic artery), right gastroepiploic artery (terminal branch of gastroduodenal artery), left gastroepiploic artery (branch of splenic artery), and short gastric arteries (branches of splenic artery)
- venous drainage: gastric veins drain directly into portal vein, short gastric arteries drain into the splenic vein which then joins the portal vein
- lymphatics: drainage via gastric and gastroepiploic lymph nodes → celiac nodes
- innervation: parasympathetic innervation via vagus nerve; sympathetic supply via celiac plexus (from T6-T9)

Table 3. Cells of the Gastric Mucosa

Cell Type	Secretory Product	Important Notes
Parietal Cells	Gastric acid (HCl)	Stimulated by histamine, ACh, gastrin
Chief Cells	Pepsinogen	Stimulated by vagal input and local acid
G-cells	Gastrin	Stimulates H^+ production from parietal cells
Superficial Epithelial Cells	Mucus, HCO_3	Protect gastric mucosa

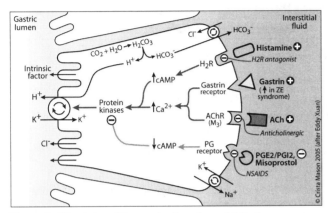

Figure 3. Stimulation of H^+ secretion from the parietal cell

Duodenum
- first part of small intestine
- neutralizes acidic components entering from stomach via secretin and bicarbonate secretion
- site of stimulation of bile secretion via CCK release
- blood supply: branches of celiac and superior mesenteric artery (SMA)
- divided into 4 parts; 1st part (bulb) is intraperitoneal; rest is retroperitoneal

Gastritis

Definition
- inflammation of the stomach; some diagnosed by endoscopy, some only by histology

Etiology
- most common causes:
  - *Helicobacter pylori* infection
  - chronic NSAID use, ethanol use
  - physiological stress-related mucosal changes
  - other: atrophic, lymphocytic, eosinophilic
- other infectious causes: TB, syphilis, CMV, fungal and parasitic infections (all rare in North America)
- systemic diseases: e.g. sarcoidosis, Crohn's disease

Clinical Features
- erosive: bleeding
- non-erosive: asymptomatic (may present with upper GI symptoms e.g. nausea, early satiety)

Table 4. Gastritis

Acute	Chronic
Self-limited syndrome caused by irritation of gastric mucosa by alcohol, corrosives, food poisoning, etc.	Diagnosed via gastric biopsy: characterized by mononuclear and polymorphonuclear (PMN) cell infiltration of mucosa, glandular atrophy and intestinal metaplasia (occasionally) Examples: Chronic Fundal Gastritis (etiology is pernicious anemia) Chronic Antral Gastritis (etiology is *H. pylori*)

Peptic Ulcer Disease (PUD)

Definition
- erosion (superficial to the muscularis mucosa, thus no scarring) or ulcer (penetrates the muscularis mucosa and can result in scarring)

Etiology

Gastric vs. Duodenal Ulcers
Gastric ulcers must always be biopsied to rule out malignancies. Duodenal ulcers are rarely malignant.

Table 5. Etiology of Peptic Ulcer Disease

	Duodenal	Gastric
***H. pylori* infection**	90%	60%
NSAIDs	7%	35%
Physiologic stress-induced	<3%	<5%
Zollinger-Ellison (ZE) syndrome	<1%	<1%

- NSAID negative, *H. pylori* negative ulcers becoming more commonly recognized
- others: CMV, ischemic, idiopathic, diet (exact role not understood)
- alcohol: damages gastric mucosa but only rarely causes ulcers
- associated with cirrhosis of liver, COPD, chronic renal failure

Clinical Features

Approach to PUD
1. Stop NSAIDs
2. Acid neutralization
3. *H. pylori* eradication
4. Quit smoking

- dyspepsia is the most common presenting symptom; however, only 20% of patients with dyspepsia have ulcers (see Table 1 for causes of dyspepsia)
- may present with complications
  - bleeding 10% (severe if from gastroduodenal artery); see *"Bleeding peptic ulcer"* section, G27
  - perforation 2% (usually anterior ulcers)
  - gastric outlet obstruction 2%
  - penetration (posterior) 2%; may also cause pancreatitis
- duodenal ulcers present with 5 classical features:
  - epigastric location
  - pain described as burning that develops 1-3 hours after meals
  - relieved by eating and antacids
  - interrupts sleep
  - periodicity (tends to occur in clusters over weeks with subsequent periods of remission)
- gastric ulcers have more atypical symptoms; a biopsy is necessary to exclude malignancy

Investigations
- endoscopy (most accurate)
- upper GI series
- *H. pylori* tests (Table 6)
- serum gastrin measurement if Zollinger-Ellison (ZE) syndrome suspected

Cigarette Smoking and PUD
- ↑ risk of ulcer
- ↑ risk of complications
- ↑ chance of death from ulcer
- impairs healing rate

Treatment
- specific management depends on etiology; refer to *H. pylori, NSAID* and *Stress Induced Ulceration*, G11-G12
- eradicate *H. pylori* if present, chief advantage is to lower ulcer recurrence rate
- stop NSAIDs if possible
- proton pump inhibitor inhibits parietal cell H^+-K^+ATPase pump which secretes acid, heals most ulcers, even if NSAIDs are continued
- other meds (e.g. histamine H2 antagonists) less effective
- discontinue tobacco
- no diet modifications required but some people have fewer symptoms if they avoid caffeine, alcohol, and spices

H. pylori-Induced Ulceration

Pathophysiology
- *H. pylori* is a gram-negative flagellated rod that resides on but does not invade the gastric mucosa
- acid secreted by parietal cell (stimulated by vagal acetylcholine, gastrin, histamine) necessary for most ulcers
- mucosal defenses moderated by PGE_2 and blood flow, mucus, etc.
- theories of how *H. pylori* causes ulcers
  - toxin production: causes gastric mucosal inflammation and necrosis
  - interference with acid regulation: *H. pylori* blocks gastrin G cells in antrum from sensing luminal acid → increased serum gastrin → increased gastric acid → ulcer

Epidemiology
- *H. pylori* is found in 20-40% of all Canadians, highest prevalence in the generation that grew up during the Depression
- infection most commonly acquired in childhood, presumably by fecal-oral route
- high prevalence in developing countries, low socioeconomic status (poor sanitation and crowding)

Symptoms
- non-erosive gastritis in 100% of patients but this does not necessarily cause symptoms
- peptic ulcer in 15% of patients, gastric malignancy (cancer and mucosal associated lymphomatous tissue lymphoma = MALT lymphoma in 0.5% of patients)
- most are asymptomatic but still worthwhile eradicating to a) lower future risk of peptic ulcer/gastric malignancy and b) prevent spread to others (mostly children <5 years of age)

Investigations

Table 6. Diagnosis of *H. pylori* infection

Test	Sensitivity	Specificity	Comments
Non-invasive Tests			
Urea breath test	90-100%	89-100%	Affected by PPI therapy
Serology	88-99%	89-95%	Remains positive
Invasive Tests (require endoscopy)			
Histology	93-99%	95-99%	Gold standard; affected by PPI therapy
Rapid urease test (on biopsy)	89-98%	93-100%	Rapid
Microbiology culture	98%	95-100%	Research only

Treatment Eradication
- *H. pylori* eradication (*Canadian Consensus Guidelines, September 2004*)
  - eradication upon documentation of *H. pylori* infection controversial since most patients will not have peptic ulcer or cancer
  - however, empiric treatment suitable for patients <50 years old with mild symptoms and no red flags
    - 1st line triple therapy; see sidebar
      - (PPI + clarithromycin 500 mg + amoxicillin 1000 mg bid) x 7-14 days (Hp - Pac™)
      - (PPI + clarithromycin + metronidazole 500 mg) x 7-14 days
      - ranitidine, bismoth-citrate + clarithromycin + amoxicillin
    - 2nd line quadruple therapy
      - PPI + BMT (bismuth + metronidazole + tetracycline) x 7 days
      - lansoprazole 500 mg bid + amoxicillin 1 g bid + PPI bid
- clarithromycin and metronidazole - resistance increasing

NSAID-Induced Ulceration

- NSAIDs cause gastric mucosal petechiae in virtually all users, erosions in most users, ulcers in some (25%) users
  - some people with NSAID erosions bleed, but usually only ulcers cause significant clinical problems
- most NSAID ulcers are clinically silent: dyspepsia is as common in patients with ulcers as in patients without ulcers
- gastric ulcers more common than duodenal ulcers
- may exacerbate underlying duodenal ulcer disease

Pathophysiology
- direct: petechiae and erosions are due to local effect of drug on gastric mucosa; drug is non-ionized (HA) in acidic gastric lumen, therefore enters gastric epithelial cell where it becomes ionized (A⁻) at intracellular neutral pH, and damages cell
- indirect: systemic NSAID effect (i.e. NSAID absorbed in upper small bowel, reaches gastric epithelial cells by arterial circulation); NSAIDs inhibit mucosal cyclooxygenase, the rate-limiting step in the synthesis of prostaglandins, which are required for mucosal integrity, leading to ulcers

Risk Factors
- age
- previous peptic ulcers/UGIB
- high dose of NSAID/multiple NSAIDs being taken

Helicobacter pylori **Management**
AJM 1998; 105:424.
For patients with PUD and *H. pylori* infection, treatment with a PPI, clarithromycin 500 mg bid, and amoxicillin 1 g bid x 14 days has approximately 90% success rate.

Meta-analysis: Sequential Therapy Appears Superior to Standard Therapy for Helicobacter pylori Infections in Patients Naive to Treatment
Ann Intern Med. 2008 May 19.
Purpose: To compare sequential therapy with standard triple therapy for *H. pylori* infection.
Study Selection: Randomized, controlled trials (RCTs) comparing sequential and standard triple therapies in treatment-naive patients with documented *H. pylori* infection. Ten RCTs involving 2747 patients were included. Standard therapy was defined as a proton-pump inhibitor and clarithromycin, with either amoxicillin or an imidazole for 7 or 10 days. Sequential therapy was defined as 5 days of treatment with a proton-pump inhibitor and 1 antibiotic (usually amoxicillin) followed by 5 day treatment with the proton-pump inhibitor and 2 other antibiotics (usually clarithromycin and a 5-nitroimidazole).
Results: Eradication rates were 93.4% (95% CI, 91.3% to 95.5%) for sequential therapy (n=1363), and 76.9% (CI, 71.0% to 82.8%) for standard therapy. Side effects were similar between therapies.
Conclusion: Sequential therapy appears superior to standard triple therapy for eradication of H. pylori infection. If RCTs in other countries confirm these findings, 10-day sequential therapy could become a standard treatment for *H. pylori* infection in treatment-naive patients.

"The David Y Graham Lecture: Use of Nonsteroidal Antiinflammatory Drugs (NSAID) in a COX-2 Restricted Environment
Am Journal Gastroenterol 2008; 103:221-227
This short article reviews the current understanding of NSAID risks, emphasizing (1) with the possible exception of naproxen, all NSAIDs increase cardiovascular/cerebrovascular risk, especially the COX-2 specific inhibitors (2) lowdose aspirin, now used widely to decrease these risks, increases the likelihood of upper GI tract bleeding and may not abrogate the cardiovascular risk of NSAIDs (3) clopidogrel is no safer than aspirin in patients with high risk of upper GI tract bleeding (4) add a proton pump inhibitor to NSAID if there is an increased risk of upper GI events."

If at high risk for recurrence of ulcers, lifelong prophylaxis with PPI may be required.

The effectiveness of five strategies for the prevention of gastrointestinal toxicity induced by non-steroidal anti-inflammatory drugs: systematic review.
BMJ. 2004;329:948.

Purpose: To assess the effectiveness of five gastroprotective strategies for people taking non-steroidal anti-inflammatory drugs (NSAIDs)-H2 receptor antagonists plus non-selective (or cyclo-oxygenase-1) NSAIDs; proton pump inhibitors plus non-selective NSAIDs; misoprostol plus non-selective NSAIDs; COX-2 selective NSAIDs; or COX-2 specific NSAIDs-in reducing serious gastrointestinal complications, symptomatic ulcers, serious cardiovascular or renal disease, and deaths, and improving quality of life.
Study Selection: The review included all studies except those that were not a randomised controlled trial; did not assess a gastroprotective strategy versus placebo; included exclusively children or healthy volunteers; lasted less than 21 days; or no review outcomes were mentioned.
Results: 112 randomised controlled trials involving 74 666 participants were included. H2 receptor antagonists were not effective for any primary outcomes (few events reported); proton pump inhibitors may reduce the risk of symptomatic ulcers (relative risk 0.09, 95% confidence interval 0.02 to 0.47); misoprostol reduces the risk of serious gastrointestinal complications (0.57, 0.36 to 0.91) and symptomatic ulcers (0.36, 0.20 to 0.67); COX-2 selectives reduce the risk of symptomatic ulcers (0.41, 0.26 to 0.65) and COX-2 specifics reduce the risk of symtomatic ulcers (0.49, 0.38 to 0.62) and possibly serious gastrointestinal complications (0.55, 0.38 to 0.80). All strategies except COX-2 selectives reduce the risk of endoscopic ulcers (at least 3 mm in diameter).
Conclusions: Misoprostol, COX-2 specific and selective NSAIDs, and probably proton pump inhibitors significantly reduce the risk of symptomatic ulcers, and misoprostol and probably COX-2 specifics significantly reduce the risk of serious gastrointestinal complications, but data quality is low. More data on H2 receptor antagonists and proton pump inhibitors are needed, as is better reporting of rare but important outcomes.

Recall MEN I (3 P's):
1. **P**ancreas (ZE, insulinoma, VIPoma)
2. **P**ituitary
3. **P**arathyroid

- concomitant corticosteroid use
- concomitant cardiovascular disease/other significant diseases

Treatment
- lower NSAID dose, or stop all together and replace with acetaminophen
- combine NSAID with PPI, or misoprostol
- enteric coating of aspirin (ECASA) provides minor benefit since this decreases incidence of erosion, not incidence of ulceration

Stress-Induced Ulceration

Definition
- ulceration or erosion in the upper GI tract of ill patients, usually in ICU; lesions most commonly in fundus of stomach

Pathophysiology
- unclear: likely involves ischemia; may occur with CNS disease, acid hypersecretion
- physiological stress (e.g. fever, severe illness, complex post-op course) causes ulcers and erosions
    - there is weak evidence linking psychological factors to ulcers

Risk Factors
- mechanical ventilation
- anti-coagulation
- multiorgan failure
- septicemia
- severe surgery/trauma
- CNS injury ("Cushing's ulcers")
- burns involving more than 35% of body surface

Clinical Features
- UGIB (see *Upper Gastrointestinal Bleeding*)
- painless

Treatment
- prophylaxis with gastric acid suppressants (H_2RA or PPI) decreases risk of UGIB, but may increase risk of pneumonia
- treatment same as for bleeding peptic ulcer but often less successful

Zollinger-Ellison (ZE) Syndrome

Definition
- rare (<1%) triad of gastric acid hypersecretion, severe peptic ulcer disease, and gastrinoma (gastrinoma: gastrin secreting tumour; most common in pancreas but 10-15% occur in duodenum)

Clinical Features
- strong family history of ZE or multiple endocrine neoplasia (MEN-I) (1/3 of patients with ZE syndrome have MEN-I)
- unusually severe symptoms of PUD
- diarrhea and malabsorption
- multiple ulcers in unusual sites; but can be just one ulcer
- refractory to treatment

Investigations
- fasting serum gastrin
- imaging of the pancreas
- high gastric acid secretion - rarely measured
- positive "secretin" test - limited availability

Treatment
- high dose PPI
- excision of gastrinoma (not found in 10-15% of patients)

Small and Large Bowel

Basic Anatomy Review

- small bowel: jejunum, ileum

Table 7. Anatomical features of the Jejunum, Ileum, and Large bowel

	Blood Supply	Structural Features	Functions
Jejunum	SMA	plicae circulares (circular folds on the interior surface), which have villi for absorption	absorption of food, salt, water and nutrients (protein, CHO, fat, folic acid, Vit B, C, and Vit A,D,E,K)
Ileum	SMA	plicae circulares	absorption of water and water soluble vitamins (incl. Vit B12) absorption of bile salts (entero-hepatic circulation)
Large bowel	branches of SMA and IMA	starts at cecum, ends at rectum tenia coli, haustra	absorption of water (5-10% of total water) bacteria: further digestion of chyme, and metabolism of undigested CHO to short chain fatty acids (SCFA); formation and storage of feces

Classification of Diarrhea

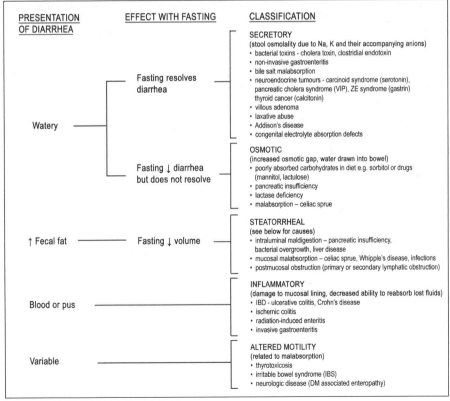

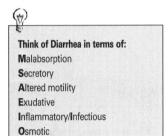

Think of Diarrhea in terms of:
Malabsorption
Secretory
Altered motility
Exudative
Inflammatory/**I**nfectious
Osmotic

Figure 4. Classification of Diarrhea

Acute Diarrhea

Definition
- passage of frequent unformed stools (>200 g of stool/24 hours) of <14 days duration

Etiology
- most commonly due to infections, many as yet undetectable pathogens
- most infections are self-limiting and resolve in less than 2 weeks

Risk Factors
- food (seafood, chicken, turkey, eggs, beef)
- medications: antibiotics, laxatives
- others
  - high risk sexual activity/homosexual contact
  - outbreaks
  - family history (inflammatory bowel disease)
  - diet (poor, changes)
  - immunosuppression
  - weight loss
  - malignancy

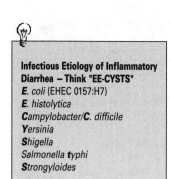

Useful Questions in Acute Diarrhea

Those Fads Wilt
Travel
Homosexual contacts
Outbreaks
Seafood
Extra-intestinal signs of IBD
Family history
Antibiotics
Diet
Steatorrhea
Weight loss
Immunosuppressed
Laxatives
Tumour history

Classification
- broadly divided and classified into inflammatory and non-inflammatory diarrhea
- mechanisms
  - in both, the diarrhea is due to molecules stimulating intestinal water secretion/inhibiting water absorption (i.e. secretory problem)
  - in inflammatory diarrhea, organisms and cytotoxins invade mucosa, killing mucosal cells, further perpetuating the diarrhea

Table 8. Classification of Acute Diarrhea

	Inflammatory	Non-Inflammatory
Definition	Disruption of intestinal mucosa	No disruption of intestinal mucosa
Site	Usually colon	Usually small intestine
Sigmoidoscopy	Usually abnormal mucosa seen	Usually normal
Symptoms	Bloody (not always) Small volume, high frequency Often lower abdominal cramping with urgency ± tenesmus May have fever ± shock	Watery, little or no blood Large volume Upper/periumbilical pain/cramp ± shock

Investigations Etiology	Fecal WBC and RBC positive
	Infectious
	• Bacterial
	  Shigella
	  Salmonella typhi
	  Campylobacter
	  Yersinia
	  E. coli (EHEC 0157:H7)
	  C. difficile
	• Protozoal
	  E. histolytica (amebiasis)
	  Strongyloides
		Fecal WBC negative
		Infectious
		• Bacterial
		  Salmonella enteritidis
		  S. aureus
		  B. cereus
		  C. perfringens
		  E. coli (ETEC, EPEC)
		  Vibrio cholerae
		• Protozoal
		  Giardia lamblia
		• Viral
		  Rotavirus
		  Norwalk
		  CMV
		
		Drugs
		  Antacids (Mg: Makes you Go)
		  Antibiotics
		  Laxatives, lactulose
		  Colchicine

Differential diagnosis	Mesenteric ischemia Radiation colitis Ulcerative colitis Crohn's disease	Chronic diarrheal illness (IBS, dietary intolerance e.g. lactose)
Significance	Higher yield with stool C&S Can progress to life-threatening megacolon, perforation, hemorrhage	Lower yield with stool C&S Chief life-threatening problem is fluid depletion and electrolyte disturbances

Infectious Etiology of Inflammatory Diarrhea — Think "EE-CYSTS"
E. coli (EHEC 0157:H7)
E. histolytica
Campylobacter/C. difficile
Yersinia
Shigella
Salmonella typhi
Strongyloides

Investigations
- stool cultures/microscopy (C&S/O&P) are not cost-effective in acute diarrhea unless inflammation (fecal WBC) present
  - C&S: easy; stool test harder to arrange and can cause delay in treatment
- diagnostic tests
  - stool WBC: stool smeared on slide and methylene blue drops added
  - postive test: >3 PMNs in 4 high power fields (HPFs)
  - usually positive for infectious but also IBD and radiation
- culture: routinely only for *Campylobacter, Salmonella, Shigella, E. Coli*
  - if you want others, order them specifically
- ova and parasites (O&P): may need more than one sample because of sporadic passage, but higher yield in first specimen
- flexible sigmoidoscopy: useful if inflammatory diarrhea suspected
  - biopsies useful to distinguish idiopathic inflammatory bowel disease (Crohn's disease and ulcerative colitis) from infectious colitis or acute self-limited colitis
- *C. difficile* toxin: indicated when recent/remote antibiotic use, hospitalization, nursing home or recent chemotherapy

Treatment
- fluid and electrolyte replacement: except in extremes of age and coma, electrolyte repletion is most important
- antimotility agents: diphenoxylate, loperamide (Imodium™); contraindicated in mucosal inflammation (controversial, may be used in non-toxic patients)
  - side effects: abdominal cramps, toxic megacolon
- absorbants: kaolin/pectin (Kaopectate™), methylcellulose, activated attapulgite
  - act by absorbing intestinal toxins/micro-organisms, or by coating/protecting intestinal mucosa
  - much less effective than antimotility agents
- modifiers of fluid transport: may be helpful, bismuth subsalicylate (Pepto-Bismol™)
- antibiotics: rarely indicated
  - risks
    - prolonged excretion of enteric pathogen
    - drug side effects (including *C. difficile* infection)
    - development of resistant strains
  - indications for antimicrobial agents in acute diarrhea
    - septicemia
    - prolonged fever with fecal blood or leukocytes
    - clearly indicated: *Shigella, V. cholerae, C. difficile*, Traveller's Diarrhea (Enterotoxigenic *E. coli* (ETEC)), *Giardia, Entamoeba histolytica, Cyclospora*
    - indicated in some situations: *Salmonella, Campylobacter, Yersinia*, non-enterotoxigenic *E. coli*
    - *Salmonella*: always treat *Salmonella typhi* (typhoid or enteric fever); treat other *Salmonella* only if there is underlying immunodeficiency, hemolytic anemia, extremes of age, aneurysms, prosthetic valve grafts/joints

Stool Osmotic Gap
Normally, and in secretory diarrhea, stool osmolality (as measured by freezing point depression; almost always about 290 mOsm/kg) is same as calculated stool osmolality (2 x stool (Na + K)) (multiplied by 2 to account for anions). In osmotic diarrhea, measured stool osmolality > calculated stool osmolality.

S. typhi has a rose spot rash (transient maculopapular rash on anterior thorax, upper abdomen).

Traveller's Diarrhea

- see Infectious Diseases

Chronic Diarrhea

Definition
- passage of frequent unformed stools (>200 mL of stool water/24 hours) for >14 days duration
- differential is similar to that of acute diarrhea, except the majority of cases are non-infectious

Investigations
- fecal fat, fecal leukocytes, ± C&S, O&P
- stool osmotic gap = OSM_{stool} (usually 290) – [2 x (Na_{stool} + K_{stool})]; only in problem cases
- history often determines investigations

Etiology/Classification
- see *Classification of Diarrhea* section, G13

Investigations
- stool analysis for:
  - WBC
  - O&P
  - sudan stain - rarely used

- blood for:
  - CBC
  - chemistry
  - C-reactive protein
  - TSH
- colonoscopy with biopsy
- small bowel biopsy
- wireless small bowel endoscopy capsule (last resort - $$ and not covered by OHIP)
- trial of lactose free diet

Maldigestion and Malabsorption

- maldigestion: inability to break down large molecules in the lumen of the intestine into their component small molecules
- malabsorption: inability to transport molecules across the intestinal mucosa to the circulation
- malassimilation: encompasses both maldigestion and malabsorption

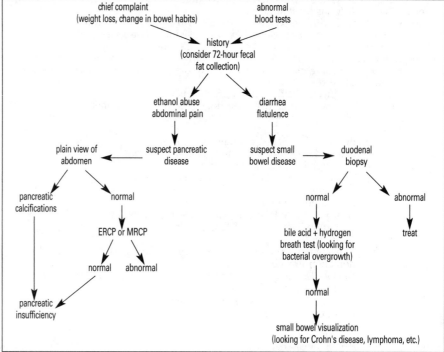

Figure 5. Approach to Malabsorption

Etiology
- maldigestion
  - inadequate mixing of food with enzymes (e.g. post-gastrectomy)
  - pancreatic exocrine deficiency
    - primary diseases of the pancreas (e.g. cystic fibrosis, pancreatitis, cancer)
  - bile salt deficiency
    - terminal ileal disease (impaired recycling), bacterial overgrowth (deconjugation of bile salts), rarely liver disease (cholestatic)
  - specific enzyme deficiencies
    - e.g. lactase
- malabsorption
  - inadequate absorptive surface (e.g. bowel resection, extensive Crohn's disease)
  - specific mucosal cell defects (e.g. abetalipoproteinemia) - very rare
  - diffuse disease
    - immunologic or allergic injury (e.g. celiac disease)
    - infections/infestations (e.g. Whipple's disease, giardiasis)
    - infiltration (e.g. lymphoma, amyloidosis)
    - fibrosis (e.g. systemic sclerosis, radiation enteritis)
- drug-induced
  - cholestyramine, ethanol, neomycin, tetracycline and other antibiotics
- endocrine
  - e.g. diabetes (complex pathogenesis)

Clinical Features
- symptoms usually vague unless disease is severe
- weight loss, diarrhea, steatorrhea, weakness, fatigue
- manifestations of malabsorption/deficiency (Table 9)

Table 9. Absorption of nutrients and fat soluble vitamins

Deficiency	Absorption	Signs and Symptoms	Investigations
Iron	duodenum, upper jejunum	hypochromic, microcytic anemia, glossitis, koilonychia (spoon nails), pica	↓ Hb, ↓ serum Fe, ↓ serum ferritin
Calcium	duodenum, upper jejunum (binds to Ca binding-protein in cells; levels ↑ by Vit D)	metabolic bone disease, may get tetany and paresthesias if serum calcium falls (see Endocrinology)	↓ serum calcium, serum magnesium, and ↑ ALP evaluate for ↓ bone mineralization radiographically (DEXA)
Folic acid	jejunum	megaloblastic anemia, glossitis ↓ red cell folate (but may see ↑ folic acid with bacterial overgrowth)	↓ serum folic acid
Vitamin B_{12}	see Figure 6	subacute combined degeneration of the spinal cord, peripheral/optic neuropathy, dementia, megaloblastic anemia, glossitis	differentiate causes by Schilling test
Carbohydrate	complex polysaccharides hydrolyzed to oligosaccharides and disaccharides by salivary and pancreatic enzymes monosaccharides absorbed in duodenum/jejunum	generalized malnutrition, weight loss, flatus and diarrhea	hydrogen breath test trial of CHO-restricted diet D-xylose test
Protein	digestion at stomach, brush border, and inside cell absorption occurs primarily in the jejunum	general malnutrition and weight loss amenorrhea and ↓ libido if severe	↓ serum albumin (low sensitivity)
Fat	lipase, colipase, phospholipase A (pancreatic enzymes) and bile salts needed for digestion products of lipolysis form micelles which solubilize fat and aid in absorption fatty acids diffuse into cell cytoplasm	generalized malnutrition, weight loss, and diarrhea foul-smelling feces + gas	Small bowel biopsy MRCP, ERCP, pancreatic function tests quantitative stool fat test (72 hr) (sudan stain of stool) (C-triolein breath test)
Vitamin A	from plants	night blindness dry skin keratomalacia	
Vitamin D	skin (via UV light) or diet	osteomalacia in adults rickets in children	
Vitamin E	from food	retinopathy, neurological problems	
Vitamin K	synthesized by intestinal flora ↑ risk of deficiency after prolonged use of broad spectrum antibiotics and/or starvation (fasting)	prolonged INR causes bleeding	

Fat Soluble Vitamins: ADEK

Vitamin K dependent coagulation factors: II, VII, IX, X, protein C, protein S

Risk factors of vitamin B$_{12}$ in patients receiving metformin
Arch Intern Med. 2006;166:1975-9.
Study: Nested case-control study.
Patients: 155 patients with metformin-related vitamin B$_{12}$ deficiency 310 matched controls
Results: Metformin patients had mean $\pm$ SD serum vitamin B$_{12}$ concentration, 148.6 $\pm$ 40.4 pg/mL; range, 50.1-203.3 pg/mL, while matched controls had mean levels of 466.1 $\pm$ 330.4 pg/mL; range, 204.6-2000.0 pg/mL. Each 1-g/d metformin dose increment conferred an odds ratio of 2.88 (95% confidence interval, 2.15-3.87) for developing vitamin B$_{12}$ deficiency (P<.001). Among those using metformin for 3 years or more, the adjusted odds ratio was 2.39 (95% confidence interval, 1.46-3.91) (P=.001) compared wth those receiving metformin for less than 3 years. After exclusion of 113 subjects with borderline vitamin B$_{12}$ concentration, dose of metformin remained the strongest independent predictor of vitamin B$_{12}$ deficiency.
Conclusion: There is an increased risk of vitamin B$_{12}$ deficiency associated with current dose and duration of metformin use despite adjustment for many potential confounders.

A case-control study on adverse effects: H2 blocker or proton pump inhibitor use and risk of vitamin B$_{12}$ deficiency in older adults
J Clin Epidemiol. 2004;57: 422-8.
Study: Case-control study in university-based geriatric primary care setting.
Patients: Patients were 65 years of age or older (mean age of 82) with documented serum vitamin B$_{12}$ studies between 1990 and 1997. Comparison was made between 53 vitamin B$_{12}$-deficient cases and 212 controls for past or current use of prescription H2RA/PPI according to information in subjects' medical records.
Results: After controlling for age, gender, multivitamin use, and *Helicobacter pylori* infection, chronic (12 months) current use of H2RA/PPI was associated with a significantly increased risk of vitamin B$_{12}$ deficiency (OR 4.45; 95% CI 1.47-13.34). No association was found between past or short-term current use of H2RA/PPI and vitamin B$_{12}$ deficiency.
Conclusion: Chronic use of H2RA/PPI by older adults is associated with the development of vitamin B$_{12}$ deficiency.

Gluten found in "BROW"
Barley
Rye
Oats (controversial)
Wheat

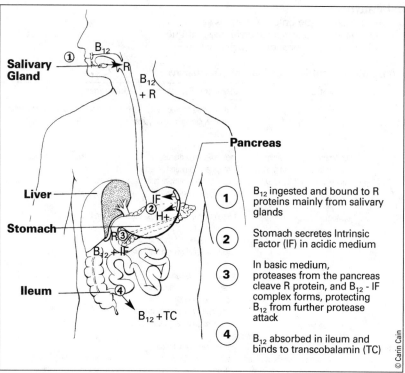

Figure 6. B$_{12}$ Absorption

① B$_{12}$ ingested and bound to R proteins mainly from salivary glands

② Stomach secretes Intrinsic Factor (IF) in acidic medium

③ In basic medium, proteases from the pancreas cleave R protein, and B$_{12}$ - IF complex forms, protecting B$_{12}$ from further protease attack

④ B$_{12}$ absorbed in ileum and binds to transcobalamin (TC)

© Carin Cain

Investigations (in malassimilation syndromes)
- 72 hour stool collection (weight, fat content)
- low serum carotene, folate, Ca, Mg, vitamin B$_{12}$, albumin, ferritin, serum iron solution, elevated INR/PTT
- stool fat globules on fecal smear - rarely used
- other tests specific for etiology

Treatment (of malassimilation syndromes)
- dependent on underlying etiology

Celiac Disease (Gluten Enteropathy/Sprue)

Definition
- abnormal small intestine mucosa due to intestinal reaction to gluten

Etiology
- only autoimmune disease in which androgen (α-gliadin) is recognized
- associated with other autoimmune diseases, especially thyroid disease
- gluten, a protein in cereal grains, is toxic factor
- HLA-DQ2 (chromosome 6) found in 80-90% of patients compared with 20% in general population; also associated with HLA-DQ8

Epidemiology
- more common in women
- family history: 15% of first-degree relatives
- may present any time from infancy (when cereals introduced), to elderly
- peak presentation in infancy and old age

Clinical Features
- classically: diarrhea, weight loss, anemia, symptoms of vitamin/mineral deficiency, failure to thrive; now more commonly bloating, gas, iron deficiency
- improves with gluten-free diet, deteriorates when gluten reintroduced
- disease is usually most severe in proximal bowel; therefore iron, calcium, and folic acid deficiency common
- gluten enteropathy may be associated with dermatitis herpetiformis skin eruption, epilepsy, myopathy, depression, paranoia, infertility, bone fractures/metabolic bone disease

Investigations

- small bowel mucosal biopsy (usually duodenum) is usually diagnostic, abnormalities seen include:
  - villous atrophy and crypt hyperplasia
  - increased number of plasma cells and lymphocytes in lamina propria
  - similar pathology in: small bowel overgrowth, Crohn's, lymphoma, *Giardia*
- small bowel follow through to exclude lymphoma
- evidence of malabsorption (localized or generalized)
  - steatorrhea
  - low levels of ferritin/iron saturation, Ca, Fe, albumin, cholesterol, carotene, B_{12} absorption
- improvement with a gluten-free diet
- serological tests
  - anti-endomysial antibody (EMA) or ELISA for IgA tissue transglutaminase (TTG)
  - anti-TTG test is 90-98% sensitive, 94-97% specific
  - IgA deficient patients have false-negative IgA anti-EMA and anti-TTG so measure serum IgA concomitantly or measure IgG EMA and IgG TTG with initial bloodwork
  - fecal fat >7% over 72 hrs

Treatment

- dietary counselling
  - gluten free diet: avoid barley, rye, wheat, maybe oats
  - rice and corn flour are acceptable
  - iron, folate supplementation (with supplementation of other vitamins as needed)
- in the event of treatment failure, consider
  - incorrect diagnosis
  - non-adherence to gluten-free diet
  - unsuspected concurrent disease (e.g. pancreatic insufficiency)
  - development of intestinal (enteropathy-associated T-cell) lymphoma (abdominal pain, weight loss, palpable mass)
  - development of diffuse intestinal ulceration, characterized by aberrant intraepithelial T-cell population, precursor to lymphoma

Prognosis

- associated with ↑ risk of lymphoma, carcinoma including small bowel and colon
- majority of patients have normal life expectancy

Bacterial Overgrowth

Definition

- syndrome caused by proliferation of bacteria in small bowel to concentrations >10^4 bacteria/mL of bowel tissue

Etiology

- anatomic factors
  - jejunal diverticulae
  - surgical blind loop
  - Crohn's & fistulas
  - strictures (regional enteritis, radiation injury)
  - obstruction
  - surgical resection of the ileocecal valve
- ↓ motility
  - scleroderma
  - diabetes, hypothyroid
  - intestinal pseudo-obstruction
- achlorhydria (often iatrogenic)
- described in elderly patients: unknown etiology

Clinical Features

- steatorrhea: bacteria deconjugate bile salts impairing micellar lipid formation
- diarrhea: bowel mucosa damaged by bacterial products, impairing absorption; altered gut motility, free bile acids stimulate colon water secretion
- megaloblastic anemia due to vitamin B_{12} malabsorption
- may be asymptomatic

A prospective, double-blind, placebo-controlled trial to establish a safe gluten threshold for patients with celiac disease.
Am J Clin Nutr. 2007;85:160-6
Study: Multicentre, double-blind, placebo-controlled, randomized trial.
Patients: 49 adults with biopsy-proven celiac disease (CD) who were being treated with a gluten-free diet (GFD) for at least 2 years. 39 patients completed the study protocol
Intervention: 0, 10, or 50 mg gluten daily for 3 months
Outcome: Small-bowel biopsies (≥4 specimens from each procedure) of the second part of the duodenum with a measurement of villous height/crypt depth (Vh/Cd) and intraepithelial lymphocyte count (IEL)
Results: One patient (challenged with 10 mg gluten) developed a clinical relapse. At 3 months, the percentage change in Vh/Cd was 9% (95% CI: 3%, 15%) in the placebo group (n=13), -1% (-18%, 68%) in the 10-mg group (n=13), and -20% (-22%, -13%) in the 50-mg group (n=13). No significant differences in the IEL count were found between the 3 groups
Conclusion: The ingestion of contaminating gluten should be kept lower than 50 mg/d in the treatment of CD

Investigations
- gold standard: mixed bacterial cultures of >10^4 CFU/mL from the jejunum
- 72-hour fecal fat collection
- bile acid breath test (^{14}C-cholyglycine) misses 1/3 of cases
- hydrogen breath test or ^{14}C-xylose breath test
- positive three stage Schilling test if done before and after treatment can be diagnostic
- low serum B_{12}, high serum folate (since folate synthesized by GI bacteria)
- small bowel follow-through to look for underlying cause
- consider small bowel biopsy to rule out primary mucosal disease as cause of malabsorption

Treatment
- treat underlying etiology if possible (e.g. prokinetic agents for small bowel motility disorder)
- symptoms relieved by a 10-14 day trial of antibiotics (best if based on culture results)
- broad-spectrum antibiotics, killing anaerobes and aerobes
  - e.g. amoxicillin + clavulinic acid 250-500 mg PO tid
    - patients may need to be treated with intermittent antibiotics indefinitely
- discontinue acid-reducing agents if possible
- consider supplemental Vit A, D, E, K, B_{12}

Inflammatory Bowel Disease (IBD)

Definition
- Crohn's Disease, Ulcerative Colitis, and Indeterminate Colitis

Pathophysiology
- poorly understood
- inappropriate response of the immune system to enteric flora in a genetically predisposed individual
- current hypothesis emphasizes that the chief problem is lack of appropriate down-regulation of immune responsiveness

Genetics
- increased risk of both ulcerative colitis and Crohn's disease in relatives of patients with either disease, especially siblings, early onset disease
  - familial risk greater if proband has Crohn's than ulcerative colitis
- probably polygenomic pattern
- 9 gene loci described to be associated
- CARD15 gene mutation associated with Crohn's (relative risk in heterozygote is 3, in homozygote is 40), especially Ashkenazi Jews, early onset disease, ileal involvement, fistulizing and stenotic disease (NOD2)
  - CARD15 gene product modulates NF_kB, which is required for the innate immune response to microbial pathogens, best expressed in monocytes-macrophages
- other gene associations described but even less well understood

Clinical Features

Table 10. Clinical Differentiation of Ulcerative Colitis from Crohn's Disease

	Crohn's Disease	Ulcerative Colitis
Location	Any part of GI tract • small bowel + colon: 50% • small bowel only: 30% • colon only: 20%	Isolated to large bowel Always involves rectum
Rectal Bleeding	Uncommon	Very common (90%)
Diarrhea	Less prevalent	Frequent small stools
Abdominal Pain	Post-prandial/colicky	Pre-defecatory urgency
Fever	Common	Uncommon
Palpable Mass	Frequent (25%), RLQ	Rare (if present, cecum full of stool)
Recurrence After Surgery	Common	None
Endoscopic Features	Discrete aphthous ulcers, patchy lesions	Continuous diffuse inflammation, erythema, friability, loss of normal vascular pattern, pseudopolyps
Histologic Features	Transmural distribution with skip lesions Focal inflammation ± noncaseating granulomas, deep fissuring & aphthous ulcerations, strictures Glands intact	Mucosal distribution Granulomas absent Gland destruction, crypt abscess
Radiologic Features	Cobblestone mucosa Frequent strictures and fistulae XR: Bowel wall thickening "string sign"	Lack of haustra Strictures rare and suggests complicating cancer
Complications	Strictures, fistulae, perianal disease, abscesses	Toxic megacolon
Colon Cancer Risk	3x that of general population	7-30x that of general population

Crohn's Disease

Definition
• chronic inflammatory disorder potentially affecting the entire gut "from gum to bum"

Epidemiology
• incidence 1-6/100,000; prevalence 10-100/100,000
• bimodal: onset before 30 years, second smaller peak age 60
• incidence of Crohn's increasing (relative to UC) especially in young females
• more common in Caucasians, Ashkenazi Jews
• M=F; smoking incidence in Crohn's patients is higher than general population

Clinical Features
• most often presents as recurrent episodes of abdominal cramps, diarrhea, and weight loss
• ileitis may present with post-prandial pain, vomiting, RLQ mass mimics acute appendicitis
• fistulae, fissures, abscesses are common
• extra-intestinal manifestations (Table 11) are more common with colonic involvement
• natural history unpredictable
• linear ulcers leading to mucosal islands and "cobblestone" appearance
• deep fissures with risk of perforation into contiguous viscera (leads to fistulae and abscesses)
• enteric fistulae may communicate with skin, bladder, vagina, and other parts of bowel
• granulomas are found in 50% of surgical specimens, 15% of mucosal biopsies

Investigations
• endoscopy with biopsy to diagnose
• C-reactive protein; can be used to rule out diagnosis & to monitor treatment response
• barium studies, CT abdomen
• bacterial cultures, O&P, *C. difficile* toxin to exclude other causes of inflammatory diarrhea

---

• nutrition
• symptomatic therapy
(e.g. loperamide, acetaminophen)

↓

• 5-ASA (mesalamine)
• antibiotics (Flagyl™, Cipro™)

↓

• corticosteroids (e.g. budesonide, prednisone)

↓

• immunosuppression
(e.g. azathioprine, 6-MP, methotrexate)

↓

• immunomodulators
(e.g. TNF-antagonists: infliximab, adalimumab)

↓

• experimental therapy or surgery

Figure 7. Traditional Graded Approach To Induction Therapy In Crohn's

Medical Management of Crohn's

	Induced Remission	Maintenance
5-ASA	+	?
Steroids	+	
Immunosuppressive	+	+
Antibiotics	+	
MTX	+	+
Infliximab	+	+

Principles of Therapy in IBD
• Aim more for clinical than histologic/endoscopic radiologic remission
• Treatment has so many side effects that, usually one disease (IBD) ends up being replaced with another (iatrogenic)
• Spend the time to lower expectations, discuss risks and expected benefits of Rx
• Don't use corticosteroids for maintenance therapy

Many patients with Crohn's suffer from vague abdominal pain and diarrhea for years before a diagnosis of Crohn's disease is considered.

Infliximab for induction of remission in Crohn's Disease
Cochrane Database of Systemic Reviews 2003, Issue 4. Art. No.: CD003574.DOI: 10.1002/14651858.CD003574.pub2.
Study: Meta-analysis of TNF blocking agents in the induction of remission of Crohn's disease.
Conclusions: There is evidence to suggest that infliximab is effective in inducing remission in patients when compared to placebo.

Infliximab for maintaining remission in Crohn's disease: the ACCENT I Trial
The Lancet 2002, 359(9317): 1541-1549
Study: Multi-centre double blind RCT evaluating the efficacy of maintenance infliximab for Crohn's Disease in patients who initially responded to infliximab.
Methods: 573 patients with active CD received an injection of 5 mg/kg at week 0 of the sudy. Responders were then randomized to three groups: I) placebo infusions, II) infliximab infusions of 5 mg/kg at 2, 6 and 8 weeks and then q8 weeks until week 46, III) 5 mg/kg infliximab at 2 and 6 weeks and then 10 mg/kg thereafter.
Results: Patients in groups II and III were 1) more likely to have sustained clinical remission throughout the 54 week trial, and 2) had significantly lower rates of corticosteriod usage during the trial. Rates of infection and serious adverse events were similar across treatment groups.
Conclusions: Infliximab is effective in maintaining remission and reducing corticosteroid use in patients who initially respond to infliximab.

Management (see Figure 7)
• Medical management (most uncomplicated cases can be managed medically)
• Diet
  ▪ fluids only during acute exacerbation
  ▪ enteral diets may aid in remission but some are not palatable
  ▪ those with extensive small bowel involvement or extensive resection need electrolyte, mineral and vitamin supplements (Vit D, Ca, Mg, zinc, Fe, B12)
• 5-ASA
  ▪ efficacy controversial, most evidence for efficacy is for mild, colonic disease
  ▪ sulfasalazine (Salazopyrin™) = a compound composed of 5-ASA bound to sulfapyridine
    ♦ hydrolysis by intestinal bacteria releases 5-ASA, the active component
    ♦ effectiveness is related to dose
  ▪ mesalamine (Pentasa™, Salofalk™, Asacol™, Mesasal™) = 5-ASA with different coatings to release 5-ASA in the ileum and colon
• Steroids
  ▪ prednisone 20-40 mg OD for acute exacerbations (but use only if symptoms are severe)
  ▪ no proven role for steroids in maintaining remissions, masks intra-abdominal sepsis
  ▪ complications of steroid therapy are dose and duration dependent
    ♦ note: budesonide has fewer side effects than prednisone
• Immunosuppressives
  ▪ 6-mercaptopurine (6-MP), azathioprine (Imuran™); methotrexate used less often
  ▪ used to treat active inflammation and to maintain remission
  ▪ most commonly used as steroid-sparing agents, i.e. to lower risk of relapse as corticosteroids are withdrawn
  ▪ may require >3 months to have beneficial effect (methotrexate works faster than azathioprine); usually continued for several years
  ▪ probably help to heal fistulae, ↓disease activity
  ▪ have important side effects (pancreatitis, bone marrow suppression, ↑ risk of cancer)
• Antibiotics
  ▪ e.g. metronidazole (20 mg/kg/d, bid or tid dosing)
  ▪ decreases disease activity and improves perianal disease
  ▪ side effects are common and reversible for metronidazole (50% have peripheral neuropathy after 6 months of treatment, may not be reversible)
  ▪ use of ciprofloxacin + metronidazole may be beneficial in Crohn's disease
• Antidiarrheal agents
  ▪ loperamide (Imodium™) > diphenoxylate (Lomotil™) > codeine (cheap but addictive)
  ▪ all work by decreasing small bowel motility
  ▪ use with caution (if colitis is severe, risk of precipitating toxic megacolon); avoid in flare-ups
• Cholestyramine
  ▪ a bile salt binding resin
  ▪ for watery diarrhea with less than 100 cm of terminal ileum diseased or resected (see below)
• Immunomodulators
  ▪ infliximab (Remicade®) or adalimumab (Humira®)= antibody to tumour necrosis factor (TNFα)
  ▪ proven effective for treatment of fistulae and patients with medically refractory Crohn's disease
  ▪ new evidence suggest first-line immunosuppressive therapy with inflixmab + immunomodulators is more effective than starting with traditional corticosteroid regimen
  ▪ often effective within days, generally well tolerated allergic reactions
  ▪ side effect → reported cases of reactivated TB, PCP, other infections, febrile neutropenia
• Surgical treatment (see General Surgery)
  ▪ surgery generally reserved for complications such as fistulae, obstruction, abscess, perforation, bleeding, and rarely for medically refractory disease
  ▪ at least 50% clinical recurrence within 5 years; 85% within 15 years; endoscopic recurrence rate even higher
  ▪ 40% likelihood of second bowel resection
  ▪ 30% likelihood of third bowel resection
  ▪ complications of ileal resection
    ♦ <100 cm resected → watery diarrhea (impaired bile salt absorption)
      – treatment: cholestyramine or anti-diarrheals e.g. loperamide
    ♦ >100 cm resected → steatorrhea (bile salt deficiency)
      – treatment: fat restriction, medium chain triglycerides

Prognosis
- highly variable course
- 10% chronic, relapsing
- 10% disabled by the disease eventually
- increased mortality, especially with more proximal disease, greatest in the first 4-5 years
- intestinal obstruction due to edema, fibrosis
- fistula formation
- intestinal perforation characteristically contained (free perforation uncommon)
- malignancy: ↑ risk especially with colonic involvement, but may not be as high as ulcerative colitis

Ulcerative Colitis (UC)

Definition
- inflammatory disease affecting colonic mucosa anywhere from rectum to cecum, but rectum always invoced

Epidemiology
- incidence 2-10/100,000; prevalence 35-100/100,000 (more common than Crohn's)
- 2/3 onset by age 30 (with second peak after 50); M=F
- small hereditary contribution (15% of cases have 1st degree relative with disease)
- risk is less in smokers
- disease limited to rectum, left colon is more common than pancolitis

Pathology
- disease can involve any portion of lower bowel from rectum only (proctitis) to entire colon (pancolitis)
- rectum always involved
- inflammation diffuse, continuous, and confined to mucosa

Clinical Features
- chronic disease characterized by rectal bleeding and diarrhea, prone to remissions and exacerbations
- severity of colonic inflammation correlates with symptoms (stool volume, amount of blood in stool)
- diarrhea, rectal bleeding most frequent, but can also have abdominal cramps/pain (especially with defecation)
- tenesmus, urgency, incontinence
- systemic symptoms: fever, anorexia, weight loss, fatigue
- extra-intestinal manifestations (Table 11)
- characteristic exacerbations and remissions; 5% of cases are fulminant

Investigations
- sigmoidoscopy with mucosal biopsy (to exclude self limited colitis) without bowel prep often sufficient for diagnosis
- colonoscopy contraindicated in severe exacerbation; helpful to determine extent of disease
- barium enema (not during acute phase or relapse)
- stool culture, microscopy, C. difficile toxin assay necessary to exclude infection
- no single confirmatory test

Management
- mainstays of treatment: 5-ASA derivatives and corticosteroids, with azathioprine used in steroid-dependent or resistant cases
- Diet of little value in decreasing inflammation but may alleviate symptoms
- Antidiarrheal medications generally not indicated in UC
- 5-ASA drugs
  - topical (suppository or enema): very effective for distal disease (no further than splenic flexure), preferable to corticosteroids
  - oral: effective for mild to moderate, but not severe colitis
  - e.g. sulfasalazine (Salazopyrin™) 3-4 g/d; mesalamine (Salofalk™, Pentasa™, Asacol™) 4 g/d
  - useful only for mild to moderate disease, not for severe disease
  - more use in maintaining remission (decreases yearly relapse rate from 60% to 15%)
  - may decrease rate of colorectal cancer
- Steroids
  - best drugs to remit acute disease, especially if severe or first attack (e.g. prednisone 40 mg PO OD)
  - limited role as maintenance therapy

Infliximab for maintaining remission of Crohn's Disease in patients with draining fistualas: the ACCENT II Trial
NEJM 2004; 350 (9) 876-896
Study: Multi-centre, double blind RCT of 306 patients with Crohn's Disease and one or more draining perianal fistulas. A total of 195 patients who responded to treatment were randomized to received placebo or 5 mg/kg of infliximab.
Results: Mean time to loss of response was significantly longer in the group that received infliximab compared to placebo (40 weeks compared to 14 weeks) p<0.001.
Conclusions: Infliximab is effective in the maintenance of remission for Crohn's patients with draining abdominal or perianal fistulas. Note: What has not been precisely defined is the infection risk associated with infliximab.

Medical Management of Ulcerative Colitis

	Induced Remission	Maintenance
5-ASA	+	+
Steroids	+	
Immunosuppressive	+	+

Infliximab for induction of remission in UC
Cochrane Database of Systematic Reviews 2006, Issue 3. Art. No.: CD005112. DOI: 10.1002/14651858.CD005112.pub2.
Conclusions: Infliximab is more useful in induction of remission (both clinical and endoscopic remission) of active UC than placebo in UC that has been refractory to BOTH corticosteriods and anti-immune medications.

Oral 5-aminosalicylic acid for maintenance of remission in ulcerative colitis.
Cochrane Database Syst Rev. 2006;(2):CD000544.
Purpose: To assess the efficacy, dose-responsiveness and safety of the newer release formulations of 5-aminosalicylic acid (5-ASA) compared to placebo or sulfasalazine (SASP) in the maintenance of remission in ulcerative colitis.
Study Selection: Randomized, double-blinded, and placebo- or SASP-controlled clinical trials of parallel design with treatment duration of at least six months.
Results: The Peto odds ratio for the failure to maintain clinical or endoscopic remission (withdrawals and relapses) for 5-ASA versus placebo was 0.47 (95% CI, 0.36 to 0.62) with an NNT of 6. In trials comparing SASP and 5-ASA, SASP was more effective, revealing an odds ratio of 1.29 (95% CI, 1.05 to 1.57), with a negative NNT vlaue (-19). SASP and 5-ASA had similar adverse event profiles, with odds ratios of 1.16(0.62 to 2.16), and 1.31(0.86 to 1.99), respectively. The NNH values were determined to be 171 and 78 respectively.
Conclusion: The newer 5-ASA preparations were superior to placebo in maintenance therapy. However, the newer preparations had a statistically significant therapeutic inferiority relative to SASP.

In UC's initial presentation, non-bloody diarrhea is frequently seen. It will however, eventually progress to bloody diarrhea.

- use suppositories for proctitis, enemas for proctosigmoiditis
- less toxic topical steroids (e.g. hydrocortison foam, budesonide enemas) have been shown to be equally effective when used as enemas/suppositories
- Immunosuppressants (steroid-sparing)
  - if severe UC is refractory to steroid therapy, add IV/oral cyclosporine: rapidly effective but has many side effects; alternative is infliximab
  - azathioprine: is too slow to rapidly resolve acute relapse but is helpful in inducing remission and sparing steroids in refractory cases
  - may be added to steroids when steroids fail, but most commonly used to maintain remission as corticosteroids withdrawn
  - infliximab entering routine clinical use
- Surgical treatment
  - early in fulminant cases and toxic megacolon
  - aim for cure with colectomy
  - indications: failure of adequate medical therapy, toxic megacolon, bleeding, pre-cancerous, dysplastic changes picked up with screening endoscopic biopsies (dysplasia)

Complications (Table 11)

- like Crohn's, except for the following:
  - more liver problems (especially primary sclerosing cholangitis (PSC) in men)
  - greater risk of colorectal cancer
    - risk increases with duration and extent of disease (5% at 10 years, 15% at 20 years for pancolitis; overall RR is 8%)
    - risk also increases with presence of sclerosing cholangitis, family history of colorectal cancer
    - therefore, regular screening colonoscopy and biopsy in pancolitis of 8 years or more is indicated
  - toxic megacolon (transverse colon diameter >6 cm on abdominal x-ray) with immediate danger of perforation (see General Surgery)

Prognosis

- chronic relapsing pattern in most patients
- 10-15% chronic continuous pattern
- >1 attack in almost all patients
- more colonic involvement in the 1st year correlates with increased severity of attacks and increased colectomy rate
- colectomy rate = 1% for all patients after the 1st year; 20-25% eventually undergo colectomy
- normal life expectancy
- if proctitis only, usually benign course

When considering complications of IBD, think:
ULCERATIVE COLITIS

Urinary Calculi
Liver problems
Cholelithiasis
Epithelial problems
Retardation of growth/sexual maturation
Arthralgias
Thrombophlebitis
Iatrogenic complications
Vitamin deficiencies
Eyes

Colorectal cancer
Obstruction
Leakage (perforation)
Iron deficiency
Toxic megacolon
Inanition (wasting)
Strictures, fistulae

Table 11. Extraintestinal Manifestations of IBD

System	Crohn's Disease	Ulcerative Colitis
Dermatologic		
Erythema Nodosum	15%	10%
Pyoderma Gangrenosum	10%	Less common
Perianal skin tags	75-80%	Rare
Oral mucosal lesions	Common	Rare
Psoriasis	statistically associated in 5-10% of those with IBD but not an EIM	
Rheumatologic		
Peripheral arthritis	15-20% of those with IBD (CD>UC)	
Ankylosing Spondylitis	10% of those with IBD (CD>UC)	
Sacroiliitis	Occurs equally in CD and UC	
Ocular (~10% of IBD)		
Uveitis (vision threatening)		
Episcleritis (benign)	3-4% of IBD patients (CD>UC)	
Hepatobiliary		
Cholelithiasis	15-35% of patients with ileal Crohn's	
Primary sclerosing cholangitis (PSC)	1-5% of IBD cases involving colon	
Fatty liver		
Urologic		
Calculi	most common in CD, especially following ileal resection	
Ureteral obstruction		
Fistulas	characteristic of Crohn's	
Others		
Thromboembolism		
Vasculitis		
Osteoporosis		
Vitamin deficiencies (B_{12}, Vit ADEK)		
Cardiopulmonary disorders		
Pancreatitis (rare)		

Irritable Bowel Syndrome (IBS)

Definition
- a form of functional bowel disease; considered a disease, not just a label for all GI symptoms that are unexplained after investigation

Epidemiology
- 20% of North Americans
- onset of symptoms usually in young adulthood
- F>M

Pathophysiology
- normal perception of abnormal gut motility
- abnormal perception of normal gut motility
- psychological: "socially acceptable vehicle for accepting care"
- behavioural: symptoms of IBS common in general population; ↑ physician seeking behaviour and expectations in small percentage reaching medical attention

Diagnosis

Table 12. Rome III Criteria for Diagnosing Irritable Bowel Syndrome

IBS Rome III Criteria
- 12 weeks or more in the past 12 months of abdominal discomfort or pain that has 2 out of 3 features:
  - relieved with defecation
  - associated with a change in frequency of stool
  - associated with a change in consistency of stool

- The following are supportive, but not essential to the diagnosis:
  - abnormal stool frequency (>3/day or <3/week)
  - abnormal stool form (lumpy/hard/loose/watery) >1/4 of defecations
  - abnormal stool passage (straining, urgency, feeling of incomplete evacuation) >1/4 of defecations
  - passage of mucus >1/4 of defecations

Diagnosis of IBS Less Likely in Presence of "Alarm" Features
- weight loss
- fever
- nocturnal defecation
- anemia
- blood or pus in stool
- abnormal gross findings on flexible sigmoidoscopy

Normal Physical Exam

Investigations
- use discretion: the more history resembles Rome III criteria or younger the patient, the less number of investigations required
- aim is to rule out:
  - enteric infections e.g. *Giardia*
  - lactose intolerance/other disaccharidase deficiency
  - Crohn's disease
  - celiac sprue
  - drug-induced diarrhea
  - diet-induced (excess tea, coffee, colas)
- CBC, TSH, albumin, C-reactive protein, TTG and serology
- stool for C&S, O&P, fat excretion if diarrhea present
- sigmoidoscopy

Management
- reassurance, realistic goals, education
- relaxation therapy, biofeedback, hypnosis, stress reduction
- no therapeutic agent consistently effective
- bran or psyllium for constipation, loperamide for diarrhea
- consider use of tricyclic antidepressants
- symptom-guided treatment
- pain predominant
  - antispasmodic medication before meals, e.g. hyosine, trimebutine
  - change diet
  - tricyclic compounds (TCA)
  - selective serotonin reuptake inhibitors (SSRI)
  - visceral antinociceptive agent
- diarrhea predominant
  - change diet
  - loperamide 2-4 mg tid/qid
  - diphenoxylate (Lomotil™)
  - cholestyramine 4 g qid
- constipation predominant
  - exercise and adequate fluid intake
  - add fibre
  - osmotic or other laxatives
  - 5-HT$_4$ receptor agonist where available

Prognosis
- 80% improve over time
- most have intermittent episodes
- normal life expectancy

Constipation

Definition
- passage of infrequent or hard stools with straining (stool water <50 mL/day); bowel frequency <3 times per week

Epidemiology
- increasing prevalence with age; F>M; rare in Africa and India where stool weight is 3-4x greater than in Western countries

Etiology
- in the absence of other clinical problems, most commonly due to lack of fibre in diet, change of diet, or poorly understood gut motility changes
- organic causes
  - medication side effects (antidepressants, codeine) most common
  - intestinal obstruction, left sided colon cancer (consider in older patients); fecal impaction
  - metabolic
    - diabetes mellitus (DM)
    - hypothyroidism
    - hypercalcemia, hypokalemia, uremia
  - neurological
    - intestinal pseudo-obstruction
    - Parkinson's disease
    - multiple sclerosis (MS)
  - collagen vascular disease
    - scleroderma
    - amyloidosis

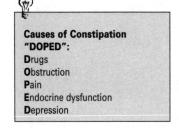

Causes of Constipation "DOPED":
Drugs
Obstruction
Pain
Endocrine dysfunction
Depression

Clinical Presentation
- IBS, depression, anorexia
- painful anal conditions (e.g. hemorrhoids)
- abdominal pain relieved by defecation, hard stools, straining and pain with defecation, flatulence, overflow diarrhea, sense of incomplete evacuation, abdominal distension <3 BM/week

Investigations
- swallow radio-opaque markers to quantify colonic transit time (normal: 70 hours)
  - normal = misperception of normal defecation
  - prolonged = "colonic inertia"
  - prolonged plus abnormal anal manometry = outlet obstruction

Treatment (in order of increasing potency)
- surface-acting (soften and lubricate)
  - docusate salts, mineral oils
- bulk-forming
  - bran 30 g/d (effective within 1 week), psyllium seed (Metamucil®), wheat fibre, sterculin, methylcellulose (ensure adequate hydration), flax seeds
- osmotic agents (effective in 2-3 days)
  - lactulose, sorbitol, magnesium citrate, magnesium sulfate, magnesium hydroxide, lactitol, milk of magnesia
- cathartics (effective in 24 hrs)
  - castor oil, senna (watch out for melanosis coli)
- enemas and suppositories (e.g. saline enema, phosphate enema, glycerin suppository)
- note: avoid senna and anthracena (↓ colon motility when used chronically)

Upper Gastrointestinal Bleeding

Definition
- bleeding proximal to the ligament of Treitz (75% of GI bleeds)
- Ligament of Treitz: suspensory ligament in the third and fourth portions of the duodenum

80% of upper GI bleeds stop spontaneously or need only supportive therapy.

Clinical Features
- in order of decreasing severity of the bleed: hematochezia > hematemesis > melena > occult blood in stool

Etiology
- above the GE junction
  - epistaxis
  - esophageal varices (10-30%)
  - esophagitis
  - esophageal cancer
  - Mallory-Weiss tear (10%)
- stomach
  - gastric ulcer (20%) (see *Peptic Ulcer Disease)*
  - gastritis (e.g. from alcohol or post surgery) (20%)
  - gastric cancer
- duodenum
  - ulcer in bulb (25%)
  - aortoenteric fistula: usually only if previous aortic graft
- coagulopathy (drugs, renal disease, liver disease)
- vascular malformation (Dieulafoy's lesion, AVM)

Management (initial)
- stabilize patient (IV fluids, cross and type, 2 large bore IVs, monitor)
- send blood for CBC, platelets, PT, PTT, electrolytes, BUN, Cr, LFTs
- keep NPO
- NG tube to determine upper vs. lower GI bleeding
- endoscopy (OGD): establish bleeding site + treat lesion
  - injection of epinephrine around bleeding points
  - injection of sclerosants (ethanol)
  - thermal hemostasis (Argon Plasma Coagulation or heater probe)
  - bipolar electrocoagulation
  - endoclips
- if stable non-variceal bleed and endoscopy is not available then PPI either IV or high dose PO
- for variceal bleeds, octreotide 50 μg loading dose followed by constant drip of 50 μg/hr is helpful prior to endoscopy
- consider IV erythromycin prior to gastroscopy to remove clots from stomach

Prognosis
- 80% stop spontaneously
- peptic ulcer bleeding: low mortality (2%) unless rebleeding occurs (25% of patients, 10% mortality)
- endoscopic predictors of rebleeding: spurt or ooze, visible vessel, fibrin clot
- H_2 antagonists have little impact on rebleeding rates and need for surgery
- esophageal varices have a high rebleeding rate (55%) and mortality (29%)

Aortoenteric Fistula is a rare and lethal cause of GI bleed, most common in patients with a history of aortic graft surgery. Therefore, perform endoscopy or surgery if suspicion arises.
Note: The window of opportunity is narrow. Suspect if abdominal pain is associated with bleeding. Act fast to prevent death.

Always ask about NSAID/aspirin intake or anticoagulant therapy in GI bleed.

Forrest Classification of Peptic Ulcers

Forrest Class	Type of lesion	Risk of Rebleed (%)
I	Arterial Bleeding (oozing/spurting)	55-100
IIa	Visible Vessel	43
IIb	Sentinel Clot	22
IIc	Hematin Covered Flat Spot	10
III	No Stigmata of Hemorrhage	5

Reference: Forrest JA, Finlayson ND, Shearman DJ. Endoscopy in Gastrointestinal Bleeding. Lancet. 1974;(17),394-397.

Bleeding Peptic Ulcer

Clinical Features
- see *PUD*, G10

Treatment
- see Figure 8

**Bleeding Peptic Ulcers;
RFs for mortality**
Co-existent illness
Hemodynamic instability
Age >60 years
Transfusion required

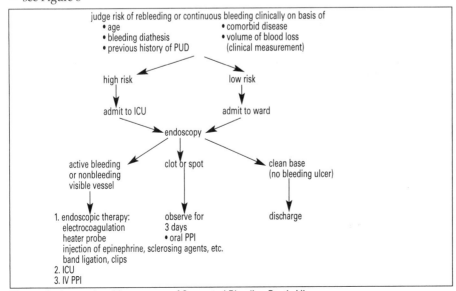

Figure 8. Approach to Management of Suspected Bleeding Peptic Ulcer

Intravenous Omeprazole vs. Placebo for Bleeding Peptic Ulcer Requiring Endoscopic Treatment
NEJM 2000; 343:310-316
Study: Randomized, double-blind placebo controlled trial.
Patients: 240 patients with actively bleeding ulcers or ulcers with non-bleeding visible vessels treated by endoscopic injection plus coagulation.
Intervention: IV omeprazole 80 mg followed by constant infusion 8 mg/h for 72 hours vs. placebo.
Main outcomes: Recurrent bleeding.
Results: Omeprazole decreased rates of recurrent bleeding (7% vs. 22%), surgery (p<0.001), all-cause mortality (p<0.001), but no statistically significant change in surgery or death.
Conclusion: Intravenous omeprazole reduces recurrent bleeding after endoscopic treatment of bleeding peptic ulcer.

Esophageal Varices

Clinical Features
- characteristically massive upper GI bleeding

Etiology
- almost always due to portal hypertension
- often accompanied by varices in stomach

Investigations
- endoscopy

Treatment
- see Figure 9

If varices isolated to stomach, think of splenic vein thrombosis.

Sclerotherapy and Octreotide for Acute Variceal Bleeding
NEJM 1995;333(9):555-60
Study: Randomized, double-blind, prospective trial.
Patients: 199 patients with cirrhosis and acute variceal bleeding
Intervention: Sclerotherapy with continuous octreotide infusion vs. sclerotherapy and placebo.
Main Outcome: Survival without rebleeding 5d after sclerotherapy
Results: After 5d, a higher proportion of patients survived without rebleeding in the octreotide group (87% vs 71%, p=0.009) and required less blood transfusions (1.2 vs. 2.0 units, p=0.006). The mean 15d cumulative survival rate was equal in both groups.
Conclusion: In patients with cirrhosis, sclerotherapy and octreotide were more effective than sclerotherapy alone in controlling acute variceal bleeding, but there was no difference in overall mortality rates.

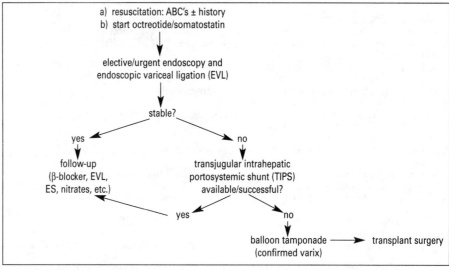

Figure 9. Management of Bleeding Esophageal Varices

Mallory-Weiss Tear

Definition
- longitudinal laceration in gastric mucosa on lesser curvature near GE junction (20% straddle junction, 5% in distal esophagus)

Etiology
- due to rapid increases in gastric pressure (i.e. retching-vomiting against a closed glottis)
- most patients abuse alcohol
- usually hiatus hernia present

Clinical Features
- hematemesis ± melena, classically following an episode of retching
- can lead to fatal hematemesis

Management
- 90% stop spontaneously; NG (if needed) and replacement of lost volume
- if persistent: endoscopy with injection ± clips or surgical repair

Variceal Ligation vs. Sclerotherapy for Acute Variceal Bleeding
J Hepatol 2006; 45(4):560-7
Study: Randomized controlled trial.
Patients: 179 patients with acute esophageal variceal bleeding and suspected cirrhosis.
Intervention: Sclerotherapy with continuous somatostatin infusion vs. variceal ligation with continuous somatostatin infusion.
Main Outcome: Therapeutic failure – failure to control acute bleeding episode or early rebleeding.
Results: Therapeutic failure occurred in 24% of patients treated with sclerotherapy compared to 10% of those treated with ligation (RR=2.4). Failure to control bleeding higher in sclerotherapy group (15% vs. 4%; p=0.02). Higher proportion of patients with sclerotherapy had serious side effects (13% vs. 4%; p=0.01).
Conclusion: The use of variceal ligation, compared to sclerotherapy as emergency endoscopic therapy for the treatment of acute variceal bleeding, significantly improves the efficacy and safety.

Lower Gastrointestinal Bleeding

Definition
- bleed distal to ligament of Treitz

Clinical Features
- hematochezia (see Figure 10)
- anemia
- occult blood in stool
- rarely melena

Etiology

- rule out upper source
- vascular
  - angiodysplasia
  - hemorrhoids
- neoplasm
  - cancer
  - polyps
- inflammation
  - colitis
  - infection

When suspecting lower GI bleed, first and foremost exclude upper GI bleeding before localizing the site of the lower GI bleed.

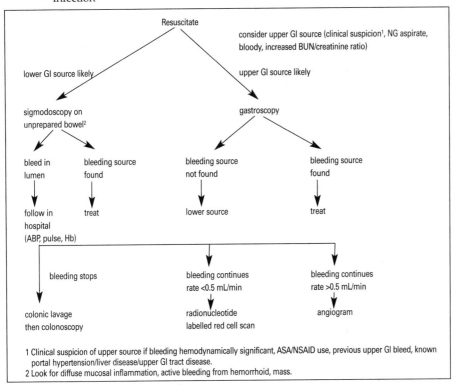

1 Clinical suspicion of upper source if bleeding hemodynamically significant, ASA/NSAID use, previous upper GI bleed, known portal hypertension/liver disease/upper GI tract disease.
2 Look for diffuse mucosal inflammation, active bleeding from hemorrhoid, mass.

Figure 10. Approach to Hematochezia

Lower GI Bleed
Most common cause of LGIB "**CHAND**":
- **C**olitis (radiation, infectious, ischemic, IBD [UC > CD])
- **H**emorrhoids/fissure
- **A**ngiodysplasia
- **N**eoplastic
- **D**iverticular disease

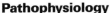

Colon Cancer

- see <u>General Surgery</u>

Etiology/Epidemiology

- environmental influences (presumed)
  - high dietary fat consumption
  - low dietary fibre consumption
- genetic influences
  - all colorectal cancers considered to have genetic component, to varying degrees
  - familial syndromes (see *Familial Colon Cancer Syndromes* section, G31)
  - multiple "step-wise" somatic mutations, contributed by environment, have been implicated
  - genetic changes implicated are
    - activation of proto-oncogenes (K-ras)
    - loss of tumour-suppressor gene activity (APC, DCC)
    - abnormalities in DNA repair genes (hMSH2, hMLH1), especially HNPCC syndromes (see *Familial Colon Cancer Syndromes* section, G31)

Some colon cancers may bleed intermittently or not at all.
No bleeding ≠ no cancer.

Melena more often seen with right-sided tumours.
Hematochezia more often seen with left-sided tumours.

Pathophysiology

- normal colon → hyperproliferative epithelium → adenoma → carcinoma

Colorectal Cancer Screening -
Canadian Association of Gastroenterology, Can J Gastroenterol 2004;18(2).

People at average risk:
>50, no family history should undergo one of:
• FOBT every 2 years
• Flexible sigmoidoscopy every 5 years
• Combined FOBT and flex sig every 5 years
• Double contrast barium enema every 5 years
• Colonoscopy every 10 years

People at above-average risk:
• HNPCC – Genetic testing + colonoscopy q 2 years beginning at age 20
• FAP – Genetic testing + sigmoidoscopy annually beginning at age 10-12
• Fam Hx of cancer/polyps but does not fit criteria for HNPCC/FAP – colonscopy q 5 years beginning at age 40, or 10 years earlier than the youngest diagnosed polyp/cancer case in the family.

Risk Factors
• 75% of new cases are in people with no known RF
• age
  ▪ 90% of cancers are in people >50 years old
  ▪ person 50 years old has 5% chance of developing colorectal cancer by 80 years old
• adenomatous polyps
• family history
  ▪ sporadic cancer
    ♦ risk increases 1.8 times for those with one affected relative, 2-6 times with two affected relatives
    ♦ risk is greater if relative has cancer diagnosed <45 years old
  ▪ familial adenomatous polyposis and Gardner's syndrome (see *Familial Colon Cancer Syndromes*, G31)
  ▪ hereditary nonpolyposis colorectal cancer (Lynch syndrome, or HNPCC) (see *Familial Colon Cancer Syndromes*, G31)
• Inflammatory Bowel Disease (IBD)
  ▪ ulcerative colitis (UC) – after 10 years with the disease, cancer risk ↑ by 1% for each additional year
  ▪ Crohn's disease - exact risk of cancer remains unclear, but many think it is similar to UC

Prevention
• some evidence to support:
  ▪ increase fibre in diet, decrease animal fat and red meat, decrease smoking and EtOH, increase exercise and decrease BMI
  ▪ secondary prevention with screening (see side bar)

Prognosis
• actuarial survival (5 year)
  ▪ stage 1 (limited to wall of bowel): 95%
  ▪ stage 2 (through wall of bowel): 80%
  ▪ stage 3 (into lymph nodes): 50%

Treatment (see General Surgery)

Colorectal Polyps

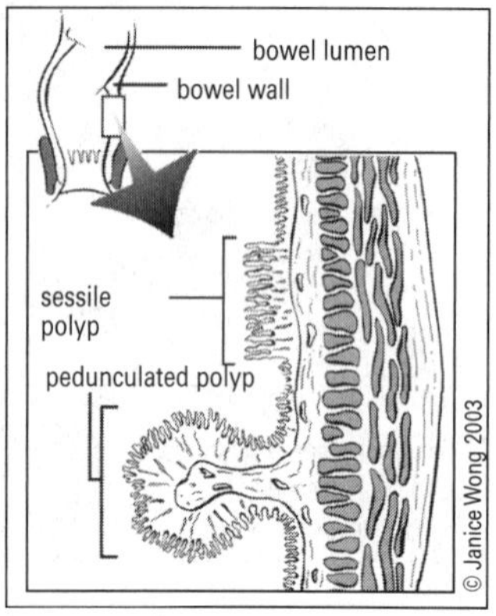

Definition
• polyp: small mucosal outgrowth into the lumen of the colon or rectum
• sessile (flat) or pedunculated (on a stalk) – see Figure 11

Epidemiology
• 30% of population have polyps by age 50, 40% by age 60, 50% by age 70

Clinical Features
• 50% in the rectosigmoid region, 50% are multiple
• usually asymptomatic, but may have rectal bleeding, change in bowel habits
• usually detected during routine endoscopy or family screening

Pathology
• hyperplastic – most common, no malignant potential
• pseudopolyps – inflammatory, associated with IBD, no malignant potential
• hamartomas: juvenile polyps (large bowel), Peutz-Jegher syndrome (small bowel)
  ▪ malignant risk due to associated adenomas (large bowel)
  ▪ low malignant potential → most spontaneously regress or autoamputate
• adenomas – premalignant, carcinoma *in situ* may occur
  ▪ some may contain invasive carcinoma ("malignant polyp" – 2.6-9.4%): invasion into muscularis
  ▪ tubular, villous, tubulovillous (see Table 13)

Figure 11. Sessile and pedunculated polyps

bowel lumen
bowel wall
sessile polyp
pedunculated polyp
© Janice Wong 2003

Table 13. Characteristics of Tubular vs. Villous Polyps

	Tubular	Villous
Incidence	Common (60% to 80%)	Less common (10%)
Size	Small (<2 cm)	Large (usually >2 cm)
Attachment	Pedunculated/sessile	Sessile
Malignant potential	Lower	Higher
Distribution	Even	Left-sided predominance

'**Amsterdam' Criteria for HNPCC diagnosis:**
• 3 relatives with colorectal cancer, where 1 is 1st degree relative of other 2
• 2 generations of colorectal cancer
• 1 colorectal cancer before age 50

Investigations
- flexible sigmoidoscope can reach 60% of polyps in men and 35% of polyps in women; if polyps detected, proceed to colonoscopy for examination of entire bowel and biopsy
- colonoscopy still the gold standard

Treatment
- endoscopic polypectomy; surgical segmental resection if unsuccessful/impossible
- follow-up for adenomas: repeat colonoscopy in 5 years, in 3 years if polyp diameter >1 cm, >3 adenomas, sessile, high grade dysplasia, villous

Familial Colon Cancer Syndromes

FAMILIAL ADENOMATOUS POLYPOSIS (FAP)

Pathogenesis
- autosomal dominant (AD) inheritance, mutation in APC gene on 5q
- plays a major role in sporadic cancer

Clinical Features
- hundreds to thousands of colonic adenomas by an average age of 40
- extracolonic manifestations:
  - carcinoma of duodenum, bile duct, pancreas, stomach, thyroid, adrenal, small bowel
  - congenital hypertrophy of retinal pigment epithelium presents early in life in 2/3 of patients
- virtually 100% lifetime risk of colon cancer (because of number of polyps)
- variants:
  - Gardner's syndrome: FAP + extraintestinal lesions (chiefly bone, desmoid tumours)
  - Turcot's syndrome: FAP + CNS tumours

Note that rectal cancers have a higher recurrence rate and lower 5-year survival rate than colon cancers. Therefore, do a rectal exam.

Investigations
- genetic testing (80-95% sensitive, 99-100% specific)
  - see sidebar for criteria for genetic screening referral
- if no polyposis found: annual flexible sigmoidoscopy from puberty to age 50, then regular screening

Treatment
- surgery indicated by age 17-20
- total proctocolectomy with ileostomy OR total colectomy with ileorectal anastomosis
- doxorubicin-based chemotherapy for intra-abdominal desmoids

Referral Criteria for Genetic Screening for APC
- To confirm the diagnosis of FAP (in patients with ≥100 colorectal adenomas)
- To provide pre-symptomatic testing for individuals at risk for FAP (1st degree relatives who are ≥10 years old)
- To confirm the diagnosis of attenuated FAP (in patients with ≥20 colorectal adenomas)

HEREDITARY NON-POLYPOSIS COLORECTAL CANCER (HNPCC)

Pathogenesis
- AD inheritance, mutation in a DNA mismatch repair gene resulting in genomic instability and subsequent mutations
- plays a minor role in sporadic cancer

Clinical Features
- early age of onset, right > left colon, synchronous and metachronous lesions
- mean age of cancer presentation is 44 years, lifetime risk 70-80% (greater for men)
  - Lynch syndrome I: hereditary site-specific colon cancer
  - Lynch syndrome II: cancer family syndrome – high rates of extracolonic tumours (endometrial, ovarian, hepatobiliary, small bowel)

Diagnosis
- diagnosis is clinical – based on Amsterdam Criteria:
  1. at least 3 relatives with colorectal cancer, and one must be 1st degree relative of the other two
  2. two or more generations involved
  3. one case must be diagnosed before 50 years old
  4. FAP is excluded

Investigations
- genetic testing (80% sensitive) – colonoscopy mandatory even if negative
  - refer for genetic screening individuals who fulfill EITHER the Amsterdam Criteria (as above) OR the revised Bethesda criteria (see sidebar)
- colonoscopy (starting age 20) every 1-2 years
- surveillance for extracolonic lesions (controversial, no guidelines available)

Revised Bethesda Criteria – Refer for genetic screening for HNPCC
- Individuals with cancer in families that meet the Amsterdam criteria
- Patients with two HNPCC-related cancers, including synchronous and metachronous colorectal cancer or associated extracolonic cancers (endometrial, ovarian, gastric, hepatobiliary, small bowel, or transitional cell carcinoma of the renal pelvis or ureter).
- Patients with colorectal cancer and a first degree relative with colorectal cancer and/or HNPCC-related extracolonic cancer and/or a colorectal adenoma with one of the cancers diagnosed before age 45 years, and the adenoma diagnosed before age 40 years.
- Patients with right-sided colorectal cancer having an undifferentiated pattern (solid/cribriform) on histopathologic diagnosis before age 45 years.
- Patients with signet-ring cell type colorectal cancer diagnosed before age 45.
- Patients with adenomas diagnosed before age 40.

Treatment
- subtotal colectomy and ileosigmoid or ileorectal anastomosis with yearly proctoscopy/sigmoidoscopy

Liver

Basic Anatomy Review

Anatomy and Physiology

* composed of 4 lobes (left, right, caudate, quadrate) and divided into 8 segments
* the liver performs several important functions including:
    * carbohydrate/lipid metabolism
    * coagulation factor production (excluding factor VIII)
    * bile production
    * drug metabolism/detoxification
* blood supply
    * arterial and venous supply:
        * hepatic artery (from celiac artery)
        * portal vein (from splenic vein and superior mesenteric vein)
    * venous drainage:
        * hepatic veins (left, middle, right which drain to inferior vena cava)

Liver Functions
* glucose homeostasis
* plasma protein synthesis
* lipid and lipoprotein synthesis
* bile acid synthesis and secretion
* vitamin A,D,E,K,B$_{12}$ storage
* biotransformation, detoxification
* excretion of endogenous and
* exogenous compounds

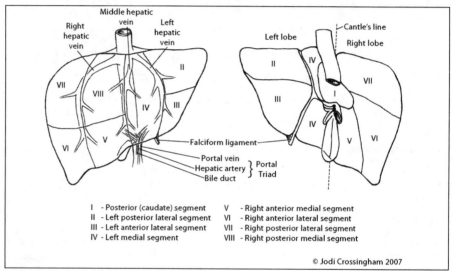

I   - Posterior (caudate) segment   V   - Right anterior medial segment
II - Left posterior lateral segment VI   - Right anterior lateral segment
III - Left anterior lateral segment   VII - Right posterior lateral segment
IV - Left medial segment   VIII - Right posterior medial segment

© Jodi Crossingham 2007

Figure 12. Liver Anatomy

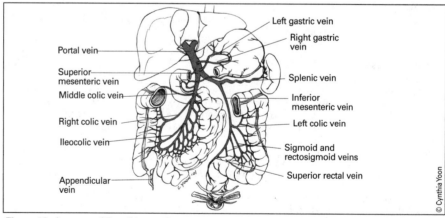

Figure 13. Anatomy of Portal Venous System

Investigations of Liver Function

Prothrombin Time (PT)
- daily marker of hepatic protein synthesis
- must exclude co-existing vitamin K deficiency

Serum Bilirubin
- product of heme metabolism in the RES of liver and spleen
- must exclude extrahepatic causes of hyperbilirubinemia

Serum Albumin Level
- detects prolonged (weeks) hepatic dysfunction
- must exclude malnutrition and renal or GI losses, acute illness

All clotting factors except factor VIII are exclusively synthesized in the liver.

Order of deterioration of Liver Function Tests:
1. ↑PT/INR
2. ↑bilirubin
3. ↓albumin

Hepatobiliary Disease Lab Tests

- ↑ AST, ALT = hepatocellular damage
  - ALT more specific to liver; AST from multiple sources
    - elevation of both highly suggestive of liver injury
  - implies hepatitis (inflammation) or vascular injury (ischemia)
  - if AST, ALT >1000, think of common bile duct stone, virus, drugs, ischemia, autoimmune hepatitis
- ↑ ALP with ↑ GGT = cholestatic disease
  - biochemical cholestasis (drugs)
  - systemic disease (e.g. sepsis), pregnancy
  - infiltrative disease (tumour, fat, lymphoma)
  - mass lesions (stone, tumour, abscess)
- Inflammatory (PBC, PSC)

Hepatitis

Etiology
- viral infection
- alcohol
- drugs
- immune-mediated
- toxins

Acute Viral Hepatitis

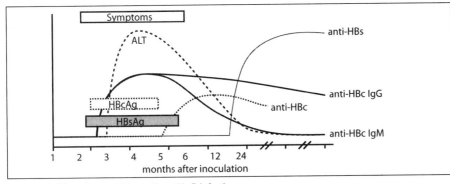

Figure 14. Time Course of Acute Hepatitis B Infection

Serum transaminases >1000 due to
- viral hepatitis
- drugs
- common bile duct stone
- hepatic ischemia
- rarely immune hepatitis

AST > ALT (usually AST/ALT >2 and AST <300) = alcoholic liver disease
ALT > AST = viral hepatitis

Fulminant Hepatic Failure

- (1) rapid (characteristically less than 8 weeks) development of hepatocellular dysfunction (usually including high bilirubin, INR)
  (2) encephalopathy (due to cerebral edema)
  (3) no prior history of liver disease
- causes: drugs, especially acetaminophen, hepatitis B (ask for serum HBV-DNA because sometimes HBsAg rapidly becomes negative), hepatitis A, exacerbation of chronic disease (Note: hepatitis C is rare in this setting); idiopathic; ischemic
- management: usually in ICU, correct hypoglycemia, monitor level of consciousness (some centres still use intracranial pressure monitoring), prevent GI bleeding with proton pump inhibitor, vigilant for infection and multiorgan failure

Risk of developing infection from needle puncture
HBV   30%
HCV   3%
HIV   0.3%

- consider liver biopsy before INR becomes too high; chief value is to exclude chronic disease, less helpful for prognosis
- liver transplant: consider early, especially if 1) rapid deterioration, 2) age <10 or >40, cause is drug or unknown, bilirubin >300, INR >3.5, creatinine >200

Chronic Hepatitis

Definition
- an increase in serum transaminases for >6 months; requires a liver biopsy to determine severity/need of treatment

Etiology
- viral (B, B+D, C, not A or E)
- drugs (methyldopa, INH, nitrofurantoin, amiodarone)
- autoimmune
- genetic (Wilson's disease, α_1-antitrypsin deficiency)
- metabolic (nonalcoholic steatohepatitis: NASH)

Clinical Features
- often asymptomatic, detected incidentally
- constitutional symptoms
- fatigue, malaise, anorexia, weight loss
- signs of chronic liver disease
- hepatomegaly (firm) and splenomegaly
- ↑ AST, ALT

Chronic Hepatitis B (HBV)

Table 14. Hepatitis B Serology

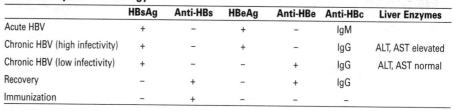

	HBsAg	Anti-HBs	HBeAg	Anti-HBe	Anti-HBc	Liver Enzymes
Acute HBV	+	–	+	–	IgM	
Chronic HBV (high infectivity)	+	–	+	–	IgG	ALT, AST elevated
Chronic HBV (low infectivity)	+	–	–	+	IgG	ALT, AST normal
Recovery	–	+	–	+	IgG	
Immunization	–	+	–	–	–	

Epidemiology
- 4 Patterns: all have positive HBsAg
  - (a) Immune Tolerance: active virus replication with high HBV-DNA, HBeAg positive, but normal ALT/AST, characteristic of perinatal infection (or 'incubation period' in adult-acquired)
  - (b) Immune Clearance: active virus replication, HBeAg positive, HBV-DNA >100,000 copies/ml, characterized by progressive disease without treatment, sometimes to cirrhosis and/or hepatocellular carcinoma; most likely to benefit from treatment
  - (c) Immune Carrier: virus slowly replicating with HBV-DNA <100,000 copies/ml, HBeAg negative, ALT/AST normal, risk of reactivation to pattern (b) especially with immunosuppression such as corticosteroids, lymphoma, reactivation clinically resembles acute hepatitis B
  - (d) Reactivation: "core or precore mutant" = active virus replication with HBV-DNA >100 copies/ml, HBeAg negative because of promoter gene mutation, ALT/AST high, tends to progress, treatment difficult therefore prognosis poor

Hepatitis D
- defective RNA virus requiring HBsAg for entry into hepatocyte, therefore infects only patients with hepatitis B, causes more aggressive disease than hepatitis B virus alone
- co-infection: acquire HDV and HBV together
  - better prognosis than superinfection
- superinfection: acquire HDV once patient already has chronic HBV
  - HDV can present as FHF and/or accelerate progression to cirrhosis

Chronic Hepatitis B + D

- low-dose interferon has limited impact, high-dose under investigation
- liver transplant more effective than in HBV alone
- liver transplant for end stage disease (reinfection rate 100% but infection usually mild)

IFN and Ribavirin for Hepatitis C
NEJM 1998;339(21): 1485-92
Study: Randomized efficacy trial.
Patients: 912 patients with chronic hepatitis C.
Intervention: IFN α-2b alone or in combination with ribavirin for 24 or 48 weeks.
Main outcomes: Efficacy as assessed by serum HCV RNA, AST/ALT, and liver biopsy.
Results: The rate of sustained virologic response (undetectable HCV RNA level 24 wks after treatment completion) was higher in the IFN + ribavirin group (31% vs. 6%, p<0.001). Drug doses had to be reduced and treatment discontinued more often in patients on combination therapy.
Conclusion: In patients with chronic hepatitis C, initial treatment with IFN + ribavirin was more effective than treatment with IFN alone.

Causes of a Spike in Serum Transaminases in Chronic Hepatitis B
- Reactivation (anti-HBe converting to HBeAg; occurs especially with immunosuppression)
- Seroconversion (HBeAg converting to anti-HBe; especially with Rx such as interferon)
- Hepatitis D
- Hepatocellular carcinoma
- Liver insult (alcohol, drugs, hepatitis A)
- Progression of disease

HDV increases severity of hepatitis but does not increase risk of progression to chronic hepatitis.

Autoimmune Chronic Active Hepatitis

- can be severe: 40% mortality at 6 months without treatment
- diagnosis of exclusion: rule out viruses, drugs, metabolic or genetic derangements
- extrahepatic manifestations
  - amenorrhea, rashes, acne, thyroiditis, Sjögren's
  - immune complex disease: arthritis, GN, vasculitis
- antibodies
  - hypergammaglobulinemia
  - ANA (antinuclear antibody homogenous), RF (rheumatoid factor), anti-smooth muscle, anti-LKM (liver kidney microsome)
  - can have false positive viral serology (especially anti-HCV)
- management: steroids (80% respond) ± azathioprine

Drug-Induced Liver Disease

Table 15. Classification of Hepatotoxins

	Direct	Indirect
Example	Acetaminophen, CCl$_4$	Phenytoin, INH
Dose-dependence	Usual	Unusual
Latent Period	Hours-days	Weeks-months
Host Factors	Not important	Very important
Predictable	Yes	No

Specific Drugs

- acetaminophen
  - metabolized by hepatic cytochrome P450 system
  - can cause fulminant hepatic failure (transaminases >1,000 U/L)
  - requires 10-15 g in normals, 4-6 g in alcoholics/anticonvulsant users
  - recent studies have emphasized liver disease in chronic users >4 g/day
  - mechanism: high acetaminophen dose saturates glucuronidation and sulfation elimination pathway → reactive metabolite is formed → covalently binds to hepatocyte membrane
  - presentation
    - first 24 hrs: nausea and vomiting usually within 4-12 hours
    - next 24-48 hrs: hepatic necrosis resulting in ↑ aminotransferases, jaundice, possibly hepatic encephalopathy, acute renal failure, death
    - after 48 hrs: continued hepatic necrosis/resolution
    - note: potential delay in presentation in sustained-release products
  - blood levels of acetaminophen correlate with the severity of hepatic injury, particularly if time of ingestion known
  - therapy
    - gastric lavage/emesis (if <2 hrs after ingestion)
    - oral charcoal
    - N-acetylcysteine (Mucomyst™) can be given PO or IV, most effective within 8-10 hours of ingestion, but should be given no matter when time of ingestion; promotes hepatic glutathione synthesis
    - no recorded fatal outcomes if NAC given before increase in transaminases
- chlorpromazine
  - cholestasis in 1% after 4 weeks; often with fever, rash, jaundice, pruritus and eosinophilia
- INH
  - 20% develop elevated transaminases but <1% develop clinically significant disease
  - susceptibility to injury increases with age
- methotrexate
  - may rarely cause cirrhosis, especially in the presence of obesity, diabetes, alcoholism
  - scarring develops without symptoms or changes in liver enzymes, therefore biopsy may be needed in long-term treatment
- amiodarone
  - can cause same histology and clinical outcome as alcoholic hepatitis
- others
  - azoles, statins, methyldopa, phenytoin, PTU, rifampin, sulfonamides, tetracyclines
- Herbs
  - chaparral, chinese herbs (e.g. germander, comfrey, bush tea)

Table 16. Characteristics of the Viral Hepatitides

Hepatitis	Clinical presentation	Definition	Communicability	Investigation	Treatment	Prognosis	Complications
Acute Viral Hepatitis	Most subclinical Prodrome: flu-like, may precede jaundice by 1-2 weeks	<6 months	variable	AST, ALT, ALP, bilirubin	Supportive (hydrate, diet) Hospitalize if: encephalopathy, coagulopathy, severe vomiting, hypoglycemia	Poor prognosis: Comorbidities, Bili, INR, ↑Alb, hypoglycemia	Hepatocellular necrosis: AST, ALT>10-20x normal, ALP and bilirubin minimally ↑ Cholestasis

Virus	Transmission	Incubation	Communicability	Serology	Management	Prognosis	Complications
Hepatitis A	Fecal-oral	2-6 weeks	2-3 weeks in late incubation to early clinical phase acute hepatitis in most adults, 10% of children		General hygiene Treat close contacts (anti-HAV Ig, 0.02 mg/kg ASAP) Prophylaxis for high-risk groups (HAV vaccine ± HAV Ig) unless immune		
Hepatitis B	Parenteral or equivalent Vertical	6 weeks – 6 months	During HBsAg+ state highly communicable ↑during T3 or early post-partum	See Table 14 HBeAg+ state	HBV vaccine and/or Hepatitis B Ig (HBIG): for needlestick, sexual contact, infants of infected mothers unless already immune	Chronicity in 5%	Serum sickness-like syndrome Glomerulonephritis Cryoglobulinemia Polyarteritis nodosa Porphyria cutanea tarda
Hepatitis C	Parenteral (transfusion, IVDU, sexual < HBV) 40% have no known risk factors	5-10 weeks		HCV RNA (detected by PCR) Anti-HCV (IgG/IgM)	Prevention (no vaccine) Rx: IFN + ribavirin	Chronicity in 80%	
Hepatitis D	Non-parenteral (close contact in endemic areas) Parenteral (blood products, IVDU)		Infectious only in presence of HBV (HBsAg required for replication)	HBsAg Anti-HDV (IgG/IgM)	Prevention HBV vaccine		Predisposes HBV carriers to severe fulminant course
Hepatitis E	Fecal-oral (endemic: Africa, Asia, central America, India, Pakistan)	2-6 weeks		Anti-HEV (IgG/IgM)	Prevention (no vaccine)		Mild, except in third trimester (10-20% fulminant liver failure)

Chronic Hepatitis	Epidemiology		Time Course	Diagnosis	Management		Prognosis
Chronic Hepatitis C	50% of chronic hepatitis Commonest indication for liver transplant		At 10 years: chronic hepatitis At 20 years: cirrhosis At 30 years: HCC	Serum HCV-RNA Anti-HCV (+)	Minimize alcohol intake Strict blood precautions Vaccinate for Hep A,B HCC screen with U/S and serum alpha fetoprotein (AFP) Rx: Pegylated interferon a2a or 2b + ribavarin		20% progress to cirrhosis 3% of cirrhotics develop HCC
Chronic Hepatitis B	1-2% of healthy adults with acute hepatitis B 90% if infected at birth		Replicative Phase (HBeAg+) - infectivity Non-reactive Phase (AntiHBe+) - ?infectivity		Limit alcohol intake Blood/sex precautions Hepatoma screen Rx: interferon, lamivudine, adefovir, entecavir, tenofivir, telbirudine		If HBV-DNA: (-) warn of reactivity (+) warn of progression into cirrhosis If ALT/AST: HCC, Hep D, reactivation, flare if known to be HBeAg (+), progression of disease, superimposed acute hepatitis
Chronic Hepatitis B+D					Liver Transplant		

Wilson's Disease

Definition
- autosomal recessive defect in copper metabolism; gene (ATP7B) has been cloned

Pathology
- ↓ rate of copper incorporation into ceruloplasmin and ↓ biliary excretion of copper

Clinical Manifestations
- slow accumulation of copper with deposition in tissues
- liver: cirrhosis, chronic active hepatitis, acute hepatitis, fulminant liver failure, low risk of HCC
- eyes: Kayser-Fleischer rings (copper in Descemet's membrane); more common in patients with CNS involvement
- CNS: basal ganglia (wing flapping tremor, Parkinsonism), cerebellum (dysarthria, dysphagia, incoordination, ataxia), cerebrum (psychosis, affective disorder)
- kidneys: Fanconi's syndrome (proximal tubule transport defects) and stones
- blood: intravascular hemolysis; may be initial presentation in fulminant hepatitis
- joints: arthritis, bone demineralization, calcifications

> **Clinical manifestions of Wilson's disease: ABCD**
> **A**sterixis
> **B**asal ganglia degeneration
> **C**eruloplasmin ↓
> **C**irrhosis
> **C**orneal deposits (KF ring)
> **C**opper ↑
> **C**horeiform movements
> **C**arcinoma (HCC)
> **D**ementia

Investigations
- suspect if increase liver function test (LFTs) with clinical manifestations; especially combination of liver disease with trauma, dystonia, psychiatric symptoms
- screening tests:
  - 1. reduced serum ceruloplasmin
  - 2. Kayser-Fleischer rings (usually require slit-lamp examination)
  - 3. increased urinary copper excretion
- gold standards:
  - 1. increased copper on liver biopsy by qualitative assay
  - 2. haplotype analysis

Treatment
- chelators (penicillamine, trientine): ↑ urinary excretion of copper
- zinc acetate
  - blocks intestinal absorption of copper
  - sequesters excess copper
- screen relatives
- liver transplant in severe cases

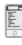

Hemochromatosis

Definition
- excess iron storage, which causes multiorgan system dysfunction with total body stores of iron ↑ to 20-40 g (normal 1 g)

Etiology
- may be primary or secondary
- primary hemochromatosis
  - due to common recessive gene (5%); 1/400 patients are homozygotes
  - results in ↑ gut absorption of iron
- secondary hemochromatosis
  - parenteral iron overload: transfusion
  - chronic hemolytic anemia: thalassemia, pyruvate kinase deficiency
  - excessive iron intake

Clinical Features
- usually presents with trivial elevation in serum transaminases or during screening
- liver: cirrhosis 30% get HCC (200x ↑ risk); most common cause of death (1/3 of patients)
- pancreas: "bronze" diabetes, chronic pancreatitis
- skin: bronze or grey (due to melanin, not iron)
- heart: dilated cardiomyopathy
- pituitary: hypogonadotropic hypogonadism (impotence, ↓ libido, amenorrhea)
- joints: arthralgia (especially MCP joints of hands), chondrocalcinosis

Investigations
- screening for individuals with clinical features and/or family history (1/4 chance of sibling having the disease)
  - transferrin saturation (free Fe/TIBC) >50%
  - serum ferritin >400
- HFE gene analysis: 90% of idiopathic hemochromatosis have Cys 282 Tyr (C282Y) gene mutation, or less frequently His 63 Asp (H63D)
- liver biopsy (to define degree of iron overload and to detect cirrhosis)
- hepatoma screening if cirrhosis

Treatment
- phlebotomy: once or twice weekly until anemia develops or serum iron and ferritin normalizes; then lifelong maintenance phlebotomies q 2-6 months
- deferoxamine if phlebotomy contraindicated (e.g. cardiomyopathy, anemia)
- primary hemachromatosis responds well to phlebotomy (secondary hemochromatosis responds poorly)

Prognosis
- normal life expectancy if treated before the development of cirrhosis or diabetes

13 g ethanol = 1 beer = 4 oz wine = 1.5 oz liquor

GI Complications of Alcohol Abuse

Esophagus:
Mallory-Weiss tear
Esophageal varices (secondary to portal hypertension)

Stomach:
Alcoholic gastritis

Pancreas:
Acute pancreatitis
Chronic pancreatitis

Liver:
Alcoholic hepatitis
Fatty liver
Cirrhosis
Hepatic encephalopathy
Portal hypertension (secondary to cirrhosis)
Ascites (secondary to cirrhosis)
Hepatoma (secondary to cirrhosis)

Biopsy + histology of alcoholic hepatitis (triad)
- hepatocyte necrosis with surrounding inflammation in zone III
- Mallory bodies (intracellular eosinophilic aggregates of cytokeratins)
- spider fibrosis (network of intralobular connective tissue surrounding cells and venules)

Alcoholic Liver Disease

Types of Lesions
- fatty liver (all alcoholics): always reversible
- alcoholic hepatitis (35% of alcoholics): usually reversible
- cirrhosis (10-15% of alcoholics): irreversible

Pathophysiology
- several mechanisms that are incompletely understood
- fatty liver related to ↑ NADPH → fatty acid and triglyceride formation
- EtOH impairs release of triglycerides causing accumulation in the liver
- acetaldehyde is probably a direct toxin
  - combines with hapten → immunological damage
- alcohol metabolism causes
  - relative hypoxia in liver zone III > zone I
  - necrosis and hepatic vein sclerosis
- alcohol causes liver cells to swell
  - turbulence in sinusoids
  - deposition of collagen in the space of Disse
  - portal hypertension

Clinical Features
- threshold for cirrhosis is >20-40 g EtOH/day in females or >60-80 g EtOH/day in males x 10-20 years; develops in >15% of those who consume this amount daily on a continuous basis
- clinical findings do not predict type of liver involvement
- fatty liver
  - mildly tender hepatomegaly; jaundice rare
  - mildly ↑ transaminases <5x normal
- alcoholic hepatitis
  - variable severity: mild to fatal liver failure
  - clinically similar to viral or toxic injury
  - constitutional symptoms ± fever, abdominal distention, jaundice, tender hepatomegaly, splenomegaly (1/3)
- blood tests are non-specific, but in general
  - AST:ALT > 2:1 (usually <300) due to B6 deficiency
  - ↑ GGT, ↑ triglycerides, ↑ INR
  - ↑ mean corpuscular volume (MCV), ↓ platelets (suggests alcohol abuse)

Treatment
- alcohol cessation (see Psychiatry)
  - Alcoholics Anonymous, disulfuram, lithium, naltrexone
- multivitamin supplements (with extra thiamine)
- caution giving drugs metabolized by the liver
- prednisone (if discriminanat function >32)
  - has been shown to decrease mortality in a severely ill subgroup with alcoholic hepatitis characterized by ↑ bilirubin, ↑ INR, encephalopathy, but no GI bleeding
- pentoxyphilline decreases TNF, shown in one trial to reduce mortality in alcoholic hepatitis, now widely used because so few side effects

Prognosis
- fatty liver: rapid and complete resolution with cessation of EtOH intake
- alcoholic hepatitis mortality
  - immediate: 5%
  - with continued alcohol: 70% in 5 years
  - with cessation: 30% in 5 years
- discriminant function (DF)
  - based on PT/INR + bilirubin

Non-Alcoholic Fatty Liver Disease (NAFLD)

Etiology/Epidemiology
- spectrum of disorders characterised by macrovesicular hepatic steatosis
- commonest cause of liver disease in North America

Pathophysiology
- pathogenesis not well elucidated; insulin resistance implicated as key mechanism, leading to hepatic steatosis
- changes indistinguishable from those of alcoholic hepatitis despite negligible history of alcohol consumption

Risk Factors
- characteristically develops in middle-aged, overweight women
- obesity (69-100% of cases)
- type II diabetes
- hypertriglyceridemia
- severe weight loss

Clinical Features/Investigations
- often asymptomatic
- may present with fatigue, malaise and vague RUQ discomfort
- elevated serum triglyceride/cholesterol levels and insulin resistance
- elevated serum AST, ALT +/- ALP; AST/ALT <1
- presents as echogenic liver texture on ultrasound
- liver biopsy diagnostic (if lack of alcohol excess can be verified) but often necessary only for prognosis

Management
- no proven effective therapy
- modification of risk factors is generally recommended, particularly gradual weight reduction
- optimization of therapy for type II diabetes recommended

Prognosis
- better prognosis than alcoholic hepatitis; fewer than 25% progress to cirrhosis over a 7-10 year period
- Risk of progression increases if inflammation or scarring alongside fat infiltration (NASH)
- clinical indicators of unfavourable prognosis: age, impaired fasting glucose and higher body mass index
- biopsy studies have revealed stabilization of disease or regression of fibrosis in up to 2/3 of patients

Cirrhosis

Definition
- diffuse, irreversible fibrosis plus hepatocellular nodular regeneration
- decompensated cirrhosis: means development of ascites +/- increased bilirubin +/- encephalopathy +/- increased INR

Etiology
- alcohol (85%)
- chronic viral hepatitis (B, B+D, C but not A nor E)
- autoimmune
- hemochromatosis
- α-1-antitrypsin deficiency
- drugs and toxins

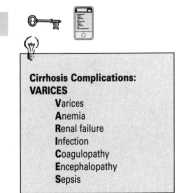

Cirrhosis Complications:
VARICES
- **V**arices
- **A**nemia
- **R**enal failure
- **I**nfection
- **C**oagulopathy
- **E**ncephalopathy
- **S**epsis

- methotrexate
- biliary cirrhosis
  - primary
  - secondary
- chronic hepatic congestion
  - cardiac cirrhosis (chronic right heart failure, constrictive pericarditis)
  - hepatic vein thrombosis (Budd-Chiari)
- idiopathic
- rare – Wilson's disease, Gaucher's

Diagnosis
- definitive diagnosis is histologic (liver biopsy)
- other tests may be suggestive:
  - blood work: liver enzymes, bilirubin, PT/PTT, increased gamma globulin, decreased albumin
  - imaging: U/S is the primary imaging modality, then CT

Management
- treat underlying disorder
- alcohol cessation
- follow patient for complications (see below)
- prognostic factors include (see Table 17)
  - nutrition (EtOH consumption)
  - ascites
  - varices
  - encephalopathy
  - labs: albumin, INR, bilirubin, creatinine
- liver transplantation for end-stage disease if no alcohold for >6 months

Complications
- hematologic changes in cirrhosis
  - pancytopenia from hypersplenism
  - ↓ clotting factors
    - fibrin, thrombin, I, II, V, VII, IX, X
- renal failure in cirrhosis
  - classifications
    - pre-renal (usually due to over diuresis)
    - acute tubular necrosis (ATN)
    - hepatorenal syndrome
  - hepatorenal syndrome can occur at any time in severe liver disease, especially after:
    - overaggressive diuresis or large volume paracentesis
    - GI bleeding
    - sepsis
  - differentiate hepatorenal syndrome from pre-renal failure
    - prerenal azotemia = hepatorenal lab findings (see <u>Nephrology</u>)
    - clinical (very difficult)
    - intravenous fluid challenge (giving volume expanders improves prerenal failure but not hepatorenal syndrome)
    - pulmonary capillary wedge pressure measurements (PCWP) (preferable)
  - differentiate hepatorenal syndrome from ATN
    - treatment for hepatorenal syndrome is generally unsuccessful
      – vasopressin, octreotide, midodrine (↑ renal blood flow by ↑ systemic vascular resistance)
    - definitive treatment is liver transplant
- hepatopulmonary syndrome (HPS)
  - present in patients with the triad of:
    1) liver disease
    2) increased alveolar-arterial gradient while breathing room air, and
    3) evidence for intrapulmonary vascular abnormalities
  - majority of cases due to cirrhosis, though can be due to other chronic liver diseases, such as noncirrhotic portal hypertension
  - thought to arise from ventilation-perfusion mismatch, intrapulmonary shunting and limitation of oxygen diffusion (failure of damaged liver to clear circulating pulmonary vasodilators, versus the production of a vasodilating substance by the liver)
  - clinical features:
    - hyperdynamic circulation with cardiac output >7 L at rest and decreased pulmonary + systemic resistance
    - dyspnea, platypnea (increase in dyspnea in upright position, improved by recumbency) and orthodeoxia (desaturation in the upright position, improved by recumbency)
  - diagnosis via contrast-enhanced echocardiography; demonstrates intrapulmonary shunting
  - only proven treatment is liver transplantation

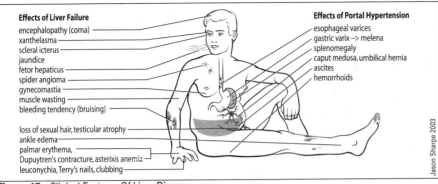

Figure 15. Clinical Features Of Liver Disease

Hepatocellular Carcinoma

- see General Surgery

Liver Transplant

- see General Surgery

Hepatic Encephalopathy

Definition
- acute neuropsychiatric syndrome secondary to liver disease

Pathophysiology
- porto-systemic shunt around hepatocytes and decreased hepatocelular function increases toxins (believed to be ammonia from gut, mercaptans, fatty acids, amino acids) to brain

Precipitating Factors
- nitrogen load (GI bleed, protein load from food intake, renal failure, constipation)
- drugs (narcotics + CNS depressants)
- electrolyte disturbance (hypokalemia, alkalosis, hypoxia, hypovolemia)
- infection (spontaneous bacterial peritonitis)
- deterioration in hepatic function or superimposed liver disease

Stages
- I: apathy, restlessness, reversal of sleep cycle, slowed intellect, impaired computational abilities, impaired handwriting
- II: asterixis, lethargy, drowsiness, disorientation
- III: stupor (rousable), hyperactive reflexes, extensor plantar responses
- IV: coma (response to painful stimuli only)

Investigations
- distinguish from non-liver-related neuropsychiatric disease in a patient with liver problems (e.g. alcohol withdrawal or intoxication, sedatives, subdural hematoma, metabolic encephalopathy)
- also distinguish from the causes of metabolic encephalopathy (e.g. renal failure, respiratory failure, severe hyponatremia, hypoglycemia); all easy to exclude/confirm
- diagnosis chiefly clinical, supported by laboratory findings, exclusion of other neuropsychiatric diseases
- only pathognomonic finding is fetor hepaticus
- characteristic EEG findings: diffuse (non-focal), slow, high amplitude waves

Treatment
- treat underlying liver disease and precipitating factors
- decrease generation of nitrogenous compounds
  - ↓ dietary protein to 50 g/day; vegetable protein is better tolerated than animal protein
  - lactulose
    - prevents diffusion of NH_3 (ammonia) from the colon into blood by lowering pH and forming non-diffusible NH_4^+ (ammonium)
    - serves as a substrate for incorporation of ammonia by bacteria, promotes growth in bowel lumen of bacteria which produce minimal ammonia
    - also acts as a laxative to eliminate nitrogen-producing bacteria from colon
- if inadequate response with lactulose, may try antibiotics
- broad-spectrum antibiotics (metronidazole, neomycin, rifaximin) eliminate ammonia-producing bacteria from bowel lumen
- neomycin is less effective than lactulose plus more side effects (ototoxicity, nephrotoxicity)

Precipitating Factors for Hepatic Encephalopathy:
Hemorrhage in GI tract/**H**yperkalemia
Excess dietary protein
Paracentesis
Acidosis/**A**nemia
Trauma
Infection
Colon surgery
Sedatives

- combination of the two may be more effective for resistant cases only
- avoid causing severe diarrhea with lactulose to decrease fluid/electrolyte problems
- best acute treatment in comatose patient is tap water enemas until clear

Portal Hypertension

Pathophysiology
- pressure = flow x resistance
- unlikely that ↑ flow alone can cause portal hypertension (although described in AV fistula or massive splenomegaly)
- 3 sites of ↑ resistance
  - pre-sinusoidal (e.g. portal vein thrombosis, schistosomiasis, sarcoidosis)
  - sinusoidal (e.g. cirrhosis, alcoholic hepatitis)
  - post-sinusoidal (e.g. right-sided heart failure, hepatic vein thrombosis, veno-occlusive disease, constrictive pericarditis)
- signs of portal hypertension: see sidebar

Management
- β-blockers (propanolol, nadolol) and nitrates decrease risk of bleeding from varices
- shunts
  - goal: decrease portal venous pressure
  - transjugular intrahepatic portosystemic shunt (TIPS): interventional radiologist creates a shunt between portal and hepatic vein via a catheter placed in the liver
  - can be used to stop acute bleeding or prevent rebleeding
  - shunt usually remains open for no longer than one year
  - other (rare): portocaval, distal spleno-renal (Warren shunt)

Portal Hypertension
Cause = ↑flow AND ↑resistance

Signs
Esophageal varices
Melena
Splenomegaly
Ascites
Hemorrhoids

Management
β-blockers
Nitrates
Shunts [e.g. Transjugular intrahepatic portosystemic shunt (TIPS)]

Table 17. Child-Pugh Classification

	1	2	3
Serum bilirubin (µmol/L)	<34	34-51	>51
Serum albumin (g/L)	>35	28-35	<28
Presence of ascites	Absent	Controllable	Refractory
Encephalopathy	Absent	Minimal	Severe
INR	<1.7	1.7-2.3	>2.3

Score: 5-6 (Child's A), 7-9 (Child's B), 10-15 (Child's C)

*Note: Child's classification is rarely used for shunting, but is still useful to quantitate the severity of cirrhosis

Ascites

Definition
- accumulation of excess free fluid in the peritoneal cavity

Etiology

Table 18. Serum-Ascites Albumin Gradient as an Indicator of the Causes of Ascites

serum [Alb] - ascitic [Alb] >11 g/L	serum [Alb] - ascitic [Alb] <11 g/L
Cirrhosis/severe hepatitis	Peritoneal carcinomatosis
Chronic hepatic congestion	TB
(right heart failure, Budd-Chiari)	Pancreatic disease
Massive liver metastases	Serositis
Myxedema	Nephrotic syndrome*

* in nephrotic syndrome: ↓ serum [Alb] to begin with therefore gradient not helpful

---

Secondary bacterial peritonitis (as opposed to primary bacterial peritonitis) usually results from a perforated viscus or surgical manipulation.

Pathogenesis of Ascites in Cirrhosis
- normal physiology
  - intravascular hydrostatic pressure (HP) and oncotic pressure (OP) are balanced (Starling forces) → preventing accumulation of extravascular fluid into peritoneal space
- in cirrhosis, HP and OP balance is disrupted, precipitating ascites by one or more of the following mechanisms:
  - fibrotic constriction of sinusoids resulting in portal HTN and increased HP → increased HP drives fluid lymphatic drainage into the abdomen across hepatic capsule and mesentery
  - renal hypoperfusion → Na and H_2O retention
  - PGE opposes sodium retention (NSAIDs may precipitate renal failure)
  - less important fact is hypoalbuminemia → decreased OP
- underfill theory
  - portal hypertension and hypoalbuminemia lead to transudation of Na and water into peritoneum causing ↓ intravascular volume and secondary renal Na and water retention via renin-angiotensin-aldosterone system

- overflow theory
  - liver disease primarily causes renal retention of Na and water which then "overflows" into peritoneal cavity
- combined theory (incorporating both above theories) is most popular
  - liver disease causes vasodilation via nitric oxide, increasing vascular capacitance
  - ↓ effective intravascular volume (i.e. volume to capacitance ratio low, but absolute volume is high)
  - secondary urinary Na and water retention

Diagnosis
- clinically detectable when >500 mL

Investigations
- diagnostic paracentesis - should be done on most patients:
  - cells and differential
  - chemistry (albumin, protein, amylase, TG)
  - C&S, gram stain
  - cytology (usually positive in peritoneal carcinomatosis)

Treatment
- therapeutic paracentesis safe, especially if albumin infusion given concomitantly
- medical
  - Na restriction
  - diuretics (spironolactone, furosemide)
  - aim for 0.5 kg loss per day to prevent ARF (this is maximum rate of ascitic fluid)
  - 1 kg loss per day if peripheral edema
- surgical
  - TIPS, liver transplantation (reserved for medically refractory cases)

Complication: Bacterial Peritonitis
- primary/spontaneous bacterial peritonitis (SBP)
  - complicates ascites, does not cause it (occurs in 10% of cirrhotic ascites)
  - 1/3 of patients are asymptomatic, thus do not hesitate to do a diagnostic paracentesis
  - fever, chills, abdominal pain, ileus, hypotension, worsening encephalopathy
  - gram negatives compose 70% of pathogens: *E. coli* (most common pathogen), *Streptococcus*, *Klebsiella*
- diagnosis:
  - absolute neutrophil count in peritoneal fluid >0.25x10^9 cells/L (250 cells/mm^3) or WBC count >0.5x10^9 cells/L (500 cells/mm^3)
  - gram stain is positive in only 10-50% of patients
  - culture is positive in only 80% of patients (not needed for diagnosis)
- treatment
  - IV antibiotics (cefotaxime is the treatment of choice until C&S is available) for 5-10 days; prophylaxis with daily norfloxacin or TMP-SMX for 5-7 days may decrease the frequency of recurrent SBP, use if GI bleeding/previous SBP
  - IV albumin decreases mortality

Biliary Tract

Basic Anatomy Review

- consists of the hepatic ducts (intrahepatic, left, right and common), gallbladder, cystic duct, common bile duct and ampulla of Vater
- gallbladder functions to store and release bile that is produced in the liver
- bile is used to emulsify fats and is composed of cholesterol, lecithin, bile acids and bilirubin
- cholecystokinin stimulates gallbladder emptying while trypsin and chymotrypsin inhibit bile release
- gallbladder blood supply: cystic artery (from the right hepatic artery) and cystic vein

Jaundice

- see Table 19, Figures 16 and 17

Definition
- yellow pigmentation of skin, sclerae and mucous membranes due to ↑ serum bilirubin (>50 umol/L or 3 mg/mL)

Signs and Symptoms
- dark urine, pale stools - suggests that bilirubin elevation is from direct fraction
- pruritus - suggests chronic problem
- abdominal pain-suggests biliary tract obstruction from stone or pancreatic tumour (obstructive jaundice)
- painless jaundice - think of pancreatic cancer

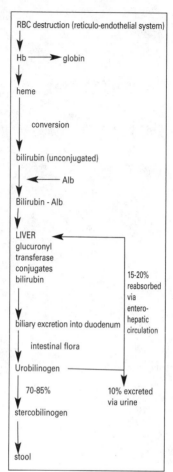

Figure 16. Production and Excretion of Bilirubin

Table 19. Classification of Jaundice

I. Predominantly Unconjugated Hyperbilirubinemia
    1. Overproduction
- Hemolysis
- Ineffective erythropoiesis (megaloblastic anemias, others)

    2. Decreased hepatic uptake
- Gilbert's syndrome
- Drugs (e.g. rifampin)

    3. Decreased conjugation
- Drug inhibition (e.g. chloramphenicol)
- Crigler-Najjar syndromes type I and II
- Neonatal jaundice
- Gilbert's syndrome

II. Predominantly Conjugated Hyperbilirubinemia
    1. Impaired hepatic secretion
- Familial disorders (e.g. Rotor syndrome, Dubin-Johnson syndrome, cholestasis of pregnancy)
- Hepatocellular disease - by far the most common
- Drug-induced cholestasis (e.g. oral contraceptives, chlorpromazine)
- Primary biliary cirrhosis (PBC)
- Primary sclerosing cholangitis (PSC)
- Sepsis
- Post-operative

    2. Extrahepatic biliary obstruction
- Intraductal obstruction
  - Gallstones
  - Biliary stricture
  - Parasites
  - Malignancy (cholangiocarcinoma)
  - Sclerosing cholangitis
- Extraductal obstruction
  - Malignancy (e.g. pancreatic cancer, lymphoma)
  - Metastases in peri-portal nodes
  - Inflammation (e.g. pancreatitis)

Investigations
- bilirubin
  - conjugated (direct) and unconjugated (indirect)
- AST, ALT, GGT, ALP
- serologic tests for hepatitis, screening tests for hemochronatosis, autoimmune liver disease, Wilson's disease
- ultrasound for evidence of bile duct obstruction
- direct duct visualization
  - endoscopic retrograde cholangiopancreatography (ERCP)
  - percutaneous transhepatic cholangiography (PTC) – only if obstruction is suspected to be periportal rather than near sphincter or if previous gastric surgery
  - magnetic resonance cholangiopancreatography (MRCP) – non-invasive
- liver biopsy

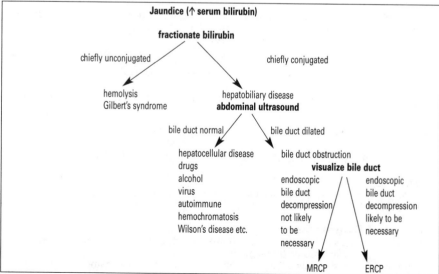

Figure 17. Approach to Jaundice

Gilbert's Syndrome

Definition
- mild decrease in glucuronyltransferase activity leading to defective conjugation of bilirubin; complete deficiency of glucuronyltransferase - Crigler-Najjar Syndrome

Etiology/Epidemiology
- some patients have ↓ hepatobiliary uptake
- affects 7% of population, especially males
- autosomal dominant

Signs and Symptoms
- presents in teens-20s, often as an incidental finding
- only manifestation is intermittent jaundice with ↑ serum unconjugated bilirubin developing most characteristically while fasting
- no treatment indicated (entirely benign)

Primary Biliary Cirrhosis (PBC)

Definition
- chronic inflammation and fibrous obliteration of intrahepatic bile ductules

Etiology/Epidemiology
- probably autoimmune (associated with Sjögren's syndrome, scleroderma, CREST syndrome, RA, thyroiditis)
- affects mainly middle-aged women (male:female ratio of 1:9)

Signs and Symptoms
- often asymptomatic
- earliest symptoms: pruritus, fatigue
- after several months-years: jaundice and melanosis (darkening skin) and other signs of cholestasis
- eventually: hepatocellular failure, portal hypertension, ascites

Investigations
- ↑ ALP, GGT
- positive anti-mitochondrial antibodies (AMA) (95% specificity)
- ↑ cholesterol → xanthelasmas, xanthomas (mild increase in LDL, larger increase in HDL)
- diagnosis based on liver biopsy and normal ERCP (i.e. rule out common bile duct (CBD) stones and sclerosing cholangitis)

Clinical Course
- may be ultimately fatal although not all asymptomatic patients progress

Treatment
- treat with ursodiol, (less frequently colchicine, methotrexate), cholestyramine (for pruritus and hypercholesterolemia), parenteral fat soluble vitamins, Vitamin D and Ca supplements
- only proven treatment is liver transplant

Secondary Biliary Cirrhosis

Definition
- results from prolonged partial or total obstruction of major bile ducts

Etiology
- acquired: post-op strictures, chronic pancreatitis, sclerosing cholangitis, rarely stone in bile duct
- congenital: cystic fibrosis (CF), congenital biliary atresia, choledochal cysts

Diagnosis
- cholangiography and liver biopsy

Treatment
- treat obstruction, give antibiotics for cholangitis prophylaxis

Ascending Cholangitis

Charcot's Triad
- RUQ pain
- Fever
- Jaundice

Raynaud's Pentad
- Charcot's triad
- hypotension
- delirium

Definition
- infection of the biliary tree secondary to stasis

Etiology
- stasis in the biliary tract due to obstruction or stricture (characteristically from previous cholecystectomy)
- infection by ascending from the duodenum or hematogenous spread from the portal vein
- bacteria
  - *E. coli, Klebsiella, Enterobacter, Enterococcus*
  - co-infection with *Bacteroides* and *Clostridia* can occur

Signs and Symptoms
- Charcot's Triad: fever, RUQ pain, jaundice (50-70%)
- Raynaud's pentad in patients with suppurative cholangitis: fever, RUQ pain, jaundice, hypotension, confusion

Diagnosis
- ↑WBC
- ↑ALP, ↑GGT, ↑bilirubin
- ↑AST, ↑ALT
- blood culture
- abdominal U/S – CBD dilation and presence of stones (sensitivity = 15%)

Treatment
- ERCP – diagnosis and therapeutic sphincterotomy, stone extraction
- antibiotic therapy – broad spectrum to cover gram negatives and enterococcus
  - ampicillin + gentamicin OR
  - 3rd generation cephalosporin OR
  - imipenem
- may consider metronidazole to cover anaerobes

Prognosis
- good with effective drainage and antibiotics in mild to moderate cases
- high mortality (~50%) in patients with Raynaud's Pentad

Sclerosing Cholangitis

PBC = intrahepatic bile duct inflammation vs. PSC = inflammation of entire biliary tree

ERCP
- absence of narrowing in PBC
- narrowing of intra and extrahepatic ducts in PSC

Definition
- inflammation of entire biliary tree (intra and/or extrahepatic bile ducts) leading to scarring and obliteration

Etiology
- primary/idiopathic
  - most common
  - associated with IBD in up to 70% (usually male)
  - one of the most common indications for transplant
- secondary - less common
  - long-term choledocholithiasis
  - cholangiocarcinoma
  - surgical/traumatic injury (iatrogenic)
  - contiguous inflammatory process
  - post ERCP
  - associated with AIDS (called "HIV cholangiopathy")

Signs and Symptoms
- often insidious, may present with fatigue and pruritus
- may present with signs of episodic bacterial cholangitis secondary to biliary obstruction

Diagnosis
- ↑ ALP, bilirubin
- minor ↑ AST, usually <300
- ERCP shows narrowing of bile ducts, both intrahepatic and extrahepatic bile ducts
- p-ANCA (30-80%), elevated IgM (40-50%)
- if just intrahepatic, do antimitochondrial antibody to rule out PBC

Treatment
- prophylactic antibiotics for bacterial cholangitis
- endoscopic sphincterotomy, biliary stent in selected cases of dominant CBD stricture
- suppurative cholangitis requires emergency drainage of pus in CBD
- liver transplantation appears the best treatment for advanced sclerosing cholangitis (nearly 90% survive 1 year; mean follow-up from time of diagnosis to need for transplant is 10 years)

Complications
- repeated bouts of cholangitis may lead to complete biliary obstruction with resultant secondary biliary cirrhosis and hepatic failure
- increased incidence of cholangiocarcinoma, 10-15%, difficult to diagnose, even more difficult to treat; serial MRCP may assist

Prognosis
- unfavourable regardless of treatment
- mean survival after diagnosis remains 4-10 years

Pancreas

Basic Anatomy Review

Anatomy and Physiology
- generally divided into 4 parts: head (includes uncinate process), neck, body, tail
- blood supply:
    - anterior/posterior superior pancreaticoduodenal artery (from the celiac trunk)
    - anterior/posterior inferior pancreaticoduodenal artery (from the superior mesenteric artery)
    - dorsal pancreatic artery (from the splenic artery)
    - pancreatic veins drain into the portal, splenic and superior mesenteric veins
- endocrine function: Islets of Langerhans produce glucagon, insulin and somatostatin (from the α, β and δ cells respectively)
- exocrine function: digestive enzymes are produced including amylase, lipase, trypsin, chymotrypsin and carboxypeptidase

Causes of ↑ Serum Amylase
- pancreatic disease
    - acute pancreatitis, chronic pancreatitis with ductal obstruction, pseudocyst, abscess, ascites, trauma, cancer
- non-pancreatic abdominal disease
    - biliary tract disease, bowel obstruction/ischemia, perforated or penetrating ulcer, ruptured ectopic pregnancy, aneurysm, chronic liver disease, peritonitis
- non-abdominal disease
    - cancer (lung, esophagus, etc.), salivary gland lesions, bulimia, renal transplant/insufficiency, burns, ketoacidosis
    - macroamylasemia
    - when serum amylase >5 times normal, the cause is almost always pancreatitis or renal disease

Pancreatic Enzymes
- amylase
- lipase
- trypsin
- chymotrypsin

Causes of Increased Serum Lipase
- pancreatic disease
    - same as above
- non-pancreatic abdominal disease (mild elevations only)
    - same as above
- non-abdominal disease
    - macrolipasemia
    - renal failure

Acute Pancreatitis

Etiology (mnemonic: I GET SMASHED)

Idiopathic: thought to be hypertensive sphincter or microlithiasis

Gallstones (45%)
Ethanol (35%)
Tumours: pancreas, ampulla, choledochocele

Scorpion stings
Microbiological
- bacterial: mycoplasma, *Campylobacter*, TB, *M. avium intracellulare*, *Legionella*, leptospirosis
- viral: mumps, rubella, varicella, viral hepatitis, CMV, EBV, HIV, Coxsackie virus, echovirus, adenovirus
- parasites: ascariasis, clonorchiasis, echinococcosis
Autoimmune: SLE, polyarteritis nodosa (PAN), Crohn's
Surgery/trauma
- manipulation of sphincter of Oddi (e.g. ERCP), post-cardiac surgery, blunt trauma to abdomen, penetrating peptic ulcer

When thinking about the causes of acute pancreatitis remember:
I GET SMASHED

Hyperlipidemia (TG >11.3 mmol/L), hypercalcemia, hypothermia
Emboli or ischemia
Drugs/toxins: azathioprine, mercaptopurine, furosemide, estrogens, methyldopa, H_2 blockers, valproic acid, antibiotics, acetaminophen, salicylates, ethanol, methanol, organophosphates, steroids (controversial)

Differential Diagnosis
- perforated peptic ulcer
- biliary colic
- acute cholangitis, acute cholecystitis
- fatty infiltration of the liver (alcohol)
- small bowel obstruction (SBO)
- perforated/ischemic bowel
- mesenteric infarction
- dissecting aneurysm
- nephrolithiasis
- acute coronary occlusion/MI

Pathology
- activation of proteolytic enzymes within pancreatic cells → local + systemic inflammatory response
- mild
    - peripancreatic fat necrosis
    - interstitial edema
- severe
    - extensive peripancreatic and intrapancreatic fat necrosis
    - parenchymal necrosis and hemorrhage → infection in 60%
    - release of toxic factors into systemic circulation and peritoneal space (causes multi-organ failure)
- severity of clinical features may not always correlate with pathology
- 3 phases:
    - local inflammation + necrosis → hypovolemia
    - systemic inflammation in multiple organs, especially in lungs, usually after IV fluids given → pulmonary edema
    - local complications 2 weeks after presentation → pancreatic sepsis/abscess

Signs and Symptoms
- clinical: patient can look well or pre-morbid
    - pain: epigastric, noncolicky, constant, can radiate to back, may improve when leaning forward (Inglefinger's sign); tender rigid abdomen; guarding
    - nausea and vomiting
    - abdominal distention from paralytic ileus
    - fever: chemical, not due to infection
    - jaundice: compression or obstruction of bile duct
    - Cullen's/Grey-Turner's signs
    - tetany: transient hypocalcemia
    - hypovolemic shock: can lead to renal failure
    - acute respiratory distress syndrome
    - coma

Investigations
- ↑ pancreatic enzymes in blood
    - ↑ amylase
    - ↑ lipase
- ALT >100 in a non-alcoholic patient strongly suggests biliary pancreatitis
- ↑ WBC
- imaging
    - x-ray: "sentinel loop" (dilated proximal jejunem), calcification and "colon cut-off sign" (colonic spasm)
    - U/S: best for evaluating biliary tree (67% sensitivity, 100% specificity)
    - CT scan with IV contrast: useful prognostic indicator because contrast seen only in viable pancreatic tissue, non-viable areas can be biopsied percutaneously to differentiate sterile from infected necrosis
    - ERCP or MRCP if no cause found, searching for duct stone, pancreatic or ampullary tumour, pancreas divisum

Prognosis
- usually a benign, self-limiting course, single or recurrent
- occasionally severe leading to:
    - shock
    - pulmonary edema
    - pancreatic abscess
    - coagulopathy
    - hyperglycemia and hypoglycemia

Increased amylase
- sensitive, not specific

Increased lipase
- higher sensitivity and specificity
- stays elevated longer

- GI ulceration due to stress
- death
- functional restitution to normal occurs if primary cause and complications are eliminated (exception: alcohol)
- occasional scarring and persistent pseudocysts
- rarely leads to chronic pancreatitis
- mortality: Ranson's ≤2 criteria = 5% mortality
  - 3-4 criteria = 15-20%
  - 5-6 criteria = 40%
  - ≥7 criteria = 99%

Treatment
- goals: (1) hemodynamic stability
  - (2) analgesia
  - (3) stop progression of damage
  - (4) treat local and systemic complications
- antibiotics controversial except in documented infection
- aspirate necrotic areas of pancreas to diagnose infection; drain if infected
- IV fluids (crystalloid or colloid)
  - beware third spacing of fluid, monitor urine output carefully
- NG suction (rests pancreas) if stomach dilated, inflammation severe or patient vomiting
- analgesics to control pain
- nutritional support: nasoenteric jejunal feeding tube or TPN if cannot tolerate enteric feeds; recent evidence supports oral or nasogastric enteral feeds
- no benefit: glucagon, atropine, trasylol, H_2 blockers, peritoneal lavage
- follow clinically and with CT/ultrasound to exclude complications
- drain abscesses (percutaneous vs. surgical)
- drain pseudocysts if large, persisting or infected
- embolize hemorrhagic vessels
- surgery for infected pancreatic necrosis (try to delay for >2 weeks to allow demarcation between viable and necrotic tissue)

Complications
- pseudocyst (cyst-like structure encapsulated with fibrous material, not epithelium)
- abscess
- lungs: pleural effusion, atelectasis, pneumonia, acute respiratory distress syndrome (ARDS)
- acute renal failure (e.g. ATN)
- CVS: pericardial effusion, pericarditis, shock
- antibiotics: especially quinolones (e.g. ciprofloxacin), imipenem (other antibiotics do not penetrate pancreas) may be useful as prophylaxis in severe pancreatitis (controversial)

Chronic Pancreatitis

Definition
- a continuing inflammatory disease of the pancreas characterized by irreversible morphological changes
- four manifestations: abdominal pain, diabetes, steatorrhea, calcification of pancreas

Etiology
- nearly always alcoholic
  - alcohol increases viscosity of pancreatic juice
  - decreases pancreatic secretion of pancreatic stone protein (lithostatin) which normally solubilizes calcium salts → precipitation of calcium within pancreatic duct
  - result is duct obstruction and subsequent gland destruction
- unusual causes:
  - cystic fibrosis
  - severe protein-calorie malnutrition
  - hereditary pancreatitis
- never gallstones - cause acute pancreatitis only

Pathophysiology
- destruction of exocrine parenchyma
- varying degrees of ductular dilatation and associated ductal strictures
- protein plugs
- calcification

Signs and Symptoms
- early stages
  - recurrent attacks of severe abdominal pain (upper abdomen and back)
  - chronic painless pancreatitis: 10%

Ranson's criteria: pancreatitis not due to gallstones (criteria slightly different for gallstone-induced pancreatitis)

At admission
G: blood glucose >11 mmol/L (with no history of hyperglycemia)
A: age >55
L: serum LDH >350 IU/L
A: AST >250 IU/L
W: WBC >16 x 10⁹/L

During first 48 hours
C: serum calcium <2 mmol/L
H: hematocrit drop >10%
O: arterial PO_2 <60 mmHg
B: base deficit >4 mmol/L
B: BUN rise >1.8 mmol/L
S: estimated fluid sequestration >6 L

- difficult course if 2+ present
- high mortality if 3+ present

What is the evidence for utilization of Ranson's Criteria?
Pancreas 2002; 25(4): 331-335
Study: 153 patients with acute pancreatitis were assessed using Ranson's Criteria, APACHE II, and APACHE III scoring systems. ROC analysis was performed for each scoring system.
Results: Sensitivity and specificity for each scoring system in identifying severe pancreatitis is listed below:
Ranson Criteria: Sens: 82%, Spec: 74%, PPV: 48%, NPV: 93%
APACHE II: Sens: 58%, Spec: 78%, PPV: 42%, NPV: 86%
APACHE III: Sens: 56%, Spec: 86%, PPV: 51%, NPV: 89%
Conclusions: The principal utility of these scales is to determine whether a patient needs to be admitted to the ICU based on their presenting characteristics. Both APACHE scoring systems require 24 hrs observation to generate a score, but Ranson criteria can be applied at the time of admission. Moreover, the test characteristics of the Ranson scale are equivalent, in some cases superior, to the more complicated APACHE scale. Of particular importance is the negative predictive value these scales (e.g. don't want to miss a patient who will need an ICU admission).

Antibiotic therapy for prophylaxis against infection of pancreatic necrosis in acute pancreatitis
Cochrane Database of Systematic Reviews 2006 Issue 4. Art. No.: CD002941.DOI: 10.1002/14651858/CD002941.pub2.
Study: Meta-Analysis of 5 RCTs which randomized 294 patients to either antibiotic prophylaxis in acute pancreatitis or placebo.
Results: Significant decrease in all cause mortality in patients receiving antibiotic prophylaxis (6% vs. 15.3%). No significant difference between the rates in infected pancreatic necrosis between the two groups. In studies evaluating beta-lactam antibiotics, significant decreases in mortality (6.3% vs. 16.7%) and infected necrosis (15.6% vs. 29.29%) were observed compared to placebo. Studies that evaluated quinolones plus imidazole, found no significant differences between mortality or infected necrosis.
Conclusions: There was a significant degree of heterogeneity between studies which makes definitive conclusions challenging (different antibiotics, dosing regimens, etc.). Therefore, the authors do not recommend routine prophylaxis. If prophylaxis is to be performed, the authors suggest starting as soon as possible and continuing for one to two weeks.

• late stages: occurs in 15% of patients
  ▪ malabsorption syndrome when >90% of function is lost, steatorrhea
  ▪ diabetes, calcification, jaundice, weight loss, pseudocyst, ascites, GI bleed
• laboratory
  ▪ increase in serum glucose
  ▪ increase in ALP (portion of common bile duct within pancreas is narrowed by pancreatic inflammation)
  ▪ serum amylase + lipase usually normal

Investigations
• flat plate (looking for pancreatic calcifications)
• ultrasound (calcification, dilated pancreatic ducts, pseudocyst)
• CT (calcification, dilated pancreatic ducts, pseudocyst)
• MRCP or ERCP (abnormalities of pancreatic ducts-narrowing and dilatation)
• trial of therapy with pancreatic enzymes
• p-aminobenzoic acid (PABA) test (exocrine function: reflects duodenal chymotrypsin activity)
• 72-hour fecal fat test (exocrine function)
• secretin test, CCK test (exocrine function)
• fecal enzyme measurement

Management
• general management
  ▪ total abstinence from alcohol
  ▪ enzyme replacement may help pain by resting pancreas via negative feedback
  ▪ analgesics
  ▪ celiac ganglion blocks
  ▪ pain decreases with time as gland burns out
• steatorrhea
  ▪ pancreatic enzyme replacement
  ▪ diet: restricted fat and protein (may also decrease pain)
• surgery
  ▪ pancreatic resection if ductal obstruction (best seen on ERCP)
  ▪ no surgical procedure can improve pancreatic function
• endoscopic
  ▪ remove pancreatic stone or insert stent if pancreatic duct obstructed

Clinical Nutrition

Determination of Nutritional Status

Investigations
• plasma proteins (albumin, pre-albumin, transferrin)
  ▪ decrease may indicate ↓ nutritional status (not very specific)
• thyroid-binding pre-albumin, retinol-binding protein
  ▪ too sensitive
• small changes in nutritional status can result in large changes in the following indices:
  ▪ hemoglobin levels
  ▪ total lymphocyte count
  ▪ cell-mediated immunity
  ▪ muscle strength (hand-grip dynamometer, electrical stimulation of adductor pollicis)
  ▪ INR: measure of vitamin K status
  ▪ creatinine-height index, compare to standard tables
  ▪ other methods are available but mainly for research (underwater weighing, total body water, total body potassium, total body nitrogen, etc.)

Table 20. Areas of Absorption of Nutrients

	Fe	CHO	Proteins, Lipids Na, H_2O	Bile Acids	Vit B_{12}
Duodenum	+++	+++	+++	+	
Jejunum		+	++	+	+
Ileum		+	++	+++	+++

Enteral Nutrition (TEN)

Definition
* enteral nutrition (tube feeding) is a way of providing food throught a tube placed in the nose, stomach or the small intestine

Indications
* oral consumption inadequate or contraindicated
* appropriate enteral feeding formula is available

Relative Contraindications
* vomiting and aspiration
* intestinal obstruction
* small bowel ileus
* enteroenteral or enterocutaneous fistulae
* uncontrolled diarrhea
* UGI bleeding

Complications
* aspiration
* diarrhea

Enteral Nutrition: Advantages Over Parenteral Nutrition
* far fewer serious complications (especially sepsis)
* nutritional requirements for enterally administered nutrition better understood
* can supply gut-specific fuels such as glutamine and short chain fatty acids
* nutrients in the intestinal lumen prevent atrophy of the gut and pancreas
* prevents gallstones by stimulating gallbladder motility
* much less expensive

Parenteral Nutrition (TPN)

Definition
* parenteral nutrition is the practice of feeding a person intravenously, bypassing the usual process of eating and digestion

Indications
* not well understood; only situations where total parental nutrition (TPN) has been well shown to increase survival are after bone marrow transplant and in short bowel syndrome, some evidence for benefit in cancer of stomach
* preoperative: only useful in severely malnourished (i.e. lost more than 15% of premorbid weight, serum albumin <28 g/L), and only if given for at least 2 weeks
* renal failure: TPN shown to increase rate of recovery from acute renal failure, but not ↑ survival
* liver disease: branched chain amino acids may shorten duration of encephalopathy, but do not increase survival
* IBD: TPN closes fistulae and heals acute exacerbations of mucosal inflammation, but effect is transient (and TEN is just as effective)
* some evidence for efficacy, but convincing data not available for:
  * radiation/chemotherapy-induced enteritis
  * AIDS
  * severe acute pancreatitis

Whenever possible, enteral nutrition is ALWAYS preferable to TPN!

Indications for routine use of TPN
* patients with inability to absorb nutrients via the GI tract
  * small bowel resection (70% resected) and inability to maintain adequate nutrition by the enteral route
  * diseases of the small intestine (e.g. scleroderma, SLE, celiac, pseudo-obstruction, multiple enterocutaneous fistulae and Crohn's disease) not responding to other treatments
  * radiation enteritis, graft vs. host disease
  * chronic severe diarrhea (e.g. primary GI disease, viral or bacterial enteritis)
  * intractable and protracted vomiting
* patients undergoing high-dose chemotherapy, radiation and bone marrow transplantation with impaired gut function
* moderate to severe acute pancreatitis with GI symptoms associated with oral ingestion of food
* severe malnutrition in the face of a non-functioning GI tract
* severely catabolic patients with or without malnutrition when GI tract is not usable within 5 days; examples include:
  * >50% body surface area burn
  * multisystem trauma
  * extensive surgery
  * sepsis
  * severe inflammatory disease

Relative Contraindications
- functional GI tract for enteral nutrition
- active infection; at least until appropriate antibiotic coverage
- inadequate venous access; triple-lumen central venous lines usually prevent this problem
- unreliable patient or clinical setting

Complications of TPN
- sepsis: most serious of the common complications
- mechanical pneumothorax from insertion of central line, catheter migration and thrombosis, air embolus
- metabolic: CHF, hyperglycemia, gallstones, cholestasis

Visualizing the GI Tract

Esophagus, Stomach, Duodenum
- consider barium swallow first if dysphagia, decreased level of consciousness, (increases risk of aspiration), inability to cooperate (increases risk of pharyngeal trauma during intubation)
- endotracheal intubation first if massive upper GI bleed, acidosis, unable to protect airway
- gastroscopy under most circumstances
- gastroscopy
  - NPO x 8 hours beforehand (min. 5 hours)
  - can be used to band varices, cauterize/clip/inject bleeding ulcers

Colon and Terminal Ileum
- usually colonoscopy, with biopsy if required, but contraindicated in acute diverticulitis, severe colitis (increased risk of perforation)
- CT colonoscopy ("virtual colonoscopy") more accurate in diagnosing diverticulosis, extrinsic pressure on colon (e.g. ovarian cancer compressing sigmoid colon), fistulae

Small Bowel
- most difficult to visualize if mucosal detail is needed
- most accurate is wireless endoscopy capsule (26 x 11 mm capsule is swallowed, transmits images to a computer; contraindicated if obstruction in bowel)
- small bowel enema (enteroclysis) more accurate than small bowel swallow, but both have low sensitivity
- CT and MRI enteroclysis more popular
- "double balloon" endoscopy (endoscope with balloons proximally and distally to propel endoscope into jejunum from mouth, into ileum from anus) may be most sensitive but currently available only in selected centres; technically demanding

Pancreatic/Biliary Duct
- MRCP (magnetic resonance cholangiopancreatography = MRI of pancreas/bile duct) as sensitive as ERCP (endoscopic retrograde cholangiopancreatography) in determining if bile duct obstruction present, but less accurate in determining cause of obstruction (tumour, stone, stricture)
- use ERCP if endoscopic draining likely to be necessary, strong suspicion of stone or ampullary tumour
- MRCP has low sensitivity in sclerosing cholangitis

Common Medications

Table 21. Common Drugs prescribed in Gastroenterology

Class	Generic Drug Name	Trade Name	Dosing Schedule	Mechanism of Action	Indications	Contraindications	Side Effects
Proton Pump Inhibitors (H^+-K^+ATPase inhibitors)	omeprazole	Losec™/Prilosec®	20 mg OD	Inhibits gastric enzymes H^+-K^+ ATPase (proton pump)	duodenal ulcer, gastric ulcer, NSAID-associated gastric and duodenal ulcers; reflux esophagitis symptomatic GERD dyspepsia Zollinger-Ellison syndrome eradication of *H. pylori* (combined with antibiotics)	hypersensitivity to drug	dizziness, headache, flatulence, abdo pain, nausea, rash, increased risk of osteoporotic fracture (secondary to impaired calcium absorption)
	lansoprazole	Prevacid™	oral therapy: 15-30 mg OD (before breakfast) IV therapy: 30 mg OD	Same as above	Same as above	Same as above	Same as above
	pantoprazole	Pantoloc® Protonix®	40 mg OD for UGIB: 80 mg bolus then 8 mg/h infusion	Same as above	Same as above and UGIB	Same as above	Same as above
	rabeprazole	Pariet™/Aciphex®	40 mg OD	Same as above	Same as above	Same as above	Same as above
	esomeprazole	Nexium®	20-40 mg OD	Same as above	Same as above	Same as above	Same as above
Histamine H_2-receptor antagonists	ranitidine	Zantac®	300 mg OD or 150 mg bid IV therapy: 50 mg q8h (but tachyphylaxis a problem)	inhibits gastric histamine H_2-receptors	duodenal ulcer, gastric ulcer, NSAID-associated gastric and duodenal ulcers; ulcer prophylaxis, reflux esophagitis, symptomatic GERD, Zollinger-Ellison syndrome	hypersensitivity to drug	confusion, dizziness, headache, arrhythmias, constipation, nausea, agranulocytosis, pancytopenia, depression
	famotidine	Pepcid®	oral therapy: duodenal/gastric ulcers: 40 mg qhs GERD: 20 mg bid IV therapy: 20 mg bid	Same as above	Same as above	Same as above	Same as above
Stool Softener	docusate sodium	Colace®	100-200 mg OD	promotes incorporation of water into stool, resulting in softer stool	relief of constipation	presence of abdo pain, fever, nausea and vomiting	throat irritation, abdo cramps, rashes
Laxative	lactulose	Lactulose/ Constulose®	constipation: 15-30 ml OD to bid encephalopathy: 15-30 ml bid to qid	is poorly absorbed in GI tract and is broken down by colonic bacteria into lactic acid into colon. ↑ osmotic pressure and acidification of colonic contents, increase stool volume	chronic constipation prevention and treatment of portal-systemic encephalopathy	patients who require a low galactose diet	flatulence, intestinal cramps, nausea, diarrhea if excessive dosage
Peristaltic Stimulant	senna	Senokot®	tablets: 1-4 at bedtime syrup: 10-15 ml at bedtime	senna glycosides are converted into aglycones in the colon and function as laxative agents by altering colonic water and electrolyte transport	relief of constipation	patients with acute abdomen	abdo cramps, discolouration of breast milk, urine, feces, melanosis coli and atonic colon from prolonged use (controversy)

Table 21. Common Drugs prescribed in Gastroenterology (continued)

Class	Generic Drug Name	Canada Name	Dosing Schedule	Mechanism of Action	Indications	Contraindications	Side Effects
Antidiarrheal Agents	loperamide	Imodium®	acute diarrhea: 4 mg initially, followed by 2 mg after each unformed stool	acts as antidiarrheal via cholinergic, noncholingeric, opiate and nonopiate receptor-medicated mechanisms; decreases activity of myenteric plexus	adjunctive therapy for acute non-specific diarrhea, chronic diarrhea associated with IBD, and for reducing the volume of discharge for ileostomies, colostomies and other intestinal resections	children <2 yrs, known hypersensitivity to drug acute dysentery characterized by blood in stools and fever, acute ulcerative colitis or pseudomembranous colitis associated with broad-spectrum antibiotics	abdo pain or discomfort, drowsiness or dizziness, tiredness, dry mouth, nausea and vomiting, hypersensitivity reaction
	diphenoxylate/ atropine	Lomotil®	5 mg tid to qid	inhibits GI propulsion via direct action on smooth muscle, resulting in a decrease in peristaltic action and in transit time	adjunctive therapy for diarrhea, as above	hypersensitivity to diphenoxylate or atropine, jaundice pseudomembranous enterocolitis, diarrhea caused by enterotoxin producing bacteria	dizziness, drowsiness, insomnia, headache, nausea, vomiting, cramps, allergic reaction
IBD Agents	mesalamine	Pentasa™ Salofalk™ Asacol™ Mesasal™	CD: 1g tid/qid Active UC: 1g qid Maintenance UC: 1.6g divided doses daily also as suppositories and enemas	5-ASA: Blocks arachidonic acid metabolism to prostaglandins and leukotrienes	IBD	hypersensitivity to mesalamine salicylates	abdo pain, constipation, arthralgia, headache
	sulfasalazine	Salazopyrin™	3-4 g/d in div doses	compound composed of 5-ASA bound to sulfapyridine, hydrolysis by intestinal bacteria releases 5-ASA, the active component	colonic disease	hypersensitivity to sulfasalazine, sulfa drugs, salicylates; intestinal or urinary obstruction, porphyria	rash, loss of appetite, nausea, vomiting, headache, oligospermia (reversible)
	prednisone		20-40 mg OD for acute exacerbation	anti-inflammatory	mod-severe CD and UC		complications of steroid therapy
Immuno-suppressive Agents	6-mercaptopurine (6-MP)	Purinethol™	CD: 1.5 mg/kg/day	immunosuppressive	IBD: active inflammation and to maintain remission	hypersensitivity to mercaptopurine, prior resistance to mercaptopurine or thioguanine history of treatment with alkylating agents, hypersensitivity to azathioprine, pregnancy	pancreatitis, bone marrow suppression, increased risk of cancer
	azathioprine	Azasan™ Imuran™	IBD: 2-3 mg/kg/day	Same as above	Same as above	Same as above	Same as above
Immunomo-dulators	infliximab	Remicade®	5-10 mg/kg IV over 2 h	antibody to tumour necrosis factor	medically refractory CD	heart failure, moderate to severe, doses greater than 5 mg/kg	reported cases of reactivated TB, PCP, other infections; lymphoma

GS General Surgery

Rubini Pathy, Theresa Pazionis and David Walmsley, chapter editors
Sami Chadi and Biniam Kidane, associate editors
Emily Partridge, EBM editor
Dr. Alexandra Easson, Dr. Darlene Fenech and Dr. Allan Okrainec, staff editors

Basic Anatomy Review

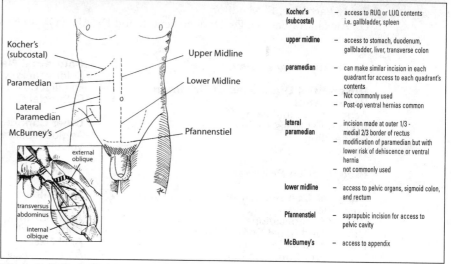

Kocher's (subcostal)	– access to RUQ or LUQ contents i.e. gallbladder, spleen
upper midline	– access to stomach, duodenum, gallbladder, liver, transverse colon
paramedian	– can make similar incision in each quadrant for access to each quadrant's contents – Not commonly used – Post-op ventral hernias common
lateral paramedian	– incision made at outer 1/3 - medial 2/3 border of rectus – modification of paramedian but with lower risk of dehiscence or ventral hernia – not commonly used
lower midline	– access to pelvic organs, sigmoid colon, and rectum
Pfannenstiel	– suprapubic incision for access to pelvic cavity
McBurney's	– access to appendix

Figure 1. Abdominal Incisions

Layers from Superficial to Deep
- skin (epidermis, dermis, subcutaneous fat)
- superficial fascia
    - Camper's fascia (fatty) → Dartos
    - Scarpa's fascia (membranous) → Colles' superficial perineal fascia
- muscle (see Figures 2 and 3)
    - external oblique → inguinal ligament → external spermatic fascia → fascia lata
    - internal oblique → cremasteric muscle/fascia
    - transversus abdominus → posterior inguinal wall
- transversalis fascia → internal spermatic fascia
- preperitoneal fat
- peritoneum → tunica vaginalis

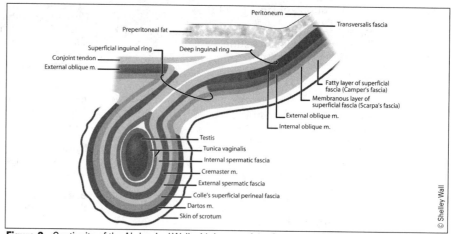

Figure 2. Continuity of the Abdominal Wall with Layers of the Scrotum and Spermatic Cord

- at midline
    - rectus abdominus muscle: in rectus sheath, divided by linea alba
    - above arcuate line (semicircular line of Douglas), which is midway between symphysis pubis and umbilicus:
        - anterior rectus sheath = external oblique aponeurosis and anterior leaf of internal oblique aponeurosis
        - posterior rectus sheath = posterior leaf of internal oblique aponeurosis and transversus muscle aponeurosis
    - below arcuate line:
        - anterior rectus sheath = aponeurosis of external, internal oblique, transversus muscles
        - posterior rectus sheath = transversalis fascia
- arteries: superior epigastric (branch of internal thoracic), inferior epigastric (branch of external iliac); both arteries anastomose and lie behind the rectus muscle

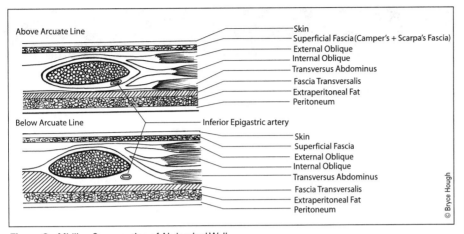

Figure 3. Midline Cross-section of Abdominal Wall

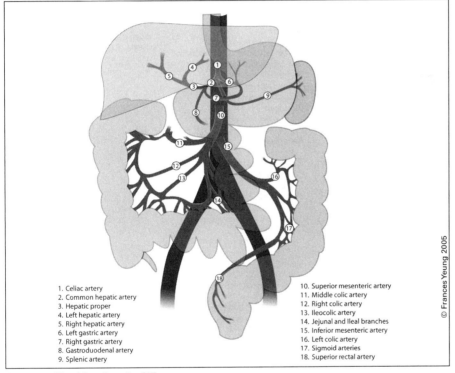

Figure 4. Blood Supply to the GI Tract

1. Celiac artery
2. Common hepatic artery
3. Hepatic proper
4. Left hepatic artery
5. Right hepatic artery
6. Left gastric artery
7. Right gastric artery
8. Gastroduodenal artery
9. Splenic artery
10. Superior mesenteric artery
11. Middle colic artery
12. Right colic artery
13. Ileocolic artery
14. Jejunal and Ileal branches
15. Inferior mesenteric artery
16. Left colic artery
17. Sigmoid arteries
18. Superior rectal artery

© Frances Yeung 2005

Organ	Arteries
Liver	Left and right hepatic (branches of hepatic proper)
Spleen	Splenic
Gallbladder	Cystic
Stomach	1) Lesser curve-right and left gastric 2) Greater curve-right and left gastroepiploic (gastro-omental) 3) Fundus-short gastrics (off splenic)
Duodenum	1) Gastroduodenal 2) Pancreaticoduodenals (off superior mesenteric)
Pancreas	1) Splenic branches 2) Pancreaticoduodenals
Small intestine	1) Superior mesenteric branches-jejunal, ileal, ileocolic
Large intestine	1) Superior mesenteric branches-right colic, middle colic 2) Inferior mesenteric branches-left colic, sigmoid, rectal

Referred Pain
Biliary colic: to right shoulder or scapula
Renal colic: to groin
Appendicitis: periumbilical to right lower quadrant (RLQ)
Pancreatitis: to back
Ruptured aortic aneurysm: to back or flank
Perforated ulcer: to RLQ (right paracolic gutter)
Hip pain: to groin

Differential Diagnoses of Common Presentations

Acute Abdominal Pain

Table 1. Differential Diagnosis of Acute Abdominal Pain

RUQ	EPIGASTRIC	LUQ
Hepatobiliary	**Cardiac**	**Pancreatic**
Biliary Colic	Aortic Dissection/Ruptured AAA	Pancreatitis (Acute vs. Chronic)
Cholecystitis	MI (ischemia)	Pancreatic Pseudocyst
Cholangitis	Pericarditis	Pancreatic Tumors (note Courvosier's Sign = painless
Mirizzi Syndrome	**Gastrointestinal**	mass + jaundice, but pain is still possible)
CBD obstruction (stone, tumor)	Gastritis	**Gastrointestinal**
Hepatitis (infection, toxic, Budd-Chiari, etc)	Peptic Ulcer Disease/Duodenal Ulcer	see 'Epigastric' causes
Hepatic Abscess	GERD/Esophagitis	Splenic flexure pathology (e.g. CRC, ischemia)
Hepatic Mass	Medications (NSAIDs, ASA, steroids,	**Splenic**
Hepatomegaly	laxatives, narcotics, some antibiotics)	Splenomegaly
Fitz-Hugh Curtis	Mallory-Weiss Tear	Splenic Rupture
Right subphrenic abscess	**Other**: hepatobiliary and pancreatic causes	Splenic Infarct/Abcess
Gastrointestinal		Splenic Aneurysm
presentation of gastric, duodenal or		**Cardiopulmonary**
pancreatic pathology (see epigastric	**DIFFUSE**	see RUQ and epigastric causes
and LUQ)	**Peritonitis**	MI (ischemia)
appendicitis in pregnancy >20 wks	hemo/pneumo/fecoperitoneum	**Genitourinary**
hepatic flexure pathology (CRC, subcostal	perforated viscus (duodenal ulcer, sigmoid	see RUQ causes
incisional hernia)	diverticulitis, meckels, appendicitis,	
Genitourinary	anastomotic leak, trauma)	
Nephrolithiasis/ Renal Colic	spontaneous bacterial peritonitis	
Pyelonephritis	post laparoscopic insufflation	
Renal: mass, ischemia, trauma	**Pancreatitis**	
Cardiopulmonary	often better on leaning forward and more	
RLL Pneumonia	of a 'retroperitoneal pain'	
RLL empyema	**Gastrointestinal**	
CHF (causing hepatic congestion and	Mesenteric Ischemia ('pain out of	
R pleural effusion)	proportion to physical findings')	
MI (ischemia)	Inflammatory Bowel Disease (Crohn's,	
Pericarditis	Ulcerative Colitis, IBD NOS)	
Pleuritis	Irritable Bowel Syndrome	
Miscellaneous	Gastroenteritis	
Herpes Zoster	Medications (i.e. stimulant laxatives,	
Trauma	chemotherapy)	
Costochondritis	Pan-colitis (pseudomembranous, ischemic,	
	infectious)	
	Constipation	
	Bowel Obstruction	
	Early appendicitis, perforated appendicitis	
	Ogilvie's Syndrome	
	Cardiovascular/Hematological	
	Aortic Dissection/ Ruptured AAA	
	Sickle Cell Crisis	
	Porphyria	
	Genitourinary/Gynecological	
	Perforated Ectopic Pregnancy	
	PID	
	Acute Urinary Retention	
	Endocrinological	
	Carcinoid Syndrome	
	Diabetic Keto-Acidosis	
	Addisonian Crisis	
	Uremia	
	Hypercalcemia	
	Psychological	
	Munchausen Syndrome	
	Depression	
	Visceral Hypersensitivity Syndrome	
	Other	
	Lead poisoning	
	Tertiary syphillis	

In all patients presenting with an acute abdomen, order the following lab tests:
1. amylase/lipase
2. urinalysis
3. β-hCG (in women)
4. consider CXR + troponins
This will help rule out "non-GI surgical" causes!

Pancreatitis can look like a surgical abdomen, but is rarely an indication for laparotomy.

Table 1. Differential Diagnosis of Acute Abdominal Pain (continued)

RLQ	SUPRAPUBIC	LLQ
Gastrointestinal Appendicitis Appendiceal Phlegmon (post perforated appendicitis) Crohn's Disease Typhlitis (in immunosuppressed/chemo patients) Tuberculosis of the ileocecal junction Cecal tumor Intussusception Mesenteric Lympadenitis Cecal Diverticulitis Cecal Volvulus Hernia: Amyands, Femoral, Inguinal Obstruction (and resulting cecal distension) **Gynecological** see 'suprapubic' **Genitourinary** see 'suprapubic' **Extraperitoneal** Abdominal wall hematoma/abscess Psoas Abscess **Hepatosplenomegaly**	**Gastrointestinal** any etiology in either of the lower quadrants acute appendicitis IBD **Gynecological** Mittelschmirtz (Ruptured Graffian Follicle) PID Ectopic Pregnancy Ovarian Torsion Hemorrhagic Fibroid Endometriosis Threatened/Incomplete Abortion Tubo-Ovarian Abcess Hydrosalphinx/Salpingitis Gynecological Tumors **Genitourinary** Cystitis (infectious, hemmorhagic) Hydroureter/Urinary Colic Epididymitis Testicular Torsion Acute Urinary Retention **Vascular** IVC thrombus **Extraperitoneal** rectus sheath hematoma (localized to midline)	**Gastrointestinal** Diverticulitis Diverticulosis Colon/ Sigmoid/Rectal Ca Fecal Impaction Proctitis (Ulcerative Colitis, infectious; i.e. gonococcus or chlamydia) Sigmoid Volvulus **See gynecological, urological, vascular and extraperitoneal as per RLQ and suprapubic**

Abdominal Mass

Table 2. Differential Diagnosis of Abdominal Mass

Right Upper Quadrant (RUQ)	Upper Midline	Left Upper Quadrant (LUQ)
gallbladder – cholecystitis, cholangiocarcinoma, cholelithiasis	transverse colon CA pancreas - pancreatic adenocarcinoma, IPMT, other pancreatic cancer, pseudocyst	spleen – splenomegaly, tumour, abscess, subcapsular splenic hemorrhage, can also present as RLQ mass if extreme splenomegaly
biliary tract – klatskin tumour	abdominal aorta – AAA (pulsatile)	stomach – tumour
liver – hepatomegaly, hepatitis, abscess, tumour (hepatocellular carcinoma, metastatic tumor, etc) colon CA - hepatic flexure	gastric tumour (adenocarcinoma, gastrointestinal stromal tumor, carcinoid tumor), MALT lympoma	Colon CA

Right Lower Quadrant (RLQ)	Lower Midline	Left Lower Quadrant (LLQ)
intestine – stool, tumour (CRC), mesenteric adenitis, appendicitis, appendicial phlegmon or other abscess, typhlitis, intussuception, Crohn's inflammation	uterus – pregnancy, leoimyoma (fibroid), uterine cancer, pyometria, hematometria	intestine – stool, tumour, abscess (see RLQ)
ovary – ectopic pregnancy, cyst (physiological vs. pathological), tumour (serous, mucinous, struma ovarii, germ cell, krukenberg	GU – bladder distention, tumour	ovary – ectopic pregnancy, cyst, tumour (see RLQ)
fallopian tube – ectopic pregnancy , tubo-ovarian abscess, hydrosalpinx, tumour		fallopian tube – ectopic pregnancy, tubo ovarian abscess, hydrosalpinx, tumour

Increased risk of perforation with distention as seen on abdo imaging:
Small bowel ≥3 cm
Distal colon ≥6 cm
Proximal colon ≥9 cm
Cecum ≥12 cm

Indications for Urgent Operation
I - **I**schemia
H - **H**emorrhage
O - **O**bstruction
P - **P**erforation

GI Bleeding

- see <u>Gastroenterology</u>

Indications for Surgery
- failure of medical management
- prolonged bleeding, significant blood loss (requiring >6 units of pRBCs in a short period of time), high rate of bleeding, associated with hypotension
- bleeding that persists despite endoscopic and angiographic therapeutic maneuvers

Surgical Management of GI Bleeding

- Upper GI Bleeding
  - bleeding from a source above the ligament of treitz
  - often presents with hematemesis and melena unless very brisk (then can present with BRBPR), hypotension, tachycardia)
  - traditionally managed by gastroenterology by endoscopy; if it fails, then consider surgery
- Lower GI Bleeding
  - bleeding from a source below the ligament of Treitz
  - often presents with BRBPR unless proximal to transverse colon (may occasionally present with melena)
  - initial management with colonoscopy to detect and potentially stop source of bleeding
  - may require more tests (angiography, RBC scan) to determine source, if no source found on above tests, then surgical intervention

Table 3. Differential Diagnosis of GI bleeding

Anatomical Source	Etiology	
Hematological	• Excess Anticoagulation (coumadin, heparin, etc)	• DIC • Congenital bleeding disorders
Nose	• Epistaxis	
Esophagus	• Esophageal Varices • Mallory-Weiss Tear	• Aorto-esophageal fistula (generally post endovascular aortic repair)* • esophagitis • esophageal cancer
Stomach	• Gastritis • Gastric Varices • Dieulafoy Lesion	• Gastric Ulcer • Gastric Cancer*
Duodenum	• Duodenal Ulcer • Perforated Duodenal Ulcer*	• Duodenal Cancer*
Jejunum		• Tumours*
Ileum and Ileocecal Junction	• Meckel's Diverticulum (rare surgical management) • Small bowel obstruction	• Crohn's Disease* • Tuberculosis of ileocecal junction
Large Intestine	• Colorectal Cancer* • Mesenteric Thrombosis/ Ischemic Bowel* • Ulcerative Colitis* (subtotal colectomy if failure of medical management) • Angiodysplasia	• Crohn's Disease (less frequently presents with bleeding)* • Pancolitis (infectious, chemotherapy or radiation induced) • Bleeding post gastrointestinal anastamosis
Sigmoid	• **Diverticulosis** (usually)* • Sigmoid Cancer*	• Polyps* (surgical management if malignant) • Bleeding post polypectomy • Inflammatory bowel disease (IBD)
Rectum and Anus	• Hemorrhoids • Fissures • Anal Varices • Rectal Cancer* • Polyps* (surgical management if malignant) • Crohn's or Ulcerative Colitis* • Solitary rectal ulcer	

*managed surgically in most cases

Jaundice

Differential Diagnosis

- **pre-hepatic:** pathology occuring prior to the liver
  - hemolysis
  - Gilbert's disease, Crigler-Najjar disease
- **hepatic:** pathology occuring at the level of the liver
  - viral hepatitis
  - alcoholic hepatitis, cirrhosis
  - drug-induced hepatitis – acetaminophen, erythromycin, isoniazid, valproic acid, phenytoin, OCP
  - Dubin-Johnson syndrome
- **post-hepatic:** pathology is located after the conjugation of bilirubin in the liver
  - choledocholithiasis, cholangitis, sclerosing cholangitis, choledochal cyst
  - benign biliary stricture
  - carcinoma – bile duct, head of pancreas, ampulla of Vater, duodenum

Bilirubin levels

	Prehepatic	Intrahepatic	Posthepatic
Serum bilirubin:			
Indirect	↑	↑	N
Direct	N	↑	↑
Urine:			
Urobilinogen	↑	↑	Absent
Bilirubin	-	+	+
Fecal:			
Urobilinogen	↑	↑	Absent

Preoperative Preparation

Considerations
- informed consent (see <u>ELOAM</u>)
- consults – anesthesia, medicine, cardiology as indicated
- NPO after midnight, AAT, (activity as tolerated), VSR (vital signs routine)
- IV – balanced crystalloid at maintenance rate (4:2:1 rule → roughly 100-125 cc/hr): normal saline or Ringer's lactate; bolus to catch up on estimated losses including losses from bowel prep
- patient's regular meds including prednisone – consider pre-op stress dose if prednisone used in past year
- prophylactic antibiotics (on call to OR): usually cefazolin (Ancef™) ± metronidazole (Flagyll™)
- bowel prep: cleans out bowel and decreases bacterial population
    - oral cathartic (e.g. fleet Phosphosoda™) + enemas (fleet/tap water) starting previous day
    - used for left-sided or rectal resections
- consider DVT prophylaxis for all inpatient surgery (heparin)
- hold ASA x 1 week preop

Investigations
- blood components: group and screen or cross and type depending on procedure
- CBC, electrolytes, BUN, creatinine
- INR/PT, PTT with history of bleeding disorder
- ABGs if predisposed to respiratory insufficiency
- CXR (PA and lateral) if >50 years old or previously abnormal within past 6 months
- ECG if >50 years old or as indicated by history

Drains
- nasogastric (NG) tube
    - indications: gastric decompression, analysis of gastric contents, irrigation/ dilution of gastric contents, feeding (only if necessary due to risk of aspiration → naso-jejunal tube preferable)
    - contraindications: suspected basal skull fracture, obstruction of nasal passages due to trauma
- Foley catheter
    - indications: to accurately monitor urine output, decompression of bladder, relieve obstruction
    - contraindications: suspected disruption of the urethra, difficult insertion of catheter

Surgical Complications

Post-Operative Fever

- fever does not necessarily imply infection
- timing of fever may help identify cause
- POD #0-2
    - usually atelectasis (most common cause of fever on POD #1)
    - early wound infection (especially *Clostridium*, Group A *Streptococcus* – feel for crepitus and look for "dishwater:"drainage)
    - aspiration pneumonitis
    - other: Addisonian crisis, thyroid storm, transfusion reaction
- POD #3
    - after day 3, infections more likely
    - UTI, wound infection, IV site infection, septic thrombophlebitis
- POD #5+
    - leakage at bowel anastomosis (tachycardia, hypotension, oliguria, abdominal pain)
    - intra-abdominal abscess (usually POD #5-10)
    - DVT/PE (can be anytime post-op, most commonly POD #7-10)
    - drug fever (POD #6-10)
- other : cholecystitis, peri-rectal abscess, URTI, infected seroma/biloma/hematoma, parotitis, *C. difficile* colitis, endocarditis

Treatment
- treat primary cause
- antipyrexia (e.g. acetaminophen)

Approach to the Critically Ill Surgical/Trauma Patient

ABC, I'M FINE
ABC (see <u>Emergency Medicine</u>)
I - IV: 2 large bore IV's with NS, wide open
M - Monitors: O$_2$ sat, ECG, BP
F - Foley catheter to measure urine output
I - Investigations: bloodwork
N - NG tube if indicated
E - "Ex" rays (abdomen 3 views, CXR), other imaging

Pre and post-op orders
A – Admit to ward X under Dr. Y
D – Diagnosis
D – Diet
A – Activity
V – Vitals
I – IV, Investigations, Ins & Outs
D – Drugs, dressings, drains
S – Special procedures

DRUGS – 5 A's
Analgesia
Anti-emetic
Anti-coagulation
Antibiotics
All other patient meds

"5 **W**'s" of post-op fever
Wind (pulmonary)
Water (urine-UTI)
Wound
Walk (DVT/PE)
Wonder drugs (drug fever)

Correlate with time spent in post-op period.

Wound Complications

WOUND INFECTION

Etiology
- *S. aureus, E. coli, Enterococcus, Streptococcus* spp., *Clostridium* spp.

Risk Factors
- type of procedure:
  - clean (elective, not emergency, not traumatic, no acute inflammation, resp/GI/biliary/GU tracts not entered): <1.5%
  - clean-contaminated (elective entering of resp/GI/biliary/GU tracts): <3%
  - contaminated (nonpurulent inflammation, gross spillage from GI, entry into biliary or GU with infected bile/urine, penetrating trauma <4 hrs old): 5%
  - dirty (purulent inflammation, pre-op perforation of resp/GI/biliary/GU tracts, penetrating trauma >4 hrs old): 33%
  - increased risk with procedures >2 h long, use of drains
- patient characteristics:
  - age, DM, steroids, immunosuppression, obesity, burn, malnutrition, patient with other infections, traumatic wound, radiation, chemotherapy
- other factors: prolonged preoperative hospitalization, reduced blood flow, break in sterile technique, multiple antibiotics, hematoma, seroma, foreign bodies (drains, sutures, grafts)

Clinical Presentation
- typically fever POD #3-6 (*Streptococcus* and *Clostridium* can present in 24 hrs)
- pain, blanchable wound erythema, induration, frank pus or purulosanguinous discharge, warmth
- complications: fistula, sinus tracts, sepsis, abscess, suppressed wound healing, superinfection, spreading infection to myonecrosis or fascial necrosis (necrotizing fasciitis), wound dehiscence evisceration

Prophylaxis
- pre-op antibiotics for all surgeries (cefazolin (Ansef™)/metronidazole (Flagyll™))
  - within 1 hour preincision; can re-dose with Ancef™ 4 hrs in the OR
- post-op antibiotics for contaminated and dirty surgeries:
  - no evidence supporting more than 24 hrs of post-op antimicrobial prophylaxis for any case
  - generally no need for post-op antibiotics unless intra-abdominal infection
- normothermia (maintain patient temperature >36°C during OR)
- hyperoxygenation consider FiO_2 >80 in OR

Treatment
- re-open affected part of incision, culture wound, pack, heal by secondary intention
- antibiotics only if cellulitis or immunodeficiency
- debride necrotic and non-viable tissue intraoperatively

WOUND HEMORRHAGE/HEMATOMA
- secondary to inadequate surgical control of hemostasis

Risk Factors
- anticoagulant therapy, myeloproliferative disorders, coagulopathies, thrombocytopenia, severe liver disease, DIC

Clinical Features
- pain, swelling, discolouration of wound edges, leakage

Treatment
- pressure dressing, if significant bleeding, may need to re-operate

WOUND DEHISCENCE
- disruption of fascial layer, abdominal contents contained by skin

Clinical Features
- typically POD #1-3, most common presenting sign is serosanguinous drainage from wound, ± evisceration (disruption of all abdominal layers and extrusion of abdominal contents – mortality of 15%)

Risk Factors
- local: technical failure of closure, increased intra-abdominal pressure (e.g. COPD, ileus, bowel obstruction), hematoma, infection, poor blood supply, radiation

Antimicrobial Prophylaxis for Surgery: An Advisory Statement from the National Surgical Infection Prevention Project – (Clin Infect Dis 2004; 38:1706.)

Level IV Evidence (Consensus)

General Recommendations from Consensus Panel:
The first antimicrobial dose should be administered via infusion within 60 minutes of the surgical incision and prophylactic antimicrobials should be discontinued within 24 hours post-operatively.
The initial dose should be based on the patient's body weight, adjusted dosing weight, or BMI. If the surgical procedure is still in progress 2 half-lives after the initial dose, another dose should be administered intraoperatively.

General Abdominal Colorectal surgery:
For parenteral antimicrobial prophylaxis, use cefoxitin OR cefotetan OR cefazolin plus metronidazole.
If the patient has a β-lactam allergy, use clindamycin combined with either gentamicin, ciprofloxacin, or aztreonam, OR metronidazole combined with either gentamicin or ciprofloxacin.

- systemic: smoking, malnutrition (hypoalbuminemia, vitamin C), connective tissue diseases, immunosuppression (disease, steroids, chemotherapy), other (age, DM, sepsis, uremia)

Treatment
- may consider conservative management
- operative closure, evisceration is a surgical emergency

Urinary and Renal Complications

URINARY RETENTION
- may occur after any operation with general anesthesia or spinal anesthesia
- more likely in older males with history of benign prostatic hyperplasia (BPH), patients on anticholinergics

Clinical Presentation
- abdominal discomfort, palpable bladder, overflow incontinence

Treatment
- bladder catheterization

OLIGURIA/ANURIA (see also Nephrology)

Etiology
- pre-renal vs. renal vs. post-renal
    - most common post-op cause is pre-renal ± ischemic ATN
        - external fluid loss: hemorrhage, dehydration, diarrhea
        - internal fluid loss: third-spacing due to bowel obstruction, pancreatitis

- urine output <0.5 cc/kg/hr, increasing Cr, increasing BUN

Treatment
- according to underlying cause; fluid deficit is treated with crystalloid

Post-Operative Dyspnea

- see *Respiratory Complications* and *Cardiac Complications*
- respiratory: atelectasis, pneumonia, pulmonary embolus (PE), acute respiratory distress syndrome (ARDS), asthma, pleural effusion
- cardiac: MI, arrhythmia, CHF
- pain

Respiratory Complications

ATELECTASIS
- comprises 90% of post-op pulmonary complications

Clinical Features
- low-grade fever on POD #1, tachycardia, crackles, decreased breath sounds, bronchial breathing, tachypnea

Risk Factors
- COPD, smoking, obesity, elderly persons
- upper abdominal/thoracic surgery, oversedation, significant post-op pain, poor inspiratory effort

Treatment
- pre-operative prophylaxis
    - smoking cessation (most beneficial if >6 weeks pre-op)
- post-operative prophylaxis
    - minimize use of respiratory depressant drugs
    - good pain control
    - incentive spirometry, deep breathing and coughing, chest physiotherapy, postural changes
    - early ambulation

PNEUMONIA/PNEUMONITIS
- may be secondary to aspiration of gastric contents during anesthetic induction or extubation, causing a chemical pneumonitis

Risk Factors
- aspiration: general anesthetic, decreased LOC, GERD, full stomach, bowel/gastric outlet obstruction + non-functioning NG tube, pregnancy, seizure disorder
- non-aspiration: atelectasis, immobility, pre-existing respiratory disease

Clinical Features
- productive cough, fever
- tachycardia, cyanosis, respiratory failure, decreased LOC
- CXR: pneumonic infiltrate

Treatment
- aspiration prophylaxis: pre-op NPO/NG tube, rapid sequence anesthetic induction
- immediate removal of debris and fluid from airway
- consider endotracheal intubation and flexible bronchoscopic aspiration
- IV antibiotics to cover oral nosocomial aerobes and anaerobes (e.g. cefotaxime, metronidazole)

PULMONARY EMBOLUS (see also Respirology)

Clinical Features
- unilateral leg swelling and pain (DVT as a source of PE), sudden onset SOB, tachycardia

Treatment
- IV heparin, long term coumadin (INR = 2-3) for 3 months
- Greenfield (IVC) filter if contraindications to anticoagulation
- prophylaxis: ambulation if possible, subcutaneous heparin or LMW heparin, compression stockings

PULMONARY EDEMA

Etiology
- cardiogenic vs noncardiogenic
- circulatory overload: excess volume replacement, LV failure, shift of fluid from peripheral to pulmonary vascular bed, negative airway pressure, alveolar injury due to toxins (e.g. ARDS), more common with pre-existing cardiac disease

Clinical Features
- SOB, crackles at lung bases

Treatment
- ABCs, O_2, diuretics, positive end-expiratory pressure (PEEP)

RESPIRATORY FAILURE

Clinical Features
- earliest manifestations – tachypnea and hypoxemia (pO_2 <60, RR >25)
- dyspnea, cyanosis, evidence of obstructive lung disease
- pulmonary edema, unexplained decrease in SaO_2

Treatment
- ABCs, O_2 ± intubation
- bronchodilators, diuretics to treat CHF
- adequate blood pressure to maintain pulmonary perfusion
- if these measures fail to keep PaO_2 >60, consider ARDS

Cardiac Complications

- abnormal ECGs common in post-op period (compare to pre-op ECG)
- common arrhythmia – supraventricular tachycardia (SVT)
- atrial fibrillation (secondary to fluid overload, PE, MI)

MYOCARDIAL INFARCTION (MI)
- surgery increases risk of MI
- incidence
  - 0.5% in previously asymptomatic men >50 years old
  - 40-fold increase in men >50 years old with previous MI

Risk Factors
- pre-op hypertension, CHF
- previous MI (highest risk if in past 6 months, but risk never returns to baseline)
- increased age
- intra-operative hypotension, operations >3 hours
- angina

Clinical Features
- majority of cases on operative day or within first 4 post-op days
- often silent without chest pain, may only present with new-onset CHF (dyspnea), arrhythmias, hypotension

Intra-abdominal Abscess

Definition
- collection of pus walled-off from rest of peritoneal cavity by inflammatory adhesions and viscera

Etiology
- usually polymicrobial: gram-negative bacteria, anaerobes
- gram-positives if coexistent cellulitis

Risk Factors
- emergency OR
- post-op contaminated OR
- GI surgery with anastomoses
- poor healing risk factors
- may occur POD #3 after laparotomy when fluid re-distribution occurs

Clinical Features
- persistent spiking fever, dull pain, weight loss
- mass difficult to palpate
- peritoneal signs if abscess perforation and secondary peritonitis
- leukocytosis or leukopenia (immunocompromised, elderly)
- co-existing effusion (pleural effusion with subphrenic abscess)
- common sites: pelvis, Morrison's pouch (space between duodenum and liver), subphrenic, paracolic gutters, lesser sac, peri-appendiceal, post-surgical anastomosis, diverticular, psoas

Investigations
- CBC, blood cultures x 2
- CT ± water-soluble contrast
- DRE (pelvic abscess)

Treatment
- drainage (percutaneous)
- debridement of infected soft tissue around infection
- antibiotics to cover aerobes and anaerobes (ampicillin/gentamicin/metronidazole or ciprofloxacin/metronidazole or clindamycin/gentamicin or cefotetan)

Paralytic Ileus

- see *Bowel Obstruction*, GS22

Delirium

- see <u>Psychiatry</u>

Thoracic Surgery

Esophagus

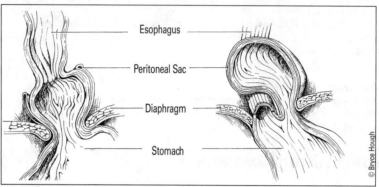

Figure 5. Types of Hiatus Hernia – Sliding (left) and Paraesophageal (right)

SLIDING HIATUS HERNIA (Type I) (see Figure 5)
- herniation of both the stomach and the gastroesophageal (GE) junction into thorax
- 90% of esophageal hernias

Risk Factors
- age
- weak myofascial structure
- increased intra-abdominal pressure (e.g. obesity, pregnancy)

Clinical Features
- majority are asymptomatic
- gastroesophageal reflux disease (GERD) – see <u>Gastroenterology</u>
  - heartburn, 1 to 3 hrs post-prandial
  - chest pain, regurgitation
  - relief with sitting, standing, water, antacids

Complications
- reflux, esophagitis, dysphagia, adenocarcinoma, chronic occult GI blood loss with anemia, ulceration, esophageal stricture, Barrett's esophagus, aspiration pneumonia, bleeding

Investigations
- upper GI series or barium swallow
- chest x-ray (CXR)
  - globular shadow with air-fluid level over cardiac silhouette
  - lateral – visible shadow in posterior mediastinum
- gastroscopy with biopsy
  - document type and extent of tissue damage
  - rule out esophagitis, Barrett's esophagus and cancer
- 24-hour esophageal pH monitoring
  - often used if atypical presentation or if considering surgery for reflux
  - gives information about frequency and duration of acid reflux and correlates symptoms with signs
- esophageal manometry
  - detects decreased lower esophageal sphincter (LES) pressure
  - may also diagnose motility disorder

Treatment
- lifestyle modification (as in GERD)
  - stop smoking, weight loss, elevate head of bed, no meals <3 hrs prior to sleeping, smaller and more frequent meals, avoid alcohol, coffee, mint and fat
- medical (as in GERD)
  - antacids
  - H_2 antagonist (e.g. cimetidine, ranitidine)
  - proton pump inhibitor (e.g. omeprazole, pantoprazole, lansoprazole)
  - adjuvant prokinetic agent (e.g. metoclopromide, domperidone)
- surgical (<15%)
  - Nissen fundoplication (laparoscopic)
    - fundus of stomach is wrapped around the lower esophagus and sutured in place
    - 90% success rate

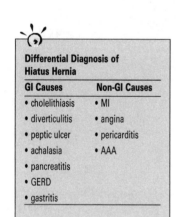

Differential Diagnosis of Hiatus Hernia

GI Causes	Non-GI Causes
• cholelithiasis	• MI
• diverticulitis	• angina
• peptic ulcer	• pericarditis
• achalasia	• AAA
• pancreatitis	
• GERD	
• gastritis	

- indications for surgery
  - complications of sliding hernia or GERD (especially stricture, severe ulceration, fibrosis, bleeding, Barrett's)
  - symptoms refractory to lifestyle modification and medical treatment
  - patient's desire not to be on lifelong medication

PARAESOPHAGEAL HIATUS HERNIA (Type II) (see Figure 5)

- herniation of all or part of the stomach through the esophageal hiatus into the thorax with an undisplaced gastroesophageal (GE) junction
- <10% of esophageal hernias (least common of types I, II, III, and IV)

Clinical Features
- usually asymptomatic due to normal GE junction
- pressure sensation in lower chest, dysphagia

Complications
- hemorrhage
- incarceration, strangulation, obstruction, gastric stasis ulcer

Treatment
- surgery to prevent severe complications
  - reduce hernia and excise hernia sac, repair defect at hiatus, and Nissen fundoplication
  - may consider suturing stomach to anterior abdominal wall (gastropexy) in some cases

MIXED HIATUS HERNIA (Type III)
- combination of Types I and II

Type IV Hernia
- herniation of other abdominal organs into thorax: colon, spleen, small bowel

ESOPHAGEAL PERFORATION

Etiology
- iatrogenic – most common
  - endoscopic, dilation, biopsy, intubation, operative, nasogastric (NG) tube placement
- barogenic
  - post-emetic (Boerhaave syndrome) with repeated, forceful vomiting
  - trauma
  - other: convulsions, defecation, labour (rare)
- foreign body
- corrosive injury
- carcinoma

> **Boerhaave's** = transmural esophageal perforation
> **Mallory-Weiss tear** = non-transmural esophageal tear
>
> Both are associated with forceful emesis

Clinical Features
- neck or chest pain, fever
- tachycardia, hypotension, dyspnea, respiratory compromise
- subcutaneous emphysema, pneumothorax, hematemesis

Investigations
- CXR
  - pneumothorax, pneumomediastinum, pleural effusion, subdiaphragmatic air
- contrast swallow
  - water-soluble then thin barium
- CT chest

Treatment
- depends on cause and location of the perforation (upper, mid, lower)
- supportive
  - drainage, NPO, vigorous fluid resuscitation, broad-spectrum antibiotics
- surgical
  - exploration and drainage
  - suture closure of major lacerations if tissue viable; may require flap if non-viable
  - cover with muscle flap

Complications
- sepsis, abscess, fistula, empyema, mediastinitis, death
- mortality 10-50% dependant on timing of diagnosis

ESOPHAGEAL CARCINOMA

Epidemiology
- 1% of all malignant lesions
- male:female = 3:1
- onset 50-60 years of age
- squamous cell carcinoma (SCC) 5x more common in African descent
- upper (20-33%), middle (33%), lower (33-50%)

Risk Factors
- obesity
- physical agents: alcohol, tobacco, nitrosamines, lye, radiation
- structural: diverticula, hiatus hernia, achalasia, GERD
- Barrett's esophagus
  - 8-10% risk of adenocarcinoma, monitor every 1-2 years by endoscopy and biopsy
- Plummer-Vinson syndrome – chronic iron deficiency

Clinical Features
- frequently asymptomatic – late presentation
- often dysphagia, first solids then liquids
- odynophagia then constant pain
- constitutional symptoms, especially weight loss and weakness
- regurgitation and aspiration (aspiration pneumonia)
- hematemesis, anemia
- tracheoesophageal or bronchoesophageal fistula
- direct, hematogenous or lymphatic spread
  - trachea (coughing), recurrent laryngeal nerves (hoarseness, vocal paralysis), aortic, liver, lung, bone, celiac and mediastinal nodes

---

Differential Diagnosis of Esophageal Carcinoma
- leiomyoma
- metastases
- lymphoma
- benign stricture
- achalasia
- GERD
- spasm

Investigations
- barium swallow to localize tumour
  - site of lesion is narrowed – shelf or annular lesion
- esophagoscopy
  - biopsy for tissue diagnosis and resectability/extent of tumour
- bronchoscopy
  - upper and mid esophageal lesions spread to tracheobronchial tree
- CT scan (chest/abdomen)
  - for local disease and staging – adrenal, liver, lung, bone metastases
- tracheoesophageal U/S
- metastatic work-up: bone scan, liver function tests, CT abdo/pelvis/chest

Treatment
- multimodal
  - combined chemotherapy, radiation and surgery
  - palliation or cure
  - survival rates higher than surgery alone
- surgery
  - esophagectomy (transthoracic or trans-hiatal approach)
    - anastomosis in chest or neck
    - stomach most often used for reconstruction
  - contraindications
    - invasion of tracheobronchial tree or great vessels
    - lesion >10 cm
  - palliation
    - resection, bypass, dilation and stent placement
    - laser ablation
- radiation
  - if unresectable, for palliation
    - relief (usually transient) of dysphagia in 2/3 of patients
- chemotherapy
  - alone, or pre- and post-operatively

Prognosis
- 5-8% operative death rate
- prognosis usually poor because presentation is usually at advanced stage

OTHER DISORDERS
- esophageal varices (see Gastroenterology)
- Mallory-Weiss tear (see Gastroenterology)

Chest Wall

CONGENITAL ABNORMALITIES
- pectus excavatum, pectus carinatum, sternal fissures
- surgery for: cosmesis, psychosocial factors, respiratory or cardiovascular insufficiency

THORACIC OUTLET SYNDROME
- impingement of subclavian vessels and brachial plexus nerve trunk

Etiology
- congenital – cervical rib
- trauma
- degenerative – osteoporosis, arthritis

Clinical Features
- neurogenic – ulnar and median nerve motor and sensory function
- arterial – fatigue, weakness, coldness, ischemic pain, paresthesia
- venous – edema, venous distention, collateral formation, cyanosis

Treatment
- conservative (50 to 90%)
    - physiotherapy, posture and behaviour modification
- surgical – if conservative treatment fails, removal of first or cervical rib (if applicable)

TUMOURS
- benign: fibrous dysplasia, eosinophilic granuloma, osteochondroma
- malignant: fibrosarcoma, chondrosarcoma, osteogenic sarcoma, Ewing's sarcoma, myeloma

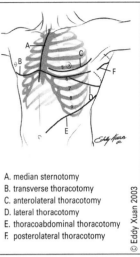

A. median sternotomy
B. transverse thoracotomy
C. anterolateral thoracotomy
D. lateral thoracotomy
E. thoracoabdominal thoracotomy
F. posterolateral thoracotomy

© Eddy Xuan 2003

Figure 6. Typical Thoracic Surgery Incisions

Pleura, Lung, and Mediastinum

- see Respirology

Stomach and Duodenum

Peptic Ulcer Disease

GASTRIC ULCERS
- see Gastroenterology

Surgical Treatment
- increasingly rare due to *H. pylori* eradication and medical treatment

Indications
- unresponsive to medical treatment (intractability)
    - always operate if fails to heal completely, even if biopsy negative – could be primary gastric lymphoma or adenocarcinoma
- dysplasia or carcinoma
    - always biopsy ulcer for malignancy
- hemorrhage – 3x greater risk of bleeding compared to duodenal ulcers
- complications: obstruction, perforation, bleeding

Procedures
- distal gastrectomy with ulcer excision – Billroth I or Billroth II (see Figure 7)
- vagotomy and pyloroplasty only if acid hypersecretion – rare
- wedge resection if possible or biopsy with primary repair

DUODENAL ULCERS
- see Gastroenterology
- most within 2 cm of pylorus (duodenal bulb)

Complications
- perforated ulcer (typically on anterior surface)
    - clinical features
        - sudden onset of pain (possibly in RLQ due to track down right paracolic gutter)
        - acute abdomen – rigid, diffuse guarding

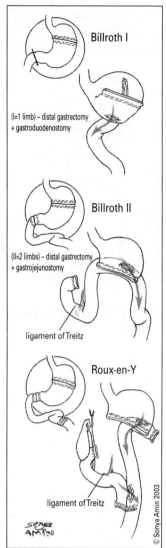

Figure 7. Billroth I & Billroth II with Roux-en-Y Reconstruction (gastrojejunostomy)

- ◆ ileus (absent bowel sounds)
- ◆ initial chemical peritonitis followed by bacterial peritonitis
  - ▪ investigations
    - ◆ CXR – free air under diaphragm (70% of patients)
  - ▪ treatment
    - ◆ oversew ulcer (plication) and omental (Graham) patch – most common treatment
- • posterior penetration
  - ▪ into pancreas → elevated amylase/lipase
  - ▪ constant mid-epigastric pain burrowing into back, unrelated to meals
- • hemorrhage (typically on posterior surface)
  - ▪ gastroduodenal artery involvement
  - ▪ treatment
    - ◆ resuscitation initially with crystalloids; blood transfusion for hypotension and hypovolemia
    - ◆ diagnostic and/or therapeutic endoscopy (laser, cautery or injection); if recurs, may have 2nd slope (NEJM 1999)
    - ◆ surgery if severe or recurrent bleeding hemodynamically unstable, or failure of endoscopy: oversewing of ulcer, pyloroplasty
- • gastric outlet obstruction
  - ▪ etiology: edema, fibrosis of pyloric channel, neoplasm
  - ▪ clinical presentation
    - ◆ nausea and vomiting (undigested food, non-bilious), dilated stomach, crampy abdominal pain
    - ◆ succession splash
    - ◆ auscultate gas and fluid movement in obstructed organ
  - ▪ treatment
    - ◆ NG decompression and correction of hypochloremic, hypokalemic metabolic alkalosis
    - ◆ medical management initially: high dose PPI therapy
    - ◆ if obstruction does not resolve, consider surgical resection: either Billroth I, pyloroplasty or gastrojejunostomy to bypass

Treatment
- • surgical indications
  - ▪ hemorrhage, rebleed in hospital, perforation, gastric outlet obstruction
    - ◆ decision to operate based on amount of blood loss (>8 units), rate of bleeding and hemodynamic stability
  - ▪ intractable despite medical management (endoscopy)
- • procedures
  - ▪ oversewing of ulcer, pyloroplasty
  - ▪ vagotomy
    - ◆ rarely done now with *H. pylori* eradication
- • complications
  - ▪ recurrent ulcer
  - ▪ retained antrum
  - ▪ fistula (gastrocolic/gastrojejunal)
  - ▪ anemia
  - ▪ dumping syndrome, postvagotomy diarrhea, afferent loop syndrome (see *Complications of Gastric Surgery* section, GS18)

Gastric Carcinoma

Epidemiology
- • male:female = 3:2
- • incidence for adenocarcinoma = 10 per 100000 incidence highest in Asia (Japan 80 times higher than in U.S.)
- • most common age group 50-59 years
- • decreased incidence by 2/3 in past 50 years

Risk Factors
- • *H. pylori*, causing chronic atrophic gastritis
- • hereditary nonpolyposis colorectal cancer (HNPCC)
- • smoking, alcohol, smoked food, nitrosamines
- • pernicious anemia associated with achlorhydria and chronic atrophic gastritis
- • gastric adenomatous polyps
- • previous partial gastrectomy (>10 years post-gastrectomy)
- • hypertrophic gastropathy
- • blood type A

Clinical Features
- clinical suspicion
  - ulcer fails to heal
  - lesion on greater curvature of stomach or cardia
- asymptomatic, insidious or late onset of symptoms
  - postprandial abdominal fullness, vague epigastric pain
  - anorexia, weight loss
  - burping, nausea, vomiting, dyspepsia, dysphagia
  - hepatomegaly, epigastric mass (25%)
  - hematemesis, fecal occult blood, melena, iron-deficiency anemia
- rare signs
  - Virchow's node – left supraclavicular node
  - Blumer's shelf – mass in pouch of Douglas
  - Krukenberg tumour – metastases to ovary
  - Sister Mary Joseph nodule - umbilical metastases
  - Irish's node - left axillary nodes
- metastasis
  - liver, lung, brain

Investigations
- oesophagogastroduodenoscopy (OGD) and biopsy
- chest/abdo/pelvis CT
- CT for metastatic work-up (see Table 4)

Table 4. Staging of Gastric and Esophageal Carcinoma

Stage	Criteria	Prognosis (5-year survival)
I	mucosa and submucosa	70%
II	extension to muscularis propria	30%
III	extension to regional nodes	10%
IV	distant metastases or involvement of continuous structures	0%
Overall		10%

Treatment
- adenocarcinoma
  - proximal lesions
    - total gastrectomy and esophagojejunostomy – Roux-en-Y (see Figure 7)
  - distal lesions
    - distal gastrectomy: wide margins, en bloc removal of omentum and lymph nodes
  - palliation
    - gastric resection to decrease bleeding and relieve obstruction, enables the patient to eat
    - radiation therapy
- lymphoma
  - chemotherapy ± radiation, surgery in limited cases (perforation, bleeding, obsruction)

Gastric Sarcoma

Gastrointestinal Stromal Tumour (GIST)
- most common mesenchymal neoplasm of GI tract
- derived from interstitial cells of Cajal (cells associated with Auerbach's plexus that have autonomous pacemaker function co-ordinate peristalsis throughout the GI tract)
- 75-80% associated with tyrosine kinase (c-KIT) mutations
- 50% in stomach, extra-gastric locations carry a higher risk of progression
- typically present with vague abdominal mass, feeling of abdominal fullness, or with secondary symptoms of bleeding and anemia
- often discovered incidentally on CT, laparotomy, endoscopy

Risk Factors
- Carney's Triad: GISTs, paraganglioma, and pulmonary chondroma
- Type IA neurofibromatosis

Prognosis
- risk of metastatic potential depends on:
  - tumour size (worse if >10 cm)
  - mitotic activity (worse if >5 mitotic figures or 50 hpf)
  - degree of nuclear pleomorphism
  - location: with identical sizes, extra-gastric location has a higher risk of progression than GISTs in the stomach

Management
- pre-operative biopsy: controversial, but useful for indeterminate lesions
  - not recommended if index of suspicion for GIST is high

- percutaneous biopsy is NOT recommended due to high friability and risk of peritoneal spread
- localized GIST: surgical resection with preservation of intact pseudocapsule
  - lymphadenectomy NOT recommended, as GISTs rarely metatasize to lymph nodes
- advanced disease: metastases to liver and/or peritoneal cavity
  - chemotherapy with imatinib mesylate (tyrosine kinase inhibitor)
  - current research looking into role of imatinib as adjuvant or neoadjuvant therapy for localized GIST

Bariatric Surgery

- weight reduction surgery for morbid obesity

Surgical Options
- malabsorptive
  - duodenal switch
    - gastrectomy, enteroenterostomy, duodenal division closure and duodenoenterostomy
- malabsorptive/restrictive
  - long-limb gastric bypass
    - staple off small gastric pouch with Roux-en-Y limb to pouch
    - laparoscopic surgery now standard of care
- restrictive
  - gastric banding
  - laparoscopic vertical banded gastroplasty
    - vertical stapled small gastric pouch with placement of silastic ring band
    - least invasive

Complications of Gastric Surgery

- most resolve within 1 year

Alkaline Reflux Gastritis
- duodenal contents (bilious) reflux into stomach causing gastritis ± esophagitis
- treatment
  - medical: H$_2$ blocker, metoclopramide, cholestyramine
  - surgical: conversion of Billroth I or II to Roux-en-Y

Afferent Loop Syndrome
- accumulation of bile and pancreatic secretions causes intermittent mechanical obstruction and distension of afferent limb
- clinical features
  - early postprandial distention, RUQ pain, nausea, bilious vomiting, anemia
- treatment: surgery (conversion to Roux-en-Y increases afferent loop drainage)

Dumping Syndrome
- early – 15 minutes post-prandial
  - etiology
    - hyperosmotic chyme released into small bowel (fluid accumulation and jejunal distention)
  - clinical features
    - post-prandial symptoms
    - epigastric fullness or pain, emesis, nausea, diarrhea, palpitations, dizziness, tachycardia, diaphoresis
  - treatment
    - small multiple low carbohydrate, low fat and high protein meals and avoidance of liquids with meals
    - last resort is interposition of antiperistaltic jejunal loop between stomach and small bowel to delay gastric emptying
- late – 3 hours post-prandial
  - etiology: large glucose load leads to large insulin release and hypoglycemia
  - treatment: small snack 2 hours after meals

Blind-Loop Syndrome
- bacterial overgrowth of colonic Gram negative bacteria in afferent limb
- clinical features
  - anemia/weakness, diarrhea, malnutrition, abdominal pain and hypocalcemia
- treatment: broad-spectrum antibiotics, surgery (conversion to Billroth I or Roux-en-y)

Postvagotomy Diarrhea
- up to 25%
- bile salts in colon inhibit water resorption
- treatment: medical (cholestyramine), surgical (reversed interposition jejunal segment)

Small Intestine

Tumours of Small Intestine

Risk Factors
- carcinogen exposure (red meat in diet)
- familial colonic polyposis, Peutz-Jegher syndrome, Gardner's syndrome
- Crohn's disease, celiac disease
- immunodeficiency, autoimmune disorders

Clinical Features
- usually asymptomatic until advanced
- most common
  - intermittent obstruction, intussusception, occult bleeding, palpable abdominal mass, abdominal pain

Benign Tumours
- usually asymptomatic until large
- 10x more common than malignant
- most common sites: terminal ileum, proximal jejunum
- polyps
  - adenomas
  - familial adenomatous polyposis (FAP) (see *Familial Colon Cancer Syndromes*, GS32)
  - malignant degeneration of polyps common
  - hamartomatous
  - juvenile polyps
- other: leiomyomas, lipomas, hemangiomas

Malignant Tumours
- usually asymptomatic until advanced stage
  - 25-30% associated with distant metastases at time of diagnosis
- adenocarcinoma
  - most common primary tumour of small intestine
  - usually 50-70 years old, male predominance
  - usually in proximal small bowel, incidence decreases distally
  - risk factors: Crohn's disease, FAP
  - early metastasis to lymph nodes – 80% metastatic at time of operation
  - investigations – CT abdo/pelvis, endoscopy
  - treatment – surgical resection ± chemotherapy
  - 5-year survival 25%
- carcinoid
  - increased incidence 50-60 years old
  - originate from enterochromaffin cell in crypts
  - most commonly 60 cm from the ileocecal (IC) valve
    - appendix 46%, distal ileum 28%, rectum 17%
  - often slow-growing
  - classified by embryological origin (correlate with morphology, biological behaviour)
    - foregut – stomach, duodenum, pancreas
    - midgut – jejunum, ileum, appendix, ascending colon
    - hindgut – transverse, descending and sigmoid colon, rectum
  - clinical features
    - usually asymptomatic, incidental finding
    - obstruction, bleeding, crampy abdominal pain, intussusception
    - carcinoid syndrome (<10%)
      - hot flashes, hypotension, diarrhea, bronchoconstriction (wheezing), tricuspid/pulmonic valve insufficiency, right heart failure
      - requires liver involvement: lesion secretes serotonin, kinins and vasoactive peptides directly to systemic circulation (normally inactivated by liver)
      - EXCEPTION: carcinoid tumours arising in the bronchi can cause carcinoid syndrome without liver involvement because of access to systemic circulation
  - investigations
    - most found at surgery for obstruction or appendectomy
    - elevated 5-HIAA (breakdown product of serotonin) in urine or increased 5-HT in blood
  - treatment
    - tumour and metastases: surgical resection ± chemotherapy
    - carcinoid syndrome: steroids, histamine, octreotide
  - prognosis
    - metastatic risk 2% if size <1 cm, 90% if >2 cm
    - 5-year survival 70%; 20% with liver metastases
- lymphoma
  - highest incidence at 70 years old, more common in males

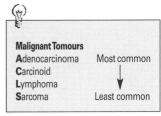

Malignant Tumours
Adenocarcinoma   Most common
Carcinoid
Lymphoma
Sarcoma   Least common

Symptoms of Carcinoid Syndrome
Flushing
Diarrhea
Right-sided heart failure

Ability of somatostatin receptor scintigraphy to identify patients with gastric carcinoids: a prospective study.
J Nucl Med 2000 41(10):1646-56
Background: Carcinoid tumours are challenging cancers to identify, with low detection rates achieved by conventional radiologic imaging modalities. Somatostatin receptor scintigraphy (SRS) is a new imaging modality which has been shown to have improved rates of detection of carcinoid tumours compared to conventional imaging studies. The purpose of this study was to determine the sensitivity and specificity of SRS in identifying gastric carcinoids.
Methods: 162 consecutive patients with Zollinger-Ellison syndrome (ZES) were studied prospectively. Patients were investigated by annual SRS with SPECT, upper gastrointestinal endoscopy, and direct biopsies of any detected gastric abnormalities, as well as random gastric tissue biopsies. Results of SRS were correlated with the gastric biopsy results.
Results: Gastric SRS localization was positive in 19 (12%) of 162 patients. Sixteen patients had a gastric carcinoid, and 12 of these patients had SRS localization. The sensitivity of SRS in localizing a gastric carcinoid was 75%, with a specificity of 95%. Positive and negative predictive values were 63% and 97%, respectively.
Conclusion: SRS is a noninvasive method which can be used to identify gastric carcinoid tumours with high specificity and reasonable sensitivity.

- usually non-Hodgkin's lymphoma
- location
  - usually distal ileum
  - proximal jejunum in patients with celiac disease
- clinical features
  - fatigue, weight loss, abdominal pain, fever, malabsorption
  - rarely – perforation, obstruction, bleeding, intussusception
- treatment
  - low grade: chemotherapy with cyclophosphamide
  - high grade: surgical resection, radiation
  - palliative: somatostatin, doxorubicin
- 5-year survival 40%
- metastatic
  - most common site for metastatic melanoma
  - hematogenous spread from breast, lung, kidney
  - direct extension from cervix, ovaries, colon
- gastrointestinal stromal tumours (GISTs)
  - most common in jejunum, ileum, Meckel's diverticulum
  - enlarge extraluminally → late obstruction

Meckel's Diverticulum

- remnant of the embryonic vitelline duct on antimesenteric border of ileum
- heterotopic – several types of mucosa including gastric, pancreatic, colonic
- most common true diverticulum of GI tract

Clinical Features
- 2% symptomatic
- GI bleed, small bowel obstruction (SBO), diverticulitis (mimics appendicitis)
- painless bleeding – ulceration caused by ectopic gastric mucosa
  - 50% of patients with this presentation are <2 years old

Investigations
- technetium-99 to identify the ectopic gastric mucosa (Meckel's scan)

Complications
- fistula: umbilicus-ileum, umbilical sinus
- fibrous cord between umbilicus and ileum
- SBO due to volvulus, intussusception, perforation

Treatment
- incidental finding – consider surgical resection
- symptomatic – fluid and electrolyte stabilization and surgical resection
- broad based – segmental resection to remove all mucosal types

Rule of 2's for Meckel's diverticulum
- **2%** of the population
- symptomatic in **2%** of cases
- found within **2** feet (10-90 cm) of the ileocecal (IC) valve
- **2** inches in length
- often present by **2** years of age

Hernia

- fascial defect → protrusion of a viscus into an area in which it is not normally contained

Epidemiology
- male:female = 9:1
- lifetime risk of developing hernia: males 5%, females 1%
- most common surgical disease of males

Clinical Features
- mass of variable size
- tenderness worse at end of day, relieved with supine position or with reduction
- abdominal fullness, vomiting, constipation
- transmits palpable impulse with coughing or straining

Investigations
- U/S ± CT

Classification
- complete – hernia sac and contents protrude through defect
- incomplete – incomplete protrusion through the defect
- internal hernia – sac is within abdominal cavity
- external hernia – sac protrudes completely through abdominal wall
- strangulated hernia – vascular supply of protruded viscus is compromised (ischemia)
- incarcerated hernia – irreducible hernia, not necessarily strangulated
- Richter's hernia – only part of circumference of bowel (usually anti-mesenteric border) incarcerated or strangulated so may not be obstructed

- a strangulated Richter's hernia may self-reduce and thus be overlooked, leaving a gangrenous segment at risk of perforation
- sliding hernia – part of wall of hernia formed by protruding viscus (usually cecum, sigmoid colon, bladder)

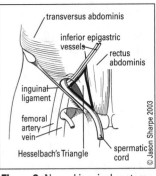

Figure 8. Normal inguinal anatomy

Anatomical Types
- groin (see Table 6)
    - indirect and direct inguinal, femoral (see Figure 10)
    - pantaloon: combined direct and indirect hernias, peritoneum draped over inferior epigastric vessels
- epigastric: defect in linea alba above umbilicus
- incisional: ventral hernia at site of wound closure, may be secondary to wound infection
- Littre's: hernia involving Meckel's diverticulum
- lumbar: defect in posterior abdominal wall (superior = Grynfeltt's, inferior = Petit's)
- obturator: through obturator foramen
- parastomal: hernia at or adjacent to an ostomy (commonly colostomy)
- Spigelian: ventral hernia through defect in linea semilunaris
- umbilical: passes through umbilical ring
    - congenital, ascites, pregnancy, obesity

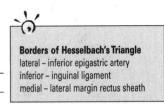

Borders of Hesselbach's Triangle
lateral – inferior epigastric artery
inferior – inguinal ligament
medial – lateral margin rectus sheath

Table 5. Superficial Inguinal Ring vs. Deep Inguinal Ring

Superficial Inguinal Ring	Deep Inguinal Ring
• opening in ext. abdominal aponeurosis; palpable superior and lateral to pubic tubercle	• opening in transversalis fascia: palpable superior to mid-inguinal ligament
• medial border: medial crus of ext. abdominal aponeurosis	• superior-lateral border: internal oblique and transversus abdominus muscles
• lateral border: lateral crus of ext. oblique aponeurosis	• medial border: inf. epigastric vessels
• roof: intercrural fibres	• inferior border: inguinal ligament

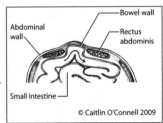

Figure 9. Richter's Hernia

Risk Factors
- activities which increase intra-abdominal pressure
    - obesity, chronic cough, pregnancy, constipation, straining on urination or defecation, ascites, heavy lifting
- congenital abnormality – e.g. patent processus vaginalis
- previous hernia repair

Complications
- incarceration: irreducible
- strangulation: irreducible with resulting ischemia
    - small, new hernias more likely to strangulate
    - intense pain followed by tenderness
    - intestinal obstruction, gangrenous bowel, sepsis
    - surgical emergency
    - do not attempt to manually reduce hernia if septic or if contents of hernial sac gangrenous

Treatment
- surgical treatment is only to prevent strangulation and evisceration or for cosmesis or symptoms; if asymptomatic can delay surgery
- repair may be done open or laparascopic and may use mesh for tension-free closure
- most repairs are now done with a plug in the hernial defect and a patch over it or patch alone

Postoperative Complications
- scrotal hematoma
    - deep bleeding – may enter retroperitoneal space and not be initially apparent
    - difficulty voiding
    - painful scrotal swelling from compromised venous return of testes
- nerve entrapment
    - ilioinguinal
    - genital branch of genitofemoral
- stenosis/occlusion of femoral vein
    - acute leg swelling
- recurrence
    - risk factors: recurrent hernia, age >50, smoking, BMI < 25, poor pre-op functional status (ASA ≥3 - see Anesthesia), associated medical conditions: type II DM, hyperlipidemia, immunosuppression, any comorbid conditions increasing intra-abdominal pressure

Groin Hernias

Contents of spermatic cord
vas deferens, testicular artery/veins, genital branch of genitofemoral nerve, lymphatics, cremaster muscle

Table 6. Groin Hernias

	Direct Inguinal	Indirect Inguinal	Femoral
Epidemiology	• 1% of all men	• most common hernia in men & women • males > females	• affects mostly females
Etiology	• acquired weakness of transversalis fascia • "wear and tear" • increased intra-abdominal pressure	• congenital persistence of processus vaginalis in 20% of adults	• pregnancy – weakness of pelvic floor musculature • increased intra-abdominal pressure
Anatomy	• through Hesselbach's triangle • medial to inferior epigastric artery • usually does not descend into scrotal sac	• originates in deep inguinal ring • lateral to inferior epigastric artery • often descends into scrotal sac (or labia majora)	• into femoral canal, below inguinal ligament but may override it • medial to femoral vein within femoral canal
Complications			• narrow neck causes incarceration (1/3) and strangulation
Treatment	• surgical repair	• surgical repair	• surgical repair
Prognosis	• 3-4% risk of recurrence	• <1% risk of recurrence	

site of deep inguinal ring

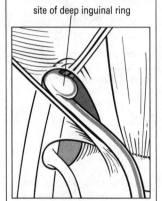

indirect hernia

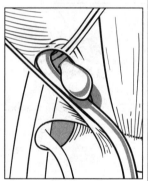

direct hernia

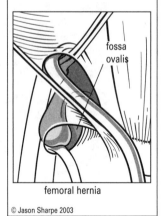

fossa ovalis

femoral hernia

© Jason Sharpe 2003

Figure 10. Schematic of Inguinal (Direct and Indirect) and Femoral Hernias

Bowel Obstruction

Differential Diagnosis
• small bowel obstruction (SBO), large bowel obstruction (LBO), pseudo-obstruction

Pathogenesis
• disruption of the normal flow of intestinal contents → proximal dilation + distal decompression
• may take 12-24 hrs to decompress, therefore passage of feces and flatus may occur after the onset of obstruction
• bowel ischemia may occur if blood supply is strangulated or bowel wall inflammation leads to venous congestion
• bowel wall edema and disruption of normal bowel absorptive function → increased intraluminal fluid → transudative fluid loss into peritoneal cavity, electrolyte disturbances

Clinical Features
• must differentiate between obstruction and ileus, and characterize obstruction as acute vs. chronic, partial vs. complete (constipation vs. obstipation), small vs. large bowel, strangulating vs. non-strangulating, and with vs. without perforation

Table 7. Bowel Obstruction vs. Paralytic Ileus

	SBO	LBO	Paralytic ileus
Nausea, vomiting	early, may be bilious	late, may be feculent	present
Abdominal pain	colicky	colicky	minimal or absent
Abdominal distention	+ (prox) → ++ (distal)	++	+
Constipation/obstipation	+	+	+
Other	± visible peristalsis	± visible peristalsis	
Bowel sounds	normal, increased absent if secondary ileus	normal, increased (borborygmi) absent if secondary ileus	decreased, absent
AXR findings	• air-fluid levels • "ladder" pattern (plicae circularis) • proximal distention (>3 cm) + no colonic gas	• air-fluid levels • "picture frame" appearance • proximal distention + distal decompression • no small bowel air if competent ileocecal valve	• air throughout small bowel and colon

Complications
• strangulating obstruction (10% of bowel obstructions) – surgical emergency
  ▪ cramping pain turns to continuous ache, hematemesis, melena (if infarction)
  ▪ fever, leukocytosis, tachycardia
  ▪ peritoneal signs, early shock
  ▪ see also *Intestinal Ischemia*, GS25
• other
  ▪ perforation: secondary to ischemia and luminal distention
  ▪ septicemia
  ▪ hypovolemia (due to third spacing)

Investigations
• radiological
  ▪ upright CXR or left lateral decubitus (LLD) to rule out free air

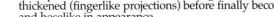

- abdominal x-ray (3 views) to determine SBO vs. LBO vs. ileus (Table 7)
  - if ischemic bowel look for: free air, pneumatosis, thickened bowel wall, air in portal vein, dilated small and large bowels, haustra become thickened (fingerlike projections) before finally becoming featureless and hoselike in appearance
- other:
  - CT provides information on level of obstruction, severity, cause
  - upper GI series/small bowel series for SBO (if no cause apparent, i.e. no hernias, no previous surgeries)
  - Hypaque™ enema for LBO (oral contrast in LBO may inspissate (thicken) and convert partial to complete LBO)
  - if suspect LBO, consider rectal contrast instead of Hypaque™ enema
  - may consider U/S in pregnant patients
- laboratory
  - may be normal early in disease course
  - BUN, creatinine, hematocrit (hemoconcentration) to assess degree of dehydration
  - fluid, electrolyte abnormalities
  - amylase elevated
  - metabolic alkalosis due to frequent emesis
  - if strangulation: leukocytosis with left shift, lactic acidosis, elevated LDH (late signs)

Small Bowel Obstruction (SBO)

Etiology
- extrinsic: **adhesions** (60%) – if previous abdo surgery > hernia (20%) > volvulus, neoplasm, annular pancreas
- intraluminal: gallstone, feces, meconium, foreign body, intussusception
- intrinsic: neoplasm (15%) > strictures (Crohn's, radiation) > congenital malformations, cystic fibrosis, superior mesenteric artery syndrome

Top 3 causes of SBO
Adhesions > **B**ulge (hernias) > **C**ancer (neoplasms)

Treatment
- consider whether complete or partial obstruction, ongoing or impending strangulation, location and cause
  - stabilize vitals, fluid and electrolyte resuscitation (with normal saline/Ringer's first, then with added potassium after fluid deficits are corrected)
  - NG tube to relieve vomiting, prevent aspiration and decompress small bowel
  - Foley catheter to monitor in/outs
  - SBO with history of abdo/pelvic surgery → conservative management (likely to resolve) → surgery if no resolution in 48-72 hrs
  - complete SBO, strangulation → urgent surgery after stabilizing patient
  - trial of medical management may be indicated in Crohn's, recurrent SBO, carcinomatosis

Prognosis
- mortality: non-strangulating <1%, strangulating 8% (25% if >36 hours), ischemic = up to 50%

Large Bowel Obstruction (LBO)

Etiology
- **colorectal carcinoma** (65%)
- diverticulitis (20%) – strictures from repeated attacks
- volvulus (5%) – sigmoid > cecum
- other causes: IBD, benign tumours, fecal impaction, foreign body, adhesions, hernia (especially sliding type), intussusception (children), endometriosis, extrinsic mass

Top 3 causes of LBO
Cancer > diverticulitis > volvulus

Clinical Features (unique to LBO)
- open loop (10-20%) (safe):
  - incompetent ileocecal valve allows relief of colonic pressure as contents reflux into ileum, therefore clinical presentation similar to SBO
- closed loop (80-90%) (dangerous):
  - competent ileocecal valve, allowing build up of colonic pressures to dangerous level
  - massive colonic distention → high risk of perforation, ischemia
    - cecum at greatest risk of perforation due to Laplace's Law (pressure = wall tension/radius)
    - suspect impending perforation in the presence of tenderness over the cecum

Treatment
- initial management: correct fluid and electrolyte imbalance, NG suction, continuous observation
- surgical correction of obstruction (usually requires resection + temporary diverting colostomy)

In a patient with clinical LBO, a cecum ≥12 cm may denote impending perforation.

- volvulus → sigmoidoscopic or endoscopic decompression followed by operative reduction if unsuccessful
    - if successful, consider sigmoid resection on same admission

Prognosis
- overall mortality: 10%
- cecal perforation + feculent peritonitis: 20% mortality

Pseudo-Obstruction

Differential Diagnosis
- acute: toxic megacolon, trauma, post-operative, neurologic disease, retroperitoneal disease
- chronic: neurologic disease (enteric, central, peripheral nervous systems), scleroderma

Toxic Megacolon

Pathogenesis
- extension of inflammation into smooth muscle layer causing paralysis
- damage to myenteric plexus and electrolyte abnormalities are not consistently found

Etiologies
- inflammatory bowel disease (ulcerative colitis > Crohn's Disease)
- infectious colitis: bacterial (*C. difficile, Salmonella, Shigella, Campylobacter*), viral (cytomegalovirus), parasitic (*E. histolytica*)
- volvulus, diverticulitis, ischemic colitis, obstructing colon cancer are rare causes

Clinical Features
- infectious colitis usually present for >1 week before colonic dilatation
- diarrhea ± blood (but improvement of diarrhea may portend onset of megacolon)
- abdominal distention, tenderness, ± local/general peritoneal signs (suggest perforation)
- triggers: hypokalemia, constipating agents (opioids, antidepressants, loperamide, anticholinergics), barium enema, colonoscopy

Be careful when giving antidiarrheals, especially with bloody diarrhea.

Diagnostic Criteria
- must have both colitis and systemic manifestations for diagnosis
- radiologic evidence of dilated colon
- three of: fever, HR >120, WBC >10.5, anemia
- one of: fluid and electrolyte disturbances, hypotension, altered LOC

Investigations
- CBC (leukocytosis with left shift, anemia from bloody diarrhea), electrolytes, elevated CRP, ESR
- metabolic alkalosis (volume contraction and hypokalemia) and hypoalbuminemia are late findings
- AXR: dilated colon >6 cm (right > transverse > left), loss of haustra
- CT: useful to assess underlying disease

Treatment
- NPO, NG tube, stop constipating agents, correct fluid and electrolyte abnormalities, transfusion
- serial AXRs
- broad-spectrum antibiotics (reduce sepsis, anticipate perforation)
- aggressive treatment of underlying disease (e.g. steroids in IBD, metronidazole for *C. difficile*)
- indications for surgery (50% improve on medical management):
    - worsening or persisting toxicity or dilation after 48-72 hrs
    - severe hemorrhage, perforation
- procedure: subtotal colectomy + end ileostomy with 2nd operation for re-anastomosis

Prognosis
- average 25-30% mortality

Paralytic Ileus

Pathogenesis
- temporary paralysis of the myenteric plexus

Associations
- post-operative, intra-abdominal sepsis, medications (opiates, anesthetics, psychotropics), electrolyte disturbances (Na, K, Ca), *C. difficile*, inactivity

Treatment
- NG decompression, NPO, fluid resuscitation, correct causative abnormalities (e.g. sepsis, meds, electrolytes), consider TPN for prolonged ileus
- post-op: gastric and small bowel motility returns by 24-48 hrs, colonic motility by 3-5 d

Ogilvie's Syndrome

- acute pseudo-obstruction
- distention of colon without mechanical obstruction
- arises in bedridden patients with serious extraintestinal illness or trauma
- first presents with abdominal distention ± tenderness
- later symptoms mimic true obstruction

Associations
- disability (long term debilitation, chronic disease, bed-bound nursing home patients, paraplegia), drugs (narcotic use, laxative abuse, polypharmacy), other (recent orthopaedic surgery, post-partum, hypokalemia, retroperitoneal hematoma, diffuse carcinomatosis)

Investigations
- AXR: cecal dilatation - if diameter >12 cm, increased risk of perforation

Treatment
- treat underlying cause
- NPO, NG tube
- decompression: rectal tube, colonoscopy, neostigmine (cholinergic drug), surgical decompression (ostomy/resection) uncommon
- surgery if perforation, ischemia or failure of conservative management (uncommon)

Prognosis
- most resolve with conservative management

Intestinal Ischemia

Etiology
- acute:
  - arterial
    - occlusive: thrombotic, embolic, extrinsic compression (e.g. strangulating hernia)
    - non-occlusive: mesenteric vasoconstriction 2° to systemic hypoperfusion (preserves supply to vital organs)
    - trauma/dissection
  - venous thrombosis (prevents venous outflow): consider hypercoagulable state, deep vein thrombosis (DVT)
- chronic: usually due to atherosclerotic disease – look for CVS risk factors

Pain "out of keeping with physical findings" is the hallmark of early intestinal ischemia.

Clinical Features
- acute: severe abdominal pain out of proportion to physical findings, vomiting, bloody diarrhea, bloating, minimal peritoneal signs early in course (difficult diagnosis to make), hypotension, shock, sepsis
- chronic: postprandial pain (fear of food), weight loss
- common sites: superior mesenteric artery (SMA) supplied territory, "watershed" areas of colon (splenic flexure, left colon, sigmoid colon)

Investigations
- labs: leukocytosis (non-specific), lactic acidosis (late finding)
  - amylase, LDH, CK, ALP can be used to observe progress
  - hypercoagulability workup if suspect venous thrombosis
- AXR: portal venous gas, intestinal pneumatosis, free air if perforation
- contrast CT: thickened bowel wall, luminal dilatation, SMA or SMV thrombus, mesenteric/portal venous gas, pneumatosis
- CT angiography – gold standard for acute arterial ischemia

Treatment
- fluid resuscitation, NPO, prophylactic broad-spectrum antibiotics
- exploratory laparotomy
- angiogram, embolectomy/thrombectomy, bypass/graft, mesenteric endarterectomy, anticoagulation therapy
- segmental resection of necrotic intestine
  - assess extent of viability; if extent of bowel viability is questionable, a second look laparotomy 12-24 hrs later is mandatory (questionable areas will declare themselves)

An acute abdomen + metabolic acidosis is bowel ischemia until proven otherwise.

Appendix

Appendicitis

Epidemiology
- 6% of population, M>F
- 80% between 5-35 years of age

Pathogenesis
- luminal obstruction → bacterial overgrowth → inflammation/swelling → increased pressure → localized ischemia → gangrene/perforation → localized abscess (walled off by omentum) or peritonitis
- etiology
  - children or young adult: hyperplasia of lymphoid follicles, initiated by infection
  - adult: fibrosis/stricture, fecolith, obstructing neoplasm
  - other causes: parasites, foreign body

Clinical Features
- most reliable feature is progression of signs and symptoms
- low grade fever (38°C), rises if perforation
- abdominal pain then anorexia, nausea and vomiting
- classic pattern: pain initially periumbilical, constant, dull, poorly localized → then well localized pain over McBurney's point
  - due to progression of disease from visceral irritation (causing referred pain from structures of the embryonic midgut, including the appendix) to irritation of parietal structures
  - McBurney's sign: tenderness 1/3 from anterior superior iliac spine (ASIS) to umbilicus
- signs:
  - inferior appendix: McBurney's sign (see above), Rovsing's sign (palpation pressure to left abdomen causes McBurney's point tenderness)
  - retrocecal appendix: psoas sign (pain on flexion of hip against resistance or passive hyperextension of hip)
  - pelvic appendix: obturator sign (flexion then external or internal rotation about right hip causes pain)
- complications:
  - perforation (especially if >24 h duration)
  - abscess, phlegmon

Investigations
- labs
  - mild leukocytosis with left shift (may have normal WBC counts)
    - higher leukocyte count with perforation
  - β-hCG to rule out ectopic pregnancy, urinalysis
- imaging

  - upright CXR, AXR: usually nonspecific – free air if perforated (rarely), calcified fecolith, loss of psoas shadow
  - U/S: may visualize appendix, but also helps rule out gynecological causes – overall accuracy 90-94%
  - CT scan: thick wall, appendicolith, inflammatory changes – overall accuracy 94-100%, optimal investigation

Treatment
- hydrate, correct electrolyte abnormalities
- surgery + antibiotic coverage
- if localized abscess (palpable mass or large phlegmon on imaging and often pain >4-5 days), consider radiologic drainage + antibiotics x 14 d + interval appendectomy in 6 weeks
- appendectomy:
  - laparoscopic or open
  - complications: spillage of bowel contents, pelvic abscess, enterocutaneous fistula

Antibiotics versus placebo for prevention of postoperative infection after appendectomy
(Cochrane Database of Systematic Reviews 2005; 3)

Study: Meta-analysis of Randomised Controlled Trials (RCTs) and Controlled Clinical Trials (CCTs), on both adults and children, in which any antibiotic regime was compared to placebo in patients undergoing appendectomy for suspected appendicitis.
Data Sources: Cochrane Central Register of Controlled Trials (2005 issue 1), PubMed (1966 to April 2005), EMBASE (1980 to April 2005), Cochrane Colorectal Cancer Group Specialised Register (April 2005), and reference lists from included studies.
Patients: Wound infection, 20 studies (n=2343). Post-operative Intra-abdominal abscess, 8 studies (n=1033).
Main Outcomes: (1) Wound infection (discharge of pus from the wounds) and (2) Postoperative intra abdominal abscess (persistent pyrexia without any other focus, after operation, palpable mass in the abdomen or discharge of pus from the rectum).
Results: Treatment with antibiotics decreased infection rates with an NNT=37 (p<0.00001). While treatment with antibiotics decreased abscess rates with an NNT=199 (p=0.03).
Conclusion: Various prophylactic antibiotic regimens are effective in preventing post-operative complications. Further studies are required to determine the ideal regiment.

Laparoscopic vs. Open Appendectomy

Laparoscopic surgery
- Intra-abdominal abscesses 3 times more likely
- Mean length of hospital stay reduced by 0.7 d
- Sooner return to normal activity, work & sport
- Costs outside hospital are reduced
- Reduced levels of pain on POD #1

Open surgery
- Wound infections 2 times as likely
- Lower operation costs

Overview
Diagnostic laparoscopy led to a large reduction in the rate of negative appendectomies, and a reduction in surgeries with unestablished diagnosis. This was especially pronounced in fertile women due to a broader differential for appendicitis.

Sauerland S, Lefering R, Neugebauer EAM. Laparoscopic versus open surgery for suspected appendicitis (Cochrane Review). In: The Cochrane Library, Issue 3, 2004. Chichester, UK: John Wiley & Sons, Ltd.

- perioperative antibiotics:
  - ◆ ampicillin + gentamicin + metronidazole (antibiotics x 24 h only if non-perforated)
  - ◆ other choices: 2nd/3rd generation cephalosporin for aerobic gut organisms

Prognosis
- morbidity/mortality 0.6% if uncomplicated, 5% if perforated

Tumours of the Appendix

CARCINOID TUMOURS (most common type)
- appendix is the most common location
- usually benign (97%)
- usually asymptomatic
- may produce carcinoid syndrome if liver function compromised (e.g. liver metastasis)
- treatment
  - appendectomy if <2 cm and not extending into serosa
  - right hemicolectomy if >2 cm, extending through the serosa, if nodal or if base of appendix involved (increased incidence of malignancy)

ADENOCARCINOMA
- 50% present as acute appendicitis
- spreads rapidly to lymph nodes, ovaries, and peritoneal surfaces
- treatment: right hemicolectomy

OTHER
- malignant mucinous cystadenocarcinoma

Inflammatory Bowel Disease (IBD)

- see also Gastroenterology

Principles of Surgical Management
- can alleviate symptoms, address complications, improve quality of life
- conserve bowel – resect as little as possible (beware short gut syndrome)
- perioperative management:
  - optimize medical status: may require TPN and bowel rest
  - hold immunosuppressive therapy pre-op, provide pre-op stress dose of corticosteroid
  - deep vein thrombosis (DVT) prophylaxis: heparin (IBD patients at increased risk of thromboembolic events)

Crohn's Disease

Treatment
- surgery is NOT curative, but over lifetime, ~70% of Crohn's patients will have surgery
- indications for surgical management
  - failure of medical management
  - complications
    - ◆ SBO (due to stricture/inflammation): indication in 50% of surgical cases
    - ◆ abscess, fistula (enterocolic, vesicular, vaginal, cutaneous abscess), quality of life
    - ◆ other: perforation, hemorrhage, chronic disability, failure to thrive (children), perianal disease

Crohn's 3 Major Patterns
- Ileocecal 40% (RLQ pain, fever, weight loss)
- (30%) small intestine (especially terminal ileum)
- Colon only 25% (diarrhea)

Procedures
• resection and anastomosis/stoma if active or subacute inflammation, perforation, fistula
  ▪ resection margin only has to be free of gross disease (microscopic disease irrelevant to prognosis)
• stricturoplasty – widens lumen in chronically scarred bowel – relieves obstruction without resecting bowel (contraindicated in acute inflammation)

Complications of Treatment
• short gut syndrome (diarrhea, steatorrhea, malnutrition)
• fistulas
• gallstones (if terminal ileum resected, decreased bile salt resorption → increased cholesterol precipitation)
• kidney stones (loss of calcium in diarrhea → increased oxalate absorption and hyperoxaluria → stones)

Prognosis
• recurrence rate at 10 years: ileocolic (25-50%), small bowel (50%), colonic (40-50%)
• re-operation at 5 years: primary resection (20%), bypass (50%), stricturoplasty (10% at 1 year)
• 80-85% of patients who need surgery lead normal lives
• mortality: 15% at 30 years

 # Ulcerative Colitis

Treatment
• indications for surgical management
  ▪ failure of medical management (including inability to taper steroids)
  ▪ complications: hemorrhage, obstruction, perforation, toxic megacolon (emergency), failure to thrive (children)
  ▪ reduce cancer risk (1-2% risk per year after 10 years of disease)

Procedures
• proctocolectomy and ileoanal anastomosis (operation of choice)
• proctocolectomy with permanent ileostomy (if not a candidate for ileoanal procedures)
• colectomy and ileal pouch-anal anastomosis (IPAA) ± rectal mucosectomy
• in emergency: total colectomy and ileostomy with Hartmann closure of the rectum, rectal preservation

Complications of Treatment
• early: bowel obstruction, transient urinary dysfunction, dehydration (high stoma output), anastamotic leak
• late: stricture, anal fistula/abscess, pouchitis, poor anorectal function, reduced fertility

Prognosis
• mortality: 5% over 10 years
• total proctocolectomy will completely eliminate risk of cancer
• perforation of the colon is the leading cause of death from ulcerative colitis

Diverticular Disease

Definitions
- diverticulum – abnormal sac or pouch protruding from the wall of a hollow organ
- diverticulosis – presence of multiple false diverticuli
- diverticulitis – inflammation of diverticuli
- right sided (true) diverticuli = contains all layers (congenital) (see Figure 11)
- left sided (false) diverticuli = contains only mucosal and submucosal layers (acquired)

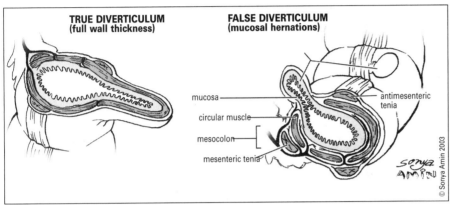

Figure 11. Diverticular Disease – Cross Sections of True and False Diverticuli

Diverticulosis

Epidemiology
- 35-50% of general population (M=F)
- increased incidence in 5th to 8th decades of life
- 95% involve sigmoid colon (site of highest pressure)
- higher incidence in Western countries, related to low fibre diet

Pathogenesis
- risk factors:
  - low-fibre diet (increases gut transit time and intraluminal pressure)
  - muscle wall weakness from aging and illness (e.g. Ehler-Danlos, Marfan's)
  - possible genetic component
- high intraluminal pressures cause outpouching to occur at area of greatest weakness: most commonly at the site of penetrating vessels at antimesenteric tenia, therefore increased risk of hemorrhage

Clinical Presentation
- uncomplicated diverticulosis: asymptomatic (70-80%)
- episodic LLQ abdominal pain, bloating, flatulence, constipation, diarrhea
- absence of fever/leukocytosis
- no physical exam findings or poorly localized LLQ tenderness
- complications:
  - diverticulitis (15-20%)
  - bleeding (5-15%): PAINLESS rectal bleeding, 2/3 of massive lower GI bleeds

Treatment
- uncomplicated diverticulosis: high fibre, education
- diverticular bleed:
  - initially work up and treat as any lower GI bleed (see Gastroenterology)
  - if hemorrhage does not stop, resect involved region

Diverticulitis ("left sided appendicitis")

- **Definition**: infection or perforation of a diverticulum

Pathogenesis
- erosion of the wall by increased intraluminal pressure (or inspissated food particles) → microperforation/macroperforation → inflammation and focal necrosis
- usually mild inflammation with perforation walled off by pericolic fat
- sigmoid colon most often involved

Clinical Features
- severity ranges from mild inflammation to feculent peritonitis
- LLQ pain/tenderness, present for several days before admission
- alternating constipation and diarrhea, urinary symptoms (dysuria if inflammation adjacent to bladder)
- palpable mass if phlegmon or abscess, nausea, vomiting
- low-grade fever, mild leukocytosis
- occult or gross blood in stool less common
- generalized tenderness suggests macroperforation and peritonitis
- complications
    - abscess – on physical exam palpable abdominal mass
    - fistula – colovesical (most common), coloenteric, colovaginal, colocutaneous
    - obstruction – due to scarring from repeated inflammation
    - macroperforation → peritonitis (feculent vs. purulent)
        - recurrent attacks RARELY lead to peritonitis

Investigations
- AXR, upright CXR:
    - localized diverticulitis (ileus, thickened wall, SBO, partial colonic obstruction)
    - free air may be seen in 30% with perforation and generalized peritonitis
- CT scan (optimal method of investigation)
    - 97% sensitive, very useful for assessment of severity and prognosis
    - very helpful in localizing an abscess
- Hypaque™ (water soluble) enema – SAFE (under low pressure)
    - saw-tooth pattern (colonic spasm)
    - may show site of perforation, abscess cavities or sinus tracts, fistulas
- barium enema: contraindicated during an acute attack
    - risk of chemical peritonitis (because of perforation)
- sigmoidoscopy/colonoscopy
    - not during an acute attack, only done on an elective basis
    - rule out other lesions, polyps, cancer, take biopsies

Treatment
- admit, NPO, fluid resuscitation, NG + suction, IV antibiotics covering *B. fragilis* (e.g. ciprofloxacin, metronidazole)
- indications for surgery:
    - unstable patient with peritonitis
    - Hinchey stage 2-4 (see Table 8)
    - after 1 attack if: (a) immunosuppressed, (b) abscess needing percutaneous drainage
    - consider after 2 or more attacks for others
    - complications: generalized peritonitis, free air, abscess fistula, obstruction, hemorrhage, inability to rule out colon cancer on endoscopy, or failure of medical management

Table 8. Hinchey Staging and Treatment for Diverticulitis

Hinchey stage	Description	Acute treatment
1	Phlegmon / small pericolic abscess	Medical
2	Large abscess / fistula	Abscess drainage, resection ± primary anastomosis
3	Purulent peritonitis (ruptured abscess)	Hartmann procedure, sometimes primary anastomosis
4	Feculent peritonitis	Hartmann procedure

Procedures
- Hartmann procedure: resection + colostomy and rectal stump → colostomy reversal in 3-6 months (see Figure 12)
- resection + primary anastomosis (± pre-op bowel prep or on-table lavage): controversial (nastomosis of inflamed tissues → ↑risk of anastomotic leakage)

Prognosis
- 13-30% recurrence after 1st attack, 30-50% risk after 2nd attack

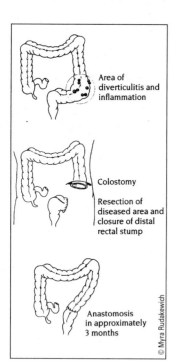

Area of diverticulitis and inflammation

Colostomy

Resection of diseased area and closure of distal rectal stump

Anastomosis in approximately 3 months

© Myra Rudakewich

Figure 12. Hartmann procedure

Colorectal Neoplasms

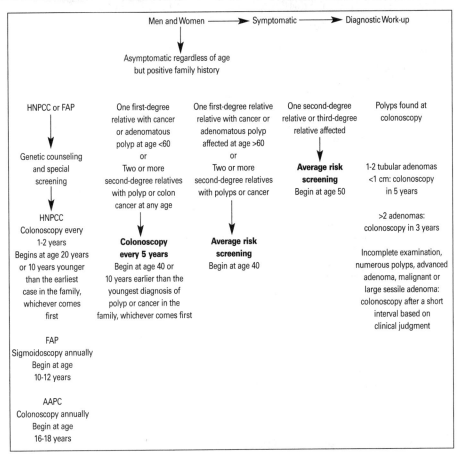

Figure 13. Approach to Higher Risk Screening. AAPC (attenuated adenomatous polyposis) FAP (familial adenomatous polyposis); HNPCC (hereditary nonpolyposis colorectal cancer); First degree relatives: parents, siblings, children; 2nd degree relatives: grandparents, aunts, uncles; 3rd degree relatives: great grandparents or cousins.
Printed with permission Canadian Journal of Gastroenterology. Reference: Volume 18 No. 2, February 2004.

Colorectal Polyps

Definition
- polyp: small mucosal outgrowth into the lumen of the colon or rectum
- sessile (flat) or pedunculated (on a stalk) (see Figure 14)

Epidemiology
- 30% of population have polyps by age 50, 40% by age 60, 50% by age 70

Clinical Features
- 50% in the rectosigmoid region, 50% are multiple
- usually asymptomatic, but may have rectal bleeding, change in bowel habits
- usually detected during routine endoscopy or familial/high risk screening

Pathology
- non-neoplastic
  - hyperplastic – most common
  - pseudopolyps – inflammatory, associated with IBD, no malignant potential
- neoplastic
  - hamartomas: juvenile polyps (large bowel), Peutz-Jegher syndrome (small bowel)
    - malignant risk due to associated adenomas (large bowel)
    - low malignant potential → most spontaneously regress or autoamputate
  - adenomas – premalignant, often carcinoma *in situ*
    - some may contain invasive carcinoma ("malignant polyp" – 2.6-9.4%): invasion into muscularis
    - tubular, villous, tubulovillous (see Table 9)

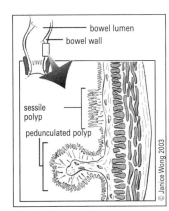

Figure 14. Sessile and pedunculated polyps

Table 9. Characteristics of Tubular vs. Villous Polyps

	Tubular	Villous
Incidence	Common (60% to 80%)	Less common (10%)
Size	Small (<2 cm)	Large (usually >2 cm)
Attachment	Pedunculated	Sessile
Malignant potential	Lower	Higher
Distribution	Even	Left-sided predominance

Investigations
- flexible sigmoidoscope can reach 60% of polyps in men and 35% of polyps in women; if polyps detected, proceed to colonoscopy for examination of entire bowel and biopsy
- colonoscopy still the gold standard

Treatment
- indications: symptoms, malignancy or risk of malignancy (i.e. adenomatous polyps)
- endoscopic removal of entire growth
- surgical resection for those invading into muscularis (high risk of malignancy) and those too large to remove endoscopically
- follow-up endoscopy 1 year later, then every 3-5 years

Familial Colon Cancer Syndromes

FAMILIAL ADENOMATOUS POLYPOSIS (FAP)

Pathogenesis
- autosomal dominant (AD) inheritance, mutation in APC gene on chromosome 5q (long arm)

Clinical Features
- hundreds to thousands of colonic adenomas usually by age of 20 (by 40's in attenuated FAP)
- extracolonic manifestations:
  - carcinoma of duodenum, bile duct, pancreas, stomach, thyroid, adrenal, small bowel
  - congenital hypertrophy of retinal pigment epithelium presents early in life in 2/3 of patients
- virtually 100% lifetime risk of colon cancer (because of number of polyps)
- variants:
  - Gardner's syndrome: FAP + extraintestinal lesions
  - Turcot's syndrome: FAP + CNS tumours

Investigations
- genetic testing (80-95% sensitive, 99-100% specific)
  - see sidebar for criteria for genetic screening referral
- if no polyposis found: annual flexible sigmoidoscopy from puberty to age 50, then regular screening
- if polyposis found: annual colonoscopy and consider surgery (see Figure 13)

Treatment
- surgery indicated by age 17-20
- total proctocolectomy with ileostomy OR total colectomy with ileorectal anastomosis
- doxorubicin-based chemotherapy for intra-abdominal desmoids

HEREDITARY NON-POLYPOSIS COLORECTAL CANCER (HNPCC)

Pathogenesis
- AD inheritance, mutation in a DNA mismatch repair gene resulting in genomic instability and subsequent mutations

Clinical Features
- early age of onset, right > left colon, synchronous and metachronous lesions
- mean age of cancer presentation is 44 years, lifetime risk 70-80% (greater for men)
  - Lynch syndrome I: hereditary site-specific colon cancer
  - Lynch syndrome II: cancer family syndrome – high rates of extracolonic tumours (endometrial, ovarian, hepatobiliary, small bowel)

Diagnosis
- diagnosis is clinical – based on Amsterdam Criteria:
  1. at least 3 relatives with colorectal cancer or HNPCC related CA
  2. 2 or more generations involved, and 1 must be 1st degree relative of the other 2

Referral Criteria for Genetic Screening for APC
- To confirm the diagnosis of FAP (in patients with ≥100 colorectal adenomas)
- To provide pre-symptomatic testing for individuals at risk for FAP (1st degree relatives who are ≥10 years old)
- To confirm the diagnosis of attenuated FAP (in patients with ≥20 colorectal adenomas)

Revised Bethesda Criteria – Refer for genetic screening for HNPCC
- Individuals with cancer in families that meet the Amsterdam Criteria
- Patients with two HNPCC-related cancers, including synchronous and metachronous colorectal cancer or associated extracolonic cancers (endometrial, ovarian, gastric, hepatobiliary, small bowel, or transitional cell carcinoma of the renal pelvis or ureter).
- Patients with colorectal cancer and a first degree relative with colorectal cancer and/or HNPCC-related extracolonic cancer and/or a colorectal adenoma with one of the cancers diagnosed before age 45 years, and the adenoma diagnosed before age 40 years.
- Patients with right-sided colorectal cancer having an undifferentiated pattern (solid/cribriform) on histopathologic diagnosis before age 45 years.
- Patients with signet-ring cell type colorectal cancer diagnosed before age 45.
- Patients with adenomas diagnosed before age 40.

3. 1 case must be diagnosed before 50 years old
4. FAP is excluded

Investigations
- genetic testing (80% sensitive) – colonoscopy mandatory even if negative
  - refer for genetic screening individuals who fulfill EITHER the Amsterdam Criteria (as above) OR the revised Bethesda Criteria (see sidebar)
- colonoscopy (starting age 20) yearly
- surveillance for extracolonic lesions

Treatment
- total colectomy and ileorectal anastomosis with yearly proctoscopy

Colorectal Carcinoma (CRC)

Epidemiology
- 3rd most common cancer (after lung, prostate/breast), 2nd most common cause of cancer death

Risk Factors
- most patients have no specific risk factors
  - FAP, HNPCC, family history of CRC
  - adenomatous polyps (especially if >1 cm, villous, multiple)
  - age >50 (dominant risk factor in sporadic cases): mean age = 70 yrs
  - IBD (especially UC: risk is 1-2%/yr if UC >10 yrs)
  - previous colorectal cancer (also gonadal or breast)
  - diet (increased fat, red meat, decreased fibre) and smoking
  - diabetes mellitus (insulin is a growth factor for colonic mucosal cells) and acromegaly

Screening Tools
- digital rectal exam (DRE): most common exam, but not recommended as a screening tool
- fecal occult blood test (FOBT):
  - proper test requires 3 samples of stool
  - still recommended annually by the World Health Organization (WHO)
  - results in 16-33% reduction in mortality in RCTs
  - Minnesota Colon Cancer Study: RCT showed that annual FOBT can ↓mortality rate by 1/3 in patients 50-80 years old
- sigmoidoscopy:
  - can identify 30-60% of lesions
  - sigmoidoscopy + FOBT misses 24% of colonic neoplasms
- colonoscopy:
  - can remove or biopsy lesions during procedure
  - can identify proximal lesions missed by sigmoidoscopy
  - used as follow-up to other tests if lesions found
  - disadvantages: expensive, not always available, poor compliance, requires sedation, risk of perforation (0.2%)
- virtual colonoscopy: 91% sensitive, 17% false positive rate
- air contrast barium enema: 50% sensitive for large (>1 cm) adenomas, 39% for polyps
- carcinogenic embryonic antigen (CEA): to monitor for recurrence q3 months

Pathogenesis
- adenoma-carcinoma sequence; rarely arise *de novo*

Clinical Features (see Table 10)
- often asymptomatic
- hematochezia/melena, abdominal pain, change in bowel habits
- others: weakness, anemia, weight loss, palpable mass, obstruction
- 3-5% have synchronous lesions

Table 10. Clinical Presentation of CRC

	Right colon	Left colon	Rectum
Frequency	25%	35%	30%
Pathology	Exophytic lesions with occult bleeding	Annular, invasive lesions	Ulcerating
Symptoms	Weight loss, weakness, rarely obstruction	Constipation ± overflow (alternating bowel patterns), abdominal pain, decreased stool caliber, rectal bleeding	Obstruction, tenesmus, rectal bleeding
Signs	Fe-deficiency anemia, RLQ mass (10%)	BRBPR, LBO	Palpable mass on rectal exam (DRE), BRBPR

Screening for colorectal cancer (asymptomatic, no history of UC, polyps, or CRC)

- Average risk individuals, at age 50 (incl. those with <2 relatives with CRC) – recommendations are variable:
- American Gastroenterology Society and American Cancer Society
  - yearly fecal occult blood test (FOBT), flexible sigmoidoscopy q5y, colonoscopy q10y
- Canadian Task Force on Preventative Health Care:
  - yearly FOBT ("A" recommendation)
  - sigmoidoscopy ("B" recommendation)
  - whether to use one or both of FOBT or sigmoidoscopy ("C" recommendation)
  - colonoscopy ("C" recommendation d/t lack of good RCTs)
- family Hx (>2 relatives with CRC/adenoma, one being a 1st degree relative):
  - start screening 10 years prior to the age of the relative's age with the earliest onset of carcinoma
- FAP genetic testing +ve:
  - yearly sigmoidoscopy starting at puberty ("B" recommendation)
- HNPCC genetic testing +ve:
  - yearly colonoscopy starting at age 20 years ("B" recommendation)

Elderly persons who present with iron-deficiency anemia should be investigated for colon cancer.

Staging for CRC

I $T_{1,2} N_0 M_0$
II $T_{3,4} N_0 M_0$
III $T_x N_x M_0$
IV $T_x N_x M_1$

- spread
  - direct extension, lymphatic, hematogenous (liver most common, lung, rarely bone and brain)
  - peritoneal seeding: ovary, Blumer's shelf (pelvic cul-de-sac)
  - intraluminal

Investigations
- colonoscopy (best), look for synchronous lesions; alternative: air contrast barium enema ("apple core" lesion) + sigmoidoscopy
- if a patient is FOBT +ve, microcytic anemia or has a change in bowel habits, do colonoscopy
- metastatic workup: CXR, abdominal CT/U/S
- bone scan, CT head only if lesions suspected
- labs: CBC, urinalysis, liver function tests, CEA (before surgery baseline)
- staging (see Table 11)

Table 11. TNM Classification System for Staging of Colorectal Carcinoma

Primary Tumour (T)	Regional Lymph Nodes (N)	Distant Metastasis (M)
T0 No primary tumour found	N0 No regional node involvement	M0 No distant metastasis
Tis Carcinoma in situ	N1 Metastasis in 1-3 pericolic nodes	M1 Distant metastasis
T1 Invasion into submucosa	N2 Metastasis in 4 or more pericolic nodes	
T2 Invasion into muscularis propria	N3 Metastasis in any nodes along the course of	
T3 Invasion through muscularis and into serosa	named vascular trunks	
T4 Invasion into adjacent structures or organs		

Treatment
- surgery (indicated in potentially curable or symplematic cases - not always in stage IV)
  - curative: wide resection of lesion (5 cm margins) with nodes and mesentery
  - palliative: if distant spread, then local control for hemorrhage or obstruction
  - 80% of recurrences occur within 2 years of resection
  - improved survival if metastasis consists of solitary hepatic mass that is resected
  - colectomy:
    - most patients get primary anastomosis (e.g. hemicolectomy, low anterior resection (LAR))
    - if cancer is below levators in rectum, patient may require an abdominal perineal resection (APR) with a permanent end colostomy, especially if lesion involves the sphincter complex
    - complications: anastomotic leak or stricture, recurrent disease, pelvic abscess, enterocutaneous fistula
- radiotherapy and chemotherapy
  - chemotherapy (5 FU based regimens): for patients with node-positive disease
  - radiation: for patients with node-positive or transmural rectal cancer (pre +/- post-op), not effective in 1° treatment of colon cancer
  - adjuvant therapy – chemotherapy (colon) and radiation (rectum)
  - palliative chemotherapy/radiation therapy for improvement in symptoms and survival

Case finding for colorectal cancer (symptomatic or history of UC, polyps, or CRC)
- surveillance (when polyps are found): colonoscopy within 3 years after initial finding
- patients with past CRC: colonoscopy every 3-5 years, or more frequently
- IBD: some recommend colonoscopy every 1-2 years after 8 years of disease (especially UC)

Follow Up
- intensive follow up improves overall survival in good risk patients
- currently there is no data suggesting optimal follow up
- combination of periodic CT chest/abdo/pelvis, CEA and colonoscopy is recommended

Other Conditions of the Large Intestine

Angiodysplasia

Definition
- vascular anomaly: focal submucosal venous dilatation and tortuosity

Clinical Features
- most frequently in right colon of patients >60 years old
- bleeding typically intermittent (melena, anemia, guaiac positive stools) and in the elderly

---

Prognosis for CRC

Stage	5 yr survival %
$T_1N_0M_0$	>90
$T_2N_0M_0$	85
$T_3N_0M_0$	70-80
$T_xN_1M_0$	35-65
$T_xN_xM_1$	5

Combined-modality treatment for resectable metastatic colorectal cancer to the liver: surgical resection of hepatic metastases in combination with continuous infusion of chemotherapy – an intergroup study.
J Clin Oncol 2002 20(6):1499-505
Background: Metastatic spread of colorectal cancer commonly targets the liver, and long-term outcome studies of surgical resection of hepatic metastases have shown high rates of treatment failure. Arterial chemotherapy regimens targeted to the liver represent a promising adjuvant treatment to reduce recurrence rates.
Methods: Patients with 1-3 resectable liver metastases were randomized preoperatively to receive no further intervention (45 patients, control group) or post-operative floxuridine and fluorouracil (30 patients).
Results: 4-year recurrence-free survival rates were 25% for the control group and 46% for the chemotherapy group (P=0.04), with liver recurrence-free rates of 43% and 67% respectively (P =0.03).
Conclusions: Adjuvant intra-arterial and intravenous chemotherapy shows promise in preventing hepatic recurrence after surgical resection of colorectal cancer hepatic metastases.

APR removes distal sigmoid colon, rectum and anus, permanent end colostomy required.
LAR removes distal sigmoid and rectum with anuscomcirois of distal colon to anus.

Investigations
- endoscopy (cherry red spots, branching pattern from central vessel)
- angiography (slow filling/early emptying mesenteric vein, vascular tuft)
- RBC technetium-99 scan
- barium enema is contraindicated (obscures other x-rays, i.e. angiogram)

Treatment
- none if asymptomatic
- cautery, right hemicolectomy, embolization, vasopressin infusion, sclerotherapy, band ligation, laser, octreotide, and rarely segmental resection if other treatments fail

Volvulus

Definition
- rotation of segment of bowel about its mesenteric axis

Risk Factors
- age (50% of patients >70 yrs: stretching/elongation of bowel with age is a predisposing factor)
- high fibre diet, elongated colon, chronic constipation, laxative abuse, pregnancy, elderly, bedridden, institutionalized (less frequent evacuation of bowels)
- congenitally hypermobile cecum

Clinical Features
- symptoms due to bowel obstruction or bowel ischemia
- sigmoid (70%), cecum (30%)

Investigations
- AXR: "omega", "bent inner-tube", "coffee-bean" signs
- barium/gastrograffin enema: "ace of spades" (or "bird's beak") appearance due to funnel-like luminal tapering of lower segment towards volvulus
- sigmoidoscopy or colonoscopy as appropriate
- CT

> **Cecal Volvulus**
> AXR: Central cleft of "coffee bean" sign points to RLQ.

> **Sigmoid Volvulus**
> AXR: Central cleft of "coffee bean" sign points to LLQ.
> Barium enema: "ace of spades" or "birds beak" sign.

Treatment
- initial supportive management with fluid, electrolyte resuscitation
- cecum:
  - nonsurgical:
    - may attempt colonoscopic detorsion and decompression
  - surgical:
    - right colectomy + ileotransverse colonic anastomosis
- sigmoid:
  - nonsurgical:
    - decompression by flexible sigmoidoscopy and insertion of rectal tube past obstruction
    - subsequent elective surgery recommended (50-70% recurrence)
  - surgical: Hartmann procedure (if urgent)
    - indications: strangulation, perforation or unsuccessful endoscopic decompression

Fistula

Definition
- abnormal communication between two epithelialized surfaces (e.g. enterocutaneous, colovesical, aortoenteric)

Etiology
- foreign object erosion (e.g. gallstone, graft)
- infection, IBD (especially Crohn's), diverticular disease
- iatrogenic/surgery
- congenital, trauma

Investigations
- contrast radiography (fistulogram)
- sonogram
- CT scan
- measure amount of drainage from fistula

> **Why fistulae stay open (FRIENDO)**
> **F**oreign body
> **R**adiation
> **I**nfection
> **E**pithelialization
> **N**eoplasm
> **D**istal obstruction (most common)
> **O**thers: increased flow; steroids (may inhibit closure, usually will not maintain fistula)

Treatment
- fluid resuscitation, manage electrolytes
- bowel rest – NPO
- drain any abscesses/control sepsis
- nutrition – elemental/low residue, TPN
- decrease secretion – octreotide/somatostatin/omeprazole
- skin care (for enterocutaneous fistula)
- surgical intervention – dependent upon etiology (for non-closing fistulas); uncertainty of diagnosis

Ostomies

Definition
- iatrogenic connection of the GI tract to abdominal wall skin
- types: colostomy vs. ileostomy, temporary vs. permanent, continent vs. incontinent, end vs. loop, ileoconduit
    - ileostomies: Brooke (incontinent, continuous drainage), Koch (continent ileostomy, manual drainage) (rarely used)
- complications (10%)
    - obstruction: herniation, stenosis (skin and abdominal wall)
    - peri-ileostomy abscess and fistula
    - skin irritation
    - prolapse or retraction

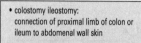

- colostomy ileostomy:
  connection of proximal limb of colon or ileum to abdomenal wall skin

- mucous fistula:
  connection of discal limb of colon to abdomenal wall skin

- ileoconduit:
  connection of colon to ureter proximally + abdomenal wall distally to drain urine

Anorectum

Hemorrhoids

Etiology
- vascular and connective tissue complexes form a plexus of dilated veins (cushion)
    - internal: superior hemorrhoidal veins, above dentate line, portal circulation
    - external: inferior hemorrhoidal veins, below dentate line, systemic circulation

Risk Factors
- increased intra-abdominal pressure: chronic constipation, pregnancy, obesity, portal hypertension, heavy lifting

Clinical Features and Treatment
- internal hemorrhoids (see Figure 15)
    - engorged vascular cushions usually at 3, 7, 11 o'clock positions (patient in lithotomy position)
    - painless rectal bleeding, anemia, prolapse, mucus discharge, pruritus, burning pain, rectal fullness
        - 1st degree: bleed but do not prolapse through the anus
            - treatment: high fibre/bulk diet, sitz baths, steroid cream, rubber band ligation, sclerotherapy, photocoagulation
        - 2nd degree: prolapse with straining, spontaneous reduction
            - treatment: rubber band ligation, photocoagulation
        - 3rd degree: prolapse requiring manual reduction
            - treatment: same as 2nd degree, but may require closed hemorrhoidectomy
        - 4th degree: permanently prolapsed, cannot be manually reduced
            - treatment: closed hemorrhoidectomy
- external hemorrhoids (see Figure 15)
    - dilated venules usually mildly symptomatic
        - pain after bowel movement, hygiene
        - medical treatment: dietary fibre, stool softeners, steroid cream (short course), avoid prolonged straining
    - thrombosed hemorrhoids are very painful
        - resolve within 2 weeks, may leave excess skin = perianal skin tag
        - treatment: consider surgical decompression within first 48 hours of thrombosis, otherwise medical treatment

Always rule out more serious causes (e.g. colon CA) in a person with hemorrhoids and rectal bleeding.

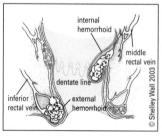

Figure 15. Hemorrhoids

Anal Fissures

Definition
- tear of anal canal below dentate line (very sensitive squamous epithelium)
- 90% posterior midline, 10% anterior midline
- if off midline: consider IBD, STIs, TB, leukemia or anal carcinoma
- repetitive injury cycle after first tear
    - spasm occurs preventing edges from healing and leads to further tearing
    - ischemia may ensue and contribute to chronicity

Etiology
- large, hard stools and irritant diarrheal stools
- tightening of anal canal secondary to nervousness/pain
- others: habitual use of cathartics, childbirth

Clinical Features
- acute fissure
    - very painful bright red bleeding especially after bowel movement
    - treatment is conservative: stool softeners, sitz baths
- chronic fissure
    - triad: fissure, sentinel skin tags, hypertrophied papillae
    - treatment
        - stool softeners, bulking agents, sitz baths
        - topical nitroglycerin or nifedipine – increases local blood flow, promoting healing and relieves sphincter spasm
        - surgery (most effective) – lateral internal sphincterotomy
            - objective is to relieve sphincter spasm → increases blood flow and promotes healing; but 5% chance of fecal incontinence therefore rarely done
        - alternative treatments
            - botulinum toxin – inhibits release of acetylcholine (ACh), stopping sphincter spasm

Anorectal Abscess

Definition
- infection in one (or more) of the anal spaces (see Figure 16)
- usually bacterial infection of blocked anal gland at the dentate line
    - *E. coli, Proteus, Streptococci, Staphylococci, Bacteroides*, anaerobes

Clinical Features
- throbbing pain that may worsen with straining and ambulation
- abscess can spread vertically downward (perianal), vertically upward (supralevator) or horizontally (ischiorectal)
- tender perianal/rectal mass on exam

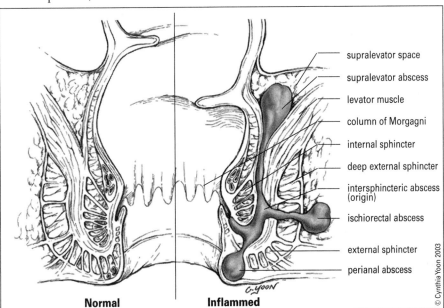

Figure 16. Schematic of Different Types of Perianal Abscesses

Treatment
- incision and drainage
  - curative in 50% of cases
  - 50% develop anorectal fistulas
- may also require antibiotics if diabetic, has heart murmur or cellulitis

Fistula-In-Ano

Definition
- a connection between two epithelialized surfaces, one must be the rectum or anus
- an inflammatory tract with internal os at dentate line, external os on skin

Etiology
- see *Fistula*
- same perirectal process as anal abscess therefore usually associated with abscess
- other causes: post-op, trauma, anal fissure, malignancy, radiation proctitis

Clinical Features
- intermittent or constant purulent discharge from peri-anal opening
- pain
- palpable cord-like tract

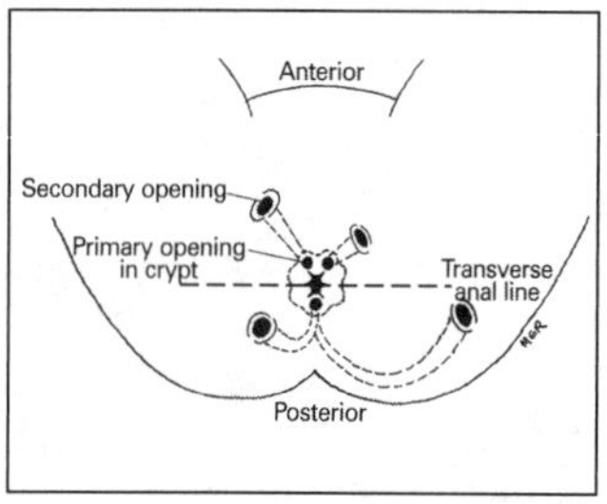

Treatment
- identification
  - internal opening
    - Goodsall's rule (see Figure 17)
      - a fistula with an external opening anterior to the transverse anal line will have its internal opening at relatively the same position (e.g. external opening at 2 o'clock = internal opening at 2 o'clock) whereas all external openings posterior to the line will tend to have their internal openings in the midline
  - fistulous tract
    - probing or fistulography under anesthesia
- surgery
  - fistulotomy: unroof tract from external to internal opening, allow drainage
  - low lying fistula (does not involve external sphincter) → primary fistulotomy
  - high lying fistula (involves external sphincter) → staged fistulotomy with seton suture placed through tract
    - promotes drainage
    - promotes fibrosis and decreases incidence of incontinence
    - delineates anatomy
    - usually for high or complicated fistula to spare muscle cutting

Post-Operative
- sitz baths, irrigation and packing to ensure healing proceeds from inside to outside

Complications
- recurrence
- rarely fecal incontinence

Pilonidal Disease

Definition
- acute abscess or chronic draining sinus in sacrococcygeal area

Etiology
- obstruction of the hair follicles in this area → formation of cysts, sinuses or abscesses

Epidemiology
- occurs most frequently in young men age 15-40 yrs

Clinical Features
- asymptomatic until acutely infected, then pain/tenderness, purulent discharge

Treatment
- acute abscess
  - incision and drainage
  - wound packed open
  - 40% develop chronic pilonidal sinuses
- chronic disease
  - pilonidal cystotomy
  - excision of sinus tract and cyst ± marsupialization

Figure 17. Goodsall's Rule

Anterior

Secondary opening

Primary opening in crypt

Transverse anal line

Posterior

Rectal Prolapse

Definition
* protrusion of full thickness of rectum through anus

Etiology
* lengthened attachment of rectum secondary to constant straining
* 3 types
  I   – false/mucosal: redundant rectal mucosa, radial furrows
  II – incomplete: rectal intussusception without sliding hernia
  III – true/complete (most common): (see Figure 18)
    * protrusion of entire rectal wall through anal orifice with herniation of pelvic peritoneum/cul de sac
    * circular furrows

Epidemiology
* extremes of ages – children <5 years old and >5th decade
* 85% women

Risk Factors
* gynecological surgery
* chronic neurologic/psychiatric disorders affecting motility

Clinical Features
* extrusion of mass with increased intra-abdominal pressure
  * straining, coughing, laughing, Valsalva
* difficulty in bowel regulation
  * tenesmus, constipation, fecal incontinence
* permanently extruded rectum with excoriation, ulceration and constant soiling
* may be associated with urinary incontinence or uterine prolapse

Treatment
* Types I and II (false/mucosal/incomplete)
  * conservative – gentle replacement of prolapsed area, especially in children
  * hemorrhoidectomy with excision of redundant mucosa, mostly in adults
* Type III (true/complete)
  * conservative treatment – reduce if possible
  * surgery – abdominal, perineal, transsacral approaches

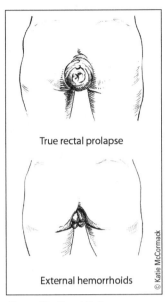

Figure 18. Rectal Prolapse (true vs. false)

Anal Neoplasms

ANAL CANAL

Squamous Cell Carcinoma of Anal Canal (above dentate line)
* most common tumour of anal canal (75%)
* anus prone to human papilloma virus (HPV) infection, therefore at risk for anal squamous intraepithelial lesions (ASIL)
  * high grade squamous intraepithelial lesion (HSIL) and low grade squamous intraepithelial lesion (LSIL) terminology used
* clinical features: anal pain, bleeding, mass, ulceration
* treatment: chemotherapy ± radiation ± surgery
* prognosis: 80% 5-year survival

Malignant Melanoma of Anal Canal
* 3rd most common site after skin, eyes
* aggressive, distant metastases common at time of diagnosis
* early radical surgery is treatment of choice
* prognosis: <5% 5-year survival

ANAL MARGIN
* clinical features and treatment as for skin tumours elsewhere
* squamous and basal cell carcinoma, Bowen's disease and Paget's disease

Liver

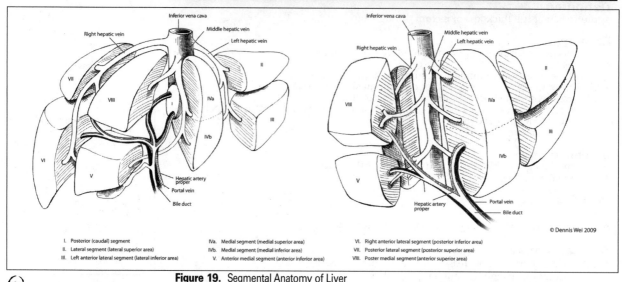

I.   Posterior (caudal) segment
II.   Lateral segment (lateral superior area)
III. Left anterior lateral segment (lateral inferior area)

IVa. Medial segment (medial superior area)
IVb. Medial segment (medial inferior area)
V.   Anterior medial segment (anterior inferior area)

VI.   Right anterior lateral segment (posterior inferior area)
VII. Posterior lateral segment (posterior superior area)
VIII. Poster medial segment (anterior superior area)

Figure 19. Segmental Anatomy of Liver

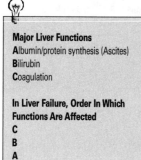

Major Liver Functions
Albumin/protein synthesis (Ascites)
Bilirubin
Coagulation

**In Liver Failure, Order In Which
Functions Are Affected**
C
B
A

Differential Diagnosis of Liver Mass
• cysts: parasitic, non-parasitic
  (choledochal, neoplastic)
• abscess: bacterial, amoebic
• neoplasm:
    • benign (hemangioma,
      adenoma, follicular nodular
      hyperplasia)
    • malignant (primary, secondary)

Liver Cysts

SIMPLE CYSTS
• clinical features
    ▪ most common type of liver cyst, may have multiple simple cysts
    ▪ usually asymptomatic, if large may present with pain or mass
• treatment: generally not required for simple cysts unless very large
• complications: intracystic hemorrhage (may then be confused with complex cysts)

POLYCYSTIC LIVER DISEASE
• progressive condition where cysts replace much of the liver
• 50% associated with polycystic kidney disease
• treatment: if symptomatic treat by partial liver resection or by creating drainage for cysts

CHOLEDOCHAL CYSTS
• congenital malformations of pancreaticobiliary tree
• 4 types with the extreme form called Caroli's disease (multiple cystic dilations in intrahepatic ducts)
• clinical features: recurrent abdominal pain, intermittent jaundice, RUQ mass
• diagnosis: U/S, transhepatic cholangiography, LFTs
• treatment
    ▪ high risk of malignancy, current treatment is complete excision of cysts
    ▪ extent of resection depends on type of cyst
    ▪ liver transplant indicated if cyst involves intrahepatic bile ducts (Caroli's disease)
• complications of chronic disease: biliary cirrhosis, portal hypertension, cholangiocarcinoma

HYDATID LIVER CYSTS (CYSTIC ECHINOCOCCOSIS)
• etiology
    ▪ infection with parasite *Echinococcus granulosus*
    ▪ endemic to Southern Europe, Middle East, Australia, South America
    ▪ associated with exposure to dogs, sheep and cattle
• clinical features
    ▪ asymptomatic mass (most often) or chronic pain, hepatomegaly
    ▪ rupture can cause biliary colic, jaundice or anaphylactic reaction
• investigations
    ▪ detection of anti-*Echinococcus* Ab (IgG) using ELISA or RIA
    ▪ US/CT: presence of mass, often calcified
    ▪ DO NOT do needle biopsy as can cause seeding of abdominal cavity or anaphylaxis

- treatment
  - medical: albendazole (anti-helminthic) – cure in up to 30%
  - surgical (risk of spillage into abdomen)
    - conservative – open endocystectomy ± omentoplasty
    - radical – partial hepatectomy or total pericystectomy

CYSTADENOMA (PREMALIGNANT)/CYSTADENOCARCINOMA
- clinical features:
  - appear as complex cysts on imaging: internal septae, papillary projections, irregular lining
- all complex, multiloculated cysts (except echinococcal) should be excised because of malignancy risk

Liver Abscesses

Etiology
- types
  - pyogenic (bacterial): most often gram negatives - *E.coli, Klebsiella, Proteus*
  - parasitic (amoebic): *Entamoeba histolytica*
  - fungal
- sources: direct spread from biliary tract infection, portal spread from GI infection, systemic infection (e.g. endocarditis)

Clinical Features
- fever, malaise, chills, anorexia, weight loss, abdominal pain, nausea
- RUQ tenderness, hepatomegaly, jaundice, pleural dullness to percussion

Investigations
- leukocytosis, anemia, elevated liver enzymes, hemagglutination titres for *Entamoeba* antibodies
- U/S, CXR (right basilar atelectasis/effusion), CT
- percutaneous aspiration and drainage

Treatment
- treat underlying cause
- surgical or percutaneous drainage and IV antibiotics

Prognosis
- overall mortality 15% – higher rate if delay in diagnosis, multiple abscesses, malnutrition

Neoplasms

BENIGN LIVER NEOPLASMS

Hemangioma (cavernous)
- pathogenesis: most common benign hepatic tumour; results from malformation of angioblastic fetal tissue
- risk factors: F:M = 6:1, steroid therapy, estrogen (exogenous, pregnancy)
- clinical features
  - usually small and asymptomatic, larger tumours may produce pain or compress nearby structures
  - shock if ruptured (very rare)
- investigations
  - contrast CT, U/S, arteriography, RBC scan
  - biopsy may result in hemorrhage
- treatment
  - usually none, unless tumour bleeds or is symptomatic, then excision by lobectomy or enucleation

Adenoma
- definition: benign glandular epithelial tumour
- risk factors: female, age 30-50, estrogen (OCP, pregnancy)
- clinical features: asymptomatic, 25% present with RUQ pain or mass
- investigations: CT, U/S, biopsy
- treatment
  - stop anabolic steroids or OCP
  - excise, especially if large (>5 cm), due to risk of malignancy and spontaneous rupture/hemorrhage

Focal Nodular Hyperplasia
- pathogenesis: thought to be due to local ischemia and tissue regeneration
- risk factors: female, middle age
- clinical features: asymptomatic, rarely grows or bleeds, no malignant potential
- investigations: central stellate scar on CT scan, technetium-99 scan is helpful
- treatment: may be difficult to distinguish from adenoma (malignant potential) → often resected

MALIGNANT LIVER NEOPLASMS

Primary
- usually hepatocellular carcinoma/hepatoma
- others include angiosarcoma, hepatoblastoma, hemangioendothelioma
- epidemiology: uncommon in North America, but represents 20-25% of all carcinomas in Asia and Africa
- risk factors
  - chronic liver inflammation: chronic hepatitis B (inherently oncogenic) and C, cirrhosis (esp. macronodular), hemochromatosis, α_1-anti-trypsin
  - meds: OCPs (3x increased risk), steroids
  - smoking, alcohol
  - chemical carcinogens (aflatoxin, vinyl chloride – associated with angiosarcoma)
- clinical features
  - RUQ discomfort, right shoulder pain
  - jaundice, weakness, weight loss, ± fever
  - hepatomegaly, bruit, rub
  - ascites with blood (sudden intra-abdominal hemorrhage)
  - paraneoplastic syndromes – e.g. Cushing's syndrome, hypoglycemia
  - metastasis: lung, bone, brain, peritoneal seeding

- investigations
  - elevated ALP, bilirubin, and α-fetoprotein (80% of patients)
  - U/S, CT, MRI (best), angiography
  - Triphasic CT characteristically shows enhancement on arterial phase and washout on portal venous phase
  - biopsy
- treatment
  - cirrhosis is a *relative* contraindication to tumour resection due to decreased hepatic reserve
  - surgical: resection (10% of patients have resectable tumours)
  - liver transplant (if cirrhosis plus solitary nodule <5 cm, or less than 3 nodules each <3 cm (Milan criteria); generally not with extrahepatic disease or vascular invasion)
  - non-surgical: percutaneous ethanol injection, transcatheter arterial chemoembolization (TACE), chemotherapy (limited efficacy)
- prognosis
  - 70% have mets to nodes and lung
  - survival without treatment: 3 months
  - 5 year survival: all patients – 5%; patients undergoing complete resection – 11-40%

Secondary
- most common hepatic malignancy
- etiology
  - GI (most common), lung, breast, pancreas, ovary, uterus, kidney, gallbladder, prostate
- treatment
  - hepatic resection if control of primary is possible, no extrahepatic or extrapulmonary metastases and if possibility of "curative" resection
  - possible chemotherapy
- prognosis: 30-40% 5-year survival with a "curative" resection; prognosis same if metastases are multilobar compared confined to one lobe

Differential Diagnosis of Metastatic Liver Mass
Some **GU** **C**ancers **P**roduce **B**umpy **L**umps:
Stomach
Genitourinary cancers – kidney, ovary, uterus
Colon
Pancreas
Breast
Lung

Liver Transplantation

Table 12. Conditions leading to Transplantation

Parenchymal disease	Cholestatic disease	Inborn errors	Tumours
Chronic hepatitis B or C*	Biliary atresia**	α_1-anti-trypsin deficiency	Hepatoma
Alcoholic cirrhosis	Primary biliary cirrhosis	Wilson's disease	
Acute liver failure	Sclerosing cholangitis	Hemochromatosis	
Budd-Chiari syndrome			
Congenital hepatic fibrosis			
Cystic fibrosis (CF)			

*leading cause in adults; ** leading cause in children

Clinical Indications
- early referral for transplant should be considered for all patients with progressive liver disease not responding to medical therapy, especially decompensated cirrhosis, unresectable primary liver cancers, and fulminant hepatic failure
- end-stage liver disease with life expectancy <1 year and if no other therapy is appropriate
- progressive jaundice, refractory ascites, spontaneous hepatic encephalopathy, recurrent sepsis, fulminant hepatic failure
- recurrent variceal hemorrhage, coagulopathy, severe fatigue

Criteria for Transplantation
- Model for End-Stage Liver Disease (MELD): considers probability of death within 3 months if patient does not receive transplant and is based on creatinine, bilirubin, INR
- Child-Turcotte-Pugh Score: patient must have 7 points (Class B) or higher (see sidebar)

Contraindications
- sepsis, HIV positive status
- active alcohol/substance abuse
- extrahepatic metastasis
- advanced cardiopulmonary disease

Post-op Complications
- primary non-function (graft failure) – urgent re-transplantation is indicated
- acute and chronic rejection, ischemia-reperfusion injury
- vascular – hepatic artery or portal vein thrombosis, IVC obstruction
- biliary complications – fever, increasing bilirubin and ALP
- recurrence of Hepatitis B
- hepatitis B virus: prophylactic medical therapy is usually effective in preventing recurrence in graft; hepatitis C anti-recurrence therapy is less effective but recurrence can be controlled medically

Prognosis
- patient survival at 1 year – 85%
- graft survival at 1 year – 60-70%, at 5 years – 40-50%

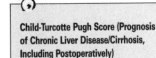

Child-Turcotte Pugh Score (Prognosis of Chronic Liver Disease/Cirrhosis, Including Postoperatively)

	1 Point	2 Points	3 Points
Albumin	>35	30-35	<28
	>3.5 g/dL	3.0-3.5	<3.0
Ascites	Absent	Easily controlled	Poorly controlled
Bilirubin	<34 umol/L	34-51	>51
	<2.0 mg/dL	2.0-3.0	>3.0
Coagulation (INR)	<1.7	1.7-2.3	>2.3
	PT 0-4s	4-6	>6
Hepatic encephalopathy	None	Minimal (Grade I-II)	Advanced (Grade III-IV)

Points	Class	One Year Survival	Two Year Survival
5-6	A	100%	85%
7-9	B	81%	57%
10-15	C	45%	35%

Biliary Tract

Cholelithiasis

Definition
- the formation of gallstones

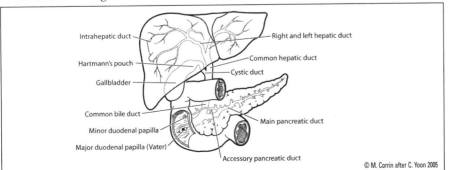

Intrahepatic duct
Hartmann's pouch
Gallbladder
Common bile duct
Minor duodenal papilla
Major duodenal papilla (Vater)
Right and left hepatic duct
Common hepatic duct
Cystic duct
Main pancreatic duct
Accessory pancreatic duct

© M. Corrin after C. Yoon 2005

Figure 20. Anatomy of biliary system

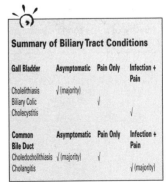

Summary of Biliary Tract Conditions

Gall Bladder	Asymptomatic	Pain Only	Infection + Pain
Cholelithiasis	√ (majority)		
Biliary Colic		√	
Cholecystitis			√

Common Bile Duct	Asymptomatic	Pain Only	Infection + Pain
Choledocholithiasis	√ (majority)	√	
Cholangitis			√ (majority)

Pathogenesis
- imbalance of cholesterol and its solubilizing agents (bile salts and lecithin)
- excessive hepatic cholesterol secretion → bile salts and lecithin are "overloaded" → supersaturated cholesterol can precipitate and form gallstones
- North America: cholesterol stones (80%), pigment stones (20%)

Risk Factors
- cholesterol stones
    - obesity, age <50
    - estrogens: female, multiparity, OCPs
    - ethnicity: First Nations heritage > Caucasian > Black
    - terminal ileal resection or disease (e.g. Crohn's disease)
    - impaired gallbladder emptying: starvation, rapid weight loss, TPN, DM type I
- pigment stones (contain calcium bilirubinate)
    - cirrhosis
    - chronic hemolysis
    - biliary stasis (strictures, dilation, biliary infection)

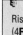

Risk factors for cholesterol stones (4F's): **F**at, **F**emale, **F**ertile, **F**orties

Clinical Features
- asymptomatic (80%)
    - most do NOT require treatment
    - consider cholecystectomy if: porcelain (calcified) gallbladder (25% risk of malignancy), sickle cell disease, pediatric patient, having bariatric surgery, diabetes, immunosuppression
- biliary colic (10-25%)
- cholecystitis
- choledocholithiasis (8-15%)
- cholangitis
- gallstone pancreatitis (see *Acute pancreatitis*, GS48)
- gallstone ileus

U/S is diagnostic procedure of choice for imaging the biliary tree.

Investigations
- U/S – diagnostic procedure of choice
    - image for signs of inflammation, obstruction, localization of stones
- ERCP (endoscopic retrograde cholangiopancreatography)
    - visualization of upper GI tract, ampullary region, biliary and pancreatic ducts
    - method for treatment of CBD stones in periampullary region
    - complications: traumatic pancreatitis (1-2%), pancreatic or biliary sepsis
- PTC (percutaneous transhepatic cholangiography)
    - injection of contrast via needle passed through hepatic parenchyma
    - useful for proximal bile duct lesions or when ERCP fails or not available
    - requires prophylactic antibiotics
    - contraindications: coagulopathy, ascites, peri/intrahepatic sepsis, disease of right lower lung or pleura
    - complications: bile peritonitis, chylothorax, pneumothorax, sepsis, hemobilia
- MRCP (magnetic resonance cholangiopancreatography)
    - same information gained as ERCP but non-invasive
    - cannot be used for therapeutic purposes
- HIDA scan
    - now used less commonly-99
    - radioisotope technetium excreted in high concentrations in bile
    - does not visualize stones, diagnosis by seeing occluded cystic duct or CBD

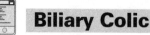

Biliary Colic

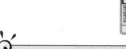
Biliary colic is a constant pain not colicky.

Pathogenesis
- gallstone transiently impacted in cystic duct, **no** infection

Clinical Features
- steady pain in epigastrium or RUQ for minutes to hours, crescendo-decrescendo pattern
- frequently occurs at night or after fatty meal
- can radiate to right shoulder or scapula
- patients often restless
- no peritoneal findings, no systemic/constitutional signs

Investigations
- normal blood work: CBC, electrolytes, LFTs, bilirubin, amylase
- U/S shows cholelithiasis, may show stone in cystic duct

Treatment
- analgesia, rehydration
- elective cholecystectomy (95% success)
  - anatomic landmarks: triangle of Calot (borders: cystic duct, common hepatic duct, cystic artery), inferior border of liver
  - complications: CBD injury (0.3-0.5%), hollow viscus injury, bile peritonitis, vessel injury

Acute Cholecystitis

Pathogenesis
- inflammation of gallbladder resulting from sustained gallstone impaction in cystic duct or Hartmann's pouch
- no cholelithiasis in 5-10% (see *Acalculous Cholecystitis*, GS46)

Clinical Features
- often have history of biliary colic
- severe constant (hours to days) epigastric or RUQ pain, anorexia, nausea, vomiting, low grade fever (<38.5°C)
- focal peritoneal findings: Murphy's sign, palpable, tender gallbladder (in 33%)

Investigation
- bloodwork: elevated WBC and left shift, mildly elevated bilirubin, AST, ALT, ALP
- U/S
  - 98% sensitive, consider HIDA scan if U/S negative
  - features on U/S
    - distended gallbladder
    - pericholecystic fluid
    - stone in cystic duct
    - thickened gallbladder wall (>3 mm)
    - sonographic Murphy's Sign – maximum tenderness on inspiration when probe over gallbladder

Complications
- gallbladder mucocele (hydrops) – long term cystic duct obstruction results in mucus accumulation in gallbladder
- gangrene, perforation – result in abscess formation or peritonitis
- empyema of gallbladder – suppurative cholecystitis, pus in gallbladder + sick patient
- cholecystoenteric fistula, from repeated attacks of cholecystitis, can lead to gallstone ileus
- emphysematous cholecystitis – bacterial gas present in gallbladder lumen, wall or pericholecystic space (risk in diabetic patient)
- Mirrizzi's syndrome – extra-luminal compression of CBD/CHD due to large stone in cystic duct

Treatment
- admit, hydrate, NPO, NG tube (if persistent vomiting from associated ileus), analgesics once diagnosis is made
- antibiotics
  - *E. coli, Klebsiella, Enterococcus* and *Clostridium* account for >80% of infections
  - ampicillin + gentamicin/ciprofloxacin + metronidazole
- cholecystectomy
  - early (within 72h) vs. delayed (after 6 weeks)
    - equal morbidity and mortality
    - early cholecystectomy preferred: shorter hospitalization and recovery time
    - emergent OR indicated if high risk, e.g. emphysematous, diabetic patient
  - laparoscopic is standard of care (convert to open for complications or difficult case)
    - laparoscopic: reduced risk of wound infections, shorter hospital stay, reduced post-op pain, increased risk of bile duct injury
- intra-operative cholangiography (IOC)
  - indications: clarify bile duct anatomy, obstructive jaundice, history of biliary pancreatitis, small stones in gallbladder with a wide cystic duct (>15 mm), single faceted stone in gallbladder, bilirubin >137 μmol/L
- percutaneous cholecystostomy tube: critically ill or if general anesthetic contraindicated

Does this patient have acute cholecystitis?
(*JAMA.* 2003; 289: 80-86)
Study: Looking at the ability of the clinical exam and basic laboratory findings to determine which patients need diagnostic imaging techniques to diagnose acute cholecystitis.
Selection criteria: Studies from 1966-2002 which evaluated the history, physical and basic laboratory tests in adult patients with abdominal pain or suspected acute cholecystitis. These studies had to have a control group with no diagnosis of acute cholecystitis. Acute cholecystitis was diagnosed through several different modalities (e.g. surgery, pathologic examination, etc). This included 17 articles.
Results: No clinical or laboratory finding was sufficient to rule in or rule out the diagnosis of acute cholecystitis. The best finding for ruling in was positive Murphy's sign (LR+ = 2.8 95% CI 0.8-86) and the best test for ruling out was absence of right upper quadrant tenderness (LR - 0.4 95% CI 0.2-1.1), but neither of these findings were statistically significant. No study looked at the combination of clinical and laboratory findings.
Conclusion: No single clinical findings or laboratory test can rule in or rule out the diagnosis of acute cholecystitis. It is through a combination of clinical findings and diagnostic imaging that the diagnosis of acute cholecystitis is made in patients presenting with abdominal pain.

Laparoscopic vs. Open Cholecystectomy

Laparoscopic Cholecystectomy
Shorter operating time
Shorter length of stay
Shorter sick leave
Shorter time to return to daily activities
Less post-operative pain*
Decreased use of post-operative analgesia*
Decreased reduction in pulmonary function*
Fewer pulmonary complications
Decreased acute phase response
Less impairment in intestinal motility*

Open Cholecystectomy
Lower conversion rates to open surgery
(for mini-laparotomies)

*NOTE:
Post-operative pain = measured on visual analog scale
Analgesic use = patient-controlled morphine consumption
Pulmonary function = O_2 consumption, spirometric parameters, arterial blood gases, and acid-base balance
Intestinal motility = auscultating intestinal peristalsis, abdominal circumference measurement, and time interval to restitution of defecation

Acute cholecystitis is treated with antibiotics and early cholecystectomy

Biliary colic is treated with analgesia and elective cholecystectomy

Acalculous Cholecystitis

Definition
• acute or chronic cholecystitis in the absence of stones

Pathogenesis
• typically due to gallbladder stasis, sludge forms in gallbladder

Risk Factors
• DM, immunosuppression, ICU stay, trauma patient, TPN, sepsis

Clinical Features
• see *Acute Cholecystitis*, GS45
• occurs in 20% of cases of acute cholecystitis

Investigations
• U/S: shows sludge in gallbladder, other U/S features of cholecystitis (see above)
• CT or HIDA scan

Treatment
• cholecystectomy or cholecystostomy if patient unstable

Choledocholithiasis

Definition
• stones in common bile duct (CBD)

Clinical Features
• 50% asymptomatic
• often have history of biliary colic
• tenderness in RUQ or epigastrium
• acholic stool, dark urine, fluctuating jaundice
• primary vs. secondary stones
  ▪ primary: formed in bile duct, indicates bile duct pathology (e.g. benign biliary stricture, sclerosing cholangitis, choledochal cyst)
  ▪ secondary: formed in gallbladder (85% of cases in U.S.)
• complications: cholangitis, pancreatitis, biliary stricture and biliary cirrhosis

Investigations
• CBC: usually normal; leukocytosis suggests cholangitis
• LFTs: increased bilirubin, ALP
• amylase/lipase: to rule out gallstone pancreatitis
• U/S: intra/extra-hepatic duct dilatation
• ERCP, PTC
• MRCP (90% sensitive, almost 100% specific, not therapeutic)

Treatment
• if no evidence of cholangitis: treat with ERCP for CBD stone extraction possibly followed by elective cholecystectomy in 25% of patients

Acute Cholangitis

Pathogenesis
• obstruction of CBD leading to biliary stasis, bacterial overgrowth, suppuration, and biliary sepsis

Etiology
• choledocholithiasis (60%), stricture, neoplasm (pancreatic or biliary), extrinsic compression (pancreatic pseudocyst or pancreatitis), instrumentation of bile ducts (PTC, ERCP), biliary stent
• organisms: *E. coli, Klebsiella, Pseudomonas, Enterococcus, B. fragilis, Proteus*

Clinical Features
• Charcot's triad – fever, RUQ pain, jaundice
• Raynaud's pentad – fever, RUQ pain, jaundice, shock, confusion
• may have nausea, vomiting, abdominal distention, ileus, acholic stools, tea-coloured urine

Charcot's triad
Fever, RUQ pain, jaundice

Investigations
- CBC: elevated WBC + left shift
- may have positive blood cultures
- LFTs: obstructive picture (elevated ALP and conjugated bilirubin, mild increase in AST, ALT)
- amylase, lipase – rule out pancreatitis
- U/S: intra/extra-hepatic duct dilatation

Raynaud's pentad
Fever, RUQ pain, jaundice, shock, confusion

Treatment
- initial: NPO, fluid and electrolyte resuscitation, ± NG tube, IV antibiotics
- decompression
  - ERCP + sphincterotomy – diagnostic and therapeutic
  - PTC with catheter drainage – if ERCP not available or unsuccessful
  - laparotomy with CBD exploration and T-tube placement if above fails
- all patients should also have a cholecystectomy, unless otherwise contraindicated

Prognosis
- suppurative cholangitis – mortality rate: 50%

Gallstone Ileus

Pathogenesis
- repeated inflammation causing a cholecystoenteric fistula (usually duodenal) → large gallstone enters the gut and impacts at or near the ileocecal valve, causing a true bowel obstruction (note: ileus is a misnomer in this context)

Clinical Features
- crampy abdominal pain, nausea, vomiting (see also *Bowel Obstruction*, GS22)

Investigations
- abdominal x-ray – dilated small intestine, air fluid level, may reveal radiopaque gallstone, air in biliary tree (40%)
- CT – biliary tract air, obstruction, gallstone in intestine

Treatment
- fluid resuscitation, NG decompression
- surgery: enterotomy and removal of stone, inspect small and large bowel for additional proximal stones
- fistula usually closes spontaneously
- elective cholecystectomy after recovery if patient experiences gallbladder symptoms

Carcinoma of the Gallbladder

Risk Factors
- chronic symptomatic gallstones (70% of cases), old age, female, gallbladder polyps, porcelain gallbladder

Clinical Features
- majority are adenocarcinoma, may be incidental finding on elective cholecystectomy (~10%)
- many patients are asymptomatic until late
- local: vague RUQ pain, ± palpable RUQ mass
- systemic: jaundice (50%) due to invasion of CBD or compression of CBD by pericholedochal nodes, weight loss, malaise, anorexia
- early local extension to liver, may extend to stomach, duodenum
- early metastasis common to liver, lung, bone

Investigations
- U/S, abdominal CT, ERCP

Treatment
- if carcinoma of the gallbladder is suspected preoperatively an open cholecystectomy should be done to avoid tumour seeding of trocar sites
- confined to mucosa (rare) – cholecystectomy
- beyond mucosa – cholecystectomy, en bloc wedge resection of 3-5 cm underlying liver, dissection of hepatoduodenal lymph nodes

Prognosis
- 5 year survival – 10% (late detection)

Cholangiocarcinoma

Definition
- malignancy of extra or intrahepatic bile ducts

Risk Factors
- age 50-70, gallstones, ulcerative colitis, primary sclerosing cholangitis, choledochal cyst, *Clonorchis sinensis* infection (liver fluke)

Clinical Features
- majority are adenocarcinoma
- 0.8% of all malignant tumors
- typically presents with gradual signs of biliary obstruction: jaundice, pruritis, dark urine, pale stool
- anorexia, weight loss, RUQ pain, Courvoisier's sign (if CBD obstructed), hepatomegaly
- early metastases are uncommon, but commonly tumour grows into portal vein or hepatic artery
- Klatskin tumour – cholangiocarcinoma located at bifurcation of common hepatic duct

Obstructive jaundice is the most common presenting symptom for cholangiocarcinoma.

Investigations
- LFTs show obstructive picture
- U/S, CT: bile ducts usually dilated, but not necessarily
- ERCP or PTC: to determine resectability, for biopsies
- CXR, bone scan

Treatment
- generally palliative
- if resectable: biliary drainage and wide excision margin
  - upper third lesions: duct resection + Roux-en-Y-hepaticojejunostomy, ± liver resection
  - middle third lesions: duct resection + Roux-en-Y-hepaticojejunostomy
  - lower third lesions: Whipple procedure
- unresectable lesions: stent or choledochojejunostomy (surgical bypass)

Prognosis
- radiotherapy useful for additional palliation, chemotherapy may be helpful
- the more proximal to the liver the worse the prognosis
- overall 5-year survival - 15%

Pancreas

Acute Pancreatitis

- see Gastroenterology for complications and other etiologies

GALLSTONE PANCREATITIS

Pathogenesis (theories)
- obstruction of pancreatic duct by large or small gallstones and biliary sludge
- backup of pancreatic enzymes can cause autodigestion of the pancreas

Clinical Features (as with pancreatitis of any etiology)
- pain (epigastric → back), nausea, vomiting, ileus, peritoneal signs, jaundice, fever
- Inglefinger's sign: pain worse when supine, better when sitting forward
- rarely may have coexistent cholangitis or pancreatic necrosis
- Ranson's criteria for determining prognosis of acute pancreatitis

Investigation
- high amylase (higher than alcoholic pancreatitis), lipase, high liver enzymes, leukocytosis
- U/S may show multiple stones (may have passed spontaneously), edematous pancreas
- CXR, AXR, CT (if severe to evaluate for complications)

Treatment
- supportive
- NPO, hydration, analgesia and antibiotics for severe cases or necrotizing pancreatitis or signs of sepsis

- stone often passes spontaneously (~90%); usually no surgical management in uncomplicated acute pancreatitis
- cholecystectomy during same admission after acute attack has subsided (25-60% recurrence if no surgery)
- may need urgent ERCP + sphincterotomy if failure of conservative management (no benefit has been shown for early ERCP + sphincterotomy if no obstructive jaundice is present)
- surgical indications in acute pancreatitis (rare):
  - debridement and drain placement for necrotizing pancreatitis if refractory to medical management, or if septic, in ICU without other sources of sepsis

Complications

- pseudocyst
- abscess/infection, necrosis
- splenic/mesenteric/portal vessel thrombosis or rupture
- pancreatic ascites/pancreatic pleural fluid effusion
- diabetes
- ARDS/sepsis/multiorgan failure
- coagulopathy/DIC
- encephalopathy
- severe hypocalcemia

RANSON'S CRITERIA
A. At admission
1) Age >55 years
2) WBC >16 x 10⁹/L
3) Glucose >11 mmol/L
4) LDH ≥350 IU/L
5) AST ≥250 IU/L
B. During initial 48 hours
1) Hct drop >10%
2) BUN rise >1.8 mmol/L
3) Arterial PO₂ <60 mmHg
4) Base deficit >4 mmol/L
5) Calcium <2 mmol/L
6) Fluid sequestration >6L
C. Interpretation
≥2 – difficult course
≥3 – high mortality

Chronic Pancreatitis

- see also Gastroenterology

Surgical Treatment

- treatment is generally medical
- indications for surgery:
  - failure of medical treatment
  - debilitating abdominal pain
  - pseudocyst complications: persistence, hemorrhage, infection, rupture
  - CBD obstruction (e.g. strictures), duodenal obstruction
  - pancreatic fistula, variceal hemorrhage secondary to splenic vein obstruction
  - rule out pancreatic cancer
  - anatomical abnormality causing recurrent pancreatitis
- pre-op CT and/or ERCP are mandatory to delineate anatomy
- surgical options:
  - drainage procedures – only effective if ductal system is dilated
    - endoscopic duct decompression
    - Puestow procedure (longitudinal pancreatojejunostomy) – improves pain in 80% of patients
  - pancreatectomy – best option in absence of dilated duct
    - proximal disease – Whipple procedure (pancreatoduodenectomy): pain relief in 80%
    - distal disease – distal pancreatectomy ± Roux-en-Y pancreatojejunostomy
    - total pancreatectomy – refractory disease
  - nerve ablation
    - celiac plexus block – lasting benefit in 30% patients, much less invasive
- pseudocyst (most resolve spontaneously with pancreatic rest)
  - cyst wall must be mature (4-6 weeks)
  - internal drainage (preferred): Roux-en-Y cyst-jejunostomy or cyst-gastrostomy
  - external drainage: may require second operation to treat pancreatic fistula
  - consider biopsy of cyst wall to rule out cystadenocarcinoma

The hallmark of chronic pancreatitis is epigastric pain radiating to the back.

Pancreatic Cancer

Epidemiology

- fourth most common cause of cancer-related mortality in both men and women in Canada in 2003
- African descent at increased risk
- male:female = 1.7:1, average age: 50-70

Risk Factors

- increased age
- smoking – 2-5x increased risk, most clearly established risk factor

Courvoisier's Sign
Palpable, nontender distended gallbladder due to CBD obstruction. Present in 33% of patients with pancreatic carcinoma. The distended gallbladder could not be due to acute cholecystitis or stone disease because the gallbladder would actually be scarred and smaller, not larger.

- high fat/low fibre diets, heavy alcohol use
- DM, chronic pancreatitis
- chemicals: betanaphthylamine, benzidine

Clinical Features (related to location of tumour)
- head of the pancreas (70%)
  - weight loss, obstructive jaundice, vague constant midepigastric pain (often worse at night, may radiate to back)
  - painless jaundice (occurs more often with peri-ampullary), Courvoisier's sign
  - palpable tumour mass → generally incurable
- body or tail of pancreas (30%)
  - tends to present later and usually inoperable
  - weight loss, vague mid-epigastric pain
  - <10% jaundiced
  - sudden onset diabetes

Investigations
- serum chemistry non-specific: elevated ALP and bilirubin >300 μmol/L
- U/S, contrast CT (also evaluates metastasis and resectability), ERCP

Pathology
- ductal adenocarcinoma – most common type (75-80%); exocrine pancreas
- intraductal papillary mucinous neoplasm (IPMN)
- other: mucinous cystic neoplasm (MCN), acinar cell carcinoma, islet-cell (insulinoma, gastrinoma)

Treatment
- resectable (20% of pancreatic cancer)
  - no involvement of liver, peritoneum or vasculature (hepatic artery, SMA, SMV, portal vein, IVC, aorta), no distant metastasis
  - Whipple procedure (pancreatoduodenectomy) for cure – 5% mortality (Figure 21)
  - distal pancreatectomy ± splenectomy, lymphadenectomy if carcinoma of midbody and tail of pancreas
- non-resectable (palliative → relieve pain, obstruction):
  - most body/tail tumours are not resectable (due to late presentation)
  - relieve biliary/duodenal obstruction with endoscopic stenting or double bypass procedure (choledochoenterostomy + gastroenterostomy)
  - chemotherapy (gemcitabine), radiotherapy – only slightly increase survival

Prognosis
- most important prognostic indicators are lymph node status, size >3 cm, perineural invasion (invasion of tumour into microscopic nerves of pancreas)
- overall 5 year survival is 10%
- average survival – 6 months if unresected, 12-18 months with curative resection

Vague abdominal pain with weight loss ± jaundice in a patient over 50 years old is pancreatic cancer until proven otherwise.

Whipple Procedure (Pancreaticoduodenectomy)

1) Removal
Choledochectomy
Cholecystectomy
Duodenectomy
Distal pancreatectomy
+/- Distal gastrectomy

2) New Connections
Hepaticojejunostomy (connect common hepatic duct to jejunum post cholecystectomy)
Pancreaticojejunostomy (connect distal pancreas remnant)
Gastrojejunostomy

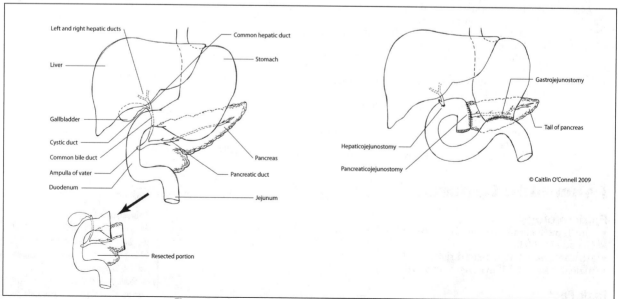

Figure 21. Schematic of Whipple resection, showing the resected components

Spleen

Splenic Trauma

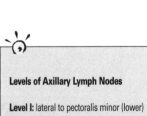

- typically from blunt trauma (esp. in people with splenomegaly)
- most common intra-abdominal organ injury in blunt trauma
- treatment:
  - in stable patients – extended bedrest with serial hematocrit levels, close monitoring
  - hemostatic control
  - splenic artery embolization
  - splenorrhaphy (suture of spleen) – if patient hemodynamically stable, patient has stopped bleeding and laceration does not involve hilum
  - partial splenectomy
  - total splenectomy if patient unstable or high-grade injury

Splenectomy

Indications
- splenic trauma (most common reason for splenectomy), hereditary spherocytosis, primary hypersplenism, chronic immune thrombocytopenia purpura (ITP), splenic vein thrombosis causing esophageal varices, splenic abscess, thrombotic thrombocytopenia purpura (TTP), non-Hodgkin's lymphoma, primary splenic tumour (rare)
- does not benefit all thrombocytopenic states (e.g. infection, most malignancies involving the bone marrow, drugs/toxins)

Complications
- short-term
  - atelectasis of left lower lung, bleeding, infection
  - injury to surrounding structures (e.g. gastric wall, tail of pancreas)
  - post-op thrombocytosis, leukocytosis
  - subphrenic abscess
- long-term
  - post-splenectomy sepsis (encapsulated organisms): 4% of splenectomized patients
    - 50% mortality
    - pre-op prophylaxis with vaccinations (pneumococcal, *H. influenzae* and meningococcus)
    - liberal use of penicillin especially in children <6 years old

Breast

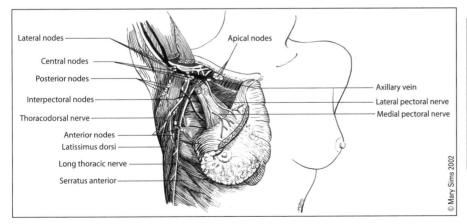

Figure 22. Anatomy of the breast

Levels of Axillary Lymph Nodes

Level I: lateral to pectoralis minor (lower)

Level II: deep to pectoralis minor

Level III: medial to pectoralis minor (higher level = worse prognosis)

Benign Breast Lesions

FIBROCYSTIC CHANGE
- benign breast condition characterized by fibrous and cystic changes in the breast
- age 30 to menopause (and after if HRT used)
- makes evaluation of mammographic malignant changes more difficult
- no increased risk of breast cancer
- clinical features:
  - breast pain, swelling with focal areas of nodularity or cysts, frequently bilateral, mobile, varies with menstrual cycle, nipple discharge (straw-like, brown or green)
- treatment:
  - evaluation of breast mass and reassurance
  - if >40 y.o.: mammography every 3 years
  - no strong evidence for avoidance of xanthine-containing products (coffee, tea, chocolate, cola)
  - analgesia (ibuprofen, ASA)
  - for severe symptoms: danazol, bromocriptine, OCP
  - evening primrose

FIBROADENOMA
- most common benign breast tumour in women under age 30
- no malignant potential
- clinical features:
  - nodules: smooth, rubbery, discrete, well-circumscribed, non-tender, mobile, hormone dependent
  - unlike cysts, needle aspiration yields no fluid
- investigations:
  - mammogram
  - U/S
  - fine needle aspiration (FNA) to rule in solid lesion, rule out cyst
- treatment:
  - generally conservative – serial observation
  - consider excision if mass rapidly growing, if >5 cm in size or if patient wants mass excised

FAT NECROSIS
- uncommon, result of trauma (may be minor, positive history in only 50%), after breast surgery (i.e. reduction)
- firm, ill-defined mass with skin or nipple retraction, ± tenderness
- regress spontaneously, but complete excisional biopsy to rule out carcinoma

INTRADUCTAL PAPILLOMA
- solitary intraductal benign polyp
- most common cause of spontaneous, unilateral bloody nipple discharge
- sometimes multiple ducts: "papillomatosis"
- 10% risk of associated malignancy/DCIS
- treatment: excision of involved duct

ABSCESS
- see Obstetrics
- unilateral localized pain, tenderness and erythema
- rule out inflammatory carcinoma, as indicated
- lactational = mastitis – *S. aureus*
  - treatment: heat or ice packs, continue nursing, oral antibiotics (dicloxacillin/cephalexin)
  - + abscess: fluctuant mass, purulent nipple discharge, fever, leukocytosis
    - D/C nursing, IV antibiotics (nafcillin/oxacillin), I&D usually required
- non-lactational – most commonly periductal
  - also subareolar pain, subareolar mass, discharge (variable colour), nipple inversion
  - may be associated with mammary duct ectasia
  - treatment: broad-spectrum antibiotics and I&D or total duct excision (definitive)
  - if mass does not resolve: fine needle aspiration (FNA) to exclude cancer, U/S to assess for presence of abscess

Differential Diagnosis for Breast Mass
- breast Ca
- fibrocystic changes
- fibroadenoma
- fat necrosis
- papilloma/papillomatosis
- galactocele
- duct ectasia
- ductal/lobular hyperplasia
- sclerosing adenosis
- lipoma
- neurofibroma
- granulomatous mastitis (e.g. Wegener's, sarcoidosis)
- abscess
- silicone implant

HYPERPLASIA
- ductal or lobular hyperplasia ± atypia
- slightly increased cancer risk if moderate or florid hyperplasia
- increased cancer risk if atypia present
- atypia may make it difficult to distinguish hyperplasia from ductal carcinoma *in situ* (DCIS) on core needle biopsy
- treatment: excision

Breast Cancer

Epidemiology
- 2nd leading cause of cancer mortality in women (1st is lung cancer)
- most common cancer diagnosis in Canadian women excluding non-melanoma skin cancer
- 1/9 women in Canada will be diagnosed with breast cancer in their lifetime
- 1/27 women in Canada will die from breast cancer

Risk Factors
- gender (99% female)
- age (80% >40 y.o.)
- prior history of breast cancer, prior breast biopsy (regardless of pathology)
- 1st degree relative with breast cancer (greater risk if relative was premenopausal)
- increased risk with nulliparity, first pregnancy >30 y.o., menarche <12 y.o., menopause >55 y.o.
- decreased risk with lactation, early menopause, early childbirth
- radiation exposure
- history of specific benign breast diseases:
  - moderate/florid hyperplasia - 2X
  - atypical hyperplasia – 4X
  - sclerosing adenosis - 1.5X
  - papilloma – 1.5X
- >5 years HRT

Gender followed by age are the two greatest risk factors for breast cancer.

Investigations
- mammography
  - indications
    - screening (see Table 13)
      - every 1-2 years for women age 50-69
      - positive FHx in 1st degree relative: every 1-2 years starting 10 years before the youngest age of presentation
      - women age 40-49 with average risk - no evidence to include or exclude a screening exam (level C evidence)
      - typical views: MLO (medio-lateral-oblique) and CC (cranial-caudal)
    - diagnostic
      - investigation of patient complaints (discharge, pain, lump)
      - metastatic adenocarcinoma of unknown primary
      - supplemental x-ray views tailored to specific problem
    - follow-up
      - after breast cancer surgery
  - findings indicative of malignancy
    - poorly defined, spiculated border
    - microcalcifications
    - architectural distortion
    - interval mammographic changes
  - normal mammogram does not rule out suspicion of cancer based on clinical findings
  - compression views to clarify results if intermediate suspicion

Any palpable dominant breast mass requires further investigation.

Diagnostic mammography is indicated even in women <50 years old.

A comparison of aspiration cytology and core needle biopsy according to tumor size of suspicious breast lesions.
Diagn Cytopathol 2008 36(1):26-31
Background: The purpose of the study was to compare the accuracy of FNAC, CNB, and combined biopsy according to tumor size of suspicious breast lesions.
Methods: Ultrasound guided FNAC and CNB were performed in 264 patients with suspicious breast lesions from August, 1997 to August, 2002. The lesions were divided in four groups according to the tumor size in the histopathology report: lesions smaller than 1 cm, between 1 and 2 cm, between 2 and 5 cm, and lesions greater than 5 cm. The final surgical histopathology results identified 222 (84%) malignant cases and benign lesions summed 42 (16%).
Results: For lesions smaller than 1 cm, FNAC, CNB, and combined biopsy were equivalent for all parameters. For lesions between 1 and 2 cm, FNAC and CNB were equivalent. Combined biopsy showed higher absolute sensitivity (P = 0.007) and lower inadequate rate (P = 0.03) when compared to FNAC. However, when combined biopsy and CNB were compared, no difference were found. For lesions between 2 and 5 cm, CNB showed higher absolute sensitivity (P <0.001) and lower inadequate rate (P < 0.007) when compared to FNAC. Combined biopsy showed higher sensitivity compared to FNAC and CNB alone (P < 0.05) in this group. For lesions greater than 5 cm, FNAC and CNB were equivalent for all parameters. Combined biopsy only showed higher absolute sensitivity (P = 0.04) when compared with FNAC alone.
Conclusions: The combination of FNAC and CNB can improve the diagnosis of suspicious breast lesions greater than 1 cm. However, for lesions smaller than 1 cm, any modality has technical limitations.

Table 13. Screening for Breast Cancer in Women of Average Risk

Test/Maneuver	Effectiveness	Level of evidence	Recommendation
Mammography, with or without clinical examination*, women aged 40-49 years	Controversial, routine mammography, with or without clinical examination, has not consistently been shown to reduce breast cancer mortality or overall mortality (7 RCTs, 7 meta-analyses)	RCTs (I)	Current evidence does not support the recommendation that screening mammography be included or excluded from the periodic health examination of women aged 40-49 with average risk of breast cancer (Grade C)
Mammography, with or without clinical examination*, women aged 50-69	Statistically significant reduction in breast cancer mortality (RR 0.76) though overall mortality not affected (7 RCTs, 5 meta-analyses)	RCTs (I)	Based on breast cancer-specific mortality, the Canadian Task Force on Preventative Health Care concluded there was good evidence for screening women aged 50-69 by mammography (and clinical breast exam).(Grade A) The best available evidence does not provide conclusive direction regarding annual versus biennial screening
Teaching of Breast Self-Examination (BSE) to women aged 40-69	Evidence of no benefit in terms of survival from breast cancer Evidence of increased number of physician visits and increased rate of benign biopsy results	RCTs (I) Non-RCTs (II-1) Cohort Studies (II-3) Case-control studies (II-3) RCTs (I) Non-RCTs (II-1)	Fair evidence of no benefit and good evidence of harm, therefore fair evidence not to recommend routine teaching of BSE from the periodic health examination (Grade D)

*   The utility of adding clinical breast examination (CBE) to mammography is unclear. Some of the 7 RCTs carried out CBE and mammography in combination and some separately. As relative contributions of mammography and clinical breast exam are unknown, both maneuvers are recommended by the Canadian Task Force on Preventative Health Care.

- **other radiographic studies**
  - U/S: differentiate between cystic and solid
  - MRI: high sensitivity, low specificity
  - galactogram (for nipple discharge): identifies lesions in ducts
  - as indicated: bone scan, abdo U/S, CXR, head CT

Diagnostic Procedures
- needle aspiration – for palpable cystic lesions; send fluid for cytology if bloody
- fine needle aspiration (FNA) – for palpable solid masses, obtains cellular material
- U/S or mammography guided core needle biopsy – larger sample than FNA, allow evaluation of invasive vs. *in situ* (most common)
- excisional biopsy – definitive method for tissue diagnosis

Genetic Screening
- consider testing for BRCA1/2 if:
  - patient diagnosed with breast AND ovarian cancer
  - strong family history of breast/ovarian cancer (e.g. among the Ashkenazi Jewish population)
  - family history of male breast cancer
- risk consultation may include: pedigree documentation, pathological review of affected family members, review of basic concepts of cancer, genetics, risk factors, limitations of testing, cost and implications of positive, negative or inconclusive testing

Staging (see Table 14)
- clinical
  - tumour size by palpation, mammogram
  - nodal involvement by palpation
  - metastasis by physical exam, CXR, abdo U/S, bone scan (usually done post-op if necessary)
- pathological
  - tumour size
  - grade: modified Bloom and Richardson score (I to III) – histologic, nuclear and mitotic grade
  - number of axillary nodes positive for malignancy out of total nodes resected, extranodal extension, sentinel node positive/negative
  - estrogen receptor (ER) + progesterone receptor (PR) testing
  - Her2Neu receptor testing
  - margins: negative, <1 mm, positive
  - lymphovascular invasion (LVI)
  - extensive *in situ* component (EIC): DCIS in surrounding tissue
  - involvement of dermal lymphatics (inflammatory) – automatically Stage IIIb

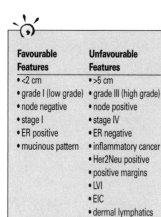

Favourable Features	Unfavourable Features
• <2 cm	• >5 cm
• grade I (low grade)	• grade III (high grade)
• node negative	• node positive
• stage I	• stage IV
• ER positive	• ER negative
• mucinous pattern	• inflammatory cancer
	• Her2Neu positive
	• positive margins
	• LVI
	• EIC
	• dermal lymphatics involved

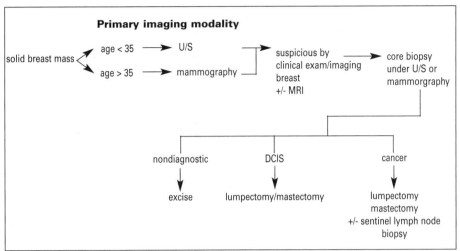

Figure 23. Management of a Solid Breast Mass by Triple Diagnosis

Table 14. Staging of Breast Cancer (American Joint Committee on Cancer)

Stage	Tumour	Nodes (regional)	Metastasis	Survival (5-year)
0	in situ	none	none	99%
I	<2 cm	none	none	94%
II A	<2 cm	mobile ipsilateral	none	85%
II B	2-5 cm	none or mobile ipsilateral	none	70%
	or >5 cm	none	none	
III A	any size	fixed ipsilateral or internal mammary	none	52%
III B	skin/chest wall invasion	any	none	48%
III C	any size	ipsilateral infraclavicular/internal mammary plus axillary nodes; ipsilateral supraclavicular node(s) ± axillary nodes	none	33%
IV	any	any	distant	18%

Etiology and Presentation
- non-invasive
  - ductal carcinoma *in situ* (DCIS)
    - proliferation of malignant ductal epithelial cells completely contained within breast ducts
    - 80% non-palpable – detected by screening mammogram
    - risk of infiltrating ductal carcinoma in same breast up to 35% in 10 years
    - histology
      - comedo vs. non-comedo: comedo tumours more frequently show tumour necrosis, high nuclear grade, association with invasive ductal carcinoma
      - often multifocal (multiple tumour foci in same quadrant of breast)
    - treatment
      - lumpectomy with wide excision margins + radiation (5-10% risk invasive cancer) – indicated if low grade, small lesion, single focus
      - mastectomy if large area of disease (risk of invasive cancer reduced to 1%)
      - possibly tamoxifen as an adjuvant treatment
      - 99% 5-year survival
      - 50% of recurrences are invasive cancer
  - lobular carcinoma *in situ* (LCIS)
    - neoplastic cells completely contained within breast lobule
    - no palpable mass, no mammographic findings, usually incidental finding on breast biopsy
    - risk of developing infiltrating ductal carcinoma in **either** breast is 20-30% at 20 years, tamoxifen prophylaxis may be beneficial
    - treatment options:
      - clinical follow-up
      - chemoprevention (tamoxifen)
      - surgery (uncommon)
- invasive
  - infiltrating ductal carcinoma (most common 80%)
    - originates from ductal epithelium and infiltrates supporting stroma
    - characteristics – hard, scirrhous, infiltrating tentacles, gritty on cross-section

- invasive lobular carcinoma (8-15%)
    - originates from lobular epithelium
    - 20% bilateral (i.e. more often than infiltrating ductal carcinoma)
    - does not form microcalcifications, harder to detect mammographically
- Paget's disease (1-3%)
    - ductal carcinoma that invades nipple with scaling, eczematoid lesion
- inflammatory carcinoma (1-4%)
    - ductal carcinoma that invades dermal lymphatics
    - most aggressive form of breast cancer
    - clinical features – erythema, skin edema, warm, swollen and tender breast ± lump
    - peau d'orange indicates advanced disease (IIIb-IV)
- male breast cancer (<1%)
    - most commonly infiltrating ductal carcinoma
    - often diagnosed at later stages
    - stage-for-stage similar prognosis to breast cancer in females
    - consider genetic testing
- other
    - papillary, medullary, mucinous, tubular cancers
    - generally better prognosis
- sarcomas
    - rare, most commonly cystosarcoma phyllodes, a variant of fibroadenoma
- lymphoma – rare

Treatment

Table 15.   Breast Cancer Treatment by Stage

Stage	Primary treatment options	Adjuvant systemic therapy
0 (*in situ*)	Breast-conserving surgery (BCS) + radiotherapy BCS alone if margins >1cm and low nuclear grade Mastectomy* +/- SLNB	None
I	BCS + axillary node dissection + radiotherapy Mastectomy* + axillary node dissection/SLNB	May not be needed; discuss risks/benefits of chemotherapy and tamoxifen
II	BCS + axillary node dissection + radiotherapy Mastectomy* + axillary node dissection/SLNB	Chemotherapy for premenopausal women or postmenopausal and estrogen receptor (ER) negative, follow by tamoxifen if ER positive
III	Likely mastectomy + axillary node dissection + radiotherapy	Neoadjuvant therapy may be considered ie. preoperative chemotherapy and/or hormone therapy. Adjuvant radiation and chemotherapy may also be appropriate (i.e. post-op)
Inflammatory	Likely mastectomy + axillary node dissection + radiotherapy	Neoadjuvant therapy
IV	Surgery as appropriate for local control	Primary treatment is systemic therapy i.e. chemotherapy and/or hormone therapy

* If no reason to select mastectomy, the choice between BCS + radiotherapy and mastectomy can be made according to patient's preference since choice of local treatment does not significantly affect survival if local control is achieved

Primary: Surgical

- breast-conserving surgery (BCS) – lumpectomy with wide local excision
    - for treatment of stage I and II disease
    - must be combined with radiation for equivalent survival as mastectomy
    - axillary lymph node dissection (ALND) or sentinel node biopsy needed
        - for staging of nodes and reduced recurrence in axilla
        - complications of ALND: arm lymphedema (10-15%), decreased arm sensation, shoulder pain
    - sentinel node biopsy
        - sentinel node: the first node(s) receiving direct lymphatic drainage from a tumour site
        - technetium-99 ± blue dye injected at tumour site to identify sentinel node(s)
        - send for frozen section, H&E and cytokeratin staining
        - ALND if any nodes positive for micrometastasis
        - false-negative rate 5%
        - uncertain if sentinel node biopsy yields comparable long-term survival to ALND
    - BCS not appropriate if:
        - factors present that increase risk of local recurrence: extensive malignant-type calcifications on mammogram, multifocal primary tumours or failure to obtain tumour-free margins after re-excision
        - contraindications to radiation therapy
        - large tumour size relative to breast
        - patient prefers mastectomy
        - patient is pregnant

- mastectomy
    - modified radical mastectomy (MRM) – removes all breast tissue, nipple-areolar complex, skin and axillary nodes
    - simple mastectomy – similar to MRM but axillary nodes not removed
    - radical mastectomy (not done anymore) – removes all breast tissue, skin, pectoralis muscle, axillary contents
    - offer breast reconstruction if mastectomy chosen (immediate or delayed)

Adjuvant/Neoadjuvant
- radiation
    - decrease risk of local recurrence, and almost always used after BCS, sometimes after mastectomy
    - axillary nodal radiation may be added if nodal involvement
    - for high-risk of local recurrence, inoperable locally advanced cancer, metastases
    - stage I/II disease: decreases local recurrence, increases disease-free survival; effect on overall survival controversial
- **hormonal**
    - indications
        - ER positive (pre-/post-menopausal) plus node-positive or high-risk node-negative
        - palliation for metastases
    - tamoxifen or aromatase inhibitors (eg. anastrozole), ovarian ablation (e.g. goserelin/GnRH agonist, oophorectomy), progestins (e.g. megestrol acetate), androgens (e.g. fluoxymesterone)
- **chemotherapy**
    - indications
        - ER negative plus node-positive/high-risk node-negative
        - ER positive and young age
        - stage I disease at high risk of recurrence (high grade, LVI)
        - palliation for metastatic disease
- **prophylactic**
    - chemoprevention – tamoxifen
    - secondary prevention – screening for early detection (see above)
    - mastectomy – high-risk women (e.g. BRCA1/2), occasionally contralateral in women with personal history of breast cancer

There is no survival benefit of mastectomy over lumpectomy plus radiation for stage I and II disease.

Post-Treatment Follow-up
- visits q3-6 months x 2 years and annually thereafter (frequency is controversial)
- annual mammography, with no other imaging unless clinically indicated
- psychosocial support and counselling
- signs of recurrence: metastasis vs. new primary
    - CXR, CT abdomen, liver enzymes, bone scan, CT brain, MRI spine, solitary lesion biopsy as indicated

Local/Regional Recurrence
- recurrence in treated breast or ipsilateral axilla
- 1% per year up to maximum of 15% risk of developing contralateral malignancy
- 5x increased risk of developing metastases

Metastasis
- bone > lungs > pleura > liver > brain
- treatment is palliative – hormone therapy, chemotherapy, radiation

Prognosis (see Table 14)
- nodal status most important prognostic feature, grade also important
- also tumour size, LVI, receptor status, cell proliferative indices, Her2Neu status

Surgical Endocrinology

Thyroid and Parathyroid

- see Endocrinology and Otolaryngology

Adrenal Gland

- see also Endocrinology
- functional anatomy:
    - cortex: glomerulosa (mineralocorticoids), fasciculata (glucocorticoids), reticularis (sex steroids)

- medulla: catecholamines (epinephrine, norepinephrine)
- types: functional (e.g. Cushing's syndrome, Conn's syndrome) or non-functional

INCIDENTALOMA - adrenal mass discovered by investigation of unrelated symptoms
- benign adenoma (38%) > metastases to adrenal (22%) >> cyst, carcinoma, pheochromocytoma, neuroblastoma
- metastasis to adrenal gland from: lung > breast, colon, lymphoma, melanoma, kidney
- peak incidence of carcinoma is 50-60 y.o. females – risk decreases with increasing age and male gender

Investigations
- MRI, CT: size >6 cm is best predictor of primary adrenal carcinoma (92% are >6 cm)
- functional study: urine and plasma steroids, urine catecholamines/metanephrines, electrolytes, suppression tests
- FNA biopsy: if suspect metastasis to adrenal (must exclude pheochromocytoma first)
    - indicated if history of cancer or patient is smoker
- iodocholesterol scintigraphy: may distinguish benign vs. malignant disease

Treatment
- functional tumour: resect
- non-functioning tumour
    - >6 cm: resect
    - 3-6 cm: MRI (T2 density, shape, margins), more likely to resect in females and if <60 y.o.
    - <3 cm: follow with repeat CT in 12-18 months

Skin Lesions

- see Dermatology

Common Medications

Antiemetics
- dimenhydrinate (Gravol™) 25-50 mg PO/IV/IM q4-6h prn
- prochlorperazine (Stemetil™) 5-10 mg IV/IM/PO bid-tid prn
- metochlopromide (Maxeran™) 10 mg IV/IM q2-3h prn, 10-15 mg PO qid (30 min before meals and qhs)
- granisetron (Kytril™) 1 mg PO bid (for nausea from chemo/radiation)

Analgesics
- acetaminophen ± codeine (Tylenol™ plain/#3) 1-2 tabs q4-6h PO/PR prn
- morphine 2.5-10 mg IM/SC q 4-6h prn + 1-2 mg IV q1h prn for breakthrough

DVT Prophylaxis
- heparin 5000 units SC bid, if cancer patient then heparin 5000 units SC tid
- dalteparin (Fragmin™) 5000 units SC OD
- enoxaparin (Lovenox™) 40 mg SC OD

Laxatives
- docusate sodium (Colace™) 100 mg PO bid
- glycerine supp 1 tab PR prn
- lactulose 15-30 ml PO qid prn
- milk of magnesia 30-60 ml PO qid prn
- bisacodyl 10-15 mg PO prn

Sedatives
- zopiclone (Imovane™) 5-7.5 mg PO qhs prn
- lorazepam (Ativan™) 0.5-2 mg PO/SL qhs prn

Antibiotics
- cefazolin (Ancef™) 1 g IV/IM on call to OR or q8h
- cefalexin (Keflex™) 250-500 mg PO qid
- ceftriaxone 1-2 g IM/IV q24h
- ampicillin 1-2 g IV q4-6h
- gentamicin 3-5 mg/kg/day IM/IV divided q8h; monitor creatinine, gentamicin levels
- ciprofloxacin 400 mg IV q12h, 500 mg PO bid
- metronidazole (Flagyl™) 500 mg PO/IV bid, (500 mg PO tid for *C. difficile*)

GM Geriatric Medicine

Andrea Herschorn and Rachel Sheps, chapter editors
Deepti Damaraju and Elliott Owen, associate editors
Erik Venos, EBM editor
Dr. Barry J. Goldlist, staff editor

Seniors in Canada and the U.S.

Health Status

Table 1. Causes of Mortality and Morbidity in Canadian and American Seniors

Mortality (Can[1]/US[2])	Morbidity[1,2]
1. Diseases of the heart and circulatory system (32.8/30.4%)	1. Hypertension
2. Malignant neoplasms (29.2/22.0%)	2. Arthritis
3. Cerebrovascular disease (6.4/7.4%)	3. Heart disease
4. Chronic lower respiratory disease (4.4//6.0%)	4. Diabetes
5. Accidents (4.5%)[1]	5. Ulcers
6. Alzheimers (3.7%)[2]	6. Stroke
	7. Asthma
	8. Allergies

[1]Statistics Canada 2000 & 2003   [2]National Center for Health Statistics 2007

Physiology and Pathology of Aging

Geriatric Giants
Falls
Incontinence
Polypharmacy
Confusion

5 I's of Geriatrics
Immobility
Intellect
Incontinence
Iatrogenesis
Impaired homeostasis

Most Common Acute Disorders in the Elderly
Cardiovascular disease (CHF, CVA, MI)
Fracture (hip, vertebrae, wrist)
Medication-related
Pneumonia
Sepsis

Most Common Chronic Disorders in the Elderly
Arthritis
Cataracts and other visual problems
COPD
Cardiovascular disease
Diabetes Mellitus (Type 2)
Hearing impairment
Hypertension
Mental disorders
Orthopaedic disorders
Sinusitis

Table 2. Changes Occurring Frequently with Aging

System	Physiological Changes	Pathological Changes
Neurologic	↓ wakefulness, decreased brain mass, cerebral blood flow	↑ insomnia, neurodegenerative disease, stroke, ↓ reflex response
Special Senses	↓ lacrimal gland secretion, lens transparency, dark adaptation, sense of smell and taste	↑ glaucoma, cataracts, macular degeneration, presbycusis, presbyopia, tinnitus, vertigo, oral dryness
Cardiovascular	↑ sBP, dBP, decreased HR, CO, vessel elasticity, cardiac myocyte size and number, β-adrenergic responsiveness	↑ atherosclerosis, CAD, MI, CHF, hypertension, arrhythmias
Respiratory	↑ tracheal cartilage calcification, mucous gland hypertrophy ↓ elastic recoil, mucociliary clearance, pulmonary function reserve	↑ COPD, pneumonia, pulmonary embolism
Gastrointestinal	↑ intestinal villous atrophy ↓ esophageal peristalsis, gastric acid secretion, liver mass, hepatic blood flow, calcium, and iron absorption	↑ cancer, diverticulitis, constipation, fecal incontinence, hemorrhoids, intestinal obstruction
Renal and Urologic	↑ proteinuria, urinary frequency ↓ renal mass, creatinine clearance, urine acidification, hydroxylation of vitamin D, bladder capacity	↑ urinary incontinence, nocturia, BPH, prostate cancer, pyelonephritis, nephrolithiasis, UTI
Reproductive	↓ androgen, estrogen, sperm count, vaginal secretion ↓ ovary, uterus, vagina, breast size	↑ breast and endometrial cancer, cystocele, rectocele, atrophic vaginitis
Endocrine	↑ NE, PTH, insulin, vasopressin ↓ thyroid and adrenal corticosteroid secretion	↑ DM, hypothyroidism, stress response
Musculoskeletal	↑ calcium loss from bone ↓ muscle mass, cartilage	↑ arthritis, bursitis, osteoporosis, polymyalgia rheumatica
Integumentary	atrophy of sebaceous and sweat glands, ↓ epidermal and dermal thickness, dermal vascularity, melanocytes, collagen synthesis	↑ lentigo, cherry hemangiomas, pruritus, seborrheic keratosis, herpes zoster, decubitus ulcers, skin cancer
Psychiatry	none	↑ depression, dementia, delirium, suicidality, substance abuse, anxiety, insomnia

Differential Diagnoses of Common Presentations

Delirium, Dementia, and Depression

- see <u>Psychiatry</u> and <u>Neurology</u>

Elder Abuse

Definition
- the definition of elder abuse includes physical abuse, sexual abuse, emotional or psychological abuse, financial abuse, abandonment, neglect and self-neglect
- elder abuse is a criminal offence under the Criminal Code of Canada
- in the U.S., most states have criminal penalties for elder abuse, laws vary from state to state

Epidemiology
- in Canada, approximately 4% of elderly persons living in private homes have suffered abuse
- in the U.S., estimates of the frequency of elder abuse range from 3-8%
- physician reporting is mandatory only in Newfoundland, Nova Scotia and PEI; in Ontario, only abuse occurring in nursing homes is mandatory to report
- insufficient evidence to include/exclude screening in the Periodic Health Exam

Risk Factors
- situational factors
  - isolation, lack of money, lack of community resources for additional care, unsatisfactory arrangements
  - shortage of beds, surplus of patients, low staff-to-patient ratio, low rates of pay for staff, low educational level of staff, staff burnout
- characteristics of the victim
  - physical or emotional dependence on caregiver, lack of close family ties, history of family violence, age over 75 years, recent deterioration in health, dementia
- characteristics of the perpetrator
  - stress caused by financial, marital or occupational factors, deterioration in health, bereavement, substance abuse, mental illness, related to victim, living with victim, long duration of care for victim (mean 9.5 years)

Management
- assess for safety and determine capacity to make decisions about living arrangements
- establish need for hospitalization or alternate accommodation, e.g. immediate risk of physical harm by self or caregiver
- involve multidisciplinary team, i.e. physician (geriatrician, psychiatrist, family physician), nurse, social worker, family members
- contact local resources, i.e. legal aid, elderly advocacy centre, crisis centre
- educate and assist caregiver, link up with community resources, i.e. personal support worker, homemaking services, caregiver support groups

Failure to Thrive (Frailty)

Definition
- declining independence and functional capacity in older adults
- not an inevitable conseqence of aging

Etiology
- four syndromes are prevalent in older patients with failure to thrive: cognitive impairment, depression, malnutrition, and impaired physical functioning

>
>
> **Red Flags for Elder Abuse**
> 1. Delay with seeking medical attention
> 2. Disparity in histories
> 3. Implausible or vague explanations
> 4. Frequent emergency room visits for exacerbations of chronic disease despite plan for medical care and adequate resources
> 5. Presentation of functionally impaired patient without designated caregiver
> 6. Lab findings inconsistent with history

>
>
> **Four Syndromes in Failure to Thrive**
> **My Pa Can't Drive**
> **M**alnutrition
> **P**hysical impairment
> **C**ognitive impairment
> **D**epression

Table 3. Common Medical Conditions Associated with Failure to Thrive

Medical Condition	Cause of Failure to Thrive
Cancer	Metastases, malnutrition, cachexia
Chronic lung disease	Respiratory failure
Chronic renal insufficiency	Renal failure
Chronic steroid use	Steroid myopathy, diabetes, osteoporosis, vision loss
Cirrhosis, hepatitis	Hepatic failure
Depression, other psychiatric disorder	Major depression, psychosis, poor functional status, cognitive loss
Diabetes	Malabsorption, poor glucose homeostasis, end-organ damage
Gastrointestinal surgery	Malabsorption, malnutrition
Hip, long bone fracture	Functional impairment
Inflammatory bowel disease	Malabsorption, malnutrition
Myocardial infarction, congestive heart failure	Cardiac failure
Recurrent UTI or pneumonia	Chronic infection, functional impairment
Rheumatologic disease (GCA, RA, SLE)	Chronic inflammation
Stroke	Dysphagia, depression, cognitive loss, functional impairment
Tuberculosis, other systemic infection	Chronic infection

Verdery RB. (1997) "Clinical evaluation of failure to thrive in older people." Clin Geriatr Med 13:769-78.

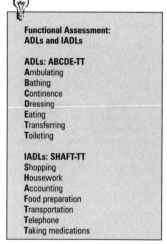

Figure 1. Evaluation of the Geriatric Patient who is Failing in the Community
Sarkisian CA, Lachs MS (1996). "Failure to thrive" in older adults. Ann Intern Med, 124:1072-1078.

Falls

Epidemiology
- 30-40% of people >65 yo, and ~50% of people >80 yo, fall each year
  - approximately 20% of falls require medical attention
  - 5% of falls lead to hospitalization
  - 5-10% with serious injuries (e.g. hip fractures, head injury, laceration)

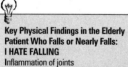

Functional Assessment:
ADLs and IADLs

ADLs: ABCDE-TT
Ambulating
Bathing
Continence
Dressing
Eating
Transferring
Toileting

IADLs: SHAFT-TT
Shopping
Housework
Accounting
Food preparation
Transportation
Telephone
Taking medications

Drugs That May Increase the Risk of Falling
Sedative-hypnotic and anxiolytic drugs (especially long-acting benzodiazepines)
Tricyclic antidepressants
Major tranquilizers (phenothiazines and butyrophenones)
Antihypertensive drugs
Cardiac medications
Corticosteroids
Nonsteroidal anti-inflammatory drugs
Anticholinergic drugs
Hypoglycemic agents
Alcohol
Fuller, George (2001) "Falls in the elderly." Am Fam Phys 61(7): 2159-2172.

Key Physical Findings in the Elderly Patient Who Falls or Nearly Falls:
I HATE FALLING
Inflammation of joints
Hypotension (orthostatic changes)
Auditory and visual abnormalities
Tremor
Equilibrium (balance) problem
Foot Problems
Arrhythmia, heart block or valvular disease
Leg-length discrepancy
Lack of conditioning (generalized weakness)
Illness
Nutrition
Gait disturbance
Fuller, George (2001) "Falls in the elderly." Am Fam Phys 61(7): 2159-2172.

- 1-2% of falls associated with hip fracture
  - 15% die in hospital, 33% 1-year mortality
- between 25-75% do not recover to previous level of ADL function
- mortality increases with age (171/100,000 in men >85 years old) and type of injury (25% with hip fracture die within 6 months)

Etiology
- commonly multifactorial
- extrinsic
  - environmental (e.g. home layout, lighting, stairs, footwear)/accidental/abuse
  - medications/substances
  - month after hospital discharge, acute/exacerbation of chronic illness
- intrinsic
  - orthostasis/syncope
  - age-related changes and diseases associated with aging: musculoskeletal/arthritis (muscle weakness), sensory (visual, proprioceptive, vestibular), cognitive (depression, dementia, delirium, anxiety), cardiovascular (CAD, arrhythmia, MI, low BP), neurologic (stroke, decreased LOC, gait disturbances/ataxia), metabolic (glucose, electrolytes)

Investigations
- directed by history and physical
- CBC, electrolytes, BUN, creatinine, glucose, Ca, TSH, B12, urinalysis, cardiac enzymes, ECG, CT head

Prevention
- multidisciplinary, multifactorial, health and environment risk factor screening and intervention programs in the community
- program of muscle strengthening, balance retraining and group exercise programs (e.g. tai chi)
- home hazard assessment and modification (e.g. remove rugs, add shower bars, etc.)
- withdrawal of psychotropic medication
- cardiac pacing for those with cardio-inhibitory carotid sinus hypersensitivity
- optimize eyesight and footwear

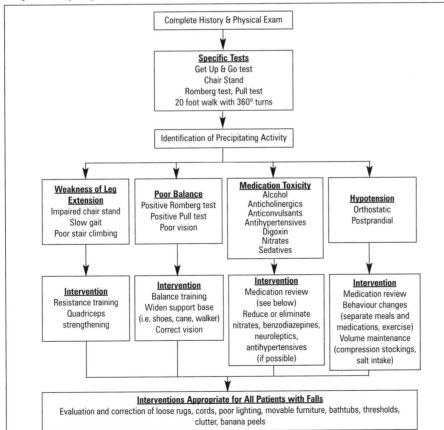

Figure 2. Approach to Falls in the Elderly
Adapted with permission from: Kiel, DP. Overview of falls in the elderly. In: UpToDate, Rose, BD (Ed), UpToDate, Waltman, MA, 2005.
For more information visit www.uptodate.com.

Fall Prevention Tips
1. Improve lighting, especially on stairs
2. Caution while adjusting to new bifocal prescription (poor depth perception)
3. Siderails in bathtubs
4. Railings on steps
5. Connect patient to lifeline button signaling systems
6. Remove loose mats or carpets, telephone cords and other tripping hazards
7. Recommend support hose for varicose veins and swelling of ankles

Goldlist B, Turpic I, Borins M. Essential Geriatrics: Managing 6 conditions: *Patient Care Canada.* 1997. 8(9).

Will my patient fall?
JAMA. 2007;297:77-86.
Purpose: To identify the prognostic value of risk factors for future falls among older patients.
Study Selection: Prospective cohort studies of risk factors for falls that performed a multivariate analysis of such factors.
Results: Clinically identifiable risk factors were identified across 6 domains: orthostatic hypotension, visual impairment, impairment of gait or balance, medication use, limitations in basic or instrumental activities of daily living, and cognitive impairment. Eighteen studies met inclusion criteria and provided a multivariate analysis including at least 1 of the risk factor domains. The estimated pretest probability of falling at least once in any given year for individuals 65 years and older was 27% (95% confidence interval, 19%-36%). Patients who have fallen in the past year are more likely to fall again [likelihood ratio range, 2.3-2.8]. The most consistent predictors of future falls are clinically detected abnormalities of gait or balance (likelihood ratio range, 1.7-2.4). Visual impairment, medication variables, decreased activities of daily living, and impaired cognition did not consistently predict falls across studies. Orthostatic hypotension did not predict falls after controlling for other factors.
Conclusions: Screening for risk of falling during the clinical examination begins with determining if the patient has fallen in the past year. For patients who have not previously fallen, screening consists of an assessment of gait and balance. Patients who have fallen or who have a gait or balance problem are at higher risk of future falls.

Medication as a risk factor for falls: Critical systematic review.
J Gerontol A Biol Sci Med Sci. 2007 Oct;62(10):1172-81.
Purpose: To systematically review all original articles examining medication use as a risk factor for falls or fall-related fractures in people aged ≥60 years.
Study Selection: Studies investigating "falls" or "accidental falls" and "pharmaceutical preparations" or specific groups of drugs were included. Studies not meeting the age criterion, not controlled with nonusers of target medicines or nonfallers, or with no clear definition of target medication were excluded.
Results: Twenty-eight observational studies and one randomized controlled trial met the inclusion criteria. The outcome measure was a fall in 22 studies and a fracture in 7 studies. The main group of drugs associated with an increased risk of falling was psychotropics: benzodiazepines, antidepressants, and antipsychotics. Antiepileptics and drugs that lower blood pressure were weakly associated with falls.
Conclusions: Central nervous system drugs, especially psychotropics, seem to be associated with an increased risk of falls. The quality of observational studies needs to be improved, for many appear to lack even a clear definition of a fall, target medicines, or prospective follow-up. Many drugs commonly used by older persons are not systematically studied as risk factors for falls.

Fecal Incontinence

Treatment of hypertension in patients 80 years of age or older
N Engl J Med. 2008 May 1;358(18):1887-98
Study: Randomized, double-blind, placebo-controlled, multicentre trial.
Patients: 3845 patients who were 80 years of age or older and had a sustained systolic blood pressure of 160 mmHg were followed for a median 1.8 years.
Intervention: Indapamide (sustained release, 1.5 mg) or matching placebo. The angiotensin-converting–enzyme inhibitor perindopril (2 or 4 mg), or matching placebo, was added if necessary to achieve the target blood pressure of 150/80 mmHg.
Primary Outcome: Fatal or nonfatal stroke.
Results: The mean age of the patients was 83.6 years and mean blood pressure while sitting was 173.0/90.8 mmHg. At 2 years, the mean blood pressure while sitting was 15.0/6.1 mm Hg lower in the active-treatment group than in the placebo group. Active treatment was associated with a 30% reduction in the rate of fatal or nonfatal stroke (95% confidence interval [CI], −1 to 51; P=0.06), a 39% reduction in the rate of death from stroke (95% CI, 1 to 62; P=0.05), a 21% reduction in the rate of death from any cause (95% CI, 4 to 35; P=0.02), a 23% reduction in the rate of death from cardiovascular causes (95% CI, −1 to 40; P=0.06), and a 64% reduction in the rate of heart failure (95% CI, 42 to 78; P<0.001). Fewer serious adverse events were reported in the active-treatment group (358 vs. 448 in the placebo group; P=0.001).
Conclusions: Antihypertensive treatment with indapamide (sustained release), with or without perindopril, in persons 80 years of age or older reduces death from stroke, death from any cause, and the incidence of heart failure.

• second leading cause of nursing home placement

Epidemiology
• pelvic floor intact
  ▪ neurologic conditions: age-related, neuropathy, multiple sclerosis, tumours, trauma
  ▪ overflow
  ▪ diarrheal conditions
• pelvic floor affected
  ▪ trauma/surgery
  ▪ nerve/sphincter damage
  ▪ malformation, ano-rectal

Etiology
• commonly multifactorial

Risk Factors
• prior vaginal delivery
• ano-rectal surgery
• pelvic radiation
• diabetes
• neurologic disease
• diarrheal conditions

Investigations
• stool studies
• endorectal ultrasound
• colonoscopy, sigmoidoscopy, anoscopy
• anorectal manometry/functional testing

Management
• disimpaction
• diet/bulking agent if stool is liquid or loose
• anti-diarrheal agents
• regular defecation program in patients with dementia
• counsel about biofeedback therapy (retraining of pelvic floor muscles)

Gait Disorders

• see Neurology

Hazards of Hospitalization

Table 4. Sequelae of Hospitalization of Older Patients - Recommendations

Sequelae	Recommendations
malnutrition	no dietary restrictions (except diabetes), assistance, dentures if necessary, eating out of bed
urinary incontinence	medication review, remove environmental barriers, discontinue use of catheter
depression	routine screening
adverse drug event	medication review
confusion/delirium	orientation, visual and hearing aids, volume repletion, noise reduction, early mobilization, medication review, remove restraints
pressure ulcers	low-resistance mattress, daily inspection, repositioning every 2 hours
infection	early mobilization, remove unnecessary IV lines, catheters, NG tubes
falls	appropriate footwear, assistive devices, early mobilization, remove restraints, medication review
hypotension/dehydration	early recognition and repletion
diminished aerobic capacity/loss of muscle strength/contractures	early mobilization
decreased respiratory function	incentive spirometry, physiotherapy

Hypertension

- see Family Medicine
- 60-80% of elderly (>65 yo) have hypertension
  - 60% of these have isolated systolic HTN
- non-pharmacologic treatments are first-line, then thiazide monotherapy is recommended (some evidence for CCB monotherapy if isolated systolic HTN)
- add ACEI/ARB if also atherosclerosis, DM, CHF or chronic kidney disease
- add β-blockers if also angina or CHF
- goal BP: sBP <140, 65<dBP<90

Immobility

Complications of Immobility
- cardiovascular: orthostatic hypotension, venous thrombosis, embolism
- respiratory: decreased ventilation, atelectasis, pneumonia
- gastrointestinal: anorexia, constipation, incontinence, dehydration, malnutrition
- genitourinary: infection, urinary retention, bladder calculi, incontinence
- musculoskeletal: atrophy, contractures, bone loss
- skin: pressure sores
- psychological: sensory deprivation, delirium, depression

Immunizations

- see Family Medicine
- the following immunizations are recommended in people over 65 years of age:
  - pneumococcus - 1 dose
  - influenza - every autumn
  - appropriate boosters (e.g. tetanus every 10 years)

Calcium Channel Blockade and Cardiovascular Prognosis in the European Trial on Isolated Systolic Hypertension
Hypertension 1998;32:410-16.
Study: Double blind, randomised, placebo controlled, multicentre study.
Patients: 4695 patients ≥60 years (mean age 70 yrs, 67% female) with baseline sBP between 160-219 mmHg, standing sBP ≥140 mmHg, and dBP<95 mmHg .
Intervention: Patients were randomized to receive either active antihypertensive medication or placebo. Active medications consisted of the CCB nitrendipine (10 to 40 mg/d) as a first-line agent with the possible addition of enalapril and/or HCTZ. The control group received matching placebos. The goal of titration and combination of medications was a reduction of >20 mmHg to achieve a sitting sBP <150 mmHg.
Primary Outcome: Cardiovascular complications.
Results: Patients taking nitrendipine alone had 25% (p=0.05) fewer cardiovascular end points when compared with the placebo group as a whole. Compared with the same control group, those requiring enalapril and/or HCTZ in addition to nitrendipine had significant decreases in mortality (40%), stroke (59%), and all cardiovascular end points (39%, p<0.01 for all). Compared with the subgroup of control patients who remained on only first-line placebo, those taking nitrendipine alone showed an almost 50% (p<0.004) reduction in total and cardiovascular mortality. A post hoc matched pairs analysis between patients taking nitrendipine monotherapy and patients drawn from the placebo group as a whole revealed significantly reduced cardiovascular mortality (41%), all cardiovascular end points (33%), and fatal and nonfatal cardiac end points (33%, p<0.05 for all) in the nitrendipine group.
Conclusions: Although not ideally designed, the results of this study suggest that monotherapy with a CCB prevents cardiovascular complications in elderly patients with isolated systolic hypertension.

Vaccines for preventing influenza in the elderly
Cochrane Database Syst Rev. 2006 Jul 19;3:CD004876.
Purpose: To review the evidence of efficacy, effectiveness and safety of influenza vaccines in individuals aged 65 years or older.
Study Selection: Randomised, quasi-randomised, cohort and case-control studies assessing efficacy against influenza (laboratory-confirmed cases) or effectiveness against influenza-like illness (ILI) or safety.
Results: Sixty-four studies were included in the efficacy/effectiveness assessment. Results were expressed as absolute vaccine efficacy (VE). In homes for elderly individuals (with good vaccine match and high viral circulation) the effectiveness of vaccines against ILI was 23% (6% to 36%) and non-significant against influenza (RR 1.04: 95% CI 0.43 to 2.51). In elderly individuals living in the community, vaccines were not significantly effective against influenza (RR 0.19; 95% CI 0.02 to 2.01), ILI (RR 1.05: 95% CI 0.58 to 1.89), or pneumonia (RR 0.88; 95% CI 0.64 to 1.20). Vaccine administration usually induced systemic side effects (general malaise, fever, nausea, headache) more frequently than placebo, but no outcome showed statistically significant results.
Conclusion: In long-term care facilities, where vaccination is most effective against complications, the aims of the vaccination campaign are fulfilled, at least in part. The usefulness of vaccines in the community is modest.

Malnutrition

Definition
- involuntary weight loss of ≥5% baseline body weight or ≥5 kg
- hypoalbuminemia, hypocholesterolemia

Etiology
- starvation
    - decreased intake: financial, psychiatric, cognitive deficits, functional deficits, anorexia associated with chronic disease
    - decreased assimilation: impaired transit, maldigestion, malabsorption
- stress
    - acute or chronic illness/infection, chronic inflammation, abdominal pain
- mechanical
    - dental problems, dysphagia
- age-related changes
    - appetite dysregulation, decreased thirst
- mixed
    - increased energy demands (e.g. hyperthyroidism), abnormal metabolism, protein-losing enteropathy

Risk Factors
- mechanical: dental problems, medical illnesses interfering with ingestion
- nutritional: medical illnesses increasing nutritional requirements or requiring dietary restrictions
- functional: difficulty shopping, preparing meals, or feeding oneself due to functional impairment
- social: economic barriers to securing food, lack of availability of high quality food
- psychological: depression, poor appetite

Clinical Features
- history
    - recent weight loss, decreased food intake, constitutional symptoms, GI symptoms, recent or chronic illness, social factors
- physical examination
    - BMI <23.5 in males, <22 in females should raise concern
    - temporal wasting, muscle wasting, presence of triceps skin fold

Investigations
- CBC, electrolytes, Ca, Mg, PO_4, Cr, LFTs (albumin, INR, bilirubin), B_{12}, folate, TSH, transferrin, lipid profile, urinalysis

Calculating Basic Caloric and Fluid Requirements
- WHO daily energy estimates for adults over 60 years of age:
    - female: 10.5 x (weight in kg) + 596
    - male: 13.5 x (weight in kg) + 487
- maintenance fluid requirements for the elderly without cardiac or renal disease:
    - 1500-2500 cc/24hrs

Osteoporosis

- see Endocrinology

Presbycusis

- see Otolaryngology

Pressure Ulcers

- see Plastic Surgery

Risk Factors
- extrinsic factors: friction, pressure, shear force
- intrinsic factors: immobility, malnutrition, moisture, sensory loss

Table 5. Classification of Pressure Ulcers

Stage I	Changes include skin temperature, tissue consistency, or sensation. An area of persistent erythema in lightly pigmented intact skin. In darker skin, it may appear red, blue or purple.
Stage II	Partial thickness skin loss involving the epidermis, dermis, or both. The ulcer is superficial and presents as an abrasion, blister, or shallow crater.
Stage III	Full thickness skin loss involving damage or necrosis of subcutaneous tissue which may extend down to, but not through, underlying fascia. Presents as a deep crater with or without undermining of adjacent tissue.
Stage IV	Full thickness skin loss with extensive destruction, tissue necrosis or damage to muscle, bone or supporting structures. May have associated undermining and/or sinus tracts.

Prevention
- pressure reduction
  - frequent repositioning
  - pressure-reducing devices (static, dynamic)
- maintaining nutrition, encouraging mobility and managing incontinence

Treatment
- continue to minimize pressure on wound (see above)
- wound debridement (mechanical, enzymatic, autolytic)
- maintain moist wound environment (to enable re-epithelialization)
- treatment of wound infections (topical gentamicin, silver sulfadiazine, mupirocin)
- analgesia
- biopsy wounds not demonstrating clinical improvement for C&S; biopsy chronic wounds to rule out malignancy
- stage IV ulcers typically warrant surgical repair
- consider other treatment options
  - negative pressure wound therapy/vacuum assisted closure (VAC)
  - biological agents: application of fibroblast growth factor, platelet-derived growth factor to wound
  - non-contact normothermic wound therapy
  - electrotherapy

A systematic review of the use of hydrocolloids in the treatment of pressure ulcers
J Clin Nurs. 2008 May;17(9):1164-73.
Purpose: To describe the current evidence in the field of pressure ulcer treatment with hydrocolloids and to give recommendations for clinical practice and further research.
Study Selection: Randomized controlled trials on the treatment of pressure ulcers with hydrocolloids.
Results: Twenty-nine publications, dealing with 28 different studies, met the inclusion criteria and were included in the review. Hydrocolloids were most frequently used on pressure ulcers grade 2-3. Concerning the healing of the pressure ulcer, hydrocolloids are more effective than gauze dressings for the reduction of the wound dimensions. The absorption capacity, the time needed for dressing changes, the pain during dressing changes and the side-effects were significantly in favour of hydrocolloids if compared to gauze dressings. Based on the available cost-effectiveness data, hydrocolloids seemed to be less expensive compared with collagen-, saline- and povidine-soaked gauze but more expensive compared to hydrogel, polyurethane foam and collagenase.
Conclusions: Based on the studies included in this review, hydrocolloids are frequently used in the treatment of grade 2 and 3 pressure ulcers and are more effective and less expensive than gauze dressings. Compared with alginates, polyurethane dressings, less-contact layers, topical enzymes and biosynthetic dressings, hydrocolloids are less effective.

Urinary Incontinence

- see Urology

Epidemiology
- 15-30% prevalence in community dwelling and at least 50% of institutionalized seniors
- morbidity: cellulitis, pressure ulcers, urinary tract infections, falls with fractures, sleep deprivation, social withdrawal, depression, sexual dysfunction
- not associated with increased mortality

Pathophysiology
- in general, with age: ↓ bladder capacity, ↑ post-void residual volume, ↑ involuntary bladder contractions (urgency incontinence)
- in elderly women: decline in bladder outlet and urethral resistance pressure promoting stress incontinence
- in elderly men: prostatic enlargement can cause overflow and urgency incontinence

Transient causes of incontinence:
DIAPERS
Delirium
Infection
Atrophic urethritis/vaginitis
Pharmaceuticals
Excessive urine output
Restricted mobility
Stool impaction

Driving Competency

Reporting Requirements

- physician reporting to the Ministry of Transportation is mandatory in all provinces and territories except in Quebec, Nova Scotia, and Alberta where it is discretionary
- in Ontario, drivers >80 years old are not automatically required to pass a road test in order to renew their driver's license unless there are indications to suggest road safety risks; all drivers >80 years old must have a vision and knowledge test and participate in a 90-minute group education session to renew their licence every 2 years
- in the U.S.: varies by states, please refer to the AMA: Physician's Guide to Assessing and Counseling Older Drivers for American recommendations, www.ama-assn.org/ama/pub/category/10791.html

Conditions That May Impair Driving

In Canada*
- alcohol
  - patients with a history of impaired driving and those deemed as having a high probability of future impaired driving should not drive any motor vehicle until further assessed
  - alcohol dependence or abuse: if suspected, should be advised not to drive
  - alcohol withdrawal seizure: must complete a rehabilitation program and remain abstinent and seizure free for 6 months before driving
- blood pressure abnormalities
  - hypertension: sustained BP >170/110 should be evaluated carefully
  - hypotension: if syncopal, discontinue until attacks are treated and preventable
- cardiovascular disease
  - suspected asymptomatic CAD or stable angina: no restrictions
  - STEMI, NSTEMI with significant LV damage, coronary artery bypass surgery: no driving for one month following hospital discharge
  - NSTEMI with minor LV damage, unstable angina: no driving for 48 hours if percutaneous coronary intervention (PCI) performed, or 7 days if no PCI performed
- cerebrovascular conditions
  - TIA: should not be allowed to drive until a medical assessment is completed
  - stroke: should not drive for at least one month; may resume driving if functionally able; no clinically significant motor, cognitive, perceptual or vision deficits; no obvious risk of sudden recurrence; underlying cause appropriately treated; no post stroke seizure
- chronic obstructive pulmonary disease
  - mild/moderate impairment: no restrictions
  - moderate or severe impairment requiring supplemental oxygen: road test with supplemental oxygen
- cognitive impairment/dementia
  - moderate to severe dementia is a contraindication to driving; defined as the "inability to independently perform 2 or more IADLs or any basic ADL"
  - patients with mild dementia should be assessed; if indicated, refer to specialized driving testing centre. If deemed fit to drive, re-evaluate patient every 6-12 months
  - poor performance on MMSE, clock drawing or Trails B suggests a need to further investigate driving ability
  - poor MMSE score alone is insufficient to determine fitness to drive
- diabetes
  - diet controlled or oral hypoglycemic agents: no restrictions in absence of diabetes complications that may impair ability to drive (i.e. retinopathy, nephropathy, neuropathy, cardiovascular or cerebrovascular disease)
  - insulin use: may drive if no complications (as above) and no severe hypoglycemic episode in the last 6 months
- drugs
  - be aware of: analgesics, anticholinergics, anticonvulsants, antidepressants, antipsychotics, opiates, sedatives, stimulants
  - degree of impairment varies: patients should be warned of the medication/withdrawal effect on driving
- hearing loss
  - effect of impaired hearing on ability to drive safely is controversial

Systematic review of driving risk and the efficacy of compensatory strategies in persons with dementia
J Am Geriatr Soc. 2007;55:878-84
Purpose: To determine whether persons with dementia are at greater driving risk and, if so, to estimate the magnitude of this risk and determine whether there are efficacious methods to compensate for or accommodate it.
Study Selection: Systematic review of the case-control studies of drivers with a diagnosis of dementia.
Results: Drivers with dementia universally exhibited poorer performance on road tests and simulator evaluations. The one study that used an objective measure of motor vehicle crashes found that the crash risk in persons with dementia was 2 to 2.5 times greater than matched controls. No studies were found that examined the efficacy of methods to compensate for or accommodate their worse driving performance.
Conclusions: Drivers with dementia are poorer drivers than cognitively normal drivers, but studies have not consistently demonstrated higher crash rates. Clinicians and policy makers must take these findings into account when addressing issues pertinent to drivers with a diagnosis of dementia.

- acute labyrinthitis, positional vertigo with horizontal head movement, recurrent vertigo: advise not to drive until condition resolves
- musculoskeletal disorders
  - physician's role is to report etiology, prognosis, and extent of disability (pain, range of motion, coordination, muscle strength)
- post-operative
  - outpatient, conscious sedation: no driving for 24 hours
  - outpatient, general anesthesia: no driving for ≥24 hours
- seizures
  - first, single, unprovoked: no driving for 3 months until complete neurologic assessment, EEG, CT head
  - epilepsy: can drive if seizure-free on medication and physician has insight into patient compliance
- sleep disorders
  - if patient is believed to be at risk due to a symptomatic sleep disorder but refuses investigation by a sleep study or refuses appropriate treatment, the patient should not drive
- visual impairment
  - visual acuity: contraindicated to drive if <20/50 with both eyes examined simultaneously
  - visual field: contraindicated to drive if <120° along horizontal meridian and 15° continuous above and below fixation with both eyes examined simultaneously

*guidelines included refer specifically to private driving; please see CMA guidelines for commercial driving

Palliative and End of Life Care

Principles and Quality of Life

- support, educate and treat both patient and family
- address physical, psychological, social and spiritual needs
- focus on symptom management
- offer therapeutic environment and bereavement support
- ensure maintenance and human dignity

Power of Attorney

- see Ethical, Legal and Organizational Aspects of Medicine

Instructional Advance Directives

- see Ethical, Legal and Organizational Aspects of Medicine

Symptom Management

Table 6. Management of Common End-of-Life Symptoms

Symptom	Non-Pharmacologic Management	Pharmacologic Management
Constipation	rule out obstruction, impaction, anorectal disease; hydration and high fibre intake; increase mobility	stop unnecessary opioids and medications with anticholinergic side effects; provide stool softener (docusate sodium), increase peristalsis (senna), alter water and electrolyte secretion (magnesium hydroxide)
Death rattle		scopolamine SC or transdermal
Dry mouth	oral hygiene q2h, ice cubes, sugarless gum	artificial saliva substitutes, bethanechol, pilocarpine 1% solution as mouthrinse
Dysphagia	frequent small feeds, ideally seated, keep head of bed elevated for 30 minutes after eating, suction as necessary	treat painful mucositis (diphenhydramine: lidocaine: Maalox™ in a 1:2:8 mixture), candidiasis (fluconazole)

Death Rattle
Noise caused by the oscillatory movement of mucous secretions in the upper airway with inspiration and expiration.

Table 6. Management of Common End-of-Life Symptoms (continued)

Symptom	Non-Pharmacologic Management	Pharmacologic Management
Dyspnea	Elevate head of bed, eliminate allergens, open window/use fan	Oxygen, bronchodilators, opioids
Hiccups	Dry sugar, breathing in paper bag	Chlorpromazine, haloperidol, metoclopramide, baclofen, marijuana
Nausea and Vomiting	Frequent and small meals, avoid offensive strong odours, treat constipation if present	Prochlorperazine, haloperidol, domperidone, dimenhydrinate, dexamethasone
Pain	Hot and cold compresses, music therapy, relaxation techniques; individualized program of physical activity should be designed to improve flexibility, strength, and endurance	Acetaminophen for mild pain, strong opioids for severe pain, around-the-clock for continuous pain, short-acting and fast-onset analgesics for breakthrough, use non-selective NSAIDs with caution, consider radiation therapy and bisphosphonates for metastatic bone pain
Pruritus	Bathing with tepid water, avoid soap, bath oils; sodium bicarbonate for jaundice	Antihistamines, phenothiazines, topical corticosteroids, calamine lotion
Weakness	Modify environment and activities to decrease energy expenditure	Treat insomnia, anemia, depression; consider psychostimulants

AGS Panel on Persistent Pain in Older Persons (2002). The management of persistent pain in older persons. *J Am Geriatr Soc*, 50(6): Supplement. Knowles, S. Symptoms management in palliative care. *On Continuing Practice*. 1993. 20(1): 20-25.

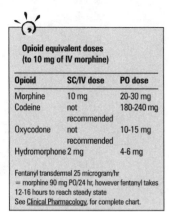

Opioid equivalent doses
(to 10 mg of IV morphine)

Opioid	SC/IV dose	PO dose
Morphine	10 mg	20-30 mg
Codeine	not recommended	180-240 mg
Oxycodone	not recommended	10-15 mg
Hydromorphone	2 mg	4-6 mg

Fentanyl transdermal 25 microgram/hr = morphine 90 mg PO/24 hr, however fentanyl takes 12-16 hours to reach steady state
See <u>Clinical Pharmacology</u>, for complete chart.

Geriatric Pharmacology

Pharmacokinetics

Serum creatinine does not reflect creatinine clearance in the elderly.
Instead, use:
CrCl (mL/min.) =
(weight in kg)(140 − age) x 1.23
(serum creatinine in μmol/L)

Multiply by 0.85 for females.

Table 7. Age-Associated Pharmacokinetics

Parameter	Age Effect	Implications
Absorption (less significant)	↑ in gastric pH; ↓ in splanchnic blood flow, GI absorptive surface, and dermal vascularity; delayed gastric emptying	Drug-drug and drug-food interactions are more likely to affect absorption.
Distribution	↑ in total body fat and α1-glycoprotein; ↓ in lean body mass, total body water, and albumin	Lipophilic drugs have a larger volume of distribution. Decrease in binding of acidic drugs. Increase in binding of basic drugs. Lower doses may be therapeutic.
Metabolism (less significant)	↓ in hepatic mass and hepatic blood flow; impaired phase I reactions (oxidative system)	
Elimination	↓ in renal blood flow, GFR, tubular secretion and renal mass	For every x% reduction in clearance, decrease the dose by x% and increase the interval by x%.

Benzodiazepines of Choice in the Elderly: LOT
Lorazepam
Oxazepam
Temazepam

Pharmacodynamics

Approach to medication review in the elderly: NO TEARS
Need and indication
Open-ended questions (to get patient's perspective on medications)
Tests and monitoring (to assess disease control)
Evidence and guidelines
Adverse events
Risk reduction (of adverse events such as falls)
Simplification or switches

Drug Sensitivity
- changes in pharmacokinetics as well as intrinsic sensitivity lead to altered drug responses
- increased sensitivity to warfarin, sedatives, and narcotics
- decreased sensitivity to β-blockers

Decreased Homeostasis
- poorer compensatory mechanisms leading to more adverse reactions (e.g. bleeding with NSAIDs/anticoagulants, altered mental status with anticholinergic/sympathomimetic/anti-Parkinsonian drugs)

Polypharmacy

Definition
- prescription, administration or use of many medications at the same time

Epidemiology
- in Canada, over 25% of elderly women and about 20% of elderly men reported using ≥3 medications
- hospitalized elderly are given an average of 10 medications over admission

Risk Factors for Non-Compliance
- risk of non-compliance correlates with medication factors, not age
  - number of medications – compliance with 1 medication is 80%, but drops to 25% with ≥6 medications
  - dosing, frequency
  - labelling, instructions, container design
  - financial constraints – medication cost and coverage (insurance, drug benefit plans)

Adverse Drug Reactions (ADRs)
- any noxious or unintended response to a drug that occurs at doses used for prophylaxis or therapy
- risk factors in the elderly
  - intrinsic: co-morbidities, age-related changes in pharmacokinetics and pharmacodynamics
  - extrinsic: number of medications, multiple prescribers, unreliable drug history
- 90% of ADRs are from: ASA, other analgesics, anticoagulants, antimicrobials, antineoplastics, digoxin, diuretics, hypoglycemics, steroids

Preventing Polypharmacy
- consider drug: safer side effect profiles, convenient dosing schedules, convenient route, efficacy
- consider patient: other medications, clinical indications, medical co-morbidities
- consider patient-drug interaction risk factors for ADRs
- review drug list regularly to eliminate medications with no clinical indication or with evidence of toxicity
- avoid treating an adverse drug reaction with another medication

Principles for prescribing in the elderly:
CARE
C – caution, compliance
A – age (adjust dosage for age)
R – review regimen regularly
E – educate

Fordyce, Moira. *Geriatric Pearls*. Philadelphia: FA Davis Company, 1999.

Adverse drug reactions in the elderly may present as delirium, falls, fractures, urinary incontinence/retention or fecal incontinence/impaction.

Inappropriate Prescribing in the Elderly

Epidemiology
- the estimated prevalence of potentially inappropriate prescribing ranges from 12-40%

Beers Criteria
- examples include long-acting benzodiazepines, strong anticholinergics, high dose sedatives
- the elderly are also often under-treated (ACEI, ASA, β-blockers, thrombolytics, warfarin)

Beers Criteria
48 medications to avoid in adults 65 and older due to safety concerns. For full list of medications, consult the following reference:
Fick DM, *et al*. (2003). Updating the Beers Criteria for potentially inappropriate medication use in older adults. *Arch Intern Med*. 163: 2716-2724.

Common Medications

Table 8. Common Medications

Drug Name	Brand Name	Dosing Schedule	Indications	Contraindications	Side Effects	Mechanism of Action
Laxatives						
bran	All-Bran™	1 cup/day	Constipation		Bloating, flatus	Bulk-forming laxative
psyllium	Metamucil™ Prodium Plain™	1 tsp PO tid	Constipation, hypercholesterolemia	N/V, fever, acute abdo, obstruction	Bloating, flatus	Bulk-forming laxative
docusate	Colace™/Docusoft™	100 mg PO bid	Constipation	Abdo pain, N/V, fever Not to be used with mineral oil	Mild cramps	Emollient, stool softener
lactulose	Chronulac™ Cephulac™ Kristalose™	15-30 cc PO daily/bid	Constipation, hepatic encephalopathy, bowel evacuation following barium exam	Patients on low galactose diets Abdo pain, N/V, fever	Flatus, cramps, nausea, diarrhea	Hyperosmolar agent, lowers pH of colon to decrease blood ammonia levels
senna	Senokot™/Ex-lax™ Glysennid™	10-15 cc PO daily/bid	Constipation	Acute abdo, abdo pain, N/V, fever	Cramps, griping, dependence	Stimulant laxative
bisacodyl	Dulcolax™	5-15 mg PO (10 mg PR)	Constipation	Ileus, obstruction, acute abdo, abdo pain, N/V, fever, severe dehydration	Cramps, pain, diarrhea	Stimulant laxative
Analgesics (Non-narcotic)						
acetaminophen	Tylenol™	325-650 mg PO q4-6h prn (up to 4 g/day)	Fever, mild pain	Lower doses for hepatic and renal disease, chronic alcoholism, known hypersensitivity	Hepatotoxicity (in overdose)	Prostaglandin-synthesis inhibition no anti-inflammatory effects
ibuprofen	Advil™, Motrin™	200-800 mg PO q4-6h prn (up to 1200 mg/day)	Mild to moderate pain, inflammatory disorders, fever	Active GI bleed/ulcer disease, known hypersensitivity, severe renal or hepatic disease Geriatrics: more susceptible to adverse effects	Dyspepsia, nausea, diarrhea, dizziness, rash, GI toxicity (ulcer, perforation, bleed)	Prostaglandin-synthesis inhibition, anti-inflammatory effects
celecoxib	Celebrex™	OA: 200 mg PO daily or 100 mg PO bid	Osteoarthritis, rheumatoid arthritis, FAP	Cardiovascular or cerebrovascular disease, CABG (peri-op), sulfonamide or ASA/NSAID allergy, active GI bleed/ulcer disease, IBD, severe renal or hepatic disease, hyperkalemia	GI symptoms (pain, diarrhea, dyspepsia, flatus), GI bleed, serious cardiovascular events	COX-2 inhibitor, analgesic, anti-inflammatory and anti-pyretic effects
Analgesics (Opioid) – refer to Clinical Pharmacology						
Anti-hypertensives						
thiazide diuretic e.g. hydrochlorothiazide	Hydrazide™	12.5-25 mg PO daily	Hypertension, edema	Anuria, hepatic coma, pre-coma, known sensitivity to thiazides	Hypotension, transient hyperlipidemia, hyperuricemia, GI symptoms	Inhibition of Na/Cl co-transporter
ACEI e.g. ramipril	Altace™	2.5-10 mg PO daily	Essential hypertension, post-MI, cardiovascular disease, renal protection in diabetic nephropathy	Known hypersensitivity, angioedema	Hypotension, cough, headache, dizziness, asthenia, chest pain, nausea, peripheral edema, somnolence, impotence, rash, arthritis, dyspnea, angioedema, hyperkalemia	Inhibition of angiotensin-converting enzyme
ARB e.g. losartan	Cozaar™	50-100 mg PO daily	Essential hypertension (+/- diabetes mellitus)	Known hypersensitivity	Dizziness, hypotension, fatigue, headache, hyperkalemia	Antagonizes angiotensin II via blockade of the angiotensin type 1 receptor
DHP CCB e.g. amlodipine	Norvasc™	5 mg PO daily	Essential hypertension, chronic stable angina	Known hypersensitivity, severe hypotension, caution in aortic stenosis	Edema, muscle cramps, dizziness, headache, constipation, heartburn	Calcium ion influx inhibition

le 8. Common Medications (continued)

Name	Brand Name	Dosing Schedule	Indications	Contraindications	Side Effects	Mechanism of Action
ng Medications						
ne	Imovane™ (Canada only)	3.75 mg PO qhs (initially)	Insomnia	Known hypersensitivity, caution in myasthenia gravis, severe hepatic disease Geriatrics: dose reduction (dose-related adverse events)	Bitter taste, palpitations, vomiting, anorexia, sialorrhea, confusion, agitation, anxiety, tremor, sweating	Short-acting hypnotic (no tolerance effects)
epam	Restoril™	15 mg PO qhs	Short-term management of insomnia	Known hypersensitivity, myasthenia gravis, sleep apnea Geriatrics: dose reduction recommended	Drowsiness, dizziness, impaired coordination, hangover, lethargy, dependence	Benzodiazepine: generalized CNS depression mediated by GABA
pam	Ativan™	0.5 mg PO qhs (initially, then increase)	Anxiety, insomnia	Known hypersensitivity, myasthenia gravis, narrow-angle glaucoma Geriatrics: dose reduction recommended	Dizziness, drowsiness, lethargy, dependence	Benzodiazepine: generalized CNS depression mediated by GABA
tive Enhancers						
ezil	Aricept™	5-10 mg PO daily	Mild to moderate dementia of Alzheimer's type	Known hypersensitivity, caution in pulmonary disease, sick sinus syndrome, seizure disorder	N/V, diarrhea, insomnia	Reversible inhibition of acetylcholinesterase
tamine	Reminyl™	8-12 mg PO bid	Mild to moderate dementia of Alzheimer's type	Known hypersensitivity, caution in sick sinus syndrome, seizure disorder, pulmonary disease, low body weight	N/V, diarrhea, anorexia	Reversible inhibition of acetylcholinesterase
igmine	Exelon™	1.5 mg PO daily (starting) up to 6 mg PO bid	Mild to moderate dementia of Alzheimer's type	Known hypersensitivity, severe hepatic disease, caution in sick sinus syndrome, pulmonary disease, seizure disorder	N/V, diarrhea, anorexia	Acetylcholinesterase inhibition
antine	Ebixa™/Namenda™ (Cdn)/(US)	5 mg PO daily (starting) up to 10 mg PO bid	Moderate to severe dementia of Alzheimer's type	Known hypersensitivity, conditions that alkalinize urine, caution in cardiovascular conditions	Agitation, fatigue, dizziness, headache, hypertension, constipation	NMDA-receptor antagonist
insonian Agents – refer to <u>Neurology</u>, N32						

Notes

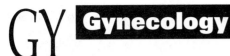

GY Gynecology

Julia Kfouri, Kelsey Mills and Jennifer Vergel de Dios, chapter editors
Justine Chan and Angela Ho, associate editors
Billie Au, EBM editor
Dr. Sari Kives, staff editor

Basic Anatomy Review

A. EXTERNAL GENITALIA (see Figure 1)
- referred to collectively as the vulva
- blood supply – internal pudendal artery
- sensory innervation – pudendal nerve
- lymphatic drainage – inguinal nodes

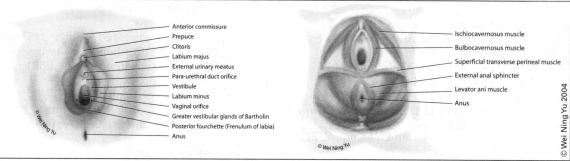

Anterior commissure
Prepuce
Clitoris
Labium majus
External urinary meatus
Para-urethral duct orifice
Vestibule
Labium minus
Vaginal orifice
Greater vestibular glands of Bartholin
Posterior fourchette (Frenulum of labia)
Anus

Ischiocavernosus muscle
Bulbocavernosus muscle
Superficial transverse perineal muscle
External anal sphincter
Levator ani muscle
Anus

© Wei Ning Yu 2004

Figure 1. Vulva and Perineum

B. VAGINA
- muscular canal extending from cervix to vulva, anterior to rectum and posterior to bladder
- lined by rugated, stratified-squamous epithelium
- upper vagina separated by cervix into anterior, posterior and lateral fornices
- blood supply – vaginal branch of internal pudendal with anastamoses from uterine, inferior vesical, and middle rectal arteries

C. UTERUS
- thick walled, muscular organ between bladder and rectum, consisting of two major parts:
  - uterine corpus
    - blood supply – uterine artery (branch of the internal iliac artery)
  - cervix
    - blood supply – cervical branch of uterine artery
- position
  - anteverted (majority)
  - retroverted
- supported by the pelvic diaphragm, the pelvic organs, and 4 paired sets of ligaments:
  - round ligaments: travel from anterior surface of uterus, through broad ligaments, through inguinal canals, and terminate in the labia majora
    - function: anteversion
  - uterosacral ligaments: arise from sacral fascia and insert into posterior inferior uterus
    - function: mechanical support for uterus and contain autonomic nerve fibres
  - cardinal ligaments: extend from lateral pelvic walls and insert into lateral cervix and vagina
    - function: mechanical support, prevents prolapse
  - broad ligaments: pass from lateral pelvic wall to sides of uterus; contains fallopian tube, round ligament, ovarian ligament, nerves, vessels, and lymphatics

Anteversion: forward tilted uterus
Anteflexion: bending of uterus so the fundus is thrust forward
Retroversion: backward tilted uterus
Retroflexion: bending of uterus so the fundus is thrust backward

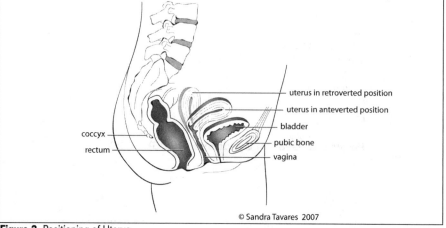

uterus in retroverted position
uterus in anteverted position
bladder
pubic bone
vagina
coccyx
rectum

© Sandra Tavares 2007

Figure 2. Positioning of Uterus

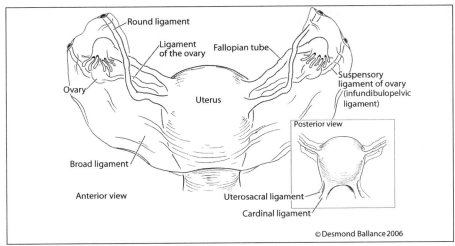

Figure 3. Internal Genital Organs

D. FALLOPIAN TUBES
- 8-14 cm muscular tubes extending laterally from the uterus
- interstitial, isthmic, ampullary and infundibular segments; end with fimbriae at the ovary
- mesosalpinx: peritoneal fold that attaches fallopian tube to broad ligament
- blood supply – uterine and ovarian arteries

E. OVARIES
- consist of cortex with ova and medulla with blood supply
- supported by infundibulopelvic ligament (suspensory ligament of ovary)
- mesovarium: peritoneal fold that attaches ovary to broad ligament
- blood supply – ovarian arteries (branch of aorta), left ovarian vein drains into the left renal vein, right ovarian vein drains into inferior vena cava

Menstruation

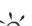

Boobs, **P**ubes, **G**row, **F**low

Stages of Puberty

- see Pediatrics
- adrenarche
    - increase in secretion of adrenal androgens usually precedes gonadarche by 2 years
- gonadarche
    - increased secretion of gonadal sex steroids; ~age 8
- thelarche
    - breast development
- pubarche
    - pubic and axillary hair development
- menarche
    - onset of menses usually follows peak height velocity and/or 2 years following breast budding

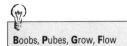

TANNER STAGE
Thelarche
I. none
II. breast bud
III. further enlargement of areola and breasts with no separation of their contours
IV. 2° mound of areola and papilla
V. areola recessed to general contour of breast = adult

Pubarche
I. none
II. downy hair along labia only
III. darker/coarse hair extends over pubis
IV. adult type covers smaller area, no thigh involvement
V. adult hair in quantity and type and extends over thighs

Menstrual Cycle

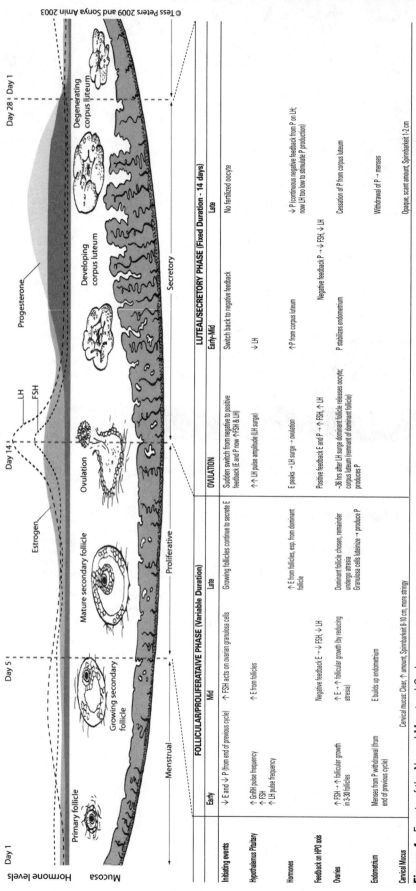

© Tess Peters 2009 and Sonya Amin 2003

Figure 4. Events of the Normal Menstrual Cycle

	FOLLICULAR/PROLIFERATIVE PHASE (Variable Duration)			LUTEAL/SECRETORY PHASE (Fixed Duration - 14 days)		
	Early	Mid	Late	OVULATION	Early-Mid	Late
Initiating events	↓ E and ↓ P (from end of previous cycle)	↑ FSH acts on ovarian granulosa cells	Growing follicles continue to secrete E	Sudden switch from negative to positive feedback (E and P now ↑FSH & LH)	Switch back to negative feedback	No fertilized oocyte
Hypothalamus Pituitary	↑GnRH pulse frequency ↑FSH ↑LH pulse frequency	↑ E from follicles		↑↑ LH pulse amplitude (LH surge)	↓ LH	
Hormones			↑ E from follicles, esp. from dominant follicle	E peaks → LH surge → ovulation	↑P from corpus luteum	↓ P (continuous negative feedback from P on LH; now LH too low to stimulate P production)
Feedback on HPO axis	Negative feedback E → ↓ FSH, ↓ LH			Positive feedback E and P → ↑ FSH, ↑ LH	Negative feedback P → ↓ FSH, ↓ LH	
Ovaries	↑FSH → ↑follicular growth in 3-30 follicles	↑E → ↑ follicular growth (by reducing atresia)	Dominant follicle chosen, remainder undergo atresia Granulosa cells luteinize → produce P	~36 hrs after LH surge dominant follicle releases oocyte; corpus luteum (remnant of dominant follicle) produces P	P stabilizes endometrium	Cessation of P from corpus luteum
Endometrium	Menses from P withdrawal (from end of previous cycle)	E builds up endometrium				Withdrawal of P → menses
Cervical Mucus		Cervical mucus: Clear, ↑ amount, Spinnbarkeit 8-10 cm, more stringy				Opaque, scant amount, Spinnbarkeit 1-2 cm

Estrogen
ESTROGEN is the main hormone in the follicular/proliferative phase. Stimulated by FSH. Follicle that will become dominant secretes greatest amount of estrogen.

Estrogen effects:
On target tissues:
1) ↓ E receptors

On the follicles in the ovaries:
1) reduces atresia

On the endometrium:
1) proliferation of glandular and stromal tissue

Progesterone
PROGESTERONE is the main hormone in the luteal/secretory phase. Stimulated by LH; progesterone mainly ↓ LH. Corpus luteum (follicle that was dominant) secretes the progesterone.

Progesterone effects:
On target tissues:
1) ↓ E receptors (the "anti-estrogen" effect)
2) ↓ P receptors

On the endometrium:
1) cessation of mitoses (stops building endometrium up)
2) "organization" of glands (initiates secretions from glands)
3) inhibits macrophages, interleukin-8 and enzymes from degrading endometrium

Characteristics
• Menarche 10-15 years
• Average 12.2 years, but onset of puberty is decreasing
• Entire cycle 28 ± 7 days with bleeding for 1-6 days
• 25-80 mL blood loss per cycle

Premenstrual Syndrome (PMS)

- synonyms: "ovarian cycle syndrome", "menstrual molimina" (moodiness)
- occurs during most menstrual cycles

Premenstrual Syndrome
Physiological and emotional disturbances which generally occur 1-2 weeks preceding menses until a few days after onset of menses. Common symptoms include depression, irritability, tearfulness, and mood swings.

Etiology
- incompletely understood, multifactorial, genetics likely play a role
- CNS-mediated neurotransmitter interactions with sex steroids (progesterone, estrogen, and testosterone)
- serotonergic dysregulation – currently most plausible theory

Diagnostic Criteria for Premenstrual Syndrome
- at least one of the following affective and somatic symptoms during the 5 days before menses in each of the three prior menstrual cycles:
    - affective – depression, angry outbursts, irritability, anxiety, confusion, social withdrawal
    - somatic – breast tenderness, abdominal bloating, headache, swelling of extremities
- symptoms relieved within 4 days of onset of menses
- symptoms present in the absence of any pharmacologic therapy, or drug or alcohol use
- symptoms occur reproducibly during 2 cycles of prospective recording
- patient suffers from identifiable dysfunction in social or economic performance

Treatment
- goal: symptom relief
- no proven beneficial treatment, suggestions include:
    - psychological support
    - diet/supplements
        - avoid sodium, simple sugars, caffeine and alcohol
        - calcium – 1,200-1,600 mg/d
        - magnesium – 400-800 mg/d
        - vitamin E – 400 IU/d
        - vitamin B_6
    - medications
        - NSAIDs for discomfort, pain
        - spironolactone for fluid retention – used during luteal phase
        - SSRI antidepressants – used during luteal phase x 14 days or continuously
        - progesterone suppositories
        - OCP (primarily beneficial for physical symptoms)
        - danazol (an androgen that inhibits pituitary-ovarian axis)
        - GnRH agonists if severe PMS unresponsive to other treatment
    - mind/body approaches
        - regular aerobic exercise
        - cognitive behavioural therapy
        - relaxation and light therapy
        - biofeedback and guided imagery
    - herbal remedies (limited value)
        - evening primrose oil, black cohosh, St. John's wort, kava, ginkgo

Premenstrual Dysphoric Disorder (PMDD)

Definition
- official diagnosis in the DSM-IV-TR
- described as a more severe form of PMS with specific diagnostic criteria
- treatment with SSRIs (first line) highly effective
- see Psychiatry

Differential Diagnoses of Common Presentations

Abnormal Uterine Bleeding (AUB)

- see *Abnormal Uterine Bleeding*, GY15
- classified as amenorrhea, oligomenorrhea, menorrhagia/hypermenorrhea, hypomenorrhea, metrorrhagia, menometrorrhagia, polymenorrhea, post-menopausal

> **Abnormal Uterine Bleeding**
> Change in frequency, duration, or amount of menstrual flow

> - **Hypomenorrhea:** regular bleeding that is decreased in amount
> - **Polymenorrhea:** vaginal bleeding occurring at intervals ≤21 days

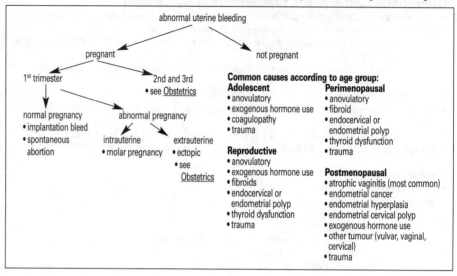

Figure 5. Approach to Abnormal Uterine Bleeding

AMENORRHEA/OLIGOMENORRHEA (see *Amenorrhea*, GY14)

- pregnancy
- hypothalamic dysfunction – low FSH/LH
    - functional – anorexia, nutritional deprivation, exercise
    - extreme stress/systemic illness
    - hypothalamic tumour, infiltrative disorder
    - congenital GnRH deficiency – e.g. Kallmann's syndrome (secondary hypogonadism characterized by anosmia/hyposmia)
- pituitary dysfunction
    - brain or pituitary tumour
    - primary hypopituitarism
    - Sheehan syndrome (hypopituitarism due to postpartum hemorrhage)
- ovarian dysfunction
    - menopause
    - radiation, chemotherapy
    - gonadal dysgenesis – e.g. Turner's syndrome (XO)
    - resistant ovary syndrome
    - chronic anovulation – e.g. PCOS, ovarian/adrenal tumour
- uterine/outflow tract defects
    - congenital Müllerian (uterine/vaginal) agenesis (e.g. Mayer-Rokitansky-Kuster-Hauser syndrome)
    - imperforate hymen
    - transverse vaginal septum
    - cervical stenosis
    - intrauterine adhesions – e.g. Asherman's syndrome
- endocrine
    - hyperprolactinemia
    - hyper/hypothyroidism
    - hyperandrogenism – e.g. PCOS, ovarian/adrenal tumour, testosterone injections
    - Cushing's disease

- other
  - androgen insensitivity syndrome (XY)
  - drugs – e.g. metoclopramide, neuroleptic antipsychotics, danazol

MENORRHAGIA
- hormonal imbalance
- leiomyomata (fibroids)
- uterine polyps
- adenomyosis
- endometritis
- copper IUD
- cancer (endometrial, cervical, ovarian, uterine sarcoma)
- ovarian cysts
- medications

> **Menorrhagia/Hypermenorrhea**
> Bleeding at regular intervals that is prolonged (>7 days) or excessive in amount (>80 cc per menstrual cycle)

METRORRHAGIA/MENOMETRORRHAGIA
- trauma, sexual abuse, foreign body
- infection – endometritis, cervicitis, vaginitis, STI
- benign growths – cervical/endometrial polyps, fibroids, ectropion
- malignant tumours – uterine, cervical, vaginal, vulvar, ovarian (granulosa-theca cell)
- pregnancy-related (bleed following a missed period)
  - implantation bleed
  - ectopic pregnancy
  - abortion (missed, threatened, inevitable, incomplete, complete; see Obstetrics chapter)
  - molar pregnancy
- PCOS
- weight loss/exercise/stress
- DUB
  - diagnosis of exclusion; 90% is anovulatory

> **Metrorrhagia**
> Bleeding at irregular intervals, particularly between expected menstrual periods
>
> **Menometrorrhagia**
> Excessive bleeding at usual time of menstrual periods and at other irregular intervals

POSTMENOPAUSAL BLEEDING
- atrophic vaginitis (most common)
- endometrial hyperplasia
- endometrial/endocervical polyps
- atrophic endometrium
- withdrawal from exogenous estrogens
- benign or malignant tumours of vulva, vagina, or cervix
- ovarian malignancy (granulosa-theca cell)
- trauma
- lichen sclerosis

> **Postmenopausal Bleeding**
> Any bleeding >1 year after menopause
>
> Postmenopausal bleeding is endometrial cancer until proven otherwise.

NON-GYNECOLOGICAL CAUSES OF AUB
- **blood dyscrasias**
  - coagulopathy – von Willebrand's Disease; more commonly diagnosed in adolescents
  - platelet abnormalities
    - immune thrombocytopenia
    - platelet function abnormality
    - thrombasthenia (Glanzman's syndrome) – rare
  - leukemia
- **hepatic disease**
  - impaired synthesis of coagulation factors
  - impaired metabolism of sex steroids (e.g. estrogen)
- **renal failure**
  - impaired excretion of estrogen
- **endocrine**
  - hyper/hypothyroid
  - adrenal insufficiency (late onset congenital adrenal hyperplasia) or excess adrenal hormones (Cushing's)
  - PCOS (insulin resistance)
  - prolactinoma

- **drugs**
  - anticoagulants
  - spironolactone
  - danazol
  - OCP/HRT – incorrectly used, or breakthrough bleeding
  - neuroleptics (interfere with dopamine and prolactin)
  - chemotherapy
  - steroids

Dysmenorrhea

- see *Dysmenorrhea*, GY16
- primary/idiopathic
- secondary (acquired)
  - endometriosis
  - adenomyosis
  - IUD - copper
  - pelvic inflammatory disease (PID)
  - ovarian cysts
  - uterine polyps
  - leiomyoma
  - foreign body
  - intrauterine synechiae
  - uterine anomalies (e.g. non-communicating uterine horn)
  - cervical stenosis
  - imperforate hymen, transverse vaginal septum

> **Dysmenorrhea**
> Painful menstruation

Vaginal Discharge/Pruritus

- see *Gynecological Infections*, GY25
- physiologic discharge and cervical mucus production
- non-physiologic
  - genital tract infection
    - vulvovaginitis: candidiasis, trichomoniasis, bacterial vaginosis (BV), polymicrobial superficial infection
    - chlamydia, gonorrhea
    - pyosalpinx, salpingitis
  - genital tract inflammation (non-infectious)
    - local – chemical irritants, douches, sprays, foreign body, trauma, atrophic vaginitis, desquamative inflammatory vaginitis, focal vulvitis
    - neoplasia – vulvar, vaginal, cervical, endometrial
    - systemic – toxic shock syndrome, Crohn's disease, collagen disease, dermatologic (e.g. lichen sclerosis)
    - IUD, OCP (secondary to progesterone)

Pelvic Pain

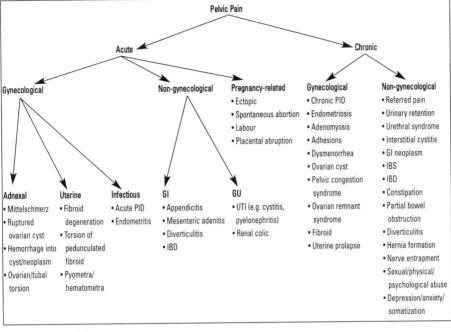

Figure 6. Pelvic Pain

Chronic Pelvic Pain (CPP)
Intermittent or constant pain of >6 months duration

20% of CPP patients have a history of previous sexual abuse/assault (remember to ask about it!)

Pyometra
Pus within the uterine cavity

Hematometra
Blood within the uterine cavity

Pelvic Mass

- **ovarian**
  - functional cysts (always benign)
    - corpus luteum cyst
    - follicular cyst
    - theca lutein cyst
    - hemorrhagic cyst
  - polycystic ovary
  - endometrioma
  - tubo-ovarian abscess
  - luteoma of pregnancy
  - benign neoplasms
    - dermoid cyst (most common)
  - malignant neoplasms
    - epithelial cell most common in >40 yrs
    - germ cell most common in <20 yrs
    - metastases (e.g. Krukenberg tumour from gastric cancer)

- **uterine**
  - symmetrical
    - pregnancy
    - adenomyosis
    - endometrial cancer
    - imperforate hymen
    - hematometra/pyometra

- **non-ovarian**
  - gynecological
    - ectopic pregnancy
    - pelvic adhesions (resulting in fluid entrapment)
    - paratubal cysts
    - pyosalpinx/hydrosalpinx
    - leiomyomata or fibroids (pedunculated)
    - primary fallopian tube neoplasms
  - gastrointestinal
    - appendiceal abscess
    - diverticular abscess
    - diverticulosis, diverticulitis
    - carcinoma of rectum/colon
  - genitourinary
    - distended bladder
    - pelvic kidney
    - carcinoma of bladder
  - lymphoma

  - asymmetrical
    - leiomyomata
    - leiomyosarcoma

Dyspareunia

- **Introital**
  - inadequate lubrication
  - vaginismus
  - rigid/intact hymen
  - vulvovaginitis
    - atrophic (hypoestrogen)
    - chemical
    - infectious (chlamydia, trichomoniasis)
  - Bartholin's or Skene's gland infection
  - lichen sclerosis

- **Midvaginal**
  - urethritis
  - short vagina
  - trigonitis
  - congenital abnormality of the vagina (e.g. vaginal septum)

Dyspareunia
Painful intercourse

- **Deep**
  - endometriosis
  - adenomyosis
  - leiomyomata
  - PID (acute vs. chronic)
    - hydrosalpinx
    - tubo-ovarian abscess
  - uterine retroversion
  - ovarian cyst

Common Investigations

Bloodwork

- CBC
  - evaluation of severity of abnormal uterine bleeding, pre-op investigation ± ferritin if anemic
- β-hCG
  - investigation of possible pregnancy or ectopic pregnancy
  - work-up for GTN/choriocarcinoma
  - monitored after the medical management of ectopic pregnancy and GTN to assess for cure or recurrence
- LH, FSH, TSH, PRL, DHEA, testosterone, estradiol, androstenedione
  - investigation of amenorrhea, menstrual irregularities, menopause, infertility

Imaging

Ultrasound (U/S)
- transabdominal or transvaginal U/S is imaging modality of choice for pelvic structures
- transvaginal U/S provides better resolution of uterus and adnexal structures
  - detects early pregnancy if β-hCG ≥1500 (β-hCG must be ≥6500 for transabdominal U/S)
- may be used to identify pelvic pathology
  - rule in or out ectopic pregnancy, intrauterine pregnancy
  - assess uterine, adnexal, cul-de-sac, ovarian masses (i.e. solid or cystic)
  - determine endometrial thickness, locate/characterize fibroids
  - monitor follicles during assisted reproduction

Check for STIs before performing SHG and HSG to prevent PID.

Sonohysterography (SHG)
- saline infusion into endometrial cavity under ultrasound visualization expands endometrial cavity, allowing visualization of uterus and fallopian tubes
- useful for investigation of
  - abnormal uterine bleeding (AUB)
  - uncertain endometrial findings on vaginal U/S
  - infertility (tubal patency)
  - congenital/acquired uterine abnormalities – rule out fibroids or endometrial polyps
- easily done, minimal cost, extremely well-tolerated, sensitive and specific
- frequently avoids need for diagnostic hysteroscopy

Hysterosalpingography (HSG)
- x-ray contrast introduced through the cervix into the uterus
- used for evaluation of size, shape, configuration of uterus, congenital uterine abnormalities, tubal patency, or obstruction
- useful for investigation of infertility

Common Procedures

Genital Tract Biopsy

Vulvar Biopsy
- performed under local anesthetic
- Keyes/punch biopsy
- hemostasis achieved with local pressure and Monsel solution (ferric sulfate) or silver nitrate, or suture (rarely)

Vaginal Biopsy and Cervical Biopsy
- generally no anesthetic used
- punch biopsy or biopsy forceps
- hemostasis with Monsel solution and pressure

Endometrial Biopsy
- performed in the office using an endometrial suction curette (pipelle) guided through the cervix to aspirate fragments of endometrium
    - pretreatment with misoprostol (Cytotec®) if nulliparous or postmenopausal
- more invasive procedure (D&C) may be done in the office or operating room ± hysteroscopy

Colposcopy

- **diagnostic use**
    - magnifies surface structures of the vulva, vagina and cervix
    - 1% acetic acid wash applied to cervix dehydrates cells and reveals white areas of increased nuclear density (abnormal) or areas with epithelial changes
    - allows biopsy of acetowhite lesions for early identification of dysplasia and neoplasia
- **therapeutic use**
    - cryotherapy: nitrous oxide or carbon dioxide freezes dysplastic lesions, genital warts
    - laser vaporization: used to treat dysplastic lesions of the exocervix and benign ectropion
    - loop electrosurgical excision procedure (LEEP): excision of transformation zone with the cervical lesion; provides a specimen for pathological examination

Dilatation and Curettage (D&C)

- dilatation of cervix with dilators of increasing diameter
- scrape entire uterine cavity with sharp curette
- anesthesia – general or local
- prior to procedure, determine depth of uterus with sound

Indications
- diagnostic (rarely done without hysteroscopy)
    - abnormal uterine bleeding (AUB)
    - dysfunctional uterine bleeding (DUB)
- therapeutic
    - removal of retained products of conception following abortion
    - therapeutic termination of pregnancy in 1st trimester
    - removal of small uterine polyps, pedunculated submucosal fibroids

Complications
- bleeding
- infection
- perforation of uterus, laceration of cervix
    - reduce risk with preoperative misoprostol inserted per vagina (Cytotec®) to soften cervix and stimulate uterine contraction
- incompetent cervix - extremely rare

Laparoscopy

- laparoscope (fiber optic camera) used to view pelvic/abdominal contents through small incisions

Indications
- diagnostic
  - evaluation of infertility, pelvic pain, pelvic masses, congenital anomalies, hemoperitoneum, and endometriosis
- therapeutic
  - tubal ligation
  - lysis of adhesions
  - excision of ectopic pregnancy
  - excision/ablation of endometriosis
  - retrieval of lost IUDs
  - cystectomies, salpingo-oophorectomy, hysterectomy, and treatment of stress incontinence
  - myomectomy

Contraindications
- bowel obstruction
- large hemoperitoneum
- clinically unstable patient
- inability to maintain pneumoperitoneum
- multiple previous abdominal surgeries

Complications
- general anesthetic
- insufflation of the preperitoneal abdominal wall
- injury to vascular structures (e.g. aorta, inferior epigastric)
- injury to viscous (bowel, bladder, ureters)
- may need to convert to laparotomy

Hysteroscopy

- flexible or rigid scope inserted through cervix, into uterus to visualize uterine cavity

Indications
- diagnostic
  - detection of uterine anomalies or pathology (i.e. infertility work-up)
  - AUB
  - DUB
- therapeutic
  - removal of uterine polyps, fibroids, adhesions, septums
  - ablation

Complications
- perforation of uterus, laceration of cervix
- bleeding
- infection
- absorption of excess distension medium → fluid overload, hyponatremia
- air emboli
- anaphylactic shock

Endometrial Ablation

- an alternative to hysterectomy for treatment of AUB
- performed as outpatient surgery
- rationale is to coagulate or resect the endometrium basalis layer to prevent monthly build-up and reduce menstrual losses
- anesthesia – usually general, may be local

Methods
- rollerball electrode coagulation or resection
- microwave endometrial ablation
- thermoablation (hot water)
- balloon ablation
- laser photocoagulation

Complications
- infection
- injury to pelvic viscera if perforated uterus
- hematometra
- absorption of excess distending media → fluid overload, hyponatremia
- failure (i.e. bleeding/menorrhagia persists)
- may eventually require hysterectomy for recurrence (~20% at 5 years)

Hysterectomy

Indications
- uterine fibroids
- endometriosis
- adenomyosis
- uterine prolapse
- pelvic pain
- AUB
- cancer (endometrium, ovaries, fallopian tubes, cervical)

Complications
- general anesthetic
- bleeding
- infection
- injury to other organs (ureter, bladder, rectum)
- loss of ovarian function (if ovaries removed)

Approaches
1) vaginal vs. abdominal
   - advantages of vaginal approach – less pain, faster recovery time, allows for simultaneous repair of rectocele/cystocele/enterocele, improved esthetics
   - indications for vaginal approach – mobile uterus, uterine size <12 weeks
2) open vs. laparoscopic
   - advantages of laparoscopy – less pain, faster recovery, improved esthetics, shorter hospital stay

Table 2. Classification of Hysterectomy

Classification	Tissues removed	Indications
Subtotal hysterectomy	Uterus	Inaccessible cervix (e.g. adhesions, disseminated ovarian cancer) Patient choice/preference
Total hysterectomy	Uterus, cervix	Uterine fibroids Endometriosis Adenomyosis Menorrhagia DUB
Total abdominal hysterectomy + bilateral salpingo-oophorectomy (TAH/BSO)	Uterus, cervix, fallopian tubes, ovaries	Malignant ovarian tumours >45 years old Consider for endometriosis
Radical abdominal hysterectomy	Uterus, cervix, fallopian tubes, ovaries, broad ligaments, parametria, upper half of vagina, regional lymph nodes	Cervical cancer (up to stage IB, see GY46)

Disorders of Menstruation

Amenorrhea

Primary Amenorrhea
No menses by age 14 in absence of 2° sexual characteristics or no menses by age 16 with 2° sexual characteristics

Secondary Amenorrhea
No menses for >6 months or 3 cycles after documented menarche

Oligomenorrhea
Episodic vaginal bleeding occurring at intervals >35 days

2° amenorrhea is pregnancy until proven otherwise.

Etiology
- see *Amenorrhea*, GY6

Clinical Features
- depends on etiology
- signs of pregnancy (see <u>Obstetrics</u>)
- hypothalamic/pituitary dysfunction – galactorrhea, headache, visual changes
- ovarian dysfunction – menopause (see *Menopause,* GY33), PCOS (see *PCOS*, GY24)
- endocrine – recent changes in weight, signs of virilization
- external genitalia and vagina – atrophy, clitoromegaly, imperforate hymen, vaginal septum, absence of vagina
- family history of delayed puberty
- prolonged intense exercise, excessive dieting
- absent puberty (e.g. Turner's syndrome)

Investigations (see Figure 7)
- β-hCG, hormonal workup (TSH, prolactin, FSH, LH, androgens, and estradiol)
- progesterone challenge to assess estrogen status
    - medroxyprogesterone acetate (Provera®) 10 mg PO OD for 10 days
    - any uterine bleed within 2-7 days after completion of Provera® is considered to be a positive test/withdrawal bleed
        - if withdrawal bleeding occurs that means there was adequate estrogen that thickened the endometrium; thus withdrawal of progesterone results in bleeding
        - if no bleeding occurs, there is inadequate estrogen (hypoestrogenism) or excessive androgens
- karyotype if indicated (if premature ovarian failure or absent puberty)
- U/S to confirm normal anatomy, PCOS

Treatment
- **hypothalamic dysfunction (low or normal FSH, LH)**
    - if low FSH/LH, consider head imaging (CT or MRI) if no obvious etiology
    - stop any medications, reduce stress, adequate nutrition, decrease excessive exercise
    - if pregnancy desired, correct underlying problem first, but may require gonadotropins to stimulate ovulation
    - otherwise OCP to induce menstruation (withdrawal bleed) - may not prevent manifestation of hypoestrogenic state
- **hyperprolactinemia**
    - bromocriptine if fertility desired; OCP if fertility not desired
    - surgery for macroadenoma (rarely)
    - consider CT of head to document presence of pituitary micro/macroadenoma
- **premature ovarian failure (high FSH, LH)**
    - treat associated autoimmune disorders (thyroid, adrenal)
    - HRT or OCP to prevent manifestations of hypoestrogenic state
    - karyotype
    - removal of gonadal tissue if Y chromosome present (at 18 years or earlier if dysgenic gonads)
- **PCOS**
    - see *Polycystic Ovarian Syndrome,* GY24

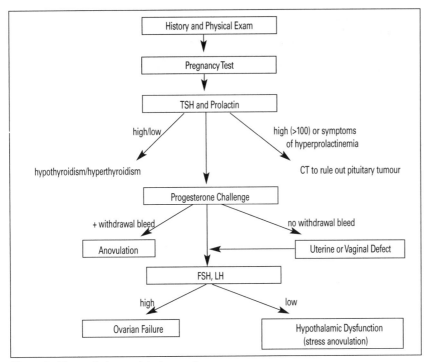

Figure 7. Diagnostic Approach to Amenorrhea

Abnormal Uterine Bleeding (AUB)

- 90% anovulatory, 10% ovulatory

Etiology
- see *Abnormal Uterine Bleeding*, GY6

Investigations
- CBC, serum ferritin
- β–hCG
- TSH
- consider according to presentation:
    - coagulation profile (esp. adolescent) - rule out von Willebrand's disease
    - prolactin if amenorrheic
    - FSH, LH
    - serum androgens (esp. free testosterone)
    - day 21 (luteal phase) progesterone to confirm ovulation
    - Pap test
    - pelvic U/S – detect polyps, fibroids; measure endometrial thickness (useful in postmenopausal women)
    - SHG – very sensitive for intrauterine pathology (polyps, submucous fibroids)
    - HSG
    - endometrial sampling – in women >40 years or at higher risk of endometrial cancer

Treatment
- treat underlying disorders
- if anatomic lesions and systemic disease have been ruled out, consider dysfunctional uterine bleeding

Dysfunctional Uterine Bleeding (DUB)

- rule out anatomic lesions and systemic disease (see *Abnormal Uterine Bleeding*, GY6)
    - blood dyscrasias, thyroid dysfunction, malignancy, PCOS, endometriosis, PID, fibroids, unopposed estrogen, polyps, or pregnancy
- 90% of DUB is due to anovulation; thus "anovulatory bleed" is often used synonymously with DUB

> **Dysfunctional Uterine Bleeding**
> Abnormal bleeding not attributable to organic (anatomic/systemic) disease. DUB is a diagnosis of exclusion.

- during anovulatory cycles, failure of ovulation results in lack of progesterone, thus endometrium is exposed to prolonged unopposed estrogen stimulation. This results in endometrial overgrowth with estrogen-dependent breakthrough bleeding that is not accompanied by premenstrual symptoms
- 10% of DUB is due to dysfunction of corpus luteum and inadequate progesterone production, or an atrophic endometrium (i.e. 2° to OCP)

> **3 Major Causes of DUB**
> **D**on't ovulate
> **U**nusual luteal activity (prolonged or insufficient luteal phase)
> **B**irth control pill

Investigations
- exclude organic (systemic/anatomic) causes first
- ensure β-hCG is negative
- CBC – rule out anemia

Treatment
- **medical**
  - mild DUB
    - NSAIDs
    - anti-fibrinolytic (e.g. Cyklokapron®) at time of menses
    - combined OCP
    - progestins (Provera®) on first 10-14 days of each month if oligomenorrheic
    - Mirena® IUD
    - danazol
  - acute, severe DUB
    - replace fluid losses/consider admission
    - medical treatment
      a) estrogen (Premarin®) 25 mg IV q4h x 24h with Gravol® 50 mg IV/PO q4h or
      b) Ovral® 1 tab PO q4h x 24h with Gravol® 50 mg IV/PO q4h
      Taper Ovral®: 1 tab tid x 2d → bid x 2d → OD
    - after (a) or (b), maintain patient on monophasic OCP for next several months or consider alternative medical treatment
  - clomiphene citrate
    - patients who are anovulatory and who wish to get pregnant
- **surgical**
  - D&C – not for treatment; diagnosis only (usually with hysteroscopy)
  - endometrial ablation; consider pretreatment with danazol or GnRH agonists
    - if finished childbearing
    - repeat procedure sometimes required
  - hysterectomy – definitive treatment

Dysmenorrhea

Definition
- see *Dysmenorrhea*, GY8

> **Primary Dysmenorrhea**
> Menstrual pain in absence of organic disease
>
> **Secondary Dysmenorrhea**
> Menstrual pain due to organic disease

Primary Dysmenorrhea
- begins 6 months - 2 years after menarche (once ovulatory cycles established)
- colicky pain in abdomen, radiating to the lower back, labia, and inner thighs beginning hours before onset of bleeding and persisting for hours or days (48-72 h)
- associated symptoms include nausea, vomiting, altered bowel habits, headaches, fatigue (prostaglandin (PG)-associated)
- likely due to frequent and prolonged PG-induced uterine contractions → decreased myometrial blood flow → ischemia
- **diagnosis:** rule out underlying pelvic pathology and confirm cyclic nature of pain
- **treatment:**
  - PG synthetase inhibitors (e.g. Anaprox®)
    - must be started before/at onset of pain
  - OCP to suppress ovulation and reduce menstrual flow

Secondary Dysmenorrhea
- menstrual pain due to organic disease
- begins in women who are in their 20s, worsens with age
- may improve temporarily after childbirth
- associated dyspareunia, abnormal bleeding, infertility
- **investigations and treatments:**
  - bimanual exam – uterine or adnexal tenderness, fixed uterine retroflexion, uterosacral nodularity, pelvic mass, or enlarged irregular uterus
  - U/S, laparoscopy and hysteroscopy may be necessary to establish the diagnosis
  - treat underlying cause

Endometriosis

Etiology
- not fully understood
- proposed mechanisms (combination likely involved)
    1. retrograde menstruation theory of Sampson
        - seeding of endometrial cells by transtubal regurgitation during menstruation
        - endometrial cells most often found in dependent sites of the pelvis
    2. immunologic theory – altered immunity may limit clearance of transplanted endometrial cells from pelvic cavity ($\downarrow$ NK cell activity?)
    3. metaplasia of coelomic epithelium
        - undefined endogenous biochemical factor may induce undifferentiated peritoneal cells to develop into endometrial tissue
    4. lymphatic flow from uterus to ovary may account for ovarian endometriosis
    5. extrapelvic disease may be due to vascular or lymphatic dissemination of cells

Epidemiology
- incidence: 15-30% of premenopausal women
- mean age at presentation: 25-30 years
- regresses after menopause

Risk Factors
- family history (7-10 fold increased risk if affected 1st degree relative)
- obstructive anomalies of the genital tract (earlier onset)
- nulliparity
- age >25 years

Sites of Occurrence
- ovaries – 60% patients have ovarian involvement
- broad ligament - vesicoperitoneal fold
- peritoneal surface of the cul-de-sac (uterosacral ligaments)
- rectosigmoid colon
- appendix

Clinical Features
- may be asymptomatic
- cyclic symptoms due to swelling and bleeding of ectopic endometrium, often precede menses and continue throughout and after flow
    - secondary dysmenorrhea
    - deep dyspareunia
    - sacral backache with menses
    - pain may eventually become constant but remains worse perimenstrually
- premenstrual and postmenstrual spotting
- infertility
    - 30-40% of patients with endometriosis will be infertile
    - 15-30% of those who are infertile will have endometriosis
- bowel and bladder symptoms
    - frequency, dysuria, hematuria
    - diarrhea, constipation, hematochezia, dyschezia
- tender nodularity of uterine ligaments and cul-de-sac felt on rectovaginal exam
- fixed retroversion of uterus
- firm, fixed adnexal mass (endometrioma)

Investigations
- definitive diagnosis requires:
    - direct visualization of lesions typical of endometriosis at laparoscopy
    - biopsy and histologic exam of specimens (2 or more of: endometrial epithelium, glands, stroma, hemosiderin-laden macrophages)
- laparoscopy
    - mulberry spots: dark blue or brownish-black implants on the uterosacral ligaments, cul-de-sac, or anywhere in the pelvis
    - endometrioma: chocolate cysts in the ovaries
    - "powder-burn" lesions on the peritoneal surface
    - early white lesions and clear blebs
    - peritoneal "platelets"
- CA-125
    - may be useful for confirming endometriosis

Endometriosis
The presence of endometrial tissue (glands and stroma) outside of the uterine cavity

Differential Diagnosis
1. chronic PID, recurrent acute salpingitis
2. hemorrhagic corpus luteum
3. benign/malignant ovarian neoplasm
4. ectopic pregnancy

Endometriosis on the ovary = endometrioma

There may be little correlation between the extent of disease and symptomatology.

Classic Triad of Endometriosis
Dysmenorrhea
Dyspareunia (cul de sac, uterosacral ligament)
Dyschezia (uterosacral ligament, cul-de-sac, rectosigmoid attachment)

A sharp, firm, and exquisitely tender "barb" on the uterosacral ligament = Sine qua non of endometriosis

Endometriosis is classified according to a scoring system standardized by the American Society for Reproductive Medicine. Score based on location and extent of disease.

Recurrence Rates
Medical therapy: 30-50%
Conservative surgery: 14-40%

Treatment

- depends on the certainty of the diagnosis, severity of symptoms, extent of disease, desire for future fertility, and threat to GI/GU systems
- **medical**
  - NSAIDs (e.g. naproxen sodium) (Anaprox®)
  - pseudopregnancy
    - cyclic/continuous estrogen-progestin (OCP)
    - medroxyprogesterone (Depo-Provera®)
  - pseudomenopause (2nd line: only short-term (<6 months) due to osteoporotic potential with prolonged use)
    - danazol (Danocrine®) = weak androgen
      - side effects: weight gain, fluid retention, acne, hirsutism, voice change
    - leuprolide (Lupron®) = GnRH agonist (suppresses pituitary)
      - side effects: hot flashes, vaginal dryness, reduced libido
      - can use ≥12 months with add-back progestin or estrogen
- **surgical**
  - laparoscopy using laser, electrocautery ± laparotomy
    - ablation/resection of implants, lysis of adhesions, ovarian cystectomy of endometriomas
  - rarely total pelvic clean-out
  - ± follow-up with medical treatment for pain control NOT preservation of fertility
  - best time to become pregnant is after surgery

Adenomyosis

Adenomyosis
Extension of areas of endometrial glands and stroma into the myometrium

- synonym: "endometriosis interna" (uterine wall may be diffusely involved)

Epidemiology

- 15% of females >35 years old
- older age group than seen in endometriosis (40-50 years)
- adenomyosis is a common histologic finding in asymptomatic patients
- found in 20-40% of hysterectomy specimens

Clinical Features

- often asymptomatic
- menorrhagia, secondary dysmenorrhea, pelvic discomfort
- dyspareunia, dyschezia
- uterus symmetrically bulky, usually <14 cm, mobility not restricted, no associated adnexal pathology
- Halban sign: tender, softened uterus on premenstrual bimanual

Investigations

- clinical diagnosis
- U/S or MRI can be helpful
- endometrial sampling to rule out other pathology and to make definitive diagnosis

Final diagnosis of adenomyosis is based on pathologic findings

Treatment

- iron supplements as necessary
- analgesics/NSAIDs
- OCP, medroxyprogesterone
- low dose danazol 100-200 mg PO OD (trial x 4 months)
- GnRH agonists (i.e. leuprolide)
- definitive – hysterectomy (no conservative surgical treatment)

Contraception

- see Family Medicine

Table 3. Classification of Contraceptive Methods

Type		Effectiveness
Physiological		
Withdrawal/coitus interruptus		77.0%
Rhythm method/calendar/mucous/symptothermal		76.0%
Lactational amenorrhea		98% (1st 6 months postpartum)
Chance – no method used		10.0%
Abstinence of all sexual activity		100.0%
Barrier Methods		
Condom alone		90.0%
Condom with spermicide		95.0%
Spermicide alone		82.0%
Sponge		90.0%
Diaphragm with spermicide		90.0%
Female condom		75.0%
Cervical cap	Parous	64.0%
	Nulliparous	82.0%
Hormonal		
OCP		98.0-99.5% (depending on compliance)
Nuvaring		98%
Skin Patch		>99%
Depo-Provera®		99%
Progestin-only pill		90-99%
Mirena® IUD		99%
Copper IUD		96-98%
Surgical		
Tubal ligation		99.6%
Vasectomy		99.8%
Emergency Postcoital Contraception (EPC)		
Yuzpe method		98% (within 24 hours)
'Plan B' levonorgestrel only		98% (within 24 hours)
Postcoital IUD		99.9%

Hormonal Methods

COMBINED ORAL CONTRACEPTIVE PILLS (OCP)
- most contain low dose ethinyl estradiol (20-35 μg) plus progestin (norethinedrone, norgestrel, levonorgestrel, desogestrel, norgestimate, drospirenone)
- failure rate (0.1% to 8%) depending on compliance
- monophasic or triphasic formulations (varying amount of progestin throughout cycle)

Mechanisms of Action
- ovulatory suppression – by inhibiting LH and FSH
- decidualization of endometrium
- thickening of cervical mucus – decreased sperm penetration

Advantages
- highly effective, reversible
- cycle regulation
- decreased dysmenorrhea and menorrhagia (less anemia)
- decreased benign breast disease and ovarian cyst development
- decreased risk of ovarian and endometrial cancer
- increased cervical mucus which may lower risk of STIs
- decreased PMS symptoms
- improved acne
- osteoporosis protection (possibly)

Common Side Effects
Estrogen-related
- nausea
- breast changes (tenderness, enlargement)
- fluid retention/bloating/edema
- weight gain
- migraine, headaches

Irregular breakthrough bleeding often occurs in the first few months after starting OCP. Usually disappears after three cycles.

Canadian Consensus Guideline on Continuous and Extended Hormonal Contraception (2007)

Definitions
*Extended use: The use of combined hormonal contraceptives with planned hormone-free intervals *Continuous Use: Uninterrupted use of combined hormonal contraceptive without hormone-free intervals

What can be used?
Oral, transdermal and vaginally administered combined hormonal contraceptives, including those originally designed for cyclic use, can be administered in a variety of Continuous and Extended (C/E) regimens.

Efficacy and Adherence
Continuous combined hormonal contraceptive regimens are as effective as cyclic regimens in preventing pregnancy.
Use of C/E combined hormonal contraceptive may be more "forgiving" about missed combined hormonal contraceptives because of the absence of a hormone-free interval.

Side Effects
The side effect profile of C/E combined hormonal contraceptive regimens is not worse than with cyclic regimens, and may be better.

Medical/Non-contraceptive Usage
For women in the perimenopausal transition who may be ovulating, C/E combined hormonal contraceptive is preferred to hormonal replacement therapy for controlling problematic bleeding and vasomotor symptoms.

http://www.sogc.org/guidelines/documents/gui1 95CPG0707_000.pdf

Missed Combined OCPs

Miss 1 pill:
• Take 1 pill as soon as patient remembers, and the next pill at the usual time; OR 2 pills at the next dose

Miss 2 pills in a row during first 2 weeks of the cycle:
• Take 2 pills the day patient remembers, and 2 pills the next day
• Then 1 pill per day until finished the pack
• Back-up method of birth control required during next 7 days

Miss 2 pills in a row during third week of the cycle OR miss 3 in a row at any time:
• Throw out pack and start a new pack immediately
• Back-up method of birth control required during next 7 days

• thromboembolic events, liver adenoma (rare)
• intermenstrual bleeding (low estradiol levels)

Progestin-related
• amenorrhea/intermenstrual bleeding
• headaches
• breast tenderness
• increased appetite
• decreased libido
• mood changes
• hypertension
• acne/oily skin*
• hirsutism*

*androgenic side effects may be minimized by prescribing a pill containing desogestrel, norgestimate, drospirenone

Drug Interactions/Risks
• rifampin, phenobarbital, phenytoin, and primidone can decrease efficacy, requiring use of back-up method
• conception despite OCP – no evidence of fetal abnormalities
• no evidence that low dose OCP is harmful to nursing infant but it may decrease milk production, therefore do not start until 6 weeks postpartum

Absolute Contraindications
• known/suspected pregnancy
• undiagnosed abnormal vaginal bleeding
• prior thromboembolic events, thromboembolic disorder (Factor V Leiden mutation; protein C, S or antithrombin III deficiency), active thrombophlebitis
• cerebrovascular or coronary artery disease
• estrogen-dependent tumours (breast, uterus)
• impaired liver function associated with acute liver disease
• congenital hypertriglyceridemia
• smoker age >35 years
• migraines with focal neurological symptoms (excluding aura)
• uncontrolled hypertension

Relative Contraindications
• migraines – nonfocal with aura <1 hour
• diabetes mellitus complicated by vascular disease
• SLE
• controlled hypertension
• hyperlipidemia
• sickle cell anemia
• gallbladder disease

Starting Oral Contraceptives
• thorough history and physical examination (including blood pressure and breast exam)
• F/U visit in 6 weeks after OCPs prescribed
• pelvic exam can be delayed until a subsequent visit

Selected Examples of OCPs

Diane 35®
• 35 μg ethinyl estradiol and 2 mg cyproterone acetate
• oral contraceptive with anti-androgen properties
• NOT approved for use solely as an oral contraceptive in North America; approved in Europe; equally effective and safe
• approved as short-term therapy for androgen-sensitive skin conditions including hirsutism and acne unresponsive to antibiotics

Yasmin®
• 30 μg ethinyl estradiol + 3 mg drospirenone (a new progestin)
• drospirenone has antimineralocorticoid activity and antiandrogenic effects
• benefits – decreased perception of cyclic weight gain, bloating; decreased PMS symptoms; improved acne
• adverse effects – hyperkalemia (rare, contraindicated in renal and adrenal insufficiency)
• check K if patient also on ACE inhibitor, ARB, K-sparing diuretic, heparin

Seasonale™/Continuous OCP
• 30 μg ethinyl estradiol + 150 μg levonorgestrel
• 84 days monophasic OCP

- withdrawal bleed only 4 times per year
- side effects similar to monthly OCP with increased spotting during first few cycles
- as effective as OCP in preventing pregnancy

Table 4. Hormonal Activity of Common Combined OCPs

	Estrogenic Activity	Progestational Activity	Androgenic Activity
low	Demulen™	Tri-cyclen™	Tri-cyclen™
	Alesse™	Alesse™	Marvelon™
	Marvelon™	Ortho 7/7/7™	Ortho 7/7/7™
	Tri-cyclen™	Ovral™	Alesse™
	Ovral™	Marvelon™	Demulen™
high	Ortho 7/7/7™	Demulen™	Ovral™

HORMONAL CONTRACEPTIVE SKIN PATCH (ORTHO EVRA™)
- continuous release of 6 mg norelgestromin + 0.60 mg ethinyl estradiol into bloodstream
- patch applied to lower abdomen, back, upper arm, buttocks, NOT breast
- patch worn weekly for 3 consecutive weeks (changed every week) with 1 week off to allow menstruation
- as effective as OCP in preventing pregnancy (>99% with perfect use)
- may be less effective in women >90 kg body weight
- 3% failure rate with typical use
- may not be covered by drug plans

HORMONAL CONTRACEPTIVE RING (NUVARING®)
- thin flexible plastic ring; releases etonogestrel 120 μg/d + estradiol 15 μg/d
- works for 3 weeks, then removed for 1 week to allow menstruation
- as effective as OCP in preventing pregnancy (98%)
- avoids first pass effect
- side effects: vaginal infection/irritation, vaginal discharge
- may have better cycle control, i.e. decreased breakthrough bleeding

PROGESTIN-ONLY METHOD
- suitable for postpartum women (does not affect breast milk supply), women with contraindications to combined OCP (e.g. thromboembolic or myocardial disease) or women intolerant of estrogenic side effects of combined OCPs
- no absolute contraindications

Mechanisms of Action
- progestin prevents LH surge
- thickening of cervical mucus
- decrease tubal motility
- endometrial suppression
- ovulation suppression - not as consistently suppressed compared to combined OCPs

Side Effects
- irregular menstrual bleeding, weight gain, headache, breast tenderness, mood changes, functional ovarian cysts

Selected Examples of Progestin-Only Methods

Progestin-Only Pill ("minipill")
- Micronor™ 0.35 mg norethindrone
- taken daily at same time of day (within 3 hours) to ensure reliable effect; no pill free interval
- higher failure rate (1.1-13% with typical use, 0.51% with perfect use) than other hormonal methods
- ovulation inhibited in 60% of women, most have regular cycles

Depo-Provera®
- injectable depot medroxyprogesterone acetate
- dose 150 mg IM q12-14wks (convenient dosing)
- initiate within 5 days of beginning of normal menses, immediately postpartum in breastfeeding and non-breastfeeding women
- irregular spotting that progresses to complete amenorrhea in 70% of women (after 1-2 years of use)
- highly effective 99%; failure rate 0.3%
- side effect – decreased bone density (may be reversible)
- disadvantage – restoration of fertility may take up to 1-2 years

ALERT
FDA recently warned that women using the US version of the patch (which contains 0.75 mg of ethinyl estradiol) are exposed to 60% more estrogen in a monthly cycle than women taking a typical 35 µg oral contraceptive. This potential for excess estrogen exposure raises concerns for an increased risk of nausea, mastalgia, and venous thromboembolism, although the degree of risk is unclear. The pharmacokinetics of the 0.60 mg patch, which is available in Canada, are less clear.

CMAJ. January 2006.

Missed Progestin-Only Pills
Use back-up contraceptive method for at least 48 hours. Continue to take remainder of pills as prescribed.

Reversibility of Depo-Provera®
[Wooltorton. Medroxyprogesterone acetate (Depo-Provera®) and bone mineral density loss. JAMC. 2005; 172(6):746]

Extended use (up to five years) of medroxyprogesterone acetate has been found to decrease spine and hip bone mineral density (BMD) by 4% to 6.9%. Two years after discontinuation, only partial recovery of BMD has been noted.

New SOGC recommendations for Depo-Provera® Users
(SOGC News Release. New recommendations from national ob/gyn society address Depo-Provera®, bone loss. May 2006. http://www.sogc.org/media/pdf/advisories/dmpa-may2006_e.pdf)

- Inform patients of potential risks and benefits at intervals throughout course of treatment.
- Recommend ways to improve bone health such as calcium, vitamin D, weight-bearing exercise, smoking cessation, decreased alcohol, and reduced caffeine.
- There is no evidence to suggest routine BMD testing.

Intrauterine Device (IUD)

Mechanism of Action
- copper-containing IUD (Nova-T®) mild foreign body reaction in endometrium which is toxic to sperm and alters sperm motility
- progesterone-releasing IUD (Mirena®) works by decidualization of endometrium and thickening of cervical mucus; may suppress ovulation
- highly effective (95-99%); failure rate 0-1.2%
- contraceptive effects last 5 years
- reversible, private, convenient
- may be used in women with contraindications to OCPs or wanting long term contraception

Absolute Contraindications
- known or suspected pregnancy
- undiagnosed genital tract bleeding
- acute or chronic PID
- lifestyle risk for STIs
- known allergy to copper (copper IUD only)
- Wilson's disease (copper IUD only)

Relative Contraindications
- valvular heart disease
- past history of PID or ectopic pregnancy
- presence of prosthesis
- abnormalities of uterine cavity, intracavitary fibroids
- severe dysmenorrhea or menorrhagia (copper IUD only)
- cervical stenosis
- immunosuppressed individuals (e.g. HIV, etc.)

Side Effects
- intermenstrual bleeding
- bloating, headache (progesterone – Mirena®)
- increased blood loss and duration of menses (copper IUD only)
- dysmenorrhea (copper IUD only)
- expulsion (5% in the first year, greatest in first month and in nulliparous women)
- uterine wall perforation (1/5000)
- if pregnancy occurs with an IUD, there is a greater chance the pregnancy will be ectopic
- increased risk of PID within first 10 days of insertion only

Emergency Postcoital Contraception (EPC)

HORMONAL METHODS

Mechanism of Action
- unknown; suggestions include:
    - suppresses ovulation or causes deficient luteal phase
    - may alter endometrium to prevent implantation
    - may affect sperm/ova transport

Side Effects
- nausea (due to estrogen; treat with Gravol®), irregular spotting

Risks/Contraindications
- pre-existing pregnancy (although not teratogenic)
- caution in women with contraindications to OCP (although NO absolute contraindications)

Yuzpe Method
- used within 72 hours of unprotected intercourse; limited evidence of benefit up to 5 days
- Ovral® 2 tablets then repeat in 12 hours (ethinyl estradiol 100 µg/levonorgestrel 500 µg)
- can substitute with any OCP as long as same dose of estrogen used
- 2% overall risk of pregnancy
- efficacy ↓ with time (e.g. less effective at 72 hours than 24 hours)

"Plan B"
- consists of levonorgestrel 750 µg q12h for 2 doses (can also take 2 doses together); taken within 72 hours of intercourse
- greater efficacy (75-95% if used within 24 h) and better side effect profile than Yuzpe method
- no estrogen thus very few contraindications/side effects (less nausea)
- efficacy ↓ with time

NON-HORMONAL METHODS

Postcoital IUD (Copper)
- insert up to 7 days postcoitus
- prevents implantation
- 1% failure rate
- usual contraindications/precautions to IUD
- can use for short duration in higher risk individuals
- Mirena® IUD cannot be used as EPC

Follow-up
- 3-4 weeks post treatment to confirm efficacy (confirm spontaneous menses or do pregnancy test)
- contraception counselling

Infertility

Epidemiology
- 10-15% of couples
- on average 75% of couples achieve pregnancy within 6 months, 85% within 1 year, 90% within 2 years
- must investigate both members of couple

> **Infertility**: the inability to conceive or carry to term a pregnancy after one year of regular, unprotected intercourse
> **Primary infertility**: infertility in the context of no prior pregnancies
> **Secondary infertility**: infertility in the context of a prior conception

Female Factor

Etiology
- **ovulatory dysfunction (15-20%)**
  - hypothalamic (hypothalamic amenorrhea)
  - pituitary
    - prolactinoma
    - hypopituitarism
  - ovarian
    - PCOS
    - premature ovarian failure
    - luteal phase defect (poor follicle production, premature corpus luteum failure, failed uterine lining response to progesterone) poorly understood
  - systemic diseases (thyroid, Cushing's syndrome, renal/hepatic failure)
  - congenital (Turner's syndrome, gonadal dysgenesis, or gonadotropin deficiency)
  - stress, poor nutrition, excessive exercise (even with presence of menstruation)
- **outflow tract abnormality**
  - tubal factors (20-30%)
    - PID
    - adhesions (previous surgery, peritonitis, endometriosis)
    - ligation/occlusion (e.g. previous ectopic)
  - uterine factors (<5%)
    - congenital anomalies (e.g. prenatal DES exposure), bicornuate uterus, uterine septum
    - intrauterine adhesions (e.g. Asherman's syndrome)
    - infection (endometritis, pelvic TB)
    - fibroids/polyps (particularly intrauterine)
    - endometrial ablation
  - cervical factors (5%)
    - hostile or acidic cervical mucus
    - anti-sperm antibodies
    - structural defects (cone biopsies, laser, or cryotherapy)
- **endometriosis**
- **multiple factors (30%)**
- **unknown factors (10-15%)**

> **Requirements for Conception**
> 1. Ovary
> 2. Tube
> 3. Cervix
> 4. Endometrium
> 5. Sperm

Investigations
- **ovulatory**
  - Day 3 FSH, LH, TSH, PRL +/- DHEA, free testosterone (if hirsute)
  - Day 21-23 serum progesterone
  - initiate basal body temperature monitoring (biphasic pattern)
  - postcoital test - evaluate mucus for clarity, pH, spinnbarkeit (rarely done)
- **tubal factors**
  - HSG (can be therapeutic – opens fallopian tube)
  - SHG
  - laparoscopy with dye insufflation

When should investigations begin?
- <35 years: after 1 year of trying to conceive
- 35-40 years: after >6 months
- >40 years: immediately
- earlier if:
  - history of PID
  - history of infertility in previous relationship
  - prior pelvic surgery
  - chemotherapy/radiation in either partner
  - recurrent pregnancy loss
  - moderate-severe endometriosis

- **peritoneal/uterine factors**
  - HSG/SHG, hysteroscopy
- **other**
  - karyotype

Treatment
- **education** – timing of intercourse in relation to ovulation (from 2 days prior to 2 days following presumed ovulation), every other day
- **medical**
  - ovulation induction
    - clomiphene citrate (Clomid®) – estrogen antagonist that causes a perceived decreased estrogen state, which results in increased pituitary gonadotropins; this causes increased FSH and LH, leading to ovulation induction (better if anovulatory)
    - human menopausal gonadotropin [HMG (Pergonal™)], urofollitropin (FSH [Metrodin®]) - FSH and LH extracted from urine of post-menopausal women
    - followed by β-hCG for stimulation of ovum release
  - may add
    - bromocriptine (dopamine agonist) if increased hyperprolactinemia
    - dexamethasone for women with hyperandrogenism (PCOS, adult onset congenital adrenal hyperplasia), metformin (PCOS)
    - luteal phase progesterone supplementation for luteal phase defect
    - ASA (81 mg PO OD) daily for women with a history of recurrent spontaneous abortions
- **surgical/procedural**
  - tuboplasty
  - lysis of adhesions
  - artificial insemination
  - sperm washing
  - IVF (in vitro fertilization)
  - intrafallopian transfers:
    - GIFT (gamete intrafallopian transfer) – immediate transfer with sperm after oocyte retrieval
    - ZIFT (zygote intrafallopian transfer) – transfer after 24 hour culture of oocyte and sperm
    - TET (tubal embryo transfer) – transfer after >24 hour culture
  - ICSI (intracytoplasmic sperm injection)
  - IUI (intrauterine insemination)
  - ± oocyte or sperm donors
  - IVM (in vitro maturation)

Male Factor

- see Urology

Etiology
- varicocele (>40%)
- idiopathic (>20%)
- obstruction (~15%)
- cryptorchidism (~8%)
- immunologic (~3%)

Investigations
- semen analysis and culture
- post-coital (Huhner) test

Normal semen analysis (WHO criteria)
- Must be obtained 48-72 hours post-abstinence
1. volume 2-5 cc
2. count > 20 million/cc
3. motility >50%
4. morphology >30% normal
5. absence of pyospermia, hyperviscosity, agglutination

NB: does not assess sperm function

Polycystic Ovarian Syndrome (PCOS)

- also called chronic ovarian androgenism

Etiology

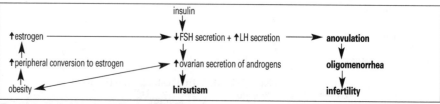

Figure 8. Pathophysiology of Polycystic Ovarian Syndrome

Clinical Signs of Endocrine Imbalance
- Menstrual disorder/amenorrhea (80%)
- Infertility (74%)
- Hirsutism (69%)
- Obesity (49%)
- Impaired glucose tolerance (35%)
- Diabetes Mellitus (10%)

Diagnosis
- 2 of 3 to make diagnosis
  1. oligomenorrhea/irregular menses for 6 months

2. clinical or lab evidence of hyperandrogenism
3. polycystic ovaries on U/S

Clinical Features
- average age 15-35 years
- anovulation, hirsutism, infertility, obesity, virilization
- acanthosis nigricans: browning of skin folds in intertriginous zones
- family history of diabetes
- insulin resistance in both lean and obese patients

Polycystic Ovarian Syndrome – HAIR-AN
Hirsutism, **H**yper**A**ndrogenism, **I**nfertility, **I**nsulin **R**esistance, **A**canthosis **N**igricans

Investigations
- transvaginal U/S – polycystic-appearing ovaries ("string of pearls")
- LH:FSH >2:1, LH is chronically high with FSH midrange or low (not part of diagnostic criteria)
- fasting glucose: insulin ratio <4.5 = insulin resistance (U.S. units)
- OGTT (particularly if obese)
- increased DHEAS, androstenedione and q2 years free testosterone (most sensitive test), decreased SHBG
- laparoscopy is not required for diagnosis; most common to see white, smooth, sclerotic ovary with a thick capsule; multiple follicular cysts in various stages of atresia; hyperplastic theca and stroma
- rule out other causes of abnormal bleeding

PCOS may be confused with:
- late onset congenital adrenal hyperplasia (21-hydroxylase deficiency)
- Cushing's syndrome
- ovarian and adrenal neoplasms
- hyperprolactinemia

Treatment
- **cycle control**
  - lifestyle modification (decrease BMI, increase exercise) to decrease peripheral estrone formation
  - OCP monthly or cyclic Provera® to prevent endometrial hyperplasia due to unopposed estrogen
  - oral hypoglycemic (metformin 500 mg PO tid, rosiglitazone, pioglitazone)
  - tranexamic acid for menorrhagia only
- **infertility**
  - medical induction of ovulation: clomiphene citrate, human menopausal gonadotropins (hMG [Pergonal®]), LHRH, recombinant FSH, and metformin
    - metformin may be used alone or in conjuction with clomiphene citrate for ovulation induction
  - ovarian drilling (perforate the stroma), wedge resection of the ovary
  - bromocriptine (if hyperprolactinemia)
- **hirsutism**
  - any OCP can be used
  - Diane 35® (cyproterone acetate) – antiandrogenic
  - Yasmin® (drospirenone and ethinyl estradiol) - spironolactone analogue (inhibits steroid receptors)
  - mechanical removal of hair
  - finasteride (5-alpha reductase inhibitor)
  - flutamide (androgen reuptake inhibitor)

Long Term Health Consequences
- hyperlipidemia
- adult-onset diabetes mellitus
- endometrial hyperplasia
- infertility
- obesity
- sleep apnea

Gynecological Infections

Physiologic Discharge

- clear, white, flocculent odourless discharge
- smear contains epithelial cells, lactobacilli
- pH 3.8-4.2
- increases with ↑ estrogen states: pregnancy, OCP, mid-cycle, PCOS or premenarchal
- if increased in perimenopausal woman, investigate for other effects of excess estrogen (e.g. endometrial cancer)

Vulvovaginitis

PREPUBERTAL VULVOVAGINITIS
- **clinical features**
  - irritation, pruritus
  - discharge
  - vulvar erythema
  - vaginal bleeding (specifically due to *Group A Streptococci* and *Shigella*)

Vulvovaginitis
Vulvar and vaginal inflammation

Most common gynecological problem in prepubertal girls is non-specific vulvovaginitis.

- differential diagnosis
  - nonspecific vulvovaginitis (25-75%)
  - infections (respiratory, enteric, systemic, sexually acquired)
  - foreign body (toilet paper most common)
  - candida (only if in diapers)
  - pinworms
  - polyps, tumour (ovarian malignancy)
  - vulvar skin disease (lichen sclerosis, condyloma acuminata)
  - trauma (accidental straddle injury, sexual abuse)
  - psychosomatic vaginal complaints (specific for vaginal discharge)
  - endocrine abnormalities (specific for vaginal bleeding)
  - blood dyscrasia (specific for vaginal bleeding)
- etiology
  - infectious:
    - poor hygiene
    - proximity of vagina to anus
    - recent infection (respiratory, enteric, systemic)
    - STI – investigate sexual abuse
  - nonspecific:
    - lack of protective hair and labial fat pads
    - lack of estrogenization
    - susceptible to chemicals, soaps (bubble baths), medications and clothing
    - enuresis
- investigations
  - vaginal swab for culture (specifically state that it is a pre-pubertal specimen)
- treatment
  - enhanced hygiene and local measures (handwashing, white cotton underwear, no nylon tights, no tight fitting clothes, no sleeper pajamas; sitz baths, avoid bubble baths; use mild detergent, eliminate fabric softener; avoid prolonged exposure to wet bathing suits; urination with legs spread apart)
  - A&D® dermatological ointment to protect vulvar skin
  - infectious: treat with antibiotics for organism identified

There is no high quality evidence showing a link between vulvovaginal candidiasis and hygienic habits or wearing tight or synthetic clothing

Table 5. Other Common Causes of Vulvovaginitis in Prepubertal Girls

	Pinworms	Lichen Sclerosis	Foreign Body
Diagnosis	Cellophane Tape test	Area of white thickening	
Treatment	Empirical treatment with mebendazole	Topical steroid creams	Irrigation of vagina with saline, may require local anesthesia

POSTMENOPAUSAL VAGINITIS/ATROPHIC VAGINITIS

- clinical features
  - dyspareunia
  - post-coital spotting
  - mild pruritus
- investigations
  - diagnosis of atrophy is usually a visual one – thinning of tissues, erythema, petechiae, bleeding points, dryness
  - rule out malignancy
- treatment
  - local estrogen replacement (ideal) – Premarin® cream, VagiFem® tablets, or Estring®
  - oral or transdermal hormone replacement therapy (if treatment for systemic symptoms is desired)
  - good hygiene

INFECTIOUS VULVOVAGINITIS

Table 6. Infectious Vulvovaginitis

	Candidiasis (Moniliasis)	Bacterial Vaginosis (BV)	Trichomoniasis
Organisms	Candida albicans (90%) Candida glabrata (<5%) Candida tropicalis (<5%)	Gardnerella vaginalis Mycoplasma hominis anaerobes: Prevotella, Mobiluncus, Bacteroides	Trichomonas vaginalis (flagellated protozoan)
Pathophysiology or Transmission	predisposing factors include: - immunosuppressed host (diabetes, AIDS, etc.) - recent antibiotic use - inc. estrogen levels, e.g. pregnancy, OCP	replacement of vaginal Lactobacillus with organisms above	sexually transmitted
Discharge	whitish, "cottage cheese", minimal	grey, thin, diffuse	yellow-green, malodorous, diffuse
Other Signs/Symptoms	- 20% asymptomatic - intense pruritus - swollen, inflamed genitals - vulvar burning, dysuria, dyspareunia	- 50-75% asymptomatic - fishy odour, esp. after coitus - absence of vulva/vaginal irritation	- 25% asymptomatic - petechiae on vagina and cervix - occasionally irritated tender vulva - dysuria, frequency
pH	≤4.5	>4.5	≥4.5

Table 6. Infectious Vulvovaginitis (continued)

	Candidiasis (Moniliasis)	Bacterial Vaginosis (BV)	Trichomoniasis
Saline Wetmount	KOH wetmount reveals hyphae and spores	1) >20% clue cells = squamous epithelial cells dotted with coccobacilli (*Gardnerella*) 2) paucity of WBC 3) paucity of *Lactobacillli* 4) positive whiff test = fishy odour with addition of KOH to slide due to formation of amines	1) motile flagellated organisms 2) many WBCs 3) inflammatory cells (PMNs)
Treatment	- recommended if uncomplicated - clotrimazole, butoconazole, miconazole, terconazole suppositories and/or creams for 1, 3, or 7-day treatments - treatment in pregnancy is usually topical treatment - fluconazole 150 mg PO in single dose	- no treatment if non-pregnant and asymptomatic unless scheduled for pelvic surgery or procedure **Oral** - metronidazole 500 mg PO bid x 7 days or metronidazole gel 0.75% x 5 day OD - clindamycin 2% 5 g intravaginally at bedtime for 7 days **Topical** - may use metronidazole in pregnancy	- treat if asymptomatic! - 2 g PO single dose metronidazole (recom.) or 500 mg bid x 7 days (alternative) - symptomatic pregnant women should be treated with 2 g metronidazole once
Other	- for repeat infections prophylaxis, treatment includes boric acid, vaginal suppositories, luteal phase fluconazole - routine treatment of partner(s) not recommended	- associated with recurrent & preterm labour, preterm birth, and postpartum endometritis in pregnancy - need to warn patients on metronidazole : do not consume alcohol (disulfiram-like action) - routine treatment of partner(s) not recommended	- warnings accompanying metronidazole use - treat partner(s)

Sexually Transmitted Infections (STIs)

- see <u>Family Medicine</u>

TRICHOMONIASIS

- see *Infectious Vulvovaginitis*, GY26

CHLAMYDIA

Etiology
- *Chlamydia trachomatis*

Epidemiology
- most common bacterial STI in Canada
- often associated with *N. gonorrheae*

Clinical Features
- asymptomatic (80% of women)
- muco-purulent endocervical discharge
- urethral syndrome: dysuria, frequency, pyuria, no bacteria
- pelvic pain
- post-coital bleeding or intermenstrual bleeding (particularly if on OCP and prior history of good cyclic control)

Investigations
- cervical culture or nucleic acid amplification test
- obligate intracellular parasite – tissue culture is the definitive standard

Treatment
- doxycycline 100 mg PO bid for 7d, or azithromycin 1 g PO in a single dose (may use in pregnancy)
- treat partners
- reportable disease
- test of cure for chlamydia required in pregnancy (cure rates lower in pregnant patients) → retest 3-4 weeks post-initiation of therapy

Screening
- high risk groups
- during pregnancy

Complications
- acute salpingitis, PID
- Fitz-Hugh-Curtis syndrome (liver capsule infection)
- arthritis, conjunctivitis, urethritis (Reactive Arthritis – male predominance, HLA-B27)

Risk Factors for STIs
- history of previous STI
- contact with infected person
- sexually active individual <25 years of age
- multiple partners
- new partner in last 3 months
- not using barrier protection
- street involvement (homelessness, drug use)

Public Health Agency of Canada: National Notifiable STIs
- AIDS
- Gonorrhea
- Chlamydia
- Syphilis
- Hepatitis B, C, D

http://dsol-smed.phac-aspc.gc.ca/dsol-smed/ndis/list_e.html

- infertility – tubal obstruction from low grade salpingitis
- ectopic pregnancy
- chronic pelvic pain
- perinatal infection – conjunctivitis, pneumonia

GONORRHEA

Etiology
- *Neisseria gonorrheae*
- symptoms and risk factors same as with chlamydia

Investigations
- Gram stain shows Gram-negative intracellular diplococci
- cervical, rectal and throat culture

Treatment
- single dose of ceftriaxone 125 mg IM, or cefixime 400 mg PO, or ciprofloxacin 500 mg PO
- **plus** doxycycline or azithromycin to treat chlamydia, because of high rate of co-infection
- if pregnant – cephalosporin regimen or 2 g spectinomycin IM (avoid quinolones)
- treat partners
- reportable disease
- screening as with chlamydia

HUMAN PAPILLOMAVIRUS (HPV)

Etiology
- most common viral STI in Canada
- >200 subtypes of which >30 are genital subtypes
- types 16, 18, 31, 33, 35, 45, 36 (and others) associated with increased incidence of cervical and vulvar intraepithelial hyperplasia and carcinoma
- HPV types 6 & 11 are classically associated with anogenital warts/condylomata acuminata
- HPV types 16 & 18 are the most oncogenic (classically associated with cervical HSIL)

Clinical Features
- latent infection
  - no visible lesions
  - detected by DNA hybridization tests
  - asymptomatic
- subclinical infection
  - visible lesion found during colposcopy, or found on Pap test
- clinical infection
  - visible wartlike lesion without magnification
  - hyperkeratotic, verrucous or flat, macular lesions
  - vulvar edema

Investigations
- cytology (see *Pap Test*, GY45)
  - koilocytosis – nuclear enlargement and atypia with perinuclear halo
- biopsy of lesions at colposcopy
- detection of HPV DNA subtype using nucleic acid probes not routinely done but can be done in presence of abnormal Pap test to guide treatment

Treatment
- patient applied
  - podofilox 0.5% solution or gel bid x 3 days in a row (4 days off) then repeat x 4 weeks
  - imiquimod (Aldara®) 5% cream 3x/wk qhs x 16wks
- provider administered
  - cryotherapy with liquid nitrogen – repeat q1-2wks
  - podophyllin resin in tincture of benzoin – weekly
  - trichloroacetic acid (TCA) or bichloroacetic acid weekly (80-90%) (safe in pregnancy)
  - surgical removal/laser
  - intralesional interferon
- **cannot** be prevented by using condoms

Prevention
- HPV types 6, 11, 16, 18 – preventable with Gardasil® (Quadrivalent HPV recombinant vaccine)

Test of cure for *C. trachomatis* and *N. gonorrheae* is not routinely indicated. Repeat testing if symptomatic, if compliance with treatment is uncertain, or if pregnant.

Genital Warts During Pregnancy
- Condylomata tend to get larger in pregnancy and should be treated early (consider excision)
- C-section only if obstruction of birth canal or risk of extensive bleeding
- Do not use imiquimod, podophyllin, or podofilox

HERPES SIMPLEX VIRUS OF VULVA (HSV)

Etiology
- 90% are HSV-2, 10% are HSV-1

Clinical Features
- may be asymptomatic
- initial symptoms
  - present 2-21 days following contact
- prodromal symptoms – tingling, burning, pruritus
- multiple, painful, shallow ulcerations with small vesicles (absent in many infected persons)
  - these lesions are infectious
  - appear 7-10 days after initial infection
- inguinal lymphadenopathy, malaise, and fever often with first infection
- dysuria and urinary retention if urethral mucosa affected
- recurrent infections – less severe, less frequent and shorter in duration

> **Classically...**
> **HSV I** – disease above the belt (oral)
> **HSV II** – disease below the belt (genital)

Investigations
- viral culture preferred in patients with ulcer present – decreased sensitivity as lesions heal
- cytologic smear
  - multinucleated giant cells
  - acidophilic intranuclear inclusion bodies
- type specific serologic tests for antibodies to HSV-1 and HSV-2 (not available routinely in Canada)
- HSV DNA PCR

> **HSV Infections During Pregnancy**
> - Antiviral suppression of women with first episode or with a history of HSV infections from 36 weeks on
> - C-section should be performed on women who have active genital lesions at time of delivery
> - Acyclovir 400 mg PO tid

Treatment
- first episode
  - acyclovir 400 mg PO tid x 7-10d (also famciclovir 250 mg PO tid x 7-10d, valacyclovir 1 g PO bid x 7-10d)
- recurrent episode
  - acyclovir 400 mg PO tid x 3-5d, or famciclovir 125 120 mg PO bid x 3-5d, or valacyclovir 500 mg PO bid x 3d
- daily suppressive therapy
  - consider if 6-8 attacks per year
  - acyclovir 400 mg PO bid, or famciclovir 250 mg bid, or valacyclovir 500 mg - 1 g PO OD
- severe disease
  - consider IV therapy acyclovir 5-10 mg/kg IV q8h x 5-7d
- education regarding transmission
- avoid contact from onset of prodrome until lesions have cleared
- use barrier contraception

SYPHILIS

Etiology
- *Treponema pallidum*

Classifications
- syphilis progresses in this order:
  - **primary syphilis**
  - 3-4 weeks after exposure
    - painless chancre on vulva, vagina or cervix
    - painless inguinal lymphadenopathy
  - serological tests usually negative
  - **secondary syphilis** (can resolve spontaneously)
    - 2-6 months after initial infection
    - nonspecific symptoms – malaise, anorexia, headache, diffuse lymphadenopathy
    - generalized maculopapular rash – palms, soles, trunk, limbs
    - condylomata lata – anogenital, broad-based fleshy grey lesions
    - serological tests usually positive
  - **latent syphilis**
    - no clinical manifestations; detected by serology only
  - **tertiary syphilis**
    - may involve any organ system

> **Epidemiology of Genital Ulcers**
> HSV   70-80%
> 1° syphilis   5%
> chancroid   <1%

- - neurological – tabes dorsalis, general paresis
    - cardiovascular – aortic aneurysm, dilated aortic root
    - vulvar gumma: nodules that enlarge, ulcerate, and become necrotic (rare)
  - **congenital syphilis**
    - may cause fetal anomalies, stillbirths, or neonatal death

Investigations
- aspirate of ulcer serum or node
- darkfield microscopy (most sensitive and specific diagnostic test for syphilis)
  - spirochetes
- non-treponemal screening tests (VDRL, RPR); nonreactive after treatment
- specific anti-treponemal antibody tests (FTA-ABS, MHA-TP, TP-PA)
  - confirmatory tests; remain reactive for life (even after adequate treatment)

Treatment
- treatment of primary, secondary, latent syphilis of <1 year duration
  - benzathine penicillin G 2.4 million units IM single dose
  - treat partners, reportable disease
- treatment of latent syphilis >1 year duration
  - benzathine penicillin G 2.4 million units IM q1wk x 3 weeks
- treatment of neurosyphilis
  - IV aqueous penicillin G 3-4 million units IM q4h for 10-14 days
- screening
  - high risk groups
  - in pregnancy

Complications
- if untreated, 1/3 will experience late complications

Bartholinitis/Bartholin Gland Abscess

Etiology
- often anaerobic and polymicrobial
- *U. urealyticum, N. gonorrheae, C. trachomatis, E. coli, P. mirabilis, Streptococcus, S. aureus* (rare)

Clinical Features
- swelling and pain in lower lateral opening of vagina
- sitting and walking may become difficult

Treatment
- sitz baths
- antibiotics
- incision and drainage using local anesthesia with placement of Word catheter (10 Fr. latex catheter) for 2-3 weeks
- marsupialization under general anesthetic – more definitive treatment
- rarely treated by removing gland

Pelvic Inflammatory Disease (PID)

- up to 20% of all gynecology-related hospital admissions

> **PID**
> Inflammation of the upper genital tract (above cervix) including endometrium, fallopian tubes, ovaries, pelvic peritoneum, ± contiguous structures

> PID accounts for up to 20% of all gyne hospital admissions.

Etiology
- causative organisms (in order of frequency)
  - *C. trachomatis*
  - *N. gonorrheae*
  - gonorrheae and chlamydia often co-exist
  - endogenous flora – anaerobic, aerobic, or both
    - *E. coli, Staphylococcus, Streptococcus, Enterococcus, Bacteroides, Peptostreptococcus, H. flu, G. vaginalis*
    - cause of recurrent PID
    - associated with instrumentation
  - *Actinomyces israelii* (Gram positive, non acid-fast anaerobe)
    - in 1-4% of PID associated with IUDs
  - others (TB, Gram-negatives, CMV, *U. urealyticum*, etc.)

Risk Factors
- age <30 years
- risk factors as for chlamydia and gonorrheae
- vaginal douching
- IUD (within first 10 days post insertion)
- invasive gynecologic procedures (D&C, endometrial biopsy)

Clinical Presentation
- up to 2/3 asymptomatic – many subtle or mild symptoms
- common
  - fever >38.3°C
  - lower abdominal pain and tenderness
  - abnormal discharge – cervical or vaginal
- uncommon
  - nausea and vomiting
  - dysuria
  - AUB
- chronic disease (often due to chlamydia)
  - constant pelvic pain
  - dyspareunia
  - palpable mass
  - very difficult to treat, may require surgery

Investigations
- bloodwork
  - β-hCG (must rule out ectopic), CBC, blood cultures if suspect septicemia
- urine R&M
- speculum exam
  - vaginal swab
  - Gram stain
  - cervical cultures for *N. gonorrheae, C. trachomatis*
  - endometrial biopsy will give definitive diagnosis (rarely done)
- ultrasound
  - may be normal
  - fluid in cul-de-sac
  - pelvic or tubo-ovarian abscess
  - hydrosalpinx
- laparoscopy (gold standard)
  - for definitive diagnosis – may miss subtle inflammation of tubes or endometritis

Treatment
- must treat with polymicrobial coverage
- **inpatient if:**
  - atypical infection
  - adnexal mass, tubo-ovarian, or pelvic abscess
  - moderate to severe illness
  - unable to tolerate oral antibiotics or failed oral therapy
  - immunocompromised
  - pregnant
  - adolescent – first episode
  - surgical emergency cannot be excluded
  - PID is secondary to instrumentation
  - recommended treatment
    - cefoxitin 2 g IV q6h (no longer available in U.S.A.) or cefotetan 2g IV q12h + doxycycline 100 mg IV/PO q12h or
    - clindamycin 900 mg IV q8h + gentamicin 2 mg/kg IV loading dose then gentamicin 1.5 mg/kg q8h maintenance dose
    - continue IV antibiotics for 24 hours after symptoms have improved then doxycycline 100 mg PO bid to complete 14 days
    - percutaneous drainage of abscess under U/S guidance
    - when no response to treatment, laparoscopic drainage
    - if failure, treatment is surgical (salpingectomy, TAH/BSO)
- **outpatient if:**
  - typical findings
  - mild to moderate illness
  - oral antibiotics tolerated
  - compliance ensured
  - follow-up within 48-72 hours (to ensure symptoms not worsening)
  - recommended treatment
    - ofloxacin 400 mg PO bid x 14d or levofloxacin 500 mg PO bid x 14d ± metronidazole 500 mg PO bid x 14d (if suspect abscess)
    - ceftriaxone 250 mg IM x 1 + doxycycline 100 mg PO bid x 14d or cefoxitin 2 g IM x 1 + probenicid 1 g PO plus doxycycline 100 mg PO bid ± metronidazole 500 mg PO bid x 14d
    - consider removing IUD after a minimum of 24 hours of treatment
    - reportable disease
    - treat partners
    - consider rescreening for *C. trachomatis* and *N. gonorrheae* 4-6 weeks after treatment if documented infection

PID Diagnosis
- *Must* have:
  - lower abdominal pain
  - cervical motion tenderness
  - adnexal tenderness
- *Plus* one or more of:
  - high risk partner
  - temperature >38°C
  - mucopurulent cervical discharge
  - positive culture for *N. gonorrheae, C. trachomatis, E. coli,* or other vaginal flora
  - cul-de-sac fluid, pelvic abscess or inflammatory mass on U/S or bimanual
  - leukocytosis
  - elevated ESR or CRP (not commonly used)

Treat PID with
FOXY DOXY
(cefoxitin + doxycycline)

PID Complications "I FACE PID"
Infertility
Fitz-Hugh-Curtis syndrome
Abscesses
Chronic pelvic pain
Ectopic pregnancy
Peritonitis
Intestinal obstruction
Disseminated infection (sepsis, endocarditis, arthritis, meningitis)

Complications of Untreated PID
- chronic pelvic pain
- abscess, peritonitis
- adhesion formation
- ectopic pregnancy
- infertility
  - 1 episode of PID → 13% infertility
  - 2 episodes of PID → 36% infertility
- bacteremia
- septic arthritis, endocarditis

Toxic Shock Syndrome

- see Infectious Diseases

> **Toxic Shock Syndrome**
> Multiple organ system failure due to
> *S. aureus* exotoxin (rare condition)

Risk Factors
- tampon use
- diaphragm, cervical cap or sponge use (prolonged use, i.e. >24 hours)
- wound infections
- post-partum infections
- early recognition and treatment of syndrome is imperative as incorrect diagnosis can be fatal

Clinical Presentation
- sudden high fever
- sore throat, headache, diarrhea
- erythroderma
- signs of multisystem failure
- refractory hypotension
- exfoliation of palmar and plantar surfaces of the hands and feet 1-2 weeks after onset of illness

Treatment
- remove potential sources of infection (foreign objects and wound debris)
- debride necrotic tissues
- adequate hydration
- penicillinase-resistant antibiotics – cloxacillin
- steroid use controversial but if started within 72 hours, may reduce severity of symptoms and duration of fever

Surgical Infections

Post Operative Infections in Gynecological Surgery
- pelvic cellulitis
  - common post hysterectomy, affects vaginal vault
  - erythema, induration, tenderness, discharge involving vaginal cuff
  - treat if fever and leukocytosis with broad spectrum antibiotics, i.e. clindamycin and gentamicin
  - drain if excessive purulence or large mass
  - can result in intra-abdominal and pelvic abscess

Sexuality and Sexual Dysfunction

SEXUAL RESPONSE
1. desire – energy that allows an individual to initiate or respond to sexual stimulation
2. arousal – physical and emotional stimulation leading to breast and genital vasodilation and clitoral engorgement
3. orgasm – physical and emotional stimulation is maximized, allowing the individual to relinquish their sense of control
4. resolution – most of the congestion and tension resolves within seconds, complete resolution may take up to 60 minutes

SEXUAL DYSFUNCTION

Etiology
- intrapsychic – patient's life experiences, value system
- relationship/interpersonal issues
- physical/organic

Classification
- lack of desire (60-70% of women)
- lack of arousal
- anorgasmia (5-10%)
  - primary anorgasmia: patient has never been able to achieve orgasm under any circumstances
  - secondary anorgasmia: patient was able to achieve orgasms before but now unable to do so
- dyspareunia (3-6%) – painful intercourse; superficial (pain with entry) or deep (pain with deeper penetration)
  - vaginismus (15%)
  - vulvodynia
  - vulvar vestibulitis: associated with history of frequent yeast infections

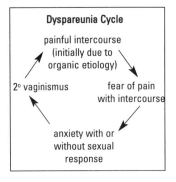

Dyspareunia Cycle

painful intercourse (initially due to organic etiology)

2° vaginismus

fear of pain with intercourse

anxiety with or without sexual response

Treatment
- lack of desire – assess factors, r/o organic causes, relationship therapy, sensate focus exercises
- anorgasmia – self-exploration/pleasuring, couple therapy if needed, bridging techniques (different sexual positions, clitoral stimulation during intercourse)
- dyspareunia
  - Kegel and reverse Kegel exercises
  - dilator treatment
  - comfort with self-exam
  - psychotherapy, other behavioural techniques
  - female on top position – allows for control of speed and duration
  - vestibulitis – remove local irritants, change in contraceptive methods, and dietary changes (↑ citrate, ↓ oxalate), vestibulectomy (rare)
  - vulvodynia – local moisturization, cold compresses, systemic nerve blocking therapy (amitriptyline, neurontin), topical anesthetic, estrogen cream

Kegel Exercises
Regular clenching and unclenching to strengthen pelvic floor muscles
Reverse Kegel Exercises
1 second contraction then 5 seconds of relaxation

Menopause

- see Family Medicine

Definitions
- types of menopause
  a) physiological; average age 51 years (follicular atresia)
  b) premature ovarian failure; before age 40 (autoimmune disorder, infection, Turner's syndrome)
  c) iatrogenic (surgical/radiation/chemotherapy)

- **menopause**: occurrence of last spontaneous menstrual period, resulting from loss of ovarian function (loss of oocyte response to gonadotropins)
- **"being in menopause"**: lack of menses for 1 yr
- **perimenopause**: period of time surrounding menopause (2-8 yrs preceding + 1 yr after last menses) characterized by fluctuating hormone levels, irregular menstrual cycles, and symptom onset

Clinical Features
- associated with estrogen deficiency
  - vasomotor instability (tends to dissipate with time)
    - hot flushes/flashes, night sweats, sleep disturbances, formication, nausea, palpitations
  - urogenital atrophy involving vagina, urethra, bladder
    - dyspareunia, vaginal itching, vaginal dryness, bleeding, urinary frequency, urgency, incontinence
  - skeletal
    - osteoporosis, joint and muscle pain, back pain
  - skin and soft tissue
    - decreased breast size, skin thinning/loss of elasticity
  - psychological
    - mood disturbance, irritability, fatigue, decreased libido, memory loss

- 85% of women experience hot flashes
- 20-30% seek medical attention
- 10% are unable to work

Investigations
- increased levels of FSH (>35 IU/L) on day 3 of cycle (if still cycling) and LH (FSH>LH)
- decreased levels of estradiol (later)

- Osteoporosis is the single most important health hazard associated with menopause
- Cardiovascular disease is the leading cause of death post-menopause

Treatment
- goal is for individual symptom management
  - vasomotor instability
    - HRT (first line), clonidine, SSRI, Effexor®, gabapentin, propanolol
  - vaginal atrophy
    - local estrogen – cream (Premarin®)/vaginal suppository (VagiFem®)/ring form (Estring®)
    - lubricants (Replens®)

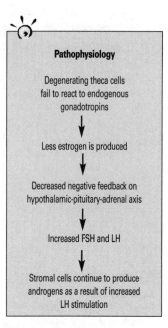

Pathophysiology

Degenerating theca cells fail to react to endogenous gonadotropins

↓

Less estrogen is produced

↓

Decreased negative feedback on hypothalamic-pituitary-adrenal axis

↓

Increased FSH and LH

↓

Stromal cells continue to produce androgens as a result of increased LH stimulation

Absolute Contraindications to HRT – "ABCD"

A: **A**cute liver disease

B: undiagnosed vaginal **B**leeding

C: **C**ancer (breast/uterine)

D: **D**VT (thromboembolic disease)

Excerpt from the SOGC 2006 Menopause Consensus Report
The primary indication for HRT is for the management of moderate to severe menopausal symptoms. HRT should be prescribed at the lowest effective dose for the appropriate duration to achieve treatment goals.

- osteoporosis
  - 1000-1200 mg calcium daily, 400-800 IU vitamin D, weight-bearing exercise, quit smoking
  - bisphosphonates (e.g. alendronate)
  - selective estrogen receptor modifiers (SERMs): raloxifene (Evista®) – mimics estrogen effects on bone, avoids estrogen-like action on breast and uterine cancer; does not help hot flashes
  - HRT – second-line treatment (unless for vasomotor instability as well)
- decreased libido
  - vaginal lubrication, sexual counseling, rarely androgen replacement (testosterone cream)
- cardiovascular disease
  - management of cardiovascular risk factors
- alternative choices (not evidence-based)
  - black cohosh, phytoestrogens, St. John's wort, gingko biloba, valerian, evening primrose oil, ginseng, Don Quai
- well-being
  - physical exercise, relaxation, yoga

Hormone Replacement Therapy (HRT)

- see Family Medicine
- for HRT regimens, see Table 7
- primary indication is treatment of menopausal symptoms (vasomotor instability)
- keep doses low (e.g. 0.3 mg Premarin®) and duration of treatment short (≤5 years)

HRT Components
- estrogen
  - oral or transdermal (e.g. patch, gel)
  - transdermal preferred for women with hypertriglyceridemia or impaired hepatic function
  - low-dose (e.g. 0.3 mg Premarin®/25 μg Estradot® patch)
- progestin
  - given in combination with estrogen for women with an intact uterus to prevent development of endometrial hyperplasia/cancer

Table 7. Examples of HRT Regimens

HRT Regimen	Estrogen Dose	Progestin Dose	Notes
Unopposed estrogen	CEE 0.625 mg PO OD	N/A	1. if no intact uterus
Standard-dose	CEE 0.625 mg PO OD	MPA 2.5 mg PO OD	1. withdrawal bleeding occurs in a spotty, unpredictable manner 2. usually abates after 6-8 months due to endometrial atrophy 3. once patient has become amenorrheic on HRT, significant subsequent bleeding episodes require evaluation (endometrial biopsy)
Standard-dose cyclic	CEE 0.625 mg PO OD	MPA 5-10 mg PO days 1-14 only	1. bleeding occurs monthly after day 14 of progestin (can continue for years) 2. PMS-like symptoms (breast tenderness, fluid retention, headache, nausea) are more prominent with cyclic HRT
Pulsatile	CEE 0.625 mg PO OD	MPA low-dose	1. 3 days on, 3 days off
Transdermal	Estroderm®-Estradiol 0.05 mg/d or 0.1 mg/d Estalis®-Estradiol® 140 μg/d or 250 μg/d	Estroderm®-MPA 2.5 mg PO OD Estalis®-NEA 50 μg/d	1. use patch twice weekly 2. can use oral progestins (Estroderm®) 3. combined patches available (Estalis®)

CEE = conjugated equine estrogen (e.g. Premarin®)   MPA = medroxyprogesterone acetate (e.g. Provera®)
NEA = norethindrone acetate
Consider lower dose regimens, PREMPRO™ 0.45/1.5 (Premarin 0.45 mg and Provera 1.5 mg recently released in the United States)

Side Effects of HRT
- abnormal uterine bleeding
- mastodynia
- edema, bloating, heartburn, nausea
- mood changes (progesterone)
- can be worse in progesterone phase of combined therapy

Contraindications to HRT
- absolute
  - acute liver disease
  - undiagnosed vaginal bleeding
  - known or suspected uterine cancer/breast cancer
  - acute vascular thrombosis or history of severe thrombophlebitis or thromboembolic disease
- relative
  - pre-existing uncontrolled hypertension
  - uterine fibroids and endometriosis
  - familial hyperlipidemias
  - migraine headaches

- family history of estrogen-dependent cancer
- chronic thrombophlebitis
- diabetes mellitus (with vascular disease)
- gallbladder disease, hypertriglyceridemia, impaired liver function (consider transdermal estrogen)
- fibrocystic disease of the breasts

WOMEN'S HEALTH INITIATIVE (WHI) (launched in 1991)

- two studies investigating health risks and benefits of hormone therapy in healthy postmenopausal women 50-79 years old; the WHI Extension Study, involving follow-up health tracking without intervention, is due to last through 2010
  - continuous combined HRT (CEE 0.625 mg + MPA 2.5 mg OD) in 16,608 women with an intact uterus
    - originally designed to run 8.5 years - stopped early after 5.2 years (July 2002) because the evidence for harm (breast cancer, CHD, stroke, PE) outweighed benefit (fracture reduction, colon cancer reduction)
  - estrogen-alone (CEE 0.625 mg) in 10,739 women with a previous hysterectomy
    - also stopped early (February 2004 instead of March 2005) because of increased stroke risk and no heart disease benefit
- benefits and risks reported as # cases per 10,000 women each year

HRT Benefits

- protective against osteoporotic fractures (recommended as 2nd line treatment only)
  - hip fractures – 5 fewer cases with combined HRT (6 fewer cases with estrogen-alone)
  - all fractures – 47 fewer cases with combined HRT
- colon cancer – 6 fewer cases with combined HRT (1 additional case with estrogen-alone)

HRT Risks

- invasive breast cancer – 8 additional cases with combined HRT
  - risk comparable to being 20% overweight, lacking regular exercise, fewer pregnancies after 30 years of age, reduced breastfeeding, excessive alcohol or cigarette use
  - NO increased risk with estrogen-alone (7 *fewer* cases)
- coronary heart disease – 7 additional MIs with combined HRT
  - no significant difference in cardiac deaths between treatment and control groups
  - NO elevated heart risks if used right after menopause (~45-55 years of age), or with estrogen-alone (5 *fewer* cases)
- DVTs or PEs – 18 additional cases with combined HRT
  - 9 additional cases for women taking estrogen-alone
- stroke – 8 additional cases with combined HRT (not statistically significant)
  - 12 additional cases with estrogen-alone
- dementia and mild cognitive impairment (WHI Memory Score)
  - women taking estrogen-alone before 65 years of age were less likely to develop dementia, *however* there was a 50% *increased* risk of developing dementia when taken after 65 years of age (those taking combined HRT were at even greater risk)
  - "window of opportunity" hypothesis: early use of estrogen (before pre-dementia changes) protects the healthy brain; in older women, where changes have already begun, use of estrogen accelerates the dementia process
- there were no significant differences in overall mortality or cause of death between treatment and placebo groups

Urogynecology

Pelvic Relaxation/Prolapse

Etiology

- relaxation, weakness, or defect in the cardinal and uterosacral ligaments which normally maintain the uterus in an anteflexed position and prevent it from descending through the urogenital diaphragm (i.e. levator ani muscles)
- related to:
  - vaginal childbirth
  - aging
  - decreased estrogen (post-menopause)
  - following pelvic surgery
  - increased intra-abdominal pressure (obesity, chronic cough, constipation, ascites, heavy lifting)
  - congenital (rarely)
  - ethnicity (white women > Asian or black women)

> **Pelvic Relaxation/Prolapse**
> Protrusion of pelvic organs into or out of the vaginal canal

GENERAL CONSERVATIVE TREATMENT
(for Pelvic Relaxation/Prolapse and Urinary Incontinence)

- Kegel exercises
- local vaginal estrogen therapy
- vaginal pessary

UTERINE PROLAPSE

Clinical Features
- protrusion of cervix and uterus into vagina
- groin/back pain (stretching of uterosacral ligaments)
- feeling of heaviness/pressure in the pelvis
  - worse with standing, lifting
  - worse at the end of the day
  - relieved by lying down
- ulceration/bleeding (particularly if hypoestrogenic)
- ± urinary incontinence

Treatment
- see General Conservative Treatment
- surgical
  - vaginal hysterectomy ± surgical prevention of vault prolapse
  - consider additional surgical procedures if urinary incontinence, cystocele, rectocele, and/or enterocele are present

VAULT PROLAPSE

Treatment
- see General Conservative Treatment
- surgical
  - sacralcolpopexy (vaginal vault suspension), sacrospinous fixation, or uterosacral ligament suspension

CYSTOCELE

Clinical Features
- frequency, urgency, nocturia
- stress incontinence
- incomplete bladder emptying ± associated increased incidence of urinary tract infections

Treatment
- see General Conservative Treatment
- surgical
  - anterior colporrhaphy ("anterior repair")
  - consider additional/alternative surgical procedure if documented urinary stress incontinence

RECTOCELE

Clinical Features
- straining/digitation to evacuate stool
- constipation

Treatment
- conservative
  - see General Conservative Treatment
  - laxatives and stool softeners
  - vaginal pessary (usually not helpful)
- surgical
  - posterior colporrhaphy ("posterior repair"), plication of endopelvic fascia and perineal muscles approximated in midline to support rectum and perineum
  - can result in dyspareunia

ENTEROCELE

Treatment
- surgical
  - similar to hernia repair
  - contents reduced, neck of peritoneal sac ligated, uterosacral ligaments, and levator ani muscles approximated

---

Uterine Prolapse Classification
- 0 = no descent
- 1 = descent between normal position and ischial spines
- 2 = descent between ischial spines and hymen
- 3 = descent within hymen
- 4 = descent through hymen
- **procidentia**: failure of genital supports and complete protrusion of uterus through the vagina

Vault Prolapse
Protrusion of apex of vaginal vault into vagina, post-hysterectomy

Cystocele
Protrusion of bladder into the anterior vaginal wall

Rectocele
Protrusion of rectum into posterior vaginal wall

Enterocele
Prolapse of small bowel in upper posterior vaginal wall

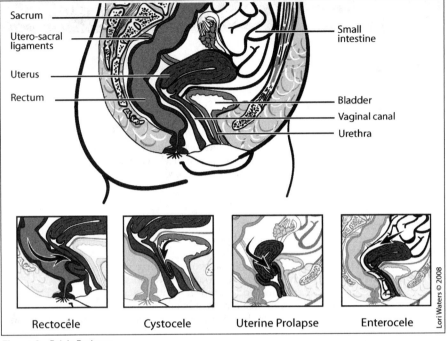

Figure 9. Pelvic Prolapse

> The only **true** hernia of the pelvis is an ENTEROCELE because peritoneum herniates with the small bowel.

Urinary Incontinence

- see Urology

STRESS INCONTINENCE

Risk Factors for Stress Incontinence in Women
- pelvic prolapse
- pelvic surgery
- vaginal delivery
- hypoestrogenic state (post-menopause)
- age
- smoking
- neurological/pulmonary disease

Treatment
- see *General Conservative Treatment*, GY36
- **surgical**
  - tension-free vaginal tape (TVT), tension-free obturator tape (TOT), prosthetic/fascial slings or retropubic bladder suspension (Burch or Marshall-Marchetti-Krantz procedures)

URGE INCONTINENCE

Definition
- urine loss associated with an abrupt, sudden urge to void
- "overactive bladder"
- diagnosed based on symptoms

Etiology
- idiopathic (90%)
- detrusor muscle overactivity ("detrusor instability")

Associated Symptoms
- frequency, urgency, nocturia, leakage

Treatment
- behaviour modification (reduce caffeine/liquid, smoking cessation, regular voiding schedule)
- Kegel exercises
- medications
  - anticholinergics – oxybutinin (Ditropan®), tolterodine (Detrol®)
  - tricyclic antidepressants – imipramine

> **Stress Incontinence**
> Involuntary loss of urine with increased intra-abdominal pressure (coughing, laughing, sneezing, walking, running)

> The gold standard diagnostic test for urinary incontinence is multi-channel urodynamics. A large proportion of cases are correctly diagnosed from clinical history alone and this can be supplemented with patient urinary and intake diaries.
> *Health Technol Assess.* 2006 Feb; 10(6):1-132.

> **Urge Incontinence**
> Urine loss associated with an abrupt, sudden urge to void

> **Must rule out anything neurological for urge incontinence**
> Multiple sclerosis
> Slipped disc
> Diabetes mellitus

Gynecological Oncology

Uterus

LEIOMYOMATA (FIBROIDS)

Leiomyomata/Fibroids
Benign smooth muscle tumour of the uterus (most common gynecological tumour)

Epidemiology
- diagnosed in approximately 40-50% of reproductive age women >35 years
- more common, larger, and occur at earlier age in black women
- most common indication for major surgery in females
- minimal malignant potential (1:1000)
- regress after menopause

Pathogenesis
- arise from smooth muscle (monoclonal proliferation)
- apoptosis is inhibited
- progesterone is most responsible for fibroid growth; estrogen causes little/no growth
- degenerative changes (occur when tumour outgrows blood supply)
    - hyaline degeneration (most common degenerative change)
    - cystic degeneration (from breakdown of hyaline)
    - red/carneous degeneration (hemorrhage into tumour, may occur with fibroid in pregnancy)
    - fatty degeneration
    - calcification
    - sarcomatous degeneration (extremely rare)
    - parasitic myoma – tumour becomes attached to omentum or small bowel mesentery, develops new blood supply, and loses connection to uterus

Clinical Features
- majority asymptomatic (60%), often discovered as incidental finding on U/S
- abnormal uterine bleeding (30%)
    - dysmenorrhea
    - menorrhagia
- pressure/bulk symptoms (20-50%)
    - pelvic pressure/heaviness
    - increased abdominal girth
    - urinary frequency and urgency
    - acute urinary retention (rare but surgical emergency!)
    - constipation, bloating (rare)
- acute pelvic pain if:
    - fibroid degeneration
    - fibroid torsion (pedunculated subserosal)
- infertility (submucosal) and pregnancy complications (difficult C-section)
- recurrent pregnancy loss

> Submucosal leiomyomata are most symptomatic (bleeding, infertility)

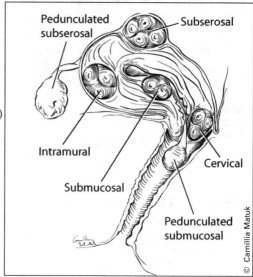

Figure 10. Possible Anatomic Locations of Uterine Leiomyomata

Investigations
- bimanual exam – uterus asymmetrically enlarged, mobile
- CBC – anemia
- ultrasound – assess location of fibroids
- sonohysterogram – useful for differentiating endometrial polyps from submucosal fibroids
- endometrial biopsy to rule out uterine cancer if abnormal uterine bleeding - especially if age >40 years
- occasionally MRI is used for prep planning

Treatment
- only if symptomatic, rapidly enlarging, or menorrhagia
- treat anemia if present
- conservative approach (watch and wait) if
    - symptoms absent or minimal
    - fibroids <6-8 cm or stable in size
    - not submucosal (i.e. submucosal fibroids are more likely to be symptomatic)
    - virtually all postmenopausal patients fall into this category
- medical approach
    - antiprostaglandins (ibuprofen)
    - tranexamic acid (Cyklokapron®)
    - OCP/Depo-Provera®
    - GnRH agonist – leuprolide (Lupron®), or androgen derivative – danazol (Danocrine®); short-term use only (6 months); often used pre-myomectomy to facilitate surgery (reduces fibroid size)
    - selective progesterone receptor modulators – currently in clinical trials; prototype is RU486 which reduces fibroid volume by 50% after 3 months without side effects of GnRH agonists
- interventional radiology approach
    - uterine artery embolization occludes both uterine arteries → shrinks fibroids by 50% at 6 months; improves menorrhagia in 90% of patients within 1-2 months (not an option in women considering childbearing)
- surgical approach
    - myomectomy (hysteroscopic, transabdominal or laparoscopic approach) – preserves childbearing capabilities
    - hysterectomy (abdominal, vaginal, or laparoscopic depending on fibroid size)
    - endometrial resection of fibroid and endometrial ablation
    - note – avoid operating on fibroids during pregnancy (due to ++ vascularity); expectant management only

ENDOMETRIAL CARCINOMA

Epidemiology
- most common gynecological malignancy in North America (40%); 4th most common cancer in women
- 2-3% of women develop endometrial carcinoma in lifetime
- mean age is 60 years
- majority are diagnosed early
- >90% 5-year survival for stage I disease
- overall 5-year survival for all stages is 60-70%

Risk Factors
- unopposed estrogen (estrogen unopposed by progesterone)
    - obesity
    - PCOS
    - HRT
- nulliparity
- late menopause
- chronic tamoxifen use
- estrogen-producing ovarian tumours (e.g. granulosa cell tumours)
- HNPCC (hereditary non-polyposis colorectal cancer)

Classification
- adenocarcinoma (most common 80%)
- adenosquamous carcinoma (15%)
- papillary serous adenocarcinoma (3-4% overall)

Clinical Features
- postmenopausal bleeding in 90%
- abnormal uterine bleeding (menorrhagia, intermenstrual bleeding)

Incidence of Malignant Gynecological Lesions
endometrium > ovary > cervix > vulva > vagina > fallopian tube

Risk Factors for Endometrial Cancer
"COLD NUT"
Cancer, (ovarian, breast, colon)
Obesity
Late Menopause
Diabetes mellitus

Nulliparity
Unopposed estrogen: PCOS, anovulation, HRT
Tamoxifen, chronic use

Postmenopausal bleeding is endometrial cancer until proven otherwise. 90% present with vaginal bleeding.

Table 8. FIGO Staging of Endometrial Cancer

Stage	Description	Stage	Description
0	carcinoma in situ	III	outside of uterus but not beyond true pelvis
		IIIA	serosal/adnexal invasion +/- cancer cells in ascites
I	confined to corpus	IIIB	vaginal metastases or direct extension
IA	tumour limited to the endometrium	IIIC	pelvic/para-aortic lymph nodes (LNs)
IB	invades through < one half of myometrium		
IC	invades through > one half of myometrium	IV	outside true pelvis
		IVA	bowel and bladder involvement
II	involves corpus and cervix	IVB	distant metastases, including metastasis to
IIA	endocervical glandular involvement only		intra-abdominal LNs, other than para-aortic and/or
IIB	cervical stromal invasion		inguinal LNs (not including metastasis to vagina,
			pelvic serosa, or adnexa)

FIGO: International Federation of Gynecology and Obstetrics

Investigations
- office endometrial biopsy
- D&C ± hysteroscopy

Spread
- most common is direct extension
- transtubal dissemination, lymphatic spread to pelvic and para-aortic nodes
- hematogenous spread (usually to lungs)

Treatment
- based on tumour grade and depth of myometrial invasion
- surgical: TAH/BSO and pelvic washings ± pelvic and periaortic node dissection
  - general trend (controversial)
        Stage 1 – TAH/BSO and washings
        Stages 2 and 3 – TAH/BSO, washings, and node dissection
        Stage 4 – no surgical option
- adjuvant radiotherapy – for selected patients based on depth of myometrial invasion, tumour grade, and/or lymph node involvement
- hormonal therapy – progestins for distant or recurrent disease
- adjuvant chemotherapy – if disease progresses

UTERINE SARCOMA
- rare – 2-6% of all uterine malignancies
- behave more aggressively and are associated with poorer prognosis
- arise from stromal components (endometrial stroma, mesenchymal or myometrial tissues)
- vaginal bleeding is most common presenting symptom
- 5-year survival – 35%

Leiomyosarcoma
- account for one third of uterine sarcomas
- benign leiomyomata (fibroids) and leiomyosarcomata often coexist in the same uterus; however, they are independent entities
- average age of presentation is 55 years
- histologic distinction (from leiomyoma)
  - ↑ mitotic count (≥10 mitoses/10 high power fields)
  - tumour necrosis
  - cellular atypia
- most are diagnosed postoperatively after uterus removed for fibroids

Clinical Features
- rapidly enlarging fibroid in a post-menopausal woman

Treatment
- TAH/BSO
- no adjuvant therapy given if disease confined to uterus and low malignant potential (mitotic index is low)
- radiation if high mitotic index
- chemotherapy (~25% response rate) if tumour spread beyond uterus

Endometrial Stromal Sarcoma
- presents mainly in perimenopausal women between age 45-50 years as abnormal uterine bleeding
- diagnosed by histology of endometrial biopsy or D&C

Treatment
- TAH/BSO, ALWAYS remove ovaries
- hormonal therapy (progestins) in low grade sarcoma ONLY

Mixed Müllerian Sarcoma (Carcinosarcoma)

- most common type of uterine sarcoma (43%)
- both epithelial and sarcomatous elements must be present
- both components may arise from a common progenitor cell that is capable of multilineage differentiation
- aggressive tumours with a propensity for extrauterine metastases
- tend to form bulky polypoid masses that often fill the uterine cavity and extend into or through the endocervical canal

Treatment
- treatment is the same as leiomyosarcoma, radiation often used

Ovary

Table 9. Ultrasound Characteristics of Benign vs. Malignant Ovarian Tumours

Benign	Malignant
<8-10 cm in diameter	>10 cm in diameter
Unilateral	Bilateral
Cystic	Solid elements (internal papillary structures/mural nodules)
Uniloculated	Multiloculated
Thin septations	Thick septations
No ascites	Ascites

BENIGN OVARIAN TUMOURS
- see Tables 10 and 11
- most are asymptomatic
- usually enlarge slowly
- may rupture or undergo torsion, causing pain
- the pain associated with torsion of an adnexal mass usually originates in the iliac fossa and radiates to the flank
- peritoneal irritation may result from an infarcted tumour - rare

MALIGNANT OVARIAN TUMOURS
- see Tables 10 and 11

Epidemiology
- lifetime risk 1.4% (1/70)
- in women >50 years, more than 50% of ovarian tumours are malignant
- causes more deaths in North America than all other gynecologic malignancies combined
- 4th leading cause of cancer death in women
- 65% epithelial; 35% non-epithelial
- 5-10% of epithelial ovarian cancers have hereditary predisposition

Risk Factors
- nulliparity
- early menarche/late menopause
- age
- family history of breast, colon, endometrial, ovarian cancer
- race – Caucasian

Protective Factors
- OCP – possibly because of ovulation suppression (even after 1 year of use)
- pregnancy/breastfeeding
- tubal ligation
- hysterectomy

Clinical Features
- usually asymptomatic until disseminated
- most present as Stage III disease (advanced)
- early
  - post-menopausal bleeding; irregular menses if pre-menopausal (rare)
  - vague abdominal symptoms (nausea, bloating, dyspepsia, anorexia, early satiety)

Risk of Malignancy Index (RMI)
RMI = U x M x CA125
ULTRASOUND FINDINGS (1 pt for each)
- multilocular cyst
- evidence of solid areas
- evidence of metastases
- presence of ascites
- bilateral lesions
U = 1 (for U/S scores of 0 or 1)
U = 3 (for U/S scores of 2-5)
MENOPAUSAL STATUS
- Postmenopausal: M = 3
- Premenopausal: M = 1
ABSOLUTE VALUE OF CA125
SERUM LEVEL
RMI>200: Gynecologic Oncology referral is recommended

BJOG. 1999. 932:448-52.

Risk/Protective Factors for Ovarian Cancer "NO CHILD"
Nulliparity
OCP, breast-feeding, tubal ligation, hysterectomy (all protective)
Caucasian
Family **H**istory
Increasing age (>40)
Late menopause
Delayed child-bearing

Any adnexal mass in postmenopausal women should be considered malignant until proven otherwise.

Most (70%) ovarian cancers present at stage III disease.

Diagnosis requires surgical pathology.

- late (due to mass effect)
  - increased abdominal girth – from ascites or tumour itself
  - urinary frequency
  - constipation
  - fluid wave

LOW MALIGNANT POTENTIAL TUMOURS
- often called "borderline" tumours
- about 15% of all epithelial type ovarian tumours
- tumour cells display malignant characteristics histologically, but no invasion is identified
- able to metastasize
- treated with surgery
- NO proven benefit of chemotherapy
- slow growing, excellent prognosis
- 5-year survival >99%
- pregnancy, OCP, and breastfeeding are found to be protective

Table 10. Benign Ovarian Tumours

Type	Description	Presentation	Ultrasound/Cytology	Treatment
Functional Tumours (all benign)				
Follicular cyst	• follicle fails to rupture during ovulation	• usually asymptomatic • may rupture, bleed, tort, infarct causing pain ± signs of peritoneal irritation	• 4-8 cm mass, unilocular, lined with granulosa cells	• if <6 cm, wait 6 weeks then re-examine as cyst usually regresses with next cycle • OCP (ovarian suppression) – will prevent development of new cysts • treatment usually laparoscopic • painful, multiloculated, or partially solid masses warrant surgical exploration
Lutein cyst	• corpus luteum fails to regress after 14 days, becoming cystic or hemorrhagic	• more likely to cause pain than follicular cyst • may delay onset of next period	• larger (10-15 cm) and firmer than follicular cysts	• same as for follicular cysts
Theca-lutein cyst	• due to atretic follicles stimulated by abnormal β-hCG levels	• associated with molar pregnancy, ovulation induction with clomiphene		• conservative • cyst will regress as β-hCG levels fall
Luteoma of pregnancy	• usually bilateral • due to prolonged elevation of β-hCG	• associated with multiple pregnancy		• same as for theca-lutein • regresses postpartum
Endometrioma	• see *Endometriosis*, GY17			
Polycystic Ovaries	• see *PCOS*, GY24			

Table 11. Neoplastic Ovarian Tumours

Type	Description	Presentation	Ultrasound/Cytology	Treatment
Benign Germ-Cell Tumours				
Benign cystic teratoma (dermoid)	• single most common solid ovarian neoplasm • elements of all 3 cell lines, contains dermal appendages (sweat and sebaceous glands, hair follicles, teeth)	• may rupture, twist, infarct • 20% bilateral • 20% occur outside of reproductive years	• smooth-walled, mobile, unilocular • ultrasound may show calcification which is pathognomonic	• cystectomy • may recur
Malignant Germ-Cell Tumours				
General	• children and young women	• aggressive, rapidly growing, 2-3% of all ovarian cancers		• surgical resection (often conservative unilateral salpingo-oophorectomy) ± chemo, ± radiation
Dysgerminoma	• produces lactate dehydrogenase (LDH)	• 10% bilateral		• usually very responsive to chemotherapy, therefore complete resection is not necessary for cure
Immature teratoma				
Yolk sac tumour	• produces alpha fetoprotein (AFP) • rare	• unilateral		
Embryonal carcinoma	• produces AFP and hCG, rare			
Choriocarcinoma	• produces hCG	• see *GTN*, GY49		
Epithelial Ovarian Tumours				
General (benign, malignant or borderline)	• derived from mesothelial cells lining peritoneal cavity • 80-85% of all ovarian neoplasms (includes malignant)		• varies depending on subtype	**Benign:** cystectomy unilateral salpingo-oophorectomy **Malignant:** 1. Early (stage 1A & 1B): TAH/BSO + omentectomy + peritoneal washings + staging (peritoneal biopsy + node dissection) 2. Advanced: cytoreductive (debulking) surgery If cannot remove, debulk to residual disease <1 cm combination (platinum + taxol)
Serous	• most common ovarian tumour • 50% of all ovarian cancers (75% of epithelial) • 70% benign	• 20-30% bilateral	• lining similar to fallopian tube epithelium • often multilocular • histologically contain Psamomma bodies (calcified concentric concretions)	

Table 11. Neoplastic Ovarian Tumours (continued)

Type	Description	Presentation	Ultrasound/Cytology	Treatment
Epithelial Ovarian Tumours				
Mucinous	• 85% benign (20% of epithelial)	• rarely complicated by *Pseudomyxoma peritonei*: implants seed abdominal cavity and produce large quantities of mucus	• resembles endocervical epithelium • often multilocular • may reach enormous size	• chemotherapy • radiation in patients with no residual disease (rare) • if mucinous - remove appendix as well
Endometrioid	• 20% of epithelial ovarian Ca • high malignant potential		• histology resembles endometrium but non-invasive (vs. endometriosis)	
Clear cell	• ≤1% of epithelial ovarian Ca • high malignant potential		• histology resembles mesonephric cells	
Brenner Tumour	• ≤1 % of epithelial ovarian Ca • majority benign		• fibrotic tumour with transitional cell–like epithelial core	
Sex Cord Stromal Ovarian Tumours				
Fibroma (benign)	• from mature fibroblasts in ovarian stroma	• non-functioning • occasionally associated with Meig's syndrome	• firm, smooth rounded tumour with interlacing fibrocytes	• surgical resection of tumour • chemotherapy not effective for cancer
Granulosa-theca cell tumours (benign or malignant)	• can be associated with endometrial cancer	• estrogen-producing → feminizing effects (precocious puberty, menorrhagia, post-menopausal bleeding)	• histologic hallmark of cancer is small groups of cells known as Call-Exner bodies	
Sertoli-Leydig cell tumours (benign or malignant)		• androgen-producing → virilizing effects (hirsutism, deep voice, recession of front hairline)		
Metastatic Ovarian Tumours				
From GI tract, breast, endometrium, lymphoma	• 4-8% of ovarian malignancies		• Krukenberg tumour = metastatic tumour from GI tract (usually stomach) with "signet-ring" cells	

Investigation of suspicious ovarian mass
- bimanual examination
- solid, irregular, fixed pelvic mass is suggestive of ovarian cancer
- bloodwork – CA-125 for baseline, CBC, liver function tests, electrolytes, creatinine
- radiology – chest x-ray, abdo/pelvic U/S ± transvaginal U/S; CT or U/S to assess urinary tract
- bone scan **not** indicated
- try to rule out primary
  - occult blood – if positive, endoscopy ± barium enema
  - if gastric symptoms, gastroscopy ± upper GI series
  - if abnormal vaginal bleed, Pap test and endometrial biopsy to rule out concurrent endometrial or cervical cancer
  - mammogram

Screening
- no effective method of mass screening
- routine CA-125 level measurements **not** recommended
- controversial in high risk groups – starting age 30, transvaginal U/S and CA-125 (no consensus on interval)
  - familial ovarian cancer (≥1 first degree relative affected, BRCA-1)
  - other cancers (i.e. endometrial, breast, colon)
  - may recommend prophylactic bilateral oophorectomy after age 35 or when child-bearing is completed (BRCA-1 or BRCA-2 mutation)

Benign Stromal Cell Tumours Meig's Syndrome
Fibroma
Ascites
Right pleural effusion

Causes of Elevated CA-125
- Age influences reliability of test as a tumour marker
- 50% sensitivity in early stage ovarian cancer

MALIGNANT
- Gyne: ovary, uterus
- Non-Gyne: pancreas, stomach, colon, rectum

NON MALIGNANT
- Gyne: benign ovarian neoplasm, endometriosis, pregnancy, fibroids, PID
- Non-Gyne: cirrhosis, pancreatitis, renal failure

CA-125 for monitoring response to treatment

Table 12. FIGO Staging for Primary Carcinoma of the Ovary (Surgical Staging)

Stage	Description
I	Growth limited to the ovaries
IA	1 ovary, no ascites
IB	2 ovaries, no ascites
IC	1 or 2 ovaries with any of the following: capsule ruptured, tumour on ovarian surface or malignant cells in ascites
II	Growth involving one or both ovaries with pelvic extension
IIA	Extension to uterus/tubes
IIB	Extension to other pelvic structures
IIC	II A/B with malignant cells in ascites or positive peritoneal washings
III	Tumour involving one or both ovaries with peritoneal implants outside the pelvis and/or positive retroperitoneal or inguinal nodes
IIIA	Microscopic peritoneal metastasis beyond pelvis
IIIB	Macroscopic peritoneal metastasis beyond pelvis <2 cm
IIIC	Implant >2 cm and/or retroperitoneal or inguinal nodes
IV	Distant metastasis beyond peritoneal cavity

> **Malignant Ovarian Tumour Prognosis 5-year survival**
> • Stage I: 75-95%
> • Stage II: 60-75%
> • Stage III: 23-41%
> • Stage IV: 11%
> • overall 5-year survival: 40% compared to 15% if >50 years of age

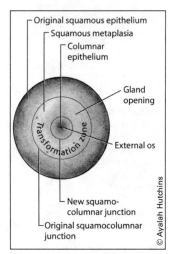

Figure 11. The Cervix

Cervix

BENIGN CERVICAL LESIONS
• Nabothian cyst/inclusion cyst
 ▪ no treatment required
• endocervical polyps
 ▪ treatment is polypectomy (office procedure)

MALIGNANT CERVICAL LESIONS
• squamous cell carcinoma (95%), adenocarcinoma (5%)
• 8,000 deaths annually in North America
• annual Pap test reduces a woman's chances of dying from cervical cancer from 4/1,000 to 5/10,000
• average age 52 years old

Etiology
• at birth, vagina is lined with squamous epithelium; columnar epithelium lines only the endocervix and the central area of the ectocervix (original squamocolumnar junction)
• during puberty, estrogen stimulates eversion of a single columnar layer (ectopy), thus exposing it to the acidic pH of the vagina, leading to metaplasia (columnar to squamous)
• metaplastic squamous epithelium covers the columnar epithelium and a new squamocolumnar junction is formed closer to the external os
• the transformation zone (TZ) is an area of squamous metaplasia located between the original and the new squamocolumnar junction (Figure 11)
• the majority of dysplasias and cancers arise in the TZ of the cervix
• must have active metaplasia and inducing agent to get dysplasia

Risk Factors
• HPV infection
 ▪ see *Sexually Transmitted Infections*, GY27
 ▪ high risk associated with types 16, 18
 ▪ low risk associated with types 6, 11
 ▪ 99% of cervical cancers contain one of the high risk HPV types
• smoking
• high risk behaviour
 ▪ multiple partners
 ▪ other STIs (HSV, trichomonas)
 ▪ early age first intercourse
 ▪ high risk male partner
• other – low socioeconomic status

> Cervical cancer is caused by HPV infection.

Prevention: Quadrivalent HPV Recombinant Vaccine (Gardasil®)
• for females 9 to 26 years of age for prevention of diseases caused by HPV types 6, 11, 16 and 18 (cervical cancer, genital warts, cervical, vulvar and vaginal dysplasias)

- for full benefit, should be administered before onset of sexual activity (i.e. before exposure to virus)
- administered IM at time 0, 2, and 6 months, may be given at the same time as Hep B or other vaccines using a different injection site
- not designed to treat active infections
- most women will not be infected with all four types of the virus at the same time, therefore vaccine is still indicated for females with history of an active or previous HPV infection
- conception should be avoided until 30 days after last dose of vaccination
- side effects – pain, swelling, erythema, low grade fever
- contraindications – pregnant women and women who are nursing (limited data)

Clinical Features
- squamous cell carcinoma (SCC)
  - exophytic, fungating tumour
- adenocarcinoma
  - endophytic, with barrel-shaped cervix
- early
  - asymptomatic
  - discharge – initially watery, becoming brown or red
  - post-coital bleeding
- late
  - 80-90% present with bleeding – either postcoital, postmenopausal or irregular bleeding
  - spontaneous irregular bleeding
  - pelvic or back pain (extension of tumour to pelvic walls)
  - bladder/bowel symptoms
- signs – friable, raised, reddened area

Pathogenesis
- dysplasia → carcinoma in situ (CIS) → invasion
- slow process (years)
- growth is by local extension
- metastasis occurs late

Cervical Screening Guidelines (Pap Test)
- endocervical and exocervical cell sampling, TZ sampling
- false positives 5-10%, false negatives 10-40%
- identifies squamous cell carcinoma, less reliable for adenocarcinoma
- all women – start screening at age 21, or 3 years after onset of vaginal intercourse
- women >30 years – If 3 normal Paps in a row, and no previous abnormal Paps, can get screened every 2-3 years (if adequate recall mechanism in place)
- women >70 years – If 3 normal Paps in a row and NO abnormal Paps in last 10 years, can discontinue screening
- pregnant women and women who have sex with women should follow the routine cervical screening regimen
- hysterectomy
  - total – discontinue screening if hysterectomy was for benign disease and NO history of cervical dysplasia or HPV infection
  - subtotal – continue screening according to guidelines
- exceptions to guidelines
  - immunocompromised (transplant, steroids, DES exposure)
  - HIV and high risk
  - unscreened patients

Table 13. Cytological Classification

Bethesda Grading System	Classic System/ Cervical Intraepithelial Neoplasia (CIN) Grading System
• within normal limits	• normal
• infection	• inflammatory atypia (organism)
• reactive and reparative changes	
• squamous cell abnormalities	
• atypical squamous cells of undetermined significance (ASCUS)	• squamous atypia of uncertain significance
• atypical squamous cells, cannot exclude HSIL (ASC-H)	
• low grade squamous intraepithelial lesion (LSIL)	• HPV atypia or mild dysplasia (CIN I)
• high grade squamous intraepithelial lesion (HSIL)	• moderate dysplasia (CIN II)
	• severe dysplasia (CIN III)
	• carcinoma in situ (CIS)
• squamous cell carcinoma (SCC)	• squamous cell carcinoma (SCC)
• glandular cell abnormalities	
• atypical glandular cells of undetermined significance (AGUS)	• glandular atypia of uncertain significance
• endocervical adenocarcinoma	• adenocarcinoma
• endometrial adenocarcinoma	
• extrauterine adenocarcinoma	
• adenocarcinoma, not otherwise specified (NOS)	

Systematic Review of RCTs for HPV Vaccination
(Rambout L, Hopkins L, Fung Kee Fung M, et al. Prophylactic vaccination against human papillomavirus infection in women: a systematic review of randomized controlled trials. CMAJ 2007;177)

Purpose: To assess the effectiveness of HPV vaccination for preventing HPV infection and precancerous cervical lesions.
Study: Systematic review of studies of prophylactic HPV vaccination.
Data Sources: MEDLINE, EMBASE, Cochrane Central Registry of Controlled Trials, and the Cochrane Library.
Patients: Of 457 hits, nine were included in the review (six of these were RCTs). A total of 40323 females were studied. All participants had received HPV vaccinations that included coverage of the HPV 16 strain.
Main outcomes: Frequency of high-grade cervical lesions, persistent HPV infection, low-grade cervical lesions, external genital lesions, adverse events, and death.
Results: HPV vaccination was associated with a reduction in the frequency of high-grade cervical lesions caused by vaccine-type HPV strains compared with control groups. The HPV vaccination was also found to be efficacious in reducing persistent HPV infection, low-grade lesions, and genital warts.
Conclusion: Prophylactic vaccination of women between 15-25 years not previously infected with vaccine-type HPV strains, has been found to be efficacious in preventing HPV infection and precancerous cervical lesions.

Liquid-based cytologic smear vs. conventional Pap smear
(Am J Obstet Gynecol 2001 Aug;185(2):308-17.)

Purpose: To assess the cytologic diagnosis and sample adequacy of liquid-based cervical cytologic smear (ThinPrep) versus conventional Papanicolaou smear.
Study: Systematic review of prospective trials comparing ThinPrep and conventional Pap smears.
Data sources: MEDLINE, PubMed, Silver Platter were searched for literature published in English between January 1990 and April 2000. Selection criteria included split-sample (SS) and direct-to-vial (DV) (case-cohort) studies.
Patients: 25 studies met the selection criteria (n=533,039 women; 221,864 in ThinPrep group; 378,659 in conventional smear group; 67,484 in both groups)
Main outcomes: (i) Frequency of diagnoses of ASCUS, LSIL, HSIL. (ii) Adequacy of sample collection (contains squamous cells, endocervical cells, and possibly metaplastic cells).
Results: Liquid-based smears (ThinPrep) had significantly improved cytologic diagnosis of LSIL (OR = 1.27 to 2.15) and diagnosis of HSIL (OR = 2.26), but no difference in rate of diagnosis of ASCUS (OR = 1.03). Liquid-based pap smear also resulted in improved sample adequacy (OR = 1.64 to 2.11).
Conclusion: Liquid-based cytologic smears resulted in better diagnosis of cervical premalignant lesions (HSIL and LSIL) and improved sampled adequacy, compared to conventional Pap smears.

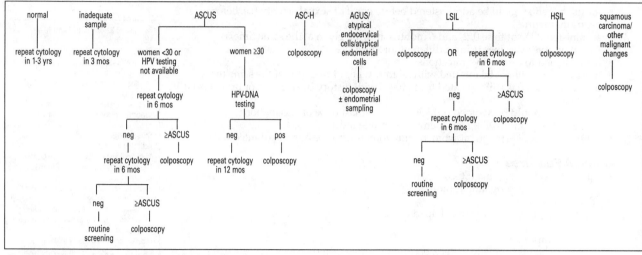

Figure 12. Decision Making Chart for Pap Test (not applicable for adolescents)
Adapted from Ontario Cervical Screening Practice Guidelines. June 2005.

The Bethesda Classification System is based on cytological results of a Pap test that permits the examination of cells but not tissue structure. The diagnosis of cervical intraepithelial neoplasia (CIN) or cervical carcinoma requires a tissue sample, obtained by biopsy of suspicious lesions (done during colposcopy), to make a histologic diagnosis.

Diagnosis
- see *Colposcopy*, GY11
- apply acetic acid and identify white lesions
- endocervical curettage (ECC) if entire lesion is not visible or no lesion visible
- cervical biopsy
- cone biopsy (under general anesthetic) if
  - lesion extends into endocervical canal
  - positive ECC
  - discrepancy between Pap test results and colposcopy
  - Pap test shows adenocarcinoma in situ
  - microinvasive carcinoma

Table 14. FIGO Staging Classification of Cervical Cancer

Stage	Description
0	carcinoma in situ (CIS)
I	confined to cervix
IA	microinvasive (diagnosed only by microscopy)
IA$_1$	stromal invasion not >3 mm deep, not >7 mm wide
IA$_2$	3-5 mm deep; not >7 mm wide
IB	clinically visible lesion confined to cervix, or microscopic lesion >IA$_2$
II	beyond uterus but not to the pelvic wall, does not involve lower 1/3 of vagina
IIA	no obvious parametrial involvement
IIB	obvious parametrial involvement
III	extends to pelvic wall and/or involves lower 1/3 of vagina and/or causes hydronephrosis or non-functioning kidney
IIIA	involves lower 1/3 vagina but no extension into pelvic sidewall
IIIB	involves lower 1/3 vagina and extends into pelvic sidewall and/or hydronephrosis or nonfunctioning kidney
IVA	beyond true pelvis ± distant spread, bladder, and/or rectum involved
IVB	distant metastases

Cervical Cancer Prognosis
5-year survival figures
- Stage 0: 99%
- Stage I: 75%
- Stage II: 55%
- Stage III: 30%
- Stage IV: 7%
- overall: 50-60%

Table 15. Treatment of Abnormal Pap Test and Cervical Cancer

	Treatment
CIN I (LSIL)	• observe with regular cytology (every 6 months) • many lesions will regress or disappear (60%) • colposcopy if positive on 2 consecutive tests • lesions which progress should have area excised by either LEEP, laser, cryotherapy or cone biopsy (with LEEP, tissues obtained for histological evaluation)
CIN II and CIN III (HSIL)	• colposcopy referral • LEEP, laser, cryotherapy, cone excision • hysterectomy – only if no desire for future childbearing
Stage 1A	• cervical conization if future fertility desired • simple abdominal hysterectomy if fertility is not an issue
Stage 1B	• radical hysterectomy and pelvic lymphadenectomy • ovaries can be spared • radiotherapy if lesion expanded beyond 4 cm
Stages 2,3,4	• radiotherapy

Abnormal Pap Tests in Pregnancy
- incidence – 1/2,200
- Pap test at all initial prenatal visits
    - if abnormal Pap or suspicious lesion, refer to colposcopy
- if a diagnostic conization is required, it should be deferred until second trimester (T2) to prevent complications (abortion)
- microinvasive carcinoma
    - followed to term and deliver vaginally or by C-section depending on degree of invasion
- stage IB carcinoma
    - depends on patient wishes
    - recommendations in T1 – external beam radiation with the expectation of spontaneous abortion
    - recommendations in T2 – delay of therapy until viable fetus and delivery
- follow-up with appropriate treatment

Vulva

BENIGN VULVAR LESIONS
- malignant potential (<5%); greatest risk when cellular atypia on biopsy

Any suspicious lesion of the vulva should be biopsied.

Non-Neoplastic Disorders of Vulvar Epithelium
- biopsy is necessary to make diagnosis
- **hyperplastic dystrophy** (squamous cell hyperplasia)
    - surface thickened and hyperkeratotic
    - pruritus most common symptom
    - post-menopausal women
    - treatment – 1% fluorinated corticosteroid ointment bid for 6 weeks
- **lichen sclerosis**
    - subepithelial fat becomes diminished, labia become thin and atrophic, membrane-like epithelium, labial fusion
    - pruritus, dyspareunia, burning
    - most common in post-menopausal women
    - treatment – ultrapotent topical steroid 0.05% clobetasol x 2-4wks then taper down
- **mixed dystrophy** (lichen sclerosis with epithelial hyperplasia)
    - hyperkeratotic areas with areas of thin, shiny epithelium
    - treatment – fluorinated corticosteroid ointment

Tumours
- papillary hidradenoma
- nevus
- fibroma
- hemangioma

MALIGNANT VULVAR LESIONS

Epidemiology
- 5% of genital tract malignancies
- 90% squamous cell carcinoma; remainder melanomas, basal cell carcinoma, Paget's disease
- 50% of invasive lesions are associated with current or previous vulvar dystrophy
- usually post-menopausal women

Risk Factors
- associated with HPV
- VIN (vulvar intraepithelial neoplasia): precancerous change which presents as multicentric white or pigmented plaques on vulva
    - progression rarely occurs
    - treatment – simple excision, superficial vulvectomy ± split thickness skin grafting
- 90% of VIN contain HPV DNA (specifically types 16, 18)

Clinical Features
- most patients asymptomatic at diagnosis
- most lesions occur on the labia majora, followed by the labia minora (less commonly on the clitoris or perineum)
- localized pruritus, lump, or mass most common

- less common – raised red, white or pigmented plaque, ulcer, bleeding, discharge, pain, dysuria
- spread
  - locally
  - ipsilateral groin nodes (superficial inguinal → pelvic nodes)
  - hematogenously

Investigations
- physical examination
- ALWAYS biopsy
- ± colposcopy

Table 16. FIGO Staging Classification and Treatment of Vulvar Cancer

Stage	Description	Treatment
0	intraepithelial neoplasia (VIN) carcinoma in situ	local excision laser superficial vulvectomy
I	<2 cm, confined to vulva or vulva and perineum no suspicious groin nodes	wide local excision simple or radical vulvectomy nodal dissection if >1 mm invasion, must do nodes
IA	≤1 mm invasion	
IB	>1 mm invasion	
II	>2 cm, confined to vulva or vulva and perineum no suspicious groin nodes	individualized local surgery ± radiation
III	local extension to adjacent structures, lower urethra, vagina, anus suspicious or positive unilateral groin nodes	as for stage II
IV	fixed bilateral groin nodes distant spread	as for stage II
IVA	spread to upper urethra, bladder, mucosa, rectum or bone	
IVB	distant mets including pelvic LN	

Prognosis
- depends on nodal involvement (single most important predictor followed by tumour size)
- lesions >3 cm associated with poorer prognosis
- overall 5-year survival rate – 79%

Vagina

BENIGN VAGINAL LESIONS
- **inclusion cysts**
  - cysts form at site of abnormal healing of laceration (e.g. episiotomy)
  - no treatment required
- **endometriosis**
  - dark lesions that tend to bleed at time of menses
  - treatment is excision
- **Gartner's duct cysts**
  - remnants of Wolffian duct, seen along side of cervix
  - treatment conservative unless symptomatic
- **urethral diverticulum**
  - can lead to recurrent urethral infection, dyspareunia
  - surgical correction if symptomatic

MALIGNANT VAGINAL LESIONS

Risk Factors
- associated with HPV
- increased incidence in patients with prior history of cervical and vulvar cancer

Investigations
- cytology (Pap test)
  - 10-20% false negative rate
- colposcopy
- Schiller test (normal epithelium takes up iodine)

Table 17. FIGO Staging Classification of Vaginal Cancer (Clinical Staging)

Stage	Description
0	intraepithelial neoplasia (VAIN) carcinoma in situ
I	limited to the vaginal wall
II	involves subvaginal tissue, NO pelvic wall extension
III	pelvic wall extension
IV	extension beyond true pelvis OR bladder/rectum involvement

- biopsy, partial vaginectomy
- staging (see Table 17)

VAIN (Vaginal Intra-Epithelial Neoplasia)
- grades: progression through VAIN1, VAIN2, VAIN3
- **treatment**
    - VAIN 1 – no treatment
    - VAIN 2 or adequately sampled VAIN 3 – laser tx
    - VAIN 3 – surgical excision

Squamous Cell Carcinoma (SCC)
- 80-90% of vaginal cancer
- 2% of gynecological malignancies
- most common site is upper 1/3 of posterior wall of vagina
- 5-year survival nyphen i.e. survival – 42%
- **clinical features**
    - asymptomatic – painless discharge and bleeding
    - vaginal discharge (often foul-smelling)
    - vaginal bleeding especially during coitus
    - urinary and/or rectal symptoms 2° to compression
- **treatment**
    - radiotherapy if primary
    - hysterectomy and vaginectomy

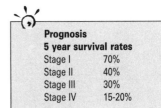

Prognosis
5 year survival rates
Stage I	70%
Stage II	40%
Stage III	30%
Stage IV	15-20%

Adenocarcinoma
- most are metastatic, usually from the cervix, endometrium, ovary, or colon
- most primaries are clear cell adenocarcinomas
- 2 types: non-DES and DES syndrome
- management as for SCC

Diethylstilbestrol (DES) Syndrome
- maternal use and fetal exposure to DES predisposes to cervical or vaginal clear cell carcinoma
- if exposed <1 in 1,000 risk of developing clear cell adenocarcinoma
- **clinical features**
    - adenosis is persistant Müllerian type glandular epithelium, only 1/1000 develop clear cell cancer
    - occurs in 30-95% of exposed females
    - DES exposure associated with malformations of upper vagina, cervix, and interior of uterus (T-shaped); cockscomb or hooded cervix, cervical collar, and pseudopolyps of cervix
    - patients with DES exposure should have annual Pap tests
        - if any abnormality, refer to colposcopy

Fallopian Tube

- least common site for carcinoma of female reproductive system (0.3%)
- usually adenocarcinoma
- more common in fifth and sixth decade

Clinical Features
- watery discharge (most important) = "hydrops tubae profluens"
- vaginal bleeding or discharge in 50% of patients
- lower abdominal pain

Treatment
- as for malignant ovarian tumours

Classic Triad
1. watery vaginal discharge
2. pelvic pain
3. pelvic mass
   (fewer than 15% of all patients)

Gestational Trophoblastic Neoplasia (GTN)

- refers to a spectrum of proliferative abnormalities of the trophoblast

Epidemiology
- 1/1000 pregnancies
- marked geographic variation, as high as 1/125 in Taiwan
- 80% benign, 15% locally invasive, 5% metastatic
- cure rate >90%

With development of hypertension early in pregnancy (i.e. <20 weeks), think gestational trophoblastic disease!

HYDATIDIFORM MOLE (Benign GTN)

- **complete mole**
    - diffuse trophoblastic hyperplasia, hydropic swelling of chorionic villi, no fetal tissues or membranes
    - most common type of hydatidiform mole
    - 2 sperm fertilize empty egg or 1 sperm with reduplication
    - 46XX or 46XY of paternal origin (90%)
    - high malignant potential (15-20%)
    - risk factors
        - maternal age >40 years
        - beta-carotene deficiency
        - vitamin A deficiency
    - clinical features
        - vaginal bleeding (97%)
        - excessive uterine size (51%)
        - theca-lutein cysts >6 cm (50%)
        - pre-eclampsia (27%)
        - hyperemesis gravidarum (26%)
        - hyperthyroidism (7%)
        - β-hCG >100, 000 mIU/mL
        - no fetal heart detected
- **partial (or incomplete) mole**
    - hydropic villi and focal trophoblastic hyperplasia are associated with fetus or fetal parts
    - often triploid (XXY, XYY, XXX)
    - single ovum fertilized by two sperm
    - no dramatic clinical features
    - low malignant potential (4%)
    - often associated with fetus that is clinically growth-restricted and has multiple congenital malformations
    - clinical features
        - similar to threatened/spontaneous/missed abortion
        - usually pathological diagnosis after D&C

Investigations

- U/S
    - if complete – no fetus (see "snow storm" due to swelling of villi)
    - if partial – molar degeneration of placenta with developing fetus/fetal parts, multiple echogenic regions corresponding to hydropic villi, and focal intra-uterine hemorrhage
- β-hCG levels
    - abnormally high (>80,000)
- features of molar pregnancies which are high risk of developing persistent GTN
    - local uterine invasion as high as 31%
    - β-hCG >100,000
    - excessive uterine size
    - prominent theca-lutein cysts

Treatment

- suction D&C with sharp curettage and oxytocin
- Rhogam if Rh negative
- hysterectomy (if patient no longer desires fertility)
- prophylactic chemotherapy (controversial)
- chemotherapy for molar pregnancies that persist after evacuation

Follow-up

- contraception to avoid pregnancy during entire follow-up period
- serial β-hCGs every week until negative x 3 (usually takes 3-10 weeks)
- then monthly for 6 months – prior to trying to conceive again
- if β-hCG plateaus or increases, patient needs chemotherapy

MALIGNANT GTN

- **invasive mole or persistent GTN**
    - diagnosis made by rising or a plateau in β-hCG, development of metastases following treatment of documented molar pregnancy
    - histology – molar tissue
    - metastases are rare (4%)
- **choriocarcinoma**
    - often present with symptoms from metastases

- highly anaplastic, highly vascular
- no chorionic villi, elements of syncytiotrophoblast and cytotrophoblast
- may follow molar pregnancy, abortion, ectopic, or normal pregnancy
- **placental-site trophoblastic tumour**
  - rare aggressive form of choriocarcinoma
  - abnormal growth of intermediate trophoblastic cells
  - low β-hCG, production of human placental lactogen (hPL), insensitive to chemotherapy
- **nonmetastatic**
  - 15% after molar evacuation
  - abnormal bleeding
  - rising or plateau of β-hCG
  - negative metastases on staging evaluation
- **metastatic**
  - 4% patients after treatment of complete molar pregnancy, mets more common with choriocarcinoma which tends toward early vascular invasion and widespread dissemination
    - hematogenous spread
    - lungs (80%) – cough, hemoptysis
    - vagina (30%) – vaginal bleeding
    - pelvis (20%) – if invades bowel, rectal bleeding
    - liver (10%) – elevated LFTs
    - brain (10%) – headaches, dizziness, symptoms of space-occupying lesion
  - highly vascular tumour → bleeding → anemia

Investigations – for staging
- when pelvic exam and chest x-ray negative, metastatic involvement uncommon
- history and physical
- bloodwork – CBC, electrolytes, creatinine, β-hCG, TSH, LFTs
- imaging – CXR, U/S pelvis, CT abdo/pelvis, CT brain
- if suspect brain mets, but CT brain negative → lumbar puncture for CSF β-hCG
  - ratio of plasma:CSF <60 indicates metastases
- classification of metastatic GTN
  - divided into good prognosis and bad prognosis
  - features of bad prognosis
    - long duration (>4 months from antecedent pregnancy)
    - high pre-treatment β-hCG titre: >100,000 IU/24h urine or >40,000 mIU/mL of blood
    - brain or liver metastases
    - significant prior chemotherapy
    - metastatic disease following term pregnancy
    - good prognostic features are the converse of each of these features

Lungs are #1 site for malignant GTN metastases.

Table 18. FIGO Staging and Management of Malignant GTN

Stage	Findings	Management

I	disease confined to uterine corpus	single agent chemotherapy if fertility desired
		  1st line – methotrexate/folinic acid (MTX-FA), 90% remission rate
		  2nd line – actinomycin D (ACT-D)
		combination chemotherapy if resistant
		PLUS hysterectomy if placental-site tumour or fertility not desired

II
III
	metastatic disease to vagina or adnexa
	metastatic disease to lungs with or without genital tract involvement
		high risk
		  combination chemotherapy: MTX-FA and ACT-D
		low risk
		  single agent chemotherapy: start with MTX-FA

IV	distant metastatic sites including brain, liver, kidney, GI tract	aggressive combination chemotherapy etoposide, MTX, ACT-D, cyclophosphamide, vincristine (EMA-CO) radiation for brain mets

Follow-up
- contraception for all stages to avoid pregnancy during entire follow-up
- stage I, II, III
  - weekly β-hCG until 3 consecutive normal results
  - then monthly x 12 months
- stage IV
  - weekly β-hCG until 3 consecutive normal results
  - then monthly x 24 months

Treatment
- chemotherapy for all stages

Common Medications

Table 19. Common Medications

Drug Name (Brand Name)	Action	Dosing Schedule	Indications	Side Effects (S/E), Contraindications (C/I), Drug Interactions (D/I)
acyclovir (Zovirax®)	Antiviral; inhibits DNA synthesis and viral replication	**First Episode:** 400 mg PO tid x 7-10d **Recurrence:** 400 mg PO tid x 5d	Genital herpes	**S/E:** headache, GI upset **D/I:** Zidovudine, Probenecid
bromocriptine (Parlodel®)	Dopaminomimetic Agonist at D_2Rx Antagonist at D_1Rx Acts directly on anterior pituitary cells to inhibit synthesis and release of prolactin	**Initial:** 1.25-2.5 mg qhs with food **Then:** 2.5 mg bid with meals	Galactorrhea + amenorrhea 2° to hyperprolactinemia Prolactin-dependent menstrual disorders and infertility Prolactin-secreting adenomas (microadenomas, prior to surgery of macroadenomas)	**S/E:** nausea, vomiting, headache, postural hypotension, somnolence **C/I:** uncontrolled hypertension, pregnancy-induced hypertension, CAD **D/I:** domperidone, macrolides, octreotide
clomiphene citrate (Clomid®)	Increases output of pituitary gonadotropins which induces ovulation	50 mg daily x 5 days Try 100 mg daily if ineffective 3 courses = adequate trial	Patients with persistent ovulatory dysfunction (e.g. amenorrhea, PCOS) who desire pregnancy	**S/E:** Common : hot flashes, abdominal discomfort, exaggerated cyclic ovarian enlargement, accentuation of Mittelschmerz Rare – ovarian hyperstimulation syndrome, multiple pregnancy, visual blurring, birth defects **C/I:** pregnancy, liver disease, hormone-dependent tumours, ovarian cyst, undiagnosed vaginal bleeding
clotrimazole (Canesten®)	Antifungal; disrupt fungal cell membrane	**Tablet:** 100 mg/d intravaginally x 7d or 500 mg x 1 dose **Cream** (1 or 2%): 1 applicator intravaginally qhs x 3-7d **Topical:** apply bid x 7	Vulvovaginal candidiasis	**S/E:** vulvar/vaginal burning
danazol (Cyclomen® - CAN) (Danocrine® - US)	Synthetic steroid that inhibits pituitary gonadotropin output & ovarian steroid synthesis Has mild androgenic properties	200-800 mg in 2-3 divided doses Used for 3-6 months Biannual hepatic U/S required if >6 month use	Endometriosis 1° menorrhagia/ DUB	**S/E:** weight gain, acne, mild hirsutism, hepatic dysfunction **C/I:** pregnancy, undiagnosed vaginal bleeding, breastfeeding, severely impaired renal/ hepatic/ cardiac function, porphyria, genital neoplasia **D/I:** warfarin, carbamazepine, cyclosporine, tacrolimus, anti-hypertensives
doxycycline	Tetracycline derivative; inhibit protein synthesis	100 mg PO bid x ≥7d	Chlamydia, gonococcal infection, syphillis	**S/E:** GI upset, hepatotoxicity **C/I:** pregnancy, severe hepatic dysfunction **D/I:** warfarin, digoxin
fluconazole (Diflucan®)	Antifungal; disrupt fungal cell membrane	150 mg PO x 1 dose	Vulvovaginal candidiasis unresponsive to clotrimazole	**S/E:** headache, rash, nausea, vomiting, abd pain, diarrhea **D/I:** terfenadine, cisapride, astemizole, hydrochlorothiazide, phenytoin, warfarin, rifampin
leuprolide (Lupron®)	Synthetic GnRH analog Induces reversible hypoestrogenic state	3.75 mg IM q1month or 11.25 mg IM q3months Usually ≤6 months, check bone density if >6 months	Endometriosis Leiomyomata DUB Precocious puberty	**S/E:** hot flashes, sweats, headache, vaginitis, reduction in bone density **C/I:** pregnancy, undiagnosed vaginal bleeding, breastfeeding
menotropin (Pergonal®)	Human Gonadotropin with FSH and LH effects; induce ovulation and stimulate ovarian follicle development	75-150 U of FSH & LH IM qd7-12 d, then 10 000 U hCG one day after last dose	Infertility	**S/E:** bloating, irritation at injection site, abd/pelvic pain, headache, nausea & vomiting **C/I:** primary ovarian failure, intracranial lesion (e.g. pituitary tumour), uncontrolled thyroid/adrenal dysfunction, ovarian cyst (not PCOS), pregnancy
metronidazole (Flagyl®)	Bactericidal; forms toxic metabolites which damage bacterial DNA	2 g PO x 1 dose or 500 mg PO bid x 7d	Bacterial vaginosis, trichomonas vaginitis	**S/E:** headache, dizziness, nausea, vomiting, diarrhea, disulfiram-like reaction (flushing, tachycardia, nausea & vomiting) **C/I:** pregnancy (1st trimester) **D/I:** cisapride, warfarin, cimetidine, lithium, alcohol
oxybutinin (Ditropan®)	Anticholinergic – relaxes bladder smooth muscle, inhibits involuntary detrusor contraction	5 mg PO bid-tid	Overactive bladder (urge incontinence)	**S/E:** dry mouth/eyes, constipation, palpitations, urinary retention **C/I:** glaucoma, GI ileus, severe colitis, obstructive uropathy, use with caution if impaired hepatic/renal function
paclitaxel (Taxol®)	Binds tubulin and inhibits disassembly of microtubules, inhibiting mitosis	175 mg/m² q3weeks	Ovarian cancer, some endometrial cancers	**S/E:** hypersensitivity, myelosuppression, peripheral neuropathy, alopecia, mucositis **C/I:** pregnancy, radiation therapy, impaired liver function
tolterodine (Detrol®)	Anticholinergic	1-2 mg PO bid	Overactive bladder (urge incontinence)	**S/E:** anaphylaxis, psychosis, tachycardia, dry mouth/eyes, headache, constipation, urinary retention, chest pain **C/I:** glaucoma, gastric/urinary retention, use with caution if impaired hepatic/renal function
tranexamic acid (Cyklokapron®)	Anti-fibrinolytic, reversibly inhibits plasminogen activation	1-1.5 g tid-qid for first 4 days of cycle Ophthalmic check if used for several weeks	Menorrhagia	**S/E:** nausea, vomiting, diarrhea, dizziness Rare cases of thrombosis **C/I:** thromboembolic disease, acquired disturbances of colour vision, subarachnoid hemorrhage, age <15 yrs
urofollitropin (Metrodin®)	FSH	75 U/d SC x 7-12 d	Ovulation induction in PCOS	**S/E:** ovarian enlargement or cysts, edema & pain at injection site, arterial thromboembolism, fever, abd pain, **C/I:** primary ovarian failure, intracranial lesion (e.g. pituitary tumour), uncontrolled thyroid/adrenal dysfunction, ovarian cyst (not PCOS), pregnancy

19. Common Medications

me (Brand Name)	Action	Dosing Schedule	Indications	Side Effects (S/E), Contraindications (C/I), Drug Interactions (D/I)
d oral contraceptive	Ovulatory suppression by inhibiting LH and FSH Decidualization of endometrium Thickening of cervical mucus to prevent sperm penetration			**S/E**: Estrogen-related: nausea, breast changes (tenderness, enlargement), fluid retention/bloating/edema, weight gain, migraines, thromboembolic events, liver adenoma, intermenstrual bleeding Progestin-related: amenorrhea/intermenstrual bleeding, headaches, breast tenderness, increased appetite, decreased libido, mood changes, hypertension, acne/oily skin, hirsutism **D/I**: rifampin, phenobarbital, phenytoin, primidone **C/I**: Absolute: known/suspected pregnancy, undiagnosed abnormal vaginal bleeding , prior thromboembolic events, thromboembolic disorder, active thrombophlebitis, cerebrovascular or coronary artery disease , estrogen-dependent tumours, impaired liver function associated with acute liver disease , congenital hypertriglyceridemia, smoker age >35 years , migraines with focal neurological symptoms (excluding aura), uncontrolled hypertension Relative: non focal migraines with aura <1 hour, diabetes mellitus complicated by vascular disease, SLE, controlled hypertension, hyperlipidemia, sickle cell anemia, gallbladder disease
ine device (IUD) JD (Nova-T®) rone-releasing ena®)	**Copper IUD**: mild foreign body reaction in endometrium which is toxic to sperm and alters sperm motility **Progesterone-releasing IUD**: decidualization of endometrium and thickening of cervical mucus, may suppress ovulation	Contraceptive effects last five years		**S/E**: intermenstrual bleeding, bloating, headache (Mirena®), increased blood loss, duration of menses and dysmenorrheal (copper IUD only), expulsion (5% in the first year, greatest in first month), uterine wall perforation (1/5000), if pregnancy occurs, there is a greater chance the pregnancy will be ectopic, increased risk of PID within first 10 days of insertion only **C/I**: Absolute: known or suspected pregnancy, undiagnosed genital tract bleeding, acute or chronic PID, lifestyle risk for STIs, known allergy to copper or Wilson's Disease (copper IUD only) Relative: valvular heart disease, past history of PID or ectopic pregnancy, abnormalities of uterine cavity, intracavitary fibroids, severe dysmenorrhea or menorrhagia (copper IUD only), cervical stenosis, immunosuppressed individuals

Notes

H

Hematology

Jack Brzezinski, Janice Kwan and Taryn Simms, chapter editors
Deepti Damaraju and Elliott Owen, associate editors
Erik Venos, EBM editor
Dr. Anne McLeod, staff editor

Basics of Hematology

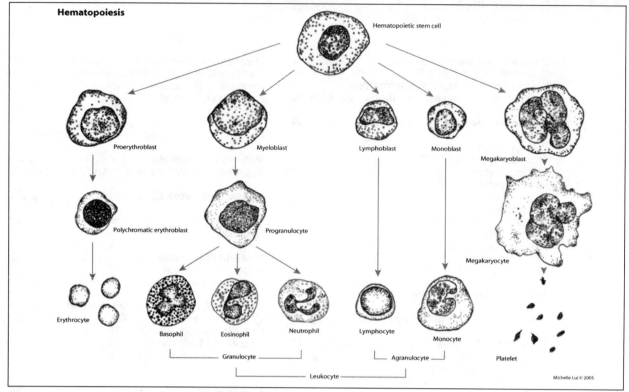

Figure 1. Hematopoiesis

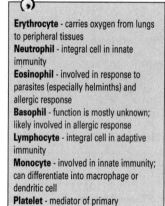

Erythrocyte - carries oxygen from lungs to peripheral tissues
Neutrophil - integral cell in innate immunity
Eosinophil - involved in response to parasites (especially helminths) and allergic response
Basophil - function is mostly unknown; likely involved in allergic response
Lymphocyte - integral cell in adaptive immunity
Monocyte - involved in innate immunity; can differentiate into macrophage or dendritic cell
Platelet - mediator of primary hemostasis

Complete Blood Count

Table 1. Common Terms Found on CBC

Test	Definition	Normal Values*
Red blood cell (RBC) count	count of actual number of RBCs per volume of blood	$4.2\text{-}6.9 \times 10^9/mm^3$
Hemoglobin (Hb)	amount of oxygen-carrying protein in the blood	130-180 g/L (13-18 g/dL) (male) 120-160 g/L (12- 16 g/dL) (female)
Hematocrit (Hct)	percentage of a given volume of whole blood occupied by packed RBCs	45%-62% (male) 37%-48% (female)
Mean corpuscular volume (MCV)	measurement of actual size of RBCs	$80\text{-}100 \ \mu m^3$
Mean corpuscular Hb (MCH)	amount of oxygen-carrying Hb inside RBCs	27-32 pg/cell
Mean corpuscular Hb concentration (MCHC)	average concentration of Hb inside RBCs	32%-36%
RBC distribution width (RDW)	measurement of variability in RBC size	11.0%-15.0%
White blood cell (WBC) count	count of actual number of WBCs per volume of blood	$4.3\text{-}10.8 \times 10^3/mm^3$
WBC differential	includes neutrophils, eosinophils, basophils, lymphocytes and monocytes	
Platelet count	count of actual number of platelets per volume of blood	$150\text{-}400 \times 10^3/mm^3$
Mean platelet volume (MPV)	measurement of actual size of platelets	
Reticulocytes	immature RBCs that contain no nucleus but have residual make up 1% of total RBC count	RNA; normally

*Every lab has its own set of normal values that may differ from these

- interpret abnormal CBC within context of individual's baseline value
    - up to 5% of population without disease may have values outside "normal" range
    - an individual may display substantial change from baseline without violating "normal" reference range

Blood Film/Bone Marrow Interpretations

RED BLOOD CELLS

Size
- microcytic (MCV<80), normocytic (MCV = 80-100), macrocytic (MCV>100)
- anisocytosis: RBCs of variable and abnormal size

Colour
- hypochromic – ↑ in the size of the central pallor (normal = less than one third of the diameter of RBC)
  - iron deficiency anemia, sideroblastic anemia
- hyperchromic – ↑ blue cells (reticulocytes)
  - ↑ RBC production by the marrow
  - bleeding, spherocytosis

Shape (see Figure 2)
- poikilocytosis: abnormal degree of variation in the shape of RBCs
- discocyte – normal (biconcave)
- spherocyte – spherical RBC (due to loss of membrane)
  - hereditary spherocytosis, immune hemolytic anemia
- elliptocyte (ovalocyte) – oval, elongated RBC
  - hereditary elliptocytosis, megaloblastic anemia
- schistocytes (helmet cells) – fragmented cells (due to traumatic disruption of membrane)
  - microangiopathic hemolytic anemia (TTP, DIC, vasculitis, glomerulonephritis), prosthetic heart valve
- sickle cell – sickle-shaped RBC (due to polymerization of hemoglobin S)
  - sickle cell disorders: HbSC, HbSS
- codocyte (target cell) – looks like "bull's eye" on dried film
  - liver disease, hemoglobin S/C, thalassemia, Fe deficiency, asplenia
- dacrocyte (teardrop cell) – single pointed end, looks like a teardrop
  - myelofibrosis
- acanthocyte (spur cell) – distorted RBC with irregularly distributed thorn-like projections (due to abnormal membrane lipids)
  - severe liver disease (spur cell anemia)
- echinocyte (burr cell) – RBC with numerous, regularly spaced, small spiny projections
  - uremia, artifact

Distribution (see Figure 2)
- rouleaux formation – aggregates of RBC resembling stacks of coins
  - artifact, paraprotein (multiple myeloma, macroglobulinemia)

Inclusion (see Figure 2)
- erythroblast (nucleated RBC)
  - immature RBC
  - extramedullary hematopoiesis, hypoxia, hemolysis
- Heinz bodies – denatured and precipitated hemoglobin
  - G6PD deficiency
- Howell-Jolly bodies – small nuclear remnant with the colour of a pyknotic nucleus
  - post-splenectomy, hyposplenism, hemolytic anemia, megaloblastic anemia
- basophilic stippling – deep blue granulations of variable size and number, pathologic aggregation of ribosomes
  - coarse: sideroblastic and megaloblastic anemia
  - fine: generally an artifact
- sideroblasts: erythrocytes with Fe containing granules in the cytoplasm

WHITE BLOOD CELLS
- lymphocytes: comprise 30-40% of white cells
  - Reed-Sternberg cell: giant, malignant and multinucleated β-lymphocyte indicative of Hodgkin's disease
    - not found on blood film; only in Hodgkin's disease
  - Smudge cells: lymphocytes damaged during preparation of the smear; indicating cell fragility, found in Chronic Lymphocytic Leukemia (CLL)
- neutrophils: only mature neutrophil and band neutrophil (immediate precursor) are normally found – neutrophils should have a 3-4 lobed nucleus
  - hypersegmented neutrophil: >5 lobes suggests megaloblastic process or iron deficiency
  - Auer rods: clumps of granular material that form long needles in the cytoplasm of myeloblasts; pathognomonic for Acute Myeloid Leukemia (AML)

PLATELETS
- small purplish anuclear cells

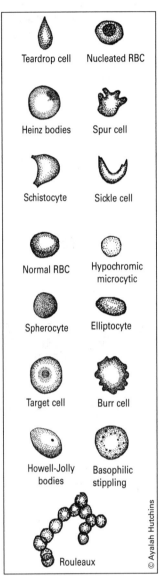

Figure 2. Morphology

Indications for Bone Marrow Biopsy and Aspirate

- unexplained anemia, leukopenia, thrombocytopenia, or pancytopenia
- diagnosis and staging of lymphoma or solid tumours
- diagnosis and evaluation of plasma cell disorders and leukemias
- evaluate iron metabolism and stores
- evaluate suspected deposition and storage disease (e.g. amyloidosis, Gaucher's disease)
- evaluate fever of undetermined origin, suspected mycobacterial, fungal or parasitic infections, or granulomatous disease
- unexplained splenomegaly
- confirm normal bone marrow in potential allogenic hematopoietic cell donor

Contraindications
- absolute: hemophilia, severe DIC, other related severe bleeding disorders
- thrombocytopenia not a contraindication - may need to transfuse platelets prior

Common Presenting Problems

Anemia

Definition
- a decrease in red blood cell (RBC) mass that can be detected by hemoglobin (Hb) concentration, hematocrit (Hct), and RBC count
    - adult males: Hb<135 g/L, 13.5 g/dL or Hct<41%
    - adult females: Hb<120 g/L, 12 g/dL or Hct<36%

Etiology and Approach
- the etiology may be obvious (e.g. following a sanguinous operation)
- in less obvious cases, consider the acuity (e.g. occult blood loss, trauma) or chronicity (e.g. congenital, anemia of chronic disease)
- differentiate anemia vs. pancytopenia (see *Pancytopenia*)
- consider decreased production vs increased destruction/loss
- in general, start with the mean corpuscular volume (MCV)
    - microcytic (MCV<80), macrocytic (MCV>100), normocytic (MCV=80-100)
- reticulocyte count helps differentiate between decreased production (↓ retics) and increased destruction/loss (↑ retics)
- causes associated with decreased production can be primary (i.e. localized to the bone marrow: aplastic anemia, myelophthisic anemia, hematologic malignancy) or systemic (e.g. chronic disease, hypothyroidism, chronic renal failure, liver disease)
- increased destruction/loss can be due to hypersplenism (sequestration and destruction), hemolytic disorders, blood loss

Reticulocytes

Reticulocytes are young erythrocytes and are markers of erythrocyte production. Any time there is a decrease in RBCs, the physiologic response is to increase production which leads to an increased reticulocyte count. A person with low hemoglobin and a normal erythropoeitic system would be expected to have a relatively high reticulocyte count. Therefore, a normal reticulocyte count in anemia should be interpreted as a sign of decreased production.

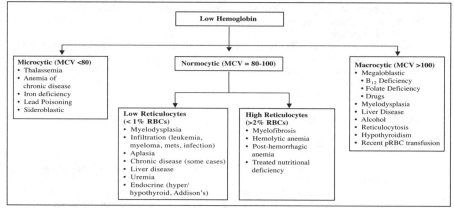

Figure 3. Approach to Anemia

Clinical Features
- presenting symptoms depend on how rapidly the anemia develops
- symptoms: fatigue, malaise, weakness, syncope, dyspnea, headache, vertigo, tinnitus
- signs
    - HEENT: pallor in mucous membranes and conjunctiva (Hb<90 g/L), ocular bruits (Hb<55 g/L)
    - CVS: tachycardia, orthostatic hypotension, systolic flow murmur, wide pulse pressure, signs of CHF
    - derm: pallor in palmar skin creases (Hb<75 g/L), jaundice (if due to hemolysis)

Investigations
- rule out dilutional anemia (low Hb due to ↑ effective circulating volume)
- CBC with differential (including MCV, RBC cell distribution width (RDW), and reticulocyte count)
- blood film
- additional laboratory investigations as indicated (see *Microcytic Anemia, Normocytic Anemia, Hemolytic Anemia* and *Macrocytic Anemia*) (H11, H14, H15, H20)

Polycythemia

Definition
- an increase in the number of RBCs: Hb>180 g/L or Hct>52% (males); Hb>160 or Hct>47% (females and black males)

Etiology
- relative/spurious erythrocytosis (↓ in plasma volume): severe dehydration, burns, "stress" (Gaisböck's syndrome)
- absolute erythrocytosis
  - primary
    - polycythemia rubra vera (PRV) – see *PRV*
  - secondary
    - poor tissue oxygenation/hypoxia
      - high altitude
      - pulmonary disease: COPD, sleep apnea, congenital
      - cardiovascular disease: R → L shunt
      - hemoglobinopathies with ↑ O_2 affinity
    - carbon monoxide poisoning
    - inappropriate production of erythropoietin
      - renal cell carcinomas, cerebellar hemangioblastoma, pheochromocytoma, hepatocellular cancer, uterine leiomyomas
    - local renal hypoxia
      - renal artery stenosis
      - benign renal cysts (compress vessels)

Clinical Features
- secondary to high red cell mass and hyperviscosity
  - headache, dizziness, tinnitus, visual disturbances
  - symptoms of angina, CHF
- thrombosis (venous or arterial) or bleeding (abnormal platelet function)
- characteristic physical findings
  - plethora (ruddy complexion) of face (70%), palms

Investigations
- principally directed at ruling out PRV
- RBC mass – normal suggests relative erythrocytosis; confirms increased red cell production; rules out ↓ plasma volume
- serum erythropoietin (Epo) – increased suggests autonomous production or hypoxia and rules out PRV
- search for tumour as source of Epo as indicated (e.g. abdominal U/S, CT head)
- arterial pO_2 – decreased suggests hypoxic etiology
- carboxyhemoglobin (hemoglobin-carbon monoxide complex) level, hemoglobin O_2 affinity

Treatment
- phlebotomy
- hydroxyurea (use if phlebotomy is unsuccessful)

Thrombocytopenia

Definition
- platelet count <150 x10^9/L

Etiology and Approach
- hemodilution (e.g. massive transfusion)
- decreased production (disease process occurs in bone marrow)
  - nutritional (e.g. severe B_{12}/folate deficiency)
  - congenital (e.g. Alport's syndrome, Fanconi's anemia)
  - marrow damage
    - injury: drugs, toxins, chemotherapy and radiation (can cause myelodysplastic syndromes (MDS))
    - invasion: malignancy, leukemia, myelofibrosis
    - failure: aplastic anemia

- increased peripheral destruction (↑ in bone marrow megakaryocytes)
- increased peripheral destruction (increase in megakaryocytes in BM)
  - immune mediated: Immune Thrombocytopenic Purpura (ITP), Heparin Induced Thrombocytopenia (HIT), drugs (e.g. thiazides, sulfa, quinidine), viral infections (e.g. HIV, HCV, CMV, EBV), systemic diseases (e.g. SLE), lymphoproliferative disorders (e.g. CLL, lymphoma), alloimmune destruction (e.g. post-transfusion, post-transplantation, neonatal)
  - non-immune mediated: Disseminated Intravascular Coagulation (DIC), Thrombotic Thrombocytopenic Purpura (TTP), Hemolytic Uremic Syndrome (HUS), Antiphospholipid Ab Syndrome (APLAS), pre-eclampsia and HELLP syndrome (see Obstetrics)
- platelet sequestration
  - any disease process that leads to splenomegaly (see H10) (up to 30% of circulating platelets are normally in the spleen at any given time)

Investigations
- CBC and differential
- blood film
  - ↓ production: blasts, hypersegmented PMNs, leukoerythroblastic changes
  - ↑ destruction: large platelets, schistocytes (only present when platelets are activated e.g. DIC)

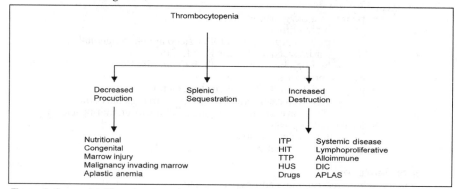

Figure 4. Approach to Thrombocytopenia

Thrombocytosis

Definition
- platelet count >500 x10^9/L
- reactive thrombocytosis – acute phase reactant (e.g. surgery, inflammation, infection, trauma, bleeding, iron deficiency, neoplasms)
- primary thrombocytosis – essential thrombocytosis, secondary to chronic myeloproliferative, myelodysplastic disorder

Clinical Features
- primary thrombocytosis more likely to cause vasomotor symptoms
- vasomotor symptoms: headache, visual disturbances, lightheadedness, atypical chest pain, acral dysesthesia, erythromelalgia
- clotting risk and rarely bleeding risk

Pancytopenia

Definition
- a decrease in all hematopoietic cell lines

Clinical Features
- anemia - fatigue
- leukopenia - recurrent infections
- thrombocytopenia - mucosal bleeding and ecchymoses

Investigations
- CBC and differential, blood film
- investigate secondary cause: HIV test, serum B_{12}, RBC folate, ANA
- often requires bone marrow biopsy to distinguish among different causes

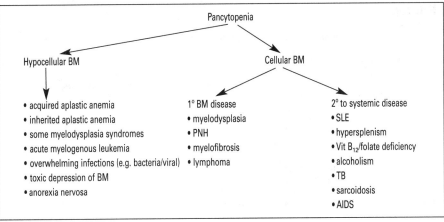

Figure 5. Approach to Pancytopenia   PNH = Paroxysmal Nocturnal Hemoglobinuria

Neutrophilia

Definition
- increase in absolute neutrophil count (ANC) above normal range ($>7.7 \times 10^9$/L)

Etiology
- primary neutrophilia
  - hereditary neutrophilia (autosomal dominant)
  - chronic idiopathic neutrophilia in otherwise healthy patients
  - chronic myelogenous leukemia (CML)
  - other myeloproliferative disorders (PRV, ET, agnogenic myeloid metaplasia)
  - leukocyte adhesion deficiency

- secondary neutrophilia
  - smoking – most common cause of mild neutrophilia
  - infection – modest leukocytosis with left shift, ± toxic granulation, Döhle bodies (intra-cytoplasmic structures composed of agglutinated ribosome); increase in inflammation, cytoplasmic vacuoles in neutrophils on blood film
  - inflammation – e.g. RA, IBD, chronic hepatitis, MI, PE, burn
  - malignancy – hematologic (i.e. marrow invaded by tumour) and nonhematologic (especially large cell lung cancer, range 12-30, can be as high as 100 due to marrow invasion and inflammation as well as solid tumours secreting substances with colony-stimulating activity)
  - stress/exercise/epinephrine – movement of neutrophils from marginated pool into circulating pool
  - medications – e.g. glucocorticoids, beta-agonists (e.g. epinephrine), lithium

Clinical Features
- look for signs and symptoms of fever, inflammation, malignancy to determine appropriate further investigations
- examine oral cavity, teeth, peri-rectal area, genitals, skin for signs of infection

Investigations
- complete blood count and blood film review → r/o spurious causes (e.g. platelet clumping, cryoglobulinemia)
- WBC differential – mature neutrophils or left shift-bands >20% of total WBC indicating infection/inflammation
- blood film – Döhle bodies, toxic granulation, cytoplasmic vacuoles if infection
- review for abnormalities in other blood counts

> Although the correct definition of "left shift" is an increase of hematopoeitic precursors in the peripheral smear, many clinicians use the term to refer to a relative neutrophilia.

Neutropenia

Definition
- **mild**: ANC $1.0\text{-}1.5 \times 10^9$/L
- **moderate**: ANC $0.5\text{-}1.0 \times 10^9$/L (risk of infection starts to increase)
- **severe**: ANC$<0.5 \times 10^9$/L

Etiology
- ↓ production
  - hematological diseases – idiopathic, aplastic anemia, myelofibrosis, BM infiltration
  - infection – TB, typhoid fever, infectious mononucleosis, malaria, viral hepatitis, AIDS
  - drug-induced – alkylating agents, antimetabolites, anticonvulsants, antipsychotics, anti-inflammatory agents, anti-thyroid drugs
  - toxic – high dose radiation, chemicals (e.g. benzene, DDT)
  - nutritional deficiency – B_{12}, folate
- peripheral destruction
  - antineutrophil antibodies
  - spleen or lung trapping
  - autoimmune disorders – RA, SLE
  - Wegener's granulomatosis
  - drugs as haptens – (e.g. α-methyldopa)
- excessive margination (transient neutropenia)
  - idiopathic (most common)
  - overwhelming bacterial infection
  - hemodialysis
  - racial variation in normal range, i.e. people of African descent commonly have mild neutropenia

Clinical Features
- fever, chills
- infection by endogenous bacteria (i.e. *S. aureus*, gram negative organisms from GI and GU tract)
- painful ulceration on skin, anus, mouth and throat following colonization by opportunistic organisms
- septicemia in later stage
- avoid digital rectal exam

Investigations
- depends on degree of neutropenia and symptoms
- ranges from observation with frequent CBCs to bone marrow aspirate and biopsy

Treatment
- regular dental care – chronic gingivitis and recurrent stomatitis major sources of morbidity
- febrile neutropenia: see <u>Infectious Diseases</u>
- in severe immune-mediated neutropenia, G-CSF may ↑ neutrophil counts
- if no response to G-CSF, then steroids and IVIG used

G-CSF = Neupogen™ = Filgrastim
GM-CSF = Leukine™ = Sargramostim

Lymphocytosis

Definition
- absolute lymphocyte count >4 x 10^9/L

Etiology
- infection
  - majority are viral infections
  - TB, pertussis, brucellosis, toxoplasmosis
- physiologic response to stress (e.g. trauma, status epilepticus)
- hypersensitivity (e.g. drugs, serum sickness)
- autoimmune (e.g. rheumatoid arthritis)
- neoplasm (e.g. ALL, CLL)

Investigations/Treatment
- peripheral smear
- "atypical lymphocytes" in EBV infection
- treat underlying cause

Lymphocytopenia

Definition
- absolute lymphocyte count <1.5 x 10^9/L

Etiology
- idiopathic CD4+ lymphocytopenia
- chemotherapeutic agents
- radiation
- malignancy
- HIV/AIDS

Clinical Features
- opportunistic infections (see <u>Infectious Diseases</u>)

Treatment
- treat/remove underlying cause
- treat opportunistic infections aggressively and consider antimicrobial prophylaxis (see <u>Infectious Diseases</u>)

Eosinophilia

- absolute eosinophil count $>0.5 \times 10^9/L$
- most common causes are parasitic (usually helminth) infections and allergic reactions to medications
- less common causes:
    - polyarteritis nodosa
    - cholesterol emboli
    - CML
    - Hodgkin's disease
    - adrenal insufficiency
- Hypereosinophilic Syndrome
    - 6 months of eosinophilia with no other detectable causes
    - can involve heart, BM, CNS

Agranulocytosis

- severe depletion of granulocytes (neutrophils, eosinophils, basophils) from the blood and granulocyte precursors from the marrow
- associated with drug use in 70% of cases: e.g. clozapine, thionamides (antithyroid drugs), sulfasalazine and ticlopidine
- pathogenesis:
    - immune-mediated destruction of circulating granulocytes by drug-induced antibodies or direct toxic effects upon marrow granulocytic precursors
- abrupt onset of
    - fever, chills and weakness
    - oropharyngeal ulcers
- highly lethal without vigorous treatment

Investigations/Treatment
- discontinue offending drug
- pan cultures if patient is febrile
- initiate broad-spectrum IV antibiotics
- G-CSF – growth factor that stimulates neutrophil production

Leukemoid Reactions

- blood findings resembling those seen in certain types of leukemia which reflect the response of healthy BM to cytokines released due to infection or trauma
- leukocytosis $>50 \times 10^9/L$, marked left shift (myelocytes, metamyelocytes, bands in peripheral blood)
- important to rule out CML
- myeloid leukemia mimicked by
    - pneumonia
    - other acute bacterial infections
    - intoxications
    - burns
    - malignant disease
    - severe hemorrhage or hemolysis
- lymphoid leukemia mimicked by
    - pertussis
    - TB
    - infectious mononucleosis
- monocytic leukemia mimicked by
    - TB

Approach to Lymphadenopathy

- lymph nodes are the site of activation of adaptive immunity
- differentiate localized from generalized lymphadenopathy

Table 2. Differential Diagnosis of Generalized Lymphadenopathy

Reactive	Inflammatory	Neoplastic	Other
Bacterial (TB)	Autoimmune (RA, SLE)	Lymphoma	Serum Sickness
Viral (EBV, CMV, HIV)	Drug hypersensitivity	Lymphocytic leukemias	Amyloidosis
Parasitic (toxoplasmosis)	Sarcoidosis, amyloidosis	Metastatic ca	Sarcoidosis
Fungal (histoplasmosis)		Histocytosis X	

- history
  - constitutional symptoms (TB, lymphoma, other malignancy)
  - signs or symptoms of infection or malignancy
  - exposures, e.g. cats (cat scratch – *Bartonella henselae*), ticks (Lyme disease), high risk behaviors (HIV)
  - medications (some cause serum sickness → lymphadenopathy)
- physical exam
  - signs of infection in region to which lymph nodes drain
  - signs of systemic disease
  - characteristics of lymph nodes
    - location
    - size (abnormal is usually >1 cm)
    - consistency (e.g. hard in cancer, rubbery in Hodgkin's)
    - fixation (normal is mobile, cancer can be fixed)
    - tenderness (suggests rapid enlargement → typically inflammatory)
- labs
  - CBC, CXR
  - +/- PPD, HIV RNA, RPR/VDRL, monospot/EBV, ANA, other imaging
  - biopsy
    - if localized and no Sx suggestive of malignancy, can observe 3-4 weeks (if no resolution by then → biopsy)
    - if generalized → lab workup, if negative → biopsy
    - if signs suggestive of malignancy, biopsy immediately
    - excisional biopsy is preferred as it preserves node architecture (essential for diagnosing lymphoma)
    - FNA (helpful for diagnosing recurrence of malignancy)

Approach to Splenomegaly

- DDx
  - hyperplastic, congestive and infiltrative causes

Table 3. Differential Diagnosis of Splenomegaly

	Increased demand for splenic function			Congestive	Infiltrative (malignant vs non-malignant)
Hematological	**Infectious**	**Autoimmune**		Cirrhosis	Amyloidosis
Spherocytosis	CMV	RA (Felty's)		Splenic vein obstruction	Gaucher's disease
Hemoglobinopathies	EBV	SLE		Portal vein obstruction	Leukemia (esp. CML)
Nutritional anemias	HIV/AIDS	Sarcoidosis		CHF	Lymphoma
	TB				Hodgkin's disease
	Malaria				Myeloproliferative disorders
	Histoplasmosis				Metastatic tumour
	Leishmaniasis				

- history
  - constitutional symptoms
  - signs or symptoms of infection or malignancy
  - history of liver disease or high risk exposures
- physical exam
  - signs of chronic liver disease
  - associated lymphadenopathy or hepatomegaly
  - jaundice, petechiae
  - signs of CHF
- labs
  - CBC and differential
  - ± reticulocyte count, haptoglobin, LDH, infectious and autoimmune workups

Microcytic Anemia

	Lab Tests				Blood Film
	Ferritin	Serum Iron	TIBC	RDW	
Iron-Deficiency Anemia	↓ ↓	↓	↑	↑(>15)	• hypochromic, microcytic
Anemia of Chronic Disease	N/↑	↓	↓	N	• normocytic/microcytic
Sideroblastic Anemia	N/↑	↑	N	↑	• dual population • basophilic stippling
Thalassemia	N/↑	N/↑	N	N/↑	• hypochromic, microcytic • basophilic stippling • poikilocytosis

Figure 6. Iron Indices and Blood Film in Microcytic Anemia (MCV<80)

Iron Metabolism

Causes of Microcytic Anemia
Thalassemia
Anemia of chronic disease
Iron deficiency
Lead Poisoning
Sideroblastic

Iron-deficiency anemia commonly co-exists with anemia of chronic disease: suggested by low serum ferritin, elevation of soluble transferrin receptor, absence of stainable iron on bone marrow aspiration/biopsy and response to a therapeutic trial of oral iron.

Iron Intake (Dietary)
• "average" North American adult diet = 10-20 mg Fe/day
• absorption = 5-10% (0.5-2 mg/day), absorption of iron enhanced by citric acid and ascorbic acid/vitamin C and reduced by polyphenols (e.g. in tea), phytate (e.g. in bran), dietary calcium, and soy protein
• males have a positive Fe balance
• up to 20% of menstruating females have a negative Fe balance

Iron Absorption
• occurs in duodenum
• can be impaired by IBD, celiac disease, etc.

Iron Transport + Cellular Absorption
• majority of non-heme Fe in plasma is bound to transferrin which:
  ▪ carries Fe from intestinal mucosal cell to RBC precursors in marrow
  ▪ carries Fe from storage pool in hepatocytes and macrophages to RBC precursors in marrow
• binding of the circulating Fe-transferrin complex to the transferrin receptor in the cell membrane leads to the absorption of Fe and release of transferrin

Iron Storage
• Fe is stored in two forms: ferritin and hemosiderin
• ferritin
  ▪ ferric iron complexed to a protein called apoferritin
  ▪ hepatocytes are main site of ferritin storage
  ▪ minute quantities are present in plasma in equilibrium with intracellular ferritin
  ▪ also an acute phase reactant so can be spuriously elevated despite low Fe stores
• hemosiderin
  ▪ aggregates or crystals of ferritin with the apoferritin partially removed
  ▪ macrophage-monocyte system is main source of hemosiderin storage

Iron Indices (see Figure 6)
• bone marrow aspirate is the gold standard test for iron stores
• serum ferritin
  ▪ single most important blood test for iron stores
  ▪ elevated in
    ♦ infection, inflammation, malignancy
    ♦ liver disease, hyperthyroidism and iron overload
• serum iron
  ▪ varies significantly daily
  ▪ a measure of all non-heme Fe present in blood
  ▪ virtually all serum iron is bound to transferrin
  ▪ only a trace of serum Fe is free or complexed in ferritin
• total iron binding capacity (TIBC)
  ▪ high specificity for decreased iron, low sensitivity
  ▪ measure of total amount of transferrin present in blood
  ▪ normally, one third of the TIBC is saturated with Fe, remainder is unsaturated
• saturation
  ▪ serum Fe divided by TIBC, expressed as a proportion or a %
  ▪ low in iron-deficiency anemia

- soluble transferrin receptor (STfR) Index
  - a new diagnostic tool
  - STfR are shortened fragments of the transmembrane transferrin receptor in the circulation
  - a quantitative determination of the functional iron status and reflects availability of iron at the tissue level
  - low in reduced erythropoiesis and iron overload, increased in Fe-deficiency anemia, ineffective or increased erythropoiesis

Iron Deficiency Anemia

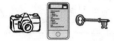
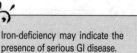

- most common cause of anemia in North America
- imbalance of intake vs requirements or loss

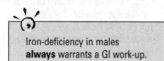

Iron-deficiency may indicate the presence of serious GI disease.

Iron-deficiency in males **always** warrants a GI work-up.

Etiology
- ↑ demand
  - ↑ physiological need for iron in the body (e.g. pregnancy)
- ↓ supply
  - dietary deficiencies (rarely the only etiology)
    - cow's milk (infant diet)
    - "tea and toast" (elderly)
  - absorption imbalances
    - post-gastrectomy
    - malabsorption (IBD of duodenum, celiac disease, autoimmune atrophic gastritis)
- ↑ loss
  - hemorrhage
    - obvious causes – menorrhagia
    - occult – peptic ulcer disease, GI tract cancer
  - intravascular hemolysis with accompanying hemoglobinuria and hemosiderinuria
    - paroxysmal nocturnal hemoglobinuria (PNH)
    - cardiac valve RBC fragmentation

Clinical Features
- iron deficiency may cause fatigue before clinical anemia develops
- symptoms due to anemia: fatigue, weakness, irritability, exercise intolerance, syncope, dyspnea, headache, palpitations, postural dizziness, tinnitus, feeling cold, confusion/loss of concentration
- brittle hair
- dysphagia (e.g. esophageal web, Plummer-Vinson ring)
- pallor – conjunctiva, palmar creases
- nails
  - brittle
  - koilonychia (spoon-shaped nails)
- glossitis
- angular stomatitis (inflammation and fissuring at the corners of the mouth)
- pica (appetite for non-food substances, e.g. ice, paint, dirt)

Investigations
- major diagnostic difficulty is to distinguish from anemia of chronic disease
- iron indices, including ferritin (Table 4), (Figure 6)
- ferritin is an acute phase protein and is stored in the liver. In patients with liver disease or infection, a serum ferritin <70 μg/L should be considered suggestive of Fe deficiency
- peripheral blood film
  - hypochromic microcytosis: RBCs are under hemoglobinized due to lack of Fe
  - pencil forms
  - target cells (thin)
- bone marrow (gold standard but not commonly done)
  - intermediate and late erythroblasts show micronormoblastic maturation
  - Fe stain (Prussian blue) shows ↓ iron in macrophages and in erythroid precursors (sideroblasts)

Table 4. The Utility of Ferritin in the Diagnosis of Iron Deficiency Anemia

Ferritin (µg/L)	Likelihood ratio for iron deficiency anemia
> 100	0.13
45-100	0.46
18-45	3.12
≤ 18	41.47

Treatment
- treat the underlying cause
- ferrous sulphate 325 mg PO tid, ferrous gluconate 300 mg PO tid, or ferrous fumarate 300 mg PO OD-bid, until anemia corrects and then for 3 months after or longer if serum ferritin has not returned to normal
- different preparations available: tablets, syrup, parenteral (if malabsorption)
- IV Venofer can be used if patient not able to tolerate or absorb oral iron

Prognosis
- reticulocytes begin to ↑ after one week
- Hb normalizes by 10 g/L per week

Anemia of Chronic Disease

Etiology
- infection; malignancy; inflammatory and rheumatologic disease; chronic renal and liver disease; endocrine disorders (e.g. diabetes mellitus, hypothyroidism, hypogonadism, hypopituitarism)

Pathophysiology
- primarily caused by a reduction in RBC production by the bone marrow
- trapping of iron in macrophages → reduced plasma iron levels making iron relatively unavailable for new hemoglobin synthesis
- erythropoietin levels are normal or slightly elevated but the marrow is unable to respond with ↑ in erythropoiesis
- a mild hemolytic component is often present
- red blood cell survival modestly ↓

Investigations
- a diagnosis of exclusion, biochemically rule out Fe deficiency
- serum iron indices (see Figure 6)
    - serum iron and TIBC low, % saturation normal
    - serum ferritin is normal or ↑
- peripheral blood
    - usually normocytic and normochromic if the anemia is mild
    - may be microcytic and normochromic if the anemia is moderate
    - may be microcytic and hypochromic if the anemia is severe but rarely <90 g/L
    - absolute reticulocyte count is frequently low, reflecting overall ↓ in RBC production
    - may have elevation in acute phase reactants (ESR, CRP, fibrinogen)
- bone marrow
    - normal or ↑ iron stores in bone marrow
    - ↓ or absent staining for iron in erythroid precursors

Treatment
- resolves if underlying disease is treated
- only treat patients who can benefit from a higher hemoglobin level
- erythropoietin may normalize the hemoglobin value (dose of erythropoietin required is higher than dose required for patients with renal disease)

Lead Poisoning

L: Lead Lines on gingivae and epiphyses of long bones on X-ray
E: Encephalopathy and Erythrocyte basophilic stippling
A: Abdominal colic and microcytic Anemia (sideroblastic)
D: Drops → wrist and foot drop. Dimercaprol and EDTA as first line of treatment

Consider lead poisoning in any child who lives in a house built before 1976 in Canada or before 1977 in the USA

Sideroblastic Anemia

Definition
- defects in the heme biosynthesis in erythroid precursors
- uncommon compared to iron deficiency anemia or anemia of chronic disease

Sideroblasts
- erythrocytes with Fe-containing (basophilic) granules in the cytoplasm
- "normal": granules randomly spread in the cell cytoplasm
    - small; found in normal individuals
- "ring": Fe build up in RBC deposits in mitochondria which form a ring around the nucleus
    - abnormal, large
    - hallmark of any sideroblastic anemia

Clinical Manifestation
- hepatosplenomegaly, Fe overload syndrome

Etiology
- hereditary (rare)
  - X-linked, median survival 10 years
- idiopathic (acquired)
  - may be a preleukemic phenomenon (10%)
  - refractory anemia with sideroblasts
- reversible
  - drugs (isoniazid, chloramphenicol), EtOH, lead, copper deficiency, zinc toxicity, hypothyroidism

Investigations
- serum iron indices and bone marrow biopsy
  - increased serum Fe, normal TIBC, increased ferritin, increased soluble transferrin receptor (STfR)
  - hypochromic, can be micro-, normo-, or macrocytic, marked variation in RBC size and shape, basophilic stippling
  - ring sideroblasts (diagnostic hallmark)
  - increased iron in bone marrow macrophages

Treatment
- X-linked: high dose pyridoxine (Vit B6) in some cases
- acquired: Epo and G-CSF
- reversible: remove precipitating cause
- transfusion for severe anemia

Thalassemia

- see *Hemolytic Anemia*, H15

Normocytic Anemia

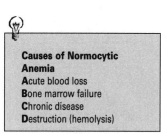

Causes of Normocytic Anemia
Acute blood loss
Bone marrow failure
Chronic disease
Destruction (hemolysis)

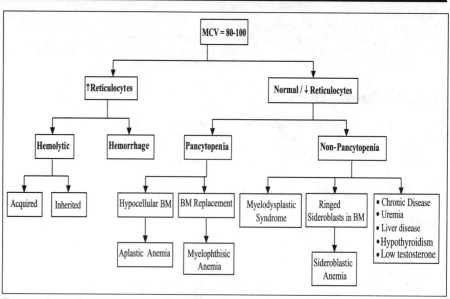

Figure 7. Approach to Normocytic Anemia (MCV = 80-100)

Aplastic Anemia

Definition
- destruction of hematopoietic cells of the bone marrow leading to pancytopenia and hypocellular bone marrow

Epidemiology
- occurs at any age
- slightly more common in males

Etiology
- congenital
  - Fanconi's anemia
  - Shwachman-Diamond syndrome (bone marrow failure and pancreatic insufficiency)
- acquired
  - idiopathic
    - often immune (T-cell mediated) – 1/2 to 2/3 of cases
  - drugs
    - dose-related (e.g. chemotherapeutic agents)
    - idiosyncratic (e.g. chloramphenicol, phenylbutazone)
  - toxins
    - benzene and other organic solvents
    - DDT and insecticides
  - ionizing radiation
  - post viral infection (e.g. parvovirus B19, EBV, HDV, HEV, HHV6, HIV)
  - autoimmune (e.g. SLE) – rare
  - Paroxysmal Nocturnal Hemoglobinuria (PNH) - associated with aplastic anemia, but not a cause

Clinical Features
- can present acutely or insidiously
- symptoms of anemia, thrombocytopenia
- presentation of neutropenia ranges from infection in the mouth to septicemia
- pallor and petechiae most common findings
- absence of splenomegaly and lymphadenopathy

Investigations
- CBC
  - anemia or neutropenia or thrombocytopenia (any combination) ± pancytopenia
  - ↓ corrected reticulocyte count <0.01 (<1% of the RBC)
- blood film
  - decreased number of normal RBCs
- bone marrow
  - aplasia or hypoplasia of marrow cells with fat replacement
  - cellularity <25%
- key: need to exclude other causes of pancytopenia first (Figure 5)

Treatment
- remove offending agents
- supportive care (red cell and platelet transfusions, antibiotics)
- immunosuppression
  - anti-thymocyte globulin – 50-60% of patients respond
  - cyclosporine
- allogenic bone marrow transplant

Hemolytic Anemia (HA)

Classification
- hereditary
  - abnormal membrane (spherocytosis, elliptocytosis)
  - abnormal enzymes (pyruvate kinase deficiency, G6PD deficiency)
  - abnormal hemoglobin synthesis (thalassemias, hemoglobinopathies)
- acquired
  - immune
    - hemolytic transfusion reaction, idiopathic or secondary autoimmune HA (AIHA), drugs (e.g. penicillin), cold agglutinins
  - non-immune
    - microangiopathic HA, PNH, hypersplenism, march hemoglobinuria (exertional hemolysis), infection (e.g. malaria)
- HA are also classified as intravascular or extravascular
  - G6PD deficiency, TTP, DIC and PNH are examples of intravascular HA
  - AIHA and hereditary spherocytosis are examples of extravascular HA

Clinical Features Specific to HA
- jaundice
- dark urine
- cholelithiasis (pigment stones)
- potential for a regenerative crisis (e.g. BM suppression in overwhelming infection)
- iron overload with extravascular hemolysis
- iron deficiency with intravascular hemolysis

Investigations
- screening tests
  - ↑ reticulocyte count
  - ↓ haptoglobin
  - ↑ unconjugated bilirubin
  - ↑ urobilinogen
  - ↑ LDH
- tests specific for intravascular hemolysis
  - RBC fragments on blood film
  - free hemoglobin in serum
  - methemalbuminemia (heme + albumin)
  - hemoglobinuria (immediate)
  - hemosiderinuria (delayed)
- tests specific for extravascular hemolysis
  - direct Coombs' test (direct antiglobulin test)
    - detects IgG or complement on the surface of RBC
    - adding anti-IgG or anti-complement antibodies to the RBCs; positive test if the RBCs agglutinate
    - indications
      - hemolytic disease of newborn
      - autoimmune hemolytic anemia (AIHA)
      - hemolytic transfusion reaction
  - indirect Coombs' test (indirect antiglobulin test)
    - detects antibodies in serum that can recognize antigens on RBC
    - mixing serum with donor RBCs and then Coombs' serum (Anti-human Ig antibodies); positive test if RBCs agglutinate
    - indications
      - cross-matching of recipient serum with donor's RBC
      - atypical blood group
      - blood group antibodies in pregnant women
      - antibodies in AIHA

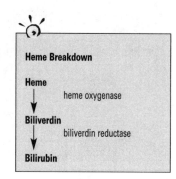

Heme Breakdown

Heme
    ↓   heme oxygenase

Biliverdin
    ↓   biliverdin reductase

Bilirubin

Thalassemia

Definition
- defects in production of α or β chains that leads to microcytosis
- clinical manifestations and treatment depends on specific gene and number of alleles affected
- common features:
  - increasing severity with increasing number of alleles involved
  - hypochromic microcytic anemia
  - basophilic stippling; abnormal shaped RBC on blood film

ThalasSEAmia – β-Thal → prevalent in Mediterranean SEA; α-Thal → prevalent in South East Asia (SEA).

Pathophysiology
- defect may be in any of the Hb genes:
  - normally 4 α genes in total, 2 on each copy of chromosome 16
  - normally 2 β genes in total, 1 on each copy of chromosome 11
  - fetal hemoglobin, HbF ($\alpha_2\gamma_2$) switches to adult forms HbA ($\alpha_2\beta_2$) and HbA$_2$ ($\alpha_2\delta_2$) at 3-6 months of life
  - HbA constitutes 97% of adult hemoglobin
  - HbA$_2$ constitutes 3% of adult hemoglobin

β-Thalassemia Minor (Thalassemia Trait)

Definition
- defect in single allele of β gene (heterozygous)
- common among people of Mediterranean and Asian descent

Microcytosis in βThal minor
Microcytosis much more profound and the anemia much milder than that of Fe deficiency.

Clinical Features
- palpable spleen (rare)

Investigations
- Hb 90-140 g/L or 9-14 g/dL, MCV<70, normal Fe
- peripheral blood film – basophilic stippling

- Hb electrophoresis
  - specific: HbA_2 ↑ to 0.025-0.05 (2.5-5%) (normal 1.5-3.5%)
  - may be masked by Fe deficiency
  - non-specific: 50% have slight ↑ in HbF

Treatment
- not necessary
- genetic counselling for patient and family

β-Thalassemia Major

Definition
- defect in both alleles of β gene (homozygous; autosomal recessive)

Pathophysiology
- ineffective chain synthesis leading to ineffective erythropoiesis, hemolysis of RBC, and ↑ in HbF

Clinical Features
- initial presentation at age 6-12 months when HbA supposed to replace HbF
- severe anemia develops in the first year of life
- jaundice
- stunted growth and development (hypogonadal dwarf)
- gross hepatosplenomegaly (extramedullary hematopoiesis)
- changes (expanded marrow cavity)
  - skull x-ray has "hair-on-end" appearance
  - pathological fractures common
- evidence of ↑ Hb catabolism (e.g. gallstones)
- death from
  - untreated anemia (transfuse)
  - infection (treat early)
  - iron overload (late, secondary to transfusions), usually 20-30 years old if untreated

Investigations
- Hb 40-60 g/L (4-6 g/dL)
- Hb electrophoresis
  - HbA: 0-0.10 (0-10%), (normal >95%)
  - HbF: 0.90-1.00 (90-100%)

Treatment
- lifelong regular transfusions
- folic acid
- Fe chelation to prevent iron overload (e.g. deferoxamine)
- bone marrow transplant

α-Thalassemia

Definition
- defect(s) in α genes
- similar distribution to β-thalassemia but a higher frequency among Asians and Africans

Clinical Features
- 1 defective α gene: clinically silent; normal Hb, normal MCV
- 2 defective α genes: ↓ MCV, normal Hb
- 3 defective α genes: HbH (β4) disease (presents in adults due to excess β chain production); ↓ MCV, ↓ Hb, splenomegaly
- 4 defective α genes: Hb Barts (γ_4) disease (hydrops fetalis, not compatible with life)

Investigations
- peripheral blood film – screen for HbH inclusion bodies with special stain
- Hb electrophoresis not diagnostic for α-thalassemia
- DNA analysis using α gene probes

Treatment
- depends on degree of anemia

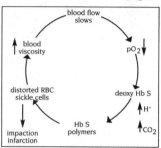

Figure 8. Pathophysiology of Sickling

Organs Affected by Vaso-Occlusive Crisis	
Organ	**Problem**
brain	seizures, stroke
eye	hemorrhage, blindness
liver	infarcts, RUQ syndrome
lung	chest syndrome, long-term pulmonary hypertension
gall bladder	stones
heart	hyperdynamic flow murmurs
spleen	enlarged (child); atrophic (adult)
kidney	hematuria; loss of renal concentrating ability
intestines	acute abdomen
placenta	stillbirths
penis	priapism
digits	dactylitis
femoral head	avascular necrosis
bone	infarction, infection
ankle	leg ulcers

Functional asplenism – ↑ susceptibility to infection by **encapsulated** organisms
- *S. pneumoniae*
- *N. meningitidis*
- *H. influenzae*
- *Salmonella* (osteomyelitis)

An Evidence-based Review for the NIH Consensus Development Conference on Hydroxyurea for the Treatment of Adults with Sickle Cell Disease.
Ann Intern Med. 2008 May 5
Objective: To synthesize the published literature on the efficacy, effectiveness, and toxicity of hydroxyurea when used in adults with sickle cell disease.
Study Selection: Randomized trials, observational studies, and case reports evaluating efficacy and toxicity of hydroxyurea in adults with sickle cell disease, and toxicity studies of hydroxyurea in other conditions that were published in English were included.
Results: In the single randomized trial, the hemoglobin level was higher in hydroxyurea recipients than placebo recipients after 2 years (difference, 6 g/L), as was fetal hemoglobin (absolute difference, 3.2%). The median number of painful crises was 44% lower than in the placebo arm. The 12 observational studies that enrolled adults reported a relative increase in fetal hemoglobin of 4% to 20% and a relative reduction in crisis rates by 68% to 84%. Hospital admissions declined by 18% to 32%. The evidence suggests that hydroxyurea may impair spermatogenesis. Limited evidence indicates that hydroxyurea treatment in adults with sickle cell disease is not associated with leukemia. Likewise, limited evidence suggests that hydroxyurea and leg ulcers are not associated in patients with sickle cell disease, and evidence is insufficient to estimate the risk for skin neoplasms, although these outcomes can be attributed to hydroxyurea in other conditions.
Conclusions: Hydroxyurea has demonstrated efficacy in adults with sickle cell disease. The paucity of long-term studies limits conclusions about toxicity.

Sickle Cell Disease

• see Pediatrics

Definition
- sickling disorders due to a mutant β globin chain, most commonly caused by a Glu→Val substitution at position 6 resulting in HbS rather than HbA
- sickle cell anemia occurs when an individual has two HbS genes (homozygous) or one HbS gene + another mutant β globin gene (compound heterozygote)

Pathophysiology (Figure 8)
- at low pO_2, deoxy HbS polymerizes, leading to rigid crystal-like rods that distort membranes → 'sickles'
- the pO_2 level at which sickling occurs is related to the percentage of HbS present
  - in heterozygotes (HbAS), sickling occurs at a pO_2 of 40 mmHg
  - in homozygotes (HbSS), sickling occurs at a pO_2 of 80 mmHg
- sickling is aggravated by ↑ H+, ↑ CO_2, ↑ 2,3-DPG, ↑ temperature and osmolality
- sickle cells are fragile and hemolyze; they also block small vessels

Clinical Features
- HbAS (heterozygous): patient will appear normal except at times of extreme hypoxia and infection (sickle cell trait)
- HbSC (most common compound heterozygote)
  - milder anemia
  - similar clinical features to HbSS although milder
  - spleen not always atrophic in adult
- HbSS (homozygous)
  - chronic hemolytic anemia
  - jaundice in the first year of life
  - may have retarded growth and development +/- skeletal changes
  - spleen enlarged in child and atrophic in adult
  - types of crises:
    I. Aplastic crises
      - toxins and infections (especially parvovirus B19) transiently suppress bone marrow activity
    II. Splenic sequestration crises
      - usually in children, with significant pooling of blood in spleen, resulting in acute ↓ Hb and shock
      - uncommon in adults because of functional asplenia from repeated infarction (adults with HbSC may not have functional asplenia)
    III. Vaso-occlusive crises (infarction) (see side bar)
      - may affect many different organs causing pain (especially in back, chest, abdomen and extremities), fever, and leukocytosis (e.g. acute chest syndrome)
      - precipitated by infections, dehydration, rapid change in temperature, pregnancy, menses and alcohol

Table 5. Investigations for Sickle Cell Disease

	HbAS	HbSS
CBC	normal	↑ reticulocyte, ↓ Hb, ↓ Hct
Peripheral blood	normal; possibly a few target cells	sickled cells
Hb electrophoresis	HbA fraction of 0.65 (65%); HbS fraction of 0.35 (35%)	No HbA, Only HbS and HbF. Proportions change with age
Other	+ve sickle cell prep (screening test)	

- Hb electrophoresis distinguishes HbAS, HbSS and other variants

Treatment
- genetic counseling
- folic acid to prevent folate deficiency
- hydroxyurea to enhance production of HbF
  - stops repression of the gene for HbF or initiates differentiation of stem cells in which this gene is active
  - presence of HbF in the SS cells ↓ polymerization and precipitation of HbS
  - note: hydroxyurea is cytotoxic and may cause bone marrow suppression
- treatment of vaso-occlusive crisis
  - oxygen (only if hypoxic)
  - hydration (reduces viscosity)
  - antimicrobials
  - correct acidosis
  - analgesics/narcotics (give enough)

- magnesium (inhibits potassium and water efflux from RBCs thereby preventing dehydration)
- indication for exchange transfusion: acute chest syndrome, stroke, bone marrow necrosis, priapism, and CNS crisis
- prevention of crises is key
  - establish diagnosis
  - avoid conditions that favour sickling (hypoxia, acidosis, dehydration, fever)
  - vaccination in childhood (e.g. pneumococcus (heptavalent AND 23-valent), meningococcus, Hib)
  - prophylactic penicillin from 3 months until at least 5 years of age
  - good hygiene, nutrition, and social support
- screening for potential complications
  - regular bloodwork (CBC, retics, iron indices, BUN, LFTs, creatinine)
  - urinalysis annually
  - transcranial doppler annually until 16 years old
  - retinal examinations annually from 8 years old
  - echocardiography every two years from 10 years old (to screen for pulmonary hypertension)

> **Acute Chest Syndrome**
> Affects 30% of patients with sickle cell disease and may be life threatening.
> Presentation includes dyspnea, chest pain, fever, tachypnea, leukocytosis, and pulmonary infiltrate on CXR.
> Caused by vaso-occlusion, infection or pulmonary fat embolus from infarcted marrow.

Autoimmune Hemolytic Anemia (AIHA)

Table 6. Classification of AIHA

	Warm	Cold
Antibody Allotype	IgG	IgM
Agglutination Temperature	37°C	4-37°C
Direct Coombs Test (direct anti-globulin test)	Positive for IgG	Positive for complement

Etiology	Idiopathic
	Secondary to lymphoproliferative disorder
	  e.g. CLL, Hodgkin's
	Secondary to autoimmune disease
	  e.g. SLE
	Drug induced
	  Type I – hapten-mediated
	    e.g. penicillin
	  Type II – immune-complex mediated
	    e.g. quinine
	  Type III – "true" anti-RBC Ab
	    e.g. methyldopa
		Idiopathic
		Secondary to infection
		  e.g. mycoplasma, EBV
		Secondary to lymphoproliferative disorder
		  e.g. macroglobulinemia, CLL

Blood Film	Spherocytes	Agglutination
Management	Treat underlying cause Corticosteroids Immunosuppression Splenectomy	Treat underlying cause Warm patient Immunosuppression Plasmapheresis

Microangiopathic Hemolytic Anemia (MAHA)

Definition
- hemolytic anemia due to intravascular fragmentation of RBCs

Etiology
- thrombotic thrombocytopenic purpura (TTP)/hemolytic uremic syndrome (HUS) (see Table 12)
- DIC
- metastatic carcinoma
- eclampsia, HELLP syndrome
- malignant hypertension
- vasculitis
- malfunctioning heart valves

Investigations
- blood film: evidence of hemolysis, schistocytes
- hemolytic work-up
- hemosiderinuria, hemoglobinuria

Hereditary Spherocytosis

- abnormality in RBC membrane proteins (i.e. spectrin)
- spleen makes defective RBCs more spherocytotic (and more fragile) by membrane removal and also acts as site of destruction
- autosomal dominant with variable penetrance
- most common type of hereditary hemolytic anemia
- investigations: blood film shows spherocytes, ↑ osmotic fragility (rarely done today), molecular analysis for spectrin gene
- treatment: splenectomy (immunize against pneumococcus, meningococcus and Hib first), but avoid in early childhood

Hereditary Elliptocytosis

- abnormality in spectrin interaction with other membrane proteins
- autosomal dominant
- 25-75% elliptocytes
- hemolysis is usually mild
- treatment: splenectomy for severe hemolysis (immunize against pneumococcus, meningococcus, and Hib first)

G6PD Deficiency

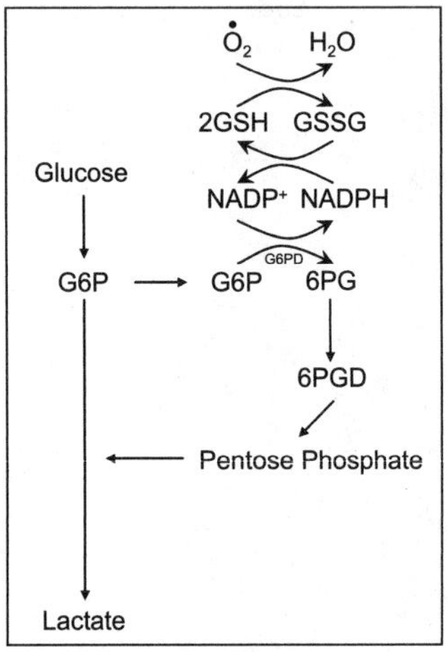

Definition
- deficiency in glucose-6-phosphate dehydrogenase (G6PD) leading to sensitivity of RBC to oxidative stress

Pathophysiology
- X-linked recessive, more prevalent in black males
- autosomal recessive, more prevalent in Mediterranean population (rare)

Clinical Features
- hemolysis precipitated by:
  - oxidative stress
  - drugs (e.g. sulfonamide, antimalarials, nitrofurantoin)
  - infection
  - food (fava beans)
- prolonged, pathologic neonatal jaundice
- chronic hemolytic anemia in autosomal recessive cases

Investigations
- neonatal screening
- high index of suspicion
- G6PD assay
  - should not be done in acute crisis when reticulocyte count is high
- blood film
  - Heinz bodies (granules in RBCs due to oxidized Hb that results in bite cells once removed by the spleen)
  - features of intravascular hemolysis (e.g. RBC fragments)

Treatment
- transfusion in severe cases
- stop offending drugs or food and avoid triggers

Figure 9. G6PD Pathway

(Figure shows: O_2, H_2O, 2GSH, GSSG, Glucose, $NADP^+$, NADPH, G6P, G6P, 6PG, G6PD, 6PGD, Pentose Phosphate, Lactate)

Macrocytic Anemia

Causes
- megaloblastic
  - vit B_{12} deficiency
  - folate deficiency
  - drugs (methotrexate, azathioprine)
- non-megaloblastic
  - reticulocytosis
  - myelodysplastic syndromes
  - liver disease
  - alcoholism
  - hypothyroidism

Table 7. Comparison Between Megaloblastic and Non-Megaloblastic Macrocytic Anemia

	Megaloblastic	Non-Megaloblastic
Morphology	Large, oval, nucleated RBC precursor Hypersegmented neutrophils	Large round RBC Normal neutrophils
Pathophysiology	Failure of DNA synthesis resulting in asynchronous maturation of RBC nucleus and cytoplasm	Reflects membrane abnormality with abnormal cholesterol metabolism

Vitamin B_{12} Deficiency

B_{12} (cobalamin)
- binds to intrinsic factor (IF) secreted by gastric parietal cells
- absorbed in terminal ileum
- total body stores sufficient for 3-4 years

Etiology
- diet
  - strict vegan (rare, more likely to present in infants and toddlers)
- gastric
  - mucosal atrophy secondary to chronic gastritis
  - pernicious anemia
  - post-gastrectomy
- intestinal absorption
  - malabsorption (e.g. Crohn's, celiac sprue, pancreatic disease)
  - stagnant bowel (e.g. blind loop, stricture)
  - fish tapeworm
  - resection of ileum
- rare genetic causes (e.g. transcobalamin II deficiency)

Pathophysiology of Pernicious Anemia
- auto-antibodies produced against gastric parietal cells leading to achlorhydria and lack of intrinsic factor secretion
- intrinsic factor is required to stabilize B_{12} as it passes through the bowel
- $\downarrow$ intrinsic factor leads to $\downarrow$ ileal absorption of B_{12}
- may be associated with other autoimmune disorders (polyglandular endocrine insufficiency)
- female:male = 1.6:1, often >60 years old

Clinical Features
- neurological
  - cerebral (common; reversible with B_{12} therapy)
    - confusion
    - delirium
    - dementia (possibly reversible)
  - cranial nerves (rare)
    - optic atrophy
  - cord (irreversible damage)
    - subacute combined degeneration
      - posterior columns – $\downarrow$ vibration sense, proprioception and 2-point discrimination
      - pyramidal tracts – spastic weakness, hyperactive reflexes
  - peripheral neuropathy (variable reversibility)
    - usually symmetrical, affecting lower limbs more than upper limbs

Investigations
- serum
  - anemia often severe ± neutropenia ± thrombocytopenia
  - MCV>120
  - low reticulocyte count relative to the degree of anemia
- serum B_{12} and RBC folate
  - caution: low serum B_{12} leads to low RBC folate because of failure of folate polyglutamate synthesis in the absence of B_{12}
- blood film
  - oval macrocytes
  - hypersegmented neutrophils
- bone marrow
  - differentiates between megaloblastic and myelodysplastic anemias
  - hypercellularity
  - failure of nuclear maturation
  - elevated unconjugated bilirubin and LDH due to marrow cell breakdown
- Schilling test to distinguish pernicious anemia from other causes (see sidebar and Gastroenterology)

Treatment
- vitamin B_{12} 100 μg IM monthly for life or 1000-1200 μg PO daily if intestinal absorption intact (see sidebar)
- less frequent, higher doses are probably as effective (e.g. 1000 μg IM q3 months)
- watch for hypokalemia and rebound thrombocytosis when treating severe megaloblastic anemia

Folate Deficiency

- uncommon due to extensive dietary supplementation in developed countries
- folate complexes with gastric R binder
- complex then binds to intrinsic factor in the duodenum
- this complex is absorbed in the jejunum
- folate stores are depleted in 3-6 months

Characteristics of megaloblastic macrocytic anemia
i) Pancytopenia
ii) Hypersegmented neutrophils
iii) Megaloblastic bone marrow

Schilling Test

Part 1
- tracer dose (1 µg) of radiolabeled B_{12} given PO
- flushing dose (1 mg) of unlabelled B_{12} IM 1 hr later to saturate tissue binders of B_{12} thus allowing radioactive B_{12} to be excreted in urine
- 24 hour urine radiolabeled B_{12} measured
- normal > 5% excretion (a normal excretion will only be seen if the low B_{12} was due to dietary deficiency)

Part 2
- same as part 1, but radiolabeled B_{12} given with oral intrinsic factor
- should be done only if first stage shows reduced excretion
- normal test result (> 5% excretion) = pernicious anemia
- abnormal test result (< 5% excretion) = intestinal causes (malabsorption)

Oral vitamin B12 versus intramuscular vitamin B12 for vitamin B12 deficiency.
Cochrane Database Syst Rev. 2005;(3):CD004655
Study: Systematic review. 2 RCTs met inclusion criteria; total 108 patients with follow-up from 90 days to 4 months
Intervention: One study evaluated 1000 µg of oral B12 compared to 1000 µg IM B12 on the same dosing schedule. The other compared 2000 µg daily oral B12 to 1000 µg IM B12 on a less frequent dosing schedule. Neurological and hematological end points were evaluated.
Results: Meta-analysis was not attempted due to study heterogeneity. Both studies reported improvements in hematological and neurological end-points in both oral and IM groups. No significant difference was observed between groups in either study.
Conclusions: High dose oral vitamin B12 (1000-2000 µg) is equivalent to IM vitamin B12 on the same or less frequent dosing schedule. This data is severely limited by small sample sizes and short follow-up periods. Insufficient numbers of patients with malabsorption conditions were included to generalize these results to the entire primary care population. Larger studies based in the primary care population are required.

Etiology
- diet (folate is present in leafy green vegetables)
  - most common cause traditionally; however with universal supplementation in foods it is now less frequent
  - seen mainly in infants, elderly, alcoholics
- intestinal
  - malabsorption
- drugs/chemicals
  - alcohol
  - anticonvulsants
  - antifolates (methotrexate)
  - birth control pills
- ↑ demand
  - pregnancy
  - prematurity
  - hemolysis
  - hemodialysis
  - psoriasis, exfoliative dermatitis

Clinical Features
- mildly jaundiced due to hemolysis of RBC secondary to ineffective hemoglobin synthesis
- glossitis and angular stomatitis
- rare
  - melanin pigmentation
  - purpura secondary to thrombocytopenia
- folate deficiency at time of conception and early pregnancy has been linked to neural tube defects

Management
- folic acid 15 mg PO OD x 3 months; then 5 mg PO OD maintenance if cause not reversible

> Never give folate alone to individual with megaloblastic anemia because it will mask B_{12} deficiency and neurological degeneration will continue.

Hemostasis

> Normal hemostasis occurs as a result of the balance between procoagulant and anticoagulant factors.

Three Phases of Hemostasis

1. Primary Hemostasis
- goal is to rapidly stop bleeding
- vessel injury results in collagen/subendothelial matrix exposure and release of vasoconstrictors
- blood flow is impeded and platelets come in contact with damaged vessel wall
  - adhesion: platelets adhere to subendothelium via vWF
  - activation: platelets are activated resulting in change of shape and release of ADP and thromboxane A_2
  - aggregation: these factors further recruit and aggregate more platelets resulting in formation of localized hemostatic plug

2. Secondary Hemostasis
- platelet plug (formed through primary hemostasis) is reinforced by production of fibrin clot in secondary hemostasis
- extrinsic pathway
  - the only way coagulation is initiated *in vivo*
- intrinsic pathway
  - allows for amplification once coagulation has started

3. Fibrin Stabilization and Fibrinolysis (resolution)
- conversion from soluble to insoluble clot
- once healing initiated, clot dissolution (anticoagulant pathway)

> **3 Phases of Hemostasis:**
>
> 1. Primary hemostasis
>   - vascular response and platelet plug formation via vWF
>
> 2. Secondary hemostasis
>   - fibrin clot formation
>
> 3. Resolution
>   - fibrinolysis

> **Tests of Secondary Hemostasis**
> PT/INR: **T**ennis is played *outside* (*Extrinsic* Pathway)
> PTT: **T**able **T**ennis is played *inside* (*Intrinsic* Pathway)

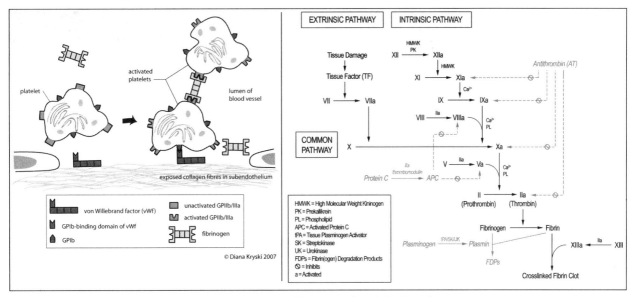

Figure 10a. Platelet Activation Cascade   **Figure 10b.** Coagulation Cascade

Table 8. Commonly Used Tests of Hemostasis

Type of Hemostasis	Test	Reference Range	Purpose	Examples of Associated Diagnoses
Primary	platelet count bleeding time	150-450 x 10⁹/L N <8 mins	- to quantitate platelet number - platelet function and vessel wall function	- low in ITP, HUS/TTP, DIC - high in severe thrombocytopenia, vWD, platelet dysfunction
Secondary	aPTT	22-35 sec	- measures intrinsic pathway (factors VIII, IX, XI, XII) and common pathway - used to monitor heparin therapy	- high in hemophilias A and B
	PT	11-24 sec	- measures extrinsic pathway (factor VII) in particular and common pathway	- high in factor VII deficiency
	INR	0.9-1.2	- permits determination of extrinsic pathway status independent of laboratory performing measurement - used to monitor warfarin therapy	

	Mixing studies		- differentiate inhibitors of clotting factor(s) from a deficiency in
			  clotting factor(s)
			- mix patient's plasma with normal plasma in 1:1 ratio and repeat
			  abnormal test
				- clotting factor(s) deficiency if test now normal
				- inhibitors of clotting factor(s) if test stilll abnormal

Fibrinolysis	euglobulin lysis time	N >9 min	- looks for accelerated fibrinolysis	- may be accelerated in DIC - low in hereditary deficiency of fibrinogen
Other	- fibrinogen - fibrinogen degradation products (FDPs), D-dimers - specific factor assays - tests of physiological inhibitors (antithrombin, protein S, protein C, hereditary resistance to APC) - tests of pathologic inhibitors (e.g. lupus anticoagulant)			

Table 9. Signs and Symptoms of Disorders of Hemostasis

	Primary (Platelet)	Secondary (Coagulation)
Surface Cuts	excessive, prolonged bleeding	normal/slightly prolonged bleeding
Onset After Injury	immediate	delayed
Site of Bleeding	superficial i.e. mucosal (nasal, gingival, GI tract, uterine), skin	deep i.e. joints, muscles, GI tract, GU tract, excessive post-traumatic
Lesions	petechiae, ecchymoses	hemarthroses, hematomas

Disorders of Primary Hemostasis

Definition
- inability to form an adequate platelet plug due to
  - disorders of blood vessels
  - disorders of platelets
    - abnormal function
    - abnormal numbers (thrombocytopenia)
  - disorders of vWF
- characterized by superficial bleeding, petechiae, ecchymoses
- life-threatening bleeding sites in thrombocytopenia: intracranial and retroperitoneal

Classification

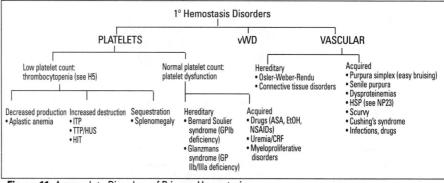

Figure 11. Approach to Disorders of Primary Hemostasis

Immune Thrombocytopenic Purpura (ITP)

Table 10. Immune Thrombocytopenic Purpura

Features	Acute ITP	Chronic ITP
Peak Age	2-6 years	20-40 years
Sex Predilection	none	F > M (3:1)
History of Recent Infection	common	rare
Onset of Bleed	abrupt	insidious
Duration	usually weeks	months to years
Spontaneous Remissions	80% or more	uncommon

ACUTE (CHILD-TYPE) ITP
- see Pediatrics

CHRONIC (ADULT-TYPE) ITP
- most common cause of isolated thrombocytopenia
- diagnosis of exclusion (i.e. isolated thrombocytopenia with no clinically apparent causes)

Pathophysiology
- anti-platelet antibodies bind to platelet surface → increased splenic destruction and clearance

Investigations
- PT and aPTT normal
- peripheral blood film: ↓ platelets, giant platelets
- bone marrow: increased number of megakaryocytes
  - critical test to rule out other causes of thrombocytopenia in people >60 years old, like myelodysplasia

Treatment
- platelet count >30 x 10^9/L, no mucosal bleeding
  - conservative
- platelet count <20-30 x 10^9/L or evidence of mucosal bleeding
  - steroids: prednisone 1-2 mg/kg/day, taper over weeks (50-75% responsive)
- if steroids fail or if significant bleeding
  - IV immunoglobulin (IVIG)
  - Anti-Rh (D) (anti-D, Win-Rho™): component of IVIG, effective only in Rh+ patients in whom the immunoglobulin binds to erythrocyte D antigen
- if steroids and IVIG fail
  - splenectomy (~65% have long-term remission)

- other: immunosuppressants (e.g. azathioprine), platelets (if life-threatening bleeding), Danazol™

Prognosis
- fluctuating course
- overall relatively benign, mortality 1-2%
- major concern is cerebral hemorrhage at platelet counts <5 x 10^9/L

Heparin-Induced Thrombocytopenia (HIT)

LMWH is also associated with HIT but the risk is less than unfractionated heparin.

Table 11. HIT-II (Heparin induced thrombocytopenia, type II)

Pathophysiology	• immune mediated • Ab recognizes a complex of heparin and platelet factor 4 (PF4) leading to platelet activation via platelet Fc receptor and activation of coagulation system
Diagnosis	50% reduction in platelets while on heparin within 5-15 days of initiation
Onset of ↓platelets	5-15 days (if previously exposed to heparin, HIT can develop in hours)
Risk of thrombosis	~30% (25% of events are arterial)
Clinical features	• bleeding complications uncommon • venous thrombosis: DVT, PE • arterial thrombosis: MI, stroke, limb and mesenteric arteries, adrenal gland involvement • heparin-induced skin necrosis • acute platelet activation syndromes: acute inflammatory reactions (e.g. fever/chills, flushing, etc.) • transient global amnesia
Specific tests	• ^{14}C serotonin release assay (uses donor platelets with ^{14}C serotonin and heparin with patient's plasma) • ELISA for HIT-Ig (↑sensitive, ↓specific than serotonin assay) • flow cytometry
Management	• clinical suspicion of HIT should prompt discontinuation of heparin (specific tests take several days) • because of 90% cross-reactivity LMWH should not be substituted • alternative agents include: Lepirudin (recombinant hirudin, avoid in renal disease), Argatroban (effective thrombin inhibitor, monitored with aPTT, use with caution in liver disease), Danaparoid

HIT Type I (Heparin-associated thrombocytopenia)
- direct heparin mediated platelet aggregation (non-immune)
- platelets >100 X 10^9/L
- self-limited (no thrombotic risk)
- may continue with heparin therapy
- onset 24-72 hours

Thrombotic Thrombocytopenic Purpura (TTP) and Hemolytic Uremic Syndrome (HUS)

Table 12. TTP and HUS

	HUS	TTP
Epidemiology	• predominantly children	• predominantly adult

Etiology	• Shiga toxin (*E.coli* serotype O157:H7)	• deficiency of metalloproteinase that breaks down ultra-large vWF multimers
		  ■ congenital (genetic absence of ADAMTS-13)
		  ■ acquired (drugs, malignancy, transplant, HIV-associated, idiopathic)

Clinical features	1. severe thrombocytopenia: (purpura, epistaxis, hematuria, hemoptysis, GI bleed) 2. microangiopathic hemolytic anemia (MAHA) 3. renal failure (abnormal urinalysis, oliguria, acute renal failure)	1. thrombocytopenia 2. microangiopathic hemolytic anemia (MAHA) 3. neurological symptoms (H/A, confusion, focal defects, seizures) 4. renal failure 5. fever
Investigations (both TTP, HUS)	• CBC and blood film: schistocytes and ↓platelets consider diagnosis • PT, aPTT, fibrinogen: normal • markers of hemolysis: ↑unconj bili., ↑LDH, ↓haptoglobin • negative Coombs' test • creatinine, urea, to follow renal function • stool C+S (HUS)	
Management (both TTP, HUS)	• plasmapheresis is the treatment of choice ± steroids • platelet transfusion is contraindicated (↑microvascular thrombosis) • plasma infusion if plasmapheresis is not immediately available •TTP mortality ~90% if untreated	

Pathophysiology of TTP
- vWF secreted by endothelial cells in a very large polymer rapidly cleaved by the ADAMTS-13 protease
- congenital TTP is deficient in ADAMTS-13
- antibodies against ADAMTS-13 present in acquired TTP

Differential diagnosis includes:
Sepsis
DIC
HELLP
Antiphospholipid Ab syndrome
Evans syndrome (autoimmune hemolytic anemia + ITP)

Von Willebrand's Disease (vWD)

Pathophysiology
- heterogeneous group of defects
- usually autosomal dominant (type 3 is autosomal recessive)
- qualitative or quantitative abnormality of vWF
  - vWF needed for platelet adhesion and acts as carrier for Factor VIII; abnormality of vWF can affect both primary and secondary hemostasis
  - vWF exists as a series of multimers ranging in size
    - the largest ones are most active in mediation of platelet adhesion
    - both large and small complex with Factor VIII
- usually mild in severity

Classification
- type 1 – mild quantitative defect (decreased amount of vWF) in 75% of cases
- type 2 – qualitative defect (dysfunctional vWF) in 20-25% of cases
- type 3 – severe total quantitative defect (no vWF produced) rare

Clinical Features
- mild
  - asymptomatic
  - mucosal and cutaneous bleeding, easy bruising, epistaxis, menorrhagia
- moderate to severe
  - as above but more severe, occasionally soft-tissue hematomas, petechiae (rare), GI bleeding, hemarthroses

Investigations
- ↑ bleeding time and PTT
- ↓ Factor VIII (5-50%)
- platelet count normal or rarely ↓
- ↓ ristocetin cofactor activity (normally causes vWF to bind platelets tightly)
- analysis of vWF multimers

Treatment
- desmopressin (DDAVP™) is treatment of choice for type I vWD
  - causes release of vWF and Factor VIII from endothelial cells
  - variable efficacy depending on disease type
  - need good response before using with further bleeding
- high-purity Factor VIII concentrate containing vWF (Hemate P™) in select cases and type 2
- conjugated estrogens (increase vWF levels)

Prognosis
- may fluctuate, often improves during pregnancy and with age

von Willebrand disease in women with menorrhagia: a systematic review.
(BJOG. 2004;111:734-40)
Purpose: To determine the prevalence of von Willebrand disease in women presenting with menorrhagia.
Study Selection: Systematic review of studies evaluating the prevalence of von Willebrand disease in women with menorrhagia.
Results: Eleven studies were included, totalling 988 women with menorrhagia. One hundred and thirty-one women were diagnosed to have von Willebrand disease with prevalences in individual studies ranging from 5% to 24%. The overall prevalence was 13% (95% CI 11–15.6%). The prevalence was higher in the European studies–18% (95% CI 15-23%) compared with that in North American studies–10% (95% CI 7.5–13%). This difference (P= 0.007) is likely to be the result of differences in the studies, which include method of recruitment of study population, method of assessing menstrual blood loss, ethnic composition of study population, criteria for diagnosis and use of race- and ABO blood group-specific values for von Willebrand factor.
Conclusions: The prevalence of von Willebrand disease is increased in women with menorrhagia and is the underlying cause in a small but significant group of women with menorrhagia across the world. Testing for this disorder should be considered when investigating women with menorrhagia, especially those of Caucasian origin, those with no obvious pelvic pathology or with additional bleeding symptoms.

Disorders of Secondary Hemostasis

Table 13. Classification of Secondary Hemostasis Disorders

Hereditary	Acquired
• Factor VIII: Hemophilia A, vWD	• liver disease
• Factor IX: Hemophilia B (Christmas Disease)	• DIC
• Factor XI	• vitamin K deficiency
• other factor deficiencies are rare	• acquired inhibitors

Hemophilia A (Factor VIII Deficiency)

Pathophysiology
- X-linked recessive, 1/5,000 males
- mild (>5% of normal factor level), moderate (1-5%), severe (<1%)

Clinical Features
See Table 9 – *Signs and Symptoms of Disorders of Hemostasis*, H23

Investigations
- prolonged aPTT, normal INR (PT)
- ↓ Factor VIII (<40% of normal)
- vWF usually normal or ↑

Hemophilia A: Five Hs
Hemarthroses
Hematomas
Hematochezia
Hematuria
Head hemorrhage

Treatment
- desmopressin (DDAVP™) in mild Hemophilia A
- recombinant Factor VIII concentrate for:
  - prophylaxis
  - minor but not trivial bleeding (e.g. hemarthroses)
  - major potentially life-threatening bleeding (e.g. multiple trauma)
- anti-fibrinolytic agents (e.g. tranexamic acid)

Hemophilia B (Factor IX Deficiency)

- a.k.a. Christmas disease
- X-linked recessive, 1/30,000 males
- clinical and laboratory features identical to Hemophilia A (except ↓ Factor IX)
- treatment: recombinant Factor IX concentrate and use of anti-fibrinolytic agents

Factor XI Deficiency

- a.k.a. Rosenthal syndrome
- autosomal recessive; more common in Ashkenazi Jews
- usually mild, often diagnosed in adulthood
- level of Factor XI does not predict bleeding risk
- treatment: fresh frozen plasma, Factor XI concentrate

Liver Disease

- pathophysiology
  - deficient synthesis of all factors except VIII
  - aberrant synthesis: fibrinogen
  - deficient clearance of hemostatic "debris" and fibrinolytic activators
  - accelerated destruction due to dysfibrinogenemias: ↑ fibrinolysis, DIC
- miscellaneous: inhibition of secondary hemostasis by FDPs
- investigations
  - peripheral blood film: target cells
  - primary hemostasis affected
    - thrombocytopenia 2° to hypersplenism, folate deficiency, EtOH intoxication, DIC
    - platelet dysfunction: e.g. EtOH abuse
  - secondary hemostasis affected
    - elevated INR (PT), aPTT and thrombin time
- treatment: supportive, fresh frozen plasma, platelets, treat liver disease

Investigations in Liver Disease
Factor V, VII, VIII. Expect decreased V and VII because they have the shortest $t_{1/2}$. Factor VIII will be normal or increased because it is produced in endothelium.

Vitamin K Deficiency

Etiology
- drugs
  - oral anticoagulants inhibit Factors II, VII, IX, X, protein C & S
  - antibiotics eradicating gut flora, which provide 50% of vitamin K supply
- poor diet (especially in alcoholics)
- biliary obstruction
- chronic liver disease (↓ stores)
- malabsorption (e.g. celiac disease)
- hemorrhagic disease of newborn, see <u>Pediatrics</u>

Vitamin K Dependent Factors
1972 Canada vs. Soviet
X, IX, VII, II protein C&S

Investigations
- INR (PT) is elevated out of proportion to the elevation of the aPTT
- ↓ Factors II, VII, IX and X (because vitamin K-dependent)

Treatment
- hold anticoagulant
- vitamin K 1 mg PO for INRs between 4.5 and 10 and not bleeding (excludes hemorrhagic disease of the newborn)
- if bleeding, give vitamin K 10 mg IV/PO and if life-threatening bleeding fresh frozen plasma (FFP)
- note: excessive amounts of vitamin K will delay therapeutic warfarin anticoagulation once re-started

PT should improve within 24 hours of vitamin K administration (onset is in 6-12 hrs). If not, search for other causes.

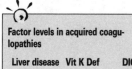

Factor levels in acquired coagulopathies

Liver disease	Vit K Def	DIC
↓V	NV	↓V
↓VII	↓VII	↓VII
↑VIII	NVIII	↓VIII

DIC is a spectrum which may include thrombosis **or** bleeding **or** both.

Important Etiologies of DIC
• trauma
• shock
• infection
• malignancy
• obstetric complications

Levels of fibrinogen can still be normal in DIC as it is an acute phase reactant.

Disseminated Intravascular Coagulation (DIC)

Definition
• uncontrolled release of plasmin and thrombin leading to uncontrolled intravascular coagulation and depletion of platelets, coagulation factors and fibrinogen subsequently giving rise to risk of life-threatening hemorrhage

Etiology
• a 2° disorder that occurs as a complication of a number of other conditions
• its unifying cause relates to widespread endothelial damage +/- extensive inflammatory cytokine release
• activation of procoagulant activity
    ▪ Antiphospholipid Antibody Syndrome
    ▪ intravascular hemolysis (incompatible blood, malaria)
    ▪ tissue injury (obstetric complications, trauma, burns, crush injuries)
    ▪ malignancy (solid tumours, hematologic malignancies especially acute promyelocytic leukemia AML-M3)
    ▪ snake venom
    ▪ fat embolism
    ▪ heat stroke
• endothelial injury
    ▪ infections/sepsis
    ▪ vasculitis
    ▪ metastatic disease (adenocarcinoma)
    ▪ aortic aneurysm
    ▪ giant hemangioma
• reticuloendothelial injury
    ▪ liver disease
    ▪ splenectomy
• vascular stasis
    ▪ hypotension
    ▪ hypovolemia
    ▪ pulmonary embolus
• other
    ▪ acute hypoxia/acidosis
    ▪ extracorporeal circulation

Clinical Features
• signs of microvascular thrombosis
    ▪ neurological: multifocal infarcts, delirium, coma, seizures
    ▪ skin: focal ischemia, superficial gangrene
    ▪ renal: oliguria, azotemia, cortical necrosis
    ▪ pulmonary: ARDS
    ▪ GI: acute ulceration
    ▪ RBC: microangiopathic hemolysis
• signs of hemorrhagic diathesis
    ▪ neurologic: intracranial bleeding
    ▪ skin: petechiae, ecchymosis, oozing from puncture sites
    ▪ renal: hematuria
    ▪ mucosal: gingival oozing, epistaxis, massive bleeding

Investigations
• primary hemostasis: ↓ platelets
• secondary hemostasis: prolonged INR (PT), aPTT, TT, ↓ fibrinogen and other factors
• fibrinolysis: ↑ FDPs or D-dimers, short euglobin lysis time (i.e. accelerated fibrinolysis)
• extent of fibrin deposition: urine output, urea, RBC fragmentation

Treatment
• recognize early
• treat underlying disorder
• individualized critical care support
• in hemorrhage: replacement of hemostatic elements with platelet transfusion, FFP, cryoprecipitate
• in thrombotic phase: LMWH (controversial)

Table 14. Screening Test Abnormalities in Coagulopathies

↑ INR Only	↑ PTT Only	↑ Both
• Factor VII def.	• Hemophilia A and B	• Prothrombin def.
• Vitamin K def.	• vWD	• Fibrinogen def.
• Warfarin	• Heparin	• Factor V and X def.
• Liver disease	• Antiphospholipid Ab	• Severe liver disease
• Factor VII inhibitors	• Factor inhibitors	• Factor V and X, prothrombin, and fibrinogen inhibitors
	• F XI/F XII deficiency	• Excessive anticoagulation

Venous Thrombosis

Definition
- the presence of a thrombus and subsequent inflammatory response in a superficial or deep vein
- thrombi propagate in the direction of blood flow (commonly originating in calf veins)
- more common in lower extremity than upper extremity
- incidence ~1% if age >60
- the most important sequelae are pulmonary embolism (~50% chance with proximal DVT) and chronic venous insufficiency

> **Virchow's Triad**
> - endothelial damage
> - stasis
> - hypercoagulability

Etiology (Virchow's Triad)
- endothelial damage
    - leads to decreased inhibition of coagulation and local fibrinolysis
- venous stasis
    - immobilization (post-MI, CHF, stroke, post-op), inhibits clearance and dilution of coagulation factors
- hypercoagulability
    - inherited (see *Hypercoagulable Disorders*, H31)
    - acquired
        - age (risk increases with age)
        - surgery (especially orthopaedic, thoracic, GI and GU)
        - trauma (especially fractures of spine, pelvis, femur, or tibia and SCI)
        - neoplasms (especially lung, pancreas, colon, rectum, kidney and prostate cancer)
        - blood dyscrasias (myeloproliferative disorders, esp. PRV, ET), PNH, hyperviscosity (multiple myeloma, polycythemia, leukemia, sickle cell)
        - prolonged immobilization (CHF, stroke, MI, leg injury)
        - hormone related (pregnancy, OCP, HRT, SERMs)
        - Antiphospholipid Antibody Syndrome (APLAS)
        - hyperhomocysteinemia
        - heart failure (risk of DVT greatest in patients with RHF and peripheral edema)
- idiopathic (10-20% are later found to have cancer)

> Folic acid 5 mg PO daily will protect against increased homocysteine levels.

Clinical Features
- absence of physical findings does not rule out disease
- unilateral leg edema, erythema, warmth and tenderness
- palpable cord (thrombosed vein)
- phlegmasia cerulea dolens and phlegmasia alba dolens with massive thrombosis
- Homan's sign (pain with foot dorsiflexion) is unreliable

Differential Diagnosis
- muscle strain or tear, lymphangitis or lymph obstruction, venous valvular insufficiency, ruptured popliteal cysts, cellulitis, arterial occlusive disease

Investigations
- D-dimer test only useful to rule out DVT if negative and low clinical suspicion of disease
- doppler ultrasound is most useful diagnostic test for DVT
    - sensitivity and specificity for proximal DVT ~95%
    - sensitivity for calf DVT ~70%
- other non-invasive tests include MRI and impedence plethysmography
- venography is the gold standard, but is expensive, invasive, and higher risk

Approach to Treatment of Venous Thrombosis

Purpose
- prevent further clot extension
- prevention of acute pulmonary embolism (occurs in ~50% of untreated patients)
- reduce the risk of recurrent thrombosis
- treatment of massive ileofemoral thrombosis with acute lower limb ischemia and/or venous gangrene (phlegmasia cerulea dolens)
- limit development of late complications, i.e. postphlebitic syndrome, chronic venous insufficiency and chronic thromboembolic pulmonary HTN

Initiating Warfarin therapy
Ann Intern Med 2003;138(9):714-9
Study: Multicentre, randomized trial.
Patients: 201 patients with acute venous thromboembolism.
Intervention: 5 mg warfarin initiation nomogram versus 10 mg nomogram.
Main outcomes: Time to therapeutic INR.
Results: Patients in the 10 mg group reached a therapeutic INR 1.4 days faster than those in the 5 mg group with no difference in major bleeds between the two groups (p<0.001).
Conclusion: Initiation of warfarin therapy with a 10 mg nomogram allows faster achievement of a therapeutic INR without increased bleeding risk.

D-Dimer in Suspected DVT
(NEJM 2003;349(13):1227-35)
Study: Multicentre, randomized trial with 16 week follow-up.
Patients: 596 patients with suspected leg DVT, stratified as either likely or unlikely to have DVT were randomized to receive or not receive D-dimer testing in addition to standard diagnostic work-ups set out by the investigators.
Results: Patients in the D-dimer tested group underwent fewer ultrasounds than those in the control group (0.78 tests per patients versus 1.34 tests per patient, p=0.008). 0.4% of patients with a negative D-dimer test and no ultrasound performed were later clinically deemed to have a DVT.
Conclusion: D-dimer testing is useful in reducing the need for ultrasound in DVT diagnosis, particularly in low-risk patients.

Duration of treatment with vitamin K antagonists in symptomatic venous thromboembolism
Cochrane Database of Systematic Reviews 2006; Issue 1
Study: Meta-analysis of 8 RCTs (2994 patients) comparing different durations of treatment with vitamin K antagonists in patients with symptomatic venous thromboembolism (VTE).
Main Results: In patients treated with vitamin K antagonists for a prolonged period, the reduction in risk of recurrent VTE remained consistent regardless of the period of time since the index event (OR 0.18, CI 0.13-0.26). In addition, there was no observed excess of VTE recurrences following cessation of prolonged vitamin K, antagonist therapy (OR 1.24, CI 0.91-1.69). However, patients who received prolonged treatment had a persistent increase in their risk of major bleeding complications (OR 2.61, CI 1.48-4.61).
Conclusion: Prolonged treatment with vitamin K antagonists leads to a consistent reduction in the risk of recurrent VTE for as long as therapy is continued. Therapy should be discontinued when the risk of harm from major bleeding (which remains constant over time) is of greater concern than the absolute risk of recurrent VTE (which declines over time). No specific recommendation was made regarding optimal duration of treatment.

Initiation of warfarin therapy requires overlap with heparin therapy for 4-5 days
• 10 mg loading dose of warfarin causes a precipitous decline in protein C levels in 1st 36 hours resulting in a transient hypercoagulable state
• warfarin decreases Factor VII levels in 1st 48 hrs → INR is prolonged (most sensitive to Factor VII levels), however full antithrombotic effect is not achieved until Factor IX, X, and II are sufficiently reduced (occurs after approx 4 days)

Low risk surgical patients: <40 yrs, no risk factors for VTE, general anesthetic (GA) <30 mins, minor elective, abdominal or thoracic surgery

Moderate risk surgical patients: >40 yrs, ≥1 risk factor for VTE, GA >30 mins

High risk surgical patients: >40 yrs, surgery for malignancy or lower extremity orthopedic surgery lasting >30 mins, inhibitors deficiency or other risk factor

High risk medical patients: heart failure, severe respiratory disease, ischemic stroke and lower limb paralysis, confined to bed and have ≥1 additional risk factor (e.g. active cancer, previous VTE, sepsis, acute neurologic disease, IBD)

Intitial Treatment
• unfractionated heparin (UFH) or low-molecular weight heparin (LMWH)
  ▪ UFH
    ♦ requires bolus (7500-10,000 IU), followed by continuous IV infusion (1000-1500 IU/h)
    ♦ weight-based heparin nomograms help to achieve proper dosing
    ♦ advantages: rapidly reversible by protamine in case of bleeding
    ♦ disadvantages: must monitor aPTT with adjustment of dose to reach therapeutic level (~2x control value); monitor platelet counts for development of thrombocytopenia (HIT)
  ▪ LMWH
    ♦ administered SC, at least as effective as UFH
    ♦ advantages: predictable dose response and fixed dosing schedule; lab monitoring not required; lower risk of HIT; safe and effective outpatient therapy
    ♦ disadvantages: only partially reversible by protamine; renally cleared, may need to adjust dose in patients with renal dysfunction
  ▪ alternatives to LMWH and UFH: heparinoids (patients with HIT), direct thrombin inhibitors (hirudin, lepirudin, argatroban), Factor Xa inhibitors (fondaparinux)
  ▪ thrombolytic (e.g. streptokinase, tPA) drugs reserved for limb/life-threatening thrombosis, recent symptoms, low bleeding risk

Long-term Treatment
• standard treatment is warfarin, which should be initiated concomitantly with heparin overlap for at least 5 days and discontinue heparin after INR>2.0 for two consecutive days (see sidebar)
• warfarin should be dosed to maintain INR at 2-3 except in select cases
• monitor INR twice weekly for 1-2 weeks, then weekly until INR stable, then every 2-4 weeks
• recent evidence suggests that a therapeutic INR can be reached quicker by using a warfarin initiation protocol that starts with 10 mg dose rather than a 5 mg dose (see sidebar, H28)
• LMWH shown to be more effective than warfarin at preventing recurrence of venous thrombosis in cancer patients
• duration of anticoagulant treatment (with warfarin unless otherwise noted):
  ▪ first episode DVT with transient risk factor: 3 months
  ▪ first episode DVT with ongoing risk factor such as cancer, or antiphospholipid antibody or more than one risk factor: consider indefinite therapy
  ▪ first episode DVT with no identifiable risk factors (idiopathic) or single inherited risk factor (i.e. Factor V Leiden etc.): 6-12 months or indefinite therapy (controversial)
  ▪ recurrent DVT (2 or more episodes): indefinite therapy
• IVC filters: useful in those with contraindications to anticoagulant therapy, recurrent thromboembolism despite adequate anticoagulation, chronic recurrent embolism with pulmonary HTN, or require emergent surgery without time to initiate anticoagulation
• pregnancy: treat with LMWH during pregnancy, then warfarin for 4-6 weeks postpartum, achieving a minimum total anticoagulation time of 3-6 months

Prophylaxis
• consider for those with a moderate to high risk of thrombosis without contraindications (see sidebar)
• non-pharmacological measures include: early ambulation; elastic compression stockings (TEDs); intermittent pneumatic compression (IPC)
• UFH 5000 IU SC bid for moderate risk
• UFH 5000 IU SC tid or enoxaparin 40 mg SC OD for high risk

Contraindications and Adverse Reactions of Anticoagulant Therapy
• see *Anticoagulation Therapy*, H48

Treatment of Pulmonary Embolism (PE)
• see Respirology

Hypercoagulable Disorders

Hypercoagulable Workup – Venous Thrombosis

- workup for malignancy or hypercoagulable state may be indicated for idiopathic VTE in presence of the following features: age <50, recurrent VTE, family history of VTE, unusual site of DVT, heparin-resistant disease (AT deficiency), warfarin-induced skin necrosis and neonatal purpura fulminans (Protein C or S deficiency)

HERITABLE CAUSES OF HYPERCOAGULABILITY LEADING TO VENOUS THROMBOEMBOLISM

Activated Protein C Resistance (Factor V Leiden)
- most common cause of hereditary thrombophilia
- 5% of general population are heterozygotes
- point mutation in the Factor V gene (Arg506Gln) results in resistance to inactivation of Factor Va by activated Protein C

Prothrombin G20210A
- G→A transposition at nucleotide position 20210 of the promoter region of the prothrombin gene results in increased levels of prothrombin subsequently leading to ↑ thrombin generation

Hyperhomocysteinemia
- both a genetic and acquired abnormality
- ↑ levels are found in vitamin B_{12}, B_6, and folate deficiencies, chronic renal failure, hypothyroidism, malignancy, methotrexate, phenytoin, theophylline
- folate 5 mg/day can ↓ plasma homocysteine by 50%, although effect on thrombosis risk reduction unclear
- also increases risk of arterial thrombosis

Protein C and Protein S Deficiency
- Protein C inactivates Factor Va and VIIIa using Protein S as a cofactor
- Protein C deficiency:
  - homozygous: neonatal purpura fulminans
  - heterozygous: type I: decreased Protein C levels; type II: decreased Protein C functional activity
  - acquired: liver disease, sepsis, DIC, warfarin
  - 1/3 of patients with warfarin necrosis have underlying Protein C deficiency
- Protein S deficiency:
  - type I: decreased free and total Protein S levels; type II: decreased Protein S functional activity; type III: decreased free Protein S levels
  - acquired: liver disease, DIC, pregnancy, nephrotic sydrome, inflammatory conditions, warfarin

Antithrombin Deficiency
- antithrombin slowly inactivates thrombin in the absence of heparin, rapidly inactivates thrombin in the presence of heparin
- autosomal dominant transmission or urinary losses in nephrotic syndrome
- type I: decreased AT levels; type II: decreased AT functional activity
- diagnosis must be made outside window of acute thrombosis and anticoagulation treatment (acute thrombosis, heparin, systemic disease all ↓ antithrombin levels)
- deficiency may result in resistance to unfractionated heparin (LMWH must be used)

Elevated Factor VIII Levels
- an independent marker of increased thrombotic risk
- genetic basis for ↑ levels poorly understood

Disorders of Fibrinolysis
- include congenital plasminogen deficiency, tissue plasminogen activator deficiency

Antiphospholipid Antibody Syndrome (APLAS)
- definition: ≥1 clinical and ≥1 laboratory criteria
- clinical: thrombosis, spontaneous abortions, fetal loss, premature birth before 34 wks
- laboratory: anticardiolipin or lupus anticoagulant antibodies
- mechanism: not well understood, interact with platelet membrane phospholipid and ↑ adhesion and aggregation; also can interfere with action of protein C&S

Common Causes of Hypercoagulability (CALMSHAPE)
C: Protein C deficiency
A: Antiphospholipid Abs
L: Factor V Leiden
M: Malignancy
S: Protein S deficiency
H: ↑ homocysteine
A: Antithrombin deficiency
P: Prothrombin G20210A
E: ↑ Factor VIII

Although lupus anti-coagulant prolongs PTT, its main clinical feature is thrombosis.

Protein C, protein S, and ATIII are decreased during acute thrombosis – therefore to test for deficiency, must be tested outside of this time period.

Causes of both venous arterial thrombosis include:
- antiphospholipid antibodies
- hyperhomocysteinemia
- myeloproliferative disorders
- heparin induced thrombocytopenia

Malignancy is a common acquired cause of hypercoagulability. Workup includes:
- complete history and physical
- routine bloodwork
- urinalysis
- CXR
- mammogram and Pap in females
- PSA in males
- colonoscopy
- close follow-up

Hematologic Malignancies

Overview

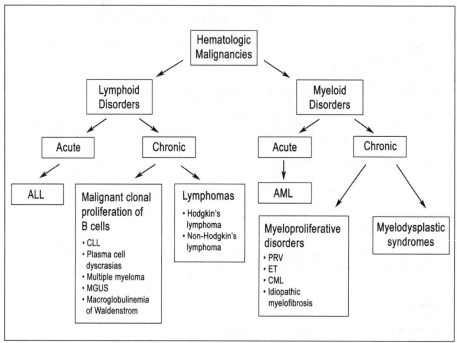

Figure 12. Overview of Hematologic Malignancies

Myeloid Malignancies

Acute Myeloid Leukemia (AML)

Definition
- rapidly progressive malignancy characterized by failure of myeloid cell to differentiate beyond blast stage

Epidemiology
- incidence ↑ with age, median age of onset is 65 years old

Risk Factors
- myelodysplastic syndromes (MDS), benzene, radiation and alkylating agents for previous malignancy

Pathophysiology
- uncontrolled growth of blasts in marrow leads to:
  - suppression of normal hematopoietic cells
  - appearance of blasts in peripheral blood
  - accumulation of blasts in other sites
  - metabolic consequences of a large tumour mass
- chronic myeloproliferative disorders and MDS can transform into AML

Clinical Features
- anemia
- thrombocytopenia (associated with DIC in promyelocytic leukemia)
- neutropenia (even with normal WBC) → infections, fever

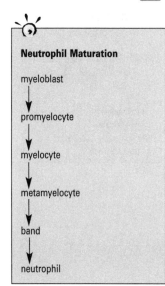

Neutrophil Maturation

myeloblast
↓
promyelocyte
↓
myelocyte
↓
metamyelocyte
↓
band
↓
neutrophil

- accumulation of blast cells in marrow
  - skeletal pain, bony tenderness, especially sternum
- organ infiltration with leukemic cells
  - gingival hypertrophy – may present to dentist first
  - splenomegaly – early satiety, LUQ fullness
  - hepatomegaly
  - lymphadenopathy (not marked)
  - skin – leukemia cutis
  - gonads
  - eyes – Roth spots, cotton wool spots, vision changes (uncommon)
- leukostasis (medical emergency)
  - patients with ↑↑ WBCs can present with symptoms of leukostasis (i.e. respiratory distress, altered mental status, bleeding)
- metabolic effects, aggravated by treatment (rare)
  - ↑ uric acid → nephropathy, gout
  - release of phosphate → ↓ Ca, ↓ Mg
  - release of procoagulants → DIC
- ↓ K before treatment, ↑ K after treatment

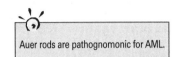

Auer rods are pathognomonic for AML.

Investigations
- CBC - anemia, thrombocytopenia, variable WBC
- peripheral blood film - circulating blasts with Auer rods (azurophilic granules)
- INR, aPTT, FDP, fibrinogen in case of DIC
- baseline RFTs, LFTs
- ↑ LDH, ↑ uric acid, ↑ PO_4 (released by leukemic blasts), ↑K
- ↓ Ca
- bone marrow aspirate
  - blast count: AML >20% (normal is <5%)
  - histologic classification (French-American-British → M0-M7; see sidebar)
  - cytogenetics, immunophenotyping
- CXR to r/o pneumonia, ECG, MUGA scan prior to chemotherapy (cardiotoxic)

FAB Classifications		
Subtype	Freq	Common Name
M0	<5%	Minimally differentiated
MI	20%	Myeloblastic without maturation
M2	25%	Myeloblastic with maturation
M3	10%	Promyelocytic (APML)
M4	20%	Myelomonocytic
M5	20%	Monocytic
M6	5%	Erythroleukemic
M7	<5%	Megakaryoblastic

Treatment
- cure: defined as survival that parallels age-matched population
- first step is complete remission – defined as normal peripheral blood film, normal bone marrow with <5% blasts, and normal clinical state
- leukemia will recur after complete remission if no further treatment given
- aims of treatment
  - eliminate abnormal clone – cytotoxic therapy
    - induction chemotherapy (daunorubicin and hydroxydoxorubicin)
    - post-induction or consolidation (BMT or chemotherapy) for younger patients
  - repopulation of marrow with normal hematopoietic cells
- consider acceleration with hematopoietic growth factors (e.g. G-CSF) if ↑ incidence of severe infection
- APML subtype (t(15;17)) responds to all-trans-retinoic acid (ATRA), which induces differentiation
- supportive care
  - screening for infection via regular C&S of urine, stool, sputum, oropharynx, catheter sites, perianal area
  - fever – C&S of all orifices, CXR, start antibiotics
  - platelet and RBC transfusions – (irradiated to prevent transfusion-related GVHD) ± erythropoietin
  - prevention and treatment of metabolic abnormalities (allopurinol should be started for prophylaxis of hyperuricemia)

Prognosis
- achievement of first remission (no visible evidence of disease and normal blood counts)
  - 70-80% if 60 years old, 50% if >60 years old
  - median survival 12-24 months
  - 5 year survival 40%
- survival may be improved by BMT – 50-60% cure rate
- adverse prognostic factors: age>60, poor performance score before treatment, AML secondary to chemotherapy or MDS/chronic myeloproliferative disorder, WBC>20 000/cm³, ↑ LDH, unfavourable cytogenetics (e.g. monosomy or deletion of chromosomes 5 or 7)

Myelodysplastic Syndromes (MDS)

Definition
- heterogeneous group of malignant stem cell disorders characterized by dysplastic and ineffective blood cell production resulting in peripheral cytopenias
- syndromes defined according to French-American-British (FAB) or World Health Organization (WHO) classifications

Pathophysiology
- ineffective hematopoiesis despite presence of adequate numbers of progenitor cells (bone marrow is usually hypercellular)
- considered preleukemic: 30-70% develop AML

Risk Factors
- elderly, post-chemotherapy, benzene or radiation exposure

Clinical Features
- insidious onset
- fatigue, weakness, pallor, infections, bruising, epistaxis, and rarely weight loss, fever, and hepatosplenomegaly

Investigations
- diagnosed by:
  - anemia ± thrombocytopenia ± neutropenia
  - bone marrow hypercellularity with trilineage dysplastic changes (dysmyelopoiesis, dyserythropoiesis, dysthrombopoiesis)
- CBC and peripheral blood film
  - RBC: usually macrocytic with oval shaped red cells (macro-ovalocytes), $\downarrow$ reticulocyte count
  - WBC: $\downarrow$ in granulocytes and abnormal morphology (e.g. bilobed or unsegmented nuclei)
  - platelets: thrombocytopenia, size and cytoplasm abnormalities (e.g. giant hypogranular platelets)
- bone marrow aspirate and biopsy with cytogenetic analysis required for definitive diagnosis

Treatment
- symptomatic: transfusion, antibiotics, antifungals
- erythropoietin SC weekly may be effective in reducing transfusion requirements in some patients
- hematopoietic growth factors (G-CSF) may $\downarrow$ risk of infection
- bone marrow transplant may be curative

Chronic Myeloproliferative Disorders

Definition
- clonal myeloid stem cell abnormalities leading to qualitative and quantitative changes in erythroid, myeloid, and platelet cells

Epidemiology
- mainly middle-aged and older patients

Clinical Features
- pruritus, bruising, thrombosis, peptic ulcer disease (histamine from basophils causes increased gastric acid secretion)

Investigations
- $\uparrow$ uric acid
- $\uparrow$ LDH
- $\uparrow$ serum B_{12}
- $\uparrow$ transcobalamin I
- $\uparrow$ eosinophils
- $\uparrow$ basophils
- $\uparrow$ serum histamine (from basophils)

WHO MDS Classification
1. Refractory anemia (RA)
2. Refractory anemia with ringed sideroblasts (RARS)
3. Refractory cytopenia with multilineage dysplasia (RCMD)
4. Refractory cytopenia with multilineage dysplasia and ringed sideroblasts (RCMD-RS)
5. Refractory anemia with excess blasts I and II
6. 5q- syndrome (MD with del(5q))
7. Myelodysplasia unclassified (seen in those cases of megakaryocyte dysplasia with fibrosis and others)

MDS is a cause of macrocytic anemia.

Basophilia is uncommon in other medical conditions

Prognosis
- may develop marrow fibrosis with time
- all disorders may progress to AML

Table 15. Chronic Myeloproliferative Disorders

	PRV	CML	IMF	ET
Hct	↑↑	↓/N	↓	N
WBC	↑	↑↑	↑/↓	N
Plt	↑	↑/↓	↑/↓	↑↑↑
Marrow fibrosis	±	±	+++	±
Splenomegaly	+	+++	+++	+
Hepatomegaly	+	+	++	–

PRV = polycythemia rubra vera   CML = chronic myeloid leukemia
IMF = idiopathic myelofibrosis   ET = essential thrombocythemia

Polycythemia Rubra Vera (PRV)

Definition
- stem cell disorder characterized by elevated RBC mass (erythrocytosis) accompanied by increased white cell and platelet production

Clinical Features
- those secondary to high red cell mass and hyperviscosity (see *Polycythemia*)
- bleeding complications: epistaxis, gum bleeding, ecchymoses, and GI bleeding
  - due to platelet abnormalities
- thrombotic complications: DVT, PE, thrombophlebitis, increased incidence of stroke, MI
  - due to ↑ blood viscosity, ↑ platelet number and/or activity
- erythromelalgia (burning pain in hands and feet)
  - associated with platelets >400 $\times 10^9$/L
  - pathognomonic microvascular thrombotic complications
- pruritus, especially after warm bath or shower (40%)
  - due to cutaneous mast cell degranulation with release of histamine
- epigastric distress, PUD
  - due to ↑ histamine from tissue basophils, alterations in gastric mucosal blood flow due to ↑ blood viscosity
- gout (hyperuricemia)
  - due to ↑ cell turnover
- characteristic physical findings
  - plethora (ruddy complexion) of face (70%), palms
  - splenomegaly (70%), hepatomegaly (40%)

> Erythromelalgia is a pathognomonic microvascular thrombotic complication in polycythemia rubra vera and essential thrombocythemia.

Investigations
- see *Polycythemia*, H5
- must rule out secondary polycythemia
- diagnosis requires presence of all 3 major criteria or first 2 major and any 2 minor criteria
- major criteria: increased red cell mass, arterial oxygen saturation ≥92%, splenomegaly
- minor criteria: increased WBCs, platelets, leukocyte alkaline phosphatase (LAP) and vitamin B_{12}
- JAK2 mutation identified in most cases

Treatment
- phlebotomy to keep hematocrit <45% in men and <42% in women
- hydroxyurea (age >65, prior thrombosis or symptoms), ^{32}P (age >80 or lifespan <10 years)
- low-dose aspirin (for erythromelalgia)
- allopurinol – as needed
- antihistamines – as needed

Prognosis
- 10-20 year survival with treatment
- complicated by thrombosis, hemorrhage, leukemic transformation (AML)

Chronic Myeloid Leukemia (CML)

Definition
- myeloproliferative disorder characterized by increased proliferation of the granulocytic cell line without the loss of their capacity to differentiate

Epidemiology
- generally presents in fourth or fifth decade of life

Pathophysiology
- Philadelphia chromosome (Ph)
  - translocation between chromosomes 9 and 22
  - the *c-abl* proto-oncogene is translocated from chromosome 9 to "breakpoint cluster region" (*bcr*) of chromosome 22 to produce bcr-abl fusion gene, an active tyrosine kinase

> Detection of the bcr-abl fusion gene is a diagnostic test for CML (present in over 90% of patients).

Clinical Features
- the disease has 3 clinical phases:
  - chronic phase – disease process easily controlled (85% diagnosed here)
  - accelerated phase – impaired neutrophil differentiation, difficult to control
  - blast crisis – more aggressive course, blasts fail to differentiate
- 20-50% of patients are asymptomatic when diagnosed (incidental lab finding)
- nonspecific symptoms
  - fatigue, weight loss, malaise, excessive sweating
- secondary to splenic involvement
  - early satiety, LUQ pain/fullness, shoulder tip pain (referred)
  - splenomegaly (most common physical finding)
- anemia
- bleeding – secondary to platelet dysfunction
- pruritus, PUD – secondary to ↑ blood histamine
- fever, weight loss – secondary to ↑ cell turnover
- leukostasis, priapism, encephalopathy (rare) – secondary to ↑↑ WBC (rare)

Investigations
- ↑↑ WBC, ↓/N RBC, ↑/↓platelets
- peripheral blood smear
  - leukoerythroblastic picture (immature cells present, e.g. myelocytes and normoblasts)
  - presence of different mid-stage progenitor cells differentiates it from AML
- bone marrow
  - myeloid hyperplasia with a left shift, ↑ megakaryocytes, mild fibrosis
- molecular and cytogenetic studies of bone marrow or peripheral blood for Philadelphia chromosome

Imatinib compared with interferon and low-dose cytarabine for newly diagnosed chronic-phase chronic myeloid leukemia.
N Engl J Med. 2003;348:994-1004.
Study: Randomized, open-label, multicenter trial.
Patients: 1106 patients with newly diagnosed chronic-phase chronic myeloid leukemia (CML).
Intervention: Imatinib (553 patients) or interferon-alfa plus low-dose cytarabine (553 patients).
Outcome: Patients were evaluated for hematologic and cytogenetic responses, toxic effects, and rates of progression.
Results: After a median follow-up of 19 months, the estimated rate of a major cytogenetic response (0 to 35%of cells in metaphase positive for the Philadelphia chromosome) at 18 months was 87.1% (95%CI, 84.1 to 90.0) in the imatinib group and 34.7%(95% CI, 29.3 to 40.0) in the group given interferon-alfa plus cytarabine (p<0.001). The estimated rates of complete cytogenetic response were 76.2% (95% CI, 72.5 to 79.9) and 14.5%(95% CI, 10.5 to 18.5), respectively (p<0.001). At 18 months, the estimated rate of freedom from progression to accelerated-phase or blast-crisis CML was 96.7% in the imatinib group and 91.5% in the combination-therapy group (p<0.001). Imatinib was better tolerated than combination therapy.
Conclusions: In terms of hematologic and cytogenetic responses, tolerability, and the likelihood of progression to accelerated-phase or blast-crisis CML, imatinib was superior to interferon-alfa plus low-dose cytarabine as first-line therapy in newly diagnosed chronic-phase CML.

Treatment
- symptomatic
  - allopurinol and antihistamines
- chronic phase
  - imatinib mesylate (Gleevec™) – inhibits proliferation and induces apoptosis by inhibiting tyrosine kinase activity in cells positive for *bcr-abl*
  - clinical success with imatinib (cytogenic remission) has resulted in fewer patients requiring bone marrow transplantation
  - interferon-α
  - hydroxyurea or occasionally busulfan
- only curative treatment is bone marrow transplantation
- stem cell transplantation may be curative

Prognosis
- 5-year survival rate of 50-60%
- chronic phase
  - normal bone marrow function
  - white blood cells differentiate and function normally
- accelerated phase
  - fever
  - marked ↑ in basophils
  - ↑ extramedullary hematopoiesis (unusual sites)
  - transformation → disease similar to idiopathic myelofibrosis
  - pancytopenia secondary to marrow aplasia
- acute phase (blast crisis – usually within 3-5 years)
  - 2/3 develop a picture similar to AML
    - unresponsive to remission induction
  - 1/3 develop a picture similar to ALL
    - remission induction (return to chronic phase) achievable

Idiopathic Myelofibrosis (IMF)

Definition
- characterized by bone marrow fibrosis, anemia, extramedullary hematopoiesis, leukoerythroblastosis, the presence of teardrop-shaped red cells in peripheral blood, and hepatosplenomegaly

Epidemiology
- rare, median age at presentation is 65

Clinical Features
- anemia (severe fatigue is most common presenting complaint, pallor on exam in >60%)
- weight loss, fever, night sweats → secondary to hypermetabolic state
- splenomegaly (90%) → secondary to extramedullary hematopoiesis; may cause early satiety
- hepatomegaly (70%) → may get portal hypertension
- bone and joint pain → secondary to osteosclerosis, gout
- signs of extramedullary hematopoiesis (depends on organ involved)

Investigations
- CBC: anemia, variable platelets, variable WBC
- biochemistry: ↑ ALP (liver involvement, bone disease), ↑ LDH ($2°$ to ineffective hematopoiesis), ↑ uric acid (↑ cell turnover), ↑ B_{12} ($2°$ to ↑ neutrophil mass), ↑ LAP
- blood film: leukoerythroblastosis with teardrop-shaped RBCs, nucleated RBCs, variable polychromasia, large platelets and megakaryocyte fragments
- bone marrow aspirate: "dry tap" in as many as 50% of patients
- bone marrow biopsy (essential for diagnosis): fibrosis, atypical megakaryocytic hyperplasia, thickening and distortion of the bony trabeculae (osteosclerosis)

Treatment
- allogeneic stem cell transplant is potentially curative
- symptomatic treatment
  - transfusion ± androgens and corticosteroids for anemia, most unresponsive to erythropoietin
  - hydroxyurea for splenomegaly, thrombocytosis, leukocytosis, systemic symptoms
  - XRT for symptomatic extramedullary hematopoiesis, symptomatic splenomegaly
  - splenectomy if symptoms refractory to hydroxyurea, and for transfusion resistant anemia (procedure is associated with high mortality and morbidity)
  - allopurinol

IMF is characterized by a dry BM aspirate and tear drop RBCs ("you cry trying to get an aspirate").

Prognosis
- median survival for patients with IMF is 3.5-5.5 years
- risk of transformation to AML

Essential Thrombocythemia (ET)

Definition
- overproduction of platelets in absence of recognizable stimulus (must rule out secondary thrombocythemia)

Epidemiology
- increases with age, F:M = 2:1 but F=M at older age

Clinical Features
- often asymptomatic
- vasomotor symptoms (40%)
  - headache (common), dizziness, syncope
  - erythromelalgia (burning pain of hands and feet, dusky color, usually worse with heat, caused by platelet activation → microvascular thrombosis)
- thrombosis (arterial and venous)
- bleeding (often GI, associated with plts>100 x 10^9/L)
- constitutional Sx, splenomegaly
- pregnancy complications; ↑ risk of spontaneous abortion
- risk of transformation to AML (0.6-5%), myelofibrosis

Etiology of secondary thrombocythemia
infection
inflammation (IBD, arthritis)
malignancy
hemorrhage
iron deficiency
hemolytic anemia
post splenectomy
post chemotherapy

Investigations
- CBC: ↑ platelets, may have abnormal platelet aggregation studies
- bone marrow hypercellularity, megakaryocytic hyperplasia, giant megakaryocytes
- ↑ K, ↑ PO_4 ($2°$ to release of platelet cytoplasmic contents)
- diagnosis: exclude other myeloproliferative disorders and reactive thrombocytosis

There is an asymptomatic "benign" form of essential thrombocythemia with a stable or slowly rising platelet count; treatment includes observation, ASA, sulfinpyrazone or dipyridamole.

Treatment
- low dose aspirin if thrombotic event, older or symptomatic
- ↓ platelets: hydroxyurea (1st line therapy), anagrelide, interferon-α, or ^{32}P (age >80 or lifespan <10 years)
- plateletpheresis in emergencies
- splenectomy not recommended (↑ risk of bleeds, thrombosis)

Lymphoid Malignancies

Acute Lymphoblastic Leukemia (ALL)

Definition
- malignant disease of the bone marrow in which early lymphoid precursors proliferate and replace the normal hematopoietic cells of the marrow

Clinical Features
- see *Acute Myeloid Leukemia* (*AML*), H32 for full list of symptoms
- distinguish ALL from AML based on Table 16
- 50% present with fever
- patients may have meningeal leukemia at the time of relapse

Investigations
- CBC: ↑ leukocytes >10 x 10^9/L (occurs in 50% of patients); neutropenia, anemia, or thrombocytopenia
- may have ↑ uric acid, K, PO$_4$, LDH
- PT, aPTT, fibrinogen, D-dimers for DIC
- leukemic lymphoblasts lack specific morphological (no granules) or cytochemical features, therefore diagnosis depends on immunophenotyping
- cytogenetics: Philadelphia (Ph) chromosome in ~25% of adult ALL cases
- CXR: patients with ALL may have a mediastinal mass
- LP prior to systemic chemotherapy to assess for CNS involvement

Treatment
- eliminate abnormal clone
    1. induction (e.g. CHOP – cyclophosphamide, hydroxydoxorubicin, vincristine (Oncovin™), prednisone)
    2. consolidation or intensification chemotherapy
    3. maintenance chemotherapy
    4. prophylaxis: CNS with radiation therapy or methotrexate (intrathecal or systemic)
- molecular targeted therapy (e.g. imatinib mesylate (Gleevec™), a selective *bcr-abl* tyrosine kinase inhibitor)

Prognosis
- depends on response to initial induction or if remission is achieved following relapse
- good prognostic factors: young, WBC<30 x 10^9/L, T-cell phenotype, absence of Ph chromosome, early attainment of complete remission
- achievement of first remission: 60-90%
- childhood ALL: 80% long term remission (>5 years)
- adult ALL: 30-40% 5-year survival

Table 16. Differentiate AML From ALL

AML	ALL
big people (adults)	small people (kids)
big blasts	small blasts
lots of cytoplasm	less cytoplasm
lots of nucleoli (3-5)	few nucleoli (1-3)
lots of granules and Auer rods	no granules
big toxicity of treatment	little toxicity of treatment
big mortality rate	small mortality rate
myeloperoxidase, Sudan black stain	PAS (periodic acid schiff)
maturation defect beyond myeloblast or promyelocyte	maturation defect beyond lymphoblast

To Differentiate AML From ALL: Remember **Big** and **SmALL** (see Table 16)

Lymphomas

- Ann Arbor staging can be used for both Hodgkin's and non-Hodgkin's lymphoma, but grade is more important for non-Hodgkin's lymphoma because it tends to present at more advanced stages

Staging (Ann Arbor Staging System)

Stage I   involvement of a single lymph node region or extralymphatic organ or site

Stage II   involvement of two or more lymph node regions or an extralymphatic site and one or more lymph node regions on same side of diaphragm

Stage III   involvement of lymph node regions on both sides of the diaphragm; may or may not be accompanied by single extra lymphatic site or splenic involvement

Stage IV   diffuse involvement of one or more extralymphatic organs including bone marrow

> Hodgkin's is distinguished from non-Hodgkin's lymphoma by the presence of Reed-Sternberg cells.

- subtypes:
  - A = absence of B symptoms
  - B = presence of B symptoms
    - unexplained fever >38°C
    - unexplained weight loss (>10% of body weight in 6 months)
    - drenching night sweats

Table 17. Chromosome Translocations

Translocation	Gene Activation	Associated Neoplasm
t(8;14)	c-myc activation	Burkitt's lymphoma
t(14;18)	bcl-2 activation	Follicular lymphoma
t(9;22)	Philadelphia chromosome (bcr-abl hybrid)	CML, ALL in adults (25% of the time)
t(11;14)	overexpression protein cyclin DI	Mantle cell lymphoma

Hodgkin's Lymphoma

Definition
- malignant proliferation of lymphoid cells with Reed-Sternberg cells (which are thought to arise from germinal center B-cells)

Epidemiology
- bimodal distribution with peaks at the age of 20 years and >50 years
- association with Epstein-Barr virus in up to 50% of cases

Clinical Features
- asymptomatic lymphadenopathy (70%)
  - non-tender, rubbery consistency
  - cervical/supraclavicular (60-80%), axillary (10-20%), inguinal (6-12%)
- mediastinal mass
  - found on routine CXR, may be symptomatic (cough)
- systemic symptoms
  - B symptoms, pruritus
- non-specific/paraneoplastic
  - alcohol induced pain in nodes, nephrotic syndrome
- starts at a single site in lymphatic system (node), spreads first to adjacent nodes

Investigations
- CBC
  - anemia (chronic disease, rarely hemolytic), eosinophilia, leukocytosis, platelets normal or ↑ early, ↓ in advanced disease
- biochemistry
  - LFTs (liver involvement)
  - RFTs (prior to initiating chemotherapy)
  - ALP, Ca (bone involvement)
  - ESR, LDH (monitor disease progression)
- imaging
  - CXR, CT chest (lymph nodes, mediastinal mass), CT abdomen/pelvis (liver or spleen involvement), gallium scan (assess treatment response), PET CT scan

- excisional lymph node biopsy confirms diagnosis
- bone marrow biopsy to assess marrow infiltration (only necessary if B symptoms, stage III or IV, bulky disease or cytopenia)

Treatment
- stage I-II: chemotherapy (ABVD) followed by involved field XRT

CHOP = cyclophosphamide, hydroxydoxorubicin (Adriamycin), vincristine (Oncovin), prednisone

VAD = vincristine, adriamycin, dexamethasone

ABVD = adriamycin, bleomycin, vinblastine, dacarbazine

BEACOPP = bleomycin, etoposide, adriamycin, cyclophosphamide, vincristine, procarbazine, and prednisone

International Prognostic Factors Project 1998

Prognostic Factors	FFP
0	84%
1	77%
2	67%
3	60%
4	51%
5-7	42%

FFP = freedom from progression at 5 years.

NHL: Associated Conditions
1. immunodeficiency (e.g. HIV)
2. autoimmune diseases (e.g. SLE)
3. infections (e.g. EBV)

- stage III-IV: chemotherapy (ABVD, BEACOPP), with XRT for bulky disease
- relapse, resistant to therapy: high dose chemotherapy, bone marrow transplant

Complications of Treatment
- cardiac disease – secondary to XRT, adriamycin is cardiotoxic
- pulmonary disease – secondary to bleomycin, which causes interstitial pneumonitis
- infertility – recommend sperm banking
- secondary malignancy
  - <2% risk of MDS, AML (secondary to treatment, usually within 8 years)
  - solid tumours of lung, breast, >10 years after treatment
  - non-Hodgkin's lymphoma
- hypothyroidism – post XRT
- infection – post splenectomy (give Pneumovax, Hib, and pneumococcal conjugate vaccines), during treatment

Prognosis
- adverse prognostic factors:
  1. serum albumin <4 g/L (4 gm/dL)
  2. hemoglobin <105 g/L (10.5 gm/dL)
  3. male
  4. stage IV disease
  5. age ≥45 years
  6. leukocytosis (WBC >1.5 x 10^9/L)
  7. lymphocytopenia (lymphocytes <0.06 x 10^9/L or <8% of WBC count or both)
- Prognostic Score (see sidebar)
  - each additional adverse prognostic factor decreases freedom from progression at 5 years

Non-Hodgkin's Lymphoma (NHL)

Definition
- malignant proliferation of lymphoid cells without Reed-Sternberg cells

Classification
- multiple classification systems exist at present and may be used at different centres
- WHO/REAL classification system
  - indolent (35-40% of NHL) – e.g. follicular lymphoma, small lymphocytic lymphoma
  - aggressive (~50% of NHL) – e.g. diffuse large B-cell lymphoma
  - highly aggressive (~5% of NHL) – e.g. Burkitt's lymphoma

Clinical Features
- painless superficial lymphadenopathy, usually >1 lymph region
- usually presents as widespread disease
- constitutional symptoms (fever, weight loss, night sweats) not as common as in Hodgkin's disease
- cytopenia: anemia ± neutropenia ± thrombocytopenia if bone marrow fails
- abdominal signs
  - hepatosplenomegaly
  - retroperitoneal and mesenteric involvement (2nd most common site of involvement)
- oropharyngeal involvement in 5-10% with sore throat and obstructive apnea
- extranodal involvement – most commonly GI tract, also testes, bone, kidney
- CNS involvement in 1% (often with HIV)

Investigations
- CBC
  - normocytic normochromic anemia
  - autoimmune hemolytic anemia
  - advanced disease: thrombocytopenia, neutropenia, and leukoerythroblastic anemia
- peripheral blood film sometimes shows lymphoma cells
- biochemistry
  - ↑ in uric acid
  - abnormal LFTs in liver metastases
  - ↑ LDH (rapidly progressing disease, poor prognostic factor)
- CXR and CT for thoracic involvement
- CT for abdominal and pelvic involvement
- gallium scan is useful for monitoring response to treatment and evaluation of residual tumour following therapy
- diagnosed by
  - lymph node biopsy
    - fine needle aspiration occasionally sufficient, core biopsy preferred
  - bone marrow biopsy

Treatment
- localized disease (e.g. GI, brain, bone, head and neck)
  - surgery (if applicable)
  - radiotherapy to primary site and adjacent nodal areas
  - adjuvant chemotherapy
- indolent lymphoma – goal of treatment is symptom management
  - watchful waiting
  - radiation therapy for localized disease
  - chemotherapy (single agent, combination or rituximab/Rituxan™, an anti-CD20 antibody)
- aggressive lymphoma
  - combination chemotherapy CHOP is mainstay plus rituximab if B-cell lymphoma
  - relapse, resistant to therapy: high dose chemotherapy, BMT

Complications
- hypersplenism
- infection
- autoimmune hemolytic anemia and thrombocytopenia
- vascular obstruction (from enlarged nodes)

Prognosis
- poor prognostic factors:
  - >60 years old
  - poor response to therapy
  - multiple nodal regions
  - elevated LDH
  - nodes >5 cm
  - previous history of low grade disease or AIDS

Malignant Clonal Proliferations of B Cells

Table 18. Characteristics of B Cell Malignant Proliferation

	CLL	Macroglobulinemia	Myeloma
Cell type	lymphocyte	plasmacytoid	plasma cell
Protein	IgM if present	IgM	IgG, A, D or E
Lymph nodes	very common	common	rare
Hepatosplenomegaly	common	common	rare
Bone lesions	rare	rare	common
Hypercalcemia	rare	rare	common
Renal failure	rare	rare	common
Immunoglobulin Complications	common	infrequent	rare

Rouleaux formation on peripheral blood smear, if not artifact, denotes hyperglobulinemia

Chronic Lymphocytic Leukemia (CLL)

Definition
- indolent disease characterized by clonal malignancy of poorly functioning B cells

Epidemiology
- most common leukemia in Western world
- mainly older patients
- M>F

Pathophysiology
- accumulation of neoplastic lymphocytes in blood, bone marrow, lymph nodes and spleen

Clinical Features
- 25% asymptomatic (incidental finding)
- 5-10% present with B symptoms (≥1 of: unintentional weight loss ≥10% of body weight within previous 6 months, fevers >38°C or night sweats for ≥2 weeks without evidence of infection, extreme fatigue)
- lymphadenopathy (50-90%), splenomegaly (25-55%), hepatomegaly (15-25%)

Investigations
- CBC: absolute lymphocytosis >10 x 10⁹/L
- peripheral blood film

Smudge cells are artifacts of damaged lymphocytes from slide preparation.

- lymphocytes are small and mature
  - smudge cells
- bone marrow aspirate
  - lymphocytes >30% of all nucleated cells
  - infiltration of marrow by lymphocytes in 3 patterns: nodular (10%), interstitial (30%), diffuse (35%, worse prognosis), or mixed (25%)

Treatment
- the gentlest treatment that will control symptoms
  - observation if early, stable, asymptomatic
  - intermittent chlorambucil
  - corticosteroids
  - radiotherapy
  - chemotherapy
- 9 year median survival, but varies greatly
- no cure

Complications
- bone marrow failure
- immune hemolytic anemia
- immune thrombocytopenia
- immune deficiency (hypogammaglobulinemia, impaired T-cell function) with recurrent infections
- polyclonal or monoclonal gammopathy (often IgM)
- hyperuricemia with treatment
- transformation to histiocytic lymphoma

Multiple Myeloma (MM)

Definition
- characterized by neoplastic proliferation of a single clone of plasma cells producing a monoclonal immunoglobulin

Epidemiology
- incidence 3 per 100,000
- ↑ frequency with age, onset between age 40-70 years

Pathophysiology
- malignant B-cells secrete one class of heavy chains and one type of light chains ("M" protein (monoclonal)), light chains only (15%; light chain disease) or IgD (1%) and IgE (rare)

Multiple Myeloma Pentad
CARLI

C ↑ Calcium
A Anemia
R Renal failure
L Lytic bone lesions
I Infections

Clinical Features and Complications
- bone disease – pain (usually back), bony tenderness, pathologic fractures
  - lytic lesions are classical (skull, spine, proximal long bones, ribs)
  - increased bone resorption secondary to osteoclast activating factors such as PTHrP
- anemia – weakness, fatigue, pallor
  - secondary to bone marrow suppression
- weight loss
- infections
  - usually *S. pneumoniae* and Gram negatives
  - secondary to suppression of normal plasma cell function
- hypercalcemia - N/V, confusion, constipation, polyuria, polydipsia
  - secondary to ↑ bone turnover
- renal disease/renal failure
  - most frequently causes cast nephropathy (see <u>Nephrology</u>)
- bleeding
  - secondary to thrombocytopenia, may see petechiae, purpura
- extramedullary plasmacytoma
  - soft tissue mass composed of monoclonal plasma cells, purplish color
- hyperviscosity - may manifest as headaches, stroke, angina, MI
  - secondary to ↑ volume of M (monoclonal) protein
- amyloidosis
  - accumulation of insoluble fibrillar protein (Ig light chain) in tissues
- neurologic disease – muscle weakness, pain, paresthesias
  - radiculopathy caused by vertebral fracture, extramedullary plasmacytoma
  - spinal cord compression (in 10-20% of pts) is a medical emergency

Investigations
- CBC
  - normocytic anemia, thrombocytopenia, leukopenia
  - rouleaux formation on peripheral smear
- biochemistry
  - ↑ Ca, ↑ ESR, ↑ Cr, proteinuria (24 hour urine collection)

Routine urinalysis will not detect light chains as dipstick detects albumin. Need sulfosalicylic acid or 24 hour urine protein.

- monoclonal proteins
    - serum protein electrophoresis (SPEP) – demonstrates monoclonal protein in serum (spike) in 80%
    - urine protein electrophoresis (UPEP) – shows urine Bence-Jones protein, immunofixation shows M protein in 75%
- bone marrow biopsy
    - often focal abnormality, greater than 10% plasma cells
- skeletal series, MRI if symptoms of cord compression
    - bone scans are not useful since they detect osteoblast activity
- β-2 microglobulin, LDH and CRP are poor prognosticators

Diagnosis
- classic diagnostic triad:
    - bone marrow containing more than 10% plasma cells or plasmacytoma
    - lytic bone lesions
    - monoclonal protein spike in serum or urine

Treatment
- autologous stem cell transplant
- chemotherapy
    - melphalan and prednisone if >75 yrs
    - melphalan, prednisone and thalidomide if 65-75 yrs
    - dexamethasone ± thalidomide if ARF
- new treatments: bortezomib, lenalidomide
- bisphosphonates
- local XRT for bone pain, spinal cord compression
- treat complications: hydration for hypercalcemia and renal failure, bisphosphonates (e.g. pamidronate) for severe hypercalcemia, prophylactic antibiotics, erothropoietin for anemia

Prognosis
- median survival 24-30 months

Light Chain Disease

- plasma cells produce only light chains
- 15% of patients with myeloma
- diagnosis
    - urine immunoelectrophoresis
    - serum studies often non-diagnostic as light chains can pass through glomerulus
- renal failure a major problem
- prognosis for survival: kappa > lambda light chains

Monoclonal Gammopathy of Unknown Significance (MGUS)

- a.k.a. benign monoclonal gammopathy
- incidence: 0.15% in general population, 5% of people >70 years of age
- asymptomatic
- diagnosis
    - presence of a serum monoclonal protein (M-protein) at a concentration ≤3g/dL
    - <10% plasma cells in bone marrow
    - absence of lytic bone lesions, anemia, hypercalcemia, and renal insufficiency related to the plasma cell proliferative process
- 1% of patients develop multiple myeloma each year in the first 3 years → monitor with annual serum protein electrophoresis

Macroglobulinemia of Waldenstrom

- uncontrollable proliferation of lymphoplasmacytoid cells (a hybrid of lymphocytes and plasma cells)
- monoclonal IgM paraprotein is produced
- symptoms: weakness, fatigue, bleeding (oronasal), weight loss, recurrent infections, dyspnea, CHF (triad of anemia, hyperviscosity, plasma volume expansion), neurological symptoms, peripheral neuropathy, cerebral dysfunction
- signs: pallor, splenomegaly, hepatomegaly, lymphadenopathy, retinal lesions
- bone marrow shows plasmacytoid lymphocytes
- bone lesions usually not present
- cold hemagglutinin disease possible
- normocytic anemia, rouleaux, high ESR if hyperviscosity not present
- watch for hyperviscosity syndrome

Management
- alkylating agents (chlorambucil), nucleoside analogues (fludarabine), rituximab, or combination therapy
- corticosteroids
- plasmapheresis for hyperviscosity

Complications of Hematologic Malignancies

Hyperviscosity Syndrome

Definition
- refers to clinical sequelae of ↑ blood viscosity (when relative serum viscosity >5-6), resulting from ↑ circulating serum Igs or from ↑ cellular blood components in hyperproliferative disorders
- macroglobulinemia of Waldenstrom accounts for 85% of cases

Clinical Features
- hypervolemia causing: CHF, headache, lethargy, dilutional anemia
- CNS symptoms due to ↓ cerebral blood flow: headache, vertigo, ataxia, stroke
- retina shows venous engorgement and hemorrhages
- bleeding diathesis
  - due to impaired platelet function, absorption of soluble coagulation factors, e.g. nasal bleeding, oozing gums
- ESR usually very low

Treatment
- plasmapheresis

Tumour Lysis Syndrome

Definition
- group of metabolic complications that result from spontaneous or treatment-related breakdown of cancer cells
- more common in diseases with large tumour burden and high proliferative rate (high grade lymphoma, leukemia)

Clinical Features
- metabolic abnormalities
  - cells lyse, releasing K, uric acid, PO_4 (↑ K, ↑ uric acid, ↑ PO_4)
  - PO_4 binds Ca (↓ Ca)
- complications
  - lethal cardiac arrhythmia (↑ K)
  - acute renal failure (urate nephropathy)

Treatment
- prevention
  - aggressive IV hydration
  - alkalinization of the urine
  - allopurinol
  - correction of pre-existing metabolic abnormalities
- dialysis

Blood Products and Transfusions

Blood Groups

- there is no universal donor
- uncrossmatched blood from the same group is safer than O–
- in emergencies, males can immediately receive O+ or O– blood; females O–

Indications for RBCs in acute blood loss
- maintain Hb >70 g/L when active bleeding
- consider maintaining a higher Hb level for patients with
  - impaired pulmonary function
  - ↑O_2 consumption
  - CAD/unstable coronary syndromes
  - uncontrolled/unpredictable bleeding
- Hb >100 g/L unlikely to benefit from transfusion

Blood Groups

Group	Antigen	Antibody
O	H	anti-A, anti-B
A	A	anti-B
B	B	anti-A
AB	A and B	nil

Red Blood Cells

Table 19. Red Cells

Product	Indication
Packed Cells (PRBCs)	symptomatic anemia, bleeding with hypovolemia
Frozen Red Cells	rare blood groups, multiple autoantibodies

Packed Cells
- stored at 4°C
- transfuse within 35 days of collection, otherwise cell lysis may result in hyperkalemia
- transfuse within 7 days of collection if renal failure or hepatic failure is present to reduce solute load
- each unit will raise Hct by about 4% or Hb by 10 g/L
- infuse each unit over 2 hours, max of 4 hours

1 unit of pRBC approximately ↑ Hb by 10 g/L or ↑ Hct by 4%.

Selection of Red Cells for Transfusion
- the donor blood should be the same ABO and Rh group as the recipient
- donor blood should be crossmatch compatible (by mixing recipient serum with donor RBC) and free of irregular blood group antibodies

Platelets

Table 20. Platelet Products

Product	Indication
Random donor (pooled)	Thrombocytopenia with bleeding
Single donor platelets	Potential BMT recipients
HLA matched platelets	Refractory to pooled or single donor platelets

- stored at 20-24°C
- random donor platelets are transfused in groups of 5 units; this should ↑ the platelet count by at least 15 x 10^9/L
- single donor platelets should ↑ the platelet count by 40-60 x 10^9/L
- if an increment in the platelet count is not seen, alloantibodies, bleeding, sepsis or hypersplenism may be present
- relative contraindications: TTP, HIT, post-transfusion purpura (PTP), HELLP

Indications for platelets transfusion

Plt (x 10⁹/L)	Indications
<10	Non-immune thrombocytopenia
<20	Procedures not associated with significant blood loss
<50	Procedures associated with blood loss or major surgery (>500 mL expected blood loss)
<100	Pre-neurosurgery or head trauma
Any	Platelet dysfunction and marked bleeding

In Canada, blood products are leukodepleted via filtration immediately after donation. Therefore it is considered:
- CMV negative (because CMV found in leukocytes)
- low in lymphokines, resulting in a lower incidence of febrile nonhemolytic transfusion reactions

Coagulation Factors

Table 21. Coagulation Factor Products

Product	Indication
Fresh Frozen Plasma (FFP)	Depletion of multiple coagulation factors (e.g. sepsis, DIC, dilution, TTP/HUS, liver disease), emergency reversal of life threatening bleeding secondary to warfarin overdose
Cryoprecipitate (enriched fibrinogen, vWF, VIII, XII)	Factor VIII deficiency von Willebrand's disease Hypofibrinogenemia
Hemate P	von Willebrand's disease
Factor VIII concentrate	Factor VIII deficiency (Hemophilia A)
Factor IX concentrate	Factor IX deficiency (Hemophilia B)
Recombinant VIIa	Factor VIII deficiency, CNS bleeds, severe trauma, F VIII inhibitors

Special Considerations
- irradiated blood products
    - prevent proliferation of donor T-cells in potential or actual BMT recipients
    - immunocompromised patients
- CMV-negative blood products
    - potential transplant recipients
    - neonates
    - AIDS patients
    - seronegative pregnant women

Acute Blood Transfusion Reactions

IMMUNE

Acute Hemolytic Transfusion Reactions (AHTR)
- ABO incompatibility resulting in intravascular hemolysis secondary to complement activation
- most commonly due to incorrect patient identification
- occurs immediately after transfusion
- risk per unit of blood is <1 in 250,000
- presents with fever, chills, hypotension, back or flank pain, dyspnea, hemoglobinuria
- acute renal failure (<24 hrs) and DIC
- treatment
    - stop transfusion
    - notify blood bank and check for clerical error
    - maintain BP with vigorous IV fluids +/- inotropes
    - maintain U/O with diuretics, crystalloids, and dopamine

Febrile Nonhemolytic Transfusion Reactions (FNHTR)
- due to alloantibodies to WBC, platelets or other donor plasma antigens and release of cytokines from blood product cells
- occurs within 0-6 hours of transfusion
- risk per unit of blood is 1 in 100
- presents with fever ± rigors, facial flushing, H/A, myalgia, hypotension
- treatment
    - R/O fever due to hemolytic reaction or infection
    - if fever <38°C, continue with transfusion but decrease rate and give antipyretics
    - if fever >38°C, stop transfusion, give antipyretics and anti-histamine

Allergic Nonhemolytic
- due to alloantibodies (IgE) to proteins in donor plasma which result in mast cell activation and release of histamine
- occurs mainly in those with history of multiple transfusions, or multiparous women
- risk per unit of blood is 1 in 100
- presents mainly as urticaria and occasionally with fever
- can present as anaphylactoid reaction with bronchospasm, laryngeal edema, and hypotension but this occurs mainly in IgA deficient patients that have anti-IgA antibodies
- treatment
    - mild: slow transfusion rate and give diphenhydramine
    - moderate to severe: stop transfusion, give IV diphenydramine, steroids, epinephrine, IV fluids and bronchodilators

Transfusion-Related Acute Lung Injury (TRALI)
- due to binding of donor antibodies to WBC of recipient and release of mediators that increase capillary permeability in the lungs
- occurs 2-4 hrs post transfusion and resolves in 24-72 hrs
- risk per unit of blood is 1 in 5000
- presents with acute respiratory distress; on CXR shows up as acute pulmonary edema
- treatment: supportive therapy (oxygen)
- inform blood bank so antibody investigation occurs

NONIMMUNE

Bacterial Infection
- Gram positive: *S. aureus, S. epidermis, Bacillus cereus*
- Gram negative: *Klebsiella, Serratia, Pseudomonas, Yersinia*
- overall risk is 1 in 100,000 for RBC and 1in 10,000 for platelets
- never store blood >4 hours after a bag has left blood bank
- treatment: stop transfusion, blood cultures, IV antibiotics, fluids

Circulatory Overload
- due to impaired cardiac function and/or excessive rapid transfusion
- presents as dyspnea, orthopnea, hypotension, tachycardia, crackles at base of lung, and increased venous pressure
- incidence is 1 in 700 of transfusions
- treatment: transfuse at lower rate, give diuretics and oxygen

Hyperkalemia
- due to K release from stored RBC
- risk increases with storage time and if blood is irradiated

- decreased risk if given fresh blood
- occurs in 5% of massively transfused patients
- treatment: see Nephrology

Citrate Toxicity
- occurs with massive transfusion in patients with liver disease
- citrate binds to Ca and causes signs and symptoms of hypocalcemia
- unable to clear citrate form blood secondary to liver disease
- treatment: IV calcium gluconate (10 ml of 10%) for every 2 units of blood

Dilutional Coagulopathy
- occurs with massive transfusion (>10 units)
- PRBC contains no clotting factors, fibrinogen, cryoprecipitate, or platelets
- treatment: FFP, platelets, and cryoprecipitate

Delayed Blood Transfusion Reactions

IMMUNE

Delayed Hemolytic
- due to alloantibodies to minor antigens such as Rh, Kell, Duff, and Kidd
- level of antibody at time of transfusion is too low to cause hemolysis; later the level of antibody increases due to secondary stimulus and causes extravascular hemolysis
- occurs 5-7 days after transfusion
- presents as anemia and mild jaundice
- treatment: no specific treatment required; important to note for future transfusion

NONIMMUNE

Iron Overload
- due to repeated transfusions over long period of time (e.g. thalassemia major)
- can cause secondary hemochromatosis
- treatment: use iron chelators after transfusion

Viral Infection Risk
- HBV <1 in 82,000
- HTLV <1 in 1,000,000
- HCV <1 in 2,800,000
- HIV <1 in 4,000,000
- other infections include EBV, CMV, WNV

Transfusion-Associated Graft Versus Host Disease (GVHD)
- transfused T-lymphocytes recognize and react against "host" (recipient)
- occurs 4-30 days following transfusion
- most patients already have severely impaired immune systems (e.g. Hodgkin's or leuken
- presents as fever, diarrhea, liver function abnormalities, and pancytopenia
- can be prevented by giving irradiated blood

Common Medications

Table 22. Drugs for Anemia

Drug	Common Formulary	Mechanism of Action	Dosing Schedule	Indications	Contraindications	Side Effects
iron	iron gluconate iron sulphate iron fumarate Palafer™ Femiron™	• synthesis of hemoglobin	2-3 mg/kg/day of elemental iron in 3 divided doses PO	• iron deficiency anemia treatment and prevention • pregnancy	• iron overload	• in children: acute iron toxicity • constipation
B$_{12}$	cyanocobalamin hydroxycobalamin Bedoz™ Cobex™	• synthesis of folic acid and DNA	up to 1000 µg/day PO	• B$_{12}$ deficiency	• hypersensitivity	• diarrhea
folic acid	folic acid Novo Folacid™ Folvite™	• synthesis of purines and thymidylate, thus DNA	up to 1 mg/day PO	• folic acid deficiency • pregnancy	• uncorrected pernicious anemia	• rash
erythropoietin	epoetin (Epogen™) Eprex™ dabrepoetin (Aranesp™)	• stimulation of RBC synthesis	50-1000 U/kg SC/IV, 3 times weekly	• renal failure • marrow failure • autologous blood donation	• uncontrolled hypertension • myelodysplastic syndrome	• hypertension

Antiplatelet Therapy

Aspirin (ASA)
- irreversibly acetylates COX, inhibiting TXA_2 synthesis, thus inhibiting platelet aggregation
- ASA is currently indicated for:
  - stroke and MI prophylaxis
  - to reduce the incidence of recurrent MI
  - to decrease mortality in post-MI patients
- dosage: single loading dose of 200-300 mg, followed by daily dose of 75-100 mg PO OD

Aggrenox™
- combination of ASA and dipyridamole
- dipyridamole ↑ intracellular cAMP levels which inhibits TXA_2 synthesis, leading to ↓ platelet aggregation
- hypothesized that these effects of dipyridamole potentiate antiplatelet actions of ASA
- Aggrenox™ is more effective than aspirin in secondary prevention of stroke
- ongoing clinical trials will determine the best indications for this agent

Clopidogrel (Plavix™)
- ADP activates GP IIb/IIIa, allowing platelets to bind to fibrinogen and aggregate
- clopidogrel and ticlopidine (Ticlid™) inhibit ADP binding to platelets, thus inhibiting aggregation
- useful for prevention of cardiovascular events in high-risk patients
- clopidogrel may cause TTP
- ticlodipine (Ticlid™) is associated with a risk of agranulocytosis and is rarely used

Glycoprotein IIb/IIIa Inhibitors
- Reopro™ (abciximab), Integrelin™ (eptifibatide), Aggrastat™ (tirofiban)
- blocking GP IIb/IIIa receptor inhibits fibrinogen and vWF binding, leading to ↓ platelet aggregation
- used most commonly in patients undergoing cardiac catheterization

Anticoagulant Therapy

- see *Approach To Treatment of Venous Thrombosis*, H29

Absolute Contraindications
- active bleeding
- severe bleeding diathesis or platelet count $<20 \times 10^9/L$ ($<20,000/mm^3$)
- intracranial bleeding, neurosurgery or ocular surgery within 10 days

Relative Contraindications
- mild-moderate bleeding diathesis or thrombocytopenia
- brain metastases
- recent major trauma
- major abdominal surgery within the past 2 days
- GI or GU bleeding within 14 days
- endocarditis
- severe hypertension (sBP >200 or BP >120)
- recent stroke

Heparin and Warfarin

Table 23. Comparison of Heparin and Warfarin

	Heparin	Warfarin
Structure	large anionic polymer, acidic	small lipid soluble molecule
Route Administration	parenteral (IV, SC)	oral (PO)
Site of Action	blood (via Antithrombin)	liver
Onset	rapid (seconds)	slow (limited by half-life of clotting factors)
Mechanism	accelerates activity of Antithrombin	Vitamin K antagonist, inhibits production of II, VII, IX, X, protein C and S
Duration of Action	acute (hours)	chronic (days)
Acute Overdose	protamine sulphate	IV Vitamin K + FFP
TREATMENT		
Monitoring	aPTT (intrinsic pathway)	PT/INR (extrinsic pathway)
Pregnancy	safe (does not cross placenta)	not used (can cross placenta), teratogenic

Aspirin plus dipyridamole versus aspirin alone after cerebral ischaemia of arterial origin (ESPRIT): randomised controlled trial.
Lancet 2006; 367:1665-73.
Study: Randomised, controlled, open-treatment, auditing-blinded trial with mean follow-up of 3.5 years.
Patients: 2739 patients within 6 months of a transient ischaemic attack or minor stroke of presumed arterial origin.
Intervention: Patients were assigned to aspirin (30-325 mg daily) with (n=1363) or without (n=1376) dipyridamole (200 mg twice daily).
Primary Outcome: The composite of death from all vascular causes, non-fatal stroke, non-fatal myocardial infarction, or major bleeding complication, whichever happened first.
Results: Primary outcome events arose in 173 (13%) patients on aspirin and dipyridamole and in 216 (16%) on aspirin alone (hazard ratio 0.80, 95% CI 0.66-0.98; absolute risk reduction 1.0% per year, 95% CI 0.1-1.8). Addition of the ESPRIT data to the meta-analysis of previous trials resulted in an overall risk ratio for the composite of vascular death, stroke, or myocardial infarction of 0.82 (95% CI 0.74-0.91). Patients on aspirin and dipyridamole discontinued trial medication more often than those on aspirin alone (470 vs 184), mainly because of headache.
Conclusion: The ESPRIT results, combined with the results of previous trials, provide sufficient evidence to prefer the combination regimen of aspirin plus dipyridamole over aspirin alone as antithrombotic therapy after cerebral ischaemia of arterial origin.

WEPT
Warfarin
Extrinsic **P**athway
↑ **PT**/INR

Comparison of Fixed-Dose Weight-Adjusted Unfractionated Heparin and LMWH for Acute Treatment of Venous Thrombembolism
JAMA 2006; 296:935-42
Study: Multicentre, randomized, open-label, adjudicator-blinded, non-inferiority trial with follow up of 3 months.
Patients: 708 adult patients (mean age 60 yrs, 55% male, mean weight 83 kg) with acute venous thrombembolism (VTE).
Intervention: Patients were randomized to receive either fixed-dose, weight-adjusted subcutaneous unfractionated heparin or LMWH (dalteparin or enoxaparin). Therapy lasted for a minimum of 5 days and continued until the INR was brought within the therapeutic range with the initiation of warfarin therapy.
Primary Outcome: Recurrent VTE over 3 months of follow up and major bleeding within 10 days of randomization.
Results: There was no significant difference in the rate of recurrent VTE in the unfractionated heparin group (13 patients, 3.8%) vs. the LMWH group (12 patients, 3.4%). There was also no significant difference in the incidence of major bleeding within 10 days of randomization in the unfractionated heparin group (4 patients, 1.1%) vs. the LMWH group (5 patients, 1.4%). In 72% of patients receiving unfractionated heparin and 68% of patients receiving LMWH, treatment was administered outside of hospital.
Conclusion: Fixed-dose, weight-adjusted, subcutaneous unfractionated heparin is as effective as standard treatment with LMWH in patients with acute VTE.

Adverse Reactions of Heparin
- hemorrhage: depends on dose, age, and concomitant use of antiplatelet agents or thrombolytics
- heparin-induced thrombocytopenia: associated with venous or arterial thrombosis (see Table 11)
- osteoporosis: with long term use

Low Molecular Weight Heparin (enoxaparin, dalteparin, tinzaparin)
- increased bioavailability compared to normal heparin
- ↑ duration of action
- SC route of administration
- do not need to monitor aPTT
- adverse reactions less common than UFH
- patients with renal failure (CrCl<30) can accumulate LMWH

Heparin Alternatives

Danaparoid
- indicated for HIT, stable patients
- inhibits Factor Xa via antithrombin III
- SC route of administration
- monitor anti-Xa levels if renal failure or extremes in weight, cannot monitor aPTT

Hirudin
- indicated for HIT+, unstable patients (ICU/CCU) requiring procedures
- direct thrombin inhibitor (natural)
- IV route of administration
- monitor aPTT levels
- risk of anti-hirudin antibodies (40-60%)
- increases INR (difficulty monitoring switch to warfarin)

Argatroban
- indicated for HIT+, renal failure and unstable patients
- direct thrombin inhibitor (synthetic)
- IV route of administration
- monitor aPTT levels
- increases INR (difficulty monitoring switching to warfarin)

Fondaparinux
- selective inhibitor of Factor Xa
- heparin pentasaccharide analogue
- one of the newer drugs for prevention and treatment of VTE

Fondaparinux vs enoxaparin for the prevention of venous thromboembolism in major orthopedic surgery: a meta-analysis of 4 randomized double-blind studies.
Arch Intern Med. 2002;162:1833-40.
Purpose: To determine whether a subcutaneous 2.5-mg, once-daily regimen of fondaparinux sodium starting 6 hours after surgery was more effective and as safe as approved enoxaparin regimens in preventing VTE.
Study Selection: Four multicenter, randomized, double-blind trials in patients undergoing elective hip replacement, elective major knee surgery, and surgery for hip fracture (n=7344).
Results: Fondaparinux significantly reduced the incidence of VTE by day 11 (182 [6.8%] of 2682 patients) compared with enoxaparin (371 [13.7%] of 2703 patients), with a common odds reduction of 55.2% (95% CI, 45.8% to 63.1%; p<.001); this beneficial effect was consistent across all types of surgery and all subgroups. Although major bleeding occurred more frequently in the fondaparinux-treated group (p=.008), the incidence of clinically relevant bleeding (leading to death or reoperation or occurring in a critical organ) did not differ between groups.
Conclusions: In patients undergoing orthopedic surgery, 2.5 mg of fondaparinux sodium once daily, starting 6 hours postoperatively, showed a major benefit over enoxaparin, achieving an overall risk reduction of VTE greater than 50% without increasing the risk of clinically relevant bleeding.

Table 24. Recommended Therapeutic INR Ranges of Common Indications for Oral Anticoagulant Therapy

Indication	INR range
Prophylaxis of venous thrombosis (high-risk surgery)	2.0-3.0
Treatment of venous thrombosis	
Most cases of thrombosis with antiphospholipid antibody syndrome	
Treatment of pulmonary embolism	
Prevention of systemic embolism	
Tissue heart valves	
AMI (to prevent systemic embolism)	
Valvular heart disease	
Atrial fibrillation	
Bileaflet mechanical valve in aortic position	
Mechanical prosthetic mitral valves (high risk)	2.5-3.5
Prophylaxis of recurrent myocardial infarction	

Chemotherapeutic Agents

Table 25. Selected Chemotherapeutic Agents

Class	Example	Mechanism of Action or Target
Alkylating Agent	• chlorambucil, cyclophosphamide, melphalan (nitrogen mustards) • carboplatin, cisplatin • dacarbazine, procarbazine • busulfan	• damage DNA via alkylation of base pairs • leads to cross-linking of bases, abnormal base-pairing, DNA breakage
Antimetabolites	• methotrexate (folic acid antagonist) • 6-mercaptopurine, fludarabine (purine antagonist) • 5-FU (pyrimidine antagonist) • hydroxyurea	• inhibit DNA synthesis
Antibiotics	• adriamycin (anthracycline) • bleomycin • mitomycin C	• interfere with DNA and RNA synthesis
Taxanes	• paclitaxel • docetaxel	• stabilize microtubules against breakdown once cell division complete
Vinca-alkaloids	• vinblastine • vincristine • vinorelbine	• inhibit microtubule assembly (mitotic spindles), blocking cell division
Topoisomerase Inhibitors	• irinotecan, topotecan (topo I) • etoposide (topo II)	• interfere with DNA unwinding necessary for normal replication and transcription
Monoclonal Antibodies	• trastuzumab (Herceptin™) • bevacizumab (Avastin™) • rituximab (Rituxan™) • cetuximab (Erbitux™)	• HER2 • VEGF • CD20 • EGFR
Small Molecule Inhibitors	• imatinib mesylate (Gleevec™) • erlotinib (Tarceva™) • gefitinib (Iressa™) • bortezomib (Velcade™) • sunitinib (Sutent™)	• Bcr-Abl • EGFR • EGFR • 26S proteasome • VEGFR, PDGFR

Infectious Diseases

Kristen Brown, Anjali Shroff and Ivan Ying, chapter editors
Deepti Damaraju and Elliott Owen, associate editors
Erik Venos, EBM editor
Dr. Wayne Gold, Dr. Jay Keystone and Dr. Sharon Walmsley, staff editors

Principles of Microbiology

Transmission of Infectious Diseases

Mechanisms
- direct contact
  - person-to-person (*S. aureus*, rhinovirus)
  - sexual (*N. gonorrheae*, *C. trachomatis*, herpes simplex virus, HIV)
  - blood-borne (HIV, hepatitis B, hepatitis C)
- respiratory droplets (*N. meningitidis*, *Bordetella pertussis*)
- aerosol: *M. tuberculosis*, varicella zoster virus, measles
- food/water borne: *Vibrio cholerae*, *Salmonella*, hepatitis A, hepatitis E
- zoonotic
  - animals (rabies, Q fever)
  - arthropods (malaria, Lyme disease)
- vertical
  - congenital syndromes (TORCH infections see <u>Obstetrics</u>)
  - perinatal (HIV, hepatitis B, group B *Streptococcus*)

Bacteriology

Bacteria Basics
- bacteria are prokaryotic cells which divide asexually by binary fission
- Gram stain divides most bacteria into two groups based on cell wall
  - Gram-positive: thick, rigid layer of peptidoglycan
  - Gram-negative: thin peptidoglycan layer + thicker outer membrane composed of lipoproteins and lipopolysaccharides
- preferred atmospheric growth conditions
  - aerobic: will not grow in the absence of oxygen
  - obligate anaerobes: growth only in complete absence of oxygen
  - facultative anaerobes: growth with or without oxygen

Gram Stain
Gram positive = blue/black
Gram negative = pink/red

Bacteria Not Seen on Gram Stain
Mycobacteria spp.
Treponema pallidum
Chlamydia spp.
Rickettsia

Acid-Fast Bacteria
Ziehl-Neelsen stain: heat or detergents are used to force dye into cell and cell cannot be decolourized by acid-alcohol e.g. *Mycobacteria*, *Nocardia*

- α-hemolytic indicates partial hemolysis
- β-hemolytic indicates complete hemolysis
- γ-hemolytic indicates no hemolysis

Table 1. Classification of Bacteria

| | Gram-positive bacteria | | Gram-negative bacteria | |
	Cocci	Bacilli (rods)	Diplococci	Bacilli (rods)
Aerobes	Staphylococcus Streptococcus Enterococcus	Bacillus Listeria Corynebacterium Nocardia	Neisseria Moraxella	Enterobacteriaceae Pseudomonas Haemophilus
Anaerobes	Peptostreptococcus	Clostridium Propionibacterium Lactobacillus Actinomyces	Veillonella	Bacteroides Fusobacterium

Mechanisms of Bacterial Disease
i) survival in the environment
  - spore formation and resistance to drying (*Clostridium*, *Bacillus*), cold growth (*Listeria*), survival in water (*Legionella*)
ii) adherence to and colonization of skin or mucous membranes
  - via fimbriae (pili): microfilaments extending through the cell wall
iii) invasion or crossing normal epithelial barriers
iv) evasion of host defense system through inhibition of:
  - phagocytic uptake: polysaccharide capsule (*S. pneumoniae*, *N. meningitidis*, *H. influenzae*) or surface proteins (*Staphylococcus*, *Streptococcus*)
  - phagocytic killing (*Listeria*, *M. tuberculosis*)
iv) toxin production
  - exotoxins are secreted by living pathogenic bacteria and cause disease even if the bacteria is not present (*Clostridium*)
  - structural endotoxins are components of the bacterial cell wall that may be shed while living or released during cell lysis
v) intracellular growth
  - *Chlamydia*, *Legionella*, *Listeria*, *Mycobacteria*, *Salmonella*

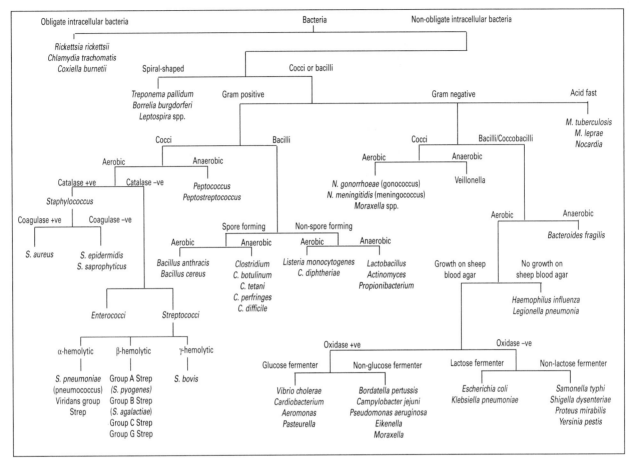

Figure 1. Laboratory Identification of Bacterial Species

Table 2. Commensal Flora

Site	Organisms
Skin	Coagulase-negative *Staphylococci, Corynebacteria, Propionibacterium acnes*
Oropharynx	*Viridans* group *Streptococci, Haemophilus, Neisseria*, anaerobes (*Peptostreptococcus, Bacteroides, Veillonella, Fusobacterium, Actinomyces, Prevotella*)
Small bowel	*E. coli*, anaerobes (low numbers)
Colon	*E. coli, Klebsiella, Enterobacter, Enterococcus*, anaerobes (*Bacteroides, Fusobacterium, Peptostreptococcus, Clostridium*)
Vagina	*Lactobacillus acidophilus, viridans* group *Streptococci*, coagulase-negative *Staphylococci*, facultative Gram-negative bacilli, anaerobes

Virology

Viral Basics
- viruses are nucleoprotein complexes which infect cells and use host metabolic processes to replicate
- virions are mature, released virus particles that can exist in the extracellular environment — they are composed of an internal nucleic acid core covered by a protein coat ± glycoprotein/lipid envelope
- host sensitivity (can the cell become infected?) governed by cell and virus surface proteins (viral tropism); receptors required like lock in key
- host permissibility (does the cell allow for production of virions?) is governed by whether or not cell machinery fulfils the virus' needs
- ___**viridae** = family, ___**virus** = genus, # = species (e.g. *Retroviridae* HIV-2)

Viral Classification

1) viral genome
   - DNA or RNA
   - double-stranded or single-stranded
   - single or multiple pieces
2) virion shape
   - helical or icosahedral or complex
   - enveloped or naked

Viral Disease Patterns

1) acute infections
   - host cells are lysed in the process of virion release (usually naked viruses i.e. adenovirus)
   - some produce acute infections with late sequelae (e.g. measles virus → subacute sclerosing panencephalitis)
2) chronic infections (>6 months)
   - host cells are hijacked to chronically release virions (usually enveloped viruses i.e. hepatitis B, HIV)
3) latent infections
   - viral genome integrated into host DNA but not actively producing virions
   - can be reactivated (usually if virus can integrate into host DNA e.g. herpes simplex virus)

Table 3. Common Viruses

Nucleic Acid	Enveloped	Virus Family	Major Viruses	Medical Importance
dsDNA	N	Adenoviridae	Adenovirus	URTI Conjunctivitis Gastroenteritis
		Herpesviridae	HHV1=HSV1 HHV2=HSV2 HHV3=VZV HHV4=EBV HHV5=CMV HHV6 HHV8=KSHV	Oral, ocular and genital herpes Genital, oral and ocular herpes Chicken pox, shingles Mononucleosis, viral hepatitis Retinitis, pneumonitis, hepatitis, encephalitis Roseola Kaposi's sarcoma
		Papovaviridae	HPV1,4 HPV6,11 HPV16,18,etc. JC virus	Plantar warts Genital warts Cervical/anal dysplasia and cancer Progressive multifocal leukoencephalopathy
	Y	Hepadnaviridae	Hepatitis B	Hepatitis
		Poxviridae	Molluscum contagiosum Variola	Molluscum contagiosum Smallpox
ssDNA	N	Parvoviridae	Parvovirus B-19	Erythema infectiosum (Fifth disease)
(+)ssRNA	N	Caliciviridae	Norwalk Hepatitis E	Gastroenteritis Acute hepatitis
		Picornaviridae	Poliovirus Echovirus Rhinovirus Coxsackie virus Hepatitis A	Poliomyelitis URTIs, viral meningitis URTIs Hand-foot-and-mouth, viral meningitis Acute hepatitis
	Y	Coronoviridae	Coronovirus	URTIs, SARS
		Flaviviridae	Yellow Fever Dengue Fever Hepatitis C West Nile	Yellow Fever Dengue Fever Hepatitis Encephalitis
		Retroviridae	HIV	AIDS
		Togaviridae	Rubella	Rubella (German measles)

Table 3. Common Viruses (continued)

Nucleic Acid	Enveloped	Virus Family	Major Viruses	Medical Importance
(-)ssRNA	Y	Arenaviridae	Lassa Fever	Lassa Fever
		Filoviridae	Ebola, Marburg	Hemorrhagic fever
		Orthomyxoviridae	Influenza A, B, C	Influenza
		Paramyxoviridae	Measles	Measles
			Mumps	Mumps
			Parainfluenza	URTIs, croup, bronchiolitis
			RSV	Bronchiolitis, pneumonia
		Rhabdoviridae	Rabies	Rabies
dsRNA	N	Reoviridae	Rotavirus	Gastroenteritis

Mycology

Fungal Basics
- fungi are strictly aerobic eukaryotic organisms with two major chemical differences from human cells
  - ergosterol is the major fungal membrane sterol (instead of cholesterol)
  - fungal cell walls contain chitin, a complex glycopolysaccharide (instead of peptidoglycans as seen in bacteria)
- two broad groups of fungi: yeast (unicellular) and molds (multicellular with hyphae)
- dimorphic fungi are generally found as mold at room temperature but grow as yeast-like forms at body temperature

Mechanisms of Fungal Disease
- primary fungal infection through
  - overgrowth of normal flora; usually yeasts or dermatophytes
  - inhalation of fungal spores
  - traumatic implantation
- toxins produced by fungi (e.g. ingestion of toxic mushrooms, aflatoxins)
- allergic reaction to fungi (e.g. bronchopulmonary aspergillosis)

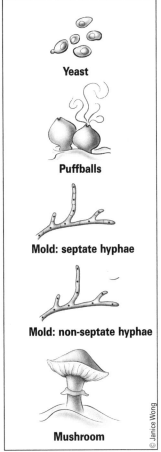

Figure 2. Common Fungus Morphology

(Yeast, Puffballs, Mold: septate hyphae, Mold: non-septate hyphae, Mushroom)
© Janice Wong

Parasitology

Parasite Basics
- a parasite is an organism that lives in or on another organism (host) and damages the host in the process
- a parasite with a complex life cycle requires more than one host to reproduce
  - reservoir host maintains a parasite and may be the source for human infection
  - intermediate host maintains the asexual stage of a parasite or allows development of the parasite to proceed to the larval stage
  - definitive host allows the parasite to develop to the adult stage where reproduction occurs
- there are 2 major groups of parasites: protozoa and helminths

Table 4. Differences Between Protozoa and Helminths

Protozoa	Helminths
unicellular	multicellular
motile trophozoite → inactive cyst	adult → egg → larva
multiplication	no multiplication
± eosinophilia	eosinophilia (proportional to extent of tissue invasion)*
indefinite life span	definite life span

*Adult ascaris, tapeworms do not cause eosinophilia

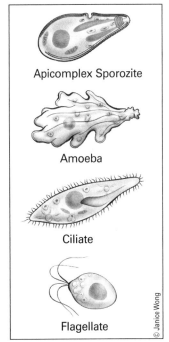

Figure 3. Basic Protozoal Morphology

(Apicomplex Sporozite, Amoeba, Ciliate, Flagellate)
© Janice Wong

Table 5. Common Parasites

Cellularity	Shape	Common Species
Protozoa	apicomplexa	*Cryptosporidia* *Microsporidia* *Cyclosporidia* *Plasmodia* (malaria)
	amoebas	*Entamoeba histolytica, Entamoeba dispar*
	ciliates	*Balantidium coli*
	flagellates	*Giardia lamblia* *Trichomonas vaginalis* *Leishmania* *Trypanomoma cruzi, gambiense, rhodiense*
Helminths	Flatworms: trematodes (unsegmented): "flukes" • use snails as intermediate hosts then infect humans via water exposure	*Clonorchis sinensis* *Schistosoma mansoni, hematobium, japonicum*

	cestodes (segmented): "tapeworms"
	• have multiple intermediate hosts
	• disease more serious in intermediate host;
	  in definitive host lives in GI tract as worm
	  measuring up to several meters
		Taenia saginata, solium
		Diphylobothrium lata

	Roundworms: nematodes (unsegmented) "roundworms" • humans are definitive host • lifecycles can be complex	roundworms: *Ascaris lumbricoides* pinworms: *Enterobius vermicularis* hookworms: *Ancyclostoma duodenale* whipworms: *Trichuris trichiura* filaria: *Wuchereria bancrofti, Onchocerca volvulus,* *Loa loa*

Parasite sampling may need to be repeated on a number of occasions before infection can be ruled out.

Characteristics of Parasitic Disease
- spectrum of disease ranging from asymptomatic to severe illness
- symptoms are usually proportional to parasite burden
- tissue damage due to the host immune response and the parasite itself
- chronic infections may occur with or without overt disease, reinfection may occur
- immunocompromised hosts are more susceptible to infection, reactivation of latent infections and more severe disease

Mechanisms of Parasitic Disease
i)   mechanical obstruction
ii) cytotoxicity leading to abscesses and ulcers
iii) inflammatory
- acute hypersensitivity (e.g. pneumonitis)
- delayed hypersensitivity (e.g. egg granulomas)
- cytokine-mediated (systemic illness)

iv) immune-mediated injury
- autoimmune (e.g. myocarditis)
- immune complex (e.g. nephritis)

Neurological Infections

Table 6. CSF Profiles for CNS Infections

	Bacterial	Viral
Appearance	Normal or cloudy	Normal or cloudy
Glucose (mmol/L)	↓	Normal
Protein (g/L)	↑↑	↑
White blood cell	~500 to 10,000 /μL	~10-500 /μL
Predominant WBC	Neutrophils	Lymphocytes

Adapted from Cecil Essentials of Medicine 6th ed.

Meningitis

- inflammation of the meninges

Etiology

Table 7. Common Organisms in Meningitis

Bacterial	Immunocompromised/ Elderly	Neonates	Viral	Fungal	Other
S. pneumoniae	S. pneumoniae	GBS	Enteroviruses	cryptococcus	Lyme disease
N. meningitidis	N. meningitidis	E. coli	HIV	coccidiodomycosis	neurosyphilis
H. influenzae	L. monocytogenes	L. monocytogenes	HSV-2	TB	
		Viral	West Nile		

Risk Factors
- hematogenous spread: respiratory tract, subacute bacterial endocarditis
- parameningeal focus (otitis media, odontogenic, sinusitis)
- penetrating head trauma
- anatomical meningeal defects
- previous neurosurgical procedures, shunts
- cancer, alcoholism and other immunodeficiency states
- contact with infected patient

Clinical Features
- neonates and children: fever, vomiting, lethargy, irritability, poor feeding
- older children and adults: fever, headache, neck stiffness, confusion, nausea and vomiting, lethargy, meningismus, altered level of consciousness, seizures, focal neurological signs (see Colour Atlas, *Infectious Diseases*)

Investigations
- CBC with differential, blood C&S, electrolytes (for SIADH)
- x-rays may indicate primary site of spread (CXR, sinuses, mastoid bone)
- LP for CSF profile (see Table 6), Gram stain, C&S, PCR ± serology (viral)
- CT, MRI, EEG if focality present

Treatment
- initial empirical antibiotics:
  - neonates (<1 month old): ampicillin + aminoglycoside
  - infants, children, adults: vancomycin 1 g IV q12h + ceftriaxone 2 g IV q12h + ampicillin 2 g IV q4h
- adjust when Gram stain, C&S results become available
- dexamethasone 10 mg IV q6h x 4 days, started before or with first dose of antibiotics in suspected bacterial meningitis with purulent CSF; most beneficial in pneumococcal meningitis
- prevention
  - children: immunization against *H. influenzae* (Pentacel™), *S. pneumoniae* (Prevnar™), *N. meningitidis* (Menjugate™, Menactra™)
  - adult: immunization against *N. meningitidis* in selected circumstances (outbreaks, travel, epidemics) and *S. pneumoniae* (Pneumovax™)
  - prophylaxis: rifampin or ciprofloxacin for household and close contacts of *H. influenzae* and *N. meningitidis* cases

---

Meningismus

Brudzinski's Sign
Passive neck flexion causes involuntary flexion of hips and knee.
Kernig's Sign
Resistance to knee extension when hip is flexed to 90°.
Jolt accentuation of H/A
Headache worsens when head turned horizontally at 2-3 rotations/sec.

Dexamethasone in adults with bacterial meningitis
NEJM 2002; 347:1549-56
Study: Randomized, double blind, placebo controlled trial.
Patients: 301 patients over the age of 17 with suspected meningitis in conjunction with cloudy CSF, positive Gram stain or >1,000 leukocytes/mm³.
Intervention: Antibiotics with dexamethasone (10 mg q6h x 4 days, first dose given within 20 minutes prior to or with first dose of antibiotics) versus antibiotics with placebo.
Main Outcome: Glasgow Outcome Scale at 8 weeks (5 is favourable outcome, 4-1 is unfavourable outcome), mortality.
Results: At 8 weeks follow up, dexamethasone group was associated with fewer unfavourable outcomes than placebo (15 vs 25%; RR=0.59, p=0.03; ARR=10%). Mortality rates were also lower in dexamethasone group than placebo (7 vs 15%; RR=0.48, p=0.04).

Does This Adult Patient Have Acute Meningitis? From The Rational Clinical Examination
JAMA July 14, 1999. Vol 281, No. 2.
Study: Systematic review of 10 studies that assessed the accuracy and precision of the clinical examination in the diagnosis of adult meningitis.
Results: Sensitivity of the clinical history is low (pooled sensitivity for headache: 50%, pooled sensitivity for nausea/vomiting: 30%, pooled sensitivity for neck pain: 28%). Two studies reported that 99-100% of patients presenting with meningitis had at least 1 of fever, neck stiffness and a change in mental status. Fever has an overall sensitivity of 85% in the diagnosis of meningitis and altered mental status had a sensitivity of 67%. The overall pooled sensitivity for neck stiffness was 70%. Kernig's and Brudzinski's signs have not been well-studied. In one study of young adults presenting with fever and headache, Kernig's sign had a sensitivity of 9% and specificity of 100% and Brudzinski's sign had a sensitivity of 15% and a specificity of 100%. Jolt accentuation of headache was assessed by one study and found to have a sensitivity of 97% and specificity of 54%. The presence of rash or focal neurological symptoms is not useful for the diagnosis of meningitis.
Conclusions: Clinical history alone is not sufficient for the diagnosis of meningitis. The absence of all three classic signs of meningitis (fever, neck stiffness, and altered mental status changes) virtually eliminates the diagnosis. Fever had the highest sensitivity among the physical signs. In patients with fever and headache, jolt accentuation of headache may be an effective maneuver in helping to distinguish which patients require a lumbar puncture. More prospective research is required to conclusively assess the accuracy of the clinical examination for meningitis.

Public Health Agency of Canada Indications for Adult Immunization
(http://www.phac.aspc.gc.ca/im/index.ht ml)

Pneumococcal polysaccharide vaccine (i.e. Pneumovax™)
• ≥ age of 65
• ≥ age of 2 with chronic cardio/respiratory/hepatic/renal disorders, asplenia, sickle cell or immunosuppression

Pneumococcal conjugate vaccine (i.e. Prevnar™)
• ≤23 mo
• < age of 5 with chronic cardio/resp/hepatic/renal disease, asplenia, sickle cell or immunosuppression

Meningococcal C-conjugate vaccine (i.e. Menjugate™)
• Asplenia
• Complement, factor D, or properdin deficiency
• HIV

Prognosis
• complications
  ▪ headache, seizures, cerebral edema, hydrocephalus, SIADH, residual neurological deficit (especially CN VIII), deafness, death
• mortality
  ▪ *S. pneumoniae* 25%; *N. meningitidis* 5-10%; *H. influenzae* 5%
  ▪ worse prognosis with extremes of age, delays in diagnosis and treatment, stupor or coma, seizures, focal neurological signs, septic shock

Encephalitis

• inflammation of brain matter

Etiology
• viral (most common)
  ▪ HSV, mumps, measles, rabies, arboviruses (e.g. West Nile), HIV, polio, CMV
• bacterial, mycobacterial and spirochetal
  ▪ *Listeria*, TB, syphilis
  ▪ rickettsial: Rocky Mountain spotted fever
• fungal (more frequently space occupying lesions)
  ▪ cryptococcosis, blastomycosis
• parasitic
  ▪ toxoplasmosis, protozoal (cysticercosis)

Pathophysiology
• an acute inflammatory disease of the brain due to direct invasion or hypersensitivity initiated by a pathogen
• some viruses reach CNS via peripheral nerves (rabies, HSV)
• herpes simplex encephalitis
  ▪ acute, necrotizing, asymmetrical hemorrhagic process with lymphocytic and plasma cell reaction which usually involves the medial temporal and inferior frontal lobes
  ▪ associated with HSV-1, but can also be caused by HSV-2

Clinical Features
• constitutional: fever, chills, malaise, nausea, vomiting
• meningeal involvement (meningoencephalitis): headache, nuchal rigidity
• parenchymal involvement: seizures, mental status changes, focal neurological signs
• herpes simplex encephalitis
  ▪ hemiparesis, focal or generalized seizures
  ▪ temporal lobe involvement: behavioural disturbance
  ▪ usually rapidly progressive over several days and may result in coma or death
  ▪ common sequelae: memory and behaviour disturbances

Investigations
• LP for CSF profile, Gram stain, C&S, PCR ± serology (viral)
• serologic studies are valuable in diagnosing some causes of encephalitis (West Nile Virus)
• CT/MRI/EEG to define anatomical sites affected
• brain tissue biopsy for culture, histological examination, and immunocytochemistry
• herpes simplex encephalitis
  ▪ CT/MRI: medial temporal lobe necrosis
  ▪ EEG: early focal slowing, periodic discharges
  ▪ PCR of CSF for HSV DNA: for rapid diagnosis
  ▪ biopsy: when diagnosis uncertain

Treatment
• general supportive care plus therapy directed against specific infecting agent
• monitor vital signs carefully
• herpes simplex encephalitis: IV acyclovir

Generalized Tetanus

Etiology and Pathophysiology
- *Clostridium tetani*: motile, spore forming, anaerobic Gram positive bacillus
- found in soil, splinters, rusty nails, GI tract (humans and animals)
- traumatic implantation into tissues with low oxygenation (e.g. puncture wound, burns, nonsterile surgeries or deliveries)
- tetanus toxin acts on anterior horn cells blocking release of GABAergic inhibitory mediators leading to sustained muscle contraction (tetanic spasms)

Clinical Features
- tetanic spasms begin in jaw area causing lockjaw (trismus) and facial grimace/smile (risus sardonicus)
- paralysis descends to involve large muscle groups (neck, abdomen)
- fever, diaphoresis, hypertension and paroxysmal tachycardia may occur (autonomic hyperactivity)
- mortality rate ~50%, secondary to paralysis of pharyngeal and respiratory muscles

Treatment
- management of infection (see Emergency Medicine)
  - clean wound
  - tetanus immune globulin (TIG) to bind exotoxin
  - metronidazole
  - supportive therapy: intubation, spasmolytic medications (benzodiazepines), quiet environment, cooling blanket
  - tetanus immunization series on discharge

Prevention
- tetanus toxoid vaccination (see Pediatrics and Family Medicine)

Rabies

Clinical Features
- incubation can be from two weeks to years, then travels to PNS and CNS
- prodrome: fever, headache, sore throat, increased sensitivity around the healed wound site
- acute encephalititis
  - hyperactivity, agitation, confusion, seizures, hypertonia
- classic brainstem encephalitis
  - cranial nerve dysfunction, painful contraction of pharyngeal muscles when swallowing liquids resulting in hydrophobia and foaming of the mouth
  - coma and death due to respiratory centre dysfunction
  - almost entirely fatal unless treated with post-exposure vaccine and immunoglobulin

Investigations
- ante-mortem: direct immunofluorescence or PCR on skin biopsy, corneal impression, saliva, viral isolation, serology
- post-mortem: direct immunofluorescence in nerve tissue, presence of Negri bodies (inclusion bodies in neurons)

Treatment and Prevention (see Emergency Medicine)
- post-exposure vaccine is effective
- treatment depends on regional prevalence (contact Public Health)
- if bitten by a possibly rabid animal (i.e. unusual behaviour or wild animals)
  - capture animal and observe for 10 days
  - sacrifice animal and examine brain for Negri bodies
  - treat immediately if the animal cannot be captured or if the animal is found to have rabies
    - clean wound
    - passive immunization with Human Rabies Ig into wound site
    - active immunization with killed rabies virus vaccine
- vaccinate animals

Respiratory Infections

Pneumonia

Definition
- infection of the lung parenchyma

Etiology and Pathophysiology
- infectious agent must overcome normal lung defences:
  - cough reflex, reflex closure of the glottis
  - tracheobronchial mucociliary transport
  - alveolar macrophages
  - inflammatory immune system response

Table 8. Common Organisms in Pneumonia

Community Acquired: Healthy Adults	Community Acquired: Elderly/Comorbidity*/Nursing Home	Nosocomial	HIV-associated	Alcoholic
S. pneumoniae	S. pneumoniae	Enteric Gram-neg rods	Pneumocystis jiroveci	Klebsiella
Mycoplasma	H. influenzae	Pseudomonas		Enteric organisms
Chlamydia	Gram-neg bacilli	S. aureus		Gram-neg bacilli
H. influenzae	S. aureus			S. aureus
Viral	Legionella			Anaerobes (aspiration)

* comorbidity includes COPD, CHF, diabetes, renal failure, recent hospitalization

Risk Factors
- increased risk when lung defences are impaired
  - smoking, toxic inhalation, aspiration, mechanical obstruction, ETT/NTT intubation, respiratory therapy
  - immunosuppression, splenectomy
- aspiration pneumonia
  - decreased level of consciousness, GERD, dysphagia secondary to stroke/multiple sclerosis/myasthenia gravis/dementia, vomiting, ETT, upper gastrointestinal endoscopy

When Klebsiella causes pneumonia, see red currant jelly sputum

3A's of Klebsiella
- Aspiration pneumonia
- Alcoholics and Diabetics
- Abscess in lungs

Clinical Features
- cough, fever, tachypnea, tachycardia are the most typical features
- fever without a concomitant rise in pulse rate may be seen in legionellosis
- elderly often present atypically; altered LOC is sometimes the only sign
- on physical exam, may hear evidence of consolidation, dullness to percussion, bronchial breath sounds, crackles, increased fremitus, and whisper pectoriloquy
- epidemiology affects clinical presentation and empiric treatment

Investigations
- routine labs: determine prognosis and need for hospitalization (along with history and physical examination)
- ABGs: assess adequacy of gas exchange and ventilatory insufficiency in more severe cases; oxygen saturation is sufficient in most
- sputum C&S and Gram stain, blood C&S, ± pleural fluid C&S, ± serology/viral detection

- CXR shows distribution (lobular consolidation or interstitial pattern), extent of infiltrate ± cavitation (see Diagnostic Medical Imaging)
- bronchoscopy ± washings for severely ill patients unresponsive to treatment and for the immunocompromised
- no organism found in >50% of cases

Treatment
Criteria for Hospitalization

Table 9. Fine Criteria, Prognosis, and Recommended Triage

Class	Score	Mortality	Suggested Triage (complement with good clinical judgement)
I	age <50, no comorbidities	<1.0%	Outpatient
II	≤ 70	<1.0%	Outpatient
III	71-90	2.8%	Brief inpatient
IV	91-130	8.2%	Inpatient
V	>130	29.2%	ICU

Calculate the Score by Adding the Points (PORT Score)

Variables	Features	Points
Demographic	men	age in years
	women	age -10
	nursing home resident	+10
Coexisting problems	neoplasm	+30
	liver disease	+20
	CVA, renal disease, CHF	+10
Exam	altered mental status	+20
	RR >30	+20
	SBP <90	+20
	Temp <35° or >40° (<95°F or >104°F)	+15
	HR >125	+10
Laboratory	pH <7.35	+30
	BUN >10.7	+20
	Na <130	+20
	glucose >13.9	+10
	hematocrit <30%	+10
	PaO_2 <60 or SaO_2 <90%	+10
	pleural effusion	+10

NEJM 1997; 336:243. Copyright 1997 Massachusetts Medical Society. All rights reserved. Adapted with permission in 2007

Table 10. DSA/ATS Community Acquired Pneumonia Treatment Guidelines 2007

Setting	Circumstances	Treatment	Example
Outpatient	- previously well - no antibiotic use in last 3 mos	macrolide OR doxycycline	clarithromycin 500 mg PO bid OR doxycycline 100 mg PO bid
	- comorbidities (listed above) - antibiotic use in last 3 mos (use different class)	respiratory fluoroquinolone (750 mg dose only) OR β-lactam + macrolide	levofloxacin 750 mg PO q24h OR amoxicillin 1000 mg PO tid + clarithromycin 500 mg PO bid
Inpatient	Ward	respiratory fluoroquinolone OR β-lactam + macrolide	levofloxacin 750 mg PO q24h OR amoxicillin 1000 mg PO tid + clarithromycin 500 mg PO bid
	ICU	β-lactam PLUS azithromycin OR a respiratory fluoroquinolone	ceftriaxone 1g IV q24h + (Azithromycin 500 mg IV q24h x 5 d) Step-down to oral therapy when tolerated

β-lactam - cefotaxime, ceftriaxone, ampicillin-sulbactam   Macrolide - azithromycin, clarithromycin, erythromycin
Respiratory fluoroquinolone - moxifloxacin, gemifloxacin, levofloxacin
http://www.thoracic.org/sections/publications/statements/pages/mtpi/idsaats-cap.html

Table 11. IDSA/ATS Hospital/Ventilator/Healthcare-Associated Pneumonia Treatment Guidelines 2005

Setting	Treatment	Example
No multi-drug resistance (MDR) risk-factors Early onset (<5 d)	ceftriaxone OR levofloxacin, moxifloxacin, or ciprofloxacin OR ampicillin/sulbactam OR ertapenem	ceftriaxone 1 g IV q24h

Risk factors for MDR:
· Antibiotic use in last 3 months
· High frequency of antibiotic resistance in the
  community or in the specific hospital unit
· Hospitalization for 2 d or more in the last 3 months
· Residence in a nursing home or extended care
  facility
· Dialysis within 30 days
· Home wound care
· Family member with multidrug-resistant pathogen
· Immunosuppressive disease and/or therapy
· Late onset (>5 d)
	antipseudomonal cephalosporin
	(cefepime, ceftazidime)
	OR
	antipseudomonal carbepenem (imipenem or meropenem)
	OR
	β-lactam/β-lactamase inhibitor (piperacillin–tazobactam)
	
	PLUS
	antipseudomonal fluoroquinolone (ciprofloxacin or levofloxacin)
	OR
	aminoglycoside (amikacin, gentamicin, or tobramycin)
	
	PLUS For MRSA
	linezolid or vancomycin
	
	PLUS for Legionella
	ensure regime includes either a macrolide or a fluoroquinolone
		piperacillin/Tazobactam 4.5 g IV q8h
		+
		ciprofloxacin 400 mg IV q12h
		
		+ vancomycin 1 g IV q12h
		for MRSA
		
		+ azithromycin 500 mg IV q24h x 7 d
		for Legionella

http://www.thoracic.org/sections/publications/statements/pages/mtpi/guide1-29.html
· Always use directed therapy against specific organism if one is found through sputum cultures, blood cultures, etc...

Evidence for Influenza Vaccination in Healthy Adults
Cochrane Database of Systematic Reviews 2007, Issue 2. Art. No.: CD001269. DOI:10.1002/14651858. CD001269.pub3
Study: Meta-analysis of 48 randomized and quasi-randomized studies evaluating influenza vaccines compared to placebo in humans.
Results: Inactivated vaccines were 80% efficacious against influenza when matched against the circulating strain and 50% when not matched. There was insufficient evidence to make firm conclusions regarding time missed from work, hospital admissions or complication rates. Common complications of parenteral vaccines included local tenderness and erythema. Parenteral vaccines were also associated with a significant increase in myalgias. Rare complications of influenza vaccines include Guillian-Barre syndrome (GBS) (estimated increased risk 1.6 cases per million vaccines), oculo-respiratory syndrome (only increased risk with trivalent inactivated split vaccines), Bell's Palsy (demonstrated increased risk with an intranasal virosomal vaccine). Attenuated vaccines have shown an increased risk of influenza-like illness.
Conclusions: The inactivated parenteral influenza vaccine has a documented efficacy of approximately 80% when matched to the strain of influenza. However, clinical effectiveness is much lower and has been estimated at approximately 15%. The authors of this review found insufficient evidence to recommend widespread vaccination of all adults. They recommend the continued vaccination of individuals in specific cases as an individual protection measure.

Influenza

Etiology
- influenza virus A & B
- type A has greatest virulence and potential epidemic/pandemic spread
- antigenic drift (minor change in antigen structure) occurs every few years in both type A and B: mutations in hemagglutinin (HA) and neuraminidase (NA) genes
- antigenic shift (genetic reassortment) occurs in type A only, associated with increased virulence: recombination of HA and NA from different strains, potentially from different species, genetic adaptation of animal strain to infect humans
- transmission: airborne spread, droplet

Clinical Features
- incubation period 1-4 days
- fever, chills, cough, myalgias, arthralgias, headache
- complications: secondary bacterial pneumonia, otitis media, sinusitis

Investigations
- culture, DFA of nasopharyngeal swabs, serology

Treatment and Prevention
- primarily supportive
- zanamivir (Relenza™) and oseltamivir (Tamiflu™) decrease the duration (by about 24 hours) and severity of symptoms if given <48 hours from onset; may be used for prophylaxis against type A and type B
- amantidine/rimantidine for treatment and prophylaxis against type A
- vaccine consisting of killed influenza A and B viruses is recommended annually for everyone
  - vaccine is reformulated each year to contain current serotypes of influenza A & B

Avian Influenza (H5N1)

- see WHO website at http://www.who.int/csr/disease/avian_influenza/en/ for more information

Epidemiology
- infection with avian influenza (H5N1) first documented in Hong Kong in 1997 with 18 human cases and 6 deaths coinciding with poultry outbreaks on farms and in live-bird markets
- WHO has confirmed human H5N1 infections in Azerbaijan, Bangladesh, Cambodia, China, Djibouti, Egypt, Indonesia, Iraq, Lao People's Democratic Republic, Myanmar, Nigeria, Pakistan, Thailand, Turkey and Vietnam (May 2008)
- 383 laboratory-confirmed cases in total with 241 (63%) resulting in death
- fatality rates have been highest among those 10-39 years old, intermediate in children less than 10 years old and lowest in those over 50

Transmission
- inhalation of infectious droplets and droplet nuclei, direct contact, possibly indirect contact (fomite) with self-inoculation of URT or conjunctiva
- bird-to-human, environment-to-human, and limited human-to-human spread

Clinical Features
- incubation period generally 2-8 days
- symptoms include high fever (>38°C), headache, myalgias, cough (± sputum). Dyspnea develops approximately 5 days into illness.
- can also have watery diarrhea, vomiting, abdominal pain, chest pain, and bleeding from the nose and gums
- almost all patients develop pneumonia but a few have no respiratory symptoms
- CXR shows infiltrates, rarely pleural effusions
- often rapidly progresses to ARDS and multi-organ failure, death from respiratory failure

Investigations
- viral isolation and viral PCR of nasopharyngeal specimens
- detection rate may be higher from pharyngeal rather than nasopharyngeal samples

Treatment
- supportive care (ventilation, ICU)
- early initiation of antivirals likely useful

- In May 2006, WHO released guidelines for the treatment and prevention of H5N1 with neuraminidase inhibitor oseltamivir. There is also weaker evidence for use of zanamivir. Amantadine or rimantadine are used where neuraminidase inhibitors are unavailable.

Prevention
- no vaccine currently available, however, at least 16 different manufacturers have an H5N1 vaccine in relatively advanced development
- contact, droplet and airborne precautions
- chemoprophylaxis with oseltamivir if unprotected exposure

Severe Respiratory Illness (SRI)

- SRI refers to severe viral pneumonias including Severe Acute Respiratory Syndrome (SARS) and influenza-like illnesses
- designated by Health Canada in order to establish surveillance for specific case definitions which will allow for implementation of infection control measures to prevent large-scale epidemics
- any person who meets the following case definitions should be reported to a local public health authority

Case Definitions
1) A person admitted to hospital with each of the following:
   - fever > 38°C AND cough or breathing difficulty
   - radiographic evidence consistent with SRI (infiltrates consistent with pneumonia or respiratory distress syndrome (RDS))
   - no alternate diagnosis within the first 72 hours of hospitalization
   - one or more of the following exposure/conditions:
     - recent travel to a potential zone of emergence/re-emergence of virus
     - close contact with a symptomatic person who has been to a potential zone of emergence/re-emergence within 10 days prior to onset of symptoms

2) A deceased person with:
   - a history of illness of fever AND cough or difficulty breathing resulting in death
   - autopsy performed with findings consistent with SRI
   - one or more of the exposures/conditions listed in 1) or the deceased person is a laboratory worker handling live SARS-CoV

- Exclusion Criteria: A person should be excluded if an alternate diagnosis can fully explain their illness

Severe Acute Respiratory Syndrome (SARS)

Definition
- rapidly progressing viral pneumonia caused by the SARS-associated coronavirus (SARS-CoV)

Epidemiology
- mutated coronavirus strain originated in China (November 2002)
- >8 000 people affected worldwide with ~ 800 deaths
- >400 people affected in Canada with > 40 deaths

Pathophysiology
- transmission by droplet spread, fomites, airborne spread in some cases
- asymptomatic infections uncommon and do not contribute to transmission
- incubation period: mean of 4-5 days with maximum of 10-14 days

Clinical Features
- difficult to differentiate SARS from other acute community-acquired pneumonias because initial symptoms are not specific
  - fever, myalgia, malaise, chills, cough, shortness of breath, tachypnea, pleurisy
  - upper respiratory symptoms are less commonly manifested
  - diarrhea
- 2/3 of patients deteriorate and experience persistent fever, increasing shortness of breath, oxygen desaturation
- 20% require ICU admission and mechanical ventilation

Investigations
- RT-PCR using respiratory specimens (sputum, nasopharyngeal aspirates and swabs), fecal specimens in viral transport media
- antibody detection via enzyme-linked immunosorbent assay
- bronchoalveolar lavage, tissues from biopsy or autopsy

Treatment
- notify the local public health authority
- detailed questioning about respiratory illness in contacts and travel history
- appropriate infection control (negative-pressure respiratory isolation, N95 Mask, gown, gloves, eye protection), see http://www.sars.gc.ca for latest recommendations
- broad-spectrum antibiotics for severe pneumonia as per the Canadian guidelines for the management of community-acquired pneumonia at presentation
- ribavirin does not appear to be effective against SARS-CoV
- steroids may inhibit damage to lungs acquired by hosts' immune response; early regimens of high-dose methylpredsnisolone were useful in some cases but clinical benefit has not been proven

Cardiac Infections

Infective Endocarditis (IE)

Definition
- infection of cardiac endothelium; previously known as acute/subacute bacterial endocarditis (SBE)
- leaflet vegetation = platelet-fibrin thrombi, WBCs and bacteria

Etiology and Pathophysiology
- predisposing conditions:
  - high risk: prosthetic cardiac valve, previous IE, congenital heart disease (unrepaired, repaired within 6 months, repaired with defects), cardiac transplant with valve disease
  - moderate risk: other congenital cardiac defects, acquired valvular dysfunction, HCM, surgically constructed systemic-to-pulmonary shunts or conduits
  - opportunity for bacteremia (IVDU, indwelling venous catheter, poor dentition, mucosal injury)
- frequency of valve involvement MV >> AV > TV > PV

Culture-negative (fastidious) gram-negative bacilli
Haemophilus
Actinobacillus
Cardiobacterium
Eikenella
Kingella

Table 12. Microbial Etiology of Infective Endocarditis Based on Risk Factors

Native Valve	IVDU	Prosthetic valve (recent surgery <1 year)	Prosthetic valve (remote surgery >1 year)
Streptococcus[1]	*S. aureus*	*S. epidermidis*	*Streptococcus*
S. aureus	*Streptococcus*	*S. aureus*	*S. aureus*
Enterococcus	Enterococcus	*Enterococcus*	*S. epidermidis*
GNB	GNB	GNB	*Enterococcus*
Other[2]	Candida	Other	Other
	Other[3]		

Notes:1. *Streptococcus* includes mainly *Viridans* group *Streptococci*; organisms in bold are the most common isolates
2. Other includes less common organisms such as
- *Strep bovis* (usually associated with underlying GI malignancy, cirrhosis)
- culture-negative organisms including nutritionally-deficient *streptococci*, HACEK, *Bartonella*, *Coxiella*, *Chlamydia*, *Legionella*, *Brucella*
- *Candida*
3. IVDU endocarditis pathogens depend on substance used to dilute the drugs (i.e. tap water → *Pseudomonas*, saliva → oral flora, toilet water → GI flora)

Clinical Features
- systemic
  - fever, chills, weakness, rigors, night sweats, weight loss, anorexia
- cardiac
  - dyspnea, chest pain, clubbing (subacute)
  - regurgitant murmur (new onset murmur or increased intensity)
  - signs of CHF (secondary to acute MR, AR)

- embolic/vascular
  - petechiae, splinter hemorrhages, Janeway lesions (painless 5 mm pink macules on soles/palms)
  - focal neurological signs (CNS emboli), headache (mycotic aneurysm)
  - splenomegaly (subacute)
  - microscopic hematuria, flank pain (renal emboli) ± active sediment
- immune complex
  - Osler's nodes (painful, raised, red/brown, 3-15 mm on digits)
  - glomerulonephritis
  - arthritis
  - Roth spots (retinal hemorrhage with pale centre)

> **Clinical Features of IE**
> **F** - fever
> **R** - roth's spots
> **O** - osler's nodes
> **M** - murmur
>
> **J** - janeway lesions
> **A** - anemia
> **N** - nail-bed hemorrhages (aka splinter hemorrhages)
> **E** - emboli

Diagnosis

Table 13. Modified Duke Criteria

Major Criteria

- Sustained bacteremia by organism known to cause endocarditis
- Endocardial involvement documented by either echocardiogram (vegetation, abscess, prosthetic valve dehiscence) or new valvular regurgitation

Minor Criteria

- Predisposing condition (abnormal heart valve, IVDU)
- Fever
- Vascular phenomena: septic arterial or pulmonary emboli, mycotic aneurysms, ICH, conjunctival hemorrhages, Janeway lesions
- Immunologic phenomena: glomerulonephritis, rheumatoid factor, Osler's nodes, Roth spots
- Positive blood culture not meeting major criteria

Definitive diagnosis if: 2 major, or 1 major + 3 minor, or 5 minor.
Possible diagnosis if: 1 major + 1 minor, or 3 minor.

Investigations

- blood work: anemia (normochromic, normocytic), ↑ESR, +RF
- urinalysis: proteinuria
- serial blood cultures: 3 sets (each containing one aerobic and one anaerobic sample) collected from different sites >1 h apart (definitive diagnosis)
  - occasionally, may collect further samples q24-48h during treatment until patient defervesces to document response
  - then samples post-treatment to document clearance of infection
- echo: vegetations, regurgitation, abscess
  - serial echo may help in assessing cardiac function
- TEE indicated if TTE is non-diagnostic or if abscess/perforation/infection suspected TTE inadequate in 20% (obesity, COPD, chest wall deformities)
- ECGs: increased PR interval may indicate perivalvular abscess

Treatment

- medical
  - IV antibiotic therapy (minimum 4 weeks)
    - empiric therapy: depending on clinical scenario and suspected organism e.g. vancomycin 1 g IV q12h + gentamicin 1 mg/kg IV q8h
  - prophylaxis only for high risk individuals listed above
    - dental/respiratory/esophageal procedures: amoxicillin 2 g PO 30-60 min prior; clindamycin 600 mg PO if pen-allergic
    - GU/GI (excluding esophageal) procedures: no longer recommended
- surgical
  - relative indications: refractory CHF, valve ring abscess, fungal etiology, valve perforation, unstable prosthesis, multiple major emboli, antimicrobial failure (persitently positive blood cultures), mycotic aneurysm

Prognosis

- adverse prognostic factors: CHF, prosthetic valve infection, valvular/myocardial abscess
- mortality up to 30%

Gastrointestinal Infections

Acute Diarrhea

Definition
- passage of frequent unformed stools, duration <14 days

Table 14. Pathogens in Infectious Diarrhea

Pathogen	Source	Incubation	Symptoms	Duration	Treatment	Miscellaneous
BACTERIA (invasive)						Dx: stool WBC+, RBC+, C&S
Campylobacter jejuni	Uncooked meat especially poultry	2-10 days	Prodrome of fever, headache, myalgia, and/or malaise precedes diarrhea, abdominal pain & fever	<1 week	Supportive (macrolide if >1 week or bloody diarrhea)	Most common bacterial cause of diarrhea in Canada
Enteroinvasive E. coli (EIEC)	Contaminated food/water	1-3 days	Fever, abdominal pain, tenesmus, scant stool containing mucus & blood	7-10 days	Supportive only, treatment hastens the resolution of symptoms, particularly in severe cases	Relatively uncommon
Salmonella typhi *S. paratyphi* (aka. Enteric Fever, Typhoid)	Fecal-oral Contaminated food/water	10-14 days	Sudden onset crampy abdo pain and diarrhea, prolonged fever (up to 4wks if untreated), headache, rash ("rose spots")	5-7 days diarrhea	Empiric treatment with ceftriaxone or azithromycin fluoroquinolone 1st-line if susceptible	Extremes of age, gallstones predispose to chronic carriage increasing quinolone resistance
Non-typhoidal Salmonellosis *S. typhimurium, S. enteritidis*	Contaminated animal food products, especially eggs, poultry, meat, milk	12-72 hrs	Nausea, vomiting, diarrhea, abdo cramping, fever >38°C	3-7 days diarrhea, <72hrs fever	Supportive ciprofloxacin - not recommended except in extremes of age, immunosuppression, aneurysms, prosthetic valve grafts/joints	
Shigella dysenteriae	Fecal-oral Contaminated food/water	1-4 days	fever, malaise, anorexia, limited watery diarrhea, progressing to frequent passage of small, bloody, mucopurulent stools	<1 week	ciprofloxacin Antidiarrheals may increase risk of toxic megacolon	Very small inoculum needed for infection Complications include toxic megacolon, HUS
Yersinia enterocolitica *Y. pseudotuberculosis*	Contaminated food Unpasteurized milk	5 days	Acute diarrhea, low-grade fever, cramping, nausea, vomiting, hematochezia	2 weeks to months	Supportive Fluoroquinolones only for septicemia, metastatic focal infections, or immunosuppression and enterocolitis	Majority cases in children 1-4 yrs Mesenteric adenitis and terminal ileitis forms without diarrhea mimicking appendicitis
BACTERIA (non-invasive/toxin-mediated)						Dx: clinical
B. cereus - Type A (emetic), (preformed exotoxin)	Rice dishes	1-6 hrs	Nausea, vomiting, cramps	<12 hrs	Symptomatic	
B. cereus - Type B (diarrheal) (secondary endotoxin)	Meats, vegetables, dried beans, cereals	8-16 hrs	Large volume watery diarrhea	<24 hrs	Symptomatic	
Enterotoxigenic E. coli (EHEC/STEC) ie: O157:H7	Verotoxin (aka Shiga-like toxin) Feco-oral, contamination of hamburger, raw milk, drinking & recreational water	3-8 days	Grossly bloody diarrhea, fever often absent	5-10 days	Supportive Monitor renal function. Antibiotics & antidiarrheals may increase risk HUS	10% develop hemolytic uremic syndrome (HUS), which, caries 3-5% mortality (especially in children & elderly)
Enterotoxigenic E. coli (ETEC) (colonization of colon + enterotoxin production)	LT and/or ST toxins Contaminated food/water	1-3 days	Watery diarrhea, cramps	3 days	Supportive loperamide (Immodium®) quinolone or azithromycin	Number 1 cause of traveller's diarrhea
Clostridium difficile	Normally present in colon in small numbers		unformed to watery or mucoid stools with characteristic odour		1st line: -metronidazole (PO/IV) 2nd line - vancomycin PO	Usually follows antibiotic treatment, (especially clindamycin), can develop pseudomembranous colitis
Clostridium perfringens (secondary enterotoxin)	Contaminated food, especially meat and poultry	8-12 hrs	Sudden onset watery diarrhea, cramps, rarely vomiting	<24 hrs	Supportive Antibiotics not effective as disease is toxin mediated	Clostridium spores are heat resistant,
Staphylococcus aureus (heat-stable preformed exotoxin)	Unrefrigerated meat and dairy products (custard, pudding, potato salad, mayo)	2-4 hrs	Sudden onset severe nausea, cramps, vomiting, prostration, diarrhea	1-2 days	Supportive ± antiemetics	
Vibrio cholerae	Contaminated food/water, especially shellfish	1-3 days	painless voluminous diarrhea without abdominal cramps or fever	3-7 days	Aggressive fluid and electrolytes resuscitation Tetracycline or quinolones (ciprofloxacin)	Massive watery diarrhea (1-3 L/d) Mortality <1% with treatment

Table 14. Pathogens in Infectious Diarrhea (continued)

Pathogen	Source	Incubation	Symptoms	Duration	Treatment	Miscellaneous
PARASITES						Dx: stool ova and parasites (O&P)
Cryptosporidium	Fecal-oral	7 days	Non-bloody, watery diarrhea, fever	1-20 days	nitazoxanide paramomycin	
Entamoeba histolytica	Worldwide endemic areas Fecal-oral	2-4 weeks	Ranges from asymptomatic to severe grossly bloody diarrhea Fever, weight loss	variable	metronidazole + iodoquinol if invasive Only iodoquinol for non-invasive	May resemble IBD If untreated, potential for liver abscess Sigmoidoscopy shows flat ulcers with yellow exudate
Entamoeba dispar						Non-pathogenic Indistinguishable from *E. histolytica* microscopically (morphological) techniques Over 100 fold more common in Ontario than *E. histolytica*
Giardia lamblia	Fecal-oral (daycare #1) Contaminated food/water (travel related "beaver fever")	1-4 weeks	Ranges from asymptomatic to acute watery diarrhea with abdo pain to protracted course of flatulence, abdominal distention, fatigue and anorexia	variable	metronidazole Treatment of asymptomatic carriers not generally recommended	May need duodenal biopsy Higher risk in men who have sex with men (MSM), Immunodeficiency (IgA decreased), and daycares/nurseries
VIRUSES						
Rotavirus	Fecal-oral	2-4 days	Watery diarrhea, vomiting, fever	3-8 days	Supportive Vaccine available, given at 2, 4 & 6 months of age	Can cause severe dehydration Virtually all children are infected by 3 years of age
Norovirus (includes Norwalk virus)	Fecal-oral	24 hrs	nausea, vomiting, abdo cramps, loose watery diarrhea	12-60 hrs	Supportive	Often causes epidemics

Approach to the Patient with Acute Diarrhea
- symptomatic treatment, fluid and electrolyte replacement for all
- thorough history including symptoms, duration of illness, antibiotic use, travel, and sick contacts
- if >1 day of symptoms get a stool sample and examine for WBC:
  - stool smeared on slide and methylene blue drops added; >3 PMNs in 4 high power fields (HPFs) = positive
  - −WBC = non-inflammatory: continue symptomatic therapy
  - + WBC = inflammatory (infectious, IBD, radiation colitis):
    - culture for *Salmonella, Shigella, C. jejuni, E. coli*
    - test for *C. difficile* cytotoxin A and B if recent/remote antibiotic use or recent chemotherapy
    - consider empiric therapy with a quinolone such as ciprofloxacin based on severity of illness
    - flexible sigmoidoscopy: biopsies useful to distinguish idiopathic inflammatory bowel disease (Crohn's disease and ulcerative colitis) from infectious colitis or acute self-limited colitis
- if >10 days consider parasitic infection *Giardia, Entamoeba histolytica* and send stool for ova & parasites
  - may need 3 stool samples because of sporadic passage
  - also consider post-infectious IBS
- antibiotics prolong excretion of non-typhoidal Salmonellosis and may cause *C. difficle* infection
  - clearly indicated: *Salmonella typhi, Shigella, V. cholera, C. difficile, Cryptosporidium, Entamoeba histolytica,* immunocompromised patients
  - indicated in some situations: Non-typhoid *Salmonella, Campylobacter, Yersinia, Giardia,* ETEC (determined by severity of illness)

Traveller's Diarrhea

Epidemiology
- up to 50% of travellers to developing countries affected in first 2 weeks and 10-20% after returning home

Etiology
- bacterial (80%): *E. coli* most common (ETEC, other *E. coli*), *Campylobacter*, *Shigella*, *Salmonella*, *Vibrio* (non-cholera)
- viral: Norwalk and Rotavirus account for about 10%
- protozoal (rarely): giardiasis, amebiasis, cryptosporidium, cyclospora

Prophylaxis
- bismuth subsalicylate (Pepto-Bismol®), 2 tablets (525 mg) qid up to 3 weeks (60% effective)
- antibiotic prophylaxis not routinely recommended except in high-risk travellers e.g. diabetes mellitus, renal failure, inflammatory bowel disease (90% effective)

Treatment
- usually self-limited; 90% last less than 1 week
- symptomatic, rehydration; ciprofloxacin in moderate-severe illness as traveller's diarrhea is primarily bacterial
- if lasts >10 days consider parasitic infection *Giardia*, *Entamoeba histolytica*, etc and send stool for ova & parasites. Also consider post-infectious IBS.

50% of MALT lymphomas will regress with treatment of *H. pylori*.

Peptic Ulcer Disease (*H. pylori*)

- see Gastroenterology

Bacterial Overgrowth

- see Gastroenterology

Acute Viral Hepatitis

Definition
- viral hepatitis lasting <6 months

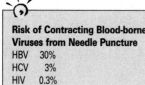

Risk of Contracting Blood-borne Viruses from Needle Puncture
HBV   30%
HCV   3%
HIV   0.3%

Etiology
- hepatitis viruses: HAV, HBV, HCV, HDV, HEV
- EBV
- CMV
- yellow fever
- HSV, VZV (immunosuppression)

Clinical Features
- most are subclinical
- prodrome may precede jaundice by 1-2 weeks
  - nausea, vomiting, anorexia, taste/smell disturbance
  - headaches, fatigue, malaise, myalgias
  - low-grade fever may be present
  - arthralgia and urticaria (especially hepatitis B)
- 50% progress to icteric (clinical jaundice) phase, lasting days to weeks
  - pale stools and dark urine 1-5 days prior to icteric phase
  - hepatomegaly plus RUQ pain
  - splenomegaly and cervical lymphadenopathy (10-20% of cases)

Table 15. Characteristics of the Viral Hepatitides

	HAV	HBV	HCV	HDV	HEV
Virus Family	Picornaviridae	Hepadnaviridae	Flaviviridae	Deltaviridae	Caliciviridae
Genome	RNA	DNA	RNA	RNA	RNA
Envelope	No	Yes	Yes	Yes	No
Transmission	Fecal-oral	Parenteral, sexual	Parenteral, sexual	Parenteral, sexual	Fecal-oral
Incubation	2-6 weeks	6 weeks – 6 months	2-26 weeks	3-13 weeks	2-8 weeks
Onset	Usually abrupt	Usually insidious	Insidious	Usually abrupt	Usually abrupt
Chronicity	None	5% adults, 90% infants	80%	5%	None
Oncogenicity	No	Yes	Yes	?	No
Mortality (acute)	0.1-0.3%	0.5-2%	1%	2-20% coinfection with HBV, 30% superinfection	1-2% overall, 10-20% in pregnancy
Immunity	Yes	Yes	?	Yes	?
Vaccine	Yes	Yes	No	No	No

Investigations
- hepatocellular necrosis causes ↑AST, ALT >10-20x normal
- ALP and bilirubin minimally elevated
- viral serology, IgM

Treatment
- see <u>Gastroenterology</u>
- supportive (hydration, diet)
- indications for hospitalization: encephalopathy, coagulopathy, severe vomiting, hypoglycemia

Prognosis
- see <u>Gastroenterology</u>
- chronicity
  - hepatitis C 80%
  - hepatitis B 5%
  - hepatitis A never becomes chronic
- poor prognostic indicators
  - comorbidities
  - persistently high bilirubin (>340 µmol/L; 20 mg/dL), ↑ INR, ↓ albumin, hypoglycemia
- cholestasis - most commonly during hepatitis A virus (HAV) infection

Prevention
- hepatitis A vaccine (Havrix™, Vaqta™, Avaxim™) in adult; given on elected date, then six months later
- hepatitis B vaccine (Recombivax HB™)
  - for routine vaccination of adolescents (age 11-15 yrs), given as two doses six months apart
  - in adults, standard dose is to give on elected date, then one and three weeks later
- combined hepatitis A and hepatitis B vaccine (Twinrix™) as for hepatitis B vaccine (0, 7, 21 days)

Chronic Hepatitis B

Epidemiology
- develops in ≤5% of healthy adults with acute HBV hepatitis and 90% of those infected at birth
- accounts for approximately 10% of chronic hepatitis in North America
- high risk groups: IVDU, chronic hemodialysis patients, men who have sex with men

Clinical Features
- many asymptomatic
- if symptomatic, generally only mild and intermittent fatigue; correlates poorly with disease severity
- signs and symptoms of liver disease: advanced histological disease

Generally liver damage is caused more by the immune response to hepatitis B virus than from the virus itself.

Types of Chronic Infection
- perinatal infection: active viral replication, normal ALT/AST, HBeAg positive, high HBV DNA
- active infection: viral replication, elevated ALT/AST, HBeAg positive, HBV DNA >100 000 copies/ml, high infectivity, ↑ liver injury
- inactive (formerly termed chronic persistent hepatitis or carrier): ALT/AST normal, HBeAg negative, anti-HBe positive, HBV DNA <100 000 copies/ml, low infectivity and minimal liver injury
  - virus reactivation can occur at any time, especially if immunosuppressed (e.g. corticosteroids, lymphoma)
  - re-activation clinically resembles acute hepatitis B
- "core or precore mutant": active virus replication with elevated HBV DNA but HBeAg negative because of promoter gene mutation
  - poor prognosis, difficult to treat

Table 16. Hepatitis B Serology

	HBsAg	Anti-HBs	HBeAg	Anti-HBe	Anti-HBc	ALT, AST
Acute HBV	+	–	+	–	IgM	elevated
Chronic active HBV (high infectivity)	+	–	+	–	IgG	elevated
Chronic inactive HBV (low infectivity)	+	–	–	+	IgG	normal
Recovery	–	+	–	+	IgG	normal
Immunization	–	+	–	–	–	normal

Treatment
- see <u>Gastroenterology</u>
- no treatment is indicated for asymptomatic, nonreplicative hepatitis B carriers
- treatment of chronic replicative hepatitis with alpha-interferon, pegylated or regular
  - 4-month course of 5 million units SC q24h or 10 million units SC 3x per week
  - increases annual rate of cessation of viral replication from 7% to 40%; loss of HBsAg less common
  - relapse after successful therapy is rare (1 to 2%)
- lamivudine (Heptovir™): resolves hepatic inflammation and leads to HBeAg negative/anti-HBe positive ("seroconversion") in > 90% of patients, but relapse when drug is stopped; drug resistance commonly develops after 1-2 years of use
- other antivirals used in hepatitis B treatment include adefovir dipivoxil, entecavir and tenofovir (nucleoside analogues used to decrease viral load)
- end-stage treatment is transplant, although acute hepatitis may recur in the transplanted liver (80-100% reinfection, but this is lowered by use of HBIg (immunoglobulin)
- ↑incidence of HCC, especially if HBeAg positive, cirrhosis, male

Hepatitis D Virus (HDV)
- requires HBsAg for replication, therefore infection only occurs in the presence of hepatitis B
- co-infection: HBV and HDV acquired at the same time
- superinfection: HBV acquired first, then HDV
- HDV increases severity of hepatitis but does not increase risk of progression to chronic hepatitis
- treatment
  - low-dose interferon has limited impact, high-dose under investigation
  - liver transplant for end-stage disease more effective than in HBV alone; reinfection rate 100% but infection usually mild

Suspect HDV superinfection if sudden worsening of chronic hepatitis B.

Chronic Hepatitis C

Epidemiology
- accounts for at least 50% of chronic hepatitis in USA
- 80% of acute HCV infections go on to become chronic; of those 20-30% go on to cirrhosis, and of those 25% per year develop hepatocellular carcinoma (HCC)
- time course:
  - clinical chronic hepatitis at 10 years
  - cirrhosis at 20 years
  - HCC at 30 years
  - time course accelerated if co-infected with HIV

Clinical Features
- usually asymptomatic
- may have non-specific symptoms: fatigue, fever, chills, night sweats, RUQ pain, nausea

Investigations
- anti-HCV: positive in chronic and resolved acute infections
- HCV RNA: positive in chronic, negative in resolved acute infections

Treatment
- see <u>Gastroenterology</u>
- pegylated interferon + ribavirin for 48 weeks
  - overall sustained remission rate of 40%
  - HCV RNA decrease of 2 log at 4-8 weeks is stronglypredictive of response to therapy
  - highest remission rate if virus genotype not 1a/1b, no cirrhosis, no underlying immunosuppression
  - multiple side effects including depression and fever/chills/malaise commonly from the interferon, hemolytic anemias commonly from the ribavirin, bone marrow suppression is uncommon
- hepatitis A and B vaccination suggested if hep C patient is not immune, because superimposed acute hepatitis A has been reported to be especially severe

Must exclude autoimmune hepatitis because interferon is detrimental.

Renal Infections

Acute Pyelonephritis

Definition
- infection of the renal parenchyma with local and systemic manifestations
- classified as uncomplicated or complicated based on absence or presence of conditions predisposing to anatomic or functional impairment of urine flow
- examples of complicated pyelonephritis include infection in the setting of renal or ureteric stones, strictures, prostatic obstruction (hypertrophy or malignancy), vesicoureteric reflux, neurogenic bladder, catheters, DM, sickle-cell disease, polycystic kidney disease, immunosuppression, post-renal transplant and during pregnancy

Etiology
- usually ascending microorganisms, most often bacteria
- causative microorganisms: *E.coli, Klebsiella, Proteus, Enterococcus, S. saphrophyticus*
- in uncomplicated pyelonephritis, *E. coli* is most common pathogen
- suspect other less common organisms if history of instrumentation
- suspect resistant GN or even fungi in hospital patients with indwelling catheters
- GP cocci (e.g *S. aureus*) in urine may represent endocarditis with septic embolization to kidney

Common Micro-organisms Responsible for UTI/Pyelonephritis
KEEPS
*K*lebsiella
E. coli
*E*nterococcus
*P*roteus
S. saphrophyticus

Clinical Features
- rapid onset (hours to a day)
- fever, chills, nausea, vomiting, myalgia, malaise
- costovertebral angle (CVA) tenderness or exquisite flank pain
- ± LUTS (urgency, frequency, dysuria)
- may have symptoms of GN sepsis
- atypical presentation in the elderly: confusion may be the only symptom

Investigations
- urine
  - dipstick: +ve for leukocytes and nitrites, possible hematuria
  - microscopy: >5 WBC/HPF in unspun urine or >10 WBC/HPF in spun urine, bacteria, ± WBC casts
  - Gram stain: GN bacilli, GP cocci

- culture and sensitivities: >10^5 colony forming units (CFU)/mL in clean catch MSU or >10^2 CFU/mL in suprapubic aspirate or catheterized specimen
- blood
  - CBC + differential: leukocytosis, high % neutrophils, left-shift
  - blood cultures: may be positive in 20% of cases
- consider investigation of complicated pyelonephritis if:
  - fever, pain, leukocytosis not resolving with treatment within 72 hours
  - male patient
  - history of urinary tract abnormalities
  - abdo/pelvic U/S, CT for renal abscess, spiral CT for stones, cystoscopy

Treatment
- 14-day course of TMP/SMX or third generation cephalosporin; 7-day course of ciprofloxacin if uncomplicated
- can treat as outpatient with PO meds if mild-moderate illness, hemodynamically stable, young, otherwise healthy, uncomplicated, tolerating PO meds and fluids, adequate follow-up arranged
- otherwise start with IV for several days and then switch to PO
- if kidney completely obscured by gas (emphysematous pyelonephritis) → emergency nephrectomy
- patient more than mildly symptomatic or complicated pyelonephritis in the setting of stone obstruction is a urologic emergency (placing patient at risk of kidney loss or septic shock)

Prognosis
- recurrent infections often constitute relapse rather than re-infection

Diabetics are predisposed to emphysematous pyelonephritis.

Bone and Joint Infections

Septic Arthritis

Routes of infection
- hematogenous (adults)
- contiguous osteomyelitis (children)
- direct inoculation via skin/trauma
- iatrogenic (surgery, arthroscopy, arthrocentesis)

Medical Emergency
Septic arthritis is a medical emergency! If untreated, rapid joint destruction will occur.

Etiology
- *N. gonorrheae*: accounts for 75% of septic arthritis in young sexually active adults
- *S. aureus*: affects all ages, rapidly destructive, accounts for most non-gonococcal cases of septic arthritis in adults (especially in those with rheumatoid arthritis)
- *Streptococci* (*pyogenes*, Group A and B)
- Gram negatives: affects neonates, elderly, IVDU, immunocompromised
- *S. pneumoniae*: affects children
- *Kingella kingae*: affects children < 2 y/o since HIB immunization
- *Salmonella* spp.: characteristic of HIV, sickle cell
- coagulase-negative Staph: prosthetic joints
- If culture negative: *Borrelia* sp. (Lyme disease) or *Tropheryma whippeli* (Whipple's disease)

Risk Factors
- extra-articular infection with hematogenous seeding
- IVDU
- chronic illness (e.g. RA, DM, malignancy)
- prior joint damage (e.g. OA, RA, prosthetic joints)

Clinical Features of Gonococcal Arthritis
- preceding bacteremia with skin lesions and migrating polyarthritis
- settles to monoarthritis, often of a large joint (most often the knee)
- systemic symptoms of sepsis: fever, malaise
- local symptoms in involved joint: swelling, warmth, pain, inability to bear weight, marked decrease in range of motion (see Rheumatology for differential diagnosis)
- gonococcal triad: migratory arthritis, tenosynovitis next to inflamed joint, pustular skin changes

Investigations
- diagnosis with high index of suspicion plus the following:
  - culture and sensitivity
    - gonococcal: in addition to blood and urine cultures, endocervical, urethral, rectal and oropharyngeal cultures
    - non-gonococcal: blood and urine
  - arthrocentesis (synovial fluid analysis) is mandatory: CBC and diff, Gram stain, culture, examine for crystals
    - infectious = opaque, ↑ WBC count (inflammatory), PMNs >85%, culture positive (see <u>Rheumatology</u>)
    - growth of GC from synovial fluid is successful in <50% of cases
  - ± plain X-ray: used to rule out osteomyelitis, provides baseline to monitor treatment

Treatment
- medical
  - start IV antibiotics empirically, delay may result in joint destruction
  - use cloxacillin or cefazolin ± ciprofloxacin or gentamicin if risk for Gram neg. (e.g. cloxacillin + ciprofloxacin in elderly) before culture results come back
  - Gram stain guides subsequent treatment
  - gonococcal: ceftriaxone 1 g q24h IM or IV; if penicillin-sensitive: ampicillin (1 g q6h IV) usually 2-4 days IV then 7 days PO
  - non-gonococcal: antibiotics against *S. aureus, Strep* x 2 wk IV then 2-4 wk PO
- surgical drainage if:
  - persistent positive joint cultures on repeat arthrocentesis
  - hip joint involvement
- daily joint aspirations until culture sterile; no need to give intra-articular antibiotics
- physiotherapy

Intra-articular steroids are contraindicated until septic arthritis has been excluded.

Prognosis
- Up to 50% morbidity (decreased joint function/motility)
- prognosis has not changed significantly despite better antimicrobials and hospital care

Diabetic Foot

- neuropathic foot ulcers that can become infected:
  - mild = superficial (no bone/joint involvement)
  - moderate = deep involving bone/joint
  - severe = moderate infection with systemic toxicity

Etiology
- mild: *S. aureus, Streptococcus* species
- mod/severe: polymicrobial with aerobes (*S. aureus, Streptococcus, Enterococcus,* GN bacilli) and anaerobes (*Peptostreptococcus, Bacteroides, Clostridium*)

Clinical Features
- ulcer with surrounding erythema/warmth and pus from ulcer or nearby sinus tract
- ± crepitus
- ± osteomyelitis
- ± systemic toxicity

Investigations
- curettage specimen or bone biopsy (superficial swabs not useful)
- blood C&S
- rule out oseteomyelitis by X-ray:
  - if initial X-ray normal, repeat 2-4 wks after initiating treatment to increase test sensitivity
  - if initial X-ray equivocal, do MRI or bone biopsy (most reliable test)

Treatment
- early surgical debridement ± revascularization or amputation
- mild: TMP/SMX-DS 2 tabs PO bid + metronidazole 500 mg PO bid x 2-3 wks
- mod: ciprofloxacin 500 mg PO bid + clindamycin 300 mg qid x 4-6 wks
- severe: same as for "moderate" or imipenem or pip-tazo

Osteomyelitis

- see <u>Orthopaedics</u>

Systemic Infections

Sepsis and Septic Shock

Definitions
- systemic inflammatory response syndrome (SIRS): 2 or more of
  (a) temperatures <36°C or >38°C
  (b) heart rate >90
  (c) respiratory rate >20
  (d) WBC <4 or >12
- sepsis: SIRS + documented infection
- septic shock: sepsis + hypotension, despite fluid resuscitation, and evidence of inadequate tissue perfusion, end-organ dysfunction and hypoperfusion

Pathophysiology
- bacteremia may or may not be present and may be primary (without identifiable focus of infection) or secondary (with extravascular focus of infection)
- circulatory insufficiency occurs when bacterial products interact with host cells and serum proteins to initiate a widespread and unregulated host response that ultimately leads to cell injury (both ischemic and directly cytopathic) and death
- septic shock develops in <50% of patients with bacteremia: ~40% of patients with Gram negative bacteremia, ~20% of patients with *S. aureus* bacteremia

Clinical Features
- history: fever, chills, SOB, cool extremities, fatigue, malaise, anxiety, confusion
- physical: vitals (fever, tachypnea, tachycardia, ↓BP), local signs of infection
- labs: CBC + diff, electrolytes, BUN, creatinine, liver enzymes, ABG, lactate, INR, PTT, FDP, blood cultures x3, urinalysis, urine C&S and culture any wounds or lines
- CXR (other imaging depends on suspicion of focus)

Treatment (also see Respirology)
- supportive: O₂, IV fluids, IV antibiotics (empirical, depends on suspected source)
- cardiovascular support: IV fluids, ± dopamine, ± norepinephrine; ICU transfer
- activated protein C
    - modulates coagulation and inflammation in severe sepsis
    - evidence suggests use in severe sepsis
- IVIg: some evidence for Streptococcal toxic shock syndrome but limited by small size of trials in literature
- hydrocortisone and fludricortisone in ACTH non-responders

Tuberculosis (TB)

Etiology
- *Mycobacterium tuberculosis*: slow growing aerobe (doubling time=18 h) that is capable of intracellular survival because it replicates in macrophages

INFECTION (Primary infection) via inhaled droplet nuclei from someone with active TB

1/3 of the world's population is infected with TB

PRIMARY TB

LATENT TB

REACTIVATION (Secondary infection) usually when immune system is weakened Only 10% of those infected will progress to active disease, of which the majority will reactivate within first 2 y of infection

ACTIVE TB

Global Epidemic of Tuberculosis
- Worldwide, TB is the second leading infectious cause of death after HIV
- WHO estimated that every year, about 9 million people develop active TB and >2 million people die from the disease

Risk Factors
- for exposure/infection
    - travel or birth in country with high TB prevalence (e.g. Asia, Sub-Saharan Africa)
    - aboriginal, crowded living conditions, low SES/homeless
    - personal or occupational contact, IVDU
- for progression from latent infection to active disease
    - immunocompromised/immunosuppressed
    - concurrent local disease process (i.e. pulmonary silicosis with latent pulmonary TB)
    - skin test conversion within past 2 years

Clinical Features
- primary infection usually asymptomatic, though increased risk of symptoms in children and HIV+
- secondary infection/reactivation usually produces constitutional symptoms (fatigue, anorexia, night sweats, weight loss) and site-dependent symptoms:
  i) pulmonary TB
      - chronic productive cough ± hemoptysis
      - CXR consolidation or cavitation, lymphadenopathy

   ii) miliary TB
- widely disseminated spread especially to lungs, abdominal organs, marrow, CNS
- CXR: multiple small 2-4 mm millet seed-like lesions

  iii) extrapulmonary TB
- lymphadenitis, pleurisy, pericarditis, hepatitis, peritonitis, meningitis, osteomyelitis (vertebral = Pott's disease), adrenal infection (causing Addison's disease), renal, ovary

Investigations
- PPD/Mantoux skin test: positive result only indicates infection, not active disease (PPD is not used to diagnose or exclude active TB)
- AM sputum on 3 consecutive days for AFB, culture ± AMTD (TB rRNA assay)
- CXR features
  - nodular or alveolar infiltrates with cavitation (middle/lower lobe if primary, apical if secondary)
  - pleural effusion (usually unilateral and exudative) may occur independently of pulmonary nodules
  - hilar/mediastinal adenopathy (90% are usually unilateral)
  - tuberculoma (semi-calcified well-defined solitary coin lesion 0.5-4 cm with adjacent satellite lesions) represents active or healed lesion
  - evidence of miliary TB: discrete nodules (2-4 mm diameter) scattered throughout lungs
  - evidence of past disease: calcified hilar and mediastinal nodes, calcified focus, pleural thickening with calcification, apical scarring

Prevention
- prevention of infection: BCG (Bacille Calmette-Guérin) vaccine
  - ~80% effective against pediatric miliary & meningeal TB
  - effectiveness in adults debated (anywhere from 0-80%)
- prevention of progression of latent to active disease (defer in pregnancy unless mother is high risk)
  - likely INH-sensitive: INH 300 mg + pyridoxine (vit B6) 50 mg PO OD x 9 mo
  - HIV+ or abnormal CXR: INH 300 mg + pyridoxine (vit B6) 50 mg PO OD x 12 mo
  - likely INH-resistant: rifampin 600 mg PO OD x 4 mo

Treatment of Active Infection
- empiric therapy: INH + rifampin + pyrazinamide + ethambutol
- pulmonary TB: INH + rifampin + pyrazinamide x 2 mos (initiation phase), then INH + rifampin x 4 mos (continuation phase), total 6 mo
- extrapulmonary TB: same regimen as pulmonary TB but increase to 9-12 mos + corticosteroids for meningitis, osteomyelitis

Leprosy (Hansen's Disease)

Etiology
- *Mycobacterium leprae:* obligate intracellular bacteria, slow-growing (doubling time 12.5d), survives in macrophages
- transmission via respiratory droplets
- invades skin and peripheral nerves leading to chronic granulomatous disease

Clinical Features
- spectrum of disease determined by host immune response to infection
  - i) paucibacillary "tuberculoid" leprosy (high cell-mediated immune response)
    - ≤5 hypesthetic lesions, usually hypopigmented, well-defined, dry
    - early nerve involvement, enlarged peripheral nerves, neuritic pain
    - either self-limited or progresses to multibacillary "lepromatous" form
  - ii) multibacillary "lepromatous" leprosy (low cell-mediated immune response)
    - ≥6 lesions, symmetrical distribution
    - leonine facies (loss of eyebrows, thickened ear lobes)
    - extensive cutaneous involvement, large nerves often better preserved
  - iii) borderline leprosy
    - lesions and progression lies between tuberculoid and lepromatous forms

Investigations
- skin biopsy or split skin smears for AFB
- histologic appearance: intracellular bacilli in spherical masses (lepra cells), granulomas involving cutaneous nerves

Tuberculous Polyserositis
= pleural + pericardial + peritoneal effusions
(usually from granuloma breakdown that spills TB into pleural cavity)

Positive PPD Test
if induration at 48-72 h
>5 mm if immunosuppressed, close contact with active TB, CXR fibrocalcific disease, with HIV or if using anti-TNF blockers
>10 mm if presence of other risk factors, recent conversion (induration ↑>10 mm in past 2 y)
>15 mm if risk factors absent
false - : anergy, malignancy, infection <10 wks ago or a very long time ago
false +: BCG <2 y ago
booster effect: initially false – result boost to a true + result by the testing procedure itself (usually if pt was infected long ago so had diminished delayed type hypersensitivity reaction or if history of BCG)
PPD: purified protein derivative

Treatment of Active TB
Rifampin
Isoniazid
Pyrazinamide
Ethambutol

Treatment
- paucibacillary: dapsone 100 mg PO OD + rifampin 600 mg monthly x 6 mos
- multibacillary: dapsone 100 mg PO OD + rifampin 600 mg monthly + ofloxacin 300 mg PO daily x 12-24 months

Prognosis
- complications: muscle atrophy, contractures, trauma/superinfection of lesions, crippling/loss of limbs, erythema nodosum leprosum

Syphilis

Etiology
- *Treponema pallidum:* thick motile spirochetes detectable by dark-field microscopy historically, although rarely done now
- transmitted sexually, vertically, or parenterally (rare)

Clinical Features
- see also <u>Dermatology</u> and <u>Gynecology</u>
- multi-stage disease (most features attributable to blood vessel involvement)
  - i) primary syphilis (3-90 days post-infection)
    - painless genital chancre and regional lymphadenopathy
    - acute disease lasts 9-90 days, 50% progress to secondary syphilis without treatment
  - ii) secondary syphilis = systemic infection (2-8 weeks following chancre)
    - maculo-papular non-pruritic rash including palms and soles
    - generalized lymphadenopathy, low grade fever, malaise, headaches, aseptic meningitis
    - condylomata lata: painless, wart-like lesion on palate, vulva or scrotum (highly infectious)
  - iii) late, latent syphilis (>1y post-infection)
    - asymptomatic disease that occurs without treatment
  - iv) tertiary syphilis (15-20 y post-infection)
    - gummatous syphilis: nodular granulomas of skin, bone, liver, testes, brain
    - aortic aneurysms and valvular disease (AI)
    - neurosyphilis – strokes, dementia, personality changes, Argyll-Robertson pupils, tabes dorsalis, Charcot joint
  - v) congenital syphilis
    - causes SA, stillbirths, congenital malformations, mental retardation, deafness
    - infants may be asymptomatic until age 2-5 then present with rhinitis, fever, lymphadenopathy, bone and cartilage degeneration (including saddle nose), hepatosplenomegaly, rash

Investigations
- screening tests: VDRL, RPR, EIA
- confirmatory tests: TPI, FTA-ABS, MHA-TP, TPPA, dark field microscopy with silver stain
- LP for 3° syphilis if: seroactive and HIV+, symptoms of neurosyphilis or receiving treatment for neurosyphilis
- LP for neurological symptoms, CD4 <350, RPR >1:32

Treatment
- for 1°, 2°, latent <1 y: PenG 2.4 million units IM x 1
  for 3°, latent (>1 y): benzathine PenG 2.4 million units IM weekly x 3
  if allergic to penicillin: doxycycline 100 mg PO bid or tetracycline 500 mg PO qid x 14 d
- neurosyphillis: aqueous PenG 18-24 million units/d IV x 10-14 d

Lyme Disease

Etiology/Epidemiology
- *Borrelia burgdorferi:* spirochete bacteria
- Lyme disease has been reported in 49 of the 50 U.S. states, but most cases occur in the Northeast, the Midwest, and Northern California
- reservoir: white-footed mouse (esp. BC's Fraser Delta + Vancouver Island; ON's north shore Lake Erie); white tailed deer
- transmitted by *Ixodes* tick
- human contact usually May-August in fields with low brush near wooded areas
- infection usually requires >36 h tick attachment

Those with untreated 1° or 2° Syphilis
1/3   cure
1/3   latent forever
1/3   3° syphillis

VDRL and RPR Test for Syphilis have a High False Positive Rate (up to 25% of all positive results)
Such false positive results can be caused by:
- Viruses (mono, hepatitis)
- Drugs and substance abuse
- Rheumatic fever and rheumatic arthritis
- Lupus and leprosy
- pregnancy
- antibody cross reactivity

Patients with 2° or 3° syphilis treated with penicillin may experience a Jarisch-Herxheimer reaction. Fever, chills, myalgia, flu-like symptoms may last up to 24 hours.

Argyll Robertson Pupil: a "prostitute's pupil" - accomodates but does not react to light. This is pathognomonic for syphilis.

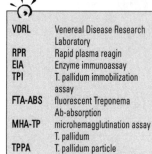

VDRL	Venereal Disease Research Laboratory
RPR	Rapid plasma reagin
EIA	Enzyme immunoassay
TPI	T. pallidum immobilization assay
FTA-ABS	fluorescent Treponema Ab-absorption
MHA-TP	microhemagglutination assay T. pallidum
TPPA	T. pallidum particle agglutination assay

Clinical Features

  i) stage 1 (early localized stage: weeks post-infection)
- malaise, fatigue, H/A, myalgias
- erythema chronicum migrans (ECM) large expanding non-pruritic bulls-eye lesion at bite (red with clear centre) on thigh/groin/axilla

  ii) stage 2 (early disseminated stage: weeks to months post-infection)
- multiple smaller ECM
- CNS: aseptic meningitis, CN palsies (CN VII), peripheral neuritis
- cardiac: transient heart block or myocarditis
- MSK: arthritis

  iii) stage 3 (chronic: months to years post-infection)
- chronic arthritis
- acrodermatitis chronicum atrophicans
- neurologic: encephalopathy, meningitis, neuropathy

Investigations
- serology: ELISA, Western Blot

Prevention
- insect repellent, inspection for ticks and swift removal of tick (vaccine exists but is currently unavailable)
- prophylaxis within 72 h of finding engorged attached nymphal tick in hyperendemic area: doxycycline 200 mg PO x 1 dose

BAKE a Key Lyme Pie: **B**ell's palsy, **A**rthritis, **K**ardiac block, **E**rythema chronicus migrans.

Treatment
- stage 1: doxycycline 100 mg PO bid x 14-21 d or amoxicillin or cefuroxime
- stage 2-3: ceftriaxone 2 g IV q24h x 2-4wks

Toxic Shock Syndrome (TSS)

Etiology
- superantigens produced by some strains of *S. aureus* or group A *Streptococcus* cause widespread T-cell activation and cytokine release (IL-1, IL-6, TNF)
- Staphylococcal TSS: toxic shock syndrome toxin 1 (TSST-1)
- Streptococcal TSS: exotoxins SPEA, SPEB, SPEC

In Toxic Shock Syndrome, blood culture can be positive for Group A Strep but not for *S. aureus*

Risk Factors
- Staphylococcal: tampon use, nasal packing, wound infections
- Streptococcal: minor trauma, preceding viral illness (chickenpox), comorbid medical conditions

Clinical Features
- acute onset, fever >38.9°C, sBP < 90mmHg
- rash with subsequent desquamation, especially on palms and soles
- renal failure, thrombocytopenia, ↑ AST/ALT/bilirubin
- Staphylococcal TSS: involvement of 3 or more organ systems: GI (vomiting, watery diarrhea), muscular (myalgia, ↑ CK), mucous membranes (hyperemia), renal, liver, heme (thrombocytopenia), CNS (disorientation)
- Streptococcal TSS: coagulopathy, respiratory failure, soft tissue necrosis (necrotizing fasciitis, myositis, gangrene)

Treatment
- supportive, fluid resuscitation
- Staphylococcal: beta-lactamase resistant anti-staphylococcal antibiotic (e.g. cloxacillin) IV x 10-14 days
- Streptococcal: high-dose penicillin and clindamycin, IVIg

Cat Scratch Disease

Etiology
- *Bartonella henselae*: intracellular parasitic bacteria
- transmitted via cat scratch

Clinical Features
- skin lesion appears 3-10 days post-innoculation
- followed by fever, tender regional lymphadenopathy, malaise, anorexia, headache
- usually self-limited

Investigations
- serology, lymph node biopsy

Treatment
- supportive in most cases
- no role for antibiotics unless immuno-compromised or asplenic

Adapted from Spira AM. Assessment of travellers who return home ill. Lancet. 2003; 361(9367): 1459-69 and Schlossberg, D, Ed. Current Therapy of Infectious Disease. 2nd Edition. Mosby Inc, St Louis, Missouri, 2001.

Important Exposures

Insect Bites	
Mosquito	*Plasmodium* spp. (Malaria) Dengue *Lymphatic filariasis* (Elephantiasis) West Nile Encephalitis Yellow Fever Japanese Encephalitis
Tick	*Borrelia burgdorferi* (Lyme Disease) *Rickettsia rickettsii* (Rocky Mountain Spotted Fever)
Fly	*Trypanosoma brucei* spp. (African sleeping sickness) *Leishmania* spp. (Leishmaniasis) *Bartonella bacilli formis* (Bartonellosis)
Flea	*Yersinia* (Plague) *Tunga penetrans* (Tungiasis)

Mammal Bites	
Dog/Cat	Rabies, *Pasteurella*, anaerobes, Strep, *Staph aureus*
Human	Strep, *Staph aureus*, oral anaerobes

Oral Exposures	
Unpasteurized Milk	*Brucella* spp., TB., *Salmonella, Shigella, Listeria*
Undercooked Meat	Enteric bacteria, helminths, protozoa
Water	Hep A/E, Norwalk, cholera, *Salmonella, Shigella, Giardia*, poliovirus, *Cryptosporidium, Cyclospora*

Environmental Exposures	
Freshwater	*Leptospira* spp., schistosomes, *Acanthamoeba, Naegleria fowleri*
Soil	Hookworms, *Toxocara* spp. (visceral larva migrans), *Leptospira interrogans* (leptospirosis)

Rocky Mountain Spotted Fever

Etiology
- *Rickettsia rickettsii*: obligate intracellular organism
- reservoir hosts: rodents, dogs
- vectors: lone star ticks (*Dermacentor* ticks)

Clinical Features
- usually occurs in summer following tick bite
- acute onset fever, headache, mylagia, N/V
- followed by macular rash and edema

Investigations
- serology

Treatment
- doxycycline

West Nile Virus

Epidemiology
- virus has been detected throughout the United States and much of southern Canada
- overall, the case-fatality rates in severe cases are ~10%

Transmission
- mostly from mosquitoes that have fed on infected birds (crows, blue jays)
- transplacental, blood products (rare), organ transplantation

Clinical Features
- most are asymptomatic
- most symptomatic cases are mild (West Nile fever)
    - acute onset of H/A, back pain, myalgia, anorexia
    - maculopapular non-pruritic rash involving chest, back, arms
- severe complications: encephalitis, meningoencelphalitis and acute flaccid paralysis (especially in those >60 years) like polio syndrome

Investigations
- CSF: elevated lymphocytes and protein
- IgM antibody in serum or CSF (cross reactivity with Yellow Fever, Dengue Fever, St. Louis encephalitis and Japanese encephalitis vaccination); may not reflect current illness as IgM antibody can last for >6 months
- viral isolation or PCR from CSF, tissue, blood and fluids (all have low sensitivity)

Treatment and Prevention
- supportive
- use of mosquito repellant (DEET), drain stagnant water, community mosquito control programs

HIV and AIDS

Epidemiology

Canadian Situation (Public Health Agency of Canada, 2007)
- 63,604 positive HIV tests reported to the Public Health Agency of Canada from 1985 – November 2007; estimated that 30% unaware of HIV positive status
- an estimated 1,225 new infections were diagnosed in Canada in the first half of 2007; men who have sex with men account for 41% of cases, IV drug users 23%, heterosexual transmission 18%

Global Situation (WHO Weekly Epidemic Update, 2007)
- estimated 33.2 million people living with HIV/AIDS at end of 2007 (1% of 15-49 year-olds worldwide) (16% lower than 2006 estimates due to improved methodology used in 2007)
- approximately 2.5 million newly infected in 2007 (approximately 68% in sub-Saharan Africa where HIV/AIDS is leading cause of death)
- every day, >6800 persons become infected with HIV and >5700 persons die from AIDS
- heterosexual transmission is dominant in many countries

- HIV-1 is the predominant strain in North America and most of the world
- HIV-2 is found mainly in West Africa
- Both lead to AIDS

Pathophysiology

- see Figure 4 for general stages of viral replication
- components of HIV virion
  - envelope: lipid bilayer derived from host cell; contains transmembrane (gp41) and surface (gp120) glycoproteins
  - matrix: composed of protein p17
  - core: contains 2 single-stranded copies of RNA genome + enzymes (reverse transcriptase, integrase, protease) surrounded by capsid made of core protein p24
- envelope glycoproteins bind to CD4 and co-receptor (CXCR4 or CCR5) on surface of T-helper lymphocytes
- virion fuses with cell and contents enter cell
- viral ssRNA is converted into dsDNA by reverse transcriptase
- viral dsDNA is combined into host genome by integrase enzyme or can be latent
- when host cell divides, viral DNA is transcribed and a polyprotein is produced
- protease enzyme cleaves polyprotein into individual proteins (Gag, Env, Pol), forming a functional virion
- new immature virus is assembled and buds out of cell, taking part of host cell membrane with it

Infection is NOT transmitted by casual contact, kissing, mosquitoes, toilet seats, shared utensils.

Modes of Transmission

- unprotected anal or vaginal intercourse, rarely oral sex
- sharing of HIV-contaminated needles and injection equipment
- vertical transmission from infected mother to child in utero, during birth, or through breastfeeding; transmission rate 25% in infants born to HIV-seropositive mothers without antiretroviral therapy or Caesarean section; reduced to <3% by prenatal and perinatal treatment of mother and postnatal treatment of infant
- transfusion of contaminated blood or blood products
- accidental parenteral exposures of health care workers; average risk of infection after HIV needlestick injury is 0.3%

For recently exposed individuals (during window period), diagnosis can be made by DNA PCR or p24 antigen; a repeat ELISA test at 6 weeks and 3 months is indicated.

Laboratory Diagnosis

- seroconversion in 2-8 weeks; rare for antibodies to be undetectable after 3 months
- ELISA (enzyme linked immunosorbent assay) detects serum antibody to HIV, sensitivity >99%, specificity approx 99%
- Western Blot confirmation by detection of antibodies to at least two different HIV protein bands (p24, gp41, gp120/160)
- PCR: detects HIV DNA in plasma for diagnosis and HIV RNA in plasma for monitoring (viral load)
- p24 antigen detection by ELISA; only positive in acute phase and late symptomatic stages

All infants born to HIV infected mothers have positive ELISA tests because of circulating maternal anti-HIV antibodies which disappear by 18 months; early diagnosis is made by detection of HIV RNA in plasma.

Natural History

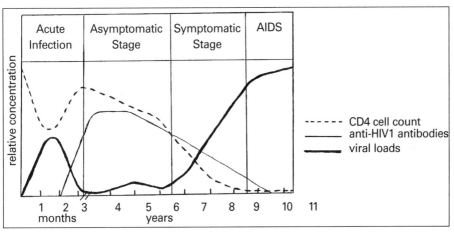

Figure 4. Relationships between CD4 T cell Count, Viral Load, and Anti-HIV Antibodies

Acute Retroviral Syndrome
- 40-70% experience a mononucleosis-like acute retroviral syndrome from 1-6 weeks after initial infection generally lasting 10-15 days
- fever, pharyngitis, lymphadenopathy, rash, myalgias, headaches, leukopenia
- aseptic meningitis is the most common neurologic presentation and occurs in 10-20% of patients; HIV RNA and/or p24 may be detected in CSF
- associated with high level plasma viremia and therefore high risk of transmission

Asymptomatic Phase
- progression of disease is highly variable: within 10 years after HIV infection, 50% of untreated individuals develop AIDS, an additional 30% have milder symptoms related to immunodeficiency, and less than 20% are persistently asymptomatic
- CD4 counts usually greater than 200 cells/mm^3
- persistent generalized lymphadenopathy occurs in 35-60% of asymptomatic patients

Symptomatic Phase
- CD4 counts <500 cells/mm^3
    - constitutional symptoms: fever, night sweats, fatigue, weight loss
    - mucocutaneous lesions: seborrheic dermatitis, HSV, VZV (shingles), oral hairy leukoplakia (EBV), candidiasis (oral, esophageal, vaginal), Kaposi's sarcoma (KS)
    - recurrent bacterial infections, especially pneumonia
    - pulmonary and extrapulmonary tuberculosis
    - lymphoma
- CD4 counts <200 cells/mm^3
    - *Pneumocystis jiroveci* pneumonia (formerly PCP)
    - visceral KS
    - local and/or disseminated fungal infections: *Cryptococcus neoformans*, *Coccidioides immitis*, *Histoplasma capsulatum*
- CD4 counts <100 cells/mm^3
    - progressive multifocal leukoencephalopathy (PML)
    - CNS toxoplasmosis
- CD4 counts <50 cells/mm^3
    - CMV infection: retinitis, colitis, cholangiopathy, CNS disease
    - *Mycobacterium avium complex* (MAC)
    - invasive aspergillosis
    - bacillary angiomatosis (disseminated *Bartonella*)
    - primary central nervous system lymphoma (PCNSL), Acquired Immunodeficiency Syndrome (AIDS)
- AIDS surveillance definition in Canada
    - HIV-positive, AND
    - one or more clinical illnesses that characterize AIDS, including:
        - opportunistic infections (e.g. PCP, esophageal candidiasis, CMV, MAC, TB, toxoplasmosis)
        - malignancy (Kaposi's sarcoma, invasive cervical cancer)
        - wasting syndrome

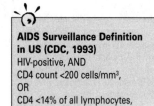

AIDS Surveillance Definition in US (CDC, 1993)
HIV-positive, AND
CD4 count <200 cells/mm^3,
OR
CD4 <14% of all lymphocytes,
OR
one or more AIDS-defining illnesses

Clinical Manifestations of HIV/AIDS

Constitutional
- fever, night sweats, weight loss, anorexia

Cutaneous
- seborrheic dermatitis: scaly eruption between the eyebrows and nasolabial folds
- herpes zoster: crops of vesicular lesions on erythematous bases in a dermatomal or multidermatomal distribution
- molluscum contagiosum: centrally umbilicated pearly papules occur in crops on face/abdomen/genitals, caused by poxvirus
- HPV: genital warts – cervical, vaginal, anal
- bacillary angiomatosis: purple-red nodules or plaques that can ulcerate and crust, caused by *Bartonella*

Oral
- candidiasis: cheesy white exudates on mucous membranes that can be scraped off easily
- oral hairy leukoplakia (OHL): white, lichenified, plaque-like lesion that cannot be scraped off
- aphthous ulcers: idiopathic ulcerative lesions
- HSV

Ophthalmologic
- CMV retinitis: causes floaters or blurred vision, fundus exam shows hemorrhages and full-thickness whitening

- herpes zoster ophthalmicus
- HIV retinopathy: cotton wool spots

Cardiac
- dilated cardiomyopathy, pericardial effusion, myocarditis, endocarditis, accelerated atherosclerosis (↑CAD, MI)

Pulmonary
- *Pneumocystis jiroveci* pneumonia: progressive dyspnea, nonproductive cough, usually normal P/E, CXR shows interstitial infiltrate, nodules, cysts, parenchymal infiltrates or may be normal
- increased risk of bacterial pneumonia, especially from encapsulated bacteria (e.g. Pneumococcus)
- *Mycobacterium tuberculosis*
- fungal pneumonia: histoplasmosis, coccidiodomycosis, aspergillosis
- nonspecific interstitial pneumonitis (NIP): similar to PCP but CD4 count >200 cells/mm^3
- HIV-related pulmonary hypertension

Gastrointestinal
- diarrhea: bacteria (*Salmonella, Shigella, Enterobacteriaceae, C. difficile*), protozoa (*G. lamblia, Cryptosporidium parvum, Isospora belli*, coccidian, microsporidia), viral (CMV), HIV-associated enteropathy, medication side effects
- HIV cholangiopathy: CMV, MAC, microsporidium, HIV itself
- proctitis: *Chlamydia*, gonococcal
- HPV-related anal carcinoma in men
- lymphogranuloma venereum

Renal
- HIV-associated nephropathy: proteinuria, progressive renal insufficiency

Genital
- HSV: recurrent genital ulcers

Vaginal and Cervical
- candidiasis: vulvovaginitis, white exudates
- HPV: cervical dysplasia and cancer

Neurological
- HIV-related dementia (subcortical): progressively poor concentration, diminished memory, slowing of thought processes, gait ataxia, spastic weakness of extremities, loss of bowel and bladder function
- focal lesions of CNS
  - *Toxoplasma gondii* encephalitis: CT with contrast dye shows multiple ring enhancing lesions
  - primary CNS lymphoma: CT frequently shows single, sometimes oligofocal enhancing lesions, often periventricularly located
  - PML: demyelinating disease caused by JC virus, leads to visual impairment/seizures/hemiparesis, multiple non-enhancing white matter lesions on MRI
- meningitis
  - cryptococcal meningitis: cryptococcal antigen in CSF, positive culture
  - *Mycobacterium tuberculosis*
  - *Treponema pallidum* (neurosyphilis)
- meningoencephalitis
  - CMV encephalitis: confusion/cranial nerve abnormalities/long tract signs, detection of CMV antigens in CSF by PCR
- peripheral neuropathy: HIV or medication-induced
- myelopathy
  - CMV, HSV, VZV
  - cord compression: epidural abscess, lymphoma
  - vacuolar myelopathy: progressive spastic paraparesis, often associated with dementia
- radiculopathy: CMV

Oncologic
- Hodgkin's and non-Hodgkin's lymphoma: increased incidence at any CD4 count, vast majority have extranodal disease
- primary CNS lymphoma: generally presents as confusion/lethargy/personality changes/memory loss (typically with CD4 <50)

Both direct neuronal destruction and effects of viral proteins on neuronal cell function contribute to nervous system complications.

- Kaposi's sarcoma:
  - caused by HHV-8
  - can occur at any CD4 count
  - mucocutaneous red-purple nodular lesions
  - pulmonary: nodular interstitial lesions, pleural effusion
  - GI: bleeding, bowel obstruction, obstructive jaundice
  - treatment: radiation/cryotherapy/intralesional vinblastine for limited disease, chemotherapy for systemic disease
- cervical and anal dysplasia/cancer: HPV-related

Management of the HIV-Positive Patient

Encourage safer sex, even with other HIV-positive individuals, to prevent spread of resistant organisms.

Reasons for Deterioration of a Patient with HIV/AIDS
Opportunistic infections
Neoplasms
Effects of medications
The disease itself
Coinfection with HCV

- confirm positive HIV test
- complete baseline history and physical examination, then follow-up every 3 months
- physical exam
  - optic fundi for hemorrhagic lesions characteristic of CMV retinitis
  - oral cavity for lesions
  - lymph node enlargement
  - hepatosplenomegaly
  - genital lesions
  - neurological exam for peripheral neuropathy, decreased global cognition
- education
  - emphasize that most patients, even without antiviral therapy, survive for 10 to 12 years after acquiring HIV infection and are asymptomatic during most of that time
  - prevention of further transmission through safer sex and clean needles for drug use
- laboratory evaluation
  - baseline plasma HIV-RNA level and CD4 count, repeat every 2-3 months
  - baseline tuberculin skin test (PPD): induration greater than 5 mm is positive
  - baseline *Toxoplasma* antibody, syphilis serology (VDRL), hepatitis A, B and C antibodies, hep B surface antigen, CMV antibody, liver enzymes, and CXR
- health care maintenance
  - assessment for ongoing counseling needs and referral for significant psychiatric or social problems
  - vaccines: influenza annually, 23-valent pneumococcal every 5 years, hepatitis B (if not immune), hepatitis A (if seronegative)
  - annual PAP test

Table 17. Prophylaxis against Opportunistic Infections in HIV-infected patients

Pathogen	Indication for prophylaxis	Prophylactic regimen
Pneumocystis jiroveci	CD4 count <200 cells/mm³ or history of oral candidiasis	TMP-SMX 1 SS or DS OD
Toxoplasma gondii	IgG antibody to *Toxoplasma* and CD4 count <100 cells/mm³	TMP-SMX 1 DS OD
Mycobacterium tuberculosis	PPD reaction >5 mm or contact with case of active TB	Isoniazid & pyridoxine x 9 months
Mycobacterium avium complex	CD4 count <50 cells/mm³	Azithro 1200 mg q week or Clarithro 500 mg bid
Varicella zoster virus	Exposure to chicken pox/shingles in previously unexposed	VZIG within ≤96 hrs of exposure

SS = single strength, DS = double strength   See 2002 USPHS/IDSA Guidelines for Preventing Opportunistic Infections Among HIV-Infected Persons.
http://aidsinfo.nih.gov/ContentFiles/OIpreventionGL.pdf

1° and 2° prophylaxis may be discontinued if CD4 count is above threshold for ≥6 months while on HAART.

Highly Active Antiretroviral Treatment (HAART)

- goals
  - reduction of HIV-related morbidity and mortality
  - improvement in quality of life and minimization of drug side effects
  - restoration and/or preservation of immunological function
  - maximal and durable suppression of viral load
  - prevention of mother-to-child transmission, sexual transmission
- decision must always be made jointly by the informed patient and physician based on the following factors:
  - comparison of potential advantages (prevention of progressive immunologic disease) vs. disadvantages (short and long term toxicities, development of antiretroviral resistance because of lapses in adherence, cost)
  - willingness, ability, and readiness of patient to begin therapy
  - likelihood of patient adherence
- perform baseline resistance testing prior to initiation of antiretroviral treatment
- three-drug combinations are recommended for the initiation of treatment to prevent development of HIV resistance against a single drug
- viral load should decrease 3-4 fold (0.5 log) within 2-8 weeks and continue to decrease thereafter; goal is have undetectable viral load (i.e. <50 copies/mL) at 6 months, although may take longer if baseline viral load >100 000 copies/mL

Table 18. Guidelines for Initiating Antiretroviral therapy in chronically HIV-infected patients

Clinical Category	Laboratory Category	Recommendation
AIDS-defining illness or severe symptoms of HIV infection	Any CD4 count	Treat
Asymptomatic	CD4 ≤350 cells/mm^3	Treat
Asymptomatic	CD4 >350 cells/mm^3	Consider treatment to decrease risk of HIV-associated complications (ie: TB, Kaposi's), decreased HIV transmission to others
HIV-associated nephropathy	Any CD4 count	Treat
Pregnant women	Any CD4 count	Treat to prevent mother-child transmission. Consider discontinuing treatment post-partum if not otherwise indicated
Persons co-infected with hepatitis B virus (HBV), when HBV treatment is indicated	Any CD4 count	Treat both HIV and HB

See 2008 OARAC Guidelines for the Use of Antiretroviral Agents in HIV-1-Infected Adults and Adolescents. http://aidsinfo.nih.gov/contentfiles/Adultand-AdolescentGL.pdf

Table 19. Antiretroviral Drugs

Class	Drugs	Mechanism	Adverse Effects
Nucleoside reverse transcriptase inhibitors (NRTIs)	zidovudine (AZT) lamivudine (3TC) stavudine (d4T) didanosine (ddl) abacavir (ABC) emtricitabine (FTC) AZT/3TC (Combivir) AZT/3TC/ABC (Trizivir) ABC/3TC (Kivexa) FTC/TDF (Truvada)	Incorporated into the growing viral DNA chain, thereby competitively inhibiting reverse transcriptase and terminating viral DNA growth	Lactic acidosis Lipodystrophy Rash N/V/diarrhea Bone marrow suppression (AZT) Peripheral neuropathy (ddl, ddC, d4T) Drug-induced hypersensitivity (ABC) Pancreatitis (ddl/d4T) Myopathy (AZT)
Nucleotide reverse transcriptase inhibitors	tenofovir (TDF)	Similar to NRTIs, except are chemically preactivated and thus require less biochemical processing in the body to become active	Renal dysfunction N/V/diarrhea
Non-nucleoside reverse transcriptase inhibitors (NNRTIs)	efavirenz nevirapine delavirdine	Non-competitively inhibit function of reverse transcriptase, thereby preventing viral RNA replication	Rash, Stevens-Johnson syndrome CNS: dizziness, insomnia, somnolence, abnormal dreams (efavirenz) Hepatotoxicity (nevirapine – avoid in females with CD4 >250, men with CD4 >400) CYP3A4 interactions
Protease inhibitors (PIs)	ritonavir saquinavir amprenavir nelfinavir indinavir atazanavir fosamprenavir lopinavir/ritonavir (Kaletra) tipranavir/ritonavir darunavir/ritonavir	Prevent maturation of infectious virions by inhibiting the cleavage of polyproteins	Lipodystrophy, metabolic syndrome N/V/diarrhea Nephrolithiasis (indinavir) Rash (APV) Hyperbilirubi-nemia (ataz, indinavir) CYP3A4 interactions Hyperlipidemia
Fusion inhibitors	enfuvirtide (T-20) maraviroc	Inhibit viral fusion with T-cells by inhibiting gp41 (Enfuvirtide) or CCR5 (Maraviroc), thus preventing infection of healthy cells	Injection site reactions
Integrase Inhibitors	raltegravir elvitegravir	Inhibits integration of HIV DNA into the human genome thus preventing HIV replication	Only available through Expanded Access Program

Lactic Acidosis
- occurs secondary to mitochondrial toxicity
- symptoms include abdominal pain, fatigue, N/V, muscle weakness

Lipodystrophy
- Body fat redistribution: dorsal fat pad, breast enlargement, increased abdominal girth, facial thinning, decreased adipose tissue in the extremities
- Metabolic abnormalities: lipids (↑ LDL, ↑TGs), glucose (insulin resistance, DM2), ↑ risk CVD

Ritonavir-boosting for Protease Inhibitors
- Ritonavir inhibits the metabolism of other PIs by inhibiting cytochrome P450 3A4 and p-glycoprotein, the enzyme systems responsible for metabolism of the PIs
- The goal of PI boosting is to increase the plasma exposure to PIs
- PI boosting is best achieved by administering low-dose ritonavir along with the PI

First Failure
- confirm adherence
- resistance testing
- construct 3-drug regimen

Subsequent Failure
- confirm adherence, resistance testing
- re-evaluate if goals are possible
- rule out opportunistic infection
- rule out marrow suppression
- try to construct regimen with 2-3 active drugs

Table 20. Recommended Regimens for Treatment of HIV-1 in Treatment-Naive Patients

	Column A (use NNRTI OR PI)		Column B (Dual NRTI)
	NNRTI	**PI**	**2-NRTI**
Preferred	Efavirenz	Atazanavir + ritonavir Fosamprenavir + ritonavir BID Lopinavir/ritonavir BID	Abacavir/Lamivudine (if negative for HLAB*5701) Tenofovir/Emtricitabine
Alternative	Nevirapine	Atazanavir (unboosted) Fosamprenavir (unboosted) Fosamprenavir + ritonavir OD Lopinavir/ritonavir OD Saquinavir + ritonavir	Zidovudine/Lamivudine Didanosine + (Emtricitabine or Lamivudine)

The revised recommendations for antiretroviral-naive patients (January 2008). Clinicians are recommended to construct a regimen by choosing one component from Column A and one component from Column B. See 2008 OARAC Guidelines for the Use of Antiretroviral Agents in HIV-1-Infected Adults and Adolescents. http://aidsinfo.nih.gov/contentfiles/AdultandAdolescentGL.pdf

Treatment Failure
- defined clinically (HIV progression), immunologically (failure to increase CD4 count by 25-50 over first year of treatment or CD4 decrease), or virologically (failure to achieve viral load <400 copies/mL after 24 wks or <50 copies/mL after 48 wks)
- ensure that viral load >50 is not just a transient viremia

Prevention of HIV Infection

- education
- safer sexual practices: condoms for vaginal and anal sex, barriers for oral sex
- harm prevention for IV drug users: avoid sharing needles
- treatment of HIV-infected women with triple therapy during the second and third trimester of pregnancy and during delivery followed by AZT treatment of the infant for 6 weeks; decreases maternal-fetal transmission from 25% to <3%
- universal blood and body precautions for health care workers
    - prophylaxis after occupational exposure with a PI-based regimen initiated immediately (<72 h) after exposure and continuing for 4 weeks

(see Updated U.S. Public Health Service Guidelines for the Management of Occupational Exposures to HIV and Recommendations for Postexposure Prophylaxis. CDC MMWR Recommendations and Reports. 2005;54(RR9);1–17) http://www.cdc.gov/mmwr/preview/mmwrhtml/rr5409a1.htm#tab1)

- screening of blood and organ donation

Fungal Infections

Skin and Subcutaneous Infections

Superficial Fungal Infections

Clinical Features
- benign skin pigmentation changes
    - i) Pityriasis versicolor (Tinea versicolor): hypo/hyperpigmented skin patches (will not tan in sun)
    - ii) Tinea nigra: dark brown-black painless patches on soles of feet and palms

Treatment
- dandruff shampoo with selenium sulfide applied to skin
- topical clotrimazole or ketoconazole (Nizoral™)
- oral ketoconazole or itraconazole

Dermatophytes

Definition
- refers to infection of keratinized tissues (in cutaneous skin layer) caused by three genera of molds
    - i) Trichophyton infects skin, nails and hair
    - ii) Microsporum infects skin and hair
    - iii) Epidermophyton infects skin and nails

Pathophysiology
- fungi secrete keratinase (thus destroying the main structural protein of skin, nails, hair) resulting in scaling of skin, loss of hair and crumbling of nails

Transmission
- most dermatophytes are highly contagious and many can be spread by person-to-person contact

Clinical Features
i)   tinea barbae ("barber's itch")
   - colonization of bearded areas of face and neck in males
   - lesions range from erythematous perifollicular papules and pustules to nodular, abscess-like lesions with associated alopecia
ii) tinea capitis
   - infection of scalp which leads to scaling and hair loss
   - usually occurs between 4-14 years of age
   - can also involve eyebrows and eyelashes
iii) tinea corporis (ring worm)
   - infection of hairless skin, can involve any area of skin
   - annular scaling plaque with erythematous border (area of inflammation) and central clearing (area of healing)
iv) tinea cruris ("jock itch")
   - sharply demarcated lesions with erythematous margins and scaling
   - usually involves genitocrural area and upper medial thigh symmetrically
   - scrotum usually not involved (unlike Candidal infection)

v) tinea pedis ("athlete's foot")
- infection of feet, usually involves webspace and soles
- associated with occlusive shoes (provides warm and moist environment needed for fungal growth) and contact with public bath or pool floors

vi) tinea unguium (onychomycosis)
- thick, discoloured, brittle nails
- confirm by KOH microscopy, culture, or histologic examination

Treatment
- topical midazoles for mild cases of tinea corporis, tinea cruris, and tinea pedis (i.e. clotrimazole, miconazole)
- oral antifungals for tinea barbae, tinea capitis and tinea unguium (i.e. terbinafine)

Subcutaneous Fungal Infection

Pathophysiology
- fungi that naturally reside in soil and enter skin via traumatic break
- *Sporothrix schenckii*: most commonly affects gardeners injured by a rose thorn or splinter
  - causes subcutaneous nodule at point of entry
  - fungi may migrate up lymphatic vessels creating nodules along the way - "nodular lymphangitis"

Treatment
- oral itraconazole
- if infection becomes disseminated use itraconazole, amphotericin B

Systemic Mycoses

Basics
- three major systemic mycoses
  - i) histoplasmosis
  - ii) blastomycosis
  - iii) coccidioidomycosis
- thermally dimorphic organisms
- infection occurs through inhalation of spores (soil, bird droppings, vegetation) or innoculation injury, not human-to-human spread
- 95% of infections are asymptomatic or cause acute self-limited pneumonia
- remaining 5% become chronic pneumonia or disseminate hematogenously
- may reactivate or cause 1° dissemination under immunocompromised conditions

Histoplasma capsulatum

Endemic Region
- river valleys in central USA, Ontario, Quebec; is widely spread

Clinical Features
i) primary pulmonary
- fever, cough, chest pain, headache, myalgia, anorexia
- CXR (acute): pulmonary infiltrates ± hilar lymphadenopathy
- CXR (chronic): pulmonary infiltrates, cavitary disease

ii) disseminated
- spread to bone marrow (pancytopenia), GI tract (ulcers), lymph nodes (lymphadenitis), skin, liver, spleen

Investigations
- fungal culture, fungal stain
- antigen detection (urinary)

Treatment
- amphotericin B, itraconazole (if progressive lung involvement)

Histoplasmosis is commonly associated with exposure to chicken coops, bird roosts and bat caves.

Blastomyces dermatitidis (Chicago or Gilchrist's Disease)

Endemic Region
- river valleys in midwest USA, Northern Ontario; not restricted to Northern Ontario

Clinical Features
i) primary
  - fever, cough, chest pain, chills, night sweats, weight loss
  - CXR (acute): lobar pneumonia
  - CXR (chronic): lobar infiltrates, fibronodular interstitial disease
ii) disseminated
  - spread to skin (ulcers, subcutaneous nodules), bones (osteolytic lesions), GU tract (prostatitis, epididymitis)

Treatment
- amphotericin B for severe disease
- itraconazole or voriconazole for mild-moderate disease

Coccidioides immitis

High Risk
1. immunocompromised (e.g. AIDS, steroids)
2. pregnancy (3rd trimester)
3. diabetes
4. Philipino

The classic exposure risk for *coccidioides* is a trip to Arizona.

Endemic Region
- deserts in southwest USA, northwest Mexico

Clinical Features
i) primary
  - "influenza-like" syndrome: fever, chills, cough, chest pain, sore throat, fatigue
  - can develop hypersensitivity with arthritis, erythema nodosum
ii) disseminated
  - spread to skin (ulcers), joints (synovitis), bones (lytic lesions), meninges (meningitis)

Treatment
- amphotericin B for severe disease
- itraconazole or fluconazole for mild-moderate disease

Opportunistic Fungi

Pneumocystis jiroveci (P. carinii)

Microbiology
- previously classified as a protozoan
- unicellular fungi

Transmission
- rarely person-to-person transmission
- believed to be acquired at an early age by the respiratory route and remain latent until immunocompromised state, although this theory has recently come into question
- common opportunistic infection in AIDS patients
  - increased disease when CD4 count $<200 \times 10^6/L$
  - 80% lifetime risk without prophylaxis in patients with CD4 count $<200 \times 10^6/L$

CXR in PCP may show anything including normal, but almost never pleural effusions.

Clinical Features
- fever, nonproductive cough, progressive dyspnea
- classic CXR = diffuse interstitial infiltrate, starts perihilar (98% bilateral)
- CXR may be normal (20-30%)

Investigations
- sputum induction, bronchoalveolar lavage, endotracheal aspirate (if intubated), for C&S and Gram stain

Treatment and Prevention
- oxygen to keep $SaO_2 > 90\%$
- antimicrobial options:
  - TMP/SMX (PO or IV)
  - dapsone and TMP
  - clindamycin and primaquine
  - pentamidine (IV)
  - atovaquone

- corticosteroids used as adjuvant therapy in those with severe hypoxia (pO_2 <70mmHg or $[A-a]O_2$ >35 mmHg)
- prophylactic TMP/SMX for those at risk (primary if CD4 <200 x 10^6/L, secondary prophylaxis for all patients with prior PCP until immune recovery)

Cryptococcus neoformans

Microbiology
- encapsulated yeast

Transmission
- inhalation of airborne yeast from soil contaminated with pigeon droppings

Clinical Features
i) pulmonary
- usually asymptomatic or self-limited pneumonitis
ii) disseminated
- CNS: meningitis (leading cause of meningitis in AIDS patients)
- skin: lesions that resemble large molluscum contagiosum

Investigations
- serum cryptococcal antigen
- CSF for meningitis: India-ink stain, cryptococcal antigen test, culture to confirm
- blood C&S, urine C&S in men

India Ink sensitivity for cryptococcus is only 50% (higher in HIV patients).

Treatment
- amphotericin B ($\pm$ flucytosine) is first-line; induction therapy x 2 weeks
- fluconazole for consolidation therapy and maintenance therapy in HIV

Candida albicans

Microbiology
- pseudohyphae and yeast forms

Transmission
- normal flora of skin, mouth, vagina and GI tract
- risk factors: immunocompromised state, broad-spectrum antibiotics, diabetes, corticosteroids, central venous catheters, TPN

Clinical Features
i) mucocutaneous
- oral thrush, esophagitis (chest pain, odynophagia), vulvovaginitis (see Gynecology), cutaneous (diaper rash, skin folds, folliculitis), chronic mucocutaneous
ii) invasive
- candidemia, endophthalmitis, endocarditis, UTI (upper tract), hepatosplenic disease

Treatment
- thrush: swish and swallow nystatin, nystatin pastilles, single dose fluconazole
- vulvovaginal candidiasis: topical imidazole or nystatin, oral fluconazole
- cutaneous infection: topical imidazole
- AIDS/opportunistic infections (thrush, esophageal, vaginal): fluconazole, itraconazole, amphotericin B, echinocandins
- systemic: amphotericin B, fluconazole, echinocandins, voriconazole
- chronic mucocutaneous: fluconazole, itraconazole or amphotericin B

Aspergillus spp.

Microbiology
- branching septate hyphae
- common species causing disease include *A. fumigatus*, *A. flavus*

Transmission
- ubiquitous in environment (everywhere in air)
- *Aspergillus* produces a toxin called aflatoxin which contaminates nuts, grains and rice

Clinical Features
i) allergic bronchopulmonary aspergillosis (ABPA)
  - IgE-mediated asthma-type reaction with dyspnea, high fever and transient pulmonary infiltrates
  - occurs more frequently in patients with asthma and allergies

ii) aspergilloma (fungus ball)
  - noninvasive ball of hyphae colonizes a preexisting lung cavity
  - ranges from asymptomatic to massive hemoptysis
  - CXR: round opacity surrounded by a thin lucent rim of air, often in upper lobes ("air crescent" sign)

iii) invasive aspergillosis
  - associated with prolonged and persistent neutropenia
  - pneumonia - invasive pulmonary aspergillosis, necrotizing pulmonary aspergillosis
  - may disseminate to other organs: brain, skin
  - severe symptoms with fever, cough, dyspnea, pleuritic pain, tends to cavitate; fatal if not treated early and aggressively
  - CXR: local or diffuse infiltrates ± pulmonary infarction

iv) mycotoxicosis
  - aflatoxin produced by *A. flavus* (nuts, grains, rice)
  - results in liver hemorrhage, necrosis and hepatoma formation

Treatment Options
- voriconazole, itraconazole, amphotericin B, echinocandins
- surgical resection for aspergilloma and hemorrhage
- steroids for allergic bronchopulmonary aspergillosis

Parasitic Infections

Protozoa

Amoebas

Entamoeba histolytica

Transmission
- reservoir: infected humans
- fecal-oral transmission of cysts in areas of poor sanitation
- seen in immigrants, travellers, institutionalized individuals, Native Canadians, men who have sex with men (MSM)

Clinical Features
i) asymptomatic carriers
ii) amoebic dysentery
  - abdominal pain, cramping, colitis, dysentery, low grade fever with bloody diarrhea secondary to local tissue destruction of large intestine
iii) amoebic abscesses
  - can occur in liver (most common); presents with RUQ pain, weight loss, fever, hepatomegaly
  - can also occur in lungs and brain

Investigations
- stool exam (for cysts and trophozoites), serology
- active disease diagnosis by RBC fragments in trophozoite
- *E. histolytica* indistinguishable microscopically from the non-pathogen *E. dispar* (serology and stool antigen detection used to distinguish)

Treatment and Prevention
- invasive: metronidazole followed by iodoquinol or paromomycin (hepatic abscesses do not need to be drained unless >3 cm)
- cyst/trophozoite passer: iodoquinol or paromomycin alone
- good personal hygiene, purification of water supply; cyst killed by boiling, filtration, not by chlorination

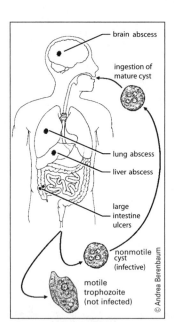

Figure 5. *Entamoeba* Life Cycle

Flagellates

Giardia lamblia

Transmission
- reservoir is infected humans and other mammals
- waterborne transmission (especially in the Rockies) and fecal-oral transmission of infectious cysts
- risk factors: institutions, daycare centres, MSM, travel

Clinical Features
- giardiasis ("beaver fever")
  - symptoms vary from asymptomatic to mild watery diarrhea to malabsorption syndrome (parasite coats small intestine and thus prevents fat absorption)
  - nausea, abdominal cramps, bloating, flatulence, fatigue, weight loss, steatorrhea
  - no hematochezia (no invasion into intestinal wall), no mucus in stool
  - no fever
  - more severe symptoms, difficult to eradicate in patients with hypogammaglobulinemia

Investigations
- multiple stool samples (daily x 3d) for concentration and stain, stool antigen used occasionally
- occasionally small bowel aspirate or biopsy for diagnosis

Treatment and Prevention
- metronidazole
- good personal hygiene and sanitation, water purification

Trichomonas vaginalis

Transmission
- sexual

Clinical Features
- males often asymptomatic; occasionally urethritis, prostatitis
- trichomonas vaginitis (see <u>Gynecology</u>)
  - malodourous (fishy) yellow-green or grey, frothy vaginal discharge, dysuria, dyspareunia

Investigations
- wet mount (motile parasites), antigen detection
- urine microscopy may show parasite in males, concentrated urine culture in males

Treatment
- metronidazole to patient and partner

Trichomonas causes 25% of vaginitis.

Trypanosoma cruzi

Transmission
- found in South and Central America
- transmission from *Reduviid* insects which defecate on skin and tryptomastigotes in the stool penetrate skin (majority of infections), placental transfer, organ donation, blood transfusion and ingestion of organism in sugar cane

Clinical Features
- American trypanosomiasis (Chagas' Disease)
  - acute: local swelling at site of inoculation (usually around one eye) with variable fever, lymphadenopathy, and hepatosplenomegaly
  - intermediate phase: asymptomatic but increasing levels of parasite and antibody in blood; most infected persons remain in this phase
  - chronic: can lead to chronic dilated cardiomyopathy, achalasia and megacolon 10-25 years after acute infection in 1/3 of infected individuals
- diagnosis: wet prep and Giemsa stain of thick and thin smear of blood, serology, PCR

Treatment and Prevention
- acute: nifurtimox or benznidazole
- intermediate: increasing trend to treat as acute
- chronic: symptomatic therapy, surgery including heart transplant as necessary
- insect control, bed nets when sleeping in adobe huts

Apicomplexa

Cryptosporidium spp.

Transmission
- reservoir: infected humans and a wide variety of young animals
- fecal-oral transmission by ingestion of cysts, waterborne
- risk factors: summer and fall, young children (daycare), men who have sex with men, contact with farm animals, HIV infection

Clinical Features
- cryptosporidiosis
  - symptoms range from self-limited watery diarrhea (immunocompetent) to chronic, severe, nonbloody diarrhea with nausea, vomiting, abdominal pain, and anorexia (immunocompromised) resulting in weight loss and death

Investigations
- modified acid-fast stain of stool specimen, stool antigen detection by direct fluorescent antibody (DFA)

Treatment and Prevention
- no treatment required for immunocompetent hosts except supportive care
- in AIDS try HAART to restore immunity; if fails, try nitazoxanide or paromomycin
- good personal hygiene, water filtration

Plasmodium spp. (malaria)

Microbiology
- species include: *P. falciparum* (most common and most lethal), *P. vivax*, *P. ovale*, *P. malariae*, *P. knowlesi* (new species isolated from primates in Malaysia, potentially fatal)
- complex life cycle: human host for asexual reproduction and mosquito for sexual reproduction
- sporozites from mosquitoes infect liver cells in which parasites multiply and are released as merozoites which infect RBCs causing disease
- *P. ovale* and *P. vivax* can produce dormant hypnozoites in the liver that may cause latent and/or recurrent malarial attacks

Transmission
- reservoir: infected human (see Figure 6)
- transmission by the night-biting female *Anopheles* mosquito, congenital and blood transfusion
- occurs in tropical and subtropical regions

Clinical Features
- flu-like prodrome
- paroxysms of high fever and shaking chills (due to synchronous systemic lysis of RBC - lasts several hours)
  - *P. vivax* and *P. ovale*: chills and fever q48h
  - *P. malariae*: chills and fever q72h
  - *P. falciparum*: less predictable fever interval
- abdominal pain, myalgia, headache, and cough
- hepatosplenomegaly

Complications
- *P. falciparum*: CNS involvement (cerebral malaria = seizures and coma), severe anemia, acute renal failure, ARDS
- *P. falciparum* is primarily responsible for fatal disease, also *P. knowlesi*, and rarely *P. vivax*

Investigations
- microscopy, blood should be examined at 12-24 hour intervals (x3) to rule out infection
  - thick smear (Giemsa stain) indicates presence of organisms
  - thin smear (Giemsa stain) for species identification and quantification of parasites
- rapid antigen detection tests (RDT)

Treatment
- *P. vivax*, *P. ovale*: chloroquine (and primaquine to eradicate liver forms); if chloroquine resistant use quinine sulfate and doxycycline or mefloquine alone + primaquine
- *P. malariae*: chloroquine only
- *P. falciparum*: most areas of world show chloroquine resistance
  - quinine plus doxycycline, or atovaquone/proguanil (Malarone™) combination
  - alternative is mefloquine alone but there is an increased risk of side effects
- *P. knowlesi*: chloroquine and primaquine

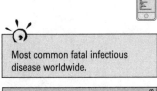

Most common fatal infectious disease worldwide.

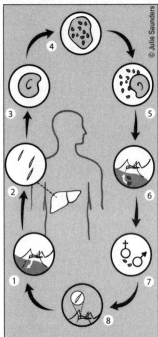

1. Sporozoites enter blood via mosquito bite, infect liver.
2. Hepatic schizont infiltration.
3. Infect red blood cells.
4. Trophozoite divides asexually many times to produce schizont (contains multinuclear merozoites).
5. Red blood cell lyses and merozoites attack other red blood cells (chills and fever).
6. Male and female gametocytes (from merozoites) ingested by mosquito during bite.
7. Male and female gametocytes (from merozoites) fuse in mosquito gut; produce ookinete.
8. Ookinete matures into sporozoite; migrates to mosquito salivary glands.

Figure 6. Life cycle of *Plasmodium* spp.

Prophylaxis/Prevention

- chloroquine (in chloroquine-sensitive areas)
  - only kills RBC stage; must continue for 4 weeks after leaving endemic region
- chloroquine sensitive areas: Haiti, Dominican, Central America, (west of Panama Canal), Egypt, parts of Middle East (not Saudi Arabia, Yemin, Iran)
- if chloroquine resistance: mefloquine, doxycycline, primaquine, atovaquone/proguanil
- borders of Thailand, Western Cambodia, South Vietnam = mefloquine and chloroquine resistance
- mosquito repellants, bed nets, screens, permethrin spray on clothes

Toxoplasma gondii

Transmission

- acquired through exposure to cat feces, ingestion of undercooked meat, vertical transmission, organ transplantation, whole blood transfusions

Clinical Features

i) congenital
- result of acute primary infection of mother during pregnancy
- stillbirth, chorioretinitis, blindness, seizures, mental retardation, microcephaly
- initially asymptomatic infant may develop reactivation of chorioretinitis as adolescent or adult → blurred vision, scotoma, ocular pain, photophobia, epiphora, hearing loss, mental retardation

ii) acquired
- usually asymptomatic or mononucleosis-like syndrome in immunocompetent patient
- infection remains latent for life unless reactivation due to immunosuppression

iii) immunocompromised (most commonly AIDS with CD4 <200)
- encephalitis with focal CNS lesions seen as single or multiple ring-enhancing masses on CT (headache and focal neurological signs)
- lymph node, liver and spleen enlargement and pneumonitis
- chorioretinitis

Investigations

- serology, CSF Wright-Giemsa stain, antigen or DNA detection (PCR); pathology provides definitive diagnosis
- immunocompromised patients: consider CT scan (ring-enhancing lesion in cortex or deep nuclei) and ophthalmologic examination
- negative serology in many AIDS patients

Treatment and Prevention

- no treatment if immunocompetent, not pregnant and no severe organ damage
- in pregnancy use spiramycin to prevent transplacental transmission or pyrimethamine + sulfadiazine (add folinic acid)
- corticosteroids for eye disease, meningitis
- cook meat thoroughly
- pregnant women to avoid undercooked meat and refrain from emptying cat litter boxes
- for prophylaxis in AIDS, see HIV section (Table 17)

Helminths

Trematodes

Schistosoma spp.

Species

- *S. mansoni, S. hematobium, S. japonicum*

Transmission

- acquired when larvae, released from snails, penetrate unbroken skin during exposure in slow-moving infested fresh water (see Figure 8)
- adult worms live in terminal venules of bladder/bowel passing eggs into urine/stool
- eggs must reach fresh water to hatch; schistosomes cannot multiply in humans
- no person-to-person transmission because snail intermediate host is required

Clinical Features

- pruritic skin rash at site of penetration (cercarial dermatitis)
- acute schistosomiasis (Katayama fever) at time of egg deposition (4-8 weeks after infection)

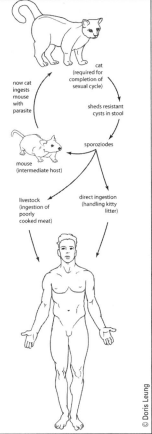

Figure 7. Life cycle of *Toxoplasma gondii*

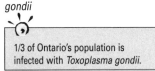

1/3 of Ontario's population is infected with *Toxoplasma gondii*.

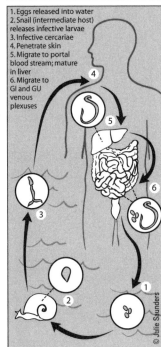

1. Eggs released into water
2. Snail (intermediate host) releases infective larvae
3. Infective cercariae
4. Penetrate skin
5. Migrate to portal blood stream; mature in liver
6. Migrate to GI and GU venous plexuses

Figure 8. Life Cycle of *Schistosoma*

- fever, hives, headache, weight loss, cough, abdominal pain, diarrhea (lasts up to 3 months), eosinophilia

Complications
- caused by granulomatous response and fibrosis secondary to egg deposition by adults in the veins surrounding the intestine or bladder
- *S. mansoni, S. japonicum*
  - worms in mesenteric vein, eggs in portal tracts of liver and bowel
  - heavy infections: intestinal polyps, portal and pulmonary hypertension, splenomegaly (2° to portal HTN)
- *S. hematobium*
  - worms in vesical plexus, eggs in distal ureter and bladder induce granulomas and fibrosis
  - terminal hematuria and rarely obstructive uropathy; associated with squamous cell bladder cancer

Investigations
- serology (very sensitive and specific), eosinophilia
- *S. mansoni, S. japonicum*: eggs in stool, liver U/S shows fibrosis, rectal biopsy
- *S. hematobium*: bladder biopsy, eggs in urine

Treatment
- praziquantel 20 mg/kg PO bid-tid x 1 d – take with food, do not cut/crush/chew
- control spread with proper disposal of human fecal waste, reduced exposure to infested water

Cestodes (flatworms)

Table 21. Cestodes (flatworms)

Nematode	Epidemiology	Transmission	Medical Importance	Treatment
Taenia solium	Developing countries	Undercooked pork (larvae), human feces (eggs)	Mild abdo symptoms. Cysticercosis: mass lesions in CNS, eyes, skin	Corticosteroids + Albendazole for cysticercosis
Taenia saginata	Developing countries	Undercooked beef (larvae)	Mild abdo symptoms	Praziquantel
Diphyllobothrium latum	Europe, North America, Asia	Raw fish	B12 deficiency leading to macrocytic anemia and posterior column deficits	Praziquantel
Echinococcus granulosus	Rural areas	Dog feces (eggs)	Liver/lung cysts (enlarge between 1-20 yrs; may cause mass effect). Risk of anaphylaxis if cystic fluid released during surgical evacuation	Albendazole alone. Surgery + perioperative albendazole. Percutaneous aspiration + perioperative albendazole

Nematodes (roundworms)

Table 22. Nematodes (roundworms)

Nematode	Epidemiology	Transmission	Medical Importance	Treatment
Ascaris lumbricoides	Tropics	Human feces	Abdo pain and intestinal obstruction from high worm burden. Cough, dyspnea, pulmonary infiltrates from larval migration through lungs (Loffler's syndrome)	Mebendazole OR Albendazole OR Pyrantel pamoate
Trichuris trichiura (whipworm)	Tropics	Ingestion of eggs in soil	Diarrhea, abdo pain, rectal prolapse, stunted growth	Mebendazole OR Albendazole
Onchocerca volvulus	Africa, Latin America	Blackfly bite	River blindness (onchocerciasis)	Ivermectin, ± doxycycline
Wuchereria bancrofti	Tropics	Mosquito bite	Damage to lymphatics resulting in lymphadenopathy and elephantiasis. Tropical Pulmonary Eosinophilia	Diethylcarbamazine, ± doxycycline
Loa Loa	Africa	Deer Fly	Subcutaneous migration of worm	Diethylcarbamazine
Enterobius vermicularis			See *Enterobius vermicularis* section	
Strongyloides stercoralis			See *Enterobius vermicularis* section	

Enterobius vermicularis (pinworm)

Transmission
- humans only host
- adult worms live in cecum and migrate at night to perianal skin to deposit eggs
- self-inoculation by fecal contaminated hand-to-mouth, person to person contact, autoinfection

Clinical Features
- asymptomatic carrier state
- severe nocturnal perianal itching
- occasionally vaginitis
- associated with *B. fragilis* (abdominal pain ± diarrhea)

Investigations
- sticky tape test (5-7 tests required to rule out infection)
- examination of perianal area at night may reveal adult worms seen with unaided eye
- usually no eosinophilia since no tissue invasion

Treatment and Prevention
- mebendazole, albendazole, pyrantel pamoate
- clean underwear change, pajamas to sleep, bathe in morning, wash hands after BM
- treat all members of family simultaneously
- reinfection common

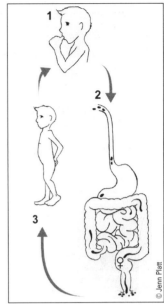

Figure 9. Life Cycle of *Enterobius*

Strongyloides stercoralis (threadworm)

Transmission
- through unbroken skin, barefoot walking in tropics/subtropics
- adult worms live embedded in mucosa of small intestine
- one of the only worms capable of multiplying in human host
- source of infection: fecal contamination of soil

Clinical Features
- mostly asymptomatic
- pruritic dermatitis at site of larval penetration
- transient pulmonary symptoms during pulmonary migration of larvae (eosinophilic pneumonitis = Löffler's syndrome – see <u>Respirology</u>)
- abdominal pain, diarrhea
- hyperinfection: occasional fatal cases caused by massive auto-infection in immunocompromised host, especially HTLV-1 (pneumonia, ARDS, multi-organ failure, enteritis, Gram negative bacteremia)

Investigations
- fecal exam for larvae (no eggs), larval culture on agar
- small bowel biopsy
- serology (most sensitive), eosinophilia (in chronic but not hyperinfection phase)

Treatment
- ivermectin, 200 mcg/kg/d PO x 2 d (albendazole 400 mg PO bid x 7 d, less effective)

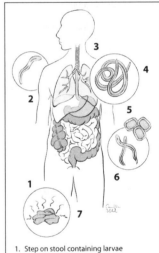

1. Step on stool containing larvae
2. Larvae migrate to lungs via bloodstream
3. Larvae crawl up trachea and down to GI tract
4. Adult worms in intestine
5. Eggs produced in bowel
6. Larvae
7. Bowel movement containing larvae

Figure 10. Life Cycle of *Strongyloides*

Infections in the Immunocompromised Host

- immunocompromised hosts have increased susceptibility to infections from pathogens that are typically low virulence, commensal, or latent
- type of immunosuppression predicts likely spectrum of agents

Factors that Compromise the Immune System
- general: age (very young or elderly), malnourishment
- immune disease: HIV/AIDS, malignancies, functional asplenia, hypogammaglobulinemia, neutropenia
- other disease: DM, malignancy, malnutrition
- iatrogenic: corticosteroids, chemotherapy, radiation treatment, anti-TNF, other immunosuppressive drugs (e.g. in transplant patients)

Table 23. Types of Immunocompromise

Type	Conditions	Vulnerable To
Cell-Mediated Immunity	HIV, Hodgkin's, hairy cell leukemia, cytotoxic drugs, SCID, DiGeorge syndrome	latent viruses fungi parasites
Humoral Immunity	CLL, lymphosarcoma, multiple myeloma, nephrotic syn, protein-losing enteropathy, burns, sickle cell anemia, asplenia, splenectomy, selective Ig deficiencies, Wiskott-Aldrich syndrome	encapsulated organisms (*S. pneumo, H. flu, N. meningitides*)
Neutrophil Function	myelodysplasia, paroxysmal nocturnal hemoglobinuria, radiation, cytotoxic drug therapy, C3, C5 deficiencies, chronic granulomatous disease	catalase-producing organisms (*Staph, Serratia, Nocardia, Aspergillus*)

Febrile Neutropenia

- fever (≥38.3°C or ≥38.0°C for ≥1 hour) and ANC (<0.5 or <1.0 but trending down to 0.5)

Pathophysiology
- decreased neutrophil production
    - marrow: infection, aplastic/myelophthisic anemia, leukemia, lymphoma, myelodysplastic syndromes
    - iatrogenic: cancer chemotherapy, radiation, drugs
    - deficiencies: vitamin B_{12}, folate
- increased peripheral neutrophil destruction
    - autoimmune: Felty's syndrome, SLE, antineutrophil antibodies
    - splenic sequestration, peripheral margination, hemodialysis, cardiopulmonary bypass

Etiology
- GN (esp. *Pseudomonas*) historically most common
- GP more common now
- fungal superinfection if neutropenia prolonged or if concurrent antibiotic use (esp. *Candida, Aspergillus*)

Investigations
- examine for potential sites of infection: mucositis and line infections are most common
- do NOT perform DRE; examine perianal region
- CXR, blood culture, urine culture, culture all in-dwelling catheter ports

Treatment
- this is one protocol, most hospitals have their own specific protocol

ANC (absolute neutrophil count) = WBC x (%neutrophils + %bands)

Usual signs and symptoms of infection may be diminished because neutrophils are required for a robust inflammatory response. Exam and X-ray findings may be more subtle.

WBC is lowest between 5-10 days after last chemo cycle.

Prophylaxis against FN with G-CSF and GM-CSF decreases hospitalization without affecting mortality (indicated if risk of FN >40% or if FN has occurred in a previous chemo cycle).

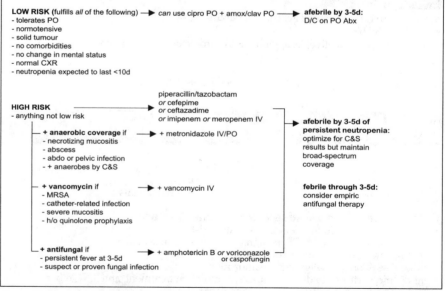

Figure 11. Example of Treatment Protocol for Febrile Neutropenia

Infections in a Transplant Patient

- infection is a leading cause of early morbidity/mortality in a transplant patient
- infection depends on degree of immunosuppression
- common infections <1 mo. post-transplant: bacterial infection of wound/lines/lungs herpetic stomatitis
- common infections >1 mo. post-transplant
    - viral (esp. CMV, EBV, VZV) (when immunosuppression is stronger)
    - fungal (especially *Aspergillus, Cryptococcus, PCP*)
    - protozoan (esp. *Toxoplasma*)
    - unusual bacterial infections (especially TB, *Nocardia, Listeria*)

Prophylactic vaccinations given before transplant

- to all transplant patients: Td, Pneumovax, hepatitis A&B vaccines
- if low titre or poor documentation: MMR, polio, varicella (0.5ml SC with booster 4-8 wks later)

Fever of Unknown Origin (FUO)

Table 24. Classification of Fever of Unknown Origin (FUO)

Classical FUO	Nosocomial FUO	Neutropenic FUO	HIV-associated FUO
• temp >38.3°C on several occasions	• temp >38.3°C on several occasions (infection not present/incubating on admission)	• temp >38.3°C on several occasions	• HIV infection
• duration >3 weeks		• neutrophil count <500/mL or is expected to fall to that level in 1-2 days	• temp >38.3°C on several occasions
• diagnosis uncertain after 3 outpatient visits or 3 days in hospital or 1 week of "intelligent and invasive" ambulatory investigation	• diagnosis uncertain after 3 days of investigation, including at least 2 days incubation of cultures	• diagnosis uncertain after 3 days of investigation, including at least 2 days incubation of cultures	• duration >4 weeks for outpatients, >3 days for hospitalized patients
			• diagnosis uncertain after 3 days of investigation, including at least 2 days incubation of cultures

Etiology Classic FUO

- infectious causes (15-25%):
    - TB – usually extra-pulmonary, miliary or pulmonary in patients with pre-existing pulmonary disease
    - abscess – usually in abdomen or pelvis; risk factors include cirrhosis, steroid or immunosuppressive medications, recent surgery, diabetes
    - osteomyelitis
    - bacterial endocarditis – cultures negative in 2-5%, especially in *Coxiella burnetii, Tropheryma whipplei, Brucella, Mycoplasma, Chlamydia*, fungi, *Legionella, Bartonella,* HACEK organisms which require either special media or longer than usual incubation
    - prostatitis, dental abscesses, sinusitis, and cholangitis are sources of occult fever
    - returning travellers/new immigrants: TB, HIV/AIDS, CMV, EBV, malaria, typhoid fever, dengue fever, hepatitis A, Lyme disease, syphilis, psittacosis (bird exposure), rat-bite fever
    - uncommonly toxoplasmosis, Leishmania, amoebiasis, histoplasmosis, Cryptococcus
- neoplastic causes (<20%)
    - most commonly lymphomas (especially non-Hodgkin's) and leukemias
    - solid tumours: RCC most common, also breast, liver, colon, pancreas or liver metastases
    - malignant histiocytosis: rare but rapidly progressive with high fever, weight loss, lymphadenopathy, hepatosplenomegaly
- collagen vascular diseases (15-25% of cases):
    - SLE, RA
    - rheumatic fever
    - vasculitis, especially temporal (giant cell) arteritis
    - JRA, Still's disease
- miscellaneous (15-20% of cases)
    - drug fever: commonly antibiotics, antihistamines, antiarrhythmics, methyldopa, phenytoin, dilantin, NSAIDs
    - sarcoidosis
    - inherited Familial Mediterranean Fever
    - factitious
    - pulmonary embolus
- unknown despite investigations

Fever Post-International Travel
Key elements in history include:
- travel location
- exposures, risk factors
- fever onset and duration
- immunization status
- antimalarial chemoprophylaxis and adherence
- presence of diarrhea and/or skin manifestations

For Nosocomial FUO, think B, C, D, E:
Bacterial and fungal infections of respiratory tract and surgical sites
Catheters (intravascular and urinary)
Drugs
Emboli

Approach to Classic FUO

- **history**: travel, environmental/occupational exposures, infectious contacts, drug medication history, immunizations, TB history, sexual history, PMHx
- thorough review of systems including complaints that disappeared before interview
- daily physical exam to assess fever pattern, paying attention to rashes, murmurs, arthritic signs, lymphadenopathy
- **initial investigations**:
  - bloodwork: CBC with differential and smear, electrolytes, BUN, Cr, calcium profile, LFTs, ESR, CRP, muscle enzymes, RF, ANA, serum protein electrophoresis, Fe, transferrin, TIBC, B12
  - cultures: blood (x 2 sets), urine, sputum, stool C&S O&P, other fluids as appropriate
  - VDRL, heterophile Ab (mononucleosis), CMV antigenemia test, HIV serology, PPD
  - CXR
- If diagnostic clues from any of the above steps, proceed with directed exam, biopsies or invasive testing as required followed by directed treatment once a diagnosis is established
- If no diagnosis with the above consider empiric therapy vs. watchful waiting
  - prognosis for most patients with FUO persisting without a diagnosis is very good without intervention
  - empiric therapies may include: anti-TB therapy, broad-spectrum antibiotics, colchicine, NSAIDS, steroids

Methicillin-Resistant Staphylococcus aureus (MRSA)

Etiology

- *Staphylococcus aureus*
  - Gram positive cocci
  - appear microscopically as grape-like clusters
  - colonizes the skin and mucous membranes of 30-50% population (nasopharynx, axilla, perineum, vagina, rectum)
- prevalence of resistant species is common; 90% of S. aureus are penicillin-resistant
- virulence of resistant species appears to be low; 10% of all S. aureus isolates in Canadian hospitals were MRSA, and <3% of clinical infections were MRSA (2003)

Risk Fastors

- ~85% MRSA in Canada is hospital-acquired (includes long-term care facilities)
- ~15% community-acquired in Canada, higher in the US
- colonized individuals are more likely to have surgical-site infection

History

- asymptomatic colonization
- skin and soft-tissue infection, infection associated with medical device (catheters, pacemakers, prosthesis, etc.), bacteremia, endocarditis, pneumonia, osteomyelitis, septic thrombophlebitis, meningitis

Investigations

- screening cultures on admission to hospital from anterior nares and perianal area
- culture of any infection site: blood, skin lesions, catheter/medical device exit site, sputum

Management
- any patients colonized or infected with MRSA should be placed on contact precautions
- severity of clinical infection may not be worse than with penicillin-sensitive *S. aureus*, but treatment options are limited with MRSA
- <u>MRSA infection</u>: vancomycin 1 g IV q12h (must adjust for renal insufficiency if CrCl <60 mL/min)
    - duration of treatment 4 weeks or more for serious infections such as endocarditis, osteomyelitis, necrotizing pneumonia or disseminated infection
    - other therapies include linezolid, daptomycin and tigecycline
- <u>decolonization</u>: 2% chlorhexidine wash daily x 7 d, AND rifampin 300 mg PO BID x 7d, AND doxycycline 100 mg PO bid x 7 d, AND 2% Mupirocin cream to anterior nares tid x 7 d

Travel Medicine

General Travel Precautions
- Vector-borne: long-sleeves, long pants, hats, repellents (permethrin containing) applied to clothes and belongings, repellents (DEET) to skin, bed nets
- Food/Water: avoid eating: raw meats/seafood, uncooked vegetables and milk/dairy products; drink only: carbonated `beverages, chlorinated water, boiled water, beer, wine
- Recreation: exercise caution when swimming in schistosomiasis-endemic regions, beaches that may contain human/animal waste products, near storm drains, after heavy rainfalls
- Prophylaxis: malaria (chloroquine, mefloquine, atovaquone + proguanil, doxycycline), traveler's diarrhea (Pepto-Bismol, fluoroquinolones)
- Vaccines: Hepatitis A, Japanese encephalitis, typhoid fever, yellow fever, rabies
- all travelers should have standard vaccines up to date (HepB, MMR, tetanus/diptheria, varicella, pertussis, polio)

Table 25. Travel Medicine by Region

	North Africa	Central/East/West Africa	Southern Africa	Caribbean	Tropical South America	Temperate South America	Mexico and Central America
Vector-borne	low risk	malaria; yellow fever; African trypanosomiasis; many other infections including dengue and West Nile fever	malaria; african tick-bite fever (Rickettsia); many other infections including dengue fever	malaria; dengue fever	malaria; dengue fever; yellow fever	low risk	malaria; dengue fever
Food/Water	dysentery/diarrhea, hepatitis A; typhoid fever; brucellosis; amebiasis	dysentery/diarrhea; hepatitis A; cholera; typhoid fever; brucellosis; amebiasis	dysentery/diarrhea; hepatitis A; typhoid fever; amebiasis	diarrhea; hepatitis A	diarrhea; hepatitis A	diarrhea; hepatitis A; typhoid fever; brucellosis; amebiasis	diarrhea; hepatitis A/E; brucellosis; typhoid fever
Airborne	TB approx 0.1%	TB >0.3%; meningococcal A; ebola	TB: 0.1-0.3%	TB: 0.1-0.3%	TB: 0.05%	TB: 0.05%	TB > 0.3%
STI	HIV: 0.1-0.5% HepB: 2-7%	HIV: 1-15% HepB: >8%	HIV: >25% HepB: >8%	HIV: 2-5% HepB: mostly <2%	HIV: 0.1-1% HepB: 2-8%	HIV: 0.1%	HIV: 0.1%
Zoonotic	rabies	rabies (dogs); Lassa fever virus (rodents)	rabies (mongoose, dogs)	low risk	rabies (bats); hantavirus (rodents);	low risk	rabies
Soil/Water	schistosomiasis	schistosomiasis; mycobacterium	schistosomiasis; leptospirosis	cutaneous larva migrans; histoplasmosis; leptospirosis	schistosomiasis; mycobacterium ulcerans; leptospirosis; histoplasmosis; paracoccidiodomycosis	histoplasmosis; coccidiodomycosis; paracoccidiodomycosis	leptospirosis
Overall	GI infection.	Risk for vector-borne and GI infection	Risk for vector-borne and GI infection	Low risk for traveler Risk of GI infection and dengue fever	Risk of malaria, dengue fever and GI infection	Low risk for traveler Risk of GI infection	Risk for GI infection, dengue fever, myiasis

	Western Europe	Eastern Europe/Northern Asia	South Asia	East Asia	South-East Asia	Middle East
Vector-borne	low risk	malaria; tick-borne encephalitis	malaria; Japanese encephalitis; dengue fever; many other infections	malaria; Japanese encephalitis; many other infections including dengue fever and spotted fever (hyperendemic)	malaria (except Singapore and Brunei); Japanese encephalitis; dengue fever (hyperendemic)	malaria; leishmaniasis
Food/Water	low risk	hepatitis A; brucellosis; typhoid fever	hepatitis A/E; typhoid/paratyphoid fever; amebiasis	diarrhea (variable); hepatitis A (excluding Japan); paragonimiasis	diarrhea; quinolone-resistant Campylobacter; cholera	diarrhea; hepatitis A; typhoid fever
Airborne	TB: 0.01-0.05%	TB: 0.1-0.3% - high rates of drug-resistant TB	TB: 0.1-0.3%	TB: 0.05-0.1% - drug-resistant TB in parts of China	TB: 0.1-0.3%	TB: 0.05%
STI	HIV: 0.3%	HIV: 1-5% HepB: 2-8%	HIV: <1% HepB: 2-7%	HIV: 0.1% HepB: >8%	HIV: 1-5% (Thailand, Burma, Cambodia); <1% elsewhere	HIV: <0.5% HepB: 2-7%
Zoonotic	tularemia; hantavirus; Q fever	rabies; tularemia	rabies; Q fever; anthrax; avian flu (H5N1)	rabies; avian flu (H5N1)	rabies (dogs); avian flu (H5N1)	rabies; Q fever; brucellosis
Soil/Water	Legionnaire's disease	low risk	leptospirosis	schistosomiasis	schistosomiasis; leptospirosis	schistosomiasis;
Overall	Low risk for traveler	Risk of GI, vector-borne and respiratory infections	Risk of GI infection, malaria, typhoid fever.	Highly variable but generally risk of respiratory infection	Risk of dengue fever, respiratory infection and GI infection	Low risk for traveler. Risk of GI infection

Antimicrobials

Antibiotics

Bactericidal Antibiotics	Bacteriostatic Antibiotics
Penicillins	Chloramphenicol
Cephalosporins	Tetracyclines
Carbapenems	Macrolides
Vancomycin	Clindamycin
Aminoglycosides	
Fluoroquinolones	
Metronidazole	

- assume no anaerobic coverage unless specifically mentioned
- assume not MRSA or VRE unless specified

Table 26. Antibiotics   (Indications and Contraindications adapted from e-CPS 2006)

Class & Drugs	Coverage	Mechanism of Action	Adverse effects	Indications	Contraindications
CELL WALL INHIBITORS					
Penicillins					
Benzyl penicillin - penicillin G IV/IM - penicillin V PO	- GP except Staphylococcus, Enterococcus - oral anaerobes except Bacteroides - Treponema	bactericidal: β-lactam inhibits penicillin binding protein (PBP) and prevents cross-linking of peptidoglycans	- immediate allergy (IgE): anaphylaxis, urticaria - late-onset allergy (IgG): urticaria, rash, serum sickness - interstitial nephritis - dose related toxicity: seizures, electrolyte disturbance, bleeding diathesis - diarrhea	mild to moderately severe infections caused by susceptible organisms including actinomycosis, streptococcal pharyngitis, streptococcal skin and soft tissue infections, syphilis	- hypersensitivity to penicillin
Aminopenicillin - ampicillin IV - amoxicillin PO (Amoxil™)	- same as penicillin - Enterococcus			bacterial meningitis and endocarditis (ampicillin); AOM, streptococcal pharyngitis, sinusitis, acute exacerbations of COPD, part of H. pylori treatment, Lyme disease, RTI , UTI (amoxicillin and ampicillin)	- hypersensitivity to penicillin or β-lactam antibiotics
Isoxozoyl penicillin - cloxacillin - methicillin - nafcillin - oxacillin	- same as penicillin - Staphylococcus			bacterial infections from susceptible penicillinase-producing staphylococci skin soft-tissue infections	- hypersensitivity to cloxacillin or any penicillin
Ureidopenicillin - piperacillin	- same as penicillin - GNB including Pseudomonas - anaerobes			Pip-tazo (Tazocin™) used for systemic and/or local bacterial infections, caused by piperacillin resistant, piperacillin/tazobactam susceptible, β-lactamase producing strains including certain abdominal, skin, and gyne infections and pneumonias	- history of allergic reactions to any penicillin, cephalosporin or β-lactamase inhibitor
Lactamase Inhibitors - amoxicillin-clavulinate (Clavulin™, Augmentin™)	- same as penicillin - Staphylococcus - H. influenzae			various infections caused by β-lactamase producing, Clavulin™ sensitive bacteria including RTI, sinusitis, AOM, skin and soft tissue infections, UTI	- hypersensitivity to penicillin or cephalosporin - pts with history of Clavulin-associated jaundice or hepatic dysfunction
- tazobactam				Pip-tazo (Tazocin™) used for systemic and/or local bacterial infections, caused by piperacillin resistant, piperacillin/tazobactam susceptible, β-lactamase producing strains including certain abdominal, skin, and gyne infections and pneumonias	- history of allergic reactions to any penicillin, cephalosporin or β-lactamase inhibitor
Carboxypenicillin - carbenicillin	- same as penicillin - extended GN coverage				

Cephalosporins

PO	IV	GP	GN			
1° cephalexin (Keflex™)	cefazolin (Ancef™)	strong except Enterococcus	only E. coli, Klebsiella, Proteus	β–lactam inhibits PBP and prevents cross-linking of peptidoglycans	- 15% penicillin allergy cross-reactivity - nephrotoxicity	skin and soft tissue infections, prevention of surgical site infections (cefazolin); infections caused by susceptible organisms - hypersensitivity to cephalosporins or other β-lactam antibiotic
2° cefuroxime (Ceftin™) cefprozil (Cefzil™)	cefuroxime (Zinacef™) cefoxitin^A	weaker activity than 1°	more coverage than 1° (^A includes anaerobes)			susceptible RTIs, soft tissue - hypersensitivity to cephalosporins or other β-lactam antibiotic
3° cefixime (Suprax™)	ceftriaxone (Rocephin™) cefotaxime (Claforan™) ceftazidime^B (Fortaz™)	S. aureus + good streptococcal coverage (^B not reliable against GP)	broad coverage (^B includes Pseudomonas)			RTI, gonorrhea, meningitis, septicemia, abdominal infections - hypersensitivity to cephalosporins or other β-lactam antibiotic
4°	cefepime (Maxipine™)	broad spectrum	broad coverage including Pseudomonas			empiric therapy for febrile neutropenia - hypersensitivity to cephalosporins or other β-lactam antibiotic

Red Man syndrome can be reduced with a slow vancomycin infusion rate.

Table 26. Antibiotics (continued)

Class & Drugs	Coverage	Mechanism of Action	Adverse effects	Indications	Contraindications
Carbapenems					
imipenem (Primaxin™)	- GP except *Enterococcus*, MRSA - GN including *Pseudomonas* + *Enterobacter* - anaerobes	β-lactam inhibits PBP and prevents cross-linking of peptidoglycans	- penicillin allergy cross-reactivity - seizures	treatment of infections caused by GNB producing extended-spectrum β-lactamases, serious infections caused by susceptible organisms	- hypersensitivity to imipenem
meropenem (Merrem™)					
vancomycin (Vancocin™)	- GP including MRSA, not VRE - *C. difficile* if PO	glycopeptide stearically inhibits addition of peptidoglycan subunits	- Red Man syndrome (histamine rxn with ↓BP) - nephrotoxicity - ototoxicity - neutropenia, thrombocytopenia	severe or life-threatening gram-positive infections, patients with beta-lactam allergy, may be taken only orally for pseudomembranous colitis	- hypersensitivity to vancomycin
teicoplanin	- GP including MRSA, not most VRE	glycopeptide sterically inhibits addition of peptidoglycan subunits			
PROTEIN SYNTHESIS INHIBITORS (50S RIBOSOME)					
Macrolides					
erythromycin (Erybid™, Eryc™)	- GP except *Enterococcus*, MRSA - GN: *Legionella, B. pertussis* - "atypicals": *Chlamydia, Mycoplasma*	inhibits 50S ribosome	- GI upset - acute cholestatic hepatitis - prolonged QT	susceptible RTI, pertussis, diphtheria, Legionnaires' Disease, skin and soft tissue infections	- hypersensitivity to erythromycin - concurrent therapy with astemizole, terfenadine
clarithromycin (Biaxin™)				susceptible RTI, skin infections, mycobacterial infections, part of *H. pylori* treatment	- hypersensitivity to macrolides - concurrent therapy with astemizole, terfenadine, or pimozide
azithromycin (Zithromax™)				susceptible pharyngitis, tonsillitis, AOM, acute exacerbations of COPD, community-acquired pneumonia, skin infections, *campylobacter* infections if treatment indicated, chlamydia	- hypersensitivity to macrolides
Lincosamides					
clindamycin (Dalacin™)	- GP except *Enterococcus*, some MRSA - anaerobes	inhibits peptide bond formation at 50S ribosome	- pseudomembranous colitis - GI upset	treatment of suspected or proven infections caused by GP, anaerobes	- hypersensitivity to clindamycin or lincomycin - infants <30 days
chloramphenicol	- GP - GN - anaerobes	inhibits peptidyl transferase action on tRNA at 50S ribosome	- aplastic anemia - grey baby syndrome	serious infections by susceptible organisms when suitable alternatives are not available	- hypersensitivity to chloramphenicol
linezolid (Zyvoxam™)	- GP including VRE + MRSA	binds 50S to prevent functional 70S initiation complex	- HTN (acts as MAOI) - risks with prolonged use: myelosuppression optic neuropathy, peripheral neuropathy	vancomycin-resistant *Enterococcus faecium* infections including intra-abdominal, skin and skin-structure, and urinary tract infections, MRSA infections as out patient therapy	- hypersensitivity to linezolid
PROTEIN SYNTHESIS INHIBITORS (30S RIBOSOME)					
Aminoglycosides					
gentamicin tobramycin[c] neomycin streptomycin amikacin (Amikin™)	- GN ([c]includes Pseudomonas)	binds 30S, causing mRNA misread	- nephrotoxicity - ototoxicity	UTIs, used in low doses for synergy with beta-lactams or with vancomycin in infective endocarditis intra-abdominal and gynecological infections, ?? sepsis	- hypersensitivity or previous ototoxic reaction to aminoglycosides
Tetracyclines					
tetracycline (Apo-Tetra™, Nu-TetraT™) minocycline (MinocinT™) doxycycline[D] (Doxycin™)	- GP - anaerobes - atypicals: Chlamydia, Mycoplasma, Rickettsia, Borrelia burgdorferi - Treponema - [D]malaria prophylaxis	blocks A site of 30S ribosome	- GI upset - hepatotoxicity - Fanconi's syndrome - photosensitivity - teratogenic - yellow teeth and stunted bone	Rickettsial infections, Chlamydia, acne (tetracycline); PID (step-down), malaria prophylaxis (doxycycline) infections growth in children	- hypersensitivity to any tetracycline - severe renal or hepatic dysfunction - pregnancy or lactation - children under 8 years

Table 26. Antibiotics (continued)

Class & Drugs	Coverage	Mechanism of Action	Adverse effects	Indications	Contraindications
TOPOISOMERASE INHIBITORS					
Fluoroquinolones					
ciprofloxacin[E] (Cipro™) norfloxacin (Apo-Norflox™) ofloxacin (Floxin™) Respiratory FQs: levofloxacin (Levaquin™) moxifloxacin[F] (Avelox™)	- poor GP activity - GN ([E] includes *Pseudomonas*) - same as above - more GP coverage than ciprofloxacin - atypicals - [F]includes anaerobes - no pseudomonas coverage	inhibits DNA gyrase	- H/A, dizziness - allergy - seizures - prolonged QT - teratogenic - dysglycemia	only use when necessary to prevent resistance; RTI, sinusitis (not ciprofloxacin unless susceptible organism isolated), UTI, prostatitis, bone and joint infections, skin and soft tissue infections, infectious diarrhea, eradication of meningococci in carriers, intra-abdominal infections, febrile neutropenia (ciprofloxacin), uncomplicated UTI (norfloxacin), pneumonia (respiratory quinolones)	- hypersensitivity to quinolones
rifampin	- GPC - *N. meningitidis* - *H. influenza* - *Mycobacteria*	inhibits RNA polymerase	- hepatic dysfunction, ↑P450 - orange tears/saliva/urine	part of treatment for active TB, alone for treatment of latent TB, part of treatment of other mycobacterial infections, endocarditis involving prosthetic valve, prophylaxis for those exposed to people with *N. meningitidis* or HiB meningitis	- jaundice - hypersensitivity to rifamycins
metronidazole (Flagyl™)	- anaerobes - Protozoa (see Table 21)	forms toxic metabolites in bacterial cell which damage microbial DNA	- disulfiram-type rxn with EtOH - seizures - peripheral neuropathy	protozoal infections (trichomonas, amebiasis, giardiasis), bacterial vaginosis, serious intra-abdominal infections	- hypersensitivity to metronidazole
ANTI-METABOLITE					
trimethoprim-sulfamethoxazole (TMP/SMX) (Septra™, Bactrim™)	- GP - GN: enteric - *Nocardia* - other: *Pneumocystis, Toxoplasmosis*	inhibits folic acid production (TMP inhibits DHFR and SMX is a competitive inhibitor of PABA)	- hepatitis - Stevens Johnson syndrome - TMP: megaloblastic anemia leuko/granulocytopenia hyperkalemia - SMX: hypersensitivity hemolysis if G6PD def interstitial nephritis BM suppression	susceptible UTI, RTI, GI infections, skin and soft tissue infections, treatment and prophylaxis of PCP	- hypersensitivity to TMP-SMX - megaloblastic anemia - hepatic parenchymal disease - blood dyscrasias, porphyria
nitrofurantoin (MacroBID™, (Macrodantin™)	- enterococcus, S. saprophyticus - GN (coliforms)	breaks bacterial DNA strands	- cholestasis, hepatitis - hemolysis in G6PD def - interstitial lung disease with chronic use	lower UTI; not pyelonephritis or bacteremia	- hypersensitivity to nitrofurantoin - anuria, oliguria or significant renal impairment - pregnant patients during labor and delivery or when labor imminent - infants under 1 month of age
ANTI-MYCOBACTERIALS					
isoniazid (INH)	- Mycobacteria	inhibits mycolic acid synthesis	- hepatitis - drug-induced SLE - peripheral neuropathy	part of treatment for active TB, alone for treatment of latent TB	- hypersensitivity to isoniazid - drug-induced hepatitis or acute liver disease
rifampin (RIF)	- GPC - *N. meningitidis* - *H. influenzae* - *Mycobacteria*	inhibits RNA polymerase	- hepatic dysfunction, ↑P450 - orange tears, saliva, urine	part of treatment for active TB, alone for treatment of latent TB, part of treatment of other mycobacterial infections, endocarditis involving prosthetic valve, prophylaxis for those exposed to people with *N. meningitidis* or HiB meningitis	- jaundice - hypersensitivity to rifamycins
ethambutol	- Mycobacteria	inhibits mycolic acid synthesis	- loss of central and colour vision	part of treatment for active TB and other mycobacterial infections	- hypersensitivity to ethambutol - optic neuritis unless benefits outweigh risk - renal failure
pyrazinamide (PZA)	- Mycobacteria	unknown	- hepatotoxicity - gout - gastric irritation	part of treatment for active TB	- hypersensitivity to pyrazinamide - severe hepatic damage or acute liver disease - patients with acute gout
Sulfones - dapsone - sulfoxone	- M. Leprae, part of treatment for PCP (with TMP), PCP prophylaxis, Toxoplasmosis prophylaxis with pyrimethamine	competitive inhibitor of PABA	- rash - drug fever - agranulocytosis		
clofazimine	- M. Leprae	binds M. leprae DNA	- skin discolouration		

Prevent INH-induced peripheral neuropathy with vitamin B6 (pyridoxine).

Reasons for Combination Therapy
- Prevention of resistance (e.g. TB, HIV)
- Synergistic action (e.g. beta-lactam and aminoglycosides for enterococci)
- Broad spectrum coverage (e.g. unidentified pathogen or polymicrobial infections)

Cephalosporin			
	GP	GN	CNS
1°	+++	+	x
2°	+	+	x
3°	+	+++	√
4°	+++	+++	√

Clindamycin has good tissue penetration, even into bone.

Chloramphenicol easily penetrates BBB.

Tetracycline and minocycline excellent secretion into dermis.

Rifampin
- good adjunct for treating prosthetic device infection (bacterial biofilm)
- always used in combination with other Abx to reduce emergence of resistance

TMP/SMX-induced granulocytopenia may be alleviated with folinic acid supplementation.

Table 27. Antibiotics for difficult bacteria

Pseudomonas	S.aureus	Enterococcus	H. Flu	Anaerobes
ciprofloxacin	cloxacillin	ampicillin	amoxicillin-clavulinate	metronidazole
tobramycin	1° cephalosporin	amoxicillin	2°/3° cephalosporin	clindamycin
piperacillin/tazobactam	clindamycin	vancomycin	macrocides	amoxicillin-clavulinate
ceftazidime	vancomycin	nitrofurantoin (UTI)	levofloxacin	cefoxitin
cefipime			moxifloxacin	cefotetan
meropenem				
imipenem				

Antivirals

Table 28. Antivirals

Class & Drugs	Coverage	Mechanism of Action	Adverse effects	Contraindications
anti-Herpesvirus				
acyclovir valacyclovir (ValtrexT™) (prodrug of acyclovir)	- HSV-1,2 - VZV	Guanosine analog inhibits viral DNA polymerase	- PO well-tolerated - IV: nephrotoxicity, CNS	- hypersensitivity to acyclovir or valacyclovir
famcilovir (Famvir™) penciclovir	- HSV-1,2 - VZV		- H/A, nausea	- hypersensitivity to famciclovir or penciclovir
ganciclovir (Cytovene™) valganciclovir (prodrug of ganciclovir)	- CMV - HSV-1,2, VZV		- Heme: neutropenia, thrombocytopenia, anemia - GI: N/V, diarrhea	- hypersensitivity to ganciclovir or valganciclovir - possible cross-hypersensitivity between acyclovir and valacyclovir
foscarnet	- CMV - Acyclovir-resistant HSV, VZV	Pyrophosphate analog inhibits viral DNA polymerase	- nephrotoxicity (reversible) - anemia, electrolyte disturbances	
other antivirals				
interferon- PEG-interferon- α 2a, 2b	- Chronic hep B, hep C - Condyloma acuminata	Inhibits viral protein synthesis	- "flu-like" syndrome - depression - bone marrow suppression	-hypersensitivity to any interferon - cannot use in combination with ribavirin if renal impairment
Ribavirin (Virazole™)	- Chronic hep C - RSV - Lassa fever	Guanosine analog with multiple postulated mechanisms of action	- hemolytic anemia - rash, conjunctivitis - highly teratogenic	- pregnancy or women who may become pregnant
lamivudine (3TC™, Heptovir™)	- Chronic hep B - HIV	See HIV/AIDS section		- hypersensitivity to lamivudine
M2 inhibitors: amantadine (Endantadine™, Symmetrel™) rimandadine	- Influenza A: treatment and prophylaxis	Inhibits viral uncoating after infection of cell	- anti-cholinergic effects - CNS: anxiety, insomnia, H/A, dizziness, difficulty concentrating	- hypersensitivity to the drug
Neuraminidase inhibitors: zanamavir oseltamavir (Tamiflu™)	- Influenza A & B: treatment and prophylaxis	Inhibits neuraminidase, an enzyme required for release of virus from infected cells and prevention of viral aggregation	- GI: N/V, diarrhea - bronchospasm in Zanamavir (rare)	- hypersensitivity to the drug

Antifungals

Table 29. Antifungals

Class & Drugs	Coverage	Mechanism of Action	Adverse effects	Contraindications
Polyenes				
amphotericin B	- systemic mycoses: *histoplasmosis, blastomycosis, coccidiomycosis* - pulmonary: *aspergillosis* - CNS: *cryptococcus*	A polyene antimicrobial: inserts into fungal cytoplasmic membrane causing altered membrane permeability and cell death	- nephrotoxicity - infusion reactions: chills, fevers, H/A - peripheral phlebitis	
nystatin	- candidiasis: mucocutaneous, GI, oral (thrush), vaginal		- GI: N/V, diarrhea	- hypersensitivity to nystatin
Imidazoles				
clotrimazole (Canesten™)	- oral and vulvovaginal candidiasis - dermatomycoses	All azoles: inhibit ergosterol synthesis and thereby alter fungal cell membrane permeability	- pruritis, skin irritation	- hypersensitivity to clotrimazole
miconazole (Monistat™, Micozole™)	- vulvovaginal candidiasis - dermatomycoses		- vaginal burning - N/V	- hypersensitivity to miconazole
ketoconazole (Apo-ketoconazole™, Nizoral™)	- dermatomycoses - seborrheic dermatitis		- pruritis, skin irritation - GI nonspecific	- hypersensitivity to ketoconazole, cross-sensitivity with other azoles possible - hepatic dysfunction - pregnant women or those that may become pregnant
Triazoles				
fluconazole (Diflucan™)	- candidiasis - cryptococcal meningitis	All azoles: inhibit ergosterol synthesis and thereby alter fungal cell membrane permeability	- elevated liver enzymes - GI nonspecific	- hypersensitivity to fluconazole, cross-sensitivity with other azoles unknown - concurrent use of terfenadine if dose of fluconazole >400 mg
itraconazole (Sporanox™)	- candidiasis - systemic mycoses: *histoplasmosis, blastomycosis, paracoccidiomycosis* - onychomycoses, coccidioidomycosis		- elevated liver enzymes - rash - GI nonspecific	- hypersensitivity to itraconazole, cross-sensitivity with other azoles unknown - severe ventricular dysfunction
voriconazole (Vfend™)	- aspergillosis - candidiasis		- visual disturbance (30%) - hepatotoxicity - rash	- hypersensitivity to voriconazole, cross-sensitivity with other azoles unknown - may avoid or alter doses if co-administered with other CYP3A4 substrates, rifampin, carbamazepine, long-acting barbiturates, ritonavir, efavirenz, sirolimus, rifabutin, ergot alkaloids
Allylamines				
terbinafine (Lamisil™)	- dermatomycoses - onychomycoses	Inhibits enzyme needed for ergosterol synthesis	- rash, local irritation - GI nonspecific	- hypersensitivity to terbinafine
Echinocandins				
caspofungin	- failed aspergillosis, candidemia, febrile neutropenia - azole-resistant Candida	Inhibits 1-3 beta-glycan synthesis	- hepatotoxicity	

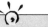

Lipid-complex or liposomal amphotericin B
For patients who are intolerant of conventional amphotericin B therapy (e.g. renal impairment)

Antiparasitics

Table 30. Antiparasitics

Class & Drugs	Coverage	Mechanism of Action	Adverse effects	Contraindications
Antimalarials				
chloroquine	- Malaria: treatment of erythrocytic phase of all five species of *Plasmodium* that infect humans Note high resistance of *P. falciparum* and *P. vivax* in certain geographic areas	Inhibit parasite heme polymerase	- CNS: blurred vision, retinopathy, dizziness - GI nonspecific (rare with prophylaxis)	- hypersensitivity to chloroquine or other 4-aminoquinoline - retinal or visual field changes due to 4-aminoquinoline
quinine	- Malaria: treatment of all four species of *Plasmodium* that infect humans, including Chloroquine-resistant *P. falciparum*		- cinchonism: ears (tinnitus, vertigo), eyes (visual disturbance), GI (N/V diarrhea), CNS (H/A, fever) - hypoglycemia	- hypersensitivity to quinine, may be cross-sensitivity with quinidine - patients with G6PD deficiency, tinnitus, optic neuritis, hypoglycemia, history of blackwater fever or thrombocytopenic purpura due to quinine use
mefloquine (Lariam™)	- Malaria: treatment and prophylaxis of all four species of *Plasmodium* that infect humans		- CNS/Psych: irritability, nightmares, psychoses, suicide, depression, seizures, H/A	- history of seizures, psychosis, severe anxiety or depression
primaquine	- Malaria: treatment of liver hypnozoites of *P. vivax* and *P. ovale*. Prophylaxis of all *Plasmodium* species - *Pneumocystis carinii* (with clindamycin)	Interferes with mitochondrial function	- hemolytic anemia in G6PD deficient - GI upset (take with food)	- GI nonspecific - G6PD deficiency - concurrent or recent use of quinacrine - pregnancy
atovaquone/proguanil (Malarone™)	- Malaria: treatment and prophylaxis of *P. falciparum*	Inhibits mitochondrial electron transport and dihydrofolate reductase	- N/V, anorexia, diarrhea, abdo pain (take with food)	- hypersensitivity to atovaquone or proguanil - severe renal impairment
doxycycline → see Antibiotics section				
Other anti-protozoal				
iodoquinol (Diodoquin™)	- Amebiasis: *E. histolytica, Dientamoeba fragilis, Balantidium coli, Blastocystis hominis*	Contact amoebicide that acts in intestinal lumen by uncertain mechanism	- GI: N/V, diarrhea, abdo pain - CNS: H/A, seizures, encephalitis	- hypersensitivity to any 8-hydroxy-quinoline or iodine - patients with hepatic damage or optic neuropathy
metronidazole → see Antibiotics section				
Anti-helminth				
praziquantel	- *Schistosomiasis* and other flukes - Tapeworms	Increases Ca permeability of helminth cell membrane, causing paralysis and detachment	- N/V, fever, dizziness	
albendazole	- intestinal roundworms - *Neurocysticercosis* - *Microsporidiosis* - *Echinococcus* → Hydatid disease	Inhibits glucose uptake into susceptible parasites	- elevated liver enzymes - alopecia - GI nonspecific - agranulocytosis	- pregnancy
mebendazole (Vermox™)	- intestinal round worms: - pinworm - whipworm - hookworm - roundworm		- GI nonspecific	- pregnancy
ivermectin	- *Strongyloidiasis* - *Onchocerciasis*			

NP Nephrology

Tamer Abdelshaheed, Warren Cheung and Ana Florescu, chapter editors
Deepti Damaraju and Elliott Owen, associate editors
Erik Venos, EBM editor
Dr. Ramesh Prasad and Dr. Martin Schreiber, staff editors

Basic Anatomy Review

Anatomy of the Kidney

- see Urology, U2

Renal Structure and Function

The Nephron
- basic structural and functional unit of the kidney, approximately 1 million per kidney
- 2 main components: glomerulus (filtration) and attached renal tubule (reabsorption/secretion)
- direction of blood flow: afferent arteriole, glomerular capillaries, efferent arteriole, vasa recta (the capillaries surrounding the tubules), renal venules
- filtration occurs across the glomerular basement membrane into Bowman's space
- reabsorption and secretion occur between the renal tubules and vasa recta (see Figure 1)

The Glomerulus
- site where blood constituents are filtered through to the kidney tubules for excretion or reabsorption
- consists of following cell types:
    - capillary endothelial cells, podocytes, mesangial cells
- functions of the cell types:
    - capillary endothelial cells and podocytes
        - support the glomerular basement membrane (GBM) and form the plasma filtration apparatus
    - mesangial cells
        - contractile properties and production of vasoactive substances help control the blood flow
    - parietal epithelium
        - covers the interior of Bowman's capsule
- filtration barrier: consists of capillary endothelium, GBM, podocyte filtration slits
    - particles are selectively filtered by size (<60 kD) and charge (negative charge repelled)

Table 1. Major Functions of the Kidneys

Function	Mechanism	Affected Elements
Waste Excretion	Glomerular filtration	Nitrogenous products of protein metabolism (urea, Cr)
	Tubular secretion	Organic acids (urate) Organic bases (Cr)
	Tubular catabolism	Drugs (antibiotics, diuretics) Peptide hormones (most pituitary hormones, insulin, glucagon)
Electrolyte Balance	Tubular NaCl absorption Tubular water reabsorption Tubular K secretion Tubular H secretion HCO_3 synthesis and reabsorption Tubular Ca, Mg, PO_4 transport	Volume status, osmolar balance Osmolar balance Potassium concentration Acid-base balance Ca, Mg, PO_4 homeostasis
Hormonal Synthesis	Erythropoietin production (cortex) Vitamin D activation Renin production (JG apparatus)	Red blood cell mass Calcium homeostasis Vascular resistance, aldosterone secretion
Blood Pressure Regulation	Altered sodium excretion Renin production	ECF volume Vascular resistance
Glucose Homeostasis	Gluconeogenesis (from lactate, pyruvate, amino acids)	Glucose supply maintained in prolonged starvation

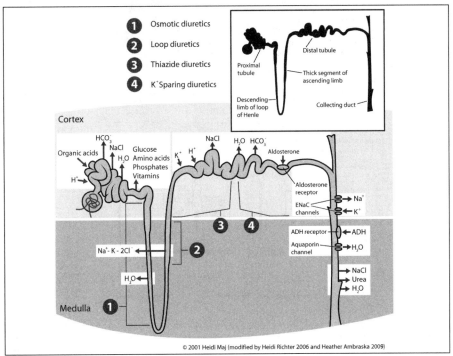

Figure 1. Nephron components

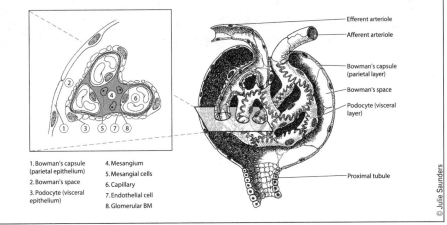

Figure 2. The Glomerulus

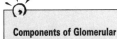

**Components of Glomerular
Filtration Barrier**
1. Capillary endothelial cells
2. Glomerular basement membrane
3. Visceral epithelial cells (podocytes)

Filtration is based on charge and pore
size.

Renal Hemodynamics

- Renal Blood Flow (RBF): 20% of cardiac output = 1000 mL/minute
- Renal Plasma Flow (RPF) = RBF x (1 – hematocrit) = 600 mL/minute
    - measured using urine and plasma para-aminohippuric acid (PAH)
    - RPF = $\dfrac{\text{urine (PAH) x urine volume}}{\text{plasma (PAH)}}$
- Glomerular Filtration Rate (GFR)
    - rate of fluid transfer between glomerular capillaries and Bowman's space
    - the result of outwardly directed net pressure governed by hydrostatic (P) and osmotic (π) pressure gradients that move fluid across the semipermeable capillary wall
    - GFR= K_f (P – π) (K_f= ultrafiltration coefficient)
    - 120 ml/min in healthy adult = 173 L/day, of which 98% is reabsorbed, giving a daily urine output 1.0-1.5 L
    - highest in early adulthood, decreasing thereafter
- renal autoregulation maintains a constant GFR over a range of mean arterial pressures (70-180 mmHg)
    - myogenic mechanism: release of vasoactive factors in response to alterations in perfusion pressure
        - rise in perfusion pressure causes afferent arteriolar constriction leading to a decrease in GFR
    - tubuloglomerular feedback: changes in Na delivery to macula densa control afferent arteriolar tone

- Filtration Fraction (FF)
  - percentage of RPF filtered across the glomeruli
  - expressed as a ratio: FF = GFR/RPF, normal = 0.2 or 20%
  - angiotensin II (AII) causes constriction of renal efferent arterioles which increases FF thereby maintaining GFR
- renin is released from juxtaglomerular apparatus in response to decreased RBF

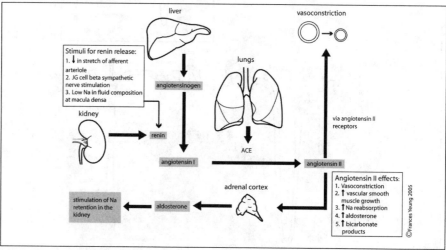

Figure 3. Stimuli for Renin Release

Differential Diagnoses of Common Presentations

Azotemia

Definition
- a higher than normal BUN and Cr usually caused by inability of the kidney to excrete urea or other nitrogen-containing compounds in the blood.

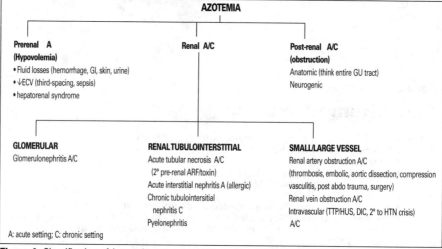

Figure 4. Classification of Azotemia

Proteinuria

- **24 hour urine protein is gold standard to assess degree of proteinuria**
- the urine albumin to creatinine ratio (ACR) is used to screen for diabetic nephropathy
  - an elevated ACR (>30 mg/mmol) is the earliest sign of diabetic nephropathy
- composition of normal total urine protein
  - 60% filtered plasma protein: (50% albumin, 15% Ig, 5% other)
  - 40% Tamm-Horsfall mucoprotein secreted from tubular cells

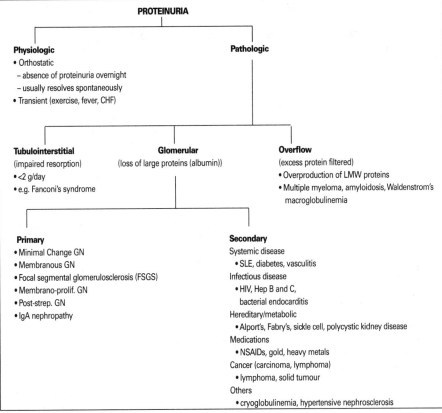

Figure 5. Classification of Proteinuria

PATHOLOGIC PROTEINURIA

1) TUBULOINTERSTITIAL
- normally low molecular weight proteins (<60 kD) pass through glomerular filtration barrier and are reabsorbed in proximal tubule
- proximal tubule dysfunction causes impaired resorption and increased excretion of LMWP
- albumin (>60 kD) is NOT affected. Thus, edema is partly secondary to salt and water retention

2) GLOMERULAR
- normally, the filtration barrier is selectively permeable to SIZE (<60 kD) and CHARGE (repels negative particles). Thus, albumin is NOT filtered through a normal glomerulus
- damage to any component of the glomerular filtration barrier results in loss of albumin and other high MW protein. Thus, edema is secondary to hypoalbuminemia (low oncotic pressure)

3) OVERFLOW
- increased production of low molecular weight proteins which exceeds the resorptive capacity of the proximal tubule
- plasma cell dyscrasias: produce light chain Ig (multiple myeloma, Waldenstrom's, monoclonal gammopathy of undetermined significance)

Table 2. Daily Excretion of Protein

Daily Excretion	Meaning
<150 mg total protein (and <30 mg albumin)	Normal
30-300 mg albumin	Microalbuminuria
>3500 mg total protein Variable amount of proteinuria	Nephrotic range proteinuria Can be seen with glomerular disease; i.e. mild glomerular disease can lead to a mild degree of proteinuria, proliferative lesions may also be associated with some degree of proteinuria
Up to 2000 mg per day	Possible with tubular disease because of failure to reabsorb filtered proteins

Investigations
- Hx and Px: look for signs and symptoms suggestive of transient physiological or secondary causes (diabetes, CHF, collagen-vascular disease, malignancy)
- urine R&M, C&S, urea, Cr
- further workup (if casts and/or hematuria):
  - CBC, glucose, electrolytes, 24hr urine protein and Cr
  - urine and serum immunoelectrophoresis, abdo/pelvic ultrasound
  - serology: ANA, RF, p-ANCA, c-ANCA, Hep B, Hep C, HIV, ASOT

Hematuria

Definition
- presence of blood or RBCs in urine
  - gross hematuria: pink, red, or tea-coloured urine
    - in gross hematuria, the urine should be centrifuged
    - it is hematuria if only the sediment is red
    - if the supernatant is red, it should be tested for heme with a dipstick
    - if +ve for heme – myoglobinuria or hemoglobinuria
    - if –ve for heme – medications (e.g. rifampin), food dyes (e.g. beets) or metabolites (e.g. porphyria)
  - microscopic hematuria: normal coloured urine, >5 RBCs/HPF on microscopy

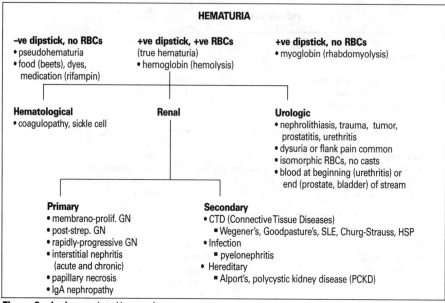

Figure 6. An Approach to Hematuria

Investigations for Hematuria
- Hx and Px: family history of nephrolithiasis, hearing loss (Alport's), cerebral aneurysm (PCKD), diet, recent URTI, dysuria
- urine R&M, C&S, urea, Cr
- 24 h urine stone workup: calcium, oxalate, citrate, magnesium, uric acid, cysteine
- further workup (if casts and/or proteinuria): CBC, electrolytes, 24 hr urine protein and Cr, serology: ANA, RF, C3, C4, p-ANCA, c-ANCA, ASOT, abdo/pelvic ultrasound, cystoscopy ± urology consult

Volume Overload

- volume overload due to renal impairment can manifest as either secondary hypertension and/or generalized edema
  - for a list of the secondary causes of hypertension, see <u>Family Medicine</u>
  - for the differential diagnosis of generalized edema, see <u>Cardiology</u>

Assessment of Renal Function

Measurement of Renal Function

- GFR = rate of filtration of plasma by the glomeruli
- most renal functions decline in parallel with a decrease in GFR
- GFR is often estimated using serum creatinine concentrations [Cr]
- creatinine (Cr) is a metabolite of creatine (intermediate in muscle energy metabolism)
- Cr is freely filtered at the glomerulus with no tubular reabsorption and minimal secretion (10%)
- rate of production determined by muscle mass
- Cr excreted = Cr filtered (at steady state)

Ways to estimate GFR
- must be in steady state – constant GFR and rate of production of Cr from muscles

1. Calculate Creatinine Clearance (CrCl)
- calculation provides reasonable estimate of GFR
- requires blood and 24 hour urine samples; measure plasma [Cr], 24 hour urine volume and urine [Cr]
  - GFR = urine [Cr] x urine volume/plasma [Cr] x duration of urine collection in minutes
  - therefore GFR is proportional to 1/plasma [Cr]
- 2 major errors limiting the accuracy of CrCl:
  - increasing Cr secretion can overestimate true GFR, particularly in azotemic patients
  - incomplete urine collection can underestimate true GFR; over-collection of urine overestimates it

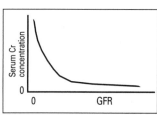

Figure 7. Serum Creatinine Concentration as a Function of GFR

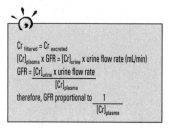

$Cr_{filtered} = Cr_{excreted}$

$[Cr]_{plasma}$ x GFR = $[Cr]_{urine}$ x urine flow rate (mL/min)

$GFR = \dfrac{[Cr]_{urine} \text{ x urine flow rate}}{[Cr]_{plasma}}$

therefore, GFR proportional to $\dfrac{1}{[Cr]_{plasma}}$

2. Cockcroft-Gault formula
- serum Cr used along with age, gender and weight (kg) to estimate GFR
  - CrCl (ml/min) = (140 – age)(weight) x 1.2 / plasma [Cr] (μmol/L)
    - the formula in US units with Cr in mg/dl:
      CrCl (mg/dl) = (140 – age)(body mass)/(plasma [Cr] x 72)
  - multiply above result by 0.85 for women
  - normal range is >90 ml/min (>1.5 ml/s)

3. MDRD (Modification of Diet in Renal Disease) formula
- most common way in which GFR is estimated
- this is a complex formula requiring information on the following variables:
  - age
  - gender
  - serum Cr
  - African descent
- most helpful way to use this formula is by entering values into online calculators (www.ukidney.com)
- GFR is reported as ml/min/1.73m^2 body surface area

Limitations of use of serum Cr measurements
1) must be in steady state
   - sudden injury may reduce GFR substantially, but it takes time for Cr to accumulate and then re-establish steady state
2) GFR must fall substantially before plasma [Cr] rises above normal laboratory range (see Figure 7)
   - with progressive renal failure, remaining nephrons compensate with hyperfiltration
   - GFR is relatively preserved despite significant structural damage
3) plasma [Cr] is influenced by the rate of Cr production
   - lower production with smaller muscle mass (i.e. female, elderly, low weight) e.g. consider plasma [Cr] of 100 μmol/L in both of these patients
     - 20 year-old man who weighs 100 kg, GFR = 144 mL/min
     - 80 year-old woman who weighs 50 kg, GFR = 30.6 mL/min
4) contribution of tubular secretion to Cr excretion is increased when GFR is low
   - CrCl overestimates GFR
   - certain drugs (cimetidine, trimethoprim) interfere with Cr secretion
5) errors in Cr measurement
   - very high bilirubin level causes [Cr] to be falsely low
   - acetoacetate (a ketone body) and certain drugs (cefoxitin) create falsely high [Cr]

Measurement of Urea Concentration
- urea is the major end product of protein metabolism
- plasma urea concentration is a measurement of renal function
- it is modified by a variety of factors and should not be used alone as a test of renal function
- urea production reflects dietary intake of protein and catabolic rate
- increased protein intake or catabolism (sepsis, trauma, GI bleed) causes urea level to rise
- ECF volume depletion causes a rise in urea independent of GFR or plasma [Cr]
- in addition to filtration, a significant amount of urea is reabsorbed along the tubule
- reabsorption is increased in sodium-avid states such as ECF volume depletion
- typical ratio of urea to [Cr] in serum is 1:20 in Canadian units (using mmol/L for urea and μmol/L for Cr), and 5:1 in US units (Cr in mg/dl)

Urinalysis

- use dipstick in freshly voided urine specimen to assess the following:

1) Specific Gravity
- ratio of the mass of equal volumes of urine/H_2O
- values <1.010 reflect dilute urine, values >1.020 reflect concentrated urine

2) pH
- urine pH is normally between 4.5-7.0; if persistently alkaline, consider:
  - renal tubular acidosis
  - UTI with urease-producing bacteria (e.g. *Proteus*)

3) Glucose
- freely filtered at glomerulus and reabsorbed in proximal tubule
- causes of glucosuria include:
  1) hyperglycemia >9-11 mmol/L (>160-200 mg/dl) exceeds tubular resorption capacity
  2) increased GFR (e.g. pregnancy)
  3) proximal tubule dysfunction (e.g. Fanconi's syndrome)

Cockcroft-Gault Formula
CrCl (ml/min) =
$\frac{(140\text{-age}) \times \text{wt (kg)} \times 1.2}{[Cr]_{plasma} \text{ (umol/L)}}$ (x 0.85 in women)

There is an inverse relationship between serum Cr concentration and CrCl at steady state.

Clinical Settings in which Urea is Affected Independent of Renal Function

Disproportionate increase in Urea
Volume depletion (prerenal azotemia)
GI hemorrhage
High protein diet
Sepsis
Catabolic state with tissue breakdown
Corticosteroid or cytotoxic agents

Disproportionate decrease in Urea
Low protein diet
Liver disease

Urine Collection
1. discard first morning specimen
2. collect all subsequent urine through the day and night
3. refrigerate between voids
4. collect second morning specimen

Last 2 digits of the specific gravity x 30 = urine osmolality approximately e.g. specific gravity of 1.020 = 600 mOsm.

4) Protein
- dipstick only detects albumin; other proteins (e.g. Bence-Jones, Ig, Tamm-Horsfall) may be missed
- microalbuminuria (defined as 30-300 mg/day) is not detected by standard dipstick (see *Diabetes and the Kidney* section, NP35)
- sulfosalicylic acid detects all protein in urine by precipitation
- gold standard is the 24 hour urine collection for total protein

5) Leukocyte Esterase
- enzyme found in WBC and detected by dipstick
- presence of WBCs indicates infection (e.g. UTI) or inflammation (e.g. AIN)
- +ve dipstick for leukocyte esterase and nitrites is 94% specific for diagnosing a UTI

6) Nitrites
- nitrates in urine are converted by bacteria to nitrites
- high specificity, low sensitivity for UTI

7) Ketones
- positive in alcoholic/diabetic ketoacidosis, prolonged starvation, fasting

8) Hemoglobin
- positive in hemoglobinuria (hemolysis), myoglobinuria (rhabdomyolysis) and true hematuria (RBCs seen on microscopy)

Urine Microscopy

- centrifuge urine specimen for 3-5 minutes, discard supernatant, resuspend sediment and plate on slide
- shaking tube vigorously may disrupt casts

1) CELLS

Erythrocytes
- normal range – 2-5 RBCs per high power field (HPF)
- hematuria = greater than 5 RBCs/HPF
- dysmorphic RBCs and/or RBC casts suggest glomerular bleeding (e.g. glomerulonephritis)
- isomorphic RBCs, no casts suggest extraglomerular bleeding (e.g. bladder Ca)

Leukocytes
- normal range – up to 3 WBCs/HPF
- pyuria = greater than 3 WBCs/HPF
- indicates inflammation or infection
- if persistent sterile pyuria present (i.e. negative culture), consider: chronic urethritis, prostatitis, interstitial nephritis, calculi, papillary necrosis, renal TB, viral infections

Eosinophils
- detected using Wright's or Hansel's stain (not affected by urine pH)
- consider allergic interstitial nephritis, atheroembolic disease

Oval Fat Bodies
- renal tubular cells filled with lipid droplets
- seen in heavy proteinuria (i.e. nephrotic syndrome)

2) CASTS
- cylindrical structures formed by intratubular precipitation of Tamm-Horsfall mucoprotein; cells may be trapped within the matrix of protein

Table 3. Interpretation of Casts

Hyaline casts	• Physiologic (concentrated urine, fever, exercise)
Red blood cell casts	• Glomerular bleeding (glomerulonephritis, vasculitis)
White blood cell casts	• Infection (pyelonephritis) • Inflammation (interstitial nephritis)
Pigmented granular casts (heme granular casts, muddy brown)	• Acute tubular necrosis • Glomerulonephritis, interstitial nephritis
Fatty casts	• Heavy proteinuria (>3.5g/day)

3) CRYSTALS
- uric acid – consider acid urine, hyperuricosuria (e.g. gout)
- calcium phosphate – alkaline urine
- calcium oxalate – consider hyperoxaluria, ethylene glycol poisoning
- sulfur – sulfa-containing antibiotics

Terminology:
Active versus Bland Sediment

	Active Sediment	Bland Sediment
Any one or more of the following seen on microscopy	• Red cell casts • White cell casts • Muddy-brown granular or epithelial cell casts • >2 red cells per high power field (hpf) • >4 white cells per hpf • Large quantities of uric acid, calcium oxalate, or calcium phosphate crystals	• Hyaline casts • <2 red cells per hpf • <4 white cells per hpf • Small quantities of crystals • Small amount of bacteria
Significance	Highly suggestive of significant pathology, casts specifically suggest renal pathology	Reduced likelihood of significant pathology, but not ruled out

Urine Electrolytes

- can use to evaluate the source of an electrolyte abnormality or grossly assess tubular function
- commonly measure: Na, K, Cl, osmolality and pH
- no 'normal' values; electrolyte excretion depends on intake and current physiological state
- therefore results must be interpreted in the context of a patient's current state, e.g.
  - (1) a patient who is clearly ECF volume depleted should have a low urine [Na] (kidneys should be retaining Na); a high urine [Na] in this setting suggests a renal problem or a diuretic; urine [Na] <10 mmol/L suggests the patient is prerenal
  - (2) daily urinary potassium excretion rate should be decreased (<20 mmol/d) in the setting of hypokalemia; if higher than 20 mmol/d, suggests renal etiology
- osmolality is useful to estimate the kidney's concentrating ability
- FE_{Na} refers to the fractional excretion of Na
  - FE_{Na} = Urine [Na] x Plasma [Cr]/{Plasma [Na] x Urine [Cr]} x 100
  - FE_{Na} <1% suggests the patient is prerenal

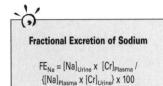

Fractional Excretion of Sodium

$$FE_{Na} = [Na]_{Urine} \times [Cr]_{Plasma} / \{[Na]_{Plasma} \times [Cr]_{Urine}\} \times 100$$

Examples of Common Urine Electrolyte Abnormalities

- high urine Na (>20 mmol/L) in the setting of acute renal failure: intrarenal disease, presence of non-reabsorbable anions (e.g. ketones), or action of diuretic including osmotic diuresis from glucose
- high urine Na (>40 mmol/L) in the setting of hyponatremia: diuretics, tubular disease (e.g. Bartter's syndrome), SIADH
- urine pH is useful to grossly assess renal acidification
  - "low" pH (<5.5) in the presence of low serum pH is an appropriate renal response
  - a high pH in this setting might indicate a renal acidification defect (e.g. RTA)

Electrolyte Disorders

Sodium Homeostasis

Introduction

- hyponatremia/hypernatremia are disorders of water balance
  - hyponatremia suggests too much water in the extracellular fluid relative to Na
  - hypernatremia is too little water in the extracellular fluid relative to Na
  - both can be associated with normal, decreased or increased total body Na
- ECF volume is determined by Na content, not Na concentration
  - Na deficiency leads to ECF volume depletion
  - Na excess leads to ECF volume expansion
- solutes (such as Na or glucose) that cannot freely traverse the plasma membrane (as does urea) contribute to effective osmolality and induce transcellular shifts of water
  - water moves out of cells in response to increased ECF osmolality
  - water moves into cells in response to decreased ECF osmolality
- clinical signs and symptoms of hyponatremia/hypernatremia are secondary to cells (especially in the brain) shrinking (hypernatremia) or swelling (hyponatremia)

Table 4. Clinical Assessment of ECF Volume (Total Body Na)

Fluid Compartment	Hypovolemic	Hypervolemic
Intravascular		
JVP	Decreased	Increased
Blood pressure	Orthostatic drop	Normal to increased
Auscultation of heart	Tachycardia	S3
Auscultation of lungs	Normal	Inspiratory crackles
Interstitial		
Skin turgor	Decreased	Normal/increased
Edema (dependent)	Absent	Present
Other		
Urine output	Decreased	Variable
Body weight	Decreased	Increased
Hct, serum protein	Increased	Decreased

Hyponatremia

- a decrease in serum [Na] to <136 mmol/L
- common clinical problem
- can be associated with increased, normal or decreased (most common) serum osmolality

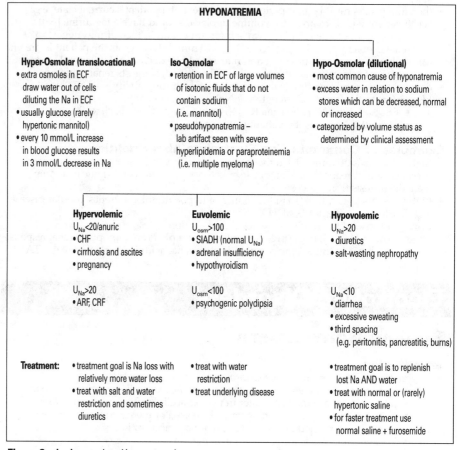

Figure 8. An Approach to Hyponatremia

Mechanisms of Hyponatremia

1. Hyponatremia despite dilute urine ($U_{osm} < 100$)
- expect urine to be dilute with hyponatremia (ADH should be suppressed)
- due to excessive water intake that overwhelms the kidneys' normal water excretion capacity
    - psychogenic polydipsia in psychiatric patients (e.g. schizophrenia)
- ability to excrete water is compromised in people with low solute excretion (particularly urea)
    - e.g. elderly women with "tea and toast" diet: low protein intake, low urea excretion

2. Hyponatremia with concentrated urine ($U_{osm} > 200$)
- if urine remains concentrated, ADH is acting when it should not be
- may be physiological (due to volume stimulus) or pathological (other reasons)
    - volume mediated ADH release can be due to true or effective volume depletion
    - causes of true volume depletion include losses from skin, GI, urine, blood or 3rd spacing
    - "effective" volume loss is seen with CHF and cirrhosis
    - pathological ADH release: SIADH and endocrine deficiency
    - adrenal insufficiency ($\downarrow$volume and co-secretion of ADH and CRH)
    - hypothyroidism ($\downarrow$cardiac output, $\downarrow$GFR)

3. Hyponatremia with no (or minimal) urine
- advanced renal failure with oliguria may be associated with hyponatremia if the patient ingests even a moderate amount of dilute fluids

---

Beware of Rapid Correction of Hyponatremia
- inadvertent rapid correction of hyponatremia can easily occur
    - e.g. patient with hyponatremia due to SIADH from nausea
    - Gravol™ given for relief of nausea
    - ADH quickly turned off in the absence of nausea, the kidneys rapidly excrete the excess free water, and the serum Na rises rapidly
    - patient at risk of osmotic demyelination
- high output dilute urine (>100 cc/hr, <100 mOsm/L) in the setting of hyponatremia is usually the first sign of dangerously rapid correction of serum sodium

Signs and Symptoms
- depend on degree of hyponatremia and more importantly, rapidity of onset
- acute hyponatremia (<24-48 hours) more likely to be symptomatic
- chronic hyponatremia (>24-48 hours) less likely to be symptomatic due to adaptation
    - adaptation: normalization of brain volume through loss of cellular electrolytes (within hrs) and organic osmolytes (within days)
    - adaptation is responsible for the risks associated with overly rapid correction
- neurologic symptoms predominate – secondary to cerebral edema
- headache, nausea, malaise, lethargy, weakness, muscle cramps, anorexia, somnolence disorientation, personality changes, depressed reflexes, decreased LOC

Complications
- seizures, coma, respiratory arrest, permanent brain damage, brainstem herniation, death
- risk of brain cell shrinkage with rapid correction of hyponatremia
    - can develop osmotic demyelination of pontine and extrapontine neurons, which may be irreversible (e.g. central pontine myelinolysis: cranial nerve palsies, quadriplegia, decreased LOC)

Patients at Particular Risk of Osmotic Demyelination
- those with associated
    - rise in serum Na with correction >8 mmol/L/d if chronic hyponatremia
    - hypokalemia
    - malnutrition
    - hyponatremia given large volume of fluid (stimulation of volume-mediated ADH release rapidly disappears causing sudden, brisk diuresis)
    - psychogenic polydipsia, deprived of water

Investigations
- ECF volume status assessment
- serum electrolytes, glucose, Cr
- serum osmolality
- urine osmolality
- urine Na <10-20 mmol/L suggests volume depletion as the cause of hyponatremia
- assess for causes of SIADH (see Table 5)
- thyroid function tests and cortisol levels
- consider CT chest if suspect pulmonary cause of SIADH

Treatment of Hyponatremia
- general measures for all patients:
    - water restrict (1 L/day)
    - treat underlying cause
    - monitor serum Na frequently to ensure correction is not occurring too rapidly
    - monitor urine output frequently: high output of dilute urine is the first sign of dangerously rapid correction of hyponatremia

Correction of sodium
Frequent monitoring of serum Na and urine output is essential when treating hyponatremia.

A. Definitely Acute (known to have developed over <24-48 hours)
- commonly occurs in hospital (dilute IV fluid + reason for ADH excess: e.g. post-operative)
- less risk to rapid correction since adaptation has not fully occurred
- if symptomatic
    - correct rapidly with 3% NaCl 1-2 cc/kg/h up to serum Na=125-130 mmol/L
    - may need furosemide to deal with volume overload
- if asymptomatic, treatment depends on severity; if there was a marked fall in plasma [Na] then patient is at high risk to become symptomatic, at low risk of harm from treatment, therefore treat as for symptomatic

B. Chronic or Unsure
1. if severe symptoms (seizures or decreased level of consciousness)
    - must partially correct acutely
    - aim for increase of Na by 1-2 mmol/L/hr for 4-6 hrs
    - limit total rise to 8 mmol/L in 24 hrs
    - IV 3% NaCl at 1-2 cc/kg/hr
    - may need furosemide
2. if asymptomatic
    - general measures as above
    - consider IV 0.9% normal saline (NS) + furosemide (reduces urine osmolality, augments excretion of electrolyte-free H_2O)
3. refractory
    - furosemide and IV NS
    - demeclocyline 300-600 mg PO bid (antagonizes effect of ADH on collecting duct)
    - extra osmoles - give oral urea (increases loss of water without Na)
    - slow rate of IV 3% NaCl (i.e. 10 cc/hr)

> **Concentration of Na in Common Infusates:**
> Na in 0.45% NaCl = 77 mmol/L
> Na in 0.9% NaCl = 154 mmol/L
> Na in 3% NaCl = 513 mmol/L
> Na in 5% NaCl = 855 mmol/L
> Na in Ringers lactate = 130 mmol/L
> Na in D5W = 0

C. Options if overly rapid correction occurs
- give water (i.e. switch to IV D5W)
- give ADH to stop water diuresis (DDAVP 5 µg SC)

Impact of IV Solution on Plasma Na
- formula to estimate the change in serum Na caused by retention of 1 L of any infusate (TBW = 0.6 x wt(kg) for men, 0.5 x wt(kg) for women)

$$\text{change in serum Na} = \frac{\text{infusate [Na]} - \text{serum [Na]}}{\text{TBW} + 1\ \text{L}}$$

- this formula assumes there are no losses of water or electrolytes

Syndrome of Inappropriate Antidiuretic Hormone Secretion (SIADH)
1. urine that is inappropriately concentrated for the serum osmolality
2. high urine sodium (>20-40 mmol/L)
3. high FE_{Na}

Table 5. Disorders Associated with SIADH

Tumour	Pulmonary	CNS	Drugs	Miscellaneous
Small cell Ca	Pneumonia	Mass lesion	**Antidepressants**	Post-op state
Bronchogenic Ca	Lung abscess	Encephalitis	TCAs	Pain
AdenoCa of pancreas	TB	Subarachnoid	SSRIs	Severe nausea
Hodgkin's disease	Acute respiratory	hemorrhage	**Antineoplastics**	HIV
Thymoma	failure	Stroke	Vincristine	
	Positive pressure	Head trauma	Cyclophosphamide	
	ventilation	Acute psychosis	**Other**	
		Acute intermittent	DDAVP	
		porphyria	Oxytocin	
			Nicotine	
			Carbamazepine	
			Barbiturates	
			Chlorpropamide	

Hypernatremia

- hypernatremia is defined as an increase in serum Na to >145 mmol/L
- too little water relative to total body Na; always a hyperosmolar state
- usually because of a net water loss, rarely due to hypertonic Na gain
- results from problems with water intake (access, thirst) and/or site of increased water loss (renal or extrarenal)
- less common than hyponatremia because protected against by thirst and release of ADH

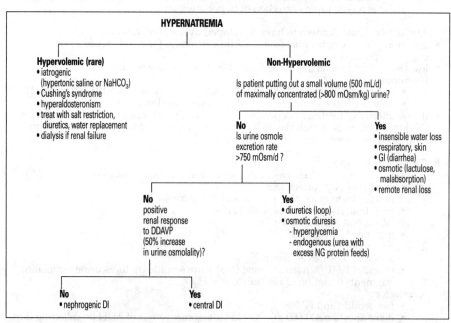

Figure 9. An Approach to Hypernatremia

Signs and Symptoms
- with acute hypernatremia no time for adaptation, therefore more likely to be symptomatic
- adaptive response: cells import and generate new osmotically active particles to normalize size
- due to brain cell shrinkage: altered mental status, weakness, neuromuscular irritability, focal neurologic deficits, seizures, coma, death; ± polyuria, thirst, signs of hypovolemia

Complications
- increased risk of vascular rupture resulting in intracranial hemorrhage
- rapid correction may lead to cerebral edema due to ongoing brain hyperosmolarity

Treatment of Hypovolemic Hypernatremia
- general measures for all patients:
    - salt restrict and give free water (oral or IV)
    - treat underlying cause
    - monitor serum Na frequently to ensure correction is not occurring too rapidly
- if evidence of hemodynamic instability, must first correct volume depletion with NS bolus
- loss of water is often accompanied by loss of Na but a proportionately larger water loss
- in patients with presumed normal total body Na, use formula to calculate water deficit:
$$H_2O \text{ deficit} = \frac{TBW \times (serum\ Na - 140)}{140} \quad (TBW = 0.6 \times wt(kg) \text{ for men}, 0.5 \times wt(kg) \text{ for women})$$
- replace free water deficit; "free water" is water without sodium
- encourage patient to drink pure water, as oral route is preferred for fluid administration
- if unable to replace PO or NG, correct H_2O deficit with hypotonic IV solution:
    - 1L D5W approximately equals 1 L free water
    - 1L 0.45% NS approximately equals 500 mL free water
- use formula (see *Hyponatremia* section, NP10) to estimate expected change in serum Na with 1L infusate
- administer fluids over appropriate time frame to lower Na by no more than 12 mmol/L in 24 hours (0.5 mmol/L/hr)
- must also provide maintenance fluids and replace ongoing losses

H_2O Deficit and TBW Equations

1) TBW = 0.6 x wt (kg) men, TBW = 0.5 x wt (kg) women

2) H_2O deficit = TBW x ([Na]$_{plasma}$- 140) / 140

Treatment of Hypervolemic Hypernatremia
- general measures as above
- hypervolemic hypernatremia: remove excess total body Na with diuresis or dialysis (if renal failure present), then replace water deficit using D5W

DIABETES INSIPIDUS (DI)
- collecting tubule is impermeable to water because of an absence of ADH or absence of response to ADH
- central defect in release of ADH (central DI) or renal responsiveness to ADH (nephrogenic DI)

Etiology
- central DI: neurosurgery, granulomatous diseases, trauma, vascular events, malignancy
- nephrogenic DI: lithium (most common), hypokalemia, hypercalcemia, congenital

Diagnosis
- urine osmolality inappropriately low (U_{osm}<750 mOsm/d)
- serum vasopressin concentration may be absent or low (central), or elevated (nephrogenic)
- dehydration test: H_2O deprivation for 12-18 h: if fails to concentrate urine, most likely DI
- administer DDAVP (exogenous ADH) (10 mg intranasally or 2 μg SC) :
    - central DI: rise in urine osmolality, fall in urine volume
        - treat with DDAVP
    - nephrogenic DI: exogenous ADH fails to concentrate urine as kidneys do not respond to ADH
        - treat with water (IV D5W or PO water), thiazides may help as well

Potassium Homeostasis

- approximately 98% of total body K stores are intracellular
- normal serum K ranges from 3.5-5.0 mEq/L
- in response to K load, rapid removal from ECF is necessary to prevent life-threatening hyperkalemia
- insulin, aldosterone, catecholamines and acid-base status influence K movement into cells
- potassium excretion is regulated at the distal nephron
    - K excretion = (urine flow rate) x (urine K concentration)

Factors which increase renal K loss

- hyperkalemia
- increased distal tubular urine flow rate and Na delivery (thiazides and loop diuretics)
- increased aldosterone via ENaC (Na in, K out)
- metabolic alkalosis
- hypomagnesemia
- increased non-reabsorbable anions in tubule lumen: HCO_3, penicillin, salicylate

Hypokalemia

- serum K <3.5 mEq/L

Approach to Hypokalemia

1. emergency measures: obtain ECG; if potentially life threatening begin treatment immediately
2. rule out transcellular shifts of K as cause of hypokalemia
3. assess contribution of dietary K intake
4. 24h K excretion or spot urine K
5. TTKG = transtubular potassium gradient = $(U_k/P_k)/(U_{osm}/P_{osm})$
6. if renal K loss, check BP and acid-base status
7. may also assess plasma renin and aldosterone levels, serum Mg

Signs and Symptoms

- usually asymptomatic, particularly when mild (3.0-3.5 mmol/L)
- nausea, vomiting, fatigue, generalized weakness, myalgia, muscle cramps, constipation
- if severe: arrhythmias, muscle necrosis, and rarely paralysis with eventual respiratory impairment
- arrhythmias occur at variable levels of K; more likely if: digoxin use, hypomagnesemia, CAD
- ECG changes are more predictive of clinical picture than K levels
    - U waves most important
    - flattened or inverted T waves
    - depressed ST segment
    - prolongation of Q-T interval
    - with severe hypokalemia: P-R prolongation, wide QRS, arrhythmias; increases risk of digitalis toxicity

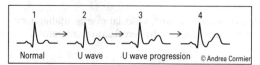

Figure 10. EKG Changes in Hypokalemia

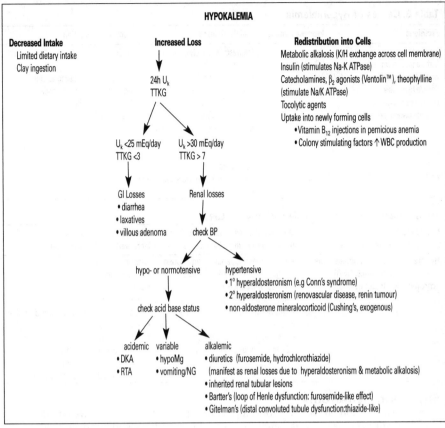

Figure 11. An Approach to Hypokalemia   *TTKG = Trans-Tubular K Gradient

Treatment

- treat underlying cause
- if urine output and renal function are impaired, correct with extreme caution
- risk of hyperkalemia especially high in elderly, diabetics, and patients with decreased renal function
- beware of excessive potassium repletion, especially if transcellular shift caused hypokalemia
- if true K deficit, potassium repletion (decrease in serum K of 1 mEq is approximately 100-200 mEq total body loss)
  - oral sources – food, tablets (K-Dur™), KCl liquid solutions
  - IV – usually KCl in saline solutions, avoid dextrose solutions (exacerbate hypokalemia via insulin release)
  - max 40 mmol/L via peripheral vein, 60 mmol/L via central vein, max infusion 20 mmol/hr
- K-sparing diuretics (triamterene, spironolactone, amiloride) can prevent renal K loss
- restore Mg if necessary

Hyperkalemia

- serum K >5.0 mEq/L

Approach to Hyperkalemia

1. emergency measures: obtain ECG, if life threatening begin treatment immediately
2. rule out factitious hyperkalemia; repeat blood test
3. hold exogenous K, and any K retaining medications
4. assess potential causes of transcellular shift
5. estimate GFR (calculate CrCl/use Cockcroft-Gault)
6. if normal GFR, calculate $TTKG = (U_k/P_k)/(U_{osm}/P_{osm})$
   - TTKG <7 = decreased effective aldosterone function
   - TTKG >7 = normal aldosterone function

Table 6. Causes of Hyperkalemia

Factitious	Increased Intake	Cellular Release	Decreased Excretion
Prolonged use of tourniquet	Diet	Intravascular hemolysis	↓GFR
Sample taken from vein	KCl tabs	Rhabdomyolysis	• renal failure
where IV KCl is running	IV KCl	Insulin deficiency	• low effective circulating volume
Sample hemolysis		Hyperosmolar states	• NSAIDs in renal insufficiency
Leukocytosis (extreme)		(e.g. hyperglycemia)	Normal GFR but hypoaldosteronism
Thrombocytosis (extreme)		Metabolic acidosis	(see Table 7)
		(except for keto- and lactic acidosis)	
		Tumour lysis syndrome	
		Drugs	
		• β-blockers	
		• Digitalis overdose (blocks Na-K ATPase)	
		• Succinylcholine	

Table 7. Causes of Hyperkalemia with normal GFR

Decreased Aldosterone stimulus (low renin, low aldosterone)	Decreased aldosterone production (normal renin, low aldosterone)	Aldosterone resistance (decreased tubular response)
Hyporeninemic, hypoaldosteronism • associated with DM2, NSAIDs, chronic interstitial nephritis, HIV	• adrenal insufficiency of any cause [e.g. Addison's disease, AIDS, metastatic cancer] • ACE inhibitors • angiotensin II receptor blockers • heparin • congenital adrenal hyperplasia with 21-hydroxylase deficiency	K-sparing diuretics • spironolactone • amiloride • triamterene Drugs which mimic K-sparing diuretics • pentamidine • trimethoprim • cyclosporine, tacrolimus Pseudohypoaldosteronism (rare inherited tubular disorders)

Signs and Symptoms
- usually asymptomatic but may develop nausea, palpitations, muscle weakness, muscle stiffness, paresthesias, areflexia, ascending paralysis, and hypoventilation
- impaired renal ammoniagenesis and metabolic acidosis
- ECG changes and cardiotoxicity (do not correlate well with K concentration)
  - peaked and narrow T waves
  - decreased amplitude and eventual loss of P waves
  - prolonged PR interval
  - widening of QRS and eventual merging with T wave (sine-wave pattern)
  - AV block
  - ventricular fibrillation, asystole

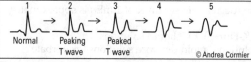

Figure 12. EKG Changes in Hyperkalemia

In patients with diabetes, increased K and hyperglycemia, often just giving insulin to restore euglycemia is sufficient to correct the hyperkalemia.

Treatment of Hyperkalemia

SEE BIG K DROP

SEE - Calcium gluconate

BIG - B-agonist, Bicarb, Insulin, Glucose

K - Kayexalate™

DROP - Diuretics, Dialysis

Treatment
- acute therapy is warranted if ECG changes present, K high, symptoms present
- tailor therapy to severity of increase in K and ECG changes
  - K <6.5 and normal ECG
    - treat underlying cause, stop K intake, increase the loss of K via urine and/or GI tract (see below)
  - K between 6.5 and 7.0, no ECG changes: add insulin to above regimen
  - K >7.0 and/or ECG changes: first priority is to protect the heart: add Ca gluconate to above

1. Protect the Heart
- Ca gluconate 1-2 amps (10 mL of 10% solution) IV
- antagonizes cardiac toxicity of hyperkalemia, protects cardiac conduction system, no effect on serum K
- onset within minutes, lasts 30-60 minutes

2. Shift K into Cells
- regular insulin (Insulin R) 10-20 units IV, with 1-2 amp D50W
  - onset of action 15-30 min, lasts 1-2 h
  - monitor blood glucose q1h
  - can repeat every 4-6 hours, or give infusion of 1 unit/hour
- NaHCO₃ 1-3 amps (given as 3 amps of 7.5% or 8.4% NaHCO₃ in 1L D5W)
  - onset of action 15-30 min, transient effect, drives K into cells in exchange for H

- β_2-agonist (Ventolin™) in nebulized form (dose = 2 cc or 10 mg inhaled) or 0.5 mg IV
  - onset of action 30-90 min, stimulates Na-K ATPase
  - caution if patient has heart disease as tachycardia may result from this high dose of β_2-agonist

3. Enhance K Removal from Body
  A. via urine
  - furosemide ($\geq$40 mg IV), may need IV NS to avoid hypovolemia
  - fludrocortisone (synthetic mineralocorticoid) if suspect aldosterone deficiency

  B. via gut
  - cation-exchange resins: calcium resonium or Kayexalate™ (less preferred because it binds Na in exchange for K) plus sorbitol PO to avoid constipation
  - Kayexalate™ enemas with tap water (not sorbitol)

  C. dialysis (renal failure, life threatening hyperkalemia unresponsive to therapy)

Acid-Base Disorders

- acid-base homeostasis influences protein function and can critically affect tissue and organ performance with consequences to cardiovascular, respiratory, metabolic and CNS function
- see Respirology, R4 for more information on respiratory acidosis/alkalosis

- normal concentration of HCO_3 = 24 mEq/L
- normal pCO_2 = 40 mmHg

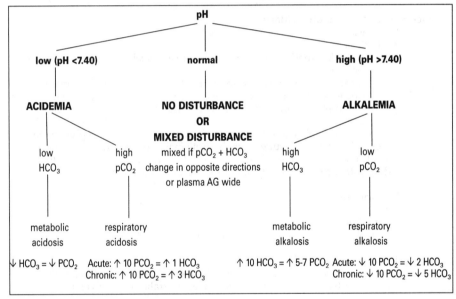

Acid-Base Equations

1) $H^+ + HCO_3^- \leftrightarrow H_2CO_3 \leftrightarrow H_2O + CO_2$

2) $[H^+] = 24\, pCO_2/[HCO_3^-]$

Figure 13. An Approach to Acid-Base Disorders

- each acid base disorder has an appropriate compensation
  - inadequate compensation or overcompensation indicates the presence of a second acid-base disorder
  - e.g. in metabolic acidosis, inadequate compensation = respiratory acidosis, overcompensation = respiratory alkalosis

Metabolic Acidosis

Approach: Identify main disturbance as in above figure, then:

1) Evaluate compensation (see Figure 13)

2) Calculate the plasma anion gap (PAG)
- $PAG = Na - (HCO_3 + Cl)$
  baseline = 12, range 10-14
- PAG can be altered by plasma albumin level: for each 10 g/L fall in albumin, lower baseline PAG by 3

3) If PAG elevated, compare increase in PAG with decrease in HCO_3
- increase in PAG < decrease in HCO_3, there is a coexisting non-AG metabolic acidosis
- if increase in PAG > decrease HCO_3, there is a coexisting metabolic alkalosis

4) Calculate osmolar gap
- osmolar gap = measured osmolality – calculated osmolality
  - calculated osmolality = $(2 \times Na)$ + urea + glucose
    (all units are in mmol/L)
  - normal osmolar gap <10
  - if gap >10, consider: methanol, ethylene glycol, end stage renal disease, alcoholic ketoacidosis, formaldehyde

Etiology and Pathophysiology

- **increased PAG metabolic acidosis** (4 types)
  1. Lactic acidosis
     - L-lactic acid:
       - **Type A**: situations of tissue hypoperfusion such as shock, septicemia, profound hypoxemia
       - **Type B**: failure to metabolize normally produced lactic acid in the liver due to severe liver disease, excessive EtOH intake, thiamine deficiency, or metformin accumulation (metformin interferes with electron transport chain)
     - D-lactic acid: rare syndrome characterized by episodes of encephalopathy and metabolic acidosis, requires carbohydrate malabsorption (i.e. short bowel syndrome), colonic bacteria that produce D-lactic acid, a carbohydrate load, diminished colonic motility and impaired D-lactate metabolism

  2. Ketoacidosis
     - diabetic
     - starvation
     - alcoholic ($\downarrow$ carbohydrate intake and vomiting)

  3. Toxins
     - methanol (toxic to retina, can cause blindness) – metabolized to formic acid
     - ethylene glycol (nephrotoxic, metabolized to oxalic acid – envelope shaped crystals in urine)
     - salicylate

  4. Advanced renal failure (e.g. serum Cr increased at least 5x above baseline – a very low GFR causes anion retention)

- **normal AG metabolic acidosis (hyperchloremic acidosis)**
  - diarrhea (HCO_3 loss from GI tract)
  - RTA (renal tubular acidosis)
    - type I RTA (distal): inability to fully excrete H load as NH_4, therefore accumulates
    - type II RTA (proximal): impaired HCO_3 reabsorption
    - type IV RTA: defective ammoniagenesis due to $\downarrow$ aldosterone or hyporesponsiveness or hyperkalemia
- to help distinguish renal causes from non-renal causes, use Urine Anion Gap = (Na + K) – Cl
- calculation establishes the presence or absence of unmeasured +ve ions (i.e NH_4) in urine
  - if <0, suggests adequate NH_4 in urine (likely nonrenal cause: diarrhea)
  - if >0, suggests problem is lack of NH_4 in urine (i.e. distal RTA)

Useful Equations

1) $PAG = [Na] - [Cl] - [HCO_3]$
(normal range = 10-14)

2) Osmolar Gap = measured osmolality - calculated osmolality (normal <10)

3) Calculated Osmolality = $2[Na] + [Urea] + [Glucose]$

Causes of Increased Anion Gap Metabolic Acidosis: MUDPILES
Methanol
Uremia
Diabetic/alcoholic/starvation ketoacidosis
Paraldehyde
Isopropyl alcohol/iron
Lactic acidosis
Ethylene glycol
Salicylates

Causes of Non-Anion Gap Metabolic Acidosis: HARDUP
Hyperalimentation
Acetazolamide
RTA
Diarrhea
Ureteroenteric fistula
Pancreaticoduodenal fistula

---

3 Clinical scenarios that produce a mixed metabolic disorder with near normal pH
(i.e. ↑PAG metabolic acidosis + resp. alkalosis)
- cirrhosis
- ASA overdose
- sepsis

Treatment of Metabolic Acidosis

- treat underlying cause (insulin for DKA, restore tissue perfusion for Type A lactic acidosis, EtOH + dialysis for methanol overdose, alkaline diuresis + possibly dialysis if level >4 mmol/L for overdose ASA)
- correct coexisting disorders of K (see *Hyperkalemia* section, NP15)
- consider treatment with exogenous alkali ($NaHCO_3$) if
  - severe reduction in [HCO_3] e.g. <8 mmol/L, especially with very low pH
  - no metabolizable anion (i.e. salicylate, formate, oxalate, sulphate)
- note: lactate and ketoacid anions can be metabolized to HCO_3
- risks of sodium bicarbonate therapy
  - hypokalemia: causes K to shift into cells (correct K deficits first)
  - ECF volume overload: Na load given with $NaHCO_3$, can exacerbate pulmonary edema
  - overshoot alkalosis: abrupt, poorly tolerated transition from overly aggressive alkali loading, partial conversion of accumulated organic anions to HCO_3 and persisting hyperventilation

Metabolic Alkalosis

Pathophysiology

- requires initiating event and maintenance factors
- initiating event
  - GI (vomiting, NG) or renal loss of H
  - exogenous alkali (oral or parenteral administration), milk alkali syndrome
  - diuretics (contraction alkalosis): ↓ excretion of HCO_3, ↓ ECF volume, therefore ↑[HCO_3]
  - posthypercapnia: renal compensation for respiratory acidosis is HCO_3 retention, rapid correction of respiratory disorder results in transient excess of HCO_3
- maintenance factors
  - volume depletion: increased proximal reabsorption of $NaHCO_3$ and increased aldosterone
  - hyperaldosteronism (1° or 2°): distal Na reabsorption in exchange for K and H excretion leads to HCO_3 generation, aldosterone also promotes hypokalemia
  - hypokalemia: transcellular K/H exchange, stimulus for ammoniagenesis and HCO_3 generation

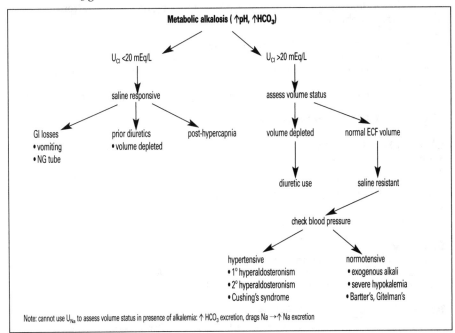

Figure 14. An Approach to Metabolic Alkalosis

Evaluate compensation (identify co-existing respiratory acid-base disorders)

- hypoventilation (an upper limit to compensation exists – breathing cannot be stopped) (see Figure 13, NP17)

Treatment

- treat underlying cause
- correct underlying disease, replenish K and Mg deficits, and possibly K-sparing diuretic

- saline sensitive metabolic alkalosis (most common)
  - treatment: volume repletion
  - ± carbonic anhydrase inhibitor (i.e. acetazolamide) to facilitate loss of HCO_3 in urine
- saline insensitive metabolic alkalosis
  - ECF volume normal or high
  - usually aldosterone or glucocorticoid excess
  - remove source of aldosterone or glucocorticoid ± spironolactone

Glomerular Disease

Terminology of Glomerular Changes

- terms applying to a population of glomeruli in the kidney:
  - diffuse: majority of glomeruli abnormal (>50%)
  - focal: some glomeruli affected
- terms applying to an individual glomerulus:
  - global: entire glomerulus abnormal
  - segmental: only part of the glomerulus abnormal

Types of Changes

- proliferation: hyperplasia of one of the glomerular cell types, with or without inflammatory cell infiltration
- membranous changes: capillary wall thickening due to immune deposits or alterations in basement membrane
- crescent formation: epithelial cell proliferation and mononuclear cell infiltration into crescent-shaped Bowman's space

Presentation of Glomerular Disease

IMPORTANT POINTS TO REMEMBER

- each glomerulonephropathy presents as one of 4 major glomerular syndromes
  - acute nephritic
  - nephrotic
  - rapidly progressive glomerulonephritis
  - asymptomatic urinary abnormalities
- each glomerulonephropathy can be caused by a primary disease OR can occur secondary to a systemic disease
- some glomerulonephropathies can present as more than one syndrome at different times

1) ACUTE NEPHRITIC SYNDROME

Features of Nephritic Syndrome
P - **P**roteinuria
H - **H**ematuria
A - **A**zotemia
R - **R**BC casts
O - **O**liguria
H - **H**ypertension

Clinical/Lab Features

- proteinuria (<3.5 g/day/1.73m²/day)
- abrupt onset hematuria (microscopic or macroscopic)
- azotemia (increased Cr and urea)
- RBC casts and/or dysmorphic RBCs in urine
- oliguria
- HTN (due to salt and water retention)

Etiology

- etiology can be divided into low and normal complement levels (see Table 8)
- frequently immune-mediated, with Ig and C3 deposits found in GBM
- outcome dependent on etiology

Table 8. Etiology of Nephritic Syndrome

	Low Complement Level	Normal Complement Level
Primary Causes	Postinfectious GN	IgA nephropathy
	Membranoprolif. GN	Anti-GBM disease
Secondary Causes	SLE	Polyarteritis nodosa
	Endocarditis	Wegener's granulomatosis
	Abscess or shunt nephritis	Henoch-Schonlein purpura
	Cryoglobulinemia	Goodpasture's syndrome

2) NEPHROTIC SYNDROME

Clinical/Lab Features
- heavy proteinuria (>3.5 g/1.73m²/d)
- hypoalbuminemia
- edema
- hyperlipidemia, lipiduria, fatty casts and oval fat bodies on microscopy
- hypercoagulable state (i.e. Protein C and Protein S urinary losses)
- glomerular pathology on renal biopsy:
    - minimal change disease (or minimal lesion disease or nil disease) – i.e. glomeruli appear normal on light microscopy
    - membranous glomerulopathy
    - focal segmental glomerulosclerosis (FSGS)
    - membranoproliferative glomerulonephritis
- each can be idiopathic or secondary to a systemic disease or drug

Table 9. Nephrotic Syndrome

	Minimal Change	Membranous Glomerulopathy	Focal Segmental Glomerulosclerosis	Membranoproliferative Glomerulonephritis
Secondary causes	DM, amyloidosis	HBV, SLE, malignancy (lung, breast, GI)	Reflux nephropathy, HIV, HBV, obesity	HCV, malaria, SLE, leukemia, lymphoma, infected shunt
Drug causes	NSAIDs	Gold, penicillamine	Heroin	N/A
Therapy	Steroids	Reduce BP, ACEI, steroids	Steroids, ACEI/ARB for proteinuria	Aspirin, ACEI, dipyridamole (Persantine™) - controversial

The Nephritic-Nephrotic Spectrum
- glomerular pathology can present with a clinical picture anywhere on a spectrum with pure nephritic and pure nephrotic syndromes at the extremes (see Figure 15)

```
Nephrotic              Intermediate                    Nephritic

                                                Hematuria, ↓GFR
 Proteinura

FSGS                   Membranoproliferative GN         Diffuse proliferative GN
Membranous glomerulopathy  Focal proliferative GN       Crescentic GN
Minimal change           • IgA nephropathy
                         • idiopathic membranoproliferative GN
                         • HBV, HCV
                         • SLE
                         • cryoglobulinemia
```

Figure 15. The Spectrum of Glomerular Pathology

3) RAPIDLY PROGRESSIVE GLOMERULONEPHRITIS (RPGN)

Clinical/Lab Features
- a subset of nephritic syndrome in which renal failure progresses in weeks to months
- usually crescent formation seen on renal biopsy
- RBC casts and/or dysmorphic RBCs in urine
- classified by immunofluorescence staining (see Table 10)
- treatment: corticosteroids + cyclophosphamide or other cytotoxic agent + plasmaphoresis in select cases
- prognosis: 50% recovery with early treatment, depends on underlying cause

Table 10. RPGN Classification

	RPGN Type I: Anti-GBM mediated	RPGN Type II: Immune Complex mediated	RPGN Type III: Non-immune mediated (i.e. pauci-immune)
% of RPGN cases	15% of cases	24% of cases	60% of cases
Immuno-fluorescence staining pattern	Linear pattern due to IgG and C3 deposition along capillary loops	Granular pattern due to subendothelial or subepithelial deposits of IgG and C3	No immune staining
Pathogenesis	Antibodies against type IV collagen in GBM	Most often 2° to systemic disease	Vasculitis of glomerular capillaries
Primary causes	Idiopathic anti-GBM disease	IgA nephropathy	Idiopathic
Secondary causes	Goodpasture's disease	Post-infectious GN, SLE, cryoglobulinemia, Henoch-Schonlein purpura	Wegener's (c-ANCA +ve), microscopic polyangiitis (p-ANCA +ve), Churg-Strauss (ANCA –ve)

4) ASYMPTOMATIC URINARY ABNORMALITIES

Clinical/Lab Features
- isolated proteinuria (usually <2 g/day) and/or isolated microscopic or macroscopic hematuria:
  - a) isolated proteinuria
    - ◆ can be postural
    - ◆ occasionally can signal beginning of more serious GN (e.g. FSGS, IgA nephropathy, amyloid, diabetic nephropathy)
  - b) hematuria with or without proteinuria
    - ◆ IgA nephropathy (Berger's disease): most common type of primary glomerular disease worldwide, usually presents after viral URTI
    - ◆ hereditary nephritis (Alport's disease): X-linked nephritis often associated with sensorineural hearing loss; proteinuria <2 g/day
    - ◆ thin basement membrane disease: usually autosomal dominant, without proteinuria, benign
    - ◆ benign recurrent hematuria: hematuria associated with febrile illness, exercise or immunization; a diagnosis of exclusion after other possibilities are ruled out

Investigations for Glomerular Disease

- blood work
  - first presentation: electrolytes, Cr, urea, albumin, fasting lipids
  - determining etiology: CBC, ESR, serum immune electrophoresis, C3, C4, ANA, p-ANCA, c-ANCA, cryoglobulins, HBV, HCV serology, ASOT (anti-streptolysin - O titres), VDRL, HIV
- urinalysis: RBCs, WBCs, casts, protein
- 24 hr urine for protein and CrCl
- radiology
  - CXR (infiltrates, CHF, pleural effusion)
  - renal ultrasound
- renal biopsy (percutaneous or open)
- urine immunoelectrophoresis
  - for Bence Jones protein if proteinuria present

Secondary Causes of Glomerular Disease

Amyloidosis
- nodular deposits of amyloid in mesangium, usually related to AL amyloid
- presents as nephrotic range proteinuria with progressive renal insufficiency
- can be primary or secondary
- secondary causes: multiple myeloma, TB, rheumatoid arthritis, malignancy

Systemic Lupus Erythematosus (see Figure 16)
- lupus nephritis can present as any of the glomerular syndromes
- nephrotic syndrome with an active sediment is most common presentation
- glomerulonephritis caused by immune complex deposition in capillary loops and mesangium with resulting renal injury
- serum complement levels are usually low during periods of active renal disease
- children and males with SLE are more likely to develop nephritis

HIV-Associated Renal Disease
1) direct nephrotoxic effect of HIV infection, antiretroviral drugs (e.g. tenofovir, indinavir) and other drugs used to treat HIV-associated infections
2) HIV-associated nephropathy
   - histology: focal and segmental glomerular collapse with mesangial sclerosis, "collapsing FSGS"
   - tubular cystic dilation and tubulo-reticular inclusions
   - clinical features: predominant in black men, heavy proteinuria, progressive renal insufficiency
   - prognosis: kidney failure within one year without treatment
   - therapy: short-term, high dose steroids, ACEI, HAART

EULAR recommendations for the management of systemic lupus erythematosus (SLE)
Ann Rheum Dis. 2008. Feb; 67:195-205
Lupus Nephritis Recommendations
Monitoring: Renal biopsy, urine sediment analysis, proteinuria, and kidney function may have independent predictive ability for clinical outcome in therapy of lupus nephritis but need to be interpreted in conjunction. Changes in immunological tests (anti-dsDNA, serum C3) have only limited ability to predict the response to treatment and may be used only as supplemental information.
Treatment: In patients with proliferative lupus nephritis, glucocorticoids in combination with immunosuppressive agents are effective against progression to end-stage renal disease. Longterm efficacy has been demonstrated only for cyclophosphamide-based regimens, which are however associated with considerable adverse effects. In short- and medium-term trials, mycophenolate mofetil has demonstrated at least similar efficacy compared with pulse cyclophosphamide and a more favourable toxicity profile: failure to respond by 6 months should evoke discussions for intensification of therapy. Flares following remission are not uncommon and require diligent follow-up.
End-stage renal disease: Dialysis and transplantation in SLE have rates for long-term patient and graft-survival comparable with those observed in non-diabetic non-SLE patients, with transplantation being the method of choice.

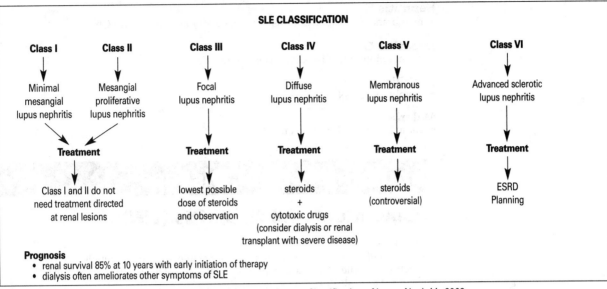

Figure 16. International Society of Nephrology/Renal Pathology Society Classification of Lupus Nephritis 2003

Henoch-Schönlein Purpura (HSP)
- disease seen most often in children
- purpura on buttocks and legs, abdominal pain, arthralgia and fever
- glomeruli show varying degrees of mesangial hypercellularity
- IgA and C3 staining of mesangium
- usually benign, self-limiting course; 10% progress to CRF

Goodpasture's Disease
- antibodies against type IV collagen present in lungs and GBM
- more common in 3rd and 6th decades of life, men slightly more affected than females
- present with RPGN type I and hemoptysis/dyspnea
- pulmonary hemorrhage more common in smokers and males
- treat with plasma exchange, cyclophosphamide, prednisone

Wegener's Granulomatosis
- 80% of patients have renal involvement
- focal segmental necrotizing RPGN with no immune staining
- majority of patients with renal disease are c-ANCA +ve
- may be indolent or fulminant in progression
- vasculitis and granulomas rarely seen on renal biopsy
- treat with cyclophosphamide, prednisone, sulfa may prevent recurrence

Cryoglobulinemia
- cryoglobulins: monoclonal IgM and polyclonal IgG
- presents as purpura, fever, Raynaud's phenomenon and arthralgias
- 50% of patients have hepatitis C
- renal disease seen in 40% of patients (isolated proteinuria/hematuria progressing to nephritic syndrome)
- most patients have ↓ serum complement (C4 initially)
- treat hepatitis C, plasmapheresis
- overall prognosis 75% renal recovery

Infections and Glomerular Disease

Shunt Nephritis
- immune-complex mediated nephritis associated with chronically infected ventriculoatrial shunts inserted for treatment of hydrocephalus
- presents as acute nephritic syndrome with ↓ serum complement
- nephrotic range proteinuria in 25% of patients

Infective Endocarditis
- manifests as mild form of acute nephritic syndrome, with ↓ serum complement
- *S. aureus* is most common infecting agent
- treatment with appropriate antibiotics usually resolves GN

Hepatitis B
- membranous GN, polyarteritis nodosa, membranoproliferative GN

Hepatitis C
- membranoproliferative GN, cryoglobulinemia

Syphilis
- membranous GN

Malaria
- variable glomerular involvement

Tubulointerstitial Disease

Tubulointerstitial Nephritis (TIN)

Definition
- cellular infiltrates affecting primarily the renal interstitium and tubule cells
- functional tubule defects are disproportionately greater than the decrease in GFR
- classified as acute or chronic

Signs and Symptoms
- manifestation of disease depends on site of tubule affected
  1) proximal tubule (e.g. multiple myeloma, heavy metals)
     - Fanconi syndrome: decreased reabsorption in proximal tubule causing glycosuria, aminoaciduria, phosphaturia
     - proximal RTA (decreased bicarbonate absorption): Type II RTA
  2) distal tubule (e.g. amyloidosis, obstruction)
     - distal RTA (Type I RTA)
     - Na-wasting nephropathy
     - ± hyperkalemia, type IV RTA
  3) collecting duct (e.g sickle cell anemia, analgesics, PCKD)
     - urine concentrating defect
     - polyuria (nephrogenic DI)

ACUTE TUBULOINTERSTITIAL NEPHRITIS

Definition
- rapid (days-weeks) decline in renal function
- 10-20% of all acute renal failure

Etiology
- hypersensitivity
  1) Antibiotics: β-lactams, sulfonamides, rifampin, quinolones, cephalosporins
  2) Other: NSAIDs, allopurinol, furosemide
- infections
  - bacterial pyelonephritis, *Streptococcus*, brucellosis, *Legionella*, CMV, EBV, toxoplasmosis, leptospirosis
- immune: SLE, acute allograft rejection, Sjögren's syndrome, sarcoidosis, mixed essential cryoglobulinemia
- idiopathic

Pathophysiology
- acute inflammatory cell infiltrates into renal interstitium

Signs and Symptoms
- acute renal failure
- if hypersensitivity reaction: may see fever, skin rash, arthralgia, serum sickness-like syndrome
- if pyelonephritis: flank pain and costo-vertebral angle (CVA) tenderness
- other signs and symptoms based on underlying etiology
- hypertension and edema are uncommon

Investigations
- urine
  - sterile pyuria, WBC casts, mild proteinuria, hematuria
  - eosinophils if allergic interstitial nephritis

- blood
  - increased Cr and urea
  - eosinophilia if drug reaction
  - non-AG metabolic acidosis (renal tubular acidosis)
  - hypophosphatemia, hyperkalemia, hyponatremia
- gallium scan shows intense signal due to inflammatory infiltrate
- renal biopsy definitive

Treatment
- treat underlying cause (e.g. stop offending medications, antibiotics if pyelonephritis)
- corticosteroids (may be indicated in allergic or immune disease)

Prognosis
- recovery within 2 weeks if underlying insult can be eliminated

CHRONIC TUBULOINTERSTITIAL NEPHRITIS

Definition
- characterized by slowly progressive renal failure, moderate proteinuria and signs of abnormal tubule function

Etiology
- persistence or progression of acute TIN
- urinary tract obstruction: most important cause of chronic TIN
- chronic pyelonephritis: due to vesicoureteral reflux or UTI with obstruction
- nephrotoxins
  - exogenous
    - analgesics (NSAIDs, phenacetin, acetaminophen)
    - cisplatin, lithium, cyclosporine, tacrolimus
    - heavy metals (lead, cadmium, copper), lithium, mercury, arsenic
    - radiation
    - Chinese herbs
  - endogenous
    - hypercalcemia, hypokalemia, oxalate, uric acid nephropathy
- vascular disease: ischemic nephrosclerosis, atheroembolic disease
- malignancies: multiple myeloma
- granulomatous: TB, sarcoidosis, Wegener's granulomatosis
- immune: SLE, Sjögren's, cryoglobulinemia, Goodpasture's, amyloidosis, renal graft rejection
- hereditary: cystic diseases of the kidney, sickle cell disease
- others: radiation, Balkan (endemic) nephropathy

Pathophysiology
- fibrosis of interstitium with atrophy of tubules, mononuclear cell inflammation

Signs and Symptoms
- tubular dysfunction (e.g. RTA, electrolyte disturbances)
- progressive renal failure and uremia
- also dependent on underlying etiology

Treatment
- stop offending agent or treat underlying disease
- supportive measures: correct metabolic disorders (Ca, PO_4) and anemia

Findings which Suggest Chronic Tubulointerstitial Nephritis
- non AG metabolic acidosis
- hyperkalemia (out of proportion to degree of renal insufficiency)
- polyuria, nocturia
- partial or complete Fanconi's syndrome
- urine: mild proteinuria, few RBCs and WBCs, no RBC casts
- ultrasound: shrunken kidneys with irregular contours

Acute Tubular Necrosis (ATN)

Definition
- abrupt and sustained decline in GFR within minutes-days after ischemic/nephrotoxic insult
- GFR shuts down to avoid life-threatening loss of electrolytes from non-functioning tubules

Etiology
- see Figure 17

Clinical Presentation
- typically presents as an abrupt rise in urea and Cr after a hypotensive episode, sepsis, rhabdomyolysis, or administration of nephrotoxic drug
- urine: high FE_{Na}, pigmented-granular casts

Complications
- hyperkalemia: can occur rapidly and cause serious arrhythmia
- metabolic acidosis, $\downarrow$Ca, $\downarrow$Na, $\uparrow PO_4$, hypoalbuminemia

Investigations
- blood: CBC, eletrolytes, Cr, urea, Ca, PO_4, blood gases
- urine: R&M, electrolytes, osmolality
- ECG
- abdominal ultrasound

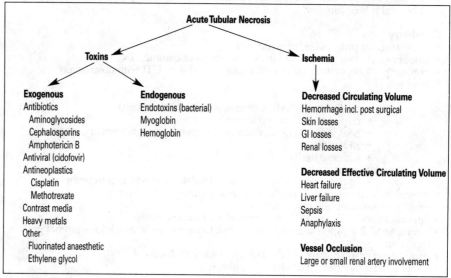

Figure 17. Etiology of ATN

Meta-analysis: effectiveness of drugs for preventing contrast-induced nephropathy.
Ann Intern Med. 2008 19;148:284-94.
Purpose: To determine the effectiveness of N-acetylcysteine, theophylline, fenoldopam, dopamine, iloprost, statin, furosemide, or mannitol on preventing nephropathy.
Study Selection: Only randomized, controlled trials that used these agents in patients receiving iodinated contrast.
Results: In the 41 RCTs included N-acetylcysteine (RR = 0.62 [0.44-0.88]) and Theophylline (RR = 0.49 [0.23-1.06]) reduced the risk of nephropathy more than saline alone. Furosemide increased the risk (RR = 3.27 [1.48-7.26]) . Other agents did not affect risk of nephropathy.
Conclusion: N-acetylcysteine is more renoprotective than hydration alone.

Therapy
- therapy for ATN is largely supportive once underlying problem is corrected
- loop diuretics may help manage volume overload and reduce tubular metabolic requirements to allow for recovery
- consider early dialysis in severe/rapidly progressing cases to prevent uremic syndrome

Prevention
- correct fluid balance before surgical procedures
- for patients with chronic renal disease requiring radiographic contrast: give N-acetylcysteine 600-1200 mg PO bid day before + day after procedure
- use renal-adjusted doses of nephrotoxic drugs in patients with renal insufficiency
- isotonic $NaHCO_3$ - 3 ml/kg bolus over 1h before procedure and 1 ml/kg/h for 6h post-procedure if not contraindicated

Analgesic Nephropathies

1) Vasomotor Acute Kidney Injury (AKI)
- normally, prostaglandins vasodilate renal arterioles to maintain blood flow
- NSAIDs act by blocking cyclooxygenase enzyme, thereby preventing prostaglandin synthesis and causing renal ischemia
- more common in elderly, underlying renal disease, hypovolemia (diuretics, CHF, cirrhosis, nephrotic syndrome)
- clinically: develop prerenal azotemia within few days of starting NSAID
- treatment: discontinue NSAID, dialysis rarely needed

2) Acute Interstitial Nephritis (AIN)

- majority due to fenoprofen (60%), ibuprofen, naproxen
- resolves eventually with discontinuation of NSAID, may require interval dialysis
- short term high dose steroids (1 mg/kg/day of prednisone) may hasten recovery

3) Chronic Interstitial Nephritis

- due to excessive consumption of antipyretics (phenacetin or acetaminophen) in combination with NSAIDs
- associated with emotional stress, psychiatric symptoms and GI disturbance
- papillary necrosis
    - gross hematuria, flank pain, declining renal function
    - calyceal filling defect seen with IVP- 'ring sign'
- increased risk of transitional cell carcinoma of renal pelvis
- good prognosis if discontinue analgesics

4) Other Effects of NSAIDs

- sodium retention (2° to reduced GFR)
- hyperkalemia, HTN (2° to hyporeninemic hypoaldosteronism)
- excess water retention (due to elimination of ADH – antagonistic effect of prostaglandins)

Vascular Diseases of the Kidney

Large Vessel Disease

1) RENAL ARTERY OCCLUSION

- important, potentially reversible cause of renal failure

Etiology

- abdominal trauma, surgery, embolism, vasculitis, extrarenal compression, hypercoaguable state, aortic dissection
- kidney transplant more vulnerable

Signs and Symptoms (depend on presence of collateral circulation)

- fever, nausea/vomiting, flank pain
- leukocytosis, elevated AST, LDH, ALP
- acute onset hypertension (activation of activation of RAAS) or sudden worsening of long-standing hypertension
- renal dysfunction (if bilateral, or solitary functioning kidney)

Investigations

- renal arteriography (more reliable but risk of contrast-mediated ATN, atheroembolic renal disease)
- enhanced CT or magnetic resonance angiography, duplex Doppler studies (operator dependent)

Treatment

- prompt localization of occlusion and restoration of blood flow
- anticoagulation, thrombolysis, percutaneous angioplasty or clot extraction, surgical thrombectomy

2) ISCHEMIC RENAL DISEASE (RENAL ARTERY STENOSIS)

- chronic renal impairment secondary to hemodynamically significant renal artery stenosis or microvascular disease
- significant cause of ESRD: 15% patients over 50 (higher prevalence if significant vascular disease)
- usually associated with large vessel disease elsewhere
- causes:
    1. atherosclerosis – more common in elderly
    2. fibromuscular dysplasia – more common in females, age 30-50

Risk Factors

- >50 yo
- smoking
- other atherosclerotic disease
- severe/refractory HTN and/or hypertensive crises
- asymmetrical renal size
- increasing Cr with ACEI/ARB
- flash pulmonary edema with normal LV function

Investigations
- must establish presence of renal vessel stenosis and prove it is responsible for renal dysfunction
- duplex Doppler U/S (kidney size, blood flow): good screening test (operator dependent)
- CT or MR angiography (effective noninvasive tests to establish presence of stenosis)
- ACE inhibitor renography (e.g. captopril renal scan)
- renal arteriography (gold standard)

Treatment
- medical therapy, percutaneous angioplasty ± stent, surgical revascularization
- little or no benefit if therapy is late

3) RENAL VEIN THROMBOSIS

Etiology
- hypercoagulable states (i.e. nephrotic syndrome, especially membranous), ECF volume depletion, extrinsic compression of renal vein, significant trauma, malignancy (i.e. RCC), sickle cell
- clinical presentation determined by rapidity of occlusion and formation of collateral circulation
- acute: nausea/vomiting, flank pain, hematuria, elevated plasma LDH, ± rise in Cr, sudden rise in proteinuria
- chronic: increasing proteinuria and/or tubule dysfunction

Investigations
- renal venography (gold standard), CT or MR angiography, duplex Doppler U/S

Treatment
- anticoagulation with heparin then warfarin (1 yr or indefinitely, depending on risk factors)

Small Vessel Disease

1) HYPERTENSIVE NEPHROSCLEROSIS
- see *Hypertension* section, NP33

2) ATHEROEMBOLIC RENAL DISEASE
- progressive renal insufficiency due to embolic obstruction of small and medium-sized renal vessels by atheromatous emboli
- spontaneous or after renal artery manipulation or surgery, angiography, percutaneous angioplasty
- anticoagulants and thrombolytics interfere with ulcerated plaque healing and can worsen disease
- presentation: acute or chronic, progressive renal dysfunction, labile hypertension, extrarenal atheroembolic disease support diagnosis (livedo reticularis is a classic sign)
- pathology: needle-shaped cholesterol clefts (due to tissue-processing artifacts) with surrounding tissue reaction in small/medium-sized vessels
- no effective treatment; avoid angiographic and surgical procedures in patients with diffuse atherosclerosis

3) THROMBOTIC MICROANGIOPATHY
- a spectrum which includes HUS, TTP, DIC, post-partum renal failure
- renal involvement more common in HUS than TTP
- renal involvement characterized by fibrin thrombi in glomerular capillary loops ± arterioles
- treatment: supportive therapy, plasma exchange, corticosteroids splenectomy, rituximab for TTP if refractory
- avoid platelet transfusions and ASA

4) SCLERODERMA
- 50% scleroderma patients have renal involvement (mild proteinuria, high Cr, HTN)
- histology: media thickened, 'onion skin' hypertrophy of small renal arteries, fibrinoid necrosis of afferent arterioles and glomeruli
- 10-15% scleroderma patients have a 'scleroderma renal crisis': malignant HTN (usually within the first few years), ARF, microangiopathy, volume overload, visual changes, HTN encephalopathy
- renal involvement usually occurs early in the course of illness
- treatment: BP control with ACEI slows progression of renal disease

5) CALCINEURIN INHIBITOR NEPHROPATHY

- cyclosporine and tacrolimus
- causes both acute reversible and chronic, largely irreversible nephrotoxicity
- acute: due to afferent and efferent glomerular capillary constriction leading to decreased GFR (tubular vacuolization)
  - pre-renal azotemia
  - treatment: calcium channel blockers or prostaglandin analogs, reduce dose of cyclosporine or switch to another immunosuppressive drug
- chronic: result of obliterative arteriolopathy causing interstitial nephritis and CRF (striped fibrosis)

Renal Failure

Presentation of Renal Failure

- signs and symptoms depend on acuity of onset, severity of insult, adaptation to nephron loss/dysfunction, treatment of reversible disease process

1) Volume Overload
- due to increase in total body Na
- weight gain, HTN, pulmonary or peripheral edema

2) Electrolyte Abnormalities
- high
  - K (decreased renal excretion, increased tissue breakdown)
  - PO_4 (decreased renal excretion, increased tissue breakdown)
  - Ca (rare; happens during recovery phase after rhabdomyolysis-induced acute kidney injury)
  - uric acid
- low
  - Na (failure to excrete excessive water intake)
  - Ca (decreased Vit D activation, hyperphosphatemia, hypoalbuminemia)
  - acidemia (especially with sepsis or severe heart failure)

3) Uremic Syndrome
- retention of urea and other metabolites and deficiencies of hormones, causing the manifestations of uremic syndrome

Signs and Symptoms:
- CNS: headache, lethargy, somnolence, confusion, asterixis, hyporeflexia
- PNS: "glove and stockings" type sensory neuropathy, wrist or foot drop
- CVS: shortness of breath, pleuritic chest pain
- GI: anorexia, nausea and vomiting, decreased taste
- Endocrine: weight loss, amenorrhea, decreased libido
- MSK: nocturnal muscle cramps, muscle weakness
- Skin: pruritis, pallor, yellow discolouration

Complications
- CNS: decreased LOC, stupor, seizure
- CVS: cardiomyopathy, CHF, arrhythmia, pericarditis, atherosclerosis
- GI: peptic ulcer disease, gastroduodenitis, colitis, AVM
- Hematologic: anemia, coagulopathy (platelet dysfunction), infections (low WBCs)
- Endocrine:
  - decreased testosterone, estrogen, progesterone
  - increased FSH, LH
- Metabolic:
  - renal osteodystrophy: secondary ↑ PTH due to ↓ Ca
    - osteitis fibrosa cystica, osteomalacia, osteoporosis
  - hypertriglyceridemia: accelerated atherogenesis
  - decreased insulin requirements, increased insulin resistance
- Dermatologic: pruritis, ecchymosis, hematoma, calciphylaxis (Ca deposition)

Acute Kidney Injury (AKI)

Definition
- abrupt decline in renal function leading to increased nitrogenous waste products
- formerly known as acute renal failure (ARF)

The 2 most common causes of acute kidney injury in hospitalized patients are prerenal azotemia and acute tubular necrosis. Remember that prerenal failure can lead to ATN.

Clues to Pre-Renal Etiology
- clinical: ↓BP, ↑HR, positive orthostatic HR & BP changes
- ↑[urea] >> ↑ [Cr]
- urine [Na] <10-20 mmol/L
- urine osmolality > 500 mOsm/kg
- fractional excretion of Na < 1%

Clues to Renal Etiology
- appropriate clinical context
- urinalysis positive for casts:
    - pigmented granular – ATN
    - WBC – AIN
    - RBC – GN

Clues to Post Renal Etiology
- known solitary kidney
- older man
- recent retroperitoneal surgery
- anuria
- palpable bladder
- ultrasound indicates hydronephrosis

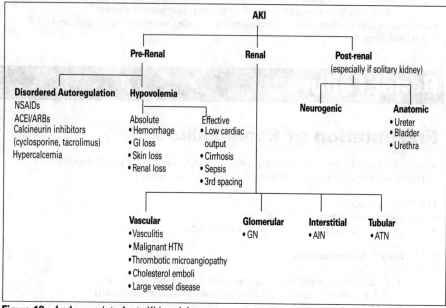

Figure 18. An Approach to Acute Kidney Injury

Clinical Features
- azotemia (increased BUN, Cr)
- abnormal urine volume (anuria, oliguria, polyuria)

Approach to AKI

Differentiating Pre-renal from ATN

	Pre-renal	ATN
Urinalysis	normal	RBC, pigmented granular casts
Urine [Na]	<20	>40 mEq/L
Urine [Cr]/[Na]	>40	<20
Urine osmolality	>500	<350 mOsm/kgH$_2$O
Fe$_{Na}$	<1	>1

Indications for Dialysis in AKI
Hyperkalemia (refractory)
Acidosis (refractory)
Volume overload (refractory)
Elevated BUN (>35 mM)
Pericarditis
Encephalopathy
Edema (pulmonary)

Investigations
- blood: CBC, electrolytes, Cr, BUN (think prerenal if increase in BUN is relatively greater than increase in Cr), Ca, PO$_4$
- urine volume, C&S, R&M: sediment, casts, crystals
- urinary indices
- foley catheterization (rule out bladder outlet obstruction)
- fluid challenge (i.e. fluid bolus to rule out most prerenal causes)
- imaging: abdo U/S (assess kidney size, hydronephrosis, post-renal obstruction)
- indications for renal biopsy:
    - diagnosis is not certain
    - prerenal azotemia or ATN is unlikely
    - oliguria persists >4 weeks

Treatment
1) preliminary measures
    - pre-renal
        - correct prerenal factors: optimize volume status and cardiac performance
    - renal
        - exclude reversible renal causes: d/c nephrotoxic drugs, treat infection, optimize electrolytes and hold ACEI/ARB
    - post-renal
        - consider obstruction: structural (stones, strictures) vs. functional (neuropathy)
        - treat with foley catheter, indwelling bladder catheter, nephrostomy, stenting
2) treat complications
    - fluid overload
        - NaCl restriction
        - high dose loop diuretics

- hyperkalemia (refer to *Treatment of Hyperkalemia* section, NP16)
- adjust dosages of medications cleared by kidney
3) definitive therapy depends on etiology
- **Note:** Renal transplant is not a therapy for AKI (unlike other organs eg: liver)

Prognosis
- high morbidity with multi-organ failure, most commonly in prerenal azotemia (ischemic insult)

Chronic Kidney Disease (CKD)

Definition
- abnormal markers (Cr, urea)
  - GFR <60 ml/min for >3 months or
  - kidney pathology seen on biopsy or
  - decreased renal size on U/S

Table 11. Stages of Chronic Kidney Disease (K/DOQI, 2002)

	Definition	GFR (mL/min/1.73m²)
Stage 1	Normal or increased GFR	≥90
Stage 2	Mild decrease in GFR	60-89
Stage 3	Moderate decrease in GFR	30-59
Stage 4	Severe decrease in GFR	15-29
Stage 5	End stage renal disease	<15 (or dialysis)

Table 12. Etiology and Incidence of Chronic Kidney Disease (CKD)

Diabetes	42.9%
Hypertension	26.4%
Glomerulonephritis	9.9%
Other/Unknown	7.7%
Interstitial nephritis/Pyelonephritis	4.0%
Cystic/Hereditary/Congenital	3.1%
Secondary GN/Vasculitis	2.4%

Management of Chronic Kidney Disease

- diet
  - protein restriction with adequate caloric intake limits endogenous protein catabolism
  - K restriction (40 mmol/day)
  - Na and water restriction
  - PO$_4$ restriction (1 g/d)
  - avoid extradietary Mg (e.g. antacids)
- medical
  - cinacalcet for hyperparathyroidism (sensitizes parathyroid to calcium → ↓PTH)
  - calcium supplements (e.g. TUMS™) treats hypocalcemia when given between meals and binds phosphate when given with meals.
  - consider calcitriol if hypocalcemic (despite normal phosphate levels)
  - sevelamer (phosphate binder) if both hypercalcemic and hyperphosphatemic
  - vitamin D analogues are being introduced in the near future
  - erythropoietin injections (Hct <30%) for anemia
  - DDAVP for prolonged bleeding time
  - ACEI for hypertension (target 130/80 or less), loop diuretics when GFR <25 mL/min
  - statins for dyslipidemia
  - adjust dosages for renally excreted medications (avoid nephrotoxic medications)
- dialysis (hemodialysis, peritoneal dialysis)
- renal transplantation

Renin angiotensin system blockade and cardiovascular outcomes in patients with chronic kidney disease and proteinuria: a meta-analysis
Am Heart J. 2008;155:791-805
Purpose: To evaluate the role of renin angiotensin system (RAS) blockade in improving cardiovascular CV outcomes in patients with chronic kidney disease.
Study Selection: Randomized controlled trials that analyzed CV outcomes in patients with chronic kidney disease (CKD)/proteinuria treated with RAS blockade (angiotensin-converting enzyme inhibitors/angiotensin receptor blockers). Renin angiotensin system blockade-based therapy was compared with placebo and control (beta-blocker, calcium-channel blockers and other antihypertensive-based therapy) therapy in the study.
Results: Twenty-five trials (N = 45758) were included. Compared to placebo, RAS blockade reduced the risk of heart failure in patients with diabetic nephropathy. In patients with non-diabetic CKD, RAS blockade decreased CV outcome compared to control therapy.
Conclusions: RAS blockade reduced CV outcomes in diabetic nephropathy as well as non-diabetic CKD.

Management of Complications of CKD
- **N** - low-nitrogen diet
- **E** - Electrolytes: monitor K
- **P** - pH: metabolic acidosis
- **H** - Hypertension
- **R** - RBCs: manage anemia with erythropoietin
- **O** - Osteodystrophy: give calcium between meals (to ↑Ca) and calcium with meals (to bind and ↓PO$_4$)
- **N** - Nephrotoxins: avoid nephrotoxic drugs (ASA, gentamicin) and adjust doses of renally excreted medications

Renal Replacement Therapy (RRT)

Dialysis

How to Write Dialysis Orders
- **Filter Type** (eg. F8O)
- **Length** (i.e. 4 h 3 times/wk or 2 h daily)
- **Q Blood Flow** (Max 500 cc/min)
- **Ultrafiltration**
  (e.g. 2L or to target dry weight)
- **Na** 140
- **K** (based on serum [K])

Serum K	Dialysate
4-6	1.5
3.5-4	2.5
< 3.5	3.5

- **Ca** 1.25
- **HCO₃** 40
- **Heparin** (none, tight [500u/h]
  or full [1000 u/h])

When to Initiate DIALYSIS

CrCl <30 mL/min
- educate patient regarding dialysis; if not a candidate for peritoneal dialysis, make arrangements for AV graft

CrCl <15 mL/min
- weigh risk and benefits or initiating dialysis

CrCl <10 mL/min
- dialysis should be initiated

NOTE
- Cockcroft-Gault equation (or Modification of Diet in Renal Disease equation) should be used to measure kidney function
- monitor for uremic complications
- significant benefits in quality of life can occur if dialysis started before CrCl <15 mL/min
- it is unclear whether patients who start dialysis early have increased survival

From: National Kidney Foundation/Kidney Disease Outcome. Quality Initiative

Indications for Dialysis in Chronic Renal Failure
- absolute indications
  - volume overload unresponsive to medication
  - hyperkalemia unresponsive to medication
  - severe metabolic acidosis unresponsive to medication
  - neurologic signs or symptoms of uremia (encephalopathy, neuropathy, seizures)
  - uremic pericarditis
  - refractory accelerated hypertension
  - clinically significant bleeding diathesis
  - persistent severe nausea and vomiting
  - plasma Cr >1060 μmol/L or BUN >36 mmol/L
- relative indications
  - anorexia
  - decreased cognitive functioning
  - profound fatigue and weakness
  - severe anemia unresponsive to erythropoietin
  - persistent severe pruritis
  - restless legs syndrome
- hemodialysis: blood is filtered across a semipermeable membrane removing accumulated toxic waste products, solutes and excess fluid and restoring buffering agents to the bloodstream
- peritoneal dialysis: peritoneum acts as a semipermeable membrane similar to hemodialysis filter
  - advantages: independence, fewer stringent dietary restrictions, better rehabilitation rates
  - available as continuous ambulatory or cyclic

Table 13. Peritoneal Dialysis vs. Hemodialysis

	Peritoneal Dialysis	Hemodialysis
Rate	Slow	Fast
Location	Home	Hospital (usually)
Ultrafiltration	Osmotic pressure via dextrose dialysate	Hydrostatic pressure
Solute removal	Concentration gradient and convection	Concentration gradient and convection
Membrane	Peritoneum	Semi-permeable artificial membrane
Method	Indwelling catheter in peritoneal cavity	Line from vessel to artificial kidney
Complications	Infection at catheter site	Vascular access (clots, collapse)
	Bacterial peritonitis	Bacteremia
	Metabolic effects of glucose	Bleeding due to heparin
	Difficult to achieve adequate	Hemodynamic stress of extracorporeal circuit
	clearance in patients with large body mass	Disequilibrium syndrome (hypotension, nausea, muscle cramps related to solute/water flux over short time)
Preferred when	Young, high functioning, residual renal function	Bed-bound, co-morbidities, no renal function

- patients with chronic kidney disease should be referred for surgery to attempt construction of a primary AV fistula when their eGFR is <30 mL/min, the serum Cr level quoted as >354 μmol/L (equal to >4.0 mg/dL), or within 1 year of an anticipated need
- refer patients with chronic renal disease to a nephrologist early on to facilitate treatment and plan in advance for RRT

Renal Transplantation

- preferred modality of RRT, best way to reverse uremic signs and symptoms
- provides maximum replacement of GFR
- only therapy shown to improve survival in patients with ESRD
- native kidneys usually left in situ
- 2 types: deceased donor, living donor (related or unrelated)
- kidney transplanted into iliac fossa, transplant renal artery anastomosed to external iliac artery of recipient
- 1 year renal allograft survival rates ≥90%

Complications
- leading causes of late allograft loss: chronic rejection and death with functioning graft
- #1 cause of mortality in transplanted patients is cardiovascular disease

Commonly Used Immunosuppressive Drugs:
- Cyclosporine
- Tacrolimus
- Mycophenolate Mofetil
- Sirolimus
- Prednisone
- Azathioprine
- Thymoglobulin
- Mycophenolic acid
- Daclizumab
- Basiliximab

- immunosuppressant drug therapy: side effects, infections, malignancy (skin, non-Hodgkin's lymphoma, post-transplant lymphoproliferative disorder)
- acute rejection; graft site tenderness, rise in Cr, oliguria, ± fever
- de novo glomerulonephritis
- new-onset diabetes mellitus (often due to prednisone use)
- cyclosporine or tacrolimus nephropathy (refer to *Small Vessel Disease*, NP28)
- chronic allograft nephropathy
  - early allograft damage caused by episodes of acute rejection and acute peritransplant injuries
  - immunologic and nonimmunologic factors (HTN, hyperlipidemia, age of donor, quality of graft, new onset diabetes)
- CMV (cytomegalovirus) infection and other opportunistic infections usually occur between 1 and 6 months post-transplant

Reduced Exposure to Calcineurin Inhibitors in Renal Transplantation (ELITE-Symphony Trial)
NEJM 2007; 257:2562-75
Study: Randomized, open-label, multi-centre study in 4 parallel groups with a 12 month follow-up period.
Patients: 1645 patients between 18 and 75 years who were scheduled to receive single organ kidney transplant. Mean age = 45.
Intervention: 4-arm trial. Arm1 - Standard cyclosporine therapy, Arm 2 - Low Dose Cyclosporine therapy with Daclizumab, Arm 3 - Low Dose Tacrolimus therapy with Daclizumab, Arm 4 - Low Dose Sirolimus therapy with Daclizumab.
Main Outcome: Primary end-point was estimated GFR 12 months after transplantation
Results: GRF was higher in patients receiving Tacrolimus (Arm 3) compared to the other arms. Acute rejection lower in the Tacrolimus group (Arm 3). Allograft survival highest in the Tacrolimus group. Serious adverse events were highest in the Sirolimus group.

Systemic Diseases and the Kidney

Hypertension (HTN)

- HTN occurs in 10-20% of population: etiology classified as "essential" (primary) or secondary
- diseases of renal parenchyma or renal vasculature can cause secondary hypertension
- conversely, hypertension due to other factors can cause renal disease (hypertensive nephrosclerosis) or worsen preexisting renal disease

Hypertensive Nephrosclerosis

Table 14. Chronic vs. Malignant Nephrosclerosis

	Chronic Nephrosclerosis	Malignant Nephrosclerosis
Histology	Slow vascular sclerosis with ischemic changes affecting intralobular and afferent arterioles	Fibrinoid necrosis of arterioles, disruption of vascular endothelium
Clinical picture	African American, underlying chronic kidney disease, chronic hypertensive disease	Acute elevation in BP (dBP>120mmHg) HTN encephalopathy
Urinalysis	Mild proteinuria, normal urine sediment	Proteinuria and hematuria (RBC casts)
Therapy	Blood pressure control, frequent follow-up	Lower dBP to 100-110 mmHg within 6 hours More aggressive treatment can cause ischemic event Identify and treat underlying cause of HTN
Prognosis	Can progress to renal failure despite patient adherence	Lower survival if renal insufficiency develops

Renovascular Hypertension

- HTN caused secondary to renovascular disease
- 1-2% of all hypertensive patients, most common cause of secondary hypertension
- suspect if:
  - negative family history of HTN
  - sudden onset or exacerbation of HTN
  - difficult to control with antihypertensive therapy
  - epigastric or flank bruit
  - spontaneous hypokalemia (renin activation from underperfused kidney)
  - history of diffuse atherosclerosis

Etiology and Classification
- decreased renal perfusion of one or both kidneys leads to increased renin release and subsequent angiotensin (AII) production.
- increased AII raises blood pressure in 2 ways:
  1) causes generalized arterioconstriction
  2) release of aldosterone increases Na and water retention
- the elevated blood pressure can in turn lead to further damage of kidneys and worsening HTN

- 2 types of renovascular HTN
  - atherosclerotic plaques: proximal 1/3 renal artery, usually males >55 years
  - fibromuscular hyperplasia: distal 2/3 renal artery or segmental branches, usually young females
- patients with bilateral renal artery stenosis are at risk of ARF with ACEI or NSAIDs
  - when there is decreased renal blood flow, GFR is dependent on AII-induced efferent arteriolar constriction which raises filtration fraction (GFR/RPF)

Investigations
- renal U/S and dopplers
- digital subtraction angiography (risks: contrast nephropathy)
- renal scan before and after ACEI (accentuates difference in GFR)
- MR angiography
- gold standard is arterial angiography

Treatment
- BP lowering medications (ACEI is drug of choice if unilateral renal artery disease but contraindicated if bilateral renal artery disease)
- surgical, angioplasty ± stent
- angioplasty for simple fibromuscular dysplasia lesion in young patients

Renal Parenchymal Hypertension

- HTN caused secondary to GN, AIN, diabetic nephropathy, or any other chronic renal disease
- mechanism of HTN not fully understood but may include:
  - excess renin-angiotensin-aldosterone system activation due to inflammation and fibrosis in multiple small intra-renal vessels
  - production of unknown vasopressors, lack of production of unknown vasodilators, or lack of clearance of endogenous vasopressor
  - ineffective sodium excretion with fluid overload

Investigations
- as well as investigations for renovascular HTN, additional tests may include:
  - 24-hour urinary estimations of Cr clearance and protein excretion
  - imaging (IVP, U/S, CT, radionuclide scan)
  - serology for collagen-vascular disease
  - renal biopsy

Treatment
- most chronic renal disease cannot be reversed but treatment of the HTN can slow the progression of renal insufficiency
- control ECF volume: Na restriction (88 mmol/day intake), diuretic, dialysis with end-stage disease
- ACE inhibitor may provide added benefit (monitor K and Cr)

Multiple Myeloma

- a malignant proliferation of plasma cells in the bone marrow with the production of immunoglobulins
- patients may present with severe bone disease and renal failure
- light chains are filtered at the glomerulus and appear as Bence-Jones proteins in the urine (monoclonal light chains)
- kidney damage can occur by several mechanisms:
  - hypercalcemia
  - hyperuricemia
  - infection
  - secondary amyloidosis
  - monoclonal Ig deposition disease (MIDD)
  - diffuse tubular obstruction
  - light chain cast nephropathy or 'myeloma kidney' (LCCN)
- LCCN
  - presents with large tubular casts in urine sediment (light chains + Tamm-Horsfall protein)
  - proteinuria and renal insufficiency, can progress rapidly to kidney failure
- MIDD
  - deposits of monoclonal Ig in kidney, liver, heart and other organs
  - mostly light chains (85-90%)
  - causes nodular glomerulosclerosis (similar to diabetic nephropathy)
- lab features: ↑ BUN, ↑ Cr, urine protein immunoelectrophoresis positive for Bence Jones protein (not detected on urine dipstick)

Features of Multiple Myeloma: CRAB

C - calcium (elevated)
R - renal failure
A - anemia
B - Bence-Jones proteins, Bone lesions

Malignancy

- cancer can have many different nephrological manifestations
    - solid tumours: mild proteinuria or membranous GN
    - lymphoma: minimal change GN or membranous GN
    - renal cell carcinoma
    - hypercalcemia
    - tumour lysis syndrome: hyperuricemia, diffuse tubular obstruction
    - chemotherapy (especially cisplatin): ATN or chronic TIN
    - pelvic tumours/mets: post-renal failure secondary to obstruction
    - 2° amyloidosis
    - radiotherapy (radiation nephritis)

Diabetes and the Kidney

- diabetic nephropathy: presence of microalbuminuria or overt nephropathy in patients with DM who lack indicators of other renal diseases
- number one cause of end-stage renal failure in North America
- 35-50% of Type 1 will develop nephropathy, unknown percentage of Type 2
- at diagnosis up to 30% of Type 2 have albuminuria (75% microalbuminuria, 25% overt nephropathy)
- microalbuminuria is a risk factor for progression to overt nephropathy and cardiovascular disease
- once proteinuria is established, renal function declines, 50% patients reach ESRD within 7-10 years
- associated with HTN and diabetic retinopathy
- indication of possible nondiabetic renal disease in diabetic patients:
    - rising Cr with little/no proteinuria
    - lack of retinopathy or neuropathy (microvascular complications)
    - persistent hematuria (microscopic or macroscopic)
    - signs or symptoms of systemic disease
    - inappropriate time course; rapidly rising Cr, short duration of DM
    - family history of nondiabetic renal disease (e.g. PCKD, Alport's)

FOUR BASIC DIABETIC RENAL COMPLICATIONS

1) Progressive Glomerulosclerosis
- classic diabetic glomerular lesion: Kimmelstiel-Wilson nodular glomerulosclerosis (15-20%)
- more common lesion is diffuse glomerulosclerosis with a uniform increase in mesangial matrix
- stage 1
    - **increased GFR** (120-150%) – compensatory hyperfiltration of remaining nephrons
    - ± slightly increased mesangial matrix
- stage 2
    - **detectable microalbuminuria** (between 0-300 mg/24hrs)
    - **Albumin-Creatinine ratio (ACR)** 2.0–20 mg/mmol in men (which is equal to 18-180 mg/g), 2.8-28 mg/mmol in women (which is 25-250 mg/g)
    - increased GFR
    - increased mesangial matrix
- stage 3
    - **macroalbuminuria** (>300 mg/24h); **ACR** in men >20 mg/mmol, (which is about >180 mg/g); in women, ACR is >28 mg/mmol (which is >250 mg/d)
    - **clinically detectable proteinuria**, +ve urine dipstick
    - normal GFR
    - very expanded mesangial matrix
- stage 4
    - **increased proteinuria** (>500 mg/24hr)
    - decreased GFR
    - <20% glomerular filtration surface area present
    - sclerosed glomeruli

2) Accelerated Atherosclerosis
- common finding
- decreased GFR
- may increase Angiotensin II production; results in increased BP
- increased risk of ATN secondary to contrast media

DM is one of the causes of ESRD that does not result in small kidneys at presentation of ESRD. The others are amyloidosis, HIV nephropathy, PCKD and multiple myeloma.

Telmisartan, Ramipril or both in patients at high risk of vascular events (ONTARGET study)
NEJM 2008; 358:1547-59
Study: Prospective, multi-centre, double-blind randomized controlled trial.
Patients: 25 577 patients followed for a median of 6 months.
Intervention: 3 arm trial. Arm 1:8576 patients receiving 10 mg of ramipril. Arm 2:8542 patients receiving 80 mg of telmisartan. Arm 3:8502 patients receiving combination therapy (ramipril and telmisartan).
Primary Outcome: Death from cardiovascular causes, myocardial infarction, stroke or hospitalization for heart failure.
Result: Mean blood pressure lower in telmisartan and combination therapy groups (compared to ramipril alone group). No difference in primary outcome amongst the three arms. Lower rates of cough and angioedema, and a higher rate of hypotensive symptoms occurred in the telmisartan group compared to ramipril. Combination therapy had higher rates of hypotensive symptoms, syncope and renal dysfunction as compared to ramipril.
Conclusion: In patients at high risk of cardiovascular events, telmisartan was as efficacious as ramipril in reducing mortality and morbidity from cardiovascular causes. Telmisartan was associated with less cough and angioedema. Combination therapy showed no increase in benefit with an increase in adverse events.

ACEI can cause hyperkalemia. Therefore, be sure to watch serum K, especially if patient has DM and renal insufficiency.

Effects of Losartan on Renal and Caridovascular Outcomes in Patients with Type 2 DM and Nephropathy
NEJM 2001;345:861-869
Study: Randomized, double-blind, placebo-controlled trial with mean follow-up of 3.4 years.
Patients: 1513 patients (mean age 60, 63% male, multi-ethnicity) with NIDDM and nephropathy (urinary albumin:Cr ≥300 and serum Cr 115-265 µmol/L) on conventional antihypertensives (CCB, diuretics, β-blockers, α-blockers, centrally acting agents).
Intervention: Losartan 50 mg PO OD (could be doubled after 4 weeks) vs. placebo
Outcomes: Primary endpoints included doubling of serum Cr, ESRD, or death. Secondary endpoints included morbidity and mortality from CVD causes.
Results: Losartan reduced incidence of doubling of serum Cr (RR 25%) and ESRD (RR 28%), but had no effect on risk of death. Benefit exceeded that attributable to BP changes alone. Secondary end points were similar, although rate of hospitalization for heart failure was significantly lower with losartan (RR 32%).
Conclusion: Losartan conferred significant renal benefits in patients with type 2 diabetes and nephropathy, and was generally well tolerated.

Effects of ACEI on Diabetic Nephropathy
NEJM 1993;329(20):1456-62
Study: Multicentre, randomized, double-blinded, placebo-controlled trial with median follow-up of 3 years.
Patients: 409 patients with Type 1 diabetes for at least 7 years, retinopathy, proteinuria, and a serum Cr less than 221.
Intervention: 25 mg captopril tid.
Main Outcomes: Doubling of baseline Cr, time to death/dialysis/transplant.
Results: 12% of patients receiving captopril experienced a doubling of their Cr, while 21% of the placebo group did as well (RR 0.52, p=0.007). Time to death/dialysis/transplant was also increased (RR 0.50, p=0.006).
Conclusion: Decline in renal function in diabetic nephropathy is slowed by captopril.

Protein restriction for diabetic renal disease
Cochrane Database Syst Rev. 2007;(4):CD002181
Purpose: To review the effects of dietary protein restriction on the progression of diabetic nephropathy.
Study Selection: Randomised controlled trials (RCTs) and before and after studies of the effects of restricted protein diet on renal function in subjects with diabetes. 12 studies were reviewed.
Results: The risk of end-stage renal disease or death was lower in patients on low-protein diet. In patients with Type 1 diabetes no effect on GFR was noted in the low-protein diet group.

3) Autonomic Neuropathy
- affects bladder; leads to functional obstruction and urinary retention
- residual urine promotes infection
- obstructive nephropathy

4) Papillary Necrosis
- Type 1 DM susceptible to ischemic necrosis of medullary papillae
- sloughed papillae may obstruct ureter
- can present as renal colic or with obstructive features ± hydronephrosis

2003 Canadian Diabetics Association Clinical Practice Guidelines on Nephropathy
- screen for microalbuminuria: random urine test for albumin to Cr ratio (ACR) and dipstick
    - annually in postpubertal who have had Type 1 DM for 5 years duration
    - Type 2 DM: at diagnosis then annually
    - must have at least 2/3 abnormal ACRs to diagnose nephropathy
- estimate CrCl: annually in those without albuminuria, at least q6mo in patients with nephropathy
- evaluate for other causes of proteinuria, rule out nondiabetic renal disease
- avoid unnecessary potential nephrotoxins (NSAIDs, aminoglycosides, dye studies)

Priorities in the Management of Patients with DM
1. vascular protection for all patients with diabetes
    - ACEI, antiplatelet therapy (as indicated)
    - BP control, glycemic control, lifestyle modification, lipid control
2. optimization of BP in patients who are hypertensive
    - treat according to hypertension guidelines
3. renal protection for DM patients with nephropathy (even in absence of HTN)
    - Type 1 DM: ACEI
    - Type 2 DM: CrCl >60 mL/min: ACEI or ARB
        - CrCl <60 mL/min: ARB
    - 2nd line agents: nondihydropyridine calcium channel blockers (diltiazem, verapamil)
    - ACEI and ARB can be safely used together (monitor for hyperkalemia)
- check serum Cr and K levels within 2 weeks of initiating ACEI or ARB
- monitor for significant worsening of renal function or development of hyperkalemia
- serum Cr can rise up to 30% with initiation of ACEI or ARB, usually stabilizes after 2-4 wks
- if >30% rise in serum Cr, or severe hyperkalemia, discontinue medication and consider 2nd line agent
- consider referral to nephrologist if ACR >75 mg/mmol (>650 mg/g)

Cystic Diseases of the Kidney

- characterized by epithelium-lined cavities filled with fluid or semisolid debris within the kidneys
- includes: simple cysts (present in 50% of population over 50), medullary cystic kidney, medullary sponge kidney, polycystic kidney disease (autosomal dominant and recessive) and acquired cystic kidney disease (in chronic hemodialysis patients)

Adult Polycystic Kidney Disease

- PKD1 (1:400), PKD2 (1:1,000), accounts for about 10% of cases of renal failure
- autosomal dominant; at least 3 genes: PKD1 (chr 16p), PKD2 (chr 4q), PKD3 (location not yet determined)
- polycystin protein from PKD1 responsible for cell-cell and cell-matrix interaction
- defect can lead to abnormal cell growth and cyst formation
- extrarenal manifestations: most common; multiple asymptomatic hepatic cysts (33%) cerebral aneurysm (10%), diverticulosis and mitral valve prolapse (25%)

- polycystic liver disease rarely causes liver failure
  - less common: cysts in pancreas, spleen, thyroid, ovary, seminal vesicles, and aorta

Signs and Symptoms
- often asymptomatic; discovered incidentally on imaging or by screening those with FHx
- acute abdominal flank pain/dull lumbar back pain
- hematuria (microscopic frequently initial sign, gross)
- nocturia (urinary concentrating defect)
- rarely extra-renal presentation (e.g. ruptured berry aneurysm, diverticulitis)
- HTN (increased renin due to focal compression of intrarenal arteries by cysts) (60-75%)
- ± palpable kidneys

Common Complications
- urinary tract and cyst infections, HTN, CRF, nephrolithiasis (5-15%), flank and chronic back pain

Clinical Course
- polycystic changes are always bilateral and can present at any age
- clinical manifestations rare before age 20-25
- kidneys are normal at birth but may enlarge to 10 times normal volume
- variable progression to renal functional impairment (ESRD in up to 50% by age 60) investigations
- radiographic diagnosis – best accomplished by renal U/S (enlarged kidneys, multiple cysts throughout renal parenchyma, increased cortical thickness, splaying of renal calyces)
- CT abdo with contrast (for equivocal cases, occasionally reveals more cystic involvement)
- gene linkage analysis for PKD1 for asymptomatic carriers
  - Cr, BUN, urine R&M (to assess for hematuria)

Treatment
- goal: to preserve renal function by prevention and treatment of complications
- educate patient and family about disease, its manifestations and inheritance pattern
- genetic counselling: transmission rate 50% from affected parent
- prevention and early treatment of urinary tract and cyst infections (avoid instrumentation of GU tract)
- TMP/SMX, ciprofloxacin: able to penetrate cyst walls, achieve therapeutic levels
- adequate hydration to prevent stone formation
- avoid contact sports due to greater risk of injury to enlarged kidneys
- screen for cerebral aneurysms if strong family history of aneurysmal hemorrhages
- monitor blood pressure and treat hypertension with ACEI
- dialysis or transplant for ESRD (disease does not recur in transplanted kidney)
- may require nephrectomy to create room for renal transplant

Medullary Sponge Kidney

- common, autosomal dominant, usually diagnosed in 4th-5th decades
- multiple cystic dilatations in the collecting ducts of the medulla
- renal stones, hematuria and recurrent UTIs are common features
- an estimated 10% of patients who present with renal stones have medullary sponge kidney
- nephrocalcinosis on abdominal x-ray in 50% patients, often detect asymptomatic patients incidentally
- diagnosis: contrast filled medullary cysts on IVP, characteristic radial pattern ("bouquet of flowers"), "swiss cheese" appearance on morphology
- treat UTIs and stone formation as indicated
- does not result in renal failure

Autosomal Recessive Polycystic Kidney Disease

- 1:20,000 incidence
- prenatal diagnosis by enlarged kidneys
- perinatal death from respiratory failure
- patients who survive perinatal period develop: CHF, HTN, chronic kidney disease
- treated with kidney and/or liver transplant

Common Medications

Table 15. Drugs in Nephrology

Classification	Examples	Site of Action	Mechanism of Action (Secondary Effect)	Indication	Dosing	Adverse Effects
Loop diuretics	furosemide (Lasix™) bumetanide (Bumex™/Buinex™) ethacrynate (Edecrin™) torsemide (Demadex™) telmisartan (Micardis™) eprosartan (Teveten™)	Thick ascending limb of Loop of Henle	↓ Na/K/2Cl transport ± renal and peripheral vasodilatory effects (K loss; ↑ H secretion; ↑ Ca excretion)	Management of edema secondary to CHF, nephrotic syndrome, cirrhotic ascites ↑free water clearance (SIADH-induced hyponatremia) ↓BP (less effective due to short action)	furosemide: edema - 20-80 mg IV/IM/PO q6-8 (max 600 mg/d) until desired response HTN - 20-80 mg/d PO OD/bid dosing telmisartan 20-80 mg PO OD eprosartan 400-800 mg PO OD	Allergy in sulfa-sensitive individuals Electrolyte abnormalities hypokalemia, hyponatremia, hypocalcemia, hypercalciuria (with stone formation) Volume depletion with metabolic alkalosis Precipitates gouty attacks
Thiazide diuretic	hydrochlorothiazide (HCTZ) chlorothiazide (Diuril™) indapamide (Lozol™, Lozide™) metolazone (Zaroxolyn™)	Distal convoluted tubule	Inhibit NaCl transporter (K loss; ↑ H secretion; ↓ Ca excretion)	1st line for essential HTN treatment of edema in states as above Idiopathic hypercalciuria + stones Diabetes Insipidus (nephrogenic)	HCTZ: edema - 25-100 mg PO OD HTN - 12.5-25 PO OD (max 50 mg/d) nephrolithiasis/hypercalciuria - 50-100 mg od	Hypokalemia Increased serum urate levels Precipitates gouty attacks, hypercalcemia Elevated lipids Glucose intolerance
Potassium-sparing	spironolactone (Aldactone™) triamterene (Dyrenium™) amiloride (Midamor™)	Cortical collecting duct Cortical collecting duct	Aldosterone antagonist ↓ Na reabsorption (K loss; ↓ H secretion) Closes apical Na channels ↓ Na reabsorption	↓K loss caused by other diuretics; can be used in combination to treat edema, HTN Severe CHF, ascites (spironolactone) CF (amiloride ↓ viscosity of secretions)	spironolactone: edema/hypervolemia - 25-200 mg/day OD/bid dosing HTN: 50-200 mg/day OD/bid dosing hyperaldosteronism - 100-400 mg/day OD/bid dosing amiloride: edema/HTN: 5-10 mg PO OD	Hyperkalemia (caution with ACE inhibitor) Gynecomastia (estrogenic effect of spironolactone) Triamterene can be nephrotoxic (rare) Nephrolithiasis
Combination agents	Dyazide™ (triamterene + HCTZ) Aldactazide™ (spironolactone + HCTZ) Moduretic™ (amiloride + HCTZ) Vaseretic™ (enalapril + HCTZ) Zestoretic™ (lisinopril + HCTZ)		Combine ACE-inhibitor with thiazide for synergistic effect	Combine K-sparing drug with thiazide to reduce hypokalemia antihypertensive effect		
Osmotic diuretics	mannitol (Osmitrol™) glycerol urea	Renal tubules (proximal and collecting duct)	Non-reabsorbable solutes increase osmotic pressure of glomerular filtrate - inhibit reabsorption of water and electrolytes	↓ intracranial or intraocular pressure Mobilization of excess fluid in renal failure or edematous states ↑ urinary excretion of toxic materials	mannitol: ↓ICP: 0.25-2 g/kg IV over 30-60 min	Transient volume expansion Electrolyte abnormalities (↓/↑ Na, ↓/↑ K)
ACEI	ramipril (Altace™) enalapril (Vasotec™) lisinopril (Prinivil™) trandolapril (Mavik™)	Lungs	Prevents angiotensin II vasodilatory action on vascular smooth muscle → ↓BP Prevents angiotensin II mediated aldosterone release from adrenal cortex and action on proximal renal tubules → ↑ Na and H₂O excretion	HTN Cardioprotective effects (see Cardiology) Renoprotective effects	ramipril: HTN - 2.5-20 mg PO OD/bid dosing renoprotective use - 10 mg PO OD trandolapril: HTN - 1-4 mg PO OD	Cough Hyperkalemia Angioedema Agranulocytosis (captopril)
ARB	losartan (Cozaar™) candesartan (Atacand™) irbesartan (Avapro™) valsartan (Diovan™) telmisartan (Micardis™) eprosartan (Teveten™)	Vascular smooth muscle, adrenal cortex, proximal tubules	Competitive inhibitor at the angiotensin II receptor: prevents angiotensin II vasodilatory action on vascular smooth muscle → ↑BP Prevents angiotensin II mediated aldosterone release from adrenal cortex and action on proximal renal tubules → ↑ Na and H₂O excretion	HTN Cardioprotective effects (see Cardiology) Renoprotective effects	HTN: losartan: 25-100 mg PO OD candesartan 8-32 mg PO OD irbesartan 150-300 mg PO OD valsartan 80-320 mg PO OD telmisartan 20-80 mg PO OD eprosartan 400-800 mg PO OD	Hyperkalemia Caution - reduce dose in hepatic impairment and in volume depletion

N Neurology

Alexandra Kuritzky, Nic Petrescu and Amol Verma, chapter editors
Deepti Damaraju and Elliott Owen, associate editors
Erik Venos, EBM editor
Dr. Cheryl Jaigobin and Dr. Liesly Lee, staff editors

Basic Anatomy Review

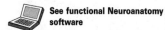

See functional Neuroanatomy software

Basic Anatomy Review

- see also Neurosurgery, NS22 for Dermatome/Myotome information

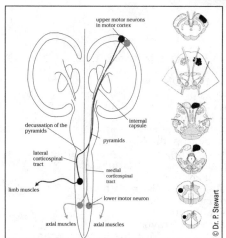

Figure 1. Corticospinal Motor Pathway

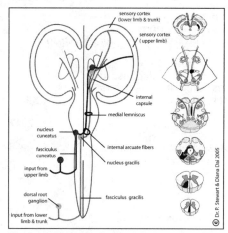

Figure 2. Discriminative Touch Pathway From Body

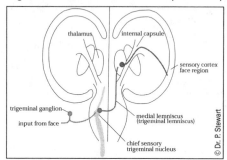

Figure 3. Discriminative Touch Pathway From Face

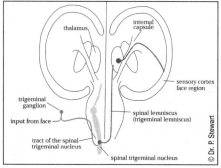

Figure 4. Spinothalamic Pain Pathway from Face

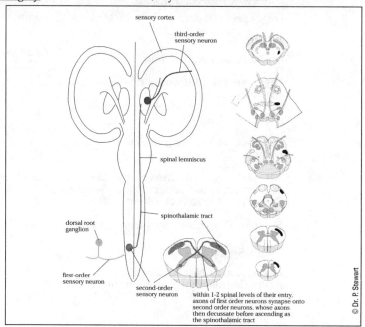

within 1-2 spinal levels of their entry, axons of first order neurons synapse onto second order neurons, whose axons then decussate before ascending as the spinothalamic tract

Figure 5. Spinothalamic Tract

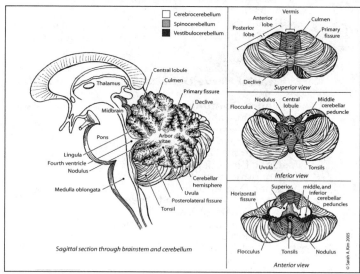

Sagittal section through brainstem and cerebellum

Figure 6. Cerebellum

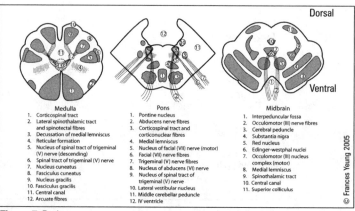

Medulla
1. Corticospinal tract
2. Lateral spinothalamic tract and spinotectal fibres
3. Decussation of medial lemniscus
4. Reticular formation
5. Nucleus of spinal tract of trigeminal (V) nerve (descending)
6. Spinal tract of trigeminal (V) nerve
7. Nucleus cuneatus
8. Fasciculus cuneatus
9. Nucleus gracilis
10. Fasciculus gracilis
11. Central canal
12. Arcuate fibres

Pons
1. Pontine nucleus
2. Abducens nerve fibres
3. Corticospinal tract and corticonuclear fibres
4. Medial lemniscus
5. Nucleus of facial (VII) nerve (motor)
6. Facial (VII) nerve fibres
7. Trigeminal (V) nerve fibres
8. Nucleus of abducens (VI) nerve
9. Nucleus of spinal tract of trigeminal (V) nerve
10. Lateral vestibular nucleus
11. Middle cerebellar peduncle
12. IV ventricle

Midbrain
1. Interpeduncular fossa
2. Occulomotor (III) nerve fibres
3. Cerebral peduncle
4. Substantia nigra
5. Red nucleus
6. Edinger-westphal nuclei
7. Occulomotor (III) nucleus complex (motor)
8. Medial lemniscus
9. Spinothalamic tract
10. Central canal
11. Superior colliculus

Figure 7. Brainstem

Differential Diagnosis of Common Presentations

1. Headache

Red Flags	No Red Flags
subarachnoid hemorrhage	migraine
meningitis	tension-type
increased intracranial pressure	cluster
temporal arteritis	

2. Paresis/Paralysis
- stroke
- tumour
- multiple sclerosis
- myasthenia gravis
- Guillain-Barré syndrome
- amyotrophic lateral sclerosis
- peripheral neuropathies
- myopathies

3. Sensory Disturbance
- stroke
- tumour
- multiple sclerosis
- peripheral neuropathies
- Vitamin B12 deficiency

4. Facial Pain
- sinusitis
- dental disease
- tic douloureux (Trigeminal Neuralgia)
- trigeminal neuropathic pain (secondary to trigeminal nerve injury or disease)
- glossopharyngeal neuralgia
- postherpetic neuralgia
- atypical facial pain
- multiple sclerosis

5. Facial Weakness
- upper motor neuron
  - TIA/stroke
  - post-ictal hemiparesis
  - tumour
  - infection: otitis media, mastoiditis, Epstein-Barr virus (EBV), herpes zoster virus (HZV), Lyme disease, HIV
- lower motor neuron
  - infection: otitis media, mastoiditis, Epstein-Barr virus (EBV), herpes zoster virus (HZV), Lyme disease, HIV
  - idiopathic (Bell's palsy)
  - sarcoid
  - neuropathy (DM)
  - parotid gland

6. Altered Mental Status
- coma

CNS (diffuse)	Metabolic	Systemic	CNS (focal structural lesion)
head trauma	diabetic ketoacidosis	liver failure	abscess
infection	hypoglycemia	renal failure	epidural/subdural hematoma
inflammation/vasculitis	electrolyte disturbance	sepsis	hemorrhage/aneurysm
global cerebral ischemia	acid-base disturbance		hydrocephalus
subclinical seizure/	thiamine deficiency		stroke
post-ictal state			tumour
hypertensive encephalopathy			venous occlusion

- acute confusional states (delirium)
  - see Psychiatry
- dementia, other psychiatric (e.g. depression)
  - see Psychiatry

7. Acute Loss of Vision

Painful	Minimal Pain
Angle Closure Glaucoma	Retinal detachment
Optic Neuritis	Central Retinal Artery Occlusion
Temporal Arteritis	TIA/Stroke
Trauma	Pseudotumour cerebri

8. Diplopia
- neuromuscular:
    - cranial nerve III/IV/VI palsies (DM, tumour, trauma, aneurysm)
    - brainstem pathology (stroke, tumour, MS)
    - myasthenia gravis
    - Wernicke's encephalopathy
    - leptomeningeal disease (e.g. meningitis)
    - Guillain-Barré syndrome (e.g. Miller-Fisher Variant)
- mechanical
    - thyroid ophthalmopathy
    - cavernous sinus pathology
    - trauma (e.g. orbital fracture)

9. Ptosis
- cranial nerve III palsy
- myasthenia gravis (uni/bilateral)
- Horner's syndrome
- congenital/idiopathic
- myotonic dystrophy (bilateral)

10. Vertigo
- brainstem lesions (stroke, MS)
- cerebellar lesions
- vertebrobasilar insufficiency
- drugs/alcohol
- peripheral causes (see Ototlaryngology)

Review of Neurological Examination

- **Vitals:** pulse (especially rhythm), BP, temperature
- **Head & Neck:** look for meningismus, bruises/injuries/trauma to head (i.e. battle sign/raccoon eyes); tongue biting may suggest seizures
- **Cardiac/Vascular:** auscultate for bruits (e.g. carotid), murmurs
- **Neurological:**
  General Approach
    1) State of Consciousness/Arousal
        - Glasgow Coma Scale (GCS) (Eye, Verbal, Motor)
        - reflexes: responses to pain may include decerebrate and decorticate posturing
        - see *Altered Level of Consciousness*
    2) Mental Status (see Psychiatry)
        - appearance, behaviour, mood, affect, speech, thought process, thought content, perceptions, insight, judgement
        - assess as is appropriate throughout the interview
    3) Cognition
        - Mini-Mental Status Exam (MMSE), clock drawing, Baycrest Neurocognitive Assessment, MOCA
        - frontal lobe testing for perseveration
    4) Cranial Nerve Examination (see Table 2)
    5) Motor Examination
        - inspection: bulk, accessory movements, tremor, fasciculations, etc.
        - tone (assess for rigidity, spasticity, clonus)
        - power (0-5, 0: no contraction, 1: flicker, 2: active movement with gravity eliminated, 3: active movement against gravity, 4-,4, 4+: active movement against gravity and resistance, 5: full power)
        - reflexes (0 – 4+, 0: absent with reenforcement, 1+: reduced, 2+: normal, 3+: increased, 4+: clonus present)
    6) Sensory Examination
        - posterior columns (vibration, proprioception, light touch)
        - spinothalamic (pain, temperature)
        - cortical sensation (graphesthesia, stereognosis, extinction, 2-point discrimination)
    7) Co-ordination
        - finger to nose, heel to shin, rapid alternating movements
    8) Stance & Gait
        - Romberg, tandem gait

Lesion Localization (*WHERE* is the lesion?)

Table 1. Anatomic Approach to Neurological Disorders, Symptoms and Signs

Location of the lesion	General Symptoms	Common Disorders
Cortex & Internal capsule	Contralateral sensory & motor deficits Cortical lesions: associated with aphasia, neglect, extinction, graphanaesthesia, astereognosia, visual loss (higher level dysfunctions) Internal capsule lesions: associated with pure motor, pure sensory losses, incoordination, absence of cortical features	Seizure disorder (cortex only) Coma Stroke
Cerebellum & Basal ganglia	Incoordination → Abnormal intentional movements for cerebellar lesions (ipsilateral) → tremor, bradykinesia, cogwheel rigidity, involuntary movements for basal ganglia lesions	Cerebellar degeneration Parkinson's disease Stroke
Brainstem (unilateral) (midbrain CN 3-4; pons CN 6-7; medulla CN 8-10)	Bilateral motor abnormalities (UMN pattern). Crossed sensory signs (ipsilateral face, contralateral body). MIDBRAIN: diplopia, ptosis, pupillary changes (large or midposition and unreactive) PONS: LMN facial weakness, quadriparesis in bilateral pontine lesions, pinpoint pupils MEDULLA: lateral or medial medullary syndromes	Cranial nerve palsies Stroke
Spinal cord (unilateral)	Ipsilateral paralysis and proprioceptive loss, contralateral pain-temperature loss below the level of the lesion – Brown-Sequard syndrome Sensory level, bowel/bladder dysfunction paraparesis	Spinal cord syndromes
Nerve root	Radicular pain + sensory/motor deficits or absent reflex	Nerve root compression Disk herniation
Peripheral nerve	Ipsilateral motor and sensory deficits along a nerve distribution. Presence of LMN signs. Polyneuropathy (distal weakness, glove and stocking distribution of sensory loss)	Neuropathies
Neuromuscular junction	Proximal & symmetrical muscle weakness without sensory loss, fatiguability Diplopia, ptosis, bulbar weakness	Myasthenia gravis Lambert-Eaton syndrome Botulism
Muscle	Proximal & symmetrical muscle weakness without sensory loss	Muscular dystrophies Myopathies including polymyositis Dermatomyositis

Table 2. Some helpful findings on physical examination

Cranial Nerves

CN1   unilateral loss of smell suggests inferior frontal lobe lesion (avoid irritative stimuli which stimulate CN5)
CN2   look at optic discs for edema and optic atrophy
CN3/4/6   look for pupillary abnormalities, ptosis, abnormal eye movements
    ***Drug reactions*:**
    bilaterally dilated fixed pupils with anticholinergics (e.g. atropine, "mushrooms"), but also seen in herniation
    bilaterally small fixed pupils with morphine and related drugs, but also seen in pontine lesion
    Horner's syndrome = ptosis, miosis (anisocoria), anhydrosis (due to interrupted sympathetic nerve supply)
    CN3 palsy = ptosis, eye is down and out, +/- impaired pupillary response (suggests a structural/compressive cause)
CN5   absent corneal reflex may be CN5 (sensory deficit) or CN7 (motor deficit)
CN7   forehead sparing = upper motor neuron lesion
CN9/10   dysarthria

Motor System

Ataxia may be due to cerebellar disease, proprioceptive abnormality
    Ataxia with eyes closed only is a positive Romberg's sign suggesting a loss of joint position sense/peripheral neuropathy
    Ataxia with eyes open or closed suggests cerebellar disease
Pronator drift suggests hemiparesis or loss of position sense
Spasticity indicates upper motor neuron disease
Atrophy and fasciculations indicates lower motor neuron disease
Cogwheel rigidity is seen in extrapyramidal processes (e.g. Parkinson's Disease)
Symmetrical weakness of proximal muscles suggests myopathy; of distal muscles suggests polyneuropathy

Sensory System

Hemisensory loss with sensory level or dissociation loss suggests spinal cord lesion
Symmetrical distal sensory loss suggests polyneuropathy
Loss of vibration sense suggests peripheral neuropathy or posterior column lesion
Impaired graphesthesia and stereognosis with intact primary sensation indicates parietal lesion

Reflexes

Increased in upper motor neuron disease
Decreased/absent in lower motor neuron disease, myopathies or neuromuscular junction disorders
Slow relaxation of ankle reflex is seen in hypothyroidism ("hung reflexes")
Pendular reflexes suggest cerebellar lesion
Babinski sign suggests an upper motor neuron lesion but may be seen following a seizure

Other

"Doll's eye" movement, if absent, suggests pons or midbrain lesion or very deep coma
Loss of vestibulo-ocular reflex with caloric stimulation suggests brain stem lesion or drug toxicity
Absence seizures can be precipitated by hyperventilation
Characteristic skin lesions are seen in neurocutaneaous syndromes (e.g. neurofibromatosis, tuberous sclerosis complex, Sturge-Weber syndrome), non-blanching petechiae are seen in meningitis, Thrombotic Thrombocytopenic Purpura (TTP)

Diagnostic Investigations

Lumbar Puncture

Indications
- **diagnostic**: CNS infection (meningitis, encephalitis), inflammatory disorder (MS, Guillain-Barré, vasculitis), sub-arachnoid hemorrhage (SAH) (CT negative), CNS neoplasm (neoplastic meningitis)
- **therapeutic**: to administer anesthesia, chemotherapy, contrast media; to decrease intracranial pressure (pseudotumour cerebri)

Contraindications
- increased intracranial pressure (ICP)
  - must do CT first to rule out mass lesion with increased intracranial pressure (ICP)
  - do not attempt if mass lesion associated with papilledema, decreased level of consciousness (LOC), or focal neurological deficit
- posterior fossa signs
  - must do MRI to rule out lesion
- coagulopathy, thrombocytopenia, anticoagulation
- infection over lumbar puncture (LP) site
- uncooperative patient

Complications
- tonsillar herniation
- post-LP headache (20-40%) – worse when upright, better supine
  - management: keep patient supine, po fluids, analgesia, blood patch
  - caffeine 300-500 mg po q4-6h
- spinal epidural hematoma
- infection

Table 3. Lumbar Puncture Interpretation

Condition	Colour	Protein	Glucose	Cells	Other
Normal	Clear	<0.45 g/L	60% of serum Glc >3.0 mmol/L	0-5 WBC, 0 RBC 0 neutrophills	
Infectious					
Viral infection	Clear or opalescent	Normal or slightly increased <0.45-1 g/L	Normal	<1000x10^6/L Lymphocytes mostly, some PMNs	
Bacterial infection	Opalescent yellow, may clot	>1 g/L	Decreased (<25% serum glc or <2.0 mmol/L)	>1000x10^6/L PMNs	
Granulomatous infection (tuberculosis, fungal)	Clear or opalescent	Increased but usually <5 g/L	Decreased (usually <2.0-4.0 mmol/L)	<1000x10^6/L Lymphocytes	Low CSF glucose in TB
Neurologic					
Guillain-Barré Syndrome	Clear or cloudy	Markedly increased	Normal	Normal	albuminocytological dissociation
Multiple Sclerosis	Clear	Normal or increased	Normal	0-20x10^6/L lymphocytes	Oligoclonal banding on protein electrophoresis
Pseudotumour Cerebri	Clear	Normal	Normal	Normal	Elevated opening pressure
Other					
Neoplasm (neoplastic meningitis)	Clear or xanthochromic	Normal or increased	Normal or decreased	Normal or increased lymphocytes	Cytology positive
Traumatic tap	Bloody, no xanthochromia	Normal	Slightly increased	RBCs = peripheral blood, less RBCs in tube 4 than tube 1	
Subarachnoid hemorrhage	Bloody, or xanthochromia after 2-8 h	Increased	Normal	WBC/RBC ratio same as blood Same number of RBCs in tubes 1 & 4	

What to send LP for
Tube #1: Cell Count and Differential
- RBCs
- WBCs and differential (normal: <3.0 x 10^6/L)
- xanthochromia (yellow in colour, from bilirubin pigmentation)
  - supernatant should be clear; if yellow, implies recent bleed into cerebrospinal fluid (CSF)

Tube #2: Chemistry
- glucose
  - must compare to simultaneously drawn serum glucose
- protein
  - CSF IgG: increased in MS and demyelinating neuropathies

Tube #3: Microbiology
- gram stain
- C&S
- specific tests depending on clinical situation/suspicion

- viral: PCR for herpes simplex virus (HSV)
- bacterial: polysaccharide antigens of *H.flu, N.meningitides, Pneumococcus*
- fungal: Cryptococcal antigen, India ink stain (cryptococcus), culture
- TB: Acid-Fast stain, TB culture, TB PCR

Tube #4: Cytology (for evidence of malignancy)
Tube #5: RBCs (cell count) – similar to tube #1
- if RBCs in tube #1 is >> RBCs in tube #5 then consider traumatic tap
- in SAH, RBCs in tubes #1 and #5 should be approximately equal

Altered Level of Consciousness

Altered Level of Consciousness/Evaluation

ALTERED LEVEL OF CONSCIOUSNESS
- see <u>Neurosurgery</u>

EVALUATION OF PATIENT

History
- previous/recent head injury (hematomas)
- sudden collapse (ICH, SAH)
- cardiovascular surgery, prolonged cardiac arrest (hypoxia)
- limb twitching, incontinence, tongue biting (seizures, post-ictal state)
- recent infection (meningitis)
- other medical problems (diabetes mellitus (DM), renal failure, hepatic encephalopathy)
- psychiatric illness (drug overdose)
- telephone witnesses, read ambulance report, check for Medic-Alert™ bracelet
- neurologic symptoms (headache, visual changes, focal weakness)

Physical Examination
- Glascow Coma Scale
- pupils – reactivity and symmetry
- fundi – papilledema (increased ICP)
- reflexes
    - corneal reflex: normal = bilateral blinking response
    - gag reflex: normal = gag
    - oculocephalic reflex (doll's eye): normal = eyes move in opposite direction of head, as if trying to maintain fixation of a point
    - vestibulocochlear response (cold caloric): normal = nystagmus fast phase away from stimulated ear
    - deep tendon reflexes
    - plantar reflex: normal = flexor plantar response
- tone
- spontaneous involuntary movements
- assess for meningeal irritation, increased temperature
- assess for head injury, battle sign, raccoon eyes, skin rashes, and joint abnormalities that may suggest vasculitis

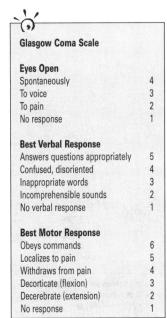

Glasgow Coma Scale

Eyes Open

Spontaneously	4
To voice	3
To pain	2
No response	1

Best Verbal Response

Answers questions appropriately	5
Confused, disoriented	4
Inappropriate words	3
Incomprehensible sounds	2
No verbal response	1

Best Motor Response

Obeys commands	6
Localizes to pain	5
Withdraws from pain	4
Decorticate (flexion)	3
Decerebrate (extension)	2
No response	1

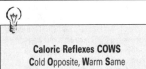

Caloric Reflexes COWS
Cold **O**pposite, **W**arm **S**ame

Coma/Vegetative State/Brain Death

COMA

Definition
- a state in which patients show no meaningful response to environmental stimuli, from which they cannot be roused; unrousable unresponsiveness

Pathophysiology
- coma can be caused by lesions affecting the cerebral cortex bilaterally, the reticular activating system (RAS) or their connecting fibres
- focal supratentorial lesions do not alter consciousness except by herniation (with compression on the brainstem or on the contralateral hemisphere) or by precipitating seizures

Classification
- structural lesions (tumor, pus, blood, infarction, CSF); 1/3 of comas
    - supratentorial mass lesion - leading to herniation as outlined above
    - infratentorial lesion - compression of or direct damage to the RAS or its projections

- metabolic disorders/diffuse hemispheric damage; 2/3 of comas
  - deficiency of essential substrates (e.g. oxygen, glucose, vitamin B12)
  - exogenous toxins (e.g. drugs, heavy metals, solvents)
  - endogenous toxins/systemic metabolic diseases (e.g. uremia, hepatic encephalopathy, electrolyte imbalances, thyroid storm)
  - infections (meningitis, encephalitis)
  - trauma (concussion, diffuse shear axonal damage)

Investigations and Management
- ABCs
- labs: electrolytes, TSH, LFTs, Cr, BUN, Ca, Mg, PO_4, tox. screen, glucose
- CT/MRI, LP, EEG
- consult neurosurgery if required

PERSISTENT VEGETATIVE STATE

Definition
- a condition of complete unawareness of the self and the environment accompanied by sleep-wake cycles with either complete or partial preservation of hypothalamic and brain stem autonomic function
- 'awake but not aware'
- follows comatose state
- diagnosis must be made with caution

Etiology/Prognosis
- most commonly caused by cardiac arrest or head injury
- due to irreversible loss of cerebral cortical function BUT with intact brainstem function
- average life expectancy 2-5 years

Seizure Disorders and Epilepsy

Seizure

Definition
- seizure = transient neurological dysfunction caused by excessive activity of cortical neurons, resulting in paroxysmal alteration in behaviour and/or EEG changes. May represent epilepsy but must be differentiated from a variety of secondary causes
- epilepsy = chronic condition characterized by recurrent, unprovoked seizure activity
- ictal = seizure
- post-ictal = state of confusion/somnolence that can occur after some seizure types
- inter-ictal = epileptic discharges that can be seen on EEG occurring between seizures

Classification
1. Epileptic Seizures
   - no identifiable cause
   - identifiable cause:
     - young: congenital brain malformation, inborn error of metabolism, febrile seizure
     - adult: intra-cranial infection, tumours, stroke, alcohol or benzodiazepine withdrawal, trauma
     - elderly: cerebral degeneration, vascular, tumours, drug reactions
     - metabolic/endocrine derangement
       - hypo/hyperthryoid
       - electrolyte disturbance: hyponatremia, hypocalcemia
       - hypoglycemia/non-ketotic hyperglycemia
       - uremia, malignant hypertension
     - hypoxemia

2. Non-epileptic seizures
   - psychogenic/psychiatric: fugue state, amnesia, conversion disorder

3. Partial (focal) seizures
   - simple partial: consciousness not impaired
     - with motor symptoms
     - with somato-sensory or special sensory symptoms
     - with autonomic symptoms/signs
     - with psychiatric symptoms
   - complex partial: impairment of consciousness
   - partial (simple or complex) evolving to secondary generalized seizure

Value of serum prolactin in the management of syncope
Emerg Med J. 2004;21:e3.

Purpose: To determine the usefulness of raised serum prolactin in diagnosing generalised tonic-clonic seizures (GTCS) in patients presenting to the accident and emergency (A&E) department after a single episode of syncope.
Study Selection: Diagnostic studies meeting the reviewers' assessment of validity.
Results: If serum prolactin concentrations three times greater than normal when drawn within one hour of syncope, the patient is nine times more likely to have suffered a GTCS as compared with a pseudoseizure positive LR = 8.92 (95% CI (1.31 to 60.91)) and five times more likely to have suffered a GTCS as compared with non-convulsive syncope positive LR 4.60 (95% CI (1.25 to 16.90)). The presence of seizures associated with alcohol withdrawal or presentations with acute medical conditions make the operating characteristics of the test less reliable.
Conclusions: A positive test result is highly predictive of a GTCS, however a negative test result does not necessarily exclude a seizure. Serum prolactin should be measured in patients presenting to the emergency department within an hour of syncopal episode, unless the cause is immediately obvious.

4. Generalized seizures
- non-convulsive
  - ◆ absence
- convulsive:
  - ◆ myoclonic
  - ◆ clonic
  - ◆ tonic
  - ◆ tonic-clonic
  - ◆ atonic

Etiology

Table 4. Classification of Seizures

	Partial	Generalized
Vascular	Cerebral hemorrhage Cortical infarct Arteriovenous malformation (AVM) Cavernous malformation Cerebral hemorrhage (subdural, epidural, intracerebral)	Cortical infarct (embolic)
Infectious/ Inflammatory	Meningitis Encephalitis Cerebral abscess Subdural empyema Syphilis Tuberculosis (TB) HIV Sarcoidosis Systemic lupus erythematosus (SLE)	Meningitis Encephalitis Neurocystercercosis
Neoplastic	Primary or metastatic CNS tumour	Primary or metastatic CNS tumour
Drug		Tricyclic antidepressants Monoamine oxidase inhibitors Neuroleptics Cyclosporine Theophylline Isoniazid Cocaine Amphetamines Alcohol withdrawal Benzodiazepine withdrawal Antiepileptic withdrawal, subtherapeutic dose
Idiopathic	Epilepsy	Epilepsy
Congenital/ Neonatal	Neonatal hypoxia, IVH	Neonatal hypoxia
Anatomic	Hippocampal sclerosis Cortical dysplasias	Diffuse cerebral damage (anoxia, storage diseases)
Traumatic	Cerebral trauma (subdural hematoma)	Cerebral trauma
Endocrine/ Metabolic		Hypoxia Electolytes- hypocalcemia, hypoglycemia, hyponatremia, hypernatremia, hyperosmolality End-stage organ failure (renal, hepatic) Porphyria

Epidemiology
- in developed countries, 2% to 4% of all persons have recurrent seizures at some period in their lives; higher incidence in developing countries (i.e. cystercercosis is one of the most common causes)
- incidence highest among young children and elderly
- age of onset: primary generalized seizures rarely begin <3 or >20 years of age
- M:F = 1.5:1
- epilepsy affects about 45 million people worldwide

Risk Factors
- stroke risk factors (see *Stroke*)
- past history of neurological insult: birth injury, head trauma, stroke, CNS infection, drug use/abuse
- past history of seizures
- family history of seizures
- malignancy

Precipitants
- sleep deprivation, drugs/alcohol, TV screen, strobe, emotional upset
- fever: febrile seizures affect 4% of children between 3 months - 5 years of age;

Signs and Symptoms (Table 5, Table 6)
- during seizure
  - unresponsiveness or impaired LOC

Stroke is the most common cause of late-onset (>50 years of age) epilepsy, accounting for 50-80% of cases.

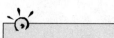

Presence of aura implies focal onset.

- nature of neurological features suggests location of focus
  - motor = frontal lobe
  - visual/olfactory/gustatory hallucinations = temporal lobe
- salivation, cyanosis, tongue biting, incontinence, loud cry
- Jacksonian march: one body part is initially affected, followed by spread to other areas (e.g. fingers to hand to arm to face)
- adversive: head or eyes are turned forcibly to the contralateral frontal eye field
- automatisms: patterns of repetitive activities that look purposeful (e.g. chewing, walking, lip-smacking)
- temporal lobe epilepsy: behavioural disturbances, automatisms, olfactory or gustatory hallucinations
- duration: ictus is seconds to minutes, post-ictus can be long (minutes to hours)
- incontinence
- after seizure
  - post-ictal symptoms: limb pains, tongue soreness, headache, drowsiness, Todd's paralysis (reversible focal weakness/numbness)

Table 5. Partial Seizures

Simple motor	• arise in precentral gyrus (motor cortex), affecting contralateral face/trunk/limbs
	• ictus
	  ▪ no change in consciousness
	  ▪ rhythmic jerking or sustained spasm of affected parts
	  ▪ characterized by forceful turning of eyes and head to side opposite the discharging focus (adversive seizures)
	  ▪ may start in one part and spread "up/down the cortex", along the homunculus (Jacksonian march)
	  ▪ duration usually seconds to minutes (Todd's paralysis may last hours)

Simple sensory	• arise in sensory cortex (postcentral gyrus), affecting contralateral face/trunk/limbs
	• somatosensory
	  ▪ numbness/tingling/"electric" sensation of affected parts
	  ▪ a "march" may occur
	• other forms include: visual, auditory, olfactory, gustatory, vertiginous (may resemble schizophrenic hallucinations but patient recognizes that the phenomenon or phenomena are not real)

Simple autonomic	• epigastric discomfort, pallor, sweating, flushing, piloerection, and pupillary dilatation
Simple psychic	• disturbance of higher cerebral function • symptoms rarely occur without impairment of consciousness and are much more commonly experienced as complex partial seizures

**Complex partial
(temporal lobe epilepsy,
psychomotor epilepsy)**
	• seizures causing alterations of mood, memory, perception
	• common form of epilepsy, with increased incidence in adolescents, young adults
	• ictus
	  ▪ automatisms occur in 90% of patients (chewing, swallowing, lip-smacking, scratching, fumbling, running, disrobing, continuing any complex act initiated prior to loss of consciousness)
	  ▪ aura of seconds-minutes
	  ▪ forms include:
	    • dysphasic, dysmnesic (déjà vu), cognitive (dreamy states, distortions of time sense)
	    • affective (fear, anger), illusions (macropsia or micropsia), structured hallucinations (music, scenes, taste, smells), epigastric fullness
	  ▪ then patient appears distant, staring, unresponsive (can be brief and confused with absence seizures)
	• recovery is characterized by confusion ± headache
	• can resemble schizophrenia, psychotic depression (if complex partial status)

Table 6. Generalized Seizures

**Absence
(Petit Mal)**
	• onset in childhood
	• hereditary
	  ▪ autosomal dominant
	  ▪ incomplete penetrance (~1/4 will get seizures, ~1/3 will have characteristic EEG findings)
	  ▪ 3 Hz spike and slow-wave activity on EEG
	• ictus
	  ▪ child will stop activity, stare, blink/roll eyes, be unresponsive; lasting approximately 5-10 seconds or so, but may occur hundreds of times/day
	  ▪ may be induced by hyperventilation
	• often associated with poor scholastic performance

Myoclonic	• ictus ▪ sudden, brief, generalized muscle contractions (rapid jerking movements) • most common disorder is juvenile myoclonic epilepsy (onset after puberty, does not remit with age) • also occurs in degenerative and metabolic disease (e.g. hypoxic encephalopathy)

**Tonic-Clonic
(Grand Mal)**
	• common
	• all of the classic features do not necessarily occur every time
	• prodrome of unease, irritability hours-days before attack
	• ictus
	  ▪ aura (if secondarily generalized from a partial onset) seconds to minutes before attack of olfactory hallucinations, epigastric discomfort, déjà vu, jerking of a limb, etc.
	  ▪ tonic phase: tonic contraction of muscles, arms flexed and adducted, legs extended, "cry" as respiratory muscles spasm and air expelled, cyanosis, pupillary dilatation, abrupt loss of consciousness, patient often "thrown" to ground; lasts 10-30 seconds
	  ▪ clonic phase: clonus involving violent jerking of face and limbs, tongue biting, and incontinence; duration variable, usually < 90 seconds
	• post-ictal phase of decreased level of consciousness, with flaccid limbs and jaw, extensor plantar reflexes, loss of corneal reflexes; lasts hours; headache, confusion, aching muscles, sore tongue, amnesia; elevated serum CK lasting for hours

Investigations
- CBC, electrolytes, glucose, Ca, Mg, Cr, BUN, LFTs
- CXR, ECG
- EEG
  - epileptiform activity: bursts of sharp and slow waves
  - secondarily generalized seizure: focal epileptiform activity
  - absence: spikes and slow waves at 3 Hz
  - interictal EEG: normal in 60% of cases
- prolactin is increased post-ictally in generalized tonic-clonic seizure (compare with baseline level)
- CT/MRI unless definite primary generalized epilepsy
- LP if signs of infection and no papilledema or midline shift of brain structures (generally done after CT or MRI, unless suspicious of meningitis)
- tox screen (alcohol, benzodiazepines, cocaine, amphetamine)

Motor and/or sensory partial seizures indicate structural disease until proven otherwise.

Differential Diagnosis
- syncope (see Table 7)
  - note: syncope may induce a seizure – this is not epilepsy
- pseudoseizure (see Table 8)
- anxiety: hyperventilation, panic disorder
- TIA
- hypoglycemia
- movement disorders: myoclonus, episodic ataxias
- alcoholic blackouts
- migraine: confusional, vertebrobasilar
- narcolepsy (cataplexy)

Table 7. Seizures versus Syncope

Characteristic	Seizure	Syncope
Time of onset	• day or night	• day
Position	• any	• upright, not recumbent
Onset	• sudden or brief	• gradual (vasodepressor)
Aura	• possible specific aura	• dizziness, visual blurring, lightheadedness
Colour	• normal or cyanotic (tonic-clonic)	• pallor
Autonomic features	• uncommon outside of ictus	• common
		• diaphoresis
Duration	• brief or prolonged	• brief
Incontinence	• common	• rare
Post-ictal symptoms	• can occur with tonic-clonic or complex partial	• rare
Motor activity	• can occur	• occasional brief jerks
Injury	• common, tongue biting	• rare, from fall
Automatisms	• can occur with absence or complex partial	• none
EEG	• frequently normal, but may be abnormal	• normal

Table 8. Seizures versus Pseudoseizures (non-epileptic "seizures"/conversion disorder)

Characteristic	Epileptic Seizure	Pseudoseizure
Age	• any • M=F	• any, less common in elderly • F>M
Triggers	• uncommon	• emotional disturbances
Duration	• brief	• may be prolonged
Motor activity	• automatisms in complex partial seizures • stereotypic • synchronous movements	• opisthotonos • rigidity • forced eye closure • irregular extremity movements • side-to-side head movements • pelvic thrusting • crying
Timing	• day or night	• usually day • usually other people present
Physical injury	• may occur	• non-serious
Incontinence	• may occur	• rare
Reproduction of attack	• spontaneous	• suggestion, or stimuli plus suggestion
EEG	• inter-ictal discharges frequent	• normal
Prolactin	• increased	• normal

Treatment

- psychosocial
  - educate patients and family
  - advise about swimming, boating, locked bathrooms, operating dangerous machinery, climbing heights, chewing gum
  - pregnancy issues: counselling and monitoring blood levels closely, teratogenicity of anticonvulsant drugs, folate 5 mg/day (three months preconceptually until 10-12 weeks post-conception, vitamin K (at time of delivery)
  - evaluate for fetal neural tube defects
  - inform of prohibition to drive and requirements to notify Ministry of Transportation
  - support groups, Epilepsy Association
  - follow-up visits to ensure compliance, evaluate changes in symptoms/seizure type (re-investigate)
- pharmacologic (Table 9)
  - begin with one major anticonvulsant with a simple dosage schedule
  - adjust dose to achieve plasma level in therapeutic range
  - if no seizure control, increase dose until maximum safe dose or side effects become intolerable
  - if still no seizure control, change to or add second drug
- non-pharmacologic treatment
  - for selected cases of complex partial epilepsy and/or identifiable focus
  - vagal nerve stimulator
  - ketogenic diet
  - surgical resection
- other adjuncts: clobazam, gabapentin, pregabalin
- newer anticonvulsants: lamotrigine, topiramate, levetiracetam

Table 9. Major Anti-Epileptic Drugs

Type of Seizure	Medication	Dosing Schedule	Therapeutic ranges
Partial or 2° generalized	carbamazepine phenytoin valproate	**carbamazepine:** start at 100-200 mg PO OD-bid, increase by 200mg/d q2d up to 800-1200 mg/d (in divided doses) if needed (mechanism: anti-convulsant, voltage dep. block of Na channels)	17-50 umol/L
1° generalized (Tonic-Clonic) (Grand Mal)	valproate	**phenytoin:** if loading necessary - 300 mg PO q4h x 3 doses, then 300 mg PO hs. Serum levels should be monitored (mechanism voltage dependant block of Na channels)	40-80 umol/L if giiven IV do not exceed 50 mg/min
		valproate: start at 15 mg/kg/d PO increasing by 5-10 mg/kg/d q weekly until seizures are controlled or intolerable side effects. Maximum daily dose is 60 mg/kg/d (mechanism unknown; GABA enhancing)	350-700 umol/L
Absence (Petit Mal)	ethosuximide valproate	**ethosuximide:** start 500 mg daily PO in divided doses, increasing by 250 mg/d q 4-7days prn up to a maximum dose of 1500 mg/d (mechanism: inhibits NADPH-linked aldehyde reductase necessary for the formation of GABA)	280-710 umol/L
Myoclonic	clonazepam valproate	**clonazepam:** 0.5 mg PO tid, increase by 0.5-1.0 mg/d q3d prn up to 20 mg/d (in divided doses) (mechanism: benzodiazepine; GABA enhancer)	

Source: Clinician's Pocket reference 9th ed. Gomella LG & Haist SA Eds, McGraw-Hill, New York, 2002.
Pharmacological Treatment of Diseases. Pressaco J & Yu H Eds, Urban Angel Medical Books, Toronto, 1996.

Status Epilepticus

- a life-threatening state (5-10% of epileptics) with either a continuous seizure lasting at least 30 minutes or a series of seizures occurring without the patient regaining full consciousness between attacks
- complications: repetitive grand mal seizures impair ventilation, resulting in anoxia, cerebral ischemia and cerebral edema; sustained muscle contraction can lead to rhabdomyolysis and renal failure
- most common cause is abrupt discontinuation of anticonvulsants from a known epileptic

Initial Management

- ABCs
  - give O_2, ensure adequate ventilation, monitor vitals, ECG, oximetry, start IV lines, blood samples (see below)
  - give 50 mL 50% glucose IV preceded by thiamine 100mg IM
  - Lorazepam 0.1 mg/kg IV at 2 mg/min
  - Phenytoin 20 mg/kg IV at maximum of 50 mg/min or fosphenytoin 20mg/kg PE IV at 150 mg/min
  - monitor cardiac rhythm and BP
- > 60 mins: if status does not stop after 20 mg/kg phenytoin
  - additional doses of phenytoin 5-10 mg/kg IV at maximum of 50 mg/min up to a total dose of 30 mg/kg or fosphenytoin (5-10 mg/kg PE IV at 150 mg/min)
  - Phenobarbital 20 mg/kg IV at 50 mg/min- watch for hypotension and respiratory depression- requires central line to monitor CVP, ventilatory assistance may be required

- if status persists, consider additional Phenobarbital 5-10 mg/kg IV at 50 mg/min or proceed with anesthesia
  - anesthesia with midazolam or propofol in ICU: vasopressors or fluid volume usually necessary, EEG should be monitored and neuromuscular blockade may be needed
- take focused history and examine patient
  - trauma
  - known seizure disorder
  - focal neurological signs
  - history or signs of medical illnesses, especially infection
  - check for neck stiffness, signs of head injury
- investigate cause of the status
  - CBC, electrolytes (including Ca), liver enzymes, Cr, BUN
  - glucose level (rule out hypoglycemia)
  - ABG
  - draw metabolic and drug screen (most common is alcohol)
  - measure anticonvulsant levels
  - CXR, EEG and consider STAT CT or MRI if first seizure or if focal neurological deficits elicited
  - LP to evaluate for infection and subarachnoid hemorrhage if CT normal

Behavioural Neurology

- see Psychiatry

Acute Confusional State/Delirium

Table 10. Clinical Features of the Acute Confusional State

Level of consciousness	• ↓ alertness, ↓ attention, ↓ concentration; fluctuating; worse at night, "sundowning"
Psychomotor status	• psychomotor retardation • psychomotor agitation
Emotional status	• anxiety/irritability • depression/apathy
Perception	• illusions and hallucinations (usually visual and tactile) • gustatory and olfactory hallucinations suggest temporal lobe epilepsy
Cognition	• memory disturbance (registration, retention, and recall) • disorientation

Delirium is a medical emergency carrying significant risks of morbidity and mortality.

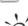

Delirium is characterized by acute onset, disorientation, marked variability, fluctuating level of consciousness, poor attention, and marked psychomotor changes.

Table 11. Selected Intracranial Causes of Acute Confusional State

	Etiology	Key Clinical Features	Investigations
Vascular	subarachnoid hemorrhage	• thunderclap headache • ↑ ICP • meningismus	• CT (non-contrast) • LP
	stroke/TIA	• focal neurological signs	• CT (non-contrast)
Infectious	meningitis	• fever, headache, nausea, photophobia • meningismus	• LP
	encephalitis	• focal neurological signs • fever, headache, ± seizure	• LP; MRI
	abscess	• ↑ ICP • focal neurological signs	• CT with contrast (often ring enhancing lesion)

Traumatic	diffuse axonal shear,
	  epidural hematoma,
	  subdural hematoma
		• trauma Hx
		• ↑ ICP
		• focal neurological signs
			• CT (non-contrast)
			• MRI

Autoimmune	acute CNS vasculitis	• skin rash, active joints	• ANA; ANCA; RF • MRI • angiography

Neoplastic	mass effect/edema,
	  hemorrhage,
	  seizure
		• ↑ ICP
		• focal neurological signs
		• papilledema
			• CT (non-contrast)
			• MRI

Seizure	status epilepticus Todd's phenomenon	• see *Seizure Disorders and Epilepsy*, N8	• EEG
Primary psychiatric	psychotic disorder mood disorder anxiety disorder	• no organic signs or symptoms	• no specific tests

Visual hallucinations more commonly indicate organic disease.

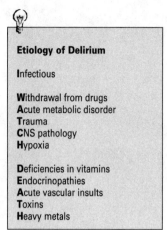

Etiology of Delirium

Infectious

Withdrawal from drugs
Acute metabolic disorder
Trauma
CNS pathology
Hypoxia

Deficiencies in vitamins
Endocrinopathies
Acute vascular insults
Toxins
Heavy metals

Table 12. Selected Extracranial Causes of Acute Confusional State – "HIT ME"

	Etiology	Key Clinical Features	Investigations
Hypoxia	respiratory failure heart failure carbon monoxide (CO) poisoning	• cyanosis, tachypnea, tachycardia • S&S of CHF • Hx CO exposure	• ABG; CXR • ABG; CXR; ECG • ABG
Infectious	septicemia pneumonia UTI	• systemic S&S septicemia • cough; respiratory distress • irritative urinary S&S	• blood C&S • CXR • urine R&M/C&S
Toxins/Meds	alcohol benzodiazepines beta-blockers anticholinergics	• see <u>Emergency Medicine</u>	• toxicology screen • drug levels
Metabolic	hepatic/renal failure electrolyte imbalance B_{12} deficiency	• S&S acute hepatic/renal failure • see <u>Gastroenterology</u> , <u>Nephrology</u> • see <u>Nephrology</u> • peripheral neuropathy; subacute combined degeneration; glossitis	• liver enzymes; LFTs • electrolytes, BUN, Cr • electrolytes • Ca panel • serum B_{12} • CBC
Endocrine	↑/↓ thyroid ↑/↓ glucose ↑/↓ cortisol	• S&S hyper/hypothyroidism • S&S DM/hypoglycemia • S&S Cushing's/Addison's disease	• TSH, T3, T4 • serum glucose • serum cortisol

Management of Acute Confusional State – General Measures
- see <u>Psychiatry</u>
- well-lit room
- hearing aids and glasses
- orienting stimuli (clocks, calendars)
- avoid restraints or catheters
- stop all unnecessary medications
- treat underlying cause, antipsycotics

Dementia

- see <u>Psychiatry</u>

Definition
- an acquired, generalized and (usually) progressive impairment of cognitive function (i.e. memory, recall, orientation, language, abstraction etc.)
- affects content, but not level of consciousness

Epidemiology
- 15% of those >65 years of age have dementia
- common etiologies: 60-80% Alzheimer's Disease (AD); 10-20% vascular dementia
- <5% reversible: hypothyroid, normal pressure hydrocephalus (NPH), nutritional deficiencies, depression and infection

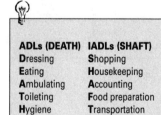

ADLs (DEATH)	IADLs (SHAFT)
Dressing	**S**hopping
Eating	**H**ousekeeping
Ambulating	**A**ccounting
Toileting	**F**ood preparation
Hygiene	**T**ransportation

History
- geriatric giants
  - incontinence, falls, polypharmacy
  - memory and safety (wandering, leaving doors unlocked, leaving stove on, losing objects)
  - behavioural (mood, anxiety, psychosis, suicidal ideation, personality changes, aggression)
- cardiovascular, endocrine, neoplastic
- EtOH, smoking
- OTCs, herbal remedies, compliance, accessibility
- collateral history is usually very helpful
- history of vascular disease

Physical Examination
- hearing and vision
- neurological exam
- as directed depending on risk factors and history
- MMSE or MOCA
  - + clock drawing
  - + frontal lobe testing (go/no-go, word lists, similarities, proverb)
  - + Baycrest Neurocognitive Assessment

Investigations

- depend on suspected etiologies (see Tables 13 and 14)
  - CBC (note MCV), glucose, TSH, B12, folate
  - electrolytes, LFTs, renal function
  - CT head
  - MRI as indicated
  - as clinically indicated – VDRL, HIV, ANA, anti-dsDNA, ANCA, ceruloplasmin, copper, cortisol, toxicology, heavy metals
- issues to consider
  - failure to cope
  - fitness to drive
  - caregiver education and stress
    - ◆ respite services and day programs
  - power of attorney
  - wills
  - advanced directives (DNR)

Table 13. Common Causes of Dementia

	Etiology	Key Clinical Features	Investigations
Primary degenerative	Alzheimer's disease	• memory impairment • aphasia, apraxia, agnosia	• CT or MRI, SPECT
	Lewy body disease	• hallucinations • parkinsonism • fluctuating cognition	• CT or MRI, SPECT
	frontotemporal dementia (e.g. Pick's disease)	• disinhibition, perseveration • ↓ social awareness • progressive non-fluent aphasia • memory relatively spared	• MRI, SPECT
	Huntington's disease	• chorea	• molecular testing
Vascular	multi-infarct dementia	• abrupt onset • stepwise deterioration • dysexecutive syndrome	• MRI, SPECT
	CNS vasculitis	• systemic S&S of vasculitis	• ANA; ANCA; RF • MRI • angiography

Table 14. Acquired Causes of Dementia

	Etiology	Key Clinical Features	Investigations
Infectious	chronic meningitis	• fever; headache; nausea • meningismus • localizing neuro deficits	• LP + investigations
	chronic encephalitis chronic abscess	• fever; headache • ↑ ICP • localizing neuro signs	• LP; MRI • CT with contrast
	HIV Creutzfelt-Jacob disease syphilis	• see <u>Infectious Diseases</u> • rapidly progressive • ataxia, myoclonus	• HIV serology • EEG • LP • VDRL
Traumatic	diffuse axonal shear, epidural hematoma, subdural hematoma	• trauma Hx • ↑ ICP, papilledema • localizing neuro signs	• CT (non-contrast)
Rheumatologic	SLE	• see <u>Rheumatology</u>	• MRI; ANA, anti-dsDNA
Neoplastic	mass effect/edema, hemorrhage, seizure	• ↑ ICP • localizing neuro signs	• CT with contrast • MRI
	paraneoplastic encephalitis	• systemic S&S of cancer	• anti-Hu antibodies

Table 15. Reversible Causes of Dementia

	Etiology	Key Clinical Features	Investigations
Toxins/Meds	Wernicke-Korsakoff	• anterograde amnesia • confabulation • ataxia, ophthalmoplegia	• no specific test • trial of thiamine
	benzodiazepines, β-blockers, anticholinergics	• see <u>Emergency Medicine</u>	• toxicology screen • drug levels
	heavy metals	• S&S heavy metal toxicity	• urine heavy metals
Metabolic	hepatic/renal failure	• S&S acute hepatic/renal failure • see <u>Gastroenterology</u>, <u>Nephrology</u>	• liver enzymes; LFT's • electrolytes, BUN, Cr
	Wilson's disease	• Kayser-Fleischer rings • hepatic failure	• serum ceruloplasmin, Cu
	B_{12} deficiency	• peripheral neuropathy; subacute combined degeneration; glossitis	• serum B_{12}
Endocrine	↑/↓ thyroid ↑/↓ glucose ↑/↓ cortisol	• S&S hyper/hypothyroidism • S&S DM/hypoglycemia • S&S Cushing's/Addison's disease	• TSH, T_3, T_4 • serum glucose • serum cortisol
Structural	NPH	• gait apraxia • incontinence • dementia	• CT • LP • measure opening pressure
Primary Psychiatric	depression (pseudodementia)	• no organic S&S	• no specific tests

Dementia DDx: VITAMIN D VEST

Vitamin deficiency (B12, folate, thiamine)
Intracranial tumour
Trauma (head injury)
Anoxia
Metabolic (diabetes)
Infection (postencephalitis, HIV)
Normal pressure hydrocephalus
Degenerative (Alzheimer's, Huntington's, CJD)
Vascular (multi-infarct dementia)
Endocrine (hypothyroid)
Space occupying lesion (chronic subdural hematoma)
Toxic (alcohol)

Alzheimer's Disease

* see Psychiatry

4 As and one **D** of AD
(**A**nterograde **a**mnesia, **A**phasia, **A**praxia, **A**gnosia, **D**isturbance in executive function)

Definition
* progressive cognitive decline interfering with social and occupational functioning characterized by the following
  1) anterograde amnesia - impaired ability to learn new information
  2) one of the following cognitive disturbance
     a. Aphasia - language disturbance
     b. Apraxia - impaired ability to carry out motor activities despite intact motor function
     c. Agnosia - failure to recognize or identify objects despite intact sensory function
     d. Disturbance in executive function - planning, organizing, sequencing, abstracting

Pathophysiology
* genetic factors
  * a minority (<7%) of AD cases are familial, autosomal dominant
  * 3 major genes for autosomal dominant AD have been identified:
    * amyloid precursor protein (chromosome 21)
    * presenilin 1 (chromosome 14)
    * presenilin 2 (chromosome 1)
  * the E4 polymorphism of apolipoprotein E is a susceptibility genotype
* pathology (although not necessarily specific for AD)
  * gross pathology
    * diffuse cortical atrophy, especially frontal, parietal, and temporal lobes
  * microscopic pathology
    * senile plaques (amyloid made from β-peptide derived from cleaved amyloid precursor protein)
    * neurofibrillary tangles (intracytoplasmic paired helical filaments with β-amyloid and hyperphosphorylated Tau protein)
  * biochemical pathology
    * 50-90% reduction in action of choline acetyltransferase

Epidemiology
* 1/12 of population 65-75 years of age
* 1/3 of population >85 years of age
* accounts for 60-80% of all dementias

Risk Factors
* FHx of AD
* head injury
* low education level
* smoking
* aluminum
* Downs syndrome

Signs and Symptoms
* cognitive impairment
  * memory impairment for newly acquired information (early)
  * deficits in language, abstract reasoning, and executive function
* psychiatric manifestations
  * major depression (5-8%)
  * psychosis (20%)
* motor manifestations (late)
  * parkinsonism (consider Lewy body disease)

Investigations
* perform investigations to rule out other causes of dementia as necessary
* EEG: generalized slowing (nonspecific)
* MRI: dilatation of lateral ventricles; widening of cortical sulci
* SPECT: hypometabolism in temporal and parietal lobes

Treatment
* acetylcholinesterase inhibitors have been shown to improve cognitive function
  * donepezil (Aricept™)
  * rivastigmine (Exelon™)
  * galantamine (Reminyl™)
* other - although efficacy not proven
  * ginkgo biloba
  * tacrine

- Vit E (caution: >400 IU/day associated with excess mortality, level 1 evidence)
- NMDA receptor agonist – memantine (Ebixa)
- symptomatic management
  - low dose neuroleptic
  - trazodone for sleep disturbance
  - antidepressants

Prognosis
- progressive
- mean duration of disease 10 years

Lewy Body Disease (LBD)

Definition
- progressive cognitive decline interfering with social or occupational function; memory loss may or may not be an early feature
- one (for possible LBD) or two (for probable LBD) of the following:
  - fluctuating cognition with pronounced variation in attention and alertness
  - recurrent visual hallucinations
  - parkinsonism

Etiology and Pathogenesis
- Lewy bodies (eosinophilic cytoplasmic inclusions) found in both cortical and subcortical structures

Epidemiology
- 15-25% of all dementias

Signs and Symptoms
- fluctuation in cognition with progressive decline
- visual hallucinations
- parkinsonism
- repeated falls
- sensitivity to neuroleptic medications (develop rigidity, neuroleptic malignant syndrome, and extrapyramidal symptoms)
- REM sleep disorder

Treatment
- acetylcholinesterase inhibitors (e.g. donepezil)

Prognosis
- typical survival 3-6 years

Frontotemporal Dementia

Definition
- progressive dementia characterized by personality change, speech disturbance, inattentiveness, and extrapyramidal signs

Etiology and Pathogenesis
- gross pathology
  - atrophy of frontal and temporal poles
- microscopic pathology
  - Pick bodies (intraneuronal inclusions containing abnormal Tau proteins)

Epidemiology
- 10% of all dementias

Signs and Symptoms
- core features
  - insidious onset and gradual progression
  - early decline in social interpersonal conduct
  - early impairment in regulation of personal conduct
  - early emotional blunting
  - early loss of insight
- behavioural disorder
  - decline in personal hygiene and grooming
  - mental rigidity/inflexibility
  - perseverative and stereotyped behaviour
- speech and language
  - altered speech output (economy or pressure of speech)
  - echolalia/perseveration

- physical signs
  - primitive reflexes (i.e. pout, grasp, palmo-mental, glabellar)
  - parkinsonism

Investigations
- MRI/SPECT – frontotemporal atrophy/hypometabolism

NPH progression of classic triad: AID
Ataxia/**A**praxia of Gait -->
Incontinence --> **D**ementia

Normal Pressure Hydrocephalus

- see Neurosurgery

Aphasia

Definition
- an acquired disturbance of language characterized by errors in speech production, writing, comprehension, or reading

Neuroanatomy of Aphasia
- Broca's area (posterior inferior frontal lobe) involved in speech production (expressive)
- Wernicke's area (posterior superior temporal lobe) used for comprehension of language
- angular gyrus is responsible for relaying written visual stimuli to Wernicke's area for reading comprehension
- the arcuate fasciculus association bundle connects Wernicke's and Broca's areas
- >99% of right-handed people have left hemisphere language representation
- 70% of left-handed people have left hemisphere language representation, 15% have right hemisphere representation, and 15% have bilateral representation

Aphasia localizes the lesion to the **dominant cerebral hemisphere.**

Assessment of Language
- assessment of context
  - handedness (writing, drawing, toothbrush, scissors)
  - education level
  - native language
  - learning difficulties
- assessment for aphasia
  1. spontaneous speech
     - fluency
     - paraphasias: semantic ("chair" for "table"), or phonemic ("clable" for "table")
  2. repetition
  3. naming
  4. comprehension (auditory and reading)
  5. writing
  6. neologisms

The left hemisphere is dominant for language in almost all right-handed people and 70% of left-handed people.

Approach to Aphasias

Table 16. Fluent Aphasias

	Wernicke's	Conduction	Anomic	Sensory Transcortical*
Lesion	• posterior superior temporal lobe (1st temporal gyrus)	• arcuate fasciculus	• numerous possible locations	1. subcortical temporoparietal 2. temporoparietal watershed between MCA and PCA territories
Comprehension	• poor	• good	• good	• poor
Repetition	• poor	• poor	• good	• good
Naming	• relatively spared	• poor	• poor	• relatively spared

*Transcortical aphasias are typically associated with cerebral anoxia (e.g. post-MI, CO poisoning, hypotension)

Table 17. Non-fluent Aphasias

	Broca's	Global	Motor Transcortical*	Mixed Transcortical*
Lesion	• posterior inferior frontal lobe	• posterior inferior frontal lobe AND posterior superior temporal lobe	a. frontal lobe watershed between MCA and ACA territories b. white matter lesions deep to (a)	• combined sensory and motor transcortical
Comprehension	• good	• poor	• good	• poor
Repetition	• poor	• poor	• good	• good
Naming	• poor	• poor	• poor	• poor

*Transcortical aphasias associated with cerebral anoxia (e.g. post-MI, CO poisoning, hypotension)

Prognosis
- most recovery from stroke-related aphasia occurs in first three months, but may continue for >1 year
- with recovery, the type of aphasia may evolve
- poor prognosis: global aphasia

Dysarthria

Definition
- inability to produce understandable speech due to impaired phonation (laryngeal sound production) and/or resonance (the alteration of sounds in the cavity between the larynx and the lips/nares) secondary to impaired motor control over peripheral speech organs

Classification of Dysarthria

Table 18. Classification of Dysarthria

Classification		Characteristics of Speech	Etiologies*
Flaccid (LMN dysarthria or bulbar palsy)		• slurred, indistinct speech • particular difficulty with vibratory "R" • difficulty with lingual consonants produced by tongue and labial consonants produced by lips	• motor neuron (e.g. ALS) • peripheral nerve (e.g. GBS) • neuromuscular junction (e.g. MG) • myopathy (e.g. Dm/Pm)
Spastic (upper motor neuron (UMN) dysarthria or pseudobulbar palsy)		• slow and monotonous • strained or strangled • harsh • low pitched	• stroke • tumour • demyelination • degeneration
Ataxic		• slow/altered rhythm • improper stress • staccato speech	• cerebellar disease • cerebellar outflow tract disease
Extrapyramidal	Hypokinetic	• low-pitched • monotonous • decrescendo volume	• Parkinson's disease • other causes of parkinsonism (see Movement Disorders)
	Hyperkinetic	Choreiform • prolonged sentence segments intermixed with silences • variable, improper stress • bursting quality Dystonic • slow speaking rate • prolonged individual phonemes	• Huntington's disease • Dystonia musculorum deformans • other hyperkinetic extrapyramidal disorders (see Movement Disorders)

*Abbreviations: ALS - amyotrophic lateral sclerosis; GBS - Guillain-Barré syndrome; MG - myasthenia gravis; DM - dermatomyositis; PM - polymyositis.

Dysphagia

- see Gastroenterology
- see Cranial Nerve X, N23

Apraxia

Definition
- inability to perform skilled voluntary motor sequences that cannot be accounted for by weakness, ataxia, sensory loss, impaired comprehension, or inattention

Clinicopathological Correlations

Table 19. Apraxia

	Description	Tests	Hemispheres
Ideomotor	• inability to perform skilled learned motor sequences	• blowing out a match; combing one's hair	• left
Ideational	• inability to sequence actions	• preparing and mailing an envelope	• right and left
Constructional*	• inability to draw or construct	• copying a figure	• right and left
Dressing*	• inability to dress	• dressing	• right

* Refers specifically to the inability to carry out the learned movements involved in construction, drawing, or dressing; not merely the inability to construct, draw, or dress. Many skills aside from praxis are needed to carry out these tasks.

Agnosia

Definition
- disorder in the recognition of the significance of sensory stimuli in the presence of intact sensation and naming

Clinicopathological Correlations

Table 20. Agnosias

	Description	Lesion
Aperceptive visual agnosia	• inability to name or demonstrate the use of an object presented visually 2° to distorted visual perception • recognition by touch remains intact	• bilateral temporo-occipital cortex
Associative visual agnosia	• inability to name an object presented visually 2° to disconnect between visual cortex and language areas • visual perception is intact as demonstrated by visual matching	• bilateral inferior temporo-occipital junction
Prosopagnosia	• inability to recognize familiar faces in the presence of intact visual perception and intact auditory recognition	• bilateral occipitotemporal areas or right inferior temporo-occipital region
Colour agnosia	• inability to perceive colour	• bilateral inferior temporo-occipital lesions
Astereognosis	• inability to identify objects by touch	• anterior parietal lobe in the hemisphere opposite the affected hand
Finger agnosia	• inability to recognize, name, and point to individual fingers	• dominant hemisphere parietal-occipital lesions

Cranial Nerve Deficits

CN I: Anosmia

Clinical Features
- absence of sense of smell
- usually associated with a loss of taste sense; if taste is intact, consider malingering
- usually not recognized by patient if it is unilateral

Classification
- nasal: odours do not reach olfactory receptors because of physical obstruction
  - heavy smoking, chronic rhinitis, sinusitis
- olfactory neuroepithelial: destruction of receptors or their axon filaments
  - influenza, herpes simplex, interferon treatment of hepatitis C virus, atrophic rhinitis (leprosy)
- central: olfactory pathway lesions
  - congenital: Kallman syndrome (anosmia and hypogonadotropic hypogonadism), albinism
  - head injury, cranial surgery, SAH, chronic meningeal inflammation
  - meningioma, aneurysm
  - Parkinson's disease

CN II: Optic Nerve

- see *Neuro-Ophthalmology*

CN III: Oculomotor Nerve Palsy

Clinical Features
- ptosis, eye is "down and out" (depressed and abducted), divergent squint, pupil dilated (mydriasis)
- pupillary constrictor fibres are on periphery of nerve
  - external compression of the oculomotor nerve results in unreactive pupil with subsequent progression to extraocular muscle paresis
  - vascular infarction results in extraocular muscle paresis with sparing of the pupil

Common Lesions
- midbrain (infarction, hemorrhage)
  - may/may not affect pupil, may be bilateral with pyramidal signs contralaterally

- posterior communicating artery aneurysm (Circle of Willis)
  - pupil involved early, headache
- cavernous sinus (internal carotid aneurysm, meningioma, sinus thrombosis)
  - CN IV, V_1 and V_2, and VI also travel in the cavernous sinus, pain and proptosis may occur
- ischemic (DM, temporal arteritis, HTN, atherosclerosis)
  - pupil often spared

Pupil sparing in CN III palsy suggests a vascular lesion.
Pupillary involvement in CN III palsy suggests external nerve compression.

CN IV: Trochlear Nerve Palsy

Clinical Features
- diplopia, especially on downward and inward gaze
- patient may complain of difficulty going down stairs or reading
- patient may hold head tilted to side opposite of palsy to minimize diplopia (Bielschowski head tilt test)

Common Lesions
- trauma
- ischemic (DM, HTN) most common
- cavernous sinus (carotid aneurysm, thrombosis)
  - CN III and VI usually involved as well
- orbital fissure (tumour, granuloma)
- at risk during neurosurgical procedures in the midbrain because of long intracranial course
- only CN that exits posteriorly and crosses midline; may get contralateral deficit

CN V: Trigeminal Nerve

Trigeminal Nerve Lesions
- **Common Lesions**
  - pons (vascular, neoplastic, demyelinating, syringobulbia)
  - petrous apex (petrositis)
  - orbital fissure, orbit, cavernous sinus (III, IV, VI also affected)
  - skull base (nasopharyngeal or metastatic carcinoma, trauma)
  - cerebellopontine angle
    - ± VII, VIII
    - acoustic neuroma, trigeminal neuroma, subacute or chronic meningitis
  - other causes (DM, SLE)
  - herpes zoster
    - usually affects ophthalmic division (V1)
    - tip of nose involvement → predictive of corneal involvement (Hutchinson's sign)

Trigeminal Neuralgia (Tic Douloureux)

Definition
- excruciating paroxysmal shooting pains in trigeminal root territory

Etiology
- redundant or tortuous blood vessel in the posterior fossa, irritating the origin of the trigeminal nerve
- tumours of cerebellopontine angle (rare)

Clinical Features
- characterized by: a series of severe, sharp, short, stabbing, unilateral shocks
  - usually in V_3 distribution ± V_1, V_2
- pain typically lasts only a few seconds to minutes, and may be so intense that the patient winces (hence the term tic)
- may be brought on by triggers: touching face, eating, talking, cold winds
- lasts for days/weeks followed by remission of weeks/months
- F > M; usually middle-aged and elderly
- physical examination is normal (if abnormal, think trigeminal neuropathy)

Investigations
- clinical diagnosis (make sure no sensory loss over CN V)
- sensory loss in trigeminal distribution suggests structural lesion (consider demyelination, tumour)

Treatment
- medical
  - carbamazepine
  - clonazepam, phenytoin, gabapentin and baclofen may also be beneficial
- surgical (all methods are 80% effective, for ~5 years)
  - microvascular decompression of redundant blood vessel at origin of trigeminal nerve
  - percutaneous thermocoagulation
  - injection of glycerol/phenol into trigeminal ganglion

CN VI: Abducens Nerve Palsy

Clinical Features
- inability to abduct the eye on the affected side
- patient complains of horizontal diplopia, which is worse on lateral gaze to the affected side

CN VI has the longest intracranial course and is vulnerable to increased ICP, creating a false localizing sign.

Common Lesions
- pons (infarction, hemorrhage, demyelination)
  - may be associated with facial weakness and contralateral pyramidal signs
- tentorial orifice (compression, meningioma)
  - may be a false localizing sign in increased ICP (i.e. mimics brainstem lesion)
- cavernous sinus (carotid aneurysm, thrombosis)
- vascular – may be secondary to DM, HTN, or temporal arteritis
- congenital – Duane's syndrome

CN VII: Facial Nerve Palsy

Clinical Features
- the entire face on ipsilateral side is weak
- taste dysfunction to ant 2/3 of tongue
- both voluntary and involuntary movements are affected
- impaired lacrimation, decreased salivation, numbness behind auricle, hyperacusis
- UMN weakness
  - weakness of contralateral lower face; frontalis is spared

Forehead is spared in a UMN CN VII lesion.

Investigations
- look for associated brainstem or cortical symptoms and signs to help localize lesion

Differential Diagnosis
- idiopathic = Bell's Palsy, 80-90% of cases
- trauma: temporal bone fracture- 90% longitudinal, 10% transverse
- infection: (otitis media, mastoiditis, Epstein-Barr virus (EBV), Ramsay-Hunt Syndrome (herpes zoster oticus, HSV)
- other
  - sarcoidosis, Group B *Streptococcus*, DM mononeuropathy, parotid gland pathology

Bell's Palsy

see <u>Otolaryngology</u>

Definition
- an idiopathic facial nerve palsy

Clinical Features
- acute onset of unilateral (rarely bilateral) LMN facial weakness
- diagnosis of exclusion
  - must rule out brainstem lesion
- etiology
  - unknown: thought to be due to swelling and inflammation of facial nerve in its canal within the temporal bone, may be due to HSV infection of CN VII
- associated features which may be present
  - pain behind ipsilateral ear (often precedes weakness)
  - prodromal viral upper respiratory tract infection (URTI)
  - hyperacusis
  - decreased taste sensation
  - abnormal tearing (decreased lacrimation)

Treatment
- patient education and reassurance
- eye protection (because of inability to close eye)
  - artificial tears, lubricating ointment
  - patch eye at night
- steroids (weigh risks and benefits)
  - start early after onset of symptoms (within 12 hours)
  - typical regime is prednisone 40-60 mg tapered over 7-10 days
- acyclovir
  - controversial but some evidence to support its use

An isolated cranial nerve defect, especially of CN VI or VII, is most likely the result of a peripheral, and not a brainstem, lesion.

Prognosis
- spontaneous recovery in 85% over weeks to months
- poor outcome
  - if complete paralysis lasts 2-3 weeks
  - if elderly or HTN
  - if symptoms of hyperacusis, abnormal tearing

Hemifacial Spasm

Definition
- segmental myoclonus of facial muscles innervated by CN VII

Clinical Features
- usually presents in the 5th or 6th decade of life
- almost always presents unilaterally, beginning as myoclonus of orbicularis oculi and can spread to other muscles after a few years
- clonic movements eventually progress to tonic contractions of involved muscles

Etiology
- majority of cases due to chronic irritation of facial nerve nucleus or nerve (causing aberrant transmission within the nerve)
- most common cause is idiopathic, caused by aberrant AICA artery compressing facial nerve within the cerebellopontine angle
- other causes
  - compressive lesions - tumour, AV malformation
  - non-compressive lesions - MS, stroke

Investigations
- EMG - observe high frequency discharges of motor unit potentials that correlate with clinically observed facial movements
- MRI - detailed analysis of posterior fossa (especially with FIESTA sequence) to obeserve aberrant blood vessels overlying the facial nerve

Treatment
- carbamazapine and benzodiazepines (i.e. clonazepam) very useful in early/mild stages
- botox injections - latency 3 - 5 days; duration 6 months
- surgery - useful when idiopathic or compressive - treat with decompression of the aberrant blood vessels - usually very favourable results

CN VIII: Vestibulocochlear Nerve

- see Otolaryngology

CN IX: Glossopharyngeal Neuralgia

Clinical Features
- brief, sharp attacks of pain affecting posterior pharynx
- pain radiates toward ear and triggered by swallowing
- taste dysfunction in post 1/3 of tongue

Treatment
- carbamazepine
- surgical lesion of CN IX

CN X: Vagus Nerve

- vagus nerve lesions result in
  - palatal weakness: affects swallowing
  - pharyngeal weakness: affects swallowing
  - laryngeal weakness: affects speech

When screening for the presence of dysphagia and assessing risk for aspiration, the presence of a gag reflex is insufficient. Rather the correct screening test is to observe the patient drinking water from a cup and looking for coughing, choking, or "wetness" of voice.

CN XI: Accessory Nerve

- accessory nerve lesions
  - this nerve is vulnerable to damage during neck surgery
  - results in shoulder drop on the affected side, and weakness when turning the head to the opposite side

CN XII: Hypoglossal Nerve

- tongue fasciculation, atrophy of affected side if chronic
- deviation towards side of lesion

Other Differentials of Lower (CN IX, X, XI and XII) Cranial Nerve Lesions

- intracranial/skull base
  - meningiomas, neurofibromas, metastases, osteomyelitis, meningitis
- brainstem
  - infarction, demyelination, syringobulbia, poliomyelitis, tumours (astrocytoma)
- neck
  - trauma, surgery, tumours

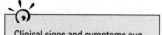

Clinical signs and symptoms suggesting lesions of both a cranial nerve and long tract signs imply a brainstem localizing disease.

Neuro-Ophthalmology

Acute Visual Loss

Etiology

- ophthalmologic (see Ophthalmology)
  - corneal edema
  - glaucoma
  - vitreous hemorrhage
  - retinal detachment
- optic nerve
  - optic neuritis
  - acute ischemic optic neuropathy (AION)
    - ◆ arteritic
    - ◆ non-arteritic
  - compression by space occupying lesion (e.g. aneurysm)
- vascular
  - TIA/amaurosis fugax
  - retinal artery occlusion
  - retinal vein occlusion
- CNS
  - infarction/hemorrhage involving occipital lobe, optic radiations in temporal/parietal lobe
  - lesions in optic tract/chiasm

Optic Neuritis

- see also *Optic Disc Edema, Multiple Sclerosis* (Ophthalmology and Neurology, N63)
- rapidly progressive loss of central vision and colour vision most commonly associated with MS

Anterior Ischemic Optic Neuropathy

- see also *Optic Disc Edema*
- painless vision loss over hours to days
- non-arteritic
  - atherosclerotic variety
  - most common in elderly
  - no evidence of systemic disease
  - diagnosis and treatment: similar to secondary stroke prevention (e.g. anti-platelet therapy, lipid lowering)
- arteritic
  - most common cause is giant cell arteritis (see Rheumatology)
  - diagnosis: elevated ESR; if suspect giant cell arteritis, must do temporal artery biopsy
  - treatment – high dose steroids
  - recovery of visual loss usually poor

If you suspect the diagnosis of Giant Cell Arteritis do not wait for biopsy results!
Begin treatment immediately!

Amaurosis Fugax

- see *Ophthalmology* and *Stroke* (Neurology, N56)
- sudden, transient monocular loss of vision secondary to vascular compromise (transient ischemic attack)

Optic Disc Edema

Table 21. Causes of Optic Disc Edema

	Optic Neuritis	Papilledema	Anterior Ischemic Optic Neuropathy	Central Retinal Vein Occlusion
Age	• <50	• any	• >50	• >50
Vision	• rapidly progressive central vision loss • acuity affected • decreased colour vision	• usually no visual loss until late • possible transient obscuration • variable acuity • normal colour vision	• acute field defects • decreased colour vision	• variable visual loss
Other symptoms	• tender globe, painful on motion • may alternate eyes in multiple sclerosis	• headache • nausea • vomiting • focal neurological deficits	• typically unilateral	• cardiovascular risk factor • usually unilateral
Pupil	• RAPD present	• no anisocoria • no RAPD	• no anisocoria • RAPD present	• no anisocoria • no RAPD
Fundus	• anterior have disc swelling • variable papillitis	• disc swelling and retinal hemorrhages • absent venous pulsations	• pale segmental disc edema with retinal dot and/or flame hemorrhages	• blood and thunder: swollen disc, venous engorgement, retinal hemorrhages
Etiologies	• MS, viral infection • associated with MS in 74% of females and 34% of males	• increased ICP (e.g. mass lesion, pseudotumour cerebri, malignant hypertension)	• giant cell arteritis	• idiopathic
Treatment	• IV methylprednisolone may shorten attacks; oral prednisone may increase relapse rate	• treat specific cause of increased ICP, consult Neurosurgery	• consider ASA for non-arteritic	• panretinal laser photocoagulation, steroids

Other Causes of Disc Edema
- central retinal vein occlusion
- systemic illness
- HTN, vasculitis, hypercapnia
- toxic/metabolic/nutritional deficiency
- infiltration
    - neoplastic: leukemia, lymphoma, glioma
    - non-neoplastic: sarcoidosis
- pseudotumour cerebri
    - idiopathic signs and symptoms of increased ICP, with a normal CT
    - usually in obese young women
- compressive
    - meningioma, hemangioma, thyroid ophthalmopathy

Abnormalities of Visual Field

Visual Field Defects
- lesions anywhere in the visual system, from the optic nerve to the occipital cortex will produce characteristic visual field defects (see Figure 8)
- several tests are used: confrontation (screening), tangent screen, Humphrey fields (computerized automated perimetry), Goldmann perimetry

Definitions
- monocular
    - scotoma: an area of absent or diminished vision within an otherwise intact visual field
- binocular
    - hemianopsia: loss of half of the visual field
    - homonymous: loss of either the right or left half of the visual field in both eyes
    - bitemporal: loss of both temporal visual fields (lesion of chiasm)
    - quadrantanopsia: loss of one quarter of the visual field

BITEMPORAL HEMIANOPSIA
- chiasmal lesion:
    - in children: craniopharyngioma
    - in middle aged: pituitary mass
    - in elderly: meningioma

HOMONYMOUS HEMIANOPSIA
- retrochiasmal lesion
- the more congruent, the more posterior the lesion
- check all hemiplegic patients for ipsilateral homonymous hemianopsia
  (e.g. left hemisphere --> right visual field defect)

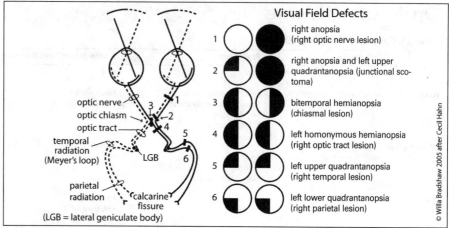

Figure 8. Characteristic Visual Field Defects with Lesions Along the Visual Pathway

Optic Disc Atrophy

- definition: damage to the optic nerve from many different kinds of pathologies. Not a disease, but rather a sign of an underlying condition
- etiologies: glaucoma, anterior ischemic optic neuropathy, tumour pressing on the optic nerve, optic neuritis, Leber's hereditary optic neuropathy, congenital
- signs and symptoms: low visual acuity, peripheral vision impairment, difficulty with colour vision, pallor of the optic disc on fundoscopy
- management: optic nerve atrophy is an irreversible condition, management of the underlying condition is crucial to prevent exacerbation

Abnormalities of Eye Movements

Disorders of Lateral Gaze

Etiology
- brainstem infarcts
- multiple sclerosis
- tumours

A lesion in a cerebral hemisphere causes eyes to "look away" from the hemiplegia.
A lesion in the brainstem causes the eyes to "look toward" the side of the hemiplegia.

Pathophysiology
- voluntary eye movements are triggered in the frontal eye fields, located anterior to the precentral gyrus, bilaterally in the frontal lobes
- each frontal eye field controls voluntary saccades to the contralateral side via connections to the contralateral paramedian pontine reticular formation (PPRF)
- a unilateral lesion in one frontal eye field: prevents voluntary saccades to the opposite side, eyes deviate toward the side of the lesion
  - can be overcome with doll's eye maneuver
- a unilateral lesion in the pons: prevents voluntary saccades to the ipsilateral side, eyes deviate away from the lesion
  - cannot be overcome with doll's eye maneuver
- seizure involving a frontal eye field: cause eye deviation towards the opposite side

Internuclear Ophthalmoplegia (INO)

Etiology
- MS (most common; see *Multiple Sclerosis*, N63)
- brain stem infarction
- neoplasm
- AV malformations
- Wernicke's encephalopathy

Pathophysiology
- results from a lesion in medial longitudinal fasciculus (MLF) which disrupts coordination between CN VI in pons and the contralateral CNIII in midbrain --> disrupts conjugate horizontal gaze

Clinical Features
- on gaze away from the side of the lesion, adduction of ipsilateral eye is impaired but there is full excursion of the contralateral eye in abduction with monocular nystagmus
    - cannot be overcome by caloric testing
    - accommodation reflex intact
- may be bilateral
- up beating nystagmus on upward gaze often present

Diplopia

Monocular
- most due to relatively benign optical problems (refractive error, cataract, functional)

Binocular
- cranial nerve palsy (see *Cranial Nerves*, N20)
    - CN III
        - diabetes, aneurysm, tumour, trauma
        - isolated CN III palsy with pupil sparing usually due to DM and most will resolve spontaneously in several months
        - isolated CN III palsy with pupil involved usually indicates compressive lesion (especially posterior communicating artery aneurysm)
    - CN IV
        - diabetes, trauma
    - CN VI
        - diabetes, tumour, trauma
    - muscle
        - thyroid eye exophthalmos
- neuromuscular junction
    - myasthenia gravis (MG) (see *Myasthenia Gravis*, N43)
        - a useful test is the Tensilon™ (edrophonium) test
        - Tensilon™ is a drug that inhibits acetylcholinesterase
        - in myasthenia gravis, Tensilon™ administration will improve muscle function immediately and transiently
- other
    - orbital trauma, tumour
    - Wernicke's encephalopathy
    - Miller-Fischer variant of GBS
    - leptomeningial disease
- clinical features
    - diplopia worse at end of the day suggests myasthenia gravis (e.g. fatiguable)
    - if only diplopia on extremes of gaze, cover each eye in isolation during extremes of gaze
        - the covered eye that makes the outermost image disappear is the one with pathology

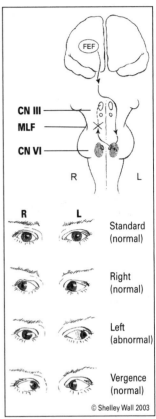

Figure 9. Internuclear Ophthalmopliegia

Nystagmus

- definition: rapid, involuntary, small amplitude movements of the eyes that are rhythmic in nature
- direction of nystagmus is defined by the rapid component of the eye movement
- can be categorized by movement type (pendular, jerking, rotatory, coarse) or as normal vs. pathological

Abnormalities of Pupils

Relative Afferent Pupillary Defect (RAPD) (Marcus-Gunn Pupil)

- see also Ophthalmology

Definition
- a failure of direct pupillary responses to light, caused by a defect in the visual afferent pathway anterior to the optic chiasm

- clinical testing
  - swinging light test
    - swing light from one eye to the other; both pupils should constrict initially
    - when normal side is illuminated, both pupils constrict
    - when damaged side is illuminated, both pupils paradoxically dilate
  - pupil reacts poorly to light, and better to accommodation
- differential diagnosis
  - optic neuritis is the most common cause of RAPD
  - other causes: optic nerve compression, large retinal detachment, central retinal artery/vein occlusion, advanced glaucoma

Horner's Syndrome

Horner's Syndrome
- Ptosis
- Miosis
- Anhydrosis

Definition
- a sympathetic defect
- clinical features: may cause partial ptosis, miosis, anhydrosis, and apparent enophthalmos occur anywhere along the sympathetic pathway on the affected side
  - 1st-order neuron (central): hypothalamus, medulla (brainstem stroke), spinal tumour, MS, intracranial tumours, syringomyelia
  - 2nd-order neuron (preganglionic): apical lung cancer (Pancoast's tumour), paravertebral mass, carotid artery dissection
  - 3rd-order neuron (postganglionic): cluster headache, cavernous sinus mass, trauma (including surgical)
- clinical confirmation with cocaine test: cocaine does not dilate a miotic Horner's pupil
- central vs. pre-ganglionic vs. post-ganglionic
  - paredrine (hydroxyamphetamine) will not dilate a post-ganglionic pupil, but will dilate a pre-ganglionic or central lesion
  - no test to differentiate central from pre-ganglionic lesion

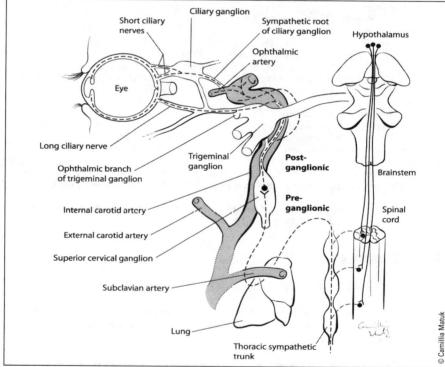

Figure 10. Sympathetic Pathway

© Camillia Matuk

Anisocoria

- definition – unequal size of the pupils
- refer to <u>Ophthalmology</u>

Movement Disorders

Localization of Extrapyramidal Disorders

Table 22. Corticospinal vs. Extrapyramidal Lesions

	Corticospinal (pyramidal)	Extrapyramidal
Muscle tone	• spastic	• rigid
Involuntary movements	• absent	• present
Tendon reflexes	• increased	• normal
Plantar reflexes	• upgoing	• downgoing
Paralysis/weakness	• present	• absent
Examples	• stroke	• Parkinson's disease

Function of the Basal Ganglia

- the globus pallidus pars interna (GPi) prevents excessive movement by tonic inhibition of the cortical motor areas via the thalamus
- net effect of striatal activity is to inhibit the GPi and thus to promote movement

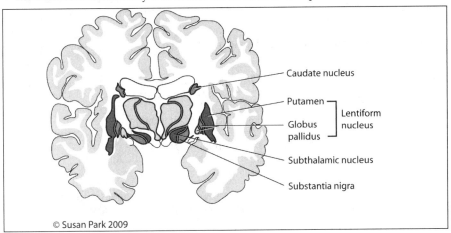

© Susan Park 2009

Figure 11. Basal Ganglia

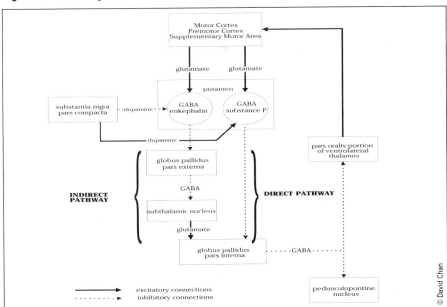

Figure 12. Neural Connections of the Basal Ganglia

The cerebral cortex initiates movement via excitatory (Glutamatergic, Glu) projections to the striatum (i.e. basal ganglia) via two pathways: direct and indirect. Final common pathway is the ventral thalamus and its projections back to the motor cortex (thalamocortical)

Indirect: Cortex → Striatum → GPe → STN → GPi → Thalamus → motor cortex   Activation of this pathway causes inhibition of the thalamus and ultimately prevents movement

Direct: Cortex → Striatum → GPe → GPi → Thalamus → motor cortex

Activation of this pathway activates STN which removes the inhibitory effect of the GPi on the thalamus, thereby allowing movement

Parkinsonism

Definition
- a set of symptoms including tremor, bradykinesia, ridigity and postural instability

Table 23. Selected Causes of Parkinsonism[+]

	1° PD**	PSP	MSA	Vascular	CBGD
L-dopa effect	+	–	±	–	–
Rest tremor	+	–	–	–	–
Postural instability	Late	Early	Early	Late	Late
Dystonia	±	± Axial	±	–	+
UMN S&S	–	+	+	+	+
Distribution	Asym	Sym; Axial	Sym; Legs>>arms	Sym	Unilateral
Dementia	±	±	-	+	–
Gaze dysfunction	–	+	±	±	+
Dysautonomia	Late	±	+ (SDS)	–	–
MRI	Normal	Midbrain atrophy	↓ striatum on T2	Multi-infarct	Parietal atrophy
Other	See below	Pseudobulbar palsy (impaired vertical gaze) postural instability	Cerebellar dysfunction (OPCA) Stridor (SND)	HTN	Alien limb phenomenon Apraxia

+ Abbreviations: PD - Parkinson's Disease; PSP - Progressive Supranuclear Palsy; MSA - Multiple System Atrophy; CBGD - Cortical Basal Ganglionic Degeneration; OPCA - Olivopontocerebellar Atrophy; SND - Striatonigral degeneration; SDS - Shy-Drager Syndrome
** Drug-induced PD can be clinically indistinguishable from primary PD

Other Important Causes of Parkinsonism
- secondary parkinsonism
  - postencephalitic
  - toxic (Mg, CO, MPTP)
  - post-traumatic
  - neuroleptics
- parkinson-plus syndromes (complex clinical presentations)
  - progressive supranuclear palsy (Steele-Richardson-Olszewski syndrome)
    - early postural instability, ophthalmoplegia, rare tremor
  - multiple-system atrophy (Shy Drager syndrome), OPCA, SND
    - autonomic symptoms/signs
  - diffuse Lewy body disease (see *Dementia*, N14)
    - presence of dementia for ≥1 year before onset of Parkinsonism
  - frontotemporal dementia (see *Dementia*, N33) – cortico-basal ganglion degeneration
- hereditary diseases
  - Wilson's disease (see *Wilson's Disease*)
  - juvenile Huntington's disease

> Ocular signs, absent rest tremor, early postural instability, and poor response to levodopa should cause one to suspect secondary parkinsonism or parkinson-plus syndromes.

Parkinson's Disease (PD)

Etiology
- genetic
  - many genes identified but account for small minority of PD
  - earlier onset → more likely genetic role
- environmental toxins
  - MPTP, pesticides
- oxidative stress/mitochondrial DNA mutations

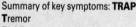

> Summary of key symptoms: **TRAP**
> **T**remor
> **R**igidity
> **A**kinesia/bradykinesia
> **P**ostural instability

Pathophysiology (Figure 12)
- ↓ striatal dopamine (DA) → disinhibition of globus pallidus pars interna and substantia nigra pars reticulata → ↑inhibition of cortical motor areas
- pathology: degeneration of dopaminergic neurons in the pars compacta of the substantia nigra
- presence of Lewy bodies in substantia nigra

Epidemiology
- 80% of all parkinsonism
- prevalence 0.5-1% in people 65-69 yrs old, 1-3% in people ≥80 yrs old
- average age of onset is 60 yrs old; M:F=1.5:1

Signs and Symptoms

- positive motor
  - rest tremor – most common initial finding
    - distal extremities; 4-5Hz
    - classic "pill-rolling" tremor of thumb and forefinger; also lips, chin, and tongue, increased with distraction, decreased with movement
  - rigidity
    - cogwheeling – ratcheting of extremity during passive motion
    - smooth – lead pipe
  - flexed posture
- negative motor
  - bradykinesia (slow movement; difficulty initiating movement; loss of automatic movement)
    - facial – hypomimia (masked facies with ↓blinking); drooling (from failure to swallow automatically); dysphagia; wide eyes
    - vocal – hypophonia (soft speech), aprosody (monotonous speech), dysarthria, and tachyphemia (inability to separate syllables clearly)
    - manual – micrographia (small and slow writing); difficulty shaving, brushing teeth, combing hair; decremental amplitude of rapid successive movements
    - gait – slow shuffling gait, short stride, ↓arm swing
  - postural instability (late sign)
    - leads to falls
    - gait
      - shuffling
      - patient moves faster so as to move feet under the flexed body's centre of gravity
  - freezing (transient inability to perform active movements)
    - commonly with walking
    - lasts a few seconds
    - triggers – beginning to walk, approaching a destination or barriers
    - overcome by visual cues
- cognitive
  - bradyphrenia – slowness in responding to questions; inability to change mental sets
  - dementia – generally occurs late
    - if occurs early (within 1 yr of diagnosis), consider Lewy body disease
- behavioural
  - changed personality (dependent, fearful, indecisive, passive)
  - ↓spontaneous speech
  - avolition and depression
  - sleep disturbances
- autonomic
  - constipation
  - inadequate bladder emptying
  - sexual dysfunction

Investigations

- the diagnosis of PD is made mostly on clinical grounds
- imaging not required in a typical presentation

Treatment

Table 24. Medical Management of Motor Symptoms of Parkinson's Disease

Mode of Action	Agents & Initial Dosages	Comments
DA precursor	*Carbidopa/Levodopa*: 25/100 mg bid-qid, increase as needed (max 200/2000 mg/d)	Mainstay of treatment, this is the most widely used formulation Excellent motor response Peripheral dopa decarboxylase inhibitor (carbidopa) decreases peripheral DA resulting in less nausea and increasing DA available in the CNS
DA agonist	*Bromocriptine*: 1.25 mg PO bid *Pergolide*: 0.05 mg PO OD, titrate q 2-3d to desired effect, usual maintenance is 3-6 mg/d in divided doses *Pramipexole*: 0.125 mg PO tid, increase to 1.5-4.5 mg/d in divided doses *Ropinirole*: 0.25 mg PO tid, increase weekly. max dose 24 g/d	Overall less effective than levodopa Longer half-life than levodopa and less likely to induce dyskinesias Used mostly as adjuvant therapy to decrease levodopa dose or to overcome fluctuations/dyskinesias Can be used as monotherapy early on
DA releaser/ NMDA antagonist	*Amantadine*: 100 mg PO OD up to 100 mg PO qid	Used in early PD Rapid action Short lived effect in advanced PD
MAO B inhibitor	*Selegeline*: 5 mg PO bid Rasagiline	Mild symptomatic effect Used in early PD Synergistic with levodopa
Anticholinergics	*Trihexyphenidyl*: 1-2 mg PO OD, then 2-5 mg PO OD-qid *Benztropine*: 0.5-6 mg/d PO in divided doses	Less effective than DA agonists Good for tremors, does not improve bradykinesia/rigidity Adverse effects include cognitive deterioration and delirium
COMT inhibitors	*Entacapone*: 200 mg administered concurrently with each levodopa/carbidopa dose to a max of 8x/d *Tolcapone*: 100 mg PO tid	Add to carbi/levo to extend pharmacokinetic half-life Used to control fluctuations Follow liver function, risk of fulminant liver failure Worsening of dyskinesia 2° to levodopa, may need to ↓dose levodopa

+Abbreviations: DA - dopamine; COMT - catechol-O-methyltransferase

Table 25. Surgical Management of Motor Symptoms of Parkinson's Disease

	Comments
Thalamotomy/thalamic stimulation*	• good for contralateral intractable tremor
Pallidotomy/pallidal stimulation*	• good for contralateral dopa-induced dystonia and chorea • also good for bradykinesia and tremor
Subthalamic stimulation	• best for contralateral bradykinesia and tremor • can allow ↓ L-dopa dose → ↓ dopa-induced complications
Embryonic dopaminergic transplantation	• for bradykinesia and rigidity in young patients

*Stimulation procedures involve permanent implantation of electrodes whose stimulation parameters can be fine-tuned to suit the patient's evolving clinical condition

Complications of Therapy

Table 26. Levodopa Related Fluctuations

	Management
Delayed onset of response	• give L-dopa before meals • reduce protein content of meals
End-of-dose deterioration ("wearing-off")*	• ↓ dose of L-dopa with dopamine agonists • slow-release carbidopa/L-dopa • COMT inhibitors
Random oscillation ("on-off")	• symptomatic relief of "off" periods with dissolved L-dopa in carbonated water (fast absorption) or injected apomorphine (soluble DA agonist) • COMT inhibitors

*Return of parkinsonian symptoms within 4 hours of last dose

Table 27. Levodopa Related Dyskinesias

	Timing	Management+
Peak-dose dyskinesias*	• at height of antiparkinsonian benefit	• ↓ size and ↑ frequency of L-dopa dosing • slow-release L-dopa • ↓ L-dopa and add Selegeline or DA agonist
Diphasic dyskinesias*	• beginning and end of dosing interval	• ↑ dose of L-dopa (but beware peak-dose dyskinesias) • use DA agonist as major antiparkinsonian with only adjunctive L-dopa
"Off" Dystonia+	• painful cramps appearing during "off" states	• limit "off" periods by using DA agonist as major antiparkinsonian with only adjunctive L-dopa

*Can be chorea, dystonia, or ballism   +Can also manage symptomatically (e.g. manage dystonia with muscle relaxant baclofen)   Abbreviations: DA - dopamine

Wilson's Disease (a.k.a. hepatolenticular degeneration)

Pathophysiology
- defect in copper metabolism resulting in accumulation of copper in brain (specifically basal ganglia, cerebellum), kidneys, liver, corneas
- autosomal recessive inheritance of mutation of ATP7B protein on chromosome 13

Signs and Symptoms
- neurological
  - movement abnormalities – parkinsonism, dysarthria, tremor (rest or action), facial dystonia, chorea, dysdiadochokinesia, incoordination, ataxia, abnormal eye movements, respiratory dyskinesia (may present as unusual cough)
- psychiatric

Diagnostic Criteria
- extrapyramidal symptoms, Kayser-Fleischer rings, low ceruloplasmin level, high serum copper, high urinary copper

Prognosis
- neurological symptoms begin to improve at 5-6 months after treatment, and do so until 2 years
- persistent neurological deficits after 2 years of treatment are likely to be permanent
- psychiatric symptoms often resolve completely
- in patients with fulminant liver failure, mortality rate up to 70%

Tremor

Table 28. Approach to Tremors

	Parkinsonian Tremor	Essential/Postural Tremor	Intention Tremor
Body Part	• distal upper extremity (head rare)	• upper extremity/head	• anywhere
Characteristics of tremor	• 3-7 Hz • pill rolling • flexion/extension • pronation/supination • at rest	• 6-12 Hz • fine tremor • with arms and hands outstretched (postural)	• <5 Hz • coarse • absent at rest • worse at end of movement
Best seen with	• hands resting in lap while concentrating on another task	• arms and hands outstretched	• finger to nose test
Associated features	• rigidity • bradykinesia • postural instability	• family history	• dysdiadochokinesia • dysmetria • dysarthria
Differential diagnosis	• primary Parkinson's disease • Wilson's Disease* • Parkinsonism	• physiological • drug-induced • hyperthyroid* • hyperglycemic*	• any cerebellar disorder* • Wilson's Disease* • pathology of the red nucleus • alcohol intoxication • multiple sclerosis
Treatment	• Levodopa/carbidopa • anti-cholinergics • pallidotomy • electrophysiologic surgery	• propranolol • anticonvulsants	• treat underlying cause

*In young patient (<45), must do TSH (thyroid disease), ceruloplasmin (Wilson's disease), CT/MRI (cerebellar disease) as indicated by type of tremor

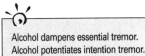

Alcohol dampens essential tremor.
Alcohol potentiates intention tremor.

Essential Tremor

Etiology and Pathogenesis
- genetic – can be autosomal dominant
- can also be sporadic
- can be physiologic or pathologic

Epidemiology and Risk Factors
- overall prevalence 1-4%; higher if >65 years old

Signs and Symptoms
- 6-12 Hz postural and kinetic tremor of the arms
- can also involve the head and voice
- tremor improves with alcohol consumptions

Treatment
- β-blockers and primidone are the mainstay of therapy
- other drugs used include clonazepam, topiramate, trihexyphenidyl
- stereotactic thalamotomy or thalamic stimulation if severe and intractable

Prognosis
- >90% never require medical attention

Chorea

Definition
- semi-purposeful flowing movements that are continuous, random, and can move from one part of the body to another

Table 29. Choreiform Disorders*

	Movement Disorder	Associated Features	Investigations
Huntington's Disease	Jerking chorea	Dementia Psychosis	Molecular testing CT (↑ ventricles, atrophy at caudate nucleus)
Neuroacanthocytosis	Mild chorea Tics Tongue biting	Peripheral neuropathy Feeding dystonia	Blood smear (acanthocytes) ↑ CK
SLE	Local chorea; periodic	see <u>Rheumatology</u>	ANA, APLA
APLA Syndrome	Chorea	Migraine Multi-infarct dementia Spontaneous abortions Thromboses Raynaud's phenomenon	↑ aPTT Lupus anticoagulant Anticardiolipin antibodies
Wilson's Disease	Arm-flapping tremor Chorea	Kayser-Fleischer rings Hepatic dysfunction	Ceruloplasmin, Cu++ Liver biopsy
Vascular Ballism	Hemiballismus		MRI – infarcts in the subthalamic nucleus
Tardive Dyskinesia	Oral- buccal dyskinesia	History of L-dopa or neuroleptic use	No specific tests
Senile Chorea	Mild chorea	Late onset No FHx No dementia	Genetic testing to rule out Huntington's disease APLA
Syndenham's chorea	Chorea	Rheumatic fever	ESR, ASOT

*Abbreviations: APLA - antiphospholipid antibody; L-dopa - levodopa

Huntington's Disease

Etiology and Pathogenesis
- genetics
    - autosomal dominant CAG-repeat disorder with anticipation of Huntington gene leading to accumulation of defective protein in neurons
- pathology
    - global cerebral atrophy with the neostriatum particularly involved

Epidemiology
- North American prevalence 4-8/100,000
- mean age onset 35-44 yrs

Signs and Symptoms
- chorea
    - purposeless and abrupt involuntary movements potentially involving any skeletal muscle
    - begin as movements of eyebrows and forehead, shrugging of shoulders, and parakinesiae (pseudopurposeful movements to mask involuntary limb jerking)

- can progress to a dance-like gait or ballism
- in the terminal stages, chorea can be replaced by dystonia and rigidity
- cognitive and psychiatric manifestations
  - dementia
    - progressive memory impairment and loss of intellectual capacity
  - mood changes
    - irritability or depression, loss of interest
    - impulsiveness and bouts of violence
  - psychosis
    - can mimic schizophrenia
- typical progression
  - onset 35-40 years (range 5-70)
  - insidious onset (clumsiness, dropping objects, fidgetiness, irritability)
  - progression over 15 years to frank dementia, psychosis, and chorea

Investigations
- MRI – enlarged ventricles, atrophy of cerebral cortex and caudate nucleus
- genetic testing

Treatment
- no disease altering treatments
- symptomatic management of depression and psychosis with antidepressants and antipsychotics
- symptomatic management of chorea with neuroleptics, benzodiazepines

Prognosis
- progressive course over 15-20 years

Dystonia

Definition
- sustained involuntary muscle contractions → twisting motions or abnormal postures
- co-contraction of agonist and antagonist muscles

Epidemiology
- most common movement disorder encountered in movement disorder clinics after parkinsonism

General Feature of Dystonias
- worsened by fatigue, stress, and emotion
- relieved by sleep (unless severe)
- can be relieved by specific tactile or proprioceptive stimuli – "geste antagoniste" (e.g. placing a hand on the side of the face in cervical dystonia)
- younger onset → more likely to progress and generalize
- leg dystonia → more likely to progress and generalize

Etiologic Classification of Dystonias
- primary dystonias
  - familial (e.g. Oppenheim dystonia)
  - sporadic (e.g. torticollis, blepharospasm, writer's cramp, etc.)
- dystonia-plus syndromes
  - dopa-responsive dystonia (DRD)
  - myoclonus-dystonia
- secondary dystonias
  - trauma/surgical (e.g. thalamotomy)
  - focal lesions (e.g. stroke, tumour, focal demyelination)
  - PNS injury (e.g. trauma, electrical injury)
  - drugs/toxins (e.g. L-dopa, neuroleptics, anticonvulsants, Mn, CO, cyanide, methanol)
- heterodegenerative dystonias
  - Parkinsonian disorders (e.g. juvenile parkinsonism, PD, PSP, MSA, CBGD)
  - metabolic disorders (e.g. Wilson's disease, Lesch-Nyhan syndrome)
  - other movement disorders (e.g. Huntington's disease)

Treatment of Dystonias
- medical
  - local
    - local injection of botulinum toxin

- systemic
  - anticholinergics (e.g. trihexyphenidyl)
  - muscle relaxants (e.g. baclofen)
  - benzodiazepines (e.g. clonazepam, diazepam)
  - antidopaminergics (e.g. reserpine, neuroleptics)
  - dopamine for DRD
- surgical
  - local
    - selective surgical denervation of affected muscles
  - systemic
    - stereotaxic thalamotomy (for unilateral dystonia)
    - posteroventral pallidotomy

Myoclonus

Definition
- brief, lightning-like involuntary muscle jerks due to either positive muscle contractions or sudden brief lapses of contraction (e.g. asterixis)

Clinical Features
- single or repetitive
- focal, segmental, or generalized
- can be stimulus sensitive (induced by noise, movement, light, visual threat, or pinprick)

Treatment
- treat underlying disorder
- symptomatic treatment – sodium valproate, clonazepam, primidone, piracetam

Normal forms of myoclonus include hiccups and muscle jerks experienced while falling asleep.

Tic Disorders

Definitions
- tic: a compulsive, rapid, repetitive, stereotyped movement or vocalization
  - simple tic: contraction of only 1 group of muscles
  - complex tic: sequence of movements or linguistically meaningful utterances

Clinical Classification of Tics
- motor tics
  - simple (blinking, head jerking)
  - dystonic (bruxism; abdominal tensing; sustained mouth opening)
  - complex (copropraxia – obscene gestures; echopraxia – imitating gestures; throwing; touching)
- vocal tics
  - simple (blowing, coughing, grunting, throat clearing)
  - complex (coprolalia – shouting obscenities; echolalia – repetition of others' phrases; palilalia – repetition of one's own phrases)

Etiologic Classification of Tic Disorders
- primary tic disorders
  - transient tic disorder (in childhood, duration < 1 year)
  - chronic tic disorder
  - Gilles de la Tourette syndrome
  - adult onset or senile tic, not otherwise specified
- secondary tic disorders
  - infections (e.g. encephalitis, Creutzfeld-Jakob disease, Sydenham's chorea)
  - head trauma
  - drugs (e.g. anticonvulsants, levodopa, stimulants, neuroleptics)
  - mental retardation syndromes (including chromosomal abnormalities)
- strong association with obsessive compulsive disorder (OCD) and ADHD

Treatment
- dopamine blockers (e.g. fluphenazine, haloperidol, clonidine tetrabenazine)

Tourette's Syndrome (a.k.a. Gilles de la Tourette's Syndrome)

Definition (DSM-IV)
1. both multiple motor and ≥1 phonic tics must be present at some time during illness, not necessarily concurrently
2. tics occur many times per day, nearly everyday or intermittently throughout a period of 1 year, with no tic-free period of 3 consecutive months
3. onset prior to 18 years of age
4. the disturbance is not due to the effects of a substance or general medical condition

Epidemiology
- prevalence among adolescents – 3-5/100,000 (M>F)

Signs and Symptoms
- tics
  - wide variety of tics that wax and wane in both type and severity
  - tics can be voluntarily repressed for a time
  - tics are preceded by an unpleasant sensation that is relieved by carrying out the tic
- psychiatric
  - compulsive ideation (often associated obsessive-compulsive disorder, ADHD)
  - hyperactive behaviour

Treatment
- clonidine
- clonazepam

Prognosis/Course
- begin at 5 years
- increase until 10 years
- decline thereafter (50% tic-free by 18 years)

Neuromuscular Disease

Overview

Table 30. Overview of Neuromuscular Diseases

		Motor Neuron Disease	Peripheral Neuropathy	Neuromuscular Junction (Myasthenia Gravis)	Myopathy
S&S	Weakness	• segmental and asymmetrical, distal → proximal	• distal (except GBS) but may be asymmetrical	• proximal and fatiguable	• proximal
	Fasciculations	• yes	• yes	• no	• no
	Reflexes	• increased	• decreased/absent	• normal	• normal (until late)
	Sensory	• no	• yes	• no	• no
	Autonomic*	• no	• yes	• no	• no
Tests	EMG	• denervation and reinnervation	• signs of demyelination ± axonal loss	• decremental response • jitter on single fibre EMG	• small, short motor potentials
	NCS	• normal	• abnormal	• normal	• normal
	Muscle Enz	• normal	• normal	• normal	• increased

*e.g. orthostatic hypotension, anhydrosis, visual blurring, urinary hesitancy or incontinence, constipation, erectile dysfunction

Abbreviations: GBS - Guillain-Barré Syndrome

Motor Neuron Disease

Amyotrophic Lateral Sclerosis (ALS)

Definition
- disease with progressive degeneration of the motor neurons featuring both upper and lower motor neuron symptoms and signs; also called Lou Gehrig's disease

Motor Neuron Diseases are characterized by UMN and/or LMN signs and symptoms.

Etiology
- genetic
    - 5-10% of ALS cases are familial (e.g. SOD1 mutation)
- indirect evidence for viral, autoimmune, paraneoplastic etiologies, and glutamate toxicity
- idiopathic

Pathology
- degeneration and loss of motor neurons with astrocytic gliosis
- Bunina bodies found in 70% of patients at autopsy
    - eosinophilic hyaline intracytoplasmic inclusions
- disorder of anterior horn cells of spinal cord and cranial nerve nuclei and corticospinal tract

Epidemiology
- frequency 5 cases per 100,000 population
- age of onset 40-60, earlier with familial form

Signs and Symptoms
- motor
    - limb findings – segmental and asymmetrical UMN and LMN signs
    - bulbar findings – dysarthria, dysphagia, tongue atrophy and fasciculations
    - ocular muscles and sphincters spared
    - death results from respiratory failure
- no sensory findings

Investigations
- bloodwork
    - CK should be normal, can be mildly elevated
- EMG
    - evidence of denervation (fibrillation, positive sharp waves, complex repetitive discharges) in 3 limbs and paraspinal muscles
    - evidence of reinnervation (↑amplitude and duration of motor units)
    - fasciculations
- muscle biopsy
    - small angulated fibres (evidence of denervation)
    - fibre type grouping
- rule out cervical cord disease/compression with CT or MRI

Management
- disease specific
    - riluzole (glutamate antagonist) prolongs survival by 3-6 months
- symptomatic
    - cramping – baclofen, quinine, phenytoin
    - sialorrhea – anticholinergics
- supportive
    - ventilatory support (e.g. BiPAP)

Prognosis
- median survival 3 years after diagnosis (can be much longer with ventilatory support)

Other Motor Neuron Diseases

Table 31. Other Motor Neuron Diseases*

	Characteristic Features
Progressive muscular atrophy/Progressive bulbar palsy	• 5-10% of patients in ALS centers • LMN S&S only • asymmetric weakness • later onset
Spinal muscular atrophy	• LMN S&S only • symmetric weakness • hypotonia, weakness, CN palsies • younger onset
Primary lateral sclerosis/ Progressive pseudobulbar palsy	• 5-10% of patients in ALS centers • UMN S&S only • later onset
Post-polio syndrome	• documented history of paralytic poliomyelitis • residual asymmetric muscle weakness, atrophy, and areflexia

*Abbreviations: ALS - amyotrophic lateral sclerosis; LMN - lower motor neuron; UMN - upper motor neuron

Peripheral Neuropathies

- see also Neurosurgery

Clinical Approach to Peripheral Neuropathies

Clinical Classification

Table 32. Anatomic Classification of Peripheral Neuropathies

Mononeuropathy	• distribution of a single peripheral nerve
Mononeuropathy multiplex	• motor, sensory, and reflex deficits affecting multiple nerves • stepwise progression; asymmetrical • can eventually summate to a symmetric stocking-glove pattern
Polyneuropathy	• diffuse, symmetric, distal stocking-glove pattern; distal hyporeflexia

> Axonal neuropathies feature ↓ amplitudes on nerve conduction studies while demyelinating neuropathies feature ↓ velocities.

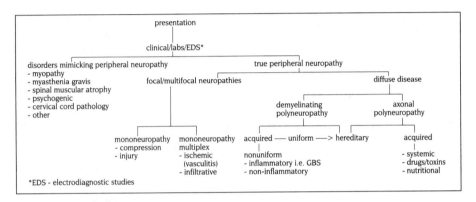

Figure 13. Classification of Peripheral Neuropathies

Mononeuropathy Multiplex

Table 33. Differential Diagnosis of Mononeuropathy Multiplex*

	Etiology	Pathophysiology	Key Investigations
Vascular	Polyarteritis nodosa	Ischemic (vasculitis)	p-ANCA LP (lymphocytosis and ↑protein) Nerve biopsy Hepatitis serology
	SLE	Ischemic (vasculitis)	ANA, anti-ds DNA Nerve biopsy
	RA	Ischemic (vasculitis)	ANA, RF Nerve biopsy
Infectious	HIV Lyme disease Syphilis	Mixed Infiltrative	HIV serology Lyme serology VDRL
Endocrine	Diabetes mellitus	Ischemic	Fasting glucose HbA1C
Immune	Chronic inflammatory demyelinating polyradiculoneuropathy	Demyelination	EMG (demyelination) LP (oligoclonal banding on electrophoresis)
	Sarcoidosis	Infiltrative	↑ serum ACE Nerve biopsy
Hereditary	Hereditary liability to pressure palsies	Demyelination	EMG - multifocal conduction block
Neoplastic	Lymphoma Paraproteinemias	Infiltrative	Imaging Nerve biopsy Serum and urine immuno electrophoresis
Toxic	Lead toxicity	NT abnormalities	Serum lead level

*Abbreviations: SLE - systemic lupus erythematosus; RA - rheumatoid arthritis; EMG - electromyography/nerve conduction studies; NT - neurotransmitter

> The top differential for mononeuritis multiplex usually includes:
> • vaculitis
> • infiltrative disease

Diffuse Symmetric Polyneuropathies

Table 34. Differential Diagnosis of Symmetric Polyneuropathy*

	Etiology+	Mechanism	Course	Modalities	Investigations
Vascular	PAN	Ischemic	Chronic	S/M	pANCA; hepatitis serology LP (↑ protein; ↑ cells) Nerve biopsy
	SLE	Ischemic	Chronic	S/M	ANA Nerve biopsy
	RA	Ischemic	Chronic	S/M	ANA, RF Nerve biopsy
Infectious	**HIV**	Axonal/demyelination	Chronic	S/A	HIV serology
	Leprosy	Infiltrative	Chronic	S/A	Leprosy serology Nerve biopsy
	Lyme	Axonal/demyelination	Chronic	M	Lyme serology
Immune	GBS	Demyelination	Acute	M	LP (↑ protein; no ↑ cells)
	CIDP	Demyelination	Chronic	S/M	LP (↑ protein)
Hereditary	HMSN	Axonal/demyelination	Chronic	S/M	Genetic testing
Neoplastic	Paraneoplastic	Axonal/demyelination	Chronic	S/M	Anti-Hu
	Osteolytic Myeloma	Axonal/demyelination	Chronic	S/M	SPEP Skeletal bone survey
	Osteosclerotic Myeloma	Demyelination	Chronic	S/M	SPEP Skeletal survey
	Lymphoma	Axonal	Chronic	M	SPEP, bone marrow biopsy
	Monoclonal gammopathy	Demyelination	Chronic	S/M	SPEP Bone marrow biopsy
Toxin	**EtOH**	Axonal	Sub-acute	S/M	GGT
	Heavy Metals	Axonal	Sub-acute	S/M	Urine heavy metals
	Medications	Axonal	Sub-acute	S/M	Drug levels
Metabolic	**Diabetes**	Ischemic/axonal	Chronic	S/A	Fasting glucose, HbA1C, 2hr OGTT
	Hypothyroidism	Axonal	Chronic	S/M	TSH, T3, T4
	Renal failure	Axonal	Chronic	S/A	Lytes, Cr, BUN
Nutritional	**B$_{12}$ Deficiency**	Axonal	Sub-acute	S/M	Vitamin B$_{12}$
Other	Porphyria	Axonal	Sub-acute	M	Urine parphyrins
	Amyloid	Axonal	Sub-acute	S	Nerve biopsy

*Abbreviations: GBS - Guillain-Barré Syndrome; PAN - polyarteritis nodosa; SLE - systemic lupus erythematosus; RA - rheumatoid arthritis; CIDP - chronic inflammatory demyelinating polyradiculoneuropathy; HMSN - hereditary motor sensory neuropathy; SPEP - serum protein electrophoresis; S - sensory; M - motor; A - autonomic
+Most common/important etiologies in boldface type

Guillain-Barré Syndrome (GBS)

Definition
- a heterogeneous set of acute, rapid evolving polyradiculoneuropathies consisting of 3 subtypes:
  1. acute inflammatory demyelinating polyneuropathy (AIDP) – 90%
  2. acute motor-sensory axonal neuropathy (AMSAN)
  3. acute motor axonal neuropathy (AMAN)

Etiology and Pathophysiology
- AIDP
  - focal inflammation and demyelination of nerve roots and distal peripheral nerve fibres resulting in conduction slowing or conduction block
- AMSAN and AMAN
  - focal inflammatory axonal degeneration of ventral (AMAN) or ventral and dorsal (AMSAN) roots

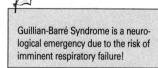

Guillian-Barré Syndrome is a neurological emergency due to the risk of imminent respiratory failure!

Epidemiology
- annual incidence 1-2/100,000
- bimodal distribution with peaks in young adulthood and elderly persons

Risk Factors

Table 35. Events Observed to Precede GBS

Viral Infections	Bacterial Infections	Vaccinations
EBV	*Campylobacter jejuni*	Rabies
CMV	*Mycoplasma pneumoniae*	Vaccinia
HIV	*Haemophilus influenzae*	Meningitis
Herpes	*Borrelia burgdorferi*	Influenza
West Nile Virus		

Signs and Symptoms
- motor
  - weakness
  - begins in muscles of lower extremities and ascends
  - loss of deep tendon reflexes (DTRs)
  - AMAN may be associated with UMN findings
- sensory
  - paresthesiae (distal and symmetric)
  - objective sensory loss (vibration and proprioception)
  - pain (deep and poorly localized)
- autonomic
  - blood pressure dysregulation (hypertension; orthostatic hypotension)
  - cardiac arrhythmias
  - bladder dysfunction
- Miller-Fisher variant
  - ophthalmoplegia
  - ataxia
  - areflexia

Investigations
- CSF analysis
  - albuminocytological dissociation ($\uparrow$ protein with normal white cell count)
  - often absent in first few days and absent in 10% of all GBS
- EMG/NCS
  - conduction block, differential slowing, or focal slowing on NCS (motor > sensory)
  - $\downarrow$ F-wave

Treatment
- supportive care (most important)
  - admit all patients with suspected GBS
    - risk of rapid deterioration
  - respiratory failure (30% of all GBS patients; due to phrenic nerve involvement)
    - monitor vital capacity and intubate if <15 ml/kg
  - dysautonomia (ICU management)
    - paroxysmal hypertension
      - short acting IV β-blockers
    - orthostatic hypotension
      - isotonic fluid replacement
    - cardiac arrhythmias
      - absence of beat-to-beat pulse variation indicates vagal denervation
      - nonsinus bradycardia $\rightarrow$ transvenous pacing
      - sinus tachycardia $\rightarrow$ fluid replacement
  - pain
    - ASA
    - antidepressants and anticonvulsants ineffective
- specific therapy
  - IVIg
  - plasmapheresis (within 1st week)
    - no effect on mortality or relapse
    - more rapid improvement, less intensive care and ventilation required

Prognosis
- typical course
  - nadir of symptoms at 2-3 weeks
  - considerable resolution at 4-6 weeks
- long term outcomes
  - 5% overall mortality (15-20% if ICU)
  - 75% recover without serious residual deficit; maximal recovery by 18 months
  - 7-15% have permanent substantial deficits (bilateral foot drop, intrinsic hand muscle weakness, sensory ataxia, dysesthesiae)

Diabetic Neuropathies

- see Endocrinology

Diabetic Distal Symmetric Polyneuropathy
- pathophysiology
  - stocking-glove "dying back" axonal neuropathy with longest nerves affected first
- clinical features - most commonly seen neuropathy
  - symptoms start in distal lower extremity
  - small sensory fibre disruption $\rightarrow$ loss of pain and temperature perception; dysesthesiae

Ototoxic drugs (e.g. aminoglycosides) should not be given to diabetics. Sensory neuropathies of the feet prevent them from adequately compensating for loss of vestibular function!

- large sensory fibre disruption → loss of proprioception, vibratory perception, and reflexes
- motor fibre disruption → intrinsic muscle weakness and wasting

Cranial Neuropathy
- pathophysiology
  - peripheral nerve ischemia
- clinical features
  - oculomotor neuropathy
    - III > IV > VI
    - pupillary sparing in 80-90% of CN III palsies (pupillary fibres are superficial and therefore not as prone to ischemia)

Focal Mononeuropathy
- pathophysiology
  - impaired glucose tolerance is associated with small fibre sensory neuropathy
  - compression/entrapment or ischemia
  - ischemia presents acutely and painfully and has poorer recovery
- clinical features
  - upper extremity
    - carpal tunnel syndrome
    - ulnar neuropathy at the elbow
  - lower extremity
    - common peroneal neuropathy at the fibular head (foot drop)

Diabetic Polyradiculopathy
- pathophysiology
  - axon loss at the root level affecting single or contiguous roots (may be inflammatory)
- clinical features – most commonly seen neuropathy
  - diabetic amyotrophy
    - L2-L4 and occasionally L5
    - rapid development of pain and weakness preferentially affecting the anterior thigh
    - wasting of the quadriceps with loss of the knee jerk
  - diabetic thoracoabdominal neuropathy
    - mid- to lower thoracic roots

Diabetic Autonomic Neuropathy
- autonomic neuropathy alone is rare
- pupils (miosis and sluggish reaction)
- CVS (resting tachycardia and orthostatic hypotension)
- GI (constipation, gastroparesis)
- GU (erectile dysfunction, ejaculation failure)

Paraneoplastic Neuropathies

Table 36. Paraneoplastic Polyneuropathies

Syndrome	Pathology	Associated Tumour	Associated Ab
Sensorimotor	• axonal/demyelination	• small cell lung	• none
Pure sensory*	• dorsal root ganglionitis	• small cell lung, breast	• anti-Hu
Pure motor	• motor neuron disease	• lymphoma	• paraprotein (IgG, IgM)

*Painful paresthesiae, sensory ataxia, and areflexia preceding tumour symptoms

Treatment
- steroids
- IVIg
- plasmapheresis
- treat underlying malignancy

Neuromuscular Junction Diseases

Clinical Approach to Disorders of the Neuromuscular Junction

Table 37. Common Disorders of the Neuromuscular Junction

	Myasthenia Gravis	Lambert-Eaton	Botulism
Ocular/bulbar paresis	+	–	++ (early)
Limb weakness	+	+	+
Fatiguability	+	+	+
Post-exercise enhancement	–	+	+
Reflexes	N	↓	↓
Autonomic anticholinergic S&S	–	+	++
Sensory S&S	–	–	–
Associated conditions	Thymoma	Small cell carcinoma	GI S&S
EMG response to repetitive stimulation	↓	↑ (rapid stimulation) ↓ (slow stimulation)	↑ (rapid stimulation) ↓ (slow stimulation)

Myasthenia Gravis

Etiology and Pathophysiology
- damage and blockade of post-synaptic acetylcholine receptors by specific antibodies
- 15% of patients with myasthenia gravis have associated thymic neoplasia, 85% have thymic hyperplasia
- autoimmune disorder

Epidemiology
- bimodal age of onset – 20's (mostly women) and 60's (mostly men)

Signs and Symptoms
- see also Table 37
- fatiguability and weakness of skeletal muscles without reflex, sensory, or coordination abnormalities
- typically ocular (diplopia/ptosis) → bulbar (dysarthria/dysphagia) → neck flexors/extensors → proximal limbs
- respiratory muscle weakness may lead to respiratory failure

Investigations
- edrophonium (Tensilon™) test – can result in respiratory difficulty so have crash cart nearby
  1. fatigue patient with easily assessed sign (ptosis, vital capacity, slurred speech)
  2. inject edrophonium
  3. assess for improvement over 2 minutes
- EMG
  - repetitive stimulation → decremental response
  - single fibre electromyography shows ↑ jitter (80-100% sensitivity)
- anti-acetylcholine receptor antibody assay (70-80% sensitivity)
- MUSK antibody, anti-agrin and anti-titin my also be seen
- CT/MRI to screen for thymoma/thymic hyperplasia

Treatment
- thymectomy
  - 85% of patients show improvement or remission
- symptomatic relief
  - acetylcholinesterase inhibitors (e.g. pyridostigmine)
  - do not affect primary pathologic process → rarely result in control of disease when used alone
- immunosuppression
  - steroids are mainstay of treatment – 70-80% remission rate
  - azathioprine, cyclophosphamide and mycophenolate as adjuncts to steroids or as steroid sparing therapy
- short-term immunomodulation (for crises)
  - IVIg and plasmapheresis

Prognosis
- 30% eventual spontaneous remission

Diseases of the neuromuscular junction typically feature prominent fatiguability.

Myasthenia Gravis is a neurological emergency due to the risk of imminent respiratory failure!

Lambert-Eaton Myasthenic Syndrome (LEMS)

Lambert-Eaton myasthenic syndrome can be differentiated from myasthenia gravis by the phenomenon of post-exercise facilitation.

Etiology and Pathophysiology
• downregulation of presynaptic voltage-gated Ca channels 2° to specific channel-binding antibody
• 50-66% are ultimately associated with small cell carcinoma of the lung

Signs and Symptoms
• weakness of skeletal muscles without sensory or coordination abnormalities
• reflexes are diminished or absent, but increase after active muscle contraction
• bulbar and ocular muscles affected in 25%
• prominent anticholinergic autonomic symptoms
  (dry mouth > impotence > constipation > blurred vision)

Investigations
• edrophonium test (see *Myasthenia Gravis*, N43) → no response
• EMG
  ▪ rapid (> 10Hz) repetitive stimulation → incremental response
• screen for malignancy, especially small cell lung cancer
• post-exercise facilitation – an incremental response to repetitive stimulation due to presynaptic calcium accumulation

Treatment
• tumour removal
• acetylcholine modulation
  ▪ ↑acetylcholine release (3-4 diaminopyridine)
  ▪ ↓acetylcholine degradation (pyridostigmine)
• immunomodulation
  ▪ steroids, plasmapheresis, IVIg

Myopathies

Clinical Approach to Muscle Diseases

Myopathies are characterized by prominent symmetric proximal weakness and absent sensory changes.

Table 38. Myopathies

	Etiology	Key Clinical Features	Key Investigations
Inflammatory	Polymyositis	Myalgias Pharyngeal involvement	↑ CK Biopsy: endomesial infiltrates; Necrosis
	Dermatomyositis	Myalgias Similar to polymyositis Characteristic rashes Can be paraneoplastic	↑ CK Biopsy: perifascicular atrophy
	Sarcoidosis	See Respirology	ACE level Biopsy: granulomas
Endocrine	Thyroid (↑ or ↓) Cushing's syndrome Parathyroid (↑ or ↓)	See Endocrinology	TSH, serum cortisol, calcium panel
Toxic	Medication Critical illness myopathy	Medication or toxin history ICU patient Hx steroids and nondepolarizing paralyzing agents Failure to wean from ventilation	Toxicology screen Biopsy: selective loss of thick Myosin filaments
Infectious	Parasitic, bacterial, or viral	Myalgias Inflammatory myopathy	↑ myoglobin
Hereditary dystrophy	Duchenne Becker	Early onset (Duchenne and Becker) Progressive proximal muscle weakness Calf pseudohypertrophy	Biopsy: abnormal dystrophin staining
	Myotonic dystrophy	Distal myopathy Myotonia Genetic anticipation	Genetic testing
Hereditary metabolic	McArdle's	Exercise-related myalgias, cramping, and myoglobuminuria	↑ lactate ↑ serum/urinary myoglobin Post-exercise
Hereditary periodic paralysis	Periodic paralysis	Episodic weakness Normal between attacks	↑ or ↓ K
Hereditary mitochondrial	MERRF MELAS Kearns Sayre	Ptosis, ophthalmoparesis common	↑ lactate Biopsy: ragged red fibres

*Abbreviations: MERRF - mitochondrial encephalomyopathy with ragged red fibers; MELAS - mitochondrial encephalomyopathy, lactic acidosis, and stroke-like episodes

Polymyositis/Dermatomyositis

- see Rheumatology

Etiology and Pathophysiology
- autoimmune: muscle microvasculature (DM); muscle fibres (PM)

Epidemiology
- cancer association
  - 9% (PM) and 15% (DM)
  - 60% of adults >40 years with DM have concomitant neoplasm
- common concurrent inflammatory disorders
  - RA, SLE, mixed connective tissue disease, Sjogren's syndrome, scleroderma

Signs and Symptoms
- myopathic features
  - myalgias and muscle tenderness
  - proximal > distal; abductors > adductors; extensors > flexors
  - dysphagia and neck flexor weakness with progression
- cutaneous features (DM)
  - photosensitive heliotrope (blue-purple) periorbital rash
  - erythematous rash on extensor surfaces of limbs and joints
  - V sign – anterior neck and chest rash
  - shawl sign – rash over shoulders
  - Gottron's papules
- systemic features
  - Raynaud's phenomenon
  - pulmonary fibrosis
  - electrocardiographic abnormalities
  - pericarditis

Investigations
- blood tests
  - CK
  - anti-nRNP; PM-Scl, antisynthetases, anti-Jo-1
  - aldolase
- EMG
  - myopathic motor units (small/short motor potentials, full interference pattern)
  - fibrillations
- muscle biopsy
  - PM: endomesial infiltrates, necrosis and atrophy
  - DM: perifascicular atrophy

Treatment
- immunosuppression
  - prednisone (mainstay)
  - azathioprine (for steroid sparing)
- immunomodulation
  - IVIg is safe and effective
  - plasmapheresis is ineffective

Prognosis
- favourable prognosis – 10 year survival up to 90%

Myotonic Dystrophy

Etiology and Pathophysiology
- unstable trinucleotide repeat in DMK gene (protein kinase) at 19q13.3
- number of repeats correlates with severity of symptoms

Epidemiology
- most common adult muscular dystrophy
- prevalence 3-5/100 000

Signs and Symptoms
- skeletal muscle
  - weakness
    - face, jaw, neck > distal extremities

- myotonia
  - delayed relaxation of muscles after exertion (elicit by tapping on thenar muscles with hammer)
  - facial (long and thin; wasted muscles of mastication → sunken cheeks; sternocleidomastoid wasting → swan neck)
- cardiac
  - 90% have conduction defects (1° heart block; atrial arrhythmias)
- respiratory (hypoventilation 2° to muscle weakness)
- ocular
  - subcapsular cataracts
  - retinal degeneration
  - ↓ intraocular pressure
- frontal balding

Investigations
- EMG
  - subclinical myotonia – long runs with declining frequency and amplitude
- muscle biopsy
  - ↑ central nuclei, nuclear chains, ringed fibres, type I fibre atrophy
- molecular diagnosis
- slit lamp examination (for cataracts)

Treatment
- no cure
- management of myotonia
  - phenytoin
- management of systemic problems
- cardiac (ECG and pacing if necessary)

Duchenne and Becker Muscular Dystrophy

- see Pediatrics

Cerebellar Disorders

Approach to Cerebellar Disorders

Clinico-Anatomic Correlations
- rostral midline → stance and gait disturbances
- caudal midline → disturbances of axial posture and equilibrium
- hemispheric → ipsilateral limb ataxia/clumsiness

Symptoms and Signs of Cerebellar Dysfunction
- nystagmus – observe on extra-ocular movement testing (most common is gaze-evoked nystagmus)
- dysarthria – ataxic dysarthria – abnormal modulation of speech velocity and volume- elicit scanning/telegraphic/slurred speech on spontaneous speech (see Dysarthria, N19)
- ataxia – broad-based, uncoordinated, lurching gait
- dysmetria – irregular placement of voluntary limb or ocular movement
- dysdiadochokinesis – unable to perform rapid alternating movements (pronation-supination task)
- postural instability – look for truncal ataxia on sitting (titubation = rhythmic rocking of trunk and head); look for difficult tandem gait and broad based gait
- intention tremor – elicit on finger-to-nose testing- typically orthogonal to intended movement, and increases as target is approached
- hypotonia – decreased resistance to passive muscular extension- occurs immediately after injury to lateral cerebellum
- reflexes: pendular patellar reflex – knee reflex causes pendular motion of leg occurs after injury to cerebellar hemispheres
- rebound phenomenon – overcorrection after displacement of a limb (with both arms extended → pushing both will cause one to rebound up if there is lesion on that side)

Acquired Cerebellar Disorders

Table 39. Acquired Cerebellar Disorders

	Onset	Etiology	Key Features	Investigations
Vascular	Acute	• infarction/TIA • hemorrhage • basilar migraine	• brainstem S&S • brainstem S&S; ↑ ICP • brainstem S&S	• CT/MRI/MRA • CT/MRI
Infectious	Subacute	• bacterial abscess • viral encephalitis	• fever • fever, neurologic abnormalities, especially personality change seizure	• CT/MRI - ring enhancing lesion • LP, CT/MRI
Toxins/Meds	(Sub)acute	• anticonvulsants • alcohol*	• drug Hx • S&S chronic EtOH	• Drug levels • liver enzymes
Autoimmune	Subacute	• multiple sclerosis • Miller-Fisher GBS	• see *Multiple Sclerosis* section • areflexia; ataxia; oculoparesis	• MRI; LP; Evoked potentials • EMG/NCS
Metabolic	Chronic	• hypothyroid • Wilson's disease • thiamine deficiency	• see Endocrinology • Kayser-Fleischer Rings • Wernicke syndrome +	• TFT • ceruloplasmin • trial of thyamine
Neoplastic	Subacute Chronic	• medulloblastoma • astrocytoma • hemangioblastoma • paraneoplastic	• children • children • VHL syndrome** • lung, breast, ovarian tumour	• MRI/CT • MRI/CT • MRI/CT • Anti-Yo Ab; CXR

*Preferentially affects gait; limb coordination preserved
+Ophthalmoparesis, gait ataxia, dementia
**Von Hippel Lindau syndrome - hemangioblastomas (cerebellum, brainstem, spinal cord, retina), renal cysts, renal cell carcinoma

Hereditary Ataxias

Friedreich's Ataxia
- onset 5-20 years
- affects cerebellum, spinal cord, peripheral nerve, and heart
- cerebellar S&S: gait ataxia progressing to limb ataxia
- leg S&S: weakness, areflexia, Babinski; impaired proprioception and vibration
- prognosis: death from cardiomyopathy or kyphoscoliotic pulmonary restriction in 10-20 years

Ataxia Telangiectasia
- onset: infancy
- multisystem disorder
- progressive cerebellar ataxia, mental retardation in 30%
- telangiectasia of conjunctiva, nose and ears develop later
- death usually occurs in 2nd or 3rd decade of life due to infection or malignancy (lymphoma, lymphocytic leukemia)

Olivopontocerebellar Atrophy (OPCA)
- onset: adulthood- mean age 53 years, M:F = 2:1 in familial, equal in sporadic
- progressive neurodegeneration of brainstem that is either familial or sporadic
- prevalance = 3-5/100,000 or approximately 5-8% of atypical parkinsonism
- cerebellar dysmetria and ataxia, abnormalities of vocal modulation, limb coordination, smooth pursuit eye movement, progressive loss of neurons in olivary nucleus of medulla, pons and cerebellum --> characteristic atrophy on CT/ MRI
- relatively refractory to levodopa treatment- differentiates from idiopathic Parkinson's

Spinocerebellar Ataxia
- onset: adult
- ataxia, dysarthria, sensory loss
- many genetic syndromes identified (most common SCA 2,3,6)
- Machado-Joseph disease (SCA3) (cerebellar, extrapyramidal, and pyramidal S&S)

Vertigo

Definition
- an illusion of movement of self (subjective) or surroundings (objective) spinning
- often associated with impulsion (sensation of body being pulled in space) or oscillopsia (visual illusion of moving back and forth)
- see Otolaryngology for further details on Etiology, Pathophysiology, Investigations, and Treatment

Etiology
- central: brainstem or cerebellar
  - vascular disease
    - vertebrobasilar insufficiency (VBI)
    - TIA
  - infection – e.g. neurosyphilis
  - inflammation – e.g. multiple sclerosis
  - neoplastic
  - drugs – anticonvulsants, hypnotics, alcohol
- peripheral
  - see Otolaryngology

Signs and Symptoms
- see Table 40

Table 40. Peripheral vs. Central Vertigo

	Peripheral	Central
Vertigo	• severe, often rotational • always present	• usually mild • often absent
Nystagmus	• horizontal, sometimes torsional • increased when looking away from the side of lesion, always 1 direction only	• vertical or rotatory • occurs in >1 direction
Caloric testing	• abnormal on side of lesion	• may be normal
Brainstem or CN signs	• absent	• often present
Hearing loss and tinnitus	• often present	• absent
Nausea and vomiting	• usually present	• usually absent, can be present if ↑ICP
Falls	• often falls toward side of lesion	• often falls toward side of lesion but may be variable in direction
Visual fixation	• inhibits nystagmus	• no change in nystagmus

Gait Disturbances

Central Motor Systems

- Three components:
  1. Pyramidal: major outflow from cortex → spinal cord. Lesions cause motor weakness, spasticity and hyperreflexia, which disturb motor function but are not true motor disorders.
  2. Extra-pyramidal: the basal ganglia and their projections receive input from cortex, and feedback to cortex via thalamus.
  3. Cerebellar: see *Cerebellar Disorders*, N46

Gait Disturbances

Approach to Gait Disturbances
1. Length of stride short
- Parkinson's (posture is stooped with no arm swing; festinating or shuffling gait)
- Marche à petit pas (Parkinson's/"Parkinson's plus" multi-infarct state)
- "magnetic gait" in NPH

2. If (1) normal, look at width of stance
- crossing over: think spastic paresis
- wide based: cerebellar ataxia
- wide with high stepping, slapping feet: sensory ataxia

3. If (1) and (2) normal, look at knees
- high knees: foot drop/ LMN

4. If (1) to (3) normal, look at pelvis and shoulders
- waddling gait (e.g. proximal muscle myopathy)
- normal pressure hydrocephalus (feet barely leave ground)

5. Look at whole movements
- disjointed movements: apraxic gait (cortical lesion from NPH, CVD)
- bizarre, elaborate and inconsistent: functional gait

6. Look for asymmetry
- think of pain (antalgic gait), bony deformity, or weakness

Disorders of Balance

Cerebellar
- etiology: see *Cerebellar Disorders*, N46
- clinical features: wide based gait, ataxia, trunk sways forward

Sensory
- etiology
  - vestibular causes (see <u>Otolaryngology</u>)
  - proprioceptive deficits (may have positive Romberg sign)
  - visual disturbances
- clinical features
  - wide based stance and gait, high steppage, positive Romberg Sign (proprioceptive)

Disorders of Locomotion

Weakness Disorders
- LMN disease
  - high steppage, distal weakness
- myopathy
  - proximal weakness with difficulty rising from chair or climbing stairs

Parkinsonism
- parkinsonian gait
  - stooped posture, shuffling gait, difficulty initiating and terminating steps, require many steps to turn

Higher Level Disorders
- hemiparesis/focal brain injury
  - spastic extended leg and flexed arm, circumduction of affected foot
- paraparesis/spinal cord injury
  - toe walking or scissoring gait, bilateral circumduction
- apraxia; hydrocephalus or frontal lobe injury
  - magnetic gait (feet barely leave ground), shuffling, difficulty initiating steps
- cerebral palsy; congenital or perinatal brain injury
  - scissoring gait, spastic extended legs and flexed arms, adventitial movements
- movement disorders (e.g. chorea, athetosis, dystonia)
  - lurching gait, may have adventitial movements

Musculoskeletal Disorders
- antalgic gait

Pain Syndromes

Approach to Pain Syndromes

Definitions

Table 41. Common Terms Used in Discussing Pain Syndromes

Term	Definition
Nociceptive pain	Pain arising from normal activation of peripheral nociceptors
Neuropathic pain	Pain arising from direct injury to neural tissue, bypassing nociceptive pathways
Spontaneous pain	Unprovoked burning, shooting, or lancinating pain
Paresthesiae	Spontaneous or evoked abnormal nonpainful sensations (e.g. tingling)
Dysesthesiae	Spontaneous or evoked pain with inappropriate quality or excessive quantity
Allodynia	A dysesthetic response to a nonnoxious stimulus
Hyperalgesia	An exaggerated pain response to a noxious stimulus

Approaches to Pain Control

Table 42. Medical Approaches to Pain Control

Role	Class	Examples
Primary analgesics	• nonopiates	• NSAIDs • acetaminophen
	• opiates	• codeine • meperidine • morphine
Adjuvant analgesics	• antidepressants	• tricyclics (nortriptyline, amitriptyline, etc.) • SSRI's (fluoxetine, paroxetine, etc.)
	• anticonvulsants	• gabapentin • carbamazepine
	• GABA agonists	• baclofen
	• oral local anesthetics	• mexiletine
	• sympatholytics	• phenoxybenzamine
	• α₂-adrenergic agonists	• clonidine • pregabalin (Lyrica™)

Table 43. Selected Surgical Procedures for Pain Control

Classification	Procedure	Principle	Selected Indications
Direct delivery of 1° analgesics	• implantable morphine pump	• deliver morphine intrathecally or epidurally to activate peripheral opiate receptors	1. failure of pain control with supratherapeutic oral meds 2. inability to tolerate systemic narcotic side effects
Central ablation	• stereotactic thalamotomy	• ablation of spinoreticular relay	• HEENT malignancy
	• spinal tractotomy*	• stereotactic radiofrequency coagulation of neural fibres in ventrolateral spinothalamic tract at C1-C2	• intractable pain in terminal malignancy
	• dorsal root entry lesions*	• ablation of dorsal roots at entry into cord	• deafferentation pain (e.g. brachial plexus avulsion)
Peripheral ablation	• nerve blocks⁺	• ablation of peripheral nerves with neurolytics (permanent) or local anesthetics (temporary)	• to provide dermatomal pain relief
	• facet joint denervation	• cut posterior ramus of spinal nerves	• degenerative back pain
Stimulatory	• deep brain stimulation	• stimulation of electrodes in periventricular gray matter, thalamus, or internal capsule	• intractable pain; central pain
	• dorsal column stimulation	• percutaneous electrodes in peridural space	• intractable pain

*Complication: ipsilateral leg weakness
+Complication: loss of motor and sympathetic function

Neuropathic Pain

Definition
• pain resulting from a disturbance of the central or peripheral nervous system

Symptoms and Signs
• hyperalgesia
• allodynia
• subjectively described as burning, heat/cold, pricking, electric shock, perception of swelling, numbness (i.e. stocking/sock distribution)
• can be spontaneous or stimulus evoked
• distribution may not fall along classical neuro-anatomical lines

Associated Issues
• sleep difficulty
• mood alteration
• anxiety
• stress
• sexual dysfunction

Causes of Neuropathic Pain
• peripheral neuropathy
    ▪ systemic disease - diabetes, thyroid disease, renal disease, rheumatoid arthritis
    ▪ nutritional/toxicity - alcoholism, pernicious anemia, chemotherapy
    ▪ infectious - HIV
    ▪ trauma - post surgical, nerve injury

- nerve root
  - post-herpetic
  - cervical and lumbar radiculopathies
  - tic douloureux (see *Trigeminal Nerve*, N21)
  - plexopathies
- central
  - MS
  - post-stroke
  - phantom limb
- Complex Regional Pain Syndrome
  - CRPS type I (reflex sympathetic dystrophy)
  - CRPS type II (causalgia)
- malignancy

TREATMENT

Pharmacotherapy
1. oral – tricyclic antidepressants (e.g. amitriptyline), antiepileptic medication (e.g. gabapentin), pregabalin (Lyrica™), duloxetine (SNRI), opioids (only long acting)
2. topical – lidocaine (if localized), or capsaicin cream
3. local
   a. intrathecal – opioids, clonidine
   b. botox injection
   c. nerve block

Surgical Therapies
1. dorsal column neurostimulator
2. deep brain stimulator (thalamus)

Other Therapies
1. neuropsychiatry – cognitive-behaviour theraphy, psychotherapy
2. rehabilitation – physiotherapy
3. CAM – acupuncture, meditation, massage therapy, TCM

Tic Douloureux

- see *Cranial Nerves*, N21

Postherpetic Neuralgia

Definition
- pain persisting beyond 3 months in the region of a cutaneous outbreak of herpes zoster

Etiology and Pathogenesis
- destruction of the sensory ganglion neurons (e.g. dorsal root, trigeminal, or geniculate ganglia) secondary to reactivation of herpes zoster infection

Epidemiology
- 10-15% of all patients with cutaneous herpes zoster
- > 80% of herpes zoster infected patients > 80 years old

Signs and Symptoms
- types of pain
  1. constant deep ache or burn
  2. intermittent spontaneous lancinating/jabbing pain
  3. allodynia
- distribution of post-herpetic neuralgia
  - thoracic > trigeminal > cervical > lumbar > sacral

Treatment
- acute herpes zoster
  - early treatment with antiviral agents (acyclovir, longer-acting famciclovir and valaciclovir more effective) may prevent PHN in patients over 50 years
- post-herpetic neuralgia – medical
  - tricyclic antidepressants, pregabalin, gabapentin
  - opiates, topical lidocaine patch
  - intrathecal methylprednisolone
- post-herpetic neuralgia – surgical
  - spinal tractotomy
  - dorsal root entry zone lesion

Complex Regional Pain Syndromes (CRPS)

Definitions
- CRPS is a pain syndrome characterized by the following:
  1. presence of an initiating noxious event
  2. continuing pain, allodynia, or hyperalgesia with pain disproportionate to inciting event
  3. evidence at some time of edema, changes in skin blood flow, or abnormal vasomotor activity
  4. absence of conditions that would otherwise account for degree of pain and dysfunction

Classification
- CRPS type I (reflex sympathetic dystrophy)
  - minor injuries of limb or lesions in remote body areas precede onset of Sx
- CRPS type II (causalgia)
  - injuries of peripheral nerve precede the onset of symptoms

Signs and Symptoms
- stage I (acute)
  - pain
    - disproportionate to initial injury
    - burning or aching
  - autonomic
    - edema
    - temperature inequality
- stage II (dystrophic)
  - pain
    - constant
    - ↑ by stimulus to affected part
  - autonomic
    - cool, hyperhydrotic skin
    - hair loss and cracked/brittle nails
    - osteoporosis
- stage III (atrophic)
  - pain
    - paroxysmal spread
  - autonomic
    - thin, shiny skin
    - thickened fascia with contractures
    - bony demineralization

Investigation
- diagnosis is clinical
- trial of differential neural blockade may be helpful

Treatment
- medical
  - phenoxybenzamine (sympatholytic)
- surgical
  - paravertebral sympathetic ganglion blockade
    - definite but transient improvement
  - paravertebral sympathetic ganglionectomy
    - for patients for whom ganglionic blocks provide only transient benefit

Thalamic Pain (Dejerine Roussy Syndrome)

Definition
- hypersensitivity to pain as a result of damage to the thalamus

Etiology and Pathogenesis
- injury to ventral posterolateral (VPL) and ventral posteromedial (VPM) nuclei of the thalamus
  - ischemic stroke
  - hypertensive vascular hemorrhage

Signs and Symptoms
- begins with hemianesthesia
- then persistent spontaneous burning contralateral to lesion
- altered response to light cutaneous and deep painful stimuli

Treatment
- medical: amitriptyline, anti-convulsants
- surgical: stereotactic thalamic stimulation (may ↑ sensory deficit)

Headache

Clinical Approach to Headaches

Table 44. Headaches - Benign

	Tension-Type	Migraine (see *Migraine*, N54)	Cluster
Prevalence	• 70%	• 12%	• <1%
Age of onset	• 15-40	• 10-30	• 20-40
Sex bias	• F > M	• F > M	• M > F
Family History	• none	• +++	• +
Location	• bilateral frontal • nuccho-occipital	• unilateral>bilateral • fronto-temporal	• retroorbital
Duration	• minutes – days	• hours – days	• 10 min – 2 hours
Onset/Course	• gradual; worse in PM	• gradual; worse in PM	• daily headache for weeks months, nocturnal
Quality	• band-like; constant	• throbbing	• constant, aching, stabbing
Severity	• mild-moderate	• moderate-severe	• severe (wakes from sleep)
Provoking	• depression • anxiety • noise • hunger • sleep deprivation	• noise • light • straining • coughing • activity	• light • EtOH
Palliating	• rest	• rest	• walking around
Associated Sx	• no vomiting • no photophobia	• nausea/vomiting • photo/phonophobia • aura	• red watery eye • stuffy nose • unilateral Horner's
Physical signs	• muscle tension in scalp/neck	• muscle tension in scalp/neck • tender scalp arteries	• red watery eye, rhinorrhea • swelling
Management	Non-pharmacological • psychological counseling • physical modalities (e.g. heat, massage) Pharmacological • simple analgesics • tricyclic antidepressants	Acute Rx • triptans ± O_2 • ergotamine Prophylaxis • Ca-channel blockers • methylsergide • lithium • prednisone	

Table 45. Headaches – Serious

	Meningial Irritation	↑Intracranial Pressure	Temporal Arteritis
Incidence	• <1%	• <1%	• <<1%
Age of onset	• any age	• any age	• >60
Sex bias	• no bias	• no bias	• no bias
Location	• generalized; stiff neck	• any location	• temporal
Duration	• variable	• chronic	• variable
Onset/Course	• meningitis: hours-days • SAH: thunderclap onset	• gradual; worse in AM	• variable
Quality	• variable	• unlike any previous headache	• throbbing
Severity	• severe	• severe	• variable; can be severe
Provoking	• head movement	• lying down • Valsalva • head low • exertion	
Palliating	• rest and immobility	• standing/sitting	
Associated Sx	• neck stiffness • photophobia • focal deficits (e.g. CN palsies)	• nausea/vomiting • focal neuro Sx • ↓ level of consciousness	• polymyalgia rheumatica • jaw/tongue claudication • visual loss
Physical signs	• Kernig's sign • Brudzinski's sign	• focal neuro Sx • papilledema	Temporal artery changes: • firm, nodular, incompressible • tender
Management	• CT/LP	• CT/MRI and treat appropriately • see also Neurosurgery	• prednisone • see also Rheumatology
Etiology	• meningitis, SAH	• tumour, IIH, malignant hypertension	• vasculitis (GCA)

SAH - subarachnoid hemorrhage; IIH - idiopathic intracranial hypertension; GCA - giant cell arteritis

Investigation
- good history and physical should be able to rule out serious causes of headache
- LP/CT if
  - new-onset headache
  - different/more severe headache (especially if the worst headache ever)
  - sudden onset ("thunderclap" headache)

The Rational Clinical Examination: Does this patient with headache have a migraine or need neuroimaging?
JAMA 2006; 296:1274-83

Does this patient with headache have a migraine?
The most useful panel of questions for diagnosing migraine is summarized by the POUNDing mnemonic:
P - Pulsatile quality
O - duration of 4-72 h**O**urs
U - Unilateral location
N - Nausea or vomiting
D - Disabling intensity
The LR for definite or possible migraine diagnosis varies with the number of features present: with ≥4, 3 and ≥2 features, the LRs are 24 (1.5-388), 3.5 (1.3-9.2) and 0.41 (0.32-0.52) respectively.

Does this patient with headache need neuroimaging?
The prevalence of significant intracranial pathology (pretest probability) varies by population. In those with chronic headache the prevalence is 1.2% (0.77-1.8%). In adult onset (>40 yrs) migraine-type headache the prevalence is 0.0% (0.0-5.3%). However, in those presenting with new or changed headache the prevalence is 3.2% (2.4-42%), and in those presenting with thunderclap headache the prevalence is 43% (20-68%). In these different populations, no clinical feature was found to be useful in ruling out significant intracranial pathology in a meaningful way. However, several individual clinical features were found to be predictive of significant intracranial pathology:

cluster-type headache	10.7 (2.2-52)
abnormal neurological exam	5.3 (2.4-12)
undefined-type headache (non-tension/migraine/cluster-type)	3.8 (2.0-7.1)
headache with aura	3.2 (1.6-6.6)
aggravated by exertion/Valsalva	2.3 (1.4-3.8)
headache with vomiting	1.8 (1.2-2.6)

S&S of **serious headaches** include 1) the sudden onset of a severe headache; 2) accompanying impaired mental status, fever, seizures, or focal neurologic deficits; or 3) new headaches beginning after age 50.

- headache associated with
  - fever
  - meningismus
  - altered level of consciousness
  - focal neurological symptoms
  - recent head injury
  - optic disc edema
  - headache worst in morning or associated with early morning nausea or vomiting

Migraine Headaches

Definition (common migraine)
- ≥5 attacks fulfilling each of the following criteria
  - 4-72 h duration
  - 2 of the following:
    - unilateral or predominantly unilateral
    - pulsating
    - moderate-severe, interfering with daily activity
    - aggravated by routine physical activity
  - 1 of the following:
    - nausea/vomiting
    - photophobia/phonophobia/osmophobia

Epidemiology
- 18% females, 6% males suffer from migraines
- frequency typically decreases with age

Etiology and Pathophysiology
- vascular theory of migraine (controversial)
  - vasoconstriction → migraine aura (2° to ischemia)
  - vasodilation → headache
- triggers
  - mood – stress, sleep excess/deprivation
  - chemical/hormonal – medications (estrogen, NTG), hormonal changes (ovulation, pregnancy)
  - diet – caffeine withdrawal, chocolate, tyramines (e.g. red wine), nitrites (e.g. processed meats)

Signs and Symptoms
- stages of uncomplicated migraine
  - i)   prodrome (hours to days before headache onset)
  - ii) aura
  - iii) headache (see Table 44 for description of typical headache)
  - iv) postdrome
- aura
  - fully reversible symptom of focal cerebral dysfunction lasting <60 minutes
  - examples:
    - homonymous visual disturbance (fortification spectra – zigzags; scintillating scotomata – spots)
    - unilateral paresthesiae and numbness
    - unilateral weakness
    - aphasia
- prodrome/postdrome
  - appetite changes
  - autonomic symptoms
  - altered mood and psychomotor agitation/retardation
- classification of migraines
  - common migraine
    - no aura
  - classic migraine
    - migraine with aura (headache follows reversible aura within 60 minutes)
  - complicated migraine
    - migraine with severe or persistent sensorimotor deficits
    - examples:
      - basilar-type migraine (occipital headache with diplopia, vertigo, ataxia, and altered level of consciousness)
      - hemiplegic/hemisensory migraine
      - ophthalmoplegic migraine

The oral contraceptive pill is contraindicated with complicated migraine due to risk of stroke.

Migraine auras can mimic other causes of transient neurological deficits (e.g. TIAs and seizures).

Pharmacological treatments for acute migraine
Pain 2002; 97:247-57

Study: Meta-analysis of 54 double-blind, placebo-controlled RCTs of pharmacologic treatment of acute migraine of moderate to severe intensity (21,022 patients in total).
Data extraction: Number of patients, dosing regimes, details of study design, and timing or type of rescue medication. Outcomes included headache relief at 1 and 2 hours, freedom from pain at 2 hours, sustained relief for 24 hours, and adverse effects within 24 hours
Main Results: Data were available for 9 oral medications, 2 intranasal medications, and subcutaneous sumatriptan. For HA relief at 2h, all interventions were effective except Cafergot™, with NNTs ranging from 2.0 for sumatriptan 6mg s.c to 5.4 for naratriptan 2.5 mg. The lowest NNT for oral medication was 2.6 for eletriptan 80mg. For patients pain free at 2h, the lowest NNT was 2.1 for sumatriptan 6mg s.c, with the lowest NNT for oral medication being 3.1 for Rizatriptan 10mg. For sustained relief over 24h NNT ranged from 2.8 for eletriptan 80 mg to 8.3 for rizatriptan 5 mg. Side effects could not be analyzed systematically. There were no drug-to-drug comparisons.
Conclusion: Overall, most treatments were effective. Subcutaneous sumatriptan and oral triptans were most effective.

- acephalgic migraine (aka migraine equivalent)
  - aura without headache

Management
- avoid triggers
- mild to moderate migraine treatment:
  - 1st line treatment: NSAIDS – ASA, ibuprofen, naproxen
- moderate to severe migraine treatment:
  - triptans (most effective):
    - oral triptans: naratriptan, rizatriptan, sumatriptan, zolmitriptan
    - sumatriptan nasal spray, sumatriptan s.c. injection
  - ergots: dihydroergotamine (DHE) nasal spray
  - acetaminophen + codeine
  - migraine prophylaxis:
    - anticonvulsants: divalproex, topiramate
    - tricyclic antidepressants: amitryptiline, nortriptyline
    - β-blockers: propranolol
    - 5-HT antagonists: methylsergide
    - calcium channel blockers: verapamil
- *Note:* A prophylactic agent is recommended only if migraine attacks are severe enough to cause impairment of a patient's quality of life or if a patient has >3 migraines/month that have not responded adequately to treatment

Source: Sliverstein SD et al. (2000) Practice parameter: Evidence-based guidelines for migraine headache (an evidence based review). *Neurology*, 55:754-63.

Episodic Tension-Type Headache

Diagnostic Criteria
1. at least 10 previous headache episodes fulfilling criteria 2 through 4; number of days with such headaches: less than 180 days per year
2. headache lasting from 30 minutes to 7 days
3. at least two of the following pain characteristics
   a. pressing or tightening (nonpulsating) quality
   b. mild or moderate intensity
   c. bilateral location
   d. no aggravation by walking stairs or similar routine physical activity
4. both of the following:
   a. no nausea or vomiting (anorexia may occur)
   b. photophobia and phonophobia are absent, or one but not the other is present

Chronic Tension-Type Headache

Diagnostic Criteria
1. average headache frequency of more than 15 days per month for more than 6 months fulfilling the following criteria:
2. at least 2 of the following pain characteristics:
   a. pressing/tightening (nonpulsating) quality
   b. mild or moderate intensity (may inhibit but does not prohibit activities)
   c. bilateral location
   d. no aggravation from climbing stairs or similar routine physical activity
3. both of the following:
   a. no vomiting
   b. no more than one of the following: nausea, photophobia, or phonophobia
4. secondary headache types not suggested or confirmed

Cluster Headache

Diagnostic Criteria
1. at least five attacks fulfilling criteria 2 to 4 below
2. severe unilateral, supraorbital and/or temporal pain lasting 15 to 180 minutes (untreated)
3. headache associated with at least one of the following on the pain side
   a. conjunctival injection or lacrimation (ipsilateral)
   b. nasal congestion or rhinorrhea
   c. forehead and facial sweating
   d. miosis or ptosis (ipsilateral)
   e. eyelid edema (ipsilateral)
   f. a sense of restlessness or agitation
4. not attributed to another disorder

- can have up to 8 attacks per day

CNS Infections

see Infectious Diseases

Spinal Cord Syndromes

see Neurosurgery

Stroke

Definition
- a clinical syndrome characterized by sudden onset of a focal neurological deficit presumed to be on a vascular basis, and without an alternative explanation

Stroke Terminology
- **Transient Ischemic Attack (TIA)**
  - stroke syndrome with neurological symptoms lasting from a few minutes to as much as 24 hours, followed by complete functional recovery
  - following TIA, between 10-15% will develop infarction in the first 3 months of follow-up, irrespective of territory involved
  - risk of infarction is greatest within 2-3 months of initial TIA
- **Amaurosis Fugax, Transient Monocular Blindness (TMB)**
  - retinal ischemia due to embolism to ophthalmic and retinal arteries resulting in a sudden, and frequently complete, transient loss of vision in one eye or an altitudinal defect (superior or inferior)
- **Reversible Ischemic Neurological Deficit (RIND)/Minor Stroke**
  - neurological abnormalities similar to acute completed stroke, but the deficit disappears after 24-36 hours, leaving few or no detectable neurological sequelae
- **Completed Stroke (CS)**
  - stroke syndrome with a persisting neurological deficit
- **Progressing Stroke (Stroke In Evolution)**
  - neurological deficits begin in a focal or restricted distribution but over the ensuing hours spread gradually in a pattern reflecting involvement of more and more of the particular vascular territory (may be due to several factors i.e. propogation of thrombus, cerebral edema, secondary hemorrhage, etc)

Risk Factors
- age
- hypertension
- smoking (risk of stroke within 3-5 years of quitting = risk of non-smoker)
- myocardial infarction
- atrial fibrillation
- diabetes mellitus
- hyperhomocysteinemia
- obesity
- hypercholesterolemia
- drugs (i.e. oral contraceptive pill, cocaine, etc.)

Differential Diagnosis – Has The Patient Had a Stroke?
- not all acute focal neurological deficits are secondary to ischemic stroke
- differential diagnosis
  - vascular
    - hypertensive encephalopathy
    - subdural hematoma, subarachnoid hemorrhage, intracranial hemorrhage
  - infectious/inflammatory
    - abscess
    - encephalitis (e.g. herpes simplex)
    - vasculitis
  - anatomic
    - demyelinating diseases (e.g. Multiple Sclerosis)
    - Bell's Palsy
    - mononeuropathy
    - plexopathies

ABCD² Score

Lancet. 2007; 369:283-92

The ABCD² score is a reliable predictor of short-term (2-day, 5-day, and 90-day) risk of stroke after presentation with a TIA. Specific cutpoints likely vary between settings and regions, but patients classified as high risk (score >5) are likely to benefit from urgent evaluation, treatment, and observation. A score of <4 was classified as low risk, and scores of 4 and 5 as medium risk (Johnston et al., 2007).

Factor	Criteria (points)
Age	>60 (1)
Blood pressure (first assessment after TIA)	SBP >140 mm Hg or DBP >90 mm Hg (1)
Clinical features of TIA	unilateral weakness (2); speech impairment without weakness (1)
Duration of TIA	>59 minutes (2); 10-59 minutes (1)
Diabetes mellitus	positive diagnosis (1)

- seizure
  - focal seizure (post ictal weakness)
- other
  - migraine, hypoglycemia
- confusion, dementia, and coma (without focal signs) are rarely modes of presentation for strokes and usually suggest diffuse disturbance of cerebral function

Signs and Symptoms – Where is the lesion and what is the blood supply? What is the lesion?

- cortical lesion (see Figure 15 and Table 46)
  - examples of cortical lesions include
    - MCA
    - ACA
    - PCA
- brainstem stroke
  - examples of syndromes include
    - Vertebrobasilar Insufficiency (VBI) - transient neurological dysfunction
      - nystagmus
      - limb and/or truncal ataxia (pt falls to one side)
      - contralateral impairment in pain + temperature sensation
      - ipsilateral limb and trunk numbness (with contralateral weakness)
      - visual field deficits (abnormal eye movements)
    - subclavian steal syndrome - VBI due to stenosis at the subclavian artery - increased arm use diverts blood down from vertebral artery into left arm
      - symptoms include vertigo, headaches, left arm claudication assoc with arm use
    - lateral medullary (Wallenberg) syndrome - infarct involving PICA or vertebral artery territory
      - ipsilateral facial pain and numbness;
      - contralateral impairment of pain and temperature sensation (body +/- face)
      - ipsilateral ataxia (pt falls to one side)
      - vertigo, N/V
      - ipsilateral Horner's syndrome
      - dysphagia, dysarthria, hiccups
    - medial medullary syndrome - infarct involving spinal artery territory
      - contralateral arm and leg weakness - sparing the face
      - contralateral impairment of proprioception and vibration
      - ipsilateral tongue weakness
    - locked-in syndrome - caused by basilar artery occlusion
      - paralysis or weakness in all four limbs (quadriplegia or quadriparesis), dysarthria or anarthria
      - horizontal gaze paresis (vertical eye movement is spared)
      - patient awake and alert because of sparing of reticular activating system but unable to respond verbally or move
  - cranial nerve findings of brainstem stroke include
    - diplopia, gaze palsy, nystagmus
    - dizziness and vertigo
    - dysarthria
    - dysphagia
  - cerebellar findings of brainstem insults include
    - ataxia
    - incoordination
  - sensory findings of brainstem insults include
    - sensory deficits on ipsilateral side of face, contralateral side of body (crossed sensory findings)
  - motor findings of brainstem insults include
    - crossed or bilateral motor deficits
  - indeterminate presentation of brainstem stroke may include
    - hemisyndromes: hemiparesis, hemisensory loss, dysarthria
- lacunar infarct
- ischemic vs. hemorrhagic
  - important to distinguish ischemic from hemorrhagic stroke (see Table 47)

Etiology – What is the Pathogenesis? (guides acute and chronic treatment)

- ischemic vs hemorrhagic

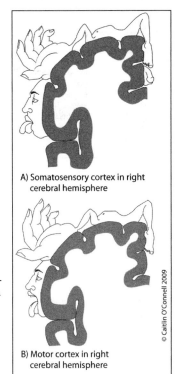

A) Somatosensory cortex in right cerebral hemisphere

B) Motor cortex in right cerebral hemisphere

© Caitlin O'Connell 2009

Figure 14. Homunculus

The National Institutes of Health Stroke Scale (NIHSS) is a widely accepted tool for clinical assessment of neurological deficits in stroke patients, and it is helpful for determining patient management and prognosis. The NIHSS form contains detailed instructions for the use of the scale. Available at: http://www.ninds.nih.gov/doctors/NIH_Stroke_Scale.pdf.

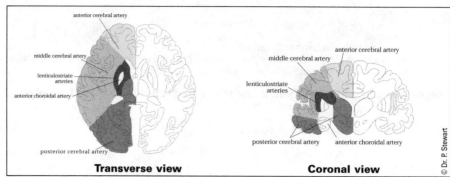

Figure 15. Vascular Territories of Major Cerebral Arteries

Table 46. Anterior vs. Middle vs. Posterior Cerebral Arteries

Anterior Cerebral Artery	Middle Cerebral Artery	Posterior Cerebral Artery
• motor ▪ contralateral hemiplegia (lower extremity) • sensory ▪ contralateral hemianesthesia (lower extremity) • gaze preference (away from hemiparesis, towards the side of the lesion) • behavioural and memory disturbances • abulia • if non-dominant hemisphere affected ▪ constructional apraxia • presence of primitive reflexes ▪ grasp, snout, palmomental	• motor ▪ contralateral hemiplegia (upper extremity and face) • sensory ▪ contralateral hemianesthesia (upper extremity and face) • homonymous hemianopsia or quadrantinopsia • if dominant hemisphere affected ▪ aphasia, Gerstmann's syndrome • if non-dominant hemisphere affected ▪ neglect	• contralateral homonymous hemianopsia, or quantrontinopsia blindness (if bilateral) • if dominant hemisphere affected with posterior corpus callosum lesion ▪ alexia without agraphia • if thalamus affected ▪ contralateral hemisensory loss ▪ spontaneous pain • if subthalamic ▪ hemiballismus • if midbrain (Weber's syndrome) ▪ ipsilateral CN III palsy ▪ contralateral motor deficits • Top of basilar syndrome (bilateral PCA intact) • If cerebral peduncle ▪ contralateral hemiparesis

Table 47. Ischemic vs. Hemorrhagic Stroke

	Ischemia	Hemorrhage
Hypertension	• often present	• usually present
Preceding TIA	• 30% of cases	• no
Course	• static (can be stepwise)	• rapidly progressive
Increased ICP?	• no	• yes
CT Scan Result	• normal, or consistent with infarct	• shows blood

Ischemic Stroke (80%)

- ischemic stroke results from focal ischemia leading to cerebral infarction
- strokes can be due to embolus from heart or large arteries, in-situ thrombosis of diseased arteries or because of hematological disease predisposing to thrombosis
- core of infarct includes electrically silent and necrotic brain tissue that cannot be revived using revascularazation
- penumbra is the tissue surrounding the infarct that contains electrically silent neurons that can be revised if revascularized (reperfused)
- surrounding region becomes edematous 2-5 days post stroke due to stasis - may lead to initial worsening of symptoms

- **cerebrovascular thrombosis (40% of all strokes)**
  - gradual, stuttering progression of S&S
  - caused by formation of in-situ clot on atherosclerotic lesion
  - may cause in-situ thrombosis or embolize to distal segment and disrupt blood flow
- **large vessel thrombosis** – occur within carotid, basilar and intracranial segments of cerebral arteries
  - risk factors
    - hypertension
    - diabates mellitus
    - cigarette smoking
    - hyperhomocysteinemia
    - hypercholesterolemia

- long term management
  - control of atherosclerotic risk factors
  - carotid endarterectomy in selected patients (if stenosis 70-99% and symptomatic)
  - antiplatelet agents - aspirin, clopidogrel (Plavix™), dipyridamole/ASA (Aggrenox™)
- **embolic origin (rapid onset of symptoms) (30% of all strokes)**
  - cardioembolic origin
    - risk factors: increased age, atrial fibrillation (most common), LV aneurysm, LV dysfunction, CHF
    - valvular etiology: valvular vegetations (i.e. infection, tumour), valvular heart disease, prosthetic valves
    - paradoxical embolus - patent foramen ovale (PFO/ASD/atrial septal aneurysm)
  - other emboli
    - air emboli: during surgery or diving
    - septic emboli
    - fat emboli (e.g. from long bone fractures)
  - long term treatment
    - risk of embolization can be decreased with anticoagulation (heparin or warfarin)
    - do CT scan prior to starting anticoagulation to exclude presence of bleeding (due to increased risk of secondary hemorrhage into a cardioembolic infarct)
    - if moderate sized infarct, delay anticoagulation
- **lacunar infarction**
  - small (< 20 mm) and deep infarcts involving penetrating branches of large cerebral artery
  - risk factors
    - HTN
    - DM
    - increasing age
  - pathology
    - lipohyalinosis of small penetrating arteries of basal ganglia and brain stem; microatheroma; junctional plaques (atherosclerosis of parent vessel blocking orifices of penetrating vessels)
  - common sites: putamen, internal capsule, thalamic, ventral pons
  - 5 characteristic syndromes

Table 48. Characteristics Lacunar Stroke Syndromes

Type	Neurological Findings
Pure Motor (66%)	Contralateral arm, leg, face weakness Dysarthria
Pure Sensory (10%)	Contralateral sensory loss in arm, leg, face of all modalities
Mixed Motor and Sensory	Contralateral sensory loss and weakness in arm, leg, face
Clumsy Hand and Dysarthria (20%)	Contralateral paresis and clumsiness of arm/hand Contralateral face/tongue weakness Dysarthria/dysphagia
Ataxic hemiparesis	Contralateral ataxia/weakness

- long term treatment
  - control risk factors
  - use antiplatelet drugs
- **other causes**
  - large artery diseases
    - vasculitis (polyarteritis nodosa, Takayasu arteritis, meningovascular syphilis)
    - other (SLE, Behcet's)
  - arterial dissection
  - hematological coagulopathy: hypercoagulable states, sickle cell anemia, homocystinuria, APLA, protein C/S deficiency
  - venous infarction (cortical vein or sinus thrombosis)
    - seen in hypercoagulable states and results in cortical infarction, often complicated by secondary hemorrhage and seizures
  - migraine
  - vasospasm (drug induced, subarachnoid hemorrhage)
  - water shed due to systemic hypoperfusion

Hemorrhagic Stroke (20%)

- see also Table 47 and Neurosurgery
- abrupt onset with focal neurological deficits, due to spontaneous (non-traumatic) bleeding into the brain
- includes ICH and SAH (90% ICH; 10% SAH)
- hemorrhage into an area of cerebral infarction is a hemorrhagic infarct which should be classified as ischemic stroke complicated by secondary hemorrhage

Symptoms
- signs of increased ICP (headaches, N/V, seizure)
- signs of meningismus
- decreased LOC
- focal neurologic deficits

Investigation of Stroke

All Patients
- CBC, electrolytes, creatinine, PT, PTT, glucose, lipids
- CT head (unenhanced CT head is imaging method of choice)
- ECG, echocardiogram
- dopplers if anterior circulation, CTA or MRA especially if posterior circulation

Selected Patients
- ischemic stroke – all patients
  - CT +/- MRI
  - assess risk factors (BP, fasting glucose, HbA1C, fasting lipids)
  - ECG, echocardiogram
  - carotid dopplers if carotid territory stroke
  - MRA if vertebrobasilar stroke, some carotid territory strokes if indicated
- hemorrhage
  - CT (noncontrast)
  - LP if suspect SAH
  - cerebral angio, CT angio, MRA if suspect aneurysm/AVM
  - for all hemorrhage, repeat CT head in 4-6 weeks to rule out underlying lesion
- ESR, VDRL, hypercoagulability work-up (Factor V Leiden, antiphospholipid antibody syndrome, protein C/S deficiency, etc.)
- MRI
- magnetic resonance angiography
- transesophageal echocardiogram
- Holter monitor

Treatment of Stroke

A) Acute Stroke Management

Goals
  - ensure medical stability
  - limit or prevent neuronal death

Practical guidelines
- general
  - ensure the ABC's, check glucose, urgent CT to rule out hemorrhage and assess infarct
  - other labs: CBC, PT, PTT, INR, ECG
- diagnosis
  - make the correct etiological diagnosis so you have a rational approach for secondary prevention of stroke
  - consider transfer to stroke center if patient seen in first few hours for neuroprotective or thrombolytic therapy (have been proven effective in clinical tests)

Thrombolysis
- rt-PA (recombinant tissue plasminogen activator) within 3 hours of acute ischemic stroke onset (NINDS trial)
  - treated patients were 30% more likely to have minimal or no disability at 3 months

- ▪ 6.4% of patients had a symptomatic intracerebral hemorrhage (0.6% in placebo group)
- ▪ treatment did not affect mortality compared to placebo but patients with severe strokes were more likely to have favourable outcomes if treated with rt-PA, benefits of rt-PA were sustained at 12 months

Anti-platelet therapy
- given at presentation
- give antiplatelet agents if ASA not suitable or if already taking ASA
  - ▪ clopidogrel (75 mg/d)
  - ▪ ASA + dipyridamole (Aggrenox™)

Blood pressure control
- **do not lower the blood pressure** unless the hypertension is severe
  - ▪ antihypertensive therapy is withheld for at least 5 days after thromboembolic stroke unless there is acute MI, renal failure, aortic dissection, or sBP above 220 mmHg, or dBP above 120 mmHg
- acutely elevated BP is necessary to maintain brain perfusion
- most patients with an acute cerebral infarct are initially hypertensive and their BP will fall spontaneously within 1-2 days
- IV labetalol is usually first line if needed

Blood sugar
- avoid hyperglycemia which will increase the infarct size

B) Other Management Issues
- prevent complications
  - ▪ NPO if swallowing difficulty
  - ▪ DVT prophylaxis if limb weakness
  - ▪ initiate rehabilitation
- therapy (see also *Primary and Secondary Prevention*)
  - ▪ investigate to determine the vascular territory and etiology, then treat accordingly
  - ▪ for carotid territory event, carotid endarterectomy benefits those with symptomatic severe stenosis (70-99%), and is less beneficial for those with symptomatic moderate stenosis (50-69%). See <u>Neurosurgery</u>
- lower temperature if febrile

PRIMARY AND SECONDARY PREVENTION

Carotid Territory Event
- carotid endarterectomy benefits those with symptomatic severe stenosis (70-99%), and is less beneficial for those with symptomatic moderate stenosis (50-69%), see <u>Neurosurgery</u>

Asymptomatic Carotid Bruit
- suggests the presence of atherosclerotic stenosis and signifies increased risk for both cerebral and myocardial infarction
- modify risk factors, ± antiplatelet therapy
- if stenosis > 60%, risk of stroke is 2% per year; carotid endarterectomy reduces the risk of stroke by 1% per year (but 5% risk of complications)

Hypertension
- primary prevention
  - ▪ antihypertensives reduce the risk of ischemic stroke in elderly patient with isolated systolic hypertension (SHEP trial)
    - ◆ ramipril 10mg OD is effective in patients at high risk for cardiovascular disease (HOPE-Stroke trial)
    - ◆ ACEI reduce the risk of stroke beyond their antihypertensive effect
- secondary prevention
  - ▪ ACEI and thiazide diuretics are useful in patients with a Hx of stroke/TIA (PROGRESS trial)

Anti-Platelet Therapy
- primary prevention
  - ▪ current evidence has not firmly established a protective role for antiplatelet agents for low-risk patients without a prior stroke/TIA

t-PA in acute stroke – NINDS trial
NEJM 1995;333:1581-7
Study: Randomized, double-blind, placebo-controlled trial (3 month follow-up).
Patients: 624 patients (mean age 76 y, 58% men, 65% white) with ischemic stroke of recent onset, and no evidence of intracranial hemorrhage on CT. Exclusions included hx of recent stroke or recent surgery, SBP≥185, DBP≥110, symptoms of SAH, recent GI or GU hemorrhage, seizure with onset of stroke, and recent use of anticoagulants.
Intervention: IV t-PA (0.9 mg/kg) or placebo within 180 minutes of the onset of symptoms.
Main outcomes: Neurologic deficit at 24 hours (NIHSS scale) and functional outcome at 3 months (composite score).
Results: There was no significant difference between groups at 24 hours. At 3 months, there were more patients in the t-PA group with minimal or no disability (50% vs. 38%, p=0.03). Intracerebral hemorrhage was more common in the t-PA group (p<0.001). There was no significant difference in mortality.
Conclusion: IV t-PA given within 3 hours of onset of acute ischemic stroke improves functional outcome at 3 months. The risk of intracerebral bleeding is increased.
Addendum: When re-assessed at 12 months from the time of treatment, patients in the t-PA group were 30% more likely to have minimal or no disability, with no significant difference in mortality or rate of recurrent stroke (*NEJM* 1999; 340:1781-7).

Aspirin and heparin in acute stroke – International Stroke Trial
Lancet 1997;349:1569-81
Study: Randomized, open trial with 6 month follow-up.
Patients: 19,435 patients (54% men) with suspected acute ischemic stroke of recent onset (less than 48 h), with no evidence of intracranial hemorrhage, and no clear indications for, or contraindications to, heparin or aspirin.
Intervention: Half the patients were allocated unfractionated heparin (5000 or 12,500 IU bid), and half were never allocated heparin; Similarly, half were allocated aspirin 300 mg daily. Thus patients were randomly assigned to receive aspirin, heparin, both, or neither.
Outcomes: Death within two weeks, and death or dependency at 6 months.
Results: For both heparin vs. no heparin and aspirin vs. no aspirin, there was no significant difference in death at 2 weeks, or death or dependency at 6 months. Both aspirin and heparin-allocated patients had significantly fewer recurrent ischaemic strokes within 14 days, but this benefit was completely offset by a similar-sized increase in hemorrhagic stroke in those receiving heparin. After adjustment for predicted prognosis, the aspirin group showed a decreased risk of death or dependence at 6 months (14 per 1000 fewer, p=0.03).
Conclusion: The IST suggests that aspirin should be started immediately after the onset of ischemic stroke.

The leading causes of death during the first month following a stroke are: pneumonia, pulmonary embolus, cardiac disease, and from the stroke itself. Leading causes of death beyond the first week are usually unrelated to the stroke itself.

ACE inhibitor in stroke prevention HOPE trial
NEJM 2000;342:145-53
Study: Randomized, blinded, placebo-controlled trial. Mean follow-up 5 years.
Patients: 9297 patients 55 years of age or older (mean age 66 y, 73% men) who had evidence of vascular disease or diabetes plus one other cardiovascular risk factor and who were not known to have a low ejection fraction or heart failure.
Intervention: Ramipril 10 mg once daily orally vs. matching placebo.
Main Outcomes: Stroke, myocardial infarction, or death from cardiovascular causes
Results:

Outcome	RRR (95%CI)	NNT (CI)
Stroke	32% (16 to 44)	67 (43 to 145)
MI, stroke, or CV mortality	22% (14 to 30)	26 (19 to 43)
All-cause mortality	16% (5 to 25)	56 (32 to 195)

Treatment with ramipril reduced the risk of stroke (3.4 percent vs. 4.9 percent; RR 0.68; p<0.001).
Conclusion: In adults at high risk for cardiovascular events, ramipril reduced the risk of stroke, as well as other vascular events and overall mortality.

Statins in stroke prevention – MRC/BHF Heart Protection Study
Lancet 2002; 360:7-22
Study: Randomized, double-blind, placebo-controlled trial with mean follow-up of 5 years.
Patients: 20 536 patients aged 40 to 80 years (28% ≥70 y of age, 75% men) with nonfasting total cholesterol ≥3.5 mmol/L, who were considered to be at substantial 5-year risk of death from coronary heart disease because of cardiovascular disease, diabetes, or treated hypertension. 16% of patients had known cerebrovascular disease. Exclusions included chronic liver disease, evidence of abnormal liver or kidney function, muscle disease, and others.
Intervention: Run-in treatment involved 4 weeks of placebo followed by 4-6 weeks of a fixed dose of 40 mg simvastatin daily. Patients were then randomized to simvastatin 40 mg/d or placebo.
Main Outcomes: Included all-cause and vascular mortality, major coronary events, and stroke.
Results:

Outcome	RRR (95%CI)	NNT (CI)
Stroke	25% (15 to 34)	73 (51 to 131)
Major coronary event	27% (21 to 33)	33 (26 to 46)
All-cause mortality	13% (6 to 19)	58 (37 to 128)

Conclusion: Simvastatin safely reduced the risk of stroke, major coronary events, and all-cause mortality in patients at significant 5 year risk of coronary heart disease.

Organized inpatient (stroke unit) care for stroke (Stroke Unit Trialists' Collaboration)
The Cochrane Database of Systematic Reviews 2001; Issue 3.
Purpose: Assess the effect of stroke unit care compared with other models of care.
Study Characteristics: 23 trials, randomized (14) or quasi-randomized studies (9) involving 4911 patients.
Participants: Patients admitted to hospital who had suffered a stroke, defined as a focal neurological deficit due to cerebrovascular disease, excluding subarachnoid hemorrhage and subdural hematoma.
Intervention: Organised inpatient stroke unit care with multidisciplinary teams that exclusively manage stroke patients in a dedicated ward, with a mobile team, or within a generic disability service, compared with alternative forms of care, usually a general medical ward.
Primary Outcomes: Death, dependency (require assistance for basic activities of daily living), and the requirement for institutional care at the end of follow-up.
Results: The NNT to prevent one death is 33 (95% CI, 20-100), to prevent one patient being unable to live at home was 20 (95% CI, 12-50), and to prevent one patient failing to regain independence was 20 (95% CI, 12-50).
Conclusions: Acute stroke patients cared for in an organized stroke unit with a multidisciplinary care team are more likely to survive their stroke, return home and make a good recovery.

- secondary prevention
    - generally ASA is chosen as the initial antiplatelet of choice for stroke prevention
    - other agents (ASA+dipyridamole; clopidogrel) are reserved for those who suffer cerebrovascular symptoms while on ASA
    - warfarin is generally reserved for specific indications in stroke prevention, dissection, cardiac/atrial fibrillation, venous thrombosis

Hypercholesterolemia
- primary prevention
    - statins reduce the risk of stroke in patients with CAD or at high risk for cardiovascular events, even with normal cholesterol (CARE study)
- secondary prevention
    - more evidence is needed for high-risk patients with symptomatic cerebrovascular disease, but statins are generally used in these patients as well

Atrial Fibrillation
- primary and secondary prevention
    - warfarin is the first-line agent

Smoking
- primary prevention
    - smoking increases risk of stroke in a dose-dependent manner
- secondary prevention
    - after smoking cessation, the risk of stroke decreases to baseline within 2-5 years

Physical Activity
- regular physical activity is an important lifestyle measure in stroke prevention and this effect has a dose-response in terms of both intensity and duration of activity

STROKE REHABILITATION
- individualized based on severity and nature of impairment, may require inpatient program and continuation through home care or outpatient services
- multidisciplinary approach includes
    - dysphagia assessment and dietary modifications
    - communication rehabilitation
    - cognitive and psychological assessments including screen for depression
    - therapeutic exercise programs
    - assessment of ambulation and evaluation of need for assistive devices, splints or bracing
    - vocational rehabilitation

Multiple Sclerosis

Definition
- a demyelinating and inflammatory disease of the CNS characterized by multiple and varied neurological signs and symptoms over time
- lesions/attacks must be separated in both space and time

Classification (based on pattern and course of illness)
- relapsing-remitting MS (80% of patients early in the course of the illness, F>M)
    - clearly defined attacks/relapses with complete recovery or some residual defect on recovery; no progression of disease between relapses
- primary progressive MS
    - progressive clinical course from onset (F=M)
- secondary progressive
    - initial relapsing-remitting course, which becomes progressive +/- occasional relapses

Etiology
- unknown; thought to involve triggering of the immune system by an agent e.g. virus (EBV), bacteria, chemicals, in genetically predisposed adults

Pathology
- multiple discrete lesions of myelin destruction (plaques)
- common plaque sites include optic nerve, periventricular areas, corpus callosum, brainstem, spinal cord

Epidemiology
- onset usually age 17-35, but can be younger or older
- F:M = 3:2
- incidence rate 1.5-11 per 100,000, may be increasing
- prevalence 50-100 per 100,000, higher prevalence in higher latitudes
- genetic predisposition: 3% risk for first degree relatives, 30% concordance for identical twins, HLA-DR2 and DW2 association

Common Features
- optic neuritis
- internuclear ophthalmoplegia (INO): demyelination in medial longitudinal fasciculus (MLF) causing failure of adduction of the ipsilateral eye and nystagmus of the abducting eye on attempted lateral gaze
- Lhermitte's sign: forward flexion of the neck causes electric shock sensation down the back to limbs, indicative of cervical cord lesion
- Uhthoff's phenomenon: worsening of symptoms with heat (e.g. hot bath, exercise)
- trigeminal neuralgia in young patient
- transverse myelitis: inflammation of spinal cord producing weakness and sensory loss (dermatomal levels)

For current MS diagnostic criteria suggested by the International Panel on MS Diagnosis please see Polman et al. (2005) in References.

Investigations
- MRI (test of choice to support a clinical diagnosis of MS)
  - demyelinating plaques appear as hyperintense lesions on T2 weighted MRI in periventricular distribution
  - contrast (gadolinium) identifies active plaque
  - classic finding of periventricular lesions in the corpus callosum (Dawson's fingers)
- CSF
  - oligoclonal Ig bands in 90% of patients with MS, increased IgG concentration, mild lymphocytosis and increased protein
- evoked potentials (visual/auditory/somatosensory)
  - delayed but well preserved wave forms may be seen

Treatment
- **patient education and counselling**
  - disclosure, future expectations, prognosis
  - refer to MS society and support groups for patient and partner/family
  - psychosocial issues - relationship distress, depression and suicidality not uncommon; refer to social work if necessary
- **acute treatment**
  - corticosteroids are indicated in the treatment of disabling relapses with objective findings of neurological impairment to speed recovery
  - IV methylprednisolone 500-1000 mg od for 3-7 days +/- short oral prednisone taper
- **disease-modifying therapy (DMT)**
  - interferon-β (Betaseron™, Avonex ™, Rebif™) and glatiramer acetate (Copaxone™), natalizumab (Tysabri™)
  - clinically isolated syndrome
    - emerging thought is that early treatment with DMT in patients with a single attack may delay second attack e.g. Avonex™ can be considered for use in patients with single attack and abnormal brain MRI
  - relapsing-remitting MS
    - interferon-β and glatiramer acetate about equally effective in reducing relapse rate by ~30%; attacks are also shorter and less disabling
  - secondary progressive MS
    - interferon-β may slow the progression of disability
  - primary progressive MS
    - immunosuppressive agents eg: methotrexate 7.5 mg q weekly
- **symptomatic treatment**
  - spasticity (baclofen, tizanidine, dantrolene, benzodiazepines)
  - bladder dysfunction (oxybutynin)
  - pain (TCA, carbamazepine, gabapentin)
  - fatigue (amantadine, modafinil, methylphenidate)
  - depression (antidepressants)
  - physiotherapy, speech therapy, occupational therapy, nutrition

Multiple Sclerosis is a common cause of internuclear ophthalmoplegia.

Prognosis
- good prognostic indicators - female, young, relapsing-remitting disease, presenting with optic neuritis, low disease burden on MRI at presentation, low rate of relapses early in course of illness
- primary progressive MS - poorest prognosis, higher rates of disability, poor response to therapy

Common Medications

Table 49. Common Medications

Mechanism of Action/Class	Generic name	Trade name	Dosing	Indications	Contraindications	Side effects
Dopamine precursor	levodopa + carbidopa	Sinemet™	Carbidopa 25 mg/levodopa 100 mg PO tid Maximum 200 mg carbidopa and 2000 mg levodopa per day	Parkinson's Disease	narrow-angle glaucoma, use of MAO inhibitor in last 14 days, history of melanoma or undiagnosed skin lesions	nausea, hypotension, hallucinations, dyskinesias
Dopamine agonist	bromocriptine	Parlodel™	1.25 mg PO bid, increase by 2.5 mg/d q2-4wks, up to 10-30 mg PO tid	Parkinson's Disease	concomitant use of potent inhibitors of CYP3A4, uncontrolled hypertension, ischemic heart disease, peripheral vascular disease. Caution with renal or hepatic disease	hypotension, nausea, dizziness, constipation, diarrhea, vomiting, abdominal cramps, headache, nasal congestion, drowsiness, hallucinations
MAO B inhibitor	selegiline	Eldepryl™	5 mg PO bid	Parkinson's Disease	concomitant use of meperidine or tricyclic antidepressants	headache, insomnia, dizziness, nausea, dry mouth, hallucinations, confusion, orthostatic hypotension, increased akinesia, risk of hypertensive crisis with tyramine-containing foods
MAO B inhibitor	pyridostigmine	Mestinon™	600 mg/d PO divided in 5-6 doses Range 60-1500 mg/d	Myasthenia Gravis	GI or GU obstruction	nausea, vomiting, diarrhea, abdominal cramps, increased peristalsis, increased salivation, increased bronchial secretions, miosis, diaphoresis, muscle cramps, fasciculations, muscle weakness
Triptan	sumatriptan	Imitrex™	25-100 mg PO prn, maximum 200 mg/d	Migraine	hemiplegic/basilar migraine, ischemic heart disease, peripheral vascular disease, cerebrovascular disease, uncontrolled hypertension, use of ergotamine/5-HT1 agonist in past 24 hours, use of MAO inhibitor in last 14 days, severe hepatic disease	dizziness, sensation of heat, hypertensive crisis, coronary artery vasospasm, cardiac arrest, nausea, vomiting, headache, hyposalivation, drowsiness
Ergot	dihydroergotamine	Migranal™	nasal spray 0.5 mg/spray, maximum 4 sprays	Migraine	hemiplegic/basilar migraine, high-dose ASA therapy, uncontrolled hypertension, ischemic heart disease, peripheral vascular disease, severe hepatic or renal dysfunction, use of triptans in last 24 hours; use of MAO inhibitors in last 14 days, concomitant	coronary artery vasospasm, transient myocardial ischemia, myocardial infarction, ventricular tachycardia, ventricular fibrillation. May cause significant rebound headache
Anticonvulsant	carbamazepine	Tegretol™ (Carbatrol, Epitol in USA)	start at 100-200 mg PO OD-bid, increase by 200 mg/d up to 800-1200 mg/d (individual doses) if needed	Epilepsy- partial +/- 2° generalization; generalized tonic-clonic	history of bone marrow depression, hepatic disease, hypersensitivity to the drug, or known sensitivity to tricyclic compounds such as amitriptyline	CNS disturbances (drowsiness, headache, unsteadiness, dizziness), nausea/vomiting, skin rash, agranulocytosis/aplastic anemia (rare)
Cholinesterase Inhibitor	donepezil	Aricept™	5 mg PO OD, may increase to 10mg PO OD after 4-6 weeks	Mild to moderate Alzheimer's Disease, Lewy Body Disease	hypersensitivity to donepezil or to piperidine derivatives	nausea, vomiting, diarrhea, insomnia, muscle cramps, fatigue, and anorexia
Immunomodulator	interferon beta-1b	Betaseron™	0.25 mg (8 MU) SC every other day	Relapsing-Remitting and Secondary Progressive Multiple Sclerosis	pregnancy, hypersensitivity to natural or recombinant interferon beta	injection site reactions; injection site necrosis, flu-like symptoms (fever, chills, myalgia) tend to decrease over time
Muscle Relaxant - Antispastic	baclofen	Lioresal, Lioresal™	Up to 20 mg PO qid, variable for intrathecal	Spasticity (i.e. MS) intrathecal route	hypersensitivity to baclofen (Spinal Cord Injury)	transient drowsiness, daytime sedation, dizziness, weakness, fatigue, convulsions, hypotonia, hypersensitivity to donepezil or to piperidine derivatives
Antispasmodic - Anticholinergic	oxybutynin chloride	Ditropan™	5 mg PO bid	Uninhibited neurogenic bladder or reflex neurogenic bladder	glaucoma, GI obstruction, megacolon, severe colitis, myasthenia gravis, obstructive uropathy, hypersensitivity to oxybutinin	headache, pain, dry mouth, constipation, urinary retention, diarrhea, nausea, dyspepsia, dizziness

Neurosurgery

Ashton Connor, Adrian Sacher and Sharmi Shafi, chapter editors
Sami Chadi and Biniam Kidane, associate editors
Emily Partridge, EBM editor
Dr. Abhaya Kulkarni and Dr. James Rutka, staff editors

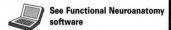 See Functional Neuroanatomy software

Basic Anatomy Review

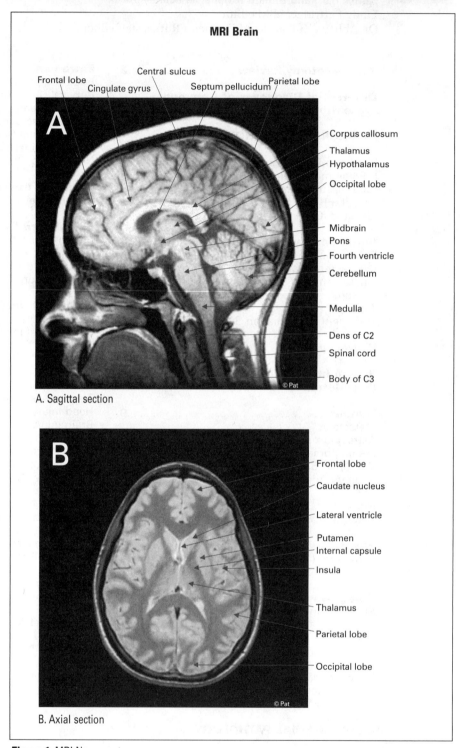

Figure 1. MRI Neuroanatomy
From Stewart P et al. Functional Neuroanatomy (Version 2.1). Health Education Assets Library, 2005.

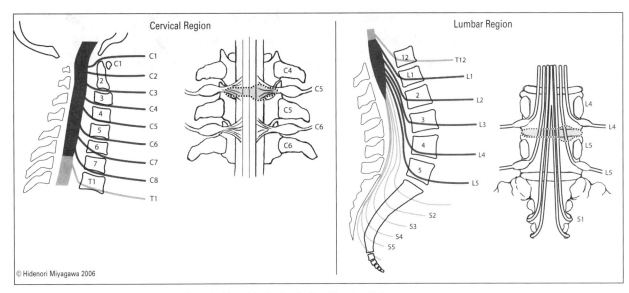

Figure 2. Relationship of Nerve Roots to Vertebral Level in the Cervical and Lumbar Spine
Note: AP views depict left-sided C4-5 and L4-5 disc herniation, and correlating nerve root impingement

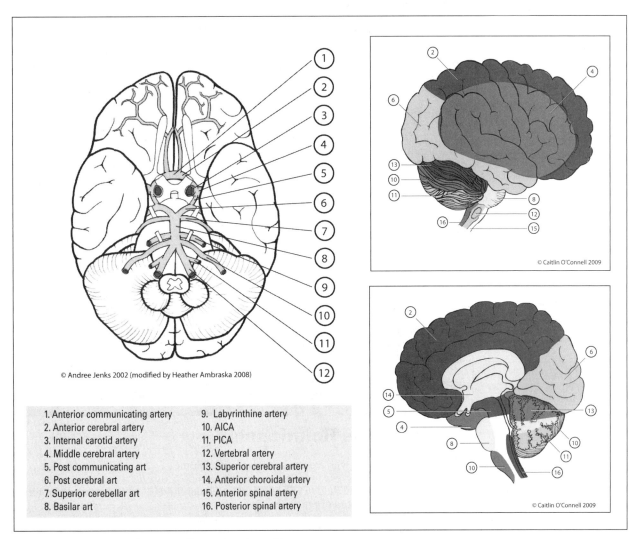

1. Anterior communicating artery
2. Anterior cerebral artery
3. Internal carotid artery
4. Middle cerebral artery
5. Post communicating art
6. Post cerebral art
7. Superior cerebellar art
8. Basilar art
9. Labyrinthine artery
10. AICA
11. PICA
12. Vertebral artery
13. Superior cerebral artery
14. Anterior choroidal artery
15. Anterior spinal artery
16. Posterior spinal artery

Figure 3. Vascular supply of the brain. Please refer to legend for artery names.
Figure 3A. Circle of Willis, most commmon variant. **Figure 3B.** Vascular territories of the brain and brainstem, sagittal view, seen laterally. **Figure 3C.** Vascular territories of the brain and brainstem, sagittal view, seen medially.

Differential Diagnoses of Common Presentations

Intracranial Mass Lesions
- tumour
  - metastatic tumours
  - astrocytoma
  - meningioma
  - vestibular schwannoma (acoustic neuroma)
  - pituitary adenoma
  - primary CNS lymphoma
- pus/inflammation
  - cerebral abscess, extradural abscess, subdural empyema
  - encephalitis (see Infectious Diseases)
  - tumefactive multiple sclerosis (MS)
- blood
  - extradural (epidural) hematoma
  - subdural hematoma
  - ischemic stroke
  - hemorrhage: subarachnoid hemorrhage (SAH), intracerebral hemorrhage (ICH), intraventricular hemorrhage (IVH)
- cyst

Disorders of the Spine
- extradural
  - degenerative: disc herniation, canal stenosis, spondylolisthesis/spondylolysis
  - infection/inflammation: osteomyelitis, discitis
  - ligamentous: ossification of posterior longitudinal ligament (OPLL)
  - trauma: mechanical compression/instability, hematoma (onset = minutes to hours)
  - tumours (55% of spinal tumours): lymphoma, metastases (lymphoma, lung, breast, prostate), neurofibroma
- intradural extramedullary
  - vascular: dural arterio-venous fistula, subdural hematoma (anticoagulation)
  - tumours (40% of spinal tumours): meningioma, schwannoma, neurofibroma
- intradural intramedullary
  - tumours (5% of spinal tumours): astrocytomas and ependymomas most common; also hemangioblastomas and dermoid
  - syringomyelia (common causes: trauma, congenital, idiopathic)
  - infectious/inflammatory: TB, sarcoid, transverse myelitis
  - vascular (AVM, ischemia)

Peripheral Nerve Lesions
- neuropathies
  - traumatic
  - entrapments
  - iatrogenic
  - inflammatory
  - tumours

INTRACRANIAL PATHOLOGY

Intracranial Pressure (ICP) Dynamics

ICP/Volume Relationship
- adult skull is rigid with a constant intracranial volume
- however, as a lesion expands, ICP does not rise initially due to:
  - cerebrospinal fluid (CSF), blood, extracellular fluid (ECF) and intracellular fluid (ICF) displaced out of the head
  - brain tissue shifts into compartments under less pressure (herniation)
- once compensation is exhausted, ICP rises exponentially
- normal ICP <15 mmHg (8-18 cm H_2O) for adult, 3-7 mmHg (4-9.5 cm H_2O) for child; varies with patient position
- waveform comprised of respiratory and blood pressure pulsations
- consider therapy for high ICP when ICP >20-25 mmHg

Primary CNS lymphoma reported in 6-20% of HIV-infected patients.

Monro-Kellie hypothesis

$$V_{brain} + V_{blood} + V_{CSF} + V_{lesion} = V_{skull} = constant$$

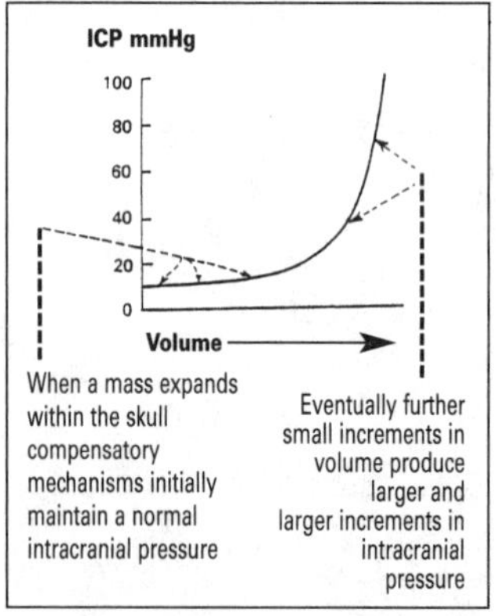

ICP mmHg

When a mass expands within the skull compensatory mechanisms initially maintain a normal intracranial pressure

Eventually further small increments in volume produce larger and larger increments in intracranial pressure

Figure 4. ICP-Volume Curve
Adapted from Lindsay KW, Bone I: Neurology and Neurosurgery Illustrated. Copyright 2004 with permission from Elsevier.

ICP Measurement

- lumbar puncture (LP) (contraindicated with known/suspected intracranial mass lesion)
- intraventricular catheter/ventriculostomy/external ventricular drain ("gold standard", permits therapeutic drainage of CSF to decrease ICP; if mass and pressure gradient present, drainage may increase gradient)
- other: fibreoptic monitor (intraventricular, intraparenchymal, subdural), subarachnoid bolt (Richmond screw), and epidural monitor

Cerebral Blood Flow (CBF)

- CBF depends on cerebral perfusion pressure (CPP) and cerebral vascular resistance
- normal CPP >50 mmHg in adults
- cerebral autoregulation maintains constant CBF by compensating for changes in CPP, unless:
    - high ICP such that CPP <60 mmHg
    - MAP >150 mmHg or MAP <50 mmHg
    - brain injury: i.e. subarachnoid hemorrhage (SAH), severe trauma

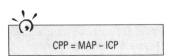

$$CPP = MAP - ICP$$

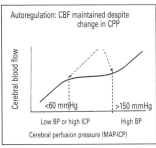

Figure 5. Cerebral Autoregulation Curve
Adapted from Lindsay et al: Neurology and Neurosurgery Illustrated. Copyright 2004 with permission from Elsevier.

Elevated ICP

Etiology of Raised ICP
- increased intracranial blood volume
    - hypoventilation → increased pCO_2/decreased pO_2 → vasodilatation
    - venous outflow obstruction (venous sinus thrombosis, superior vena cava (SVC) syndrome)
    - cranial dependency, Valsalva
- cerebral edema: vasogenic (vessel damage), cytotoxic (cell death), osmotic (acute hyponatremia, hepatic encephalopathy)
- hydrocephalus
- intracranial mass lesion (tumour, pus, blood, depressed skull fracture, foreign body)
- tension pneumocephalus
- status epilepticus
- hypertensive encephalopathy (loss of autoregulation and cerebral edema)

CLINICAL FEATURES

Acute Raised ICP
- headache (H/A)
- nausea and vomiting (N/V)
- decreased level of consciousness (LOC) if ICP = diastolic BP or midbrain compressed
- drop in Glasgow Coma Scale (GCS) → best index to monitor progress and predict outcome of acute intracranial process (see *Neurotrauma*)
- papilledema ± retinal hemorrhages (may take 24-48 hours to develop)
- abnormal extra-ocular movements (EOM)
    - CN VI palsy → often falsely localizing (causative mass may be remote from nerve)
    - upward gaze palsy (especially in children with obstructive hydrocephalus)
- herniation syndromes (see *Herniation Syndromes*)
- focal signs/symptoms due to lesion

Cushing's Triad of Acute Raised ICP
Full triad seen in 1/3 of cases
1. hypertension
2. bradycardia (late finding)
3. abnormal respiratory pattern

Chronic Raised ICP
- H/A
    - postural: worsened by coughing, straining, bending over (Valsalva)
    - morning/evening H/A → vasodilatation due to increased CO_2 with recumbency
- visual changes
    - due to papilledema
    - enlarged blind spot, if advanced → episodic constrictions of visual fields ("grey-outs")
    - optic atrophy/blindness
    - differentiate from papillitis (usually unilateral with decreased visual acuity)

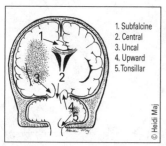

1. Subfalcine
2. Central
3. Uncal
4. Upward
5. Tonsillar

© Heidi Maj

Figure 6. Herniation Types

Herniation Syndromes

Subfalcine (Cingulate) Herniation

- **definition**: cingulate gyrus herniates under falx
- **etiology**: lateral supratentorial lesion
- **clinical features**:
  - usually asymptomatic, pathological/radiological observation
  - warns of impending transtentorial herniation, risk of ACA compression

Central Tentorial (Axial) Herniation

- **definition**: displacement of diencephalon and midbrain through tentorial notch
- **etiology**: supratentorial midline lesion, diffuse cerebral swelling, late uncal herniation
- **clinical features**:
  - rostral to caudal deterioration (sequential failure of diencephalon → medulla)
  - decreased LOC (midbrain compressed)
  - EOM/upward gaze impairment ("sunset eyes")
  - brainstem hemorrhage ("Duret's" secondary to shearing of basilar artery perforating vessels)
  - diabetes insipidus (traction on pituitary stalk and hypothalamus) → end stage sign

Lateral Tentorial (Uncal) Herniation

- **definition**: uncus of temporal lobe herniates down through tentorial notch
- **etiology**: lateral supratentorial lesion (often rapidly expanding traumatic hematoma)
- **clinical features**:
  - ipsilateral non-reactive dilated pupil (earliest, most reliable sign), EOM paralysis (CN III compressed)
  - decreased LOC (midbrain compressed)
  - contralateral hemiplegia, ± extensor (upgoing) plantar response
  - ± "Kernohan's notch": contralateral cerebral peduncle compressed due to shift of brain → ipsilateral hemiplegia (a false localizing sign)

Upward Herniation

- **definition**: cerebellar vermis herniates through tentorial incisura, compressing midbrain
- **etiology**: large posterior fossa mass causing herniation of cerebellum rostrally, common after VP shunting
- **clinical features**:
  - superior cerebellar artery (SCA) compression → cerebellar infarct
  - compression of cerebral aqueduct → hydrocephalus

Tonsillar Herniation ("Coning")

- **definition**: cerebellar tonsils herniate through foramen magnum
- **etiology**: infratentorial lesion or following central tentorial herniation
- **clinical features**:
  - compression of cardiovascular and respiratory centers in medulla (rapidly fatal)
  - may be precipitated by LP in presence of space occupying lesion (particularly in the posterior fossa)

Treatment of Herniation Syndromes

- goals: keep ICP <20 mmHg, CPP >60-70 mmHg

General Measures
- elevate head of bed at 30-45° → increases intracranial venous outflow
- prevent hypotension with fluid and pressors prn
- ventilate to normocarbia (pCO_2 35-40 mmHg) → prevents vasodilatation
- oxygen prn to maintain pO_2 >60 mmHg → prevents hypoxic brain injury
- CT or MRI to identify etiology, assess for midline shift/herniation

Specific Measures (proceed stepwise prn)
- mannitol (20% IV solution 1-1.5 g/kg, then 0.25 g/kg q6h)
  - can give rapidly, acts in 30 minutes, must maintain sBP >90 mmHg
- hyperventilate to pCO_2 30-35 mmHg

- sedation ("light" e.g. codeine → "heavy" e.g. fentanyl/MgSO$_4$ ± paralysis with vecuronium → reduces sympathetic tone, HTN induced by muscle contraction)
- corticosteroids
  - decreases edema over subsequent days around brain tumour, abscess, blood
  - no proven value in head injury or stroke
- surgery
  - drain 3-5 ml CSF via ventricles, assess each situation independently
  - remove mass lesion, insert external ventricular drain (if acute) or shunt
  - decompressive craniectomy is a last resort

Hydrocephalus

Definition
- increased CSF volume

Etiology
- decreased CSF absorption (majority)
- increased CSF production (rarely) – e.g. choroid plexus papilloma (0.4-1% of intracranial tumours)

Epidemiology
- estimated prevalence 1-1.5%; incidence of congenital hydrocephalus ~1-2/1000 live births

Classification

1. Obstructive (Non-Communicating) Hydrocephalus
- absorption blocked within ventricular system proximal to the arachnoid granulations
- acquired causes:
  - acquired aqueductal stenosis (adhesions following infection, hemorrhage)
  - intraventricular lesions (tumours – e.g. 3rd ventricle colloid cyst, hematoma)
  - mass causing tentorial herniation, aqueduct/4th ventricle compression
  - others: neurosarcoidosis, abscess/granulomas, arachnoid cysts
- congenital causes:
  - aqueductal stenosis, Dandy-Walker malformation, Chiari malformation (see *Pediatric Neurosurgery*)
- CT findings:
  - ventricular enlargement proximal to block

2. Non-Obstructive (Communicating) Hydrocephalus
- CSF absorption blocked at extraventricular site = arachnoid granulations
- causes:
  - post-infectious (#1 cause) → meningitis, cysticercosis
  - post-hemorrhagic (#2 cause) → SAH, IVH, traumatic
  - choroid plexus papilloma (rare, causes ↑ CSF production)
  - idiopathic → normal pressure hydrocephalus
- CT findings:
  - all ventricles dilated

3. Normal Pressure Hydrocephalus (NPH)
- gradual onset of classic triad developing over weeks or months
  - gait disturbance (ataxia and apraxia usually initial symptoms)
  - urinary incontinence
  - dementia
- CSF pressure within clinically "normal" range, but symptoms abate with CSF shunting
- idiopathic etiology
- CT/MRI - enlarged ventricles without increased prominence of cerebral sulci

4. Hydrocephalus Ex Vacuo
- enlargement of ventricles and sulci secondary to cerebral atrophy, not hydrocephalus
- usually a function of normal aging, also in Alzheimer's, Creutzfeldt-Jacob Disease

Clinical Features (see *Pediatric Neurosurgery* for infant/child)
- Acute Hydrocephalus
  - signs and symptoms of acute raised ICP (see *Elevated ICP*)
  - impaired upward gaze ("sunset eyes") and/or CN VI palsy
- Chronic Hydrocephalus
  - similar to NPH (see above)

Investigations
- CT/MRI
  - ventricular enlargement, may see prominent temporal horns
  - periventricular hypodensity (transependymal migration of CSF forced into extracellular space)
  - narrow/absent sulci
- ultrasound (through anterior fontanelle in infants)
- ICP monitoring (e.g. LP) may be used to investigate NPH, test response to shunting (lumbar tap test)
- radionuclide cisternography can test CSF flow and absorption rate (unreliable)

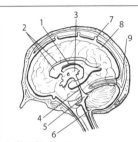

1. Choroid plexus
2. Lateral ventricles
3. Third ventricle
4. Cerebral aqueduct (of Sylvius)
5. Fourth ventricle
6. Foramen Luschka and Magendie
7. Arachnoid granulations
8. Subarachnoid space
9. Sagittal sinus

© Kari Francis 2004

Figure 7. The Flow of CSF

CSF produced by choroid plexuses, flows to: → ventricles → foramina of Luschka and Magendie → subarachnoid space → absorbed by arachnoid villi/granulations into venous sinuses.

Luschka = **l**ateral, **M**agendie = **m**edial

NPH Progression "AID" =
Ataxia/**A**praxia of gait → **I**ncontinence → **D**ementia

CSF production = CSF reabsorption = ~ 500ml/day in normal adults

Normal CSF volume ~ 150 ml
(50% spinal, 50% intracranial → 25 cc intraventricular, 50 cc subarachnoid)

Treatment
- surgical removal of obstruction (if possible) or excision of choroid plexus papilloma
- shunts:
  - ventriculoperitoneal (VP) – most common
  - ventriculo-atrial (VA) – not first choice because of ↑ infections, shunt emboli
  - ventriculopleural
  - lumboperitoneal – for communicating hydrocephalus and pseudotumour cerebri
- third ventriculostomy (for obstructive hydrocephalus) via ventriculoscopy
- LPs (for transient, IVH in premature infants, etc.)

Shunt Complications
- obstruction (most common cause of shunt malfunction)
  - **etiology**: obstruction by choroid plexus, buildup of proteinaceous accretions, blood, cells (inflammatory or tumour), infection, disconnection or damage
  - **clinical features**: acute hydrocephalus, increased ICP
  - **investigations**: "shunt series" (plain x-rays of entire shunt that only rule-out disconnection, break, tip migration), CT, radionuclide "shuntogram"
  - shunt tap and surgical exploration prn
- infection (3-6%)
  - **etiology**: S. epidermidis, S. aureus, P. acnes, Gram-negative bacilli
  - **clinical features**: fever, N/V, anorexia, irritability, meningitis, peritonitis, signs and symptoms of shunt obstruction, shunt nephritis (VA shunt)
  - **investigations**: CBC, blood culture, tap shunt for C&S (LP usually NOT recommended)
- overshunting (10% over 6.5 years)
  - ± slit ventricle syndrome (collapse of ventricles leading to occlusion of shunt ports by ependymal lining)
  - ± subdural effusion, hematoma (collapsing brain tears bridging veins, especially in NPH patients)
  - ± secondary craniosynostosis (children)
  - ± low pressure headache
- seizures (5.5% risk in 1st year, 1.1% after 3rd year)
- inguinal hernia (17% incidence with VP shunt inserted in infancy), skin breakdown over hardware

Benign Intracranial Hypertension (Pseudotumour Cerebri)

Definition
- raised intracranial pressure and papilledema without evidence of any mass lesion, hydrocephalus, infection or hypertensive encephalopathy (a diagnosis of exclusion)

Etiology
- unknown (majority), but associated with
  - lateral venous sinus thrombosis
  - habitus/diet: obesity, hyper/hypovitaminosis A
  - endocrine: reproductive age, menstrual irregularities, Addison's/Cushing's disease, thyroid irregularities
  - hematological: iron deficiency anemia, polycythemia vera
  - drugs: steroid administration or withdrawal, tetracycline, nalidixic acid, etc.
- risk factors overlap with those of venous sinus thrombosis and similar to those for gallstones

Epidemiology
- incidence ~0.5/100,000/year
- usually in 3rd and 4th decade (F>M)

Clinical Features
- symptoms and signs of raised ICP (H/A in >90%, pulsatile intracranial noise), but NO decreased LOC or diplopia
- ↓ visual acuity, papilledema, visual field defect, optic atrophy (key morbidity, preventable cause of often permanent blindness)
- usually self-limited, recurrence is common, chronic in some patients
- risk of blindness is not reliably correlated to symptoms or clinical course

Investigations
- CT: normal
- CSF studies: normal
- MRI: must look for venous sinus thrombosis

Treatment
- R/O conditions that cause intracranial hypertension
- D/C offending medications, encourage weight loss, fluid/salt restriction
- pharmacotherapy: acetazolamide (decreases CSF production), thiazide diuretic or furosemide
- if above fail → serial LPs, shunt
- optic nerve sheath decompression (if progressive impairment of visual acuity)
- 2-year follow-up with imaging to rule out occult tumour, ophthalmology follow-up

Tumour

Definition
- **classification**: primary vs. metastatic, intra-axial (parenchymal) vs. extra-axial, supratentorial vs. infratentorial, adult vs. pediatric
- **benign**: non-invasive, but can be devastating due to expansion of mass in fixed volume of skull
- **malignant**: implies rapid growth, invasiveness, but rarely extracranial metastasis
- **four basic types:**
  - **glioma**: astrocytomas, oligodendrogliomas, ependymomas
  - **neuronal**: ganglion cell tumours, cerebral neurocytomas/neuroblastomas
  - **meningeal**: meningioma
  - **poorly differentiated neoplasms**: medulloblastoma, atypical teratoid/rhabdoid
  - **other**: primary CNS lymphoma, primary brain germ cell tumours, pineal tumours

Important features to note on CT and MRI (± contrast enhancement)
- lesions (± edema, necrosis, hemorrhage)
- midline shifts and herniations
- effacement of ventricles and sulci (often ipsilateral), basal cisterns
- single or multiple (multiple implies metastasis)

Table 1. Tumour Types: Age, Location

Age	Supratentorial	Infratentorial (posterior fossa)
<15 years • incidence: 2-5/100,000/year • 60% infratentorial	- astrocytoma (all grades) (50%) - craniopharyngioma (5-10%) - others: pineal region tumours, choroid plexus tumours, ganglioglioma, DNET	- medulloblastoma (15-20%) - cerebellar astrocytoma (15%) - ependymoma (9%) - brainstem astrocytoma
>15 years • 80% supratentorial	- high grade astrocytoma (e.g. glioblastoma multiforme (GBM) (12-15%) - metastasis (15-30%, includes infratentorial) - meningioma (15-20%) - low grade astrocytoma (8%) - pituitary adenoma (5-8%) - oligodendroglioma (5%) - other: colloid cyst, CNS lymphoma, dermoid/epidermoid cysts	- metastasis - acoustic neuroma (schwannoma) (5-10%) - hemangioblastoma (2%) - meningioma

DDx for ring enhancing lesion on CT with contrast: "MAGICAL DR"
- ***M**etastases
- ***A**bscess
- ***G**lioblastoma (high grade astrocytoma)
- **I**nfarct
- **C**ontusion
- **A**IDS (toxoplasmosis)
- **L**ymphoma
- **D**emyelination
- **R**esolving hematoma

[* by far the 3 most common Dx's]

Clinical Features
- **progressive neurological deficit** (70%) – usually motor weakness, ± CN deficits, sensory, cognitive, personality, endocrine deficits may localize lesion
- **H/A** (50%) ± raised ICP (acute or chronic depending on growth rate), H/A classically worse in am but non-specific (likely hypoventilation during sleep causing vasodilatation →↑ ICP), also may worsen with bending forward/Valsalva
- **N/V** (40%)
- **seizures** (25%)
- papilledema, obscured vision
- symptoms suggestive of TIA (ictal, post-ictal, or ischemic 2° to "steal phenomenon")
- rarely presents with hemorrhage
- familial syndromes associated with CNS tumours:
  - von Hippel-Lindau (hemangiomas)
  - tuberous sclerosis (astrocytomas)
  - neurofibromatosis type 1 and 2 (astrocytomas, acoustic neuromas respectively)
  - Li-Fraumeni (astrocytomas)
  - Turcot syndrome (GBMs)
  - multiple endocrine neoplasia type 1 (pituitary adenoma)

Primary Sources of Metastatic Brain Tumours

Lung	44%
Breast	10%
Kidney (RCC)	7%
GI	6%
Melanoma	3%

Investigations
- CT, MRI, stereotactic biopsy (tissue diagnosis), metastatic work-up prn

Treatment
- conservative – serial Hx, Px, imaging for slow growing/benign lesions
- medical – corticosteroids to reduce cytotoxic cerebral edema, pharmacological (see *Pituitary Adenoma*)
- surgical – total or partial excision (decompressive, palliative), shunt if hydrocephalus
- radiotherapy – conventional fractionated radiotherapy (XRT), stereotactic radiosurgery (Gamma Knife™)
- chemotherapy – e.g. alkylating agents (temozolomide)

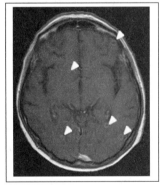

Figure 8. Multiple Brain Metastases

Metastatic Tumours

- **most common brain tumour seen clinically**
- 15-30% of cancer patients present with cerebral metastatic tumours
- usually spread hematogenously

Location
- 80% are hemispheric, often at grey-white matter junction or junction of temporal-parietal-occipital lobes (likely emboli spreading to terminal MCA branches)

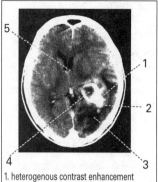

1. heterogenous contrast enhancement
2. ill-defined borders (infiltrative)
3. peritumour edema
4. central necrosis
5. compression of ventricles, midline shift

Figure 9. High Grade Astrocytoma on CT

Investigations
- metastatic work-up (CXR, CT chest/abdo, abdominal U/S, bone scan, mammogram)
- CT with contrast → round, well-circumscribed, often ring enhancing, ++ edema, often multiple
- MRI more sensitive, especially for posterior fossa
- consider biopsy in unusual cases

Treatment
- medical
  - phenytoin for seizure prophylaxis if patient presents with seizure
  - dexamethasone to reduce edema (often significant cause of symptoms), given with ranitidine
  - chemotherapy (small cell lung cancer)
- radiation
  - whole brain radiation therapy (WBRT) can help reduce symptoms in inoperable cases (some tumours respond poorly e.g. melanoma), typically the sole treatment if multiple lesions
  - post-op WBRT is commonly used
  - stereotactic radiosurgery
  - multiple lesions:
    1. metastatic work-up negative → brain biopsy
    2. metastatic work-up positive → biopsy affected sites other than the brain
- surgical
  - single/solitary lesions → surgery + radiation
- prognosis: median survival without treatment once symptomatic is ~1 month, with optimal treatment 6-9 months but varies depending on primary

Astrocytoma

- **most common primary intra-axial brain tumour**

Table 2. Astrocytoma Grading System (one of many schemes)

World Health Organization (WHO)	Typical CT/MRI Findings	Survival
I – pilocytic astrocytoma	+/- mass effect, +/- enhancement	>10 years, cure if gross total resection
II – low grade/diffuse	Mass effect, no enhancement	5 years
III – anaplastic	Complex enhancement	1.5-2 years
IV – glioblastoma multiforme	Necrosis (ring enhancement)	8-10 months, 10% at 2 years

Clinical Features
- **epidemiology**: most common in fourth to sixth decades
- **sites**: cerebral hemispheres >> cerebellum, brainstem, spinal cord
- **symptoms**: recent onset of new/worsening H/A, N/V, seizure, ± focal deficits or symptoms of increased ICP

Investigations
- CT with contrast → variable appearance depending on grade (see Table 2)
- tissue biopsy: WHO grade and histology correlates with prognosis, but 25% chance of sampling error due to tumour heterogeneity

Treatment
- low grade diffuse astrocytoma:
  - close follow-up, radiation, chemotherapy, surgery all valid options
  - surgery: not curative, trend towards better outcomes
  - radiotherapy alone or post-op prolongs survival (retrospective evidence)
  - chemotherapy – usually reserved for tumour progression
- high grade astrocytomas (comprised of anaplastic astrocytoma and glioblastoma multiforme (GBM))
  - surgery: gross total removal with radiation to tumour bed ± WBRT is the standard treatment unless: extensive dominant lobe GBM, significant bilateral involvement, end of life near, extensive brainstem involvement
  - aim to prolong "quality" survival
  - chemotherapy: ~20% response rate, temozolomide (agent of choice)
- multiple gliomas: WBRT ± chemotherapy

Radiotherapy plus concomitant and adjuvant temozolomide for glioblastoma
NEJM 2005 352:987-996
Background: The current standard of treatment for newly diagnosed glioblastoma multiforme (GBM) includes gross surgical resection followed by adjuvant radiotherapy. Here, the safety and efficacy of temozolomide, an oral alkylating agent, is studied following tumour resection and adjuvant radiotherapy.
Methods: Patients with histologically-confirmed GBM were randomized to receive radiotherapy alone (total dose 60 Gy over 6 weeks) or radiotherapy plus temozolomide (continuous daily temozolomide during radiotherapy, followed by 6 cycles of adjuvant temozolomide). Primary end point: Overall survival. Secondary end points: Progression-free survival, safety.
Results: 573 patients were randomized to receive radiotherapy (n=286) or radiotherapy plus temozolomide (n=287). Epidemiologic and clinical characteristics of the two groups were well balanced. At the time of follow-up (median 28 months), survival rates were significantly increased in the temozolomide group compared to control patients (14.6 months [95% CI 13.2 to 16.8] vs 12.1 months [95% CI 11.2 to 13.0]). The median period of progression-free survival was also prolonged in the temozolomide group (6.9 months [95%CI 5.8 to 8.2] vs 5.0 months [95% CI 4.2 to 5.5]. 7% of patients treated with temozolomide developed grade 3 or 4 hematologic toxic effects (neutropenia, leucopenia and thrombocytopenia); no grade 3 or 4 hematologic toxic effects were observed in the control cohort. Thromboembolic events were not significantly different between the two treatment arms (observed in 0.06% of radiotherapy patients and 0.04% of temozolomide patients).
Conclusions: The addition of temozolomide to adjuvant radiotherapy treatment for histologically-confirmed, newly-diagnosed GBM resulted in a statistically significant survival benefit. Adverse events were within acceptable limits for patient safety. Temozolomide is the first chemotherapeutic agent with demonstrable efficacy in the treatment of GBM.

Meningioma

- mostly benign (1% malignant), slow-growing, extra-axial, circumscribed (non-infiltrative), arise from arachnoid membrane
- often cause hyperostosis of adjacent bone, often calcified, classically see Psammoma bodies on histology

Common Locations
- parasagittal convexity or falx (70%), sphenoid wing, tuberculum sellae, foramen magnum, olfactory groove

Clinical Features
- middle aged, slight female preponderance (male:female = 3:2), high progesterone receptors (increase in size with pregnancy), symptoms of increased ICP, focal deficits, usually solitary (10% multiple, likely with loss of NF2 gene/22q12 deletion)

Investigations
- CT with contrast: homogeneous, densely enhancing, along dural border ("dural tail"), well circumscribed (see Figure 10)
- contrast enhanced MRI provides better detail
- angiography: most are supplied by external carotid feeders (meningeal vessels)
    - also assesses venous sinus involvement, "tumour blush" commonly seen (prolonged contrast image)

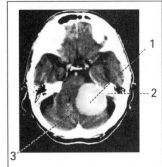

1. homogenous contrast enhancement
2. dural attachment
3. distinct margins

Figure 10. Meningioma on CT

Treatment
- conservative management for non-progressive, asymptomatic lesions
- surgery is treatment of choice if symptomatic or progression on sequential imaging (curative if complete resection)
- stereotactic radiosurgery (SRS) may be an option for lesions <3 cm
- endovascular embolization to facilitate surgery
- SRS or XRT for recurrent atypical/malignant meningiomas

WHO classification of meningioma (by histology)
Grade 1: low risk of recurrence
Grade 2: intermediate risk of recurrence
Grade 3: high risk of recurrence

Prognosis
- >90% 5-year survival, recurrence rate variable (often ~10-20%)
- depends on extent of resection (Simpson's classification)

Vestibular Schwannoma ("Acoustic Neuroma")

- progressive unilateral or asymmetrical sensorineural hearing loss = acoustic neuroma until proven otherwise (earliest symptom)
- slow-growing (average of 1 mm/yr), benign posterior fossa tumour
- arises from vestibular component of CN VIII in internal auditory canal, expanding into bony canal and cerebello-pontine angle (CPA)
- if bilateral, diagnostic of neurofibromatosis type II
- epidemiology: all age groups affected, peaks at fourth to sixth decades

Clinical Features
- compression of structures in CPA, often CN VIII (hearing loss 98%, tinnitus, dysequilibrium), then V, then VII
- ataxia and raised ICP are late features

Investigations
- MRI with gadolinium or T2 FIESTA sequence (>98% sensitive/specific), CT with contrast 2nd choice
- audiogram, brainstem auditory evoked potentials, caloric tests

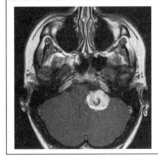

Figure 11. Vestibular Schwannoma (tumour in cerebello-pontine angle)

Treatment
- conservative: serial imaging
- radiation: stereotactic radiosurgery is the treatment of choice
- surgery if: 1. lesion >3 cm; 2. brainstem compression; 3. edema; 4. hydrocephalus
    - several routes, curable if complete resection (almost always possible)
    - operative complications: CN VII, VIII dysfunction (only significant disability if bilateral), CSF leak

Pituitary Adenoma

- primarily from anterior pituitary, 3rd-4th decade, M=F
- incidence in autopsy studies approximately 20%
- **classification**:
    - microadenoma <1 cm in diameter; macroadenoma ≥1 cm in diameter
    - endocrine active (functional/secretory), endocrine inactive (non-functional)

Clinical Features
- **mass effects**
  - H/A
  - bitemporal hemianopsia (compression of optic chiasm) (see <u>Neurology</u> for details of visual field deficit)
  - CN III, IV, V_1, V_2, VI palsy (compression of cavernous sinus)
- **endocrine effects**
  - hyperprolactinemia (prolactinoma) → infertility, amenorrhea, galactorrhea, decreased libido
  - ACTH production → Cushing's disease, hyperpigmentation
  - GH production → acromegaly/gigantism
  - panhypopituitarism (hypothyroidism, hypoadrenalism, hypogonadism)
  - associated MEN 1 syndrome
  - diabetes insipidus
- **pituitary apoplexy**
  - apoplexy (sudden expansion of mass due to hemorrhage or necrosis)
  - abrupt onset H/A, visual disturbances, ophthalmoplegia, and reduced mental status, and panhypopituitarism
  - CSF rhinorrhea and seizures (rare presenting signs of pituitary tumour)
  - signs and symptoms of SAH (rare)

Investigations
- formal visual fields, CN testing, endocrine tests (PRL level, TSH, 8 a.m. cortisol, fasting glucose, FSH/LH, IGF-1), electrolytes, urine electrolytes and osmolarity, imaging (MRI with and without contrast)

Differential
- parasellar tumours (e.g. craniopharyngioma, tuberculum sellae meningioma), carotid aneurysm

Treatment
- **medical**
  - rapid corticosteroid administration ± surgical decompression for apoplexy
  - dopamine agonists (e.g. bromocriptine) for prolactinoma
  - serotonin antagonist (cyproheptadine), inhibition of cortisol production (ketoconazole) for Cushing's
  - somatostatin analogue (octreotide) ± bromocriptine for acromegaly
  - endocrine replacement therapy
- **surgical**
  - trans-sphenoidal, transethmoidal, transcranial approaches

> **Go Look For The Adenoma Please –**
> GH, LH, FSH, TSH, ACTH, Prolactin
> A compressive adenoma in the pituitary will impair hormone production in this order (i.e. GH-secreting cells are most sensitive to compression)

Pus

Sources of Pus/Infection
- four routes of microbial access to CNS
  - hematogenous spread (**most common**): arterial and retrograde venous
    - adults: chest is #1 source (lung abscess, bronchiectasis, empyema)
    - children: congenital cyanotic heart disease with R to L shunt
    - immunosuppression (AIDS – toxoplasmosis)
  - direct implantation: with dural disruption due to trauma, iatrogenic (e.g. following LP, post-op), or congenital defect (e.g. dermal sinus)
  - contiguous spread (adjacent infection): from air sinus, naso/oropharynx, surgical site (e.g. otitis media, mastoiditis, sinusitis, osteomyelitis, dental abscess)
  - spread from PNS (e.g. viruses: rabies, HVZ)
- common examples:
  - epidural abscess: associated with osteomyelitis, in cranial and spinal epidural space, surgical emergency if cord compression, treatment: immediate drainage and antibiotics
  - subdural empyema: bacterial/fungal infection, due to contiguous spread from bone or air sinus, progresses rapidly, treatment: surgical drainage and antibiotics, 20% mortality
  - meningitis, encephalitis (see <u>Infectious Diseases</u>)
  - cerebral abscess (see *Cerebral Abscess* below)

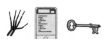

Cerebral Abscess

Definition
- pus in brain substance, surrounded by tissue reaction (capsule formation)

Etiology
- modes of spread: see above, 10-60% of patients have no cause identified
- pathogens
  - *Streptococcus* (**most common**), often anaerobic or microaerophilic

- *Staphylococcus* (penetrating injury)
- Gram negatives, anaerobes (*Bacteroides, fusobacterium*)
- in neonates: proteus and citrobacter (exclusively)
- immunocompromised: fungi and protozoa: *Toxoplasma, Nocardia, Candida albicans, Listeria monocytogenes, Mycobacterium* and *Aspergillus*

Risk Factors
- lung abnormalities (infection, AV fistulas (especially Osler-Weber-Rendu syndrome))
- CCHD: R to L shunt bypasses pulmonary filtration of micro-organisms
- bacterial endocarditis
- penetrating head trauma
- Immunosuppression (e.g. AIDS)

Clinical Features
- focal neurological signs and symptoms
- mass effect, increased ICP and sequelae (cranial enlargement in children)
- hemiparesis and seizures in 50%
- ± signs of systemic infection (mild fever, leukocytosis)

Complications
- with abscess rupture: ventriculitis, meningitis, venous sinus thrombosis
- CSF obstruction
- transtentorial herniation

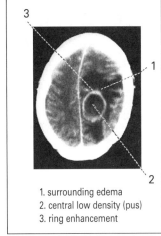

1. surrounding edema
2. central low density (pus)
3. ring enhancement

Figure 12. Brain Abscess on CT

Investigations
- WBC/ESR may be normal, blood cultures rarely helpful and LP contraindicated if large mass
- CSF: nonspecific (high ICP, high WBC, high protein, normal carbohydrate), rarely helpful, usually negative culture
- CT scan often 1st test in emergency department
- MRI
  - imaging of choice
  - diffusion/apparent diffusion coefficient (ADC) used to differentiate abscess (black) from tumour (white)

Treatment
- multiple aspiration ± excision and send for Gram stain, acid fast bacillus (AFB), C&S, fungal culture
- excision preferable if location suitable
- antibiotics
  - empirically: vancomycin + ceftriaxone + metronidazole or chloramphenicol or rifampin (6-8 weeks therapy)
  - revise antibiotics when C&S known
- anti-convulsants (1-2 years)
- follow up CT is critical (do weekly initially, more frequent if condition deteriorates)

Prognosis
- mortality with appropriate therapy ~10%, permanent deficits in ~50%

Blood

Extradural ("Epidural") Hematoma

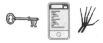

Etiology
- temporal-parietal skull fracture → 85% are due to ruptured middle meningeal artery. Remainder of cases are due to bleeding from middle meningeal vein, or dural sinus, or bone/diploic veins

Epidemiology
- young adult, male > female = 4:1. Rare before age of 2 or after age 60

Clinical Features
- in 60%, there is lucid interval of several hours between concussion and coma
- then, obtundation, hemiparesis, ipsilateral pupillary dilatation
- signs and symptoms depend on severity but can include H/A, N/V, amnesia, altered LOC, HTN and respiratory distress. Deterioration can take hours to days

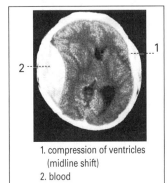

1. compression of ventricles (midline shift)
2. blood

Figure 13. Extradural Hematoma on CT

Investigations
- CT without contrast → high density biconvex mass against skull, "lenticular-shaped," usually with uniform density and sharp margins, usually limited by suture lines

Treatment
- admit, observe, head elevation, mannitol pre-op, craniotomy to evacuate clot, follow up CT. Optional: steriods for several days, then taper

Prognosis
- good with prompt management, as the brain is often not damaged. Bilateral babinski or decerebration pre-op--worse prognosis. Death is usually due to respiratory arrest from uncal herniation causing injury to the midbrain.

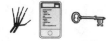

Subdural Hematoma

ACUTE SUBDURAL HEMATOMA

Etiology
- rupture of vessels that bridge the subarachnoid space (e.g. cortical artery, large vein, or venous sinus) or cerebral laceration

Risk Factors
- anticoagulants, EtOH, cerebral atrophy

Clinical Features
- no lucid period, signs and symptoms can include altered LOC, pupillary irregularity, hemiparesis

Investigations
- CT – high density concave mass, "crescentic" usually less uniform, less dense and more diffuse than extradural hematoma

Treatment
- craniotomy for subdurals greater than 1cm, optimal if surgery <4 hrs from onset

Prognosis
- poor overall since the brain is often injured (mortality range is over 50%)

CHRONIC SUBDURAL HEMATOMA

Etiology
- many start out as acute subdurals. Blood within the subdural space evokes an inflammatory response. Within days, fibroblasts invade the clot and form neomembranes. This is followed by growth of neocapillaries, fibrinolysis and liquefaction of blood clot. Course is determined by the balance of rebleeding from neomembranes and resorption of fluid

Risk Factors
- older, alcoholic, patients with CSF shunts, anticoagulants, coagulopathies

Clinical Features
- often due to minor injuries or no history of injury
- may present with minor H/A, confusion, language difficulties, TIA-like symptoms
- or symptoms of raised ICP ± seizures, progressive dementia, gait problem
- obtundation disproportionate to focal deficit; "the great imitator" of dementia, tumours

Investigations
- CT → hypodense (liquefied clot), crescentic mass

Treatment
- seizure prophylaxis used by some
- coagulopathies should be reversed
- burr hole drainage as clot liquefies, craniotomy if recurrent

Prognosis
- good overall as brain usually undamaged, but may require repeat drainage

CT density and MRI appearance of blood			
Time	CT	MRI -T1	MRI -T2
Acute (<72h)	Hyper.	Grey	Black
Subacute (<4w)	Iso.	White	White
Chronic (>4w)	Hypo.	Black	Black

MRI-T1: "**G**eorge **W**ashington **B**ridge"
MRI-T2: "Oreo" cookie – Black/White/Black

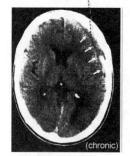

old blood

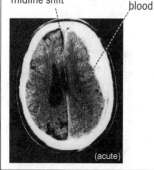

compression of ventricles
midline shift

blood

(chronic)

(acute)

Figure 14. Subdural Hematoma on CT

Cerebrovascular Disease

Ischemic Cerebral Infarction (80%)
- embolic (heart, carotid artery, aorta) or thrombosis of intracerebral arteries (see *Carotid Stenosis* section, and <u>Neurology</u>)

Intracranial Hemorrhage (20%)
- subarachnoid hemorrhage (SAH), spontaneous intracerebral hemorrhage (ICH), intraventricular hemorrhage (IVH)

Subarachnoid Hemorrhage (SAH)

Definition
- bleeding into subarachnoid space (intracranial vessels between arachnoid and pia)

Etiology
- **trauma (most common)**
- spontaneous
  - **aneurysms** (75-80%)
  - idiopathic (14-22%)
  - AVMs (5%)
- coagulopathies (iatrogenic or primary), vasculitides, tumours (<5%)

Epidemiology
- ~10-28/100,000 population/year
- peak age 55-60, 20% of cases occur under age 45

Risk Factors
- hypertension
- pregnancy/parturition in patients with pre-existing AVMs, eclampsia
- oral contraceptive pill
- substance abuse (cigarette smoking, cocaine, alcohol (debatable))
- conditions associated with high incidence of aneurysms (see *Intracranial Aneurysms* section)

Clinical Features of Spontaneous SAH
- sudden onset (seconds) of severe/thunderclap headache usually following exertion and described as the "worst headache of my life" (up to 97% sensitive, 12-25% specific)
- nausea/vomiting, photophobia
- meningismus (neck pain/stiffness, positive Kernig's and Brudzinski's sign)
- decreased LOC (can include raised ICP, ischemia, seizure)
- focal deficits: cranial nerve palsy (e.g. III, IV), hemiparesis
- ocular hemorrhage in 20-40% (due to sudden raised ICP compressing central retinal vein); subhyaloid/pre-retinal hemorrhages
- reactive hypertension
- sentinel bleeds
  - SAH-like symptoms lasting <1 day ("thunderclap H/A")
  - may have blood on CT or LP
  - ~50% of patients with full blown SAH give history suggestive of a warning leak within past 3 weeks
- **differential diagnosis of severe H/A, onset within seconds**: SAH; sentinel bleed; dissection/thrombosis of aneurysm; venous sinus thrombosis; benign exertional H/A

Investigations
- non-contrast CT (see Figure 15)
- 98% sensitive within 12h, 93% within 24h; 100% specificity
- may be negative if small bleed or presentation delayed several days
- acute hydrocephalus, IVH, ICH, infarct or large aneurysm may be visible
- CT may suggest site of aneurysm but CTA/MRA/angio more appropriate for localization
- positive history for SAH with negative CT – MUST do LP to look for blood or xanthochromia (may be negative <12h)

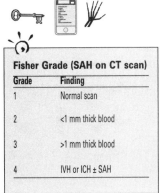

Fisher Grade (SAH on CT scan)

Grade	Finding
1	Normal scan
2	<1 mm thick blood
3	>1 mm thick blood
4	IVH or ICH ± SAH

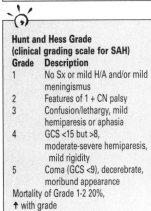

Hunt and Hess Grade (clinical grading scale for SAH)

Grade	Description
1	No Sx or mild H/A and/or mild meningismus
2	Features of 1 + CN palsy
3	Confusion/lethargy, mild hemiparesis or aphasia
4	GCS <15 but >8, moderate-severe hemiparesis, mild rigidity
5	Coma (GCS <9), decerebrate, moribund appearance

Mortality of Grade 1-2 20%, ↑ with grade

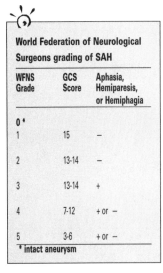

World Federation of Neurological Surgeons grading of SAH

WFNS Grade	GCS Score	Aphasia, Hemiparesis, or Hemiphagia
0 *		
1	15	–
2	13-14	–
3	13-14	+
4	7-12	+ or –
5	3-6	+ or –

* intact aneurysm

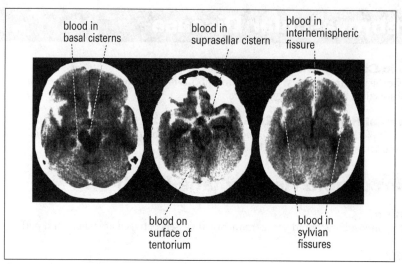

Figure 15. Diagnosis of SAH

- lumbar puncture (LP) – findings (highly sensitive):
  - elevated opening pressure (>18 cm H_2O)
  - bloody initially, xanthochromic supernatant with centrifugation ("yellow") by ~12h, lasting 2 weeks
  - spectrophotometry is most sensitive for xanthochromia
  - RBC count usually >100,000/mm³ without significant drop from 1st to last tube as in traumatic tap
  - protein elevated due to blood breakdown products
- cerebral angiography ("gold standard for aneurysms")
  - demonstrates source of SAH in 80-85% of cases
  - "angiogram negative SAH": repeat angiogram in 7-14 days, if negative → "perimesencephalic SAH"
- magnetic resonance angiography (MRA) and CT angiography
  - sensitivity may be up to 95% for aneurysms

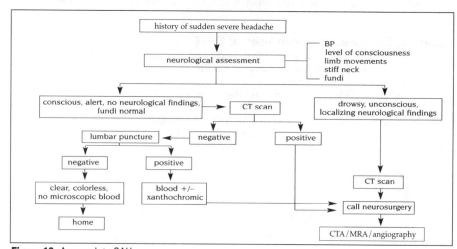

Figure 16. Approach to SAH

Treatment
- admit to ICU or NICU
- oxygen/ventilation prn
- NPO, bed rest, elevate head of bed 30°, minimal external stimulation, neurological vitals q1h
- aim to maintain sBP = 120-150 (balance of vasospasm prophylaxis, risk of re-bleed, risk of hypotension since CBF autoregulation impaired by SAH)
- IV NS with 20 mmol KCl/L at 125-150 cc/h
- phenytoin if seizure or temporal lobe clot
- mild sedation prn
- nimodipine for vasospasm neuroprotection → 21 days

- cardiac rhythm monitor
- Foley prn, strict ins & outs
- 4 vessel angiography, early surgery or coiling to prevent rebleed

Complications

- vasospasm
    - definition: constriction of blood vessels in response to arterial blood clot outside vessels at the base of the brain
    - clinical features: confusion, ↓ LOC, focal deficit (speech or motor)
    - onset: 4-14 days post SAH (if deterioration within first 3 days, MUST look for other cause)
    - "radiographic" vasospasm in 30-70% of arteriograms performed 7 days following SAH (peak incidence)
    - "symptomatic" vasospasm in 20-30% of SAH patients
    - detect clinically and/or with angiogram or transcranial Doppler (increased velocity of blood flow), CBC/electrolytes/CT urgently to r/o other causes
    - risk factors: large amount of blood on CT (high Fisher grade), smoking, ↑age, prior HTN
    - risk of cerebral infarct and death (biggest cause of morbidity and mortality in patients who reach hospital)
    - treatment
        - "triple H" therapy (hypertension, hypervolemia, hemodilution) using fluids and pressors (examples: norepinenphrine, phenylephrine)
        - angioplasty for refractory cases
- hydrocephalus (15-20%) – due to blood obstructing arachnoid granulations or subarachnoid space
    - can be acute or chronic – requiring extraventricular drain (EVD) or shunt respectively
- neurogenic pulmonary edema
- hyponatremia – (SIADH, cerebral salt wasting)
- diabetes insipidus
- cardiac – arrhythmia (>50% have ECG changes), MI, CHF

> **"Triple H" Therapy for Vasospasm**
> - **H**ypertension
> - **H**ypervolemia
> - **H**emodilution

Prognosis

- 10-15% mortality before reaching hospital, overall 50% mortality (majority within first 2-3 weeks)
- 30% of survivors have moderate → severe disability
- a major cause of mortality is rebleeding, for aneurysms:
    - risk of rebleed: 4% on first day, 15-20% within 2 weeks, 50% by 6 months
    - if no rebleed by 6 months risk decreases to same incidence of unruptured aneurysm (2%)
    - only prevention is early clipping or coiling of "cold" aneurysm
    - rebleed risk for "perimesencephalic SAH" is ~ same as for general population

Intracerebral Hemorrhage (ICH)

Definition

- hemorrhage within brain parenchyma, accounts for ~10% of strokes
- can dissect into ventricular system (IVH) or through cortical surface (SAH)

Etiology

- hypertension (usually at putamen, thalamus, pons and cerebellum)
- hemorrhagic transformation (reperfusion post stroke, surgery, strenuous exercise, etc.)
- vascular anomalies
    - aneurysm, AVMs and other vascular malformations (see *Vascular Malformations*)
    - venous sinus thrombosis
    - arteriopathies (cerebral amyloid angiopathy, lipohyalinosis, vasculitis)
- tumours (1%) – often malignant (e.g. GBM, lymphoma, metastases)
- drugs (amphetamines, cocaine, EtOH, etc.)
- coagulopathy (iatrogenic, leukemia, TTP, aplastic anemia)
- CNS infections (fungal, granulomas, herpes simplex encephalitis)
- post trauma (immediate or delayed, frontal and temporal lobes most commonly injured via coup/contre-coup mechanism)
- eclampsia
- post-operative (carotid endarterectomy, craniotomy)
- idiopathic

Epidemiology
- 12-15 cases/100,000 population/year

Risk Factors
- increasing age (mainly >55 years)
- male gender
- hypertension
- Black/Asian > Caucasian
- previous CVA of any type (23x risk)
- both acute and chronic heavy EtOH use, cocaine, amphetamines
- liver disease

Clinical Features
- TIA-like symptoms often precede ICH, can localize to site of impending hemorrhage
- location: basal ganglia/internal capsule (50%), thalamus (15%), cerebral white matter (15%), cerebellum/brainstem (15%)
- gradual onset of symptoms over minutes to hours, usually during activity
- H/A, vomiting, decreased LOC are common
- specific symptoms/deficits depend on location of ICH

Investigations
- high density blood on CT without contrast

Treatment
- medical:
  - decrease BP to pre-morbid level or by ~20%; check PTT, INR, and correct coagulopathy (stop anticoagulation for 1-2 weeks)
  - control raised ICP (see *Intracranial Pressure Dynamics* section)
  - phenytoin for seizure prophylaxis
  - follow electrolytes (SIADH common)
  - angiogram to R/O vascular lesion UNLESS >45 yrs, known HTN, and putamen/thalamic/posterior fossa ICH (yield ~ 0%)
- surgical:
  - craniotomy with evacuation of clot under direct vision, resection of source of ICH (i.e. AVM, tumour, cavernoma), ventriculostomy to treat hydrocephalus
  - indications:
    - symptoms appear related to raised ICP or mass effect
    - rapid deterioration (especially with signs of brainstem compression)
    - favourable location, e.g. cerebellar, non-dominant hemisphere
    - young patient (<50 y.o.)
    - if tumour, AVM, aneurysm, or cavernoma suspected (resection or clip to decrease risk of rebleed)
  - contraindications:
    - small bleed: minimal symptoms, GCS >10 (not necessary)
    - poor prognosis: massive hemorrhage (especially dominant lobe), low GCS/coma, lost brainstem function
    - medical reasons (e.g. very elderly, severe coagulopathy, difficult location (e.g. basal ganglia, thalamus))

Prognosis
- 30-day mortality rate is 44%, mostly due to cerebral herniation
- rebleed rate is 2-6%, higher if HTN poorly controlled

Intracranial Aneurysms

Epidemiology
- prevalence ~5% (20% are multiple)
- female > male; age 35-65 years

Risk Factors
- autosomal dominant polycystic kidney disease (15%)
- fibromuscular dysplasia (7-21%)
- AVMs
- connective tissue diseases (Ehlers-Danlos, Marfan's)
- FHx
- bacterial endocarditis
- Osler-Weber-Rendu syndrome
- atherosclerosis and HTN
- trauma

International Subarachnoid Aneurysm Trial (ISAT) of neurological clipping vs. endovascular coiling in 2143 patients with ruptured intracranial aneurysms: a randomized trial
Lancet 2002; 360:1267-74
Introduction: This randomized control trial aimed to compare endovascular detachable coil treatment against craniotomy and clipping for ruptured intracranial aneurysms in patients who were considered eligible for either modality of therapy.
Methods: 2143 patients were randomized to neurosurgical clipping (n=1070) vs. treatment by endovascular coil (n=1073). The primary clinical outcome was assessment using the modified Rankin scale for a score of 3-6 (dependency or death) at 1 year.
Results: Patients in this trial tended to be of good clinical grade prior to intervention and a majority of aneurysms were in the anterior circulatory system. 190 out of 801 (23.7%) patients who completed follow up in the endovascular treatment were dependent or dead at 1 year compared with 243 of 793 (30.6%) in the neurosurgical treatment group (p=0.0019). This showed a relative risk reduction of 22.6% (95% CI 8.9-34.2) and an absolute risk reduction of 6.9 (95 CI 2.5-11.3) when comparing endovascular to neurosurgical therapy.
Conclusion: In patients with a ruptured intracranial aneurysm who are suitable for either endovascular coiling or neurosurgical clipping, the outcome of dependency or death at one year favours the endovascular coiling therapy. Further neuropsychological assessment is being planned in subgroups to allow for subtle outcomes to be detected. Further follow up for dependency death is planned as well.

Types
- **saccular (berry)**
  - most common type
  - located at branch points of major cerebral arteries (Circle of Willis)
  - 85-95% in carotid system, 5-15% in vertebrobasilar circulation
- **fusiform**
  - atherosclerotic
  - more common in vertebrobasilar system, rarely rupture
- **mycotic**
  - secondary to any infection of vessel wall, 20% multiple
  - 60% *Streptococcus* and *Staphylococcus*
  - 3-15% of patients with SBE

Clinical Presentation
- rupture (90%), most often SAH, but 30% ICH, 20% IVH, 3% subdural bleed
- sentinel hemorrhage ("thunderclap H/A") → requires urgent clipping/coiling to prevent catastrophic bleed
- mass effect (giant aneurysms)
  - internal carotid or anterior communicating aneurysm may compress:
    - the pituitary stalk or hypothalamus causing hypopituitarism
    - the optic nerve or chiasm producing a visual field defect
  - basilar artery aneurysm may compress midbrain, pons (limb weakness), or CN III
  - posterior communicating artery aneurysm may produce CN III palsy
  - intracavernous aneurysms (CN III, IV, V_1, V_2, VI)
- small infarcts due to distal embolization (amaurosis fugax etc.)
- seizures
- headache (without hemorrhage)
- incidental CT or angiography finding (asymptomatic)

Investigations
- CT angiogram (CTA), magnetic resonance angiography (MRA), angiogram

Treatment
- **ruptured aneurysms**:
  - overall trend towards better outcome with early surgery or coiling (48-96 hours after SAH)
  - choice of surgery vs. coiling not yet well defined, morphology/location can aid decision
  - treatment options: surgical placement of clip across aneurysm neck, trapping (clipping of proximal and distal vessels), thrombosing using Gugliemi detachable coils (coiling), wrapping as last resort
- **unruptured aneurysms**:
  - 1% annual risk of rupture: risk dependent on size and location of aneurysm
  - no clear evidence on when to operate: need to weigh life expectancy
  - risk of morbidity/mortality of SAH (20%/50%) vs. surgical risk (2%/5%)
  - generally treat unruptured aneurysms >10 mm
  - consider treating when aneurysm 7-9 mm in middle-aged, younger patients or patients with a family history of aneurysms
  - follow smaller aneurysms with serial angiography

Carotid Stenosis

Definition
- narrowing of the internal carotid artery lumen due to atherosclerotic plaque formation, usually near common carotid bifurcation into internal and external carotids

Risk Factors
- for atherosclerosis: : HTN, smoking, DM, CVD or CAD, dyslipidemia

Clinical Features
- may be asymptomatic
- symptomatic stenosis may present as transient ischemic attack (TIA), reversible ischemic neurologic deficit (RIND), or stroke
- retinal insufficiency or infarct due to emboli occluding central retinal artery or branches permanently or temporarily (amaurosis fugax)
- middle cerebral artery (MCA) occlusive symptoms

Carotid System Aneurysms	
%	**Aneurysm Site**
30	ACom, ACA
25	PCom
20	MCA

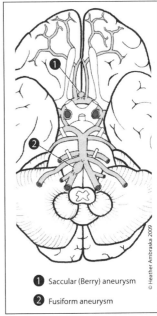

1 Saccular (Berry) aneurysm

2 Fusiform aneurysm

Figure 17. Berry and Fusiform Aneurysms of the Circle of Willis

Prevention of disabling and fatal strokes by successful carotid endarterectomy in patients without recent neurological symptoms: randomised controlled trial
Lancet 2004; 363:1491-1502

Study: Asymptomatic Carotid Surgery Trial (ACST), a randomized, controlled trial with follow-up at 5 years.
Patients: 3120 asymptomatic patients with significant carotid artery stenosis were randomized equally between immediate carotid endarterectomy (CEA) and indefinite deferral of CEA and were followed for up to 5 years (mean 3.4 years).
Main Outcome: Any stroke (including fatal or disabling).
Results: The risk of stroke or death within 30 days of CEA was 3.1% (95% CI 2.3-4.1). Comparing all patients randomized to immediate CEA vs. deferral, the 5-year stroke risks were 3.8% vs. 11% (gain 7.2% [95% CI 5.0-9.4], p<0.0001). This gain primarily involved ischemic strokes in the carotid artery territory (2.7% vs. 9.5%; gain 6.8% [4.8-8.8], p<0.0001), of which half were disabling or fatal (1.6% vs. 5.3%; gain 3.7% [2.1-5.2], p<0.0001). Combining the perioperative and the non-perioperative strokes, the net 5-year risks were 6.4% vs. 11.8% for all strokes (gain 5.4% [3.0-7.8], p<0.0001), 3.5% vs. 6.1% for fatal or disabling strokes (gain 2.5% [0.8-4.3], p=0.004), and 2.1% vs. 4.2% for fatal strokes (gain 2.1% [0.6-3.6], p=0.006).
Conclusions: In asymptomatic patients with significant carotid artery stenosis, immediate CEA reduced the net 5-year stroke risk from about 12% to about 6%. Half of this 5-year benefit involved disabling or fatal strokes.

Endarterectomy for Asymptomatic Carotid Artery Stenosis
JAMA 1995; 273:1421-1428.

Study: Asymptomatic Carotid Atherosclerosis Study (ACAS), a prospective, randomized, multi-centre trial.
Patients: 1662 patients with asymptomatic carotid artery stenosis of 60% or greater were randomized. Follow-up data are available on 1659. Recognized risk factors for stroke were similar between the two groups at baseline.
Intervention: Daily aspirin administration and medical risk factor management for all patients and carotid endarterectomy for patients randomized to receive surgery.
Main outcome: TIA or cerebral infarction occurring in the carotid artery territory and any TIA, stroke, or death occurring in the perioperative period.
Results: The risk for ipsilateral stroke and any perioperative stroke or death based on a 5-year follow-up (median of 2.7 years) was estimated to be 5.1% for surgical patients and 11.0% for patients treated medically (aggregate risk reduction of 53% (95% CI=22-72%)).
Conclusions: Patients with asymptomatic carotid artery stenosis of 60% or greater that are good candidates for elective surgery will have a reduced 5-year risk of ipsilateral stroke if carotid endarterectomy is performed in addition to aggressive management of modifiable risk factors.

Investigations
- CBC, PTT, INR (hypercoagulable states)
- fundoscopy → cholesterol emboli in retinal vessels (Hollenhorst plaques)
- auscultation over carotid bifurcation for bruits
- carotid duplex Doppler ultrasound: determines size of lumen and blood flow velocity, safest but least accurate, unable to scan above mandible
- angiogram: "gold standard" but invasive and 1/200 risk of stroke (not for screening)
- MRA: safer than angiogram, may overestimate stenosis

Treatment
- control of HTN, lipids, diabetes (risk factor management)
- antiplatelet agents (ASA ± dipyridamole, clopidogrel) ~25% relative risk reduction
- carotid endarterectomy (generally if symptomatic and >70% stenosis, see Prognosis)
- endovascular angioplasty ± stenting (utility being evaluated)

Prognosis

Table 3. Symptomatic Carotid Stenosis: North American Symptomatic Carotid Endarterectomy Trial (NASCET)

% Stenosis on Angiogram	Risk of Major Stroke or Death	
	Medical Rx	**Medical + Surgical Rx**
70-99 %	26% over 2 years	9% over 2 years
50-69%	22% over 5 years	16% over 5 years
<50%	Surgery has no benefit with 5% complication rate	

Table 4. Asymptomatic Carotid Stenosis: Asymptomatic Carotic Atherosclerosis Study (ACAS) and Asymptomatic Carotid Surgery Trial (ACST)

% Stenosis on Angiogram	Risk of Major Stroke or Death	
	Medical Rx	**Medical + Surgical Rx**
60-99%	11% over 5 years	5.1% over 5 years (ACAS)
70-99%	11.8% over 5 years	6.4% over 5 years (ACST)

Vascular Malformations

Types
- arteriovenous malformations (AVMs)
- cavernous malformations (cavernoma, cavernous hemangioma/angioma)
- venous angioma
- capillary telangiectasias
- arterio-venous fistula (AVF) (carotid-cavernous fistula, dural AVF, vein of Galen aneurysm)
- "angiographically occult vascular malformations" (any type, 10% of malformations)
- clinical significance:
  - principally AVMs and cavernous malformations produce intracranial hemorrhages and seizures

Arteriovenous Malformations (AVMs)

Spetzler-Martin AVM Grading Scale

Item	Score
Size	
0–3 cm	1
3.1–6.0 cm	2
>6 cm	3
Location	
Noneloquent	0
Eloquent	1
Deep venous drainage	
Not present	0
Present	1

AVM grades calculated by adding the 3 individual Spetzler-Martin Scale scores from the above table.

Definition
- tangle of abnormal vessels/arteriovenous shunts, with no intervening capillary beds or brain parenchyma
- congenital

Epidemiology
- prevalence ~0.14%, male:female = 2:1, average age at diagnosis = 33 years
- 15-20% of patients with Osler-Weber-Rendu syndrome will have cerebral AVMs

Clinical Features
- hemorrhage (40-60%) – small AVMs are more likely to bleed due to direct high pressure AV connections
- seizures (50%) – more common with larger AVMs
- mass effect
- focal neurological signs secondary to ischemia (high flow → "steal phenomena")

- localized headache, increased ICP
- bruit (especially with dural AVMs)
- may be asymptomatic ("silent")

Investigations
- MRI (flow void), MRA
- angiography (7% will also have one or more associated aneurysm)

Treatment
- decreases risk of future hemorrhage and seizure
  - surgical excision is treatment of choice for AVMs
  - endovascular embolization (glue, balloon) can facilitate surgery or stereotactic radiosurgery (SRS) for suitable grade II to V lesions
  - SRS is treatment of choice for small (~3 cm in diameter) or very deep
  - surgery alone is unsuitable for grade IV and V lesions
- conservative (e.g. palliative embolization, seizure control if necessary)

Prognosis
- 10% mortality, 30-50% morbidity (serious neurological deficit) per bleed
- risk of major bleed: 2-4% per year (untreated AVMs)

Cavernous Malformations

Definition
- benign vascular hamartoma consisting of irregular sinusoidal vascular channels located within the brain without intervening neural tissue or associated large arteries/veins

Epidemiology
- 0.1-0.2%, both sporadic and hereditary forms described
- several genes now described: CCM1, CCM2

Clinical Features
- seizures (60%), progressive neurological deficit (50%), hemorrhage (20%), H/A
- often an incidental finding
- hemorrhage risk less than AVM, usually minor bleeds

Investigations
- T2WI MRI (non-enhancing), gradient echo sequencing (best for diagnosis)
- usually not seen with angiography or CT

Treatment
- surgical excision – depending on presentation and location (supratentorial lesions are less likely to bleed than infratentorial lesions)
  - only appropriate for symptomatic lesions that are surgically accessible (not for asymptomatic lesions or for diagnosis)

Important Dermatomes and Myotomes
C2 – angle of jaw
C4 – collar of shirt
"C3,4,5 keeps the diaphragm alive"
T4 – nipple line
T6 – xiphoid
T10 – umbilical
T12 – suprapubic
"L3 above the knee"
"S2,3,4 – keeps your stool off the floor"

Myotomes
C5 – Shoulder abduction/elbow flexion
C6 – Wrist extensors
C7 – Elbow extension
C8 – Squeeze hand
T1 – Abduct fingers
T2-9 – Intercostal (Abdominal reflexes)
T9-10 – Upper abdominals
T11-12 – Lower abdominals
L2 – Flex hip
L3 – Hip adduction
L4 – Knee extension & ankle dorsiflexion
L5 – Ankle dorsiflexion & big toe extension
S1 – Plantarflex foot

Reflexes
1, 2 tie my shoe › S1-2 Ankle jerk
3, 4 kick the door › L3-4 Knee
5, 6 pick up sticks › C5-6 Biceps/Brachioradialis
7, 8 lay them straight › C7-8 Triceps

RED FLAGS for back pain
Concern for Cauda Equina
urinary retention or incontinence, fecal incontinence or loss of anal sphincter tone, saddle anesthesia, uni/bilateral, leg weakness/pain
Concern for Malignancy
age >50, previous hx of cancer, pain unrelieved by bed rest, constitutional symptoms
Concern for Infection
increased ESR, IV drug use, immunosuppressed, fever
Concern for Compression fracture
age >50, trauma, prolonged steroid use

RED FLAGS REDUX
Bowel/Bladder (retention or incontinence)
Anesthesia (saddle)
Cosntitutional symptoms
Khronic disease
Parasthesia
Age >50 or <20
IV drug use
Neuromator deficits

EXTRACRANIAL PATHOLOGY

Dermatomes/Myotomes

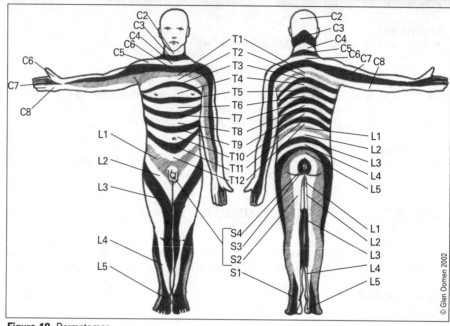

Figure 18. Dermatomes

Approach to Limb/Back Pain

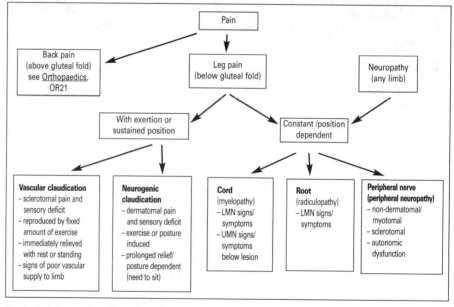

Figure 19. Approach to Limb/Back Pain

Extradural Lesions

Root Compression

Differential Diagnosis
- herniated disk
- neoplasm (neurofibroma, schwannoma)
- synovial cyst, abscess
- hypertrophic bone/spur

Cervical Disc Syndrome

Etiology
- nucleus pulposus herniates through annulus fibrosis and impinges upon nerve root

Epidemiology
- **most common levels C6-C7 (C7 root) > C5-C6 (C6 root)**

Clinical Features
- pain down arm in nerve root distribution, worse with neck extension, ipsilateral rotation and lateral flexion (all compress the ipsilateral neural foramen)
- LMN signs/symptoms
- central cervical disc protrusion causes myelopathy as well as nerve root deficits

Investigations
- C-spine x-ray, CT, MRI (procedure of choice), EMG, nerve conduction studies

Treatment
- conservative
  - no bedrest unless severe radicular symptoms
  - activity modification, patient education (reduce sitting, lifting)
  - physiotherapy (PT), exercise programs
  - analgesics, collar, traction may help
- surgical indications
  - intractable pain despite adequate conservative treatment for >3 months
  - progressive neurological deficit
  - anterior cervical discectomy is usual surgical choice

Prognosis
- 95% improve spontaneously in 4-8 weeks

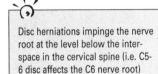

Disc herniations impinge the nerve root at the level below the interspace in the cervical spine (i.e. C5-6 disc affects the C6 nerve root)

Table 5. Lateral Cervical Disc Syndromes

	C4-5	C5-6	C6-7	C7-T1
Root Involved	C5	C6	C7	C8
Incidence	2%	19%	69%	10%
Sensory	Shoulder	Thumb	Middle finger	Ring finger, 5th finger
Motor	Deltoid, biceps, supraspinatus	Biceps	Triceps	Digital flexors, intrinsics
Reflex	No change	Biceps, Brachioradialis	Triceps	Finger jerk

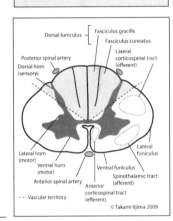

Figure 20A. Axial section of Cervical Spine with Vascular and Functional Territories

Cervical Stenosis (Cervical Spondylosis)

Cervical Spondylosis
- cervical spondylosis is chronic disc degeneration and associated facet arthropathy.
- resultant syndromes include mechanical neck pain, radiculopathy (root compression), myelopathy (spinal cord compression) and combinations
- **epidemiology**: typically begins at age 40-50, is seen in men > women, and most commonly occurs at the C5-C6 > C6-C7 levels
- **pathogenesis**: with neck extension, the cervical cord is pinched. With neck flexion, the canal dimensions increase slightly to relieve pressure on the cervical cord

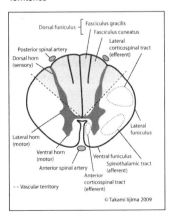

Figure 20B. Axial section of Thoracic Spine with Vascular and Functional Territories

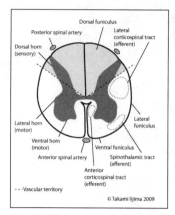

Figure 20C. Axial section of Lumbar Spine with Vascular and Functional Territories

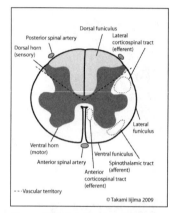

Figure 20D. Axial section of Sacral Spine with Vascular and Functional Territories

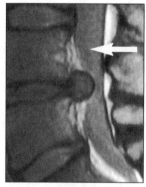

Figure 21. T_2-weighted MRI of Lumbar Disc Herniation

- **clinical features:**
  - insidious onset of mechanical neck pain exacerbated by excess vertebral motion (particularly rotation and lateral bend with a vertical compressive force-Spurling's test)
  - occipital headache is common
  - radiculopathy may involve 1 or more roots, and symptoms include neck, shoulder and arm pain, paresthesias and numbness
  - cervical myelopathy may be characterized by weakness (upper > lower extremity), decreased dexterity and sensory changes. UMN findings such as hyperreflexia, clonus, babinski reflex may be present. The most worrisome complaint is lower extremity weakness (corticospinal tracts)
  - myelopathy may be associated with funicular pain, characterized by burning and stinging ± Lhermitte's sign (lightning-like sensation down the back with neck flexion)
- **investigations:** x-ray of cervical spine ± flexion/extension or oblique views (studied for changes in Luschka and facet joints, osteophytes and disc space narrowing), MRI, CT, EMG
- **treatment:**
  - NSAIDS, moist heat, strengthening and range of motion exercises, analgesics, cervical collar, cervical traction
  - surgery – indications: myelopathy with motor impairment, progressive neurologic impairment, intractable pain

Lumbar Disc Syndrome

Etiology
- laterally herniated lumbar disc compresses nerve root, central herniation causes cauda equina or lumbar stenosis (neurogenic claudication)

Epidemiology
- **common (>95% of herniated lumbar disks) – L5 and S1 roots**

Clinical Features
- leg pain > back pain
- limited back movement (especially forward flexion) due to pain
- motor weakness, dermatomal sensory changes, reflex changes
- exacerbation with coughing, sneezing or straining. Relief with flexing the knee or thigh
- nerve root tension signs:
  - straight leg raise (SLR: Lasegue's test) or crossed SLR (pain should occur at less than 60 degrees) suggest L5, S1 root involvement
  - femoral stretch suggest L2, L3 or L4 root involvement

Investigations
- MRI, CT
- x-ray spine (only to rule out other lesions)
- myelogram and post-myelogram CT (if surgery contemplated and plain CT not conclusive)

Treatment
- conservative (same as cervical disc disease)
- surgical indications
  - same as cervical disc + cauda equina syndrome

Prognosis
- 95% improve spontaneously within 4 to 8 weeks

Table 6. Lateral Lumbar Disc Syndromes

	L3-4	L4-5	L5-S1
Root Involved	L4	L5	S1
Incidence	<10%	45%	45%
Pain	Femoral pattern	Sciatic pattern	Sciatic pattern
Sensory	Medial leg	Dorsal foot to hallux Lateral leg	Lateral foot
Motor	Tibialis anterior (dorsiflexion)	Extensor hallucis longus (hallux extension)	Gastrocnemius, soleus (plantar flexion)
Reflex	Knee jerk	Medial hamstrings	Ankle jerk

Cauda Equina Syndrome

Etiology
- compression or irritation of lumbosacral nerve roots below conus medullaris (below L2 level)
- Decreased space in the vertebral canal below L2. Common causes include herniated disk ± spinal stenosis, vertebral fracture and tumor

Speed of Onset
- usually acute (develops in less than 24 hours); rarely subacute or chronic

Clinical Features
- motor (LMN signs)
  - weakness/paraparesis in multiple root distribution
  - reduced deep tendon reflexes (knee and ankle)
- autonomic
  - urinary retention (or overflow incontinence) and/or fecal incontinence due to loss of anal sphincter tone
- sensory
  - low back pain radiating to legs (sciatica) aggravated by Valsalva maneuver and by sitting; relieved by lying down
  - bilateral sensory loss or pain: depends on the level of cauda equina affected
  - saddle area (S2-S5) anesthesia (most common sensory deficit)
  - sexual dysfunction (late finding)

Treatment
- requires urgent investigation (MRI) and decompression (<48 hrs) to preserve bowel and bladder function and/or to prevent progression to paraplegia

Prognosis
- markedly improves with surgical decompression. Without surgery, greater chance of persistent problems with bladder function, severe motor deficits, pain and sexual dysfunction. Recovery correlates with function at initial consult: if patient is ambulatory, likely to continue to be ambulatory; if unable to walk, unlikely to walk after surgery

Lumbar Spinal Stenosis

Etiology
- congenital narrowing of spinal canal combined with degenerative changes (herniated disk, hypertrophied facet joints and hypertrophied ligamentum flavum)

Clinical Features
- symptomatic stenosis produces gradually progressive back and leg pain with standing and walking that is relieved by sitting or lying (neurogenic claudication – 60% sensitive)
- neurologic exam may be normal, including straight leg raise test

Spinal cord ends at L1-2; dura ends at S1-2

Investigations
- spine x-ray, CT, MRI, myelogram

Treatment
- conservative – NSAIDs, analgesia
- surgical – laminectomy with root decompression

Neurogenic Claudication

Etiology
- ischemia of lumbosacral nerve roots secondary to vascular compromise and increased demand from exertion, often associated with lumbar stenosis

Clinical Features
- dermatomal pain/paresthesia/weakness of buttock, hip, thigh, or leg initiated by standing or walking
- slow relief with postural changes (sitting >30 min), NOT simply exertion cessation
- induced by variable degree of exercise or standing
- may be elicited with lumbar extension, but may not have any other neurological findings, no signs of vascular compromise (e.g. ulcers, poor capillary refill, etc.)

Key Features of Neurogenic vs. Vascular Claudication
Neurogenic Claudication: dermatomal distribution with positional relief occurring over minutes
Vascular Claudication: sclerotomal distribution with relief occurring with rest over seconds

Investigations
- bicycle test may help distinguish neurogenic claudication (NC) from vascular claudication (with the waist flexed individuals with NC can last longer)

Treatment
- same as for lumbar spinal stenosis

Intradural Intramedullary Lesion

Syringomyelia

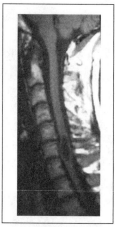

Figure 22. T$_1$ weighted MRI of Syringomyelia

- **definition**: cystic cavitation of the spinal cord. Presentation is highly variable, usually progresses over months to years. Initially, pain, weakness, atrophy and loss of pain and temperature sensation in the upper extremities is common
- **etiology**: 70% are associated with Chiari I malformation. May also be posttraumatic or associated with tumor
- **clinical features** (nonspecific features for any intramedullary spinal cord pathology):
  - sensory loss similar to central cord syndrome
  - dissociated pain and temperature loss with preserved touch and joint position sense in a cape-like distribution at level of cervical syrinx
  - dysesthetic pain often occurs in the distribution of the sensory loss
  - LMN arm/hand weakness or wasting
  - painless arthropathies (Charcot's joints), especially in the shoulder and neck due to loss of pain and temperature sensation (seen in less than 5%)
- **investigations**: MRI is best method, myelogram with delayed CT
- **treatment**:
  - treat underlying cause (e.g. posterior fossa decompression for Chiari I, surgical removal of tumour if causing a syrinx)

Spinal Cord Syndromes

- see Neurology for Spinal Cord Anatomy

Complete Spinal Cord Lesion
- bilateral loss of motor/sensory and autonomic function at ≥4 segments below lesion/injury, with UMN signs. About 3% of patients with complete injuries will develop some recovery within 24 hours. Beyond 24 hours, no distal function will recover

Compartmentalize **spinal cord syndromes** anatomically by location.

Incomplete Spinal Cord Lesion
- any residual function at ≥4 segments below lesion
- signs include sensory/motor function in lower limbs and "sacral sparing" (perianal sensation, voluntary rectal sphincter contraction)
- syndromes include Brown-Sequard's, central cord, anterior cord and posterior cord

Brown-Séquard Syndrome

- hemisection of spinal cord (lateral compression of one half of spinal cord)
- **common causes:**
  - trauma, tumour (extrinsic compression)

Signs and Symptoms
- motor
  - ipsilateral loss of voluntary motor function (due to corticospinal tract lesion) below level of lesion with UMN signs
  - ipsilateral LMN signs at level of lesion
- sensory
  - ipsilateral loss of vibration and proprioception (posterior column function)
  - contralateral loss of pain and temperature (spinothalamic tract lesion) beginning 1-2 segments below
  - preserved light touch due to redundant ipsilateral and contralateral paths (anterior spinothalamic tracts)
- prognosis
  - best prognosis of cord injuries (90% ambulate independently and have good sphincter control)

Anterior Cord Syndrome

- **common causes**
    - anterior spinal artery territory compression or occlusion (anterior spinal artery supplies anterior 2/3 of cord)

Signs and Symptoms
- motor
    - bilateral paraplegia (UMN below and LMN at level of lesion)
    - sphincter dysfunction (urinary retention)
- sensory
    - dissociated sensory loss
        - bilateral loss of pain and temperature below level of lesion (spinothalamic tract lesion)
        - preserved light touch, vibration and proprioception (posterior column function)

Central Cord Syndrome

- **most common incomplete spinal cord injury syndrome**
- **common causes:**
    - syringomyelia (progressive central cord cavitation), central tumours, spinal hyperextension injuries (e.g blow to the upper face or forehead due to MVA, forward fall, sporting accidents)

Signs and Symptoms
- motor
    - bilateral motor weakness; upper (LMN lesion) > lower (UMN lesion) extremities; more pronounced in the hands
- sensory
    - variable bilateral suspended sensory loss (dissociated sensory loss – pain and temperature loss greater than vibration and proprioception loss)
    - intact sensation above and below affected dermatomes; sacral sparing
- other
    - bowel and/or bladder dysfunction usually urinary retention is commonly a late manifestation
- prognosis
    - 50% recover enough lower extremity function to ambulate, 90% ambulate within 5 days, hand recovery variable

The pattern of impairment in Central Cord Syndrome is
"MUD":
Motor > sensory loss
Upper > lower extremity
Distal > proximal

Posterior Cord Syndrome

- **common causes**
    - posterior spinal artery infarction, trauma

Signs and Symptoms
- motor
    - preserved motor function
- sensory
    - bilateral loss of vibration and proprioception below level of lesion
    - preserved pain and temperature
- prognosis
    - more favourable than anterior cord syndrome

Peripheral Nerves

Clinical Features
- peripheral polyneuropathy vs. peripheral nerve injury (entrapment/trauma)
- sclerotomal distribution (non-dermatomal/myotomal)
- loss of sensation, paraesthesia, motor weakness
- denervated limb: muscle atrophy/fibrosis, joint stiffness, trophic changes (cold extremities, cutaneous hair loss, brittle nails)
- autonomic changes: local vasoconstriction (hypohidrosis) → edema → vasodilation (hyperhidrosis)

Peripheral Nerve Injury

Classification and Clinical Course
- neuropraxia: nerve intact but fails to function, recovery within hours to months
- axonotmesis: axon disrupted but nerve sheath intact → Wallerian degeneration (of axon segment distal to injury) → axonal recovery ~1 inch/month, max at 1-2 years
- neurotmesis: nerve completely severed, need surgical repair for recovery

Causes
- **DDx: DANG THERAPIST** (see sidebar)
- **trauma**: lacerations, contusion, stretch, compression
- **infectious**: diphtheria, mumps, influenza, malaria, syphilis, typhoid, typhus, dysentery, TB, gonorrhea
- **toxic/metabolic**: DM, rheumatic fever, gout, leukemia, PAN, vitamin deficiency, drug reaction, heavy metals, carbon monoxide

Investigations
- radiologic (C-spine, chest/bone x-rays, myelogram, CT, MRI), bloodwork (CSF)
- electrophysiological studies (EMG, nerve conduction velocities (NCV)) may be helpful in assessing nerve integrity and monitoring recovery, not helpful 2-3 weeks post-injury

Complications
- **neuropathic pain**: with neuroma formation
- **Complex Regional Pain Syndrome**: with sympathetic nervous system involvement

Treatment
- **of laceration**:
    - surgical repair of nerve sheath unless known to be intact (suture nerve sheaths directly if ends approximate or nerve graft (usually sural nerve))
    - clean laceration: early exploration and repair
    - contamination/associated injuries: tag initially with nonabsorbable suture, reapproach within 10 days
- **of stretch/contusion**:
    - follow-up clinically for recovery; exploration if no recovery in 3 months
- **of axonometric**:
    - if no evidence of recovery, resect damaged segment
- prompt physical therapy and rehabilitation to increase muscle function, maintain joint range of motion, and maximize return of useful function
- recovery usually incomplete

Differential Diagnosis for Peripheral Neuropathy – "DANG THERAPIST"
Diabetes or Drugs
Alcohol or AIDS
Nutritional (B$_{12}$ deficiency)
Guillain-Barré Syndrome
Traumatic
Hereditary (Refsum's)
Endocrine or Entrapment
Renal (uremia)
Amyloid
Porphyria
Infectious
Sarcoid
Toxins

Nerve Entrapment

- **definition**: nerve compressed by nearby anatomic structures, often secondary to localized, repetitive mechanical trauma with additional vascular injury to nerve
- **clinical features**: sensory loss in nerve distribution (often discriminative touch lost first)

Carpal Tunnel Syndrome (CTS)
- see Plastic Surgery

Ulnar Nerve Entrapment at Elbow
- **etiology**: may be entrapped at several locations:
    - behind medial epicondyle
    - at medial intermuscular septum
    - distal to elbow at cubital tunnel
- **epidemiology**: second most common entrapment neuropathy
- **clinical features**
    - sensory: pain, numbness in ulnar 1.5 fingers
    - wasting of interossei (especially first dorsal interosseous)
    - weakness (especially abduction of index finger) – Wartenberg's sign
    - claw hand
    - ± Tinel's sign from percussion of elbow (does not localize site of entrapment)
    - dislocation of ulnar nerve may be palpated at medial epicondyle with elbow flexion/extension
- **investigations**: NCV → conduction delay across elbow

- treatment
  - conservative: prevent repeated minor trauma (e.g. leaning on elbow or sleeping with hand under head), elbow pads, NSAIDs
  - surgical: nerve decompression and transposition anterior to medial epicondyle

Less Common Entrapments

- **brachial plexus**
  - Erb's palsy ("Bellhop's tip position"): C5-6 injury; arm hangs at side, internally rotated, extension at elbow
  - Klumpky's palsy: C8-T1 injury; clawed hand and wasting of small muscles of hand, ± flexed elbow
- **thoracic outlet syndrome**
  - compression of the lower portion of the brachial plexus (which supplies the ulnar nerve) as it emerges from the axilla, through a narrow passage beneath the clavicle and between the anterior and middle scalene muscles, while resting on the first rib
  - CXR to rule out Pancoast tumour (associated with Horner's syndrome) as this may mimic thoracic outlet syndrome, congenital cervical rib
- **radial nerve ("Saturday Night Palsy")**
  - more often a pressure palsy (compression of axilla)
  - weakness of wrist and finger extensors (normal triceps)
- **motor branch of ulnar nerve at wrist (Guyon's canal)**
  - same as ulnar nerve entrapment but no sensory deficit on dorsum of hand
- **common peroneal nerve**
  - superficial and fixed behind fibular neck (sensitive to trauma, e.g. fracture)
  - motor: decreased foot and toe extension ("foot drop"), decreased ankle eversion
  - sensory: decreased lateral foot and dorsum (less common)
- **lateral cutaneous femoral nerve of the thigh ("meralgia paraesthetica")**
  - pain over anterior/lateral aspect of thigh
  - common in obese people, patients post-iliac bone grafts
- **posterior tibial nerve ("tarsal tunnel")**
  - pain/paresthesia in toes and sole of foot ± clawing of toes (Tinel's sign over medial malleolus)

SPECIALTY TOPICS

Neurotrauma

Trauma Management (see also <u>Emergency Medicine</u>)

Indications for intubation in trauma

1. depressed level of consciousness (patient cannot protect airway): usually GCS less than 8
2. need for hyperventilation
3. severe maxillofacial trauma: patency of airway is doubtful
4. need for pharmacologic paralysis for evaluation or management
   - if basal skull fracture is possible, avoid nasotracheal intubation, instead use orotracheal intubation
   - intubation prevents patient's ability to verbalize for determining GCS

Trauma Assessment

INITIAL MANAGEMENT

ABC's of trauma management take priority

- see <u>Emergency Medicine</u>

Glasgow Coma Scale		
Eye Response	**Verbal Response**	**Motor Response**
4 spontaneous	5 oriented	6 obeys commands
3 opens eyes to voice	4 confused	5 localizes to pain
2 opens eye to pain	3 inappropriate words	4 withdraws from pain
1 no eye opening	2 incomprehensible sounds	3 flexion to pain (decorticate posturing)
	1 no response	2 extension to pain (decerebrate posturing)
		1 no response

Assessment of Spine CT/Xray (parasagittal view) - "ABCDS"
Alignment (Columns: anterior vertebral line, posterior vertebral line, spinolaminar line, posterior spinous line)
Bone (vertebral bodies, facets, spinous processes)
Cartilage
Disc (disc space and interspinous space)
Soft tissues

NEUROLOGICAL ASSESSMENT

Mini-History
- period of LOC, post traumatic amnesia, loss of sensation/function, type of injury/accident

Neurological Exam
- Glasgow Coma Scale (GCS)
- head and neck (lacerations, bruises, basal skull fracture signs, facial fractures, foreign bodies)
- spine (palpable deformity, midline pain/tenderness)
- eyes (pupillary size and reactivity)
- brainstem (breathing pattern, CN palsies)
- cranial nerve exam
- motor exam, sensory exam (only if GCS is 15), reflexes
- sphincter tone
- record and repeat neurological exam at regular intervals

Investigations
- spinal injury precautions (cervical collar) are continued until c-spine is cleared
- C,T,L-spine x-rays
  - AP, lateral, odontoid views for C-spine (must see from C1 to T1 (swimmer's view if necessary) or CT
  - rarely done: oblique views looking for pars interarticularis fracture ("Scottie dog" sign)
- CT head and upper C-spine (whole C-spine if patient unconscious) look for fractures, loss of mastoid or sinus air spaces, blood in cisterns, pneumocephalus
- cross and type, ABG, CBC, drug screen (especially alcohol)
- chest and pelvic x-ray as indicated

TREATMENT

Treatment for Minor Head Injury
- see also Canadian CT Head Rule sidebar, <u>Emergency Medicine</u>)
- observation over 24-48 hours
- wake every hour
- judicious use of sedatives or pain killers during this monitoring period

Admitting orders for Minor head injury (GCS>14)
1. activity: bed rest with head of bed elevated to 30-45 degrees
2. neuro checks q1-2h. Contact physician for neurologic deterioration. Admit to ICU for GCS less than 13
3. NPO until alert; then clear liquids
4. Isotonic IVF (eg NS with 20 meq KCl/L) run at maintenance (eg 100 cc/hr)
5. mild analgesics: acetaminophen (PO or PR if NPO), codeine if necessary
6. anti-emetic: give infrequently to avoid excessive sedation, use trimethobenzamide 200 mg IM q8h prn for adults, avoid phenothiazine anti-emetics as they lower seizure threshold

Treatment for Severe Head Injury (GCS ≤8)
- clear airway and ensure breathing (intubate if necessary)
- secure C-spine
- maintain adequate BP
- monitor to detect complications (GCS, CT, ICP)
- monitor and manage increased ICP if present (see *Herniation Syndromes*)
- rarely done:
  - pharmacotherapy: anticonvulsants x 7 days, calcium channel blocker (CCB) for adult cases only
  - repair dural tears (>7 days)

Which patients should be admitted to hospital?
- skull fracture
- indirect signs of basal skull fracture
- confusion, impaired consciousness
- focal neurological signs
- extreme headache, vomiting
- seizures
- concussion with >5 minutes amnesia
- unstable spine

Which patients need CT head or transfer to a neurosurgical center?
- remains unconscious after resuscitation
- focal neurological signs
- deteriorating

- use of alcohol
- poor social support (i.e. no friend/relative to monitor for next 24 hours)
- if there is any doubt, especially with children

KEY POINTS
- never do lumbar puncture in head injury
- all patients with head injury have C-spine injury until proven otherwise
- don't blame coma on alcohol – there may also be a hematoma
- low BP after head injury means injury elsewhere
- must clear spine both radiologically AND clinically (will require re-assessment if/when patient improves clinically)

Head Injury

Epidemiology
- male to female: 2-3:1

Head Injury can involve:
Scalp, Skull, Meninges, Brain

Pathogenesis
- acceleration/deceleration: direct impact (contusions), subdural hematoma, axon and vessel shearing/mesencephalic hematoma
- impact: skull fracture, concussion, epidural hematoma
- penetrating: high and low velocity types (> and < 300 feet/second), worse with high velocity and/or high missile mass
  - low velocity: highest damage to structures on entry/exit path
  - high velocity: highest damage away from missile tract

Etiologies:
- MVA (30-55%)
- Falls (15-35%)
- Gun Shot Wound (5-20%)

Scalp Injury
- rich blood supply
- considerable blood loss (vessels contract poorly when ruptured)
- minimal risk of infection due to rich vascularity

Skull Fractures
- depressed fractures → double density on skull x-ray (outer table of depressed segment below inner table of skull), CT with bone windows is gold standard
- simple fractures (closed injury) → no need for antibiotics, no surgery
- compound fractures (open injury) → increased risk of infection, surgical debridement within 24 hours is necessary
  - internal fractures into sinus → meningitis, pneumocephalus, risk of operative bleed may limit treatment to antibiotics
- basal skull fractures → not readily seen on x-ray, rely on clinical signs
  - retroauricular ecchymoses (Battle's sign)
  - periorbital ecchymoses (raccoon eyes)
  - hemotympanum
  - CSF rhinorrhea, otorrhea (suspect CSF if halo or target sign present) suspect with Lefort II or III midface fracture (seen on imaging)

Layers of Scalp – "SCALP"
Skin
Connective tissue (dense)
Aponeurosis (galea)
Loose connective tissue
Periosteum

Cranial Nerve Injury
- most traumatic causes of cranial nerve injury do not warrant intervention and have at least minimal improvement
- surgical intervention:
  - CN II – local eye/orbit injury
  - CN III, IV, VI – if herniation secondary to mass
  - CN VIII – repair of ossicles
- CN injuries that improve:
  - CN I – recovery may occur in a few months; most do not improve
  - CN III, IV, VI – majority recover
  - CN VII – recovery with delayed lesions
  - CN VIII – vestibular symptoms improve over weeks, deafness usually permanent (except when resulting from hemotympanum)

Arterial Injury
- e.g. carotid-cavernous (C-C) fistula, carotid/vertebral artery dissection

Intracranial Bleeding
(see *Blood* and *Cerebrovascular Disease*)

AAN Classification
Grade 1: altered mental status <15 min
Grade 2: altered mental status > 15 min
Grade 3: any loss of consciousness

Management Associated with AAN Concussion Grades	
AAN Grade	**Management Options**
1	Examine 15min for amnesia and other symptoms
	Return to normal activity if symptoms clear within 15 mins
2	Remove from activity for 1 day, then reexamine
	CT or MRI if H/A or other symptoms worsen or last >1 week
	Return to normal activity after 1 week without symptoms
3	Emergent neuro exam + imaging
	If initial exam is normal, may go home with close follow up
	Admit if any signs of pathology or persistent abnormal mental status
	CT or MRI if H/A or other symptoms
	If brief concussion (<1 min), return to normal activity after 1 week without symptoms
	If prolonged concussion (>1 min), return to normal activity only after 2 weeks without symptoms

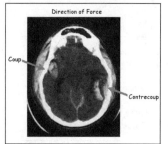

Figure 23. CT Showing Coup-Contre-Coup Injury

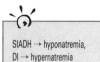

SIADH → hyponatremia,
DI → hypernatremia

Brain Injury

Primary Impact Injury
- mechanism of injury determines pathology: penetrating injuries, gunshot wounds
  - low velocity → local damage
  - high velocity → distant damage possible (due to wave of compression), concussion
- American Academy of Neurology (AAN) definition of concussion: "a trauma-induced alteration in mental status that may or may not involve loss of consciousness"
  - AAN Classification:
    - Grade 1: altered mental status <15 min
    - Grade 2: altered mental status >15 min
    - Grade 3: any loss of consciousness
  - no parenchymal abnormalities on CT
- coup (damage at site of blow)
- contre-coup (damage at opposite site of blow)
  - acute decompression causes cavitation followed by a wave of acute compression
- contusion (hemorrhagic)
  - high density areas on CT ± mass effect
  - commonly occurs with brain impact on bony prominences (inferior frontal lobe, pole of temporal lobe)
- diffuse axonal injury/shearing
  - may tear blood vessels → hemorrhagic foci
  - wide variety of damage results
  - all brain injury causes shear
  - often the cause of decreased LOC if no space occupying lesion on CT

Secondary Pathologic Processes
- same subsequent biochemical pathways for each traumatic etiology
- 1/3 of in-hospital mortalities following head injury were able to talk after the injury
- delayed and progressive injury to the brain due to:
  - high glutamate release → NMDA → cytotoxic cascade
  - cerebral edema
  - intracranial hemorrhages
  - ischemia/infarction
  - raised ICP, intracranial HTN
  - hydrocephalus

Extracranial Conditions
- hypoxemia
  - trauma: chest, upper airway, brainstem
  - exceptionally damaging to traumatized brain cells
  - leads to ischemia, raised ICP
- hypercarbia
  - leads to raised ICP (secondary to vasodilation)
- systemic hypotension
  - caused by blood loss, not by head injury (e.g. ruptured spleen)
  - cerebral autoregulation lost in trauma
  - leads to decreased CPP, ischemia
- hyperpyrexia
  - leads to increased brain metabolic demands → ischemia
- fluid and electrolyte imbalance
  - iatrogenic (most common)
  - syndrome of inappropriate antidiuretic hormone (SIADH) secretion (from head injury)
  - diabetes insipidus (DI) from head injury
  - may lead to cerebral edema and raised ICP
- coagulopathy

Intracranial Conditions
- raised ICP due to traumatic cerebral edema OR traumatic intracranial hemorrhage

Brain Injury Outcomes
- **mildly traumatic (GCS 13-15):** post-concussive symptoms: H/A, fatigue, dizziness nausea, blurred vision, diploplia, memory difficulty, tinnitus, irritability, low concentration; 50% at 6 weeks, 14% at 1 year
- **moderately traumatic (GCS 9-12):** proportional to age (>40) and CT findings; 60% good recovery, 26% moderately disabled, 7% severely disabled, 7% vegetative/dead
- **severe (GCS < 8):** difficult to predict, proportional to post-resuscitation GCS (especially motor) and age

Late Complications of Head/Brain Injury

- seizures:
  - 5% of head injury patients develop seizures
  - incidence related to severity and location of injury → increased with local brain damage or intracranial hemorrhage
  - post-traumatic seizure may be immediate, early, or late
  - presence of early (within first week) post-traumatic seizure raises incidence of late seizures to 25%
- meningitis: associated with CSF leak from nose or ear
- hydrocephalus: acute hydrocephalus or delayed normal pressure hydrocephalus (NPH)

Spinal Cord Injury

- see Orthopaedics and Emergency Medicine

Spinal Shock
This term is often used in 2 completely different senses:
1. Hypotension (shock) that follows spinal cord injury (SBP usually equal to or less than 80 mmHg) caused by
   - interruption of sympathetics (leaving parasympathetics unopposed with loss of vascoconstrictors) below the level of injury
   - loss of muscle tone due to skeletal muscle paralysis below level of injury results in venous pooling and thus a relative hypovolemia
   - blood loss from associated wounds – true hypovolemia

2. Transient loss of all neurologic function below the level of the spinal cord injury, causing flaccid paralysis and areflexia for varying periods

Whiplash-associated disorders
- **definition**: traumatic injury to the soft tissue structures in the region of the cervical spine due to hyperflexion, hyperextension or rotational injury to the neck

Initial management of spinal cord injury
- the major causes of death in spinal cord injury (SCI) are aspiration and shock
- any of the following patients should be treated as having a SCI until proven otherwise:
  - all victims of significant trauma
  - minor trauma patients with decreased LOC or complaints referable to neck or back pain or SCI (weakness, abdominal breathing, numbness or tingling, priapism-sign of autonomic dysfunction)

Stabilization and initial evaluation in the hospital
1. **Immobilization**: maintain backboard/head-strap and use log-rolling during transfers
2. **Hypotension**: maintain sBP greater than 90 mmHg with:
   - pressors if necessary: dopamine is agent of choice (avoid phenylephrine-causes bradycardia)
   - careful hydration (cautiously to prevent pulmonary edema)
   - atropine (for bradycardia associated with hypotension)
3. **Oxygenation**
4. **NG tube to suction**: prevents nausea and vomiting, decompresses abdomen to facilitate breathing
5. **Foley catheter** to urometer (to monitor ins and outs)
6. **DVT prophylaxis**
7. **Temperature regulation**
8. **Monitor electrolytes**
9. **Focused history:**
   - mechanism of injury (hyperflexion, extension, axial loading, etc),
   - weakness/numbness/tingling in extremities
10. **Palpate spine for:**
    - point tenderness
    - a "step-off" deformity
    - widened interspinous space
11. **Motor level assessment:**
    - skeletal muscle exam (to assess myotome power)
    - rectal exam for voluntary anal sphincter contraction

12. **Sensory level assessment:**
   - sensation to pinprick – tests spinothalamic tract to localize dermatome
   - test sensation in face – spinal trigeminal tract can sometimes descend as low as C4
   - light touch – tests anterior spinothalamic tract (anterior cord)
   - proprioception/joint position sense (tests posterior columns)
13. **Evaluation of reflexes**
14. **Signs of autonomic dysfunction:** altered levels of perspiration, bowel or bladder incontinence, persistent penile erection (priapism)
15. **Radiographic evaluation:**
   - 3 view C-spine x-rays (AP, lateral and odontoid) to adequately visualize C1 to C7-T1 junction
   - oblique views to assess integrity of articular masses and lamina
   - flexion – extension views to disclose occult instability
   - CT scan – helpful in identifying bony injuries
   - MRI – utility limited to specific situations
16. **Medical management specific to spinal cord injury:** Methylprednisolone (given within 8 hours of injury is an option)

Fractures of the Spine

Fractures and fracture-dislocations of the thoracic, thoracolumbar and lumbar spine
- assess ligamentous instability using flexion/extension x-ray views of C-spine ± MRI
- thoracolumbar spine unstable if 4/6 segments disrupted (3 columns divided into left and right)
   - anterior column: anterior half of vertebral body, disc and anterior longitudinal ligament
   - middle column: posterior half of vertebral body, disc and posterior longitudinal ligament
   - posterior column: posterior arch, facet joints, pedicle, lamina and supraspinous, interpinous and ligamentum flavum ligaments

Types of injury
- burst fracture:
   - stable: anterior and middle columns parted with bone retropulsed close to spinal cord (seen on x-ray and CT); posterior column is uninjured
   - unstable: same as the stable but with posterior column disruption; hallmark is pedicle widening on AP X-ray
- compression fracture
   - produced by flexion
   - posterior ligament complex (supraspinous and interspinous ligament, ligamentum flavum and intervertebral joint capsules) remain intact
   - fractures are stable but lead to kyphotic deformity

- **Investigations:** AP and lateral X-rays of the spine, CT scan, MRI

- **Treatment:**
   - minor stable fractures without neurologic involvement
      - bed rest (few days) with minimal analgesia
      - Jewett brace to immobilize fractured segments
      - early flexion-extension physiotherapy with brace
      - early ambulation
   - fractures that are unstable and/or with neurologic deficit
      - consider surgery (ORIF, decompression ± fusion)

Fractures of the Cervical Spine
- C1 vertebral fracture (Jefferson fracture):
   - vertical compression force can push the occipital condyles of the skull down on C1 vertebral (atlas), thus pushing lateral masses of the atlas outward and disrupt ring of the atlas
   - same mechanism can produce an occipital condylar fracture
- odontoid process fracture:
   - causes C1 and odontoid of C2 to move independently of C2 body
   - this occurs because:
      - normally C1 vertebra and odontoid of C2 are a single functional unit
      - alar and transverse ligaments on posterior aspect of odontoid most commonly remain intact following injury
   - patients often report feeling of instability and present by holding their head with their hands
- C2 vertebral fracture (hangman fracture, traumatic spondylolisthesis of axis):
   - bilateral fracture through the pars interarticularis of C2 with subluxation of C2 on C3
   - usually neurologically intact

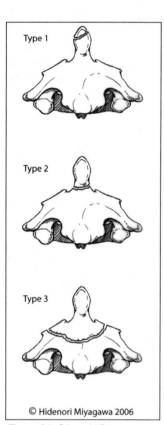

Type 1

Type 2

Type 3

© Hidenori Miyagawa 2006

Figure 24. Odontoid Fracture Classification

- clay shoveler's fracture:
  - avulsion of spinous process, usually C7
- **Imaging**: AP spine X-ray (open-mouth and lateral view), CT
- **Treatment**:
  - immobilization in cervical collar or halo vest until healing occurs, usually in 2-3 months
  - Type II and III odontoid fractures
    - ◆ consider surgical fixation for comminution, displacement or inability to maintain alignment with external immobilization
  - confirm stability after recovery with flexion-extension X-rays

Neurologically Determined Death

Definition
- irreversible and diffuse brain injury resulting in absence of clinical brain function
- cardiovascular activity may persist for up to two weeks

Criteria of Diagnosis
- prerequisites: no CNS depressant drugs/neuromuscular blocking agents, no drug intoxication/poisoning, temperature >32°C, no electrolyte/acid-base/endocrine disturbance
- absent brainstem reflexes:
  - absent pupillary light reflex
  - absent corneal reflexes
  - absent oculocephalic response
  - absent caloric responses (e.g. no deviation of eyes to irrigation of each ear with 50cc of ice water – allow 1 min after injection, 5 min between sides)
  - absent pharyngeal and tracheal reflexes
  - absent cough with tracheal suctioning
  - absent respiratory drive at $PaCO_2$ >60mmHg or >20mmHg above baseline (apnea test)
- 2 evaluations separated by time, usually performed by two specialists (e.g. neurologist, anesthetist, neurosurgeon)
- confirmatory testing: flat EEG, absent perfusion assessed with cerebral angiogram

Pediatric Neurosurgery

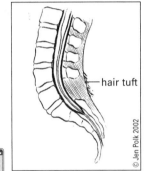

Figure 25. Spina Bifida Occulta

Spinal Dysraphism

Spina Bifida Occulta
- **definition**:
  - congenital absence of a spinous process and variable amounts of lamina
  - no visible exposure of meninges or neural tissue
- **epidemiology**: 15-20% of the general population; most common at L5 or S1
- **etiology**: failure of fusion of the posterior neural arch
- **clinical features**:
  - no obvious clinical signs
  - presence of lumbosacral cutaneous abnormalities (dimple, sinus, port-wine stain, or hair tuft) should increase suspicion of an underlying anomaly (lipoma, dermoid, diastomatomyelia)
- **investigations**:
  - plain film – absence of the spinous process along with minor amounts of the neural arch
  - U/S or MRI to exclude spinal anomalies
- **treatment**: requires no treatment

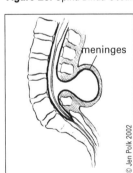

Figure 26. Meningocele

Meningocele (Spina Bifida Aperta)
- **definition**: a defect consisting of a herniation of meningeal tissue and CSF through a defect in the spine, but not neural tissue
- **etiology**:
  - primary failure of neural tube closure
- **clinical features**:
  - most common in lumbosacral area
  - usually no disability, low incidence of associated anomalies and hydrocephalus
- **investigations**: plain films, CT, MRI, U/S, echo, genitourinary (GU) investigations
- **treatment**: surgical excision and tissue repair (excellent results)

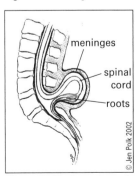

Figure 27. Myelomeningocele

Myelomeningocele
- **definition**: a defect consisting of a herniation of meningeal tissue and CNS tissue through a defect in the spine
- **etiology**: same as meningocele
- **clinical features**:
  - sensory and motor changes distal to anatomic level producing varying degrees of weakness
  - urine and fecal incontinence
  - 65-85% of patients with myelomeningocele have hydrocephalus
  - most have Type II Chiari malformation
- **investigations**: plain films, CT, MRI, U/S, echo, GU investigations
- **treatment**: surgical closure
  - indications: preserve neurologic status, prevent CNS infections
- **prognosis**:
  - operative mortality close to 0%, 95% 2-year survival
  - 80% have IQ >80 (but most are 80-95), 40-85% ambulatory, 3-10% have normal urinary continence
  - most common cause of early mortality are complications from Chiari malformation (respiratory arrest and aspiration), whereas late mortality is due to shunt malfunction

Intraventricular Hemorrhage (IVH)

- see Pediatrics

Hydrocephalus in Pediatrics

Etiology
- congenital
  - aqueductal anomalies, primary aqueductal stenosis in infancy
  - secondary gliosis due to intrauterine viral infections (mumps, varicella, TORCH)
  - Dandy-Walker malformation (2-4%)
  - Chiari malformation, especially Type II
  - myelomeningocele
- acquired
  - post meningitis
  - post hemorrhage (SAH, IVH)
  - masses (vascular malformation, neoplastic)

Clinical Features
- symptoms and signs of hydrocephalus are age related in pediatrics
- increased head circumference (HC), bulging anterior fontanelle, widened cranial sutures
- irritability, lethargy, poor feeding and vomiting
- "cracked pot" sound on cranial percussion
- scalp vein dilation (increased collateral venous drainage)
- sunset sign – forced downward deviation of eyes
- episodic bradycardia and apnea

Investigations
- skull x-ray, U/S, CT, MRI, ICP monitoring

Treatment
- similar to adults (see *Hydrocephalus*)

Dandy-Walker Malformation

Definition
- atresia of foramina of Magendie and Luschka, resulting in:
  - complete or incomplete agenesis of the cerebellar vermis with widely separated, hypoplastic cerebellar hemisphere
  - posterior fossa cyst, enlarged posterior fossa
  - dilatation of 4th ventricle (also 3rd and lateral ventricles)

- associated anomalies
  - hydrocephalus (90%)
  - agenesis of corpus callosum (17%)
  - occipital encephalocele (7%)

Epidemiology
- 2-4% of pediatric hydrocephalus

Clinical Features
- 20% are asymptomatic, seizures occur in 15%
- symptoms and signs of hydrocephalus combined with a prominent occiput in infancy
- ataxia, spasticity, poor fine motor control common in childhood

Investigations
- skull x-ray, CT

Treatment
- asymptomatic patients require no treatment
- associated hydrocephalus requires surgical treatment
- supratentorial lateral ventricular or cystoperitoneal shunt

- **Prognosis**: 75-100% survival, 50% have normal IQ

Chiari Malformations

Definition
- malformations at the medullary-spinal junction

Etiology
- unclear, likely maldevelopment/dysgenesis during fetal life

Categories
- **Type I (cerebellar ectopia):**
  - definition: cerebellar tonsils lie below the level of the foramen magnum
  - epidemiology: average age at presentation 41 years
  - clinical features:
    - many are asymptomatic
    - scoliosis
    - brain compression
    - **central cord syndrome** (65%)
    - syringomyelia (50%)
    - foramen magnum compression syndrome (22%)
    - cerebellar syndrome (11%)
    - hydrocephalus (10%)
- **Type II:**
  - definition: part of cerebellar vermis, medulla and 4th ventricle extend through the foramen magnum often to midcervical region
  - epidemiology: present in infancy
  - clinical features: findings due to brainstem and lower cranial nerve dysfunction
    - syringomyelia, hydrocephalus in >80%

Investigations
- MRI or CT myelography

Treatment
- indications for surgical decompression:
  - Type I: symptomatic patients (early surgery recommended; <2 years post symptom onset) → suboccipital craniectomy, duroplasty
  - Type II: neurogenic dysphagia, stridor, apneic spells → cervical laminectomy, duroplasty

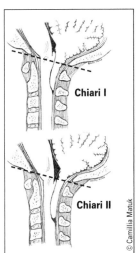

Figure 28. Chiari Malformations

Craniosynostosis

Definition
- premature closure of the cranial suture(s)

Classification
- **sagittal (most common)**: long narrow head with ridging sagittal suture (scaphocephaly)
- coronal: expansion in superior and lateral direction (brachiocephaly)
- metopic (trigonocephaly)
- lambdoid: least common

Epidemiology
- 0.6/1,000 live births, most cases are sporadic, familial incidence is 2% of sagittal and 8% of coronal synostosis

Clinical Features
- skull deformity, raised ICP, ± hydrocephalus
- ophthalmologic problems due to increased ICP or bony abnormalities of the orbit

Investigations
- plain radiographs, CT scan

Treatment
- parental counseling about nature of deformity, difficulty growing up as "cone head", associated neurological symptoms
- surgery for cosmetic purposes, except in cases of elevated ICP (≥2 sutures involved)

Pediatric Brain Tumours

Relative frequency of pediatric brain tumours	
Tumour type	**Percent**
Astrocytoma, low-grade	40
Supratentorial	(23)
Infratentorial	(17)
Medulloblastoma	20
Brainstem glioma	8
Ependymoma	8
Malignant glioma	6
Craniopharyngioma	6
PNET	4
Pineal, germ cell tumour	3
Other	5

Reprinted from Pediatric Clinics of North America, Vol. 44(4), Kun LE, Brain Tumors: challenges and directions, pp. 907-17. Copyright 1997, with permission from Elsevier.

- see also *Tumour*

Epidemiology
- 20% of all pediatric cancers (second only to leukemia)
- **60% of pediatric tumours are infratentorial**
- pediatric brain tumours arise from various cellular lineages:
  - glia: **low-grade astrocytoma** (supra- or infratentorial), anaplastic astrocytoma, glioblastoma multiforme (largely supratentorial) (see *Astrocytoma* for details)
  - primitive nerve cells: supratentorial (primitive neuroectodermal tumour, PNET) 90% of neonatal brain tumours), infratentorial (medulloblastoma), pineal gland (pineoblastoma)
  - non-neuronal cells: germ cell tumour, craniopharyngioma, dermoid, meningioma, neurinoma, pituitary adenoma, others

Clinical Features
- vomiting, seizure, macrocrania, hydrocephalus
- developmental delay, poor feeding, failure to thrive
- often escape diagnosis initally due to expansile cranium and neural plasticity in children

Functional Neurosurgery

Surgical Treatment of the following disorders (see Neurology for details)
- Parkinson's disease and tremor
- spasticity (including dystonias)
- surgical management of pain

Common Medications

The following are guidelines ONLY; follow clinical judgment and up-to-date prescription recommendations in practice; dosages refer to adults unless otherwise specified

Table 8. Common Medications

Drug Name	Dosing Schedule	Indications	Side Effects	Common Interactions	Contraindications	Comments
lorazepam (Ativan™)	4 mg IV over 2 minutes, q10-15 minutes (do not exceed 8 mg/12hr)	Status epilepticus	• drowsiness, sedation	• other CNS depressants, digoxin (increases digoxin levels)		• start phenytoin loading simultaneously
carbamazepine (Tegretol™)	**Tic douloureux** (Trigeminal neuralgia): 100 mg PO bid, increase by 200 mg/day up to a maximum of 1,200 mg/day 200 mg tid) **Seizures:** 200 mg PO bid, increase by 200 mg (inpatient: q3 days; outpatient: q7 days) until therapeutic level achieved (usual optimum dosage: 800-1,200 mg/day; range: 600-2,000 mg/day)	Tic douloureux (Trigeminal neuralgia) Seizures	• worsening of seizures, heart failure, arrhythmias, AV block, aplastic anemia, agranulocytosis, thrombocytopenia, hepatitis, erythema multiforme, Stevens-Johnson syndrome	• lithium (increases lithium toxicity), MAOI other meds may increase carbamazepine levels or have decreased effects	• hypersensitivity to TCAs, previous bone marrow suppression, MAOI in past 14 days	• monitor CBC (potential hematological toxicity)
phenytoin (Dilantin™)	**Seizures:** Loading dose: 18mg/kg slow IV or 300-600 mg PO/day divided bid/tid, Maintenance: 200-500 mg IV/day (max. rate: <40-50 mg/min or 300 mg PO q4h); average maintenance dose: 300 mg/day PO **Status epilepticus:** 200 mg IV over 30 minutes (~ 20 mg/kg; if not taking regularly), or 500 mg IV over 10 minutes (if already on phenytoin)	Seizures Status epilepticus	• thrombocytopenia, leukopenia, agranulocytosis, pancytopenia, toxic hepatitis, Stevens-Johnson syndrome, toxic epidermal necrolysis	• other meds may increase phenytoin levels and toxicity or have decreased effects	• bradyarrhythmias, heart block	• important to give over time to prevent causing a cardiac arrest
dexamethasone (Decadron™)	Loading dose: 10-20 mg IV; Maintenance: 4-6 mg IV/day divided qid (may be PO)	Cerebral edema (e.g. secondary to tumour, head injury, pseudotumour cerebri) Preoperative preparation for patients with increased ICP secondary to brain neoplasms	• pseudotumour cerebri, seizures, heart failure, arrhythmias, thromboembolism, pancreatitis, acute adrenal insufficiency; avoid abrupt withdrawal	• aminoglutethimide, antidiabetics, ASA, NSAIDs, barbituates, phenytoin, rifampin, cardiac glycosides, cyclosporine, ephedrine, oral anticoagulants, potassium-depleting drugs, salicylates, skin-testing antigens, toxoids, vaccines	• systemic fungal infections, immunosuppressive dose with live virus vaccines	• no longer used in acute spinal cord injury
mannitol	1-1.5 g/kg IV rapid infusion (350 mL of 20% solution) followed by 0.25 g/kg IV q6h	Raised ICP	• seizures, heart failure	• lithium (increases excretion of lithium)	• anuria, severe pulmonary congestion, frank pulmonary edema, severe heart failure, severe dehydration, metabolic edema, progressive renal disease or dysfunction, active intracranial bleeding except during craniotomy	• effect occurs in 1-5 mins, maximal at 20-60 mins • often alternated with furosemide 10-20 mg IV q6h • indwelling urinary catheter to measure ins and outs
nimodipine (Nimotop™)	60 mg PO/NG q4h x 21 days started within 96 hours of SAH	Vasospasm in SAH	• decreased blood pressure, tachycardia, dyspnea	• antihypertensives (may increase hypotensive effects), CCB (may increase effects), cimetidine (increases nimodipine bioavailability)	• none known	• causes vasodilation • only calcium channel blocker (CCB) to cross BBB (blood brain barrier) • use half the normal dose for liver failure; monitor BP always

Notes

OB — Obstetrics

Priscilla Che, Annie Keeler and Melissa Vyvey, chapter editors
Justine Chan and Angela Ho, associate editors
Billie Au, EBM Editor
Dr. Filomena Meffe, staff editor

Basic Anatomy Review

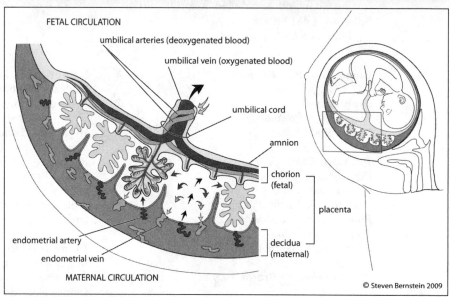

Figure 1. Placenta Blood Flow

Pregnancy

Diagnosis of Pregnancy

History

- obstetrical and gynecological history
  - obtain the year, location, mode of delivery, duration of labour, sex, gestational age, weight at birth and complications of every pregnancy; organize into **GTPAL** format:
    - Gravidity (G)
      - total number of pregnancies of any gestation
      - includes current pregnancy, abortions, ectopic pregnancies, and hydatidiform moles (twins = one pregnancy)
    - Parity (TPAL)
      - **T**: number of term infants delivered (>37 weeks)
      - **P**: number of premature infants delivered (20-37 weeks)
      - **A**: number of abortions (loss of intrauterine pregnancy prior to viability of fetus <20 weeks and/or <500 g fetal weight) – induced (therapeutic) and spontaneous (miscarriage)
      - **L**: number of living children
- symptoms: amenorrhea, nausea and/or vomiting, breast tenderness, urinary frequency, fatigue

Physical Signs

- Goodell's sign: softening of the cervix (4-6 weeks)
- Chadwick's sign: bluish discolouration of the cervix and vagina due to pelvic vasculature engorgement (6 weeks)
- Hegar's sign: softening of the cervical isthmus (6-8 weeks)
- uterine enlargement

Investigations

- β-hCG: peptide hormone composed of alpha and beta subunits produced by placental trophoblastic cells – maintains the corpus luteum during pregnancy
  - positive in serum 9 days post-conception, positive in urine 28 days after last menstrual period (LMP)
  - plasma levels double every 1-2 days, peak at 8-10 weeks, then fall to a plateau until delivery
    - levels less than expected by dates suggest ectopic pregnancy, abortion, or wrong dates
    - levels higher than expected suggest multiple gestation, molar pregnancy, trisomy 21, or wrong dates

---

Trimesters
- T1 (first trimester): 0-12 wks
- T2 (second trimester): 12-28 wks
- T3 (third trimester): 28-40 wks
- Normal pregnancy term: 37-42 wks

β-hCG Rule of 10s
10 IU at time of missed menses
100000 IU at 10 weeks (peak)
10000 IU at term

- U/S
  - transvaginal
    - 5 weeks: gestational sac visible (β-hCG $\geq$ 1200-1500 mIU/ml)
    - 6 weeks: fetal pole seen
    - 7-8 weeks: fetal heart tones visible
  - transabdominal
    - 6-8 weeks: intrauterine pregnancy visible (β-hCG $\geq$ 6500 mIU/mL)

Maternal Physiology

Table 1. Physiologic Changes During Pregnancy

Skin	• ↑ pigmentation of perineum and areola, chloasma (pigmentation changes under eyes and on bridge of nose), linea nigra (midline abdominal pigmentation) • other: spider angiomas, palmar erythema due to increased estrogen striae gravidarum due to connective tissue changes
Cardiovascular	• hyperdynamic circulation ↑ CO, HR and blood volume ↓ BP due to ↓ PVR • enlarging uterus compresses IVC and pelvic veins ↓ venous return leads to risk of hypotension ↑ venous pressure leads to risk of varicose veins, hemorrhoids, leg edema
Hematologic	• hemodilution causes causes physiologic anemia and apparent ↓ in hemoglobin and hematocrit • ↑ leukocyte count but impaired function leads to improvement in autoimmune diseases • gestational thrombocytopenia: mild (platelets >70000/μL) and asymptomatic, normalizes within 2-12 weeks following delivery • hypercoagulable state: ↑ risk of DVT and PE but also ↓ bleeding at delivery • resetting of the osmostat under the influence of beta-hCG leads to non-pathological hyponatremia in pregnancy
Respiratory	• ↑ incidence of nasal congestion and epistaxis • ↑ O2 consumption to meet increased metabolic requirements • elevated diaphragm i.e. patient appears more "barrel-chested" • ↑ minute ventilation leads to ↓ CO_2 with a resulting mild respiratory alkalosis that helps CO2 diffuse across the placenta and be eliminated from the fetus • no change VC and FEV1 • decreased TLC, FRC, and RV
Gastrointestinal	• GERD due to ↑ intra-abdominal pressure + progesterone (causing decreased sphincter tone and delayed gastric emptying • ↑ gallstones due to progesterone causing ↑ gallbladder stasis • constipation and hemorrhoids due to progesterone causing ↓ GI motility • atypical appendicitis presentation due to upward displacement of appendix
Genitourinary	• ↑ urinary frequency due to increased total urinary output • ↑ incidence of UTI and pyelonephritis due to urinary stasis (see *Urinary Tract Infection* section, OB22) • glycosuria: can be physiologic, must test for gestational diabetes mellitus (GDM) • ureters and renal pelvis dilation (R>L) due to progesterone-induced smooth muscle relaxation and uterine enlargement • ↑ CO and thus ↑ GFR leads to ↓ creatinine (normal in pregnancy **35-44 mmol/L**), uric acid, and BUN
Neurologic	• ↑ incidence of carpal tunnel syndrome and Bell's palsy
Endocrine	• thyroid: moderate enlargement and increased basal metabolic rate ↑ total thyroxine and thyroxine binding globulin (TBG) free thyroxine index and TSH levels are normal • adrenal: maternal cortisol rises throughout pregnancy (total and free) • calcium: ↓ total maternal Ca due to ↓ albumin free ionized Ca (i.e. active) proportion remains the same due to parathyroid hormone (PTH) which results in ↑ bone resorption and gut absorption ↑ bone turnover but no loss of bone density because estrogen inhibits resorption

Prenatal Care

- Antenatal Records 1 & 2:
  http://www.health.gov.on.ca/english/public/forms/form_menus/pubh_fm.html

Preconception Counselling

Advise all women capable of becoming pregnant to supplement their diet with 0.4 mg/day of folic acid (CTFPHC Grade II-2- A Evidence).

Foods rich in folic acid include: spinach, lentils, chick peas, asparagus, broccoli, peas, Brussels sprouts, corn and oranges.

- 3-8 weeks gestational age (GA) is a critical period of organogenesis, so early preparation is vital
- past medical history: optimize medical illnesses and necessary medications prior to pregnancy (see *Medical Conditions in Pregnancy* section, OB11 and *Drugs in Pregnancy* section, OB56)
- supplementation
  - encourage diet rich in folic acid and supplement folic acid 8-12 wks preconception to prevent neural tube defects (NTDs) (0.4-1 mg daily in all women, 5 mg if past NTD, anti-epileptic medications, diabetes mellitus or BMI >35 kg/m²) and continue for first trimester of pregnancy
  - iron supplementation (especially if anemic), prenatal vitamins
- risk modification (see Antenatal Records 1 and 2 for details)
  - lifestyle: balanced nutrition and physical fitness
  - infection screening: rubella, HBsAg, VDRL, Pap smear, gonorrhea/chlamydia, HIV, toxoplasmosis, CMV, TB, varicella
  - genetic testing as appropriate for high risk groups (e.g. Tay-Sachs, sickle cell, thalassemia)
  - social: alcohol, smoking, drug use, domestic violence – use Antenatal Psychosocial Health Assessment (ALPHA) form to screen for antenatal risk factors associated with poor postpartum family outcomes (woman abuse, child abuse, postpartum depression, marital dysfunction and increased physical illness)

Initial Prenatal Visit

- within 12 weeks of the LMP or earlier if <20 or >35 years old
- fill out antenatal forms 1 and 2

History

Ask every woman about abuse – not just those whose situations raise suspicion of abuse AND ask as early as possible in pregnancy.

- gestational age by dates from the first day of the LMP
- if LMP unreliable, get a dating ultrasound (see below)
- estimated date of confinement (EDC) using **Naegle's Rule**
  - **1st day of LMP + 7 days – 3 months**
  - e.g. LMP = 1 Apr 2001, EDC = 8 Jan 2002 (modify if cycle >28 days by adding number of days >28)
- history of present pregnancy (any problems)
- history of all previous pregnancies: GTPAL/year/sex/weight/gestational age/mode of delivery/length of labour/complications
- gynecological, past medical history
- prescription and non-prescription drugs
- family history: genetic disease, birth defects, multiple gestation
- social history: smoking, alcohol, drug use, domestic violence (use ALPHA form)

Physical Examination

- complete exam to obtain baseline
- BP and weight important for interpreting subsequent changes
- pelvic exam

Investigations

- bloodwork
  - CBC, blood group and type, Rh antibodies, infection screening as per preconception counselling
- urine R&M, C&S
  - bacteriuria & proteinuria
- pelvic exam
  - Pap smear (unless done within last 6-12 mo), culture for *N. gonorrheae* (GC) and *C. trachomatis,* bacterial vaginosis (BV) swab

Counselling

- exercise
  - under physician guidance
  - absolute contraindications:
    - ◆ ruptured membranes, preterm labour, hypertensive disorders of pregnancy, incompetent cervix, IUGR, multiple gestation (>3), placenta previa after 28th week, persistent 2nd or 3rd trimester bleeding, uncontrolled type I diabetes, thyroid disease, or other serious cardiovascular, respiratory, or systemic disorder
  - relative contraindications:
    - ◆ previous spontaneous abortion, previous preterm birth, mild/moderate cardiovascular or respiratory disorder, anemia (Hb ≤100 g/L), malnutrition or eating disorder, twin pregnancy after 28th week, other significant medical conditions
- nutrition
  - Canada's Food Guide to Healthy Eating suggests:
    - ◆ 3-4 servings of milk products daily (greater if multiple gestation)
    - ◆ a daily caloric increase of ~100 cal/d in the 1st trimester, ~300 cal/d in the second and third trimesters and ~450 cal/d during lactation
  - daily multivitamin should be continued in the second trimester for women who do not consume an adequate diet (avoid excess vitamin A)
  - iron is the only known nutrient for which requirements during pregnancy can not be met by diet alone (see *Iron Deficiency Anemia* section, OB11)
- nutrients important during pregnancy
  - folate – supports maternal increase in blood volume, growth of maternal and fetal tissue, decreases incidence of neural tube defects
    - ◆ 0.4-5 mg per day
  - calcium – maintains integrity of maternal bones, skeletal development of fetus, breast milk production
    - ◆ 1200-1500 mg per day
  - vitamin D – absorption of calcium
    - ◆ 200 IU or 5 μg per day
  - iron – supports maternal increase in blood cell mass, supports fetal and placental tissue
    - ◆ 0.8 mg/d in T1, 4-5 mg/d in T2 and >6 mg/d in T3
    - ◆ amounts exceed normal body stores and typical intake, and therefore should give supplemental iron
  - essential fatty acids (EFA) – supports fetal neural and visual development
    - ◆ contained in vegetable oils, margarines, peanuts, fatty fish
- weight gain: optimal gain depends on pre-pregnancy weight (varies from 6.8-18.2 kg)
- work: strenuous work, extended hours and shift work during pregnancy may be associated with greater risk of low birth weight, prematurity, and spontaneous abortion
- travel: not harmful per se, but stress related to travel may be associated with preterm labour
- air travel is acceptable in the second trimester but discouraged after 36 weeks
- sexual intercourse: may continue except in patients at risk for abortion, preterm labour, or placenta previa. Breast stimulation may induce uterine activity and is discouraged in high-risk patients near term
- address social issues including physical or sexual abuse
- smoking: assist/encourage all who smoke to reduce or quit
- alcohol: encourage avoidance of alcohol during pregnancy
- genetic screening must be offered to all women (see *Prenatal Screening* section, OB8 and *Chromosomal Screening* section, OB10)

Vital nutrients during pregnancy:
- Folate*
- Calcium
- Vitamin D
- EFA
- Iron*

*Nutrients that require supplementation

Expected weight gain:

BMI (kg/m²)	Weight (kg)
< 19	12.7-18.2
19-25	11.3-15.9
>25	6.8-11.3

General Rule: 1-3.5 kg during T1, then 0.45 kg/week until delivery

Subsequent Prenatal Visits

Timing
- for uncomplicated pregnancies, q4-6 weeks until 28 weeks, q2 weeks from 28 to 36 weeks and q weekly from 36 weeks until delivery

Assess at Every Visit
- history: estimate GA; history of present pregnancy: fetal movements, uterine bleeding, leaking, cramping
- physical exam: BP, weight gain, symphysis fundal height (SFH), Leopold's maneuvers (T3) for lie, position and presentation of fetus
- investigations: urinalysis for glucosuria, ketones, proteinuria; fetal heart tones starting at 12 weeks using Doppler U/S

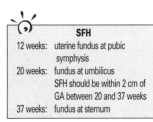

SFH	
12 weeks:	uterine fundus at pubic symphysis
20 weeks:	fundus at umbilicus
	SFH should be within 2 cm of GA between 20 and 37 weeks
37 weeks:	fundus at sternum

Leopold's Manoeuvers
- first manoeuver: to determine which fetal part is lying furthest away from the pelvic inlet
    - palpate upper abdomen with both hands; the consistency, mobility, and and shape of the form palpated is noted
    - head: moves independently of the trunk, is round and firm
    - buttocks: moves with the trunk, is softer and has bony processes
- second manoeuver: to determine the location of the fetal back
    - one hand remains steady on a side of the abdomen while the other hand palpates the other side
    - the fetal back will feel smooth, while the limbs will feel like protrusions
- third manoeuver (Pawlick's Grip): to determine which fetal part is lying above the pelvic inlet
    - palpate the lower abdomen with thumb and fingers
    - should validate findings from the first manoeuver
- fourth manoeuver: to locate the fetal brow
    - examiner faces patient's feet
    - brow is located on the side where there is greatest resistance when fingers are moved down the side of the uterus towards the symphysis pubis
    - fetal head flexed: brow and back on opposite sides
    - fetal head extended: brow and back on the same side

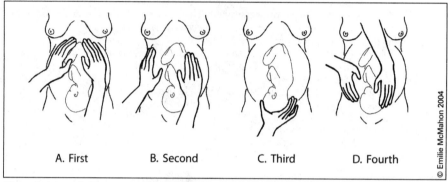

A. First   B. Second   C. Third   D. Fourth

© Emilie McMahon 2004

Figure 2. Leopold's Manoeuvers (Third Trimester)
Reprinted with permission from Essentials of Clinical Exam Handbook, 4th ed. Butalia, Ko, Lam, Tan.

Prenatal Fetal Monitoring

Fetal Movements
- first noticed by 18-20 wks (primigravidas), 14-16 wks (multigravidas)
- if mother concerned about ↓ movement: mother chooses a time when fetus is normally active to count movements
    - if <6 movements in 2 hours, try drinking juice, eating, changing position or moving to a quiet room and count for another 2 hours
    - if decreased movement persists, notify MD

NON-STRESS TEST (NST)

Definition
- fetal heart rate (FHR) tracing using an external Doppler to assess FHR and its relationship to fetal movement (see *Fetal Monitoring in Labour* section, OB36)

Indication
- any suggestion of uteroplacental insufficiency or suspected fetal distress

Operating Characteristics
- false positive rate depends on duration; false negative rate = 0.2-0.3%

Interpretation
- reassuring NST (normal result): at least 2 accelerations of FHR >15 bpm from the baseline lasting ≥15 seconds, in 20 minutes
- non-reassuring NST (abnormal/positive result): <2 such FHR accelerations in 40 minutes
    - if no observed accelerations or fetal movement in the first 20 minutes, stimulate fetus (fundal pressure, acoustic/vibratory stimulation) and continue monitoring for 30 minutes
    - if NST nonreactive, then perform biophysical profile (BPP)

DDx of Decreased Fetal Movements
DASH:
Death of fetus
Amniotic fluid decreased
Sleep cycle of fetus
Hunger/Thirst

Table 2. Classifying NST Results

Parameter	Normal NST (Previously "Reactive")	Atypical NST (Previously "Non-Reactive")	Abnormal NST (Previously "Non-Reactive")
Baseline	110-160 bpm	100-110 bpm >160 bpm for <30 min Rising baseline	Bradycardia <100 bpm Tachycardia >160 for >30min Erratic baseline
Variability	6-25 bpm (moderate) ≤5 (absent or minimal) for <40 min	5 (absent or minimal) for 40-80 min 25 bpm for >10 min.	≤5 for = 80 min Sinusoidal
Decelerations	None or occasional variable <30 sec	Variable decelerations 30-60 sec duration	Variable decelerations >60 sec duration Late deceleration(s)
Accelerations in Term Fetus	2 accelerations with acme of ≥15 bpm, lasting 15 sec. over <40 min of testing	2 accelerations with acme of ≥15 bpm, lasting 15 sec. in 40-80 min	<2 accelerations with acme of 15 bpm, lasting 15 sec. in >80 min
Accelerations in Preterm Fetus (<32 weeks)	>2 accelerations with acme of >10 bpm, lasting 10 sec. in <40 min	<2 accelerations with acme of >10 bpm, lasting 10 sec. in 40-80 min	<2 accelerations with acme of >10 bpm lasting 10 sec. in >80 min
Action	FURTHER ASSESSMENT OPTIONAL, based on total clinical picture	FURTHER ASSESSMENT REQUIRED	URGENT ACTION REQUIRED An overall assessment of the situation and further investigation with U/S or BPP is required. Some situations will require delivery.

Reprinted with permission from SOGC, Fetal Health Surveillance: Antepartum and Intrapartum Consensus Guideline., September 2007.

BIOPHYSICAL PROFILE (BPP)

Definition
• consists of a 30 minute U/S assessment of the fetus (see Table 3) ± NST

Indication
• non-reassuring NST
• BPP is the test of choice for:
  ▪ non-reassuring NST
  ▪ post-term pregnancy
  ▪ ↓ fetal movement
  ▪ any other suggestion of fetal distress or uteroplacental insufficiency

Operating Characteristics
• false positive rate = <30%, false negative rate = 0.1%

Interpretation
• 8: perinatal mortality rate 1:1000; repeat BPP as clinically indicated
• 6: perinatal mortality 31:1000; repeat BPP in 24 hours
• 0-4: perinatal mortality rate 200:1000; deliver fetus if benefits of delivery > risk

Table 3. Scoring of the Biophysical Profile

Parameter	Reassuring (2 points)	Non-Reassuring (0 points)
AFV*	Fluid pocket of 2 cm in 2 axes	Oligohydramnios
Breathing	At least one episode of breathing lasting at least 30 seconds	No breathing
Limb Movement	Three discrete movements	Two or less
Fetal Tone	At least one episode of limb extension followed by flexion	No movement

*Amniotic fluid volume (AFV) is a marker of chronic hypoxia, all other parameters indicate acute hypoxia

Prenatal Screening

Table 4. Gestation-Dependent Screening Investigations

Gestational Age (weeks)	Investigation
8-12	Dating U/S
10-12	Chorionic Villus Sampling (CVS)
11-14	First Trimester Screening
	Integrated Prenatal Screening Part 1
11-13	Nuchal Translucency U/S
14-18 to term	Fetal Movements (Quickening)
15-16 to term	Amniocentesis
15-18	Integrated Prenatal Screening Part 2
16-18	Maternal Serum Screen
18-20	U/S for dates, structural assessment
24-28	50 g oral glucose challenge test (OGCT)
28	Repeat CBC
	RhIG for all Rh negative women
36	Rh antibody screen if indicated
	Group B Streptococcus (GBS) screen
6 weeks postpartum	Discuss contraception
	Breast & pelvic exam incl. Pap smear
	Depression/mental health

> **DDx of increased MSAFP:**
> - incorrect GA
> - >1 fetus (e.g. twins)
> - fetal demise,
> - oNTD
> - abdominal wall defects (e.g. omphalocele)
>
> **DDx of decreased MSAFP:**
> - incorrect GA
> - gestational trophoblastic neoplasia
> - missed abortion
> - chromosomal anomalies
> - maternal DMI/DMII

Ultrasound Screening

- dating ultrasound best between 8-12 weeks GA
  - measurement of crown-rump length (margin of error ± 3 days)
- nuchal translucency ultrasound (NTUS) at 11-14 weeks GA
  - measures the amount of fluid behind the neck of the fetus
  - early screen for serious congenital anomalies (Down syndrome)
- fetal growth and anatomy ultrasound routinely done at 18-20 weeks GA (margin of error ± 7 days)
- earlier or subsequent ultrasounds performed when medically indicated

Table 5. Comparison of FTS, MSS and IPS

First Trimester Screen (FTS)	Maternal Serum Screen (MSS)	Integrated Prenatal Screen (IPS)

• 11-14 wks
• measures
  1. nuchal translucency on U/S
  2. β-hCG
  3. pregnancy-associated plasma protein A (PAPP-A)
	• 15-18 wks
	• measures
	  1. maternal serum α-fetoprotein (MSAFP)
	  2. β-hCG
	  3. unconjugated estrogen (estriol or uE3)
		• nuchal translucency on 12 wk U/S
		• FTS at 11-14 wks
		• MSS at 15-18 wks

• risk estimate for
  1. Down syndrome (Trisomy 21): increased NT, increased β-hCG, decreased PAPP-A
	• risk estimate for
	  1. open neural tube defect (oNTD) ↑ MSAFP (sensitivity 80-90%)
	  2. Trisomy 21: ↓MSAFP, ↑β-hCG, ↓μE3 (sensitivity 65%)
	  3. Trisomy 18: ↓MSAFP, ↓β-hCG, ↓μE3 (sensitivity 80%)
		• risk estimate for oNTD, Trisomy 21, Trisomy 18

• useful where patient wants results within the first trimester • more accurate estimate of Down syndrome risk than MSS, sensitivity ~85% (when combined with age) • 5% false positive rate • patients with positive screen should be offered CVS or amniocentesis	• only offered alone if patient missed the time window for IPS or FTS • 8% baseline false positive rate for t21, lower for oNTD and t18 • patients with positive screen should be offered U/S or amniocentesis	• sensitivity ~85% • 2% false positive rate • patients with positive screen should be offered U/S and/or amniocentesis

> **Risk Factors for Neural Tube Defects (GRIMM)**
> - **G**enetics: family history of NTD (risk of having second child with NTD is increased to 2-5%), consanguinity, chromosomal (characteristic of trisomy 13, 18, and 21)
> - **R**ace: European Caucasians > than African Americans, 3-fold higher in Hispanics
> - **I**nsufficient vitamins: zinc and folate
> - **M**aternal chronic disease (e.g. diabetes)
> - **M**aternal use of anti-epileptic drugs
>
> (*general population risk for NTD is 0.1%)

ISOIMMUNIZATION SCREENING

Definition
- isoimmunization: antibodies (Ab) produced against a specific RBC antigen (Ag) as a result of antigenic stimulation with RBC of another individual

Etiology
- maternal-fetal circulation normally separated by placental barrier, but sensitization can occur (see below) and can affect the current pregnancy, or more commonly, future pregnancies
- in pregnancy, anti-Rh Ab produced by a sensitized Rh-negative mother can lead to fetal hemolytic anemia
- overall risk of isoimmunization of an Rh-negative mother with an Rh-positive ABO-compatible infant is 16% (2% antepartum, 7% within 6 months of delivery, and 7% in the second pregnancy)

- sensitization routes
  - incompatible blood transfusions
  - previous fetal-maternal transplacental hemorrhage (e.g. ectopic pregnancy)
  - invasive procedures in pregnancy (e.g. prenatal diagnosis, cerclage, D&C)
  - any type of abortion
  - labour and delivery

Investigations
- routine screening at first visit for blood group, Rh status, and antibodies are measured by the indirect Coombs test
- if Rh positive with antibodies present, the severity of fetal anemia is determined primarily by antibody concentration:
  - Ab titres <1:16 considered benign
  - Ab titres >1:16 necessitates amniocentesis to determine severity of fetal anemia (which correlates with the amount of biliary pigment in amniotic fluid from 27 wks +)
  - a positive titre means that the fetus is at risk of hemolytic anemia, not that it has occurred or will develop
- Kleihauer-Betke test used to determine extent of fetomaternal hemorrhage
  - fetal red blood cells identified on a slide treated with citrate phosphate buffer because adult hemoglobin elutes through cell membrane in presence of acid more readily
- detailed U/S for hydrops fetalis

Prophylaxis
- exogenous Rh IgG (Rhogam™ or WinRho™) binds to Rh Ag of fetal cells and prevents it from contacting maternal immune system
- Rhogam™ (300 μg) given to all Rh negative women in the following scenarios:
  - routinely at 28 weeks GA
  - within 72 hours of the birth of an Rh positive fetus
  - with a positive Kleihauer-Betke test
  - with any invasive procedure in pregnancy
  - in ectopic pregnancy
  - with miscarriage or therapeutic abortion (only 50 μg required)
  - with an antepartum hemorrhage
- if Rh negative and Ab screen positive, follow mother with serial monthly Ab titres throughout pregnancy ± serial amniocentesis as needed (Rhogam™ has no benefit)

Investigations
- bilirubin is measured by serial amniocentesis to assess the severity of hemolysis
- cordocentesis for fetal Hb; should be used cautiously, not first line

Treatment
- falling biliary pigment warrants no intervention (usually indicative of fetus which is unaffected or mildly affected)
- intrauterine transfusion of O-negative pRBCs may be required for severely affected fetus or early delivery of the fetus for exchange transfusion

Complications
- anti-Rh IgG can cross the placenta and cause fetal RBC hemolysis resulting in fetal anemia, CHF, edema, ascites
- severe cases can lead to hydrops fetalis (edema in at least two fetal compartments due to fetal heart failure secondary to anemia) or erythroblastosis fetalis (moderate to severe immune-mediated hemolytic anemia)

GROUP B STREPTOCOCCUS (GBS) SCREEN

Epidemiology
- 15-40% vaginal carrier rate

Risk Factors (for neonatal disease)
- GBS bacteriuria during current pregnancy even if treated
- previous infant with invasive GBS infection
- preterm labour <37 weeks
- amniotic membrane rupture >18 hours
- intrapartum maternal temperature >38°C
- positive GBS screen during current pregnancy

Clinical Features
- not harmful to mother
- danger of vertical transmission (neonatal sepsis, meningitis or pneumonia)

Hydrops fetalis = abnormal edema in 2 or more fetal compartments e.g. ascites, pericardial effusion. Classified as immune (caused by isoimmunization) or non-immune (caused by many different end-stage fetal diseases)

Screening vs. risk-based approach for GBS prevention in newborns
(N Engl J Med 2002; 347:233-9.)
Study: Large retrospective cohort study comparing the effectiveness of screening and risk-based approaches in preventing early-onset GBS disease (within 7 days of birth).
Patients: From a stratified random sample of 629,912 live births in areas where there was active surveillance for GBS infection, the records for 5144 live births (screened group: n=2628; risk-based group: n=2515) were randomly selected to be reviewed, including all births where newborns had early-onset disease (n=312).
Intervention: Screening approach (routine screening with cultures for GBS between 35-37 wks GA, and offering intrapartum antibiotic prophylaxis to carriers) vs. risk-based approach (offering intrapartum antibiotic prophylaxis to women presenting at time of labour with clinical risk factors for GBS transmission – fever, prolonged ROM, preterm delivery, etc.).
Main outcome: Early-onset GBS disease
Results: Infants of women in the screened group had a significantly lower risk of early-onset disease compared to those in the risk-based group (RR=0.46; 95% CI=0.36 to 0.60). The greatest risk factors for early-onset disease were (a) intrapartum fever (RR=5.99; 95% CI=4.28-8.38) and (b) history of a previous child with GBS disease (RR=3.79; 95% CI=1.30-11.11).
Conclusion: Routine screening for GBS during pregnancy is more effective for preventing GBS infection in newborns than the risk-based approach.

Indications for GBS Intrapartum Prophylaxis
- GBS bacteriuria during current pregnancy (rectovaginal culture at 35-37 wks GA not required)
- GBS status unknown within six weeks of delivery and any of the following:
  - <37 weeks GA and C/S not planned
  - Prolonged ROM (18 hours before delivery)
- Maternal temp of 38.0°C or greater and no evidence of chorioamnionitis
- Positive maternal GBS culture at 35-37 weeks GA during current pregnancy
- Previous newborn with GBS-invasive disease
If GBS status unknown (or no GBS culture in past six weeks) recommended treatment is:
- Obtain rectovaginal GBS culture, and
- Start GBS prophylaxis and, if no culture growth in 48 hours, stop Abx
Schrag S, et al. Prevention of perinatal group B streptococcal disease. Revised guidelines from CDC. MMWR Morb Mortal Wkly Rep 2002; 51 (RR-11):1-22.

Investigations
- SOGC recommends: offer screening for all women at 35-37 weeks with vaginal and anorectal swabs (vaginal done first, then rectal) for C&S

Treatment
- treatment of maternal GBS at delivery decreases neonatal morbidity and mortality
- indications for antibiotic prophylaxis: positive GBS screen or GBS status unknown and one of the risk factors (see above)
- antibiotics for GBS prophylaxis
  - penicillin G 5 million U IV then 2.5 million U IV q4h until delivery
  - penicillin allergic but not at risk for anaphylaxis – cefazolin 2 g IV then 1 g q8h
  - penicillin allergic and at risk for anaphylaxis – clindamycin 900 mg IV q8h or erythromycin 500 mg IV q6h
- if fever, broad spectrum antibiotic coverage is advised

Chromosomal Screening

Indications
- maternal age >35 (increased risk of chromosomal anomalies)
- risk factors in current pregnancy
  - teratogen exposure
  - abnormal U/S
  - abnormal prenatal screen (FTS, MSS or IPS)
- past history/family history of:
  - previous pregnancy with chromosomal anomaly or genetic disease
  - either parent a known carrier of a genetic disorder or balanced translocation
  - family history of chromosomal anomaly, genetic disorder, birth defect, or undiagnosed mental retardation
  - consanguinity
  - three or more spontaneous abortions

AMNIOCENTESIS
- U/S-guided transabdominal extraction of amniotic fluid

L/S Ratio (Lecithin/sphingomyelin ratio)
Lecithin levels increase rapidly after 35 weeks gestation, whereas sphingomyelin levels remain relatively constant. The L/S ratio is a measure of fetal lung maturity - less than 2:1 indicates pulmonary immaturity. Presence of blood or meconium in the amniotic fluid can affect the ratio.

Indications
- identification of genetic anomalies (15-16 weeks gestation) as per indications above
- assessment of fetal lung maturity (T3) via the L/S ratio (lecithin:sphingomyelin)
  - if >2:1, respiratory distress syndrome (RDS) is less likely to occur
- assessment of amniotic fluid bilirubin concentration in Rh-isoimmunized pregnancies

Advantages
- also screens for oNTD (acetylcholinesterase and amniotic AFP) – 96% accurate
- in women >35 years, the risk of chromosomal anomaly (1/180) is greater than the increased risk of miscarriage from the procedure
- more accurate genetic testing than CVS

Disadvantages
- 0.5% risk of spontaneous abortion and risk of fetal limb injury
- results take 14-28 days

CHORIONIC VILLUS SAMPLING (CVS)
- biopsy of fetal-derived chorion using a trans-abdominal needle or trans-cervical catheter at 10-12 weeks

Advantages
- enables pregnancy to be terminated earlier than with amniocentesis
- rapid karyotyping and biochemical assay within 48 hours, incl. FISH analysis
- high sensitivity and specificity

Disadvantages
- 1-2% risk of spontaneous abortion and risk of fetal limb injury
- does not screen for neural tube defects
- 1-2% incidence of genetic mosaicism → false negative results

Table 6. Characteristics of Amniocentesis and CVS

Characteristic	Amniocentesis	CVS
Accuracy of prenatal cytogenetic diagnosis	99.8%	97.5%
Detection of cytogenetic abnormality	3.4%	5.6%
Laboratory failure	0.1%	2.3%
Risk of spontaneous abortion	0.5%	1-2%

Termination of Pregnancy

Definition
- active termination of a pregnancy before fetal viability (usually <500 g or 20 weeks GA)

Indications
- inability to carry a pregnancy to term due to medical or social reasons (including patient preference)

Management
- medical:
  - <9 weeks: methotrexate + misoprostol
  - >12 weeks: prostaglandins (intra- or extra-amniotically or IM) or misoprostol
- surgical:
  - <12-16 weeks: dilatation + vacuum aspiration ± curettage
  - >16 weeks: dilatation and evacuation, early induction of labour
  - common complications: pain or discomfort
  - less common complications: hemorrhage, perforation of uterus, laceration of cervix, risk of sterility, infection/endometritis, Asherman's syndrome (adhesions within the endometrial cavity causing amenorrhea/infertility), retained products of conception
- counselling:
  - supportive services
  - future contraception plans
  - ensure follow-up

Medical Conditions in Pregnancy

Iron Deficiency Anemia

- iron requirements increase during pregnancy due to
  - fetal/placental growth (500 mg), increased maternal RBC mass (500 mg) and losses (200 mg) – more needed for multiple gestations
  - mother needs 1 g of elemental iron per fetus; this amount exceeds normal stores + dietary intake

Etiology
- inadequate iron intake (diet)
- decreased iron absorption (malabsorption syndrome, antacid use)
- increased losses (vaginal bleeding, other source of bleeding)
- increased requirement (fetal growth, multiple gestation)

Epidemiology
- responsible for 80% of causes of nonphysiologic anemia during pregnancy

Clinical Features
- same as in non-pregnant states
  - non-specific symptoms: pallor, fatigue, palpitations, tachycardia, dyspnea
  - severe anemia: angular stomatitis, glossitis

Investigations
- serum iron, serum ferritin, blood smear – do not include total iron binding capacity (TIBC) since it is increased during normal pregnancy

Complications
- maternal complications: angina, CHF, infection, slower recuperation, preterm labour

CMA policy (1988)
"Induced abortion should be uniformly available to all women in Canada" and "there should be no delay in the provision of abortion services".

Induced Abortion Statistics:
* Rate per 1,000 women (all ages): 13.7
* Rate per 1,000 women (age 20-24): 27.7
* Ratio of induced abortions per 100 live births (all ages): 28.3
* Ratio of induced abortions per 100 live births (age 20-24): 54.9
* 31.4% of all abortion services are assessed by women aged 20-24
Adapted from Statistics Canada, 2005, Induced Abortion Statistics, 82-223-XWE, page 16 of 32.

- fetal complications: decreased oxygen carrying capacity leading to fetal distress, IUGR, low birth weight and hydrops

Management
- prevention: 150 mg ferrous sulfate OD, 300 mg ferrous gluconate OD or 30 mg of ferrous iron OD for all pregnant women in 2nd and 3rd trimester
- if anemic: 1 g ferrous sulfate OD (180 mg elemental Fe)

Folate Deficiency Anemia

- most often associated with iron deficiency anemia
- folic acid is necessary for closure of neural tube during early fetal development (by day 28 of gestation)

Etiology
- nutritional: decreased intake
- non-nutritional factors: multiple gestation, drugs (phenytoin, methotrexate), chronic hemolytic anemia, malabsorption entities (celiac sprue)

Epidemiology
- incidence varies from 0.5-25% depending on region, population, diet
- takes approximately 18 weeks of a folate deficient diet to produce anemia
- minimum daily requirement is 0.4 mg

Clinical Features
- non-specific symptoms: anorexia, nausea, vomiting, diarrhea, depression, pallor, UTI, sore mouth or tongue
- complications
  - maternal: decreased blood volume, nausea, vomiting, anorexia
  - fetal: neural tube defects in first trimester, low birth weight, prematurity

Investigations
- RBC and serum folate, blood smear

Management
- prevention
  - 0.4-1 mg folic acid PO daily for 1-3 months preconceptually and throughout T1
  - 5 mg folic acid per day with past history of oNTD, diabetes or anti-epileptic medication use

Diabetes Mellitus (DM)

Classification of Diabetes Mellitus
- Type 1 and Type 2 DM (see Endocrinology)
- gestational dependent diabetes mellitus (GDM): onset of diabetes mellitus during pregnancy

Etiology
- Type 1 and Type 2 DM (see Endocrinology)
- GDM: around 24-28 weeks GA, anti-insulin factors produced by placenta & high maternal cortisol levels create increased peripheral insulin resistance → higher fasting glucose → leading to GDM and/or exacerbating pre-existing DM

Epidemiology
- 2-4% of pregnancies are complicated by DM

Risk Factors
- Type 1 and Type 2 DM (see Endocrinology)
- GDM:
  - age >25
  - obesity
  - certain ethnicities (Aboriginal, Hispanic, Asian, African)
  - family history of DM
  - previous history of GDM
  - previous child with birthweight >4.0 kg

MANAGEMENT

A. TYPE I AND TYPE 2 DM

Preconception
- pre-plan and refer to high-risk clinic
- optimize glycemic control
- counsel patient re: potential risks and complications
- evaluate for diabetic retinopathy, neuropathy, coronary artery disease

Pregnancy
- may consider continuing Glyburde or Melformin +/- adding insulin; teratogenicity unknown for other oral anti-hyperglycemics
- tight glycemic control
  - diet management first line therapy
  - if blood glucose not well controlled, initiate insulin therapy
  - insulin dosage may need to be adjusted in T2 due to increased demand and increased insulin resistance
- monitor as for normal pregnancy plus initial 24-hr urine protein and creatinine clearance, retinal exam, HbA1c
  - HbA1c: >140% of pre-pregnancy value associated with ↑ risk of spontaneous abortion and congenital malformations
- increased fetal surveillance (BPP, NST)

Target Blood Glucose Values in Pregnancy (mmol/L)
Fasting Blood Glucose ≤ 5.3
1-Hour Post Prandial Blood Glucose ≤ 7.8
2-Hour Post Prandial Blood Glucose ≤ 6.7

Labour
- timing of delivery depends on fetal and maternal health and risk factors (i.e. must consider size of baby, lung maturity, maternal glucose and blood pressure control)
- can wait for spontaneous labour if glucose well-controlled and BPP normal
- induce by 40 weeks
- type of delivery
  - increased risk of cephalopelvic disproportion (CPD) and shoulder dystocia with babies >4,000 g (8.8 lbs)
  - elective C/S for predicted birthweight >4,500 g (9.9 lbs) (controversial)
- monitoring
  - during labour monitor blood sugars q1h with patient on insulin and dextrose drip
  - aim for blood sugar between 3.5 to 6.5 mmol/L to reduce the risk of neonatal hypoglycemia

Postpartum
- insulin requirements dramatically drop with expulsion of placenta (source of insulin antagonists)
- no insulin is required for 48-72 hours postpartum in most Type 1 DM
- monitor glucose q6h, restart insulin at two-thirds pre-pregnancy dosage when glucose >8 mmol/L

B. GESTATIONAL DIABETES MELLITUS

Screening
- at 24-28 weeks GA
- pregnant females age >25 or age <25 years old with ≥1 risk factor listed above
- 1-hour, 50 g Oral Glucose Challenge Test (OGCT)
  - plasma glucose (PG) <7.8 mmol/L → no GDM
  - PG ≥7.8 and <10.3 mmol/L → do 2-hour 75 g oral glucose tolerance test (OGTT) for diagnosis
  - PG ≥10.3 mmol/L → GDM established

Diagnosis
- fasting plasma glucose (FPG) and 2-hour, 75 g OGTT
  - 2/3 of the following = GDM
  - 1/3 of the following = impaired glucose tolerance (IGT)
    - FPG ≥5.3 mmol/L
    - PG 1-hour, 75 g OGTT ≥10.6
    - PG 2-hour, 75 g OGTT ≥8.9

Management
- treat both GDM and IGT
- tight glycemic control optimal as in Type 1 and Type 2 DM (see above)
- monitoring and timing of delivery as for Type 1 and Type 2 DM (see above)
- stop insulin and diabetic diet postpartum
- follow-up with 2-hour, 75 g OGTT 6 weeks-6 months postpartum

Prognosis
- most maternal and fetal complications are related to hyperglycemia and its effects

Table 7. Complications of DM in Pregnancy

Maternal	Fetal
Obstetric Hypertension/pre-eclampsia (especially if pre-existing nephropathy/proteinuria): insulin resistance is implicated in etiology of hypertension Polyhydramnios: maternal hyperglycemia leads to fetal hyperglycemia, which leads to fetal polyuria (a major source of amniotic fluid)	**Growth Abnormalities** Macrosomia: maternal hyperglycemia leads to fetal hyperinsulinism resulting in accelerated anabolism Intrauterine growth retardation (IUGR): due to placental vascular insufficiency
Diabetic Emergencies Hypoglycemia Ketoacidosis Diabetic coma	**Delayed Organ Maturity** Fetal lung immaturity: hyperglycemia interferes with surfactant synthesis (respiratory distress syndrome)
End-organ involvement or deterioration **(occur in DM1 and DM2, not in GDM)** Retinopathy Nephropathy	**Congenital Anomalies** **(occur in DM1 and DM2, not in GDM)** 2-7x increased risk of cardiac (VSD), NTD, GU (cystic kidneys), GI (anal atresia), MSK (sacral agenesis) anomalies due to hyperglycemia Note: Pregnancies complicated by GDM do not manifest an increased risk of congenital anomalies because GDM develops after the critical period of organogenesis (in T1)
Other Pyelonephritis/UTI: glucosuria provides a culture medium for *E. coli* and other bacteria Increased incidence of spontaneous abortion (in DM1 and DM2, not in GDM): related to pre-conception glycemic control	**Labour and Delivery** Preterm labour/prematurity: most commonly in patients with hypertension/pre-eclampsia. Preterm labour is associated with poor glycemic control but the exact mechanism is unknown. Increased incidence of stillbirth Birth trauma: due to macrosomia, can lead to difficult vaginal delivery and shoulder dystocia
	Neonatal Hypoglycemia: due to pancreatic hyperplasia and excess insulin secretion in the neonate Hyperbilirubinemia and jaundice: due to prematurity and polycythemia Hypocalcemia: exact pathophysiology not understood, may be related to functional hypoparathyroidism Polycythemia: hyperglycemia stimulates fetal erythropoietin production

Long Term Maternal Complications
- Type 1 and Type 2 DM: risk of progressive retinopathy and nephropathy
- GDM: 50% risk of developing Type 2 DM in next 20 years

Hypertension in Pregnancy

Table 8. Classification of Hypertensive Disorders of Pregnancy

Classification	Definition
A. Pre-existing hypertension	Diastolic hypertension that predates pregnancy or is diagnosed before 20 weeks gestation. In most cases hypertension persists >42 d postpartum. It may be associated with proteinuria.
1. Essential	Primary hypertension
2. Secondary	Secondary to such conditions as renal disease, pheochromocytoma and Cushing syndrome
B. Gestational hypertension	Diastolic hypertension develops after 20 weeks gestation. In most cases it resolves <42 d postpartum.
1. Without preeclampsia	Protein excretion in 24 hour urine collection is <0.3 g/d. No adverse conditions
2. With preeclampsia	Further classified as: a) with new proteinuria (protein excretion in 24 hour urine ≥ 3 g/d) b) with one or more adverse conditions
C. Pre-existing hypertension + preeclampsia	Pre-existing hypertension (as defined in A) associated with one or more of the following after 20 weeks a) resistant hypertension b) new or worsening proteinuria c) one or more adverse conditions
D. Unclassifiable antenatally	Hypertension with or without systemic manifestations if blood pressure was first recorded after 20 weeks gestation. Reassessment is necessary at or after 42 d postpartum. If the hypertension has resolved by then, the condition should be reclassified as gestational hypertension with or without proteinuria; if the hypertension has not resolved by then, the condition should be reclassified as pre-existing hypertension
E. Severe preeclampsia	Severe preeclampsia defined as: a) onset before 34 wks gestation b) heavy proteinuria (3-5 g/d in 24hr urine) OR with one or more adverse conditions

SOGC. Diagnosis, Evaluation, and Management of the Hypertensive Disorders of Pregnancy. *Journal of Obstetrics and Gynecology of Canada.* March 2008 (Vol 30, no 3)

> **Adverse conditions in hypertensive disorders of pregnancy**
> 1. convulsions (eclampsia)
> 2. very high diastolic pressure (>100 mmHg)
> 3. thrombocytopenia (platelet count <100,000 x 10⁹/L)
> 4. oliguria (<500 mL/d)
> 5. pulmonary edema
> 6. elevated LFTs
> 7. severe nausea and vomiting
> 8. frontal headache
> 9. visual disturbances
> 10. persistent abdominal pain in RUQ
> 11. chest pain or shortness of breath
> 12. suspected abruptio placentae
> 13. HELLP syndrome
> 14. intrauterine growth retardation
> 15. oligohydramnios
> 16. absent or reversed umbilical artery end diastolic flow as determined by Doppler velocitometry

PRE-EXISTING HYPERTENSION

Definition
- HTN (>140/90) prior to 20 weeks GA (unless a gestational trophoblastic neoplasia (GTN)), persisting postpartum
- essential hypertension associated with an increased risk of gestational HTN, abruptio placenta, IUGR and IUD

Management
- α-methyldopa 250-500 mg PO tid/qid or labetalol 100-300 mg PO bid/tid
- no ACE inhibitors, diuretics or propranolol (teratogens)
- monitor progress with serial U/S

GESTATIONAL HYPERTENSION

Etiology
- imbalance of thromboxane (vasoconstrictor) and prostaglandin (vasodilator), arteriolar constriction, capillary damage, protein extravasation, and hemorrhage
- in patients with trophoblastic diseases (hydatidiform mole, hydrops, choriocarcinoma), occurs earlier than 20 weeks GA, otherwise occurs after 20 weeks

Risk Factors
- maternal factors
  - primigravida (80-90% of gestational HTN)
  - first conception with a new partner
  - PMHx or FHx of gestational HTN
  - DM, chronic HTN, or renal insufficiency
  - antiphospholipid antibody syndrome (APLA)
  - extremes of maternal age (<18 or >35)
- fetal factors
  - IUGR or oligohydramnios, GTN, multiple gestation, fetal hydrops

Clinical Evaluation of Gestational Hypertension

- in general, clinical evaluation should include the mother and fetus
- evaluation of mother
  - right upper quadrant pain, headache, and visual disturbances are potentially ominous symptoms requiring immediate assessment
  - central nervous system
    - presence and severity of headache
    - visual disturbances – blurring, scotomata
    - tremulousness, irritability, somnolence
    - hyperreflexia
  - hematologic
    - bleeding
    - petechiae
  - hepatic
    - RUQ or epigastric pain
    - severe nausea and vomiting
  - renal
    - urine output
    - urine colour
  - non-dependent edema (i.e. hands and face)
- evaluation of fetus
  - fetal movement
  - fetal heart rate tracing – NST
  - ultrasound for growth
  - biophysical profile
  - Doppler flow studies

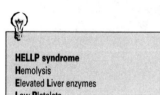

Preeclampsia investigations:

CBC	LDH
LFT's	Albumin
INR and aPTT	Bilirubin
Cr	Urine (dip +/- 24
Uric Acid	hour collection)

Laboratory Evaluation of Gestational Hypertension

- hemoglobin, platelets, blood film
- PTT, INR, fibrinogen, D-dimer – especially if surgery or regional anesthetics are planned
- ALT, AST, LDH
- proteinuria, creatinine, uric acid
- 24 hour urine collection for total protein and creatinine clearance

Management of Gestational Hypertension

- Gestational hypertension without preeclampsia
  - bed rest in left lateral decubitus position (LLDP), normal salt and protein intake
  - avoid diuretics and anti-hypertensives
  - monitor for progression
  - if ≥37 weeks GA, consider induction of labour (see *Induction of Labour* section, OB39)

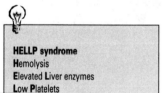

HELLP syndrome
Hemolysis
Elevated **L**iver enzymes
Low **P**latelets

- Gestational hypertension with preeclampsia
  - for discussion of HELLP, see *Jaundice in Pregnancy* section, OB18
  - stabilize and deliver; only "cure" is delivery, independent of gestational age (vaginal delivery preferred)
  - ↑ maternal monitoring to hourly input and output, urine dip q12h and neurological vitals q hourly
  - ↑ fetal evaluation to include continuous monitoring
  - anticonvulsant therapy
    - raises seizure threshold
    - Mg sulfate (4 g IV bolus over 20 min) followed by maintenance of 2-4 g/hour
    - monitor for signs of Mg toxicity: depressed deep tendon reflexes, ↓RR, anuric, hypotonic, CNS or cardiac depression
    - antagonist to Mg sulfate: calcium gluconate (10%) 10 mL (1 g) IV over 2 minutes
  - antihypertensive therapy
    - lowering BP decreases the risk of stroke
    - hydralazine 5-10 mg IV bolus over 5 minutes q15-30 minutes as necessary
    - labetalol 20-50 mg IV q10 minutes
    - 2nd line: nifedipine 10-20 mg PO q20-60 minutes
    - ACE-inhibitors are contraindicated
  - postpartum management
    - risk of seizure highest in first 24 hours postpartum, thus continue Mg sulfate for 12-24 hours
    - vitals q1h
    - consider HELLP syndrome in toxic patients
    - most return to a normotensive BP within 2 weeks

Management of Gestational Hypertension with Seizures
- ABC's
- seizure control and prevention

Complications
- maternal
  - hemorrhagic stroke (50% of deaths)
  - left ventricular failure/pulmonary edema
  - liver and renal dysfunction
  - abruption
  - seizure
  - DIC (release of placental thromboplastin → consumptive coagulopathy)
  - HELLP syndrome: **H**emolysis, **E**levated **L**iver enzymes, **L**ow **P**latelets
    - treat with FFP infusion or plasma exchange
- fetal (2° to placental insufficiency):
  - fetal loss, IUGR, prematurity, abruptio placentae

PRE-EXISTING HYPERTENSION + PREECLAMPSIA
- 2-7 fold increased likelihood of developing preeclampsia/eclampsia if pre-existing maternal hypertension
- occurs early, tends to be severe (often with IUGR) and to recur with subsequent pregnancies

Hyperemesis Gravidarum

Definition
- intractable nausea and vomiting, severe enough to cause weight loss, dehydration, ketonuria, electrolyte imbalance, acid-base disturbances and if severe, hepatic and renal damage
- usually presents in T1 then diminishes; persists throughout pregnancy in a minority

Etiology
- multifactorial with hormonal, immunologic and psychologic components
- rapidly rising β-hCG ± estrogen levels may be implicated

Epidemiology
- ~1% of pregnancies
- nausea and vomiting affect at least 50% of pregnant women ("morning sickness"), most common in T1 and early T2

Investigations
- diagnosis of exclusion: rule out GI inflammation, pyelonephritis, thyrotoxicosis, multiple gestation, GTN, HELLP syndrome
- CBC, electrolytes, BUN, creatinine, LFTs, urinalysis
- ultrasound

Management
- supportive
  - if severe, admit to hospital
  - NPO initially, then small frequent meals of appealing foods
  - correct hypovolemia, electrolyte imbalance and ketosis
  - thiamine supplementation may be indicated
  - TPN if severe to reverse catabolic state
- pharmacological options
  - Diclectin™ (10 mg doxylamine succinate with vitamin B6) can be started at 2 tablets qhs + 1 tablet qAM + 1 tablet qPM. Dosage can be increased up to 8 tablets per day
  - Gravol™ can be safely used as an adjunct to Diclectin™ (1 suppository bid or 25 mg PO qid)
- non-pharmacological options (controversial)
  - rest
  - avoid triggers (i.e. certain smells)
  - acupressure at inner aspect of the wrists, just proximal to the flexor crease has been shown to significantly reduce symptoms
  - studies suggest ginger ingestion daily is effective (tea or tablet extracts; 100 mg/d), but teratogenic effect unknown

Complications
- maternal:
    - dehydration, electrolyte and acid-base disturbances
    - Mallory-Weiss tear
    - Wernicke's encephalopathy, if protracted course
    - death
- fetal: usually none, IUGR is 15x more common in women losing >5% of pre-pregnancy weight

Jaundice in Pregnancy

Epidemiology
- affects 1 in 1500 pregnancies

Etiology
- viral hepatitis (most common)
- unique to pregnancy
    - cholestatic jaundice of pregnancy
    - HELLP syndrome
    - hepatic rupture, hematoma and infarct
    - acute fatty liver of pregnancy (AFLP)
    - hyperemesis gravidarum (rarely causes hepatic dysfunction)
- pre-existing conditions: chronic hepatitis, cirrhosis, familial hyperbilirubinemia, Budd-Chiari syndrome, Wilson's disease, hepatic tumours, intrahepatic cholestasis, biliary obstruction, PBC, PSC

HELLP SYNDROME

Definition
- syndrome characterized by hemolysis, elevated liver enzymes and low platelets
- pathogenesis unknown

Epidemiology
- affects 20% of women with severe pre-eclampsia
- presents >27th week gestation (11% sooner); up to 30% of cases present AFTER delivery and with no signs of hypertension at delivery

Clinical Features
- epigastric, RUQ or chest pain, N/V, symptoms of pre-eclampsia (headache, blurred vision, thirst)
- atypical presentations: asymptomatic reduction in platelet count, "flu-like" symptoms

Laboratory Findings and Investigations
- AST (70-663 U/L), total bilirubin slightly ↑, platelet count (7-99), elevated LDH
- may exhibit: elevated D-dimers, tissue polypeptide antigen (TPA) and fibronectin, fragmented RBCs on smear
- liver biopsy: rarely done, demonstrates periportal hemorrhage and fibrin deposition with periportal necrosis; macro- and microvesicular fatty deposits (NOT pericentral as in AFLP)
- DDx: ITP, TTP, APLA, acute fatty liver of pregnancy (AFLP)

Management
- supportive care (in ICU) and prompt delivery

Complications
- sepsis, multi-system organ failure, hepatic failure, DIC, death (rare)

CHOLESTATIC JAUNDICE OF PREGNANCY

Definition
- clinical syndrome characterized by intense pruritus that precedes jaundice by 7-14 days

Pathogenesis
- unknown, but may be due to increased sensitivity to high levels of estrogen or abnormal progestational steroids

- risk of decreased vitamin K absorption (thus increased incidence of postpartum hemorrhage)

Epidemiology
- 17-29 weeks GA
- high incidence in Chile and Scandinavia; rare in Asian and African populations
- selenium may be protective against cholestasis
- strong familial predisposition
- correlates with oral contraceptive sensitivity
- episode predisposes to cholestasis on subsequent gestations

Clinical Features and Laboratory Findings
- intense pruritis ± icterus (1-2 weeks later)
- ALT <500 IU, ALP and GGT markedly elevated (to levels consistent with moderate to severe cholestasis)
- steatorrhea unusual

Management
- ursodeoxycholic acid (20-25 mg/kg/day) (well tolerated by mother and fetus)
- pruritus: cholestyramine (worsens steatorrhea)
- prophylactic vitamin K before delivery
- consider induction of labour (see *Induction of Labour* section, OB39)

HEPATIC INFARCT, HEMATOMA, AND RUPTURE

- a rare consequence of pre-eclampsia typically occuring in T3
- vasospasm-induced hepatic infarction can lead to hematoma formation
- hematoma can rupture

Presentation
- hepatic rupture: RUQ abdominal pain, abdominal distention, nausea/vomiting, and hypertension, followed by shock

Diagnosis
- hemoperitoneum (paracentesis, U/S, CT, MRI showing ruptured liver)

Management
- aggressive: rapid delivery + trauma surgery to repair liver

Complications
- death (mother and fetus) if untreated

ACUTE FATTY LIVER OF PREGNANCY (AFLP)

Definition
- form of hepatic failure with coagulopathy and encephalopathy that is characterized by microvesicular fatty infiltrates in liver parenchyma
- pathogenesis unknown

Epidemiology
- 1 in 6659 deliveries
- 3rd trimester (28-40 week GA)
- maternal mortality as high as 75%; resolution of hepatic function with delivery or termination of pregnancy

Risk Factors
- primigravidas
- male gestations (2.7 times higher vs. female gestations)
- long-chain acyl-CoA dehydrogenase (LCHAD) deficiency with at least one allele for the G1528 mutation in either mother or fetus
- no recurrence with subsequent pregnancies

Clinical Features
- acute nausea, vomiting, severe upper abdominal pain preceding jaundice
- confusion
- pre-eclampsia

- pruritus
- range in presentation:
  - mild
  - fulminant: GI bleeding, hepatic coma, renal failure and true hepatic failure (coagulopathy and encephalopathy)

Diagnosis
- elevated PTT and low serum fibrinogen
- AST>ALT (moderate increase)
- hypoglycemia
- pre-eclampsia and HELLP features frequently present
- liver biopsy to establish diagnosis
  - microvesicular fatty infiltrates of the central zone hepatocytes
  - Oil Red O stain on frozen tissue
  - electron microscopy on glutaraldehyde fixed tissue
- U/S, MRI, CT: not consistently useful in confirming AFLP, but if liver biopsy is not possible (i.e. with coagulopathy, impending hepatic rupture, Reye's syndrome), CT is most helpful showing reduced attenuation of the liver that is compatible with AFLP

Management
- early diagnosis with prompt delivery followed by maximal supportive care
  - ABC; mechanical ventilation, transfusion of blood products
  - hepatic encephalopathy treatment – lactulose, catharsis
  - treat hypoglycemia

Prognosis
- recovery begins with delivery
- persistent or increasing hyperbilirubinemia and complications:
  - should not be interpreted as indications for liver transplantation
  - continue aggressive supportive measures

Infections During Pregnancy

- see Table 9

Table 9. Infections During Pregnancy * indicates TORCH infection

Infection	Agent	Source of Transmission	Greatest Transmission Risk to Fetus	Effects on Fetus	Effects on Mother	Diagnosis	Management
Chicken Pox	Varicella zoster virus (herpes family)	Direct, respiratory, transplacental	13-30 weeks GA, and 5d pre- to 2d post-delivery	Congenital varicella syndrome (limb aplasia, chorioretinitis, cataracts, cutaneous scars, cortical atrophy, IUGR, hydrops), preterm labour (PTL)	Fever, malaise, vesicular pruritic lesions	Clinical, ± vesicle fluid culture, ± serology	VZIG for mother if exposed, decreases congenital varicella syndrome. Do not administer vaccine during pregnancy (live attenuated)
***CMV**	DNA virus (herpes family)	Blood/organ transfusion, sexual contact, breast milk, transplacental, during delivery	T1-T3	5-10% develop CNS involvement (mental retardation, cerebral calcification, hydrocephalus, microcephaly, deafness, chorioretinitis)	Asymptomatic or flu-like	Serologic screen; isolate virus from urine or secretion culture	No specific treatment; maintain good hygiene and avoid high risk situations
Erythema Infectiosum (Fifth Disease)	Parvovirus B19	Respiratory, infected blood products, transplacental	10-20 weeks GA	Spontaneous abortion (SA), stillbirth, hydrops in utero	Flu-like, rash, arthritis; often asymptomatic	Serology, viral PCR, maternal AFP; if IgM present, follow fetus with U/S for hydrops	If hydrops occurs, consider fetal transfusion
Hepatitis B	DNA virus	Blood, saliva, semen, vaginal secretions, breast milk, transplacental	T3 10% vertical transmission if asymptomatic HBsAg +ve; 85-90% if HBsAg and HBeAg +ve	Prematurity, low birth weight, neonatal death	Fever, N/V, fatigue, jaundice, elevated liver enzymes	Serologic screening for all pregnancies	Rx neonate with HBIG and vaccine (at birth, 1, 6 mo); 90% effective
***Herpes Simplex Virus**	DNA virus	Intimate mucocutaneous contact, transplacental, during delivery	Delivery (if genital lesions present); less commonly in utero	Disseminated herpes (20%); CNS sequelae (35%); self-limited infection	Painful vesicular lesions	Clinical diagnosis	Acyclovir for symptomatic women, suppressive therapy at 36 wks controversial; C/S if active genital lesions, even if remote from vulva
HIV	RNA retrovirus	Blood, semen, vaginal secretions, breast milk, during delivery, in utero	1/3 in utero, 1/3 at delivery, 1/3 breastfeeding	IUGR, preterm labour, premature rupture of membranes	See Infectious Diseases	Serology, viral PCR. All pregnant women are offered screening	Triple antiretroviral therapy decreases transmission to <1%; Elective C/S: no previous antiviral Rx or monotherapy only, viral load unknown or >500 RNA copies/ml, unknown prenatal care, patient request
***Rubella**	ssRNA togavirus	Respiratory droplets (highly contagious), transplacental	T1	SA or congenital rubella syndrome (hearing loss, cataracts, CV lesions, MR, IUGR, hepatitis, CNS defects, osseous changes)	Rash (50%), fever, posterior auricular or occipital lymphadenopathy, arthralgia	Serologic testing; all pregnant women screened (immune if titre >1:16); infection if IgM present or >4x increase in IgG	No specific treatment; offer vaccine following pregnancy. Do not administer during pregnancy (live attenuated)
Syphilis	Spirochete (*Treponema pallidum*)	Transplacental	T1-T3	Risk of PTL, multisystem involvement, fetal death	See Infectious Diseases	VDRL screening for all pregnancies; if positive, requires confirmatory testing	Pen G 2.4 M U IM 1 dose if early syphilis 3 doses if late syphilis monitor VDRL monthly
***Toxoplasmosis**	Protozoa (*Toxoplasma gondii*)	Raw meat, unpasteurized goat's milk, cat feces/urine, transplacental	T3 (but most severe if infected in T1); only concern if primary infection during pregnancy	Congenital toxoplasmosis (chorioretinitis, hydrocephaly, intracranial calcification, MR, microcephaly) NB: 75% initially asymptomatic at birth	Majority subclinical; may have flu-like symptoms	IgM and IgG serology PCR of amniotic fluid	Self-limiting in mother; spiramycin decreases fetal morbidity, not rates of transmission

Urinary Tract Infection (UTI)

Etiology
- increased urinary stasis from mechanical and hormonal (progesterone) factors
- organisms are the same as in non-pregnant woman, and also GBS

Epidemiology
- most common medical complication of pregnancy
- asymptomatic bacteriuria in 2-7% of pregnant women depending on parity and socioeconomic factors

Clinical Features
- may be asymptomatic
- dysuria, urgency, and frequency in cystitis
- fever, flank pain, costovertebral angle tenderness in pyelonephritis

Investigations
- urinalysis, urine C&S
- VCUG, cystoscopy, and renal function tests in recurrent infections

Treat asymptomatic bacteriuria in pregnancy because of increased risk of progression to cystitis, pyelonephritis and probable increased risk of **PRETERM LABOUR.**

Management
- uncomplicated UTI
    - first line: amoxicillin (250-500 mg PO q8h x 7 days)
    - alternatives: TMP-SMX (Septra™) or nitrofurantoin (avoid sulpha drugs during last 6 weeks of pregnancy due to displacement of bilirubin from albumin and increased kernicterus in the newborn)
    - follow with monthly urine cultures
- pyelonephritis
    - hospitalization and IV antibiotics

Prognosis
- complications: acute cystitis, pyelonephritis, and possible preterm premature rupture of membranes (PPROM)
- recurrence common

Venous Thromboembolism (VTE)

Epidemiology
- incidence 0.5-3/1,000 pregnancies occurring with approximately equal frequency in all three trimesters and postpartum

Risk Factors
- previous VTE, age >35, obesity, infection, bedrest/immobility, shock/dehydration, thrombophilias (congenital and acquired)

Table 10. Risk Factors for VTE Specific to Pregnancy

Hypercoagulability	Stasis	Endothelial

Increased factors:
   II, V, VII, VIII, IX, X, XII, fibrinogen
 Increased platelet aggregation
 Decreased protein S, tPA, factors XI, XIII
 Increased resistance to activated protein C
 Antithrombin can be normal or reduced
	Increased venous distensibility
	 Decreased venous tone
	 50% decrease in venous flow in lower extremity by T3
	 Uterus is mechanical impediment to venous return
		Vascular damage at delivery
		   (C/S or SVD)
		 Uterine instrumentation
		 Peripartum pelvic surgery

Clinical Features
- most DVTs occur in the iliofemoral or calf veins with a predilection for the left leg
- signs of a pulmonary embolism, as in non-pregnant patients, are non-specific
- unexplained spontaneous fetal loss

Investigations
- duplex venous Doppler sonography for DVT
- CXR and V/Q scan for PE

Management

- before initiating treatment, obtain a baseline CBC, including platelets, and aPTT
- warfarin is contraindicated during pregnancy due to its potential teratogenic effects
- unfractionated heparin
  - bolus of 5000 IU followed by an infusion of ~30 000 IU/24 hours
  - measure the aPTT six hours after the bolus
  - maintain the aPTT at a therapeutic level (1.5-2 times normal)
  - repeat q24h once therapeutic
  - heparin-induced thrombocytopenia (HIT) uncommon (3%) but serious complication
- compression stockings
- poor evidence to support a recommendation for or against avoidance of prolonged sitting
- prophylaxis
  - women on long-term anticoagulation: full therapeutic anticoagulation throughout pregnancy and for 6-12 weeks postpartum
  - women with a non-active PMHx of VTE: unfractionated heparin regimens suggested
- routine prophylaxis
  - insufficient evidence in pregnancy to recommend routine use of LMWH
  - current prophylaxis regimens for acquired thrombophilias, such as APLA syndrome, include the use of low dose aspirin in conjunction with prophylactic heparin

Bleeding in Pregnancy

First and Second Trimester Bleeding

Differential Diagnosis
- physiologic bleeding: spotting, due to implantation of placenta – reassure and check serial β-hCGs
- abortion (threatened, inevitable, incomplete, complete) (see Table 11)
- abnormal pregnancy (ectopic, molar) (see <u>Gynecology</u> for molar pregnancy)
- trauma (post-coital)
- genital lesion (e.g. cervical polyp, neoplasms)

Spontaneous Abortions

Table 11. Classifications of Spontaneous Abortions

Type	History	Clinical	Management (± Rhogam™)
Threatened	Vaginal bleeding ± cramping	Cervix closed and soft U/S shows viable fetus	Watch and wait <5% go on to abort
Inevitable	Increased bleeding and cramps ± rupture of membranes	Cervix closed until products start to expel, then external os opens	a) watch and wait b) Misoprostol 400-800 ug PO/PV c) D&C +/- oxytocin
Incomplete	Extremely heavy bleeding and cramps ± passage of tissue noticed	Cervix open	a) watch and wait b) Misoprostol 400-800 ug PO/PV c) D&C +/- oxytocin
Complete	Bleeding and complete passage of sac and placenta	Cervix open	No D&C – expectant management
Missed	No bleeding (fetal death in utero)	Cervix closed U/S may show SGA	a) watch and wait b) Misoprostol 400-800 ug PO/PV c) D&C +/- oxytocin
Habitual	3+ consecutive spontaneous abortions		Evaluate mechanical, genetic, environmental and other risk factors
Septic	Contents of uterus infected – infrequent		D&C IV broad spectrum antibiotics

- see *Termination of Pregnancy* for therapeutic abortions

Etiology of Recurrent Pregnancy Loss (MAKE ME)
Mechanical: uterine anatomy, cervical incompetence (T2)
Autoimmune: antiphospholipid antibody syndrome, lupus anticoagulant
Karyotype: both parents
Endocrine: hypothyroidism, diabetes mellitus
Maternal infection
Environment: smoking, alcohol, drugs, radiation

Approach to the patient with bleeding in T1/T2
- History: risk factors for ectopic pregnancy (previous ectopic pregnancies, history of STI/PID, IUD use, previous pelvic surgery, & smoking), previous SA, recent trauma, characteristics of the bleeding (including any tissue passed), characteristics of the pain (cramping pain suggests SA), history of coagulopathy, gynecological/obstetric history, dizziness (significant blood loss, may be associated with ruptured ectopic), fever (may be associated with septic abortion)
- Physical: vitals (including orthostatic changes), abdomen (SFH, tenderness, presence of contractions), perineum (signs of trauma, genital lesions), speculum exam (cervical os open or closed, presence of active bleeding/clots/tissue), pelvic exam (uterine size, adnexal mass, uterine/adnexal tenderness)
- Investigations: ß-hCG (lower than expected for GA in SA/ectopic), U/S (to confirm intrauterine pregnancy), CBC, group & screen
- Treatment: IV resuscitation for hemorrhagic shock. Treat the underlying cause.

Management of Abortions
- *Always* rule out an ectopic
- *Always* check Rh status before D/C
- *Always* ensure patient is hemodynamically stable

Antepartum Hemorrhage

Definition
- vaginal bleeding from 20 weeks to term

Differential Diagnosis
- bloody show (shedding of cervical mucous plug) – most common etiology in T3
- placenta previa
- abruptio placentae - most common pathological etiology in T3
- vasa previa
- marginal sinus bleeding
- cervical lesion (cervicitis, polyp, ectropion, cervical cancer)
- uterine rupture
- other: bleeding from bowel or bladder, placenta accreta, abnormal coagulation

PLACENTA PREVIA

Definition
- abnormal location of the placenta near, partially or completely over the cervical os

Etiology
- idiopathic

Epidemiology
- incidence = 0.5-0.8% of all pregnancies

Risk Factors
- history of placenta previa (4-8% recurrence risk)
- multiparity
- increased maternal age
- multiple gestation
- uterine tumour (e.g. fibroids) or other uterine anomalies
- uterine scar due to previous abortion, C/S, D&C, myomectomy

Clinical Features
- classification
  - total: placenta completely covers the internal os
  - partial: placenta partially covers the internal os
  - marginal: within 2 cm of os but does not cover any part of os – causes potential risk of hemorrhage during cervical effacement and dilatation
  - low lying (NOT a previa): placenta in lower segment but clear of os (can also bleed, but usually in labour)
- history
  - **PAINLESS** bright red vaginal bleeding (recurrent), may be minimized and cease spontaneously, but can become catastrophic
  - mean onset of bleeding is 30 wks GA, but onset depends on degree of previa (complete bleed earlier, marginal bleed at onset of labour)
- physical exam
  - uterus soft and non-tender
  - presenting part high or displaced
- complications
  - fetal
    - perinatal mortality low but still higher than with a normal pregnancy
    - prematurity (bleeding often dictates early C/S)
    - intrauterine hypoxia (acute or IUGR)
    - fetal malpresentation
    - PPROM
    - risk of fetal blood loss from placenta, especially if incised during C/S
  - maternal
    - <1% maternal mortality
    - hemorrhage and hypovolemic shock, anemia, acute renal failure, pituitary necrosis (Sheehan syndrome)
    - placenta accreta – especially in previous uterine surgery; anterior placenta previa
    - hysterectomy

Placenta Previa
PAINLESS
NO tenderness
Uterus SOFT
No uterine irritability/contractions
Malpresentation and/or high presenting part
Fetal heart usually NORMAL
Shock and anemia CORRESPOND to apparent blood loss
Coagulopathy very UNCOMMON initially

Do NOT perform a vaginal exam until placenta previa has been ruled out by U/S.

Placenta Accreta – Placental tissue invades superficially into myometrium (most common)
Placenta Increta – Deep into myometrium
Placenta Percreta – Through the myometrium

Investigations

- ultrasound diagnosis (transabdominal ultrasound has 95% accuracy)
- due to development of lower uterine segment, 90-95% of previas diagnosed in T2 resolve by T3 – (repeat U/S at 30-32 weeks for partial or total previas, repeat U/S for low-lying not indicated unless recurrent bleeding)

Management

- goal: keep pregnancy intrauterine until the risk of delivery < risk of not delivering
- stabilize and monitor
    - maternal stabilization: large bore IV with hydration; O_2 for hypotensive patients
    - maternal monitoring: vitals, urine output, blood loss, bloodwork (hematocrit, CBC, INR/PTT, platelets, fibrinogen, FDP, type and cross match)
    - electronic fetal monitoring
    - U/S assessment: when fetal and maternal condition permit, determine fetal viability, gestational age and placental status/position
- Rhogam™ if mother is Rh negative
    - Kleihauer-Betke test to determine extent of fetomaternal transfusion so that appropriate dose of Rhogam can be given
- GA <37 weeks and minimal bleeding – expectant management
    - admit to hospital
    - limited physical activity, no douches, enemas, or sexual intercourse
    - consider corticosteroids for fetal lung maturity
    - delivery when fetus is mature or hemorrhage dictates
- GA >36 weeks, profuse bleeding or L/S ratio is >2:1 – deliver by C/S

Kleihauer-Betke Test
Quantifies fetal cells in the maternal circulation.

ABRUPTIO PLACENTAE

Definition

- premature separation of a normally implanted placenta after 20 weeks gestation

Etiology

- most are idiopathic

Epidemiology

- incidence: 1-2% of all pregnancies

Risk Factors

- previous abruption (recurrence rate 5-16%)
- maternal hypertension (essential or gestational HTN in 50% of abruptions) or vascular disease
- cigarette smoking (>1 ppd), excessive alcohol consumption, cocaine
- multiparity, maternal age >35 (felt to reflect parity)
- PPROM
- rapid decompression of a distended uterus (polyhydramnios, multiple gestation)
- uterine anomaly, fibroids
- trauma (e.g. motor vehicle collision, maternal battery)

Abruptio Placenta
Abdominal PAIN and/or backache
Uterine TENDERNESS
INCREASED uterine tone
Uterine IRRITABILITY/CONTRACTIONS
Usually NORMAL fetal presentation
FHR may be ABSENT or Non-reassuring
Shock and anemia OUT OF
    PROPORTION to apparent blood loss
May have COAGULOPATHY

Clinical Features

- classification
    - total (fetal death inevitable) vs. partial
    - external/revealed/apparent: blood dissects downward toward cervix
    - internal/concealed (20%): blood dissects upward toward fetus
    - most are mixed
- presentation
    - **PAINFUL** vaginal bleeding, uterine tenderness, uterine contractions
    - pain: sudden onset, constant, localized to lower back and uterus
    - ± fetal distress, fetal demise (15% present with demise), bloody amniotic fluid

Complications

- fetal complications: perinatal mortality 25-60%, prematurity, intrauterine hypoxia
- maternal complications: <1% maternal mortality, DIC (in 20% of abruptions); (placental abruption is the most common cause of DIC in pregnancy), acute renal failure, anemia, hemorrhagic shock, pituitary necrosis (Sheehan syndrome), amniotic fluid embolus

Investigations

- clinical diagnosis: ultrasound not sensitive for abruption (sensitivity = 15%) – may see clot

Table 12. Grades of Abruptio Placentae

Grade	Uterine Irritability	Maternal Hemodynamics	Maternal Fibrinogen	FHR
Mild	Mild	Normal	Normal	Normal
Moderate	Moderate-severe ± tetany	BP with postural drop ↑ HR	↓	Distress: ↓ variability Late decelerations
Severe	Tetany	↓ BP, ↓ HR	↓↓	Absent

Management

- maternal stabilization: large bore IV with hydration; O_2 for hypotensive patients
- electronic fetal monitoring
- maternal monitoring: vitals, urine output, blood loss, bloodwork (hematocrit, CBC, PTT/PT, platelets, fibrinogen, FDP, type and cross match)
- blood products on hand (red cells, platelets, cryoprecipitate) because of DIC risk
- Rhogam™ if Rh negative
    - Kleihauer-Betke test may confirm abruption
- **Mild Abruption**
    - GA <36 weeks: use serial Hct to assess concealed bleeding, deliver when fetus is mature or hemorrhage dictates
    - GA >36 weeks: stabilize and deliver
- **Moderate to Severe Abruption**
    - hydrate and restore blood loss and correct coagulation defect if present
    - vaginal delivery if no evidence of fetal or maternal distress and if cephalic presentation OR with dead fetus
    - C/S if live fetus and fetal or maternal distress develops with fluid/blood replacement, labour fails to progress or non-cephalic fetal presentation

VASA PREVIA

Definition
- unprotected fetal vessels pass over the cervical os; associated with velamentous insertion of cord into membranes of placenta or succenturiate lobe

Epidemiology
- 1 in 5,000 deliveries – higher in twin pregnancies

Clinical Features
- **PAINLESS** vaginal bleeding and fetal distress (tachy- to bradyarrhythmia)
- 50% perinatal mortality, increasing to 75% if membranes rupture (most infants die of exsanguination)

Investigations
- **Apt test** (NaOH mixed with the blood) can be done immediately to determine if the source of the bleeding is fetal (supernatant turns pink) or maternal (supernatant turns yellow)
- **Wright stain** on blood smear and look for nucleated red blood cells (in cord, not maternal blood)

Management
- emergency C/S (since bleeding is from fetus, a small amount of blood loss can have catastrophic consequences)

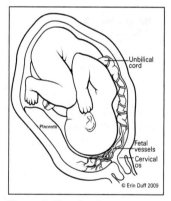

Figure 3. Vasa Previa

Ectopic Pregnancy

Definition
- embryo implants outside of the endometrial cavity

Epidemiology
- 1/100 pregnancies
- fourth leading cause of maternal mortality, leading cause of death in first trimester
- increase in incidence over the last 3 decades

Etiology
- 50% due to damage of fallopian tube cilia from PID
- intrinsic abnormality of the fertilized ovum
- conception late in cycle
- transmigration of fertilized ovum to contralateral tube

> **DDx of Lower Abdominal Pain**
> Urinary tract: UTI, kidney stones
> GI: diverticulitis, appendicitis
> Gyne: endometriosis, PID, fibroid (degenerating, infarcted, torsion), ovarian torsion, ovarian neoplasm, ovarian cyst, pregnancy-related

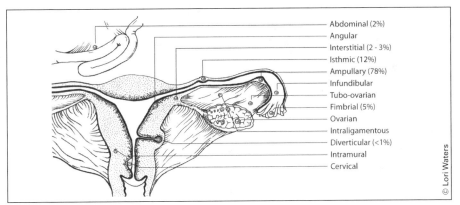

Abdominal (2%)
Angular
Interstitial (2 - 3%)
Isthmic (12%)
Ampullary (78%)
Infundibular
Tubo-ovarian
Fimbrial (5%)
Ovarian
Intraligamentous
Diverticular (<1%)
Intramural
Cervical

© Lori Waters

Figure 4. Sites of Implantation

Risk Factors
- <50% of patients have any risk factors
- demographics: older women, black women
- smoking
- endometriosis
- gynecologic:
    - IUD use – although decreased pregnancy rate, if pregnancy occurs there is increased risk of ectopic
    - history of PID (especially infection with *C. trachomatis*), salpingitis
    - infertility
    - clomiphene citrate (for induction of ovulation)
- previous procedures:
    - any surgery on fallopian tube (for previous ectopic, tubal ligation, etc.)
    - abdominal surgery for ruptured appendix, etc.
    - IVF pregnancies following ovulation induction (7% ectopic rate)
- structural:
    - uterine leiomyomas
    - adhesions
    - abnormal uterine anatomy (e.g. T-shaped uterus)
- prior ectopic pregnancy

Clinical Features
- temperature >38°C (20%)
- abdominal tenderness (90%) ± rebound (45%)
- bimanual examination
    - cervical motion and adnexal (usually unilateral) tenderness
    - palpable adnexal mass (50%) (half have contralateral mass due to lutein cyst)
- other signs of pregnancy (e.g. Chadwick's sign, Hegar's sign)
- if ectopic pregnancy ruptures
    - acute abdomen with increasing pain
    - abdominal distention
    - symptoms of shock

Investigations

- serial β-hCG levels; normal doubling time with intrauterine pregnancy is 1.6-2.4 days in early pregnancy
    - rise of <20% of β-hCG is 100% predictive of a nonviable pregnancy
    - prolonged doubling time, plateau or decreasing levels before 8 weeks implies non-viable gestation but does not provide information on location of implantation
- ultrasound
    - U/S is only definite if fetal cardiac activity is detected in the tube or uterus
    - intrauterine sac should be visible when serum β-hCG is
        - >1500 mIU/mL (transvaginal)
        - >6000 mIU/mL or 6 weeks gestational age (transabdominal)
    - specific finding on transvaginal U/S is a tubal ring
- culdocentesis (rarely done)
- laparoscopy (for definitive diagnosis)

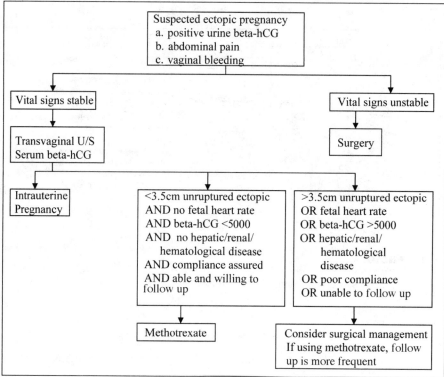

Figure 5. Algorithm for Suspected Ectopic Pregnancy

Treatment

- goals of treatment: be conservative (preserve tube if possible)
- surgical (laparoscopy)
    - linear salpingostomy if tube salvageable
    - salpingectomy if tube damaged or ectopic is ipsilateral recurrence
    - 15% risk of persistent trophoblast; must monitor β-hCG titres weekly until they reach non-detectable levels
    - if patient is Rh negative give anti-D gamma globulin (Rhogam™)
    - may require laparotomy
- medical = methotrexate
    - use 50 mg/m² body surface area; given in a single IM dose
    - this is 1/5 to 1/6 chemotherapy dose, therefore minimal side effects (reversible hepatic dysfunction, diarrhea, gastritis, dermatitis)
    - follow β-hCG levels weekly until β-hCG is non-detectable
        - plateau or rising levels are evidence of persisting trophoblastic tissue: requires further medical or surgical therapy
    - success 67%; as many as 25% will require a 2nd dose
    - tubal patency following methotrexate treatment approaches 80%

Prognosis

- 9% of maternal deaths
- 40-60% of patients will become pregnant again after surgery
- 10-20% will have subsequent ectopic gestation

Multiple Gestation

Epidemiology
- incidence of twins is 1/80 and triplets 1/6400 in North America
- 2/3 of twins are dizygotic (i.e. fraternal)
- monozygous twinning occurs at a constant rate worldwide (1/250)
- determine zygosity by number of placentas, thickness of membranes, sex, blood type

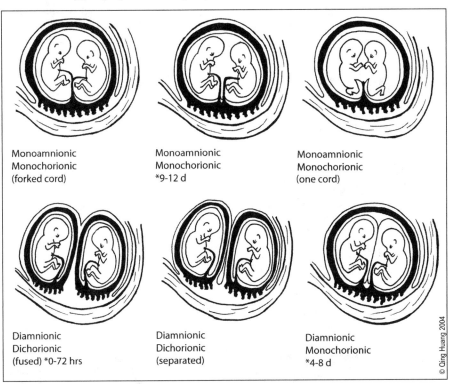

Monoamnionic
Monochorionic
(forked cord)

Monoamnionic
Monochorionic
*9-12 d

Monoamnionic
Monochorionic
(one cord)

Diamnionic
Dichorionic
(fused) *0-72 hrs

Diamnionic
Dichorionic
(separated)

Diamnionic
Monochorionic
*4-8 d

© Qing Huang 2004

Figure 6. Classification of Twin Pregnancies   *indicates time of cleavage

Clinical Features

Table 13. Complications Associated with Multiple Gestation

Maternal	Utero-placental	Fetal
Hyperemesis gravidarum	↑ PROM/PTL	Prematurity*
GDM	Polyhydramnios	IUGR
Gestational HTN	Placenta previa	Malpresentation
Anemia	Placental abruption	Congenital anomalies
↑ physiological stress on all systems	PPH (uterine atony)	Twin-twin transfusion
↑ compressive symptoms	Umbilical cord prolapse	↑ perinatal morbidity and mortality
C/S	Cord anomalies (velamentous insertion, 2 vessel cord)	Twin interlocking (twin A breech, twin B vertex)
		Single fetal demise

*Most common cause of perinatal mortality in multiple gestation

Management
- U/S determination of chorionicity must be done within the first trimester (ideally 8-12 weeks GA)
- increased antenatal surveillance
  - nonstress test (NST) weekly from 24 weeks GA
  - serial U/S q 2-3 weeks from 28 weeks GA to assess growth
  - Doppler flow studies weekly if discordant fetal growth
  - BPP as needed
- vaginal examinations in third trimester to check for cervical dilatation
- may attempt vaginal delivery if twin A presents as vertex, otherwise C/S (40-50% of all twin deliveries, 15% of cases have twin A delivered vaginally and twin B delivered by C/S)
- mode of delivery depends on fetal weight, GA, presentation

Twin-Twin Transfusion Syndrome

Epidemiology
- 10% of monochorionic twins

Etiology
- arterial blood from donor twin passes through placenta into vein of recipient twin

Clinical Features
- donor twin: IUGR, hypovolemia, hypotension, anemia, oligohydramnios
- recipient twin: hypervolemia, hypertension, CHF, polycythemia, edema, polyhydramnios, kernicterus in neonatal period

Investigations
- detected by U/S screening, Doppler flow analysis

Management
- therapeutic serial amniocentesis to decompress polyhydramnios of recipient twin and decrease pressure in cavity and on placenta
- laparoscopic occlusion of placental vessels

Growth Discrepancies

Intrauterine Growth Restriction (IUGR)

Differential Diagnosis of Incorrect Uterine Size for Dates:
- **Inaccurate dates**
- **Maternal:** diabetes mellitus
- **Maternal-fetal:** polyhydramnios, oligohydramnios, multiple gestation
- **Fetal:** abnormal karyotype, IUGR, macrosomia, fetal anomaly, abnormal lie

Definition
- infant weight <10th percentile for a particular GA
- weight not associated with any constitutional or familial causes

Etiology/Risk Factors
- maternal causes:
  - malnutrition, smoking, drug abuse, alcoholism, cyanotic heart disease, Type 1 DM, SLE, pulmonary insufficiency, previous IUGR
- maternal-fetal:
  - any disease causing placental insufficiency
  - includes gestational HTN, chronic HTN, chronic renal insufficiency, gross placental morphological abnormalities (infarction, hemangiomas)
- fetal causes: TORCH infections, multiple gestation, congenital anomalies

Clinical Features
- symmetric/Type I (20%):
  - occurs early in pregnancy
  - inadequate growth of head and body
  - head:abdomen ratio may be normal
  - usually associated with congenital anomalies or TORCH infections
- asymmetric/Type II (80%)
  - occurs late in pregnancy
  - brain is spared, therefore head:abdomen ratio increased
  - usually associated with placental insufficiency
  - more favorable prognosis than Type I
- complications
  - prone to meconium aspiration, asphyxia, polycythemia, hypoglycemia, and mental retardation
  - greater risk of perinatal morbidity and mortality

Investigations
- symphysis-fundus height (SFH) measurements at every antepartum visit
- if mother at high risk or SFH lags >2 cm behind GA:
  - Anatomy U/S exam should include assessment of biparietal diameter (BPD), head and abdomen circumference, femur length and fetal weight, amniotic fluid volume (↓ associated with IUGR)
  - ± BPP
  - Doppler analysis of umbilical cord blood flow as needed

Management
- prevention via risk modification prior to pregnancy is ideal
- modify controllable factors: smoking, alcohol, nutrition and treat maternal illness
- bed rest in LLDP
- serial BPP (monitor fetal growth)
- determine cause of IUGR, if possible
- delivery when extrauterine existence is less dangerous than continued intrauterine existence or if GA >34 weeks with significant oligohydramnios
- liberal use of C/S since IUGR fetus withstands labour poorly

Macrosomia

Definition
- infant weight >90th percentile for a particular GA or >4,000 g

Etiology/Risk Factors
- maternal obesity, gestational diabetes mellitus, past history of macrosomic infant, prolonged gestation, multiparity

Clinical Features
- increased risk of perinatal mortality
- cephalopelvic disproportion (CPD) and birth injuries (shoulder dystocia, fetal bone fracture) more common
- complications of DM in labour (see *Medical Conditions in Pregnancy* section, OB11)

Investigations
- serial SFH
- further investigations if mother at high risk or SFH >2 cm ahead of GA (same as above for suspected IUGR)
- U/S predictors:
  - polyhydramnios
  - third trimester abdominal circumference (AC) >1.5 cm/week
  - head circumference (HC)/AC ratio <10th percentile
  - femur length (FL)/AC ratio <20th percentile

Management
- prophylactic c-section is a reasonable option where estimated fetal weight (EFW) >5000 g in nondiabetic women and EPW >4500 g in diabetic women
- there is no evidence that prophylactic c-section improves outcomes
- induction of early labour is not recommended

Polyhydramnios

Definition
- amniotic fluid volume (AFV) >2,000 cc at any stage in pregnancy
- U/S criteria: >8 x 8 cm (3.1 x 3.1 in) pocket of amniotic fluid

Etiology
- idiopathic: most common (40%)
- maternal:
  - Type 1 DM: causes abnormalities of transchorionic flow
- maternal-fetal:
  - chorioangiomas
  - multiple gestation
  - hydrops fetales (↑ erythroblastosis)
- fetal:
  - chromosomal anomaly (up to 2/3 of fetuses with severe polyhydramnios)
  - respiratory: cystic adenomatoid malformed lung
  - CNS: anencephaly, hydrocephalus, meningocele
  - GI: tracheoesophageal fistula, duodenal atresia, facial clefts (interfere with swallowing)

Epidemiology
- incidence: 1/250 deliveries

Clinical Features
- pressure symptoms from overdistended uterus (dyspnea, edema, hydronephrosis)
- uterus large for dates, difficulty palpating fetal parts and hearing fetal heart tones

Complications
- cord prolapse, placental abruption, malpresentation, preterm labour, uterine dysfunction and postpartum hemorrhage (PPH)
- increased perinatal mortality rate

Management
- determine underlying cause
  - screen for maternal disease/infection
  - complete fetal U/S evaluation
- depends on severity
  - mild to moderate cases require no treatment
  - if severe, hospitalize and consider therapeutic amniocentesis

Oligohydramnios

Definition
- amniotic fluid index of 5 cm (2 in) or less
- an important sign of chronic placental insufficiency

Etiology
- early onset oligohydramnios
  - decreased production: renal agenesis or dysplasia, urinary obstruction, posterior urethral valves (male), chronic hypoxemia leading to IUGR results in shunting away from the kidneys to ensure profusion of the brain
  - increased loss: prolonged amniotic fluid leak (although most often labour ensues)
- late onset oligohydramnios
  - amniotic fluid normally decreases after 35 weeks
  - common in post-term pregnancies
  - U/S doppler studies (umbilical cord and uterine artery dopplers)

Epidemiology
- occur in ~ 4.5% of all preganancies
- severe form in <0.7%
- common in pregnancies >41 weeks (~12%)

Clinical Features
- cord compression
- early onset:
  - 15-25% have fetal anomalies
  - amniotic fluid bands (T1) can lead to Potter's facies, limb deformities, abdominal wall defects
- late onset:
  - pulmonary hypoplasia
  - marker for infants who may not tolerate labour well

Investigations
- always warrants admission and investigation:
  - rule out rupture of membranes (ROM)
  - fetal monitoring (NST, CTG, BPP)
  - U/S doppler studies (umbilical cord and uterine artery dopplers)

Management
- maternal hydration with oral or IV fluids to help increase amniotic fluid
- vesicoamniotic shunt: if etiology is related to fetal obstuctive uropathy, however, pulmonary function not may be restored with restoration of amniotic fluid.
- injection of fluid via amniocentesis will improve condition for ~ 1 wk - may be most helpful for visualizing any associated fetal anomalies
- consider delivery if at term
- amnio-infusion may be considered during labour via intra-uterine catheter, evidence to show improved fetal outcomes is equivocal

Prognosis
- poorer with early onset
- high mortality related to congential malformations and pulmonary hypoplasia when diagnosised during T2

Normal Labour and Delivery

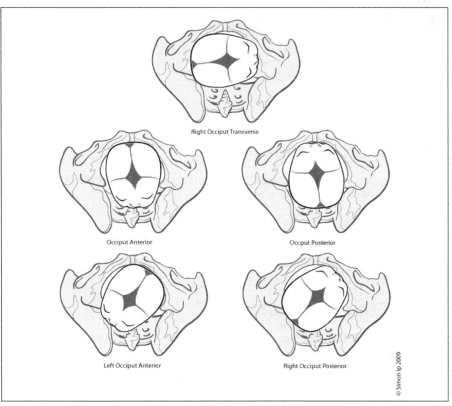

Figure 7. Fetal Positions

The Fetus

- fetal lie
    - orientation of the long axis of the fetus with respect to the long axis of the uterus (longitudinal, transverse, oblique)

- fetal presentation
    - fetal part presenting at pelvic outlet
        - breech (complete, frank, footling) – see Figure 9
        - cephalic (vertex, face, asynclitic)
        - transverse (shoulder)
        - compound (fetal extremity prolapses along with presenting part)
    - all except vertex are considered malpresentations (see *High Risk Labour and Delivery* section, OB41)

- fetal position
    - position of presenting part of the fetus relative to the maternal pelvis
        - occiput anterior (OA): most common presentation ("normal") – left OA most common
        - occiput posterior (OP): most rotate spontaneously to OA; may cause prolonged second stage of labour
        - occiput transverse (OT): leads to arrest of dilatation
    - normally, fetal head enters maternal pelvis and engages in OT position
    - subsequently rotates to OA position or (in a small percentage of cases) OP

- attitude
    - flexion/extension of fetal head relative to shoulders
        - brow presentation: head partially extended (requires C/S)
        - face presentation: head fully extended
            - mentum posterior always requires C/S, mentum anterior will deliver vaginally

- station
    - position of presenting part relative to ischial spines - determined by vaginal exam

Presenting Parts include:
Occiput for vertex
Sacrum for breech
Mentum for face

♦ at ischial spines = station 0 = engaged
♦ cm above (–5 → –1) or cm below (+1 → +5)

The Cervix

- dilatation: latent phase: 0-3 cm; active phase: 4-10 cm
- effacement: thinning of the cervix by percentage or length of cervix (cm)
- consistency: soft vs. hard
- position: posterior vs. anterior
- application: contact between the cervix and presenting part i.e. well or poorly applied
- for Bishop score, see Table 17

Definition of Labour

- regular, painful contractions associated with progressive **dilatation** and **effacement** of cervix and **descent** of presenting part, or **station**
  - preterm (>20 but <37 weeks GA)
  - term (37-42 weeks GA)
  - post-term (>42 weeks GA)
- Braxton-Hicks contractions ("false labour")
  - irregular, occur throughout pregnancy and not associated with any dilatation, effacement or descent

Four Stages of Labour

First Stage of Labour
- latent phase:
  - uterine contractions typically infrequent and irregular
  - slow cervical dilatation (usually to 3-4 cm) and effacement
- active phase:
  - rapid cervical dilatation to full dilatation (nulliparous ~1.2 cm/h, multiparous ~1.5 cm/h)
  - phase of maximum slope on cervical dilatation curve (see Figure 10)
  - painful, regular contractions ~q2 min, lasting 45-60 seconds
  - contractions strongest at fundus, weakest at lower segment

Second Stage of Labour
- from full dilatation to delivery of the baby
- mother feels a desire to bear down and push with each contraction
- women may choose a comfortable position that enhances pushing efforts and delivery
  - upright (semi-sitting, squatting) and LLDP have studies supporting their favour
- progress measured by descent

Third Stage of Labour
- separation and expulsion of the placenta
- can last up to 30 minutes before intervention indicated
- start oxytocin IV drip or give 10 U IM after delivery of anterior shoulder in anticipation of placental delivery
- routine oxytocin administration in third stage of labour can reduce the risk of PPH by >40%

Fourth Stage of Labour
- first postpartum hour
- monitor vital signs and bleeding
- repair lacerations
- ensure uterus is contracted (palpate uterus and monitor uterine bleeding)
- inspect placenta for completeness and umbilical cord for presence of 2 arteries and 1 vein
- 3rd and 4th stages of labour most dangerous to the mother (i.e. hemorrhage)

Signs of Placental Separation
1. gush of blood
2. lengthening of cord
3. uterus becomes globular
4. fundus rises

Table 14. Course of Normal Labour

Stage	Nulliparous	Multiparous
First	6-18 hours	2-10 hours
Second	30 min-3 hours	5-30 minutes
Third	5-30 minutes	5-30 minutes

The Cardinal Movements of the Fetus during Delivery

- engagement
- descent
- flexion
- internal rotation (to OA position ideally)
- extension (delivery of head)
- external rotation (restitution); head rotates in line with the shoulders
- expulsion (delivery of shoulders and body)

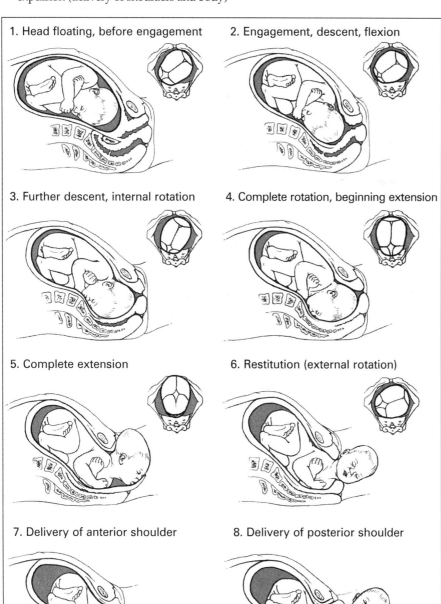

1. Head floating, before engagement
2. Engagement, descent, flexion
3. Further descent, internal rotation
4. Complete rotation, beginning extension
5. Complete extension
6. Restitution (external rotation)
7. Delivery of anterior shoulder
8. Delivery of posterior shoulder

©Danielle Bader

Figure 8. Cardinal Movements of Fetus during Delivery
(adapted from illustration in Williams Obstetrics, 19th Ed.)

Fetal Monitoring in Labour

Vaginal Exam
• membrane status
• cervical effacement (thinning), dilatation, consistency, position, application
• fetal presenting part, position, station
• bony pelvis size and shape
• monitor progress of labour at regular intervals and document in a partogram

Intrapartum Fetal Cardiotocography (CTG)
• intermittent fetal auscultation with Doppler device q15-30 minutes for one minute in first stage active phase following a contraction, q5 minutes during second stage when pushing has begun
• continuous electronic FHR monitoring reserved for non-reassuring auscultation, prolonged labour, and labour which is induced or augmented
    ▪ routine use of continuous electronic monitoring shown to lead to higher intervention rates and no improvement in outcome for the neonate
    ▪ techniques for continuous monitoring include external (Doppler) vs. internal (fetal scalp electrode) monitoring
• fetal scalp sampling should be used in conjunction with electronic monitoring (CTG) to resolve the interpretation of non-reassuring patterns

Electronic Fetal Heart Rate (FHR) Monitoring
• measured by tocometer
• described in terms of baseline FHR, variability (short term, long term) and periodicity (accelerations, decelerations)

• Baseline FHR
    ▪ normal range is 110-160 bpm
    ▪ parameter of fetal well-being vs. distress

• Variability
    ▪ physiologic variability is a normal characteristic of fetal heart rate
    ▪ effect of vagus nerve on fetal heart
    ▪ demonstrable fetal heart rate variability indicates fetal acid-base status is acceptable
    ▪ variability decreases intermittently even in healthy fetus
    ▪ can only be assessed by electronic fetal monitoring (CTG)
    ▪ if absent or decreased variability lasts more than 40 min, need to assess fetal well being
    ▪ causes of absent or decreased fetal heart rate variability: persistant hypoxia causing acidosis, fetal sleep, narcotics, sedatives, β-blockers, $MgSO_4$, preterm fetus, fetal tachycardia, congenital anomalies

• Periodicity
    ▪ accelerations: increase of ≥15 bpm lasting ≥15 seconds, in response to fetal movement or uterine contraction
    ▪ decelerations: 3 types, described in terms of shape, onset, depth, duration, recovery, occurrence, and impact on baseline FHR and variability

Continuous cardiotocography (CTG) as a form of electronic fetal monitoring (EFM) for fetal assessment during labour.
Cochrane Database of Systematic Reviews 2006, Issue 3.

Purpose: To examine the effectiveness of continuous fetal heart monitoring (cardiotocography) during labour on improving health outcomes.
Methods: Systematic review of randomized and semi-randomized trials comparing continuous fetal monitoring with no monitoring, intermittent auscultation, and intermittent monitoring. Trials were identified from the Cochrane Pregnancy and Childbirth Group Trials Register (March 2006), CENTRAL (*The Cochrane Library 2005, Issue 4*), MEDLINE (1966 to December 2005), EMBASE (1974 to December 2005), Dissertation Abstracts (1980 to December 2005) and the National Research Register (December 2005).
Results: 12 trials (37 000 women) meeting search criteria were identified, of which 2 trials were high quality. Continuous electronic fetal heart monitoring did not have an effect on overall perinatal death rate compared to intermittent auscultation, with a relative risk (RR) or 0.85, 95% CI 0.59-1.23. Continuous monitoring also lead to increased incidence of C-section (RR 1.66, 95% CI 1.30 to 2.13, n=18,761, 10 trials) and instrument assisted vaginal delivery (RR 1.16, 95% CI 1.01 to 1.32, n = 18,151, nine trials). These results appeared consistent regardless if pregnancy was high risk, low risk, or pre-term.
Summary: Continuous fetal cardiotocography does not significantly improve infant mortality or other standards of infant well-being. It increases the incidence of C-section and instrument assisted vaginal delivery.

Table 15. Factors Affecting Fetal Heart Rate

	Fetal Tachycardia (FHR >160)	Fetal Bradycardia (FHR <110)	Decreased Variability
Maternal Factors	Fever Hyperthyroidism Anemia	Hypothermia Hypotension Hypoglycemia	Infection Dehydration
Fetal Factors	Arrhythmia Anemia	Rapid descent Dysrhythmia Heart block	CNS anomalies Dysrhythmia Inactivity/sleep cycle
Drugs	Sympathomimetics	β-blockers Anesthetics	Narcotics Magnesium sulphate
Uteroplacental	Early hypoxia (abruption, HTN) Chorioamnionitis	Late hypoxia (abruption, HTN) Acute cord prolapse Hypercontractility	Hypoxia

Table 16. Comparison of Decelerations

Early Decelerations

- uniform shape with onset early in contraction; returns to baseline by end of contraction
- gradual deceleration
- often repetitive; no effect on baseline FHR or variability
- due to vagal response to head compression
- benign, usually seen with cervical dilatation of 4-7 cm
- **management:**
  no action (normal response)

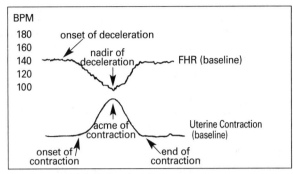

CTG Tracing of Early Deceleration

Variable Decelerations

- variable in shape, onset, and duration
- most common type of periodicity seen during labour
- may or may not be repetitive
- often with abrupt drop in FHR; usually no effect on baseline FHR or variability
- due to cord compression or, in second stage, forceful pushing with contractions
- benign unless repetitive, with slow recovery, or when associated with other abnormalities of FHR
- **management if non reassuring:**
  - intrauterine resuscitation
  - amnioinfusion
  - confirm fetal well being
  - consider operative delivery (vacuum, forceps, C/S)

CTG Tracing of Variable Deceleration

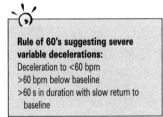

Rule of 60's suggesting severe variable decelerations:
Deceleration to <60 bpm
>60 bpm below baseline
>60 s in duration with slow return to baseline

Late Decelerations

- uniform shape with onset late in contraction, lowest depth after peak of contraction, and return to baseline after end of contraction
- may cause decreased variability and change in baseline FHR
- must see 3 in a row, all with the same shape to define a late deceleration
- due to fetal hypoxia and acidemia, maternal hypotension or uterine hypertonus
- usually a sign of uteroplacental insufficiency (an ominous sign)
- **management if persistent:**
  - intrauterine resuscitation
  - confirm fetal well being
  - consider operative delivery
  - see fetal blood sampling

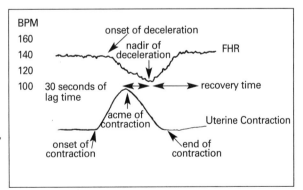

CTG Tracing of Late Deceleration

Approach to the Management of Abnormal FHR:
Ensure fetal tracing
Call for help
Change position to LLDP
100% O₂ by mask
Stop oxytocin
Correct maternal hypotension
Fetal scalp pH/fetal scalp electrode
Vaginal exam to rule out cord prolapse
Rule out fever, dehydration, drug effects, prematurity
Amnioinfusion or tocolytics in selected cases
C/S when necessary

Fetal Scalp Blood Sampling

- indicated when non-reasssuring fetal heart rate (NRFHR) is suggested by clinical parameters including heavy meconium or moderately to severely abnormal FHR patterns, including unexplained absent baseline variability, repetitive late decelerations, complex variable decelerations, fetal cardiac arrythmias
  - pH ≥7.25: normal, repeat if abnormal FHR persists
  - pH 7.21-7.24: repeat assessment in 30 minutes or consider delivery if rapid fall since last sample
  - pH ≤7.20: indicates fetal acidosis, delivery is indicated
- contraindications
  - known or suspected fetal blood dyscrasia (hemophilia, von Willebrand)
  - active maternal infection (HIV, genital herpes)

Fetal Oxygenation

- uterine contractions during labour decrease uteroplacental blood flow, which results in reduced oxygen delivery to the fetus
- most fetuses tolerate this reduction in flow and have no adverse effects
- distribution of oxygen to the fetus depends on maternal, uteroplacental and fetal factors
- maternal factors
  - decreased maternal oxygen carrying capacity
    - significant anemia (iron deficiency, hemoglobinopathies)
    - carboxyhemoglobin (smokers)
  - decreased uterine blood flow
    - hypotension (blood loss, sepsis)
    - regional anesthesia
    - maternal positioning
  - chronic maternal conditions
    - vasculopathies (lupus, Type 1 DM, chronic HTN)
    - antiphospholipid syndrome
    - cyanotic heart disease
    - COPD
- uteroplacental factors
  - uterine hypertonus
    - hyperstimulation secondary to oxytocin, prostaglandins or normal labour
    - placental abruption
  - uteroplacental dysfunction
    - placental abruption
    - placental infarction (dysfunction marked by IUGR, oligohydramnios, abnormal doppler studies)
    - chorioamnionitis
    - placental edema (diabetes, hydrops)
    - placental senescence (post dates)
- fetal factors
  - cord compression
    - oligohydramnios
    - cord prolapse or entanglement
  - decreased fetal oxygen carrying capability
    - significant anemia (isoimmunization, feto-maternal bleed)
    - carboxyhemoglobin (exposure to smokers)
- fetal response to hypoxia/asphyxia
  - decreased movement, tone, and breathing activities
  - redistribution of fetal blood flow
    - increased flow to brain, heart, and adrenals
    - decreased flow to kidneys, lungs, gut, liver, and peripheral tissues
    - increase in blood pressure
  - transient fetal bradycardia followed by fetal tachycardia
  - anaerobic metabolism (decreased pH)

Induction of Labour

Definition
- artificial initiation of labour before its spontaneous onset for the purpose of delivery of the fetus and placenta

Prerequisites for Labour Induction
- capability for C/S if necessary
- maternal
  - short, thin, soft, anterior cervix with open os ("inducible" or "ripe")
  - if cervix is not ripe, use prostaglandin vaginal insert (Cervidil™), prostoglandin gel (Prepidil™), or Foley catheter
- fetal
  - reassuring fetal heart tracing
  - cephalic presentation
  - adequate fetal monitoring available
- likelihood of success determined by Bishop score (see Table 17)
  - cervix considered unfavourable if <6
  - cervix favourable if >6
  - score of 9-13 associated with high likelihood of vaginal delivery

Induction is indicated when the risk of continuing pregnancy exceeds the risks associated with induced labour and delivery.

Table 17. Bishop Score

Cervical characteristic	0	1	2	3
Position	Posterior	Mid	Anterior	–
Consistency	Firm	Medium	Soft	–
Effacement (%)	0-30	40-50	60-70	>80
Dilatation (cm)	0	1-2	3-4	≥5
Station of fetal head	–3	–2	–1	+1

Indications
- maternal factors
  - significant antepartum hemorrhage
  - gestational HTN
  - other maternal medical problems, e.g. diabetes, renal or lung disease
- maternal-fetal factors
  - isoimmunization, PROM, chorioamnionitis, post-term pregnancy
- fetal factors
  - suspected fetal jeopardy as evidenced by biochemical or biophysical indications
  - fetal demise, severe IUGR

Consider the following before induction
- indication for induction
- contraindications
- GA
- cervical favourability
- fetal presentation
- potential for CPD
- fetal well-being/FHR
- membrane status

Risks
- failure to achieve labour and/or vaginal birth
- uterine hyperstimulation and fetal compromise
- uterine rupture
- uterine atony and PPH
- maternal side effects to medications

Contraindications
- maternal
  - prior classical or inverted-T incision or uterine surgery (e.g. myomectomy)
  - unstable maternal condition
  - gross CPD (although diagnosis cannot be made until active labour)
  - active maternal genital herpes
  - invasive cervical carcinoma
  - pelvic structure deformities
- maternal-fetal
  - placenta previa or vasa previa
  - cord presentation
- fetal
  - fetal distress, malpresentation, preterm fetus without lung maturity

Induction Methods

CERVICAL RIPENING

Definition
- use of medications or other means to soften, efface and dilate cervix to increase likelihood of induction success
- ripening of an unfavourable cervix (Bishop score <6) is warranted prior to induction of labour

Methods
- intravaginal prostaglandin PGE_2 gel (Prostin® gel): long and closed cervix with no ROM
    - recommended dosing interval of prostaglandin gel is every 6 to 12 hours up to 3 doses
- intravaginal PGE_2 (Cervidil™): long and closed cervix, may use if ROM, continuous release, can be removed if needed
    - controlled release PGE_2
- misoprostol: synthetic methylated PGE_1 (not commonly used)
- Foley catheter placement to mechanically dilate the cervix
- hydroscopic dilators, osmotic dilators (laminaria)

Evidence for Cervical Ripening Methods (SOGC Guidelines)
- meta-analysis of five trials has concluded that the use of oxytocin to ripen the cervix is not effective
- since the best dose and route of misoprostol for labour induction with a live fetus are not known and there are concerns regarding hyperstimulation, misoprostol's use for induction of labour should be within clinical trials only (Level Ib evidence) or in cases of intrauterine fetal death to initiate labour

INDUCTION OF LABOUR

Amniotomy
- artificial rupture of membranes (amniotomy) to stimulate PG synthesis and secretion; may try this as initial measure if cervix is dilated
- few studies address the value of amniotomy alone for induction of labour
- amniotomy plus intravenous oxytocin: more women delivered vaginally at 24 hours than amniotomy alone (relative risk = 0.03) and had fewer instrumental vaginal deliveries (relative risk = 5.5)

Oxytocin
- oxytocin (Pitocin™): 10 U in 1L NS, run at 0.5-2 mU/min IV increasing by 1-2 mU/minute q20-60 min to a max of 36-48 mU/min
- oxytocin alone reduced the rate of unsuccessful vaginal deliveries within 24 hours (8.3% vs 54%, RR 0.16). The ideal dosing regime of oxytocin is not known. It is currently recommended to use the minimum dose to achieve active labour with an increase every 30 minutes or more. Reassessment should occur once a dose of 20 mU/min is reached
- potential complications
    - hyperstimulation/tetanic contraction (may cause fetal distress or rupture of uterus)
    - uterine muscle fatigue, uterine atony (may result in PPH)
    - vasopressin-like action causing anti-diuresis

Augmentation of Labour

- augmentation of labour is used to promote adequate contractions when spontaneous contractions are inadequate and cervical dilatation or descent of fetus fails to occur
- oxytocin (0.5-2 mU/min IV increasing by 1-2 mU/minute q20-60 min to a max of 36-48 mU/min)

Use of Prostaglandins in Cervical Ripening and Induction
Intravenous prostaglandin for induction of labour. Cochrane Review. *The Cochrane Library.* 2000 Issue 2

- Prostaglandin E2 and F2 alpha can be used for cervical ripening and induction of labour. A meta-analysis comparing intravenous prostaglandin with oxytocin concluded that intravenous prostaglandin was no more likely to result in vaginal delivery (RR 0.85). Prostaglandins were associated with significantly more maternal side effects including gastrointestinal problems, thrombophlebitis and pyrexia. Currently, there is not enough evidence to draw any conclusions about the relative effects of prostaglandins vs. oxytocin and the choice is between the patient and the physician.
- Intravaginal prostaglandins are associated with higher rate of uterine hypertonus, uterine hyperstimulation, and fetal heart rate abnormalities.
- Prostaglandins are associated with reduced rate of C/S, instrumental vaginal delivery, and failed induction.

Intravaginal PGE_2 (Cervidil™) Compared to Intravaginal Prostaglandin Gel
4 RCTs have compared the two with varying results, depending on the dosing regime of gel used. Theoretical advantages of Cervidil™:
- insertion without a speculum
- slow, continuous release
- only one dose required
- ability to use oxytocin 30 min. after removal
- ability to remove insert if required (i.e. excessive uterine activity)

Oxytocin $t_{1/2}$ = 3-5 minutes.

High Risk Labour and Delivery

Preterm Labour (PTL)

Definition
- labour occurring between 20 and 37 weeks gestation

Etiology
- idiopathic (most common)
- maternal: infection (recurrent pyelonephritis, untreated bacteriuria, chorioamnionitis), genital infection (bacterial vaginosis is associated with a twofold increase in relative risk of preterm birth), HTN, DM, chronic illness, mechanical factors, previous obstetric, gynecological and abdominal surgeries, socio-environmental (poor nutrition, smoking, drugs, alcohol, stress)
- maternal-fetal: PPROM (a common cause), polyhydramnios, placenta previa or abruption, placental insufficiency
- fetal: multiple gestation, congenital abnormalities of fetus, fetal hydrops
- uterine: incompetent cervix, excessive enlargement (hydramnios), malformations (leiomyomas, septate)

Epidemiology
- preterm labour complicates about 10% of pregnancies

Risk Factors and Prediction of PTL
- maternal risk scoring using above etiologies fails to identify up to 70% of preterm deliveries and is therefore of limited use
- most important risk factor is prior history of spontaneous PTL
- cervical length – measured by TVUS. Cervical length >30 mm has high negative predictive value for PTL before 34 weeks
- identification of bacterial vaginosis (Rx - metronidazole) and *Ureaplasma urealyticum* (Rx - erythromycin) infections – routine screening not supported by current data but it is reasonable to screen high risk women
- fetal fibronectin – a glycoprotein in amniotic fluid and placental tissue functioning to maintain integrity of chorionic-decidual interface in asymptomatic women, a positive fetal fibronectin in cervicovaginal fluid (>50 ng/mL) @ 24 weeks gestation predicted spontaneous PTL @ <34 weeks with sensitivity of 23%, specificity of 97%, PPV of 25%, NPV of 96%
- in symptomatic women (i.e. preterm contractions) fetal fibronectic is most effectively combined with U/S detecting cervical length; if cervical length is not short and fetal fibronectic is negative, preterm labour is highly unlikely, thus preventing unnecessary admissions or transfers to higher level facilities

Clinical Features
- regular contractions (2 in 10 minutes)
- cervix >2 cm dilated or 80% effaced OR documented change in cervix

Management
A. Initial
- transfer to appropriate facility if stable
- hydration (NS @ 150 mL/hour)
- bed rest in LLDP
- sedation (morphine)
- avoid repeated pelvic exams (increased infection risk)
- U/S examination of fetus (for GA, BPP, position, placenta location, estimated fetal weight (EFW))
- prophylactic antibiotics; controversial but may help delay delivery, important to consider if PPROM

B. Suppression of Labour – Tocolysis
- does not inhibit preterm labour completely, but may buy time to allow Celestone™ use/transfer to appropriate centre
- requirements – all must be satisfied
    - preterm labour
    - live, immature fetus, intact membranes, cervical dilatation of ≤4 cm
    - absence of maternal or fetal contraindications

- contraindications
  - maternal
    - bleeding (placenta previa or abruption), maternal disease (hypertension, diabetes, heart disease), pre-eclampsia or eclampsia, chorioamnionitis
  - fetal
    - erythroblastosis fetalis, severe congenital anomalies, fetal distress/demise, IUGR, multiple gestation (relative)
- tocolytic procedure
  - ensure availability of necessary personnel and equipment to assess mother and fetus during labour and care for baby of the predicted GA if therapy fails
  - if no contraindications present, agent used depends on clinical situation
  - proven efficacy
    - calcium channel blockers: nifedipine
    - prostaglandin (PG) synthesis inhibitors (2nd line agent): indomethacin
    - beta-mimetics: ritodrine, terbutaline (rarely used)
    - should be used only for ≤48 hr, and/or transfer to an appropriate facility
  - no proven efficacy
    - nitroglycerin patch: vasodilator and smooth muscle relaxant that may delay delivery by 24-48h
    - magnesium sulfate (if diabetes or cardiovascular disease present)

C. Enhancement of Fetal Pulmonary Maturity
- betamethasone valerate (Celestone™) 12 mg IM q24h x 2 or dexamethasone 6 mg IM q12h x 4
  - 28-34 weeks GA: reduces incidence of respiratory distress syndrome (RDS)
  - 24-28 weeks GA: reduces severity of RDS, overall mortality and rate of intraventricular hemorrhage (IVH)
  - specific maternal contraindications: active TB, viral keratosis, maternal DM

D. Cervical Cerclage
- definition: placement of cervical sutures, wires or synthetic tape at the level of the internal os, usually at the end of the first trimester and removed in the third trimester
- indications
  - cervical incompetence (CI) - cervical dilation and effacement in the absence of increased uterine contractility
- diagnosis of CI
  - obstetrical Hx: silent cervical dilation
  - ability of cervix to hold an inflated Foley catheter during a hysterosonogram
- proven benefit in the prevention of PTL in women with primary structural abnormality of the cervix (e.g. conization of the cervix, connective tissue disorders)
- benefit is variable in those with secondary cervical incompetence causing premature ripening of the cervix (e.g. infection, abnormal placentation)
- contraindication: preterm labour; cerclage must be removed in presence of labour

Prognosis
- prematurity is the leading cause of perinatal morbidity and mortality
  - 30 weeks or 1500 g (3.3 lbs) = 90% survival
  - 33 weeks or 2000 g (4.4 lbs) = 99% survival
- morbidity due to asphyxia (may lead to cerebral hemorrhage), hypoxia (may lead to necrotizing enterocolitis), sepsis, respiratory distress syndrome (RDS), intraventricular hemorrhage, thermal instability, retinopathy of prematurity, bronchopulmonary dysplasia (see *Paediatrics* chapter)

Prevention of Preterm Labour
- currently there are no agents approved by Health Canada to arrest preterm labour
- preventative measures: good prenatal care, identify pregnancies at risk, treat silent vaginal infection or UTI, patient education
- transvaginal ultrasound of cervical length is not supported for routine prenatal care; however, it is recommended for high-risk pregnancies: cervical length of >30 mm has a high negative predictive value for delivery before 34 weeks (this measurement can be used to avoid unnecessary intervention)

Premature Rupture of Membranes (PROM)

Definitions
- premature ROM (PROM or amniorrhexis): rupture of membranes prior to labour at any GA
- prolonged ROM: >24 hours elapse between rupture of membranes and onset of labour

- preterm ROM: ROM occurring before 37 weeks gestation (associated with PTL)
- preterm premature ROM (PPROM): rupture of membranes before 37 weeks AND prior to onset of labour

Risk Factors
- maternal: multiparity, cervical incompetence, infection (cervicitis, vaginitis, STI, UTI), family history of PROM, low socioeconomic class/poor nutrition
- fetal: congenital anomaly, multiple gestation
- other risk factors associated with PTL

Clinical Features
- history of fluid gush or continued leakage

Investigations
- sterile speculum exam (avoid introduction of infection)
  - pooling of fluid in the posterior fornix
  - may observe fluid leaking out of cervix on cough/Valsalva ("cascade")
- amniotic fluid turns nitrazine paper blue (low specificity as can be positive with blood, urine or semen)
- ferning (high salt in amniotic fluid evaporates, looks like ferns under microscope)
- U/S to rule out fetal anomalies, assess GA and BPP

Management
- admit and monitor vitals q4h, daily BPP and WBC count
- avoid introducing infection with examinations (do **NOT** do a bimanual exam)
- cultures (cervix for GC, lower vagina for GBS)
- assess fetal lung maturity by L/S ratio of amniotic fluid
  - consider administration of betamethasone valerate (Celestone™) to accelerate maturity if <32 weeks and no evidence of infection
  - consider tocolysis for 48h to permit administration of steroids if PPROM
- weigh degree of prematurity vs. risk of amnionitis and sepsis by remaining in utero
  - <24 weeks consider termination (poor outlook due to pulmonary hypoplasia)
  - 26-34 weeks: expectant management as prematurity complications are significant
  - 34-36 weeks: "grey zone" where risk of death from RDS and neonatal sepsis is the same
  - >36 weeks: induction of labour since the risk of death from sepsis is greater than RDS
- if not in labour or labour not indicated, consider antibiotics (controversial)
  - studies show broad spectrum coverage increases the time to onset of labour from PROM by 5-7 days with no increase in maternal or neonatal morbidity or mortality
- deliver urgently if evidence of fetal distress and/or chorioamnionitis

Prognosis
- varies with gestational age
  - 90% of women with PROM at 28-34 weeks GA go into spontaneous labour within 1 week
  - 50% of women with PROM at <26 weeks GA go into spontaneous labour within 1 week
- complications: cord prolapse, intrauterine infection (chorioamnionitis), premature delivery, limb contracture

Breech Presentation

Definition
- fetal buttocks or lower extremity is the presenting part (see Figure 9)
- complete (10%): flexion at hips and knees
- frank (60%): flexion at hips, extension at knees
  - most common type of breech presentation
  - most common breech presentation to be delivered vaginally
- footling (30%): may be single or double with extension at hip(s) and knee(s) so that foot is the presenting part

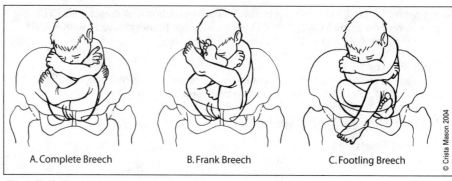

Figure 9. Types of Breech Presentation

Epidemiology
- occurs in 3-4% of pregnancies at term (25% before 28 weeks)

Risk Factors
- maternal risk factors
  - pelvis (contracted)
  - uterus (shape abnormalities, intrauterine tumours, fibroids)
  - extrauterine tumours causing compression
  - grand multiparity
- maternal-fetal
  - placenta (previa)
  - amniotic fluid (poly/oligohydramnios)
- fetal
  - prematurity
  - multiple gestation
  - congenital malformations (found in 6% of breeches; 2-3x the incidence in vertex presentations)
  - abnormalities in fetal tone and movement
  - aneuploidy

Clinical Features
- noted by Leopold's maneuvers (see Figure 2) and U/S – PPV of Leopold's maneuvers is only 30%

Management
- external cephalic version
  - repositioning of fetus within uterus
  - overall success rate of 65%
  - criteria: >37 weeks, singleton, unengaged presenting part, reactive NST
  - contraindications: previous T3 bleed, prior classical C/S, previous myomectomy, oligohydramnios, PROM, placenta previa, abnormal U/S, suspected IUGR, hypertension, uteroplacental insufficiency, nuchal cord
  - risks: abruption, cord compression
  - method: tocometry, followed by ultrasound guided transabdominal manipulation of fetus with consistent fetal heart monitoring via real-time sonography
  - if patient Rh negative, give Rhogam™ prior to procedure
  - good prognostic factors (for a successful version)
    - multiparous
    - good fluid volume
    - small baby
    - skilled obstetrician
- criteria for vaginal delivery (only if desired – see box)
  - frank or complete breech, GA >36 weeks
  - EFW 2500-3800 g based on clinical and U/S assessment (5.5–8.5 lb)
  - fetal head flexed
  - continuous fetal monitoring
  - maternal pelvis adequately large (clinically, or "proven" by previous delivery)
  - 2 experienced obstetricians, assistant, and anesthetist present
- C/S for all other presentations
  - recommended if the breech has not descended to the perineum in the second stage of labour after 2 hours, in the absence of active pushing, or if vaginal delivery is not imminent after 1 hour of active pushing

---

Planned Caesarean Section for Term Breech Delivery

Planned caesarean section for term breech delivery (Cochrane Review). In: *The Cochrane Library*, Issue 4, 2003. Chichester, UK: John Wiley & Sons, Ltd.

Study: 3 randomized control trials included from a search of the Cochrane Pregnancy and Childbirth Group trials register and the Cochrane Central Register of Controlled Trials.
Patients: 2396 women with breech presentation considered suitable for vaginal delivery.
Intervention: Comparison of planned Caesarean section for singleton breech presentation at term with planned vaginal birth.
Main Outcomes: Perinatal or neonatal death or serious neonatal morbidity and maternal death or maternal morbidity.
Results: Caesarean delivery occurred in 550/1227 (45%) of women allocated to a vaginal delivery protocol. Perinatal or neonatal death (excluding fatal anomalies) or serious neonatal morbidity was reduced (relative risk (RR) 0.33, 95% confidence interval (CI) 0.19 to 0.56) with planned Caesarean section. Planned Caesarean section was associated with modestly increased short-term maternal morbidity (RR 1.29, 95% CI 1.03 to 1.61). At 3 months after delivery, women allocated to the planned Caesarean section group reported less urinary incontinence (RR 0.62, 95% CI 0.41 to 0.93); more abdominal pain (RR 1.89, 95% CI 1.29 to 2.79); and less perineal pain (RR 0.32, 95% CI 0.18 to 0.58).

- recent RCT has demonstrated that for women with frank or complete breech presentations, perinatal mortality, neonatal mortality, and serious neonatal morbidity is significantly lower for those with planned C/S over those with planned vaginal birth, with no significant difference in maternal complications

Prognosis
- regardless of route of delivery, breech infants have lower birth weights and higher rates of perinatal mortality, congenital anomalies, abruption and cord prolapse

Vaginal Birth After Caesarean (VBAC)

- recommended after previous low transverse incision
- success rate varies with indication for previous C/S (generally 60-80%)
- risk of uterine rupture (<1% with low transverse incision)

Contraindications
- previous classical, inverted-T, or unknown uterine incision, or complete transection of uterus (6% risk of rupture)
- history of hysterotomy or previous uterine rupture
- multiple gestation
- estimated fetal weight >4000 g (9 lbs)
- non-vertex presentation or placenta previa
- inadequate facilities or personnel for emergency C/S

> **Vaginal Delivery After C-Section (VBAC)**
> Safety of vaginal birth after caesarean section: a systematic review. *Obstet Gynecol.* 2004. Mar; 103(3):420-9
>
> - rate of VBAC ranges from 60-82%
> - no significant difference in maternal deaths or hysterectomies between VBAC or C-section
> - uterine rupture more common in VBAC group
> - evidence regarding fetal outcome is lacking

Prolonged Pregnancy

Definition
- pregnancy beyond 42 weeks GA

Epidemiology
- 41 weeks GA: up to 27%
- 42 weeks GA: 4-14%

Etiology
- most cases idiopathic
- anencephalic fetus with no pituitary gland
- placental sulfatase deficiency (X-linked recessive condition in 1/2000-1/6000 infants)

Clinical Features
- risks increase with increasing GA: intrauterine infection, asphyxia, meconium aspiration syndrome, placental insufficiency, placental aging and infarction, macrosomia, dystocia, fetal distress, operative deliveries
- postmaturity syndrome: 10-20% of post-term pregnancies (fetal weight loss, reduction in subcutaneous fat, scaling, dry skin from placental insufficiency, long thin body, open-eyed, alert and worried look, long nails, palms and soles wrinkled)

Management
- GA 40-41 weeks – expectant management
    - there is no evidence to support induction of labour (IOL) or C/S unless other risk factors for morbidity are present (see prognosis)
- GA >41 weeks – offer induction of labour (IOL) if vaginal delivery is not contraindicated
    - IOL shown to decrease C/S, fetal heart rate changes, meconium staining, macrosomia and death when compared with expectant management at GA >41
- GA >41 weeks and expectant management elected – serial fetal surveillance:
    - fetal movement count by the mother
    - AFV ± NST (modified BPP)

Prognosis
- if >41 weeks, perinatal mortality 2-3x higher (due to progressive uteroplacental insufficiency)
- morbidity increased with hypertension/preeclampsia, DM, abruption, IUGR and multiple gestation

Intrauterine Fetal Death

Definition
- fetal death in utero after 20 weeks GA

Epidemiology
- 1% of pregnancies

Etiology
- 50% idiopathic
- 50% – HTN, DM, erythroblastosis fetalis, congenital anomalies, umbilical cord or placental complications, intrauterine infection, APLA syndrome

Clinical Features
- decreased perception of fetal movement by mother
- SFH and maternal weight not increasing
- absent fetal heart tones (not diagnostic)
- high MSAFP

Management
- diagnosis: absent cardiac activity and fetal movement on U/S required for diagnosis
- to determine secondary cause:
    - maternal: HbA1c, Kleihauer-Betke, VDRL, ANA, antibody screens, INR/PTT, serum/urine toxicology screens, cervical and vaginal cultures, TORCH screen
    - fetal: chromosomes, cord blood, skin biopsy, genetics evaluation, autopsy
    - placenta: pathology, bacterial cultures

Treatment
- induction of labour
- monitor for maternal coagulopathy - 10% risk of disseminated intravascular coagulation (DIC)
- address psychologic aspects of fetal loss including anxiety and depression
- f/u visit to discuss cause of death (if desired), risk of recurrence and counselling for future pregnancies

Complications of Labour and Delivery

Meconium in Amniotic Fluid

Epidemiology
- usually not present early in labour
- in general, meconium may be present in up to 25% of all labours; usually NOT associated with poor outcome, but extra care is required at time of delivery to avoid aspiration

Etiology
- likely cord compression ± uterine hypertonus
- may indicate undiagnosed breech
- increasing meconium during labour may be a sign of fetal distress

Clinical Features
- timing: early (prior to ROM) or late (after ROM with clear fluid)
- consistency
    - thin meconium: light green or yellow, not usually associated with poor outcome
    - thick meconium: dark green or black, pea-soup consistency, associated with lower APGARs and increased risk of meconium aspiration

---

DIC: Generalized coagulation and fibrinolysis leading to depletion of coagulation factors

Obstetrical causes:
- Abruption
- PIH
- Fetal demise
- PPH

DIC-specific bloodwork
- platelets
- aPTT and PT
- FDP (fibrin degradation products)
- fibrinogen

Treatment:
- treat underlying cause
- supportive
    - Fluids
    - Blood products
        - FFP, platelets, cryoprecipitate
- consider anti-coagulation as VTE prophylaxis

Dark green or black meconium is associated with lower APGARs and increased risk of meconium aspiration.

Treatment
- call pediatrics to delivery room
- oropharynx suctioning upon head expulsion if baby not breathing spontaneously
- consider amnioinfusion of ~800 mL of IV NS over 50-80 min during active stage of labor and a maintenance dose of ~3 mL/min until delivery
- closely monitor FHR for signs of fetal distress

Abnormal Progression of Labour (Dystocia)

Definition
- expected patterns of descent of the presenting part and cervical dilatation fail to occur in the appropriate time frame; can occur in all stages of labour (see Figure 10)
- during active phase: >4 hrs of <0.5 cm/hr
- during 2nd phase: >1 hr with no descent during active pushing

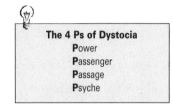

The 4 Ps of Dystocia
Power
Passenger
Passage
Psyche

Etiology
- **P**ower (leading cause): contractions (hypotonic, incoordinate), inadequate maternal explusive efforts
- **P**assenger: fetal position, attitude, size, anomalies (hydrocephalus)
- **P**assage: pelvic structure (cephalopelvic disproportion), maternal soft tissue factors (tumours, full bladder or rectum, vaginal septum)
- **P**syche: hormones released in response to stress can bring about dystocia
    - psychological and physiological stress should be evaluated as part of the management once dystocia has been diagnosed

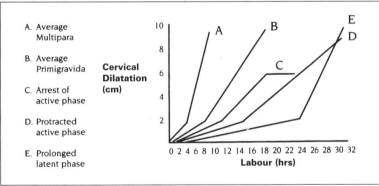

Figure 10. Normal and Abnormal Courses of the First Stage of Labour

Arrest Disorder (Curve C)
- arrest of dilatation
    - dilatation progress does not occur for ≥2 hours in a patient who has entered the active phase
    - arrest usually occurs at a cervical dilatation of 5-8 cm
- arrest of descent
    - no progress in station for >1 hour during second stage
    - should search for factors causing CPD (nearly 50% require C/S)
    - CPD diagnosed if adequate contractions measured by intrauterine pressure catheter (IUPC) with no descent/dilatation for >2 hours
    - if CPD ruled out, IV oxytocin and amniotomy can be attempted

Protraction Disorders (Curve D)
- protraction of dilatation: slope of cervical dilatation is <1.2 cm/h in primigravidas or <1.5 cm/hr in multigravidas
- protraction of descent: a rate of descent of <1.0 cm/h in primigravidas or 2.0 cm/h in multigravidas
- treatment: oxytocin augmentation if contractions are inadequate ± amniotomy

- 1/3 of protraction disorders develop into 2° arrest of dilatation due to CPD
- 2/3 of protraction disorders progress through labour to vaginal delivery

Prolonged Latent Phase (Curve E)
- ≥20 hrs in primigravidas or ≥14 hrs in multigravidas during which labour has not progressed to the active phase
- most often due to false labour (avoid amniotomy for fear of false labour and increased risk of intrauterine infection)
- premature or excessive use of sedation or analgesia may play a role

- careful search for factors of CPD should be made
- management: oxytocin augmentation if diagnosis of labour is certain, otherwise rest ± sedation

Risks of Dystocia
- inadequate progression of labour is associated with an increased incidence of:
    - maternal stress
    - maternal infection
    - postpartum hemorrhage
    - need for neonatal resuscitation

Umbilical Cord Prolapse

Definition
- descent of the cord to a level adjacent to or below the presenting part causing cord compression between presenting part and pelvis

Etiology/Epidemiology
- increased incidence with prematurity/PROM, fetal malpresentation (~50% of cases), low-lying placenta, polyhydramnios, multiple gestation, CPD
- incidence: 0.17-0.63%

Clinical Features
- visible or palpable cord
- FHR changes (variable decelerations, bradycardia or both)

Treatment
- emergency C/S: "code pink"
- O_2 to mother, monitor fetal heart
- alleviate pressure of the presenting part on the cord by placing digit in vagina - maintain position until C/S
- keep cord warm and moist by replacing it into the vagina ± applying warm saline soaks
- position mother in Trendelenburg or knee-to-chest position
- if fetal demise or too premature (<22 weeks), allow labour and delivery

Shoulder Dystocia

Definition
- impaction of anterior shoulder of fetus against symphysis pubis after fetal head has been delivered
- life threatening emergency

Etiology/Epidemiology
- incidence 0.15-1.4% of deliveries
- occurs when breadth of shoulders is greater than biparietal diameter of the head

Risk Factors
- maternal: obesity, diabetes, multiparity
- fetal: prolonged gestation, macrosomia
- labour:
    - prolonged 2nd stage
    - prolonged deceleration phase (8-10 cm)
    - instrumental midpelvic delivery

Clinical Features
- "turtle sign" (head delivered but retracts against inferior portion of pubic symphysis)
- complications
    - chest compression by vagina or cord compression by pelvis can lead to hypoxia
    - danger of brachial plexus injury (Erb palsy: C5-C7; Klumpke's palsy: C8-T1) – 90% resolve within 6 months
    - fetal fracture (clavicle, humerus, cervical spine)
    - maternal perineal injury, may result in PPH
    - intrapartum fetal hypoxia or trauma

Treatment
- goal: to displace anterior shoulder from behind symphysis pubis; follow a stepwise approach of maneuvers until goal achieved (see box)

Approach to the Management of Shoulder Dystocia:
ALARMER

Apply suprapubic pressure and ask for help

Legs in full flexion (McRobert's maneuver)

Anterior shoulder disimpaction (suprapubic pressure)

Release posterior shoulder by rotating it anteriorly with hand in the vagina under adequate anesthesia

Manual corkscrew i.e. rotate the fetus by the posterior shoulder until the anterior shoulder emerges from behind the maternal symphysis

Episiotomy

Rollover (on hands and knees)

- other options when ALARMER fails:
    - cleidotomy (deliberate fracture of neonatal clavicle)
    - Zavanelli maneuver: replacement of fetus into uterine cavity and emergent C/S
    - symphysiotomy
    - abdominal incision and shoulder disimpaction via hysterotomy – subsequent vaginal delivery

Prognosis
- 90% of shoulder dystocias will resolve with McRobert's maneuver and suprapubic pressure
- 1% risk of long term disability for infant

Uterine Rupture

Etiology/Epidemiology
- associated with previous uterine scar (in 40% of cases), hyperstimulation with oxytocin, grand multiparity and previous intrauterine manipulation
- generally occurs during labour, but can occur earlier with a classical incision
- 0.5-0.8% incidence, up to 12% with classical incision

Clinical Features
- acute onset abdominal pain
- hyper or hypotonic uterine contractions
- abnormal fetal heart rate, often bradycardia
- vaginal bleed

Treatment
- rule out placental abruption
- immediate delivery for fetal survival
- maternal stabilization (may require hysterectomy)

Complications
- maternal mortality 1-10%
- maternal hemorrhage and shock
- DIC
- amniotic fluid embolus
- hysterectomy required
- fetal distress, 50% mortality

Amniotic Fluid Embolus

Definition
- amniotic fluid debris in maternal circulation triggering an anaphylactoid-like immunologic response

Etiology/Epidemiology
- rare intrapartum or immediate postpartum complication
- 60-80% maternal mortality rate, accounts for 10% of all maternal deaths
- leading cause of maternal death in induced abortions and miscarriages
- 1/8000-1/80 000 births

Risk Factors
- placental abruption
- rapid labour
- multiparity
- uterine rupture
- amniocentesis or uterine manipulation

Differential Diagnois
- pulmonary embolus, drug-induced anaphylaxis, septic shock, eclampsia, HELLP syndrome, abruption, chronic coagulopathy

Clinical Features
- sudden onset of respiratory distress, cardiovascular collapse (hypotension, hypoxia) and coagulopathy
- seizure in 10%
- ARDS and left ventricular dysfunction seen in survivors

Management
- supportive measures (high flow O_2, ventilation support, fluid resuscitation, inotropic support, ± intubation), coagulopathy correction
- ICU admission

Chorioamnionitis

Definition
- infection of the chorion, amnion and amniotic fluid typically due to ascending infection by organisms of normal vaginal flora

Etiology/Epidemiology
- incidence 1-5% of term pregnancies and up to 25% in preterm deliveries
- may result from hematogenous spread or more commonly, ascending from vagina
- predominant microorganisms include GBS, *Bacteroides* and *Prevotella* species, *E. coli* and anaerobic *Streptococcus*

Risk Factors
- prolonged ROM, long labour, multiple vaginal exams during labour, internal monitoring
- bacterial vaginosis and other vaginal infections

Clinical Features
- maternal fever, maternal or fetal tachycardia, uterine tenderness, foul and purulent cervical discharge

Investigations
- CBC – look for ↑ WBC
- blood and amniotic fluid: leukocytes or bacteria in amniotic fluid

Treatment
- IV antibiotics (ampicillin and gentamicin and anaerobic coverage if C/S)
- expedient delivery regardless of gestational age

Complications
- bacteremia of mother or fetus, wound infection if C/S, pelvic abscess, infant meningitis

> - RCTs indicate that forceps delivery is associated with more maternal perineal and vaginal trauma while vacuum extraction causes more neonatal injury.

Operative Obstetrics

Operative Vaginal Delivery

Definition
- operative vaginal delivery is a forceps or vacuum extraction

Indications
- fetal
  - non-reassuring fetal status
  - consider if second stage is prolonged as this may be due to poor contractions or failure of fetal head to rotate
- maternal
  - need to avoid voluntary expulsive effort (cardiac/cerebrovascular disease)
  - exhaustion, lack of cooperation and excessive analgesia may impair pushing effort

Forceps

Outlet Forceps Position
- head visible between labia in between contractions
- sagittal suture in or close to AP diameter
- rotation cannot exceed 45 degrees

Low Forceps Position
- presenting part at station +2 or greater
- subdivided based on whether rotation less than or greater than 45 degrees

Mid Forceps Position
- presenting part below spines but above station +2

Types of Forceps
- Simpson forceps for OA presentations
- rotational forceps (Kielland) when must rotate head to OA
- Piper forceps for breech
- see Figure 11

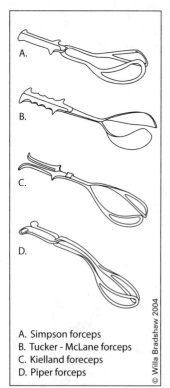

A. Simpson forceps
B. Tucker - McLane forceps
C. Kielland forceps
D. Piper forceps

© Willa Bradshaw 2004

Figure 11. Types of Forceps

Complications
- maternal: anesthesia risk, lacerations, injury to bladder, uterus, bone, pelvic nerve damage, PPH, infections
- fetal: fractures, facial nerve palsy, trauma to face/scalp, intracerebral hemorrhage (ICH), cephalohematoma, cord compression

Vacuum Extraction

- traction instrument used as alternative to forceps delivery; aids maternal pushing

Advantages
- easier to apply
- less anesthesia required
- less maternal soft-tissue injury compared to forceps
- will lose suction and dislodge if unrecognized CPD present

Disadvantages
- contraindicated if fetus at risk for coagulation defect
- suitable only for vertex presentations
- maternal pushing required
- contraindicated in preterm delivery
- EFW must be ≥2500 g
- increased incidence of cephalohoematomata and retinal hemorrhages compared to forceps

Specific Complications of Vacuum Extraction for Fetus
- subglial hemorrhage
- subaponeurotic hemorrhage
- soft tissue trauma
- retinal hemorrhage

Lacerations

- first degree: involves skin and vaginal mucosa but not underlying fascia and muscle
- second degree: involves fascia and muscles of the perineal body but not the anal sphincter
- third degree: involves the anal sphincter but does not extend through it
- fourth degree: extends through the anal sphincter into the rectal mucosa

Episiotomy

Definition
- incision in the perineal body at the time of delivery
  - midline: incision through central tendinous portion of perineal body and insertions of superficial transverse perineal and bulbocavernosus muscle; better healing but increased risk of deep tear
  - mediolateral: incision through bulbocavernosus, superficial transverse perineal muscle, and levator ani; reduced risk of extensive tear but poorer healing and more pain

Indications
- to prevent a tear (episiotomy is easier to repair)
- to relieve obstruction of the unyielding perineum
- instrumental delivery
- controversy over whether it is preferable to make a cut, or let the perineum tear as needed; current evidence suggests letting perineum tear and then repair as needed

Complications
- infection, hematoma, extension into anal musculature or rectal mucosa, fistula formation

Prerequisites for Operative Vaginal Delivery: ABCDEFGHIJK
Anesthesia
Bladder empty
Cervix fully dilated and effaced with ROM
Determine position of fetal head
Equipment ready (including facilities for emergent C/S)
Fontanelle (posterior fontanelle midway between shanks, fenestration barely palpable)
Gentle traction
Handle elevated
Incision (episiotomy)
once **J**aw visible remove forceps
Knowledgeable operator

Limits for trial of vacuum
- 3 pulls
- 3 pop-offs
- 20 minutes with no delivery

Restrictive vs. Routine Episiotomies with Vaginal Births
Episiotomy for vaginal birth. *The Cochrane Library*, Issue 3, 2003. Oxford: Update Software
Study: 6 Randomized control trials included from a search of the Cochrane Pregnancy and Childbirth Group trials register.
Patients: Of the 2409 patients in the routine episiotomy group, 1752 (72.7%) women had episiotomies. In the restrictive episiotomy group, 673 (27.6%) of the 2441 women had episiotomies.
Intervention: Use of restrictive (only done for fetal indications or if severe perineal trauma was judged to be imminent) vs. routine (liberally done to prevent any tear) episiotomy in women undergoing vaginal birth.
Main Outcomes: Anterior and posterior perineal trauma, need for suture repair and healing complications.
Results: Restrictive episiotomies appear to have less posterior perineal trauma (RR 0.88), less suturing (RR 0.74) and fewer complications (RR 0.69) compared to routine episiotomies. There is no difference for pain measures, dyspareunia, urinary incontinence, and severe vaginal or perineal trauma, but there was an increased risk of anterior perineal trauma (RR 1.79) with restrictive episiotomy. The two studies examining benefit of mediolateral vs. midline episiotomies were excluded due to poor methodological quality.

Caesarean Delivery

Epidemiology
- incidence 20-25%

Indications
- maternal: obstruction, active herpetic lesion on vulva, invasive cervical cancer, previous uterine surgery, underlying maternal illness (eclampsia, HELLP syndrome, heart disease)
- maternal-fetal: failure to progress, placental abruption or previa
- fetal: NRFHR, malpresentation, cord prolapse, certain congenital anomalies

Types of Caesarean Incisions
- skin
    - vertical midline
        - rapid peritoneal entry and increased exposure
        - increased dehiscence
    - transverse
        - decreased exposure and slower entry
        - improved strength and cosmesis
- uterine
    - low transverse (most common) – in noncontractile segment – decreased chance for rupture in subsequent pregnancies
    - low vertical – used for very preterm infants, poorly developed maternal lower uterine segment
    - classical (rare) – in thick, contractile segment – used for transverse lie, fetal anomaly, >2 fetuses, lower segment adhesions, obstructing fibroid

Risks/Complications
- anesthesia
- hemorrhage (average blood loss ~1000 cc)
- infection (UTI, wound, endometritis)
- injury to surrounding structures (bowel, bladder, uterus) → a single-dose prophylactic antibiotic should be used (cefazolin 1-2 g)
- thromboembolic phenomena
- increased recovery time/hospital stay
- maternal mortality (<0.1%)

Puerperium

Definition
- 6-week period of adjustment after pregnancy when pregnancy-induced anatomic and physiologic changes are reversed

Postpartum Care

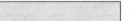

The acronym "**BUBBLE**" for what to ask about when rounding on postpartum care. Modify this for C/S or vag delivery
B = **b**aby care and breast feeding (how's the latch? Amount etc.?)
U = **u**terus. Is it firm or boggy?
B = **b**ladder function? Urinating? Dysuria etc...
B = **b**owel function? Passing gas or stool? Constipated etc...
L = **l**ochia or discharge? Any blood?
E = **e**pisiotomy

The 10 Bs
- Be careful: do not use douches or tampons for 4-6 weeks post-delivery
- Be fit: encourage gradual increases in walking, Kegel exercises
- Birth control: breastfeeding is NOT an effective method of birth control
- Bladder: maintain high fluid intake
- Bleeding: (see *Lacerations* section, OB51), 300 μg of RhIG should be given if Rh+ fetus and Rh– mother or extensive bleeding at delivery
- Blood pressure: especially if gestational HTN
- Blood tests: glucose
- Blues: (see *Postpartum Mood Alterations* section, OB56)
- Bowel: fluids and high-fibre foods, bulk laxatives may be helpful; for hemorrhoids/perineal tenderness: pain meds, doughnut cushion, Sitz baths, ice compresses
- Breast: encourage breast-feeding if no contraindications (see <u>Pediatrics</u>) – watch for Staphyloccoccal or Streptococcal mastitis/abscess

Uterus
- uterus weight rapidly diminishes through catabolism, cervix loses its elasticity and regains firmness
- should involute ~1 cm (1 finger breadth) below umbilicus per day in first 4-5 days – involution then slows down; reaches non-pregnant state in 4-6 weeks postpartum

Ovarian Function
- ovulation resumes in ~45 days for nonlactating women and within 3-6 months for lactating women

Lochia
- normal vaginal discharge postpartum
- decreases and changes colour from red (lochia rubra; due to presence of erythrocytes) → yellow (lochia serosa) → white (lochia alba; residual leukorrhea) over 3-6 weeks
- foul smelling lochia suggests endometritis

Puerperal Complications

Postpartum Hemorrhage (PPH)

Definition
- loss of >500 mL of blood at the time of vaginal delivery, or >1000 mL with C/S
- early – within first 24h postpartum
- late – after 24h but within first 6 weeks

Epidemiology
- incidence 5-15%

Etiology (4 Ts)
1. Tone
   - uterine atony
     - most common cause of PPH
     - avoid by giving oxytocin with delivery of the anterior shoulder
     - occurs within first 24 hours
   - due to:
     - labour (prolonged, precipitous, induced, augmented)
     - uterus (infection, over-distention)
     - placenta (abruption, previa)
     - maternal factors (grand multiparity, gestational HTN)
     - halothane anesthesia
2. Tissue
   - retained placenta
   - retained blood clots in an atonic uterus
   - gestational trophoblastic neoplasia
3. Trauma
   - laceration (vagina, cervix, uterus), episiotomy, hematoma (vaginal, vulvar, retroperitoneal), uterine rupture, uterine inversion
4. Thrombin
   - coagulopathy
     - most identified prior to delivery (low platelets increases risk)
     - includes hemophilia, DIC, aspirin use, ITP, TTP, vWD (most common)
     - do not forget therapeutic anti-coagulation

Investigations
- assess degree of blood loss and shock by clinical exam
- explore uterus and lower genital tract for evidence of tone, tissue or trauma
- may be helpful to observe red-topped tube of blood – no clot in 7-10 minutes indicates coagulation problem

Management
- ABCs
- 2 large bore IVs and crystalloids
- CBC, coagulation profile, cross and type 4 units pRBCs
- treat the cause

Uterine atony is #1 cause of PPH.

DDx of Early PPH:
1. Atony
2. Retained placenta
3. Laceration
4. Uterine inversion
5. Coagulopathy

DDx of Late PPH:
1. Retained products
2. +/- endometritis
3. Sub-involution of uterus

Medical Therapy
- oxytocin 20 U/L NS or RL IV continuous infusion – in addition can give 10 U intramyometrial (IMM) after delivery of the placenta
- methylergonavine maleate (ergotamine) 0.25 mg IM/IMM q5min up to 1.25 mg; can be given as IV bolus of 0.125 mg (may exacerbate HTN)
- carboprost (Hemabate™) (synthetic PGF-2 alpha analog) 0.25 mg IM/IMM q15 min to max 2 mg (major prostaglandin side effects and contraindicated in CV, pulmonary, renal and hepatic dysfunction)

Local Control
- bimanual compression: elevate the uterus and massage through patient's abdomen
- uterine packing (mesh with antibiotic treatment)
- intrauterine Senstaken-Blakemore catheter for balloon tamponade - may slow hemorrage enough to allow time for correction of coagulopathy or for preparation of an OR

Surgical Therapy (Intractable PPH)
- D&C (beware of vigorous scraping which may cause Asherman's syndrome)
- laparotomy with bilateral ligation of uterine artery (may be effective), internal iliac artery (not proven), ovarian artery, or hypogastric artery
- hysterectomy (last option) with angiographic embolization if post-hysterectomy bleeding

Retained Placenta

Definition
- placenta undelivered after 30 minutes postpartum

Etiology
- placenta separated but not delivered
- abnormal placental implantation i.e. placenta accreta, placenta increta, placenta percreta (see box, OB24)

Risk Factors
- placenta previa, prior C/S, post-pregnancy curettage, prior manual placental removal, uterine infection

Clinical Features
- incomplete placenta removed
- risk of postpartum hemorrhage and infection

Investigations
- explore uterus
- assess degree of blood loss

Management
- 2 large bore IVs, type and screen
- Brant maneuver (firm traction on umbilical cord with one hand applying suprapubic pressure to hold uterus in place)
- oxytocin 10 IU in 20 mL NS into umbilical vein
- manual removal if above fails
- D&C if required

Uterine Inversion

Definition
- uterine prolapse through cervix ± vaginal introitus

Etiology/Epidemiology
- often iatrogenic (excess cord traction with fundal placenta)
- excessive use of uterine tocolytics
- more common in grand multiparous (lax uterine ligaments)
- 1/1500-1/2000 deliveries

Clinical Features
- can cause profound vasovagal response with vasodilation and hypovolemic shock
- shock may be disproportionate to maternal blood loss

Management
- urgent management essential, call anesthesia
- ABCs – initiate IV crystalloids
- can use tocolytic drug (e.g. terbutaline) or nitroglycerin IV to relax uterus and aid replacement
- replace uterus without removing placenta
- remove placenta manually and withdraw slowly
- IV oxytocin infusion (only after uterus replaced)
- re-explore uterus
- may require GA ± laparotomy

Postpartum Pyrexia

Definition
- fever >38.0°C on any 2 of the first 10 days postpartum, except the first day

Etiology
- **W**ind (atelectasis, pneumonia), **W**ater (UTI), **W**ound (C/S incision or episiotomy site), **W**alking (pelvic thrombophlebitis, DVT), **B**reast (engorgement, mastitis – *S. aureus*), **W**omb (endometritis)

Investigations
- appropriate clinical exam and relevant cultures
- for endometritis: blood and genital cultures

Treatment
- empiric treatment for wound infections: clindamycin + gentamicin
- prophylaxis against post-C/S endometritis: begin antibiotic immediately after cord clamping and administer only 1-3 doses – cefazolin is most common choice

> **Etiology of post-partum pyrexia: B-5W:**
> **B**reast: engorgement, mastitis
> **W**ind: atelectasis, pneumonia
> **W**ater: UTI
> **W**ound: episiotomy/C/S site infection
> **W**alking: DVT, thrombophlebitis
> **W**omb: endometritis

Mastitis

- rule out inflammatory carcinoma, as indicated

Table 18. Lactational versus Non-Lactational Mastitis

	Lactational	Non-Lactational
Epidemiology	• more common than non-lactational • often 2-3 wks postpartum	• periductal mastitis most commonly • mean age 32 y
Etiology	• *S. aureus*	• may be sterile • may be infected with *S. aureus* or anaerobes • smoking is risk factor • may be associated with mammary duct ectasia
Symptoms	• unilateral localized pain • tenderness • erythema	• subareolar pain • may have subareolar mass • discharge (variable colour) • nipple inversion
Treatment	• heat or ice packs • continued nursing • antibiotics (dicloxacillin/cephalexin)	• broad-spectrum antibiotics and I&D • total duct excision (definitive)
Abscess	• fluctuant mass • purulent nipple discharge • fever, leukocytosis • d/c nursing, IV antibiotics (nafcillin/oxacillin), I&D usually required	• if mass does not resolve, FNA to exclude cancer and U/S to assess presence of abscess • treatment includes antibiotics, aspiration or I&D (tends to recur); may develop mammary duct fistula • a minority of non-lactational abscesses may occur peripherally in breast with no associated periductal mastitis (usually *S. aureus*)

- mammary duct ectasia = mammary duct(s) beneath nipple clogged and dilated ± ductal inflammation ± nipple discharge (thick, grey to green), often postmenopausal women

Postpartum Mood Alterations

POSTPARTUM BLUES
- 85% of new mothers, onset day 3-10; extension of the "normal" hormonal changes and adjustment to a new baby
- self-limited, does not last more than 2 weeks
- manifested by mood lability, depressed affect, increased sensitivity to criticism, tearfulness, fatigue, irritability, poor concentration/despondency

POSTPARTUM DEPRESSION (PPD)
- definition: major depression occurring in a woman within 6 months of childbirth (see Psychiatry)
- epidemiology: 10-20%, risk of recurrence 50%
- risk factors
    - personal or family history of depression (including PPD)
    - prenatal depression or anxiety
    - stressful life situation
    - poor support system
    - unwanted pregnancy
    - colicky or sick infant
- clinical features: suspect if the "blues" last beyond 2 weeks, or if the symptoms in the first two weeks are severe (e.g. extreme disinterest in the baby, suicidal or homicidal ideation)
- treatment: antidepressants, psychotherapy, supportive care, ECT if refractory
- prognosis: interferes with bonding and attachment between mother and baby so it can have long term effects

POSTPARTUM PSYCHOSIS
- definition: presents as an acute psychotic episode, or in the context of depression – abrupt onset of symptoms over 24-72 hours within first month post-partum
- epidemiology: rare (0.2%)
- treatment: (see Psychiatry)

Drug and Food Safety During Pregnancy

- most drugs cross the placenta to some extent
- use any drug with caution and only if necessary

Antibiotics

Drug Resources during Pregnancy and Breastfeeding
- Motherisk at the Hospital for Sick Children in Toronto
  416-813-6780
  www.motherisk.org
- Hale, T. *Medications and Mothers' Milk*, 11th Edition. Pharmasoft Publishing, 2004.

- safest: ampicillin, cephalosporins
- erythromycin: maternal liver damage (acute fatty liver)
    - used only if contraindication to penicillin use
- tetracyclines: stain children's teeth
- sulpha drugs: anti-folate properties, therefore theoretical risk in T1
    - risk of kernicterus in T3
- metronidazole: anti-metabolite, therefore theoretical risk in T1
- chloramphenicol: grey baby syndrome
    - fetal circulatory collapse 2° to toxic accumulation
- fluoroquinolones: risk of cartilage damage (in dog and rat studies)

Other Medications & Substances

- ACE inhibitors: fetal renal defects, IUGR, oligohydramnios
- anticonvulsants:
    - phenytoin associated with fetal hydantoin syndrome in 5-10% (IUGR, MR, facial dysmorphogenesis, congenital anomalies)
    - valproate associated with oNTD in 1%
    - carbamazepine associated with oNTD in 1-2%
    - generally recommended to remain on the lowest dose anticonvulsant appropriate for their condition
- DES (and other estrogenic or androgenic compounds): vaginal adenosis, adenocarcinoma, uterine malformation in females exposed to DES in utero
- lithium: Ebstein's cardiac anomaly, goitre, hyponatremia
- misoprostol: Mobius syndrome (congenital facial paralysis with or without limb defects)
- retinoids (e.g. Accutane™): CNS, craniofacial, cardiovascular, and thymic anomalies

- warfarin: ↑ incidence of spontaneous abortion, stillbirth, prematurity, IUGR
  - fetal warfarin syndrome (nasal hypoplasia, epiphyseal stippling, optic atrophy, MR, intracranial hemorrhage)
- alcohol: ↑ incidence of abortion and stillbirth, congenital anomalies
  - fetal alcohol syndrome (growth retardation, CNS involvement and facial anomalies)
- cigarette smoke: ↓ birth weight, placenta previa/abruption, ↑ spontaneous abortion, preterm labour, stillbirth
- cocaine: microcephaly, growth retardation, prematurity, MR

Immunizations

Intrapartum
- administration is dependent on the risk of infection vs. risk of immunization complications
- safe: tetanus toxoid, diphtheria, influenza, hepatitis B
- avoid live vaccines (risk of placental and fetal infection): polio and mumps, varicella
- contraindicated: rubella, oral typhoid

Postpartum
- rubella as needed
- hepatitis B vaccine should be given to infant within 12h of birth if maternal status unknown or positive – follow-up doses at 1 and 6 months

Breastfeeding and Drugs

- safe
  - penicillins, aminoglycosides, cephalosporins
  - oral contraceptive use (low dose) – OCP will decrease quantity but not affect composition of breast milk
  - medroxyprogesterone acetate
- avoid
  - chloramphenicol (bone marrow suppression)
  - metronidazole (mutagenic in vitro)
  - sulphonamides (hemolysis with G6PD deficiency)
  - nitrofurantoin (hemolysis with G6PD deficiency)
  - tetracycline (stains teeth and bones)
  - lithium
  - anti-neoplastics and immunosuppressants
  - psychotropic drugs (relative)

Breast Feeding: Contraindicated Drugs
BREAST:
Bromocriptine/ **B**enzodiazepines
Radioactive isotopes/ **R**izatriptan
Ergotamine/ **E**thosuximide
Amiodarone/ **A**mphetamines
Stimulant laxatives/ **S**ex hormones
Tetracycline/ **T**retinoin

Food

Caffeine
- caffeine has diuretic and stimulant properties
- no known adverse effects on pregnancy or fetus
- consumption should be limited to no more than 400-450 mg per day from all sources during pregnancy and lactation

Sources of caffeine
400-450 mg of caffeine:
<2.5 cups of percolated or filter drip coffee
<3.5 cups strong tea
7–16 cans of cola
16 cups of hot cocoa
10 dark regular chocolate bars

Herbal Teas and Preparations
- not enough scientific information about the safety of various herbs and herbal products to recommend their general use during pregnancy and lactation
- some herbal teas can have toxic or pharmacological effects on the mother or fetus
- chamomiles have been reported to exhibit adverse effects on the uterus

Food Borne Illnesses
- microbiological contamination of food may occur through cross-contamination and/or improper food handling
  - listeriosis (*Listeria monocytogenes*) and toxoplasmosis (*Toxoplasma gondii*) are of concern during pregnancy
  - avoid consumption of raw meats, fish, poultry, raw eggs, and unpasteurized dairy products
  - wash all raw fruit and vegetables thoroughly
  - soft cheeses and patés may be sources of *Listeria* and should be avoided during pregnancy
- chemical contamination of food
  - current guideline for mercury of 0.5 ppm in fish is considered protective for the general population, including pregnant women
  - Health Canada advises pregnant women to limit consumption of top predator fish such as shark, swordfish and fresh/frozen tuna (not canned tuna) to one meal per month

Herbal teas considered safe in moderation (2-3 cups/day)
citrus peel
ginger
lemon balm
linden flower – not with prior cardiac condition
orange peel
rose hip

Common Medications

Table 19. Common Medications

Drug Name (Brand Name)	Dosing Schedule	Indications/Comments
betamethasone valerate (Celestone™)	12 mg IM q24h x 2 doses	Enhancement of fetal pulmonary maturity for PTL
carboprost (Hemabate™)	0.25 mg IM/IMM q15min; max 2 mg	Treatment of uterine atony
dexamethasone	6 mg IM q12h x 4 doses	Enhancement of fetal pulmonary maturity for PTL
dinoprostone (Cervidil™ - PGE$_2$ impregnated thread)	10 mg PV (remove after 12h) max of 3 doses	Induction of labour Advantage: can remove if uterine hyperstimulation
doxylamine succinate (Diclectin™)	2 tabs qhs + 1 tab qAM + 1 tab qPM max of 8 tabs/day	Each tablet contains 10 mg doxylamine succinate with vitamin B6 Used for hyperemesis gravidarum
folic acid	0.4-1.0 mg PO OD x 1-3 mo preconception and T1 4.0 mg PO OD with past Hx of NTD	Prevention of oNTD
methotrexate	50 mg/m^2 IM or 50 mg po x 1 dose	For ectopic pregnancy or medical abortion
methylergonavine maleate (Ergotamine™)	0.25 mg IM/IMM q5min up to 1.25 mg or IV bolus 0.125 mg	Treatment of uterine atony
misoprostol (Cytotec™)	800-1000 µg pr x 1 dose 400 µg po x 1 dose or 800 µg pv x 1 dose, 3 to 7 days after methotrexate	For treatment of PPH For medical abortion Also used for NSAID-induced ulcers (warn female patients of contraindications)
oxytocin (Pitocin™)	0.5-2.0 mU/min IV, or 10 U/L N/S incr. by 1-2 mU/min q20-60min max of 36-48 mU/min	Augmentation of labour (also induction of labour)
	10 U IM @ delivery of ant shoulder	Prevention of uterine atony
	20 U/L NS or RL IV continuous infusion	Treatment of uterine atony
PGE$_2$ gel (Prostin® gel)	0.5 mg PV q6-12h; max of 3 doses	Induction of labour
Rh IgG (Rhogam™)	300 µg IM x 1 dose	Given to Rh negative women: routinely at 28 wks GA within 72 hrs of birth of Rh +ve fetus positive Kleihauer-Betke test with any invasive procedure in pregnancy ectopic pregnancy antepartum hemorrhage miscarriage or TA (dose: 50 µg IM only)

Misoprostol (Cytotec®) is also indicated to protect against NSAID-induced gastric ulcers. The use of misoprostol for cytoprotection is contraindicated in pregnancy. Warn female patients of this contraindication.

OP Ophthalmology

Malcolm C. W. Gooi, Silvia Odorcic, Dominik W. Podbielski and Fereshte N. Samji, chapter editors
Justine Chan and Angela Ho, associate editors
Billie Au, EBM editor
Dr. Wai-Ching Lam, staff editor

Basic Anatomy Review

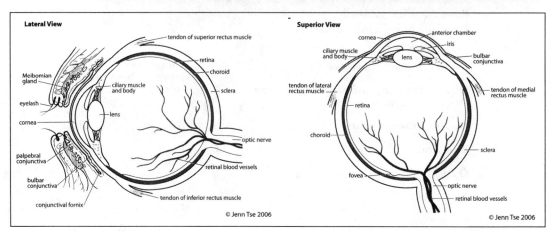

Figure 1. Anatomy of the Eye

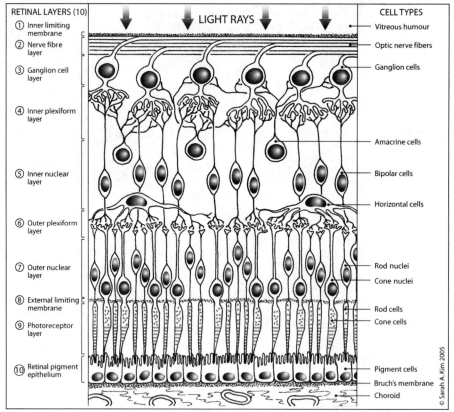

Figure 2. Layers of the Retina

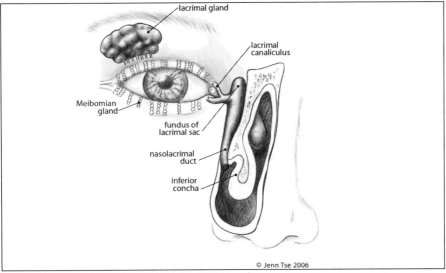

Figure 3. Tear Drainage from the Eye (Lacrimal Apparatus)

Differential Diagnoses of Common Presentations

Transient Loss of Vision (lasting seconds to hours)
- transient ischemic attack (TIA)
- migraine with aura
- papilledema

Acute Loss of Vision (occurring in seconds to days)

Cornea/Anterior Segment
- corneal edema
- hyphema
- acute angle-closure glaucoma
- trauma/foreign body

Cortical/Other
- occipital infarction/hemorrhage
- cortical blindness
- functional (non-organic, diagnosis of exclusion)

Vitreous/Retina/Optic Nerve
- vitreous hemorrhage
- retinal detachment
- retinal artery/vein occlusion
- acute macular lesion
- optic neuritis
- temporal arteritis
- anterior ischemic optic neuropathy (AION)

> **Top 3 in DDx of Acute Loss of Vision**
> 1. trauma/foreign body
> 2. retinal artery/vein occlusion
> 3. retinal detachment

Chronic Loss of Vision (occurring over weeks to months)

Cornea/Anterior Segment
- corneal dystrophy, scarring, edema
- refractive error
- cataract
- glaucoma

Vitreous/Fundus/Optic Nerve
- age-related macular degeneration (ARMD)
- diabetic retinopathy
- retinal vascular insufficiency
- compressive optic neuropathy (intracranial mass, orbital mass)
- intraocular neoplasm
- retinitis pigmentosa (RP)

Cortical/Other
- pituitary adenoma
- medication-induced (sildenafil, amiodarone)
- nutritional deficiency
- pituitary adenoma

> **Top 3 in DDx of Chronic Loss of Vision**
> **Reversible:**
> 1. cataract
> 2. refractive error
> 3. corneal dystrophy
>
> **Irreversible:**
> 1. age-related macular degeneration
> 2. glaucoma
> 3. diabetic retinopathy

Red Eye
- lids/orbit/lacrimal system
  - hordeolum/chalazion
  - blepharitis
  - foreign body/laceration
  - dacryocystitis/dacryoadenitis
- conjunctiva/sclera
  - subconjunctival hemorrhage
  - conjunctivitis
  - dry eyes
  - pterygium/pinguecula
  - episcleritis/scleritis
  - preseptal/orbital cellulitis

- cornea
  - foreign body
  - keratitis
  - abrasion, laceration
  - ulcer
- anterior chamber
  - uveitis (iritis, iridocyclitis)
  - acute angle-closure glaucoma
  - hyphema
  - hypopyon
- endophthalmitis

Table 1. Common Differential Diagnosis of Red Eye

	Conjunctivitis	Acute Iritis	Acute Angle Closure Glaucoma	Keratitis
Discharge	Bacteria: purulent Virus: serous Allergy: mucous	No	No	Profuse tearing
Pain	No	++ (tender globe)	+++ (nauseating)	++ (on blinking)
Photophobia	No	+++	+	++
Blurred Vision	No	++	+++	Varies
Pupil	Normal	Smaller	Fixed in mid-dilation	Same or smaller
Injection	Conjunctiva with limbal pallor	Ciliary flush	Diffuse	Diffuse
Cornea	Normal or opacified	Keratic precipitates	Steamy	Infiltrate, edema, epithelial defects
Intraocular pressure	Normal	Varies	Increased markedly	Normal or increased
Anterior chamber	Normal	Cells + flare	Shallow	Cells + flare or normal
Other	Large, tender preauricular node if viral	Posterior synechiae	Coloured halos Nausea and vomiting	

> Not every red eye has conjunctivitis.

Ocular Pain
- differentiate from ocular ache: eye fatigue (asthenopia)
- herpes zoster prodrome
- trauma/foreign body
- keratitis
- corneal abrasion, corneal ulcer
- acute angle-closure glaucoma
- acute uveitis
- scleritis, episcleritis
- optic neuritis
- ocular migraine

Floaters
- vitreous syneresis (shrinkage and collapse of vitreous gel)
- posterior vitreous detachment (PVD)
- vitreous hemorrhage
- retinal tear/detachment
- posterior uveitis

Flashes of Light (Photopsia)
- posterior vitreous detachment (PVD)
- retinal tear/detachment
- migraine with aura

Photophobia (Severe Light Sensitivity)
- corneal abrasion, corneal ulcer
- keratitis
- acute angle-closure glaucoma
- iritis
- meningitis, encephalitis
- migraine

Diplopia (Double Vision)
- binocular diplopia: strabismus, CN palsy (III, IV, VI) secondary to ischemia, diabetes, tumour, trauma, myasthenia gravis, muscle restriction/entrapment, thyroid ophthalmopathy, internuclear ophthalmologia (INO) secondary to multiple sclerosis, brainstem infarct
- monocular diplopia: refractive error, strands of mucus in tear film, keratoconus, cataract, dislocated lens, peripheral iridotomy

Ocular Problems in the Elderly
- blepharitis, ptosis, entropion, ectropion
- dry eyes, epiphora
- presbyopia, cataracts
- glaucoma
- age-related macular degeneration
- retinal artery/vein occlusion
- temporal arteritis (arteritic ischemic optic neuropathy)

Ocular Problems in the Contact Lens Wearer
- superficial punctate keratitis (SPK)/dry eyes
- solution hypersensitivity
- tight lens syndrome
- corneal abrasion
- giant papillary conjunctivitis
- sterile corneal infiltrates (immunologic)
- infected ulcers (*Pseudomonas, Acanthamoeba*)

Ocular Emergencies

These Require Urgent Consultation to an Ophthalmologist for Management

Sight Threatening
- lid/globe lacerations
- corneal ulcer
- gonococcal conjunctivitis
- acute iritis
- acute angle-closure glaucoma
- central retinal artery occlusion (CRAO)
- intraocular foreign body
- retinal detachment (especially macula threatening)
- endophthalmitis

Life Threatening
- proptosis (rule out cavernous sinus fistula or thrombosis)
- CN III palsy with dilated pupil (intracranial aneurysm or neoplastic lesion)
- papilledema (must rule out intracranial mass lesion)
- orbital cellulitis
- giant cell (temporal) arteritis
- leukocoria - white pupil (must rule out retinoblastoma)

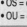

- OD = oculus dexter = right eye
- OS = oculus sinister = left eye
- OU = oculus uterque = both eyes

The Ocular Examination

Note: Sometimes vision may be blurry secondary to eye drops/ointment/mucus → ask patient to blink a few times

VISION ASSESSMENT

- always test visual acuity first, especially in emergency room
- test best corrected vision (with corrective lenses) whenever possible
- assess both distance (Snellen chart) and near vision (Rosenbaum pocket screener)
- test right eye first, then left. Cover eye not being tested
- improvement of visual acuity using a "pinhole test" indicates an uncorrected refractive error

Visual Acuity – Distance
- Snellen Fraction (Figure 4) = testing distance (usually 20 feet or 6 metres) / smallest line patient can read on the chart
- e.g. 20/40 = what the patient can see at 20 feet (numerator), a "normal" person can see at 40 feet (denominator)
- testing hierarchy for low vision: Snellen acuity (20/x) → counting fingers at x distance (CF) → hand motion (HM) → light perception with projection (LP with projection) → light perception (LP) → no light perception (NLP)
- legal blindness is best corrected visual acuity that is worse or equal to 20/200 in the better eye, or a limit to the binocular central field of vision of <20 degrees

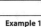

A Snellen visual acuity of 20/20 equates to "normal" vision.

Example 1

$\overline{SC}$

V 20/40 -1
20/80 + 2 → 20/25 PH

Example 2

$\overline{CC}$

V CF 3'
HM

Note: RIGHT EYE visual acuity always listed on top.

V	Vision
$\overline{SC}$	Without correction
$\overline{CC}$	With correction
20/40-1	All except one letter of 20/40
20/80+2	All of 20/80 plus two letters of 20/70
PH	Visual acuity with pinhole correction
CF	Counting fingers at 3 feet
HM	Hand motion

Figure 4. Ophthalmology Nomenclature for Visual Acuity

- minimum visual requirements to operate a non-commercial automobile in Ontario are, with both eyes open and examined together, 20/50 best corrected visual acuity, a visual field of 120 continuous degrees along the horizontal meridian, and a visual field of 15 continuous degrees above and below fixation
- note that each province/state has different regulations

Visual Acuity – Near
- use pocket vision chart (e.g. Rosenbaum Pocket Vision Screener)
- record Jaeger (J) or Point number and testing distance (usually 30 cm), e.g. J2 @ 30 cm
- conversion to distance visual acuity can be made when distance vision cannot be tested (e.g. immobile patient, no distance chart available)

Visual Acuity for infants, children non-English speakers, and dysphasics
- newborns
    - visual acuity cannot be tested
- 3 mos-2 yrs (can only assess visual function, not acuity)
    - test each eye for fixation and maintaining fixation using an interesting object
    - noted as "CSM" = central, steady and maintained
- 2 years until alphabet known
    - picture chart/card (child names simple objects presented at different sizes)
    - tumbling "E" chart (child indicates direction of "E")
    - Sheridan-Gardiner matching test

Colour Vision
- test with Ishihara Pseudoisochromatic Plates (usually referred to as Ishihara plates)
- record number correct out of total plates presented to each eye
- important for testing optic nerve function (e.g. optic neuritis, chloroquine use)

VISUAL FIELDS
- test "visual fields by confrontation" (4 quadrants, each eye tested separately) for estimate of visual field loss (Figure 5)
- accurate, quantifiable assessment done with automated visual field testing (Humphrey or Goldmann) or Tangent Screen
- use Amsler grid (each eye individually) to test for central or paracentral scotomas (island-like gaps in the vision), especially for patients with AMD

PUPILS
- use reduced room illumination with patient focusing on distant object to prevent "near reflex"
- examine pupils for shape, size, symmetry and reactivity to light (both direct and consensual response)
- test for relative afferent pupillary defect (RAPD) with swinging flashlight test
- test pupillary constriction portion of near reflex by bringing object close to patient's nose
- "normal" pupil testing often noted as "PERRLA" = pupils equal, round, and reactive to light and accommodation

ANTERIOR CHAMBER DEPTH
- shine light tangentially from temporal side
- shallow anterior chamber (AC): >2/3 of nasal side of iris in shadow (Figure 7)

EXTRAOCULAR MUSCLES

Alignment
- Hirschberg corneal reflex test
    - examine in primary position of gaze (e.g. straight ahead) with patient focusing on distant object (to eliminate accommodative convergence)
    - shine light into patient's eyes from ~30 cm away
    - corneal light reflex should be symmetric and at same position on each cornea
- strabismus testing as indicated (cover test, cover-uncover test, prism testing) (see *Strabismus* section, OP41)

Movement
- examine movement of eyeball through six cardinal positions of gaze (Figure 6) (with six muscles responsible for extra-ocular movement)
- ask patient if diplopia is present in any position of gaze

Infant and Child Visual Acuity
- 6-12 months - 20/120
- 1-2 years - 20/80
- 2-4 years - 20/20

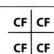

RIGHT EYE fields drawn on right side; LEFT EYE fields drawn on left side (as if seen through patient's eyes).

CF Able to count fingers in specified quadrant with peripheral vision

Gross visual field deficit in specified quadrant using peripheral vision

Figure 5. Ophthalmology Nomenclature for Visual Fields by Confrontation

For patients with dark irises, test the pupils using an ophthalmoscope focused on the red reflex. This will provide a better view than using a penlight.

Changing fixation from distance to near results in the "near reflex":
1. eye convergence
2. pupil constriction
3. lens accommodation

- CN III - Superior, Medial and Inferior Rectus, Inferior Oblique
- CN IV - Superior Oblique (SO)
- CN VI - Lateral Rectus (LR)

- observe for horizontal, vertical or rotatory nystagmus (rhythmic, oscillating movements of the eye)
- resolving horizontal nystagmus at end gaze is usually normal
- cranial nerve III: superior rectus (SR), medial rectus (MR), inferior rectus (IR), inferior oblique (IO)
- cranial nerve IV: superior oblique (SO)
- cranial nerve VI: lateral rectus (LR)

EXTERNAL EXAMINATION

- the four L's
  - lymph nodes (preauricular, submandibular)
  - lids
  - lashes
  - lacrimal system

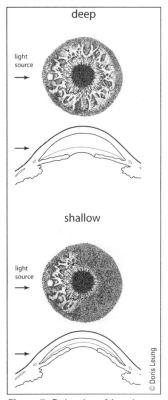

Figure 6. Diagnostic Positions of Gaze to Isolate Primary Action of Each Muscle

Figure 7. Estimation of Anterior Chamber Depth

Schematic drawing of the slit lamp

1 Power switch (on/off)
2 Slit lamp joystick control
3 Locking knob
4 Ocular
5 Magnification adjustment knob
6 Brightness adjustment lever
7 Slit beam height adjustment knob
8 Slit beam width adjustment knob
9 Patient-positioning frame
10 Forehead strap
11 Patient chin rest
12 Chin rest height adjustment knob

© Janice Wong and Danielle Bader

The ophthalmology note: Slit lamp exam

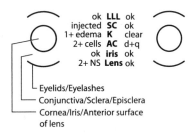

ok	**LLL**	ok
injected	**SC**	ok
1+ edema	**K**	clear
2+ cells	**AC**	d+q
ok	**iris**	ok
2+ NS	**Lens**	ok

— Eyelids/Eyelashes
— Conjunctiva/Sclera/Episclera
— Cornea/Iris/Anterior surface of lens

Note: RIGHT EYE drawn on the left, LEFT EYE drawn on the right (as if looking at patient's face).

LLL Lids, lashes, lacrimal
SC Sclera, conjunctiva
K Cornea
AC Anterior chamber
d+q Deep (not shallow) and quiet (no cells in AC)
NS Nuclear sclerosis (cataract)

Any abnormality or pathology is drawn on the sketch in the appropriate location, and is labelled (e.g. trichiasis, conjunctivitis/episcleritis/scleritis, corneal abrasion/ulcer, foreign body, etc).

Figure 8. Slit-Lamp

Central Corneal Thickness
Average CCT = 550 μm
A thick cornea overestimates IOP by GAT
A thin cornea underestimates IOP by GAT

Note: RIGHT EYE intraocular pressure (IOP) always listed on top.

Always note which method used to measure IOP (Goldmann, Tonopen, airpuff).

Figure 9. Tonometry

Desired Myers Pattern on GAT

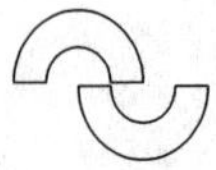

Note: Thick Myers underestimate the IOP and are a result of excess fluorescein.

Quick Tips on Direct Ophthalmoscopy
1. Examine in a dark room
2. Ask patient to focus on a distant object
3. Match ophthalmoscope light aperture to size of pupil (i.e. smaller aperture for undilated eye)
4. Use moderate light intensity
5. Use your left/right eye and hand to examine patient's left/right eye respectively
6. Get in close! Proximity to patient's eye is key with hand resting on patient's cheek

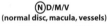
Ⓝ D/M/V
(normal disc, macula, vessels)

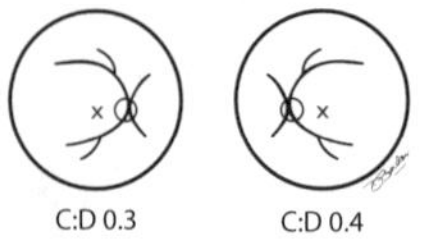

C:D 0.3   C:D 0.4

Note: RIGHT EYE drawn on the left, LEFT EYE drawn on the right (as if looking at patient's face).

C:D Cup:Disc ratio
x   Fovea

Any abnormality or pathology of the fundus is drawn on the sketch in the appropriate location, and is labelled (e.g. hemorrhages, neovascularization, cotton-wool spots, drusen, retinal tear/detachment, etc.).

Figure 10. Fundus

SLIT-LAMP EXAMINATION
- systematically examine all structures of the anterior segment + anterior vitreous
    - lids (including upper lid eversion if necessary), lashes, and lacrimal system
    - conjunctiva and sclera
    - cornea
    - iris
    - anterior chamber (for depth, cells, and flare)
        - to observe cells and flare: 1. Dark room 2. High power beam 3. 1 mm beam height 4. Thin beam 5. Highest magnification 6. Approach at angle and focus on anterior chamber (space between cornea and lens)
    - lens
    - anterior vitreous
- when necessary, use
    - fluorescein dye – stains Bowman's membrane in de-epithelialized cornea, appearing green with cobalt blue filtered light
    - Rose Bengal dye – stains devitalized corneal epithelium
- special lenses (78 or 90 diopter (D)) used with the slit-lamp allow a binocular, stereoscopic view of the fundus and vitreous

TONOMETRY
- measurement of intraocular pressure (IOP) (Figure 9)
- normal range is 10-21.5 mmHg, with a mean of 15 mmHg
- commonly measured by
    - Goldmann applanation tonometry (GAT) – gold standard, performed using slit-lamp with special tip (prism)
    - Tonopen – benefit is portability and use of disposable probe tip. Use when cornea is scarred/assymetric, rendering GAT inaccurate
    - air puff (non-contact and least reliable readings)
- use topical anesthetic for Goldmann and Tonopen

OPHTHALMOSCOPY/FUNDOSCOPY
- can be performed with
    - direct ophthalmoscope (monocular with small field of view, only posterior pole visualized)
    - slit-lamp with 78D or 90D lens (binocular view, visualization to mid-periphery of retina)
    - indirect ophthalmoscopy with headlamp and 20D or 28D lens (binocular view, visualization of entire retina to ora serrata/edge of retina)
- assess red reflex
    - light reflected off the retina produces a "red reflex" when viewed from ~ 1 foot away
    - anything that interferes with the passage of light will diminish the red reflex (e.g. large vitreous hemorrhage, cataract)
- examine the posterior segment of the eye (Figure 10)
    - vitreous
    - optic disc (colour, cup/disc ratio, sharpness of disc margin)
    - macula (~2 disc diameters temporal to disc), fovea (foveal light reflex)
    - retinal vessels
    - retinal background
- best peformed with pupils fully dilated (see Table 8 for list of mydriatics and cycloplegics)
- contraindications to pupillary dilatation
    - shallow anterior chamber - can precipitate acute angle closure glaucoma
    - iris-supported anterior chamber lens implant
    - potential neurologic abnormality requiring pupil evaluation
    - use caution with cardiovascular disease – mydriatics may cause tachycardia

Optics

EMMETROPIA
- no refractive error
- image of distant objects focus exactly on the retina (Figure 11)

MYOPIA
- "nearsightedness"
- prevalence of 30-40% in U.S. population

HYPEROPIA
- "farsightedness"
- may be developmental or due to any etiology that shortens the globe

PRESBYOPIA
- normal aging process (especially over 40 years)

ASTIGMATISM
- light rays not refracted uniformly in all meridians due to non-spherical surface of cornea or non-spherical lens (e.g. football-shaped)

ANISOMETROPIA
- difference in refractive error between eyes
- second most common cause of amblyopia in children

REFRACTION
- determining the lens parameters needed to correct the refractive errors of the eye
- two techniques used
  - Flash/Streak Retinoscopy – refractive error determined objectively by use of lenses and retinoscope
  - Manifest – subjective trial using phoropter (device the patient looks through that is equipped with lenses)
- a typical lens prescription would contain
  - sphere power in diopters (D), negative lens for myopes, positive lens for hyperopes
  - cylinder power in D to correct astigmatism (always positive value)
  - axis of cylinder (in degrees)
  - "add" (bifocal/progressive reading lens) for presbyopes
  - e.g. -1.50 + 1.00 x 120 degrees, add +2.00

REFRACTIVE EYE SURGERY
- permanently alters corneal refractive properties by ablating tissue to change curvature of the cornea
- used for correction of myopia, hyperopia, and astigmatism
- common types include photorefractive keratectomy (PRK) and laser-assisted in-situ keratomileusis (LASIK)
- potential risks/side-effects: infection, undercorrection/overcorrection, decreased night vision, corneal haze, dry eyes, regression, corneal flap completely cut (LASIK only)

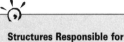

Structures Responsible for Refractive Power
1. cornea (2/3)
2. lens (1/3)

Diopter (D) = measurement of refractive power of a lens
- "negative" lens = concave, corrects for myopia
- "positive" lens = convex, corrects for hyperopia

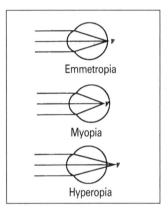

Figure 11. Emmetropia and Refractive Errors

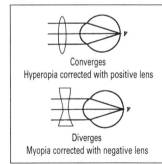

Figure 12. Correction of Refractive Errors

Table 2. Optics

	Pathophysiology	Clinical Features	Treatment	Complications
Myopia	• globe too long relative to refractive mechanisms, or refractive mechanisms too strong • light rays from distant object focus in front of retina --> blurring of distant vision (Figure 11)	• usually presents in 1st or 2nd decade, stabilizes in 2nd and 3rd decade; rarely begins after 25 years of age except in patients with diabetes or cataracts • blurring of distant vision; near vision usually unaffected	• correct with negative diopter/concave/ "negative" lenses to diverge light rays (see Figure 12) • refractive eye surgery – see *Refractive Eye Surgery* section	• retinal tear/detachment, macular hole, open angle glaucoma, complications not prevented with refractive correction
Hyperopia	• globe too short relative to refractive mechanisms, or refractive mechanisms too weak • light rays from distant object focus behind retina --> blurring of near +/- distant vision (see Figure 11)	• youth: usually do not require glasses (still have sufficient accommodative ability to focus image on retina), but may develop accommodative esotropia (see *Strabismus*) • 30s-40s: blurring of near vision due to decreased accommodation, may need reading glasses • >50s: blurring of distance vision due to severely decreased accommodation	• when symptomatic, correct with positive Diopter/convex/"plus" lenses to converge light rays (see Figure 12) • refractive eye surgery – see *Refractive Eye Surgery* section	• angle-closure glaucoma, particularly later in life as lens enlarges
Astigmatism	• two types of astigmatism • regular – curvature uniformly different in meridians at right angles to each other • irregular – distorted cornea, caused by injury, keratoconus (cone-shaped cornea), corneal scar, or severe dry eye	• affects approximately 30% of population, with prevalence increasing with age • mild astigmatism unnoticeable • higher amounts of astigmatism may cause blurry vision, squinting, asthenopia, or headaches	• correct with cylindrical lens (if regular), try contact lens (if irregular) • refractive eye surgery – see *Refractive Eye Surgery* section	
Presbyopia	• hardening/reduced deformability of the lens results in decreased accommodative ability • near images cannot be focused onto retina (focus is behind retina as in hyperopia)	• if initially emmetropic, person begins to hold reading material further away, but distance vision remains unaffected • if initially myopic, person begins removing distance glasses to read • if initially hyperopic, symptoms of presbyopia occur earlier	• correct vision with positive diopter/convex/"plus" lenses for reading	

The Orbit

Exophthalmos (Proptosis)

- anterior displacement (protrusion) of the globe
- investigate with CT/MRI head/orbits, ultrasound orbits, thyroid function tests
- exophthalmos generally refers to an endocrine etiology (e.g. Graves' disease) or protrusion of the globe by >18 mm
- proptosis generally refers to other etiologies (e.g. cellulitis) or protrusion <18mm

Etiology
- Graves' disease (unilateral or bilateral, most common cause in adults)
- orbital cellulitis (unilateral, most common cause in children)
- primary or secondary orbital tumours
- orbital/retrobulbar hemorrhage
- cavernous sinus thrombosis or fistula

Enophthalmos

- posterior displacement (retraction) of the globe
- investigate with CT/MRI orbits

Etiology
- "blow-out" fracture (see *Ocular Trauma* section, OP45)
- orbital fat atrophy
- congenital abnormality

Preseptal Cellulitis

- infection of soft tissue **anterior** to orbital septum

Etiology
- usually follows periorbital trauma or dermal infection

Clinical Features (Table 3)
- tender, swollen and erythematous lids
- may have low-grade fever
- normal visual acuity, pupils, extraocular movements (EOM)
- no exophthalmos or RAPD

Treatment
- systemic antibiotics (suspect *H. influenzae* in children; *S. aureus* or *Streptococcus* in adults)
- warm compresses

Orbital Cellulitis

- OCULAR and MEDICAL EMERGENCY
- inflammation of orbital contents posterior to orbital septum
- common in children, but also in the elderly and immunocompromised

Etiology
- usually secondary to sinus/facial/tooth infections or trauma

> Orbital cellulitis is life-threatening if untreated (mortality of 17-20% without antibiotic use). Thus, it needs to be diagnosed and treated promptly.

Clinical Features (Table 3)
- decreased visual acuity, as well as pain, red eye, headache, fever
- lid erythema, tenderness, and edema with difficulty opening
- conjunctival injection and chemosis (conjunctival edema)
- proptosis, limitation of ocular movements (ophthalmoplegia) and pain with movement
- RAPD, optic disc swelling

Treatment
- admit, IV antibiotics, commonly ceftriaxone + vancomycin or equivalent for 1 week, blood cultures, orbital CT
- surgical drainage of abscess and follow closely

Complications
- cavernous sinus thrombosis, meningitis, brain abscess, optic nerve inflammation with possible loss of vision, death

Table 3. Differentiating Between Preseptal and Orbital Cellulitis

Finding	Preseptal Cellulitis	Orbital Cellulitis
Fever	May be present	+
Lid edema	Moderate to severe	Severe
Chemosis	– or mild	Marked
Proptosis	–	+
Pain on eye movement	–	+
Ocular mobility	Normal	Decreased
Vision	Normal	Diminished ± diplopia
RAPD	Absent	May be seen
Leukocytosis	Moderate	Marked
ESR	Normal or elevated	Elevated
Additional findings	Skin infection	Sinusitis, dental abscess

Lacrimal Apparatus

- tear film made up of three layers
  - an outer oily layer (reduces evaporation) secreted by the Meibomian glands
  - a middle watery layer (forms the bulk of the tear film) constant secretion from conjunctival glands and reflex secretion by lacrimal gland with ocular irritation or emotion
  - an inner mucinous layer (aids with tear adherance to cornea) secreted by conjunctival goblet cells
- tears drain from eye through upper and lower lacrimal puncta → superior and inferior canaliculi → lacrimal sac → nasolacrimal duct → nasal cavity behind inferior concha (Figure 3)

Dry Eye Syndrome (Keratoconjunctivitis Sicca)

Etiology
- idiopathic – tear production normally decreases with aging
- blepharitis
- ectropion – downward and outward turning of lower eyelid
- decreased blinking (CN VII palsy)
- diminished corneal sensitivity (e.g. neurotrophic keratitis)
- systemic diseases: rheumatoid arthritis, Sjögren's syndrome, sarcoidosis, amyloidosis, leukemia, lymphoma
- medications: anticholinergics, diuretics, antihistamines, oral contraceptives
- vitamin A deficiency

Clinical Features
- dry eyes, red eyes, foreign body sensation, blurred vision, tearing
- slit-lamp exam: decreased tear meniscus, decreased tear break up time (TBUT, normally should be 10 seconds), superficial punctate keratitis (SPK)
- stains with fluorescein/Rose Bengal
- Schirmer's test: measures tear quantity on surface of eye in 5 minute time period (<10 mm of paper strip wetting in 5 minutes is considered a dry eye)

Complications
- erosions and scarring of cornea

Treatment
- nonpreserved artificial tears up to q1h and ointment at bedtime (preservative toxicity becomes significant if used more than q4h)
- punctal occlusion (punctal plug insertion), lid taping, tarsorrhaphy (sew lids together) if severe
- treat underlying cause

Epiphora (Excessive Tearing)

Etiology
- emotion
- environmental stressor (cold, wind, pollen, sleep deprivation)
- ectropion/entropion/trichiasis
- conjunctivitis
- corneal foreign body/keratitis
- dry eyes (reflex tearing)
- lacrimal drainage obstruction (aging, rhinitis, dacryocystitis, congenital failure of canalization)
- paradoxical lacrimation (crocodile tears)

Excessive tearing can be caused by dry eyes – if the tear quality is insufficient, "reflex tearing" may occur.

Investigations
- using fluorescein dye, examine for punctal reflux by pressing on canaliculi
- Jones dye test – irrigate dye through punctum into nose, noting resistance/reflux

Treatment
- lid repair for ectropion/entropion
- eyelash removal for trichiasis
- punctal irrigation
- nasolacrimal duct probing (infants)
- tube placement: temporary (Crawford) or permanent (Jones)
- surgical: dacryocystorhinostomy (DCR) – forming a new connection between the lacrimal sac and the nasal cavity

Dacryocystitis

- acute or chronic infection of the lacrimal sac
- most commonly due to obstruction of the nasolacrimal duct
- commonly associated with *S. aureus, S. pneumoniae, Pseudomonas* species

Clinical Features
- pain, swelling, redness over lacrimal sac at medial canthus
- tearing, crusting, fever
- digital pressure on the lacrimal sac may extrude pus through the punctum
- in the chronic form, tearing may be the only symptom

Treatment
- warm compresses, nasal decongestants, systemic and topical antibiotics
- if chronic, obtain cultures by aspiration
- once infection resolves, consider dacryocystorhinostomy (DCR)

Dacryoadenitis

- inflammation of the lacrimal gland (outer third of upper eyelid)
- acute causes: *S. aureus*, mumps, EBV, herpes zoster, *N. gonorrheae*
- chronic causes: lymphoma, leukemia, sarcoidosis, tuberculosis, thyroid ophthalmopathy

Clinical Features
- pain, swelling, tearing, discharge, redness of the outer region of the upper eyelid
- chronic form is more common and may present as painless enlargement of the lacrimal gland

Treatment
- supportive: warm compresses, oral NSAIDs
- systemic antibiotics if bacterial cause
- if chronic, treat underlying disorder

Lids and Lashes

Lid Swelling

Etiology
- commonly due to allergy, with shrivelling of skin between episodes
- dependent edema on awakening (e.g. CHF, renal or hepatic failure)
- orbital venous congestion due to mass or cavernous sinus fistula
- dermatochalasis: loose skin due to aging
- lid cellulitis, thyroid disease (e.g. myxedema), trauma, chemosis

Ptosis

- drooping of upper eyelid

Etiology
- aponeurotic: disinsertion or dehiscence of levator aponeurosis
  - most common cause
  - associated with advancing age, trauma, surgery, pregnancy, chronic lid swelling
- mechanical
  - eyelid prevented from opening completely by mass or scarring
- neuromuscular
  - poor levator function associated with myasthenia gravis (neuromuscular palsy), myotonic dystrophy
  - CN III palsy
  - Horner's syndrome
- congenital
- pseudoptosis (e.g. dermatochalasis, enophthalmos, contralateral exophthalmos)

Treatment
- surgery

Trichiasis

- eyelashes turned inwards
- may result from chronic inflammatory lid diseases (e.g. blepharitis), Stevens-Johnson syndrome, trauma, burns, etc.
- patient complains of red eye, foreign body sensation, tearing
- may result in corneal ulceration (detected with fluoroscein staining at the slit lamp)

Treatment
- topical lubrication, eyelash plucking, electrolysis, cryotherapy

Entropion

- lid margin turns in towards globe causing tearing, foreign body sensation and red eye
- most commonly affects lower lid
- may cause abrasions with secondary corneal scarring

Etiology
- involutional (aging)
- cicatricial (herpes zoster, surgery, trauma, burns)
- orbicularis oculi muscle spasm
- congenital

Treatment
- lubricants, evert lid with tape, surgery

Testing for Entropion
Forced lid closure (Ask patient to tighten lid then open. In entropion, lid rolls inwards)

Testing for Ectropion
Snapback test (Pull eyelid inferiorly. In ectropion, lid remains away from globe)

Ectropion

- lid margin turns outward from globe causing tearing and possibly exposure keratitis

Etiology
- involutional (weak orbicularis oculi)
- paralytic (CN VII palsy)
- cicatricial (burns, trauma, surgery)
- mechanical (lid edema, tumour, herniated fat)
- congenital

Treatment
- topical lubrication, surgery

Hordeolum (Stye)

- acute inflammation of eyelid gland – either Meibomian glands (internal lid) or glands of Zeis (modified sweat gland) or Moll (modified sebaceous gland) (external lid)
- infectious agent is usually *S. aureus*
- painful, red swelling of lid

Treatment
- warm compresses, lid care, gentle massage
- topical antibiotics (e.g. erythromycin ointment bid)
- usually resolves in 2-5 days

Chalazion

- chronic granulomatous inflammation of Meibomian gland (often preceded by an internal hordeolum
- acute inflammatory signs are usually absent
- differential diagnosis: basal cell carcinoma, sebaceous cell adenoma, Meibomian gland carcinoma

Treatment
- warm compresses
- if no improvement after 1 month, consider incision and curettage
- chronic, recurrent lesion must be biopsied to rule out malignancy

Blepharitis

- inflammation of lid margins

Etiology
- staphylococcal (*S. aureus*): ulcerative, dry scales
- seborrheic: no ulcers, greasy scales

Clinical Features
- itching, tearing, foreign body sensation
- thickened, red lid margins, crusting, discharge with pressure on lids ("toothpaste sign")

Complications
- recurrent chalazia
- conjunctivitis
- keratitis (from poor tear film)
- corneal ulceration and neovascularization

Treatment
- warm compresses and lid scrubs with diluted "baby shampoo"
- topical or systemic antibiotics as needed
- if severe, an ophthalmologist may prescribe a short course of topical corticosteroids

Xanthelasma

- eyelid xanthoma (lipid deposits in dermis of lids)
- appear as pale, slightly elevated yellowish plaques or streaks
- most commonly on the medial upper lids, often bilateral
- associated with hyperlipidemia (approximately 50% of the time)
- common in the elderly, more concerning in the young

Treatment
- excision for cosmesis only, recurrences common

Conjunctiva

- thin, vascular mucous membrane/epithelium
- bulbar conjunctiva: lines sclera to limbus (junction between cornea and sclera)
- palpebral conjunctiva: lines inner surface of eyelid

 # Pinguecula

- yellow-white subepithelial deposit of hyaline and elastic tissue adjacent to the nasal or temporal limbus
- associated with sun and wind exposure, aging
- common, benign, sometimes enlarge slowly
- surgery for cosmesis only

 # Pterygium

- fibrovascular triangular encroachment of epithelial tissue onto the cornea, usually nasal
- may induce astigmatism, decrease vision
- excision for chronic inflammation, threat to visual axis, cosmesis
- one-third recur after excision
- much decreased recurrence with conjunctival autograft (5%)

 # Subconjunctival Hemorrhage

- blood beneath the conjunctiva, otherwise asymptomatic
- idiopathic or associated with trauma, Valsalva maneuver, bleeding disorders, hypertension
- give reassurance if no other ocular findings, resolves in 2-3 weeks
- if recurrent, consider medical/hematology work-up

 # Conjunctivitis

Etiology
- infectious
    - bacterial, viral, chlamydial, fungal, parasitic
- non-infectious
    - allergy: atopic, seasonal, giant papillary conjunctivitis (in contact lens wearers)
    - toxic: irritants, dust, smoke, irradiation
    - secondary to another disorder such as dacryocystitis, dacryoadenitis, cellulitis, Kawasaki's disease

Clinical Features
- red eye, itching, foreign body sensation, chemosis (conjunctival edema), tearing, discharge, crusting of lashes in the morning
- lid edema, conjunctival injection often with limbal pallor, preauricular node, subepithelial infiltrates
- follicles: pale lymphoid elevations of the conjunctiva
- papillae: fibrovascular elevations of the conjunctiva with central network of finely branching vessels (cobblestone appearance)

- enlarged lymph nodes suggest infectious etiology, especially viral or chlamydial conjunctivitis
- temporal conjunctival lymphatics drain to preauricular nodes, and nasal to submandibular nodes

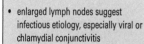

- follicles are seen in viral and chlamydial conjunctivitis
- papillae are seen in allergic and bacterial conjunctivitis

ALLERGIC CONJUNCTIVITIS

Atopic
- associated with rhinitis, asthma, dermatitis, hay fever
- small papillae, chemosis, thickened, erythematous lids, corneal neovascularization
- treatment: cool compresses, antihistamine, mast cell stabilizer
- seasonal (pollen, grasses, plant allergens)

Giant Papillary Conjunctivitis (GPC)
- immune reaction to mucus debris on lenses in contact lens wearers
- large papillae form on superior palpebral conjunctiva
- specific treatment: clean, change or discontinue use of contact lens

Vernal Conjunctivitis
- large papillae (cobblestones) on superior palpebral conjunctiva with corneal ulcers, keratitis
- seasonal (warm weather)
- occurs in children, lasts for 5-10 years and then resolves
- specific treatment: consider topical steroid, cyclosporine (not in primary care)

VIRAL CONJUNCTIVITIS
- serous discharge, lid edema, follicles, subepithelial corneal infiltrates
- may be associated with rhinorrhea
- preauricular node often palpable and tender
- initially unilateral, often progresses to the other eye
- mainly due to adenovirus – highly contagious for up to 12 days

Treatment
- cool compresses, topical lubrication
- usually self-limiting (7-12 days)
- proper hygiene is very important
- may develop corneal epithelial defects and subepithelial infiltrates requiring specific treatment

BACTERIAL CONJUNCTIVITIS
- purulent discharge, lid swelling, papillae (often), conjunctival injection, chemosis
- common agents include *S. aureus*, *S. pneumoniae*, *H. influenzae* and *M. catarrhalis*
- in neonates and sexually active people must consider *N. gonorrheae* (invades cornea to cause keratitis)
- *Chlamydia trachomatis* is the most common cause in neonates

Treatment
- topical broad-spectrum antibiotic
- systemic antibiotics if indicated, especially in children
- usually a self-limited course of 10-14 days if no treatment, 1-3 days with treatment

CHLAMYDIAL CONJUNCTIVITIS
- caused by *Chlamydia trachomatis*
- affects neonates on day 3-5, sexually active people
- causes trachoma, inclusion conjunctivitis

Trachoma
- leading infectious cause of blindness in the world
- severe keratoconjunctivitis leads to corneal abrasion, ulceration, and scarring
- initially, follicles on superior palpebral conjunctiva
- treatment: topical and systemic tetracycline

Inclusion Conjunctivitis
- chronic conjunctivitis with follicles and subepithelial infiltrates
- most common cause of conjunctivitis in newborns
- prevention: topical erythromycin at birth
- treatment: topical and systemic tetracycline, doxycycline or erythromycin

Types of Discharge
Allergic: mucoid
Viral: watery
Bacterial: purulent
Chlamydial: mucopurulent

Sclera

- the white fibrous outer protective coat of the eye
- continuous with the cornea anteriorly and the dura of the optic nerve posteriorly
- episclera is a thin layer of vascularized tissue between the sclera and conjunctiva

Episcleritis

- immunologically mediated inflammation of episclera
- one-third bilateral; simple (80%) or nodular (20%)
- more frequent in women than men (3:1)

Etiology
- mostly idiopathic
- in 1/3 of cases, associated with collagen vascular diseases, infections (herpes zoster, herpes simplex, syphilis), IBD, rosacea, atopy

Clinical Features
- asymptomatic usually, may have mild pain and red eye
- sectoral or diffuse injection of radially-directed vessels, chemosis, small mobile nodules
- blanches with topical phenylephrine (constricts superficial conjunctival vessels)

Treatment
- generally self limited, recurrent in 2/3 of cases
- topical steroid for 3-5 days if painful (prescribed and monitored by ophthalmologist)

Scleritis

- usually bilateral: diffuse, nodular or necrotizing
- anterior scleritis: may cause scleral thinning
- posterior scleritis: may cause exudative retinal detachment
- more common in women and elderly

Etiology
- half are a manifestation of systemic disease
- collagen vascular disease (e.g. systemic lupus erythematosus (SLE), rheumatoid arthritis (RA), ankylosing spondylitis (AS))
- granulomatous (e.g. tuberculosis (TB), sarcoidosis, syphilis)
- metabolic (e.g. gout, thyrotoxicosis)
- infectious (e.g. *S. aureus*, *S. pneumoniae*, *P. aeruginosa*, herpes zoster)
- chemical or physical agents (e.g. thermal, alkali or acid burns)
- idiopathic

Clinical Features
- severe pain, photophobia, red eye, decreased vision
- pain is best indicator of disease progression
- inflammation of scleral, episcleral and conjunctival vessels
- may have anterior chamber cell/flare, corneal infiltrate, scleral thinning
- sclera may have a blue hue best seen in natural light by gross inspection because of scleral thinning and visualization of underlying choroid pigment
- scleral edema or thinning
- failure to blanch with topical phenylephrine

Treatment
- systemic NSAID or steroid (topical steroids are not effective)
- treat underlying etiology

To differentiate between episcleritis and scleritis, place a drop of phenylephrine 2.5% (Mydfrin®; AK-Dilate®) in the affected eye. Re-examine the vascular pattern 10-15 minutes later. Episcleral vessels should blanch. Scleral vessels do not.

Scleromalacia Perforans
- anterior necrotizing scleritis without inflammation and asymptomatic
- strongly associated with rheumatoid arthritis
- may result in scleral thinning
- traumatic perforation can easily occur – examine eye very gently

Cornea

- function
    - transmission of light
    - refraction of light (2/3 of total refractive power of eye)
    - barrier against infection, foreign bodies
- transparency due to avascularity, uniform structure and deturgescence (relative dehydration)
- 5 layers (anterior to posterior): epithelium, Bowman's membrane, stroma, Descemet's membrane, endothelium (dehydrates the cornea; dysfunction = corneal edema)
- extensive sensory fibre network (V_1 distribution); therefore abrasions and inflammation (keratitis) are very painful
- two most common corneal lesions: abrasions and foreign bodies

Foreign Body

- foreign material in or on cornea
- may have associated rust ring if metal
- patients may note tearing, photophobia, foreign body sensation, redness
- signs include foreign body, conjunctival injection, epithelial defect that stains with fluorescein, corneal edema, anterior chamber cells/flare

> Foreign body behind lid may cause multiple vertical corneal epithelial abrasions due to blinking.

Complications
- abrasion, infection, scarring, rust ring, secondary iritis

Treatment
- remove under magnification using local anesthetic and sterile needle or refer to ophthalmology (depending on depth and location)
- treat as per corneal abrasion (below)

Corneal Abrasion

- epithelial defect usually due to trauma (e.g. fingernails, paper, twigs), contact lens (see Figure 13)

> Topical analgesics should only be used to facilitate examination. They should NEVER be used as treatment for any ocular problem.

Clinical Features (Table 4)
- pain, redness, tearing, photophobia, foreign body sensation
- de-epithelialized area stains with fluorescein dye
- pain relieved with topical anesthetic

> NEVER patch abrasion if patient wears contact lenses (prone to *Pseudomonas* infection).

Complications
- infection, ulceration, recurrent erosion, secondary iritis

Treatment
- topical antibiotic (drops or ointment)
- consider topical NSAID, cycloplegic (relieves pain and photophobia by paralyzing ciliary muscle), tight patch
- pressure patch alone is not effective
- most abrasions clear spontaneously within 24-48 hours

> Corneal abrasions from organic matter (e.g. twig, finger nail, etc.) have higher recurrence, even years later.

Recurrent Erosions

- recurrent episodes of pain, photophobia, foreign body sensation with a spontaneous corneal epithelial defect
- usually occurs upon awakening
- associated with improper adherence of epithelial cells to the underlying basement membrane

> **Corneal Abrasion: To Patch or Not to Patch**
> Patching for corneal abrasion. *Cochrane Review* 2006.
>
> Patching is not indicated for simple corneal abrasions, measuring less than 10 mm². There is no improvement in healing rates on days 1-3, no changes in reported pain and no difference in the use of antibiotics between the patch and non-patch groups.

Etiology
- previous traumatic corneal abrasion
- corneal dystrophy
- idiopathic

Treatment
- as for corneal abrasion until re-epithelialization occurs
- topical hypertonic saline ointment, topical lubrication
- bandage contact lens, anterior stromal puncture or phototherapeutic keratectomy for chronic recurrences

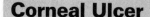

Abrasion vs. Ulcer on Slit Lamp
An abrasion appears clear while an ulcer is more opaque.

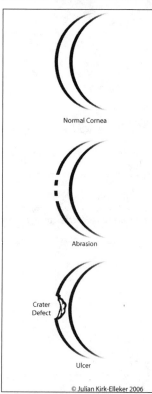

Normal Cornea

Abrasion

Crater Defect

Ulcer

© Julian Kirk-Elleker 2006

Figure 13. Corneal Abrasion vs. Ulcer

Corneal Ulcer

Etiology
- local necrosis of corneal tissue due to infection (Figure 13)
- infection is usually bacterial, rarely viral, fungal or protozoan (*acanthamoeba*)
- secondary to corneal exposure, abrasion, foreign body, contact lens use (50% of ulcers)
- also associated with conjunctivitis, blepharitis, keratitis, vitamin A deficiency

Clinical Features
- pain, photophobia, tearing, foreign body sensation, decreased visual acuity (if central ulcer)
- corneal opacity that necroses and forms an excavated ulcer with infiltrative base
- overlying corneal epithelial defect that stains with fluorescein
- may develop corneal edema, conjunctival injection, anterior chamber cell/flare, hypopyon, corneal hypoesthesia (in viral keratitis)
- bacterial ulcers may have purulent discharge, viral ulcers may have watery discharge

Complications
- decreased vision, corneal perforation, iritis, endophthalmitis

Treatment
- urgent referral to ophthalmology
- culture first
- topical antibiotics every hour
- must treat vigorously to avoid complications

Table 4. Corneal Abrasion vs. Corneal Ulcer

	Abrasion	Ulcer
Time course	Acute (instantaneous)	Subacute (days)
History of trauma	Yes	Not usually
Cornea	Clear	White, necrotic area
Iris detail	Clear	Obscured
Corneal thickness	Normal	May have crater defect/thinning
Extent of lesion	Limited to epithelium	Extension into stroma

Herpes Simplex Keratitis

- usually HSV type 1 (90% of population are carriers)
- may be triggered by stress, fever, sun exposure, immunosuppression

Clinical Features
- pain, tearing, foreign body sensation, redness, may have decreased vision, eyelid edema
- corneal hypoesthesia
- dendritic (thin and branching) lesion in epithelium that stains with fluorescein

Complications
- corneal scarring (can lead to loss of vision)
- chronic interstitial keratitis due to penetration of virus into stroma
- secondary iritis

Treatment
- topical antiviral such as trifluridine, consider systemic antiviral such as acyclovir
- dendritic debridement
- NO STEROIDS initially – may exacerbate condition
- ophthalmologist must exercise caution if adding topical steroids for chronic keratitis or iritis

Steroid treatment for ocular disorders should only be prescribed and supervised by an ophthalmologist, as they can impair corneal healing and exacerbate herpetic keratitis.

Herpes Zoster Keratitis

- dermatitis of the forehead (the CN V_1 territory) may involve the globe (Figure 14)
- Hutchinson's sign: if tip of nose is involved (nasociliary branch of V_1) then eye will be involved in approximately 75% of cases
- if no nasal involvement, the eye is involved in 1/3 of patients

Clinical Features
- pain, tearing, photophobia, red eye
- corneal edema, pseudodendrite, superficial punctate keratitis
- corneal hypoesthesia

Complications
- corneal keratitis, ulceration, perforation and scarring
- iritis, secondary glaucoma, cataract
- muscle palsies (rare) due to CNS involvement
- occasionally severe post-herpetic neuralgia

Treatment
- oral antiviral (acyclovir, valcyclovir or famciclovir)
- topical steroids as indicated for keratitis, iritis (prescribed by an ophthalmologist)
- cycloplegic, antibiotic if indicated

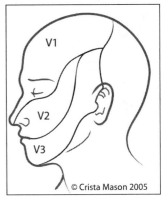

Figure 14. Trigeminal Distribution

Keratoconus

- bilateral paracentral thinning and bulging (ectasia) of the cornea to form a conical shape
- familial occurrence: associated with Down's syndrome and atopy
- associated with breaks in Descemet's and Bowman's membrane
- results in irregular astigmatism, scarring, stromal edema
- blurring of visual acuity is the only symptom

Treatment
- attempt correction with spectacles or contact lens
- penetrating keratoplasty (corneal transplant) 90% successful
- post-operative complications: endophthalmitis, graft rejection, graft dehiscence

To detect keratoconus, look for bulging of the lower eyelid when the patient looks downward (Munson's sign)

Arcus Senilis

- hazy white ring in peripheral cornea, <2 mm wide, clearly separated from limbus
- common, bilateral, benign corneal degeneration due to lipid deposition, part of the aging process
- may be associated with hypercholesterolemia if age <40 years, therefore check lipid profile
- no associated visual symptoms, no complications, no treatment necessary

Kayser-Fleischer Ring

- brown-yellow-green pigmented ring in peripheral cornea, starting inferiorly
- due to copper pigment deposition in Descemet's membrane
- present in 95% of Wilson's disease (hepatolenticular degeneration)
- no associated symptoms or complications of ring
- treat underlying disease

The Uveal Tract

- uveal tract = iris, ciliary body, and choroid
- vascularized, pigmented middle layer of the eye, between the sclera and the retina

Uveitis

- may involve one or all three parts of the tract
- idiopathic or associated with autoimmune, infectious, granulomatous, malignant causes
- should be managed by an ophthalmologist

Anterior Uveitis (Iritis)

- inflammation of iris, usually accompanied by cyclitis (inflammation of ciliary body), when both = iridocyclitis
- usually unilateral

Etiology
- usually idiopathic
- connective tissue diseases:
    - HLA-B27 (usually anterior uveitis): Reiter's syndrome, ankylosing spondylitis (AS), psoriasis, inflammatory bowel disease (IBD)
    - Non-HLA-B27: juvenile rheumatoid arthritis (JRA)
- infectious: syphilis, Lyme disease, toxoplasmosis, TB, HSV, herpes zoster
- other: sarcoidosis, trauma, large abrasion, post ocular surgery

Clinical Features
- photophobia (from reactive spasm of inflamed iris muscle), ocular pain, tenderness of the globe, brow ache (ciliary muscle spasm), decreased visual acuity, tearing
- ciliary flush (perilimbal conjunctival injection), miosis (spasm of sphincter muscle) (Figure 15)
- anterior chamber "cells" (WBC in anterior chamber due to anterior segment inflammation) and "flare" (protein precipitates in anterior chamber secondary to inflammation), hypopyon (collection of neutrophilic exudates inferiorly in the anterior chamber)
- occasionally keratitic precipitates (clumps of cells on corneal endothelium)
- iritis typically reduces intraocular pressure because ciliary body inflammation causes decreased aqueous production; however, severe iritis, or iritis from herpes simplex and zoster may cause an inflammatory glaucoma

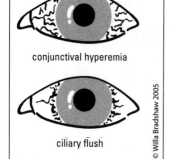

conjunctival hyperemia

ciliary flush

© Willa Bradshaw 2005

Figure 15. Conjunctival hyperemia vs ciliary flush

Complications
- inflammatory glaucoma
- posterior synechiae
    - adhesions of posterior iris to anterior lens capsule
    - indicated by an irregularly shaped pupil
    - if occurs 360°, entraps aqueous in posterior chamber, iris bows forward "iris bombé" → angle closure glaucoma
- peripheral anterior synechiae (PAS) (rare): adhesions of iris to cornea → glaucoma
- cataracts
- band keratopathy (with chronic iritis)
    - superficial corneal calcification keratopathy
- macular edema with chronic iritis

Treatment (by Ophthalmologists)
- mydriatics: dilate pupil to prevent formation of posterior synechiae and to decrease pain from ciliary spasm
- steroids: topical, subconjunctival or systemic
- systemic analgesia
- medical workup may be indicated to determine etiology

Posterior Uveitis (Choroiditis)

- inflammation of the choroid

Etiology
- bacterial: syphilis, tuberculosis
- viral: herpes simplex virus, cytomegalovirus in AIDS
- fungal: histoplasmosis, candidiasis
- parasitic: toxoplasmosis (the most common cause), toxocara
- immunosuppression may predispose to any of the above infections
- autoimmune: Behçet's disease (triad of oral ulcers, genital ulcers, and posterior uveitis)
- malignancies (masquerade syndrome): metastatic lesions, malignant melanoma

Clinical Features
- painless as choroid has no sensory innervation
- frequently no conjunctival or scleral injection present
- decreased visual acuity
- floaters (debris and inflammatory cells)
- vitreous cells and opacities
- hypopyon formation

Treatment
- steroids: retrobulbar or systemic if indicated (e.g. threat of vision loss)

Lens

- consists of an outer capsule surrounding a soft cortex and a firm inner nucleus

Cataracts

- any opacity of the lens
- most common cause of reversible blindness worldwide
- types: nuclear sclerosis, cortical, posterior subcapsular (Figure 16)

Etiology
- acquired
  - age-related (over 90% of all cataracts)
  - cataract associated with systemic disease (may have juvenile onset)
    - diabetes mellitus
    - metabolic disorders (e.g. Wilson's disease, galactosemia, homocystinuria)
    - hypocalcemia
  - traumatic (may be rosette shaped)
  - intraocular inflammation (e.g. uveitis)
  - toxic (steroids, phenothiazines)
  - radiation
- congenital
  - present with altered red reflex or leukocoria
  - treat promptly to prevent amblyopia

Clinical Features
- gradual, painless, progressive decrease in visual acuity
- glare, dimness, haloes around lights at night, monocular diplopia
- "second sight" phenomenon – patient is more myopic than previously noted, due to increased refractive power of the lens (in nuclear sclerosis only)
  - patient may read without previously needed reading glasses
- diagnose by slit-lamp exam, and by noting changes in red reflex using ophthalmoscope
- may impair view of retina during fundoscopy

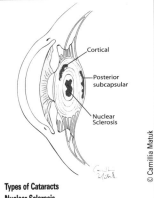

Types of Cataracts
Nuclear Sclerosis
- yellow to brown ("brunescent") discoloration of the central part of the lens
- age-related

Cortical
- radial or spoke-like opacification in the cortex of the lens, either anteriorly or posteriorly
- associated with age and diabetes

Posterior Subcapsular
- usually in the posterior of the lens, adjacent to the capsule
- associated with steroid use, intraocular inflammation, diabetes, trauma, radiation, aging

Figure 16. Types of Cataracts

Treatment
- medical: attempt correction of refractive error
- surgical: definitive treatment is via surgical removal of cataract
  - indications for surgery
    - to improve visual function in patients whose visual loss leads to functional impairment (patients may be inclined to postpone surgery as long as one eye has sufficient vision)
    - to aid management of other ocular disease (e.g. cataract that prevents adequate retinal exam or laser treatment of diabetic retinopathy)
    - congenital or traumatic cataracts
  - phacoemulsification (phaco = lens)
    - most commonly used surgical technique
    - ultrasonic needle is used to emulsify and aspirate nucleus and cortex
    - synthetic intraocular lens (usually a posterior chamber IOL) is placed in bag formed by empty capsule
  - post-operative complications
    - retinal detachment, endophthalmitis, dislocated IOL, macular edema, glaucoma
    - with new foldable IOL's that have truncated edges, <10% of patients get posterior capsular opacification (PCO), which is treated with YAG laser

Prognosis
- excellent if not complicated by other ocular disease

Dislocated Lens (Ectopia Lentis)

Etiology
- associated with Marfan's Syndrome, Ehlers-Danlos type VI, homocystinuria, syphilis, lens coloboma (congenital cleft due to failure of ocular adnexa to complete growth)
- traumatic

Clinical Features
- decreased visual acuity
- may get unilateral diplopia
- iridodenesis (quivering of iris with movement)
- direct ophthalmoscopy may elicit abnormal red reflex

Complications
- cataract, glaucoma, uveitis

Treatment
- surgical correction ± lens replacement

Vitreous

- clear gel (99% water plus collagen fibrils, glycosaminoglycans and hyaluronic acid) that fills the posterior segment of eye
- normally adherent to optic disc, pars plana, and along major retinal blood vessels
- central vitreous commonly shrinks and liquefies with age (syneresis)
- during syneresis, the molecules that held water often condense, causing vitreous floaters
- floaters are usually harmless, but retinal tear/detachment and hemorrhagic diseases must be ruled out

> **Floaters** = "bugs," "cobwebs" or "spots" that change with eye position

Posterior Vitreous Detachment (PVD)

Etiology
- normal aging process of vitreous liquification (syneresis)
- liquid vitreous moves between posterior vitreous gel and retina
- vitreous is peeled away and separates from the retina

> **Weiss' Ring** – glial tissue around the optic disc remains attached to PVD.

Clinical Features
- floaters, flashes of light

Complications
- traction to areas of abnormal vitreoretinal adhesions may cause retinal tears/detachment
- retinal tears/detachment may cause vitreous hemorrhage if tear bridges blood vessel
- complications more common in high myopes and following ocular trauma (blunt or perforating)

> New or a marked increase in floaters and/or flashes of light requires a dilated fundus exam to rule out retinal tears/detachment.

Treatment
- acute onset of PVD requires a dilated fundus exam to rule out retinal tears/detachment
- no specific treatment available for floaters/flashes of light symptoms

Vitreous Hemorrhage

- bleeding into the vitreous cavity

Etiology
- proliferative diabetic retinopathy (PDR)
- retinal tear/detachment
- posterior vitreous detachment (PVD)
- retinal vein occlusion
- trauma

> Any time a vitreous or retinal hemorrhage is seen in a child, it is important to rule out child abuse.

Clinical Features
- sudden loss of visual acuity
- may be preceded by many floaters and/or flashes of light
- ophthalmoscopy: no red reflex if large hemorrhage, retina not visible due to blood in vitreous

Treatment
- ultrasound (B-scan) to rule out retinal detachment
- expectant: in non-urgent cases (e.g. no retinal detachment), blood usually resorbs in 3-6 months
- surgical: vitrectomy ± retinal detachment repair ± retinal endolaser to possible bleeding sites/vessels

> Common causes of vitreous hemorrhage are proliferative diabetic retinopathy and retinal tears.

Endophthalmitis and Vitritis

- intraocular infection: acute, subacute or chronic

Etiology
- most commonly a postoperative complication; risk following cataract surgery is <0.1%
- also due to penetrating injury to eye (risk is 3-7%) and endogenous spread
- etiology usually bacterial, may be fungal

> Remember to inquire about tetanus status in post-traumatic endophthalmitis.

Clinical Features
- very painful, red eye, photophobia, discharge
- severely reduced visual acuity, lid edema, proptosis, corneal edema, anterior chamber cells/flare, hypopyon, reduced red reflex
- may have signs of a ruptured globe (severe subconjunctival hemorrhage, hyphema, decreased intraocular pressure, etc.)

Treatment
- OCULAR EMERGENCY: presenting vision best indicates prognosis
- LP or worse → admission, immediate vitrectomy and intravitreal antibiotics to prevent loss of vision
- HM or better → vitreous tap for culture and intravitreal antibiotics
- topical fortified antibiotics

> **Endophthalmitis Vitrectomy Study**
> For treatment of post-cataract surgery endophthalmitis:
>
> - Intravitreal antibiotics preferred over systemic antibiotics
>
> - Vitrectomy indicated only if vision LP or worse
>
> Endophthalmitis Vitrectomy Study Group. Results of the Endophthalmitis Vitrectomy Study. *Archives of Ophthalmology* 1995;113 (12):1479-96.

Retina

- composed of two parts (Figure 2)
  - neurosensory retina – comprises 9 of the 10 retinal layers, including the photoreceptors and the ganglion cell layer
  - retinal pigment epithelium (RPE) layer – external to neurosensory retina
- macula: rich in cones (for colour vision); most sensitive area of retina; looks darker due to lack of retinal vessels and thinning of retina in this region; 15° temporal and slightly below the optic disc
- fovea: centre of macula; responsible for the most acute, fine vision
- optic disc: slightly oval vertically, pinkish colour with centrally depressed yellow cup (normal cup/disc (C:D) ratio is <0.5), retinal artery and vein pass through cup
- ora serrata: irregularly-shaped, anterior margin of the retina (can only be visualized with indirect ophthalmoscopy of the far peripheral retina, or through a Goldmann 3 mirror lens)

Central Retinal Artery Occlusion (CRAO)

Etiology
- emboli from carotid arteries or heart (e.g. arrhythmia, endocarditis, valvular disease)
- thrombus
- temporal arteritis

Clinical Features
- sudden, painless (except in temporal arteritis), severe monocular loss of vision
- relative afferent pupillary defect (RAPD)
- patient will often have experienced transient episodes in the past (amaurosis fugax)
- fundoscopy
  - "cherry-red spot" at centre of macula (visualization of unaffected highly vascular choroid through the thin fovea)
  - retinal pallor
  - narrowed arterioles, boxcarring (segmentation of blood in arteries)
  - cotton-wool spots (retinal infarcts)
  - cholesterol emboli (Hollenhorst plaques) – usually located at arteriole bifurcations
  - after ~6 weeks: cherry-red spot recedes and optic disc pallor becomes evident

Treatment for a central retinal artery occlusion (CRAO) must be initiated within 2 hours of symptom onset for any hope of restoring vision.

Treatment
- OCULAR EMERGENCY: attempt to restore blood flow within 2 hours
- the sooner the treatment = better prognosis (irreversible retinal damage if >90 min of complete CRAO)
  - massage the globe (compress eye with heel of hand for 10 s, release for 10 s, repeat for 5 min) to dislodge embolus
  - decrease intraocular pressure
    - topical β-blockers
    - inhaled oxygen – carbon dioxide mixture
    - IV Diamox™ (carbonic anhydrase inhibitor)
    - IV mannitol (draws fluid from eye)
  - drain aqueous fluid – anterior chamber paracentesis (carries risk of endophthalmitis)
  - treat underlying cause to prevent CRAO in fellow eye
- follow up 1 month to rule out neovascularization

Branch Retinal Artery Occlusion (BRAO)

- only part of the retina becomes ischemic resulting in a visual field loss
- more likely to be of embolic etiology than CRAO; need to search for source
- management: ocular massage to dislodge embolus if visual acuity is affected

Central/Branch Retinal Vein Occlusion (CRVO/BRVO)

- second most frequent "vascular" retinal disorder after diabetic retinopathy
- usually a manifestation of a systemic disease (e.g. hypertension, diabetes mellitus)
- thrombus occurs within the lumen of the blood vessel

Predisposing Factors
- arteriosclerotic vascular disease
- hypertension
- diabetes mellitus
- glaucoma
- hyperviscosity (e.g. polycythemia rubra vera, sickle-cell disease, lymphoma, leukemia)
- drugs (oral contraceptive pill (OCP), diuretics)

Clinical Features
- painless, monocular, gradual or sudden visual loss
- +/- relative afferent pupillary defect (RAPD)
- fundoscopy
  - "blood and thunder" appearance
  - diffuse retinal hemorrhages, cotton-wool spots, venous engorgement, swollen optic disc, macular edema
- two fairly distinct groups
  - venous stasis/non-ischemic retinopathy
    - no RAPD, VA approximately 20/80
    - mild hemorrhage, few cotton wool spots
    - resolves spontaneously over weeks to months
    - may regain normal vision if macula intact
  - hemorrhagic/ischemic retinopathy
    - usually older patient with deficient arterial supply
    - RAPD, VA approximately 20/200, reduced peripheral vision
    - more hemorrhages, cotton wool spots, congestion
    - poor visual prognosis

Complications
- degeneration of retinal pigment epithelium
- neovascularization of retina and iris (secondary rubeosis), leading to secondary glaucoma
- vitreous hemorrhage
- macular edema

Treatment
- no treatment available to restore vision in CRVO
- treat underlying cause/contributing factor
- fluorescein angiography to determine extent of retinal non-perfusion = risk of neovascularization
- retinal laser photocoagulation to reduce neovascularization and prevent neovascular glaucoma

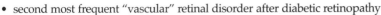

> **Branch Vein Occlusion Study (BVOS)**
> BVOS showed that argon laser treatment improves sight significantly in patients with macular edema following BRVO. The treatment also decreases the risk of vitreous hemorrage.
>
> Branch Vein Occlusion Study Group: Argon laser photocoagulation for macular edema in branch vein occlusion. *Am J Ophthalmol* 98: 271-282, 1984.

> 8-10% risk of developing CRVO or BRVO in other eye.

> The "blood and thunder" appearance on fundoscopy is very characteristic of a central retinal vein occlusion (CRVO).

Retinal Detachment (RD)

- cleavage in the plane between the neurosensory retina and the retinal pigment epithelium (RPE)
- three types
  - rhegmatogenous
    - most common type of RD
    - caused by a tear or hole in the neurosensory retina, allowing fluid from the vitreous to pass into the subretinal space
    - tears may be caused by posterior vitreous detachment (PVD), degenerative retinal changes, trauma or iatrogenically
    - incidence increases with advancing age, and more likely to occur spontaneously in high myopes, or after ocular surgery/trauma
  - tractional
    - caused by traction (due to vitreal, epiretinal or subretinal membrane) pulling the neurosensory retina away from the underlying RPE
    - found in conditions such as diabetic retinopathy, CRVO, sickle cell disease, retinopathy of prematurity (ROP), and ocular trauma

> Superotemporal retina most common site for horseshoe tears.

- exudative
  - caused by damage to the RPE resulting in fluid accumulation in the subretinal space
  - main causes are intraocular tumours, posterior uveitis, central serous retinopathy

Clinical Features
- sudden onset
- flashes of light
  - due to mechanical stimulation of the retinal photoreceptors
- floaters
  - hazy spots in the line of vision which move with eye position, due to drops of blood in the vitreous (blood vessels tear as the retina tears)
- curtain of blackness/peripheral field loss
  - darkness in one field of vision when the retina detaches in that area
- loss of central vision
  - visual acuity dramatically drops if the macula becomes detached
- decreased IOP (usually 4-5 mmHg lower than the other, normal eye)
- ophthalmoscopy: detached retina is grey with surface blood vessels, loss of red reflex
- +/- relative afferent pupillary defect (RAPD)

Treatment
- prophylactic: a symptomatic tear (flashes or floaters) can be sealed off with laser or cryotherapy, with the goal of preventing progression to detachment
- therapeutic
  - rhegmatogenous retinal detachment
    - scleral buckle (a band is secured on the outside of the globe that indents the eye wall, thereby relieving tension on the retina around any tears/holes, allowing the tears/holes to remain sealed)
    - pneumatic retinopexy (intraocular injection of air or an expandable gas in order to tamponade the retinal break)
    - both above treatments are used in combination with localization of retinal tears/holes and subsequent treatment with diathermy, cryotherapy or laser to create adhesions between the RPE and the neurosensory retina
    - vitrectomy plus injection of silicone oil in cases of recurrent detachment
  - tractional retinal detachment:
    - vitrectomy +/- membrane removal/scleral buckling/injection of intraocular gas as necessary
  - exudative
    - treatment of underlying cause

Complications
- loss of vision, vitreous hemorrhage, recurrent retinal detachment
- a retinal detachment should be considered an emergency, especially if the macula is still attached
- prognosis for visual recovery varies inversely with the amount of time the retina is detached and whether the macula is attached or not

Shaken Baby Syndrome
Syndrome of findings characterized by no external signs of abuse and respiratory arrest, seizures, and coma. Ocular exam findings are important diagnostically for Shaken Baby Syndrome. These findings include extensive retinal and vitreous hemorrhages that occur during the shaking process and are extremely rare in accidental trauma. Thus a detailed fundoscopic exam or an Ophthalmology referral should be conducted for all infants in whom abuse is suspected.

Retinitis Pigmentosa

- worldwide incidence between one per 3500 and one per 7000
- many forms of inheritance, most commonly autosomal recessive (60%)
- hereditary degenerative disease of the retina manifested by rod > cone photoreceptor degeneration and retinal atrophy
- symptoms: night blindness, decreased peripheral vision, decreased central vision (macular changes), glare (from cataract)
- fundoscopy: areas of "bone-spicule" pigment clumping in mid-periphery of retina, narrowed retinal arterioles, pale optic disc
- electrophysiological tests (ERG, EOG) assist in diagnosis
- management: no treatments available to reverse the condition; cataract extraction improves visual function

Triad of Retinitis Pigmentosa – "Apo":
Arteriolar narrowing
Perivascular bony-spicule pigmentation
Optic disc pallor

Age-Related Macular Degeneration (ARMD)

- leading cause of blindness in the western world, associated with increasing age, usually bilateral
- 10% of people >65 years old have some degree of ARMD, female > male
- degenerative changes are concentrated at the macula thus only central vision is lost
- peripheral vision (important for navigation) is maintained so patients can usually maintain an independent lifestyle

Classification
- **Non-Exudative/"Dry" (Non-Neovascular) ARMD**
  - most common type of ARMD (90% of cases)
  - slowly progressive loss of visual function
  - drusen: pale, yellow-white deposits of membranous vesicles and collagen deposited between the retinal pigment epithelium (RPE) and Bruch's membrane (area separating inner choroidal vessels from RPE)
  - RPE atrophy: coalescence of depigmented RPE, clumps of focal hyperpigmentation or hypopigmentation
  - may progress to neovascular ARMD

- **Exudative/"Wet" (Neovascular) ARMD**
  - 10% of ARMD, but 80% of ARMD resulting in severe visual loss
  - choroidal neovascularization: drusen predispose to breaks in Bruch's membrane causing subsequent growth and proliferation of choroidal capillaries
  - may get serous detachment of overlying RPE and retina, hemorrhage and lipid precipitates into subretinal space
  - can also get an elevated subretinal mass due to fibrous metaplasia of hemorrhagic retinal detachment
  - leads to disciform scarring and severe central visual loss

Risk Factors
- female
- increased age
- family history
- smoking
- Caucasian race
- blue irides

Clinical Features
- variable amount of progressive central visual loss
- metamorphopsia (distorted vision characterized by straight parallel lines appearing convergent or wavy) due to macular edema

Investigations
- Amsler Grid: held at normal reading distance with glasses on, assesses macular function
- fluorescein angiography (FA): assess degree of neovascularization – pathologic new vessels leak dye

Treatment
- non-neovascular ARMD (dry)
  - monitor, Amsler grid allows patients to check for metamorphopsia
  - low vision aids (e.g. magnifiers, closed-circuit television)
  - anti-oxidants, green leafy vegetables
  - sunglasses/visors
  - see sidebar on AREDS
- neovascular ARMD (wet)
  - see *Common Medications*, OP49
  - laser photocoagulation for neovascularization
  - 50% of choroidal neovascularization cannot be treated initially
  - no definitive treatment for disciform scarring
  - photodynamic therapy (PDT) with verteporfin (Visudyne®)
    - IV injection of verteporfin followed by low intensity laser to area of choroidal neovascularization
  - intravitreal injection of anti-angiogenesis growth factor (anti-vascular endothelial growth factor/anti-VEGF)
    - pegaptanib (Macugen®), ranibizumab (Lucentis®), bevacizumab (Avastin®)
- treatment of ARMD with Photodynamic Therapy Study Group indicated that for patients with subfoveal lesions in ARMD with predominantly classic choroidal neovascularization, verteporfin treatment can reduce the risk of moderate vision loss for at least 2 years; this therapy cannot stop or reverse vision loss in all patients with ARMD

Age-related Eye Disease Study (AREDS)
AREDS studied the effect of high-dose combination of vitamin C, vitamin E, beta-carotene, and zinc in patients with and without ARMD. Those who are already affected by ARMD showed 19% decrease in risk of further visual loss, whereas this treatment showed no benefit in patients with early or no ARMD.

The Age-Related Eye Disease Research Group: A randomized, placebo-controlled, clinical trial of high-dose supplementation with vitamins C and E, beta-carotene, and zinc for age-related macular degeneration and vision loss. AREDS Report No. 8. Arch Ophthalmol 119: 1417-1436, 2001.

Wet ARMD Lesions on FA
Classic: well-defined leakage
Occult: mottled or ill-defined leakage

Drusen vs Exudate
Drusen: hyaline material secreted by RPE seen frequently in ARMD typically in peri-macular region
Hard/Soft Exudates: lipid deposits in the retina associated with diabetic retinopathy and hypertension

Anti-angiogenic therapy with anti-vascular endothelial growth factor modalities for neovascular age-related macular degeneration.
Cochrane Database of Systematic Reviews 2008, Issue 2

Study: Cochrane systemic review of RCTs investigating the use of anti-VEGF (vascular endothelial growth factor) modalities for the treatment of wet age-related macular degeneration (ARMD).
Patients: Classic or occult wet type ARMD.
Interventions: Pegaptanib/Macugen™ (aptamer comprised of ribonucleic acids that bind VEGF), ranibizumab/Lucentis™ (anti VEGF fragment antibody) and verteporfin/Visudyne™ photodynamic therapy (PDT).
Results: The MARINA trial showed that the pooled relative risk (RR) for a gain of 15 or more letters of visual acuity was 5.81 for ranibizumab versus placebo, while the FOCUS trial showed that the pooled RR for a gain of 15 or more letters at one year was 4.44 for a combination of ranibizumab + verteporfin PDT versus verteporfin PDT alone.
Conclusions: Pegaptanib and ranibizumab are of significant benefit for the treatment of wet ARMD with significant improvements in best corrected visual acuity at one year.

Glaucoma

Definition

- progressive optic neuropathy involving characteristic structural changes to optic nerve head with associated visual field changes
- commonly associated with high intraocular pressure (IOP) although not required for diagnosis

Background

- aqueous is produced by the ciliary body and flows from the posterior chamber to the anterior chamber through the pupil, and drains into the episcleral veins via the trabecular meshwork and the canal of Schlemm (see Figure 17)
- an isolated increase in IOP is termed ocular hypertension (or glaucoma suspect) and these patients should be followed for increased risk of developing glaucoma (~10% if IOP = 20-30 mmHg; 40% if IOP = 30-40 mmHg; and most if IOP >40 mm Hg)
- average IOP is 15 ± 3 mm Hg (diurnal variation, higher in a.m.)
- pressures >21 mmHg more likely to be associated with glaucoma; however, up to 50% of patients with glaucoma do not have IOP >21mmHg
- normal C:D (cup:disc) ratio <0.4
- be suspicious of glaucoma if C:D ratio >0.6, C:D ratio difference between eyes >0.2 or cup approaches disc margin
- loss of peripheral vision most commonly precedes central loss
- sequence of events: gradual pressure rise, followed by increased C:D ratio, followed by visual field loss
- screening tests should include:
  - medical and family history
  - visual acuity testing
  - slit lamp exam to assess anterior chamber depth
  - ophthalmoscopy to assess the disc features
  - tonometry by applanation or indentation to measure the IOP
  - visual field testing

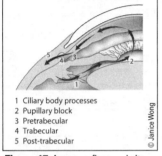

1 Ciliary body processes
2 Pupillary block
3 Pretrabecular
4 Trabecular
5 Post-trabecular

© Janice Wong

Figure 17. Aqueous flow and sites of potential resistance

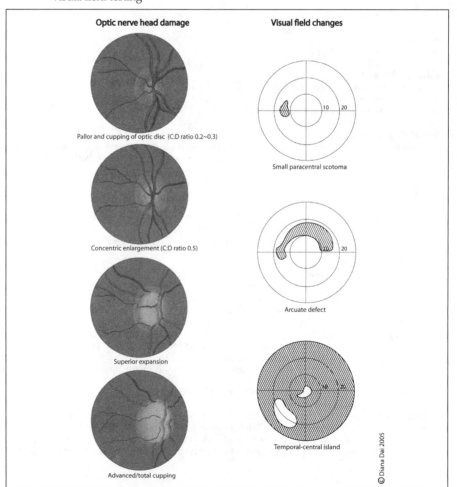

Figure 18. Glaucomatous Damage

Primary Open Angle Glaucoma (POAG)

- most common form, >95% of all glaucoma cases
- due to obstruction of aqueous drainage within the trabecular meshwork and its drainage into the Canal of Schlemm
- insidious and asymptomatic, so screening is critical for early detection

Major Risk Factors
- elevated intraocular pressure (>21 mm Hg)
- age: prevalence in 40 y.o. is 1-2% and in 80 y.o. 10%
- black race
- familial (2-3x increased risk); polygenic

Minor Risk Factors
- myopia
- hypertension
- diabetes
- hyperthyroidism (Graves' disease)
- chronic topical ophthalmic steroid use on eyes in steroid responders – yearly eye exams recommended if >4 weeks of steroid use
- previous ocular trauma
- anemia/hemodynamic crisis (ask about blood transfusions in past)

Clinical Features
- asymptomatic initially
- insidious, painless, gradual rise in IOP due to restriction of aqueous outflow
- bilateral, but usually asymmetric
- earliest signs are optic disc changes (safe to dilate pupil)
  - increased cup to disc ratio (vertical C:D >0.6)
  - significant C:D asymmetry between eyes (>0.2 difference)
  - thinning, notching of the neuroretinal rim
  - flame shaped disc hemorrhage
  - 360° of peripapillary atrophy
  - nerve fibre layer defect
  - large vessels become nasally displaced
- visual field loss
  - slow, progressive, irreversible loss of peripheral vision
  - paracentral defects, arcuate scotoma and nasal step are characteristic
  - late loss of central vision if untreated

Treatment
- principles: decrease IOP by increasing the drainage and/or decreasing the production of aqueous
- medical treatment (see *Glaucoma Medications*, Table 9, OP48):
  - increases aqueous outflow
    - topical cholinergics
    - topical prostaglandin analogues
    - topical alpha-adrenergics
  - decreases aqueous production
    - topical beta-blockers
    - topical and oral carbonic anhydrase inhibitor
    - topical alpha-adrenergics
- laser trabeculoplasty, cyclophotocoagulation = selective destruction of ciliary body (for refractory cases)
- microsurgery: trabeculectomy (filtering bleb) - shunts fluid from AC to under conjunctiva and fibrosis prevented with mitomycin C or 5-FU injection during surgery; if extensive fibrosis after surgery can use tube shunt placement as alternative
- optic nerve head examination, IOP measurement and visual field testing to monitor course of disease

Normal Pressure Glaucoma

- POAG with IOP in normal range
- often found in women >60 but may occur earlier
- damage to optic nerve may be due to vascular insufficiency

Treatment
- treat any causative underlying medical condition and lower the IOP further

Open- and Closed-Angle Glaucoma

POAG	PACG
• common (95%)	• rare (5%)
• chronic course	• acute onset
• painless eye without redness	• painful red eye
• moderately ↑ IOP	• extremely ↑ IOP
• normal cornea and pupil	• hazy cornea
• no N/V	• mid-dilated pupil unreactive to light
• no halos around light	• ± nausea and vomiting
	• halos around light

Risk factors for POAG: "A FIBT"
Age
Family History
IOP
Black race
Thin Cornea

Contraindications to dilating:
- neurological abnormality requiring pupil assessment
- shallow chamber
- iris supported anterior chamber IOL

Reduction of Intraocular Pressure and Glaucoma Progression
Arch Ophthalmol 2002; 120:1268-1279
Study: Randomized controlled clinical trial.
Patients: 255 participants, mainly selected through a population screening protocol, aged 50-80 with newly detected open-angle glaucoma, visual field defects, and a median intraocular pressure (IOP) of 20 mm Hg.
Intervention: Participants were randomized to either topical beta-blocker (betaxolol) plus argon laser trabeculoplasty or no initial treatment, with close observation for both groups. Median follow-up was 6 years.
Main Outcome: Glaucoma progression as defined by visual field and optic disc abnormalities.
Results: IOP was reduced by 25% (mean 5.1 mm Hg) in the treatment group. Glaucoma progression was evident in 62% of individuals in the control group vs. only 45% in the treatment group (p=0.007). The progression was significantly later in the treatment group vs. the controls.

Secondary Open Angle Glaucoma

- increased IOP secondary to ocular/systemic disorders that clog the trabecular meshwork

Steroid-induced Glaucoma
- due to topical/systemic corticosteroid use
- develop in 25% (higher in extended use) of general population (responders) after 4 weeks (or less) of QID topical steroid use
- 5% of population are super-responders

Traumatic Glaucoma
- hyphema-induced increase in IOP
- angle recession glaucoma occurs with blunt, non-penetrating trauma to globe and orbit, causing tears in trabecular meshwork and ciliary body with secondary scarring

Pigmentary Dispersion Syndrome
- iris pigment clogs trabecular meshwork
- typically seen in younger myopes

Pseudoexfoliation Syndrome
- systemic disease, abnormal basement membrane-like material clogs trabecular meshwork
- seen mostly in the elderly

Primary Angle Closure Glaucoma (PACG)

- 5% of all glaucoma cases
- peripheral iris bows forward in an already susceptible eye with a shallow anterior chamber obstructing aqueous access to the trabecular meshwork
- sudden shifting forward of the lens-iris diaphragm = pupillary block, results in inability of the aqueous to flow from the posterior chamber to the anterior chamber and a sudden rise in IOP (Figure 19)

Risk Factors
- hyperopia: small eye, big lens – large lens crowds the angle
- age >70
- female
- family history
- more common in Asians and Inuits
- mature cataracts
- shallow anterior chamber
- pupil dilation (topical and systemic anticholinergics, stress, darkness)

Clinical Features
- unilateral, but other eye predisposed
- red, painful eye = RED FLAG
- decreased visual acuity, vision acutely blurred from corneal edema
- halo around lights
- nausea and vomiting, abdominal pain
- fixed mid-dilated pupil
- corneal edema with conjunctival injection
- marked increase in IOP even to palpation (>40 mmHg)
- shallow anterior chamber ± cells in anterior chamber

Complications
- irreversible loss of vision within hours to days if untreated
- permanent peripheral anterior synechiae

Treatment
- refer to ophthalmologist
  - laser iridotomy
  - aqueous suppressants and hyperosmotic agents
- immediate treatment important to
  - preserve vision
  - prevent adhesions of peripheral iris to trabecular meshwork (peripheral anterior synechiae) resulting in permanent closure of angle

---

Rule of Fours
1/4 of general population after using 4 weeks of topical steroid 4x/day will develop an increase in IOP.

Medical Interventions for primary open angle glaucoma and ocular hypertension.
Cochrane Database of Systematic Reviews 2007, Issue 4.

Study: Cochrane systematic review of 26 trails and meta-analysis of 10 trails investigating the effectiveness of topical pharmacological therapies for primary open angle glaucome (POAG) or ocular hypertension (OHT).
Patients: 4979 participants randomized in 26 trails. Patients had ocular hypertension with intraocular pressure (IOP) >21 mmHg or open angle glaucoma.
Intervention: topical eye medications, including beta-blockers, dorzolamide, brimonidine, pilocarpine and epinephrine versus each other and placebo.
Main outcome: Reduction of progression or prevention of onset of visual field defects.
Results: Meta-analysis on all trails that tested drugs against placebo or untreated controls demostrated that lowering IOP reduces incidence of glucomatous visual field defects, with an odds ratio of 0.62 (95% CI 0.47-0.81). However, this result is of limited practical use since different therapies were pooled. No single indivual drug demonstrated significant visual field protection. However, as a class, beta-blockers showed borderline significance in reducing onset of glaucoma in patients with OHT when compared to placebo, with an OR of 0.67 (95% CI 0.45-1.00).
Conclusions: Lowering IOP can reduce progression of visual field defects in patients with OHT.

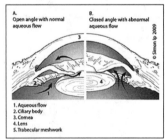

A. Open angle with normal aqueous flow
B. Closed angle with abnormal aqueous flow

1. Aqueous flow
2. Ciliary body
3. Cornea
4. Lens
5. Trabecular meshwork

© Simon Ip 2009

Figure 19. Normal open angle versus angle closure glaucoma

Angle Closure Glaucoma – "BACH"
Tx with miotics and beta-**B**lockers, **A**drenergics, **C**holinergics, **H**yperosmotic agents.

- medical treatment: see *Glaucoma Medications,* Table 9
    - miotic drops (pilocarpine) to reverse pupillary block
    - ↓ IOP
        - topical β-blockers
        - topical adrenergics
        - topical cholinergics
            - pilocarpine 1-4% q15min, up to q5min
        - systemic carbonic anhydrase inhibitors
            - IV acetazolamide 250-500 mg
        - systemic hyperosmotic agents
            - oral glycerine, 1.0 g/kg
            - mannitol IV 1.0 g/kg

Secondary Angle Closure Glaucoma

Uveitis
- inflamed iris adheres to lens (posterior synechiae)

Neovascular Glaucoma
- abnormal blood vessels develop on surface of iris (rubeosis iridis), into the angle, and within the trabecular meshwork
- due to retinal ischemia associated with proliferative diabetic retinopathy and CRVO
- treatment with laser therapy to retina reduces neovascular stimulus to iris vessels

Pupils

- pupil size is determined by the balance between the sphincter muscle and the dilator muscle
- sphincter muscle is innervated by the parasympathetic nervous system (PNS)
    - carried by CN III: pre- and post-ganglionic fibres synapse in ciliary ganglion, and use acetylcholine as the neurotransmitter
- dilator muscle is innervated by the sympathetic NS
    - first order neuron = hypothalamus → brainstem → spinal cord
    - second order/preganglionic neuron = spinal cord → sympathetic trunk via internal carotid artery → superior cervical ganglion in neck
    - third order/postganglionic fibres originate in the superior cervical ganglion, neurotransmitter is noradrenaline
        - as a diagnostic test, 4% cocaine prevents the re-uptake of noradrenaline, and will cause dilatation of normal pupil, but not one with loss of sympathetic innervation (Horner's Syndrome)

5 Targets of Retinal Signals
- Pre-tectal nucleus (pupillary reflex/eye movements)
- Lateral geniculate body of thalamus
- Superior colliculus (eye movements)
- Suprachiasmatic nucleus (optokinetic)
- Accessory optic system (circadian rhythm)

Pupillary Light Reflex

- light shone directly into eye travels along optic nerve to optic tracts to both sides of midbrain
- impulses enter both sides of midbrain via pretectal area and Edinger-Westphal nuclei
- nerve impulses then travel down both CN III nerves to reach the ciliary ganglia, and finally to the iris sphincter muscle, which results in direct and consensual light reflex

Pupil Abnormalities

Denervation Hypersensitivity
- when post-ganglionic fibres are damaged, understimulated end-organ develops an excess of receptor and becomes hypersensitive
- postganglionic parasympathetic lesions (i.e. Adie's pupil)
    - pupil will constrict with 0.125% pilocarpine (cholinergic agonist), whereas a normal pupil will not
- postganglionic sympathetic lesions (i.e. Horner's Syndrome)
    - pupil will dilate with 0.125% adrenaline, whereas a normal pupil will not; this test is used to differentiate between pre- and post-ganglionic lesions in Horner's syndrome

Local Disorders of Iris
- posterior synechiae (adhesions between iris and lens) due to iritis and presents as an abnormally shaped pupil margin
- ischemic damage
    - i.e. post-acute angle closure glaucoma (ACG)

> ▪ ischemic damage usually at 3 and 9 o'clock positions results in vertically oval pupil that reacts poorly to light
- trauma (i.e. post intraocular surgery)

Anisocoria
- unequal pupil size
- idiopathic anisocoria
  - ▪ round, regular, <1 mm difference
  - ▪ pupils reactive to light and accommodation
  - ▪ responds normally to mydiatrics/ miotics
- see Table 5 for other causes of anisocoria

Table 5. Summary of Conditions Causing Anisocoria

	Features	Site of Lesion	Light and Accommodation	Anisocoria	Mydriatics Miotics	Effect of Pilocarpine
ABNORMAL PUPIL MIOTIC (impaired pupillary dilation)						
Argyll-Robertson pupil	Irregular, usually bilateral	Midbrain	Poor to light; better to accommodation		Dilates / Constricts	
Horner's Syndrome	Round, unilateral, ptosis, anhidrosis pseudoenophthalmos	Sympathetic system	Both brisk	Greater in dark	Dilates / Constricts	
ABNORMAL PUPIL MYDRIATIC (impaired pupillary constriction)						
Adie's Tonic pupil	Irregular, larger in bright light	Ciliary ganglion	Poor to light, better to accommodation	Greater in light	Dilates / Constricts	Constricts (hypersensitivity to dilute pilocarpine)
CNIII Palsy	Round	CN III	± fixed (acutely) at 7-9mm	Greater in light	Dilates / Constricts	Constricts
Mydriatic pupil	Round, uni- or bilateral	Iris sphincter	Fixed at 7-8mm	Greater in light	No effect	Will not constrict

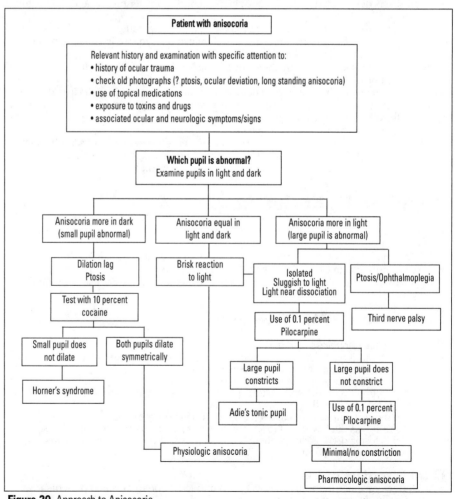

Figure 20. Approach to Anisocoria
Reproduced with permission from: Kedar S, Biousse V, Newman NJ. Approach to the patient with anisocoria. In: UpToDate, Rose, BD (ed), UpToDate, Waltham, MA, 2008. Copyright 2008 UpToDate, Inc. For more information visit www.uptodate.com.

Dilated Pupil (Mydriasis)

Physiologic Anisocoria
- occurs in 20% of population
- difference <1-2 mm, most pronounced in low light
- normal light reactivity, may vary from day to day

Sympathetic Stimulation
- fight or flight response
- mydriatic drugs: epinephrine, dipivefrin (Propine™), phenylephrine

Parasympathetic Understimulation
- cycloplegics/mydriatics: atropine, tropicamide, cyclopentolate (parasympatholytic)
- CN III palsy
  - eye deviated down and out with ptosis present
  - etiology includes stroke, neoplasm, aneurysm, acute rise in ICP, diabetes mellitus (may spare pupil), trauma
  - CN III palsy will respond to drugs (e.g. pilocarpine), unlike a pupil dilated from medication (mydriatics)

Acute Angle Closure Glaucoma
- fixed, mid-dilated pupil

Adie's Tonic Pupil
- 80% unilateral, females > males
- pupil is tonic or reacts poorly to light (both direct and consensual) but constricts with accommodation
- if ↓ deep tendon reflexes = Adie's syndrome
- caused by benign lesion in ciliary ganglion; results in denervation hypersensitivity of parasympathetically innervated constrictor muscle
  - dilute (0.125%) solution of pilocarpine will constrict tonic pupil but have no effect on normal pupil
- pupil eventually gets smaller than that in the unaffected eye

Trauma
- damage to iris sphincter from blunt or penetrating trauma
- iris transillumination defects may be apparent using ophthalmoscope or slit lamp
- pupil may be dilated (traumatic mydriasis) or irregularly shaped from tiny sphincter ruptures

> In a CN III palsy, if the pupil is involved, consider the possibility of a posterior communicating artery aneurysm. The pupillomotor fibers run on the outside of the nerve and are most susceptible to compression. Ischemic changes are more likely to cause a palsy without pupillary involvement.

Constricted Pupil (Miosis)

Physiologic Anisocoria
- see *Dilated Pupil* section, OP35

Senile Miosis
- decreased sympathetic stimulation with age

Parasympathetic Stimulation
- local or systemic medications such as
  - cholinergic agents: pilocarpine, carbachol
  - cholinesterase inhibitor: phospholine iodide
  - opiates, barbiturates

Horner's Syndrome
- lesion in sympathetic pathway
- difference in pupil size greater in dim light, due to decreased innervation of adrenergics to iris dilator muscle
- associated with ptosis, anhydrosis of ipsilateral face/neck
- application of cocaine 4% to eye does not result in pupil dilation (vs. physiologic anisocoria)
- hydroxyamphetamine 1% will dilate preganglionic lesion, not postganglionic lesion
- postganglionic lesions result in denervation hypersensitivity, which will cause pupil to dilate with 0.125% adrenaline, whereas normal pupil will not
- causes: aneurysm of carotid or subclavian, brainstem infarct, demyelinating disease, cervical or mediastinal tumour, apical lobe bronchogenic CA, goiter, cervical lymphadenopathy, surgical sympathectomy, Lyme disease, cervical ribs, tabes dorsalis, cervical vertebral fractures

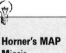

Horner's MAP
Miosis
Anhydrosis
Ptosis

Argyll Robertson Pupil (ARP)
Accomodation **R**eflex **P**resent
Pupillary **R**eflex **A**bsent

Dense cataracts never produce a relative afferent pupillary defect.

It is possible to have RAPD and normal vision at the same time.
For example, in damaged superior colliculus caused by thalamic hemorrhage.

When assessing for an RAPD, a slight dilatation after inital constriction is normal when swinging from eye to eye.

Iritis
- miotic pupil initially
- later, may be irregularly shaped pupil due to posterior synechiae
- does not react to light in later stages

Argyll Robertson Pupil
- both pupils irregular and <3 mm in diameter, may have ptosis
- does not respond to light stimulation
- does respond to accommodation (light-near dissociation)
- suggestive of CNS syphilis or other conditions (DM, encephalitis, MS, chronic alcoholism, CNS degenerative diseases)

Relative Afferent Pupillary Defect (RAPD)

- see Neurology
- also known as Marcus Gunn pupil
- lesion in visual afferent (sensory) pathway anterior to optic chiasm
- differential diagnosis: large retinal detachment, BRAO, CRAO, CRVO, advanced glaucoma, optic nerve compression, optic neuritis
- does not occur with media opacity (e.g. corneal edema, cataracts)
- test: swinging flashlight
  - if light is shone in the affected eye, direct and consensual response to light is decreased
  - if light is shone in the unaffected eye, direct and consensual response to light is normal
  - if the light is moved quickly from the unaffected eye to the affected eye, "paradoxical" dilation of both pupils occurs
  - observe red reflex, especially in patients with dark iris

Malignancies

- uncommon site for primary malignancies
- eye usually affected secondarily by cancer or cancer treatments
- see *Retinoblastoma* section, OP44

Lid Carcinoma

Etiology
- basal cell carcinoma (90%)
  - spread via local invasion, rarely metastasizes
  - rodent ulcer, indurated base with pearly rolled edges, telangiectasia
- squamous cell carcinoma (<5%)
  - spread via local invasion, may also spread to nodes and metastasize
  - ulceration, keratosis of lesion
- sebaceous cell carcinoma (1-5%)
  - often masquerades as chronic blepharitis or recurrent chalazion
  - highly invasive, metastasize
- Kaposi's sarcoma, malignant melanoma, Merkel cell tumour, metastatic tumour

Treatment
- incisional or excisional biopsies
- may require cryotherapy, radiotherapy, chemotherapy, immunotherapy
- surgical reconstruction

Malignant Melanoma

- most common **primary** intraocular malignancy in adults
- more prevalent in Caucasians
- arise from uveal tract
- hepatic metastases predominate

Treatment
- choice is dependent on the size of the tumour
- radiotherapy, enucleation (removal of globe from eye socket), limited surgery

Metastases

- most common intraocular malignancy in adults
- most common from breast and lung in adults, neuroblastoma in children
- usually infiltrate the choroid, but may also affect the optic nerve or extraocular muscles
- may present with decreased or distorted vision, irregularly shaped pupil, iritis, hyphema

Treatment
- local radiation, chemotherapy
- enucleation if blind painful eye

Ocular Manifestations of Systemic Disease

HIV / AIDS

- up to 75% of patients with AIDS have ocular manifestations

External Ocular Signs
- Kaposi's sarcoma
    - affects conjunctiva of lid or globe
    - numerous vascular skin malignancies
    - DDx: subconjunctival hemorrhage (non-clearing), hemangioma
- multiple molluscum contagiosum
- herpes simplex keratitis
- herpes zoster

Retina
- HIV retinopathy (most common)
    - cotton wool spots in >50% of HIV
    - intraretinal hemorrhage
- cytomegalovirus (CMV) retinitis
    - ocular opportunistic infection that develops in late stages of HIV when severely immunocompromised (CD4 count ≤50)
    - a necrotizing retinitis, with retinal hemorrhage and vasculitis, brushfire or pizza pie appearance
    - symptoms and signs: scotomas related to macular involvement and retinal detachment, blurred vision, and floaters
    - untreated infection will progress to other eye in 4-6 weeks
    - treat with virostatic agents gancyclovir or foscarnet via IV or intravitreal injection
- necrotizing retinitis
    - from herpes simplex virus, herpes zoster, *Pneumocystis carinii*, toxoplasmosis
- disseminated choroiditis
    - *Pneumocystis carinii, Mycobacterium avium intracellulare, Candida*

Other Systemic Infections

- herpes zoster (see *Herpes Zoster Keratitis* section, OP21)
- candidal endophthalmitis
    - fluffy, white-yellow, superficial retinal infiltrate that may eventually result in vitritis
    - may see inflammation of the anterior chamber
    - treatment: systemic amphotericin B
- toxoplasmosis
    - focal, grey-yellow-white, chorioretinal lesions with surrounding vasculitis and vitreous infiltration (vitreous cells)
    - can be congenital (transplacental) or acquired, (caused by *Toxoplasma gondii* protozoa transmitted through raw meat and cat feces)
    - congenital form more often visual impairing as more likely to involve macula
    - treatment: pyrimethamine, sulfonamide, folinic acid, steroids

Diabetes Mellitus (DM)

- see <u>Endocrinology</u>
- most common cause of blindness in young people in North America
- blurring of distance vision with rise of blood sugar

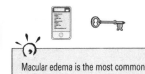

Macular edema is the most common cause of visual loss in patients with background DR.

- consider DM if unexplained retinopathy, cataract, EOM palsy, optic neuropathy, sudden change in refractive error
- loss of vision due to
  - progressive microangiopathy, leading to macular edema
  - progressive diabetic retinopathy → neovascularization → traction → retinal detachment and vitreous hemorrhage
  - rubeosis iridis (neovascularization of the iris) leading to neovascular glaucoma (poor prognosis)
  - macular ischemia

DIABETIC RETINOPATHY (DR)
- background:
  - altered vascular permeability (loss of pericytes, breakdown of blood-retinal barrier, thickening of basement membrane)
  - retinal vessel closure

Classification
- **non-proliferative**: increased vascular permeability and retinal ischemia
  - dot and blot hemorrhages
  - microaneurysms
  - hard exudates (lipid deposits)
  - macular edema
- **advanced non-proliferative (or pre-proliferative):**
  - non-proliferative findings plus
  - venous beading (in 2 of 4 retinal quadrants)
  - intraretinal microvascular anomalies (IRMA) in 1 of 4 retinal quadrants
    - IRMA: dilated, leaky vessels within the retina
  - cotton wool spots (nerve fibre layer infarcts)
- **proliferative**
  - 5% of patients with diabetes will reach this stage
  - neovascularization: iris, disc, retina to vitreous
  - neovascularization of iris (rubeosis iridis) can lead to neovascular glaucoma
  - vitreous hemorrhage from bleeding fragile new vessels, fibrous tissue can contract causing tractional retinal detachment
  - increased risk of severe visual loss

Screening Guidelines for Diabetic Retinopathy
- Type 1 DM
  - screen for retinopathy beginning annually 5 years after disease onset
  - screening not indicated before the onset of puberty
- Type 2 DM
  - initial examination shortly after diagnosis, then repeat annually
- pregnancy
  - ocular exam in 1st trimester, close follow-up throughout as pregnancy can exacerbate DR
  - gestational diabetics not at risk for retinopathy

Treatment
- Diabetic Control and Complications Trial (DCCT) (see side bar)
  - tight control of blood sugar decreases frequency and severity of microvascular complications
- blood pressure control
- focal laser for clinically significant macular edema
- panretinal laser photocoagulation, for proliferative diabetic retinopathy, reduces neovascularization, hence reducing the angiogenic stimulus from ischemic retina by decreasing retinal metabolic demand → reduces risk of blindness
- vitrectomy for vitreous hemorrhage and retinal detachment in proliferative diabetic retinopathy which is complicated by non-clearing vitreous hemorrhage or retinal detachment
- the diabetic retinopathy vitrectomy study indicated that vitrectomy before vitreous hemorrhage does not improve the visual prognosis

Lens Changes
- earlier onset of senile nuclear sclerosis and cortical cataract
- may get hyperglycemic cataract, due to sorbitol accumulation (rare)
- sudden changes in refraction of lens: changes in blood glucose levels (poor control) may cause refractive changes by 3-4 diopters

Macular edema is the most common cause of visual loss in patients with background DR.

Presence of DR in:
Type 1 DM
25% after 5 years
60% after 10 years
>80% after 15 years[1,2]
Type 2 DM
20% at time of diagnosis[1]
60% after 20 years[3]

1. Complications: Your eyes & diabetic retinopathy. *Canadian Diabetes Association* Nov 2003.
2. Diabetic Retinopathy. *Diabetes Care* 1998; 21(1): 143-156.
3. Diabetes in Ontario: an ICES Practice Atlas. *ICES* June 2003.

Clinically significant macular edema is defined as thickening of the retina at or within 500 μm of the centre of the macula

Diabetic Control and Complication Trial
New England Journal of Medicine, 329(14), September 30, 1993.

DCCT trial shows intensive glycemic control will reduce the risk of diabetic retinopathy by 76%, and reduce the risk of worsening diabetic retinopathy by 54%.

Early Treatment Diabetic Retinopathy Study
ETDRS demonstrates
- no benefit of aspirin in reduction in risk of progression of diabetic retinopathy, however no increased risk of hemorrhage either
- early treatment using panretinal photocoagulation reduces the risk of visual loss
- clinically significant macula edema should be treated by focal laser
Early Treatment Diabetic Retinopathy Study Investigators: Aspirin effects on mortality and morbidity in patients with diabetes mellitus. ETDRS Report 14. JAMA 268: 1292-1300, 1992. And other publications by the same group.

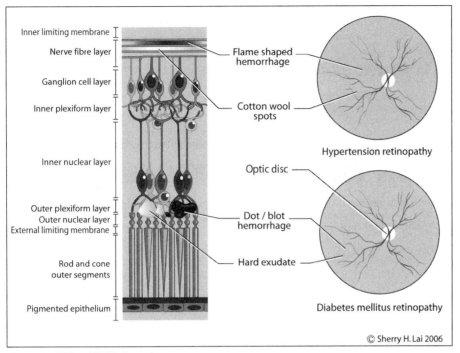

Figure 21. DM vs. HTN Retinopathy

Extra Ocular Muscle (EOM) Palsy
- usually CN III infarct
- pupil usually spared in diabetic CN III palsy, but get ptosis
- may involve CN IV and VI
- usually recover within few months

Optic Neuropathy
- visual acuity loss due to infarction of optic disc/nerve

Hypertension

- retinopathy is the most common ocular manifestation of hypertension
- key features of **chronic** HTN retinopathy: AV nicking, blot retinal hemorrhages, microaneurysms, cotton wool spots
- key features of **acute** HTN retinopathy: retinal arteriolar spasm, superficial retinal hemorrhage, cotton-wool spots, optic disc edema

Table 6. Keith-Wagener-Barker Classification

Group 1	Mild to moderate narrowing or sclerosis of the arterioles
Group 2	Moderate to marked narrowing of the arterioles Local and/or generalized narrowing of arterioles Exaggeration of the light reflex Arteriovenous crossing changes
Group 3	Retinal arteriolar narrowing and focal constriction Retinal edema Cotton-wool patches Hemorrhage
Group 4	Same as group 3, plus papilledema

Multiple Sclerosis (MS)

- see Neurology

Clinical Features
- blurred vision and decreased colour vision: secondary to optic neuritis
- central scotoma: due to damage to papillomacular bundle of retinal nerve fibres
- diplopia: secondary to internuclear ophthalmoplegia (INO)
- RAPD, ptosis, nystagmus, uveitis, optic atrophy, optic neuritis
- white matter demyelinating lesions of optic nerve on MRI

Optic Neuritis Treatment Trial (ONTT)
Optic Neuritis Study Group: The Optic Neuritis Treatment Trial. Three-year follow-up results. Arch Ophthalmol 113: 136-137, 1995

ONTT recruited patients with acute new onset optic neuritis and studied outcome of three treatment regimes: oral steroid x 14d, IV steroid x 3d + oral steroid x 11d, and placebo x 14d. They found that oral steroid actually increases risk of recurrence, IV + oral steroid expedite recovery, and "no treatment" a viable therapeutic option. IV + oral steroid does not decrease risk of recurrence.
Another finding from ONTT is that brain MRI is most valuable in prediction of onset of MS.

The most common cause of unilateral or bilateral proptosis in adults is Graves' disease.

Progression of signs and symptoms of Graves Ophthalmopathy: NO SPECS

No signs/symptoms
Only signs (lid retraction, lid lag)
Soft tissue swelling (periorbital edema)
Proptosis (exophthalmos)
Extraocular muscle weakness (causing diplopia)
Corneal exposure
Sight loss

ESR in GCA
males > age/2
females > (age + 10) /2

Does this patient have GCA?
JAMA 2002; 287:92-101.

Rule in: jaw claudication and diplopia on history, temporal artery beading, prominence of the artery and tenderness over the artery on exam.
Rule out: no temporal artery abnormalities on exam, normal ESR.

Treatment
- IV steroids for optic neuritis
  - NOT oral steriods as these increase likelihood of developing MS later

TIA/Amaurosis Fugax

- sudden, transient blindness from intermittent vascular compromise; ipsilateral carotid most frequent embolic source
- typically monocular, lasting <5-10 minutes
- may be associated with paresthesia/weakness in contralateral limbs
- Hollenhorst plaques (glistening microemboli seen at branch points of retinal arterioles)

Graves' Disease

- ophthalmopathy occurs despite control of thyroid gland status.
- ocular manifestations occur secondary to sympathetic overdrive and/or specific inflammatory infiltrate of the orbital tissue

Clinical
- see sidebar
- initial inflammatory phase is followed by a quiescent cicatricial phase

Treatment
- treat hyperthyroidism
- monitor for corneal exposure and maintain corneal hydration
- manage diplopia, proptosis and compressive optic neuropathy with one or a combination of:
  - steroids (during acute phase)
  - orbital bony decompression
  - external beam radiation of the orbit
- consider strabismus and/or eyelid surgical procedures once acute phase subsides

Connective Tissue Disorders

- RA, juvenile rheumatoid arthritis (JRA), SLE, Sjogren's syndrome, ankylosing spondylitis, polyarteritis nodosa (PAN)
- most common ocular manifestation: dry eyes (keratoconjunctivitis sicca)

Giant Cell/Temporal Arteritis (GCA)

- see Rheumatology
- women>men, >60 y.o.

Clinical
- common in women >60 y.o.
- abrupt monocular loss of vision, pain over the temporal artery, jaw claudication, scalp tenderness, polymyalgia rheumatica, constitutional symptoms
- ischemic optic atrophy
  - 50% lose vision in other eye if untreated

Diagnosis
- temporal arterial biopsy + ↑ESR (ESR can be normal, but likely 80-100 in first hour)
- if biopsy of one side is negative, biopsy the other side

Treatment
- high dose corticosteroid to relieve pain and prevent further ischemic episodes
- if diagnosis of GCA is suspected clinically: start treatment + within 1 week perform temporal artery biopsy to confirm diagnosis (DO NOT WAIT TO TREAT)

Sarcoidosis

- granulomatous uveitis with large "mutton fat" keratitic precipitates and posterior synechiae
- neurosarcoidosis: optic neuropathy, oculomotor abnormalities, visual field loss

Treatment
- steroids and mydriatics

Pediatric Ophthalmology

Strabismus

- ocular misalignment, found in 3% of children
- object not visualized simultaneously by fovea of each eye
- often presents with parental concern about a wandering eye, crossing eye, or poor vision
- types: heterotropia (paralytic or non-paralytic), heterophoria
- complications: amblyopia, cosmetic

HETEROTROPIA

- manifest deviation
- deviation not corrected by the fusion mechanism (i.e. deviation is apparent when the patient is using both eyes)

Types

- exo- (lateral deviation), eso- (medial deviation)
- hyper- (upward deviation), hypo- (downward deviation)
- esotropia = "crossed-eyes"; exotropia = "wall-eyed"
- pseudoesotropia: epicanthal folds give appearance of esotropia but Hirschberg test is normal, more common in Asians

Tests

- Hirschberg test (corneal light reflex): positive if the light reflex in the cornea of the two eyes is asymmetrical
    - light reflex lateral to central cornea indicates esodeviation; light reflex medial to central cornea indicates exodeviation
    - false positives occur if visual axis and anatomic pupillary axis of the eye are not aligned (angle kappa)
- cover test (Figure 22)
    - ask patient to fixate on target
    - cover the fixating eye, the deviated eye will then move to fixate on the target
    - if deviated eye moves inward = exotropia
    - if deviated eye moves outward = esotropia
- the deviation can be quantified using prisms

HETEROPHORIA

- latent deviation
- deviation corrected in the binocular state by the fusion mechanism (i.e. deviation not seen when patient is using both eyes)
- Hirschberg test will be normal (light reflexes symmetrical)
- very common – majority are asymptomatic
- may be exacerbated or become manifest with asthenopia (eye strain, fatigue)

Tests

- cover-uncover test (Figure 22)
    - placing a cover over an eye with a phoria causes a breakdown of fixation of that eye, which allows it to move to a misaligned position
    - uncovering the covered eye will allow it to return to a normal central position
    - covered eye moves inward on removing cover = exophoria
    - covered eye moves outward on removing cover = esophoria
- alternate cover test
    - alternating the cover between both eyes reveals the total deviation, both latent and manifest
    - maintain cover over one eye for 2-3 seconds before rapidly shifting to other eye

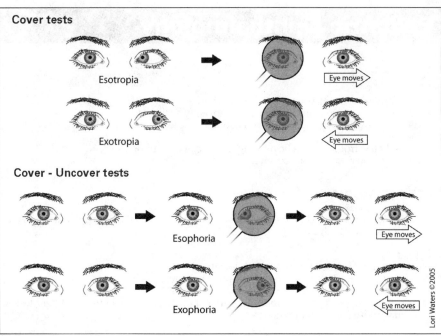

Figure 22. Cover and Cover-Uncover Tests for Detection of Tropias and Phorias

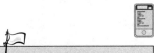

All children with strabismus and/or possible reduced vision require prompt referral to an ophthalmologist.

PARALYTIC STRABISMUS
- incomitant strabismus (i.e. deviation varies in different positions of gaze)
- reduction or restriction in range of eye movements

Etiology
- neural (CN III, IV, VI): ischemia (e.g. DM), MS, aneurysm, brain tumour, trauma
- muscular: myasthenia gravis (neuromuscular junction pathology), Graves' disease
- structural: restriction/entrapment of extraocular muscles due to orbital inflammation, tumour, fracture of the orbital wall

Clinical Features
- mostly in adults, acquired
- present mainly with diplopia
- greatest deviation in field of action of the weakened muscle
- visual acuity is usually unaffected in either eye, unless CN II is involved

NON-PARALYTIC STRABISMUS
- concomitant strabismus (i.e. deviation equal in all directions of gaze)
- no restriction in range of eye movements
- monocular, alternating, or intermittent

Clinical Features
- usually begins in infancy, up to age 8-10
- usually no diplopia (child suppresses the image from the misaligned eye)
- deviated eye may become amblyopic if not treated when the child is young (see *Amblyopia* section, OP43)
- amblyopia treatment rarely successful after age 8-10
- amblyopia usually does not develop if child has alternating strabismus or intermittency – allows neural pathways for both eyes to develop

Accommodative Esotropia
- normal response to approaching object is the triad of the near reflex: convergence, accommodation and miosis
- hyperopes must constantly accommodate – excessive accommodation can lead to esotropia in young children via over-activation of the near reflex
- average age of onset is 2.5 years
- usually reversible with correction of refractive error

Non-accommodative Esotropia
- accounts for 50% of childhood strabismus
- most are idiopathic
- may be due to monocular visual impairment (i.e. cataract, corneal scarring, anisometropia, retinoblastoma) or divergence insufficiency (ocular misalignment that is greater at distance fixation than at near fixation)

Amblyopia

Definition
- reduction of best-corrected visual acuity due to cortical suppression of sensory input from an eye that is receiving blurred or conflicting visual information, leading to disruption of the normal development of visual pathways serving that eye

Detection
- "Holler Test": young child upset if good eye is covered
- quantitative visual acuity by age 3-4 years using picture charts and/or matching game (Sheridan-Gardiner), testing each eye separately
- amblyopia treatment rarely successful after age 8-10 years, but a trial should be given no matter what age
- prognosis: 90% will have good vision restored and maintained if treated <4 years old

Etiology and Management
- strabismus
  - correct with glasses for accommodative esotropia (50% of children experience relief of their esotropia with glasses and will not require surgery)
  - occlusion of unaffected eye forces brain to use previously strabismic eye; aims to bring vision in previously suppressed eye to normal before surgery
  - surgery: recession (weakening) = moving muscle insertion further back on the globe; or resection (strengthening) = shortening the muscle
  - botulinum toxin for single muscle weakening
  - after ocular alignment is restored (glasses, surgery, botulinum toxin), patching is frequently necessary to maintain vision until approximately age 8
- refractive errors
  - anisometropia (difference in refractive power between the eyes)
    - amblyopia usually in the more hyperopic eye
  - the less hyperopic eye receives a clear image while the more hyperopic eye receives a blurred image; input from the blurred eye is cortically suppressed and visual pathway fails to develop normally
  - treat with glasses to correct refractive error
  - patching is required if visual acuity difference persists after 4-8 weeks of using glasses
- deprivation amblyopia
  - occlusion due to ptosis, cataract, retinoblastoma, corneal opacity
  - occlusion amblyopia: prolonged patching of good eye may cause it to become amblyopic

General Treatment
- correct the underlying cause
- occlusion therapy (patching) or atropine cycloplegia (optical degradation therapy) of the good eye

Leukocoria

- white pupil (red reflex is absent)

Differential Diagnosis
- cataract
- retinoblastoma
- retinal coloboma
- retinopathy of prematurity (ROP)
- persistent hyperplastic primary vitreous (PHPV)
- Coat's disease (exudative retinitis)
- toxocariasis
- retinal detachment

Retinoblastoma

- most common primary intraocular malignancy in children
- incidence: 1/1000; sporadic or genetic transmission; screening of siblings/offspring vital
- unilateral or bilateral (in 1/3 of cases)
- malignant – direct or hematogenous spread
- diagnosis
  - may be detected by leukocoria (white pupil) in infant
  - CT scan: dense radiopaque appearance (contains calcium)

Treatment
- radiotherapy, enucleation or both

Retinopathy of Prematurity (ROP)

- vasoproliferative retinopathy that is a major cause of blindness in the developed world

Risk Factors
- non-black race (black infants have lower risk of developing ROP)
- low gestational age, birth weight (<1500 g)
- high oxygen exposure after birth

Classification (according to CRYO-ROP study)
- stage 1: demarcation line between vascular and avascular retina
- stage 2: ridge of tissue with a width and height
- stage 3: extraretinal fibrovascular proliferation extending into vitreous
- threshold disease: stage 3+ in zones 1 or 2 (defined by CRYO-ROP study) with either (1) 5 contiguous clock hours, or (2) 8 cumulative clock hours of ROP involvement
  Note: "+" or plus disease = dilatation and tortuosity of retinal vessels
  - significance: treatment of threshold disease within 72 hours significantly reduced adverse outcome including retinal detachment; the goal is to halt progression beyond threshold or to cause regression of ROP
- stage 4: partial retinal detachment (4A: macula "on" or attached, 4B: macula "off" or detached)
- stage 5: total retinal detachment

Management
- threshold disease is treated with cryotherapy or laser (laser is now the standard treatment, with better refractive outcome)
- ROP beyond threshold level is either watched carefully (usually stage 4A) or treated with vitrectomy/scleral buckle

Prognosis
- higher incidence of myopia among ROP infants, even if treated successfully
- stage 4B and 5 have poor prognosis for visual outcome despite treatment

Nasolacrimal System Defects

- congenital obstruction of the nasolacrimal duct (failure of canalization)
- usually spontaneously open by 1-2 months of age
- increased tearing, crusting, discharge, recurrent conjunctivitis
- can have reflux of mucopurulent material from lacrimal punctum when pressure is applied over lacrimal sac
- treatment: massage over lacrimal sac at medial corner of eyelid bid to qid
- consider referral for duct probing if no spontaneous resolution by 9-12 months

Ophthalmia Neonatorum

- newborn conjunctivitis (in first month of life)
- toxic: silver nitrate, erythromycin
- infectious: bacterial (e.g. *N. gonorrheae* – most common), herpes simplex virus (HSV), *Chlamydia trachomatis*
- gonococcal infection is the most serious threat to sight, because it can rapidly penetrate corneal epithelium causing corneal ulceration
- diagnose using stains and cultures

- treat with systemic antibiotics with possible hospitalization if infectious etiology
- topical prophylaxis, most commonly with erythromycin (or silver nitrate), is required by law at birth

Congenital Glaucoma

- due to inadequate development of the filtering mechanism of the anterior chamber angle

Clinical Features
- cloudy cornea, increased IOP
- photophobia, tearing
- buphthalmos (large "ox eye"), blepharospasm

Treatment
- filtration surgery is required soon after birth to prevent blindness

Ocular Trauma

Blunt Trauma

- caused by blunt object such as fist, squash ball
- history: injury, ocular history, drug allergy, tetanus status
- exam: VA first, pupil size and reaction, EOM (diplopia), external and slit lamp exam, ophthalmoscopy
- if VA normal or slightly reduced, globe less likely to be perforated
- if VA reduced, may be perforated globe, corneal abrasion, lens dislocation, retinal tear
- bone fractures
  - blow out fracture: restricted EOM, diplopia, enophthalmos (sunken eye)
  - ethmoid fracture: subcutaneous emphysema of lid
- lids: swelling, laceration, emphysema
- conjunctiva: subconjunctival hemorrhage
- cornea: abrasions – detect with fluorescein staining and cobalt blue filter in ophthalmoscope or slit lamp
- anterior chamber: assess depth, hyphema, hypopyon
- iris: prolapse, iritis
- lens: cataract, dislocation
- retinal tear/detachment

Always test visual acuity (VA) first – medicolegal protection.

Refer if you observe any of these signs:
- decreased VA
- shallow anterior chamber
- hyphema
- abnormal pupil
- ocular misalignment
- retinal damage

Penetrating Trauma

- include ruptured globe ± prolapsed iris, intraocular foreign body (FB)
- rule out intraocular foreign body, especially if history of "metal striking metal" do orbit CT
- initial management: refer immediately!!
  - ABCs
  - don't press on eyeball!
  - don't check IOP if possibility of globe rupture
  - check vision, diplopia
  - apply rigid eye shield to minimize further trauma
  - keep head elevated 30-45° to keep IOP down
  - keep NPO
  - tetanus status
  - give IV antibiotics

Management of suspected globe rupture: CAN'T forget
CT orbits
Ancef IV
NPO
Tetanus status

Hyphema

- bleed into anterior chamber, often due to damage to root of the iris
- may occur with blunt trauma

Treatment
- refer to Ophthalmology
  - shield and bedrest x 5 days or as determined by ophthalmologist
  - sleep with head upright
- may need surgical drainage if hyphema persists or if re-bleed occurs

Complications
- risk of re-bleed highest on days 2-5, resulting in secondary glaucoma, corneal staining, and iris necrosis
- never prescribe aspirin as it will increase the risk of a re-bleed

Blow-Out Fracture

- see Plastic Surgery
- blunt trauma causing fracture of orbital floor and orbital contents to herniate into maxillary sinus
- orbital rim remains intact
- inferior rectus and/or inferior oblique muscles may be incarcerated at fracture site
- infraorbital nerve courses along the floor of the orbit and may be damaged

Clinical Features
- pain and nausea at time of injury
- diplopia, restriction of EOM
- infraorbital and upper lip paresthesia (CN V_2)
- enophthalmos (sunken eye), periorbital ecchymoses

Classic Signs of Blow-Out
Enophthalmos
Decreased upgaze (IR trapped)
Cheek anesthetized (infraorbital nerve trapped)

Investigations
- plain films: Waters' view and lateral
- CT: anteroposterior and coronal view of orbits

Treatment
- refrain from coughing, blowing nose
- systemic antibiotics may be indicated
- surgery if fracture >50% orbital floor, diplopia not improving, or enophthalmos >2 mm
- may delay surgery if the diplopia improves

Chemical Burns

Fluorescein lights up alkali so you can detect it and assess whether it has been removed.

- alkali burns have a worse prognosis vs. acid burns because acids coagulate tissue and inhibit further corneal penetration
- poor prognosis if cornea opaque, likely irreversible stromal damage
- even with a clear cornea initially, alkali burns can progress for weeks (thus, very guarded prognosis)

Treatment
- irrigate at site of accident immediately, with water or buffered solution
  - IV drip for at least 20-30 minutes with eyelids retracted in emergency department
  - swab upper and lower fornices to remove possible particulate matter
- do not attempt to neutralize because the heat produced by the reaction will damage the cornea
- cycloplegic drops to decrease iris spasm (pain) and prevent secondary glaucoma (due to posterior synechiae formation)
- topical antibiotics and patching
- topical steroids (not in primary care) to decrease inflammation, use for less than two weeks (in the case of a persistent epithelial defect)

Ocular Drug Toxicity

Table 7. Drugs with Ocular Toxicity

Amiodarone	Corneal microdeposits and superficial keratopathy (vortex keratopathy) rare: ischemic optic neuropathy
Atropine, benztropine	Pupillary dilation (risk of angle closure glaucoma)
Bisphosphonates (Fosamax™, Actonel™)	Inflammatory eye disease (iritis, scleritis, episcleritis)
Chloroquine, hydroxychloroquine	Bull's eye maculopathy Vortex keratopathy
Chlorpromazine	Anterior subcapsular cataract
Contraceptive pills	Decreased tolerance to contact lenses Migraine Optic neuritis Central vein occlusion
Digitalis	Yellow vision Blurred vision
Ethambutol	Optic neuropathy
Haloperidol (Haldol™)	Oculogyric crises Blurred vision
Indomethacin	Superficial keratopathy
Isoniazid	Optic neuropathy
Nalidixic acid	Papilledema
Steroids	Posterior subcapsular cataracts Glaucoma Papilledema (systemic steroids) Increased severity of HSV infections (geographic ulcers) Predisposition to fungal infections
Sulphonamides, NSAIDS	Stevens-Johnson syndrome
Tamsulosin (Flomax™)	Intraoperative Floppy Iris Syndrome (IFIS), which can complicate cataract surgery
Tetracycline	Papilledema (associated with pseudotumour cerebri)
Thioridazine	Pigmentary degeneration of retina
Vigabatrin	Retinal deposition with macular sparing, peripheral visual field loss
Vitamin A intoxication	Papilledema
Vitamin D intoxication	Band keratopathy

Common Medications

TOPICAL OCULAR DIAGNOSTIC DRUGS

Fluorescein Dye
- water soluble orange-yellow dye
- green under cobalt blue light – ophthalmoscope or slit lamp
- absorbed in areas of epithelial loss (ulcer or abrasion)
- also stains mucus and contact lenses

Rose Bengal Stain
- stain devitalized epithelial cells and mucus

Anesthetics
- e.g. proparacaine HCl 0.5%, tetracaine 0.5%
- indications: removal of foreign body and sutures, tonometry, examination of painful cornea
- toxic to corneal epithelium (inhibit mitosis and migration) and can lead to corneal ulceration and scarring with prolonged use, therefore NEVER prescribe

Mydriatics
- dilate pupils
- two classes
  - cholinergic blocking
    - dilation plus cycloplegia (lose accommodation) by paralysis of iris sphincter and the ciliary body
    - e.g. tropicamide (Mydriacyl™)
    - indications: refraction, ophthalmoscopy, therapy for iritis
  - adrenergic stimulating
    - stimulate pupillary dilator muscles, no effect on accommodation
    - e.g. phenylephrine HCl 2.5% (duration: 30-40 minutes)
    - usually used with tropicamide for additive effects
    - side effects: hypertension, tachycardia, arrhythmias

Table 8. Mydriatic Cycloplegic Drugs and Duration of Action

Drugs	Duration of action
Tropicamide (Mydriacyl™) 0.5%, 1%	4-5 hours
Cyclopentolate HCL 0.5%, 1%	3-6 hours
Homatropine HBr 1%, 2%	3-7 days
Atropine sulfate 0.5%, 1%	1-2 weeks
Scopolamine HBr 0.25%, 5%	1-2 weeks

GLAUCOMA MEDICATIONS

Table 9. Glaucoma Medications

Drug Category	Dose	Effect	Comment/Side Effects
Alpha-agonist • epinephrine HCl 1% (Epifrin™) • dipivalyl epinephrine 0.1% (Propine™) • brimonidine 0.2% (Alphagan™) • apraclonidine 0.5% (Lopidine™)	1 gtt OS/OD BID/TID	1. Non-selective – ↓ aqueous production + ↑TM outflow 2. Selective – ↓ aqueous production + ↑ uveoscleral outflow non-selective = Epifrin™, Propine™ α_2 selective = Alphagan™, Lidopine™	1. Non-selective – mydriasis, macular edema, tachycardia 2. Selective – contact allergy, hypotension in children
β-blocker • timolol (Timoptic™) • levobunolol (Betagan™) • betaxolol (Betoptic™)	1 gtt OS/OD OD/BID	↓ aqueous production β non-selective =Timoptic™, Betagan™ β_1 selective = Betoptic™	Bronchospasm **(watch in asthma/COPD)** ↑ CHF Depression Bradycardia Heart block Hypotension Impotence
Carbonic Anhydrase Inhibitor • acetazolamide (Diamox™) • dorzolamide (Trusopt™) • brinzolamide (Azopt™)	1 gtt OS/OD TID	↓ aqueous production	****Must ask about sulfa allergy!** Generally local side effects with topical preparations

Table 9. Glaucoma Medications (continued)

Drug Category	Dose	Effect	Comment/Side Effects	
Parasympathmimetic (cholinergic stimulating) • pilocarpine (Pilopine™) • carbachol (Isopto Carbachol™)	1-2 gtts OS/OD TID/QID	↑ TM outflow ↓ night vision	Miosis Headache ↑ GI motility	Brow ache ↓ heart rate
Prostaglandin Analogues • latanoprost (Xalatan™) • travaprost (Travatan™) • bimatoprost (Lumigan™)	1 gtt OS/OD qhs	↑ uveoscleral outflow (uveoscleral responsible for 20% of drainage)	Iris colour change, periorbital skin pigmentation Lash growth Conjunctival hyperemia	

Cosopt™ = timolol + dorzolamide;　Xalacom™ = timolol + lantanoprost;　Combigan™ = timolol + brimonidine; DuoTrav™ = tinolol + travaprost

gtt = drop, gtts = drops

WET AGE-RELATED MACULAR DEGENERATION MEDICATIONS

Vascular Endothelial Growth Factors (VEGF) Inhibitors
• block vascular endothelial growth factor which prevents ocular angiogenesis and further development of choroidal neovascularization
• administered via intravitreal injections
• e.g. pegaptanib (Macugen®), ranibizumab (Lucentis®) and bevacizumab (Avastin®)
• bevacizumab is only FDA approved for metastatic breast cancer, colorectal cancer and non-small cell lung cancer

TOPICAL OCULAR THERAPEUTIC DRUGS

NSAIDs
• used for less serious chronic inflammatory conditions
• e.g. ketorolac (Acular™) drops, diclofenac (Voltaren™) drops

Anti-Histamines
• used to relieve red and itchy eye, often in combination with decongestants
• sodium cromoglycate (stabilizes membranes)

Corticosteroids
• e.g. fluorometholone (FML™), betamethasone, dexamethasone (Maxidex™), prednisolone (Predsol™ 0.5%, Pred Forte™ 1%), rimexolone (Vexol™)
• primary care physicians should avoid prescribing topical corticosteroids due to risk of glaucoma, cataracts, and reactivation of HSV keratitis
• complications:
  ▪ potentiates herpes simplex keratitis and fungal keratitis as well as masking symptoms (within days)
  ▪ posterior subcapsular cataract (within months)
  ▪ increased IOP, more rapidly in steroid responders (within weeks)

Decongestants
• weak adrenergic stimulating drugs (vasoconstrictor)
• e.g. naphazoline, phenylephrine (Isopto Frin™)
• rebound vasodilation with overuse; rarely can precipitate angle closure glaucoma

Antibiotics
• indications: bacterial conjunctivitis, keratitis, or blepharitis
• commonly as topical drops or ointments, may give systemically
• e.g. sulfonamide (sodium sulfacetamide, sulfisoxazole), gentamicin (Garamycin™), erythromycin, tetracycline, bacitracin, polymyxin B, fluoroquinolomes (Ciloxan™, Ocuflox™, Vigamox™, Zymar™)

Notes

OR Orthopaedics

Winston Bharat, Amir Khoshbin and Timothy Leroux, chapter editors
Sami Chadi and Biniam Kidane, associate editors
Emily Partridge, EBM editor
Dr. Peter Ferguson, Dr. William Kraemer, Dr. Markku Nousiainen and Dr. Herbert von Schroeder, staff editors

Basic Anatomy Review

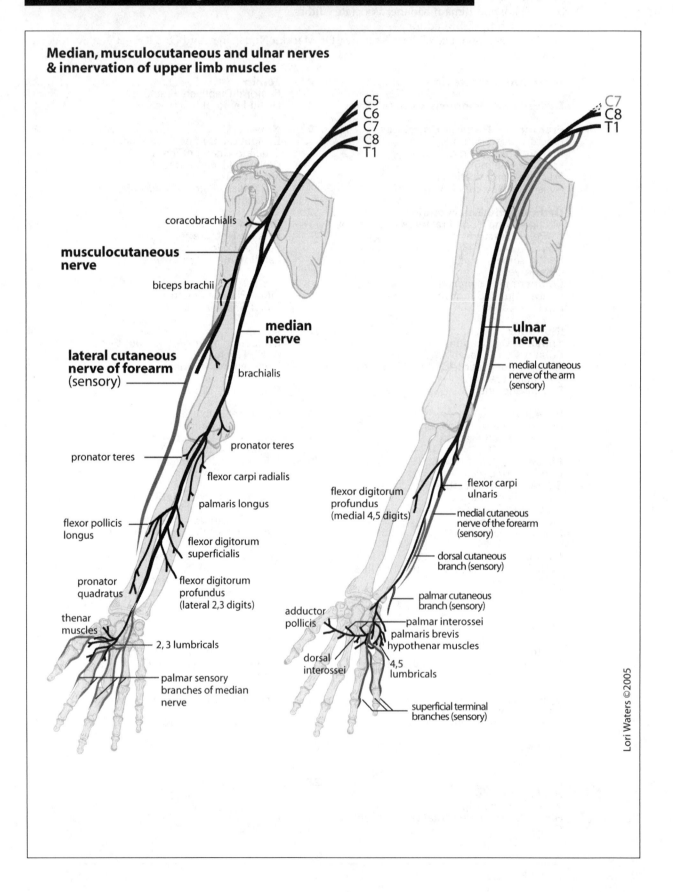

Median, musculocutaneous and ulnar nerves & innervation of upper limb muscles

C5
C6
C7
C8
T1

C7
C8
T1

coracobrachialis

musculocutaneous nerve

biceps brachii

median nerve

ulnar nerve

lateral cutaneous nerve of forearm (sensory)

brachialis

medial cutaneous nerve of the arm (sensory)

pronator teres

pronator teres

flexor carpi radialis

flexor carpi ulnaris

palmaris longus

flexor pollicis longus

flexor digitorum profundus (medial 4,5 digits)

medial cutaneous nerve of the forearm (sensory)

flexor digitorum superficialis

dorsal cutaneous branch (sensory)

pronator quadratus

flexor digitorum profundus (lateral 2,3 digits)

palmar cutaneous branch (sensory)

thenar muscles

adductor pollicis

palmar interossei
palmaris brevis
hypothenar muscles

2, 3 lumbricals

dorsal interossei

4,5 lumbricals

palmar sensory branches of median nerve

superficial terminal branches (sensory)

Lori Waters ©2005

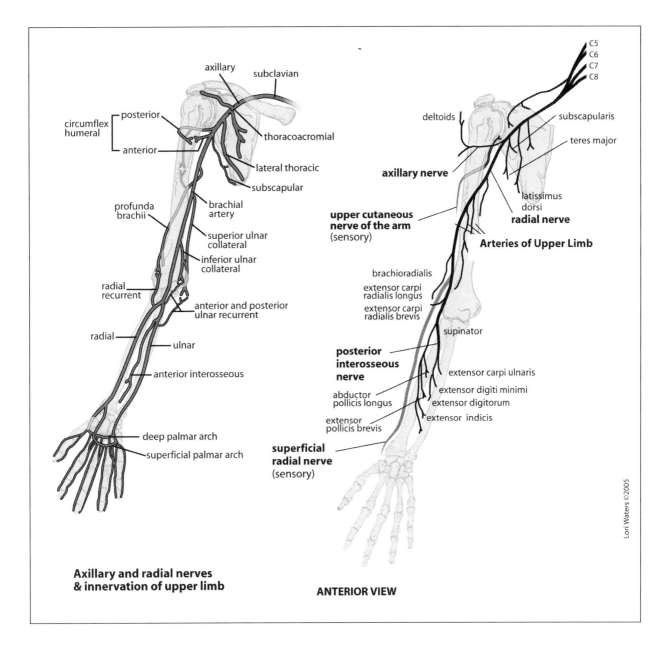

Axillary and radial nerves & innervation of upper limb

ANTERIOR VIEW

Lori Waters ©2005

S = sensory innervation
M = motor innervation

- **Axillary**
  - S: lateral upper arm (sergeant's patch)
  - M: deltoid
- **Musculocutaneous**
  - S: lateral forearm
  - M: elbow flexion (biceps, brachialis)
- **Radial**
  - S: dorsum of hand (1st web space)
  - M:
    - ◆ proximal: triceps, wrist extension
    - ◆ distal: PIN – thumb and finger extension
- **Median**
  - S: volar thumb to ½ ring finger
  - M: most selective abductor and opponens pollicus
- **Ulnar**
  - S: small and ½ of ring
  - M: hand intrinsics

Quick Nerve Exam
- **"thumbs up"**
  - PIN (radial nerve)
- **"OK sign"**
  - AIN (median nerve)
- **"spread fingers"**
  - ulnar

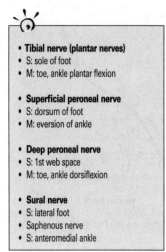

- **Tibial nerve (plantar nerves)**
- S: sole of foot
- M: toe, ankle plantar flexion

- **Superficial peroneal nerve**
- S: dorsum of foot
- M: eversion of ankle

- **Deep peroneal nerve**
- S: 1st web space
- M: toe, ankle dorsiflexion

- **Sural nerve**
- S: lateral foot
- Saphenous nerve
- S: anteromedial ankle

Nerves and arteries of lower limbs

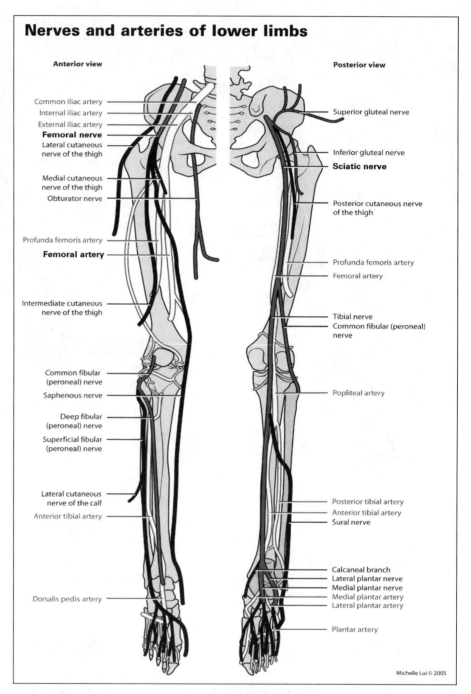

Anterior view

Common iliac artery
Internal iliac artery
External iliac artery
Femoral nerve
Lateral cutaneous nerve of the thigh
Medial cutaneous nerve of the thigh
Obturator nerve
Profunda femoris artery
Femoral artery
Intermediate cutaneous nerve of the thigh
Common fibular (peroneal) nerve
Saphenous nerve
Deep fibular (peroneal) nerve
Superficial fibular (peroneal) nerve
Lateral cutaneous nerve of the calf
Anterior tibial artery
Dorsalis pedis artery

Posterior view

Superior gluteal nerve
Inferior gluteal nerve
Sciatic nerve
Posterior cutaneous nerve of the thigh
Profunda femoris artery
Femoral artery
Tibial nerve
Common fibular (peroneal) nerve
Popliteal artery
Posterior tibial artery
Anterior tibial artery
Sural nerve
Calcaneal branch
Lateral plantar nerve
Medial plantar nerve
Medial plantar artery
Lateral plantar artery
Plantar artery

Michelle Lui © 2005

Differential Diagnosis of Joint Pain

Extrinsic
- neurologic (nerve root compression, herpes zoster, etc.)
- generalized (fibromyalgia, polymyalgia rheumatica, sickle cell (ischemic), dermato/polymyositis)
- referred pain
- pain originating from surrounding organs

Intrinsic
- articular
  - arthritis (degenerative, rheumatoid, crystal-induced, septic, avascular necrosis)
  - neoplastic
  - traumatic (fracture, soft tissue damage, neuropathic arthropathy)
- non-articular
  - bursa, tendons, ligaments, muscle (bursitis, tendonitis, myositis)

Fractures – General Principles

Fracture Description

1. Integrity of skin/soft tissue
- closed: skin/soft tissue over and near fracture is intact
- open: skin/soft tissue over and near fracture is lacerated or abraded, fracture exposed to outside environment, continuous bleeding from puncture site or fat droplets in blood suggest communication with fracture

2. Location
- epiphyseal: end of bone, forming part of the adjacent joint
- metaphyseal: the flared portion of the bone at the ends of the shaft
- diaphyseal: the shaft of a long bone (proximal, middle, distal)
- physis: growth plate

3. Orientation/Fracture Pattern
- transverse: perpendicular fracture line, direct force, high energy
- oblique: angular fracture line, angular or rotational force
- butterfly: slight comminution at the fracture site which looks largely like a butterfly
- segmental: a separate segment of bone bordered by fracture lines - high energy
- spiral: complex, multi-planar fracture line, rotational force - low energy
- comminuted: more than 2 fracture fragments
- intra-articular: fracture line crosses articular cartilage and enters joint
- compression/impacted: impaction of bone, e.g. vertebrae, proximal tibia
- torus: a buckle fracture of one cortex, often in children
- green-stick: an incomplete fracture of one cortex, often in children
- pathologic: fracture through bone weakened by disease/tumour

4. Displacement
- nondisplaced: fracture fragments are in anatomic alignment
- displaced : fracture fragments are not in anatomic alignment
- distracted: fracture fragments are separated by a gap
- angulated: direction of fracture apex, e.g. varus/valgus
- translated: percentage of overlapping bone at fracture site
- rotated: fracture fragment rotated about long axis of bone

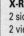

X-Ray rule of 2's
2 sides = bilateral
2 views = AP + lateral
2 joints = joint above + below
2 times = before + after reduction

Varus/valgus displacement
Varus = Apex away from midline
Valgus = Apex torward midline

NOTE: displacement refers to direction of distal fragment.

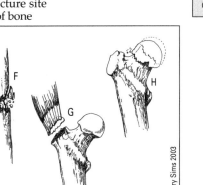

Figure 1. Fracture Types

A. Transverse   B. Oblique   C. Butterfly   D. Segmental   E. Spiral   F. Comminuted   G. Avulsion   H. Impacted

© Mary Sims 2003

Management of Fractures

- ABCs, primary survey and secondary survey (ATLS protocol)
  - rule out other fractures/injuries
  - rule out open fracture
- AMPLE history – **A**llergies, **M**edications, **P**ast medical history, **L**ast meal, **E**vents surrounding injury
  - consider pathologic fracture with history of only minor trauma
- Additional History/Physical:
  - 1) Baseline Functional Status - Handedness (upper extremity) vs. Ambulatory ability (lower extremity - note distances; stairs; and use of assistive devices such as canes, walkers, wheelchairs, etc)
  - 2) Occupation
  - 3) Mechanism of Injury
  - 4) Past Medical History (*note any contraindications to surgery or general anaesthetic)

Indications for Open Reduction NO CAST
N: non-union
O: open fracture
C: neurovascular compromise
A: intra-articular fracture
S: Salter-Harris 3,4,5
T: polytrauma

- ▪ 5) Neurovascular Status
- analgesia
- imaging
- splint extremity

1) Obtain the reduction
  - ▪ closed reduction
    - ◆ apply traction in the long axis of the limb
    - ◆ reverse the mechanism that produced the fracture
    - ◆ reduce under fluoroscopy with IV sedation and muscle relaxation
  - ▪ indications for open reduction – NO CAST (see side bar, OR5)
  - ▪ other indications include
    - ◆ failed closed reduction
    - ◆ cannot cast or apply traction due to site (e.g. hip fracture)
    - ◆ pathologic fractures
    - ◆ potential for improved function with open reduction and internal fixation (ORIF)
  - ▪ potential complications of open reductions
    - ◆ infection
    - ◆ non-union
    - ◆ implant failure
    - ◆ new fracture
  - ▪ re-check neurovascular status after reduction and obtain post-reduction x-ray

2) Maintain the reduction:
  - ▪ external stabilization – splints, casts, traction, external fixator
  - ▪ internal stabilization – percutaneous pinning; extramedullary fixation (screws, plates, wires); intramedullary fixation (rods)
  - ▪ follow-up – evaluate bone healing

3) Rehabilitate: to regain functioning and avoid joint stiffness

Fracture Healing

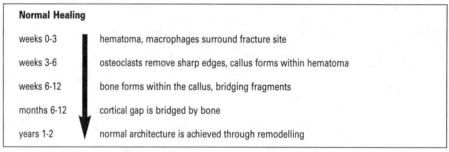

Normal Healing	
weeks 0-3	hematoma, macrophages surround fracture site
weeks 3-6	osteoclasts remove sharp edges, callus forms within hematoma
weeks 6-12	bone forms within the callus, bridging fragments
months 6-12	cortical gap is bridged by bone
years 1-2	normal architecture is achieved through remodelling

Figure 2. Stages of Bone Healing

Evaluation of Healing: Tests of Union
- clinical: no longer tender to palpation or angulation stress
- x-ray: trabeculae cross fracture site, visible callus bridging site

Fracture Complications

Table 1. Fracture Complications

	Early	Late
Local	compartment syndrome	mal/nonunion
	neurological injury	avascular necrosis (AVN)
	vascular injury	osteomyelitis
	infection	heterotopic ossification (HO)
	implant failure	post-traumatic arthritis
	fracture blisters	reflex sympathetic dystrophy (RSD)
Systemic	sepsis	
	deep vein thrombosis (DVT)	
	pulmonary embolus (PE)	
	acute respiratory distress syndrome (ARDS)	
	hemorrhagic shock	

Heterotrophic Ossification
The formation of bone in abnormal locations (e.g. in muscle), secondary to pathology.

Avascular Necrosis (AVN; Osteonecrosis)

Definition
- disruption of blood supply to bone resulting in ischemia
- occurs in bones extensively covered in cartilage which rely on intra-osseous blood supply (femoral head) or in bones with a distal → proximal blood supply (proximal pole of scaphoid, body of talus, femoral head)

Risk Factors
- steroid use
- chronic alcohol use
- post-traumatic fracture/dislocation
- septic arthritis
- sickle cell disease
- storage disease (e.g. Gaucher's disease)
- dysbarism (Caisson's disease "the bends")
- idiopathic (Chandler's disease)

X-Ray Features of AVN:
- reactive sclerosis of adjacent bone
- subchondral fracture
- flattening of weightbearing zones with eventual collapse
- see atlas for image

MRI is more sensitive than x-rays at diagnosing early AVN.

Orthopaedic Emergencies

Multiple Long Bone Fractures and Unstable Pelvic Fracture

Etiology
- high energy trauma
- generally multiple lower extremity and/or pelvic fractures
- may be associated with spinal injuries or life threatening injuries

Clinical Presentation
- local swelling, tenderness, deformity of the hips and instability of the pelvis with palpation

Investigations
- routine views of pelvis: AP inlet and outlet; if acetabular fracture, AP and Judet (see Table 13 for classification of pelvic fractures)
- x-ray AP and lateral of all long bones suspected to be injured

Management
- ABCs
- assess genitourinary injury (rectal exam/vaginal exam mandatory)
- external or internal fixation of all fractures
- DVT prophylaxis

Complications
- **hemorrhage – life threatening** (may produce signs and symptoms of hypovolemic shock)
- acute respiratory distress syndrome (ARDS)
- fat embolism syndrome
- venous thrombosis - DVT and PE
- bladder/bowel injury
- neurological damage
- obstetrical difficulties in future
- persistent sacro-iliac joint pain
- post-traumatic arthritis of the hip with acetabular fractures
- sepsis, if missed open fracture

Orthopaedic Emergencies
VON CHOP
V: Vascular compromise
O: Open fracture
N: Neurological compromise/Cauda equina syndrome
C: Compartment Syndrome
H: Hip dislocation
O: Osteomyelitis/Septic arthritis
P: Unstable pelvic fracture

Open Fractures

Definition
- fractured bone in communication with the external environment

Emergency Measures
- removal of obvious foreign material
- cover wound with sterile dressings
- tetanus status
- IV antibiotics (see Table 2)

- splint fracture
- NPO and prepare for OR (bloodwork, consent, ECG, CXR)
  - operative irrigation and debridement within 6-8 hours to decrease risk of infection
  - traumatic wound usually left open to drain
  - re-examine with repeat I&D in 48 hrs

Complications
- osteomyelitis
- soft tissue injury
- neurovascular injury
- blood loss
- nonunion

Table 2. Gustillo Classification of Open Fractures

Gustilo Grade	Length of Open Wound	Description	Antibiotic Regimen
I	<1 cm	Minimal contamination and soft tissue injury Simple or minimally comminuted fracture	First generation cephalosporin (cefazolin) for 48 hours
II	1-10 cm	Moderate contamination Soft tissue injury Fracture comminution	Gram negative coverage (gentamicin) for at least 72 hours
III	>10 cm	Gross contamination Severe soft tissue injury Fracture comminution	*For soil contamination, penicillin is provided for *clostridial* coverage

* Any high energy injury, comminuted fracture, shotgun blast, farmyard/soil contamination, or fracture more than 8 hrs old is immediately classified as Grade III

Septic Joint

Etiology
- most commonly caused by *Staph. aureus* in adults
- consider coagulase - negative staph in patients with prior joint replacement
- consider *Neisseria gonorrheae* in sexually active adults
- most common route of infection is hematogenous

Clinical Presentation
- inability/refusal to bear weight, localized joint pain, erythema, warmth, swelling with pain on active and passive ROM, ± fever

Investigations
- x-ray (to r/o fracture, tumour, metabolic bone disease), ESR, CRP, WBC, blood cultures
- joint aspirate (WBC >80,000 with >90% neutrophils, protein level >4.4 mg/dL; glucose level << blood glucose level, no crystals, positive gram stain results)

Management
- IV antibiotics
- for small joints: needle aspiration, serial if necessary, until sterile; major joints such as knee, hip, or shoulder should be decompressed and drained surgically in emergent fashion

Serial C-reactive protein (CRP) can be used to monitor response to therapy.

Osteomyelitis

Etiology
- most common organism is *Staph. aureus*
- consider *Salmonella typhi* in patients with sickle cell disease
- neonates and immunocompromised patients are susceptible to gram-negative organisms

Clinical Presentation
- localized extremity pain, ± fever, 1 to 2 weeks after respiratory infection or infection at another non-bony site

Investigations
- blood culture, aspirate cultures, ESR, CBC (leukocytosis)
- x-ray, bone scan (increased uptake), MRI most sensitive/specific

Plain Film Findings of Osteomyelitis
1. soft tissue swelling
2. lytic bone destruction
3. periosteal reaction (formation of new bone, esp. in response to #)

Management
- IV antibiotics, empiric therapy, adjust pending blood and aspirate cultures
- surgical decortication and drainage ± local antibiotics (i.e. antibiotic beads) if MRI suggests an abscess or if patient does not improve after 36 hours on IV antibiotics

Acute osteomyelitis is a medical emergency.

Compartment Syndrome

Definition
- increased interstitial pressure in an anatomical "compartment" (forearm, calf) where muscle and tissue are bounded by fascia and bone (fibro-osseous compartment) with little room for expansion
- interstitial pressure exceeds capillary perfusion pressure leading to muscle necrosis (in 4-6 hrs) and eventually nerve necrosis

Etiology
- intracompartmental: fracture (particularly tibial fractures, pediatric supracondylar fractures, and forearm fractures), crush injury, revascularization
- extracompartmental: constrictive dressing (circumferential cast), circumferential burn

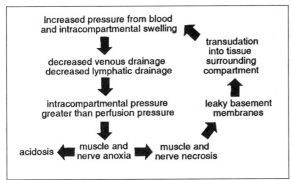

Figure 3. Pathogenesis of Compartment Syndrome

Physical Examination
- pain with passive stretch
- 5 P's –> late sign

Clinical Features
- pain with active contraction of compartment
- pain with passive stretch
- swollen, tense compartment
- suspicious history

Investigation
- usually not necessary as compartment syndrome is a clinical diagnosis
- in children or unconscious patients where clinical exam is unreliable, compartment pressure monitoring with catheter, AFTER clinical diagnosis is made (normal = 0 mmHg; elevated ≥30 mmHg or within 30 mmHg of diastolic BP)

Treatment
- remove constrictive dressings (casts, splints)
- elevate limb
- definitive treatment: fasciotomy to release compartments

Complications
- rhabdomyolysis, renal failure secondary to myoglobinuria, Volkmann's ischemic contracture (ischemic necrosis of muscle, followed by secondary fibrosis and finally calcification; esp. following supracondylar # of humerus)

Cauda Equina Syndrome

- see <u>Neurosurgery</u>

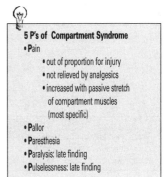

5 P's of Compartment Syndrome
- **Pain**
  - out of proportion for injury
  - not relieved by analgesics
  - increased with passive stretch of compartment muscles (most specific)
- **Pallor**
- **Paresthesia**
- **Paralysis:** late finding
- **Pulselessness:** late finding

Most important sign is increased pain with passive stretch. Most important symptom is pain out of proportion to injury.

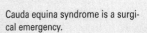

Cauda equina syndrome is a surgical emergency.

Hip Dislocation

- also see *Hip Dislocation after THA*
- reduce hip dislocations ASAP (ideally within 6 hours) to ↓ risk of AVN of the femoral head

ANTERIOR HIP DISLOCATION (rare)
- mechanism: posteriorly directed blow to knee with hip widely abducted
- clinical features: shortened, abducted, externally rotated limb
- treatment
  - closed reduction under GA
  - post-reduction CT to assess joint congruity

POSTERIOR HIP DISLOCATION
- mechanism: severe force to knee with hip flexed and adducted (e.g. knee into dashboard in motor vehicle accident (MVA))
- clinical features: shortened, adducted and internally rotated limb
- treatment
  - closed reduction under GA
  - ORIF if unstable, intra-articular fragments or posterior wall fracture
  - post-reduction CT to assess joint congruity and fractures
  - if reduction is unstable put in traction x 4-6 weeks

CENTRAL HIP DISLOCATION
- mechanism: traumatic injury where femoral head is pushed through acetabulum toward pelvic cavity

COMPLICATIONS FOR ALL HIP DISLOCATIONS
- post-traumatic arthritis
- AVN
- fracture of femoral shaft or neck
- sciatic nerve palsy in 25% (10% permanent)
- heterotopic ossification (HO)
- damage to femoral head

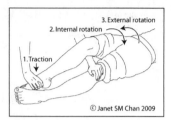

Figure 4. Rochester Method

Rochester Method
- patient lying supine with hip & knee flexed on injured side
- surgeon stands on patient's injured side
- surgeon passes one arm under patient's flexed knee, reaching to place that hand on patient's other knee (thus supporting patient's injured leg)
- with other hand, surgeon grasps patient's ankle on injured side, applying traction
- reduction via traction, int. rotation, then ext. rotation once femoral head clears acetabular rim

There are 4 joints in the shoulder: glenohumeral, acromioclavicular (AC), sternoclavicular (SC), scapulothoracic

Factors causing shoulder instability
- shallow glenoid
- loose capsule
- large mobility

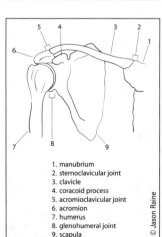

1. manubrium
2. sternoclavicular joint
3. clavicle
4. coracoid process
5. acromioclavicular joint
6. acromion
7. humerus
8. glenohumeral joint
9. scapula

Figure 5. Shoulder Joints

Shoulder

Shoulder Dislocation

- the glenohumeral joint is the most commonly dislocated joint in the body since stability is sacrificed for motion

Prognosis
- recurrence rate depends on age of 1st dislocation: <20 yrs = 65-95%; 20-40 yrs = 60-70%; >40 yrs = 2-4%

Complications
- tuberosity fracture, glenoid rim fracture
- rotator cuff tear, shoulder stiffness
- injury to axillary nerve/artery, brachial plexus injury
- recurrent/unreduced dislocation

ANTERIOR SHOULDER DISLOCATION (>90%)

Mechanism
- abducted and externally rotated arm or blow to posterior shoulder

Clinical Features
- pain
- arm held in slight abduction, external rotation; internal rotation is blocked
- "squared off" shoulder
- +ve apprehension test: apprehension with shoulder abduction and external rotation to 90° since humeral head is pushed anteriorly and recreates feeling of anterior dislocation

- +ve relocation test: a posteriorly directed force applied during the apprehension test relieves apprehension since anterior subluxation is prevented
- +ve sulcus sign: presence of subacromial indentation with distal traction on humerus indicates inferior shoulder instability
- neurovascular exam including:
  - axillary nerve (sensory patch over deltoid and deltoid contraction)
  - musculocutaneous nerve (sensory patch on lateral forearm and biceps contraction)

Table 3. An EBM Perspective on Tests of Anterior Shoulder Instability

	Apprehension	Relocation	Surprise
Sensitivity	52.78%	45.83%	63.89%
Specificity	98.91%	54.35%	98.91%
PPV	97.73%	43.86%	98.22%
NPV	72.82%	56.26%	77.86%

An Evaluation of the Apprehension, Relocation, and Surprise Tests for Anterior Shoulder Instability. The American Journal of Sports Medicine 32:301-307 (2004).

Investigations
- x-rays: AP, trans-scapular, axillary

X-Ray Findings
- dislocation
  - axillary view: humeral head is anterior
  - trans-scapular view: humeral head is anterior to the centre of the "Mercedes-Benz sign"
- ± Hill-Sachs lesion: divot in posterior humeral head due to forceful impaction of an anteriorly dislocated humeral head against the glenoid rim
- ± bony Bankart lesion: avulsion of the anterior glenoid labrum (with attached bone fragments) from the glenoid rim

Treatment
- closed reduction with IV sedation and muscle relaxation
- 2 methods:
  - Traction-countertraction: assistant stabilizes torso with a folded sheet wrapped across the chest while the MD applies gentle steady traction
  - Stimson: while patient lies prone with arm hanging over table edge, hang a 5 lb weight on wrist for 15-20 min
- obtain post-reduction x-rays
- check post-reduction neurovascular status (NVS)
- sling x 3 weeks, followed by shoulder rehabilitation

POSTERIOR SHOULDER DISLOCATION (5%)
- often missed due to poor physical exam and radiographs

Mechanism
- adducted, internally rotated, flexed arm
- fall on an outstretched hand (FOOSH)
- 3 E's (epileptic seizure, EtOH, electrocution)
- blow to anterior shoulder

Clinical Features
- arm is held in adduction and internal rotation; external rotation is blocked
- anterior shoulder flattening, prominent coracoid
- posterior apprehension ("jerk") test: with patient supine, flex elbow 90° and adduct, internally rotate the arm while applying a posterior force to the shoulder; patient will "jerk" back with the sensation of subluxation

Investigation
- x-rays: AP, trans-scapular, axillary

X-Ray Findings
  - dislocation
    - AP view: partial vacancy of glenoid fossa (vacant glenoid sign) and >6 mm space between anterior glenoid rim and humeral head (positive rim sign)
    - axillary view: humeral head is posterior

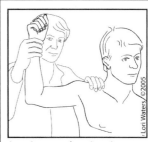

Anterior apprehension sign

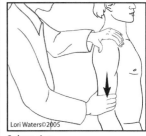

Sulcus sign

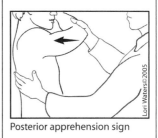

Posterior apprehension sign

Figure 6. Apprehension Tests

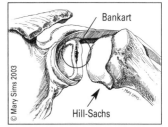

Figure 7. Anterior Dislocation Causing Hill-Sachs and Bankart Lesions

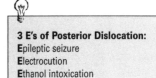

3 E's of Posterior Dislocation:
Epileptic seizure
Electrocution
Ethanol intoxication

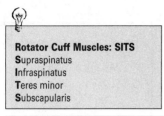

Rotator Cuff Muscles: SITS
Supraspinatus
Infraspinatus
Teres minor
Subscapularis

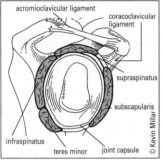

Figure 8. Muscles of the Rotator Cuff

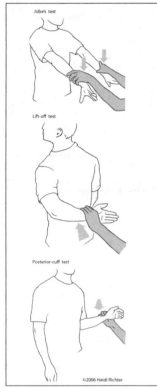

Figure 9. Rotator Cuff Tests

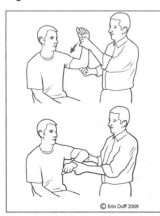

Figure 10. Hawkins Test

   ◆ trans-scapular view: humeral head is posterior to center of "Mercedes-Benz sign"
  ▪ reverse Hill-Sachs lesion: divot in anterior humeral head
  ▪ reverse bony Bankart lesion: avulsion of the posterior glenoid labrum from the bony glenoid rim

Treatment
- closed reduction: inferior traction on a flexed elbow with pressure on the back of the humeral head
- obtain post-reduction x-rays
- check post-reduction neurovascular status
- sling x 3 weeks, followed by shoulder rehabilitation

Rotator Cuff Disease

- rotator cuff consists of 4 muscles that act to stabilize humeral head within the glenoid

Table 4. Rotator Cuff Muscles

Muscle	Muscle attachments	Nerve supply	Muscle function
Supraspinatus	Scapula → greater tuberosity of humerus	Suprascapular nerve	Abduction
Infraspinatus	Scapula → greater tuberosity of humerus	Suprascapular nerve	External rotation
Teres minor	Scapula → greater tuberosity of humerus	Axillary nerve	External rotation
Subscapularis	Scapula → lesser tuberosity of humerus	Subscapular nerve	Internal rotation and adduction

SPECTRUM OF DISEASE: IMPINGEMENT, TENDONITIS, MICRO OR MACRO TEARS

Etiology
- compression of rotator cuff tendons (primarily supraspinatus) and subacromial bursa between the head of the humerus and the acromion; leads to bursitis, tendonitis and, if left untreated, can lead to rotator cuff thinning and tear
- anything that leads to a narrow subacromial space
  1. glenohumeral muscle weakness leading to abnormal motion of humeral head
  2. scapular muscle weakness leading to abnormal motion of acromion
  3. acromial abnormalities such as congenital narrow space or osteophyte formation

Clinical Features
- night pain and difficulty sleeping on affected side
- trouble with overhead activities
- tenderness to palpation over greater tuberosity
- Jobe's test (supraspinatus): weakness with active resistance when examiner pushes arms to ground at 90° forward flexion in scapular plane with forearm pronated suggests supraspinatus tear
- Lift-off test (subscapularis): internally rotate arm so dorsal surface of hand rests on lower back. Inability to actively lift hand away from back against resistance indicates subscapularis tear
- Posterior-cuff (infraspinatus and teres minor): weak resisted active external rotation with elbow flexed 90° and at patient's side indicates posterior cuff tear
- +ve Neer's test: pain with passive shoulder flexion between 130-170°
- +ve Hawkins' test: pain with shoulder flexion and passive internal rotation
- +ve painful arc: pain with active abduction between 60-120°

Investigations
- x-rays: AP view may show high riding humerus relative to glenoid, evidence of chronic tendonitis
- U/S: see large cuff tears
- arthrogram: see full thickness tear
- MRI arthrogram: geyser sign (injected dye leaks out of joint through rotator cuff tear)

Treatment and Prognosis
- mild ("wear")
  - treatment is non-operative (physiotherapy, NSAIDs)
- moderate ("tear")
  - non-operative treatment ± steroid injection
- severe ("repair")
  - impingement that is refractory to 2-3 months physio and 1-2 injections
  - may require surgical repair; i.e. acromioplasty, rotator cuff repair

Warning
Repeated steroid injections can ultimately accelerate propagation of rotator cuff tear. Patients should never receive more than 3 subacromial injections.

Acromioclavicular (AC) Joint Pathology

- 2 main ligaments attach clavicle to scapula: acromioclavicular (AC) and coracoclavicular (CC) ligaments

Mechanism
- fall onto shoulder with adducted arm (fall onto tip of shoulder)

Clinical Features
- palpate step deformity between distal clavicle and acromion (with dislocation)
- pain with adduction/limited ROM

Investigations
- X-rays: AP, Zanca view (10-15° cephalic tilt), axillary ± stress views (10 lbs. weight in patient's hand)

Management
- usually non-operative: sling 1-3 weeks, ice, analgesia
- consider operative management (excision of lateral clavicle with AC/CC ligament reconstruction) if
  - 1) AC and CC ligaments are both torn AND/OR
  - 2) clavicle displaced posteriorly

Clavicular Fracture

- incidence: proximal (5%), middle (80%), or distal (15%) third of clavicle
- common in children (unites rapidly without complications)

Mechanism
- fall on shoulder, FOOSH, direct trauma to clavicle

Clinical Features
- pain and tenting of skin
- arm is clasped to chest to prevent movement
- evaluate neurovascular status of entire upper limb

Treatment
- proximal and middle third clavicular fractures
  - sling x 1-2 weeks
  - early ROM and strengthening once pain subsides
  - if ends overlap >2 cm, consider ORIF
- distal third clavicular fractures
  - undisplaced (with ligaments intact): sling x 1-2 weeks
  - displaced (CC ligament injury): ORIF or excision

Complications
- cosmetic bump usually only complication
- nonunion/malunion
- shoulder stiffness
- pneumothorax, injuries to brachial plexus and subclavian vessel (all very rare)

Frozen Shoulder (Adhesive Capsulitis)

Definition
- disorder characterized by progressive pain and stiffness of the shoulder usually resolving spontaneously after 18 months

Mechanism
- primary adhesive capsulitis
  - idiopathic, usually associated with diabetes mellitus
  - may resolve spontaneously in 9-18 months
- secondary adhesive capsulitis
  - due to prolonged immobilization
  - shoulder-hand syndrome - type of reflex sympathetic dystrophy characterized by arm and shoulder pain, decreased motion and diffuse swelling
  - following myocardial infarction, stroke, shoulder trauma

Clinical Features
- aching arm and shoulder with:
  - decreased active and passive ROM
  - increased pain: often prevents sleeping on affected side
  - increased stiffness as pain subsides: continues for 6-12 months after pain has disappeared

Investigations
- x-rays may be normal, or may show demineralization from disease

Treatment
- active and passive ROM (physiotherapy)
- NSAIDs and steroid injections if limited by pain
- MUA (manipulation under anesthesia) or arthroscopy for debridement/decompression

Humerus

Proximal Humeral Fracture

Mechanism
- young: high energy trauma (MVA)
- older: FOOSH from standing height in osteoporotic individuals

Investigations
- x-rays: AP, trans-scapular, axillary are essential
- CT scan: in complex cases

Classification
- Neer classification is based on 4 fracture fragments: head, greater tuberosity, lesser tuberosity, shaft
- can be
  - nondisplaced: displacement <1 cm and/or angulation <45°
  - displaced: displacement >1 cm and/or angulation >45°
  - dislocated/subluxed: humeral head dislocated/subluxed from glenoid

Treatment
- non-operative
  - sling immobilization (nondisplaced): begin ROM in 7-10 days to prevent stiffness
  - closed reduction (minimally displaced)
- operative
  - ORIF (displaced, dislocated): hemiarthroplasty may be necessary

Complications
- AVN, axillary nerve palsy, nonunion/malunion, shoulder stiffness, post-traumatic arthritis

Anatomic neck fractures disrupt blood supply to the humeral head and avascular necrosis (AVN) of the humeral head may ensue.

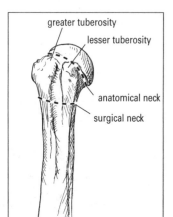

Figure 11. Fractures of the Proximal Humerus

Humeral Shaft Fracture

Mechanism
- FOOSH, MVA, direct blows, twisting injuries, metastasis (in elderly)

Clinical Features
- pain, swelling, ± shortening, motion/crepitus at fracture site
- must test radial nerve function before and after treatment

Risk of radial n. and brachial a. injury!

Investigations
- x-rays: AP and lateral full length views of humerus

Treatment
- in general humeral shaft #'s are treated conservatively; "If both ends are in the same room, they'll heal"
- non-operative (most common)
    - ± reduction – can accept deformity due to compensatory range of motion of shoulder
    - hanging cast (weight of arm in cast provides traction across fracture site) with sling immobilization x 7-10 days then Sarmiento functional brace
- operative
    - indications: open fracture, neurovascular injury, unacceptable fracture alignment, polytrauma, segmental fracture, pathological fracture, "floating elbow" (simultaneous unstable humeral and forearm fractures), intra-articular
    - procedure: compression plating (most common), intramedullary rod insertion, external fixation

Complications
- radial nerve injury: expect spontaneous recovery in 3-4 months, otherwise send for electromyography (EMG)
- non/malunion
- decreased ROM
- compartment syndrome

Elbow

General Principles

- articulation between distal humerus, proximal ulna, proximal radius (humeroradial, humeroulnar and radioulnar joints)
- fractures and dislocations of the elbow are evident on AP, lateral and oblique radiographs

Supracondylar Fracture

- most common in pediatric population (peak age ~7 years old), seldomly seen in adults
- anterior interosseous nerve (AIN) injury commonly associated with extension type

Mechanism
- >96% are extension injuries via FOOSH; <4% are flexion injuries

Clinical Features
- pain, swelling, point tenderness ± neurovascular injury

Investigations
- x-rays: AP, lateral of elbow

Treatment
- undisplaced: cast in flexion for 3 weeks
- displaced
    - closed reduction alone usually unstable
    - requires percutaneous pinning followed by limb cast with elbow flexed >90°
    - in adults, ORIF is necessary

Complications
- joint stiffness, brachial artery injury, median or ulnar nerve injury, heterotopic ossification, malunion, compartment syndrome (leads to Volkmann's ischemic contracture), malalignment cubitus varus (distal fragment tilted into varus)

Radial Head Fracture

- a common fracture of the upper limb in young adults

Mechanism
- FOOSH with elbow extended and forearm pronated

Clinical Features
- marked local tenderness on palpation over radial head (lateral elbow)
- decreased ROM at elbow, mechanical block to forearm pronation and supination
- pain on pronation/supination

Terrible Triad
1. Radial head fracture
2. Coronoid fracture
3. Elbow dislocation

Investigations
- x-ray: enlarged anterior fat pad ("sail sign") or the presence of a posterior fat pad indicate occult radial head fractures

Table 5. Classification and Treatment of Radial Head Fractures

Mason Class	Radiographic Description	Treatment
1	undisplaced fracture	elbow slab or sling x 3-5 days with early ROM
2	displaced fracture	ORIF if: angulation >30°; involves ≥1/3 of the radial head; or if ≥3 mm of joint incongruity exists
3	comminuted fracture	radial head excision ± prosthesis
4	comminuted fracture with posterior elbow dislocation	radial head excision ± prosthesis

Complications
- joint stiffness, myositis ossificans, recurrent instability (if medial collateral ligament injured and radial head excised)

Olecranon Fracture

Mechanism
- direct trauma to posterior aspect of elbow (fall onto the point of the elbow)

Do not immobilize elbow joint >2-3 weeks to avoid stiffness

Clinical Features
- ± loss of active extension due to avulsion of triceps tendon

Treatment
- undisplaced (<2 mm, stable): cast 3 wks (elbow in 45° flexion) then gentle ROM
- displaced: ORIF (plate and screws or tension band wiring) and early ROM if stable

Elbow Dislocation

- third most common joint dislocation after shoulder and patella
- most commonly occurs in young people (5-25 years) in sporting events or high speed MVAs, dislocation of ulna
- 90% are posterior/posterolateral, anterior are rare
- collateral ligaments disrupted

Mechanism
- elbow hyperextension via FOOSH or valgus/supination stress during elbow flexion

Clinical Features
- elbow pain, swelling, deformity
- flexion contracture
- ± absent radial or ulnar pulses

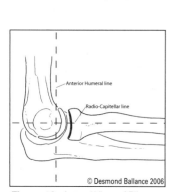

Figure 12. Lateral View of Elbow

Treatment
- closed reduction under anesthesia (post-reduction x-rays required)
- long-arm splint with forearm in neutral rotation and elbow in 90° flexion
- early ROM (<2 weeks)

Complications
- stiffness (loss of extension), intra-articular loose body, neurovascular injury (ulnar nerve, median nerve, brachial artery), heterotopic bone formation, radial head fracture

Epicondylitis

- lateral epicondylitis = "tennis elbow", inflammation of the common extensor tendon as it inserts into the lateral epicondyle
- medial epicondylitis = "golfer's elbow", inflammation of the common flexor tendon as it inserts into the medial epicondyle

Mechanism
- repeated or sustained contraction of the forearm muscles

Clinical Features
- point tenderness over humeral epicondyle
- pain upon resisted wrist extension (lateral epicondylitis) or wrist flexion (medial epicondylitis)

Treatment
- rest, ice, NSAIDs
- use brace/strap
- PT, stretching and strengthening
- corticosteroid injection
- surgery: percutaneous release of common tendon from epicondyle (only after 6-12 months of conservative therapy)

Forearm

Both Bones Fracture (Radius and Ulna)

Mechanism
- commonly a FOOSH or direct blow

Investigations
- x-ray
  - AP and lateral of forearm
  - AP, lateral, oblique of elbow and wrist
- CT if fracture is close to joint

Treatment
- goal is anatomic reduction since imperfect alignment significantly limits forearm pronation and supination
- ORIF with compresion plates and screws

Complications
- compartment syndrome
- non-union
- malunion

Monteggia Fracture

Definition
- fracture of the proximal ulna with radial head dislocation

Mechanism
- direct blow on the posterior aspect of the forearm
- hyperpronation
- fall on the hyperextended elbow

Clinical Features
- decreased rotation of forearm ± palpation lump at the radial head
- ulna angled apex anterior and radial head dislocated anteriorly (rarely the reverse deformity occurs)

Treatment
- ORIF of ulna with indirect radius reduction in 90%
- splint and early post-op ROM if elbow completely stable; otherwise immobilization in plaster with elbow flexed for 6 weeks

Complications
- compartment syndrome
- radial/posterior interosseous nerve (PIN) injury
- nonunion/malunion
- decrease ROM

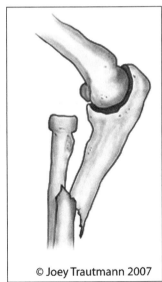

© Joey Trautmann 2007

Figure 13. Monteggia Fracture

In all isolated ulna fractures, assess proximal radius to rule out a Monteggia fracture.

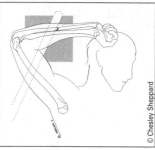

Figure 14. Nightstick Fracture

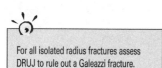

For all isolated radius fractures assess DRUJ to rule out a Galeazzi fracture.

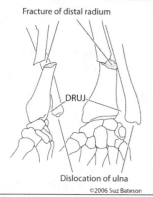

Fracture of distal radium

DRUJ

Dislocation of ulna

©2006 Suz Bateson

Figure 15. Galeazzi Fracture

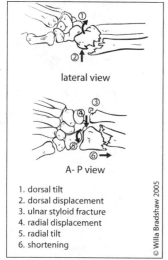

lateral view

A-P view

1. dorsal tilt
2. dorsal displacement
3. ulnar styloid fracture
4. radial displacement
5. radial tilt
6. shortening

© Willa Bradshaw 2005

Figure 16. Colles' Fracture and Associated Bony Deformity

Nightstick Fracture

Definition
- isolated fracture of ulna

Mechanism
- direct blow to forearm (holding arm up to protect face)

Treatment
- non-displaced: below elbow cast (10 days) followed by forearm brace (~8 weeks)
- displaced: ORIF if >50% shaft displacement or >10° angulation

Galeazzi Fracture

Definition
- fracture of the distal radial shaft with disruption of the distal radioulnar joint (DRUJ)
- most commonly in the distal 1/3 of radius near junction of metaphysis/diaphysis

Mechanism
- usual cause is fall on the hand (mechanical axial loading of pronated forearm)

Investigations
- x-rays
  - shortening of distal radius >5 mm relative to the distal ulna
  - widening of the DRUJ space on AP
  - dislocation of radius with respect to ulna on true lateral

Treatment
- ORIF of radius
- if DRUJ is stable, splint with early ROM
- if DRUJ is unstable, DRUJ pinning and long arm cast in supination x 6 weeks

Wrist

Colles' Fracture

Definition
- transverse distal radius fracture (about 2 cm proximal to the radiocarpal joint) with dorsal displacement ± ulnar styloid fracture

Epidemiology
- most common fracture in those >40 years, especially in women and those with osteoporotic bone

Mechanism
- FOOSH

Clinical Features
- "dinner fork" deformity
- swelling, ecchymosis, tenderness

Investigations
- findings on x-ray (see Figure 16)

Treatment
- goal is to restore radial height, radial inclination (22°) and volar tilt (11°)
- closed reduction (think opposite of the deformity):
  - hematoma block (sterile prep and drape, local anesthetic injection directly into # site) or conscious sedation
  - closed reduction - traction with extension (exaggerate injury), then traction with ulnar deviation, pronation, flexion of distal fragment – not at wrist)
  - dorsal slab/below elbow cast for 5-6 weeks
  - x-ray q1 week to ensure reduction is maintained
- obtain post-reduction films immediately – repeat reduction if necessary, consider external fixation or ORIF

Smith's Fracture

Definition
- volar displacement of the distal radius (i.e. reverse Colles' fracture)

Mechanism
- fall onto the back of the flexed hand

Treatment
- usually unstable and needs ORIF
- if patient is poor operative candidate, may attempt non-operative treatment
- closed reduction with hematoma block (reduction opposite of Colles')
- long-arm cast in supination x 6 weeks

Complications of Wrist Fractures

- most common complications are poor grip strength, stiffness, and radial shortening
- distal radius fractures in individuals <40 years of age are usually highly comminuted and are likely to require ORIF
- 80% have normal function in 6-12 months
- early
    - difficult reduction ± loss of reduction
    - compartment syndrome
    - extensor pollicis longus (EPL) tendon rupture
    - acute carpal tunnel syndrome
    - finger swelling with venous or lymphatic block
- late
    - malunion, radial shortening
    - painful wrist secondary to ulnar prominence
    - frozen shoulder ("shoulder-hand syndrome")
    - post-traumatic arthritis
    - carpal tunnel syndrome
    - reflex sympathetic dystrophy (RSD)

Scaphoid Fracture

Epidemiology
- common in young men; not common in children or in patients beyond middle age

Mechanism
- FOOSH resulting most commonly in a transverse fracture through the waist (middle) of the scaphoid

Clinical Features
- pain on wrist movement
- tenderness in scaphoid region (anatomical "snuff box")
- usually undisplaced

Investigations
- x-ray (AP/lat/scaphoid views with wrist exended and ulnar deviation) q2 weeks
- ± bone scan
- ± CT
- **Note**: a fracture may not be radiologically evident up to 2 weeks after acute injury, so if a patient complains of wrist pain and has anatomical snuff box tenderness but a negative x-ray, treat as if positive for a scaphoid fracture and repeat x-ray 2 weeks later to rule out a fracture

Treatment
- non-displaced = long-arm thumb spica cast x 4 weeks then short arm cast until radiographic evidence of healing is seen (2-3 months)
- displaced = open (or percutaneous) screw fixation

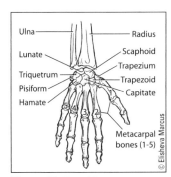

Figure 17. Carpal Bones

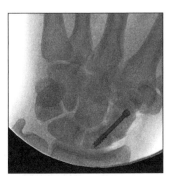

Figure 18. ORIF left scaphoid

Complications
- delayed union
- non-union (must use bone graft to heal)
- AVN of the proximal fragment (since the scaphoid has distal to proximal blood supply, the more proximal the fracture, the greater the incidence of AVN)
- osteoarthritis

Prognosis
- fractures of the proximal third of the scaphoid have >40% rate of nonunion or AVN
- waist fractures have healing rates of 80-90%
- distal third fractures have healing rates close to 100%

Spine

- cross-sectional anatomy of the spine is divided into 3 columns (see Figure 19):
- if more than one column involved in fracture, then instability of spine usually ensues

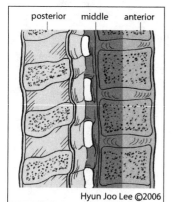

Figure 19. Three-Column Concept of Spinal Stability

Table 6. Spinal Columns

Anterior column	Anterior longitudinal ligament
	Anterior aspect of vertebral body
	Anterior aspect of annulus fibrosis
Middle column	Posterior longitudinal ligament
	Posterior aspect of vertebral body
	Posterior aspect of annulus fibrosis
Posterior column	Pedicle
	Facet joint
	Neural arch
	Ligamentum flavum
	Interspinous ligament
	Supraspinous ligament

- there are 4 main types of fractures:

Table 7. Fracture Type and Column Involvement

Fracture Type	Column Failure	Stable/Unstable	Mechanism
Compression	Anterior	Stable	Compression
Burst	Anterior, middle	± Unstable	High-energy axial loading + flexion
Flexion-distraction (Chance fracture)	Middle, posterior	± Unstable	MVA (lap belt only) causing flexion and distraction
Fracture-dislocation	Anterior, middle, posterior	Unstable	Significant force applied to spine (flexion, extension, distraction, rotation, shear or axial load)

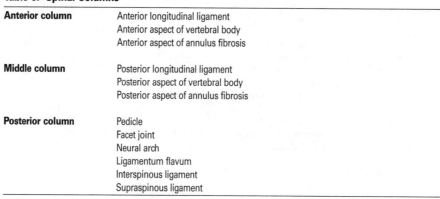

Figure 20. Burst, Compression and Dislocation Fracture

Cervical Spine

General Principles
- C1 = atlas: no vertebral body, no spinous process
- C2 = axis: odontoid = dens
- 7 cervical vertebrae; 8 cervical nerve roots
- nerve root exits above vertebra (i.e. C4 nerve root exits above C4 vertebra)
- radiculopathy = impingement of nerve root
- myelopathy = impingement of spinal cord

ROM
- flexion: chin to chest
- extension: look at ceiling
- rotation: chin in line with shoulder
- lateral bend: 45° to each side

Special Testing
- compression test: pressure on head worsens radicular pain
- distraction test: traction on head relieves radicular symptoms
- Valsalva test: Valsalva maneuver increases intrathecal pressure and causes radicular pain

Table 8. Cervical Radiculopathy/Neuropathy

Root	C5	C6	C7	C8
Motor	Deltoid Biceps Wrist extension	Biceps Brachioradialis	Triceps Wrist flexion Finger extension	Interossei Digital flexors
Sensory	Axillary nerve (patch over lateral deltoid)	Thumb and index finger	Middle finger	Ring and little finger
Reflex	Biceps	Biceps Brachioradialis	Triceps	Finger jerk

X-rays for C-Spine
- AP: alignment
- AP odontoid: atlantoaxial articulation
- lateral
  - vertebral alignment: posterior vertebral bodies should be aligned (translation >3.5 mm is abnormal)
  - angulation: between adjacent vertebral bodies (>11° is abnormal)
  - disc or facet joint widening
  - anterior soft tissue space (at C3 should be ≤3 mm; at C4 should be ≤8-10 mm)
- oblique: evaluate pedicles and intervertebral foramen
- ± swimmer's view: lateral view with arm abducted 180° to evaluate C7-T1 junction if lateral view is inadequate (must see C7-T1 in all trauma situations)
- ± lateral flexion/extension view: evaluate subluxation of cervical vertebrae

Differential Diagnosis of C-Spine Pain
- trapezial sprain, whiplash, cervical spondylosis, cervical stenosis, rheumatoid arthritis (spondylitis), traumatic injury

C-SPINE INJURY

Etiology
- high energy accidents (MVA, diving, fall); must protect the C-spine at all times

Investigations
- cross table lateral C-spine x-ray (patient secured to spine board)
- neurological exam
- spinal cord injuries can be complete or incomplete (central cord, anterior cord, Brown-Sequard, posterior cord)
- for details of spinal cord injuries, see Neurosurgery

Thoracolumbar Spine

General Principles
- spinal cord terminated at conus medullaris (L1)
- individual nerve roots exit below pedicle of vertebra (i.e. L4 nerve root exits below L4 pedicle)

Special Tests
- straight leg raise (SLR): passive lifting of leg reproduces radicular symptoms of pain radiating down post/lat leg to knee, ± into foot
- Lasegue maneuver: dorsiflexion of foot during SLR makes symptoms worse or if leg is less elevated, dorsiflexion will bring on symptoms
- femoral stretch test: with patient prone, flexing the knee of the affected side and passively extending the hip results in radicular pain

Red Flags for Back Pain:
B: bowel or bladder dysfunction
A: anesthesia (saddle)
C: constitutional symptoms/malignancy
K: chronic disease
P: paresthesias
A: age >50
I: IV drug use
N: neuromotor deficits

Use Canadian C-spine Rule (CCR) or National Emergency X-Radiography Utilization Study (NEXUS) to guide imaging if suspected C-spine injury

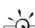

Immediate immobilization of C-spine at scene of accident with spine board, C-collar and sandbags.

In many spinal conditions, imaging may reveal significant lesions in asymptomatic patients. This is not necessarily an indication for intervention.

Table 9. Lumbar Radiculopathy/Neuropathy

Root	L4	L5	S1
Motor	Quadriceps (knee extension, hip adduction) Tibialis anterior (ankle inversion + dorsiflexion)	EHL (extensor hallucis longus) Gluteus medius (hip abductor)	Peroneus longus + brevis (ankle eversion) Gastrocnemius, soleus (plantarflexion)
Sensory	Medial leg	1st dorsal webspace and Lateral leg	Lateral foot
Reflex	Knee	Medial hamstring*	Ankle
Test	Femoral stretch	Straight leg raise	

* Unreliable

Differential Diagnosis of Back Pain

- degenerative (90% of all back pain)
  - mechanical (degenerative, facet)
  - spinal stenosis (congenital, osteophyte, central disc)
  - peripheral nerve compression (disc herniation)
- cauda equina syndrome
- neoplastic: primary, metastatic
- trauma
  - fracture (compression, distraction, translation, rotation)
- spondyloarthropathies (i.e. ankylosing spondylitis)
- referred
  - aorta, renal, ureter, pancreas

DEGENERATIVE BACK PAIN

- loss of vertebral disc height with age results in
  - bulging and tears of annulus fibrosus
  - change in alignment of facet joints
  - osteophyte formation
- can cause back-dominant pain
- management
  - non-operative
    - modified activity
    - back strengthening
    - NSAIDs
    - do not treat with opioids
  - operative - rarely indicated
    - decompression ± fusion
    - no difference in outcome between non-operative and surgical management in 2 years

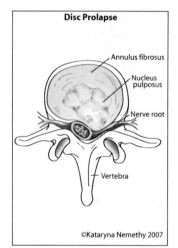

Disc Prolapse

Annulus fibrosus

Nucleus pulposus

Nerve root

Vertebra

©Kataryna Nemethy 2007

Figure 21. Disc Herniation

Table 10. Types of Low Back Pain

	Mechanical Back Pain		Direct Nerve Root Compression	
	Disc Origin	Facet Origin	Spinal Stenosis	Root Compression
Pain dominance	Back	Back	Leg	Leg
Aggravation	Flexion	Extension Standing, walking	Exercise, extension, walking, standing	Flexion
Onset	Gradual	More sudden	Congenital or acquired	Acute leg ± back pain
Duration	Long (weeks, months)	Shorter (days, weeks)	Acute or chronic history (weeks to months)	Short episodes Attacks (minutes)
Treatment	Relief of strain, exercise	Relief of strain, exercise	Relief of strain, exercise	Relief of strain, exercise + surgical decompression if progressive or severe deficit

SPINAL STENOSIS

- definition: narrowing of spinal canal <10 mm
- etiology: congenital (idiopathic, osteopetrosis, achondroplasia) or acquired (degenerative, iatrogenic – post spinal surgery, ankylosing spondylosis, Paget's disease, trauma)
- clinical features
  - ± bilateral back and leg pain
  - neurogenic claudication (Table 11)
  - ± motor weakness
  - normal back flexion; difficulty with back extension

- investigations: CT/MRI reveals narrowing of spinal canal, but gold standard
  = CT myelogram
- treatment
  - non-operative: vigorous PT (flexion exercises, stretch/strength exercises),
    NSAIDs, lumbar epidural steroids
  - operative: decompression surgery if conservative methods failed >6 months

Table 11. Differentiating Claudication

	Neurogenic	Vascular
Aggravation	With standing or exercise Walking distance variable	Walking set distance
Alleviation	Change in position (usually flexion, sitting, lying down)	Stop walking
Time	Relief in ~10 min	Relief in ~2 min
Character	Neurogenic ± neurological deficit	Muscular cramping

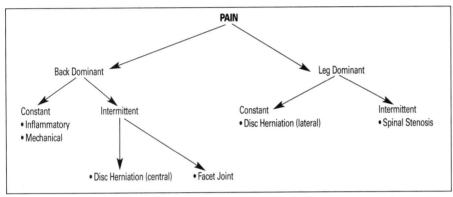

Figure 22. Approach to Back Pain

MECHANICAL BACK PAIN
- definition: back pain NOT due to prolapsed disc or any other clearly defined
  pathology
- clinical features
  - dull backache aggravated by activity
  - morning stiffness
  - no neurological signs
- treatment: symptomatic (analgesics, PT)
- prognosis: symptoms may resolve in 4-6 weeks, others become chronic

Loss of sphincter tone or urinary retention are signs of cauda equina syndrome & represent a surgical emergency

LUMBAR DISC HERNIATION
- definition: tear in annulus fibrosis allows protrusion of nucleus pulposus causing either
  a central, posterolateral or lateral disc herniation, most commonly at L5-S1 > L4-5 >
  L3-4
- etiology: usually a history of flexion-type injury which tears the annulus fibrosis
  allowing for protrusion of the nucleus pulposus
- clinical features
  - back dominant pain (central herniation) or leg dominant pain (lateral
    herniation)
  - tenderness between spines at affected level
  - muscle spasm ± loss of normal lumbar lordosis
  - neurological disturbance is segmental and varies with level of central herniation
    - motor weakness (L4, L5, S1)
    - diminished reflexes (L4, S1)
    - diminished sensation (L4, L5, S1)
  - +ve SLR
  - +ve Lasegue test
  - bowel or bladder symptoms, decreased rectal tone suggests cauda equina
    syndrome due to central disc hernation – surgical emergency
- investigations: MRI

- treatment
  - symptomatic:
    - extension protocol (PT)
    - NSAIDs
    - 90% resolved in 3 months
  - surgical discectomy reserved for progressive neurological deficit, failure of symptoms to resolve within 3 months or cauda equina syndrome due to central disc herniation

ANKYLOSING SPONDYLITIS

- see Rheumatology

SPONDYLOLYSIS

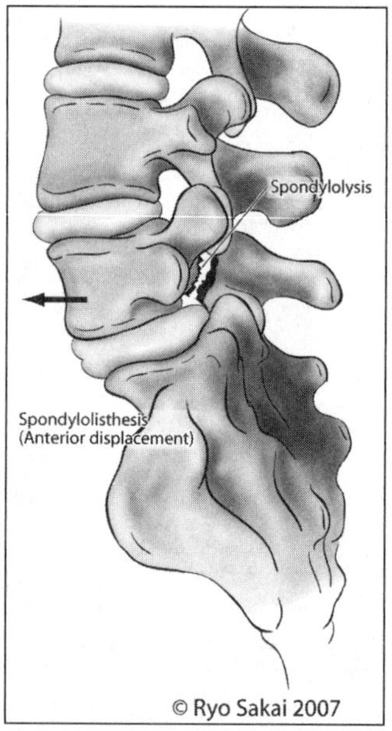

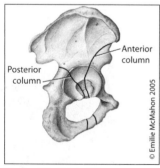

- definition: defect in the pars interarticularis with no movement of the vertebral bodies
- etiology
  - trauma: gymnasts, weightlifters, backpackers, loggers, labourers
- clinical features: activity related back pain
- investigations
  - oblique x-ray: "collar" break in the "Scottie dog's" neck
  - bone scan
  - CT
- treatment: activity restriction, brace, stretching exercise

SPONDYLOLISTHESIS

- definition
  - defect in pars interarticularis causing a forward slip of one vertebrae on another usually at L5-S1, less commonly at L4-5
- etiology: congenital (children), degenerative (adults), traumatic, pathological
- clinical features: lower back pain radiating to buttocks

Table 12. Classification and Treatment of Spondylolisthesis

Class	Percentage of slip	Treatment
1	0-25%	Symptomatic operative fusion only for intractable pain
2	25-50	
3	50-75	Spinal fusion
4	75-100	
5	>100	

Complications
- may present as cauda equina syndrome due to roots being stretched over the edge of L5 or sacrum

Pelvis

Pelvic Fracture

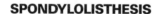

Mechanism
- high energy trauma, either direct or by force transmitted longitudinally through the femur

Clinical Features
- local swelling, tenderness
- deformity of hips
- pelvic instability
- only a management problem if they cause instability of the bony ring of the pelvis

Investigations
- x-ray: AP, Judet (inlet and outlet)

Figure 23. Spondylolysis, Spondylolisthesis

Figure 24. Pelvic Columms

Classification

Table 13. Tile Classification of Pelvic Fractures

Type	Stability	Description
A	Rotationally stable Vertically stable	A1: fracture not involving pelvic ring A2: minimally displaced fracture of pelvic ring (e.g. ramus fracture)
B	Rotationally unstable Vertically stable	B1: open book B2: lateral compression – ipsilateral B3: lateral compression – contralateral
C	Rotationally unstable Vertically unstable	C1: unilateral C2: bilateral C3: associated acetabular fracture

Treatment
- ABCs
- assess genitourinary injury (rectal exam, vaginal exam) – if involved, the fracture is considered open
- Type A: bedrest, mobilize with walking aids
- Types B & C: external or internal fixation (refer to *Orthopaedic Emergencies*)

Complications
- **hemorrhage (life threatening) - 1500-3000ml blood loss**
- bladder/urethral injury
- neurological damage
- obstetrical difficulties
- persistent sacroiliac (SI) joint pain
- post-traumatic arthritis of the hip with acetabular fractures
- injury to rectum

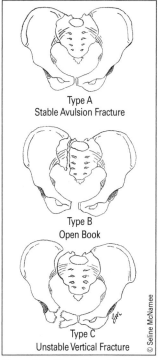

Type A
Stable Avulsion Fracture

Type B
Open Book

Type C
Unstable Vertical Fracture

© Seline McNamee

Figure 25. Illustration of the Tile Classification of Pelvic Fractures

Hip

Hip Fracture

FEMORAL NECK (SUBCAPITAL) FRACTURE

Definition
- intracapsular fracture of the femoral neck

Mechanism
- young = MVA, fall from height; older = simple fall onto hip usually rotational force

Clinical Features
- acute onset of hip pain
- unable to weight bear
- shortened, externally rotated leg
- painful ROM

Investigations
- x-ray: AP hip, pelvis, lateral hip

Classification
- Garden classification

X-ray Features of Subcapital Hip Fractures
- Disruption of Shenton's line (a radiographic line drawn along the upper margin of the obturator foramen, extending along the inferomedial side of the femoral neck)
- Altered neck-shaft angle (normal is 120-130°)

Table 14. Garden Classification of Femoral Neck Fractures

Type	Displacement	Extent	Alignment	Trabeculae
1	None	Incomplete	Valgus	Malaligned
2	None	Complete	Neutral	Aligned
3	Some	Complete	Varus	Malaligned
4	Complete	Complete	Varus	Aligned

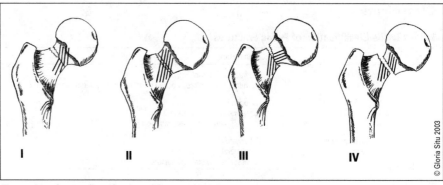

Figure 26. Garden Classification of Femoral Neck Fractures

Treatment
- type of treatment depends on displacement and patient age
    - undisplaced (Garden 1,2): internal fixation to prevent displacement
    - displaced (Garden 3,4): depends on patient age and function
    - older patient → hemiarthroplasty
    - young patient, high function → reduction with internal fixation within 12 hrs of fracture

Complications
- AVN of femoral head: vascular supply is distal to proximal inside the capsule of the femoral neck, so a fracture of the neck will disrupt the blood supply to the head and increase the risk of AVN
- nonunion
- DVT

INTERTROCHANTERIC FRACTURES

Definition
- extracapsular fracture including the greater and lesser trochanters and transitional bone between the neck and shaft

Mechanism
- direct or indirect force transmitted to the intertrochanteric area

Clinical Features
- acute onset hip pain
- unable to weight bear
- shortened, externally rotated leg
- ecchymosis at back of upper thigh

Classification
- stable vs. unstable
    - stable = intact posteromedial cortex
    - unstable = non-intact posteromedial cortex fractures

Investigations
- AP pelvis, AP/lateral hip

Treatment
- DVT prophylaxis
- obtain a closed reduction under fluoroscopy
- after reduction obtained, internal fixation with dynamic hip screw or intramedullary nail

Complications
- varus displacement of the proximal fragment
- malrotation deformity
- nonunion
- failure of fixation device

DVT Prophylaxis in Hip Fractures
enoxaparin 30 mg SC BID start on admission, do not give <12 hrs before surgery.

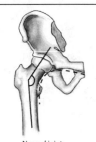

Normal joint

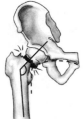

Subcapital fracture

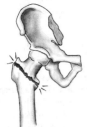

Intertrochanteric fracture

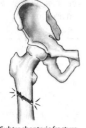

Subtrochanteric fracture

Figure 27. Subcapital, Intertrochanteric, Subtrochanteric Fractures

SUBTROCHANTERIC FRACTURES

Definition
- fracture begins at or below the lesser trochanter and involves the proximal femoral shaft

Mechanism
- young = high energy trauma
- older = osteopenic bone + fall, pathological fracture

Clinical Features
- similar to intertrochanteric fractures

Investigations
- AP pelvis, AP/lateral hip and femur

Treatment
- DVT prophylaxis
- obtain a good closed reduction under fluoroscopy
- after reduction obtained, internal fixation with intramedullary nail or plating

Complications
- malalignment
- nonunion
- wound infection

Arthritis of the Hip

Etiology
- osteoarthritis (OA), inflammatory arthritis, post-traumatic arthritis, late effects of congenital hip disorders or septic arthritis

Clinical Features
- pain (groin, medial thigh) and stiffness aggravated by activity
- morning stiffness, multiple joint swelling, hand nodules (RA)
- decreased ROM (internal rotation is lost first)
- crepitus
- ± fixed flexion contracture leading to apparent limb shortening (Thomas test)
- ± Trendelenberg sign

Investigations
- x-ray
  - OA: joint space narrowing, subchondral sclerosis, subchondral cysts, osteophytes
  - RA: osteopenia, joint space narrowing
- bloodwork: ANA+ve, RF+ve (RA)

Treatment
- conservative: weight reduction, activity modification, PT, analgesics, walking aids
- operative: realign = osteotomy; replace = arthroplasty; fuse = arthrodesis
- complications with arthroplasty: component loosening, dislocation (see below), heterotopic bone formation, thromboembolus, infection, neurovascular injury
- arthroplasty is standard of care in most patients with hip arthritis

> **DVT Prophylaxis in Elective THA**
> (continue 2-3 weeks post op)
> Fragmin™ 5000 units SC bid start 12 hrs before surgery and continue 12-24 hrs post-op
> or
> Warfarin to target INR of 2.5

Hip Dislocation after THA

Etiology
- total hip arthroplasty (THA) is unstable when hip is flexed and internally rotated (avoid crossing legs)

Epidemiology
- occurs in 1-4% of primary THA and 10-16% of revision THAs
- risk factors: posterior approach with no soft tissue repair, female, neurological impairment

Treatment
- external abduction splint to prevent hip adduction
- constrained acetabular component for recurrent dislocation

Complications
- fracture of femoral shaft or neck
- sciatic nerve palsy in 25% (10% permanent)
- heterotopic ossification (HO)

Femur

Femoral Diaphysis Fracture

Mechanism
- high energy trauma (MVA, fall from height, gunshot wound)
- in children, can result from low energy trauma (spiral fracture)

Clinical Features
- shortened, externally rotated leg
- inability to weight bear
- often open injury, always a Gustillo 3

Investigations
- AP pelvis, AP/lateral hip, femur, knee

Complications
- hemorrhage requiring transfusion
- fat embolism leading to ARDS
- extensive soft tissue damage
- ipsilateral hip dislocation
- nerve injury
- infection
- malunion
- nonunion
- knee stiffness

Treatment
- stabilize patient
- immobilize leg
- ORIF with intramedullary nail within 24 hours
- early mobilization and strengthening

Distal Femoral Fracture

Mechanism
- direct high energy force or axial loading
- three types (Figure 28)

Clinical Features
- direct high energy force or axial loading
- extreme pain
- knee effusion (hemarthrosis)
- shortened, externally rotated leg if displaced

Treatment
- ORIF
- early mobilization and strengthening

Complications
- femoral artery tear
- extensive soft tissue injury
- angulation deformities
- post-traumatic arthritis
- nerve injury

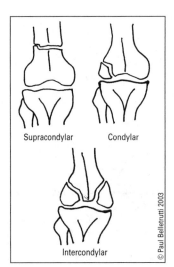

Supracondylar   Condylar

Intercondylar

© Paul Belletrutti 2003

Figure 28. Distal Femoral Fractures

Knee

Evaluation of Knee Complaints

History
- general orthopaedic history
- also inquire about common knee symptoms
  - locking: mechanical block to extension
    - torn meniscus/loose body in joint
  - pseudo-locking: limited ROM without mechanical block
    - effusion, muscle spasm after injury, arthritis
  - painful clicking (audible)
    - torn meniscus
  - giving way: instability
    - cruciate ligament or meniscal tear, patellar dislocation

Physical Examination
- general orthopaedic physical exam (do not forget to evaluate hip)

Special Tests of the Knee (see Table 15)
- **anterior and posterior drawer tests**
  - demonstrate torn ACL and PCL, respectively
  - knee flexed at 90°, foot immobilized, hamstrings released
  - if able to sublux tibia anteriorly then ACL may be torn
  - if able to sublux tibia posteriorly then PCL may be torn
- **Lachmann test**
  - demonstrates torn ACL
  - hold knee in 10-20° flexion, stabilizing the femur
  - try to sublux tibia anteriorly on femur
  - similar to anterior drawer test, more reliable due to less muscular stabilization
- **posterior sag sign**
  - demonstrates torn PCL
  - may give a false positive anterior draw sign
  - flex knees and hips to 90°, hold ankles and knees
  - view from the lateral aspect
  - if one tibia sags posteriorly compared to the other, its PCL is torn
- **pivot shift sign**
  - demonstrates torn ACL
  - start with the knee in extension
  - internally rotate foot, slowly flex knee while palpating and applying a valgus force
  - normal knee will flex smoothly
  - if incompetent ACL, tibia will sublux anteriorly on femur at start of maneuver. During flexion, the tibia will reduce and externally rotate about the femur (the "pivot")
  - reverse pivot shift (start in flexion, externally rotate, apply valgus and extend knee) suggests torn PCL
- **collateral ligament stress test**
  - palpate ligament for "opening" of joint space while testing
  - with knee in full extension apply valgus force to test MCL, apply varus force to test LCL
  - repeat tests with knee in 20° flexion to relax joint capsule
  - opening only in 20° flexion due to MCL damage only
  - opening in 20° of flexion and full extension is due to MCL, cruciate, and joint capsule damage
- **tests for meniscal tear**
  - crouch compression test
    - joint line pain when squatting (anterior pain suggests patellofemoral pathology)
  - McMurray's test useful collaborative information
    - with knee in flexion palpate joint line for painful "pop/click"
    - internally rotate foot, varus stress, and extend knee to test lateral meniscus
    - externally rotate foot, valgus stress, and extend knee to test medial meniscus

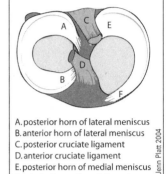

A. posterior horn of lateral meniscus
B. anterior horn of lateral meniscus
C. posterior cruciate ligament
D. anterior cruciate ligament
E. posterior horn of medial meniscus
F. anterior horn of medial meniscus

© Jenn Platt 2004

Figure 29. Diagram of the Right Tibial Plateau

6 Degrees of Freedom of the Knee
1) Flex. & ext.
2) Ext. & int. rotation
3) Varus & valgus angulation
4) Ant. & post. glide
5) Med. & lat. shift
6) Compression & distraction

Knee History - CLIPS
Clicking
Locking
Instability
Pain (location)
Swelling

Physical examination difficult in acute knee injuries. Immobilize leg and re-examine in one week.

X-Rays
- AP standing, lateral
- skyline – tangential view with knees flexed at 45° to see patellofemoral joint
- 3-foot standing view – useful in evaluating leg length and varus/valgus alignment

Cruciate Ligament Tears

- ACL tear much more common than PCL tear

Table 15. Comparison of ACL and PCL Injuries

	Anterior Cruciate Ligament	Posterior Cruciate Ligament
Mechanism	Sudden deceleration	Sudden posterior displacement of tibia when knee is flexed or
	Hyperextension and internal rotation of tibia on femur	hyperextended (dashboard MVA injury)
History	Audible "pop"	Audible "pop"
	Immediate swelling	Immediate swelling
	Knee "giving way"	Pain with push off
	Inability to continue activity	Can't descend stairs
Physical	Effusion (hemarthrosis)	Effusion (hemarthrosis)
	Posterolateral joint line tenderness	Anteromedial joint line tenderness
	Positive anterior drawer	Positive posterior drawer
	Positive Lachmann	Posterior sag
	Pivot shift	Reverse pivot shift
	Test for MCL, meniscal injuries (see Clinical Pearl)	Other ligamentous, bony injuries
Treatment	Stable knee with minimal functional impairment: immobilization 2-4 weeks with early ROM and strengthening	
	Unstable knee or young person/high-demand lifestyle: ligament reconstruction	

O'Donahue's unhappy triad: ACL, MCL, medial meniscal tears commonly occur simultaneously so if you see one, look for the other two.

Tissue Sources for ACL Reconstruction
1) Hamstring
2) Middle 1/3 patellar tendon (bone-patellar-bone)
3) Allograft

Collateral Ligament Tears

- MCL tear more common than LCL tear

Mechanism
- valgus force to knee = medial collateral ligament
- varus force to knee = lateral collateral ligament

Clinical Features
- swelling/effusion
- tenderness above and below joint line medially (MCL) or laterally (LCL)
- joint laxity with varus or valgus force to knee
    - laxity with endpoint suggests partial tear
    - laxity with no endpoint suggests a complete tear
- test for other injuries (e.g. O'Donahue's triad), common peroneal nerve injury

Partial ligamentous tears are much more painful than complete ligamentous tears.

Treatment
- partial tear: immobilization x 2-4 weeks with early ROM and strengthening
- complete tear or multiple ligamentous injuries: surgical repair of ligaments

Meniscal Tears

- medial tear much more common than lateral tear

Mechanism
- twisting force on knee when it is partially flexed (e.g. stepping down and turning)
- requires moderate trauma in young person but only mild trauma in elderly due to degeneration

Clinical Features
- immediate pain, difficulty weight bearing, instability and clicking
- increased pain with squatting and/or twisting
- effusion (hemarthrosis) with insidious onset (24-48 hrs after injury)
- joint line tenderness medially or laterally
- locking of knee (if portion of meniscus mechanically obstructing extension)

Investigations
- MRI, arthroscopy

Treatment
- if not locked: ROM and strengthening
- if locked or failed above: arthroscopic repair/partial meniscectomy

Quadriceps/Patellar Tendon Rupture

Mechanism
- sudden forceful contraction of quadriceps during an attempt to stop
- more common in obese patients and those with pre-existing degenerative changes in tendon
  - DM, SLE, RA, steroid use, renal failure on dialysis

Clinical Features
- inability to extend knee
- patella in lower or higher position with palpable gap above or below patella respectively
- may have an effusion

Investigations
- knee x-ray to rule out patellar fracture

Treatment
- surgical repair of tendon

Dislocated Knee

Mechanism
- high energy trauma
- by definition, caused by tears of multiple ligaments

Clinical Features
- classified by relation of tibia with respect to femur
  - anterior, posterior, lateral, medial, rotary
- knee instability
- effusion, pain

Investigations
- x-rays: AP, lateral, skyline
  - associated radiographic findings include tibial plateau fracture dislocations, proximal fibular fractures and avulsion of fibular head
- arteriogram if abnormal vascular exam

Treatment
- urgent closed reduction
  - complicated by interposed soft tissue
- assessment of peroneal nerve, tibial artery, and ligamentous injuries
- repair of associated injuries; if vascular repair undertaken, also need decompressive fasciotamy
- knee immobilization x 6-8 weeks

Complications
- high incidence of associated injuries
  - popliteal artery tear
  - peroneal nerve injury
  - capsular tear
- chronic: instability, stiffness, post-traumatic arthritis

Patella

Patellar Fracture

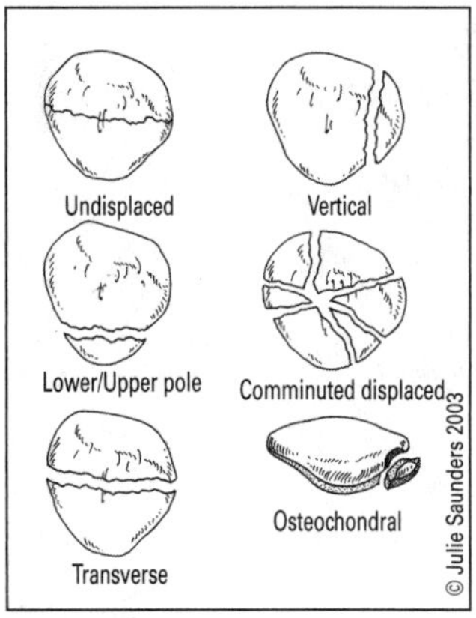

Mechanism
- direct blow to the patella
- indirect trauma by sudden flexion of knee against contracted quadriceps

Clinical Features
- marked tenderness
- inability to extend knee or straight leg raise
- proximal displacement of patella
- patellar deformity
- +/- effusion

Investigations
- x-rays: AP, lateral, skyline
- consider bipartite patella: congenitally unfused ossification centres with smooth margins on x-ray

Treatment
- non-displaced (<2 mm)
  - straight leg immobilization 6-8 weeks
  - PT: quadriceps strengthening
- displaced: ORIF (>2 mm)
- comminuted: ORIF; may require partial/complete patellectomy

Figure 30. Types of Patellar Fractures

Undisplaced / Vertical / Lower/Upper pole / Comminuted displaced / Osteochondral / Transverse

© Julie Saunders 2003

Patellar Dislocation

Mechanism
- lateral displacement of patella after contraction of quadriceps against a flexed knee

Risk Factors
- young, female
- obesity
- high-riding patella (patella alta)
- knock-knees (genu valgum)
- Q angle (quadriceps angle) increased
- shallow intercondylar groove
- weak vastus medialis
- tight lateral retinaculum

Clinical Features
- knee catches or gives way with walking
- severe pain, tenderness anteromedially from rupture of capsule
- weak knee extension or inability to extend leg unless patella reduced
- +ve patellar apprehension test
  - patient apprehensive when examiner laterally displaces patella
- often recurrent, self-reducing

Investigations
- x-rays: AP, lateral, skyline view of patella
  - check for fracture of medial patella and lateral femoral condyle

Treatment
- non-operative first
  - knee immobilization x 4-6 weeks
  - progressive weight bearing and isometric quadriceps strengthening
- if recurrent
  - surgical tightening of medial capsule and release of lateral retinaculum

Figure 31. Q Angle

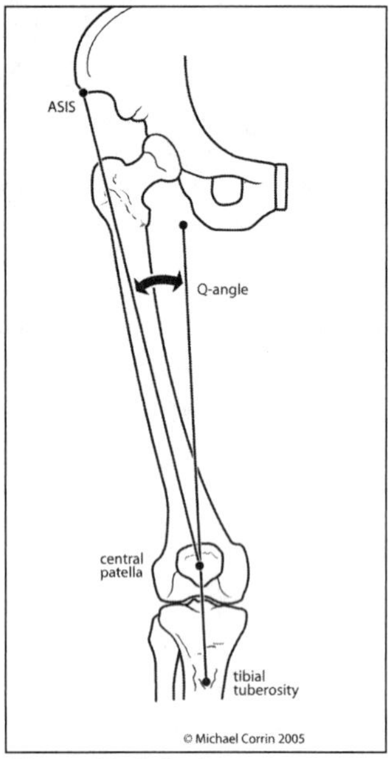

ASIS / Q-angle / central patella / tibial tuberosity

© Michael Corrin 2005

Patellofemoral Syndrome (Chondromalacia Patellae)

Mechanism
- softening, erosion and fragmentation of articular cartilage, predominantly medial aspect of patella
- commonly seen in active young females
- predisposing factors

Pain with firm compression of patella into medial femoral groove is pathognomonic of chondromalacia patellae.

- malalignment causing patellar maltracking (patellofemoral syndrome)
- post-trauma
- deformity of patella or femoral groove
- recurrent patellar dislocation, ligamentous laxity
- excessive knee strain (athletes)

Clinical Features
- deep, aching anterior knee pain
  - exacerbated by prolonged sitting (theatre sign), strenuous athletic activities, stair climbing, squatting
- sensation of instability, pseudolocking
- tenderness to palpation of underside of medially displaced patella
- pain with extension against resistance through terminal 30-40°
- swelling rare, minimal if present

Investigations
- x-rays: AP, lateral, skyline

Treatment
- non-operative
  - continue non-impact activities
  - NSAIDs
  - PT: quadriceps strengthening
- surgical with refractory patients
  - tibial tubercle elevation
  - arthroscopic shaving/debridement
  - lateral release of retinaculum

Tibia

Tibial Plateau Fracture

Mechanism
- axial loading (e.g. fall from height)
- femoral condyles driven into proximal tibia
- can result from minor trauma in osteoporotics

Clinical Features
- lateral fractures more common than medial

Investigations
- x-rays: AP, lateral, skyline

Treatment
- if depression on x-ray is <3 mm
  - straight leg immobilization x 4-6 weeks with progressive ROM weight bearing
- if depression is >3 mm
  - ORIF often requiring bone grafting to elevate depressed fragment

Complications
- ligamentous injuries
- meniscal lesions
- delayed union
- AVN
- infection
- decreased knee mobility/stiffness
- post-traumatic arthritis

Tibial Shaft Fracture

Mechanism
- numerous, including MVA, falls, sporting injuries

Clinical Features
- open vs. closed
- amount of displacement
- neurovascular status
- most commonly fractured long bone
- most common open fracture

Tibial shaft fractures have high incidence of compartment syndrome.

Investigations
- x-rays: AP, lateral, skyline

Treatment
- closed
  - minimally displaced: straight leg cast x 4-6 weeks with early weight bearing
  - displaced: ORIF with reamed IM nail
- open
  - external fixation or IM nail
  - vascularized coverage of soft tissue defects (often heal poorly)

Complications
- high incidence of neurovascular injury and compartment syndrome
- poor soft tissue coverage
- non/malunion

Ankle

Evaluation of Ankle and Foot Complaints

Special Tests
- anterior drawer: examiner attempts to displace the foot anteriorly against a fixed tibia
- talar tilt: foot is stressed in inversion and angle of talar rotation is evaluated by x-ray

X-ray
- AP, lateral
- mortise view: ankle at 15° of internal rotation
  - gives true view of ankle joint
  - joint space should be symmetric with no talar tilt
- Ottawa Ankle Rules should guide use of x-ray (see side bar)
- ± CT to better characterize fractures

Ankle Fracture

Mechanism
- pattern of fracture depends on the position of the ankle when trauma occurs
- generally involves
  - ipsilateral ligamentous tears or transverse bony avulsion
  - contralateral shear fractures (oblique or spiral)
- classification systems
  - Danis-Weber (see below)
  - Lauge-Hansen

Danis-Weber Classification (see Figure 32)
- based on level of fibular fracture relative to syndesmosis
- **Type A** (infra-syndesmotic)
  - pure inversion injury
  - avulsion of lateral malleolus below plafond or torn calcaneofibular ligament
  - ± shear fracture of medial malleolus
- **Type B** (trans-syndesmotic)
  - external rotation and eversion (most common)
  - ± avulsion of medial malleolus or rupture of deltoid ligament
  - spiral fracture of lateral malleolus starting at plafond
- **Type C** (supra-syndesmotic)
  - pure external rotation
  - avulsion of medial malleolus or torn deltoid ligament
  - ± posterior malleolus may be avulsed with posterior tibio-fibular ligament
  - fibular fracture is above plafond (called Maisonneuve fracture if at proximal fibula)
  - frequently tears syndesmosis

Treatment
- undisplaced: non-weight bearing below knee cast
- indications for ORIF
  - all fracture-dislocations
  - most of type B, and all of type C
  - trimalleolar (medial, posterior, lateral) fractures
  - talar tilt >10°
  - open fracture/open joint injury
- high incidence of post-traumatic arthritis

Ottawa Ankle Rules
X-rays are only required if:
pain in the malleolar zone AND bony tenderness over the posterior aspect of the medial or lateral malleolus OR inability to weight bear both immediately after injury and in the E.R.

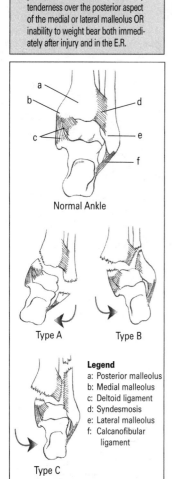

a
b
c
d
e
f

Normal Ankle

Type A   Type B

Legend
a: Posterior malleolus
b: Medial malleolus
c: Deltoid ligament
d: Syndesmosis
e: Lateral malleolus
f: Calcanofibular ligament

Type C

Figure 32. Ring Principle of the Ankle and Danis-Weber Classification

Ligamentous Injuries

Medial Ligament Complex (deltoid ligament)
- eversion injury
- usually avulses medial or posterior malleolus and strains syndesmosis

Lateral Ligament Complex (ATF, CF, PTF)
- inversion injury
- ATF most severely injured if ankle is plantar flexed
- swelling and tenderness anterior to lateral malleolus
- ++ecchymoses
- +ve ankle anterior drawer
- may have significant medial talar tilt on inversion stress x-ray

Treatment
- microscopic tear (Grade I)
  - rest, ice, compression, elevation (RICE)
- macroscopic tear (Grade II)
  - strap ankle in dorsiflexion and eversion x 4-6 weeks
  - PT: strengthening and proprioceptive retraining
- complete tear (Grade III)
  - below knee walking cast 4-6 weeks
  - PT: strengthening and proprioceptive retraining
  - surgical intervention may be required if chronic symptomatic instability develops

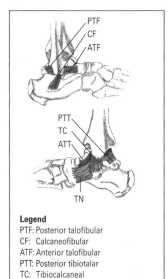

Legend
PTF: Posterior talofibular
CF: Calcaneofibular
ATF: Anterior talofibular
PTT: Posterior tibiotalar
TC: Tibiocalcaneal
ATT: Anterior tibiotalar
TN: Tibionavicular

Figure 33. Ankle Ligament Complexes

Foot

Talar Fracture

Mechanism
- axial loading or hyperdorsiflexion (MVA, fall from a height)
- 60% of talus covered by articular cartilage
- tenuous blood supply runs distal to proximal along talar neck
  - high risk of AVN with displaced fractures

Investigations
- x-rays: AP, lateral
- CT to better characterize fracture
- MRI can clearly define extent of AVN

Treatment
- undisplaced: non-weight bearing below knee cast x 20-24 weeks
- displaced: ORIF (high rate of nonunion, AVN)

With a history of trauma from axial loading of lower limb always consider spinal injuries, femoral neck, tibial plateau, talar/calcaneal fractures.

Calcaneal Fracture

Mechanism
- axial loading: fall from a height onto heels
- 10% of fractures associated with compression fractures of thoracic or lumbar spine
- 5% are bilateral

Physical Examination
- swelling, bruising on heel/sole
- wider, shortened, flatter heel when viewed from behind

Investigations
- x-rays: AP, lateral, oblique (Broden's view)
- loss of Bohler's angle
- CT – assess intraarticular extension

Treatment
- closed vs. open reduction is controversial
- non-weight bearing cast 20-24 weeks with early ROM and strengthening

Achilles Tendonitis

Mechanism
- chronic inflammation from activity or poor-fitting footwear
- may also develop heel bumps (retrocalcaneobursitis)

Physical Examination
- pain, stiffness and crepitus with ROM
- thickened tendon, palpable bump

Treatment
- rest, NSAIDs
- gentle stretching, deep tissue calf massage
- orthotics, open back shoes
- DO NOT inject steroids (risk of tendon rupture)

Achilles Tendon Rupture

The most common site of Achilles tendon rupture is 2-6 cm from its insertion where the blood supply is the poorest.

Mechanism
- loading activity, stop-and-go sports (e.g. squash, tennis, basketball)
- secondary to chronic tendonitis, steroid injection

Clinical Features
- audible pop, sudden pain with push off movement
- sensation of being kicked in heel when trying to plantarflex
- palpable gap
- apprehensive toe off when walking
- weak plantar flexion, +ve Thompson test: with patient prone, squeezing the calf muscles should passively plantar flex the foot to demonstrate intact Achilles tendon. +ve test = no passive plantar flexion = ruptured tendon

Treatment
- low demand or elderly: cast foot in plantar flexion (to relax tendon) x 8-12 weeks
- high demand: surgical repair, then cast as above x 6-8 weeks

Plantar Fasciitis (Heel Spur Syndrome)

Mechanism
- repetitive strain injury causing microtears and inflammation of plantar fascia
- female:male = 2:1
- common in athletes
- also associated with obesity, DM, seronegative and seropositive arthritis

Clinical Features
- morning pain and stiffness
- intense pain when walking from rest that subsides as patient continues to walk
- swelling, tenderness over sole
- greatest at medial calcaneal tubercle and 1-2 cm distal along plantar fascia
- pain with toe dorsiflexion (stretches fascia)

Investigations
- plain radiographs to rule out fractures
- often see exostoses (heel spurs) at insertion of fascia into medial calcaneal tubercle
- spur is reactive to inflammation, not the cause of pain

Treatment
- rest, ice, NSAIDs, steroid injection
- PT: stretching, ultrasound
- orthotics with heel cup
  - to counteract pronation and disperse heel strike forces
- endoscopic surgical release of fascia in refractory cases
  - spur removal is not required

Bunions (Hallux Valgus)

Mechanism
- valgus alignment on 1st MTP (hallux valgus) causes eccentric pull of extensor and intrinsic muscles
- reactive exostosis forms with thickening of the skin creating a bunion
- most often associated with poor-fitting footwear but can be hereditary
- 10x more frequent in women

Clinical Features
- painful bursa over medial eminence of 1st metatarsal head
- pronation (rotation inward) of great toe
- numbness over medial aspect of great toe

Treatment
- cosmetic and to relieve pain
- non-operative first
  - properly fitted shoes (low heel) and toe spacer
- surgical
  - osteotomy with realignment of 1st MTP joint

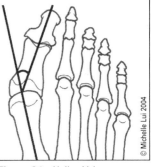

Figure 34. Hallux Valgus

Metatarsal Fracture

- as with the hand, 1st, 4th, 5th metatarsals (MT) are relatively mobile, while the 2nd and 3rd are fixed (Table 16)
- use Ottawa foot rules to determine need for x-ray (see sidebar)

Table 16. Types of Metatarsal Fractures

Fracture Type	Mechanism	Clinical	Treatment
Avulsion of base of 5th MT	Sudden inversion followed by contraction of peroneus brevis	Tender base of 5th MT X-ray foot	Requires ORIF if displaced
Midshaft 5th MT (Jones fracture)	Stress injury	Painful shaft of 5th MT	*NWB BK cast x 6 wks ORIF if athlete
Shaft 2nd, 3rd MT (March fracture)	Stress injury	Painful shaft of 2nd or 3rd MT	Symptomatic
1st MT	Trauma	Painful 1st MT	ORIF if displaced otherwise NWB BK cast x3 wks then walking cast x2 wks
Tarso-MT fracture- dislocation (Lisfranc fracture)	Fall onto plantar flexed foot or direct crush injury	Shortened forefoot prominent base	ORIF

* Non weight bearing, Below knee cast

Ottawa Foot Rules
X-rays only required if:
pain in the midfoot zone AND bony tenderness over the navicular or base of the fifth metatarsal OR inability to weight bear both immediately after injury and in the E.R.

Pediatric Orthopaedics

Fractures in Children

Greenstick fractures are easy to reduce but can redisplace while in cast due to intact periosteum.

- type of fracture
  - usually greenstick or buckle because periosteum is thicker and stronger
  - adults fracture through both cortices
- epiphyseal growth plate
  - plate often mistaken for fracture and vice versa
  - x-ray opposite limb for comparison
  - mechanism which causes ligamentous injury in adults causes growth plate injury in children
  - intra-articular fractures have worse consequences in children because they usually involve the growth plate
- anatomic reduction
  - gold standard with adults
  - may cause limb length discrepancy in children (overgrowth)
  - accept greater angular deformity in children (remodelling)
- time to heal
  - shorter in children
- always be aware of the possibility of child abuse
  - make sure mechanism compatible with injury
  - high index of suspicion, look for other signs, including x-ray evidence of healing fractures at other sites

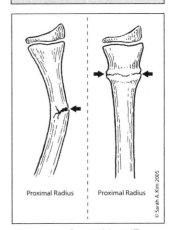

Figure 35. Greenstick and Torus Fractures

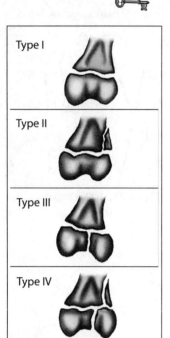

Figure 36. Salter-Harris Classification

Stress Fractures

Mechanism
- insufficiency fracture
    - stress applied to a weak or structurally deficient bone
- fatigue fracture
    - repetitive, excessive force applied to normal bone
- most common in adolescent athletes
- tibia is most common site

Diagnosis and Treatment
- localized pain and tenderness over the involved bone
- plain films may not show fracture for 2 weeks
- bone scan +ve in 12-15 days
- treatment is rest from strenuous activities to allow remodeling (can take several months)

Evaluation of the Limping Child

- see Pediatrics

Epiphyseal Injury

Table 17. Salter-Harris Classification of Epiphyseal Injury

SALT(E)R-Harris Type	Description	Treatment
I (**S**table)	transverse through growth plate	closed reduction and cast immobilization heals well, 95% do not affect growth
II (**A**bove)	through metaphysis and along growth plate	
III (**L**ow)	through epiphysis to plate and along growth plate	anatomic reduction by ORIF to prevent growth arrest
IV (**T**hrough)	through epiphysis and metaphysis	
V (**R**am)	crush injury of growth plate	high incidence of growth arrest; no specific treatment

Slipped Capital Femoral Epiphysis (SCFE)

- type I Salter-Harris epiphyseal injury
- most common adolescent hip disorder, peak at pubertal growth spurt
- risk: male, obese, hypothyroid
- acute (sudden displacement) and chronic (insidious displacement) forms

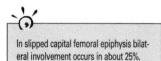

In slipped capital femoral epiphysis bilateral involvement occurs in about 25%.

Etiology
- multifactorial
    - genetic: autosomal dominant, blacks > caucasians
    - cartilaginous physis thickens rapidly under growth hormone (GH) effects
    - sex hormone secretion, which stabilizes physis, has not yet begun
    - overweight: mechanical stress
    - trauma: causes acute slip

Clinical Features
- acute: sudden, severe pain with limp
- chronic: limp with medial knee or anterior thigh pain
- tender over joint capsule
- restricted internal rotation, abduction, flexion
    - Whitman's sign: with flexion there is an obligate external rotation of the hip
- pain at extremes of ROM

Investigations
- x-rays: AP, frog-leg, lateral radiographs
    - posterior and medial slip
    - if mild slip, AP view may be normal or show slightly widened growth plate compared with opposite side

Treatment and Complications
- mild/moderate slip: stabilize physis with pins in current position
- severe slip: ORIF or pin physis without reduction and osteotomy after epiphyseal fusion
- complications: AVN (most common), chondrolysis, pin penetration, premature OA, loss of ROM

Developmental Dysplasia of the Hip (DDH)

- formerly called congenital dysplasia of the hip (CDH)
- due to ligamentous laxity, muscular underdevelopment, and abnormal shallow slope of acetabular roof
- spectrum of conditions
  - dislocated femoral head completely out of acetabulum
  - dislocatable head in socket
  - head subluxates out of joint when provoked
  - dysplastic acetabulum, more shallow and more vertical than normal
- painless
- if painful suspect septic dislocation

5 **F**'s that predispose to developmental dysplasia of the hip:
Family history
Female
Frank breech
First born
Le**F**t hip

Physical Examination
- diagnosis is clinical
  - limited abduction of the flexed hip (<50-60°)
  - affected leg shortening results in asymmetry in skin folds and gluteal muscles, wide perineum
  - Barlow's test (for dislocatable hip)
    - flex hips and knees to 90° and grasp thigh
    - fully adduct hips, push posteriorly to try to dislocate hips
  - Ortolani's test (for dislocated hip)
    - initial position as above but try to reduce hip with fingertips during abduction
    - palpable clunk if reduction is a positive test (reduction is felt, not heard)
  - Galeazzi's Sign
    - knees at unequal heights when hips and knees flexed
    - dislocated hip on side of lower knee
    - difficult test if child <1 year
  - Trendelenburg test and gait useful if older (>2 years)

Investigations
- U/S in first few months to view cartilage
- follow up radiograph after 3 months

Treatment and Complications
- 0-6 months: reduce hip using Pavlik harness to maintain abduction and flexion
- 6-18 months: reduction under GA, hip spica cast x 2-3 months (if Pavlik harness fails)
- >18 months: open reduction; pelvic and/or femoral osteotomy
- complications
  - redislocation, inadequate reduction, stiffness
  - AVN of femoral head

Legg-Calve-Perthes Disease

- self-limited AVN of femoral head, presents at 4-10 years of age
- etiology unknown, 20% bilateral, males > females, 1/10,000
- associations
  - family history
  - low birth weight
  - abnormal pregnancy/delivery
  - history of trauma to affected hip
- key features
  - AVN of proximal femoral epiphysis, abnormal growth of the physis, and eventual remodelling of regenerated bone

Clinical Features
- child with hip pain and limp
- tender over anterior thigh
- flexion contracture: decreased internal rotation, abduction of hip

Investigations
- x-rays
  - may be negative early
  - eventually, characteristic collapse of femoral head (diagnostic)
    - subchondral fracture
    - metaphyseal cyst

Treatment
- goal is to preserve ROM and preserve femoral head in acetabulum
- PT: ROM exercises
- brace in flexion and abduction x 2-3 years
- femoral or pelvic osteotomy
- prognosis better in
    - males <5 years old, <50% of femoral head involved, abduction >30°
- 50% of involved hips do well with conservative treatment
- complicated by early onset osteoarthritis and decreased ROM

Osgood-Schlatter Disease

Mechanism
- repetitive tensile stress on insertion of patellar tendon over the tibial tuberosity causes minor avulsion at the site and subsequent inflammatory reaction
- most common in adolescent athletes, especially jumping sports

Clinical Features
- tender lump over tibial tuberosity
- pain on resisted leg extension
- anterior knee pain exacerbated by jumping or kneeling, relieved by rest

Investigations
- x-rays: fragmentation of the tibial tubercle, ± ossicles in patellar tendon

Treatment
- benign, self-limited condition
- may restrict activities such as basketball or cycling
- flexibility, strengthening exercises

Congenital Talipes Equinovarus (Club Foot)

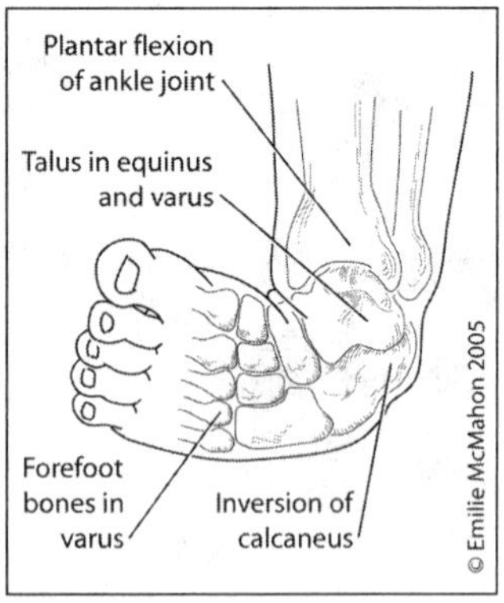

- fixed deformity
- 3 parts to deformity
    - talipes: talus is inverted and internally rotated
    - equinus: ankle is plantar flexed
    - varus: heel and forefoot are in varus (supinated)
- may be idiopathic, neurogenic, or syndrome-associated
- 1-2/1,000 newborns, 50% bilateral, occurrence M>F, severity F>M

Physical Examination
- examine hips for associated DDH
- examine knees for deformity
- examine back for dysraphism (unfused vertebral bodies)

Treatment
- correct deformities in the following order (Ponseti Technique):
    - forefoot adduction, ankle inversion, equinus
        - change strapping/cast q1-2 weeks
    - surgical release in refractory case (50%)
        - delayed until 3-4 months of age
- 3 year recurrence rate = 5-10%
- mild recurrence common; affected foot is permanently smaller/stiffer than normal foot with calf muscle atrophy

Scoliosis

Definition
- lateral curvature of spine with vertebral rotation

Epidemiology
- age: 10-14 years
- more frequent and more severe in females

Plantar flexion
of ankle joint

Talus in equinus
and varus

Forefoot
bones in
varus

Inversion of
calcaneus

© Emilie McMahon 2005

Figure 37. The Club Foot – depicting the gross and bony deformity

Etiology
- idiopathic: most common (90%)
- congenital: vertebrae fail to form or segment
- neuromuscular: UMN or LMN lesion, myopathy
- other: osteochondrodystrophies, neoplastic, traumatic
- postural: leg length discrepancy, muscle spasm

Clinical Features
- ± back pain
- 1° curve where several vertebrae affected
- 2° curves above and below fixed 1° curve to try and maintain normal position of head and pelvis
- asymmetric shoulder height when bent forward
- Adam's test: rib hump when bent forward
- prominent scapulae, creased flank, asymmetric pelvis
- associated posterior midline skin lesions in non-idiopathic scolioses
  - café-au-lait spots, dimples, neurofibromas
  - axillary freckling, hemangiomas, hair patches
- associated pes cavus or leg atrophy
- apparent leg length discrepancy

X-Rays
- 3-foot standing
  - measure curvature
  - may have associated kyphosis

Treatment
- based on degree of curvature
  - <20°: observe for changes
  - >20° or progressive: bracing (many types)
  - >40°, cosmetically unacceptable or respiratory problems: surgical correction (spinal fusion)

Bone Tumours

- primary bone tumours are rare after 3rd decade
- metastases to bone are relatively common after 3rd decade

Diagnosis
- pain, swelling, tenderness, rarely regional adenopathy
- routine x-ray
  - location (which bone, diaphysis, metaphysis, epiphysis)
  - size
  - lytic/lucent vs. sclerotic
  - involvement (cortex, medulla, soft tissue)
  - matrix (radiolucent, radiodense or calcified)
  - periosteal reaction
  - margin (geographic vs. permeative)
  - any pathological fracture
  - soft tissue swelling
- malignancy is suggested by rapid growth, warmth, tenderness, lack of sharp definition
- staging should include
  - bloodwork including liver enzymes
  - CT chest
  - bone scan
  - bone biopsy
    - should be referred to specialized centre prior to biopsy
    - classified into benign, benign aggressive, and malignant
  - MRI of affected bone

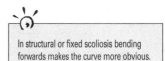

In structural or fixed scoliosis bending forwards makes the curve more obvious.

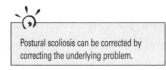

Postural scoliosis can be corrected by correcting the underlying problem.

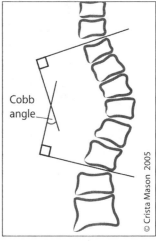

Figure 38. Cobb Angle – used to monitor the progression of the scoliotic curve

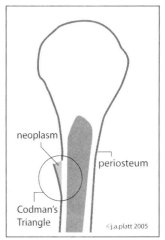

Figure 39. Codman's Triangle – a radiographic finding in malignancy, where the partially ossified periosteum is lifted off the cortex by neoplastic tissue

Benign Active Bone Tumours

1. Osteoid Osteoma
- peak incidence in 2nd and 3rd decades, M:F = 3:1
- small, round radiolucent nidus (<1 cm) surrounded by dense bone
    - tibia and femur most common
- produces severe intermittent pain, mostly at night
- characteristically relieved by NSAIDs

2. Osteochondroma
- 2nd and 3rd decades, M:F = 1.8:1
- metaphysis of long bone
    - cartilage-capped bony spur on surface of bone ("mushroom" on x-ray)
    - may be multiple (hereditary, autosomal dominant form) – higher risk of malignant change
- generally asymptomatic unless impinging on neurovascular structure
- malignant degeneration occurs in 1-2%

3. Enchondroma
- 2nd and 3rd decades
- 50% occur in the small tubular bones of the hand and foot; others in femur, humerus, ribs
- benign cartilagenous growth, develops in medullary cavity
    - single/multiple enlarged rarefied areas in tubular bones
    - lytic lesion with sharp margination and central calcification
- malignant degeneration occurs in 1-2%

4. Cystic Lesions
- includes unicameral/solitary bone cyst (most common), fibrous cortical defect
- children and young adults
- local pain, pathological fracture or incidental detection
    - lytic translucent area on metaphyseal side of growth plate
    - cortex thinned/expanded; well defined lesion
- treatment of unicameral bone cyst with steroid injections ± bone graft

Treatment
- treatment only necessary if symptomatic
- osteochondroma: resection
- cystic lesions: currettage and bone graft

Benign Aggressive Bone Tumours

1. Giant Cell Tumours/Aneurysmal Bone Cyst/Osteoblastoma
- affects patients of skeletal maturity, peak 3rd decade
- distal femur, proximal tibia, distal radius, sacrum, tarsal bones, spinal (osteoblastoma)
- cortex appears thinned, expanded; well-demarcated sclerotic margin
- local tenderness and swelling
- aggressively destroy bone
- 15% recur within 2 years of surgery
- giant cell tumour occasionally metastasizes (1-2%)

Treatment
- intralesional currettage + bone graft or cement
- wide local excision of expendable bones

Malignant Bone Tumours

Table 18. Most Common Malignant Tumour Types for Age

Age	Tumour
<1	Neuroblastoma
1-10	Ewing's of tubular bones
10-30	Osteosarcoma, Ewing's of flat bones
30-40	Reticulum cell sarcoma, fibrosarcoma, periosteal osteosarcoma, malignant giant cell tumour, lymphoma
>40	Metastatic carcinoma, multiple myeloma, chondrosarcoma

1. Osteosarcoma
- mostly frequently diagnosed in 2nd decade of life (60%)
- history of Paget's disease radiation
- predilection for distal femur (45%), proximal tibia (20%) and proximal humerus (15%)
  - invasive, variable histology; frequent metastases without treatment
- painful, poorly defined swelling, decreased ROM
- x-ray shows Codman's triangle (Figure 39)
  - characteristic periosteal elevation and spicule formation representing tumour extension into periosteum
- treatment: complete resection (limb salvage, rarely amputation), neo-adjuvant chemo
- survival – 70%

2. Chondrosarcoma
- primary
  - previous normal bone, patient over 40; expands into cortex to give pain, pathological fracture, flecks of calcification
- secondary
  - malignant degeneration of pre-existing cartilage tumour such as enchondroma or osteochondroma
- most commonly occurs in pelvis, femur, ribs, scapula, humerus
- unresponsive to chemotherapy, treat with aggressive surgical resection + reconstruction

3. Ewing's Sarcoma
- most occur between 5-20 years old
- florid periosteal reaction in diaphysis of long bone
  - moth-eaten appearance with periosteal lamellated pattern (onion-skinning)
- present with mild fever, anemia, leukocytosis and ↑ ESR
- metastases frequent without treatment
- treatment – resection, chemotherapy, radiation
- survival – 70%

4. Multiple Myeloma
- most common primary malignant tumour of bone in adults
- 90% occur in people >40 years old
- present with anemia, anorexia, renal failure, nephritis, ↑ ESR, bone pain, compression fractures, hypercalcemia
- diagnosis
  - punched-out lytic lesions on x-ray at multiple bony sites
  - serum/urine protein electrophoresis
- treatment: chemotherapy, radiation, surgery for symptomatic lesions or impending fractures
- see Hematology

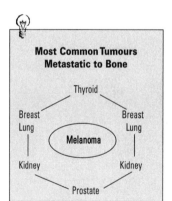

Most Common Tumours Metastatic to Bone

Thyroid

Breast
Lung

Melanoma

Breast
Lung

Kidney

Kidney

Prostate

5. Bone Metastases
- 2/3 from breast or prostate; also consider thyroid, lung, kidney
- usually osteolytic; prostate occasionally osteoblastic
- bone scan, MRI may be helpful
- stabilization of impending fractures
  - internal fixation, IM rods
  - bone cement

Articular Cartilage Defects

Properties of Articular Cartilage
- lacks blood supply and does not have innervation or lymphatic drainage
- varies in thickness from 2 mm to 4 mm and is thickest at periphery of concave surfaces and central portions of convex surfaces
- composed of type 2 collagen, water, proteoglycans, and chondrocytes
- collagen provides resistance against tensile stresses and transmits vertical loads
- water and proteoglycans provide turgor and elasticity and help to limit friction
- chondrocytes synthesize the cartilage matrix and control matrix turnover rate

Etiology
- overt trauma or repeated minor trauma; most commonly from sports injuries
- early stage osteoarthritis
- genetic degenerative diseases such as osteochondritis dissecans

Clinical Features
- very similar to symptoms of osteoarthritis (joint line pain with possible effusion, etc.)
- often have predisposing factors such as ligament injury, malalignment of the joint (varus/valgus), obesity, bone deficiency (avascular necrosis, osteochondritis dissecans, ganglion bone cysts), inflammatory arthropathy, and familial osteoarthropathy
- may have symptoms of locking or catching related to the torn/displaced cartilage

Investigations
- arthroscopy to visualize focal pathology and guide treatment strategy
- MRI may also be used to visualize the defect

Table 19. Outerbridge Classification of Chondral Defects

Grade	Chondral Damage
I	Softening and swelling of cartilage
II	Fragmentation and fissuring <1/2 inch (1.27 cm) in diameter
III	Fragmentation and fissuring >1/2 inch (1.27 cm) in diameter
IV	Erosion of cartilage down to bone

Treatment
- arthroscopic lavage and debridement of the joint
- marrow stimulation techniques (microfracture, drilling, abrasion arthroplasty)
  - involves creating a site of bleeding where new growth/healing can take place
- osteochondral grafts; also known as the OATS procedure or mosaicplasty
  - involves transferring osteochondral fragments from non-weightbearing surface to area of defect
- autologous chondrocyte implantation (ACI)
  - currently only available in the U.S. and Europe
  - involves harvesting patient's cartilage, growing it in culture medium outside of the patient, then reinserting the newly cultured chondrocytes back to fill the chondral defect
- osteochondral allograft; only used in limited circumstances when defect is very large

Common Medications

Table 20. Common Medications

Drug Name	Dosing Schedule	Indications	Comments
cefazolin (Ancef™)	1-2 g IV q8h	Prophylactically before orthopaedic surgery	First generation cephalosporin; do not use with penicillin allergy
heparin	5000 IU SC q12h	To prevent venous thombosis and pulmonary emboli	Monitor platelets, follow PTT which should rise 1.5-2x
LMWH dalteparin (Fragmin™) enoxaparin (Lovenox™) fondaparinux (Arixtra™)	5000 IU SC OD 30 mg SC bid 2.5 mg SC OD	DVT prophylaxis esp. in hip and knee surgery	Fixed dose, no monitoring, improved bioavailability, ↑ bleeding rates
midazolam (Versed™)	0.02 mg/kg IV	Conscious sedation for short procedures	Medications used together during fracture reduction – monitor for respiratory depression
fentanyl (Sublimaze™)	0.5-3 ug/kg IV	Conscious sedation for short procedures	Short acting anesthetic used in conjunction with midazolam (Versed™)
triamcinolone (Aristocort™) – an injectable steroid	0.5-1 mL of 25 mg/mL	Suspension (injected into inflamed joint or bursa)	Potent anti-inflammatory effect Increased pain for 24 hours, rarely causes fat necrosis and skin depigmentation
naproxen (Naprosyn™)	250-500 mg bid	Pain due to inflammation, arthritis, soft tissue injury	NSAID, may cause gastric erosion and bleeding
misoprostol (Cytotec™)	200 µg qid	Prophylaxis of heterotopic ossification after THA	Use with indomethacin
indomethacin (Indocid™)	25 mg PO tid	Prophylaxis of heterotopic ossification after THA	Use with misoprostol

OT Otolaryngology – Head and Neck Surgery

Nayha Mody and Indra Rasaratnam, chapter editors
Justine Chan and Angela Ho, associate editors
Billie Au, EBM editor
Dr. Jonathan Irish and Dr. Blake Papsin, staff editors

Basic Anatomy Review

Ear

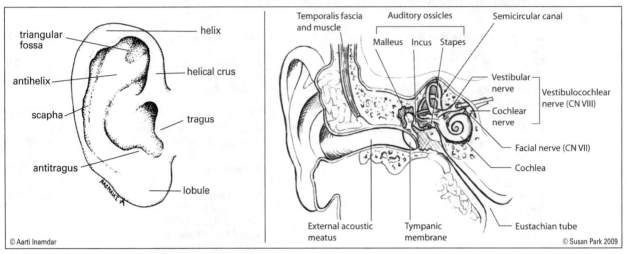

© Aarti Inamdar

© Susan Park 2009

Figure 1. Surface Anatomy of the External Ear and Inner Ear

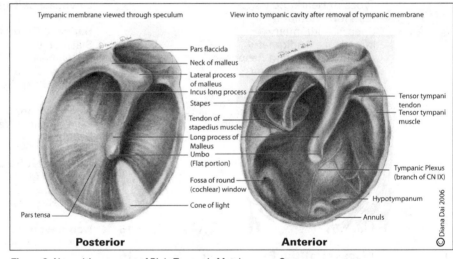

Tympanic membrane viewed through speculum   View into tympanic cavity after removal of tympanic membrane

© Diana Dai 2006

Figure 2. Normal Appearance of Right Tympanic Membrane on Otoscopy

Nose

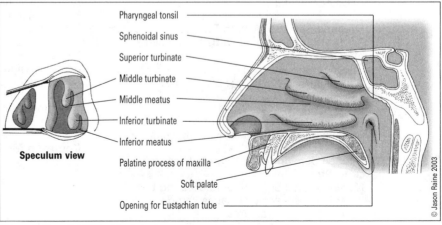

© Jason Raine 2003

Figure 3. Superficial Nasal Anatomy

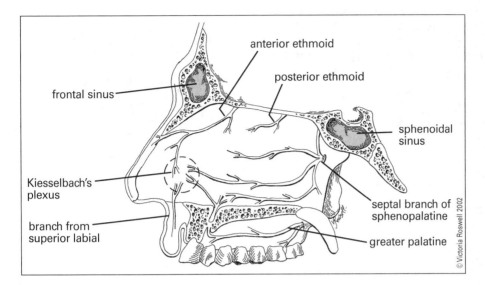

Figure 4. Nasal Septum and its Blood Supply

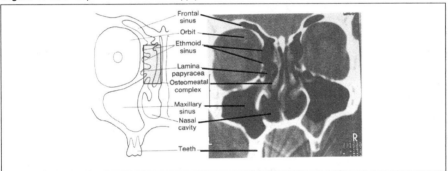

Figure 5. Anatomy of Paranasal Sinuses. There are four paranasal sinuses: maxillary, ethmoid, sphenoid, and frontal Reprinted from Dhillon R.S, and East CA. Ear, Nose and Throat and Head and Neck Surgery, 2nd ed. Copyright 1999, with permission from Elsevier.

Throat

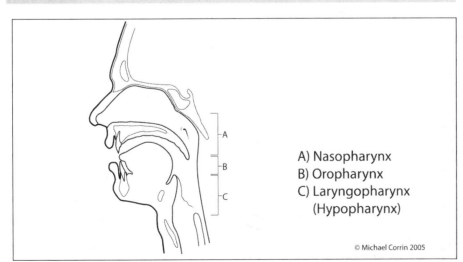

A) Nasopharynx
B) Oropharynx
C) Laryngopharynx
    (Hypopharynx)

© Michael Corrin 2005

Nasopharynx: skull base to soft palate
Oropharynx: soft palate to hyoid bone
Laryngopharynx: hyoid bone to inferior cricoid cartilage

Figure 6. Sagittal Section with Divisions of Nasopharynx, Oropharynx, Hypopharynx

Branches of Facial Nerve
(in order from superior to inferior)
"**T**en **Z**ebras **B**roke **M**y **C**ar"

Function of Facial Nerve
"ears, tears, face, taste"
ears – stapedius muscle
tears – lacrimation and salivation (parotid)
face – muscles of facial expression
taste – sensory anterior 2/3 of tongue

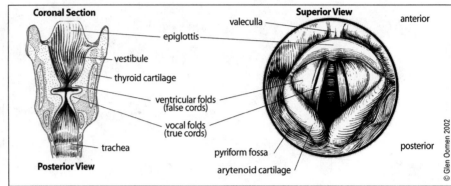

Figure 7. Anatomy of a Normal Larynx

Head & Neck

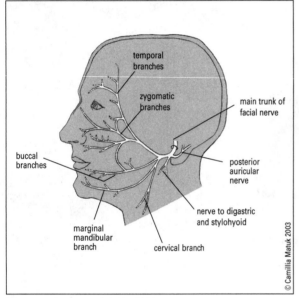

Figure 8. Anatomy of the Facial Nerve

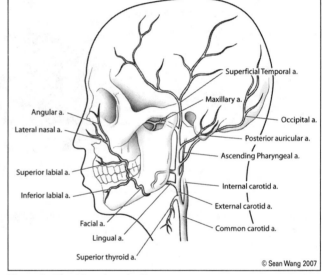

Figure 9. Blood Supply to the Face

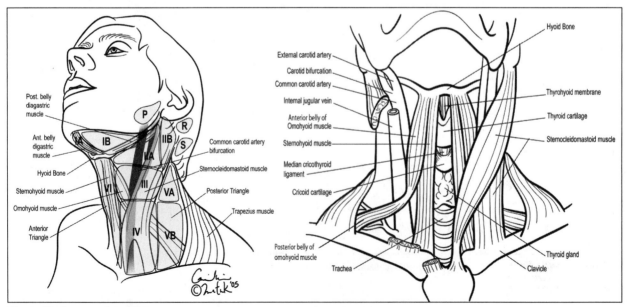

Figure 10. Anatomy of the Neck

Anatomical Triangles of the Neck

- **anterior triangle**
    - bounded by anterior border of sternocleidomastoid (SCM), midline of neck, and lower border of mandible
    - divided into
        - **submental triangle**: bounded by both anterior bellies of digastrics and hyoid bone
        - **digastric triangle**: bounded by anterior and posterior bellies of digastric, and inferior border of mandible
        - **carotid triangle**: bounded by sternocleidomastoid, anterior belly of omohyoid, and posterior belly of digastric
            - contains: tail of parotid, submandibular gland, hypoglossal nerve, carotid bifurcation, and lymph nodes
- **posterior triangle**
    - bounded by posterior border of sternocleidomastoid, anterior border of trapezius, and middle third of clavicle
    - divided into
        - **occipital triangle**: superior to posterior belly of the omohyoid
        - **subclavian triangle**: inferior to posterior belly of omohyoid
    - contains: spinal accessory nerve and lymph nodes

Table 1. Lymphatic Drainage of Nodal Groups and Anatomical Triangles of Neck

Nodal Group/Level	Location	Drainage
1. Suboccipital (S)	Base of skull, posterior	Posterior scalp
2. Retroauricular (R)	Superficial to mastoid process	Scalp, temporal region, ext. auditory meatus, post. pinna
3. Parotid-preauricular (P)	In front of ear	External auditory meatus, anterior pinna, soft tissues of frontal and temporal regions, root of nose, eyelids, palpebral conjunctiva
4. Submental (Level IA)	(Midline) Anterior bellies of digastric muscles, tip of mandible, and hyoid bone	Floor of mouth, anterior oral tongue, anterior mandibular alveolar ridge, lower lip
5. Submandibular (Level IB)	Anterior belly of digastric muscle, stylohyoid muscle, body of mandible	Oral cavity, anterior nasal cavity, soft tissues of the mid-face, submandibular gland
6. Upper jugular (Levels IIA and IIB)	Skull base to inferior border of hyoid bone along SCM muscle	Oral cavity, nasal cavity, naso/oro/hypopharynx, larynx, parotid glands
7. Middle jugular (Level III)	Inferior border of hyoid bone to inferior border of cricoid cartilage along SCM muscle	Oral cavity, naso/oro/hypopharynx, larynx
8. Lower jugular (Level IV)	Inferior border of cricoid cartilage to clavicle along SCM muscle	Hypopharynx, thyroid, cervical esophagus, larynx
9. Posterior triangle* (Levels VA and VB)	Posterior border of SCM, anterior border of trapezius, from skull base to clavicle	Nasopharynx and oropharynx, cutaneous structures of the posterior scalp and neck
10. Anterior compartment** (Level VI)	(Midline) Hyoid bone to suprasternal notch between the common carotid arteries	Thyroid gland, glottic and subglottic larynx, apex of piriform sinus, cervical esophagus

* Includes some supraclavicular nodes
**Contains Virchow, pretracheal, precricoid, paratracheal, and perithyroidal nodes

> **Left-sided enlargement** of a supraclavicular node (Virchow's node) may indicate an abdominal malignancy; **right-sided enlargement** may indicate malignancy of the mediastinum, lungs, or esophagus.
>
> Enlargement of the occipital and/or posterior auricular nodes may be a sign of rubella.

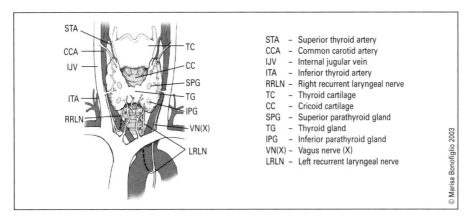

STA – Superior thyroid artery
CCA – Common carotid artery
IJV – Internal jugular vein
ITA – Inferior thyroid artery
RRLN – Right recurrent laryngeal nerve
TC – Thyroid cartilage
CC – Cricoid cartilage
SPG – Superior parathyroid gland
TG – Thyroid gland
IPG – Inferior parathyroid gland
VN(X) – Vagus nerve (X)
LRLN – Left recurrent laryngeal nerve

© Marisa Bonofiglio 2003

Figure 11. Anatomy of Thyroid Gland

Differential Diagnosis of Common Presenting Problems

Dizziness/Vertigo

If caused by a peripheral lesion, true nystagmus and vertigo will never last longer than a couple of weeks because compensation occurs; such is not true for a central lesion.

4 D's of Vertebrobasilar Insufficiency
Drop attacks
Diplopia
Dysarthria
Dizziness

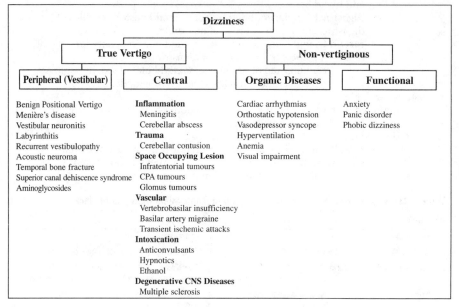

Figure 12. Differential Diagnosis of Dizziness

Otalgia

1. Local Causes

Table 2. Differential Diagnosis of Otalgia - Local Causes

Etiology	External Ear Pain	Middle and Inner Ear Pain
Infection	a. Otitis externa	a. Acute otitis media
	b. Herpes simplex/Zoster	b. Otitis media with effusion
	c. Auricular cellulitis	c. Mastoiditis, myringitis, skull base infections
	d. External canal abscess	(malignant otitis in diabetics)
Trauma	frostbite, burns, hematoma, lacerations	traumatic perforation, barotrauma
Other	neoplasm of external canal, foreign body, cerumen impaction	neoplasm, Wegener's, cholesteatoma

2. Referred Pain (from CN V, IX, & X) - Ten T's + 2
- Eustachian Tube
- TMJ Syndrome (pain in front of the ears)
- Trismus (spasm of masticator muscles; early symptom of tetanus)
- Teeth
- Tongue
- Tonsil (tonsillitis, tonsillar cancer, post-tonsillectomy)
- Tic (glossopharyngeal neuralgia)
- Throat (cancer of larynx)
- Trachea (foreign body; tracheitis)
- Thyroiditis
- Geniculate herpes and Ramsey Hunt Syndrome
- +/- CN VII palsy (Bell's Palsy)

Hearing Loss

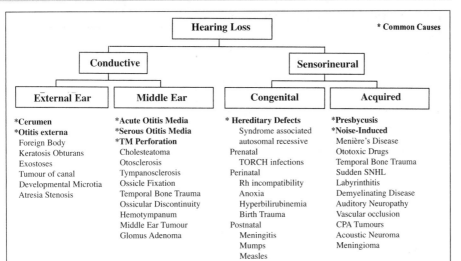

Figure 13. Differential Diagnosis of Hearing Loss

The incidence of Menière's disease has decreased since the introduction of H. flu & S. pneumo vaccines.

Tinnitus

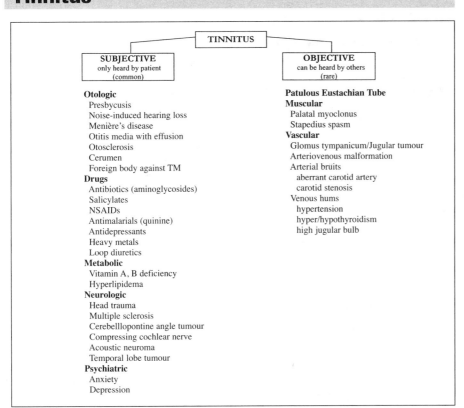

Figure 14. Differential Diagnosis of Tinnitus

Tinnitus is most commonly associated with SNHL, although the exact mechanism is unknown.

Nasal Obstruction

Table 3. Differential Diagnosis of Nasal Obstruction

Acquired	Congenital

Nasal cavity
• Rhinitis
  ▪ acute/chronic
  ▪ vasomotor
  ▪ allergic
• Polyps
• Foreign bodies
• Enlarged turbinates
• Tumour
  ▪ Benign – inverting papilloma
  ▪ Malignant
    ♦ squamous cell carcinoma (SCC)
    ♦ esthesioneuroblastoma
    ♦ adenocarcinoma
	• Nasal dermoid
	• Encephalocele
	• Glioma
	• Choanal atresia

Nasal septum • Septal deviation • Septal hematoma/abscess • Dislocated septum	

Nasopharynx
• Adenoid hypertrophy
• Tumour
  ▪ Benign – juvenile nasopharyngeal angiofibroma (JNA)
  ▪ Malignant – nasopharyngeal carcinoma	

Functional Tunnel Nose Syndrome: absence of feeling in nose prevents the sensation of aeration through nostrils	

Hoarseness

Table 4. Differential Diagnosis of Hoarseness

Infectious	• acute/chronic laryngitis • laryngotracheobronchitis (croup)	• bacterial tracheitis
Inflammatory	• gastro-esophageal reflux (GERD), smoking, chronic sinusitis with PND or muscle tension dystonia, overuse • vocal cord polyps • Reinke's edema (polypoid corditis) • contact ulcers or granulomas • vocal cord nodules	
Trauma	• external laryngeal trauma	• endoscopy and endotracheal tube

Neoplasia	• **benign tumours**
	  ▪ vocal cord polyps
	  ▪ papillomas (HPV infection)
	  ▪ chondromas, lipomas, hemangiomas
		• **malignant tumours**
		  ▪ early leukoplakic lesions
		  ▪ squamous cell carcinoma (SCC)
		  ▪ Kaposi's sarcoma

Cysts	• retention cysts	• laryngoceles

Systemic	• **endocrine**
	  ▪ hypothyroidism
	  ▪ virilization
		• **connective tissue disease**
		  ▪ rheumatoid arthritis (RA)
		  ▪ SLE
		  ▪ angioneurotic edema

Neurologic
(vocal cord paralysis due to superior ± recurrent laryngeal nerve injury)
	• **central lesions**
	  ▪ cerebrovascular accident (CVA)
	  ▪ head injury
	  ▪ multiple sclerosis (MS)
	  ▪ Arnold-Chiari
	  ▪ skull base tumours
	• **peripheral lesions**
	  ▪ **unilateral**
	    ♦ most common cause of vocal cord paralysis = lung malignancy
	    ♦ neck, chest, laryngeal trauma
	    ♦ thoracic aneurysm
	    ♦ neoplasms: glomus jugulare, thyroid, bronchogenic, esophageal, neural
	    ♦ iatrogenic injury – thyroid, parathyroid surgery, carotid endarterectomy. Anterior approach to cervical spine disc surgery
	    ♦ radiation induced fibrosis
	    ♦ degenerative neural disorders: bulbar palsies (e.g. polio), demyelinating disease, vascular syndromes (Wallenberg's)
	    ♦ cardiac: left atrial enlargement, aneurysm of aortic arch
	  ▪ **bilateral**
	    ♦ iatrogenic injury: bilateral thyroid surgery
	  ▪ **neuromuscular**
	    ♦ myasthenia gravis
	    ♦ presbylaryngeus/presbyphonia (↓ tone of vocalis muscle with age)
	    ♦ spasmodic dysphonia	

Functional	• psychogenic aphonia (hysterical aphonia) • habitual aphonia • ventricular dysphonias • catatonic state	
Congenital	• webs, atresia	• laryngomalacia

Neck Mass

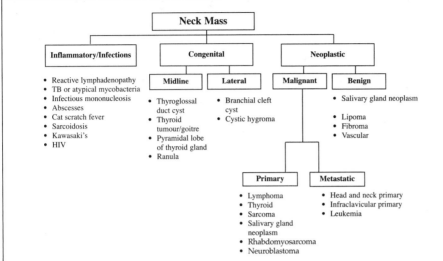

Figure 15. Differential Diagnosis of a Neck Mass

DDx Neck Mass
K - congenital
I - infectious/inflammatory
T - trauma
T - toxins
E - endocrine
N - neoplasm
S - systemic

Hearing Loss

Types of Hearing Loss

1. Conductive Hearing Loss (CHL)
- the conduction of sound to the cochlea is impaired
- can be caused by external and middle ear disease

2. Sensorineural Hearing Loss (SNHL)
- due to a defect in the conversion of sound into neural signals or in the transmission of those signals to the cortex
- can be caused by disease of the cochlea, acoustic nerve (CN VIII), brainstem, or cortex

3. Mixed Hearing Loss
- the conduction of sound to the cochlea is impaired, as well as transmission through the cochlea to the cortex

Auditory Acuity
- mask one ear and whisper into the other
- tuning fork tests (see Table 5) (audiogram of greater utility)
- sensitivity depends on which tuning fork used (256 Hz, 512 Hz, 1024 Hz)
  - Rinne test
    - 512 Hz tuning fork is struck and held firmly on mastoid process to test bone conduction (BC). The tuning fork is then placed beside the pinna to test air conduction (AC)
    - If AC >BC → positive Rinne, which is normal
  - Weber test
    - 512 Hz tuning fork is held on vertex of head and patient states whether it is heard centrally (Weber negative) or is lateralized to one side (Weber right, Weber left)
    - can place vibrating fork on patient's chin while they clench their teeth, or directly on teeth to elicit more reliable response
    - will only lateralize if difference in hearing loss between ears is >6 dB

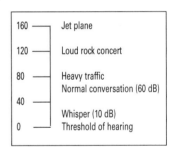

160 —	Jet plane
120 —	Loud rock concert
80 —	Heavy traffic Normal conversation (60 dB)
40 —	
0 —	Whisper (10 dB) Threshold of hearing

Frequency of Tuning Fork (Hz)	Minimum hearing loss to have NEGATIVE Rinne (BC > AC) (dB)
256	15
512	30
1024	45

Table 5. The Interpretation of Tuning Fork Tests

Examples	Weber	Rinne
Normal or bilateral sensorineural hearing loss	Central	AC>BC (+) bilaterally
Right-sided conductive hearing loss, normal left ear	Lateralizes to Right	BC>AC (–) right
Right-sided sensorineural hearing loss, normal left ear	Lateralizes to Left	AC>BC (+) bilaterally
Right-sided severe sensorineural hearing loss or dead right ear, normal left ear	Lateralizes to Left	BC>AC (–) right *

* a vibrating tuning fork on the mastoid stimulates the cochlea bilaterally, therefore in this case, the left cochlea is stimulated by the Rinne test on the right, i.e. a false negative test
These tests are not valid if the ear canals are obstructed with cerumen (i.e. will create conductive loss)

Weber Test Lateralization = Ipsilateral conductive hearing loss or Contralateral sensorineural hearing loss

Pure Tone Audiometry

- threshold is the lowest intensity level at which a patient can hear the tone 50% of the time
- thresholds are obtained for each ear for frequencies 250 to 8000 Hz
- air conduction thresholds are obtained with headphones and measure outer, middle, inner ear, and auditory nerve function
- bone conduction thresholds are obtained with bone conduction oscillators which bypass the outer and middle ear

Degree of Hearing Loss
- determined on basis of the pure tone average (PTA) at 500, 1000, and 2000 Hz

Sound Characteristics

Intensity/Loudness = amplitude of sound waves in decibels (dB)

Pitch/Tone = frequency of vibration in Hertz (Hz)

Timbre/Quality = overtones superimposed on the pure tone

Range of frequencies audible to human Ear → 20 to 20,000 Hz
Most sensitive frequencies → 1,000 to 4,000 Hz
Range of human speech → 500 to 2,000 Hz

Hearing loss most often occurs at higher frequencies. Noise-induced (occupational) HL is seen at 4000 Hz. HL associated with otosclerosis is seen at 2000 Hz (Carhart's notch).

Air conduction thresholds can only be equal to or greater than bone conduction thresholds.

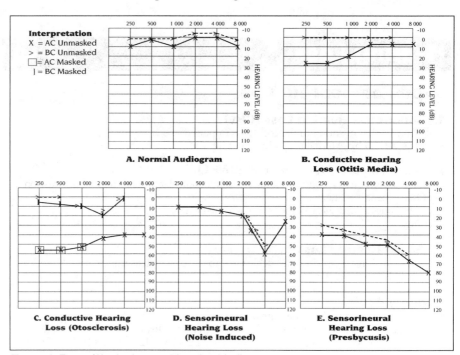

Figure 16. Types of Hearing Loss and Associated Audiograms

PURE TONE PATTERNS

1. Conductive Hearing Loss (CHL) (Figure 16B)
- bone conduction (BC) in normal range
- air conduction (AC) outside of normal range
- gap between AC and BC thresholds >10 dB (an air-bone gap)

2. Sensorineural Hearing Loss (SNHL) (Figure 16D)
- both air and bone conduction thresholds below normal
- gap between AC and BC <10 dB (no air-bone gap)

3. Mixed Hearing Loss
- both air and bone conduction thresholds below normal
- gap between AC and BC thresholds > 10 dB (an air-bone gap)

Degree of Hearing loss

Decibel loss	Degree of Hearing loss
0 to 15 dB	Normal
16 to 25 dB	Slight
26 to 40 dB	Mild
41 to 55 dB	Moderate
56 to 70 dB	Moderate - Severe
71 to 90 dB	Severe
≥91 dB	Profound

Speech Audiometry

Speech Reception Threshold (SRT)
- lowest hearing level at which patient is able to repeat 50% of two syllable words which have equal emphasis on each syllable (spondee words)
- SRT and best pure tone threshold in the 500 to 2000 Hz range (frequency range of human speech) usually agree within 5 dB. If not, suspect a retrocochlear lesion or functional hearing loss
- used to assess the reliability of the pure tone audiometry

Speech Discrimination Test
- percentage of words the patient correctly repeats from a list of 50 monosyllabic words
- tested at a level 35 to 50 dB > SRT, therefore degree of hearing loss is taken into account
- patients with normal hearing or conductive hearing loss score >90%
- score depends on extent of SNHL
- a decrease in discrimination as sound intensity increases is typical of a retrocochlear lesion (rollover effect)
- investigate further if scores differ more than 20% between ears
- used as best predictor of hearing aid response

| Speech Discrimination ||
% of words identified	Speech Discrimination
90 to 100%	Excellent
80 to 90%	Good
60 to 80%	Fair
40 to 60%	Poor
<40%	Very poor

Impedance Audiometry

Tympanogram
- the eustachian tube equalizes the pressure between external and middle ear
- tympanograms graph the compliance of the middle ear system against pressure gradient ranging from to –400 to +200 mmH$_2$O
- tympanogram peak occurs at the point of maximum compliance where the pressure in the external canal is equivalent to the pressure in the middle ear
- normal range: –100 to +50 mm H$_2$O

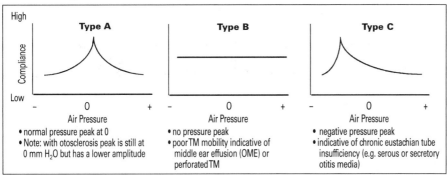

Figure 17. Tympanograms

Static Compliance
- volume measurement reflecting overall stiffness of the middle ear system
- normal range: 0.3 to 1.6 cc
- negative middle ear pressure and abnormal compliance indicate middle ear pathology

Acoustic Stapedial Reflexes
- stapedius muscle contracts 2° to loud sound
- **acoustic reflex thresholds** = 70 to 100 dB greater than hearing threshold; if hearing threshold >85 dB, reflex likely absent
- stimulating either ear causes bilateral and symmetrical reflexes
- for reflex to be present, CN VII must be intact and no conductive hearing loss in monitored ear
- if reflex is absent without conductive or severe sensorineural loss → suspect CN VIII lesion
- **acoustic reflex decay test** = ability of stapedius muscle to sustain contraction for 10 s at 10 dB
- normally, little reflex decay occurs at 500 and 1000 Hz
- with cochlear hearing loss, acoustic reflex thresholds = 25 to 60 dB
- with retrocochlear hearing loss (acoustic neuroma) → absent acoustic reflexes or marked reflex decay (>50%) within 5 seconds

Auditory Brainstem Response (ABR)

- measures neuroelectric potentials (waves) in response to a stimulus in five different anatomic sites. This test can be used to map the lesion according to the site of the defect
- delay in brainstem response suggests cochlear or retrocochlear abnormalities (tumour or multiple sclerosis)
- does not require volition or co-operation of patient

This objective test can be used to screen newborns or to uncover normal hearing in malingering patients.

Otoacoustic Emissions

- objective test of hearing where a series of clicks is presented to the ear and the cochlea generates an echo which can be measured
- often used in newborn screening

Aural Rehabilitation

- dependent on degree of hearing loss, communicative requirements, motivation, expectations, age, physical, and mental abilities
- negative prognostic factors
  - poor speech discrimination
  - narrow dynamic range (recruitment)
  - unrealistic expectations
  - cosmetic concerns
- types of hearing aids
  - behind the ear
  - all in the ear
  - bone conduction – bone anchored hearing aid (BAHA): applied to the skull and attached to the skull
  - contralateral routing of signals (CROS)
- assistive listening devices
  - direct/indirect audio output
  - infrared, FM radio, or induction loop systems
  - telephone, television, or alerting devices
- cochlear implants
  - electrode is inserted into the cochlea to allow direct stimulation of the auditory nerve
  - for profound bilateral sensorineural hearing loss not rehabilitated with conventional hearing aids
  - established indication: post-lingually deafened adults, pre- and post-lingually deaf children

Pre-lingual deaf infants are the best candidates for aural rehabilitation because they benefit from developmental plasticity.

Vertigo

Evaluation of the Dizzy Patient

- vertigo: an illusion of rotary movement of self or environment, made worse in the absence of visual stimuli
  - produced by peripheral (inner ear) or central (brainstem-cerebellum) stimulation
- it is important to distinguish vertigo from other disease entities that may present with similar complaints (e.g. cardiovascular, psychiatric, neurological, aging)

Vertigo Symptom Description
- dizziness
- spinning
- lightheadedness
- giddiness
- unsteadiness

Table 6. Peripheral vs. Central Vertigo

Symptoms	Peripheral	Central
Imbalance	Mild-Moderate	Severe
Nausea and vomiting	Severe	Variable
Auditory symptoms	Common	Rare
Neurologic symptoms	Rare	Common
Compensation	Rapid	Slow
Nystagmus	Unidirectional	Bidirectional
	Horizontal	Horizontal or vertical

Table 7. Differential Diagnosis of Vertigo Based on History

Condition	Duration	Hearing Loss	Tinnitus	Aural Fullness	Other Features
Benign paroxysmal positional vertigo (BPPV)	seconds	–	–	–	
Menière's disease	minutes to hours precedes attack	uni/bilateral	+	pressure/warmth	
Recurrent vestibulopathy	minutes to hours	–	–	none	
Vestibular neuronitis	hours to days	unilateral	–	–	
Labyrinthitis	days	unilateral	whistling	–	recent AOM
Acoustic neuroma	chronic	progressive	–	–	ataxia CN VII palsy

Benign Paroxysmal Positional Vertigo (BPPV)

Definition
- acute attacks of transient vertigo lasting seconds to minutes initiated by certain head positions, accompanied by nystagmus

Etiology
- due to migration of an otolith (cupulolithiasis) into posterior semicircular canal where it stimulates one of the semicircular canals
    - causes: head injury, viral infection (URTI), degenerative disease, idiopathic
    - results in slightly different signals being received by the brain from the two balance organs resulting in sensation of movement

Diagnosis
- history and positive Dix-Hallpike maneuver

Dix-Hallpike Positional Testing
- the patient is rapidly moved from a sitting position to a supine position with the head hanging over the end of the table, turned to one side at 45° holding the position for 20 seconds
- onset of vertigo is noted and the eyes are observed for nystagmus
- 5 key points of the Dix-Hallpike maneuver
    - geotropic rotatory nystagmus
    - fatigues with repeated maneuver
    - reversal of nystagmus upon sitting
    - latency of 20 seconds
    - crescendo-decrescendo vertigo – 20 seconds

Treatment
- reassure patient that process resolves spontaneously
- particle repositioning maneuvers
    - Epley's maneuver (performed by MD)
    - Brandt-Daroff exercises (performed by patient)
- surgery for refractory cases
- anti-emetics for nausea / vomiting
- drugs to suppress the vestibular system delay eventual recovery and are therefore not used

BPPV is the most common cause of episodic vertigo.

5 signs of BPPV seen with Dix-Hallpike Maneuver
- geotropic rotatory nystagmus
- fatigues with repeated maneuver
- reversal of nystagmus upon sitting up
- latency of ~20 seconds
- crescendo/decrescendo vertigo ~20 seconds

Patients can wear Frenzel's magnifying eyeglasses during the Dix-Hallpike Maneuver for better visualization of the eyes.

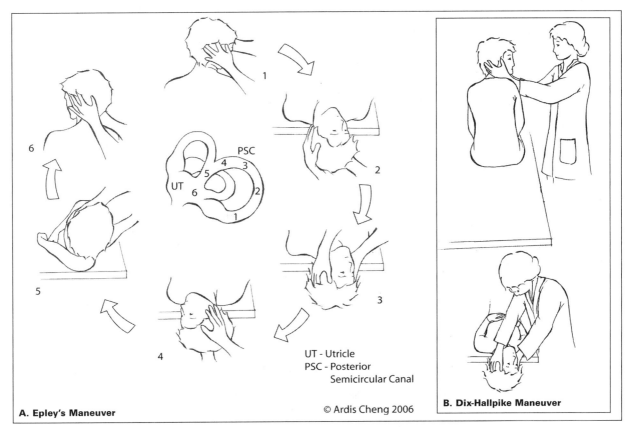

UT - Utricle
PSC - Posterior Semicircular Canal

A. Epley's Maneuver   © Ardis Cheng 2006   B. Dix-Hallpike Maneuver

Figure 18. Epley's and Dix-Hallpike Maneuvers

Menière's Disease (Endolymphatic Hydrops)

Definition
- episodic attacks of tinnitus, hearing loss, aural fullness, and vertigo lasting minutes to hours

Proposed Etiology
- inadequate absorption of endolymph leads to endolymphatic hydrops (over accumulation) that distorts the membranous labyrinth

Epidemiology
- peak incidence 40 to 60 years
- bilateral in 35% of cases

Clinical Features
- syndrome characterized by vertigo, fluctuating hearing loss, tinnitus, and aural fullness
- ± drop attacks (Tumarkin crisis), ± nausea and vomiting
- vertigo disappears with time (minutes to hours), but hearing loss remains
- early in the disease, fluctuating sensorineural hearing loss
- later stages are characterized by persistent tinnitus and low-frequency hearing loss
- attacks come in clusters and may be very debilitating to the patient
- may be triggered by stress

Treatment
- acute management may consist of bed rest, antiemetics, antivertiginous drugs (e.g. betahistine (Serc™)), and low molecular weight dextrans (not commonly used)
- long term management may include
  - medical
    - low salt diet, diuretics (e.g. hydrochlorothiazide, triamterene, amiloride)
    - local application of gentamicin to destroy vestibular end-organ
    - Serc™ prophylactically to decrease intensity of attacks
  - surgical – selective vestibular neurectomy or transtympanic labyrinthectomy
- may recur in opposite ear after treatment

Triad of Meniere's Disease
Vertigo, Tinnitus and Hearing Loss

Drop Attacks (Tumarkin's Otolithic Crisis) are sudden falls occurring without warning and without LOC.

Before proceeding with gentamicin treatment, perform a CT Head to rule out CPA tumour as the cause of symptoms.

Recurrent Vestibulopathy

- peak age 30 to 50 years old, M=F
- episodic vertigo lasting minutes to hours
- no hearing loss, tinnitus, or focal neurological deficit
- etiology unknown (?post-traumatic, ?post-viral, ?deafferentation of CN VIII)
- treatment: symptomatic, most eventually go into remission

Vestibular Neuronitis

Definition
- acute onset of disabling vertigo often accompanied by nausea, vomiting and imbalance without hearing loss that resolves over days leaving a residual imbalance that lasts days to weeks

Etiology
- thought to be due to a viral infection (e.g. measles, mumps, herpes zoster)
- ~30% of cases have associated URTI symptoms
- other possible etiologies: microvascular events, diabetes, autoimmune process
- considered to be the vestibular equivalent of Bell's palsy, sudden hearing loss, and acute vocal cord palsy

Clinical Features
- acute phase
  - severe vertigo with nausea, vomiting, and imbalance lasting 1 to 5 days
  - irritative nystagmus (fast phase towards the offending ear)
  - patient tends to veer towards affected side
- convalescent phase
  - imbalance and motion sickness lasting days to weeks
  - spontaneous nystagmus away from affected side
  - gradual vestibular adaptation requires weeks to months
- incomplete recovery likely with the following risk factors: elderly, visual impairment, poor ambulation
- repeated attacks can occur

Treatment
- acute phase
  - bed rest, vestibular sedatives (dimenhydrinate (Gravol™), diazepam)
- convalescent phase
  - progressive ambulation especially in the elderly
  - vestibular exercises: involve eye and head movements, sitting, standing, and walking

Labyrinthitis

Definition
- acute infection of the inner ear resulting in vertigo and hearing loss

Etiology
- may be serous (viral), or purulent (bacterial)
- occurs as a complication of acute and chronic otitis media, bacterial meningitis, cholesteatoma, and temporal bone fractures
- bacterial: *S. pneumoniae, H, influenzae, M. catarrhalis, P. aeruginosa, P. mirabilis*
- viral: rubella, CMV, measles, mumps, varicella zoster

Clinical Features
- sudden onset of vertigo, nausea, vomiting, tinnitus, and unilateral hearing loss, with no associated fever or pain
- meningitis is a serious complication

Investigations
- CT head
- if meningitis is suspected: lumbar puncture, blood cultures

Treatment
- treat with IV antibiotics, drainage of middle ear ± mastoidectomy

Acoustic Neuroma

Definition
- schwannoma of the vestibular portion of CN VIII

Pathogenesis
- starts in the internal auditory canal and expands into cerebellar pontine angle (CPA), compressing cerebellum and brainstem
- when associated with type 2 neurofibromatosis (NF2): bilateral tumours of CN VIII, café-au-lait skin lesions, multiple intracranial lesions

Acoustic neuroma is the most common intracranial tumour causing hearing loss and the most common cerebellopontine angle tumour.

Clinical Features
- usually presents with unilateral sensorineural hearing loss or tinnitus
- dizziness and unsteadiness may be present, but true vertigo is rare as tumour growth occurs slowly
- facial nerve palsy and trigeminal (V_1) sensory deficit (corneal reflex) are late complications

In the elderly, unilateral tinnitus or SNHL is acoustic neuroma until proven otherwise.

Diagnosis
- MRI with gadolinium contrast is the gold standard
- audiogram – sensorineural hearing loss
- poor speech discrimination and stapedial reflex absent or significant reflex decay
- acoustic brainstem reflexes (ABR) – increase in latency of the 5th wave

Treatment
- expectant management if tumour is very small, or in elderly
- definitive management is surgical excision
- other options: gamma knife, radiation

Tinnitus

Definition
- an auditory perception in the absence of an acoustic stimuli, likely related to loss of input to neurons in central auditory pathways and resulting in abnormal firing

History
- subjective vs. objective (see Figure 14)
- continuous vs. pulsatile (vascular in origin)
- unilateral vs. bilateral
- associated symptoms: hearing loss, vertigo, aural fullness, otalgia, otorrhea

Investigations
- audiology
- if unilateral
    - ABR, MRI/CT to exclude a retrocochlear lesion
    - CT to diagnose glomus tympanicum
    - MRI or angiogram to diagnose AVM
- if suspect metabolic abnormality: lipid profile, TSH

Treatment
- if a cause is found, treat the cause (e.g. drainage of middle ear effusion, embolization or excision of AVM)
- with no treatable cause, 50% will improve, 25% worsen, 25% remain the same
- avoid loud noise, ototoxic meds, caffeine, smoking
- tinnitus workshops
- identify situations where tinnitus is most bothersome (e.g. quiet times), mask tinnitus with soft music or "white noise"
- hearing aid if coexistent hearing loss
- tinnitus instrument
    - combines hearing aid with white noise masker
- trial of tocainamide

Glomus Tympanicum/Jugular Tumour signs and symptoms:
- soft blowing tinnitus
- hearing loss
- blue mass behind TM

Diseases of the External Ear

Cerumen Impaction

Cerumen impaction is the most common cause of conductive hearing loss in 15 to 50 year olds.

Etiology
- ear wax is a mixture of secretions from ceruminous and pilosebaceous glands, squames of epithelium, dust, and debris

Risk Factors
- hairy or narrow ear canals, in-the-ear hearing aids, cotton swab usage, osteomata

Clinical Features
- hearing loss (conductive)
- ± tinnitus, vertigo, otalgia, aural fullness

Treatment
- ceruminolytic drops (bicarbonate solution, olive oil, glycerine, Cerumenol™, Cerumenex™)
- syringing
- manual debridement (by MD)

Exostoses

Definition
- bony protuberances in the external auditory canal composed of lamellar bone

Etiology
- believed to be associated with swimming in cold water

Clinical Features
- usually an incidental finding
- if large, they can cause cerumen impaction or otitis externa

Treatment
- no treatment required unless symptomatic

SYRINGING

Indications
- totally occlusive cerumen with pain, decreased hearing, or tinnitus

Contraindications
- non-occlusive cerumen
- previous ear surgery
- only hearing ear
- TM perforation

Complications
- failure
- otitis externa
- TM perforation
- trauma
- pain
- vertigo
- tinnitus
- otitis media

Method
- establish that TM is intact
- gently pull the pinna up and back
- using warm water, aim the syringe nozzle upwards and posteriorly to irrigate the ear canal

Otitis Externa (OE)

Etiology
- bacteria (~90% of OE): *Pseudomonas aeruginosa, Pseudomonas vulgaris, E. coli, S. aureus*
- fungus: *Candida albicans, Aspergillus niger*

Risk Factors
- associated with swimming ("swimmer's ear")
- mechanical cleaning (Q-tips™), skin dermatitides, aggressive scratching
- devices that occlude the ear canal: hearing aids, headphones, etc.

Clinical Features
- acute
    - pain aggravated by movement of auricle (traction of pinna or pressure over tragus)
    - otorrhea (sticky yellow purulent discharge)
    - conductive hearing loss ± aural fullness 2° to obstruction of external canal by swelling and purulent debris
    - post-auricular lymphadenopathy
    - complicated OE exists if the pinna and/or the periauricular soft tissues are erythematous and swollen
- chronic
    - pruritus of external ear ± excoriation of ear canal
    - atrophic and scaly epidermal lining, ± otorrhea, ± hearing loss
    - wide meatus but no pain with movement of auricle
    - tympanic membrane appears normal

Treatment
- clean ear under magnification with irrigation, suction, dry swabbing, and C&S
- bacterial etiology
    - antipseudomonal otic drops (e.g. gentamicin, ciprofloxacin) or a combination of antibiotic and steroid (e.g. Garasone™ or Cipro HC™)
    - do not use aminoglycoside if the tympanic membrane (TM) is perforated because of the risk of ototoxicity
    - introduction of fine gauze wick (pope wick) if external canal edematous
    - ± 3% acetic acid solution to acidify ear canal (low pH is bacteriostatic)
    - systemic antibiotics if either cervical lymphadenopathy or cellulitis
- fungal etiology
    - repeated debridement and topical antifungals (gentian violet, Mycostatin™ powder, boric acid, Locacorten™, Vioform™ drops)
- ± analgesics
- chronic otitis externa (pruritus without obvious infection) → corticosteroid alone e.g. diprosalic acid

> Otitis externa has two forms: a benign infection of the outer canal that could occur in anybody and a potentially lethal disease which usually occurs in elderly, immunosuppressed or diabetic patients.

> Pulling on the pinna is extremely painful in otitis externa, but is usually well tolerated in otitis media.

Malignant (Necrotizing) Otitis Externa/ Skull Base Osteomyelitis

Definition
- osteomyelitis of the temporal bone

Epidemiology
- occurs in elderly diabetics and immunocompromised patients

Etiology
- rare complication of otitis externa
- *Pseudomonas* infection in 99% of cases

Clinical Features
- otalgia and purulent otorrhea that is refractory to medical therapy
- granulation tissue on the floor of the auditory canal

Complications
- lower cranial nerve palsies
- systemic infection, death

Management
- imaging: high resolution temporal bone CT scan, gadolinium scan, technetium scan
- requires hospital admission, debridement, IV antibiotics , hyperbaric O_2
- may require OR for debridement of necrotic tissue/bone

> **Gallium and Technetium Scans**
> Gallium scans are used to show sites of active infection. Gallium is taken up by PMNs and therefore only lights up when active infection is present. It will not show the extent of osteomyelitis. Technetium scans provide information about osteoblastic activity and as such are used to demonstrate sites of osteomyelitis. Technetium scans help with diagnosis whereas gallium scans are useful in follow-up.

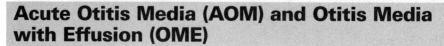

Diseases of the Middle Ear

Acute Otitis Media (AOM) and Otitis Media with Effusion (OME)

(see *Pediatric ENT*, OT38)

Cholesteatoma

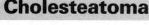

Definition
- a cyst composed of keratinizing squamous epithelium in an abnormal place (e.g. middle ear, mastoid, temporal bone)

Congenital
- presents as a "small white pearl" behind an intact tympanic membrane or as a conductive hearing loss
- believed to be due to aberrant migration of external canal ectoderm during development
- not associated with otitis media

Acquired (more common)
- generally occurs as a consequence of otitis media and chronic eustachian tube dysfunction
- frequently associated with retraction pockets in the pars flaccida and marginal perforations of the tympanic membrane
- the associated chronic inflammatory process causes progressive destruction of surrounding bony structures

> **Mechanisms of Acquired Cholesteatoma Formation**
> 1. Epithelial migration through TM perforation
> 2. Invagination of TM
> 3. Metaplasia of middle ear epithelium
> 4. Basal cell hyperplasia

Clinical Features
- symptoms
  - history of otitis media (especially if unilateral), ventilation tubes, ear surgery
  - progressive hearing loss (predominantly conductive although may get sensorineural hearing loss in late stage)
  - otalgia, aural fullness, fever
- signs
  - retraction pocket in TM, may contain keratin debris
  - TM perforation
  - granulation tissue, polyp visible on otoscopy
  - malodorous, unilateral otorrhea

Complications

Table 8. Complications of Cholesteatoma

Local	Intracranial
• ossicular erosion: conductive hearing loss	• meningitis
• sensorineural hearing loss from inner ear erosion	• sigmoid sinus thrombosis
• dizziness from inner ear erosion or labyrinthitis	• intracranial abscess (subdural, epidural, cerebellar)
• temporal bone infection: mastoiditis, petrositis	
• facial paralysis	

Investigations
- audiogram and CT scan

Treatment
- there is no conservative therapy for cholesteatoma
- surgical: mastoidectomy ± tympanoplasty ± ossicle reconstruction

Mastoiditis

Definition
- infection (usually subperiosteal) of mastoid air cells, most commonly seen approximately two weeks after onset of untreated or inadequately treated acute suppurative otitis media

> Mastoiditis is now rare due to rapid and effective treatment of acute otitis media with antibiotics.

Etiology
- acute mastoiditis caused by the same organisms as AOM: *S. pneumoniae, S. pyogenes, S. aureus, H. influenzae*

Clinical Features
- classic triad
    - otorrhea
    - tenderness to pressure over the mastoid
    - retroauricular swelling with protruding ear
- fever, hearing loss, ± TM perforation (late)
- radiologic findings: opacification of mastoid air cells by fluid and interruption of normal trabeculations of cells

Treatment
- IV antibiotics with myringotomy and ventilating tubes - usually all that is required acutely
- cortical mastoidectomy
    - debridement of infected tissue allowing aeration and drainage
    - requires lifelong care
- indications for surgery
    - failure of medical treatment after 48 hours
    - symptoms of intracranial complications
    - aural discharge persisting for 4 weeks and resistant to antibiotics

Otosclerosis

Definition
- fusion of stapes footplate to oval window so that it cannot vibrate

Etiology
- autosomal dominant, variable penetrance approximately 40%
- female > male, progresses during pregnancy (hormone responsive)

Otosclerosis is the second most common cause of conductive hearing loss in 15 to 50 year olds (after cerumen impaction).

Clinical Features
- progressive conductive hearing loss first noticed in teens and 20's (may progress to sensorineural hearing loss if cochlea involved)
- ± pulsatile tinnitus
- tympanic membrane normal ± pink blush (Schwartz's sign) associated with the neovascularization of otosclerotic bone
- characteristic dip at 2,000 Hz (Carhart's notch) on audiogram (Figure 16C)

Treatment
- monitor with serial audiograms if coping with loss
- hearing aid
- stapedectomy or stapedotomy (with laser or drill) with prosthesis is definitive treatment

Diseases of the Inner Ear

Congenital Sensorineural Hearing Loss

Hereditary Defects
- genetic factors are being identified increasingly among the causes of hearing loss
- non-syndrome associated (70%) (often idiopathic, autosomal recessive), connexin 26 (GJB2) most common
- syndrome associated (30%)
    - Waardenburg's – white forelock, heterochromia iridis, wide nasal bridge and increased distance between medial canthi
    - Pendred's – deafness associated with thyroid gland disorders, SLC26A4 gene, enlarged vestibular aqueducts
    - Treacher-Collins – first and second branchial cleft anomalies
    - Alport's – hereditary nephritis

Congenital SNHL is decreasing in incidence due to the availability of vaccines & improved neonatal care.

Prenatal TORCH Infections
- toxoplasmosis, rubella, cytomegalovirus (CMV), herpes simplex, others (e.g. HIV)

Perinatal
- Rh incompatibility
- anoxia
- hyperbilirubinemia
- birth trauma (hemorrhage into inner ear)

Postnatal
- meningitis
- mumps
- measles

High Risk Registry (For Hearing Loss in Newborns)
- risk factors (no longer of clinical significance with advent of universal newborn screening)
  - low birth weight/prematurity
  - perinatal anoxia (low APGARs)
  - kernicterus – bilirubin >25 mg/dL
  - craniofacial abnormality
  - family history of deafness in childhood
  - 1st trimester illness – CMV, rubella
  - neonatal sepsis
  - ototoxic drugs
  - perinatal infection, including post-natal meningitis
  - consanguinity
- 50 to 75% of newborns with sensorineural hearing loss have at least one of the above risk factors, and 90% of these have spent time in the NICU
- presence of any risk factor: auditory brainstem response (ABR) study performed before leaving NICU and at 3 months adjusted age
- early rehabilitation improves speech and school performance

Presbycusis

Definition
- sensorineural hearing loss associated with aging (5th and 6th decades)

Presbycusis is the most common cause of sensorineural hearing loss.

Etiology
- hair cell degeneration
- age related degeneration of basilar membrane
- cochlear neuron damage
- ischemia of inner ear

Clinical Features
- progressive, gradual bilateral hearing loss initially at high frequencies, then middle frequencies (see Figure 16E)
- loss of discrimination of speech especially with background noise present – patients describe people as mumbling
- recruitment phenomenon: inability to tolerate loud sounds
- tinnitus

Recruitment Phenomenon results in a large rise in sensitivity to loud noises with relatively small changes in sound intensity.

Treatment
- hearing aid if patient has difficulty functioning, hearing loss >30-35 dB
- ± lip reading, auditory training, auditory aids (doorbell and phone lights)

Sudden Sensorineural Hearing Loss

Clinical Features
- presents as a sudden onset of significant hearing loss (usually unilateral) ± tinnitus, aural fullness
- usually idiopathic, rule out other causes:
  - autoimmune causes – ESR, rheumatoid factor, ANA
  - MRI to rule out tumour and/or CT to rule out ischemic/hemorrhagic stroke if associated with any other focal neurological signs (e.g. vertigo, ataxia, abnormality of CN V or VII, weakness)

Sudden sensory neural hearing loss may easily be confused with ischemic brain events. It is important to keep a high index of suspicion especially with elderly patients presenting with sudden sensory neural hearing loss as well as vertigo.

Treatment
- treat with oral corticosteroids within 3 days of onset: prednisone 1-2 mg/kg/day, tapering over 2 weeks

Prognosis (depends on degree of hearing loss and other factors)
- 70% resolve spontaneously within 10 to 14 days
- 20% experience partial resolution
- 10% experience permanent hearing loss

Drug Ototoxicity

Aminoglycosides
- toxic to hair cells by any route: oral, IV, and topical (only if the TM is perforated)
- destroys sensory hair cells – outer first, inner second
- high frequency hearing loss develops earliest
- ototoxicity occurs days to weeks post-treatment
- streptomycin and gentamicin (vestibulotoxic), kanamycin and tobramycin (cochleotoxic)
- must monitor with peak and trough levels when prescribed, especially if patient has neutropenia, history of ear or renal problems
- q24h dosing, with amount determined by creatinine clearance, not serum creatinine

- aminoglycoside toxicity displays saturable kinetics therefore once daily dosing presents less risk than divided daily doses
- duration of treatment is the most important predictor of ototoxicity
- treatment: immediately stop aminoglycosides

Salicylates
- hearing loss with tinnitus, reversible if discontinued

Antimalarials (Quinine)
- hearing loss with tinnitus
- reversible if discontinued but can lead to permanent loss

Others
- many antineoplastics agents are ototoxic (weigh risks vs. benefits)
- loop diuretics

Noise-Induced Sensorineural Hearing Loss

Pathogenesis
- 85 to 90 dB over months or years causes cochlear damage
- early-stage hearing loss at 4000 Hz (because this is the resonance frequency of the temporal bone), extends to higher and lower frequencies with time (see Figure 16D)
- speech reception not altered until hearing loss >30 dB at speech frequency, therefore considerable damage may occur before patient complains of hearing loss
- difficulty with speech discrimination, especially in situations with competing noise

Phases of Hearing Loss
- dependent on intensity level and duration of exposure
- temporary threshold shift
  - when exposed to loud sound, decreased sensitivity or increased threshold for sound
  - may have associated aural fullness and tinnitus
  - with removal of noise, hearing returns to normal
- permanent threshold shift
  - hearing does not return to previous state

Short exposures to louder sounds can cause significant SNHL

Treatment
- hearing aid
- prevention
  - ear protectors: muffs, plugs
  - machinery which produces less noise
  - limit exposure to noise with frequent rest periods
  - regular audiologic follow-up

Limits of Noise Causing Damage
- continuous sound pressure >85 dB
- single sound impulse >135 dB

Inner Ear Diseases that cause Vertigo

- (see *Vertigo* section, OT12)
  - benign paroxysmal positional vertigo (BPPV)
  - Menière's disease (endolymphatic hydrops)
  - recurrent vestibulopathy
  - vestibular neuronitis
  - labyrinthitis
  - acoustic neuroma (AN)

Temporal Bone Fractures

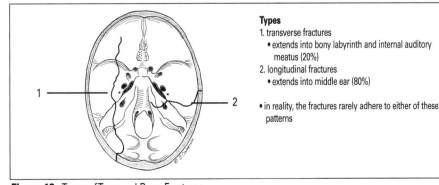

Types
1. transverse fractures
   - extends into bony labyrinth and internal auditory meatus (20%)
2. longitudinal fractures
   - extends into middle ear (80%)

- in reality, the fractures rarely adhere to either of these patterns

© Teddy Cameron 2002

Figure 19. Types of Temporal Bone Fractures

Table 9. Features of Temporal Bone Fractures (see Figure 19)

	Transverse	Longitudinal
Incidence	10 to 20%	70 to 90%
Etiology	frontal/occipital trauma	lateral skull trauma
CN pathology	CN VII palsy (50%)	CN VII palsy (10 to 20%)
Hearing loss	sensorineural loss due to direct cochlear injury injury	conductive hearing loss secondary to ossicular
Vestibular symptoms	sudden onset vestibular symptoms due to direct semicircular canal injury (vertigo, spontaneous nystagmus)	rare
Other features	• intact external auditory meatus, tympanic membrane ± hemotympanum • spontaneous nystagmus • CSF leak in eustachian tube to nasopharynx ± rhinorrhea (risk of meningitis)	• torn tympanic membrane or hemotympanum • bleeding from external auditory canal • step formation in external auditory canal • CSF otorrhea • Battle's sign = mastoid ecchymoses • Raccoon eyes = periorbital ecchymoses

Signs of Basilar Skull Fracture
• Battle's Sign: ecchymosis of the mastoid process of the temporal bone
• Racoon Eyes
• CSF Rhinorrhea/Otorrhea
• Cranial Nerve involvment (facial palsy - CN VII, nystagmus - CN VI, facial numbness - CN V)

The halo sign is the double ringed appearance of CSF fluid on white filter paper as it separates out from blood.

Hemotympanum can also be indicative of temporal bone trauma.

Diagnosis
• otoscopy
• do not syringe or manipulate external auditory meatus due to risk of inducing meningitis via TM perforation
• CT head
• audiology, facial nerve tests (for transverse fractures), Schirmer's test, stapedial reflexes if CN VII palsy
• if suspecting CSF leak: look for halo sign, send fluid for beta-2-transferrin

Treatment
• ABC's
• medical – expectant, prevent otogenic meningitis
• surgical – explore temporal bone, indications are
  ▪ CN VII palsy (complete)
  ▪ gunshot wound
  ▪ depressed fracture of external auditory meatus
  ▪ early meningitis (mastoidectomy)
  ▪ bleeding intracranially from sinus
  ▪ CSF otorrhea (may resolve spontaneously)

Complications
• acute otitis media ± labyrinthitis ± mastoiditis
• meningitis/epidural abscess/brain abscess
• post-traumatic cholesteatoma

Facial Nerve Paralysis

Etiology
• supranuclear and nuclear (MS, poliomyelitis, cerebral tumours)
• infranuclear – see chart

Treatment
• treat according to etiology plus provide corneal protection with artificial tears, nocturnal lid taping, tarsorrhaphy, gold weighting of upper lid

Table 10. Differential Diagnosis of Peripheral Facial Paralysis (PFP)

Etiology	Incidence	Findings	Investigations	Treatment, Follow-up , and Prognosis
Bell's Palsy • idiopathic, (HSV) infection of the facial nerve • diagnosis of exclusion	• 80 to 90% of PFP **Risk Factors:** • diabetes • pregnancy • viral prodrome (50%)	**Hx:** • acute onset • **numbness of ear** face or neck (50%) • Schirmer's test - measures lacrimation • recurrence (12%) - + FHx (14%) - hyperacusis (30%) **P/E:** • paralysis or paresis of all muscle groups on one side of the face • absence of signs of CNS disease • absence of signs of ear or CPA diseases	1. stapedial reflex absent 2. audiology normal (or baseline) 3. electromyogram (EMG) – best measure for prognosis 4. topognostic testing 5. MRI w/ gadolinium - enhancement of CN VII & VIII 6. high resolution CT	**Rx:** 1. protect the eye to prevent exposure keratitis with patching or tarsorraphy 2. systemic steroids may lessen degeneration and hasten recovery 3. consider antiviral (acyclovir) **F/U:** • spontaneous remission should begin within 3 weeks of onset • delayed (3 to 6 months) recovery portends at least some functional loss **Px:** 1. 90% recover spontaneously and completely overall; 95 to 100% if incomplete paralysis 2. poorer px if hyperacusis, >60 yrs, diabetes, HTN, severe pain
Ramsay-Hunt Syndrome (Herpes Zoster Oticus) varicella zoster infection of CN VII/VIII	4.5 to 9% of PFP **Risk Factors:** • >60 years • impaired immunity • cancer • radiotherapy • chemotherapy	**Hx:** • hyperacusis • sensorineural HL • severe pain of pinna, mouth, or face **P/E:** • vesicles on pinna, ext. canal (erupt 3-7 days after onset of pain) • associated herpes zoster ophthalmicus (uveitis, keratoconjunctivitis, optic neuritis, or glaucoma)	1. stapedial reflex absent 2. audiology – sensorineural loss 3. viral ELISA studies to confirm 4. MRI w/ gadolinium (86% of facial nerves enhance)	**Rx:** 1. pt. should avoid touching lesions to prevent spread of infection 2. systemic steroids can relieve pain, vertigo, avoid postherpetic neuralgia 3. acyclovir may lessen pain, aid healing of vesicles **F/U:** 2 to 4 weeks **Px:** • poorer prognosis than Bell's palsy; 22% recover completely, 66% incomplete paralysis, 10% complete
Temporal Bone Fracture **– Longitudinal** (90%)	• 20% have PFP	**Hx:** • blow to side of head **P/E:** • trauma to side of head • neuro findings consistent with epidural/ subdural bleed	1. skull X-rays 2. CT head	**Px:** • injury usually due to stretch or impingement; may recover with time
– Transverse (10%)	• 40% have PFP	**Hx:** • blow to frontal or occipital area **P/E:** • trauma to front or back of head	1. skull X-rays 2. CT head	**Px:** • nerve transection more likely
Iatrogenic	• ?	• variable (depending on level of injury)	1. wait for lidocaine to wear off 2. EMG	**Rx:** • exploration if complete nerve paralysis • no exploration if any movement at all

Source: Paul Warrick. http://icarus.med.utoronto.ca/carr/manual/afnptable.html

Rhinitis

Definition
• inflammation of the lining (mucosa) of the nasal cavity

Table 11. Classification of Rhinitis

Inflammatory	Non-Inflammatory

• perennial non-allergic
  ▪ asthma, ASA sensitivity
• allergic
  ▪ seasonal
  ▪ perennial
• atrophic
  ▪ primary: *Klebsiella ozena* (especially in elderly)
  ▪ acquired: post-surgery if too much mucosa or turbinate has been resected
• infectious
  ▪ viral: e.g. rhinovirus, influenza, parainfluenza, etc.
  ▪ bacterial: e.g. *S. aureus*
  ▪ fungal
  ▪ granulomatous: TB, syphilis, leprosy
• non-infectious
  ▪ sarcoidosis
  ▪ Wegener's granulomatosis
• irritant
  ▪ dust
  ▪ chemicals
  ▪ pollution
	• rhinitis medicamentosa
	  ▪ topical decongestants
	• hormonal
	  ▪ pregnancy
	  ▪ estrogens
	  ▪ thyroid
	• idiopathic vasomotor

Rhinitis Medicamentosa is rebound congestion due to the overuse of intranasal vasoconstrictors. For prevention, use of these medications for only 5-7 days is recommended.

Table 12. Nasal Discharge: Character and Associated Conditions

Character	Associated Conditions
Watery/mucoid	Allergic, viral, vasomotor, CSF leak (halo sign)
Mucopurulent	Bacterial, foreign body
Serosanguinous	Neoplasia
Bloody	Trauma, neoplasia, bleeding disorder, hypertension/vascular disease

Allergic Rhinitis (Hay Fever)

Definition
- rhinitis characterized by an IgE-mediated hypersensitivity to foreign allergens
- acute-and-seasonal or chronic-and-perennial
- perennial allergic rhinitis often confused with recurrent colds

Etiology
- when allergens contact the respiratory mucosa, specific IgE antibody is produced in susceptible hosts
- concentration of allergen in the ambient air correlates directly with the rhinitis symptoms

Epidemiology
- age at onset usually <20 years
- more common in those with a personal or family history of allergies/atopy

Clinical Features
- nasal: obstruction with pruritus, sneezing
- clear rhinorrhea (containing increased eosinophils)
- itching of eyes with tearing
- frontal headache and pressure
- mucosa – swollen, pale, lavender colour, and "boggy"
- seasonal (summer, spring, early autumn)
  - pollens from trees
  - lasts several weeks, disappears and recurs following year at same time
- perennial
  - inhaled: house dust, wool, feathers, foods, tobacco, hair, mould
  - ingested: wheat, eggs, milk, nuts
  - occurs intermittently for years with no pattern or may be constantly present

Complications

- chronic sinusitis/polyps
- serous otitis media

Diagnosis
- history
- direct exam
- allergy testing

Treatment
- education: identification and avoidance of allergen
- nasal irrigation with saline
- antihistamines e.g. diphenhydramine, fexofenadine
- oral decongestants e.g. pseudoephedrine, phenylpropanolamine
- topical decongestant may lead to rhinitis medicamentosa
- other topicals: steroids (fluticasone), disodium cromoglycate, antihistamines, ipratropium bromide
- oral steroids if severe
- desensitization by allergen immunotherapy

Vasomotor Rhinitis

- neurovascular disorder of nasal parasympathetic system (vidian nerve) affecting mucosal blood vessels
- nonspecific reflex hypersensitivity of nasal mucosa
- caused by
  - temperature change
  - alcohol, dust, smoke
  - stress, anxiety, neurosis
  - endocrine – hypothyroidism, pregnancy, menopause
  - parasympathomimetic drugs
  - beware of rhinitis medicamentosa: reactive vasodilation due to prolonged use (>5 days) of nasal drops and sprays (Dristan™, Otrivin™)

Congestion reduces nasal airflow and allows the nose to repair itself. Treatment should focus on the initial insult rather than target this defense mechanism.

Clinical Features
- chronic intermittent nasal obstruction, varies from side to side
- rhinorrhea: thin, watery
- nasal allergy must be ruled out
- mucosa and turbinates: swollen, pale between exposure
- symptoms are often more severe than clinical presentation suggests

Treatment
- elimination of irritant factors
- parasympathetic blocker (Atrovent™ nasal spray)
- steroids (e.g. beclomethasone, fluticasone)
- surgery (often of limited lasting benefit): electrocautery, cryosurgery, laser treatment or removal of inferior or middle turbinates
- vidian neurectomy (rarely done)
- symptomatic relief with exercise (increased sympathetic tone)

Sinusitis

Development of Sinuses
- sinus pneumatization begins in 3rd-4th month of fetal life. Maxillary sinus first to develop
- neonate – clinically significant ethmoid and maxillary buds present
- age 9 – maxillary full grown; frontal and sphenoid cells starting
- age 18 – frontal and sphenoid cells full grown

Drainage of Sinuses
- frontal, maxillary, anterior ethmoids: middle meatus
- posterior ethmoid: superior meatus
- sphenoid: sphenoethmoidal recess

Pathogenesis of Sinusitis
- inflammation of the mucosal lining of the paranasal sinuses
- anything that blocks mucus from exiting the sinuses predisposes them to inflammation

Definition
- inflammation of the mucosal lining of the sinuses

Classification
- acute: <4 weeks
- subacute: 4 weeks to 3 months
- chronic: >3 months

FESS = functional endoscopic sinus surgery
Opening of the entire osteomeatal complex in order to facilitate drainage while sparing the sinus mucosa.

Table 13. Etiologies of Sinusitis

Ostial obstruction	Inflammation:	• URTI
		• allergy
	Mechanical:	• septal deviation
		• turbinate hypertrophy
		• polyps
		• tumours
		• adenoid hypertrophy
		• foreign body
		• congenital abnormalities i.e. cleft palate
Non-ostial obstruction	Immune:	• Wegener's granulomatosis
		• lymphoma, leukemia
		• immunosuppressed patients e.g. neutropenics, diabetics, HIV
	Systemic:	• cystic fibrosis
		• immotile cilia (Kartagener's)
Direct extension	Dental:	• infection
	Trauma:	• facial fractures

Source: Dr. J. Chapnik. http://icarus.meds.utoronto.ca/otolaryngology/OTL300/sinusitis.pdf

Acute Suppurative Sinusitis

Definition
- acute infection and inflammation of the paranasal sinuses

Etiology
- viral vs. bacterial
- children are more prone to a bacterial etiology than adults, but viral is still more common
- maxillary sinus most commonly affected
- must rule out fungal causes (mucormycosis) in immunocompromised hosts
- organisms
  - Viral (most common): rhinovirus, influenza, parainfluenza
  - Bacterial: *S. pneumoniae* (35%), *H. influenzae* (35%), *M. catarrhalis*, anaerobes (dental)

Clinical Features
- sudden onset of:
  - nasal blockage/congestion and/or
  - nasal discharge/posterior nasal drip
- +/- facial pain or pressure, hyposmia
- signs more suggestive of a bacterial etiology are erythematous nasal mucosa, mucopurulent discharge, pus originating from the middle meatus and the presence of nasal polyps of a deviated septum
- acute viral rhinosinusitis lasts <10 days. If symptoms increase after 5 days or last longer than 10 days, consider a bacterial etiology

Management
- anterior rhinoscopy
- xray/CT scan not recommended unless complications are suspected
- symptoms improving within 5 days: symptomic relief and expectant management
- moderate symptoms that worsen or persist beyond 5 days: institute an intranasal corticosteroid spray and continue for 14 days if symptomic relief is noted within 48hrs
- severe symptoms that worsen or persist beyond 5 days and retractory to INCS: amoxicillin therapy +/- INCS +/- referral to a specialist
- surgery if medical therapy fails: FESS

Acute Sinusitis Complications
Consider hospitalization if any of the following are suspected

1. Orbital (Chandler's classification)
   a. periorbital cellulitis
   b. orbital cellulitis
   c. subperiosteal abscess
   d. orbital abscess
   e. cavernous sinus thrombosis

2. Intracranial
   a. meningitis
   b. abscess

3. Bony
   a. subperiosteal frontal bone abscess ("Pott's Puffy Tumour")
   b. osteomyelitis

4. Neurologic
   a. superior orbital fissure syndrome (CN III/IV/VI palsy, immobile globe, dilated pupils, ptosis, V1 hypoesthesia)
   b. orbital apex syndrome (as "a" above, plus neuritis, papilledema, decreased acuity)

Chronic Sinusitis

Definition
- inflammation of the paranasal sinuses lasting >3 months

Etiology
- can result from any of the following:
  - inadequate treatment of acute sinusitis
  - untreated nasal allergy
  - allergic fungal rhinosinusitis
  - anatomic abnormality e.g. deviated septum (predisposing factor)
  - underlying dental disease
  - ciliary disorder e.g. cystic fibrosis, Kartagener's
  - chronic inflammatory disorder e.g. Wegener's
- organisms
  - bacterial: *S. pneumoniae*, *H. influenzae*, *M. catarrhalis*, *S. pyogenes*, *S. aureus*, anaerobes
  - fungal: *Aspergillus*

Clinical Features (similar to acute, but less severe)
- chronic nasal obstruction
- purulent nasal discharge
- pain over sinus or headache
- halitosis
- yellow-brown post-nasal discharge
- chronic cough
- maxillary dental pain

Treatment
- antibiotics for 3 to 6 weeks for infectious etiology
  - augmented penicillin (Clavulin™), macrolide (clarithromycin), fluoroquinolone (levofloxacin), clindamycin, Flagyl™
- topical nasal steroid, saline spray
- surgery if medical therapy fails or fungal sinusitis

Allergic fungal rhinosinusitis is a chronic sinusitis affecting mostly young, immunocompetent, atopic individuals. Treatment options include FESS +/- intranasal topical steroids, antifungals and immunotherapy.

Chronic Sinusitis Complications
1. Polyps
2. Mucocele (frontal and ethmoid)

Surgical Treatment

- removal of all diseased soft tissue and bone, post-op drainage and obliteration of pre-existing sinus cavity
- functional endoscopic sinus surgery

Epistaxis

Blood Supply to the Nasal Septum

1. Superior posterior septum
  - internal carotid → ophthalmic → anterior/posterior ethmoidal

2. Posterior septum
  - external carotid → internal maxillary → sphenopalatine artery → nasopalatine

3. Lower anterior septum
  - external carotid → facial artery → superior labial artery → nasal branch
  - external carotid → internal maxillary → descending palatine → greater palatine

- these arteries all anastomose to form Kiesselbach's plexus, located at Little's area (anterior portion of the cartilaginous septum), where 90% of nosebleeds occur
- bleeding from above middle turbinate is internal carotid, and from below is external carotid

Table 14. Etiology of Epistaxis

Type	Causes	
Local	Trauma (most common) • fractures: facial, nasal • self-induced: digital, foreign body Iatrogenic: nasal, sinus, orbit surgery Barometric changes Nasal dryness: dry air, ± septal deformities Septal perforation Chemical: cocaine, nasal sprays, ammonia, etc.	Tumours • benign: polyps, inverting papilloma, angiofibroma • malignant: squamous cell carcinoma, esthesioneuroblastoma Inflammation • rhinitis: allergic, non-allergic • infections: bacterial, viral, fungal Idiopathic
Systemic	Coagulopathies • meds: anticoagulants, NSAIDs • hemophilias, von Willebrand's • hematological malignancies • liver failure, uremia Vascular: hypertension, atherosclerosis, Osler-Weber-Rendu Others: Wegener's, SLE	

Investigations

- CBC, PT/PTT (if indicated)
- x-ray, CT as needed

Treatment

- aim is to localize bleeding and achieve hemostasis

1. First-aid

- ABC's
- patient leans forward to minimize swallowing blood
- constant firm pressure applied for 20 min on soft part of nose (not bony pyramid)

2. Assess Blood Loss (can be potentially fatal hemorrhage)

- pulse, blood pressure, and other signs of shock
- IV NS, cross match for 2 units packed RBCs if significant

3. Determine Site of Bleeding

- insert cotton pledget of 4% topical lidocaine ± topical decongestant cocaine, visualize nasal cavity with speculum and aspirate excess blood and clots
- anterior/posterior hemorrhage defined by location in relationship to bony septum
- if suspicion, coagulation studies

4. Control the Bleeding

- first line topical vasoconstrictors (Otrivin™, cocaine)
- if first line fails and bleeding adequately visualized, cauterize with silver nitrate
- do not attempt to cauterize both sides of the septum at one time due to risk of septal perforation from loss of septal blood supply

Special Cases
- Adolescent male with unilateral recurrent epistaxis consider juvenile nasopharyngeal angiofibroma (JNA). This is the most common benign tumour of the nasopharynx

- Thrombocytopenic patients – use resorbable packs to avoid risk of re-bleeding caused by pulling out the removable pack.

A. Anterior hemorrhage treatment
  - if fail to achieve hemostasis with cauterization
  - anterior pack with half inch Vaseline™ and ribbon gauze strips or absorbable packing (i.e. Gelfoam™) layered from nasal floor toward nasal roof extending to posterior choanae for 2 to 3 days
  - can also attempt packing with Merocel™ or nasal tampons of different shapes

B. Posterior hemorrhage treatment
  - if unable to visualize bleeding source, then usually posterior source
  - different ways of placing a posterior pack with a Foley catheter, gauze pack or Epistat™ balloon
  - bilateral anterior pack is layered into position
  - antibiotics for any posterior pack or any pack in longer than 48 hours
  - admit to hospital with packs in for 3 to 5 days
  - watch for complications: hypoxemia (naso-pulmonic reflex), toxic shock syndrome (Rx: remove packs immediately), pharyngeal fibrosis/stenosis, alar/septal necrosis, aspiration

C. If anterior/posterior packs fail to control epistaxis
  - selective catheterization and embolization of branches of external carotid artery
  - ± septoplasty
  - vessel ligation of
    - anterior/posterior ethmoid artery
    - internal maxillary
    - external carotid

5. Prevention
- prevent drying of nasal mucosa with humidifiers, saline spray, or topical ointments
- avoidance of irritants
- medical management of hypertension and coagulopathies

Hoarseness

If hoarseness present for >2 weeks in a smoker, laryngoscopy must be done to rule out malignancy.
Acute <2 weeks, chronic >2 weeks.

Definitions
- **hoarseness**: change in voice quality, ranging from voice harshness to voice weakness reflects abnormalities anywhere along the vocal tract from oral cavity to lungs
- **dysphonia**: a general alteration in voice quality
- **aphonia**: no sound is emanated from vocal folds

Acute Laryngitis

Etiology
- viral: influenza, adenovirus
- bacterial: Group A Streptococcus
- acute voice strain → submucosal hemorrhage → vocal cord edema → hoarseness
- toxic fume inhalation

Clinical Features
- URTI symptoms, hoarseness, aphonia, cough attacks, ± dyspnea
- true vocal cords erythematous/edematous with vascular injection and normal mobility

Treatment
- self-limited, resolves within ~1 week
- voice rest
- humidification
- hydration
- avoid irritants (e.g. smoking)
- treat with antibiotics if there is evidence of coexistent bacterial pharyngitis

Vocal Cord Paralysis
Unilateral – affected cord lies in the parmedian position, inadequate glottic closure during phonation → weak, breathy voice
Bilateral – cords rest in midline therefore voice remains good but respiratory function is compromised and may present as stridor
Treatment options – voice therapy, injection laryngoplasty (collagen, fat), cord medialization

Chronic Laryngitis

Definition
- long standing inflammatory changes in laryngeal mucosa

Etiology
- repeated attacks of acute laryngitis
- chronic irritants (dust, smoke, chemical fumes)
- chronic voice strain

- chronic sinusitis with postnasal drip (PND)
- chronic alcohol use
- esophageal disorders: GERD, Zenker's diverticulum, hiatus hernia
- systemic: allergy, hypothyroidism, Addison's

Clinical Features
- chronic dysphonia – rule out malignancy
- cough, globus sensation, frequent throat clearing 2° to GERD
- cords erythematous, thickened with ulceration/granuloma formation and normal mobility

Treatment
- remove offending irritants
- treat related disorders e.g. antisecretory therapy for GERD
- speech therapy with voice rest
- ± antibiotics, ± steroids to decrease inflammation

Vocal Cord Polyps

Definition
- structural manifestation of vocal cord irritation
- acutely, polyp forms 2° to capillary damage in the subepithelial space during extreme voice exertion

Etiology
- voice strain (muscle tension dysphonia)
- laryngeal irritants (GERD, allergies, tobacco)
- most common benign tumour of vocal cords

Epidemiology
- 30 to 50 years of age
- M>F

Clinical Features
- hoarseness, aphonia, cough attacks ± dyspnea
- pedicled or sessile polyp on free edge of vocal cord
- typically asymmetrical, soft and smooth
- more common on the anterior 1/3 of the vocal cord
- intermittent respiratory distress with large polyps

Treatment
- avoid irritants
- endoscopic laryngeal microsurgical removal

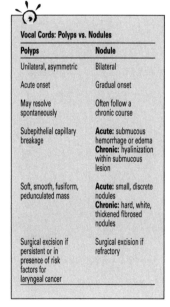

Vocal Cords: Polyps vs. Nodules

Polyps	Nodule
Unilateral, asymmetric	Bilateral
Acute onset	Gradual onset
May resolve spontaneously	Often follow a chronic course
Subepithelial capillary breakage	**Acute:** submucous hemorrhage or edema **Chronic:** hyalinization within submucous lesion
Soft, smooth, fusiform, pedunculated mass	**Acute:** small, discrete nodules **Chronic:** hard, white, thickened fibrosed nodules
Surgical excision if persistent or in presence of risk factors for laryngeal cancer	Surgical excision if refractory

Vocal Cord Nodules

Definition
- vocal cord callus
- "screamer's or singer's nodules"

Etiology
- early nodules occur 2° to submucous hemorrhage
- mature nodules result from hyalinization which occurs with long term voice abuse
- chronic voice strain
- URTI, smoke, alcohol

Epidemiology
- frequently in singers, children, bartenders, and school teachers
- F>M

Clinical Features
- hoarseness worst at end of day
- on laryngoscopy:
    - red, soft nodules
    - often bilateral
    - at the junction of the anterior 1/3 and posterior 2/3 of the vocal cords – point of maximal cord vibration
- chronic nodules may become fibrotic, hard, and white

Treatment
- voice rest
- hydration
- speech therapy
- avoid irritants
- surgery rarely indicated for refractory nodules

Benign Laryngeal Papillomas

Etiology
- human papilloma virus (HPV) types 6, 11
- ?hormonal influence, ?acquired during delivery

Epidemiology
- biphasic distribution – 1) birth to puberty (most common laryngeal tumour) and 2) adulthood

Clinical Features
- hoarseness/"frog voice" and airway obstruction
- can seed into tracheobronchial tree
- highly recurrent
- some juvenile papillomas resolve spontaneously at puberty
- papillomas in adults may undergo malignant transformation
- laryngoscopy shows wart-like lesions in supraglottic larynx and trachea

Treatment
- CO_2 laser and microsurgery
- adjuvants under investigation: interferon, cidofovir, acyclovir
- Gardasil HPV vaccine may prevent/decrease the incidence but more research is needed

Laryngeal Carcinoma

- see *Neoplasms of the Head and Neck* section, OT34

Salivary Glands

Sialadenitis

Definition
- inflammation of salivary glands

Etiology
- viral most common (mumps)
- bacterial causes: *S. aureus, S. pneumoniae, H. influenzae*
- obstructive vs. non-obstructive
- obstructive infection involves salivary stasis and bacterial retrograde flow

Predisposing Factors
- HIV
- anorexia/bulimia
- Sjogren's syndrome
- Cushing's, hypothyroidism, DM
- hepatic/renal failure
- meds that increase stasis: diuretics, TCAs, β-blockers, anticholinergics, antibiotics

Clinical Features
- acute onset of pain and edema of parotid or submandibular gland that may lead to marked swelling
- ± fever
- ± leukocytosis
- ± suppurative drainage from punctum of the gland

Mumps usually presents with bilateral parotid enlargement, ± sensorineural hearing loss, ± orchitis.

Investigations
- U/S imaging to differentiate obstructive vs. non-obstructive sialadenitis

Treatment
- bacterial: treat with cloxacillin ± abscess drainage
- viral: no treatment

Sialolithiasis

Definition
- ductal stone (mainly hydroxyapatite) leading to chronic sialadenitis
- 80% in submandibular gland, <20% in parotid gland, ~1% in sublingual gland

Risk Factors
- any condition causing duct stenosis or a change in salivary secretions
  (e.g. dehydration, diabetes, EtOH, hypercalcemia)

Clinical Features
- pain and tenderness over involved gland
- intermittent swelling related to meals
- digital palpation reveals presence of calculi

Investigations
- sialogram

Treatment
- may resolve spontaneously
- encourage salivation to clear calculus
- remove calculi by dilating duct and orifice or excision through floor of mouth
- if calculus is within the gland parenchyma then the whole gland must be excised

Enlargement of the parotid glands may be a manifestation of a systemic disease, such as Sjögren's or bulimia.

Salivary Gland Neoplasms

Etiology
- anatomic distribution
  - parotid gland: 70 to 85%
  - submandibular gland: 8 to 15%
  - sublingual gland: 1%
  - minor salivary glands, most concentrated in hard palate: 5 to 8%
- malignant (see Tables 16 and 19)
- benign
  - benign mixed (pleomorphic adenoma): 80%
  - Warthin's tumour (5 to 10% bilateral, M>F): 10%
  - cysts, lymph nodes and adenomas: 10%
  - oncocytoma: <1%

Epidemiology
- 3 to 6% of all head and neck neoplasms in adults
- mean age at presentation: 55 to 65
- M=F

A mass sitting above an imaginary line drawn between the mastoid process and angle of the mandible is a parotid neoplasm until proven otherwise.

Parotid Gland Neoplasms

Clinical Features
- 80% benign (pleomorphic adenoma most common), 20% malignant (mucoepidermoid most common)
- painless slow-growing mass
- if bilateral, suggests benign process (Warthin's tumour, Sjögren's, bulimia, mumps) or possible lymphoma

Investigations
- fine needle aspiration biopsy
- CT or MRI to determine extent of tumour

DDx Parotid Tumour
Benign
1. pleomorphic adenoma
2. Warthin's tumour
3. cyst

Malignant
1. mucoepidermoid
2. adenoid cystic carcinoma
3. acinic cell carcinoma

Treatment
- treatment of choice is surgery for all salivary gland neoplasms – benign and malignant
- benign tumours are excised due to risk of malignant transformation
  - pleomorphic adenoma → carcinoma ex-pleomorphic adenoma
- superficial lesion
  - superficial parotidectomy above plane of CN VII, ± radiation
  - incisional biopsy contraindicated
- deep lesion
  - near-total parotidectomy sparing as much of CN VII as possible
  - if CN VII involved then it is removed and cable grafted
- complications of parotid surgery
  - hematoma, infection, salivary fistula, temporary facial paresis, Frey's syndrome (gustatory sweating)

Prognosis
- benign: excellent, <5% of pleomorphic adenomas may recur

Neck Masses

Approach to a Neck Mass

- ensure that the neck mass is not a normal neck structure (hyoid, transverse process of C1 vertebra)

Zones of Injury to the Neck
- Clavicle → inferior border of cricoid cartilage
  - injuries here have highest mortality
  - angiography, esophagoscopy
- Cricoid → angle of mandible
  - most common site, lower mortality due to good accessibility
  - to OR for surgical exploration
- Angle of mandible → skull base
  - angiography

Table 15. Acquired Causes of Neck Lumps According to Age

Age (yrs)	Possible Causes of Neck Lump
<20	• inflammatory neck nodes (tonsillitis, infectious mononucleosis, Kawasaki's) • lymphoma
20-40	• HIV • salivary gland (calculi, infection, tumour) • thyroid (goitre, infection, tumour) • granulomatous disease (TB, sarcoidosis)
>40	• primary or secondary malignant disease

Rule of 7s for Duration of Symptoms of a Neck Mass
7 days: inflammatory
7 months: neoplastic
7 year: congenital

Evaluation

Investigations
- history and physical (including nasopharynx and larynx)
- laboratory investigations
  - WBC – infection vs. lymphoma
  - Mantoux TB test
  - thyroid function tests and scan
- imaging
  - neck U/S
  - CT scan
  - angiography – vascularity and blood supply to mass
  - radiologic exam of stomach, bowel and sinuses
- biopsy – for histologic examination
  - fine needle aspiration (FNA) – least invasive
  - needle biopsy
  - open biopsy – for lymphoma
- identification of primary tumour
  - panendoscopy: nasopharyngoscopy, laryngoscopy, esophagoscopy, bronchoscopy with washings, and biopsy of suspicious lesions
  - biopsy of normal tissue of nasopharynx, tonsils, base of tongue, and hypopharynx
  - primary identified 95% of time → stage and treat
  - primary occult 5% of time – excisional biopsy of node for histologic diagnosis → manage with radiotherapy and/or neck dissection (squamous cell carcinoma)

Inflammatory vs. Neoplastic Neck Masses

	Inflammatory	Neoplastic
History		
painful	Y	N
H&N infection	Y	N
fever	Y	N
weight loss	N	Y
CA risk factors	N	Y
age	younger	older
Physical		
tender	Y	N
rubbery	Y	occ.
rock hard	N	Y
mobile	Y	±fixed
size	<2cm	>2cm

Congenital Neck Masses in Detail

Branchial Cleft Cysts/Fistulae

Embryology
- at 6th week of development, the 2nd branchial arch grows over the 3rd and 4th arches and fuses with the neighbouring caudal pre-cardial swelling forming the cervical sinus
- 3 types of malformations:
  1) branchial fistula – persistent communication between skin and GI tract
  2) branchial sinus – blind-ended tract opening to skin
  3) branchial cyst – persistent cervical sinus with no external opening

Clinical Features
- 2nd branchial cleft malformations most common
  - fistulas present in infancy as a small opening anterior to the sternocleidomastoid muscle
  - cysts present as a smooth, painless, slowly enlarging lateral neck mass, often following an URTI
- 1st branchial groove malformations present as pre-auricular pit/sinus

Treatment
- surgical removal of cyst or fistula tract
- if infected – allow infection to settle before removal

Thyroglossal Duct Cysts

Embryology
- thyroid originates as ventral midline diverticulum of floor of pharynx caudal to junction of 3rd and 4th branchial arches (foramen cecum)
- thyroid migrates caudally along a tract then curves underneath and down to cricoid; thyroglossal duct cysts are vestigial remnants of tract

Clinical Features
- usually presents in the 2nd to 4th decades as a midline cyst that elevates with swallowing and tongue protrusion

Treatment
- pre-operative antibiotics to reduce inflammation
- potential for neoplastic transformation so complete excision of cyst and tract up to foramen cecum at base of tongue with removal of central portion of hyoid bone (Sistrunk procedure)

Cystic Hygroma

Definition
- lymphangioma arising from vestigial lymph channels of neck

Clinical Features
- usually presents by age 2
- thin-walled cyst extending from floor of mouth to mediastinum, usually in posterior triangle or supraclavicular area
- usually painless, soft, compressible
- infection causes a sudden increase in size

Treatment
- surgical excision if it fails to regress – difficult dissection due to numerous cyst extensions

Neoplasms of the Head and Neck

Pre-Malignant Disease
- leukoplakia
  - hyperkeratosis
  - risk of malignant tranformation 5 to 20%
- erythroplakia
  - red superficial patches adjacent to normal mucosa
  - commonly associated with epithelial dysplasia
  - associated with carcinoma in situ or invasive tumour in 40% of cases
- dysplasia
  - histopathologic presence of mitoses and prominent nucleoli
  - involvement of entire mucosal thickness = carcinoma in situ
  - associated progression to invasive cancer in 15 to 30% of cases

Investigations
- initial metastatic screen includes chest x-ray
- scans of liver, brain, and bone only if clinically indicated
- TNM (tumour, nodes, metastases) classification varies slightly depending on the specific type of head and neck tumour (see Table 17)
- TNM classification widely used for staging in order to:
  - guide treatment
  - indicate prognosis
  - evaluate results of treatment
  - facilitate accurate exchange of information
- CT scan is superior to MRI for the detection of pathologic nodal disease and bone cortex invasion
- MRI is superior to discriminate tumour from mucus and to detect bone marrow invasion

Treatment
- treatment depends on
  - histologic grade of tumour
  - stage
  - physical and psychological health of patient
  - facilities available
  - expertise and experience of the medical and surgical oncology team
- in general
  - 1° surgery for malignant oral cavity tumours with radiotherapy reserved for salvage or poor prognostic indicators
  - 1° radiotherapy for nasopharynx, oropharynx, hypopharynx, larynx malignancies with surgery reserved for salvage
  - palliative chemotherapy for metastatic or incurable disease
  - concomitant chemotherapy or alternating chemoradiotherapy may ↑ survival in resectable/unresectable disease
  - chemotherapy has a role as induction therapy prior to surgery and radiation
- panendoscopy to detect primary disease when lymph node metastasis is identified

Prognosis
- synchronous tumours occur in 9 to 15% of patients
- late development of 2nd primary most common cause of post-treatment failure after 36 months

Detection of cervical lymph nodes on physical examination:
False negative rate 15 to 30%
False positive rate 30 to 40%

Pathological lymphadenopathy defined radiographically as:
1. a node >1.5 cm in diameter
2. a node of any size which contains central necrosis

Common sites of distant metastases for head and neck neoplasms:
lungs > liver > bones

Table 16. Quick Look-Up Summary of Head and Neck Malignancies – Etiology and Epidemiology

Etiology	Epidemiology	Risk Factors
Oral Cavity		
95% SCC	50% on anterior 2/3 of tongue	smoking/EtOH
others : sarcoma, melanoma,	mean age: 50 to 60	poor oral hygiene
minor salivary gland tumour	M>F	leukoplakia, erythroplakia
	most common site of H&N cancers	UV light - lip
Nose and Paranasal Sinus		
75 to 80% SCC	mean age: 50 to 70	wood/shoe/textile industry
then adenoCA and mucoepidermoid	rare tumours	hardwood dust (nasal / ethmoid sinus)
99% in maxillary / ethmoid sinus	↓incidence in last 5 to 10 years	nickel, chromium (maxillary sinus)
10% arise from minor salivary glands		air pollution
		chronic sinusitis
		HPV infection – role unclear
Carcinoma of the Pharynx – Subtypes (Nasopharynx, Oropharynx, Hypopharynx and Larynx)		
Nasopharynx		
90% SCC	incidence 0.8 per 100,000	Epstein-Barr virus (EBV)
~10% lymphoma	100x ↑ in southern Chinese	salted fish
	M:F= 2.4:1	nickel exposure
	mean age: 50 to 59	poor oral hygiene
		southern Chinese
Oropharynx		
95% SCC - poorly differentiated	M:F = 4:1	smoking/EtOH
	mean age: 50 to 70	
Hypopharynx		
95% SCC	M>F	smoking/EtOH
3 sites - piriform sinus (60%)	mean age: 50 to 70	
- post-cricoid (30%)	8 to 10% of all H&N cancer	
- post pharyngeal wall (10%)		
Larynx		
SCC most common	45% of all H&N cancer	smoking/EtOH
3 sites - supraglottic (30 to 35%)	M:F = 10:1	
- glottic (60 to 65%)	mean age: 45 to 75	
- subglottic (1%)		
Salivary Gland (see *Salivary Gland* section)		
40% mucoepidermoid	rate of malignancy:	
30% adenoid cystic	parotid 15 to 25%	
5% acinic cell	submandibular 37 to 43%	
5% malignant mixed	minor salivary >80%	
5% lymphoma	3 to 6% of all H&N cancer	
	mean age: 55 to 65	
	M=F	
Thyroid (90% benign – 10% malignant)		
60 to 70% papillary	children	radiation exposure
15 to 20% follicular	adults <30 or >60	family history – papillary CA or multiple
2 to 5% anaplastic	nodules more common in females	endocrine neoplasia (MEN) II
2 to 5% medullary	malignancy more common in males	older age
1 to 5% Hurthle cell		male
3% lymphoma		papillary – Gardner's, Cowden's,
1 to 2% metastatic		familial adenomatous polyposis (FAP)
Parathyroid		
	rare tumour	
	mean age: 44 to 55 years	

Table 17. TNM Classification of Head and Neck Cancers

Tumour size		Nodal Status		Distant Metastasis	
Tis	Tumour in situ	Nx	Unable to assess regional lymph nodes	Mx	Unable to assess metastasis
T1	Tumour <2 cm	N0	No palpable lymph nodes (clinically node negative)	M0	No metastasis
T2	Tumour >2 cm and <4 cm	N1	Metastasis to ipsilateral node <3 cm	M1	Evidence of metastasis
T3	Tumour >4 cm	N2a	Metastasis to single ipsilateral node 3 to 6 cm		
T4	Tumour >4 cm with local	N2b	In greatest diameter		
	extension into other tissues		Metastasis to multiple ipsilateral nodes <6 cm		
		N2c	Metastasis to bilateral or contralateral nodes <6 cm		
		N3	Metastasis to node >6 cm in greatest dimension		

Table 18. TNM Classification of Laryngeal Cancer

Supraglottis		Glottis		Subglottis	
T1	Limited to one subsite, with normal vocal cord mobility	T1	Limited to the vocal cord(s), with normal mobility	T1	Limited to the subglottis
T2	Invades mucosa > 1 adjacent subsite of supraglottis or glottis or a region outside the supraglottis, without fixation of larynx	T1a	Limited to one vocal cord	T2	Extends to the vocal cord(s) with normal/impaired mobility
		T1b	Limited to both vocal cords	T3	Limited to the larynx with vocal cord fixation
		T2	Extends to the supraglottis and/or subglottis, and/or with impaired cord mobility		
T3	Limited to larynx with vocal cord fixation and/or invasion of postcricoid area, pre-epiglottic tissues, paraglottic space, and/or minor thyroid cartilage erosion	T3	Limited to the larynx with vocal cord fixation	T4a	Invades the cricoid or thyroid cartilage and/or tissues beyond the larynx
		T4a	Invades through the thyroid cartilage and/or tissues beyond the larynx		
T4a	Invades through the thyroid cartilage and/or tissues beyond the larynx	T4b	Invades the prevertebral space, encases the carotid artery, or invades the mediastinal structures	T4b	Invades the prevertebral space, encases the carotid artery, or invades the mediastinal structures
T4b	Invades prevertebral space, encases the carotid artery, or invades the mediastinal structures				

Table 19. Quick Look-Up Summary of Head and Neck Malignancies – Diagnosis and Treatment

Clinical Features	Investigations	Treatment	Prognosis
Oral Cavity asymptomatic neck mass (30%) non-healing ulcer ± bleeding dysphagia, sialorrhea, dysphonia oral fetor, otalgia leukoplakia or erythroplakia (pre-malignant changes or CIS)	biopsy CT	1° surgery local resection ± neck dissection ± reconstruction 2° radiation	5 year: T1/T2: 75% T3/T4: 30 to 35% poor prognostic indicators: depth of invasion, close surgical margins location (tongue worse than floor of mouth) cervical nodes, extra capsular spread
Nose and Paranasal Sinus **Early symptoms:** unilateral nasal obstruction epistaxis, rhinorrhea **Late symptoms:** 2° to invasion of nose, orbit, nerves, oral cavity, skin, skull base, cribriform plate	CT/MRI biopsy	surgery and radiation chemoradiotherapy for unresectable disease	5 year: 30 to 60% poor prognosis 2° to late presentation
Carcinoma of the Pharynx - Subtypes **Nasopharynx** cervical nodes (60 to 90%) nasal obstruction, epistaxis unilateral AOM ± hearing loss CN III to VI, IX to XII (25%) proptosis, voice change, dysphagia	nasopharyngoscopy biopsy CT/MRI	1° radiation 2° surgery	5 year survival I: 79% II: 72% III 50 to 60% IV: 36 to 42%
Oropharynx odynophagia, otalgia ulcerated/enlarged tonsil fixed tongue/trismus/dysarthria oral fetor, bloody sputum cervical lymphadenopathy (60%) distal mets : lung/bone/liver (7%)	biopsy CT	1° radiation 2° surgery local resection ± neck dissection ± reconstruction	base of tongue - control rates T1: >90% T4: 13 to 52% tonsils - cure rate T1/T2: 90 to 100% T4: 15 to 33%
Hypopharynx dysphagia, odynophagia otalgia, hoarseness cervical lymphadenopathy	pharyngogoscopy biopsy CXR r/o lung mets CT	1° radiation 2° surgery	T2/T3 cure rate: 60% T4/5 year survival: 25 to 40%
Larynx dysphagia, odynophagia, globus otalgia, hoarseness, dyspnea/stridor cough/hemoptysis cervical nodes (rare w/glottic CA)	laryngoscopy CT/MRI	1° radiation 2° surgery 1° surgery for bulky T4	5 year T4 >40% (surgery w/ radiation) control rate early lesions >90% (radiation) 10 to 12% of small lesions fail radiotherapy

The smaller the salivary gland the greater the likelihood that a mass in the gland is malignant.

Table 19. Quick Look-Up Summary of Head and Neck Malignancies – Diagnosis and Treatment (continued)

Clinical Features	Investigations	Treatment	Prognosis
Salivary Gland			
painless mass	fine needle aspirate	surgery	**Parotid** 10-year survival:
CN VII - parotid mass	CT	benign & malignant	85, 69, 43, and 14% for stages I to IV
cervical lymphadenopathy		lymph node sampling	**Submandibular**
rapid growth		post-op radiotherapy	2 year: 82%, 5 year: 69%
invasion of skin		chemo if unresectable	**Minor salivary gland**
constitutional signs/symptoms			10 year: 83, 52, 25, 23% for stages I to IV
Thyroid			
thyroid mass, cervical nodes	FNA	1° surgery	Recurrences occur within 5 years
vocal cord paralysis	U/S	I¹³¹ for metastatic deposits	Need long-term f/u: clinical exam, TSH
hyper/hypothyroidism	thyroid scan	post-op TSH suppression	
dysphagia	(See Table 22)		
Parathyroid			
↑ serum Ca		wide surgical excision	Recurrence rates: 1-year 27%
neck mass		post-op monitoring of serum Ca	5-year 82%
bone disease, renal disease			10-year 91%
pancreatitis			Mean survival: 6 to 7 years

Table 20. Cytology results of FNA Samples

Category	Characteristics
Non-diagnostic	
Benign	Macrofollicular or colloid adenomas, chronic autoimmune (Hashimoto's) thyroiditis
Suspicious or indeterminate	Microfollicular or cellular neoplasm
Malignant	

Thyroid Carcinoma

Table 21. Thyroid Carcinoma

	Papillary	Follicular	Medullary	Anaplastic	Lymphoma
Incidence (% of all thyroid cancers)	70 to 75 %	10%	3 to 5% (10% familial 90% sporadic)	2 to 5%	<1% 2% of extranodal lymphomas
Route of Spread	lymphatic	hematogenous	lymphatic & hematogenous		
Histology	Orphan Annie nuclei Psammoma bodies	capsular/blood vessel invasion influences prognosis	amyloid may secrete calcitonin, prostaglandins, ACTH, serotonin, kallikrein or bradykinin	giant cells spindle cells	
Other	**P's** - papillary cancer **P**opular (most common) **P**alpable lymph nodes **P**ositive I¹³¹ uptake **P**ositive prognosis **P**ost-op I¹³¹ scan to diagnose treatments	**F's** - follicular cancer **F**ar away mets **F**emale (3:1) **F**NA, NOT (can't be diagnosed by FNA) **F**avourable prognosis	**M's** - medullary cancer **M**ultiple endocrine neoplasia (MEN IIa or IIb) **a**Myloid **M**edian node dissection	more common in elderly 70% in women 20 to 30% have Hx of differentiated thyroid Ca (mostly papillary) or nodular goitres rapidly enlarging neck mass	usually non-Hodgkin's rapidly enlarging goitre Hashimoto's thyroiditis ↑ risk 60x 4:1 female predominance dysphagia, dyspnea, stridor, hoarseness, neck pain, facial edema accompanied by "B" symptoms *
Prognosis	98% at 10 years	92% at 10 years	50% at 10 years 20% at 10 years if detected when clinically palpable	20 to 35% at 1 year 13% at 10 years	5 year survival Stage IE 55%-80% Stage IIE 20%-50% Stage IIE/IV 15%-35%
Treatment	**small tumours:** near total thyroidectomy or lobectomy **diffuse/bilateral:** total thyroidectomy post-op I¹³¹ tx	**small tumours:** near total thyroidectomy/lobectomy/ isthmectomy **large/diffuse tumours:** total thyroidectomy	total thyroidectomy median lymph node dissection if lateral cervical nodes +ve modified neck dissection post-op thyroxine tracheostomy screen asymptomatic relatives	**small tumours:** total thyroidectomy ± external beam	non-surgical combined radiation chemotherapy (CHOP**)

*B symptoms = fever, night sweats, weight loss >10% in 6 mos   ** CHOP = cyclophosphamide, adriamycin, vincristine, prednisone

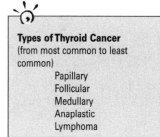

Types of Thyroid Cancer
(from most common to least common)
       Papillary
       Follicular
       Medullary
       Anaplastic
       Lymphoma

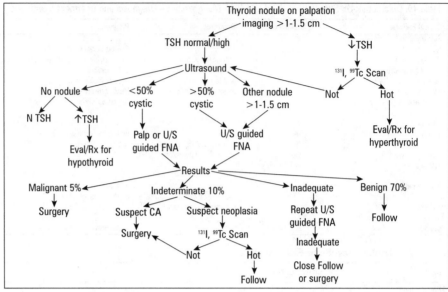

Figure 20. Approach to Thyroid Nodule

Table 22. Investigation of the Thyroid Nodule

Lab Tests	Imaging	Invasive Tests
TSH and T_4	U/S*	FNA
Thyroglobulin and anti-thyroid peroxidase antibody	Thyroid scan	

Table 23. Management of the Thyroid Nodule

Treatment	Indications
Radioiodine therapy	Hyperthyroid with suspicious solid mass, that is HOT on thyroid scan
Chemotherapy and / or radiotherapy	Anaplastic Ca or thyroid lymphoma
Surgical excision	Recurrent cyst that is "suspicious" on FNA or if patient is extremely anxious Malignancy other than anaplastic CA or thyroid lymphoma Solid "suspicious" mass that is "cold" on thyroid scan (excise to r/o capsular invasion) Hyperthyroid with suspicious solid mass, that is HOT on thyroid scan

*U/S findings: cystic: risk of malignancy < 1%, solid: risk of malignancy approx. 10%, solid with cystic components: risk of malignancy same as if solid

Pediatric Otolaryngology

Acute Otitis Media (AOM)

Definition
- acute inflammation of middle ear

Epidemiology
- 60 to 70% of children have at least 1 episode of AOM before 3 years of age
- 18 months to 6 years most common age group
- peak incidence January to April
- one third of children have had 3 or more episodes by age 3

Etiology
- *S. pneumoniae* – 35% of cases (incidence decreasing due to pneumococcus vaccine)
- *H. influenzae* – 25% of cases
- *M. catarrhalis* – 10% of cases
- *S. aureus* and *S. pyogenes* (all β-lactamase producing)
- anaerobes (newborns)
- gram negative enterics (infants)
- viral

Predisposing Factors
- eustachian tube dysfunction/obstruction
  - swelling of tubal mucosa
    - upper respiratory tract infection (URTI)
    - allergies/allergic rhinitis
    - chronic sinusitis
  - obstruction/infiltration of eustachian tube ostium
    - tumour – nasopharyngeal carcinoma (adults)
    - adenoid hypertrophy (not due to obstruction but by maintaining a source of infection)
    - barotrauma (sudden changes in air pressure)
  - inadequate tensor palati function – cleft palate (even after repair)
  - abnormal spatial orientation of eustachian tube
    - Down's syndrome (horizontal position of eustachian tube), Crouzon's, and Apert's syndrome
- disruption of action of:
  - cilia of eustachian tube – Kartagener's syndrome
  - mucus secreting cells
  - capillary network that provides humoral factors, PMNs, phagocytic cells
- immunosuppression/deficiency due to chemotherapy, steroids, diabetes mellitus, hypogammaglobulinemia, cystic fibrosis

Risk Factors
- bottle feeding, pacifier use
- passive smoke
- crowded living conditions (day care/group child care facilities) or sick contacts
- male
- family history (presumably due to eustachian tube or middle ear anatomy)

Pathogenesis
- obstruction of eustachian tube → air absorbed in middle ear → negative pressure (an irritant to middle ear mucosa) → edema of mucosa with exudate/effusion → infection of exudate from nasopharyngeal secretions

Clinical Features
- triad of otalgia, fever (especially in younger children), and conductive hearing loss
- rarely tinnitus, vertigo, and/or facial nerve paralysis
- otorrhea if tympanic membrane perforated
- pain over mastoid
- infants/toddlers
  - ear-tugging
  - hearing loss, balance disturbances (mild)
  - irritable, poor sleeping
  - vomiting and diarrhea
  - anorexia
- otoscopy of tympanic membrane
  - hyperemia
  - bulging
  - loss of landmarks: handle and short process of malleus not visible

Treatment
- antibiotic treatment hastens resolution – 10 day course
  - 1st line:
    - amoxicillin 40 mg/kg/day divided into two doses – safe, effective, and inexpensive
    - if penicillin allergic: macrolide (clarithromycin, azithromycin), trimethoprim-sulphamethoxazole (Bactrim™)
  - 2nd line (for amoxicillin failures):
    - double dose of amoxicillin (80 mg/kg/day), amoxicillin-clavulinic acid (Clavulin™)
    - cephalosporins: cefuroxime axetil (Ceftin™), ceftriaxone IM (Rocephin™), cefaclor (Ceclor™), cefixime (Suprax™)
  - AOM deemed unresponsive if clinical signs/symptoms and otoscopic findings persist beyond 48 hours of antibiotic treatment
- symptomatic therapy
  - antipyretics/analgesics (e.g. acetaminophen)
  - decongestants – may relieve nasal congestion but does not treat AOM
- prevention
  - parent education about risk factors (see above)
  - antibiotic prophylaxis – amoxicillin or macrolide shown effective at half therapeutic dose
  - pneumococcal and influenza vaccine

Antibiotics for acute otitis media in children
Cochrane Database of Systematic Reviews 2004;1
Study: Meta-analysis of Randomized Controlled Trials (RCTs) on children (>6 mo) with acute otitis media comparing any antibiotic regime to placebo.
Data Sources: Cochrane Central Register of Controlled Trials (2003 issue 1), MEDLINE (January 2000 to March 2003), and EMBASE (January 1990 to March 2003) without language restrictions.
Main Outcomes: 1) Pain at 24 hours, and 2-7 days. 2) Hearing measured by tympanometry at 1 and 3 months. Patients: Pain: 24 hours, 4 studies (n=717); 2-7 days 9 studies (n=2287). Hearing: 1 month, 3 studies (n=472); 3 months, 2 studies (n=370).
Results: Treatment with antibiotics had no significant impact on pain at 24 hours. However, pain at 2-7 days was lower in the antibiotic groups with an NNT of 16 (p<0.00001). Antibiotics had no significant effect on hearing.
Conclusion: The role of antibiotics is largely restricted to pain control. This can also be achieved by analgesics. Therefore, parents should be counseled that other analgesics may be a safer option.

- surgery
  - choice of surgical therapy for recurrent AOM depends on whether local factors (eustachian tube dysfunction) are responsible (use ventilation tubes), or regional disease factors (tonsillitis, adenoid hypertrophy, sinusitis) are responsible

Indications for Myringotomy and Tympanostomy tubes in Recurrent AOM and OME (tubes are more commonly inserted for OME, rarely for AOM)
- persistent effusion >3 months (OME)
- lack of response to >3 months of antibiotic therapy (OME)
- persistent effusion for ≥3 months after episode of AOM (OME)
- recurrent episodes of AOM (>7 episodes in 6 months)
- bilateral conductive hearing loss of >20 dB (OME)
- chronic retraction of the tympanic membrane or pars flaccida (OME)
- bilateral OME lasting >4 to 6 mos
- craniofacial anomalies predisposing to middle ear infections (e.g. cleft palate) (OME)
- complications of AOM

McIsaac WJ. Coyte PC. Croxford R. Asche CV. Friedberg J. Feldman W. Otolaryngologists' perceptions of the indications for tympanostomy tube insertion in children. *CMAJ*. 162(9):1285-8, 2000 May 2.
Myringotomy and tympanostomy tubes. In: 2000 clinical indicators compendium. Alexandria (VA): American Academy of Otolaryngology-Head and Neck Surgery; 1999.

Complications of AOM
- otologic
  - TM perforation
  - chronic suppurative OM
  - ossicular necrosis
  - cholesteatoma
  - persistent effusion (often leading to hearing loss)
- CNS
  - meningitis
  - brain abscess
  - facial nerve paralysis
- other
  - mastoiditis
  - labyrinthitis
  - sigmoid sinus thrombophlebitis

<aside>
Complications of Tympanostomy Tubes
Early
- extrusion
- blockage
- persistent otorrhea

Late
- myringosclerosis
- persistent TM perforation
- cholesteatoma
</aside>

Otitis Media with Effusion (OME)

Definition
- presence of fluid in the middle ear without signs or symptoms of ear infection

Epidemiology
- not exclusively a pediatric disease
- follows AOM frequently in children:
  - middle ear effusions have been shown to persist following an episode of AOM for 1 mos in 40% of children, 2 mos in 20% and 3+ mos in 10%

Risk Factors
- same as AOM

Clinical Features
- fullness – blocked ear
- hearing loss ± tinnitus
  - confirm with audiogram and tympanogram (flat) (see Figure 16B and 17B)
- ± pain, low grade fever
- otoscopy of tympanic membrane
  - discolouration – amber or dull grey with "glue" ear
  - meniscus fluid level
  - air bubbles
  - retraction pockets/TM atelectasis
  - most reliable finding with pneumotoscopy is immobility

Treatment
- expectant – 90% resolve by 3 months
- document hearing loss
- no statistical proof that antihistamines, decongestants, antibiotics clear disease faster
- surgery: myringotomy ± ventilating tubes ± adenoidectomy (if enlarged)
- ventilating tubes to equalize pressure and drain ear

Complications of Otitis Media with Effusion (OME)
- hearing loss, speech delay, learning problems in young children
- chronic mastoiditis
- ossicular erosion

- cholesteatoma especially when retraction pockets involve pars flaccida or postero-superior TM
- retraction of tympanic membrane, atelectasis, ossicular fixation

Adenoid Hypertrophy

- size peaks at age 5 and resolves by 12 to 18 years of age
- increase in size with repeated URTI and allergies

Clinical Features
- nasal obstruction
    - adenoid facies (open mouth, flat midface, dark circles under eyes)
    - hypernasal voice
    - history of snoring
    - long term mouth breather; minimal air escape through nose
- choanal obstruction
    - chronic sinusitis/rhinitis
    - obstructive sleep apnea
- chronic inflammation
    - nasal discharge, post-nasal drip, and cough
    - cervical lymphadenopathy

Diagnosis
- enlarged adenoids on direct/indirect nasopharyngeal exam
- enlarged adenoid shadow on lateral soft tissue x-ray
- lateral view of the nasopharynx may show a large pad of adenoidal tissue

Complications
- eustachian tube obstruction leading to serous otitis media
- interference with nasal breathing, necessitating mouth-breathing
- malocclusion
- sleep apnea/respiratory disturbance
- orofacial developmental abnormalities

Indications for Adenoidectomy
- chronic upper airway obstruction with sleep disturbance/apnea ± cor pulmonale
- chronic nasopharyngitis resistant to medical treatment
- chronic serous otitis media and chronic suppurative otitis media (after 2-3 sets of tubes)
- recurrent acute otitis media resistant to antibiotics
- suspicion of nasopharyngeal malignancy
- persistent rhinorrhea

Contraindications for Adenoidectomy
- bleeding disorders
- recent pharyngeal infection
- short or abnormal palate (cleft or false palate, zona pellucidum)

Complications of Adenoidectomy
- bleeding, infection
- velopharyngeal insufficiency with speech defect ± nasal regurgitation
- scarring of Eustachian tube orifice

Acute Tonsillitis

Etiology
- Group A β-hemolytic streptococcus and Group G streptococcus
- *S. pneumoniae, S. aureus, H. influenzae, M. catarrhalis*
- Epstein-Barr virus (EBV)

Clinical Features
- symptoms
    - sore throat
    - dysphagia, odynophagia, trismus
    - malaise, fever
    - otalgia (referred)

Trismus: motor disturbance of the trigeminal nerve, leading to spasm of masticatory muscles, with difficulty in opening the mouth (lock-jaw).

- signs
  - tender cervical lymphadenopathy especially submandibular, jugulodigastric
  - tonsils enlarged, inflammation ± exudates/white follicles
  - strawberry tongue, scarletiniform rash (scarlet fever)
  - palatal petechiae (infectious mononucleosis)

Investigations
- CBC
- swab for C&S
- latex agglutination tests
- Monospot – less reliable children <2 years old

Treatment
- bed rest, soft diet, ample fluid intake
- gargle with warm saline solution
- analgesics and antipyretics
- antibiotics
  - only after appropriate swab for C&S
  - 1st line penicillin or amoxicillin (erythromycin if penicillin allergic) x 10 days
  - rheumatic fever risk emerges approximately 9 days after the onset of symptoms: antibiotics are utilized mainly to avoid this serious sequela and to provide earlier symptomatic relief
  - no evidence for the role of antibiotics in the avoidance of post-streptococcal glomerulonephritis

Complications
- deep neck space infection
- abscess: peritonsillar, intratonsillar
- sepsis
- glomerulonephritis

DDx Sore Throat:
Streptococcal pharyngitis
viral pharyngitis
infectious mononucleosis
tonsilitis
peritonsillar abscess
foreign body/trauma
leukemia
Hodgkin's disease

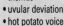

Complications of tonsillitis
(now uncommon due to antibiotics):
• rheumatic heart disease
• arthritis
• scarlet fever
• quinsy (peritonsillar abscess)

Peritonsillar Abscess (Quinsy)

Definition
- cellulitis of space behind tonsillar capsule extending onto soft palate leading to abscess

Etiology
- bacterial: Group A strep (GAS) (50% of cases), *S. pyogenes*, *S. aureus*, *H. influenzae*, and anaerobes

Epidemiology
- can develop from acute tonsillitis with infection spreading into plane of tonsillar bed
- unilateral, most common in 15 to 30 year old age group

Clinical Features
- fever and dehydration
- sore throat, dysphagia and odynophagia
- extensive peritonsillar swelling but tonsil may appear normal
- edema of soft palate
- uvular deviation
- involvement of motor branch of CN V → can lead to increased salivation and trismus
- dysphonia with "hot potato" voice (edema → failure to elevate palate) 2° to CN X involvement
- unilateral referred otalgia
- cervical lymphadenitis

Complications
- aspiration pneumonia 2° to spontaneous rupture of abscess
- airway obstruction
- lateral dissection into parapharyngeal and/or carotid space
- bacteremia

Treatment
- secure airway

Quinsy Triad:
• trismus
• uvular deviation
• hot potato voice

- surgical drainage (incision or needle aspiration) with C&S
- warm saline irrigation
- IV penicillin G x 10 days if cultures positive for GAS
- add oral/IV metronidazole or clindamycin x 10 days if culture +ve for *Bacteroides*
- possible tonsillectomy 6 weeks later with interim oral antibiotic prophylaxis for high risk individuals

Other parapharyngeal space infection
- pharyngitis
- parotitis (see *Salivary Gland* section)
- otitis
- mastoiditis (Bezold's abscess)
- odontogenic infection

Tonsillectomy

Absolute Indications
- acute airway obstruction ± cor pulmonale
- suspected malignancy, especially if unilateral tonsillar hypertrophy (lymphoma/squamous cell carcinoma)
- acute hemorrhage

Relative Indications
- age 1 to 4 years: tonsillar hypertrophy leading to
  - sleep apnea → cor pulmonale
  - mouth breathing → malocclusion
  - difficulty swallowing → FTT
- school age: chronic recurrent tonsillitis if >5 episodes
- any complication of tonsillitis
  - quinsy, parapharyngeal abscess, retropharyngeal abscess
  - strep bacteremia: rheumatic heart disease, nephritis, arthritis
  - strep carrier: infective or halitosis

Airway Problems in Children

DIFFERENTIAL DIAGNOSIS BY AGE GROUP

Neonates (obligate nose breathers)
- extralaryngeal
  - choanal atresia
  - nasopharyngeal dermoid, glioma, encephalocele
  - glossoptosis – Pierre-Robin sequence, Down syndrome, lymphangioma, hemangioma
- laryngeal
  - laryngomalacia – most common cause of stridor in children
  - laryngocele
  - vocal cord palsy (Arnold-Chiari malformations)
  - glottic web
  - subglottic stenosis
  - laryngeal cleft
- tracheal
  - tracheoesophageal fistula
  - tracheomalacia
  - vascular rings

2 to 3 Months
- congenital
  - laryngomalacia
  - vascular: subglottic hemangioma (more common), innominate artery compression, double aortic arch
  - laryngeal papilloma
- acquired
  - subglottic stenosis – post intubation
  - tracheal granulation – post intubation
  - tracheomalacia – post tracheotomy and tracheoesophageal fistula (TEF) repair

Infants – Sudden Onset
- foreign body aspiration
- croup
- bacterial tracheitis
- caustic ingestion
- epiglottitis

Children and Adults
- infection
  - Ludwig's angina
  - peritonsillar-parapharyngeal abscess
  - retropharyngeal abscess
- neoplastic
  - squamous cell carcinoma (SCC) (adults): larynx, hypopharynx
  - retropharyngeal: lymphoma, neuroblastoma
  - nasopharyngeal: carcinoma, rhabdomyosarcoma
- allergic
  - angioneurotic edema
  - polyps (suspect cystic fibrosis in children)
- trauma
  - laryngeal fracture, facial fracture
  - burns and lacerations
  - post-intubation
  - caustic ingestion
- congenital
  - lingual thyroid/tonsil

Signs of Airway Obstruction

Symptoms and signs of airway obstruction require a full assessment to diagnose potentially serious causes.

Stridor
- note quality, timing
- body position important
  - lying prone: subglottic hemangioma, double aortic arch
  - lying supine: laryngomalacia, glossoptosis
- site of stenosis
  - vocal cords or above: inspiratory stridor
  - subglottis and extrathoracic trachea: biphasic stridor
  - distal tracheobronchial tree: expiratory stridor

Respiratory Distress
- nasal flaring
- supraclavicular and intercostal indrawing
- sternal retractions
- use of accessory muscles of respiration
- tachypnea
- cyanosis
- altered LOC

Feeding Difficulty and Aspiration
- supraglottic lesion
- laryngomalacia
- vocal cord paralysis
- post laryngeal cleft → aspiration pneumonia
- tracheoesophageal fistula

Acute Laryngotracheobronchitis (Croup)

- inflammation of tissues in subglottic space ± tracheobronchial tree
- swelling of mucosal lining and associated with thick, viscous, mucopurulent exudate which compromises upper airway (subglottic space narrowest portion of upper airway)
- normal function of ciliated mucous membrane impaired

Etiology
- viral: parainfluenzae I (most common), II, III, influenza A, and B, RSV

Signs of Croup – the 3 S's
Stridor
Subglottic swelling
Seal bark cough

Clinical Features
- age 4 months to 5 years
- preceded by URTI symptoms
- generally occurs at night
- biphasic stridor and croupy cough (loud, sea-lion bark)
- appear less toxic than with epiglottitis
- supraglottic area normal
- rule out foreign body and subglottic stenosis
- "steeple-sign" on AP x-ray of neck
- if recurrent croup, think subglottic stenosis

Treatment
- racemic epinephrine via nebulizer q1 to 2h, prn
- systemic corticosteroids (e.g. dexamethasone, prednisone)
- adequate hydration
- close observation for 3 to 4 hours
- intubation if severe
- hospitalize if poor response to steroids after 4 hours and persistent stridor at rest
- consider alternate diagnosis if poor response to therapy (e.g. bacterial tracheitis)

Acute Epiglottitis

- acute inflammation causing swelling of supraglottic structures of the larynx without involvement of vocal cords

Etiology
- *H. influenzae* type B
- relatively uncommon condition due to HiB vaccine

When managing epiglottitis, it is important not to agitate the child, as this may precipitate complete obstruction.

Clinical Features
- any age, most commonly 1 to 4 years
- rapid onset
- toxic-looking, fever, anorexia, restlessness
- cyanotic/pale, inspiratory stridor, slow breathing, lungs clear with decreased air entry
- prefers sitting up, open mouth, drooling, tongue protruding, sore throat, dysphagia

Investigations and Management
- investigations and physical examination may lead to complete obstruction, thus preparations for intubation or tracheotomy must be made prior to any manipulation
- stat ENT/anesthesia consult(s)
- lateral neck radiograph – cherry-shaped epiglottic swelling ("thumb sign") – only if stable
- WBC (elevated), blood and pharyngeal cultures after intubation

Treatment
- secure airway
- IV access with hydration
- antibiotics – IV cefuroxime, cefotaxime, or ceftriaxone
- moist air
- extubate when leak around tube occurs and afebrile
- watch for meningitis

Subglottic Stenosis

Congenital
- diameter of subglottis <4 mm in neonate (due to thickening of soft tissue of subglottic space or maldevelopment of cricoid cartilage)

Acquired
- following nasotracheal intubation due to
  - long duration
  - trauma of intubation
  - large tube size
  - infection

Clinical Features
- biphasic stridor
- respiratory distress
- recurrent/prolonged croup

Diagnosis
- laryngoscopy
- CT

Treatment
- if soft tissue – laser and steroids
- if cartilage – laryngotracheoplasty (LTP)

Acquired subglottic stenosis is now rare due to the use of smaller, softer tubes and secure taping to prevent movement.

Laryngomalacia

- elongated omega-shaped epiglottis, short aryepiglottic fold, pendulous mucosa
- caused by indrawing of supraglottis on inspiration

Clinical Features
- high-pitched crowing inspiratory stridor at 1 to 2 weeks
- constant or intermittent and more pronounced supine
- usually mild but when severe can be associated with feeding difficulties, leading to failure to thrive

Treatment
- observation is usually sufficient as symptoms usually spontaneously subside by 12 to 18 months
- in the case of severe laryngomalacia, division of the aryepiglottic folds provides relief

Laryngomalacia is the most common cause of stridor in infants.

Foreign Body

Ingested
- usually stuck at cricopharyngeus
- coins, toys
- presents with drooling, dysphagia, stridor if very large

Aspirated
- usually stuck at right mainstem bronchus
- peanuts, carrot, apple core, popcorn, balloons
- presentation
  - stridor if lodged in trachea
  - unilateral "asthma" if bronchial, therefore often misdiagnosed as asthma
  - if impacts to totally occlude airway: cough, lobar pneumonia, atelectasis, mediastinal shift, pneumothorax

Foreign body inhalation is the most common cause of accidental death in children.

Diagnosis and Treatment
- inspiration-expiration chest x-ray (if patient is stable)
- bronchoscopy and esophagoscopy with removal
- rapid onset, not necessarily febrile or elevated WBC

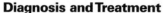

Common Medications

Table 24. Antibiotics

Generic Name (Brand Name)	Dosing Schedule	Indications	Comments
amoxicillin (Amoxil™; Amoxi ™; Amox™)	500 mg PO tid	*Streptococcus, Pneumococcus, H. influenzae, Proteus* coverage	In patients with infectious mononucleosis, may cause rash
piperacillin with tazobactam (Zosyn™)	3 g PO q6h	Gram-positive and negative aerobes and anaerobes plus *Pseudomonas* coverage	May cause pseudomembranous colitis
ciprofloxacin (Cipro™; Ciloxan™)	500 mg PO bid	*Pseudomonas, Streptococci*, MRSA, and most gram-negative; no anaerobic coverage	Do not give quinolones to children
erythromycin (Erythrocin™, EryPed™; Staticin™; T-Stat™; Erybid ™; Novorythro Encap ™)	500 mg PO qid	Alternative to penicillin	Ototoxic

Table 25. Otic Drops

Generic Name (Brand Name)	Dose	Indications / Notes
ciprofloxacin (Cipro HC™)	5 gtt in affected ear bid	For complications of otitis media *Pseudomonas, Streptococci*, MRSA, and most gram-negative; no anaerobic coverage
neomycin, polymyxin B sulfate, and hydrocortisone (Cortisporin Otic™)	5 gtt in affected ear tid	For otitis externa Used for inflammatory conditions which are currently infected or at risk of bacterial infections May cause hearing loss if placed in inner ear
hydrocortisone and acetic acid (VoSol HC™)	5-10 gtt in affected ear tid	Bactericidal by lowering pH
tobramycin and dexamethasone (TobraDex™)	5-10 gtt in affected ear bid	For chronic suppurative otitis media Risk of vestibular or cochlear toxicity

Table 26. Nasal Sprays

Generic Name (Brand Name)	Indications	Notes: General
STEROID		
flunisolide (Rhinalar™)	Allergic rhinitis	Requires up to four weeks of consistent use to have effect
budesonide (Rhinocort™)	Chronic sinusitis	Long term use
triamcinolonoe (Nasacort™)		Dries nasal mucosa; get minor bleeding
beclomethasone (Beconase™)		Patient should stop if epistaxis
mometasone furoate, monohydrate (Nasonex™)		May sting
		Flonase™ and Nasonex™ not absorbed systemically
ANTIHISTAMINE		
levocarbastine (Livostin™)	Allergic rhinitis	Immediate effect If no effect by 3 days then discontinue Use during allergy season
DECONGESTANT		
xylometazoline (Otrivin™)	Acute sinusitis	Careful if patient has hypertension
oxymetazoline (Dristan™)	Rhinitis	Short term use (<5 days)
phenylephrine (Neosynephrine™)		If long term use, can cause decongestant addiction i.e. rhinitis medicamentosa
ANTIBIOTIC / DECONGESTANT		
framycetin, gramicidin, phenylephrine (Soframycin™)	Acute sinusitis	
ANTICHOLINERGIC		
ipratropium bromide (Atrovent™)	Vasomotor rhinitis	Careful not to spray into eyes Increased rate of epistaxis when combined with topical nasal steroids
LUBRICANTS		
saline; Rhinaris™; Secaris™; Polysporin™, Vaseline™	Dry nasal mucosa	Use prn Rhinaris™ and Secaris™ may cause stinging

Source: Dr. M.M. Carr http://icarus.med.utoronto.ca/carr/manual/sprays.html

Notes

P

Pediatrics

Kate Hanneman, Karen Jang and Jennifer Lam, chapter editors
Justine Chan and Angela Ho, associate editors
Billie Au, EBM editor
Dr. Hosanna Au, Dr. Stacey Bernstein, Dr. Rayfel Schneider and Dr. Michael Weinstein, staff editors

Pediatric Quick Reference Values 3

Primary Care Pediatrics 4
Regular Visits
Developmental Milestones
Immunization
    Routine Immunization
    Other Vaccines
Nutrition
Normal Physical Growth
Dentition
Failure to Thrive (FTT)
Obesity
Colic
Milk Caries
Injury Prevention Counselling
Sudden Infant Death Syndrome (SIDS)
Circumcision
Toilet Training
Approach to the Crying/Fussing Child

Abnormal Child Behaviours 13
Elimination Disorders
Sleep Disturbances
Breath-Holding Spells

Child Abuse and Neglect 15

Adolescent Medicine 16
Normal Sexual Development
Normal Variation in Puberty

Cardiology 18
Heart Murmurs
Congenital Heart Disease (CHD)
    Acyanotic CHD
    Cyanotic CHD
Congestive Heart Failure (CHF)
Infective Endocarditis
Dysrhythmias

Dermatology ....D

Development 25
Developmental Delay
Mental Retardation (MR)
Learning Disorders
Language Delay
Fetal Alcohol Spectrum Disorder

Endocrinology 27
Diabetes Mellitus (DM)
Diabetes Insipidus
Syndrome of Inappropriate Antidiuretic
    Hormone (SIADH)
Hypercalemia/Hypocalcemia/Rickets
Hypothyroidism
Hyperthyroidism
Ambiguous Genitalia
Congenital Adrenal Hyperplasia
Precocious Puberty
Delayed Puberty
Short Stature

Growth Hormone Deficiency
Tall Stature

Gastroenterology 34
Vomiting
    Vomiting in the Newborn Period
    Vomiting After the Newborn Period
Acute Diarrhea
Chronic Diarrhea
    Chronic Diarrhea Without Failure to Thrive
    Chronic Diarrhea With Failure to Thrive
Constipation
Acute Abdominal Pain
Chronic Abdominal Pain
Abdominal Mass
Upper Gastrointestinal Bleeding
Lower Gastrointestinal Bleeding

Genetics, Dysmorphisms, and Metabolism ..42
Approach to the Dysmorphic Child
Genetic Syndromes
Muscular Dystrophy (MD)
 Associations
    VACTERL
    CHARGE
Metabolic Disease
    Phenylketonuria
    Galactosemia

Hematology 46
Anemia
    Physiologic Anemia
    Iron Deficiency Anemia
    Anemia of Chronic Disease
    Hemoglobinopathies
Bleeding Disorders
    Immune Thrombocytopenic Purpura (ITP)
    Hemophilia
    von Willebrand's Disease

Infectious Diseases 50
Fever
Acute Otitis Media (AOM)
Meningitis
HIV Infection
Pharyngitis and Tonsillitis
    Streptococcal (GAS) Pharyngitis
    Infectious Mononucleosis
Pertussis
Varicella (Chickenpox)
Roseola
Measles
Mumps
Rubella
Reye Syndrome
Erythema Infectiosum
Urinary Tract Infection

Toronto Notes 2009   Pediatrics P1

Pediatrics

Pediatric Quick Reference Values

Table 1. Average Vitals at Various Ages

Age	Pulse (bpm)	Resp. Rate (br/min)	sBP (mmHg)
Birth	120 – 160	35 – 50	70
Preschool	70 – 140	20 – 30	80 – 90
Adolescent	60 – 120	15 – 20	90 – 120

Table 2. Average Blood Chemistry at Various Ages

Test	Birth	Preschool	Adolescent
Sodium (mmol/L)	133 – 142	135 – 143	135 – 145
Potassium (mmol/L)	4.5 – 6.5	3.5 – 5.2	3.5 – 5.2
Chloride (mmol/L)	96 – 106	99 – 111	98 – 106
Serum Creatinine (μmol/L)	< 441	< 44	< 106
BUN (mmol/L)	2.9 – 10	1.8 – 5.4	2.9 – 7.1
Glucose (fasting; mmol/L)	> 2.5	2.8 – 6.1	3.3 – 6.1
Glucose (fasting; mg/dL)	> 45	50 – 110	60 – 110
pH (arterial)	7.30 – 7.40	7.35 – 7.45	7.35 – 7.45
pCO_2 (mmHg)	30 – 50	30 – 42	33 – 46
pO_2 (mmHg)	50 – 60	80 – 100	80 – 100
Bicarbonate (mmol/L)	16 – 22	18 – 24	20 – 28
ALT (U/L)	< 60	< 40	< 40
AST (U/L)	< 110	< 45	< 36

Table 3. Average Hematological Labs at Various Ages

Test	2 Days	1 Week	1 Month	1-5 Yrs	6-14 Yrs
Hemoglobin (g/L)	150 – 250		115 – 180	110 – 140	120 – 160
Hemoglobin (g/dL)	15 – 20		11.5 – 18	11 – 14	12 – 16
Hematocrit	0.46 – 0.74		0.35 – 0.54	0.33 – 0.42	0.36 – 0.48
RBC count (x 10^{12}/L)	3.5 – 6.0		3.5 – 5.5	4.0 – 5.0	4.5 – 5.5
Reticulocytes (x 10^9/L)	< 5.0		< 5.0	10.0 – 100.0	10.0 – 100.0
MCV (fL)		110	90	80 – 94	80 – 94
MCH (pg)			24 – 34	24 – 31	24 – 31
MCHC (g/L)	320 – 360	320 – 360	320 – 360	320 – 360	320 – 360
WBC (x 10^9/L)	20 – 40	5 – 21		5 – 12	4 – 10
Polymorphs (x 10^9/L)	6 – 26	1.5 – 10		1.5 – 8.5	1.5 – 7.5
Bands (x 10^9/L)	0 – 4.5	0 – 4.5		0	0
Lymphocytes (x 10^9/L)	2.0 – 11.0	2.0 – 11.0		2.0 – 8.0	1.5 – 7.0
Platelets (x 10^9/L)	150 – 450	150 – 450	150 – 450	150 – 450	150 – 450
INR	0.9-2.7	0.9-2.7	0.8-1.2	0.8-1.2	0.8-1.2
PTT (s)	25 – 60	25 – 60	25 – 60	25 – 40	25 – 40
TSH (mU/L)	1-38.9		1.7-9.1	0.7-6.4	0.7-6.4

Primary Care Pediatrics

Regular Visits

- usual schedule: newborn, within 1 week post-discharge, 1, 2, 4, 6, 9, 12, 15, 18, 24 months
  - yearly until age 6, then every other year
  - yearly again after age 11
- history
- physical exam
- immunization (see *Immunization*)
- counselling/anticipatory guidance (see *Nutrition, Colic, Sudden Infant Death Syndrome (SIDS)*, and *Injury Prevention Counselling*)

Developmental Milestones

Table 4. Developmental Milestones

Age	Gross Motor	Fine Motor	Speech and Language	Adaptive and Social Skills
6 weeks	prone-lifts chin intermittently			social smile
2 months	prone-arms extended forward	pulls at clothes	coos	recognizes parents
4 months	prone-raises head + chest, rolls over, no head lag	reach and grasp, objects to mouth	responds to voice, laughs	
6 months	prone-weight on hands, tripod sit	ulnar grasp, transfers objects from hand to hand	begins to babble, responds to name	stranger anxiety beginning of object permanence
9 months	pulls to stand, crawls	finger-thumb grasp	"mama, dada" - appropriate, imitates 1 word	plays games, plays peek-a-boo separation/stranger anxiety
12 months	walks with support	pincer grasp, throws	2 words, follows 1-step command	drinks with cup, wave bye-bye
15 months	walks without support	draws a line	jargon	points to needs
18 months	up steps with help	tower of 3 cubes, scribbling	10 words, follows simple commands	uses spoon, points to body parts
24 months	up 2 feet/step, runs, kicks ball walks up and down steps	tower of 6 cubes, undresses	2-3 words phrases, uses " I, me, you", 50% intelligible	parallel play, helps to dress
3 years	tricycle, up 1 foot/step, down 2 feet/step, stands on one foot, jumps	copies a circle and a cross, puts on shoes	prepositions, plurals, counts to 10, 75% intelligible	dress/undress fully except buttons, knows sex, age
4 years	hops on 1 foot, down 1 foot/step	copies a square, uses scissors	tells story, knows 4 colours, speech intelligible, uses past tense	cooperative play, toilet trained, buttons clothes, knows names of body parts
5 years	skips, rides bicycle	copies a triangle, prints name, ties shoelaces	fluent speech, future tense, alphabet	

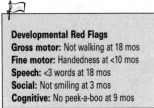

Pediatric Developmental Milestones
1 year:
  -**single** words
2 years:
  -**2** word sentences
  -understands **2** step commands
3 years:
  -**3** word combos
  -repeats **3** digits
  -rides **tri**cycle
4 years:
  -draws **square**
  -counts **4** objects

Developmental Red Flags
Gross motor: Not walking at 18 mos
Fine motor: Handedness at <10 mos
Speech: <3 words at 18 mos
Social: Not smiling at 3 mos
Cognitive: No peek-a-boo at 9 mos

Primitive Reflexes

- reflexes seen in normal newborns; may indicate abnormality (e.g. cerebral palsy) if persist after 4-6 months
- Moro reflex
  - infant is placed semi-upright, head supported by examiner's hand, sudden withdrawal of supported head with immediate resupport elicits reflex
  - reflex consists of abduction and extension of the arms, opening of the hands, followed by flexion and adduction of arms
  - absence of Moro suggests CNS injury; asymmetry suggests focal motor lesions (e.g. brachial plexus injury)
- Galant reflex
  - infant is held in ventral suspension and one side of the back is stroked along paravertebral line; the pelvis will move in the direction of stimulated side
- Grasp reflex: flexion of fingers with the placement of a finger in the infant's palm
- Tonic neck reflex: turning the head results in the "fencing" posture (extension of ipsilateral leg and arm)
- Placing and stepping reflex ("primitive walking"): infant places foot on a surface when it is brought into contact with it
- Rooting reflex: infant pursues tactile stimuli near the mouth
- Parachute reflex: tilting the infant to the side while in a sitting position results in ipsilateral arm extension (appears by 6-8 months)
- upgoing plantar reflexes (Babinski sign) is normal in infants (i.e. < 2 yrs)

Immunization

Routine Immunization

Table 5. Routine Immunization Schedule

Vaccine	Schedule	Route	Reaction	Contraindications
DTaP-IPV	2, 4, 6, 18 mos 4-6 yrs	IM	@ 24-48 hrs • Minor: fever, local redness, swelling, irritability • Major: prolonged crying (1%), hypotonic unresponsive state (1:1750), seizure (1:1950) on day of vaccine • Prophylaxis: acetaminophen 10-15 mg/kg given 4 hrs prior to injection and q4h afterwards	Previous anaphylactic reaction to vaccine; evolving unstable neurologic disease; hyporesponsive/hypotonic following previous vaccine; anaphylactic reaction to neomycin or streptomycin
Hib	2, 4, 6, 18 mos	IM	• Minor: fever, local redness, swelling, irritability	
Pneu-C	2, 4, 6, 15 mos	IM	• Minor: fever, local redness, swelling, irritability	
MMR	12, 18 mos	SC	@ 7-14 days • Fever, measle-like rash • Lymphadenopathy, arthralgia, arthritis, parotitis (rare)	Pregnancy, immunocompromised infants (except healthy HIV positive children), anaphylactic reaction to gelatin
Men-C	2, 4, 6 mos OR 12 mos	IM	redness/swelling (<50%), fever (9%), irritability (<80%), rash (0.1%)	
Var	15 mos	SC	Mild local reaction (20% but higher in immunocompromised) Mild varicella-like papules or vesicles (5%) Low-grade fever (15%)	Pregnant or planning to get pregnant within next 3 months; anaphylactic reaction to gelatin
Hep B	3 doses: initial, then 1 month later, then at 6 months-grade 7 administered in schools (can be given at birth or in school)	IM	• Local redness, swelling	Anaphylactic reaction to Baker's yeast
dTap	start at 14-16 yrs	IM	Anaphylaxis (very rare)	Pregnancy (1st trimester)
Td	adult yrs, q10 yrs	IM	Local erythema and swelling (70%)	
Flu**	every autumn 6 mos - 23 mos	IM	Local tenderness at injection site Fever, malaise, myalgia, rash, febrile seizures Hypersensitivity reactions	Anaphylactic reaction to eggs, <6 mos of age

DTaP - IPV - diptheria, tetanus, acellular pertussis, inactivated polio vaccine (for children under 7 yrs)
MMR - measles, mumps, rubella
Hib - *Hemophilus influenzae* type b conjugate vaccine
Men-C - meningococcal C conjugate vaccine
Hep B – Hepatitis B vaccine
Td – tetanus and diphtheria adult type formulation

Vaccine/Pneu-C – pneumococcal 7-valent conjugate vaccine
Var – varicella vaccine
dTap – diphtheria, tetanus, acellular pertussis vaccine (adolescent/adult formulation)
Flu – influenza vaccine

Adapted from: National Advisory Committee on Immunization. Recommended Immunization Schedule for Infants, Children and Youth (updated March 2005)

*If varicella vaccine and MMR vaccine not given during the same visit, they must be administered at least 28 days apart.
**For children with severe or chronic disease, e.g. cardiac, pulmonary, or renal disease, sickle cell disease, diabetes, endocrine disorders, HIV, immunosuppressed, long-term aspirin therapy, or those who visit residents of chronic care facilities

> **Safety of MMR Vaccine**
> According to the CDC, the weight of currently available scientific evidence does not support the hypothesis that MMR vaccine causes either autism or IBD.
> http://www.cdc.gov/nip/vacsafe/concerns/autism/autism-mmr.htm#2
> (see website for more details)

Administration of Vaccines
- injection site
  - infants (<12 months old): anterolateral thigh
  - children: deltoid
- DTaP+IPV+Hib (Pentacel™, Pentavax™): 5 vaccines given as one IM injection
- two live vaccines (varicella, MMR) must be given either at the same visit or separated by 4 weeks or more

Contraindications to Any Vaccine
- moderate to severe illness ± fever (no need to delay vaccination for mild URTI)
- allergy to vaccine component

Possible Adverse Reactions
- any vaccine
  - local: induration or tenderness (MMR is especially painful!)
  - systemic: fever, rash
  - allergic: urticaria, rhinitis, anaphylaxis
- specific vaccine reactions (see Table 5)

Other Vaccines

Hepatitis A
- inactivated monovalent hepatitis A vaccine (Havrix™, Vaqta™, Avaxim™, Epaxal Berna™)
- given as a series of 2 vaccinations 4-6 months apart (cost ~$50 total)
- recommended for pre-exposure prophylaxis for individuals at increased risk of infection (e.g. travel to endemic countries, residents of communities with high endemic rates, IV drug use, etc.)
- can also be given as a combination vaccine with Hep B (Twinrix™)
- immunoglobulin can be used for short-term protection in infants and immunocompromised patients

Hepatitis B
- set of 3 vaccinations given in infancy (0, 1, 6 months) or mid-childhood to early teens (in Ontario, given in grade 7)
- if mother is HBsAg +ve, give HBIg at birth and Hep B vaccine at birth, 1 mo, 6 mos

BCG Vaccine
- infants of parents with infectious TB at time of delivery
- groups/communities with high rates of disease/infection (offered to aboriginal children on reserves), health care workers at risk
- only given if patient has a negative TB skin test
- side effects: erythema, papule formation 3-6 weeks after intradermal injection, enlargement of regional lymph nodes

TB Skin Test (Mantoux)
- screen high risk populations only (family history, HIV, immigrants from countries with increased incidence, substance abuse in family, homeless, aboriginal)
- intradermal injection of 5TU (0.1 ml) of tuberculous antigen (purified protein derivative), read result at 48 hrs
- TB test should be postponed for 4-6 weeks after administration of live BCG vaccine due to risk of false negative result
- test interpretation
    - check area of raised INDURATION (not just area of erythema) at 48-72 hours
    - positive result if:
        - >15 mm: children >4 years with no risk factors
        - >10 mm: children <4 years, at risk for environmental exposure
        - >5 mm: children with close TB contact, immunosuppressed
- BCG history irrelevant – does not usually give positive response (unless <6 weeks previously)
- positive reaction means active disease or previous contact with TB

Human papillomavirus vaccine (Gardasil™) – see Gynecology
- given in grades 7-8 in some provinces

Quadrivalent Meningococcal Vaccine (Menactra™)
- given in some provinces in Grade 9
- protects against Neisseria meningitidis strains A, C, W-135, and Y
- in Canada, currently recommended for patients with asplenia, travelers to endemic areas (such as the Hajj in Mecca), laboratory workers, and military recruits

Rotavirus Vaccine (RotaTeq™)
- oral vaccine given in 3 doses with first at age 6-12 weeks
- shown to reduce viral gastroenteritis in infants
- not currently covered in Canada

Nutrition

Breast Feeding
- colostrum for first few days = clear fluid with nutrients (high protein, low fat) and immunoglobulins
- full milk production by 3-7 days; mature milk by 15-45 days
- support for mothers who want to breast feed should start while in hospital
- signs of inadequate intake: <6 wet diapers per day after first week, sleepy or lethargic, <7 feeds per day, sleeping throughout the night, weight loss >10% of birth weight, jaundice
    - rule of thumb: ~ 1 stool/day of age for first week
- feeding schedule (newborn baby needs 120 kcal/kg/day)
    - premature infants: q2-3 hours
    - term infants: q3.5-4 hours, q5 hours at night until about 2-3 months of age

- breast-fed babies require the following supplements
    - vitamin K (given IM at birth)
    - vitamin D 400 IU/d (Tri-Vi-Sol™ or Di-Vi-Sol™); especially during winter months
    - fluoride (after 6 months if not sufficient in water supply)
    - iron: from 4 months to 12 months (iron fortified cereals or ferrous sulphate solution)
- **contraindications to breast feeding**
    - mother receiving chemotherapy or radioactive compounds
    - mother with HIV/AIDS, active untreated TB, herpes in breast region
    - mother using >0.5 g/kg/d alcohol and/or illicit drugs (decrease milk production and/or directly toxic to baby)
    - mother taking certain medications e.g. antimetabolites, bromocriptine, chloramphenicol, high dose diazepam, ergots, gold, metronidazole, tetracycline, lithium, cyclophosphamide
    - Note: oral contraceptive pills (OCP) not a contraindication to breast feeding. (estrogen may decrease lactation but is not dangerous to infant)

Advantages of Breast Feeding
- "Breast is Best" – exclusive breastfeeding during the first 4 months of life is recommended by Health Canada, the Dietitians of Canada, and the Canadian Pediatric Society
- breast milk is easily digested and has a low renal solute load
- immunologic:
    - IgA, macrophages, active lymphocytes, lysozyme, lactoferrin (lactoferrin inhibits *E. coli* growth in intestine)
    - protection is greatest during early months, but is cumulative with increased duration of breastfeeding
    - lower allergenicity than cow's milk protein (decreased cow's milk protein allergy and eczema)
    - lower pH promotes growth of lactobacillus in the gastrointestinal tract (protective against pathogenic intestinal bacteria)
- parent-child bonding, economical, convenient

Complications of Breast Feeding
- mother
    - sore/cracked nipples: treat with warm compresses, massage, frequent feeds, soothing barrier creams (Desitin™, Vaseline™), proper latching technique
    - breast engorgement (usually in first week): continue breast feeding and/or pumping
    - mastitis (usually due to *S. aureus*): treat with cold compresses between feeds, cloxacillin for mother, continue nursing, ± incision and drainage
- infant
    - breast feeding jaundice (first 1-2 weeks): due to lack of milk production and subsequent dehydration (see *Jaundice*)
    - breast milk jaundice: rare (0.5% of newborns); due to substances in breast milk that inhibit conjugation of bilirubin (persists up to 4-6 months)
    - poor weight gain: consider dehydration or failure to thrive
    - oral candidiasis (thrush): check baby's mouth for white cheesy material that does not scrape off; treat baby with antifungal such as nystatin (Mycostatin™) (treat mother topically to prevent transmission)

Alternatives to Breast Feeding

Table 6. Infant Formulas

Type of Formula	Indication(s)	Content (compared to breast milk)
Breast milk	Most babies	70:30 whey:casein ratio Fat from human butterfat Carbohydrate from lactose
Cow's milk based (Enfamil™, Similac™)	Premature babies Transitional Contraindication to breastfeeding	Plant fats instead of human butterfat Lower whey: casein ratio
Fortified formula	Low birth weight Premature babies	More calories Higher amounts of vitamins A, D, K, C May only be used in hospital due to risk of fat-soluble vitamin toxicity
Soy protein (Isomil™, Prosobee™)	Galactosemia Lactose intolerance	Corn syrup solids or sucrose instead of lactose

Infant growth and health outcomes associated with 3 compared with 6 mo of exclusive breastfeeding
The American Journal of Clinical Nutrition 78: 291-295, 2003
Purpose: To compare differences in growth and health in infants exclusively breastfed for 3 versus 6 months.
Study: Observational cohort study with 3483 term newborns
Results: The rate of gastrointestinal infections was significantly reduced in the group of infants who were exclusively breastfed for 6 months. This finding was limited to the period between 3 and 6 months of age (adjusted IDR 0.35 (95% CI: 0.13, 0.96). The breastfed babies were smaller at 6 months but there was no different in growth between the two groups by 12 months. No significant association was found between breastfeeding and the rate of eczema or respiratory infections.
Conclusions: There is an association between breastfeeding and a lower incidence of gastrointestinal infections in term infants.

Term newborn should gain 20-30 g/day
"1 oz. per day except on Sunday"

To estimate weight of child >1 year (kg)
~ Age x 2 + 8

Head Circumference
Remember 3, 9, and multiples of 5:
Newborn **35** cm
3 mos **40** cm
9 mos **45** cm
3 yrs **50** cm
9 yrs **55** cm

Table 6. Infant Formulas (continued)

Type of Formula	Indication(s)	Content (compared to breast milk)
Partially hydrolyzed proteins (Good Start™)	Delayed gastric emptying Risk of cow's milk allergy	Protein is 100% whey with no casein
Protein hydrolysate (Nutramigen™, Alimentum™, Pregestimil™, Portagen™)	Malabsorption Food allergy	Protein is 100% casein with no whey Corn syrup solids, sucrose, OR tapioca starch instead of lactose
Amino acid (Neocate™)	Food allergy Short gut	No proteins, just free amino acids Corn syrup solids instead of lactose Very expensive
Metabolic	Inborn errors of metabolism	Various different compositions for children with galactosemia, propionic acidemia, etc.

Most formulas contain 680 calories per litre; "fortified" formulas for premature babies may contain more calories
Formula may also be supplemented with specific nutrients in babies with malabsorption syndromes
True lactose intolerance is extremely rare in children under age 5

Infant Feeding

Table 7. Dietary Schedule for Infants

Age	Food	Comments
0 to 4-6 months	Breast milk, formula	
6 to 9 months	Iron enriched cereals	Rice cereals first because less allergenic
	Pureed vegetables	Yellow/orange vegetables first and green last (more bulky) Avoid vegetables with high nitrite content (beets, spinach, turnips) Introduce vegetables before fruit (alternate yellow and green vegetables daily)
	Pureed fruits and juices Pureed meats, fish, poultry, egg yolk	No egg white until 12 months (risk of allergy)
9 to 12 months	Finger foods, peeled fruit, cheese and cooked vegetables, homo milk	No honey until >12 months (risk of botulism) No peanuts or raw, hard vegetables until age 3 to 4 years No added sugar, salt, fat or seasonings

- do not delay introduction of solid foods beyond 9 months
- introduce 2-3 new foods per week (easier to identify adverse reactions) and allow a few days between each introduction
- avoid excessive milk/juice intake when >1 year

Normal Physical Growth

- newborn size influenced by maternal factors (placenta, in utero environment)
- premature infants (<37 weeks): use corrected gestational age until 2 years
- not linear: most rapid growth during first two years; growth spurt at puberty
- different tissue growth at different times
  - first two years: CNS
  - mid-childhood: lymphoid tissue
  - puberty: gonadal maturation (testes, breast tissue)
- body proportions: upper/lower segment ratio – midpoint is symphysis pubis
  - newborn 1.7; adult male 0.97; adult female 1.0
  - poor correlation between birth weight and adult weight

Table 8. Average Growth Parameters

Birth	Normal	Growth	Comments
Weight	3.25 kg (7 lbs)	2 x birth wt by 4-5 mos 3 x birth wt by 1 year 4 x birth wt by 2 years	Wt. loss (up to 10% of birth wt) in first 7 days of life is normal Neonate should regain wt by 10 days of age
Length/Height	50 cm (20 in)	25 cm in 1st year 12 cm in 2nd year 8 cm in 3rd year then 4-7 cm/year until puberty 1/2 adult height at 2 years	Measure supine length until 2 years of age, then measure standing height
Head Circumference	35 cm (14 in)	2 cm/month for 1st 3 mos 1 cm/month at 3-6 mos 0.5 cm/month at 6-12 mos	Measure around occipital, parietal, and frontal prominences to obtain the greatest circumference

Dentition

- primary dentition (20 teeth)
    - first tooth at 5-9 months (lower incisor), then 1 per month until 20 teeth
    - 6-8 central teeth by 1 year
- secondary dentition (32 teeth)
    - first adult tooth is first molar at 6 years, then lower incisors
    - 2nd molars at 12 years, 3rd molars at 18 years

Failure to Thrive (FTT)

Table 9. Failure to Thrive Patterns

Growth Parameters			Suggestive Abnormality	
decreased Wt	normal Ht	normal HC	• caloric insufficiency • decreased intake	• hypermetabolic state • increased losses
decreased Wt	decreased Ht	normal HC	• structural dystrophies • endocrine disorder	• constitutional growth delay • familial short stature
decreased Wt	decreased Ht	decreased HC	• intrauterine insult	• genetic abnormality

(HC = head circumference; Ht = height; Wt = weight)

Definition
- weight <3rd percentile, or falls across two major percentile curves, or <80% of expected weight for height and age
- inadequate caloric intake most common factor in poor weight gain
- may have other nutritional deficiencies (e.g. protein, iron, vitamin D)
- **history:**
    - duration of problem and growth history
    - detailed dietary and feeding history, appetite, behaviour before and after feeds, bowel habits
    - pregnancy, birth, and postpartum history; developmental and medical history (including medications); social and family history (parental height, weight, growth pattern)
    - assess 4 areas of functioning: child's temperament, child-parent interaction, feeding behaviour and parental psychosocial stressors
- **physical exam:**
    - height (Ht), weight (Wt), head circumference (HC), arm span, upper-to-lower (U/L) segment ratio
    - assessment of nutritional status, dysmorphism, Tanner stage, evidence of chronic disease
    - observation of a feeding session and parent-child interaction
    - signs of abuse or neglect
- **investigations:** as indicated by clinical presentation
    - CBC, blood smear, electrolytes, urea, ESR, T4, TSH, urinalysis
    - bone age x-ray (left wrist – compared to standardized wrist x-rays)
    - karyotype in all short girls and in short boys where appropriate
    - any other tests indicated from history and physical exam: renal or liver function tests, venous blood gases, ferritin, immunoglobulins, sweat chloride, fecal fat

Organic FTT
- inability to feed
    - insufficient breast milk production
    - poor retention (GERD, vomiting)
    - CNS, neuromuscular, mechanical problems with swallowing, sucking
    - anorexia (associated with chronic disease)
- inadequate absorption (see *Pediatric Gastroenterology*)
    - malabsorption: celiac disease, cystic fibrosis (CF), pancreatic insufficiency
    - loss from the GI tract: chronic diarrhea, vomiting
- inappropriate utilization of nutrients
    - renal loss: e.g. tubular disorders
    - inborn errors of metabolism
    - endocrine: type 1 diabetes, diabetes insipidus (DI), hypopituitarism, congenital hypothyroidism
- increased energy requirements
    - pulmonary disease: CF
    - cardiac disease
    - endocrine: hyperthyroidism, DI, hypopituitarism
    - malignancies

Energy Requirements
- 0-10 kg: 100 cal/kg/day
- 0-20 kg: 1,000 cal + 50 cal/kg/day for each kg >10
- +20 kg: 1,500 cal + 20 cal/kg/day for each kg >20

Clinical signs of FTT (SMALL KID):
S - subcutaneous fat loss
M - muscle atrophy
A - alopecia
L - lethargy
L - lagging behind normal
K - Kwashiorkor
I - infection (recurrent)
D - dermatitis

- chronic infections
  - inflammatory: systemic lupus erythematosus (SLE)
- decreased growth potential
  - specific syndromes, chromosomal abnormalities, GH deficiency
  - intrauterine insults: fetal alcohol syndrome (FAS), TORCH infections
- treatment: cause-specific

Non-Organic FTT
- often due to malnutrition, inadequate nutrition, poor feeding technique, errors in making formula
- these children may present as picky eaters, with poor emotional support at home or poor temperemental "fit" with caregiver
- may have delayed psychomotor, language, and personal/social development
- emotional deprivation, poor parent-child interaction, dysfunctional home
- child abuse and/or neglect
- parental psychosocial stress, personal history of suffering abuse or neglect
- treatment: most are managed as outpatients with multidisciplinary approach
  - primary care physician, dietitian, psychologist, social work, child protection services

Obesity

- prevalence of childhood obesity in Canada has tripled (1981-1996)

Geographic and demographic variation in the prevalence of overweight Canadian children
Obesity Research. 11(5):668-73, 2003 May
Purpose: To determine geographic and demographic variation in the prevalence of overweight Canadian children
Study: Assessment of trends in BMI using data from the 1981 Canadian Fitness Survey and the 1996 National Longitudinal Survey of Children and Youth.
Main Outcomes: The prevalence of overweight and obese children age 7 to 13 years, secular trends from 1981 to 1996 by province, and provincial variation after adjusting for socioeconomic and demographic characteristics.
Results: In 1996, 33% of boys and 26% of girls were classified as overweight, and 10% of boys and 9% of girls were classified as obese. The odds ratio associated with the 1981 to 1996 change in the prevalence of overweight children was 3.24 (95% CI, 2.83-3.70) for Canada as a whole. There are clear regional differences, with those in Atlantic Canada more likely to be overweight and Prairie children less likely. These differences were not sufficiently accounted for by differences in socioeconomic circumstances.
Conclusions: The prevalence of childhood obesity is increasing in all areas of Canada, although more so in Atlantic Canada.

Definition
- weight >95th percentile for age and height, or BMI >30, or weight >20% greater than expected for age and height
- caused by a chronically positive energy balance (intake exceeds expenditure)

Risk Factors
- genetic predisposition:
  - if 1 parent is obese – 40% chance of obese child
  - if both parents are obese – 80% chance of obese child
- genetic heritability accounts for 25-40% of juvenile obesity

Clinical Presentation
- history: diet, activity, family heights and weights, growth curves
- body mass index (BMI) tends not to be used by pediatricians prior to adolescence
- physical examination: may suggest secondary cause, e.g. Cushing syndrome
- organic causes are rare (<5%)
  - genetic: e.g. Prader-Willi, Carpenter, Turner syndromes
  - endocrine: e.g. Cushing syndrome, hypothyroidism
- complications
  - childhood obesity is an unreliable predictor of adult obesity
    - unless >180% of ideal body weight
    - however, 70% of obese adolescents become obese adults
  - association with: hypertension, dyslipidemia, slipped capital femoral epiphysis, type 2 diabetes, asthma, obstructive sleep apnea
  - boys: gynecomastia; girls: polycystic ovarian disease, early menarche, irregular menses
  - psychological: teasing, decreased self-esteem, unhealthy coping mechanisms, depression
- management
  - encouragement and reassurance; engagement of entire family
  - diet: qualitative changes; do not encourage weight loss but allow for linear growth to catch up with weight; special diets used by adults are not encouraged
  - evidence against very low calorie diets for preadolescents
  - behaviour modification: increase activity, change eating habits/meal patterns
  - insufficient evidence for or against exercise, family programs for obese children
  - education: multidisciplinary approach, dietitian, counselling
  - surgery and pharmacotherapy are not used in children

Colic

- rule of 3's: unexplained paroxysms of irritability and crying for >3 hours/day and >3 days/week for >3 weeks in an otherwise healthy, well-fed baby
- occurs in 10% of infants

- etiology: generally regarded as a lag in the development of normal peristaltic movement in gastrointestinal tract, other theories suggest a lack of self-soothing mechanisms
- other reasons why babies cry: wet, hunger or gas pains, too hot or cold, overstimulated, need to suck or be held
- timing: onset 10 days to 3 months of age; peak 6-8 weeks
- child cries, pulls up legs and passes gas soon after feeding
- management
  - parental relief, rest and reassurance
  - hold baby, soother, car ride, music, vacuum, check diaper
  - medications (Ovol™ drops, gripe water) of no proven benefit
  - if breast feeding, elimination of cow's milk protein from mother's diet (effective in very small percentage of cases)
  - try casein hydrosylates formula (Nutramigen™)

Milk Caries

- decay of superior front teeth and back molars in first 4 years of life
- often occur in children put to bed with a bottle of milk or juice
- can also be caused by breast-feeding (especially prolonged night feeds)
- prevention
  - no bottle at bedtime (unless plain water)
  - use water as thirst quenchers during the day, do not sweeten pacifier
  - can clean teeth with soft damp cloth or toothbrush and water
  - avoid fluoridated toothpaste until able to spit (>3 years) because of fluorosis risk (stains teeth)
  - Canadian Dental Association recommends assessment by dentist 6 months after eruption of first tooth, or by 1 year of age

Injury Prevention Counselling

- injuries are the leading cause of death in children >1 year of age
- main causes: motor vehicle crashes, burns, drowning, falls, choking, infanticide

Table 10. Injury Prevention Counselling

0-6 months	6-12 months	1-2 years	2-5 years

• do not leave infant alone on bed, on change table or in tub
• keep crib rails up
• check water temp. before bathing
• do not hold hot liquid and infant at the same time
• turn down hot water heater
• check milk temp. before feeding
• have appropriate car seats – required before allowed to leave hospital
  • <9 kg: rear-facing
  • 10-18 kg: front-facing
  • 18-36.4 kg: booster seat
	• install stair barriers
	• discourage use of walkers
	• avoid play areas with sharp-edged tables and corners
	• cover electrical outlets
	• unplug appliances when not in use
	• keep small objects, plastic bags, cleaning products, and medications out of reach
	• supervised during feeding
		• never leave unattended
		• keep pot handles turned to back of stove
		• no nuts, raw carrots, etc. due to choking hazard
		• no running while eating
			• bicycle helmet
			• never leave unsupervised at home, driveway or pool
			• teach bike safety, stranger safety, and street safety
			• swimming lessons, sunscreen, toddler seats in the car, fences around pools, dentist by age 3

• always have Poison Control number by telephone • have smoke and carbon monoxide detectors in the house and check yearly			

Sudden Infant Death Syndrome (SIDS)

Definition
- sudden and unexpected death of an infant <12 months of age in which the cause of death cannot be found by history, examination or a thorough postmortem and death scene investigation

Epidemiology
- 0.5/1,000 (leading cause of death between 1-12 months of age); M:F = 3:2
- more common in children placed in prone position
- in full term infants, peak incidence is 2-4 months, 95% of cases occur by 6 months
- increase in deaths during peak respiratory syncytial virus (RSV) season
- most deaths occur between midnight and 8 AM

Risk Factors
- more common in prematurity, if smoking in household, minorities (higher incidence in aboriginals and African Americans), socially disadvantaged
- risk of SIDS is increased 3-5 times in siblings of infants who have died of SIDS

Prevention – "Back to Sleep, Front to Play"
- place infant on back, NOT in prone position when sleeping
- allow supervised play time daily in prone position
- alarms/other monitors not recommended – increase anxiety and do not prevent life-threatening events
- avoid overheating and overdressing
- appropriate infant bedding (use firm mattress, avoid loose bedding)
- avoid smoking
- pacifiers appear to have a protective effect; do no reinsert if falls out

Circumcision

- elective procedure to be performed only in healthy, stable infants
- contraindicated when genital abnormalities present (hypospadias, etc.) or known bleeding disorder
- usually performed for social or religious reasons (not covered by OHIP)
- complications (<1%): local infection, bleeding, urethral injury
- medical benefits include prevention of phimosis, slightly reduced incidence of UTI, balanitis, cancer of the penis
- 2 recent RCTs (Lancet 369, Feb 2007) suggested that routine circumcision significantly reduced HIV transmission; these results are controversial and they have not been replicated in Western populations
- routine circumcision is not recommended by the CPS or AAP

Toilet Training

- 90% of kids attain bowel control before bladder control
- generally females train earlier than males
- 25% by 2 years old (in North America), 98% by 3 years old have daytime bladder control
- signs of toilet readiness
    - ambulating independently, stable on potty, desire to be independent or to please caregivers (i.e. motivation), sufficient expressive and receptive language skills (2-step command level), can stay dry for several hours (large enough bladder)

Approach to the Crying/Fussing Child

History
- description of infant's baseline feeding, sleeping, crying patterns
- infectious symptoms – fever, tachypnea, rhinorrhea, ill contacts
- feeding intolerance – gastroesophageal reflux with esophagitis
- nausea, vomiting, diarrhea, constipation
- trauma
- recent immunizations (vaccine reaction) or medications (drug reactions), including maternal drugs taken during pregnancy (neonatal withdrawal syndrome), and drugs that may be transferred via breast milk
- inconsistent history, pattern of numerous emergency department (ED) visits, high-risk social situations all raise concern of abuse

Physical Examination
- perform a thorough head-to-toe exam with the child completely undressed

Table 11. The Physical Examination of the Crying/Fussing Child

Organ System	Examination Findings	Possible Diagnosis	
HEENT	Bulging fontanelle	Meningitis Shaken baby syndrome	
	Blepharospasm, tearing	Corneal abrasion	
	Retinal hemorrhage	Shaken baby syndrome	
	Oropharyngeal infections	Thrush	Gingivostomatitis
		Herpangina	Otitis media
Neurologic	Irritability or lethargy	Meningitis Shaken baby syndrome	
Cardiovascular	Poor perfusion	Sepsis	Anomalous coronary artery
		Meningitis	Myocarditis
		Congestive Heart Failure (CHF)	
	Tachycardia	Supraventricular tachycardia	
Respiratory	Tachypnea	Pneumonia	CHF
	Grunting	Respiratory disease	Response to pain
Abdomen	Mass, empty RLQ	Intussusception	
Genitourinary	Scrotal swelling	Incarcerated hernia	Testicular torsion
	Penile/clitoral swelling	Hair tourniquet	
Rectal	Anal fissure	Constipation or diarrhea	
	Hemoccult positive stool	Intussusception	Necrotizing Enterocolitis
		Volvulus	
Musculoskeletal	Point tenderness or decreased movement	Fracture	Syphilis
		Osteomyelitis	Toe/finger hair tourniquet

Abnormal Child Behaviours

Elimination Disorders

ENURESIS
- involuntary urinary incontinence by day (>4 years old) and/or night (>6 years old)
- treatment should not be considered until 6 years of age; high rate of spontaneous cure
- should be evaluated if >6 years old; dysuria; change in gross colour, odour, stream; secondary or diurnal

Primary Nocturnal Enuresis
- wet only at night during sleep, can be normal up to age 6
- prevalence: 10% of 6-year olds, 3% of 12-year olds, 1% of 18-year olds
- developmental disorder or maturational lag in bladder control while asleep
- more common in boys, family history common
- treatment:
  - time and reassurance (~20% resolve spontaneously each year), bladder retention exercises, scheduled toileting
  - conditioning: "wet" alarm wakes child upon voiding (70% success rate)
  - medications: DDAVP by nasal spray or oral tablets, oxybutynin (Ditropan™), imipramine (Tofranil™) (rarely used)

Secondary Enuresis
- develops after child has sustained period of bladder control (3 months or more)
- nonspecific regression in the face of stress or anxiety (e.g. birth of sibling, significant loss, family discord)
- may also be secondary to urinary tract infection (UTI), diabetes mellitus (DM), diabetes insipidus (DI), neurogenic bladder, cerebral palsy (CP), sickle cell disease, seizures, pinworms
- may occur if engrossed in other activities
- treatment depends on cause

Diurnal Enuresis
- daytime wetting (60-80% also wet at night)
- timid, shy, temperament problems
- rule out structural anomaly (e.g. ectopic ureteral site, neurogenic bladder)
- treatment: depends on cause, remind child to go to toilet, focus on verbal expression of feelings, positive attitudes and support

ENCOPRESIS
- fecal incontinence in a child >4 years old, at least once per month for 3 months
- prevalence: 1-1.5% of school-aged children (rare in adolescence); M:F = 6:1
- usually associated with chronic constipation
- must exclude medical causes (e.g. Hirschsprung disease, hypothyroidism, hypercalcemia, spinal cord lesions, anorectal malformations)

Retentive Encopresis (Psychogenic Megacolon)
- causes
  - physical: anal fissure (painful stooling)
  - emotional: disturbed parent-child relationship, coercive toilet training, social stressors
- history
  - child withholds bowel movement, develops constipation, leading to fecal impaction and seepage of soft or liquid stool (overflow incontinence)
  - crosses legs or stands on toes to resist urge to defecate
  - distressed by symptoms, soiling of clothes
  - toilet training coercive or lacking in motivation
  - may show oppositional behaviour
- physical exam
  - digital rectal exam: large fecal mass in rectal vault
  - anal fissures (result from passage of hard stools)
- treatment
  - diet modification (see *Pediatric Gastroenterology*)
  - toilet schedule and positive reinforcement
  - complete clean-out of bowel
    - stool softeners (e.g. Colace™, Lactulose™, Lansoyl™ regularly)
    - enemas and suppositories
- complications: continuing cycle, toxic megacolon (requires >3-12 months to treat), bowel perforation

Non-Retentive Encopresis
- continuous: present from birth (never gained primary control of bowel function)
  - bowel movement randomly deposited without regard to social norms
  - family structure usually does not encourage organization and skill training
  - child has not had adequate consistent bowel training
  - treatment: consistent toilet training
- discontinuous: previous history of normal bowel control
  - bowel movements as an expression of anger or wish to be seen as a younger child
  - breakdown occurs in face of stressful event, regression
  - displays relative indifference to symptoms
  - treatment: psychotherapy if persistent for many weeks

Sleep Disturbances

Daily Sleep Requirement
- <6 months   16 hours
- 6 months   14.5 hours
- 12 months   13.5 hours
- 2 years   13 hours
- 4 years   11.5 hours
- 6 years   9.5 hours
- 12 years   8.5 hours
- 18 years   8 hours

Nap Patterns
- 2/day at 1 year
- 1/day at 2 years: 2-3 hours
- 0.5/day at 5 years: 1.7 hours

Nightmares
- prevalence: common in boys, 4-7 years old
- associated with REM sleep (anytime during night)
- upon awakening, child is alert and clearly recalls frightening dream
- may be associated with daytime stress/anxiety
- treatment: reassurance

Night Terrors
- prevalence: 15% of children have occasional episodes
- abrupt sitting up, eyes open, screaming
- panic and signs of autonomic arousal
- occurs in early hours of sleep, non-REM, stage 4 of sleep
- no memory of event, parents unable to calm child
- stress/anxiety can aggravate them
- course: remits spontaneously at puberty
- treatment: reassurance

Breath-Holding Spells

- occur in 0.1-5% of healthy children 6 months-4 years of age
- spells usually start during first year of life
- 2 types
  - anger/frustration → blue/cyanotic (more common)
  - pain/surprise → white/pallid
- child is provoked (usually by anger, injury or fear), starts to cry and then becomes silent
- spell resolves spontaneously or the child may lose consciousness; rarely progresses to seizures
- treatment
  - behavioural – help child control response to frustration and avoid drawing attention to spell
- avoid being too permissive in fear of precipitating a spell

Child Abuse and Neglect

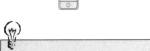

Definition
- an act of commission (abuse – physical, sexual, or psychological) or omission (neglect) by a caregiver that harms a child

> "If no cruising, no bruising."

Legal Duty to Report
- upon reasonable grounds to suspect abuse and/or neglect, physicians are required by law to contact the Children's Aid Society (CAS) personally to disclose all information
- duty to report overrides patient confidentiality; physician is protected against liability
- ongoing duty to report: if there are additional reasonable grounds to suspect abuse and/or neglect, a further report to the CAS must be made

Risk Factors
- environmental factors
  - social isolation
  - poverty
  - domestic violence
- caregiver factors
  - parents were abused as children
  - psychiatric illness
  - substance abuse
  - single parent family
  - poor social and vocational skills, below average intelligence
- child factors
  - difficult temperament
  - disability, special needs (e.g. developmental delay)
  - premature

Presentation of Physical Abuse
- history inconsistent with physical findings, or history not reproducible
- delay in seeking medical attention
- injuries of varied ages, recurrent or multiple injuries
- distinctive marks: belt buckle, cigarette burns, hand prints
- patterns of injury: bruises on the face, abdomen, buttocks, genitalia, upper back, posterior rib fractures, immersion burns (i.e. hot water)
- altered mental status: head injury, poisoning
- physical findings not consistent with any underlying medical condition
- shaken baby syndrome
  - violent shaking of infant resulting in intracranial hemorrhages, retinal hemorrhages, and fractures (e.g. posterior rib fractures)
  - diagnosis confirmed by head CT or MRI, ophthalmologic exam, skeletal survey/bone scan
  - head trauma is the leading cause of death in child maltreatment

Presentation of Neglect
- Failure to thrive, developmental delay
- Inadequate or dirty clothing, poor hygiene
- Child exhibits poor attachment to parents, no stranger anxiety

Sexual Abuse
- prevalence: 1 in 4 females, 1 in 10 males
- peak ages at 2-6 and 12-16 years
- most perpetrators are male and known to child
  - in decreasing order: family member, non-relative known to victim, stranger
- presentation
  - disclosure: diagnosis usually depends on child telling someone
  - psychosocial: specific or generalized fears, depression, nightmares, social withdrawal, lack of trust, low self-esteem, school failure, sexually aggressive behaviour, advanced sexual knowledge, sexual preoccupation or play
  - physical signs: recurrent UTIs, pregnancy, STIs, vaginitis, vaginal bleeding, pain, genital injury, enuresis
- investigations depend on presentation, age, sex, and maturity of child
  - sexual assault examination kit within 24 hours if prepubertal, within 72 hours if pubertal
  - rule out STI, UTI, pregnancy (consider STI prophylaxis or morning after pill)
  - rule out other injuries (vaginal/anal/oral penetration, fractures, head trauma)

Management of Child Abuse and Neglect
- history
  - from child and each caregiver separately (if possible)
- physical exam
  - head to toe (do not force)
  - emotional state
  - development
  - document and/or photograph all injuries: type, location, size, shape, colour, pattern
  - be aware of "red herrings" (e.g. Mongolian blue spots vs. bruises)
- investigations
  - blood tests to rule out medical causes (e.g. thrombocytopenia or coagulopathy)
  - STI work-up
  - skeletal survey/bone scan
  - CT/MRI
  - ophthalmology exam
- report all suspicions to Children's Aid Society; request emergency visit if imminent risk to child or any siblings in the home
- acute medical care: hospitalize if indicated or if concerns about further or ongoing abuse
- arrange consultation to social work and appropriate follow-up
- may need to discharge child directly to CAS or to responsible guardian under CAS supervision

Adolescent Medicine

Normal Sexual Development

- puberty occurs with the maturation of the hypothalamic–pituitary–gonadal axis
- increases in the pulsatile release of gonadotropin hormone (GnRH) → increased release of LH and FSH → maturation of gonads and release of sex steroids → secondary sexual characteristics
- also requires adrenal production of androgens

Females
- occurs between age 7-13 years (may start early as 6 years in African-American girls)
- usual sequence
  - thelarche: breast budding (breast asymmetry may occur as one breast may grow faster than the other; becomes less noticeable as maturation continues)
  - adrenarche: axillary hair, body odour, mild acne
  - growth spurt
  - menarche: mean age 13 years; occurs 2 years after breast development and indicates that growth spurt is almost complete (Tanner Stage 4)
- early puberty is common and often constitutional, late puberty is rare

Males
- occurs between age 9-14 years (starts 2 years later than in girls)
- usual sequence
  - testicular enlargement
  - penile enlargement: occurs at Tanner Stage 4
  - adrenarche: axillary and facial hair, body odour, mild acne
  - growth spurt: occurs later in boys (Tanner Stage 4)
- early puberty is uncommon (need to rule out organic disease) but late puberty is common and often constitutional

Table 12. Tanner Staging (Sexual Maturity Rating)

| Stage | FEMALE | | MALE | |
	Breast	Pubic Hair	Genitalia	Pubic Hair
1	–	–	–	–
2	bud	sparse labial hair	scrotal/testes enlargement	sparse hair at base of penis
3	bud enlarges	hair over pubis	increase in length of penis	hair over pubis
4	areola + papilla secondary mound	coarse adult hair	further increase in length and breadth of penis	coarse adult hair
5	areola recedes adult size and shape	extends to medial thigh	adult size and shape	extends to medial thigh

Normal Variation in Puberty

Premature Thelarche
- isolated breast tissue development in girls 6 months to 2 years
- requires careful history and physical to ensure no other estrogen effects or other signs of puberty (e.g. growth spurt)
- may be due to increased sensitivity to estrogen
- requires observation and periodic examinations every 6-12 months to ensure no further signs of puberty

Physiologic Leukorrhea
- occurs in the 6 months prior to menarche; scant mucoid, clear to milky vaginal discharge, not associated with pruritis or foul odour
- due to stimulation of endometrial glands by estrogen

Irregular Menstruation
- menses may be irregular in duration and length of cycle
- on average it takes 18 months to go through the first 12 periods
- birth control pills should be avoided as treatment

Premature Adrenarche
- usually develops in boys and girls before the age of 6, benign self-limiting condition
- adrenal production of DHEAS (precursor of androstenedione, testosterone and estrogen) reaches pubertal levels at an earlier age
- pubic and axillary hair, body odour, mild acne
- determine whether other signs of puberty are present (girls - thelarche; boys - testicular enlargement)
- exclude androgen secreting tumours (investigations: DHEAS levels, androstenedione, testosterone, bone age)

Gynecomastia
- transient development of breast tissue in boys
- common self-limited condition seen in 50% of male adolescents during puberty
- must distinguish true breast tissue from fat: 1-3 cm round, mobile, sometimes tender, firm mass under areola
- discharge from nipple or fixed mass should be investigated

Other Adolescent Medicine Topics
- Substance Abuse – see Psychiatry
- Eating Disorders – see Psychiatry
- Depression/Suicide – see Psychiatry
- Sexually Transmitted Infections – see Gynecology

Cardiology

Heart Murmurs

- 50-80% of children have audible heart murmurs at some point in their childhood
- most childhood murmurs are functional (i.e. "innocent") without associated structural abnormalities and have normal ECG and radiologic findings
- in general, murmurs can become audible or accentuated in high output states, e.g. fever, anemia

Table 13. Differentiating Innocent and Pathological Heart Murmurs

	Innocent	Pathological
History and Physical	Asymptomatic	Symptoms and signs of cardiac disease (FTT, exercise intolerance)
Timing	Systolic ejection murmur (SEM)	All diastolic, pansystolic, or continuous (except venous hum)
Grade	<3/6	≥3/6 (palpable thrill)
Splitting	Physiologic S2	May have fixed split or single S2
Extra sounds/Clicks	None	May be present
Change of Position	Murmur varies	Unchanged

Table 14. Five Innocent Heart Murmurs

Type	Description	Age	Differential Diagnosis
Peripheral Pulmonic Stenosis	Neonates, low-pitched, radiates to axilla and back	neonates, usually disappears by 3-6 mos	Patent Ductus Arteriosus (PDA) Pulmonary stenosis
Still's Murmur	Vibratory, lower left sternal border (LLSB) or apex, SEM	3-6 yrs	Subaortic stenosis Small ventricular septal defect (VSD)
Venous Hum	Infraclavicular hum, continuous, R>L	3-6 yrs	PDA
Pulmonary Ejection	Soft, blowing, upper left sternal border (ULSB), SEM	8-14 yrs	Atrial septal defect (ASD) Pulmonary stenosis
Supraclavicular Arterial Bruit	Low intensity, above clavicles	any age	Aortic stenosis Bicuspid aortic valve

Congenital Heart Disease (CHD)

Prenatal Circulation

Fetal circulation is designed so that oxygenated blood is preferentially delivered to the brain and myocardium.

Before Birth:
- fetal lungs bypassed by flow through fetal shunts:
  - shunting deoxygenated blood
    - ductus arteriosus: connection between pulmonary artery and aorta
  - shunting oxygenated blood
    - foramen ovale: connection between R and L atria
    - ductus venosus: connecting between umbilical vein and IVC
- circulation:
  - placenta (oxygenated blood) > umbilical vein > ductus venosus > IVC > R atrium > oxygenated blood shunted through foramen ovale > L atrium > L ventricle > aorta > brain/myocardium/upper extremities
  - deoxygenated blood returns via SVC to R atrium > 1/3rd of blood entering R atrium does not flow through foramen ovale and flows to the R ventricle > pulmonary arteries > ductus arteriosus > aorta > systemic circulation > placenta for reoxygenation

At birth:
- with first breath, lungs open up and pulmonary resistance decreases allowing pulmonic blood flow
- with separation of low resistance placenta, systemic circulation becomes a high resistance system
- with closure of the fetal shunts and changes in pulmonic/systemic resistance, infant circulation assumes normal adult flow
- increasing pulmonic flow increases left atrial pressures leading to foramen ovale closure
- increased oxygen concentration in blood after first breath leads to decreased prostaglandins leading to closure of the ductus arteriosus
- as the umbilical cord is clamped, the umbilical vein closes, systemic vascular resistance increases and the ductus venosus closes

Embryologic Development
- most critical period of fetal heart development is between 3-8 weeks gestation
- single heart tube grows rapidly forcing it to bend back upon itself and begin to assume the shape of a 4 chambered heart
- insults at this time are most likely to lead to CHD

Epidemiology
- 8/1,000 live births can present with heart murmur, heart failure, or cyanosis
- at birth, ventricular septal defect is the most common lesion

Table 15. Risk Factors for Common CHD

Infant factors/Genetic conditions		Maternal factors	
Abnormality	**Dominant cardiac defect**	**Abnormality (% risk)**	**Dominant cardiac defect**
Prematurity	PDA	Prior child with CHD (2-4% risk)	
CHARGE association	TOF, AVSD, ASD, VSD	Torch esp. rubella (35%)	PDA, PS
DiGeorge	Aortic arch anomalies	Diabetes Mellitus (2-3%)	TGA, coarctation, VSD
Down syndrome	AVSD, VSD, ASD, TOF	PKU (25-50%)	TOF
Ehlers-Danlos	Mitral prolapse, dilated aortic root	SLE (20-40%)	Complete heart block
Kartagener's	Dextrocardia	Alcohol (25-30%)	ASD, VSD
Marfan	Mitral prolapse, aortic dissection or insufficiency, dilated aortic root		
Noonan	Pulmonary stenosis, ASD	Medications: Phenytoin	VSD, ASD, PS, AS, coarctation
Osteogenesis Imperfecta	Aortic incompetence	Valproate	Coarctation, HLHS, AS, VSD
Turner	Coarctation, bicuspid aortic valve	Retinoic acid	Aortic arch abnormalities

VSD = ventricular septal defect; ASD = atrial septal defect; PDA = patent ductus arteriosus; TOF = tetralogy of Fallot;
TGA = transposition of great arteries; PS = pulmonary stenosis; AS = aortic stenosis; HLHS = hypoplastic left heart syndrome
AVSD = atrioventricular septal defect

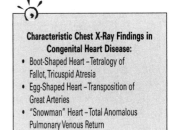

Characteristic Chest X-Ray Findings in Congenital Heart Disease:
- Boot-Shaped Heart – Tetralogy of Fallot, Tricuspid Atresia
- Egg-Shaped Heart – Transposition of Great Arteries
- "Snowman" Heart – Total Anomalous Pulmonary Venous Return

Investigations
- Echo, ECG, CXR

CYANOTIC VS. ACYANOTIC CONGENITAL HEART DISEASE
- cyanosis: blue mucous membranes, nail beds, and skin secondary to an absolute concentration of deoxygenated hemoglobin of at least 3 g/dL
- **cyanotic heart disease:** (i.e. R > L shunt) blood bypasses the lungs > no oxygenation occurs > high levels of deoxygenated hemoglobin enters the systemic circulation > cyanosis
- **acyanotic heart disease:** (i.e. L > R shunt, obstruction occurring beyond lungs) blood passes through pulmonic circulation > oxygenation takes place > low levels of deoxygenated blood in systemic circulation > no cyanosis

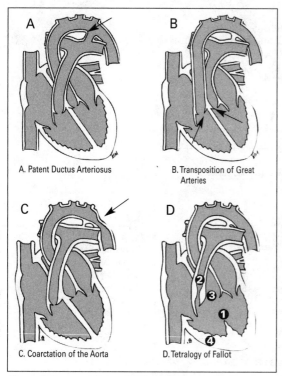

A. Patent Ductus Arteriosus

B. Transposition of Great Arteries

C. Coarctation of the Aorta

D. Tetralogy of Fallot

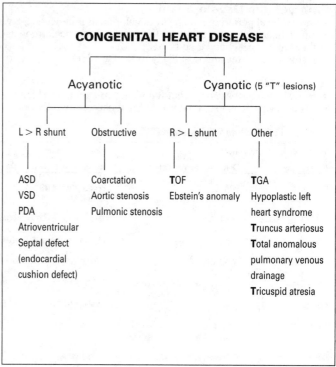

CONGENITAL HEART DISEASE

Acyanotic		**Cyanotic** (5 "T" lesions)	
L > R shunt	Obstructive	R > L shunt	Other
ASD	Coarctation	**T**OF	**T**GA
VSD	Aortic stenosis	Ebstein's anomaly	Hypoplastic left
PDA	Pulmonic stenosis		heart syndrome
Atrioventricular			**T**runcus arteriosus
Septal defect			**T**otal anomalous
(endocardial			pulmonary venous
cushion defect)			drainage
			Tricuspid atresia

Figure 1. Common Congenital Heart Diseases

Acyanotic Congenital Heart Disease

1. LEFT TO RIGHT SHUNT LESIONS
- extra blood is displaced through a communication from the left to the right side of the heart → increased pulmonary blood flow → increased pulmonary pressures
- shunt volume dependent upon three factors: size of defect, pressure gradient between chambers or vessels, peripheral outflow resistance
- untreated shunts can result in pulmonary vascular disease, right ventricular hypertension and hypertrophy (RVH), and eventually R→L shunts

Atrial Septal Defect (ASD)
- three types: ostium primum (common in Down syndrome), ostium secundum (most common type, 50-70%), sinus venosus (defect located at entry of superior vena cava (SVC) into right atrium)
- epidemiology: 6-8% of congenital heart lesions
- natural history: 80-100% spontaneous closure rate if ASD diameter <8 mm
- if remains patent, congestive heart failure (CHF) and pulmonary hypertension can develop in adult life
- history: often asymptomatic in childhood
- physical exam: grade 2-3/6 pulmonic outflow murmur (SEM), a mid-diastolic rumble at the left lower sternal border, and a widely split and fixed S2
- investigations:
    - ECG: right axis deviation (RAD), mild RVH, right bundle branch block (RBBB)
    - CXR: increased pulmonary vasculature
- treatment: elective surgical or catheter closure between 2-5 years of age

Ventricular Septal Defect (VSD)
- most common congenital heart defect (30-50% of CHD)

Small VSD (majority)
- history: asymptomatic, normal growth and development
- physical exam: early systolic to holosystolic murmur, best heard at left lower sternal border (LLSB)
- investigations: ECG and CXR are normal
- treatment: most close spontaneously, do not need surgical closure even if remains patent

Moderate-to-large VSD
- natural history: secondary pulmonary hypertension, CHF by 2 months of age
- history: delayed growth and development, decreased exercise tolerance, recurrent URTIs or "asthma" episodes, CHF

- physical exam: holosystolic murmur at LLSB with thrill, mid-diastolic rumble at apex, size of VSD is inversely related to intensity of murmur
- investigations:
  - ECG: left ventricular hypertrophy (LVH), left atrial hypertrophy (LAH), RVH
  - CXR: increased pulmonary vasculature, cardiomegaly, CHF
- treatment: treatment of CHF and surgical closure by 1 year of age

Patent Ductus Arteriosus (PDA)
- patent vessel between descending aorta and left pulmonary artery
- epidemiology
  - functional closure within first 15 hours of life, anatomical closure within first days of life
  - 5-10% of all congenital heart defects
  - common in premature infants (1/3 of infants <1750 grams)
  - natural history: spontaneous closure common in premature infants, less common in term infants
- history: may be asymptomatic or have apneic or bradycardic spells, poor feeding, accessory muscle use
- physical exam: tachycardia, bounding pulses, hyperactive precordium, wide pulse pressure, continuous "machinery" murmur, best heard at left infraclavicular area
- investigations:
  - ECG: may show LAH, LVH, BVH
  - CXR: normal to mildly enlarged heart, increased pulmonary vasculature, prominent pulmonary artery
  - diagnosis by echocardiography (Echo)
- treatment:
  - indomethacin (Indocid™) – PGE1 antagonist (PGE1 maintains ductus arteriosus patency) in premature infants if necessary
  - catheter or surgical closure if PDA is contributing to respiratory compromise or persists beyond 3rd month of life

Endocardial Cushion Defect (Atrioventricular [AV] Canal)
- spectrum from endocardial cushion VSD and ostium primum ASD to complete AV canal with common AV valve
- commonly associated with Down syndrome
- treatment:
  - natural history depends on size of defect and valvular involvement, and should be repaired by age 6 months to prevent development of pulmonary hypertension
  - complete AV canal requires early complete surgical repair, preferably before 3 months of age

2. OBSTRUCTIVE LESIONS
- present with pallor, decreased urine output, cool extremities and poor pulses

Coarctation of the Aorta
- narrowing of aorta almost always at the level of the ductus arteriosus
- commonly associated with bicuspid aortic valve (50%); Turner syndrome (35%)
- few have high BP in infancy (160-200 mmHg systolic) but this decreases as collaterals develop
- if severe, presents with shock in the neonatal period when the ductus closes
- history: often asymptomatic
- physical exam: upper extremity systolic pressures of 140-145 mmHg, decreased blood pressure and weak/absent pulses in lower extremities, radial-femoral delay, absent or systolic murmur with late peak at apex, left axilla, and left back
- investigations: ECG - RVH early in infancy, LVH later in childhood
- prognosis and treatment
  - if associated with other lesions (e.g. PDA, VSD) can cause CHF
  - complications: hypertension
  - management: balloon arterioplasty or surgical correction in symptomatic neonate, give prostaglandins to open up PDA for stabilization

Aortic Stenosis
- valvular (75%), subvalvular (20%), supravalvular and idiopathic hypertrophic subaortic stenosis (IHSS) (5%)
- history: often asymptomatic but may be associated with CHF, exertional chest pain, syncope or sudden death
- physical exam: SEM at upper right sternal border (URSB) with aortic ejection click at the apex

- treatment
    - surgical repair if infant with critical aortic stenosis or older child with symptoms or peak gradient >50 mmHg
    - exercise restriction required

Pulmonary Stenosis
- valvular (90%), subvalvular, or supravalvular
- usually part of other congenital heart lesions (e.g. Tetralogy of Fallot) or in association with other syndromes (e.g. congenital rubella, Noonan syndrome)
- critical pulmonic stenosis: inadequate pulmonary blood flow, dependent on ductus for oxygenation, progressive hypoxia and cyanosis
- history: spectrum from asymptomatic to CHF
- physical exam: wide split S2 on expiration, SEM at ULSB, pulmonary ejection click
- investigations:
    - ECG: RVH
    - CXR: dilated post-stenotic pulmonary artery
- treatment: surgical repair if critically ill or severe PS, or if presence of symptoms in older infants/children

Cyanotic Congenital Heart Disease

- systemic venous return re-enters systemic circulation directly
- most prominent feature is cyanosis (O_2 sat <75%)
- differentiate between cardiac and other causes of cyanosis with hyperoxic test
    - obtain preductal, right radial ABG in room air, repeat ABG after the child inspires 100% oxygen
    - if PaO_2 improves to greater than 150 mmHg, cyanosis less likely cardiac in origin
- survival depends on mixing via shunts (e.g. ASD, VSD, PDA)

1. RIGHT TO LEFT SHUNT LESIONS

Tetralogy of Fallot
- 10% of all CHD, most common cyanotic heart defect diagnosed beyond infancy
- embryologically, a single defect with hypoplasia of the conus causing:
    - VSD
    - right ventricle (RV) outflow tract obstruction (RVOTO)
    - overriding aorta
    - RVH
- degree of RVOTO directly determines the direction and degree of shunt and therefore the extent of clinical cyanosis and degree of RVH
- infants may initially have a L→R shunt and therefore are not cyanotic but the RVOTO is progressive, resulting in increasing R→L shunting with hypoxemia and cyanosis
- history: hypoxic "tet" spells
    - primary pathophysiology is hypoxia, leading to increased pulmonary vascular resistance (PVR) and decreased systemic resistance, occurring in exertional states (e.g. crying, exercise)
    - paroxysm of rapid and deep breathing, irritability and crying
    - hyperpnea, increasing cyanosis often leading to deep sleep and decreased intensity of murmur (decreased flow across RVOTO)
    - peak incidence at 2-4 months of age
        - if severe may lead to seizures, loss of consciousness, death (rare)
        - management: O_2, knee-chest position, fluid bolus, morphine sulfate, propanolol
- physical exam: single loud S2 due to severe pulmonary stenosis (i.e RVOTO)
- investigations:
    - ECG: RAD, RVH
    - CXR: boot shaped heart (small PA, RVH), decreased pulmonary vasculature, right aortic arch (in 20%)
- treatment: surgical repair within first two years of life, or earlier if marked cyanosis, "tet" spells, or severe RV outflow tract obstruction

Ebstein's Anomaly
- congenital defect of the tricuspid valve in which the septal and posterior leaflets are malformed and displaced into the RV leading to variable degrees of RV dysfunction, TS, TR or functional pulmonary atresia if RV unable to open pulmonic valves
- RA massively enlarged, interatrial communication (PFO) often exists allowing R → L shunting

Tetralogy of Fallot
1. Ventricular septal defect (VSD)
2. Right ventricular outflow tract obstruction (RVOTO)
3. Aortic root "overriding" VSD
4. Right ventricular hypertrophy
See Figure 1

- TR and accessory conduction pathways (WPW) are often present
- cause: unknown, associated with maternal lithium and benzo use in 1st trimester
- treatment:
  - in newborns, consider closure of tricuspid valve + aortopulmonary shunt, or transplantation
  - in older children, tricuspid valve repair or valve replacement + ASD closure

2. OTHER CYANOTIC CONGENITAL HEART DISEASES

Transposition of the Great Arteries (TGA)
- 3-5% of all congenital cardiac lesions
- parallel pulmonary and systemic circulations
  - systemic: body → RA → RV → aorta → body
  - pulmonary: lungs → LA → LV → pulmonary artery → lungs
- physical exam:
  - no murmur if no VSD
  - newborn presents with progressive cyanosis unresponsive to oxygen therapy as the ductus arteriosus closes and mixing between the two circulations diminishes; severe hypoxemia, acidosis, and death can occur rapidly
  - if VSD present, cyanosis is not prominent and infant presents with CHF after a few weeks of life
- investigations:
  - ECG: RAD, RVH
  - CXR: egg-shaped heart with narrow mediastinum ("egg on a string")
- treatment:
  - prostaglandin E_1 (Prostin VR™) infusion to keep ductus open until septostomy or surgery (arterial switch procedure)
  - infants without VSD must be repaired within 2 weeks to avoid weak LV muscle

Hypoplastic Left Heart Syndrome
- 1-3% of all congenital cardiac lesions; most common cyanotic CHD in the neonate
- a spectrum of hypoplasia of left ventricle, atretic mitral and/or aortic valves, small ascending aorta, coarctation of the aorta with resultant systemic hypoperfusion
- most common cause of death from congenital heart disease in first month of life
- systemic circulation is dependent on ductus patency; upon closure of the ductus, infant presents with circulatory shock and metabolic acidosis
- treatment
  - intubate and correct metabolic acidosis
  - IV infusion of PGE_1 to keep ductus open
  - surgical correction (overall survival 50% to late childhood) or heart transplant

Hypoplastic LHS:
Hypoplastic LV
Narrow mitral/aortic valves
Small Ascending Aorta
Contracted Aorta

Univentricular Heart (single ventricle)
- spectrum of anomalies in which the heart has only one effective pumping chamber (usually hypoplastic RV), e.g. tricuspid atresia
- both AV valves are committed to the dominant chamber, giving rise to the name "double inlet left ventricle"
- TGA is usually present, so the LV pumps directly into the PA and via the VSD into the aorta
- treatment: surgical therapy if progressive cyanosis and/or to prevent pulmonary vascular disease

Double Outlet Right Ventricle
- a complex spectrum of lesions in which one great artery and more than 50% of the other arise from the RV, with LV outflow through a VSD
- classified by the location of the VSD – subpulmonic, subaortic, doubly committed (lies beneath both valves), or noncommitted
- treatment: surgical repair if progressive cyanosis or refractory CHF

Total Anomalous Pulmonary Venous Connection
- only 1-2% of CHD
- characterized by all of the pulmonary veins draining into the right-sided circulation (supracardiac – SVC or innominate vein, infracardiac – hepatic/portal vein or IVC, intracardiac – coronary sinus or RA)
- no direct oxygenated pulmonary venous return to left atrium
- often associated with obstruction at connection sites
- an ASD must be present to allow blood to shunt into the LA and systemic circulation
- treatment: surgical repair if severe cyanosis or CHF related to pulmonary venous obstruction

Truncus Arteriosus
- a single great vessel arising from the heart which gives rise to the aorta, PA, and coronary arteries
- the truncal valve overlies a large VSD
- treatment: surgical repair within first 6 months of life to prevent development of pulmonary vascular disease

Congestive Heart Failure (CHF)

- see Cardiology

Etiology
- congenital heart disease (CHD)
- arteriovenous malformations (AVMs)
- cardiomyopathy
- arrhythmias
- acute hypertension
- anemia
- cor pulmonale
- myocarditis

Symptoms
- infant: feeding difficulties, easy fatiguability, exertional dyspnea, diaphoresis when sleeping or eating, respiratory distress, lethargy, cyanosis, FTT
- child: decreased exercise tolerance, fatigue, decreased appetite, failure to thrive, respiratory distress, frequent URTIs or "asthma" episodes
- orthopnea, paroxysmal nocturnal dyspnea, pedal/dependant edema are all uncommon in children

Physical Findings
- four key features: tachycardia, tachypnea, cardiomegaly, hepatomegaly
- failure to thrive (FTT)
- respiratory distress, gallop rhythm, wheezing, crackles, cyanosis, clubbing (with CHD)
- alterations in peripheral pulses, four limb blood pressures (in some CHDs)
- dysmorphic features associated with congenital syndromes
- CXR – cardiomegaly, pulmonary venous congestion

Management
- correction of underlying cause
- general: sitting up, O_2, sodium and water restriction, increased caloric intake
- pharmacologic: diuretics, digoxin, afterload reducers

4 Key Features of CHF
2 tachy's and 2 megaly's
Tachycardia
Tachypnea
Cardiomegaly
Hepatomegaly

Pharmacologic Management of CHF
3 D's
Diuretics
Digoxin
Afterload Decreasers

Infective Endocarditis

- see Infectious Diseases
- 70% *Streptococcus*, 20% *Staphylococcus* (*aureus, epidermidis*)
- serial positive cultures are needed for definitive diagnosis, but rely on clinical suspicion and other investigations if initially negative (i.e. use Echo to look for vegetations)
- 10-15% of cases are culture negative, this is a risk factor for poor prognosis
- Osler's nodes, Janeway's lesions, splinter hemorrhages are late findings in children
- antibiotic prophylaxis is necessary for all patients with:
  - congenital heart disease (except for isolated secundum ASD or 6 mos post repair of ASD, VSV,PDA)
  - rheumatic valve lesions (except if no valve dysfunction)
  - prosthetic heart valves
  - surgical shunts
  - previous endocarditis
  - pacemaker leads
- SBE prophylaxis: amoxicillin 50 mg/kg 1 hour before procedure, or if allergic clindamycin 20 mg/kg
- high risk patients for GI/GU procedures may receive 2 doses amp + gent IV (30 min before procedure and 6 hours later)

Dysrhythmias

- see Cardiology
- can be transient or permanent, congenital (structurally normal or abnormal) or acquired (toxin, infection, infarction)

Sinus Arrhythmia
- phasic variations with respiration
- present in almost all normal children

Premature Atrial Contractions (PACs)
- may be normal variant or can be caused by electrolyte disturbances, hyperthyroidism, cardiac surgery, digitalis toxicity

Premature Ventricular Contractions (PVCs)
- common in adolescents
- benign if single, uniform, disappear with exercise, and no associated structural lesions
- if not benign, may degenerate into more severe dysrhythmias

Supraventricular Tachycardia (SVT)
- most frequent sustained dysrhythmia in children
- not life-threatening but can lead to symptoms
- caused by re-entry via accessory connection (atrioventricular (AV) node most common site)
- characterized by a rate of greater than 210 bpm
- treatment
    - stable (alert, normal BP)
        - vagal maneuvres
        - adenosine
        - synchronized cardioversion
    - unstable (decreased LOC, decreased BP)
        - immediate synchronized cardioversion

> **Pediatric vs Adult ECG**
> Pediatric ECG findings that may be normal:
> - HR > 100bpm
> - Shorter PR, QT intervals and QRS duration
> - Inferior and lateral small Q waves
> - RV larger than LV in neonates, so normal to have:
>   - right axis deviation
>   - large precordial R waves
>   - upright T waves

Complete Heart Block
- congenital heart block can be caused by maternal Rho antibody (e.g. in mothers with lupus)
- clinical symptoms related to level of block (the lower the block, the greater the symptoms of inadequate cardiac output)
- symptomatic patients need a pacemaker

Development

Developmental Delay

- developmental delay is defined as performance significantly below average in a given area
- causes:
    1. global delay
        - environmental neglect (under stimulation)
        - chromosome disorders (trisomy 21)
        - CNS abnormalities/prenatal exposures (fetal hyponia, fetal-alcohol syndrome, viral infections)
        - other (inborn errors of metabolism, hypothyroidism, anemia, lead, idiopathic)
    2. speech/language delay
    3. motor delay
- neglect and lack of stimulation is also a major cause of developmental delay

Mental Retardation (MR)

Epidemiology
- 1% of general population; M:F = 1.5:1
- psychiatric comorbidity
    - 3-4 times greater vs. general population
    - ADHD, mood disorders, PDD, stereotypic movement disorders

Etiology
- genetic: Down syndrome, Fragile X, PKU
- prenatal: rubella, fetal alcohol syndrome, prenatal exposure to heroin, cocaine, TORCH infections, HIV; maternal DM; toxemia; maternal malnutrition; birth trauma/hypoxia
- perinatal: prematurity, low birth weight, cerebral ischemia, intracranial hemorrhage, maternal deprivation
- childhood: intracranial infection, head trauma, FTT, lead poisoning
- psychosocial factors: mild MR associated with low socioeconomic status (SES), limited parental education, parental neglect, teen pregnancy, family instability

Diagnosis

- below average general intellectual functioning as defined by an IQ of approximately 70 or below (2 standard deviations below the mean)
- deficits in adaptive functioning in at least two of:
  - communication, self-care, home-living, social skills, self-direction, academic skills, work, leisure, health, safety
- onset before 18 years of age

Table 16. Classification of Mental Retardation

Severity	% Cases of MR	IQ
Mild	85%	50-70
Moderate	10%	35-49
Severe	3-4%	20-34
Profound	1-2%	<20

Treatment

- main objective: enhance adaptive functioning level
- emphasize community-based treatment vs. institutionalization and early intervention
- education: life skills, vocational training, communication skills, family education
- therapy: individual/family therapy; behaviour modification (to decrease aggressive/distracting behaviours)
- support of parents and respite care

Learning Disorders

Definition

- a significant discrepancy between a child's intellectual ability and his or her academic performance

Epidemiology

- prevalence: 2-10%
- psychiatric comorbidity = 10-25% of individuals with dysthymia, conduct disorder (CD), major depressive disorder (MDD), oppositional defiant disorder (ODD), attention deficit hyperactivity disorder (ADHD)

Diagnosis

- categorized by
  - individual scores on achievement tests in reading, mathematics or written expression (WISC III, WRAT) significantly below (>2 SD) that expected for age, education, and IQ
  - interferes with academic achievement or ADLs that require reading, mathematics, or writing skills
- types: reading, mathematics, disorders of written expression
- rule out occult seizure disorder, sensory impairments

Complications

- low self-esteem, poor social skills
- 40% school drop-out rate

Language Delay

Differential Diagnosis

- hearing impairment
  - spectrum of impairment – slight to profound loss
  - language development may seem normal for up to 6 months (including cooing and babbling) but may regress due to lack of feedback
  - risk factors for sensorineural hearing loss (≥1 risk factor warrants infant screening, if newborn screening not available in jurisdiction for all newborns):
    - genetic syndromes/family history
    - congenital (TORCH) infections
    - craniofacial abnormalties
    - <1,500 g birthweight
    - hyperbilirubinemia/kernicterus
    - asphyxia/low APGAR scores
    - bacterial meningitis, viral encephalitis
  - to evaluate hearing loss in children:
    - <6 months old: auditory brainstem response (ABR): tympanometry (impedence testing), evoked potentials
    - >6-8 months old: behaviour audiometry
    - >3-4 years old: pure tone audiometry

- cognitive disability
  - global developmental delay, mental retardation
  - both receptive and expressive language components affected
  - child often has interest in communication
- pervasive developmental disorder (PDD), including autism
  - poor social interaction and language impairment, stereotypical behaviours
- selective mutism
  - a childhood anxiety disorder with onset age 5-6
  - only speaks in certain situations, usually at home
  - healthy children with no hearing impairment
  - often above-average intelligence
- Landau-Kleffner syndrome (acquired epileptic aphasia)
  - presents in late preschool to early school age years, may be similar to autism
  - child begins to develop language normally, then sudden regression of language
  - child has severe aphasia with EEG changes, often has overt seizure activity
- mechanical problems
  - cleft palate
  - cranial nerve palsy
- social deprivation

Management
- ENT and dental referral if mechanical cause
- speech therapy in disorders of fluency, receptive or expressive language
- psychiatric consultation in selective mutism, PDD

Fetal Alcohol Spectrum Disorder (FASD)

- this disorder refers to the full range of problems resulting from the use of alcohol during pregnancy, including Fetal Alcohol Syndrome (FAS) and Fetal Alcohol Effects (FAE)

No "safe" level of alcohol consumption during pregnancy has been established.

Fetal Alcohol Syndrome
- prevalence of FAS: 1 in 300
- not known how much alcohol is harmful during pregnancy
- criteria for Diagnosis of Fetal Alcohol Syndrome
  - a) growth deficiency – low birth weight and/or length at birth that continues through childhood
  - b) abnormal craniofacial features – small head, short palpebral fissures, long smooth philtrum, thin upper lip
  - c) central nervous system dysfunction – microcephaly and/or neurobehavioural dysfunction (e.g. hyperactivity, fine motor problems, attention deficits, learning disabilities, cognitive disabilities)
  - d) strong evidence of maternal drinking during pregnancy
- cardiac and renal defects, hypospadias may occur
- FASD is one of the most common causes of mental retardation in the world

Fetal Alcohol Spectrum Disorder
- prevalence of FAE: 1 in 200
- child born to a mother who was known to be drinking heavily during pregnancy
- child has some but not all of physical characteristics of FAS; often missed diagnosis as features are subtle
- most children with FASD have normal stature and do not have microcephaly, however, they may show milder forms of the facial features present in FAS
- if present, short stature and microcephaly will persist through adolescence, while facial features will become more subtle with age

Endocrinology

Diabetes Mellitus (DM)

- see Endocrinology

TYPE 1 DIABETES (Insulin-Dependent DM)

Epidemiology
- insulin dependent, most common type in childhood
- prevalence: 1 in 400-500 children under 18 years of age
- can present at any age; bimodal peaks 5-7 years and puberty
- classic presentation: polyuria, polydipsia, abdominal pain, weight loss, and fatigue
- 25% present with diabetic ketoacidosis (DKA)

Etiology
- genetic predisposition and environmental trigger
  - autoimmune destruction of β-cells of the pancreas (antibodies directed towards

Diagnostic Criteria for Diabetes Mellitus
Symptoms (polyuria, polydipsia, weight loss) + random glucose ≥11.1 mmol/L (200 mg/dL)
OR
Fasting glucose ≥7.0 mmol/L (126 mg/dL)
OR
2hr glucose during OGTT ≥11.1 mmol/L (200 mg/dL)
OGTT=oral glucose tolerance test

        glutamic acid decarboxylase have been identified)
- a non-immune variation has been described
- diseases of pancreas (i.e. cystic fibrosis) and long term corticosteroids

Management of Uncomplicated Diabetes
- meal plan, exercise, education, psychosocial support
- insulin injections 2-3 times per day, blood glucose monitoring
- young children more susceptible to CNS damage with hypoglycemia with fewer benefits from tight control, hence target glucose range higher at 6-12 mmol/L (110-220 mg/dL)
- increasingly tighter control in older children, 4-8 mmol/L (70-140 mg/dL)
- continuous subcutaneous insulin infusion (CSII) pump
  - contains a cartridge full of short-acting insulin (Lispro™) or a syringe connected to a catheter that is inserted into the subcutaneous tissue
  - continuously delivers predetermined basal rates to meet nonprandial insulin requirements
  - bolus infusion to cover mealtime or snack time insulin requirements
  - requires as much or more blood glucose monitoring when compared to injections ± ketone monitoring - patients must be highly motivated
  - allows for tighter glycemic control
  - risk of DKA with operator or mechanical failure (catheter occlusion, battery failure, depleted insulin)

Complications of Type 1 Diabetes
- hypoglycemia
  - cause: missed/delayed meals, excess insulin, increased exercise, illness
  - complications: seizures, coma
  - must have glucagon kit for quick injections
  - infants may not show classic catecholaminergic signs with hypoglycemia
- hyperglycemia
  - cause: infection, stress, diet-to-insulin mismatch, eating disorder
  - complications: risk of DKA, long-term end-organ damage
- DKA
  - cause: new-onset diabetes, missed insulin doses, infection
  - medical emergency: most common cause of death in children with diabetes (attributed to cerebral edema)
- long-term complications (retinopathy, nephropathy, neuropathy)
  - usually not seen in childhood (often begins 5 years after presentation or 3-5 years after puberty)
- metabolic syndrome
- other auto-immune conditions (e.g. celiac disease, hypothyroidism)

TYPE 2 DIABETES
- these tend to be obese and present with glycosuria without ketonuria, absent or mild polydipsia and polyuria, little weight loss
- especially prevalent among North American Aboriginals, Africans, Asians, Hispanics
- onset >10 and in middle to late puberty
- may present in DKA or HONK states

Treatment
- ill child with ketosis - insulin
- well child without ketosis - diet, exercise, oral agents
- metformin is used in children because it does not cause hypoglycemia

Diabetes Insipidus (DI)

- DI is the inability of the kidneys to concentrate urine
- central:
  - due to decreased ADH production from the brain (genetic, due to trauma, surgery, radiation, neoplasm, meningitis)
  - presents with polyuria, polydipsia, enuresis
- nephrogenic:
  - renal unresponsiveness to ADH (genetic, drug-induced)
  - x-linked recessive condition that affects males in early infancy
  - polyuria, FTT, hyperpyrexia, vomiting, hypernatremic dehydration

Diagnosis
- symptoms: polyuria, enuresis, nocturia, polydipsia, dehydration
- labs: dilute urine (SG<1.010), hypernatremia, elevated serum osmolality, low urine osmolality
- water deprivation test; central cause if >50% change in urine osmolality after ADH administration

Management
- central: DDAVP intranasally, SC, or PO
- nephrogenic: low-solute diet, thiazide diuretics

If a child presents with polyuria and polydipsia, dip urine for glucose and ketones.

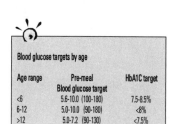

Blood glucose targets by age

Age range	Pre-meal Blood glucose target	HbA1C target
<6	5.6-10.0 (100-180)	7.5-8.5%
6-12	5.0-10.0 (90-180)	<8%
>12	5.0-7.2 (90-130)	<7.5%

Syndrome of Inappropriate Antidiuretic Hormone (SIADH)

- etiology: intracranial, malignancy, pulmonary disease, psychiatric disease, drugs
- common in hospitalized patients (associated with post-op pain and nausea)
- symptoms: asymptomatic, oliguria, volume expansion, or hyponatremic symptoms (nausea, vomiting, H/A, seizure, coma)
- labs: hyponatremia, urine Osm > plasma Osm, urine Na > 20mmol/L
- management: fluid restriction, 3% NaCl for symptomatic hyponatremia

Hypercalcemia/Hypocalcemia/Rickets

- see Endocrinology

Hypothyroidism

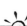

- see Endocrinology

Congenital Hypothyroidism
- incidence: 1 in 4000 births; F:M=2:1
- usually caused by malformation of the thyroid gland (agenesis or ectopic) also maternal factors – iodine deficiency, prenatal exposure to antithyroid medications or radioiodine
- diagnosis through newborn screening of TSH or T4
- usually asymptomatic in neonatal period because maternal T4 crosses the placenta but may have the following symptoms:
  - prolonged jaundice
  - constipation
  - sluggish, hoarse cry, lethargy, poor feeding
  - macroglossia, coarse facial features, large fontanelles, umbilical hernia
- prognosis
  - excellent if treatment started within 1-2 months of birth
  - if treatment started after 3-6 months of age may result in permanent developmental delay and/or mental retardation (mild to profound)
- management: thyroxine replacement

Acquired Hypothyroidism
- most commonly Hashimoto's thyroiditis (autoimmune destruction of the thyroid)
- signs and symptoms similar to hypothyroidism in adults, but also:
  - delayed bone age, decline in growth velocity, short stature, goiter
  - sexual pseudoprecocity: early sexual development with short stature and delayed bone age
  - does not cause permanent developmental delay
- treated with L-thyroxine 10 μg/kg/day

> Thyroid neoplasms that develop in childhood have a higher rate of malignancy; be suspicious of rapid and painless enlargement of the thyroid gland.

Hyperthyroidism

- see Endocrinology

Congenital Hyperthyroidism
- results from transplacental passage of maternal thyroid stimulating antibodies (mother with Graves' disease)
- clinical manifestations in the neonate may be masked by transplacental maternal antithyroid medication
- presentation: tachycardia with congestive heart failure, irritability, craniosynostosis, poor feeding, failure to thrive, heart murmur
- spontaneous resolution by 2-3 months of life as antibodies cleared
- management: propylthiouracil until antibodies cleared

Graves' Disease
- peak incidence in adolescence; F:M = 5:1
- may exhibit classic signs and symptoms of hyperthyroidism, but also personality changes, school difficulty, mood instability
- management similar to adults: anti-thyroid drugs (propylthiouracil, methimazole), radioiodine reserved for older teens, surgical thyroidectomy
- children with a solitary thyroid nodule require prompt evaluation as 30-40% have carcinoma; the remainder have an adenoma, abscess, cyst, or multinodular goiter

Juvenile Graves' Disease
- gradual onset over 6-12 months of diffuse goiter, ophthalmopathy, dermopathy
- increased appetite, weight loss or maintenance, fatigue, myopathy, sweating, menstrual irregularities
- treatment is propylthiouracil and propranolol
- thyroidectomy is sometimes performed

Ambiguous Genitalia

Etiology
- male pseudohermaphrodite (XY)
  - inborn error of testosterone biosynthesis or Leydig cell hypoplasia
  - 5-α-reductase deficiency, androgen receptor deficiency or insensitivity
  - luteinizing hormone (LH)/hCG unresponsiveness
  - small phallus, hypospadias, undescended testicles
- female pseudohermaphrodite (XX)
  - virilizing congenital adrenal hyperplasia (CAH) (most common)
  - maternal source: virilizing ovarian or adrenal tumours, untreated maternal CAH, placental aromatase deficiency
  - virilization of external genitalia – clitoral hypertrophy, labioscrotal fusion
- mixed pattern
- true hermaphrodite
  - both ovarian follicles and seminiferous tubules in the same patient with a 46XX karyotype
  - increased risk of malignant transformation of gonad tissue
- mixed gonadal dysgenesis

Investigations
- history: pregnancy (hormones and medications), family history
- physical exam: palpation of gonads, rectal exam
- investigations
  - karyotype
  - electrolytes and renin (evidence of salt-wasting in CAH)
  - measurement of 17-OH-progesterone (must wait until day 3 of life), androgens, follicle stimulating hormone (FSH) and luteinizing hormone (LH)
  - pelvic U/S to look for uterus, testicles, ovaries

Clinical Presentation
- depends on the degree and the specific deficiency
- infants may present with FTT, salt-wasting (adrenal crisis due to lack of aldosterone), hyperpigmentation (genital, areola), clitoral hypertrophy, fused labia
- hypertension is rare (usually seen in the 11-hydroxylase variant)
- adult onset (11-hydroxylase variant) more insidious, may present as hirsutism
- female: ambiguous genitalia to complete virilization, amenorrhea
- male: precocious puberty, with early adrenarche, dehydration
- accelerated linear bone growth in early years, but premature epiphyseal closure due to high testosterone, resulting in decreased adult height
- possible Addisonian picture (adrenal insufficiency) if adrenal output of cortisol severely compromised

Congenital Adrenal Hyperplasia (CAH)

- occurs in 1/15000 live births and is the most common cause of ambiguous genitalia
- autosomal recessive condition causing partial or total enzyme defect
- 21-hydroxylase deficiency causes 95% of CAH cases; this causes decreased cortisol and aldosterone with shunting toward overproduction of androgens
- cortisol deficiency leads to elevated ACTH, which causes adrenal hyperplasia
- clinical presentation depends on the specific deficiency and the cause
- high ACTH, increased 17-OH progesterone, increased testosterone, DHEAS, urinary 17-ketosteroids, advanced bone age

Late-Onset 21-Hydroxylase Deficiency
- allelic variant of classic 21-hydroxylase deficiency – mild enzymatic defect
- girls present with amenorrhea
- boys present with precocious puberty with early adrenarche, dehydration
- accelerated linear growth in early puberty but early fusion of epiphyses leading to decreased adult height
- diagnosis
  - increased plasma 17-OH-progesterone after ACTH stimulation test
- treatment
  - dexamethasone, spironolactone (anti-androgen)
  - mineralocorticoid replacement is not needed

Salt-wasting 21-hydroxylase deficiency CAH (2/3 of cases)
- infants present with FTT, low Na, high K, low Cl, low glucose, high ACTH
- adrenal insufficiency
- hyperpigmentation of genitals and areola

Simple virilizing 21-hydroxylase deficiency
- virilization in girls

11-hydroxylase deficiency
- sexual ambiguity in females
- may have insidious onset; may present with hirsuitism, occasionally hypertension

17-hydroxylase deficiency
- sexual ambiguity in males

Investigations
- low Na, high K, low cortisol, high ACTH if both glucocorticoid and mineralocorticoid deficiency
- increased serum 17-OH-progesterone (substrate for 21-hydroxylase)
- increased testosterone, DHEAS, urinary 17-ketosteroids
- advanced bone age

Treatment
- glucocorticoid replacement to lower ACTH
- in salt-wasting type mineralcorticoids given as well
- spironolactone is used in late-onset 21-hydroxylase deficiency as anti-androgen
- surgery to correct ambiguous genitalia

The salt-wasting form of CAH is a medical emergency – babies can die of vomiting, dehydration and shock at 2-4 weeks of age; order glucose and electrolytes; replace fluids and electrolytes, manage hypoglycemia, and start the child on lifelong hydrocortisone.

Table 17. Clinical Features of CAH Based on Enzyme Defect

Enzyme Defect	Sexual Ambiguity		Postnatal Virilization	Salt Wasting	Hypertension
	Female	Male			
21-hydroxylase					
salt-wasting	–	–	+	+	–
simple virilizing	+	–	+	–	–
late onset	–	–	+	–	–
11-hydroxylase	+	–	+	–	+
17-hydroxylase	–	+	–	–	+

Precocious Puberty

- secondary sexual development <8 years in girls, <9 years in boys
  - incidence: 1 in 10,000
  - more common in females; more worrisome in males (higher incidence of pathology)
- indications for medical intervention to delay progression of puberty are male sex, age <6, bone age advancing more quickly than height age, and psychological issues
- GnRH agonists such as leuprolide are most effective at delaying central precocious puberty
- medications used in peripheral precocious puberty include ketoconazole (to block steroid production), 5-□reductase blockers (finasteride), steroid receptor blockers (spironolactone), Aromatase blockers (testolactone, anastrozole)

A child with proven central precocious puberty should receive an MRI of the brain.

True (Central) Precocious Puberty
- hypergonadotropic hypergonadism, hormone levels as in normal puberty
- premature activation of the hypothalamic-pituitary-gonadal axis
- much more common in females than males – 9:1
- differential diagnosis
  - idiopathic or constitutional (most common, especially females)
  - CNS disturbances: tumours, hamartomas, post-meningitis, increased ICP, radiotherapy
  - neurofibromatosis (NF), primary severe hypothyroidism

Pseudo (Peripheral) Precocious Puberty
- hypogonadotropic hypergonadism
- differential diagnosis
  - adrenal disorders: CAH, adrenal neoplasm
  - testicular/ovarian tumour
  - gonadotropin secreting tumour: hepatoblastoma, intracranial teratoma, germinoma

- exogenous steroid administration
- McCune-Albright syndrome: endocrine dysfunction resulting in precocious puberty, café-au-lait spots, and fibrous dysplasia of skeletal system

Investigations
- history: symptoms of puberty, family history of puberty onset, medical illness
- physical exam: growth velocity, Tanner staging, neurological exam
- estradiol, testosterone, LH, FSH, TSH, GnRH test
- bone age (often advanced)
- consider CT or MRI of head, U/S of adrenals, pelvis

Treatment
- GnRH analogs, GnRH agonist (Lupron™) – negative feedback to downregulate GnRH receptors
- medroxyprogesterone – slows breast and genital development
- treat underlying cause

Heterosexual Precocious Puberty
- development of secondary sexual characteristics opposite to genotypic sex
- e.g. virilizing tumour (ovarian, adrenal), CAH, exogenous androgen exposure

Delayed Puberty

- see Gynecology
- absence of pubertal development by age 13 in girls and age 14 in boys
- more common in males, more suggestive of pathology in females

Central Causes
- delay in activation of hypothalamic-pituitary-gonadal axis
- hypogonadotropic hypogonadism
- differential diagnosis
  - constitutional (bone age delayed) – most common (>90%)

Peripheral Causes
- hypergonadotropic hypogonadism (e.g. primary gonadal failure)
- differential diagnosis
  - genetic (e.g. Turner syndrome, Klinefelter syndrome)
  - gonadal damage – infection, radiation, trauma
  - gonadal dysgenesis
  - hormonal defect – androgen insensitivity, 5-α-reductase deficiency

Investigations
- history: weight loss, short stature, family history of puberty onset, medical illness
- physical exam: growth velocity (minimum 4 cm/year), Tanner staging, neurological exam, complete physical exam
- hormone levels: estradiol, testosterone, LH, FSH, TSH, GnRH, test bone age
- consider CT or MRI of head, ultrasound of adrenals, pelvis
- karyotype in girls <3rd percentile in height (rule out Turner syndrome)

Management
- identify and treat underlying cause
- hormonal replacement: cyclic estradiol and progesterone for females, testosterone for males

Short Stature

Table 18. Short Stature

NORMAL GROWTH VELOCITY (non-pathological short stature)	DECREASED GROWTH VELOCITY (pathological short stature)

• **Constitutional Growth Delay**
  - delayed puberty
  - may have family history of delayed puberty
  - may require short-term therapy with androgens/estrogens
  - delayed bone age
  - often mid-parental height is normal
	• **Primordial** (height, weight, and HC are affected)
	  - chromosomal (e.g. Turner, Down syndrome, dysmorphic features)
	  - skeletal dysplasias
	  - intrauterine growth restriction (IUGR) (teratogen, placental insufficiency, infection)

• **Familial**
  - normal bone age
  - treatment not indicated
  - family Hx of short stature
	• **Endocrine** (height affected more than weight) – "short and fat"
	  - GH deficiency (slow growth velocity, decreased bone age, delayed puberty)
	  - hypothyroidism
	  - hypercortisolism (Cushing syndrome) (exogenous and endogenous)
	  - hypopituitarism

	• **Chronic disease** (weight affected more than height) – "short and skinny"
	  - cyanotic congenital heart disease
	  - celiac disease, inflammatory bowel disease, cystic fibrosis
	  - chronic infections
	  - chronic renal failure (often height more affected)

	• **Psychosocial neglect** (psychosocial dwarfism) - usually decreased height and weight (decreased head circumference if severe)

Short Stature DDx: ABCDEFG
Alone (neglected infant)
Bone dysplasias (rickets, scoliosis, mucopolysaccharidoses)
Chromosomal (Turner, Down)
Delayed growth
Endocrine (low growth hormone, Cushing, hypothyroid)
Familial
GI malabsorption (celiac, Crohn)

4 questions to ask when evaluating short stature
1. Was there IUGR?
2. Is the growth proportionate?
3. Is the growth velocity normal?
4. Is bone age delayed?

calculate mid-parental height (predicted adult height) ± 8 cm for 2 SD ranges
• check the mid-parental height for percentile of adults
• boy = [father height (cm) + mother height (cm) + 13 cm]/2
• girl = [father height (cm) + mother height (cm) – 13 cm]/2

- special growth charts available for Turner, Achondroplasia, Down syndrome (DS); these children grow along percentiles specific to their condition and growth velocity is often normal
- children are usually in a percentile between their parents' height
- decreased growth velocity may be more worrisome than actual height

Assessment of Short Stature
- height <3rd percentile, height crosses 2 major percentile lines, low growth velocity (<25th percentile)
- history: perinatal history, growth pattern, medical history, parental height and age of pubertal growth spurt
- physical exam: growth velocity (over 6 month period), sexual development
- growth hormone (GH) deficiency accounts for a small minority of children with short stature

Investigations
- bone age (anteroposterior x-ray of left hand and wrist)
- karyotype in girls to rule out Turner syndrome or if dysmorphic features present
- other tests as indicated by history and physical exam

Management
- depends on severity of problem as perceived by parents/child
- no treatment for non-pathological short stature
- GH therapy if requirements met (see *Growth Hormone Deficiency*)

Growth Hormone (GH) Deficiency

- GH important for chondrocyte proliferation and IGF-1 release
- GH has little effect on fetal growth (maternal IGF-1, uterine factors more important)
- IGF-1 acts at long bones, liver, negative feedback

Etiology
- congenital GH deficiency
  - idiopathic
  - embryologic CNS malformation: associated midface anomalies, neurologic defects, and micropenis in males
  - perinatal asphyxia
  - rare mutations
- acquired GH deficiency
- tumours (e.g. craniopharyngioma), trauma, cranial infection, irradiation, post-surgical

Clinical Presentation
- infantile features and fat distribution (short and chubby), delayed puberty, hypoglycemia, high-pitched voice

Investigations
- testing for GH Deficiency (Stimulation Testing) only performed when:
  - height <3rd percentile
  - decreased growth velocity
  - midline craniofacial anomalies
  - episodes of hypoglycemia
  - delayed bone age, puberty
- physiologic increase in GH with: arginine, clonidine, insulin, dopamine, or propranolol
- positive test if failure to raise GH >8-10 ng/mL post-stimulation

Treatment
- GH Therapy if the following criteria are met:
  - GH shown to be deficient by 2 different stimulation tests
  - patient is short, insufficient growth velocity, <3rd percentile
  - bone age x-rays show unfused epiphyses
  - Turner syndrome, Noonan syndrome, chronic renal failure

Tall Stature

- constitutional tall stature is advanced height and bone age during childhood but not necessarily associated with tall adult height (obesity can contribute to this by causing bone age to advance more rapidly)

Etiology
- constitutional/familial: most common, advanced bone age/physical development in childhood but normal once adulthood reached
- endocrine: hypophyseal (pituitary) gigantism, precocious puberty, thyrotoxicosis, Beckwith-Wiedemann syndrome
- genetic: Marfan, Klinefelter syndromes, Sotos syndrome, homocystinuria

> **Upper to lower (U/L) segment ratio is...**
> **Increased** in achondroplasia, short limb syndromes, hypothyroid, storage diseases.
> **Decreased** in Marfan, Klinefelter, Kallman, testosterone deficiency.

Investigations
- history and physical examination: differentiate familial from other causes
- calculate mid-parental height (predicted adult height)
- look for associated abnormalities (e.g. hyperextensible joints, long fingers in Marfan syndrome)

Treatment
- depends on etiology
- treatment only required in pituitary gigantism
- estrogen used in females to cause epiphyseal fusion (rarely indicated)

Gastroenterology

Vomiting

- investigations (based on history and physical exam)
  - bloody emesis: investigate for causes of upper gastrointestinal (GI) bleed
  - bilious emesis: rule out obstruction (upper GI series, U/S)
  - evaluate for gastroesophageal reflux (24-hour esophageal pH probe)
  - CBC, electrolytes, BUN, creatinine, ESR, venous blood gases, amylase, lipase
  - urine, blood, stool C&S
  - abdominal x-ray, U/S, contrast radiology, endoscopy
  - consider head imaging
- management
  - rehydration (see *Pediatric Nephrology*)
  - treat underlying cause

> **Vomiting**: forceful expulsion of stomach contents through the mouth
> **Regurgitation**: the return of partly digested food from the stomach to the mouth

Vomiting in the Newborn Period

Tracheoesophageal Fistula (TEF)
- incidence: 1:3,000-1:4,500
- clinical presentation (vary with type of fistula)
    - may have history of maternal polyhydramnios
    - may present after several months, if no associated esophageal atresia, with vomiting, coughing, and gagging
    - cyanosis with feeds, respiratory distress, recurrent pneumonia
    - frothy bubbles of mucus in mouth and nose that return after suctioning
    - associated anomalies in 50%: VACTERL association (see *Pediatric Genetics, Dysmorphisms, and Metabolism*)
    - x-ray: anatomic abnormalities, NG tube curled in pouch
- management
    - investigate for other congenital anomalies
    - early repair by surgical ligation to prevent lung damage and maintain nutrition and growth
- complications
    - pneumonia, sepsis, reactive airways disease
    - following repair: esophageal stenosis and strictures at repair site, gastroesophageal reflux and poor swallowing (i.e. dysphagia, regurgitation)

Duodenal Atresia
- incidence: 1:10 000, 50% are born prematurely
- clinical features
    - bile-stained vomiting if atresia distal to bile duct
    - no abdominal distention
    - dehydration
    - associated with Down syndrome, prematurity
    - may have history of maternal polyhydramnios
- abdominal x-ray: air-fluid levels on upright film; "double bubble" sign (dilated stomach and duodenum)
- differential diagnosis: annular pancreas, aberrant mesenteric vessels, pyloric stenosis
- treatment
    - decompression with NG tube
    - correction of metabolic abnormalities
    - surgical correction

Pyloric Stenosis
- incidence: 1:500, M:F = 4:1, onset common in first-born males, positive FH
- clinical features
    - non-bilious projectile vomiting that occurs after feeding
    - usually starts at 2-4 weeks of age
    - infant hungry and alert, will re-feed
    - constipation, FTT, wasting
    - dehydration, may lead to prolonged jaundice
    - gastric peristalsis goes from left upper quadrant (LUQ) to epigastrium
    - "olive sign": olive-shaped mass at margin of right rectus abdominus muscle
    - hypochloremic metabolic alkalosis
- diagnosis: clinical, abdominal U/S and x-ray
- treatment: surgical (pyloromyotomy)

> **Pyloric stenosis 3 P's:**
> **P**alpable mass
> **P**eristalsis visible
> **P**rojectile vomiting (2-4 weeks after birth)

Malrotation of the Intestine
- incidence: 1:500
- 80% experience symptoms in first two months of life
- 3 presentations
    - recurrent vomiting (bilious intermittently)
    - FTT with vomiting
    - sudden onset abdominal pain and then shock (if vomiting with bilious material, malrotation with volvulus until proven otherwise)
- clinical features
    - distended abdomen
    - vomiting due to volvulus and bands across duodenum
- diagnosis: abdominal U/S and upper GI series
- treatment: NG tube decompression and surgery
- complications: volvulus is a surgical emergency as it can result in bloody stools, perforation, and peritonitis

Vomiting After the Newborn Period

Infectious and Inflammatory
- GI causes: gastroenteritis, peritonitis, appendicitis, hepatitis, ulcers, pancreatitis, cholecystitis
- non-GI causes: urinary tract infection (UTI), pyelonephritis, nephrolithiasis, otitis media, labyrinthitis, meningitis, pneumonia, increased ICP

Anatomic
- GI tract obstruction
    - intussusception, volvulus
    - foreign body (e.g. bezoar)

Gastroesophageal Reflux
- extremely common in infancy (up to 50%): thriving baby requires no investigation
- vomiting typically soon after feeding, non-bilious, rarely contains blood, small volume (<1 oz)
- investigations required if: FTT, recurrent cough, pneumonia or bronchospasm, GI blood loss, symptoms persist after 18 months
    - 24-hour pH probe, UGI series to rule out anatomical cause, upper endoscopy and esophageal biopsy for suspected esophagitis
- management
    - conservative: thickened feeds, frequent and smaller feeds, elevate bed to 45°
    - medical:
        - short-term parenteral feeding to enhance weight gain
        - ranitidine, omeprazole: to decrease gastric acidity, decrease esophageal irritation
        - domperidone: to improve gastric emptying and GI motility
    - surgical: indicated for failure of medical therapy (Nissen fundoplication)
- complications: esophagitis, strictures, Barrett's esophagus, FTT, aspiration

Central Nervous System
- increased intracranial pressure (ICP) (e.g. hydrocephalus, neoplasm)
- drugs/toxins
- migraine, cyclic vomiting

Other
- metabolic/endocrine: DKA, inborn errors of metabolism, liver failure
- poisons/drugs: lead, digoxin, erythromycin, theophylline
- psychogenic: rumination syndrome, anorexia/bulimia
- food allergy
- overfeeding
- pregnancy

Acute Diarrhea

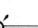

Diarrhea is defined as an increase in frequency and/or decreased consistency of stools compared to normal.

Normal stool volume:
Infants: 5-10g/kg
Children: 200g/day

Table 19. Causes of Acute Diarrhea

Infectious			Non-Infectious
Viral	Bacterial	Parasitic	Antibiotic-induced
• Rotavirus	• Salmonella	• Giardia lamblia	Non-specific: associated with systemic infection
• Norwalk	• Campylobacter	• Entamoeba histolytica	Hirschsprung's disease
• Enteric Adenovirus	• Shigella		Toxin ingestion
	• pathogenic E. coli		Primary disaccharide deficiency
	• Yersinia		
	• C. difficile		

VIRAL INFECTION
- most common cause of gastroenteritis in Canada and worldwide
- Rotaviruses are the most common agent, often seen in winter months in temperate climates
- Astroviruses are the second most important etiological agent, common in both developing and developed nations
- Norwalk virus is the third most common agent, it typically affects older children and adults
- clinical features:
    - associated with URTIs
    - resolves in 3-7 days
    - slight fever, malaise, vomiting, vague abdominal pain

BACTERIAL INFECTION
- clinical features: severe abdominal pain, high fever, bloody diarrhea
- risk factors: travel, poorly cooked meat, poorly refrigerated foods

Investigations
- history and physical examination critical to determine degree of dehydration (see *Pediatric Nephrology* Table 42)
- rectal exam for fecal consistency and for microscopy (leukocytes suggestive of invading pathogen)
- stool for culture and sensitivity (C&S), ova and parasites (O&P), electron microscopy for viruses
- if severe: routine blood work, blood and urine cultures

Treatment
- prevention and treatment of dehydration is most important (see *Dehydration* P72)
- oral rehydration therapy with frequent small volumes of pediatric rehydration solutions, IV may be required, see *Fluid & Electrolyte Therapy* P73
- early refeeding advisable, start with small amounts of easily digested carbohydrates, postpone dairy and fibrous vegetables
- antibiotic therapy when indicated, antidiarrheal medications not indicated
- notify Public Health authorities if appropriate

Chronic Diarrhea

Investigations
- perform serial heights, weights, growth percentiles
- if child is growing well and thriving, minimal workup is required
- investigations depending on suspected diagnosis:
    - stool: consistency, pH, reducing substances, microscopy, occult blood, O&P, C&S, *C. difficile* toxin, 3-day fecal fat
    - urinalysis
    - CBC, differential, ESR, smear, electrolytes, total protein, albumin
    - absorptive and nutritional status: albumin, carotene, Ca, PO_4, Mg, Fe, ferritin, folate, fat-soluble vitamins, PTT, INR
    - sweat chloride, thyroid function tests, urine vanillyl mandellic acid (VMA) and homovanillic acid (HVA), HIV test, lead levels
    - CXR, upper GI series and follow-through
    - specialized tests: endoscopy, small bowel biopsy

Chronic diarrhea: three or more loose, watery stools per day, lasting >14 days

Table 20. Causes of Chronic Diarrhea

0-3 months	3 months-3 years	3 years-18 years	Uncommon causes
GI infection	Toddler's diarrhea	GI infection	Constipation with overflow diarrhea
Disaccharidase deficiency	GI infection	Celiac disease	Drug induced
Cow's milk intolerance	Celiac disease	IBD	UTI
Cystic fibrosis			Short bowel syndrome

4F's Diet for Chronic Diarrhea
- adequate Fibre
- normal Fluid intake
- 35-40% Fat
- discourage excess Fruit juice

Chronic Diarrhea Without Failure to Thrive

Infectious
- bacterial: *Campylobacter, Salmonella*
- antibiotic-induced: *C. difficile* colitis
- parasitic: *Giardia lamblia*
- post-infectious: secondary lactase deficiency

Toddler's Diarrhea
- epidemiology
    - most common cause of chronic diarrhea during infancy
    - onset between 6-36 months of age, ceases spontaneously between 2-4 years
- clinical presentation
    - diagnosis of exclusion in thriving child (no weight loss/FTT, no fluid or electrolyte abnormalities)
    - diet history: too much juice overwhelms small bowel resulting in disaccharide malabsorption
    - stool may contain undigested food particles, 4-6 bowel movements (BM's)/day
    - excoriated diaper rash
- management
    - reassurance, self-limiting
    - four F's (adequate Fibre, normal Fluid intake, 35-40% Fat, discourage excess Fruit juice)

Lactase Deficiency (Lactose Intolerance)
- clinical features
    - chronic, watery diarrhea
    - abdominal pain, bloating associated with dairy intake
- primary lactose intolerance: crampy abdominal pain with loose stool (older children, usually of East Asian and African descent)
- secondary lactose intolerance: older infant, persistent diarrhea (post viral/bacterial infection, celiac disease, or IBD)
- diagnosis
    - trial of lactose-free diet
    - watery stool, acid pH, positive reducing sugars
    - positive breath hydrogen test if >6 years
- management
    - lactose-free diet, soy formula
    - lactase-containing tablets/capsules/drops (e.g. Lacteeze™, Lactaid™)

Irritable Bowel Syndrome
- diagnosis of exclusion in older child/adolescent; may be similar to recurrent abdominal pain
- management
    - encourage high fibre diet
    - reassurance
    - medications (cAMP inhibitors) for refractory cases

Chronic Diarrhea With Failure to Thrive

1. INTESTINAL CAUSES

Celiac Disease
- 1:250 - 1:100 incidence
- also known as "gluten-sensitive enteropathy", caused by a reaction to gliaden (a gluten protein)
- T cell mediated inflammation → damage to enterocytes
- defect in mucosa: immune-mediated inflammation and destruction of absorptive villi
- clinical features
    - presents at any age, usually 6-24 months with the introduction of gluten in the diet
    - FTT with poor appetite, irritability, apathy
    - anorexia, nausea, vomiting, edema, anemia, abdominal pain
    - wasted muscles, distended abdomen, flat buttocks, clubbing of fingers
    - rickets
    - non-GI manifestations: dermatitis herpetiformis, dental enamel hypoplasia, osteopenia/porosis, short stature, delayed puberty
    - associated with other auto-immune disorders
- diagnosis
    - anti-transglutaminase (tTG), antigliadin, antiendomysial antibodies (anti-EMA), low D-xylose absorption
    - fat malabsorption studies
    - small bowel biopsy (gold standard): total villous atrophy with resolution after trial of gluten-free diet
- treatment
    - gluten-free diet for life
- complications if untreated
    - small bowel lymphoma
    - malnutrition, FTT

Celiac disease diet must avoid gluten present in "**BROW**" foods
Barley
Rye
Oats
Wheat

Celiac disease is associated with an increased prevalence of IgA deficiency. Since tTG is an IgA-detecting test, you must order an accompanying IgA level!

Milk Protein Allergy
- immune-mediated mucosal injury
- up to 50% of children intolerant to cow's milk may be intolerant to soy protein as well
- often history of atopy
- 2 scenarios
    - enterocolitis: vomiting, diarrhea, anemia, hematochezia
    - enteropathy: chronic diarrhea, hypoalbuminemia
- treatment: casein hydrosylate formula (dairy-free e.g. Nutramigen™, Pregestimil™)

Inflammatory Bowel Disease (IBD) (see Gastroenterology)
- incidence: 15-30:100 000, increasing in North America, mostly older children and teenagers

Other
- specific enzyme deficiencies
- liver disease, biliary atresia
- α-β-lipoproteinemia
- short gut toxic or immunologic reaction
- blind loop syndrome
- giardiasis

2. PANCREATIC INSUFFICIENCY

Cystic Fibrosis (CF) (see *Pediatric Respirology*)

Schwachman-Diamond Syndrome
- incidence: 1:20,000, autosomal recessive
- pancreatic insufficiency, cyclic neutropenia, and anemia
- skeletal abnormalities (metaphyseal dysostosis leading to short stature)
- recurrent pyogenic infections
- distinguished from CF by normal sweat chloride test, characteristic metaphyseal lesions, fatty pancreas on CT

3. OTHER

- diets rich in sorbitol, fructose (poorly absorbed carbohydrates)
- metabolic/endocrine
    - thyrotoxicosis, Addison's disease, galactosemia
- immune defects
    - IgA deficiency, hypogammaglobulinemia, severe combined immunodeficiency (SCID), AIDS
- neoplastic
    - pheochromocytoma, lymphoma of small bowel, carcinoid tumours, secretory tumours
- food allergy
- laxative abuse

Constipation

Functional Constipation
- 99% of cases of constipation
- lack of fibre in diet or change in diet, poor fluid intake
- infants: often when introducing cow's milk after breast milk because increased fat and solute amounts, lower water content
- toddlers/older children: can occur during toilet training, or due to pain on defecation, stool withholding
- complications
    - pain retention cycle: anal fissures and pain → withhold passing stool → chronic dilatation and overflow incontinence
- treatment
    - adequate fluid intake (if <6 months, 150 ml/kg/day)
    - adequate dietary fibre, mineral oil, gentle laxatives occasionally (chronic use not recommended)
    - appropriate toilet training technique

Constipation
Decreased stool frequency (<3 stools/week) and/or stool fluidity

As many as 20% of children <5 years of age experience constipation.

Hirschsprung's Disease (congenital aganglionic megacolon)
- failure of normal innervation of the distal colon by the ganglion cells of the myenteric plexus
- colon remains contracted and impairs fecal movement
- incidence: M:F = 3:1; 1 in 5,000 live births
- clinical features
    - typically only rectosigmoid involvement but may extend to entire colon
    - no meconium within first 24 hours
    - palpable stool on abdominal exam with empty rectum on digital rectal exam
    - intermittent diarrhea, BM only with rectal stimulation
    - constipation, abdominal distention, vomiting, failure to thrive
- complications
    - enterocolitis: may be fatal, peak incidence 2-3 months of age
    - toxic megacolon and perforation
- diagnosis
    - barium enema: proximal dilatation due to functional obstruction, empty rectum
    - manometric studies: shows failure of anal sphincter relaxation, may have false positives
    - rectal biopsy: definitive diagnosis (absent ganglion cells)
- treatment
    - nonsurgical if short segment: increase fibre and fluid intake, mineral oil
    - surgical: colostomy and re-anastomosis

Other Organic Disorders Causing Constipation
- endocrine: hypothyroidism, diabetes mellitus (DM), hypercalcemia
- neurologic: spina bifida
- anatomic: bowel obstruction, anus (imperforate, atresia, stenosis)
- drugs: lead, chemotherapy, opioids

Acute Abdominal Pain

Table 21. Differential Diagnosis for Acute Abdominal Pain

Gastrointestinal	Other Systems
gastroenteritis	UTI
incarcerated hernia, volvulus, intussusception	Henoch-Schönlein Purpura (HSP)
appendicitis	sickle cell crisis
malrotation	pneumonia
mesenteric adenitis	DKA
cholecystitis	nephrolithiasis
Meckel's diverticulitis	gynecological (ectopic pregnancy, PID, endometriosis, menstruation)

Assessment
- description of pain (location, radiation, duration, constant vs. colicky, relativity to meals)
- associated symptoms: nausea, vomiting, diarrhea, fever
- physical examination: peritoneal signs, bowel sounds, rectal exam
- labs: CBC, differential, urinalysis to rule out urinary tract infection (UTI)

Appendicitis
- see General Surgery
- most common cause of acute abdomen after 5 years of age
- clinical features
  - low grade fever, anorexia
  - nausea, vomiting (after onset of pain)
  - abdominal pain, peritoneal signs
  - generalized peritonitis is a common presentation in infants/young children
- treatment: surgical
- complications: perforation, abscess

Intussusception - Classic Triad
Abdominal pain
Palpable mass
Red current jelly stools

Intussusception
- 90% idiopathic, children with CF or GJ tube at significantly increased risk
- 50% between 3-12 months, 75% before 2 years of age
- telescoping of segment of bowel into distal segment → ischemia and necrosis
- usual site: ileocecal junction; jejunum in children with GJ tubes
- lead point of telescoping segment may be swollen Peyer's patches, Meckel's diverticulum, polyp, malignancy, Henoch-Schönlein Purpura
- clinical features
  - "classic triad"
    - abdominal pain
    - palpable sausage-shaped mass: upper to mid-abdomen
    - "red currant jelly" stools (only in 10-15% of patients)
  - sudden onset of recurrent, paroxysmal, severe periumbilical pain with pain-free intervals
  - later vomiting and rectal bleeding
  - shock and dehydration
- diagnosis and treatment
  - U/S
  - air enema diagnostic, can be therapeutic (reduce intussusception in 75% of cases)
  - reduction under hydrostatic pressure
  - surgery rarely needed

Chronic Abdominal Pain

- 10-15% of children
- definition "rule of 3s"= 3 episodes of pain severe enough to affect activities, occurring in a child >3 years of age over a period of 3 months
- distinguish organic from non organic

Chronic Abdominal Pain- Rule of 3's
3 episodes of severe pain
Child > 3 years old
Over 3 month period

Organic (<10%)
- gastrointestinal
  - constipation (cause vs. effect), infectious
  - IBD, esophagitis, peptic ulcer disease, lactose intolerance
  - anatomic anomalies, masses
  - pancreatic, hepatobiliary
- genitourinary causes
  - recurrent urinary tract infections, nephrolithiasis, chronic PID, mittelschmerz
- neoplastic

Functional/Recurrent Abdominal Pain (RAP) (90%)

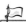

- school age, peak 8-10 years
- prevalence: 10% of school children, F>M
- characteristics
  - vague, crampy periumbilical or epigastric pain, vivid imagery to describe pain, clustering of episodes
  - seldom awakens child from sleep
  - aggravated by exercise, alleviated by rest
- psychological factors related to onset and/or maintenance of pain, school avoidance
- psychiatric comorbidity: anxiety, somatoform, mood, learning disorders, sexual abuse, eating disorders, elimination disorders
- diagnosis by exclusion of organic disorders
- investigations as indicated
  - CBC, ESR, urinalysis, stools for O&P, C&S, occult blood
- treatment
  - continue to attend school
  - manage any emotional or family problems, counselling
  - trial of high fibre diet, trial of lactose-free diet
  - reassurance
- prognosis
  - pain resolves in 30-50% of kids within 2-6 weeks of diagnosis
  - 30-50% of kids with RAP have functional pain as adults (e.g. irritable bowel syndrome)

> **Red flags for organic etiology of chronic abdominal pain**
> - age <5 years old
> - fever
> - localizes pain away from midline
> - anemia
> - rectal bleeding
> - rash
> - pain awakens child at night
> - travel history
> - prominent vomiting, diarrhea
> - weight loss or failure to gain weight
> - joint pain

Abdominal Mass

Table 22. Differential Diagnosis for Abdominal Mass

	Benign	Malignant
Renal	hydronephrosis polycystic kidney disease (PCKD) hamartoma	nephroblastoma (Wilms) renal cell carcinoma (RCC)
Adrenal		neuroblastoma
Ovarian	ovarian cysts	ovarian tumours
Other	splenomegaly pyloric stenosis abdominal hernia teratoma	lymphoma rhabdomyosarcoma retroperitoneal

- 50% of abdominal masses in the newborn are renal in origin

Upper Gastrointestinal Bleeding

- see Gastroenterology

Lower Gastrointestinal Bleeding

- see Gastroenterology

ETIOLOGY

Acute
- infectious
- bacterial, parasitic, antibiotic-induced (*C. difficile*)
- anatomic
  - malrotation/volvulus, intussusception
  - Meckel's diverticulitis
  - anal fissures, hemorrhoids
- vascular/hematologic
  - Henoch-Schönlein Purpura (HSP)
  - hemolytic uremic syndrome (HUS)
  - coagulopathy

Chronic
- anal fissures (most common)
- colitis
- inflammatory bowel disease (IBD)

- allergic (milk protein)
- structural
  - polyps (most are hamartomas)
  - neoplasms (rare)
- coagulopathy

Assessment
- hemodynamic status, evidence of FTT, fever
- anal and rectal exam
  - tags, fissures, anal fistulas, polyps
  - foreign body
  - blood
  - stool appearance
- NG aspirate
  - lower GI bleed may present as melena (if it involves the small bowel) or hematochezia
- stool cultures (*C. difficile*)
- urinalysis and microscopy
- CBC, smear, differential, platelets, ESR, electrolytes, urea, creatinine, INR, PTT, albumin, iron studies, amoeba titers
- radiologic investigations
  - abdominal x-ray (AXR) to rule out obstruction

Treatment
- acute stabilization: ABCs, volume and blood replacement, bowel rest (NPO, NG tube)
- once stable, endoscopy and surgery as indicated

Genetics, Dysmorphisms, and Metabolism

- minor anomaly = an unusual anatomic feature that is of no serious medical or cosmetic consequence to the patients
- major anomaly
  - 1°
    - malformation - results from an intrinsically abnormal developmental process (e.g. polydactyly)
  - 2°
    - disruption - results from the extrinsic breakdown of, or an interference with, an originally normal developmental process (e.g. amniotic band disruption sequence)
    - deformation - results from mechanical forces (e.g. potter deformation sequence)

Definitions
association = non-random concurrence of independent malformations whose etiology is unknown (e.g. VACTERL association)
sequence = pattern of multiple anomalies derived from a single known or presumed prior anomaly or mechanical factor (e.g. oligohydramnios sequence)
syndrome = recognized pattern of developmentally independent malformations having one known etiology (e.g. Down syndrome)

Mendelian Inheritance
- disorders caused by mutation of one or both copies of a gene, inherited in one of several patters:
  - Autosomal - encoded by genes on one of 22 pairs of autosomes
    - autosomal dominant (AD) = disorder is expressed in a heterozygote (inheritance is 'vertical', both males and females are affected and can transmit the trait); e.g. Neurofibromatosis type I
    - autosomal recessive (AR) = disorder is manifest only in homozygotes (inheritance is 'horizontal', disease not found in multiple generations, parents of an affected child are usually normal); e.g. cystic fibrosis
  - X-linked - encoded by a gene on the X chromosome
    - males have a single X chromosome and are affected, females have two X chromosomes, and recessive X-linked disorders are rarely expressed in females; i.e. Duchenne Muscular Dystrophy (DMD)

Approach to the Dysmorphic Child

- 2-3% of infants are born with a serious congenital defect, 1% of newborns have a monogenetic disease, 0.5% have a chromosomal disorder and 1-3% have a multifactorial illness
- genetic disorders are the most common cause of infant death in developed countries
- diagnosis of syndromes is based on pattern of dysmorphic features and organ involvement

History
- prenatal/obstetrical history (see Obstetrics)
- complete 3 generation family pedigree: consanguinity, stillbirths, neonatal deaths, specific illnesses, mental retardation (MR), multiple miscarriages, ethnicity

Physical Examination
- growth parameters and pattern: head circumference (HC), height (Ht), and weight (Wt)
- skull: contour and symmetry
- hair: texture and pattern
- neck: look for redundant nuchal skin/webbed neck
- facial gestalt: compare with siblings and parents
- ears: structure, size, placement and rotation
- eyes and adnexa: distance apart, orientation, eyebrows and eyelashes, any folds or creases, coloboma, fundus
- nose: nasal bridge, nostrils
- philtrum: length and shape
- mouth: lips, palate, tongue and teeth
- chin: size and position
- thorax: shape, size, and nipple spacing
- hands and feet: creases, structure (e.g. overlapping fingers/toes), and nails
- limbs: proportions and amputations
- spine: scoliosis, kyphosis
- genitalia: ambiguous
- skin: hair tufts, sacral dimples/sinus

Investigations
- ask for serial photographs if child is older, family pictures
- x-rays if bony abnormalities or if suspect a congenital infection
- cytogenetic/chromosome studies ± skin fibroblasts
- biochemistry: specific enzyme assays
- genetic probes now available e.g. Fragile X, microdeletion 22; in the future, microarray techniques
- prenatal counselling and recurrence risk assessment
- skin fibroblasts if mosaicism suspected

Genetic Syndromes

Table 23. Common Genetic Syndromes

	Trisomy 21	Trisomy 18	Trisomy 13
Disease	Down syndrome	Edwards syndrome	Patau syndrome
Incidence	• 1:600-800 births • most common abnormality of autosomal chromosomes • rises with advanced maternal age from 1:2000 at age 20 to 1:20 by age 45	• 1:6000 live births • female : male = 3:1	• 1:10 000 live births
Cranium / brain	• Mild microcephaly, flat occiput, 3rd fontanelle, brachycephaly	• Microcephaly, prominent occiput	• Microcephaly, sloping forehead, occipital scalp defect, holoprosencephaly
Eyes	• Upslanting palpebral fissures, inner epicanthal folds, speckled iris (Brushfield spots), refractive errors (myopia), acquired cataracts, nystagmus and strabismus	• Microopthalmia, hypotelorism, iris coloboma, retinal anomalies	• Microopthalmia, corneal abnormalities
Ears	• Low-set, small, overfolded upper helix, frequent AOM, hearling loss	• Low-set, malformed	• Low-set, malformed
Facial features	• Protruding tongue, large cheeks, low flat nasal bridge, small nose	• Cleft lip/palate • Small mouth, micrognathia	• 60- 80% Cleft lip and palate
Skeletal/ MSK	• Short stature • Excess nuchal skin • Joint hyperflexibility (80%) including dysplastic hips, vertebral anomalies, atlantoaxial instability	• Short stature • Clenched fist with overlapping digits, hypoplastic nails, clinodactyly, polydactyly	• Severe growth retardation • Polydactyly, clenched hand
Cardiac defect	• 40%, particularly AVSD	• 60% (VSD, PDA, ASD)	• 80% (VSD, PDA, ASD)
GI	• Duodenal/esophageal/anal atresia, TE fistula, Hirschsprung disease, chronic constipation	• Hernia	
GU	• Cryptorchidism, rarely fertile	• Polycystic kidneys, cryptorchidism	• Polycystic kidneys
CNS	• Hypotonia at birth • Low IQ, developmental delay, hearing problems • Onset of Alzheimer's disease in 40's	• Hypertonia	• Hypo- or hypertonia • Seizures, deafness • Severe developmental delay
Other features	• Simian (transverse palmar) crease, clinodactyly and absent middle phalanx of the 5th finger • 1% lifetime risk of leukemia • polycythemia • Hypothyroidism	• Small for gestational age (SGA) • Rocker-bottom feet	• Single umbilical artery • Midline anomalies: scalp, pituitary, palate, heart, umbilicus, anus
Prognosis / Management	• Prognosis: long-term Management: • Recommend chromosomal analysis • Echo, thyroid test, atlanto-occipital x-ray at 2 & 12 years (controversial), hearing test, ophthalmology assessment • Early intervention programs help children reach full potential	• 44% die in 1st month • 10% survive past 1 year (profound MR in survivors)	• 33% die in 1st month, 50% by 2nd month, 90% by 1 year from FTT • profound MR in survivors

Table 23. Common Genetic Syndromes (continued)

Most Common Sex Chromosome Disorders

	Turner syndrome	Noonan syndrome	Klinefelter syndrome	Fragile X syndrome
Genotype	• 45X (most common) • Mosaic: 46XX with p deletion, 45XO/47XXX	• 46XX and 46XY • Autosomal dominant with variable expression • Higher transmission of affected maternal gene	• 47 XXY (most common) • 48XXXY, 49XXXXY	• X-linked • Genetic anticipation • CGG trinucleotide repeat on X chromosome confers easy breakage of chromosome
Incidence	• 1:4000 live female births • Risk not increased with advanced maternal age	• 1:2000 male and female live births	• 1:1000 live male births • Increased risk with advanced maternal age	• 1:3600 males • 1:6000 females • Most common genetic cause of MR in boys
Phenotype	• Short stature, short webbed neck, low posterior hair line, wide carrying angle • Broad chest, widely spaced nipples • Lymphedema of hands and/or feet, cystic hygroma in newborn with polyhydraminins, lung hypoplasia • Coarctation of aorta, bicuspid aortic valve • Renal and cardiovascular abnormalities, increased risk of HTN • Less severe spectrum with mosaic	• Certain phenotypic features similar to females with Turner syndrome • Short stature, webbed neck, triangular facies, hypertelorism, low set ears, epicanthal folds, ptosis • Pectus excavatum • Right-sided congenital heart disease, pulmonary stenosis	• Tall, slim, underweight • No features prepuberty • Postpuberty : male may suffer from developmental delay, long limbs, gynecomastia, lack of facial hair	Overgrowth: • Prominent jaw, forehead, and nasal bridge • Long, thin face with large protuberant ears, macroorchidism • Hyperextensibility, high arched palate Complications: • Seizures, scoliosis, mitral valve prolapse
IQ & behavior	• Mildly deficient to normal intelligence	• Moderate MR in 25% of patients	• Mild MR • Behavioural or psychiatric disorders – anxiety, shyness, aggressive behaviour, antisocial acts	• Mild to moderate MR, 20% of affected males have normal IQ • ADHD and/or autism • Female carriers may show intellectual impairment
Gonad & reproductive function	• Streak ovaries with deficient follicles, infertility, primary amenorrhea, impaired development of secondary sexual characteristics	• Delayed puberty	• Infertility due to hypogonadism/ hypospermia	
Diagnosis/ Prognosis/ Management	• Normal life expectancy if no complications • Increased risk of X-linked diseases (same as males) Management: • Echo, ECG to screen for cardiac malformation • GH therapy for short stature • Estrogen replacement at time of puberty for development of secondary sexual characteristics	Management: • Affected males may require testosterone replacement therapy at puberty • Echo, ECG	Management: • Testosterone in adolescence	Diagnosis: • Cytogenetic studies: region on Xq which fails to condense during mitosis, fragile X marker • Molecular testing: overamplification of the trinucleotide repeat, length of segment is proportional to severity of clinical phenotype (genetic anticipation)

Other genetic syndromes

	DiGeorge syndrome	Prader-Willi syndrome	Angelman Syndrome
Genotype	• Microdeletions of 22q11	• Lack of paternally imprinted genes on chromosome 15q11 • Due to deletion of paternal chromosome 15q11 or two maternal chromosome 15s (maternal uniparental disomy)	• Lack of maternally imprinted genes on chromosome 15q11
Incidence	• Second most common genetic diagnosis (next to Down syndrome)	• 1:15000	
Clinical features	**"CATCH 22"** • **C**yanotic CHD (may account for up to 5% of all cases of CHD) • **A**nomalies: craniofacial anomalies typically micrognathia and low set ears • **T**hymic hypoplasia "immunodeficiency" recurrent infections • **C**ognitive impairment • **H**ypoparathyroidism, hypocalcemia • **22**q11 microdeletions	"H3O": hypotonia and weakness, hypogonadism, obsessive hyperphagia, obesity • Short stature, almond-shaped eyes, small hands and feet with tapering of fingers • Development delay (variable) • Hypopigmentation, DM II	• Severe MR, seizures, tremulousness, hypotonia • Midface hypoplasia, fair hair, uncontrollable laughter

Muscular Dystrophy (MD)

• a group of inherited diseases characterized by progressive skeletal and cardiac muscle degeneration

Duchenne Muscular Dystrophy (DMD)

• 1:4,000 males, 1/3 spontaneous mutations, 2/3 X-linked recessive
• missing structural protein dystrophin → muscle fibre fragility → fibre breakdown → necrosis and regeneration
• clinical features
  ▪ proximal muscle weakness by age 3; Gower's sign (i.e. child uses hands to "climb up" the legs to move from a sitting to a standing position); waddling gait; toe walking common
  ▪ hypertrophy of calf muscles and wasting of thigh muscles
  ▪ decreased reflexes
  ▪ dystrophin is expressed in the brain, and boys with DMD may have delayed motor and cognitive development; this is not progressive

Causes of increased CK
Prolonged exercise (5-10x increase)
Trauma
Rheumatoid arthritis
DMD (increase from birth)

- - cardiomyopathy
  - moderate intellectual compromise
- diagnosis
  - family history (pedigree analysis)
  - increased CK (50-100x normal) and lactate dehydrogenase
  - muscle biopsy, electromyography (EMG)
- complications
  - patient usually wheelchair-bound by 12 years of age
  - early flexion contractures, scoliosis, develop osteopenia of immobility, increased risk of fracture
  - death due to pneumonia/respiratory failure or CHF in 2nd-3rd decade
- treatment
  - supportive (i.e. physiotherapy, wheelchairs, braces), prevent obesity
  - surgical (for scoliosis)
  - use of steroids (e.g. prednisone or deflazacort)
  - gene therapy trials underway

Becker's Muscular Dystrophy

- X-linked recessive, due to a mutation in dystrophin gene with some protein production
- symptoms similar to Duchenne but onset is later in childhood and progression is slower
- death due to respiratory failure in 4th decade

Associations

- Associations are a non-random occurrence of multiple malformations with unknown etiology, while syndromes are a pattern of anomalies that have a known etiology
- two common associations are VACTERL and CHARGE
- **VACTERL** should be suspected when a child is found to have tracheo-esophageal fistula:

V	Vertebral dysgenesis (70%)
A	Anal atresia (imperforate anus) ± fistula (80%)
C	Cardiac anomalies – VSD (53%)
T-E	TracheoEsophageal fistula ± esophageal atresia (70%)
R	Renal anomalies (53%)
L	Limb anomalies – radial dysplasia, pre-axial polydactyly, syndactyly (65%)

  - may also present with a single umbilical artery or FTT
  - prognosis: may have normal health and mental development with aggressive treatment of abnormalities
- **CHARGE**

C	Coloboma
H	congenital Heart disease
A	Choanal Atresia
R	mental Retardation
G	GU anomalies
E	Ear anomalies

  - etiology thought to be due to abnormal development rather than a genetic mechanism

Metabolic Disease

- an inherited disorder of intermediary metabolism; often autosomal recessive
- infants and older children may present with failure to thrive (FTT) or developmental delay
- currently in Canada and the United States, newborns may be tested for CAH, congenital hypothyroidism, galactosemia, sickle cell disease (in certain ethnic groups), PKU, maple syrup urine disease, homocystinuria, and biotinidase deficiency

Metabolic disease must be ruled out in any newborn who becomes acutely ill after a period of normal behaviour and development or with a family history of early infant death.

Clinical Manifestations

- vomiting and acidosis after feeding initiation (amino acid or carbohydrate metabolic disorder)
- hepatosplenomegaly (metabolites accumulate in the liver)
- neurologic syndrome: acute and chronic encephalopathy, MR, megalencephaly (mucopolysaccharide disorders)
- severe acidosis (aminoaciduria), hyperammonemia (urea cycle and organic acid disorders)
- growth retardation, seizures, coma, hypoglycemia
- autonomic manifestations (e.g. pallor, sweating, tremor)

Physical Exam

- odour: burnt sugar, sweaty feet, musty, ammonia-like
- skin: hypo/hyperpigmentation, rash, xanthomas
- hair: alopecia, hirsutism, abnormal architecture, fair colouring
- eyes: cornea (clouding, crystals), lens (cataracts, dislocation), retina (macular cherry red spot, pigment retinopathy, optic atrophy)

Initial Investigations
- electrolytes, ABGs (calculate anion gap, rule out acidosis)
- CBC with differential and smear
- blood glucose (hypoglycemia seen with organic acidemia, fatty acid oxidation defects and glycogen storage diseases)
- lactate, ammonium (hyperammonemia with urea cycle defects), plasma Ca and Mg
- routine urinalysis: ketonuria must be investigated
- others: urate, urine nitroprusside, amino acid screen, CSF glycine, free fatty acids (3-β-hydroxybutyrate ratio >4 in fatty acid oxidation defect)
- storage diseases: urine mucopolysaccharide and oligosaccharide screen

Phenylketonuria (PKU)

- incidence: 1 in 10,000
- screened in all newborns
- etiology: deficiency of phenylalanine hydroxylase prevents conversion of phenylalanine to tyrosine leading to build up of toxic metabolites
- mothers who have PKU may have infants with congenital abnormalities
- presentation
    - baby is normal at birth then develops a musty odour, eczema, hypertonia, tremors, and mental retardation
    - hypopigmentation due to low tyrosine (fair hair, blue eyes)
- treatment
    - PKU screening at birth
    - dietary restriction of phenylalanine starting within the first 10 days of life
    - duration of dietary restriction controversial – lifelong or until end of puberty, recommended during pregnancy

Galactosemia

- incidence: 1 in 60,000, autosomal recessive disease
- most commonly due to deficiency of galactose-1-phosphate uridyltransferase leading to an inability to process lactose/galactose
- increased risk of sepsis
- if the diagnosis is not made at birth, liver and brain damage may become irreversible
- features: neonate who ingests lactose/galactose exhibits signs of liver and renal failure, FTT and cataracts
- treatment
    - elimination of galactose from the diet (i.e. dairy, breast milk)
    - most infants are fed a soy-based diet

Hematology

Anemia

- see Hematology

Physiologic Anemia

- high hemoglobin (>170 g/L) and reticulocyte count at birth as a result of relatively hypoxic environment in utero
- after birth, levels start to fall due to shorter fetal RBC lifespan, decreased RBC production (during first 6-8 weeks of life virtually no erythropoiesis due to new O_2 rich environment) and increasing blood volume secondary to growth
- lowest levels about 100 g/L at 8-12 weeks age (earlier and more exaggerated in premature infants); levels rise spontaneously with activation of erythropoiesis
- no treatment usually required

Iron Deficiency Anemia

- most common cause of childhood anemia (most often between 6-24 months)
- full term infants exhaust iron reserves by 6 months age, preterm infants have lower reserves – exhaust by 2-3 months of age
- common diagnosis between 6 months-3 years and 11-17 years: periods of rapid growth and increased iron requirements; adolescents also have poor diet and menstrual losses
- can cause irreversible effects on development if untreated (behavioural and intellectual deficiencies) in infancy

Normal Hg Values by Age	
Age	Hg Range (g/L)
Newborn	137-201
2 weeks	130-200
3 months	95-145
6 months-6 years	105-140
7-12 years	110-160
Adult female	120-160
Adult male	140-180

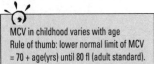
MCV in childhood varies with age
Rule of thumb: lower normal limit of MCV
= 70 + age(yrs) until 80 fl (adult standard).

Iron deficiency is rare in childen
<6 months in the absence of blood loss
or prematurity.

- presentation: usually asymptomatic until marked anemia, pallor, fatigue, pica (eating non-food materials), tachycardia, systolic murmur
- complications: angular cheilitis, glossitis, koilonychia

Ferritin is an acute phase reactant, therefore, normal or high ferritin does not exclude iron deficiency anemia during an infection.

Investigations
- CBC: low MCV & MCH, reticulocyte count normal or high (absolute number low), normal WBC
- Blood smear: hypochromic, microcytic RBCs, pencil shaped cells, poikylocytosis
- Iron studies: low ferritin, low iron, high TIBC
- Initial therapy: trial of iron

Etiology
- dietary risk factors
  - "milk baby" – baby (9-24 months old) receiving large volumes (>20 oz per day) of cow's milk by bottle leading to poor intake of iron-rich foods
  - formula without iron
  - delayed introduction of iron fortified infant cereal
- blood loss
  - iatrogenic: repeated blood sampling (especially in hospitalized neonates)
  - true cow's milk allergy: occult bleeding and protein-losing enteropathy secondary to GI inflammation

Prevention
- breast-fed full-term infants: after 6 months, give iron-fortified cereals and iron-rich foods
- non-breast-fed infants: give iron-fortified formula from birth
- premature infants: give iron supplements from 1 month to 1 year of age

Management
- encourage diverse, balanced diet, limit homogenized milk to 16-20 oz/day
- oral iron therapy – 6 mg/kg/day elemental iron, divided BID to TID for 3 months to replete iron stores
  - increased reticulocyte count in 2-3 days (peaks day 5-7)
  - increased hemoglobin in 4-30 days
  - repletion of iron stores in 1-3 months
  - re-check hemoglobin levels after 1 month of treatment
- poor response to oral iron therapy: non-compliance, ongoing blood loss, incorrect diagnosis, insufficient duration of therapy, high gastric pH (antacid use)

Anemia of Chronic Disease

- most often normocytic, normochromic (microcytic, hypochromic may occur with chronic infection/malignancy)
- multi-factoral in origin
- chronic inflammatory states including juvenile idiopathic arthritis (JIA), chronic infections, chronic renal failure, and malignancies
- iron stores are variable and ferritin levels are unreliable (acute phase reactant) therefore bone marrow assessment may be necessary for diagnosis
- anemia of chronic renal failure predominantly caused by decreased EPO production
  - treatment with erythropoietin

Hemoglobinopathies

SICKLE CELL DISEASE
- see Hematology
- identification of specific genotypes important due to differences in frequency, type and severity of clinical complications (most severe: SS, less severe: SC, S-beta thalassemia, rare: SD)

8% African Americans carry the HbS trait, 0.2% have the disease.
Heterozygotes (trait) are relatively malaria resistant.

Pathophysiology
- caused by a genetic defect in β-globin genes
  - HgS: single amino acid replacement (glutamic acid → valine)
- red blood cells sickle under conditions of stress (low pO_2, dehydration, fever, acidosis)
- acute intravascular sickling results in infarction of tissue (capillary occlusion and thrombosis – spleen, lungs, bones, brain, digits)
- hemolysis causes chronic, well-compensated normochromic normocytic anemia (Hb 60-90 g/L)
- increased incidence in people of African and Mediterranean heritage
- greatest cause of mortality is infection

Presentation
- newborns from high-risk families undergo screening; may be part of provincial newborn screening program
- clinical disease presents after 5-6 months of age after fall in fetal Hb
- anemia, fever, jaundice, splenomegaly, crisis (dactylitis is often the first presentation)
- sickle cell trait: asymptomatic (may have microscopic hematuria)

Types of Crises
- vaso-occlusive crisis
  - due to obstruction of blood vessels by rigid, sickled cells → tissue hypoxia → cell death; presents as fever and pain in any organ; most commonly in long bones of arms and legs, chest, abdomen, CNS (stroke), dactylitis (in young children), priapism
  - acute chest crisis: fever, chest pain, progressive respiratory distress, increased WBC count, pulmonary infiltrates
- aplastic crisis – depression of erythropoiesis (decreased reticulocyte count to <1%, decreased Hb), generally associated with infection (especially parvovirus B19)
- acute splenic sequestration – sudden massive pooling of red cells in spleen, splenomegaly, tender spleen, acute fall in hemoglobin, shock, increased reticulocyte count

Functional Asplenia
- splenic dysfunction usually by 5 years of age secondary to autoinfarction
- susceptible to infection by encapsulated organisms (especially *S. pneumoniae*)
- requires prophylactic antibiotics, pneumococcal/meningococcal/*H. influenzae* type b vaccination, and immediate evaluation of any fever

Other Manifestations
- increased incidence of osteomyelitis (especially due to *Salmonella*)
- growth delay, bony abnormalities – e.g. avascular necrosis (AVN) of femoral head, gallstones, retinopathy, restrictive lung disease

Management
- acute crises
  - admit for supportive and symptomatic treatment
  - fluids (1.5x maintenance; 1x maintenance only if in chest crisis), analgesia (morphine), antibiotics (e.g. 3rd gen. cephalosporins), incentive spirometry to decrease risk of chest crisis
  - straight transfusions for symptomatic/significant anemia (e.g. aplastic crisis), evolving chest crisis
  - RBC exchange transfusion for impending stroke, severe chest crisis, persistent priapism
  - O_2 if respiratory distress or chest crisis (with incentive spirometry)
  - cultures and CBC if febrile, reticulocyte counts, CXR or LP if indicated
- chronic
  - early aggressive treatment of infections, prophylactic antibiotics (daily oral penicillin)
  - pneumococcal, meningococcal, hepatitis B, Hib, and influenza vaccines
  - folate supplementation if folate deficient
  - hydroxyurea if frequent crises (raises HbF level)
  - transcranial doppler ultrasound to assess risk of stroke
  - chronic transfusion program if history of stroke or abdominal transcranial doppler
  - genetic counselling and education
  - annual ophthalmologic exam (after 10 years old)
  - referral to hematology

SPHEROCYTOSIS
- red cell membrane protein abnormality, causes a sphering of RBCs which are removed by the spleen
- genetics
  - autosomal dominant (positive family history in 75%)
  - high spontaneous mutation rate (no family history in 25%)
- wide range of clinical severity from well-compensated, mild hemolytic anemia to severe hemolytic anemia with growth failure, splenomegaly, gallstones, neonatal jaundice and chronic transfusion requirements in infancy
- diagnosis: spherocytes (circular RBCs) on blood smear, osmotic fragility test
- management
  - transfusion, splenectomy as needed
  - genetic counselling

GLUCOSE-6-PHOSPHATE DEHYDROGENASE (G6PD) DEFICIENCY

- X-linked recessive; the most common enzyme deficiency worldwide
- higher prevalence in Mediterraneans, African Americans, Asians
- enzyme-deficient RBC unable to defend against oxidative stress (infection, drugs) → form Heinz bodies (Hb precipitates within RBCs) → phagocytosed by splenic macrophages creating "bite cells" (RBCs that appear to have bites taken out of them, also known as "cookie cells")
- presents with acute hemolytic anemia (hemoglobinuria, decreased haptoglobin, increased LDH, and elevated indirect bilirubin) with jaundice, pallor and dark urine (rarely causes chronic anemia)
- management: supportive, hydration, transfusion, phototherapy
- prevention: avoid known oxidants (e.g. fava beans, antimalarials (primiquine), sulfonamides)

> G6PD deficiency protects against parasitism of RBC's (i.e. malaria).

Bleeding Disorders

- see Hematology

Coagulation Defects
- characterized by bleeding into joints (hemarthroses) and muscles
- large spreading ecchymoses and hematomas

Platelet Abnormalities
- characterized by petechiae, purpura, bruises, mucocutaneous bleeding (i.e. epistaxis, gingival bleeding), menorrhagia, prolonged bleeding from superficial cuts

Table 24. Classification of Bleeding Disorders

Site of pathophysiology	Mechanism	Examples
Blood Vessels	Vasculitis	Henoch-Schönlein purpura
Platelets	Decreased production	Drugs, marrow infiltration, leukemia/lymphoma
	Increased destruction	Immune thrombocytopenic purpura, infection, drugs
	Increased consumption	DIC, giant hemangioma, hypersplenism
	Dysfunctional	von Willebrand disease, drugs (ASA), uremia
Coagulation Pathway	Vitamin K deficiency	Hemorrhagic disease of the newborn
	Factor VIII deficiency	Hemophilia A
	Factor IX deficiency	Hemophilia B
	Abnormal vWF	von Willebrand disease

Immune Thrombocytopenic Purpura (ITP)

- most common cause of thrombocytopenia in childhood
- peak age: 2-6 years, M=F
- incidence 5 in 100,000 children per year
- caused by antibodies that bind to platelet membranes → splenic uptake (Fc-receptor mediated) → destruction of platelets
- presentation and course
  - 50% presents 1-3 weeks after viral illness (URTI, chicken pox)
  - sudden onset of petechiae, purpura, epistaxis in an otherwise well child
  - no lymphadenopathy, no hepatosplenomegaly
  - labs: thrombocytopenia with normal RBC, WBC
  - if atypical presentation (≥1 cell line abnormal, hepatosplenomegaly), do bone marrow to rule out leukemia
  - differential diagnosis: leukemia, drug-induced thrombocytopenia, HIV, infection (viral), SLE
  - highest risk of bleeding in first 1-2 weeks
- management
  - self-limited in children; spontaneous recovery in >80% of cases
  - usually choose to treat because spontaneous recovery takes a few months, and risk of bleeding (especially intracranial hemorrhage with platelets <20)
  - IVIG or oral prednisone (mainstays of treatment), IV anti-D (if blood group Rh positive)
  - splenectomy (only for life-threatening bleeding)
  - avoid ASA/NSAIDS
  - no contact sports
  - reassurance: very low risk of serious hemorrage(3%), and CNS hemorrage rare (<0.5%)

Corticosteroids versus intravenous immune globulin for the treatment of acute immune thrombocytopenic purpura in children: a systematic review and meta-analysis of randomized controlled trials
J Pediatr 2005 Oct;147(4):521-7
Study: Meta-analysis of 10 RCTs from 1985-2003. RCTs compared corticosteroids and IVIG in the treatment of pediatric ITP, and had to include patient platelet counts.
Patients: 586 children 3 months to 18 years of age who were presenting for the first time with primary acute ITP, with no other underlying condition.
Intervention: Corticosteroids and IVIG at any dose. Corticosteroid treatments included methyl-prednisolone 10 - 30mg/kg/d and prednisone 2 - 4g/kg/d. IVIG dosing ranged from 0.5 - 1g/kg/d. Treatment durations ranged from 1-5 days.
Main Outcome: Primary outcome was platelet levels > 20,000/mm³ (20x10⁹/L) at 48 hours after treatment. (This outcome was chosen because intracranial hemorrhage rarely occurs at platelet above 20). Secondary outcomes included incidence of ICH.
Results: The relative risk (RR) of reaching a platelet count >20,000/mm³ at 48 hours was 0.74 (95%CI 0.65-0.85) for corticosteroids versus IVIG (at any dose), with a NNT of 4.55 (95%CI 3.23-7.69). Subgroup analyses by dosing favoured IVIG in 6/10 dose comparisons. Only 3/586 children developed ICH - two were treated with corticosteroids and one with IVIG.
Summary: Children treated with corticosteroids are less likely to have a platelet count >20,000/mm³ than children treated with IVIG after 48 hours of therapy. However, optimal dosing of IVIG is unclear, and impact of IVIG versus corticosteroids on ICH and mortality are unclear.

Hemophilia

- see Hematology

von Willebrand's Disease

- see Hematology

Table 25. Evaluation of Abnormal Bruising/Bleeding

	BT	PT	PTT	VIII:C	vWF	Platelets	Fibrinogen
Hemophilia A	N	N	↑	↓	N	N	N
Hemophilia B	N	N	↑	N	N	N	N
von Willebrand's	↑	N	N or ↑	↓	↓	N	N
DIC	N or ↑	↑	↑	↓	N	↓	↓
Vit. K deficiency	N	↑	↑	N	N	N	N
Thrombocytopenia	↑	N	N	N	N	↓	N

BT = Bleeding Time, VIII:C = Factor VIII Coagulant Activity, vWF = von Willebrand's Factor, DIC = Disseminated Intravascular Coagulation

> Extensive bruising in the absence of lab abnormalities: consider child abuse.

Infectious Diseases

Table 26. Antibiotic Treatment of Pediatric Bacterial Infections

Infection	Pathogens	Treatment
Meningitis Sepsis		
• Neonatal	GBS, E.coli, Listeria, gram negative bacilli	• ampicillin + aminoglycoside (gentamicin or tobramycin)
• 1-3 months	same pathogens as above and below	• ampicillin + cefotaxime ± cloxacillin if risk of S. aureus • ampicillin + cefotaxime ± vancomycin (meningitis)
• >3 mos	S. pneumococcus, meningococcus, H. influenzae type b (>5 yrs)	• cefuroxime (sepsis) • ceftriaxone + vancomycin (meningitis)
Otitis Media		
• 1st line	S. pneumoniae, H. influenzae type b, M. Catarrhalis	• amoxicillin
• 2nd line		• high dose amoxicillin or clavulin
• Treatment Failure		• high dose clavulin or cefuroxime or ceftriaxone
Strep Pharyngitis		
	group A β-hemolytic Streptococcus	• penicillin/amoxicillin or erythromycin (pencillin allergy)
UTI		
	E. Coli, Klebsiella, Proteus, H. Influenzae, Pseudomonas, S. saprophyticus, Enterococcus, GBS	• cephalexin, cefixime (uncomplicated) or • IV ampicillin and gentamycin • ampicillin and gentamycin (neonates)
Pneumonia (Community Acquired, Bacterial)		
• 1-3 mos	S. pneumoniae, C. trachomatis, B. pertussis, S. aureus, H. influenzae	• cefuroxime ± macrolide (erythromycin) or • ampicillin ± macrolide
• 3 mos-5 yrs	S. pneumoniae, S. aureus, H. influenzae, Mycoplasma pneumoniae	• ampicillin/amoxicillin or clavulin or cefuroxime
• >5 years	as above	• macrolide (1st line) or cefuroxime or ampicillin/amoxcillin or clavulin

> **Rochester Criteria** – developed to identify infants ≤60 days of age with fever (rectal temperature ≥38°C) at low risk of serious bacterial infection
>
> | | |
> |---|---|
> | Clinically | Well |
> | WBC count | 5-15 x 10⁹/L |
> | Bands | <1.5 x 10⁹/L |
> | Urinalysis | 10 WBC/HPF |
> | Stool (if diarrhea) | 5 WBC/HPF |
> | Past Health | Born >37wk
Home with/before mom
No hospitalizations
No prior antibiotics use
No treated unexplained hyperbilirubinemia
No chronic disease |

Fever

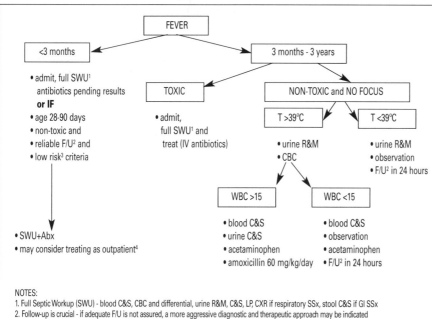

NOTES:
1. Full Septic Workup (SWU) - blood C&S, CBC and differential, urine R&M, C&S, LP, CXR if respiratory SSx, stool C&S if GI SSx
2. Follow-up is crucial - if adequate F/U is not assured, a more aggressive diagnostic and therapeutic approach may be indicated
3. Low-Risk (Rochester) Criteria
4. Considerable practice variation exists in terms of empirical Abx treatment
5. Important Principles - the younger the child, the greater the difficulty to clinically assess the degree of illness

Figure 2. Approach to the Febrile Child

Febrile infants at low risk for serious bacterial infection – an appraisal of the Rochester criteria and implications for management
Febrile Infant Collaborative Study Group. Pediatrics. 1994; 94(3):390 – 396

Purpose: To test the hypothesis that infants unlikely to have serious bacterial infection (SBI) can be correctly identified using the Rochester criteria.
Study Characteristics: Prospective study with 1057 infants.
Participants: Febrile infants less than 60 days old.
Intervention: Application of Rochester criteria.
Main Outcomes: Culture of speciments of blood, cerebrospinal fluid and urine for bacteria.
Results: Of the 1057 febrile infants that were involved, 931 were well-looking and 437 met the remaining low risk criteria. The negative predictive value of the low risk criteria was 98.9% (95% CI, 97.2%-99.6%) for SBI.
Conclusions: Low risk Rochester criteria are useful in identifying infants at decreased risk of SBI and antibiotic use may be delayed in these patients.

Observation option only appropriate if follow-up can be ensured if persistent symptoms.

Acute Otitis Media (AOM)

Epidemiology
- peak incidence 3 mos-3 yrs

Etiology
- bacterial (70%) – *S. pneumoniae* (25-40%), non-typable *H. influenzae* (10-30%), *M. catarrhalis* (5-15%), Group A *Streptococcus* (3%), *S. aureus*
- viral (20%) – commonly RSV, influenza, parainfluenza, adenovirus

Definitions
- **certain diagnosis**: 1) recent, usually abrupt, onset of signs and symptoms of middle ear inflammation and effusion 2) presence of middle ear effusion (MEE) 3) middle ear inflammation (MEI)
- **uncertain diagnosis**: does not meet all three criteria
- **severe illness**: moderate to severe otalgia or fever >39°C
- **non-severe illness**: mild otalgia and fever <39°C

History
- otalgia, tugging at ears, otorrhea, decreased hearing
- irritability, fever, URI symptoms
- nausea, vomiting, diarrhea
- risk factors: bottle feeding, passive smoking, daycare, low SES, cleft lip, Down syndrome, previous/recurrent AOM, family history of recurrent OM, prematurity, male gender, siblings in household
- risk of drug resistance: previous antibiotic therapy in past month, history of AOM, daycare attendance, age 18-24 months, recent hospitalization
- recurrent AOM – 3 episodes in 6 months or 4 episodes in 1 year

Physical Examination
- febrile
- MEE indicated by any of the following on otoscopy: loss of landmarks, bulging tympanic membrane (TM), opaque erythematous TM, yellow fluid behind TM, decreased TM mobility, air-fluid levels behind the TM, otorrhea (if TM perforated)
- MEI indicated by either: distinct erythema of the TM or distinct otalgia (discomfort clearly referable to the ear(s) that results in interference with normal activity or sleep)

A review of Antibiotics for AOM in children comparing any antibiotic against observation indicates that antibiotic use has no significant impact on pain at 24 hours and no significant effect on hearing
Cochrane 2004

In older children >6 years, it is appropriate to consider a "wait and see prescription", with instructions for re-evaluation if the child has not improved significantly within 72 hours.

In children <2 years with bilateral AOM or AOM with otorrhea, antibiotics are recommended by a recent meta-analysis. (Rovers MM, Glasziou P, Appelman CL, et al, Antibiotics for acute otitis media: a meta-analysis with individual patient data. Lancet 2006; 368:1429-1435.)

The concept and practice of a wait-and-see approach to acute otitis media
Current Opinion in Pediatrics, 2008, 20:72-78

Purpose: To summarize recent AOM trials comparing antibiotics versus a "wait and see prescription".
Study Characteristics: Guidelines formulated based on evidence from three recent clinical trials.
Recommendations:
Treat immediately with antibiotics when:
- age <6 months
- ill appearance (shock, unresponsive)
- recurrent AOM
- suspicion of another concurrent bacterial illness (e.g. pneumonia)
- recent treatment with antibiotics (within last 7 days)
- perforated TM (including tympanostomy tubes)
- immunocompromised
- craniofacial abnormalities
- poor access to medical care

Management
- 80% of AOM in children self-resolve without antibiotic therapy, therefore controversy exists surrounding antibiotic use in AOM management
- antibiotics:
    - non-severe: amoxicillin, 40-50 mg/kg/day divided tid
    - severe: amoxicillin 80-90 mg/kg/day
- treatment failure 48-72 hr. after initial antibiotic use in severe AOM: ceftriaxone cefuroxime, or amoxicillin 80-90 mg/kg/day + clavulin 6.4 mg/kg/day
- analgesics: acetaminophen or ibuprofen for pain management
- see Otolaryngology

Observation option only appropriate if follow-up can be ensured if persistent symptoms. Consider a safety-net antibiotic prescription.

Table 27. Treatment of AOM

Age	Certain Diagnosis	Uncertain Diagnosis
<6 mos	Antibacterial therapy x 10d	Antibacterial therapy x 10d
6 mos to 2 yrs	Antibacterial therapy x 10d	Severe illness: antibacterial therapy x 10d Non-severe illness: observation option
≥2 yrs	Antibacterial therapy if severe illness x 5d; observation option if nonsevere illness	Observation option

Meningitis

- peak age: 6-12 months; 90% occurs in <5 years old

Risk Factors
- immunocompromised (e.g. HIV, asplenia, prematurity)
- neuroanatomical defects (e.g. dermal sinus, neurosurgery)
- parameningeal infection (e.g. sinusitis, mastoiditis, orbital cellulitis)
- environmental (e.g. day-care centres, household contact)

Etiology
- 0-3 months: Group B *Strep.*, *E. coli*, *L. monocytogenes*, viral (HSV, enteroviruses)
- 3 months-3 years: *S. pneumoniae*, *N. meningitidis*, *H. influenzae*, TB, viral (enteroviruses, herpes virus 6, HSV)
- 3-18 years: *S. pneumoniae*, *N. meningitidis*, *H. influenzae*, viral (enteroviruses, adenoviruses, herpes viruses)

Pathophysiology
- URTI → compromise in integrity of mucosa → blood stream invasion from respiratory tract → hematogenous seeding of meninges → meningeal and CNS inflammation

Clinical Presentation
- toxic
- ± URTI prodrome
- fever, lethargy, irritability, photophobia, nausea/vomiting, headache, stiff/sore neck
- younger infants: may not demonstrate localizing signs, may have non-specific symptoms (poor feeding, irritability, lethargy), bulging fontanelle, increasing head circumference
- signs of meningismus
    - Brudzinski's sign: reflex flexion of hips and knees upon active flexion of the neck
    - Kernig's sign: reflex contraction and pain in hamstrings upon extension of leg that is flexed at the hip
    - opisthotonos: spasm in which head and heels are bent backward and body bowed forward
    - nuchal rigidity
- signs of increased ICP: headache, diplopia, ptosis, CN VI palsy, bradycardia with hypertension, apnea, papilledema is uncommon
- seizure in 20-30% of patients with bacterial meningitis
- petechial rash (meningococcemia): associated with poor prognosis

Signs of meningismus
BONK on the head
Brudzinski's sign
Opisthotonos
Nuchal rigidity
Kernig's sign

Diagnosis
- lumbar puncture (LP) for cerebrospinal fluid (CSF)
    - raised opening pressure (norms: recumbent and relaxed, less flexed position <160 mm H_2O, flexed lateral decubitus position = 100-280 mm H_2O)
    - cloudy in bacterial infection
- CSF examination: WBC, protein, glucose, Gram stain, C&S, latex agglutination tests (if partially treated bacterial meningitis), Ziehl-Neilson stain (if TB suspected)
- viral versus bacterial meningitis (see Table 28)
- bloodwork: CBC, blood cultures (positive in 90% cases), blood glucose, electrolytes (to monitor for SIADH)

Table 28. CSF Findings of Meningitis

Component	Normal child	Normal newborn	Bacterial meningitis	Viral meningitis	Herpes meningitis
WBC (/µL)	0-6	0-30	>1000	100-500	10-1000
Neutrophils (%)	0	2-3	>50	<40*	<50
Glucose (mg/dL)	40-80	32-121	<30	>30	>30
Protein (mg/dL)	20-30	19-149	>100	50-100	>75
RBC (/µL)	0-2	0-2	0-10	0-2	10-500

[Modified from Smith A. (1993) *Peds in Review* 14:11-18 and Ahmed A. et al (1996) *Ped Inf Dis J* 15:298-303]   * lymphocytes predominate

Complications
- mortality: neonate 15-20%, children <1-8%; pneumococcus > meningococcus > Hib
- morbidity: up to 50% may have neurobehavioural morbidity, severe neurodevelopmental sequelae in 10-20%
- acute
  - SIADH → hyponatremia → brain edema → seizures
  - subdural effusion/empyema
  - brain abscess, disseminated infection (osteomyelitis, septic arthritis, abscess)
  - shock/DIC
- chronic
  - hearing loss
  - mental retardation, learning disability
  - neurological deficit, seizure disorder
  - hydrocephalus

Treatment
- isolation with appropriate infection control procedures until 24hr after culture-sensitive antibiotic therapy
- bacterial: empiric antibiotics, see Table 26
- viral: supportive, acyclovir for HSV meningitis
  - most cases of viral meningitis can be sent home (except HIV)
  - if neonatal, use high dose ampicillin as part of regimen until GBS and *Listeria* ruled out
- monitor: glucose, acid-base and volume status
- anticonvulsants may be needed to treat seizures
- prophylaxis
  - *H. influenzae* type b vaccine – routine
  - meningococcal vaccine – asplenism, complement deficiency, for outbreaks, routine in some provinces
  - pneumococcal vaccine – immunocompromised, asplenism, routine in some provinces
  - BCG vaccine – if born in TB-endemic area
  - antibiotic prophylaxis for contacts and index case
    - *H. influenzae* – rifampin
    - *N. meningitidis* – rifampin, ceftriaxone or ciprofloxacin
- report to public health: acute meningitis (bacterial, viral, other)

HIV Infection

- see Infectious Diseases

Epidemiology
- risk of vertical transmission 20-30% born to untreated HIV infected women (risk decreases from 25% to <1% with antiretroviral treatment during pregnancy)
- transmission:
  - infants and children: **transplacental** (most common), maternal blood, breast milk
  - adolescents: sexual intercourse, needles (IV drug use and tattoos), blood products

Risk Factors
- HIV positive mother
- IV drug use (IVDU)
- mother is with HIV positive partner
- unprotected sex
- receipt of blood products (rare)
- sexual abuse

Incubation
- time from contracting infection to developing symptoms is usually <2 years, but can be several years

Clinical Features of AIDS in Infants and Children
- signs and symptoms occur often within the first year, most within two years of age
  - encephalopathy
  - recurrent/persistent thrush
  - chronic interstitial pneumonitis (relatively common); *Pneumocystis jiroveci pneumonia* (PJP) infection (formerly PCP)
  - hepatomegaly
  - FTT, opportunistic infections, lymphadenopathy

HIV Testing
- should be offered to all women as early as possible in pregnancy (requires consent)
- 1st step: screening for HIV Ab with ELISA.
- if positive do 2nd step: confirmatory test for Ab using Western blot or immunofluorescence (sensitivity and specificity of 99%)
  - maternal HIV antibodies can persist up to 18 months (can result in a false positive HIV test), typically test every 6 months from 0-18 months if asymptomatic
  - if child breastfeeding, repeat test 3 months after stopping breastfeeding
- other tests: viral nucleic acid by PCR, viral culture, viral antigen
- if sexually active, must re-test 6 months after 1st test (if negative)

Management
- adequate nutrition (breast feeding contraindicated in developed countries)
- prompt treatment of infections
- prophylaxis
  - TMP/SMX for PJP
  - azithromycin for mycobacterium avium complex (MAC)
  - nystatin, ketoconazole, acyclovir if indicated
- ± IVIG
- immunizations
  - all routine immunizations (including MMR and varicella if well)
  - avoid OPV, BCG and yellow fever
  - pneumococcal, influenza, and varicella vaccines
- suppression of HIV
  - HAART (highly active anti-retroviral therapy)
- HIV positive pregnant women should be offered antiretroviral therapy along with resources for formula feeding to decrease perinatal transmission
  - consider elective C-section if not on therapy, or if significant viral load

Pharyngitis and Tonsillitis

Etiology
- viral (adenoviruses, enteroviruses, EBV virus) – 80%
- bacterial (Group A *Streptococcus*) – 20%
- others: fungal (*Candida*), Kawasaki's, retropharyngeal/peritonsillar abscess, epiglottitis, bacterial tracteitis
- cannot be reliably distinguished on clinical features alone

Clinical Features
- refer to Table 32
- exudative tonsillitis: GAS, adenovirus, EBV, diphtheria
- soft palate petechiae: GAS, EBV

Table 29. Clinical Features of Pharyngitis

	Viral	Bacterial
Age	<3	>3
Onset	Gradual	Abrupt
Fever	Low-grade	>38°C
Clinical Features	Sore throat Rhinorrhea/cough Conjunctivitis Hoarseness Rash	Sore throat NO rhinitis/cough Nausea Abdominal discomfort HEENT findings: red pharynx, tender cervical nodes, tonsillar exudates palatal petechiae

Streptococcal (GAS) Pharyngitis

Clinical Features
- Group A *Streptococcus* (GAS) infection
- most commonly school aged (4-13 yrs), uncommon in children <3 yrs
- McIsaac Criteria: no cough, tender anterior cervical lymphadenopathy, erythematous tonsils with exudate, fever >38°C, age 3-14
  - score 0-1: no culture, no antibiotic; 2-3: culture, treat if positive; 4: antibiotics

Management
- >2 years old, culture before treatment or do rapid *Strep* antigen test
  - rapid strep test only 70-90% sensitive (pick up 20% of carriers of GAS), culture if negative (throat swab for culture is gold standard, sensitivity 90-95%)
- symptomatic
  - if 1 symptom, no culture or antibiotics
  - if >1 symptom, culture → antibiotics
    - penicillin V or amoxil 40 mg/kg/day PO divided bid x 10 days
    - erythromycin 40 mg/kg/day PO divided tid x 10 days if allergic to penicillin
    - acetaminophen for discomfort
  - can prevent rheumatic fever if treated within 9-10 days
  - antibiotics do not alter the risk of post-streptococcal glomerulonephritis
  - tonsillectomy for proven, recurrent streptococcal tonsillitis
- complications
  - if untreated, can lead to
    - suppurative complications: otitis media, sinusitis, cervical adenitis, pneumonia, mastoiditis
    - direct extension: retropharyngeal/peritonsillar abscess
    - scarlet fever, rheumatic fever
    - hematogenous spread: bone/joint infection, meningitis, SBE
  - acute glomerulonephritis (irrespective of antibiotic treatment)
  - invasive GAS disease: illness associated with isolation of GAS from normally sterile sites (blood, CSF, or pleural fluid)
- treatment of invasive GAS disease
  - admit
  - IV clindamycin 40 mg/kg divided into 3-4 doses + IV penicillin 250 000-400 000 U/kg/day divided into 6 doses
- other illnesses caused by strep: impetigo, cellulitis, bacteremia, vaginitis, toxic shock syndrome
- streptococcal toxic shock: illness associated with isolation of GAS from normally sterile sites (blood, CSF, or pleural fluid) + hypotension, renal impairment, coagulopathy, liver impairment, RDS, rash, soft tissue necrosis (necrotizing fasciitis, myositis, or gangrene)

SCARLET FEVER
- erythrogenic strain of Group A *Streptococcus*
- acute onset of fever, sore throat, strawberry tongue
- 24-48 hours after pharyngitis, rash begins in the groin, axillae, neck, antecubital fossa
- within 24 hours, "sandpaper" rash becomes generalized with perioral sparing, non-pruritic, non-painful
- rash fades after 3-4 days, may be followed by peeling
- treatment: penicillin, amoxicillin or erythromycin (if penicillin allergic) x 10 days

RHEUMATIC FEVER
- Jones Criteria (revised)
  - requires 2 major OR 1 major and 2 minor PLUS evidence of preceding strep infection (history of scarlet fever, group A streptococcal pharyngitis culture, rapid Ag detection test (only useful if positive), anti-streptolysin O titers (ASOT)
  - major criteria: "**SPACE**"
    - **s**ubcutaneous nodules, pea-sized firm, non-tender nodules typically on extensor surfaces
    - **p**ancarditis involving pericardium, myocardium, endocardium
    - **a**rthritis (migratory): very tender, red, warm, swollen joints, affects mostly large joints
    - **c**horea (Sydenham's): may be characterized by clumsiness, difficulty with handwriting
    - **e**rythema marginatum: begins as pink macules on trunk with central blanching; non-pruritic
  - minor criteria
    - previous history of rheumatic fever or rheumatic heart disease
    - polyarthralgia
    - fever
    - elevated ESR or C-reactive protein or leukocytosis
    - prolonged PR interval

McIsaac Criteria
Hot LACE
Fever >38°C
Lymphadenopathy- anterior, tender, cervical
Age 3-14
No **C**ough
Erythematous, exudative tonsils

Scarlet Fever
4 S and 4 P
Sore throat
Strawberry tongue
Sandpaper rash
Perioral Sparing
Non-Pruritic
Non-Painful
Peeling

- treatment
  - penicillin or erythromycin for acute course x 10 days
  - ASA for arthritis
  - prednisone if severe carditis
- secondary prophylaxis with daily penicillin or erythromycin; course depends on:
  - without carditis: 5 years or until 21 years old, whichever is longer
  - with carditis but no residual heart disease (no valvular disease): 10 years or longer
  - carditis and residual heart disease (persistant valvular disease): at least 10 years since last episode, sometimes life long prophylaxis
- complications
  - acute: myocarditis, conduction system (sinus tachycardia, atrial fibrillation), valvulitis (acute MR), pericarditis
  - chronic: rheumatic valvular heart disease – mitral and/or aortic insufficiency/stenosis, increased risk of infectious endocarditis ± thromboembolic phenomenon
  - onset of symptoms usually after 10-20 year latency from acute carditis of rheumatic fever

Infectious Mononucleosis

- the "great imitator": systemic viral infection that affects many organ systems
- Epstein-Barr virus (EBV): a member of herpesviridae
- incubation: 1-2 months
- spread through saliva ("kissing disease"), sexual activity

Clinical Features
- prodrome: 2-3 days of malaise, anorexia
- infants and young children: often asymptomatic or mild disease
- older children and young adults: may develop typical infectious mononucleosis syndrome
  - fever, tonsillar exudate, generalized lymphadenopathy, pharyngitis
  - ± hepatosplenomegaly
  - ± rash (rash more frequent with patients treated with amoxicillin/ampicillin)
  - any "-itis" (including arthritis, hepatitis, nephritis, myocarditis)
  - chronic fatigue
- resolves over 2-3 weeks although fatigue may persist for several months
- administration of amoxicillin results in rash in >90% of cases

Complications
- aseptic meningitis, encephalitis, Guillain-Barré, splenic rupture, agranulocytosis, myocarditis (rare)

Diagnosis
- heterophil antibody test (Monospot™ test) 85% sensitive in adults and older children, only 50% sensitive <4 yrs of age
- false positive results with HIV, SLE, lymphoma, rubella, parvovirus
- EBV titres
- CBC + differential: atypical lymphocytes, lymphocytosis, Downey cells, ± anemia, ± thrombocytopenia

Treatment
- throat culture to rule out streptococcal pharyngitis
- supportive care (bed rest, fluids, saline gargles for sore throat, acetaminophen)
- if airway obstructed secondary to node and/or tonsillar enlargement, admit to hospital, steroids
- patients with splenic enlargement often not apparent clinically so all patients should avoid contact sports for 6-8 weeks
- acyclovir not useful

Pertussis

- *Bordetella pertussis*, whooping cough, "100-day cough"
- incubation: 6-20 days; infectivity: 1 week before paroxysms to 3 weeks after
- increase in number of reported cases since early 1990's
- spread: highly contagious; via air droplets released during intense coughing
- greatest incidence among children <1 year and adolescents

Clinical Presentation
- prodromal catarrhal stage
  - 1-2 weeks, most contagious
  - coryza, mild cough
- paroxysmal stage
  - 2-4 weeks
  - paroxysms of cough, sometimes followed by inspiratory whoop (whoop may be absent in children <6 months or adults)
  - infants may present with apnea
  - ± vomiting with coughing spells
  - onset of attacks precipitated by yawning, sneezing, eating, physical exertion
  - can have severe symptoms for 6 weeks, cough for 6 months
  - pressure effect – subconjunctival hemorrhage, rectal prolapse, hernias, epistaxis
- convalescent stage
  - 1-2 weeks, noninfectious
  - occasional paroxysms of cough, but decreased frequency and severity, lasts up to 6 months

Diagnosis
- clinical: URTI symptoms followed by paroxysms of cough in an afebrile child
- lymphocytosis
- PCR of nasopharyngeal swab or aspirate

Complications
- otitis media
- respiratory complications
  - sinusitis, secondary pneumonia, atelectasis, pneumomediastinum, pneumothorax, interstitial or subcutaneous emphysema secondary to ruptured alveoli
- neurological complications
  - seizures, encephalopathy (1:100,000), intracranial hemorrhage

Treatment
- supportive care
- hospitalize if paroxysms of cough are associated with cyanosis and/or apnea, (give O_2)
- erythromycin 40 mg/kg/day x 10 days started within 3 weeks after onset of cough
  - isolate until 5 days of treatment
  - treatment will decrease infectivity but not change course of illness
  - shortens period of communicability
- antibiotic prophylaxis: erythromycin for all household contacts
- prevention: acellular pertussis vaccine (Pentacel™) in infants and children, and pertussis booster (Adacel™) in adolescents and adults

Varicella (Chickenpox)

- varicella-zoster virus (VZV)
- incubation: 10-21 days, infectivity: 1-2 days pre-rash until vesicles have crusted over
- transmission rate is 86% in household contacts, via respiratory secretions (airborne) and vesicular fluid
- primary infection with virus usually results in life-long immunity: >95% of young adults with varicella are immune
- maternal infection in first or early second trimester (<2% risk) can cause congenital varicella syndrome (low birth weight, CNS abnormalities, digit/limb abnormalities, cutaneous scarring, eye defects)
- maternal infection 5 days before to 2 days after delivery can lead to severe varicella of neonate

Clinical Presentation
- 1-3 day prodrome: fever and respiratory symptoms
- characteristic polymorphous rash
  - very pruritic
  - crops of red macules which quickly become vesicles surrounded by erythema
  - "dewdrop on erythematous base"
  - vesicles burst and lesions crust over
  - on trunk, face, scalp, conjunctivae, vagina, oral mucosa, palms and soles
  - new crops usually stop forming after 5-7 days

Complications
- **secondary bacterial infection** (most common)
  - infection with staph, GAS
  - presents as impetigo, abscesses, cellulitis, necrotizing fasciitis, sepsis
- cerebellar ataxia, pneumonia, hepatitis, encephalitis
- immunocompromised patients: varicella may be life-threatening

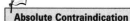

Absolute Contraindication
Do not use ASA in children with chickenpox due to the risk of Reye syndrome (see P59).

> **Complications of VZV**
> **2-HAP-E**
> **2**ndary bacterial infection
> **H**epatitis
> Cerebellar **A**taxia
> **P**neumonia
> **E**ncephalitis

- neonates born to mothers who develop varicella from 5 days before to 2 days after delivery are considered high risk
  - must administer varicella-zoster immune globulin (VZIG) and follow for signs of infection/sepsis
- virus latent in sensory ganglia and reappears as herpes zoster in 68/100,000 individuals
  - incidence is increased in immunocompromised patients

Treatment
- supportive (hydration, acetaminophen, antipruritics, AVOID salicylates)
- proper hygiene, discourage scratching
- acyclovir for severe disease, immunocompromised patients, neonates
- avoid contact with others until lesions are dry and crusted and no new ones are appearing

Prophylaxis and Prevention
- immunization (see *Pediatric Immunization*)
- VZIG for post-exposure in high risk susceptible patient (within 96 hours of exposure)

Roseola

- human herpes virus 6
- incubation: 5-15 days; infectivity and spread: unknown
- typically affects children <3 years

Clinical Presentation
- high fever (>39.5) lasting 3-5 days, cough, respiratory symptoms, nasal congestion
- pharynx, tonsils and tympanic membranes are erythematous
- cervical, posterior cervical lymphadenopathy, bulging anterior fontanelle (if CNS involvement)
- fever ceases before rash appears
  - pink non-pruritic macules and maculopapules
  - macules coalesce and disappear in 1-2 days

Treatment
- supportive (acetaminophen)

Complications
- febrile seizures
- encephalitis

Measles

- morbillivirus
- incubation: 10-14 days; infectivity: 4 days pre-rash, spread by airborne route

Clinical Presentation
- prodrome: "3 C's" – **c**ough, **c**oryza, **c**onjunctivitis, fever, eyelid edema
- **Koplik spots** (1-2 days before and after rash): small white papules on red base on buccal mucosa
- maculopapular rash spreads over face and hairline spreading in a descending fashion over the body over 3 days

Diagnosis
- clinical examination and positive serology for measles IgM

Treatment
- supportive and symptomatic (appropriate treatment of secondary bacterial infection)
- prophylactic immunoglobulin to prevent disease if administered within 6 days of exposure
- vitamin A supplementation in selected children

Complications
- secondary bacterial infection (laryngotracheobronchitis, otitis media, sinusitis), bronchopneumonia, croup
- encephalitis (1:1,000): ataxia, vomiting, seizures, coma
- subacute sclerosing panencephalitis (1:100,000): slow measles virus infection of brain manifesting years later, characterized by progressive cerebral deterioration with myoclonic jerks, fatal within 6-12 months

Mumps

- paramyxovirus
- incubation: 12-25 days; infectivity: 7 days pre-parotitis to 7 days post-parotitis, spread by droplets
- diagnosis: urine or saliva for viral serology

Clinical Presentation
- fever, headache, **parotitis** (bilateral; pushes earlobes up and out), myalgia, malaise
- 30-40% of cases are subclinical with minimal symptoms

Treatment
- supportive

Complications
- meningoencephalomyelitis: over 10% of patient with parotitis
- orchitis, epididymitis, infertility
- pancreatitis: may see elevated serum amylase without symptoms
- other: ocular complications, thyroiditis, hearing impairment, myocarditis, arthritis, thrombocytopenia, cerebellar ataxia, glomerulonephritis

Rubella

- rubivirus
- incubation:14-21 days
- infectivity: 7 days pre-rash to 5 days post-rash, spread by droplets
- diagnosis: serology for rubella IgM; may not be detected 4-5 days after rash onset

Clinical Presentation
- prodrome of nonspecific respiratory symptoms and suboccipital adenopathy
- rash
    - maculopapular, initially on face, then spreading to entire body
    - pruritic, disappearing by fourth day
- congenital rubella syndrome (CRS)
    - mother infected in first 4 months of pregnancy (highest risk)
    - infection in utero, failure of rubella vaccine is <5% and rarely results in CRS
    - cataracts/congenital glaucoma, congenital heart disease, hearing impairment (common), purpura ("blueberry muffin baby"), hepatosplenomegaly, jaundice, microcephaly, developmental delay, radiolucent bone disease
    - prevention: routine childhood immunization, assure immunity of women of childbearing age with vaccination

Treatment
- symptomatic

Prognosis
- excellent prognosis in patients with acquired disease
- irreversible defects in congenitally infected patients

Complications
- arthritis/arthralgia: polyarticular (fingers, wrists, knees), lasts days to weeks
- encephalitis

Reye Syndrome

- acute hepatic encephalopathy and noninflammatory fatty infiltration of liver and kidney
- mitochondrial injury of unknown etiology results in reduction of hepatic mitochondrial enzymes, diagnosis by liver biopsy
- associated with aspirin ingestion by children with varicella or influenza infection
- 40% mortality

Clinical Presentation
- vomiting
- hyperventilation, tachycardia, decerebrate posturing
- respiratory failure
- agitated delirium, coma, death

Treatment
- should be tailored based on severity of presentation
- IV glucose (to counteract effects of glycogen depletion)
- fluid restriction, mannitol (if cerebral edema)
- prevention: avoid aspirin with viral illness

Erythema Infectiosum

- parvovirus B19, "fifth disease"
- incubation: 4-14 days; infectivity: prior to onset of rash

Clinical Presentation
- initial 7-10 days: flu-like illness with fever
- day 10-17: rash appears (immune response)
  - raised maculopapular lesions on cheeks ("slapped cheek" appearance), forehead, chin, circumoral sparing
  - warm, nontender, may be pruritic, may also appear on extensor surfaces, trunk, neck, buttocks
- days to weeks: rash fades, may reappear with local irritation (heat, sunlight)

Treatment
- supportive
- blood transfusions for some with aplastic crisis

Complications
- arthritis (10%, pain and stiffness in peripheral joints), vasculitis, fetal loss in pregnancy
- aplastic crisis: reticulocytopenia occurs for 1 week during illness, unnoticed in normal individuals, but severe anemia in patients with chronic hemolytic anemia

Urinary Tract Infection

Definition
- urine specimen with >10^5 colonies/ml of a single organism

Epidemiology and Etiology
- 3-5% of girls, 1% of boys
  - <1 yr: more common in boys
  - >1yr F:M = 10:1
- *E.coli* (80-90%), *Klebsiella*, *Proteus* (especially boys), *S. saprophyticus*, *Enterococcus*, and *pseudomonas*
- risk factors: female, vesicoureteral reflux (VUR), diabetes, immunocompromised, urinary stasis (neurogenic bladder), voiding dysfunction, wiping from back to front

Symptoms and Diagnosis
- cystitis: dysuria, urgency, frequency, suprapubic pain, incontinence, malodorous urine
- pyelonephritis: abdominal or flank pain, fever, malaise, nausea, vomiting (may present as non-specific illness in newborn)
- sterile specimen required: suprapubic aspiration, transurethral catheter, clean catch
- dipstick for nitrates, leukocytes, and blood, urine C&S (definitive diagnosis)
- if systemically ill: CBC, electrolytes, Cr, BUN, blood cultures

Radiologic Evaluation
- U/S to assess for renal growth, hydronephrosis, or structural anomalies and voiding cystourethrography (VCUG) to assess for VUR for all children <2 yrs presenting with febrile UTI
- dimercaptosuccinic acid (DMSA) if VCUG abnormal or history of pyelonephritis to assess for renal scarring
- nuclear studies to follow VUR or assess function

Treatment
- duration 7-14 days
- encourage fluid intake (promotes urinary flow)
- uncomplicated UTI: oral cephalexin, TMP-SMX, amoxicillin, or nitrofurantoin x 7d
- complicated UTI (acutely ill, <2-3 months, vomiting, immunocompromised): admit for hydration, IV ampicillin and aminoglycoside
- prophylaxis: TMP-SMX for all kids with reflux, awaiting investigations and/or >3 UTIs/yr, Trimethoprim alone if <2mos
- follow up:
  - if no clinical response within 48 hrs re-culture urine

Complications
- long term morbidity: focal renal scarring may lead to hypertension and end-stage renal disease

---

Bagged specimen not useful for ruling in UTI (high false + >85%) but useful for ruling out UTI (high sensitivity).

Sensitivity and specificity of urine dip in children

	Sensitivity	Specificity
Leukocytes	62%	70%
Nitrates	50%	92%
Both	46%	94%

*Walter, et al. The urine dipstick test useful to rule out infections. A meta-analysis of the accuracy. BMC Urol. 2004; 4: 4.

Neonatology

Normal Baby at Term

- RR: 40-60 breaths/min
- HR: 120-160 beats/min when awake
- sBP: 50-80 mmHg; dBP: 30-40 mmHg
- weight: 2,500-4,500 g
- glucose: >2.2 mmol/L (40 mg/dL)

Gestational Age (GA) and Size

Definitions
- classification by gestational age (GA)
  - pre-term: <37 weeks
  - term: 37-42 weeks
  - post-term: >42 weeks
- classification by birth weight
  - small for gestational age (SGA): 2 SD < mean weight for GA or <10th percentile
  - appropriate for gestational age (AGA): within 2 SD of mean weight for GA
  - large for gestational age (LGA): 2 SD > mean weight for GA or >90th percentile
- methods for determining postnatal GA using Dubowitz/Ballard scores:
  - assessment at delivery of physical maturity (e.g. plantar creases, lanugo, ear maturation) and neuromuscular-maturity (e.g. posture, arm recoil)

Table 30. Abnormalities of Gestational Age and Size

Features	Causes	Problems
Pre-term infants <37 weeks	• Infections (TORCH) • Maternal pathology • Drugs/EtOH, smoking • Chromosomal • Multiple pregnancy • Placental insufficiency	• Respiratory distress syndrome, recurrent apnea, bronchopulmonary dysplasia • Feeding difficulties, necrotizing enterocolitis (NEC) • Hypocalcemia, hypoglycemia, hypothermia • Anemia, jaundice • Retinopathy of prematurity • Intracranial/intraventricular hemorrhage
Post-term infants • Wizened-looking, leathery skin • Meconium staining		• Severe asphyxia, meconium aspiration • Hypoglycemia • Birth trauma

SGA infants
• Asymmetric (head-sparing):
  late onset, growth arrest
 	
• Symmetric:
  early onset, lower growth potential
	• Extrinsic causes:
	  poor nutrition, hypertension, multiple pregnancies,
	  drugs, EtOH, smoking
	
	• Intrinsic causes:
	  infections (TORCH), congenital abnormalities,
	  syndromal, idiopathic
		• Perinatal asphyxia
		• Hypoglycemia, hypocalcemia, hypothermia
		• Hyperviscosity (polycythemia)
		• Hypomotility
		• Patent ductus arteriosus (PDA)

LGA infants	• Maternal diabetes • Racial or familial factors	• Birth trauma, perinatal asphyxia, meconium aspiration, respiratory distress syndrome, transient tachypnea of newborn (TTN), persistent pulmonary hypertension (PPHN) • Jaundice, hypoglycemia, hypocalcemia, polycythemia

Routine Neonatal Care

- performed in delivery suite
- erythromycin ointment – applied to both eyes for ophthalmia neonatorum (gonorrhea, chlamydia) prophylaxis
- vitamin K IM – to avoid hemorrhagic disease of newborn
- screening tests
  - varies across Canada and United States (see NNSGRC websites)
  - new tandem mass spectrometry (MS/MS) can detect 25 inborn errors of metabolism (IEM) in a single process (replaced old Guthrie method for PKU and TSH screening)
    - 100% sensitivity and 83-99% specificity depending on IEM
  - in Ontario, newborn screening tests for:
    - endocrine disorders (congenital adrenal hyperplasia, congenital hypothyroidism, cystic fibrosis)
    - hemoglobinopathies (HbSS, HbSc, sBthal)
    - inborn errors of metabolism (22 in total)
      - 3 categories: fatty acid oxidation defects, aminoacidopathies, organic acid defects
      - others: biotinidase deficiency and galactosemia
  - if mother Rh negative: blood group, direct antiglobulin test
  - if indicated: G6PD deficiency testing
- if mother hepatitis B positive: HBIg and start hepatitis B vaccine series

Approach to the Depressed Newborn

- between 5-10% of newborn babies require assistance with breathing after delivery
- a depressed newborn lacks one or more of the following characteristics for a normal newborn:
  - completely pink in appearance
  - pulse >100 bpm
  - cries when stimulated
  - actively moves all extremities
  - has a good strong cry

Table 31. Etiology of Respiratory Depression in the Newborn

Etiology	Examples
Respiratory problems	• Respiratory Distress Syndrome/Hyaline Membrane Disease • Asphyxia or CNS depression • Meconium aspiration • Pneumonia • Pneumothorax
Anemia (severe)	• Erythroblastosis fetalis • Secondary hydrops fetalis
Maternal causes	• Drugs • Diabetes mellitus • Pregnancy-induced hypertension
Congenital malformations/Birth injury	
Shock/Cyanosis/Congenital heart disease	
Other	• Hypothermia • Hypoglycemia • Trauma

Diagnosis
- vital signs
- take a good maternal history
  - include illnesses, use of drugs, labour, previous high risk pregnancies, infections during pregnancy, current infections, duration of ruptured membranes, blood type and Rh status, amniotic fluid status, gestational age, meconium, Apgar scores
- clinical findings (observe for signs of respiratory distress: cyanosis, tachypnea, retractions, and grunting)
- laboratory results (CBC, ABG, pH, blood type)
- transillumination or chest x-ray (if suspecting pneumothorax)

Management
- suction and postural drainage (if clinically indicated)
- apply vigorous tactile stimulation (do not 'spank')
- provide air/oxygen and assisted ventilation if needed
- monitor oxygen saturation and heart rate (if pulse <60 bpm, start CPR)
- treat the underlying cause
- counsel and provide explanation and support to family

Neonatal Resuscitation

- assess Apgars at 1 and 5 minutes
- if <7 at 5 minutes then reassess q5 min, until >7

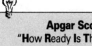

Apgar Score
"How Ready Is This Child?"
See Table 32

Table 32. Apgar Score

Sign	0	1	2
Heart Rate	Absent	<100/min	>100/min
Respiratory Effort	Absent	Slow, irregular	Good, crying
Irritability	No response	Grimace	Cough/cry
Tone	Limp	Some flexion of extremities	Active motion
Colour	Blue, pale	Body pink, extremities blue	Completely pink

Initial Resuscitation

- anticipation – know maternal history, history of pregnancy, labour, and delivery
- steps to take for all infants ("before ABC's")
    - provide warmth: warm (radiant heater, warm towels), dry (remove wet towels)
    - position & clear airway: "sniffing" position
    - stimulate infant (if needed): rub back gently or flick soles of feet EXCEPT if meconium present
- **Airway**
    - gentle suction of mouth then nose
    - if meconium is present and:
        - baby is vigorous (strong respiratory effort, good muscle tone, HR >100): suction nasopharynx after delivery of head
        - baby is not vigorous: free flow O_2, intubate and suction trachea
- **Breathing**
    - if HR <100 or apneic apply positive pressure ventilation (PPV)
    - PPV at rate of 40-60/min 100% O_2 with enough pressure to see visible chest expansion
- **Circulation**
    - if HR <60, apply chest compressions ("60 or less, compress")
    - chest compressions at lower 1/3 of the sternum at 1/3 of the AP depth at a rate of 120 events/min (3 compressions: 1 ventilation = 90 compressions/min: 30 breaths/min)

Table 33. Drugs Used in Neonatal Resuscitation

Drug Name	Schedule	Indications	Comments
epinephrine (adrenalin)	(0.1-0.3 ml/kg/dose of 1:10,000 IV/intratracheal q3-5 min prn	HR <60	Side effects: tachycardia, hypertension, cardiac arrhythmias
sodium bicarbonate	2-4 mL/kg/dose of 4.2% solution IV push over 2 min	Prolonged CPR that does not respond to other treatment Later used for metabolic acidosis or hyperkalemia	
calcium gluconate	2-4 mL/kg of 10% solution	Evidence of hypocalcemia	
naloxone (Narcan™)	0.1 mg/kg of a 0.4 mg/mL solution (= 0.25 mL/kg/dose) IV/IM/SC	Newborn with respiratory depression and maternal narcotic use 4 hours before delivery	May cause withdrawal symptoms including hypertension, irritability, poor feeding
fluid bolus (NS, whole blood, Ringer's lactate)	10 mL/kg/dose over 5-10 min	Evidence of hypovolemia	

Sepsis in the Neonate

Table 34. Sepsis Considerations in the Neonate

Early Onset (0-8 days)	Late Onset (8-28 days)

• begins in utero, 95% present within 24 hr
• risk factors:
  ▪ maternal infection: UTI, GBS positive
  ▪ maternal fever/leukocytosis/chorioamnionitis
  ▪ prolonged rupture of membranes, chorioamnionitis
  ▪ prematurity
  ▪ can be acquired postnatally e.g. RSV infection in NICU
• pathogens: GBS, *E. coli, Listeria*
	• Acquired after birth
	• Usually healthy, full-term
	• Same pathogens plus:
	  Streptococcus, Meningococcus,
	  Staphylococcus

Chronic Non-bacterial Perinatal Infections (TORCHES)
Toxoplasmosis
Others
Rubella virus
Cytomegalovirus, chickenpox, coxsackievirus
Herpes simplex virus, HIV, Hepatitis B
Erythema infectiosum (parvovirus B 19), Epstein-Barr virus
Syphilis

Signs of Sepsis

- no reliable absolute indicator of occult bacteremia in infants <3 months, most consistent result has been WBC >15
- temperature instability (hypo/hyperthermia)
- respiratory distress, cyanosis, apnea
- tachycardia/bradycardia
- lethargy, irritability
- poor feeding, vomiting, abdominal distention, diarrhea
- hypotonia, seizures, confusion, lethargy, coma
- jaundice, hepatomegaly, petechiae, purpura

Cyanosis

- peripheral cyanosis
    - can be normal transiently but may indicate sepsis, temperature instability
- central cyanosis
    - due to poor oxygenation – decreased SaO_2, decreased PaO_2
    - secondary to
        - respiratory insufficiency
        - cardiac (congenital heart disease, PPHN)
        - CNS (asphyxia)
        - hematologic (polycythemia)
        - sepsis

Management
- ABGs or capillary blood gas
- hyperoxic test (to rule out CHD): get baseline pO_2 in room air, then pO_2 on 100% O_2 x 10-15 min
    - pO_2 <150 mmHg: suggests congenital heart disease (see *Pediatric Cardiology*)
    - pO_2 >150 mmHg: suggests respiratory (airway, chest, lungs), brain or blood problems

Apnea

- periodic breathing is a normal respiratory pattern seen in newborns during sleep in which periods of rapid respiration are alternated with apneic spells lasting 5-10 seconds
- absence of respiratory gas flow for more than 15-20 seconds (less if associated with bradycardia or cyanosis)
    - central: no chest wall movement
    - obstructive: chest wall movement continues
    - mixed: combination of central and obstructive apnea

Differential Diagnosis
- in term infants, apnea always requires full work-up
- apnea <24 hrs – strongly associated with sepsis
- apnea >24 hrs
    - CNS:
        - apnea of prematurity: combination of CNS prematurity and obstructive apnea, resolves by 36 weeks GA, diagnosis of exclusion
        - seizures
        - intracranial hemorrhage (ICH)
        - hypoxic injury
    - infectious: sepsis, meningitis, necrotizing enterocolitis
    - GI: gastroesophageal reflux disease (GERD), aspiration with feeding
    - metabolic: hypoglycemia, hyponatremia, hypocalcemia
    - cardiovascular: low and high blood pressure, anemia, hypovolemia, PDA, heart failure
    - drugs: morphine

Management
- correct underlying cause, monitor
- O_2, continuous positive airway pressure (CPAP), ventilation
- tactile stimulation
- medications
    - methylxanthines (caffeine) stimulate the CNS and diaphragm

Respiratory Distress in the Newborn

Clinical Presentation
- tachypnea: RR >60/min; tachycardia: HR >160/min
- grunting/intercostal indrawing/nasal flaring
- duskiness/central cyanosis
- decreased air entry, crackles on auscultation

Differential Diagnosis of Respiratory Distress
- pulmonary
    - respiratory distress syndrome (RDS)
    - transient tachypnea of the newborn (TTN)
    - meconium aspiration syndrome (MAS)
    - pleural effusions, pneumothorax
    - congenital lung malformations

- infectious
  - sepsis
  - pneumonia (GBS + others)
- cardiac
  - congenital heart disease (cyanotic, acyanotic)
  - persistent pulmonary hypertension (PPHN)
- hematologic
  - blood loss
  - polycythemia
- anatomic
  - tracheoesophageal fistula
  - congenital diaphragmatic hernia
  - upper airway obstruction (see <u>Otolaryngology</u>)
    - choanal atresia
    - Pierre-Robin sequence (retrognathia and/or micrognathia plus cleft palate, and glossoptosis)
    - laryngeal (malacia)
    - tracheal (malacia, vascular ring)
    - mucous plug
    - cleft palate
- metabolic
  - hypoglycemia
  - inborn errors of metabolism (amino acidemia, organic acidemia, urea cycle disturbance, galactosemia, 1° lactic acidosis)
- neurologic
  - CNS damage (trauma, hemorrhage)
  - drug withdrawal syndromes

Investigations
- CXR, ABG or capillary blood gas, CBC, blood glucose
- blood cultures
- ECHO, ECG if indicated

Respiratory Distress Syndrome (RDS)

- also known as "hyaline membrane disease"

Pathophysiology
- surfactant deficiency → poor lung compliance due to high alveolar surface tension and atelectasis → decreased surface area for gas exchange → hypoxia + acidosis → respiratory distress
- surfactant decreases alveolar surface tension, improves lung compliance and maintains functional residual capacity

> RDS is the most common cause of respiratory distress in the pre-term infant.

Risk Factors
- premature babies: rare at term, risk is inversely proportional to birth weight and GA, sufficient surfactant production usually by 36 weeks
- infants of diabetic mothers (IDM): insulin inhibits the cortisol surge necessary for surfactant synthesis
- C-section without labour
- asphyxia, acidosis, sepsis, meconium aspiration
- males > females
- hypothermia

Clinical Presentation
- symptoms of respiratory distress
- onset within first few hours of life, worsens over next 24-72 hours
- infants may develop respiratory failure and require ventilation
- CXR: decreased aeration and lung volumes, reticulonodular pattern throughout lung fields with air bronchograms, atelectasis; may resemble pneumonia, if severe can see white-out

> "Ground glass" appearance of lungs is pathognomonic of RDS.

Prevention
- steroid therapy (e.g. Celestone™) for mothers (12 mg q24h x 2 doses) prior to delivery of premature infants
- monitor lecithin:sphingomyelin (L/S) ratio with amniocentesis, L/S >2:1 indicates lung maturity

Treatment
- supportive
  - O₂, assisted ventilation (PEEP, CPAP, or intubation), and nutrition
  - administer fluids cautiously to avoid pulmonary edema
- endotracheal surfactant administration (4 ml/kg/dose, can repeat q6-12h x 2 doses)

Prognosis
- in severe prematurity and/or prolonged ventilation, increased risk of bronchopulmonary dysplasia (BPD)

Complications
- bronchopulmonary dysplasia
- pulmonary air leaks (pneumothorax)

Transient Tachypnea of the Newborn (TTN)

- also known as "wet lung syndrome" and respiratory distress syndrome type II

Pathophysiology
- delayed resorption of fetal lung fluid → accumulation of fluid in peribronchial lymphatics and vascular spaces → tachypnea

Risk Factors
- full term or slightly premature infant
- no labour/short labour (hypothesized lack of catecholamine release)
- C-section (lungs are not compressed during passage through pelvic floor)
- diabetic mother

Clinical Presentation
- tachypnea within the first few hours of life, mild retractions, grunting, nasal flaring, without signs of severe respiratory distress
- usually resolves in 24-72 hours
- CXR: fluid in fissures, increased vascularity, slight cardiomegaly

Treatment
- supportive: O_2, nutrition, careful fluid administration
- full recovery expected within 2-5 days

Meconium Aspiration Syndrome (MAS)

- 10-15% of all infants are meconium stained at birth, ~5% of meconium stained infants get MAS (higher incidence with thick meconium)
- usually associated with fetal distress in utero, or post-term infant

Clinical Presentation
- respiratory distress within hours of birth
- small airway obstruction, chemical pneumonitis → tachypnea, barrel chest with audible crackles
- CXR: hyperinflation, streaky atelectasis, patchy infiltrates
- 10-20% have pneumothorax

Complications
- hypoxemia, hypercapnea, acidosis, PPHN, pneumothorax, pneumomediastinum, pneumonia, sepsis, respiratory failure, death

Treatment
- supportive care and ventilation
- may benefit from surfactant replacement (surfactant function is inhibited by meconium irritation)
- inhaled NO, extracorporeal membrane oxygenation

Prevention
- in utero: careful monitoring
- after delivery of the head: suction naso/oropharynx
- at birth: intubate and suction below cords

Pneumonia

- see *Pediatric Respirology*
- consider in infants with prolonged or premature rupture of membranes (PROM), maternal fever, or if mother GBS positive, baby has fever
- suspect if temperature unstable, WBC elevated, or low if patient is neutropenic
- symptoms may be non-specific
- CXR: hazy lung + distinct infiltrates (may be difficult to differentiate from RDS)

Diaphragmatic Hernia

- if resuscitation required at birth, DO NOT bag because air will enter stomach and compress lungs

Clinical Presentation
- respiratory distress, cyanosis
- scaphoid abdomen and barrel-shaped chest
- affected side dull to percussion and breath sounds absent, may hear bowel sounds instead
- asymmetric chest movements, trachea deviated away from affected side
- resultant pulmonary hypoplasia
- may present outside of neonatal period
- often associated with other anomalies (cardiovascular, CNS lesions)
- CXR: portion of GI tract in thorax (usually left side), displaced mediastinum

Treatment
- surgery

Persistent Pulmonary Hypertension of the Newborn (PPHN)

Pathophysiology
- severe hypoxemia due to persistence of fetal circulation
- R to L shunt through PDA, foramen ovale, intrapulmonary channels $\rightarrow$ decreased pulmonary blood flow and hypoxemia $\rightarrow$ further pulmonary vasoconstriction

Risk Factors
- asphyxia, MAS, RDS, sepsis, structural abnormalities (e.g. diaphragmatic hernia)

Investigations
- echocardiogram reveals increased pulmonary artery pressure and a R $\rightarrow$ L shunt, also used to rule out other cardiac defects

Treatment
- O_2 given early and tapered slowly, minimize stress and hypoxia, alkalinization, inotropes (to make systemic pressure greater than pulmonary pressure)
- mechanical ventilation, high frequency oscillation (HFO), extracorporeal membrane oxygenation (ECMO)

Bronchopulmonary Dysplasia (BPD)

- usually after prolonged intubation/ventilation with high pressures and high O_2 concentration (often after ventilation for RDS)
- O_2 requirement at 28 days/36 wks GA and abnormal CXR findings (lung opacification, then cysts with sites of over distention and atelectasis, appears spongy)
- chronic respiratory distress leads to pulmonary hypertension, poor growth, right-sided heart failure

Treatment
- gradual wean from ventilator, optimize nutrition, stress avoidance, diuretics, bronchodilators
- dexamethasone may help decrease inflammation and encourage weaning

Hypoglycemia

- glucose <2.2 mmol/L (40 mg/dL) in full term infant; <2.6-2.8 mmol/L (47-51 mg/dL) in preterm

Etiology
- decreased carbohydrate stores (premature, IUGR)
- infant of a diabetic mother (IDM): maternal hyperglycemia $\rightarrow$ fetal hyperglycemia and hyperinsulinism $\rightarrow$ hypoglycemia in the newborn infant because of high insulin levels
- sepsis
- endocrine: hyperinsulinism due to islet cell hyperplasia (e.g. Beckwith-Wiedemann syndrome), panhypopituitarism
- inborn errors of metabolism: fatty acid oxidation defects, galactosemia

Clinical Findings
- signs often non-specific and subtle: lethargy, poor feeding, irritability, tremors, apnea, cyanosis, seizures

Management
- identify and monitor infants at risk, (pre-feed blood glucose checks)
- begin oral feeds within first few hours of birth
- if hypoglycemic, provide glucose IV (D10, D12.5)
- if persistent hypoglycemia (past day 3), hypoglycemia unresponsive to IV glucose, and/or no predisposing cause for hypoglycemia, send the following "critical bloodwork" during an episode of hypoglycemia
  - insulin
  - cortisol
  - growth hormone (GH)
  - β-hydroxybutyrate
  - lactate
  - ammonia
  - free fatty acids (FFA's)
  - ABG
- treat hyperinsulinism with diazoxide, glucagon

Jaundice

- jaundice visible at serum bilirubin levels of 85-120 μmol/L (5-6 mg/dL)
- look at sclera, mucous membranes, palmar creases, tip of nose
- jaundice more severe/prolonged (due to increased retention of bilirubin in the circulation) with:
  - prematurity
  - acidosis
  - hypoalbuminemia
  - dehydration

> Jaundice is very common – 60% of term newborns develop visible jaundice.

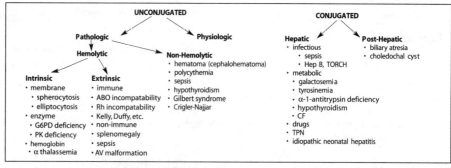

Figure 3. Approach to Neonatal Hyperbilirubinemia

PHYSIOLOGIC JAUNDICE

Epidemiology
- term infants: onset 2-3 days of life, resolution by 7 days of life
- premature infants: higher peak and longer duration

> Jaundice in the first 24 hours is always pathological.

Pathophysiology
- increased hematocrit and decreased RBC lifespan
- immature glucuronyl transferase enzyme system (slow conjugation of bilirubin)
- increased enterohepatic circulation

Table 35. Risk Factors

Maternal factors	Perinatal factors	Neonatal factors
• Ethnic group (e.g. Asian, native American) • Complications during pregnancy (infant of diabetic mother, Rh or ABO incompatibility) • Breast feeding	• Birth trauma (cephalohematoma, ecchymoses) • Infection	• Prematurity • Genetic factors • Polycythemia • Drugs • Low intake breast milk

Breast Feeding Jaundice
- common
- due to lack of milk production and subsequent dehydration, leading to exaggerated physiologic jaundice

Breast Milk Jaundice
- rare (1 in 200 breast-fed infants)
- inhibitor of glucuronyl transferase found in breast milk
- onset 7 days of life, peak at 2nd to 3rd week of life

Table 36. Causes of Neonatal Jaundice by Age

<24 hours	24-72 hours	72-96 hours	Prolonged (>1 week)
ALWAYS PATHOLOGIC	• Physiologic, polycythemia • Dehydration (breast feeding jaundice)	• Physiologic ± breast feeding jaundice	• Breast milk jaundice • Prolonged physiologic jaundice in preterm

• Hemolysis
  - Rh or ABO incompatibility
	• Hemolytic
	  - G6PD deficiency
	  - Pyruvate kinase deficiency
		• Sepsis	• Hypothyroidism
			 • Neonatal hepatitis
			 • Conjugation dysfunction

• Sepsis
  - GBS
  - Congenital infection
    (TORCH)
	- Spherocytosis
	  - Bruising hemorrhage, hematoma
			- e.g. Gilbert syndrome, Crigler-Najjar
			    syndrome

	• Sepsis/congenital infection		• Inborn errors of metabolism
			  - e.g. galactosemia
			 • Biliary tract obstruction
			  - e.g. biliary atresia

PATHOLOGIC JAUNDICE
- must be investigated if:
  - jaundice at <24 hours of age
  - serum unconjugated bilirubin rises rapidly or is excessive for patient's age and weight (>85 μmol/L per day or >220 μmol/L before 4 days of age)
  - conjugated bilirubin >35 μmol/L (2.0 mg/dL)
  - persistent jaundice lasting beyond 1-2 weeks of age
- investigations
  - hemolytic work-up: CBC, blood group (mother and infant), peripheral blood smear, Coombs test, bilirubin (conjugated, unconjugated)
  - if baby is unwell or has fever, septic work-up: CBC + differential, blood and urine cultures, CXR ± LP
  - other: TSH, G6PD screen (in males)
  - conjugated hyperbilirubinemia: consider liver enzymes (AST, ALT), coagulation studies (PT, PTT), serum albumin, ammonia, TSH, TORCH screen, septic work-up, galactosemia screen (erythrocyte galactose-1-phosphate uridyltransferase levels), metabolic screen, abdominal U/S, HIDA scan, sweat chloride

TREATMENT OF UNCONJUGATED HYPERBILIRUBINEMIA
- to prevent kernicterus (see below)
- breast feeding does not need to be discontinued, ensure adequate feeds and hydration
- get lactation consultant support, mother to pump after feeds
- treat underlying causes (e.g. sepsis)
- phototherapy
  - insoluble unconjugated bilirubin is converted to excretable form via photoisomerization
  - serum bilirubin should be monitored during and immediately after therapy (risk of rebound because photoisomerization reversible when phototherapy discontinued)
  - contraindicated in conjugated hyperbilirubinemia: results in "bronzed" baby
  - side effects: hypernatremic dehydration, eye damage, skin rash, diarrhea
- exchange transfusion
  - prevents toxic effects of bilirubin by removal from body
  - indications: depending on level and rate of rise of bilirubin
  - most commonly performed for hemolytic disease (G6PD)

Kernicterus
- unconjugated bilirubin concentrations exceed albumin binding capacity and bilirubin enters and is deposited in the brain resulting in permanent damage (often basal ganglia or brainstem)
- incidence increases as serum bilirubin levels increase above 340 μmol/L (19.8 mg/dL)
- can occur at lower levels in presence of sepsis, meningitis, hemolysis, hypoxia, hypothermia, hypoglycemia and prematurity
- up to 15% of infants have no obvious neurologic symptoms
- acute form
  - first 1-2 days: lethargy, hypotonia, poor feeding, high-pitched cry, emesis, seizures
  - middle of first week: hypertonia, opisthotonic posturing, fever, bulging fontanelle, pulmonary hemorrhage
- chronic form (first year and beyond)
  - hypotonia, delayed motor skills, extrapyramidal abnormalities (choreoathetoid cerebral palsy), gaze palsy, MR, sensorineural hearing loss
- treatment: exchange transfusion
- complications: sensorineural deafness, choreoathetoid cerebral palsy (CP), gaze palsy, mental retardation

BILIARY ATRESIA
- atresia of the extrahepatic bile ducts
- cholestasis and ↑ conjugated bilirubin after the first week of life
- incidence: 1/10,000-15,000 live births

Clinical Presentation
- dark urine, pale stool, jaundice (persisting for >2 weeks), abdominal distention, hepatomegaly

Diagnosis
- HIDA scan

Treatment
- surgical drainage procedure
- hepatoportoenterostomy (Kasai procedure most successful if before 8 weeks of age)
- usually requires liver transplantation
- Vitamins A, D, E, and K. Diet should be enriched with medium-chain triglycerides to ensure adequate fat ingestion

Bleeding Disorders in Neonates

Differential Diagnosis
- increased platelet destruction: maternal ITP, neonatal alloimmune thrombocytopenia purpura (NATP), infection, DIC, drugs, extensive localized thrombosis, critically ill infants, giant hemangiomas, maternal lupus
- decreased platelet production: bone marrow replacement, pancytopenia, Fanconi anemia, trisomy 13 & 18
- mechanism undetermined: inborn error of metabolism, congenital thyrotoxicosis
- hemorrhage disease of the newborn

Neonatal Alloimmune Thrombocytopenia Purpura (NATP)
- development of maternal antibodies against antigens on fetal platelets that are shared with father and seen as foreign by maternal immune system
- platelet equivalent of Rh disease of the newborn
- incidence: 1/4000-5000 live births
- clinical features: maternal serum (with immunoglobins) react with father's or child's platelets
- diagnosis: check for the presence of maternal alloantibodies against father's platelets
- treatment: IVIG to mother prenatally, starts in second trimester; transfusion of infant with washed maternal platelets

Autoimmune Thrombocytopenia
- caused by antiplatelet antibodies from maternal ITP or SLE
- similar presentation to NATP but must distinguish; if infant is transfused with maternal platelets, the transfused platelets will also be destroyed
- treatment: steroids to mother x 10-14 days prior to delivery, or IVIG to mother before delivery or to infant after delivery

Hemorrhagic Disease of the Newborn
- caused by vitamin K deficiency
- factors II, VII, IX, X are vitamin K-dependent, therefore both PT and PTT are abnormal
- presents at 2-7 days of life with GI hemorrhage, intracranial hemorrhage, bleeding from circumcision or umbilical stump
- prevention: vitamin K IM administration at birth to all newborns

Necrotizing Enterocolitis (NEC)

- intestinal inflammation associated with focal or diffuse ulceration and necrosis
- primarily affecting terminal ileum and colon
- affects 1-5% of all newborns admitted to NICU

Pathophysiology
- postulated mechanism of bowel ischemia → mucosal damage, and enteral feeding providing a substrate for bacterial growth and mucosal invasion, leading to bowel necrosis or gangrene and perforation

Risk Factors
- prematurity (immature defenses)
- asphyxia, shock (poor bowel perfusion)
- enteral feeding with formula (breast milk can be protective)
- sepsis

Clinical Presentation
- distended abdomen

Differential Diagnosis of Pneumatosis Intestinalis
NEC
Hirschsprung disease
Pseudomembranous enterocolitis
Neonatal ulcerative colitis
Ischemic bowel disease

- increased amount + bile stained gastric aspirate/vomitus
- frank or occult blood in stool
- feeding intolerance
- diminished bowel sounds
- signs of bowel perforation – sepsis, shock, peritonitis, DIC

Investigations
- abdominal x-ray: intramural air ("train tracks"), free air, fixed loops, thickened bowel wall, portal venous gas
- CBC, ABG, blood culture (25% will be positive at time of diagnosis)
- high WBC, low platelets, electrolyte imbalance, acidosis, hypoxia, hypercapnea

Treatment
- NPO (minimum 2-3 weeks), vigorous IV fluid resuscitation, NG decompression
- TPN
- antibiotics for infection (triple therapy given empirically: ampicillin, gentamicin, metronidazole x 7-10 days)
- serial abdominal x-rays detect early perforation
- surgical resection of necrotic bowel and surgery for complications (e.g. perforation, strictures)

Intraventricular Hemorrhage (IVH)

- intracranial hemorrhage originating in the periventricular subependymal germinal matrix (GM)
- incidence and severity inversely proportional to GA

Risk Factors
- extreme prematurity, birth asphyxia, need for vigorous resuscitation at birth, pneumothorax, ventilated preterm infants, seizures, sudden increase in arterial blood pressure with volume expansion, hypotensive event, hypertension, RDS

Clinical Presentation
- may be asymptomatic
- subtle symptoms and signs: bulging fontanelle, drop in hematocrit, apnea, bradycardia, acidosis, seizures, and decreased muscle tone or level of consciousness

Classification
- screening and diagnosis by U/S on first day of life if risk factors present (50% of IVH occurs during the first 6-12 hours of life) ± CT/MRI at 4-7 days of life (detects 90-100% of all hemorrhages)
  - grade I: GM hemorrhage
  - grade II: IVH without ventricular dilatation
  - grade III: IVH with ventricular dilatation
  - grade IV: GM hemorrhage or IVH with parenchymal involvement

Management of Acute Hemorrhage
- supportive care to maintain blood volume and acid-base status
- avoid fluctuations in blood pressure and cerebral blood flow
- follow-up with serial imaging

Prognosis
- short-term outcomes: mortality and posthemorrhagic hydrocephalus (PHH)
- long-term major neurological sequelae: cerebral palsy, cognitive deficits, motor deficits, visual and hearing impairment

Table 37. Prognosis of IVH

Classification	Mortality	PHH rate	Neurological sequelae
mild to moderate IVH	5-10%	5-20%	5-15%
severe IVH	20%	55%	30-40%
severe IVH and parenchymal involvement	~50%	~80%	as high as 100%

Retinopathy of Prematurity (ROP)

- interruption in the progression of developing retinal vessels

Pathophysiology
- early vasoconstriction and obliteration of the capillary bed → neovascularization → detachment of the retina → blindness

Risk Factors
- association with period of high oxygen concentrations is now not so clear
- extreme prematurity is the most significant risk factor

- maternal complications, apnea, sepsis, hyper- and hypocapnea, vitamin E deficiency, intraventricular hemorrhage, anemia, exchange transfusion, hypoxia, lactic acidosis, and bright light

Clinical Presentation
- ROP is classified by stage (I → V)
- see Ophthalmology

Assessment
- ophthalmoscopic examination
  - infants weighing ≤1500 g or ≤28 weeks GA: starting at 4-6 weeks of chronologic age or at 32 weeks corrected age (whichever is later) with exams q2-3 weeks until retinal maturity with no disease
  - infants with ROP or very immature vessels: exams q1-2 weeks

Management
- cryotherapy or laser photocoagulation
- follow-up eye examinations for myopia, strabismus, amblyopia, glaucoma, and late detachment

Prognosis
- stage I and II: 90% spontaneous regression
- stage III+: ~50% spontaneous regression; with treatment, incidence of severe visual impairment reduces by ~50%

Common Neonatal Skin Conditions

Table 38. Common Neonatal Skin Conditions

Neonatal Skin Conditions	Description
Vasomotor Response (Cutis Marmorata, acrocyanosis)	Transient mottling when exposed to cold; usually normal, particularly in prems
Vernix Caseosa	Soft creamy white layer covering baby at birth
Slate-grey nevus of childhood ('Mongolian spots')	Bluish grey macules over lower back and buttocks (may look like bruises); common in dark skinned infants
Capillary Hemangioma	Raised red lesion which increases in size after birth and involutes; 50% resolved by 5ys, 90% by 9 yrs
Erythema Toxicum	Erythematous vesiculo-pustular rash, lesions disappear and reappear in minutes to hours, resolves by 2 weeks
Milia	Lesions 1-2mm firm white pearly papules on nasal bridge, cheeks, and palate; self-resolving
Pustular melanosis	Brown macular base with dry vesicles, seen more commonly in African American infants
Angiomatous lesions (Salmon patch)	Transitory macular capillary hemangiomas of the eyelids and neck ("Angel Kiss" & "Stork Bite"); usually disappears with age
Neonatal Acne	Self-resolving

Nephrology

Dehydration

Table 39. Assessment of Dehydration

Point of Assessment	Method
Volume deficit	History, physical examination
Osmolar disturbance	Serum Na
Acid-base disturbance	Blood pH, pCO_2, bicarbonate
Potassium	Serum K
Renal function	BUN, creatinine, urine specific gravity/osmolality, urine sediment

Table 40. Assessment of Severity of Dehydration

	Mild	Moderate	Severe
Pulse (HR)	normal, full	rapid	rapid, weak
Blood Pressure (BP)	normal	normal-low	shock – ↓BP
Urine Output (UO)	decreased	markedly decreased	anuria
Oral Mucosa	slightly dry	dry	parched
Anterior Fontanelle	normal	sunken	markedly sunken
Eyes	normal	sunken	markedly sunken
Skin Turgor	normal	decreased	tenting
Capillary Refill	normal (<3 sec)	normal to ↑	↑ (>3 sec)
% loss of Pre-Illness Body Weight			
≤2 years	5%	10%	15%
>2 years	3%	6%	9%

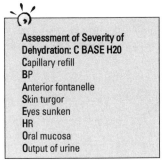

Assessment of Severity of
Dehydration: C BASE H20
Capillary refill
BP
Anterior fontanelle
Skin turgor
Eyes sunken
HR
Oral mucosa
Output of urine

Fluid and Electrolyte Therapy

Principles of Treatment
- provision of maintenance daily fluid and electrolyte requirements (see Table 41)
- PLUS replacement of deficit fluids and electrolytes (see Table 42)
- PLUS replacement of ongoing losses

Table 41. Maintenance Fluid and Electrolyte Requirements

Body Weight	100:50:20 Rule	4:2:1 Rule
	(24-hour maintenance fluids)	(hourly rate of maintenance fluids)
1-10 kg	100 cc/kg/day	4 cc/kg/hr
11-20 kg	50 cc/kg/day	2 cc/kg/hr
>20 kg	20 cc/kg/day	1 cc/kg/hr
Electrolyte Requirements		
Na:	3 mEq/kg/day	
K:	2 mEq/kg/day	
Cl:	3 mEq/kg/day	

Table 42. Correction of Fluid and Electrolyte Deficits

Dehydration[1]	5%	10%	Rate
Isotonic (80%)	Na 4-5 mmol/kg K 4-5 mmol/kg	Na 8-10 mmol/kg	1/2 total replacement over 1st 8 hours, then 1/2 over 16 hours
Hypotonic[2] (5%) (Na <130 mmol/L)	Na 5-6 mmol/kg K 3 mmol/kg	Na 10-12 mmol/kg K 5 mmol/kg	If Na ≥105, correct as above If Na <105, correct by 20 mmol/L maximum over 0.5-4 hours with hypertonic saline
Hypertonic (15%) (Na >150 mmol/L)	Na 2-4 mmol/kg K 2-4 mmol/kg	Na 2-4 mmol/kg K 2-4 mmol/kg	Correct over 48-72 hours Do not allow serum Na to drop faster than 10-15 mmol/L/day[3]

Note: [1]For all types dehydration, H_2O for 5% dehydration = 50mL/kg; for 10% dehydration = 100 mL/kg
                 [2]To calculate exact deficit: [Na] deficit = ([Na]target – [Na]actual) x body weight (kg) x total body water (L)
                 [3]To lower serum Na by a predictable amount, remember: 4 mL/kg of free H2O lowers serum Na by 1 mmol/L

Common IV Fluids
- first month of life: D5W/0.2 NS + 20 mEq KCl/L (only add KCl if voiding well)
- children: D5W/0.9 NS + 20mEq KCl/L or D5W/0.45 NS + 20mEq KCl/L
- NS: as bolus to restore circulation in dehydrated children

Table 43. Common Manifestations of Renal Disease

Neonate	Differential Diagnosis
Flank Mass	Dysplasia, polycystic disease, hydronephrosis, tumour
Hematuria	Asphyxia, malformation, trauma, renal vein thrombosis
Anuria/oliguria	Agenesis, obstruction, asphyxia
Child and Adolescent	**Differential Diagnosis**
Cola/red-coloured urine	Hemoglobinuria (hemolysis) Myoglobinuria (rhabdomyolysis) Hematuria (e.g. glomerulonephritis), pigmenturia
Gross Hematuria	Glomerulonephritis, benign hematuria, trauma, cystitis, tumour, stones
Edema	Nephrotic syndrome, nephritis, acute/chronic renal failure (also consider cardiac or liver disease)
Hypertension	Acute glomerulonephritis, renal failure, dysplasia (also consider coarctation of aorta, drugs, endocrine causes)
Polyuria	DM, central and nephrogenic diabetes insipidus, hypercalcemia, polyuric renal failure
Oliguria	Dehydration, acute tubular necrosis (ATN), interstitial nephritis
Urgency	Urinary tract infection (UTI), vaginitis

Hematuria

- 0.5-2% prevalence of asymptomatic microscopic hematuria in school-aged children
- history of prior acute infection (upper respiratory, skin or GI)
- family history: dialysis, transplant, SLE, familial hematuria
- physical exam: BP, edema, rashes, arthritis

Causes of coloured urine (negative dipstick): beets, lead, rifampin, urates, nitrofurantoin, ibuprofen.

False positive dipstick (positive dipstick, but no RBCs): myoglobinuria (rhabdomyolysis), hemoglobinuria (intravascular hemolysis, intravascular coagulation).

Etiology
- nephrologic
    - glomerular disease:
        - recurrent gross hematuria: IgA nephropathy, benign familial hematuria, Alport syndrome
        - post-streptococcal GN, lupus nephritis, HSP, HUS, Goodpasture disease (rare in childhood)
    - tubulointersitial: ATN, interstitial nephritis, pyelonephritis, hypercalciuria
- infection: bacterial, TB, viral, UTI, pyelonephritis
- hematologic: coagulopathies, thrombocytopenia, sickle cell disease or trait, renal vein thrombosis
- nephrolithiasis
- anatomic abnormalities: congenital, trauma, polycystic kidneys, vascular abnormalities, tumours (Wilms)
- other: exercise, drugs

Asymptomatic Microscopic Hematuria
- definition: 5-10 RBC/HPF of centrifuged urine
- usually found on routine screening
- dipsticks are very sensitive, but have a high false positive rate
    - 5% of school-aged children on single test but <1% on repeated testing
- benign familial hematuria in 2/3 of cases
    - sporadic or familial
    - no associated proteinuria

Gross Hematuria
- urinalysis (U/A)
    - renal source
        - cola/tea-coloured urine
        - casts, proteinuria, dysmorphic RBCs
        - associated symptoms and signs (e.g. edema, azotemia, hypertension)
    - post-renal source
        - bright red urine, initial and terminal stream hematuria, clots
        - normal RBC morphology, <2+ proteinuria, no casts
        - very large renal bleeding can look like a lower urinary tract bleed

Investigations
- CBC, urine dip and culture, creatinine, BUN, 24hr urine collection for creatinine, protein, Ca, serum C3 and C4 level
- other if suspected: antistreptolysin O titer, ANA, throat swab
- if above do not yield a diagnosis, consider U/S ± Doppler to rule out structural anomalies

- treat underlying cause if applicable
  - supportive treatment (e.g. anthihypertensives, fluid restriction, dietary modifications
  - referral to pediatric rephrologist, may warrant renal biopsy depending on findings

Proteinuria

- a small amount of protein is found in the urine of healthy children <4 mg/m²/h or <100 mg/m²/d
- definition
  - qualitative: 1+ (30 mg/dL) in dilute, 2+ (100 mg/dL) in concentrated urine (specific gravity >1.015)
  - quantitative: >4 mg/m²/h on timed urine (>40 mg/m²/h is nephrotic range)
- urine dipstick is the least accurate (false positives if urine pH >8 or SG >1.025)
- protein/creatinine ratio on spot urine is more accurate (normal <0.5 if 6 mos-2 yrs; <0.2 if over 2 yrs)
- 24-hour protein is the most accurate (normal <100 mg/m²/day)
- microalbuminuria assesses risk of progressive glomeronephropathy in diabetes (normal <30 mg albumin/gram creatinine on first morning void)
- progressive proteinuria is the best predictor of renal disease
- transient proteinuria: due to fever (>38.3°C/101°F), dehydration, exercise, seizures, stress
- persistent proteinuria (≥1+ on dipstick)
  - orthostatic (more common in adolescents – usually benign): elevated protein excretion when upright and normal when recumbent; rarely exceeds 1 g/m²/day
  - glomerular (e.g. nephrotic syndrome, glomerulonephritis)
  - tubulointerstitial (e.g. Fanconi syndrome, ATN)
  - structural abnormalities of urinary tract (e.g. hydronephrosis)

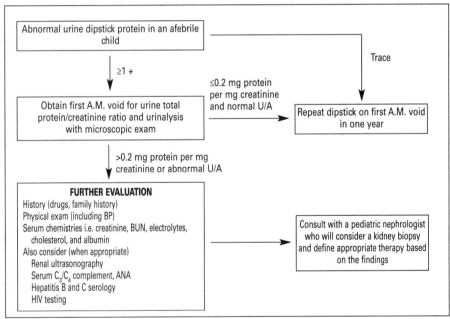

Figure 4. Evaluation of Persistent Proteinuria in Children/Adolescents
Hogg R.J. et al. (2000) Paediatrics - Vol. 105: 1242-49.

Hemolytic Uremic Syndrome (HUS)

Epidemiology
- most common cause of acute renal failure in children
- more common from 6 months to 4 years of age

Pathophysiology
- *E. coli* O157:H7 verotoxin ("hamburger disease") or shiga toxin
  - toxin binds, invades and destroys colonic epithelial cells, causing bloody diarrhea
  - toxin enters the systemic circulation, attaches and injures endothelial cells (especially in kidney) causing a release of endothelial products (e.g. von Willebrand factor, platelet aggregating factor)

- form platelet/fibrin thrombi in multiple organ systems (e.g. renal, pancreas, brain) resulting in thrombocytopenia
- RBCs are forced through occluded vessels resulting in fragmented RBC (schistocytes) and removed by the reticuloendothelial system (hemolytic anemia)
- other, rare forms of HUS in childhood are due to bacteria (e.g. *S. pneumoniae*), viruses, familial inheritance, or drugs

Clinical Presentation
- triad: acute renal failure, thrombocytopenia, microangiopathic hemolytic anemia
- initial presentation of abdominal pain and diarrhea, followed by bloody diarrhea
- within 5-7 days the patient begins to show signs of anemia, thrombocytopenia and renal insufficiency
    - history: weakness, lethargy, oliguria
    - physical exam: pallor, jaundice (hemolysis), edema, petechiae, hypertension
- investigations: CBC, platelets, blood smear, urinalysis, BUN, creatinine
- prognosis: 5-10% mortality, 10-30% kidney damage
- supportive treatment; nutritional support; monitor electrolytes; dialysis if electrolyte abnormality cannot be corrected, fluid overload, or BUN >100 mg/dL; PRBC for symptomatic anemia
- steroids not helpful; antibiotics not indicated

Nephritic Syndrome

- acute, subacute or chronic
    - hematuria with RBC casts, proteinuria (<50 mg/kg/day, not nephrotic-range), azotemia, hypertension
    - renal failure (oliguria)

Post-Streptococcal Glomerulonephritis
- antigen-antibody mediated complement activation
- most common in children, especially in 4-8 year olds, M > F
- occurs 1-3 weeks following group A β-hemolytic streptococcal infection of skin or throat
- diffuse, proliferative glomerulonephritis
- diagnosed by elevated serum antibody titres against strep antigens (ASOT, anti-DNAse B)
- 95% of children recover completely within 1-2 weeks
- 5-10% have persistent hematuria
- management:
    - symptomatic treatment: fluid restriction, antihypertensives, diuretics
    - in severe cases: hemodialysis or peritoneal dialysis may be necessary
    - eradication of infection (penicillin or erythromycin)

Nephritic syndrome: PHAROH
Proteinuria (<50 mg/kg/d)
Hematuria
Azotemia
RBC casts
Oliguria
Hypertension

Table 44. Major Causes of Acute Glomerulonephritis

	↓C3	Normal C3
Renal	Post-infectious GMN Membranoproliferative Type I (50-80%) Type II (>80%)	IgA Nephropathy Idiopathic rapidly progressive GMN Anti-GBM disease
Systemic	SLE SBE Shunt nephritis Cryoglobulinemia	Polyarteritis nodosa Wegener's granulomatosis Goodpasture's syndrome Henoch-Schönlein purpura (HSP)

Nephrotic Syndrome

Clinical Presentation
- severe proteinuria (>50 mg/kg/day or > 40 mg/m²/hr)
- hypoalbuminemia <20 g/L (<2.0 g/dL)
- edema (usually first sign, initially see facial swelling, especially periorbital, and pretibial edema)
- hyperlipidemia >5.17 mmol/L (200 mg/dL)
- secondary findings: hypocalcemia, hyperkalemia, hyponatremia (likely a dilutional effect), hypercoagulability (decreased PTT)

Etiology
Primary NS
- minimal change disease (MCD) (76%)
    - peak occurrence between 2-6 years of age, more common in boys than girls (2:1)

PALE
Proteinuria (>50 mg/kg/d)
hypo**A**lbuminemia (<20g/L)
hyper**L**ipidemia
Edema

- often treated empirically with steroids without kidney biopsy, 90% steroid responsive
- membranous glomerulonephritis (8%)
- focal segmental glomerular sclerosis (FSGS) (7%)
- membranoproliferative glomerulonephritis (5%)

Secondary NS
- vasculitis
- infections (e.g. hepatitis B & C, syphilis, HIV)
- medications (e.g. captopril, penicillamine, NSAIDs, anticonvulsants)
- malignancy
- hereditary (e.g. sickle cell disease, Alport syndrome)
- metabolic, inflammatory (e.g. lupus nephropathy, rheumatoid arthritis)

Complications
- risk of infections (e.g. spontaneous peritonitis, cellulitis, sepsis)
- hypercoagulability due to decreased intravascular volume and antithrombin III depletion (pulmonary embolism, renal vein thrombosis)
- side effects of drugs (diuretics, steroids, immunosuppressants)
- hypotension, shock, renal failure

Investigations
- to rule out secondary causes of NS: serum complement levels, BUN, Cr, serum chemistries, ANA, antistreptolysin O titre, in certain cases HIV, Hep B/C and syphilis titers
- consider kidney biopsy if:
  - HTN (higher risk of focal segmental glomenlosclerosis(FSGS)), steroid resistant, frequent relapses (>2 relapses in 6 month period), low serum complement, decreased renal function
  - presentation before first year of life (high likelihood of congenital nephrotic syndrome)
  - presentation after 10 years of age to rule out more serious renal pathology than MCD

Management
- salt and water restriction, diuretic may be required
- optimal nutrition, including high-quality protein
- daily weights to assess therapeutic progress
- varicella antibody titre if not immune
- pneumococcal vaccine after remission (avoid live vaccines)
- initial treatment of MCD:
  - oral prednisone (or equivalent) 60 mg/m^2/day in divided doses (max. dose 80 mg/day) for up to 12 weeks
  - a negative tuberculin skin test should be performed before starting steroid medications
  - a measurable decrease in protein excretion may take at least 7 to 10 days following initiation of treatment, and proteinuria clears by third week of oral prednisone
  - up to 2/3 of patients experience relapses
- if unresponsive to steroids, frequent relapses or steroid-resistant (proteinuria continues beyond 3 months):
  - consider renal biopsy or treat with cytotoxic agent (i.e. cyclophosphamide or chlorambucil), immunomodulating agents such as levamisole and cyclosporine A, and high-dose pulse corticosteroid with guidance of a pediatric nephrologist

Hypertension in Childhood

Etiology
- consider white coat hypertension for all ages

Table 45. Etiology of Childhood Hypertension by Age Group

<1 year	renal artery/vein thrombosis, congenital renal disease, coarctation of the aorta bronchopulmonary dysplasia, hypercalcemia
1-6 years	renal artery stenosis, renal parenchymal disease, Wilm's tumor, neuroblastoma, coarctation of aorta
7-12 years	renal parenchymal disease, abnormalities of renal vasculature, endocrine causes (hyperthyroid, hyperparathyroid, Cushing, primary hyperaldosteronism), essential hypertension
>13 years	essential hypertension, renal parenchymal disease, endocrine cause

Investigations
- labs:
  - urine dipstick for blood and protein (suggests renal disease)
  - urine catecholamines and their metabolites (may suggest pheochromocytoma)
  - electrolytes, creatinine, catecholamines, renin, aldosterone
- imaging:
  - echocardiography
  - abdominal U/S
  - doppler studies, angiography, or radionuclide imaging of renal arteries

Management
- treat underlying cause
- weight reduction, reduction in salt intake, exercise
- first line antihypertensives are thiazide diuretics, but none of the antihypertensives have been formally studied in children
- referral to specialist
- medications used in hypertensive emergencies: nifedipine, hydralazine, labetalol, sodium nitroprusside
- assessment and management of end organ damage (e.g. retinopathy, LVH)

Table 46. 95th Percentile Blood Pressures (mmHg)

Age (Years)	Female		Male	
	50th percentile for height	75th percentile for height	50th percentile for height	75th percentile for height
1	104/58	105/59	102/57	104/58
6	111/73	112/73	114/74	115/75
12	123/80	124/81	123/81	125/82
17	129/84	130/85	136/87	138/88

Adapted from "Update on the 1987 Task Force Report on High Blood Pressure in Children and Adolescents working group report from the National High Blood Pressure Education Program".

Neurology

Seizure Disorders

- see Neurology

Differential Diagnosis of Seizures in Children
- benign febrile seizure (most common)
- hypoxic ischemic encephalopathy ("asphyxia")
- intracranial hemorrhage, trauma
- metabolic causes (e.g. hypoglycemia, hypocalcemia, hyponatremia)
- CNS infection
- idiopathic epilepsy and epileptic syndromes
- neurocutaneous syndromes
- CNS tumour
- arteriovenous malformationingestions/drug withdrawal
- rule out conditions that mimic seizure:
  - breath holding
  - night terror
  - benign paroxysmal vertigo
  - narcolepsy
  - pseudoseizure
  - syncope
  - tic
  - hypoglycemia
  - TIA

Investigations
- CBC, electrolytes, calcium, magnesium, glucose
- toxicology screen if indicated
- EEG, CT, LP, if indicated
  - EEG may be indicated for first-time non-febrile seizure (predict
  - EEG/CT not indicated for benign febrile seizures recurrence risk, determine seizure type, or epileptic syndrome)

Heart problems such as long QT syndrome and hypertrophic cardiomyopathy are often misdiagnosed as epilepsy. Include cardiac causes of syncope in your differential diagnosis, particularly when the episodes occur during physical activity.

Childhood Epileptic Syndromes

- infantile spasms
  - onset 4-8 months
  - brief, repeated symmetric contractions of neck, trunk, extremities (flexion and extension) lasting 10-30 seconds
  - occur in clusters; often associated with developmental delay
  - 20% unknown etiology; may have good response to treatment
  - 80% due to metabolic or developmental abnormalities, encephalopathies, or are associated with neurocutaneous syndromes; these have poor response to treatment
  - can develop into West syndrome (infantile spasms, psychomotor developmental arrest, and hyperarrythmia) or Lennox Gastaut
  - typical EEG: hypsarrhythmia (high voltage slow waves, spikes and polyspikes, background disorganization)
  - treatment: ACTH, vigabatrin, benzodiazepenes
- Lennox-Gastaut
  - onset commonly 3-5 years of age
  - characterized by triad of 1) multiple seizure types, 2) diffuse cognitive dysfunction and 3) slow generalized spike and slow wave EEG
  - seen with underlying encephalopathy and brain malformations
  - treatment: valproic acid, benzodiazepines and ketogenic diet; however, response often poor
- juvenile myoclonic epilepsy (Janz)
  - adolescent onset (12-16 years of age); autosomal dominant with variable penetrance
  - myoclonus particularly in morning; frequently presents as generalized tonic-clonic seizures
  - typical EEG: 3.5-6 Hz irregular spike and wave, increased with photic stimulation
  - requires lifelong treatment (valproic acid); prognosis excellent
- childhood absence epilepsy
  - multiple absence seizures per day that may generalize in adolescence or resolve spontaneously
  - peak age of onset 6-7, F>M, strong genetic predisposition
  - each seizure is less than 30 seconds, no post-ictal state, may have multiple seizures per day
  - typical EEG: 3/sec spike and wave
  - treatment valproic acid or ethosuximide
- benign focal epilepsy of childhood with Rolandic/centrotemporal spikes
  - onset peaks at 5-10 years of age, 16% of all non-febrile seizures
  - focal motor seizures involving tongue, mouth, face, upper extremity usually occuring in sleep-wake transition states
  - remains conscious but aphasic post-ictally
  - remits spontaneously in adolescence; no sequelae
  - typical EEG: repetitive spikes in centrotemporal area with normal background
  - treatment: frequent seizures controlled by carbamazepine, no medication if infrequent seizures

Treatment

- anticonvulsants often initiated if >2 unprovoked afebrile seizures within 6-12 months
- treat with drug appropriate to seizure type
- start with one drug and increase dosage until seizures controlled
- if no effect, switch over to another before adding a second anticonvulsant
- ketogenic diet (high fat diet) – used in patients who do not respond to polytherapy or who do not wish to take medication (valproic acid contraindicated in conjunction with ketogenic diet because may increase hepatotoxicity)
- education for patient and parents
  - privileges and precautions in daily life (e.g. buddy system, showers instead of baths)
- continue anticonvulsant treatment until patient free of seizures for 2 years or more, then wean medications over 4-6 months
- legal obligation to report to Ministry of Transportation if patient wishes to drive, Ministry will determine if driver's license is permitted

Generalized and Partial Seizures

- see Neurology

If a febrile seizure lasts >15 minutes, suspect meningitis or a toxin.

Randomized, controlled trial of ibuprofen syrup administered during febrile illnesses to prevent febrile seizure recurrences
(van Stuijvenberg M et al. Pediatrics. 102(5):E51, 1998 Nov)
Purpose: To assess the efficacy of intermittent antipyretic treatment in the prevention of febrile seizure recurrences.
Study: Double blind RCT with 220 children and 2 year follow-up.
Participants: Children age 1-4 with febrile seizure within the last month, and at least one risk factor for febrile seizure recurrence: either family history of febrile seizures, previous recurrent febrile seizures, temperature <40.0 C at the initial seizure, or multiple type initial seizure.
Interventions: Ibuprofen 5 mg/kg every 6 hours during fever (rectal T >38.4 C) or placebo.
Main Outcomes: First recurrence of febrile seizure.
Results: On an intention-to-treat analysis, the 2-year recurrence probabilities were 32% in the ibuprofen group and 39% in the placebo group, with a non-significant risk reduction of 0.9 (95% CI, 0.6-1.5).
Conclusions: There is no evidence to support intermittent antipyretic therapy in preventing febrile seizures.

Benign Febrile Seizures

- most common cause of seizure in children
- 3-5% of all children, M>F

Characteristics
- age 6 months-6 years
- thought to be associated with initial rapid rise in temperature
- no neurologic abnormalities or developmental delay before or after seizure
- no evidence of CNS infection/inflammation before or after seizure
- no history of non-febrile seizures
- most common seizure type is generalized tonic-clonic

Simple Febrile Seizure
- duration <15 minutes (95% <5 minutes)
- generalized, symmetric
- does not recur in a 24-hour period

Complex Febrile Seizure
- any one of the following features:
  - focal onset, focal features during the seizure, or neurological deficit after
  - duration >15 minutes
  - recurrent seizures (>1 in 24-hour period)
  - previous neurological impairment

Risk Factors for Recurrence
- 33% chance of recurrence, 75% recur within 1 year
  - 50% chance of recurrence if <1 year of age
  - 28% chance of recurrence if >1 year of age
- family history of febrile seizures or epilepsy
- risk factors include developmental or neurological abnormalities of child prior to seizures, family history of non-febrile seizures and an atypical initial seizure, multiple simple febrile seizures

Workup
- history: determine focus of fever, description of seizure, meds, trauma history, development, family history
- exam: LOC, signs of meningitis, neurological exam
- septic work-up including LP if suspecting meningitis (if child <12 months, strongly consider doing an LP; if child is 12-18 months, consider including an LP; if child >18 months, do LP if meningeal signs)
- EEG not warranted unless complex febrile seizure or abnormal neurologic findings
- if simple febrile seizure, investigations unnecessary except for determining focus of fever

Management
- counsel and reassure patient and parents (febrile seizures do not cause brain damage, very small risk of developing epilepsy; 9% in child with multiple risk factors; 2% in child with febrile simple seizures compared to 1% in general population)
- antipyretics (e.g. acetaminophen) and fluids for comfort (neither prevent seizure)
- prophylaxis not recommended
- if high risk for recurrent or prolonged seizures, have rectal or sublingual lorazepam at home (danger of lorazepam is that it may hide signs of a CNS infection)
- treat underlying cause of fever (e.g. otitis media)

Recurrent Headache

- see <u>Neurology</u>

Assessment
- if unremarkable history, and neurological and general physical exam is negative, likely diagnosis is migraine or tension-type headache
- obtain CT or MRI if history or physical reveals red flags
- inquire about level of disability, academic performance, after-school activities

Differential Diagnosis
- primary headache: tension, migraine, cluster
- secondary headache: see <u>Neurology</u>

MIGRAINE
- 4-5% of school aged children
- prevalence F:M = 2:1 after puberty
- heterogeneous autosomal dominant inheritance with incomplete penetrance (majority of patients have a positive family history)

Types
- common (without aura) - most common in children, associated with intense nausea and vomiting
- classic (with aura)
- complicated: e.g. basilar, ophthalmoplegic, confusional, hemiplegic

Clinical Features
- in infancy, symptoms include spells of irritability, sleepiness, pallor, and vomiting
- in a young child, symptoms include periodic headaches with nausea and vomiting; relieved by rest
- usually unilateral throbbing headaches in kids with photophonia or phonophobia

Prognosis and Treatment
- over 50% of children undergo spontaneous prolonged remission after 10 years of age
- early analgesia (Ibuprofen) and rest in quiet, dark room
- non-pharmacological treatment and prophylaxis: avoid triggers (poor sleep, stress, cheese, chocolate, caffeine), biofeedback techniques, exercise
- pharmacological prophylaxis: β-blockers (propranolol), antihistamines, antidepressants (e.g. amitryptiline), calcium-channel blockers, anticonvulsants (e.g. divalproex sodium)
- children >12 years can use sumatriptan nasal spray, other tryptans

TENSION HEADACHES
- usually consists of bilateral pressing tightness anywhere on the cranium or suboccipital region, usually frontal, hurting or aching quality, non-throbbing
- lasts 30 minutes to days, waxes and wanes, may build in intensity during the day
- no nausea/vomiting, not aggravated by routine physical activity
- most children have insight into the origin of headache: poor self-image, fear of school failure
- red flags: sudden mood changes, disturbed sleep, fatigue, withdrawal from social activities, chronic systemic signs (e.g. weight loss, fever, anorexia, focal neurological signs)
- treatment
  - reassurance and explanation about how stress may cause a headache
  - mild analgesia (NSAIDs, acetaminophen)
  - supportive counselling

ORGANIC HEADACHES
- organic etiology often suggested with occipital headache
- with increased ICP
  - etiology: brain tumours, hydrocephalus, meningitis, encephalitis, cerebral abscess, pseudotumour cerebri, subdural hematoma
  - characteristics: diffuse early morning headaches, early morning vomiting, headache worsened by increased ICP (cough, sneeze, Valsalva); as ICP increases, headache is constant and child is lethargic and irritable
- without increased ICP
  - etiology: cerebral arteriovenous malformation (AVM), aneurysm, collagen vascular diseases, subarachnoid hemorrhage, stroke

Hypotonia

- decreased resistance to movement – "floppy baby"
- proper assessment of tone requires accurate determination of gestational age
- evaluate:
  - spontaneous posture (spontaneous movement, movement against gravity, frog-leg position) important in evaluation of muscle weakness
  - joint mobility (hyperextensibility)
  - muscle bulk, presence of fasiculations
- postural maneuvers
  - traction response – pull to sit, look for flexion of arms to counteract traction and head lag
  - axillary suspension – suspend infant by holding at axilla and lifting; hypotonic babies will slip through grasp because of low shoulder girdle tone

- ventral suspension – infant is prone and supported under the abdomen by one hand; infant should be able to hold up extremities; inverted "U" posturing demonstrates hypotonia, i.e. baby will drape self over examiner's arms
- investigations will depend on history and physical exam
  - rule out systemic disorders
  - blood glucose
  - enhanced CT of brain
  - peripheral CK, EMG, muscle biopsy
  - chromosome analysis, genetic testing
- treatment: counsel parents on prognosis and genetic implications; refer patients for specialized care, refer for rehabilitation, OT, PT, assess feeding ability

Differential Diagnosis
- central
  - chromosomal (e.g. Down syndrome, Prader-Willi, Fragile X)
  - metabolic (e.g. hypoglycemia, kernicterus)
  - perinatal problems (e.g. asphyxia, ICH)
  - endocrine (e.g. hypothyroidism, hypopituitarism)
  - infections (e.g. TORCH)
  - CNS malformations
  - dysmorphic syndromes
- peripheral
  - motor neuron (e.g. spinal muscular atrophy, polio)
  - peripheral nerve (e.g. Charcot-Marie-Tooth syndrome)
  - neuromuscular junction (e.g. myasthenia gravis)
  - muscle fibres (e.g. mitochondrial myopathy, muscular dystrophy, myotonic dystrophy)

Cerebral Palsy (CP)

- a symptom complex, not a disease
- nonprogressive central motor impairment syndrome due to insult to or anomaly of the immature CNS, extent of intellectual impairment varies
- incidence: 1.5-2.5:1,000 live births (developing countries)
- life expectancy is dependent on the degree of mobility and intellectual impairment, not on severity of CNS lesion

Etiology
- often obscure, no definite etiology identified in 1/3 of cases
  - only 10% related to intrapartum asphyxia
  - 10% due to postnatal insult (infections, asphyxia, prematurity with intraventricular hemorrhage and trauma)
  - association with low birth weight babies

Clinical Presentation

Table 47. Types of Cerebral Palsy

Type	% of total CP	Characteristics	Area of Brain Involved
Spastic	70-80%	Truncal hypotonia in 1st year ↑ tone, ↑ reflexes, clonus Affects one limb (monoplegia), one side of body (hemiplegia), both legs (diplegia), both arms and legs (quadriplegia)	UMN of pyramidal tract • diplegia associated with periventricular leukomalacia (PVL) in premature babies • quadriplegia associated with HIE (asphyxia) , associated with higher incidence of MR
Athetoid/Dyskinetic	10-15%	Athetosis (involuntary writhing movements) ± chorea (involuntary jerky movements) Can involve face, tongue (results in dysarthria)	Basal ganglia (may be associated with kernicterus)
Ataxic	<5%	Poor coordination, poor balance (wide based gait) Can have intention tremor	Cerebellum
Atonic	<5%	Marked hypotonia, hyperreflexia, severe cognitive delay	
Mixed	10-15%	More than one of the above motor patterns	

Other Signs
- swallowing incoordination – aspiration
- microcephaly (25%)
- seizures
- mental retardation, learning disabilities
- delay in motor milestones

Investigations
- may include metabolics, chromosome studies, serology, neuroimaging, EMG, EEG (if seizures), ophthalmology, audiology

Treatment
- maximize potential through multidisciplinary services; important for family to be connected with various support systems
- orthopaedic management (e.g. dislocations, contractures, rhizotomy)
- management of symptoms: spasticity (baclofen, botox), constipation (stool softeners)

Neurocutaneous Syndromes

- characterized by tendency to form tumours of CNS, PNS, viscera and skin

Neurofibromatosis Type I (NF-1)
- autosomal dominant but 50% are the result of new mutations
- also known as von Recklinghausen disease
- incidence 1:3000, mutation in NF1 gene on 17q11.2 (codes for neurofibromin protein)
- learning disorders, abnormal speech development, and seizures are common
- diagnosis of NF-1 requires 2 or more of:
  - ≥6 café-au-lait spots (>5 mm if prepubertal, >1.5 cm if postpubertal)
  - ≥2 neurofibromas of any type or one plexiform neurofibroma
  - ≥2 Lisch nodules (hamartomas of the iris)
  - optic glioma
  - freckling in the axillary or inguinal region
  - a distinctive bony lesion (e.g. sphenoid dysplasia, cortical thinning of long bones)
  - a first degree relative with confirmed NF-1

In neurocutaneous syndromes, the younger the child at presentation, the more likely they are to develop mental retardation.

Neurofibromatosis Type II (NF-2)
- autosomal dominant
- incidence 1:33 000
- characterized by predisposition to form intracranial, spinal tumours
- diagnosed when either bilateral vestibular schwannomas found, or a first-degree relative with NF-2 and either a neurofibroma, meningioma, glioma, or schwannoma
- also associated with posterior subcapsular cataracts
- treatment consists of monitoring for tumour development and surgery

Sturge-Weber Syndrome
- port-wine nevus syndrome in V_1 distribution with associated angiomatous malformations of brain causing contralateral hemiparesis and hemiatrophy, also associated with seizure, glaucoma and mental retardation

Tuberous Sclerosis
- autosomal dominant inheritance; 50% new mutations
- adenoma sebaceum (angiokeratomas on face, often in malar distribution), Shagreen patch (isolated raised plaque over lower back, buttocks), "ash leaf" hypopigmentation seen with Wood's lamp (UV light)
- cardiac rhabdomyomas, kidney angiomyolipoma, mental retardation and seizures
- cerebral cortex tubers (areas of cerebral dysplasia); subependymal nodules (SEN) may evolve into giant cell astrocytomas (may cause obstructive hydrocephalus)
- calcifications within the SEN are seen on CT, MRI (especially around the foramen of Munroe); these may obstruct the foramen and cause hydrocephalus

Oncology

- cancer is second most common cause of death in children after 1 year of age (injuries are first)
- cause is rarely known, but increased risk with
  - chromosomal syndromes
  - prior malignancy
  - neurocutaneous syndromes
  - immunodeficiency syndromes
  - family history
  - exposure to radiation, chemicals, biologic agents
- leukemias are the most common type of pediatric malignancy (40%), followed by brain tumours (20%), and lymphomas (15%)
- some malignancies are more prevalent in certain age groups
  - newborns: neuroblastoma, other embryonal tumours e.g. Wilms' tumour (nephroblastoma), retinoblastoma
  - infancy and childhood: leukemia, neuroblastoma, Wilms' tumour, retinoblastoma
  - adolescence: lymphoma, gonadal tumours, bone tumours
- unique treatment considerations because radiation, chemotherapy, and surgery can impact growth and development, endocrine function and fertility
- most children do survive – treatments have led to remarkable improvements in overall survival and cure rates for many pediatric cancers

Leukemia

- see Hematology

Epidemiology
- mean age of diagnosis 2-5 years but can occur at any age
- heterogenous group of diseases:
  - acute lymphoblastic leukemia (ALL) (75%)
  - acute myeloblastic leukemia (AML) (10%)
  - chronic myelogenous leukemia (CML) (5%)
  - unclear type (10%)
- children with Down syndrome are 15 times more likely to develop leukemia

Etiology
- mostly unknown; retrovirus (HTLV) may be associated with T cell leukemia

Clinical Presentation
- infiltration of leukemic cells into bone marrow results in bone pain, and subsequent bone marrow failure (anemia, neutropenia, thrombocytopenia, purpura, petechiae)
- infiltration into tissues results in: lymphadenopathy, hepatosplenomegaly, CNS manifestations
- fever, fatigue, weight loss

Prognosis
- 80-90% 5-year event-free survival for ALL, 50% for AML

Lymphoma

- see Hematology

Hodgkin's Lymphoma
- incidence is bimodal-peaks at age 15-34 and 50+
- similar to adult Hodgkin's
- most common presentation is persistent, painless, firm, cervical or supraclavicular lymphadenopathy
- can present as persistent cough (secondary to mediastinal mass) or less commonly as splenomegaly, axillary or inguinal lymphadenopathy
- constitutional symptoms (B symptoms) in 30% of children

'B Symptoms' = fever, night sweats, unexplained weight loss

Non-Hodgkin's Lymphoma
- incidence peaks 7-11 years
- lymphoblastic, small non-cleaved cell (Burkitt) large cell
- rapidly growing tumour with distant metastases which differs from adult non-Hodgkin lymphoma
- signs and symptoms related to disease site, most commonly abdomen, chest (mediastinal mass), head and neck region

Etiology
- mostly unknown; EBV associated with African Burkitt lymphoma

Treatment
- aggressive multidrug chemotherapy with radiation and surgery to debulk large tumour masses
- 80-90% 5-year survival in Hodgkin's; 50-75% in non-Hodgkin's

Brain Tumours

- see Neurosurgery
- classified by location and histology
- location: 60% infratentorial (cerebellum, midbrain, brainstem) versus supratentorial
- histology: glial (cerebellar astrocytomas most common), primitive neuroectodermal (medulloblastoma), neuronal, pineal

Clinical Presentation
- infratentorial: increased ICP (obstruction of 4th ventricle), vomiting, morning headache, increased head circumference, VI nerve palsy, upward-gazing eyes, ataxia, cranial nerve palsies
- supratentorial: focal deficits, seizures, long tract signs, visual field defects
- evaluation
    - history, physical exam including complete neurological exam
    - CT and/or MRI of head

Wilms' Tumour (Nephroblastoma)

- usually diagnosed between 2 and 5 years of age
    - most common primary renal neoplasm of childhood
    - M=F
    - 5-10% of cases both kidneys are affected (simultaneously or in sequence)
- differential diagnosis
    - hydronephrosis, polycystic kidney disease, renal cell carcinoma, neuroblastoma

Clinical Presentation
- 80% present with asymptomatic, unilateral abdominal mass
- may also present with hypertension, gross hematuria, abdominal pain, vomiting
- may have pulmonary metastases at time of primary diagnosis (respiratory symptoms)

Associated Congenital Abnormalities
- WAGR syndrome (**W**ilms' tumour, **A**niridia, **G**enital anomalies, mental **R**etardation) with 11p13 deletion
- Beckwith-Wiedemann syndrome
    - characterized by enlargement of body organs, hemihypertrophy, renal medullary cysts, and adrenal cytomegaly
    - also at increased risk for developing hepatoblastoma, adrenocortical tumours, rhabdomyosarcomas, and pancreatic tumours
- Denys-Drash syndrome
    - characterized by gonadal dysgenesis and nephropathy leading to renal failure

Management
- nephrectomy
- staging, chemotherapy, radiation

Prognosis
- 90% long-term survival

Neuroblastoma

Epidemiology
- most common cancer occurring in first year of life
- neural crest cell tumour arising from sympathetic tissues (neuroblasts)
    - adrenal medulla (45%)
    - sympathetic chain (25% retroperitoneal, 20% posterior mediastinal, 4% pelvis, 4% neck)

Clinical Presentation
- can originate from any site in sympathetic nervous system, presenting as mass in neck, chest or abdominal mass (most common site is adrenal gland)
- signs and symptoms of disease vary with location of tumour
    - thoracic: dyspnea, Horner's syndrome
    - abdomen: palpable mass

- metastases are common at presentation (>50% present with advanced stage disease)
    - usually to bone or bone marrow (presents as bone pain, limp)
        - can also present with periorbital ecchymoses, abdominal pain, emesis, fever, weight loss, anorexia, hepatomegaly, "blueberry muffin" skin nodules
- paraneoplastic: hypertension, palpitations, sweating (from excessive catecholamines), diarrhea, FTT (from VIP secretion), opsomyoclonus

Investigations
- CBC, electrolytes, LFTs, renal function tests, LDH, Ca, Mg, serum ferritin
- urine VMA, HVA levels
- CT scan of chest, abdomen and pelvis, bone scan
- bone marrow analysis – neuroblastoma cells in "rosettes"
- tissue biopsy

Good Prognostic Factors
- "age and stage" are important determinants of better outcome
    - <1 year old
    - stage I, II, IV-S disease
- primary site: posterior mediastinum and neck
- low serum ferritin
- specific histology
- tumour cell markers
    - aneuploidy
    - absent N-*myc* oncogene amplification

Management
- surgery, radiation, chemotherapy ± bone marrow transplantation
- prognosis is often poor as it is found at an advanced stage

Rhabdomyosarcoma

- third most common extracranial solid tumour of children (after neuroblastoma and Wilms' tumour)
- no clear predisposing risk factors
- common sites of origin are structures of the head and neck, GU tract and extremities
- presentation: firm, painless mass
- metastases to lung, bone marrow and bones
- evaluation: MRI or CT scan of primary site, CT chest, bone scan, bilateral bone marrow aspirates and biopsies
- treatment: multidrug chemotherapy and surgery

Generalized Lymphadenopathy

- features of malignant lymphadenopathy (LAD): firm, discrete, non-tender, enlarging, no associated erythema, warmth, fluctuance, ± suspicisous mass/imaging findings, ± 'B' symptoms

Differential Diagnosis
- Infection:
    - viral - URTI, EBV, CMV, Adenovirus, HIV
    - bacterial - S. aureus, GAS, anaerobes, Mycobacterium, cat scratch disease
    - other: fungal, protozoan, rickettsia
- Auto-immune: rheumatoid arthritis, SLE, serum sickness
- Malignancy: lymphoma, leukemia, metastatic solid tumors
- Storage diseases: Niemann-Pick, Gauchers
- Other: sarcoidosis, Kawasaki Disease, histiocytoses

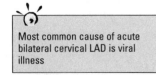

Most common cause of acute bilateral cervical LAD is viral illness

Investigations
- Generalized LAD:
    - CBC & differential, blood culture
    - Uuric acid, LDH
    - ANA, RF, ESR
    - EBV/CMV/HIV serology
    - toxoplasma titre
    - fungal serology
    - CXR
    - PPD
    - biopsy
- Regional LAD:
    - period of observation in an asymptomatic child
    - trial of oral antibiotics
    - biopsy (especially if persistent >6 weeks and/or 'B' symptoms)

Respirology

Approach to Dyspnea

- see Table 1 "Average Vitals at Various Ages"

	Pulmonary		Cardiac	Other
Upper Airway • Foreign body • Croup • Laryngeal edema • Epiglottitis • Retropharyngeal abscess	**Lower airway** • Tracheitis • Bronchiolitis • Pneumonia • Atelectasis • Asthma	**Pleura** • Pleural effusion • Empyema • Pneumothorax	• CHF • Cardiac tamponade • Pulmonary embolus	• ↑ICP • Ascites • Scoliosis

Figure 5. Approach to Dyspnea in Childhood

Upper Respiratory Tract Diseases

- see <u>Otolaryngology</u>
- disease above the thoracic inlet characterized by inspiratory stridor, hoarseness, and suprasternal retractions
- differential diagnosis of stridor:
    - croup
    - bacterial tracheitis
    - epiglottitis
    - foreign body aspiration
    - subglotic stenosis: congenital or iatrogenic
    - laryngamalacia/tracheomalacia – collapse or epiglottis cartilage on inspiration

Table 48. Common Upper Respiratory Tract Infections

	Croup (Laryngotracheobronchitis)	Bacterial tracheitis	Epiglottitis
Anatomy	Subglottic laryngitis	Subglottic tracheitis	Supraglottic laryngitis
Epidemiology	Common 6 months-4 years Peak incidence: fall and early winter	Rare All age groups	Rare Usually older (2-6 years)
Etiology	*Parainfluenza* (75%) Influenza A and B RSV Adenovirus	*S. aureus* *H. influenza* Alpha-hemolytic strep Pneumococcus *Moraxella catarrhalis*	*H. influenza* β-hemolytic strep
Clinical Presentation	Hoarse voice Barking cough Stridor Worse at night	Similar symptoms as croup but more rapid deterioration with high fever Toxic appearance Does not respond to croup treatments	Toxic appearance Rapid progression Severe airway obstruction Drooling Stridor Tripod position Sternal recession Anxious
Investigations	Clinical diagnosis CXR in atypical presentation: "steeple sign" from sublogottic narrowing	Clinical diagnosis Endoscopy: definitive diagnosis	Clinical diagnosis Avoid examining the throat to prevent further respiratory exacerbation
Treatment	Humidified O$_2$ Dexamethasone: PO 1 dose Racemic epinephrine: nebulized, 1-3 doses, q1-2h Intubation if unresponsive to treatment	Start therapy for croup Usually required intubation Antibiotics	Intubation Antibiotics Prevented with Hib vaccine

Lower Respiratory Tract Diseases

- obstruction of airways below thoracic inlet, produces more expiratory sounds
- classic symptom: **wheezing**

Differential Diagnosis of Wheezing
- common
    - asthma: recurrent wheezing episodes, identifiable triggers
    - bronchiolitis: first episode of wheezing

- recurrent aspiration: often neurological impairment
  - pneumonia: fever, cough, malaise
- uncommon
  - foreign body: acute wheezing and coughing
  - cystic fibrosis: prolonged wheezing, unresponsive to therapy
  - bronchopulmonary dysplasia: often develops after prolonged ventilation in the newborn
- rare
  - congestive heart failure
  - mediastinal mass
  - bronchiolitis obliterans
  - tracheobronchial anomalies

Pneumonia

- inflammation of pulmonary tissue, associated with consolidation of alveolar spaces

Clinical Presentation
- incidence is greatest in first year of life
- viral cause is more common in children <5 years old
- viral
  - cough, wheeze, stridor
  - CXR – diffuse, streaky infiltrates bilaterally
- bacterial
  - cough, fever, chills, dyspnea
  - CXR – lobar consolidation, possibly pleural effusion

Etiology and Management
- supportive therapy: hydration, antipyretics, humidified O_2

Table 49. Common Causes and Treatment of Pneumonia at Different Ages

Age	Bacterial	Viral	Atypical bacteria	Treatment
Neonates	GBS E. Coli Listeria	CMV Herpes virus Enterovirus	*Mycoplasma hominis* *Ureaplasma urealyticum*	ampicillin + tobramycin (add erythromycin if suspect *Chlamydia*)
1-3 months	S. aureus H. influenzae S. pneumoniae B. pertussis	CMV, RSV Influenza virus Parainfluenza virus	*Chlamydia trachomatis* *Ureaplasma*	cefuroxime OR ampicillin ± erythromycin OR clarithromycin
3 months - 5 years	S. pneumoniae S. aureus H. influenzae GAS	RSV Adenovirus Influenza virus	*M. pneumoniae*, TB	ampicillin OR cefuroxime Mild: PO amoxicillin
>5 years	S. pneumoniae H. influenzae S. aureus	Influenza virus Varicella Adenovirus	*Mycoplasma pneumoniae* (most common) *Chlamydia pneumoniae* TB Legionella pneumophila	erythromycin OR clarithromycin (1s line) OR ampicillin OR cefuroxime

Bronchiolitis

- defined as the first episode of wheezing associated with URTI and signs of respiratory distress

Epidemiology
- common, affects 50% of children in first 2 years of life
- peak incidence at 6 months, winter or early spring
- occurs in children prone to airway reactivity, increased incidence of asthma in later life

Etiology
- respiratory syncytial virus (RSV) (>50%)
- parainfluenza, influenza, rhinovirus, adenovirus, rarely *M. pneumoniae*

Clinical Presentation
- prodrome of URTI with cough and fever
- feeding difficulties, irritability
- wheezing, respiratory distress, tachypnea, tachycardia, retractions, poor air entry lasting for 5-6 days
- children with chronic lung disease, severe CHD and immunodeficiency have a more severe course of the illness

Investigations
- CXR (only needed in severe disease, poor response to therapy, chronic episode)
    - air trapping, peribronchial thickening, atelectasis, increased linear markings
- nasopharyngeal swab
    - direct detection of viral antigen (immunofluorescence)
- WBC usually normal

Treatment
- mild distress
    - supportive: oral or IV hydration, antipyretics for fever
    - humidified O_2 (maintain O_2 sat >92%)
    - inhaled bronchodilator (Ventolin™) 0.03 cc in 3 ml NS by mask, q20 min, and then q1 hour – stop if no response
- moderate to severe distress
    - as above - rarely, intubation and ventilation
    - ipratropium (Atrovent™) and steroids are not effective
    - consider rebetol (Ribavirin™) in high risk groups: bronchopulmonary dysplasia, CHD, congenital lung disease, immunodeficient
- monthly RSV-Ig or palivizumab (monoclonal antibody against the F-glycoprotein of RSV) may offer some protection against severe disease in high risk groups
    - case fatality rate <1%
- antibiotics have no therapeutic value unless there is secondary bacterial pneumonia
- indications for hospitalization
    - hypoxia: O_2 saturation <92% on initial presentation
    - persistent resting tachypnea >60/minute and retractions after several salbutamol (Ventolin™) masks
    - past history of chronic lung disease, hemodynamically significant cardiac disease, neuromuscular problem, immunocompromised
    - young infants <6 months old (unless extremely mild)
    - significant feeding problems
    - social problem (e.g. inadequate care at home)

Asthma

- see Respirology
- characterized by airway hyperreactivity, bronchospasm and inflammation, reversible small airway obstruction
- very common, presents most often in early childhood
- associated with other atopic diseases such as allergic rhinitis or atopic dermatitis

Clinical Presentation
- episodic bouts of
    - wheezing
    - dyspnea
    - cough: at night, early morning, with activity, with cold exposure
    - tachypnea
    - tachycardia
    - post-tussive emesis
- physical exam may reveal hyper-resonant chest, prolonged expiration, wheeze

Triggers
- URI (viral or *Mycoplasma*)
- weather (cold exposure, humidity changes)
- allergens (pets), irritants (cigarette smoke)
- exercise, emotional stress
- drugs (aspirin, β-blockers)

Classification
- mild asthma
    - occasional attacks of wheezing or coughing (<2 per week)
    - symptoms respond quickly to inhaled bronchodilator
- moderate asthma
    - more frequent episodes with symptoms persisting and chronic cough
    - decreased exercise tolerance
- severe asthma
    - daily and nocturnal symptoms
    - frequent ER visits and hospitalizations

Management
- acute
  - O_2 to keep O_2 saturation >92%
  - fluids if dehydrated
  - β_2-agonists: salbutamol (Ventolin™) 0.03 cc/kg in 3 cc NS q20 minutes by mask until improvement, then masks hourly if necessary
  - ipratropium bromide (Atrovent™) if severe: 1 cc added to each of first 3 salbutamol masks
  - steroids: prednisone (2 mg/kg in ER, then 1 mg/kg PO OD x 4 days) or dexamethasone (0.3 mg/kg/day PO)
    - in severe disease, give steroids immediately since onset of action is slow (4 hours)
- indications for hospitalization
  - pre-treatment O_2 saturation <92%
  - past history of life-threatening asthma (ICU admission)
  - unable to stabilize with q4h masks
  - concern over environmental issues or family's ability to cope
- chronic
  - education, emotional support, avoidance of environmental allergens or irritants, development of an "action plan"
  - exercise program (e.g. swimming)
  - monitoring of respiratory function with peak flow meter (improves compliance and allows modification of medication)
  - PFTs for children >6 years
  - patients with moderate or severe asthma will need regular prophylaxis in addition to bronchodilators (e.g. daily inhaled steroids, long-acting β-agonists, anticholinergics, sodium cromoglycate, theophylline, leukotriene receptor antagonist)

Cystic Fibrosis (CF)

- see Respirology
- autosomal recessive, CFTR gene found on chromosome 7 (ΔF508 mutation in 70%, over 800 different mutations identified)
- 1 in 3,000 live births, mostly Caucasians
- mutation in transmembrane conductance regulator of chloride – causes cells to be impermeable to Cl which increases the reabsorption of Na
- leads to relative dehydration of airway secretions, resulting in impaired mucociliary transport and airway obstruction

CF Presenting Signs
CF PANCREAS:
Chronic cough and wheezing
Failure to thrive
Pancreatic insufficiency (symptoms of malabsorption like steatorrhea)
Alkalosis and hypotonic dehydration
Neonatal intestinal obstruction (meconium ileus)/ **N**asal polyps
Clubbing of fingers/ **C**hest radiograph with characteristic changes
Rectal prolapse
Electrolyte elevation in sweat, salty skin
Absence or congenital atresia of vas deferens
Sputum with *Staph* or *Pseudomonas* (mucoid)

Clinical Presentation
- neonatal
  - meconium ileus
  - prolonged jaundice
  - antenatal bowel perforation
- infancy
  - pancreatic insufficiency with steatorrhea and FTT (despite voracious appetite)
- childhood
  - anemia, hypoproteinemia, hyponatremia
  - heat intolerance
  - wheezing or chronic cough
  - recurrent chest infections (*S. aureus, P. aeruginosa, H. influenzae*)
  - hemoptysis
  - nasal polyps (associated with milder disease)
  - distal intestinal obstruction syndrome, rectal prolapse
  - clubbing of fingers
- older patients
  - chronic obstructive pulmonary disease (COPD)
  - infertility

Investigations
- sweat chloride test x 2 (>60 mEq/L)
  - false positive tests: malnutrition, celiac disease, adrenal insufficiency, anorexia nervosa, hypothyroidism, nephrogenic diabetes insipidus, nephrotic syndrome
  - false negative tests: peripheral edema, cloxacillin, glycogen storage disease, hypoparathyroidism, atopic dermatitis, Klinefelter syndrome, hypogammaglobulinemia
- pancreatic dysfunction – determined by 3-day fecal fat collection
- genetics – useful where sweat chloride test is equivocal

Treatment
- nutritional counselling
  - high calorie diet
  - pancreatic enzyme replacements
  - fat soluble vitamin supplements
- management of chest disease
  - physiotherapy, postural drainage
  - exercise
  - bronchodilators
  - aerosolized DNAase
  - antibiotics: depends on sputum C&S (e.g. cephalosporin, cloxacillin, ciprofloxacin, inhaled tobramycin)
  - lung transplantation
- genetic counselling

Complications
- respiratory failure
- pneumothorax (poor prognostic sign)
- cor pulmonale (late)
- pancreatic fibrosis with diabetes mellitus
- gallstones
- cirrhosis with portal hypertension
- infertility
- early death (current median survival is 30 years)

Rheumatology

Evaluation of Limb Pain

Table 50. Differential Diagnosis of Limb Pain

Cause	<3 years	3-10 years	>10 years
Trauma	x	x	x
Infectious			
• septic arthritis	x	x	x
• osteomyelitis	x	x	x
Inflammatory			
• transient synovitis	x	x	
• JIA	x	x	x
• seronegative spondyloarthropathy			x
• SLE			x
• dermatomyositis (DMY)			x
• HSP		x	
Anatomic/Orthopedic			
• Legg-Calve-Perthes disease		x	x
• slipped capital femoral epiphysis			x
• Osgood-Schlatter disease			x
Neoplastic			
• leukemia	x	x	x
• neuroblastoma	x	x	x
• bone tumours		x	x
Hematologic			
• hemophilia (hemarthosis)	x	x	x
• sickle cell anemia	x	x	x
Pain Syndromes			
• growing pains		x	
• fibromyalgia			x
• reflex sympathetic dystrophy			x

Investigations
- CBC, differential, blood smear, ESR
- x-rays of painful joints/limbs
- as indicated: blood C&S, ANA, RF, PTT, sickle cell prep, viral serology, immunoglobulins, complement, urinalysis, synovial analysis and culture, TB test, ASOT, slit lamp

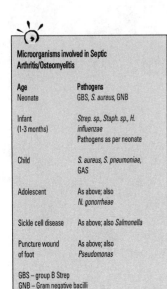

Microorganisms involved in Septic
Arthritis/Osteomyelitis

Age	Pathogens
Neonate	GBS, *S. aureus*, GNB
Infant (1-3 months)	*Strep. sp., Staph. sp., H. influenzae* Pathogens as per neonate
Child	*S. aureus, S. pneumoniae*, GAS
Adolescent	As above; also *N. gonorrheae*
Sickle cell disease	As above; also *Salmonella*
Puncture wound of foot	As above; also *Pseudomonas*

GBS – group B Strep
GNB – Gram negative bacilli
GAS – group A Strep

Septic Arthritis

- medical emergency
- hematogenous osteomyelitic spread seen most commonly in neonates and infants
- clinical presentation: acute monoarthritis with erythema, warmth, swelling, intense pain on passive movement (pain may be so severe that it causes pseudoparalysis of involved limb), fever & chills
- definitive test: joint aspirate and culture
- management: proper antibiotic selection requires knowledge of likely bacterial pathogen at various ages

Growing Pains

- age 2-12 years, M=F
- diagnosis
    - intermittent, well between episodes
    - poorly localized pain in the legs
    - usually bilateral
    - occurs in evening or awakens child at night
    - responds to reassurance, massage or analgesics
    - resolves completely in the morning
- no associated systemic symptoms (e.g. fever)
- possible family history of growing pains
- normal physical examination
- lab investigations not necessary if typical presentation

Transient Synovitis

- age 3-10 years, M>F
- benign, self limited disorder, usually occurs after upper respiratory tract infection, pharyngitis, bronchitis, otitis media
- clinical presentation – afebrile or low-grade fever, pain typically occurs in hips, knees, painful limp but still capable of ambulating
- symptoms resolve over 7-10 days
- lab investigations (ESR, WBC) within normal limits
- x-ray is typically normal
- U/S may show joint effusion
- must exclude septic arthritis, osteomyelitis, AVN, SCFE
- treatment: symptomatic and anti-inflammatory medications

Juvenile Idiopathic Arthritis (JIA)

- formerly known as Juvenile Rheumatoid Arthritis (JRA)
- a heterogenous group of conditions characterized by persistent arthritis in children under 16 years
- diagnosis: arthritis in ≥1 joint lasting >6 weeks in child <16 years with exclusion of other causes of arthritis
- classification defined by features/number of joints affected in the first 6 months of onset:
    - systemic: arthritis, fever and other systemic features
    - oligoarticular: ≤4 joints (most common)
    - polyarticular: ≥5 joints
    - enthesitis-related arthritis
    - psoriatic arthritis
    - unclassified

Systemic Arthritis (Still's disease)
- high spiking fever (38.5°C) for at least 2 weeks
- extra-articular features: erythematous "salmon-coloured" maculopapular rash, lymphadenopathy, hepatosplenomegaly, leukocytosis, thrombocytosis, anemia, serositis (pericarditis, pleuritis)
- onset at any age, M=F
- arthritis may occur weeks to months later
- high ESR, CRP, WBC, platelet count

Oligoarticular Arthritis (arthritis of 1-4 joints in the first 6 months)
- persistent – affects no more than 4 joints during the disease course
- extended – affects more than 4 joints after the first six months
- onset 1-3 years of age, F > M
- typically affects large joints – knees > ankles, elbows, wrists, hip involvement unusual
- ANA positive ~80%, rheumatoid factor (RF) negative
- screening eye exams for asymptomatic anterior uveitis (occurs in ~20%)
- complications: knee flexion contracture, quadriceps atrophy, leg-length discrepancy, growth disturbances

Polyarticular Arthritis (arthritis of 5 or more joints)
- RF negative
  - often involves large and small joints of hands and feet, temporomandibular joint, cervical spine
  - patients, especially those who are ANA positive, are prone to chronic uveitis
- RF positive
  - similar to the aggressive form of adult rheumatoid arthritis
  - severe, rapidly destructive, symmetrical arthritis of large and small joints
  - may have rheumatoid nodules at pressure points (elbows, knees)
  - unremitting disease, persists into adulthood

Enthesitis-Related Arthritis
- arthritis or enthesitis or both with at least two of:
  - sacroiliac tenderness and/or inflammatory spinal pain
  - HLA B27 positive
  - family history of confirmed HLA B27 –associated disease in a 1st or 2nd degree relative
  - symptomatic (acute) anterior uveitis
  - onset of arthritis in a boy >8 years

Psoriatic Arthritis
- arthritis and psoriasis or arthritis and at least two of:
  - dactylitis, nail abnormalities, or family history of psoriasis in a 1st degree relative

Unclassified
- arthritis of unknown cause that persists for 6 weeks and either does not fulfill criteria for any category or fulfills criteria for more than one category

Management
- children may complain very little about their pain and disability
- exercise to maintain range of motion (ROM) and muscle strength
- multidisciplinary approach with OT/PT, social work, orthopaedics, ophthalmology, rheumatology
- first line drug therapy: NSAIDs, intra-articular corticosteroids
- 2nd line:
  - DMARDs – methotrexate, sulfasalazine
  - other corticosteroids – intra-articular, systemic for systemic onset of JIA, topical eye drops for uveitis
  - biologic agents – etanercept (Enbrel™): binds TNF and blocks its interaction with cell surface receptors

Systemic Lupus Erythematosus (SLE)

- see Rheumatology
- autoimmune illness affecting multiple organ systems
- incidence 1:1000; more commonly age >10, F:M= 10:1

Reactive Arthritis

- arthritis follows bacterial infection especially, with *Salmonella, Shigella, Yersinia, Campylobacter, Chlamydia,* and *Streptococcus* (post-streptococcal reactive arthritis)
- prognosis:
  - typically resolves
  - may progress to chronic illness or Reiter's syndrome (urethritis, conjunctivitis)

Lyme Arthritis

- see Infectious Diseases
- caused by spirochete *Borrelia burgdorferi*
- incidence highest among 5-10 year olds
- arthritis begins months after initial infection (late Lyme disease)
- typically involves large joints, especially knees (affected in >90 % of cases)
- large, expanding erythematous macule with fever = erythema migrans of Lyme arthritis
- management: doxycycline or amoxicillin for 30 days; do not treat children <8 years old with doxycycline as it may cause permanent discolouration of teeth

Vasculitides

HENOCH-SCHÖNLEIN PURPURA (HSP)
- most common vasculitis of childhood
- vasculitis of small vessels
- peak incidence 4-10 years, M:F= 2:1
- recurrence in about one third of patients
- often have history of URTI 1-3 weeks before onset of symptoms

Clinical Presentation
- skin: palpable, non-thrombocytopenic purpura in lower extremities and buttocks, edema, scrotal swelling
- joints: arthritis/arthralgia involving large joints
- GI: abdominal pain, GI bleeding, intussusception
- renal: IgA nephropathy, hematuria, proteinuria, hypertension, renal failure in <5%

Management
- symptomatic, corticosteroids may relieve abdominal pain
- monitor for renal disease, may develop late
- immunosuppressive therapy for severe renal disease

Prognosis
- self-limited disease in 90%

Kawasaki Disease

- acute vasculitis of unknown etiology
- mainly affecting medium-size arteries
- most common cause of acquired heart disease in children
- peak age <5 years ; East Asians > Blacks > Caucasians

> **Diagnostic Criteria for Kawasaki Disease: "Warm CREAM"**
> **Fever** ≥5 days
> **C**onjunctivitis
> **R**ash
> **E**dema/**E**rythema (hands and feet)
> **A**denopathy
> **M**ucosal involvement

Diagnostic Criteria
- fever persisting 5 days or more AND
- 4 of the following features:
    1. bilateral nonpurulent conjunctivitis
    2. red fissured lips, strawberry tongue, erythema of oropharynx
    3. changes of the peripheral extremities
        - acute phase: erythema, edema of hands and feet
        - subacute phase: peeling from tips of fingers and toes
    4. polymorphous rash
    5. cervical lymphadenopathy >1.5 cm in diameter
- exclusion of other diseases (e.g. scarlet fever, measles)
- atypical Kawasaki disease: less than 5 of 6 diagnostic features but coronary artery involvement

Associated Features
- acute phase (as long as fever persists, about 10 days)
    - most of diagnostic criteria present
    - irritability, aseptic meningitis, myocarditis, pericarditis, CHF
    - diarrhea, gallbladder hydrops, pancreatitis, urethritis, arthritis
- subacute phase (resolution of fever, peeling of skin, elevated ESR and platelets, usually days 11-21)
    - arthritis
- convalescent phase (lasts until ESR and platelets normalize, >21 days)
    - coronary artery aneurysms, aneurysm rupture, myocardial infarction (MI), CHF

Management
- high (anti-inflammatory) dose of ASA while febrile
- low (anti-platelet) dose of ASA in subacute phase until platelets normalize or longer if coronary artery involvement
- IV immunoglobulin (2 g/kg) reduces risk of coronary aneurysm formation
- baseline 2D-echo and follow up periodic 2D-echocardiograms (usually at 6 weeks)

Complications
- coronary artery vasculitis with aneurysm formation occurs in 20-25% of untreated children, <5% if receive IVIG within 10 days of fever
  - 50% of aneurysms regress within 2 years
  - anticoagulation for multiple or large coronary aneurysms
- risk factors for coronary disease: male, age <1 or >9 years, fever >10 days

Commonly Used Medications in Pediatrics

Table 51.

Drug Name	Dosing Schedule	Indications	Comments
acetaminophen (Tylenol ®)	10-15 mg/kg/dose PO/PR q4-6h prn	analgesic, antipyretic	
amoxicillin (Amoxil ®)	80-90 mg/kg/day PO divided q8h	otitis media	
dexamethasone	0.6 mg/kg IV x 1 OR 1 mg/kg PO x 1 0.3 mg/kg/day PO	croup acute asthma	
fluticasone (Flovent ®)	moderate dose – 250-500 µg/day divided bid high dose – >500 µg/day divided bid	asthma	
ibuprofen (Advil ®)	5-10 mg/kg/dose PO q6-8h	analgesic, antipyretic	cautious use in patients with asthma
iron	6 mg/kg/day elemental iron bid-tid	anemia	side effects: dark stool, constipation, dark urine
predisone	1-2 mg/kg/day PO x 5 days	asthma	
salbutamol (Ventolin ®)	0.01-0.03 mL/kg/dose in 3 mL normal saline via nebulizer q1/2-4h prn 100-200 µg/dose prn, max frequency q4h	acute asthma maintenace of asthma	

[From Kowalczyk A. (2005) The 2004-2005 Formulary - The Hospital for Sick Children].

Notes

Plastic Surgery

Heather Baltzer and Michelle Lin, chapter editors
Sami Chadi and Biniam Kidane, associate editors
Emily Patridge, EBM editor
Dr. Arnis Freiberg and Dr. Nancy McKee, staff editors

Basic Anatomy Review

Skin

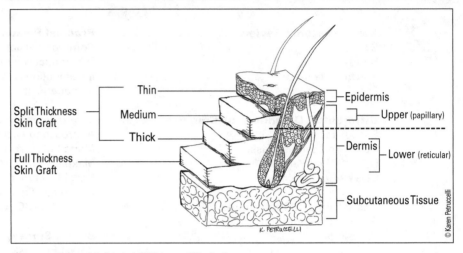

Figure 1. Split and Full (whole) Thickness Skin Grafts

Hand

BONES AND NERVES

Carpal Bone Mnemonic
(in order: proximal then distal row, radial then ulnar side)
Some – scaphoid
Lovers – lunate
Try – triquetrum
Positions – pisiform
That – trapezium
They – trapezoid
Cannot – capitate
Handle – hamate

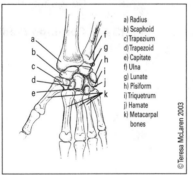

a) Radius
b) Scaphoid
c) Trapezium
d) Trapezoid
e) Capitate
f) Ulna
g) Lunate
h) Pisiform
i) Triquetrum
j) Hamate
k) Metacarpal bones

Figure 2. Carpal Bones

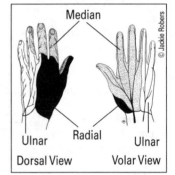

Figure 3. Sensory Distribution in the Hand

Table 1. Peripheral Nerve Examination of the Hand

	Median	Ulnar	Radial
Sensory (see Figure 3)	radial aspect of index finger pad	ulnar aspect of little finger pad	dorsal webspace of thumb
Motor extrinsic	flex distal IP joint of index finger (flexor digitorum profundus)	flex distal IP joint of little finger (flexor digitorum profundus)	extend wrist and thumb (extensor pollicis longus, extensor carpi radialis)
Motor intrinsic	thumb to ceiling with palm up (abductor pollicis brevis)	abduct index finger	none (first dorsal interosseous)

TENDONS

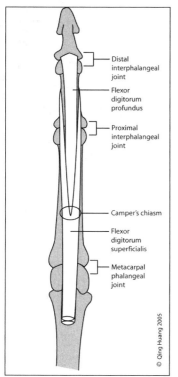

Figure 4. Flexor Tendon Insertion at PIP and DIP

Distal interphalangeal joint
Flexor digitorum profundus
Proximal interphalangeal joint
Camper's chiasm
Flexor digitorum superficialis
Metacarpal phalangeal joint

© Qing Huang 2005

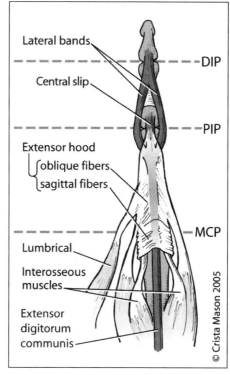

Figure 5. Extensor Mechanism of Digits

Lateral bands
Central slip
Extensor hood
- oblique fibers
- sagittal fibers
Lumbrical
Interosseous muscles
Extensor digitorum communis

DIP
PIP
MCP

© Crista Mason 2005

Flexor Tendons
Almost all require OR repair.

Extensor Tendons
ER repair unless proximal/multiple tendons.

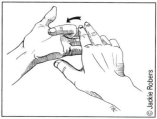

Figure 6. Testing Profundus (FDP)

© Jackie Robers

Figure 7. Testing Superficialis (FDS)

© Jackie Robers

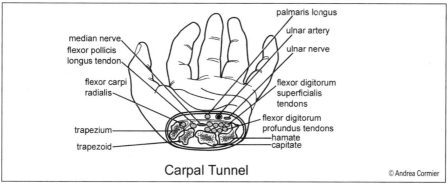

median nerve
flexor pollicis longus tendon
flexor carpi radialis
trapezium
trapezoid

palmaris longus
ulnar artery
ulnar nerve
flexor digitorum superficialis tendons
flexor digitorum profundus tendons
hamate
capitate

Carpal Tunnel

© Andrea Cormier

Figure 8. Carpal Tunnel

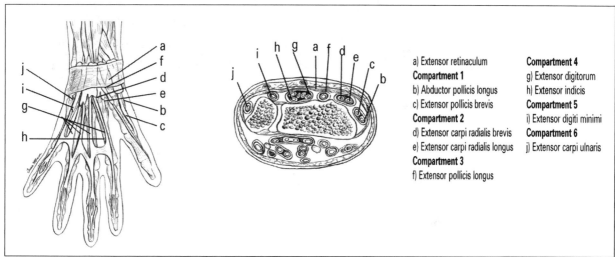

a) Extensor retinaculum
Compartment 1
b) Abductor pollicis longus
c) Extensor pollicis brevis
Compartment 2
d) Extensor carpi radialis brevis
e) Extensor carpi radialis longus
Compartment 3
f) Extensor pollicis longus

Compartment 4
g) Extensor digitorum
h) Extensor indicis
Compartment 5
i) Extensor digiti minimi
Compartment 6
j) Extensor carpi ulnaris

Figure 9. Extensor Compartments of the Wrist (dorsal view and cross-sectional view)

Brachial Plexus

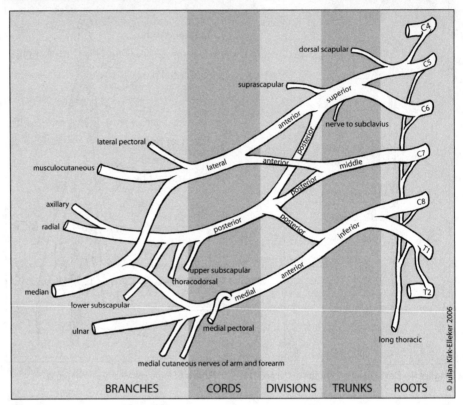

Figure 10. Brachial Plexus Anatomy

Face

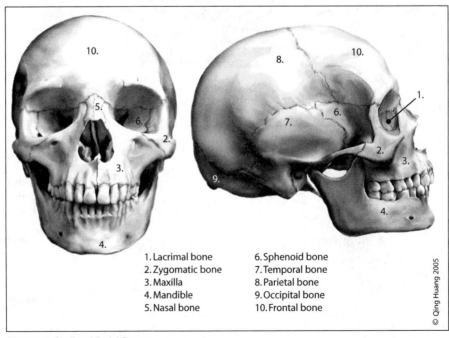

1. Lacrimal bone
2. Zygomatic bone
3. Maxilla
4. Mandible
5. Nasal bone
6. Sphenoid bone
7. Temporal bone
8. Parietal bone
9. Occipital bone
10. Frontal bone

Figure 11. Skull and Facial Bones

Differential Diagnoses of Common Presentations

DDx Skin Lesions/Mass

A. ON THE SKIN

Benign
- epidermal lesions: nevi, seborrheic keratosis, lentigo
- dermal lesions: pyogenic granuloma, dermatofibroma, neurofibroma
- dermal appendages
- calcifying epithelioma of Malherbe
- cyclindroma ("tomato tumour")
- sebaceous adenoma

Premalignant
- actinic keratosis → squamous cell carcinoma
- lentigo maligna → melanoma
- dysplastic nevi → melanoma

Malignant
- malignant melanoma
- squamous cell carcinoma
- basal cell carcinoma
- Kaposi's sarcoma
- dermatofibrosarcoma protuberans

B. IN THE SKIN
- cysts: epidermal inclusion cyst, dermoid cyst

C. UNDER THE SKIN
- lipoma
- ganglion
- lymph node
- calcifying epithelioma
- arteriovenous/lymphatic malformations
- nerve tumours
- muscle masses
- bony masses

DDx of Wrist Pain

Bone/Joints
- fracture, osteoarthritis (OA), rheumatoid arthritis (RA)

Ligamentous
- triangular fibrocartilage complex (TFCC) tear, distal radioulnar joint (DRUJ) instability, other intercarpal ligamentous injuries, e.g. scapholunate ligament

Tendonous
- tendonitis (consider in suspected repetitive use population: musicians, typists, etc.)

Nervous
- Carpal Tunnel Syndrome (CTS); associated with numbness and tingling in the median nerve distribution, ulnar nerve entrapment

DDx of Hand Pain

Bone/Joints
- fracture, osteoarthritis, OA (Heberden's and Bouchard's nodes), RA

Ligamentous
- PIP/DIP/MCP dislocation, Gamekeeper's thumb

Tendonous
- De Quervain's Tenosynovitis (thumb tendon sheath), Ganglion Cyst
- flexor tendons: Stenosing tenosynovitis ("trigger finger")

Nervous
- carpal tunnel syndrome, ulnar nerve entrapment

Vascular
- embolus, Raynaud disease, thoracic outlet syndrome

Basic Surgical Techniques

Sutures and Suturing

ANESTHESIA
- inject anesthetic before final debridement and irrigation
- lidocaine ± epinephrine (vasoconstrictor, limits bleeding)
  - toxic limit and duration of action (1 cc of 1% solution contains 10 mg lidocaine):
    - without epinephrine: 5 mg/kg, lasts 46-60 min
    - with epinephrine: 7 mg/kg, lasts 1.5-2 hrs
  - signs of toxicity: CNS excitation followed by CNS, respiratory, and cardiovascular depression

IRRIGATION AND DEBRIDEMENT
- clean surrounding skin, do not use antiseptic solutions in the wound as they are toxic to exposed tissue
- irrigate copiously with a physiologic solution such as Ringer's lactate or normal saline to remove surface clots, foreign material, and bacteria
- debride all obviously devitalized tissue, irregular or ragged wounds may be excised to produce sharp wound edges that will reduce scarring when approximated

SUTURES (see Table 2)
- use of a particular suture material is highly dependent on surgeon preference
- subsequent bacterial infection: monofilament < multifilament (braided)
- dehiscence occurs more with absorbable than nonabsorbable

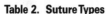

Table 2. Suture Types

Type	Trademark	Description	Characteristics	Wound Support: Absorption Time (days)	Indications
Absorbable					
Surgical gut (plain or chromic)	N/A	Natural, twisted fibre formed from collagen	Poor knot security, low memory	Plain – 8 : 70 Chromic – 15 : 90	Subcutaneous closure and vessel ligation
Polyglycolic Acid	Dexon®	Synthetic multifilament	Good knot security, good handling	21 : 90	Skin and subcuticular closure
Polygalactin 910	Vicryl® Ethicon®	Coated, synthetic multifilament	Poor knot security, good handling	21 : 90	Skin and subcuticular closure
Polydioxanone	PDSII®	Synthetic monofilament	Stiff, poor knot security, poor handling	60 : 210	Contaminated wounds, or buried suture in wounds requiring prolonged dermal support
Polyglecaprone	Monocryl®	Synthetic monofilament	Pliable, good handling, good knot security	20 : 100	Buried suture in wounds that do not require prolonged dermal support
Non-Absorbable					
Nylon	Ethilon® Nurolon®	Synthetic monofilament Synthetic multifilament	Good elasticity, good memory	N/A	Skin closure
Polypropylene	Prolene®	Synthetic monofilament	Good elasticity, slippery, poor knot security	N/A	General skin ± soft tissue approximation, even in contaminated wounds
Silk	Mersilk® Virgin silk	Natural multifilament	Good handling	N/A	Skin closure

BASIC SUTURING TECHNIQUES

Basic Principles
- minimize tissue trauma: follow curve of needle, handle wound edges gently (use toothed forceps), use just enough tension to approximate edges (do not strangulate)
- use the finest needle and suture possible
- to ensure good cosmesis:
  - evert skin edges when closing
  - avoid tension on skin (close in layers)
  - ensure equal width and depth of tissue on both sides
  - remove sutures within 7-10 days (5 days for the face; 14 days if over a joint)

Basic Suture Methods (Figure 12)
- simple interrupted – can be used in almost all situations
- intra cuticular – good cosmetic result; weak, used in combination with deep sutures
- vertical mattress – for areas difficult to evert (e.g. dorsum of the hand)
- horizontal mattress – everting, time saving
- continuous over and over – time saving

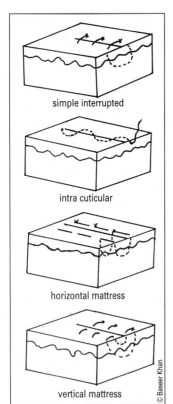

simple interrupted

intra cuticular

horizontal mattress

vertical mattress

© Baseer Khan

Figure 12. Basic Suture Methods

Approximate, don't strangulate!

Sutures that are too tight can create ischemia within the tissue, leading to a potential necrosis or infection.

Other Skin Closure Materials

- tapes – sterile adhesive tape (e.g. Steri-Strips) is the skin closure of choice for clean or contaminated wounds, as they minimize infection by separating skin surface from wound dead space. Tape cannot be used on actively bleeding wounds, or wounds with complex surfaces. Placed across the incision; will prevent surface marks and can be used primarily or after surface sutures have been removed. Tape burns may occur if there is excessive tension or swelling around the incision
- skin adhesives – e.g. 2-octylcyanoacrylate (e.g. Dermabond™) works well on small areas without much tension or shearing. Advisable in children
- staples – steel-titanium alloys that incite minimal tissue reaction (healing is comparable for wounds closed by suture or staples)

Dressings

- goals: protection, environment for healing (absorption), immobilization, cosmesis, compression
- "wet-to-dry" dressing (for dirty or infected wounds): dressing cleans wound and prevents build-up of exudates. Exudates, debris and nonviable tissue adhere to gauze and are removed with dressing change
- wet dressing: for healing uninfected wounds; doesn't debride wound
- 1st layer (contact layer): Moisture Balance (see Table 3)
    - clean wounds (heal by re-epithelialization)
        - protect new epithelium
        - use "wet-to-wet" dressing, non-adherent (e.g. Mepitel) impregnated gauze (e.g. Jelonet, Bactigras™) or antibiotic ointment
    - chronic/contaminated wounds:
        - mechanically debride nonviable tissue
        - use "wet-to-dry" dressing (e.g. adherent saline or betadine soaked gauze)
        - decrease local bacterial load with anti-infective agents (see Table 3)
- 2nd layer (absorbent layer): saline soaked gauze, to encourage exudate into dressing by "wick" effect
- 3rd layer (protective layer): dry gauze held in place with roller gauze or tape

Excision

- incise along relaxed skin tension lines (Langer's) to minimize appearance of scar
- use spindle shaped incision to prevent "dog ears" (heaped up skin at end of incision)
- if needed, undermine skin edges to decrease wound tension
- use layered closure including dermal sutures when necessary (decreases tension)

Microsurgery

- requires specialized surgical instruments, microsutures, and an operating microscope or loupes
- necessary for vascular anastamosis, nerve coaptation, and nerve grafting

VASCULAR

- to provide blood flow to flaps, or following damage to a blood vessel, vascular anastamoses are utilized
- blood vessels may be joined in end-to-end or in end-to-side orientations
- flaps must be carefully monitored for arterial or venous insufficiency, with immediate return to the OR for failing inflow or outflow

NERVES

- ideally, nerve repair brings together viable nerve ends with good alignment of fascicles
- nerve graft(s) or a conduit should be used if there is excess tension

Nerve Grafting

- normally utilizes the sural, superficial radial or medial antebrachial cutaneous nerves as donor grafts

Neurotization

- nerve transfer procedure
- transferring a nerve from an area of some redundancy to an area of no innervation to improve function
- e.g. restoring elbow flexion by transferring the medial pectoral/thoracodorsal nerve to the musculocutaneous nerve

Table 3. Wound Care Products

Local bacterial load reduction

1. Bacteriocidal
- Products containing iodized silver: ACTICOAT™, Aquacel Ag®
- Cadexamer Iodine: Iodosorb™, Iodoform
- Chlorhexidine: Bactigras™

2. Bacteriostatic
- Antibiotic creams/ointments: Fucidic acid, Flamazine™, Bactigras™

Improves epithelialization

1. Moisture Balance
- Foams: Allevyn™
- Hydrofibres: Aquacel®
- Alginates: Algisite™
- Hydrocolloids: CombiDERM®
- Films: Tegaderm™
- Gels: Intrasite™

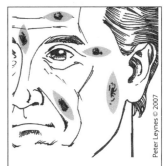

Grey regions indicate areas of skin to be excised.

Peter Leynes © 2007

Figure 13. Incision of lesions along Langer's lines

Wounds

Causal Conditions

Consider the mechanism of injury. Lacerations are often non-contaminated wounds whereas crush and puncture wounds are more likely to be contaminated (esp. bites).

- laceration – cut or torn tissue
- abrasion – superficial skin layer is removed, variable depth
- contusion – injury caused by forceful blow to the skin and soft tissue; entire outer layer of skin intact yet injured
- avulsions – tissue/limb ripped off; either partially or fully
- puncture wounds – opening relatively small as compared with depth (e.g. needle)
  - bite wounds – humans, animals (domestic, non-domestic); heavily contaminated by bacteria, viruses etc.
- crush injuries – caused by compression
- thermal and chemical wounds

Principles of Wound Healing

- wound: disruption of the normal anatomical relationships of tissue as a result of injury

STAGES OF WOUND HEALING

- see Figure 14
- growth factors released by tissues play an important role

Myofibroblasts are the cells responsible for wound contraction. They do this at a rate of less than 0.75 mm/day.

PHASE	PROCESS
1. Inflammatory (Reactive)	1) Hemostasis – vasoconstriction + PLT plug
• 0-4 days	2) Chemotaxis – migration of macrophages and PMN
• limits damage, prevents further injury	
• debris and organisms cleared via inflammatory response, e.g. leukocytes, macrophages	
• finite time (approx. 4 days) in 1° intention healing; continues until wound is closed in 2° and 3° intention healing	
2. Proliferative (Regenerative)	1) Collagen synthesis (mainly type III)
• collagen and fibroblastic phase: 5-42 days	2) Angiogenesis
• reparative process: re-epithelialization, matrix synthesis, neovascularization (relieves ischemia)	3) Epithelialization
• fibroblasts synthesize collagen at ↑ rate for 42-60 days → rapid gain in tensile strength of wound	
• granulation tissue formed with neovascularization	
3. Remodeling (Maturation)	1) Contraction
• 6 weeks-1 year	2) Scarring
• remodeling of collagen via intramolecular cross-links → flatter, paler scar, little ↑ in tensile strength	3) Remodeling of scar
• dynamic (collagenolysis and collagen synthesis); ongoing; requires approx. 9-12 months (longer in children)	

Figure 14. Stages of Wound Healing

FACTORS INFLUENCING WOUND HEALING

Local (reversible/controllable):
- mechanical (local trauma, tension)
- blood supply (ischemia/circulation)
- temperature
- technique and suture materials
- retained foreign body
- infection
- hematoma/seroma (↑ infection rate)
- tissue irradiation

General (often irreversible):
- age
- nutrition (protein, vit. C, O_2)
- smoking
- chronic illness (e.g. diabetes, cancer, CVD)
- venous hypertension
- immunosuppression (steroids, chemo, radiation)
- peripheral vascular disease
- collagen vascular disease

ABNORMAL HEALING

Hypertrophic scars resolve with time.
Keloid scars do not resolve spontaneously.

Hypertrophic Scar
- scar remains roughly within boundaries of original injury
- red, raised, widened, frequently pruritic

- common sites: back, shoulder, sternum
- treatment: conservative (silicone sheets), improves with time, rarely improved by surgical revision

Keloid Scar
- scar extends beyond boundaries of original injury
- frequently pruritic, often painful; collagen in whorls rather than bundles
- common sites: sternum, deltoid, earlobe; more common in darker skinned people
- treatment: pressure dressings, silicone sheets, topical steroids, intralesional steroid injection, surgical resection (intralesional excision ± steroids used as it may recur/become worse with surgical revision), radiation therapy

Chronic Wound
- fails to heal within 3 months (e.g. diabetic, pressure and venous stasis ulcers)
- treatment: may heal with meticulous wound care; many require surgical intervention
- Marjolin's ulcer: squamous cell carcinoma arising in a chronic wound (e.g. chronic burn scars and pressure sores) secondary to genetic changes caused by chronic inflammation → consider biopsy of chronic wound)

WOUND CLOSURE

Primary (1°) Closure (First Intention)
- definition: wound closure by direct approximation of edges within hours of wound creation (i.e. with sutures, staples, skin graft, etc.)
- indication: recent (<6 hrs, longer with facial wounds), clean wounds
- contraindications: animal/human bites, crush injuries, infection, long time lapse since injury (>6 hrs, longer for facial wounds), retained foreign body, too much tension on wound

Secondary (2°) Closure / Spontaneous Healing (Second Intention)
- definition: wound left open to heal spontaneously (epithelialization 1 mm/day from wound margins in concentric pattern), contraction (myofibroblasts) and granulation – maintained in inflammatory phase until wound closed; requires dressing changes; inferior cosmetic result
- indication: when 1° closure not possible or indicated (see *Primary Closure*, above)

Tertiary (3°) Closure (Delayed Primary Closure, Third Intention)
- definition: intentionally interrupt healing process (e.g. with packing), then wound is usually closed at 4-10 days post-injury after granulation tissue has formed and there is <10^5 bacteria/gram of tissue
- indication: contaminated (high bacterial count), long time lapse since initial injury, severe crush component with significant tissue devitalization
- prolongation of inflammatory phase decreases bacterial count and lessens chance of infection after closure

Contaminated Wounds

Definition
- a contaminated wound contains >100,000 bacteria/gram

Acute Contaminated Wound (<24 hr)
- cleanse and irrigate open wound with physiologic solution (NS or RL) – don't use irritants (soap, alcohol, etc.)
- debridement: removal of foreign material, devitalized tissue, old blood
  - surgical debridement: blade and irrigation
  - gauze debridement: wet to dry dressings
- evaluate for injury to underlying structures (vessels, nerve, tendon and bone)
- control active bleeding
- systemic antibiotics: wound older than 8 hours, severely contaminated, immunocompromised, involvement of deeper structures (e.g. joints, fracture), obvious infection
- ± tetanus toxoid (Td) 0.5 ml IM ± tetanus immunoglobulin 250 U deep IM (see Tables 4 and 5)

> **Wound Tips 101**
> **1.** Golden period for treating wound = 8 hours (12-24 hours if wound was washed and dressed), if not, need to debride and allow for healing by secondary intention.
> **2.** Infection with GBS a concern regardless of amount present in wound.
> **3.** Human Bites = mixed aerobic (*S. aureus, S. epidermitis, Strep*) and anaerobic (*Eikenella corrodens, Bacteroides, Peptostreptococci, Peptococci*), Cat and Dog Bites = *S. aureus, S. epidermitis, Pasturella multocida*.
> **4.** Prior to wound closure, examine all patients thoroughly for evidence of injuries involving important underlying structures (tendons, nerves, etc.).
> **5.** In all cases of human bites, or punctures caused by a syringe needle or contaminated object, elicit information about HIV and hepatitis status. Investigate HIV and hepatitis status where appropriate and treat accordingly.

Table 4. Risks for Tetanus

Wound Characteristics	Tetanus-Prone	Not Tetanus-Prone
Time since injury	>6 hrs	<6 hrs
Depth of injury	>1 cm	<1 cm
Mechanism of Injury	Crush, burn, gunshot, frostbite, puncture through clothing, farming injury	Sharp cut (e.g. clean knife, clean glass)
Devitalized tissue	Present	Not present
Contamination (e.g. soil, dirt, saliva, grass)	Yes	No
Retained foreign body	Yes	No

Table 5. Tetanus Immunization Recommendations

History of Tetanus	Clean, minor wounds		All other wounds	
Immunization	Td or Tdap*	Tig**	Td or Tdap	Tig
Uncertain or <3 doses of immunization	Yes	No	Yes	Yes
3 doses received in immunization series	No~	No	No§	No¶

* 0.5 ml of Combined tetanus and diptheria toxoids ± acellular pertussis.
** Tetanus immune globulin, 250 U given at a separate site from Td/Tdap
~ Yes, if > 10 years since last booster
§ Yes, if > 5 years since last booster.
¶ Yes, if immunocomprimised.

- ± postexposure treatment of:
    - hepatitis B, hepatitis C, HIV
- re-evaluate in 24-48 hours for signs of deep infection
    - open infected portion of wound by removing sutures

Chronic Contaminated Wounds (e.g. lacerations >24 hours, ulcers)
- irrigation and debridement: surgical or mechanical (e.g. wet-to-dry dressings)
- topical antibacterial creams (e.g. bacitracin, Neosporin™) – avoid inhibitors of epithelialization
- systemic antibiotics are indicated if there is concern of inflammation/infection of the surrounding tissue
- closure: final closure via secondary intention (most common), delayed wound closure (3° closure), skin graft or flap; successful closure depends on ↓ bacteria count to ≤100,000/gram prior to closure and frequent dressing changes

BITES

Dog bites to the hand have an infection rate of 30%. Cat bites carry a 50% infection rate.

Dog and Cat Bites
- **pathogens**: *Pasteurella multocida, S. aureus, S. viridans*
- **investigations**; same as for human bites; see below
- **treatment**: Clavulin™ (500 mg PO q8h started immediately – amoxil + clavulinic acid)
    - consider rabies prophylaxis if animal has symptoms of rabies
        - ± rabies Ig (20 IU/kg around wound, or IM) and 1 of the 3 types of rabies vaccines (1.0 ml IM in deltoid, repeat on days 3, 7, 14, 28)
    - debridement
    - secondary closure for small wounds, loose approximation and insertion of drains for large wounds (see <u>Emergency Medicine</u>)

Suspect a human bite when the laceration is above the MCP of patient's hand. This can lead to rapid septic arthritis. Must ask patient if they have punched another person in the mouth (houses oral bacteria).

Human Bites (*Staph > α-hemolytic Strep > Eikenella corrodens > Bacteroides*)
- **mechanism**: most commonly over dorsum of MCP from a punch in mouth; "fight-bite"
- serious, as mouth has 10^9 microorganisms/mL, which get trapped in joint space when fist unclenches and overlying skin forms an air-tight covering ideal for anaerobic growth – can lead to septic arthritis
- **investigations**:
    - radiographs prior to therapy to rule out foreign body (tooth)/fracture
    - culture for aerobic and anaerobic organisms, gram stain
- **treatment**:
    - **urgent surgical exploration** of joint, drainage and debridement of infected tissue
    - wound must be copiously irrigated
    - Clavulin™ 500 mg PO q8h, clindamycin 300 mg PO q6h + ciprofloxacin 500 mg PO q12h (if allergic to penicillin) + secondary closure (see <u>Emergency Medicine</u>)

Reconstruction

SKIN GRAFTS

Definition
- a segment of skin detached from its blood supply at the donor site and dependent on revascularization from the recipient site

Donor Site Selection
- must consider size, hair pattern, texture, thickness of skin, and colour (facial grafts best if taken from above clavicle)
- usually taken from inconspicuous areas (e.g. buttocks, lateral thighs, etc.)

Graft Survival
- 3 phases of skin graft "take":
  1. plasmatic imbibition – diffusion of nutrition from recipient site (first 48 hours)
  2. inosculation – vessels in graft connect with those in recipient bed
  3. neovascular ingrowth – graft revascularized (day 3-5)
- requirements for survival
  - bed: well-vascularized (unsuitable: bone, tendon, heavily irradiated, infected wounds, etc.)
  - contact between graft and recipient bed: fully immobile ($\downarrow$ shearing and hematoma formation)
  - staples, sutures, splinting, and appropriate dressings (pressure) are used to prevent movement of graft and hematoma or seroma formation
  - site: low bacterial count ($<10^5$, to prevent infection)

Classification
(i) by species – autograft: from same individual
  – allograft (homograft): from same species, different individual
  – xenograft (heterograft): from different species (e.g. porcine)
(ii) by thickness: (see Table 6)

Table 6. Skin Grafts

	Split Thickness Skin Graft (STSG)	Full Thickness Skin Graft (FTSG)
Definition	Epidermis and part of dermis	Epidermis and all of dermis
Donor site	More sites	Limited donor sites (full thickness skin loss, must be closed 1° or with STSG)
Healing of donor site	Re-epithelialization via dermal appendages in graft and wound edges	Primary closure or split thickness skin graft
Re-harvesting	~10 days (faster on scalp)	N/A
Graft take	Easier; shorter nutrient diffusion distance (better with thinner graft)	Lower rate of survival (thicker, slower vascularization)
Contraction	Less 1° contraction, greater 2° contraction (less with thicker graft)	Greater 1° contraction, less 2° contraction
Sensation	Poor	Better than STSG
Aesthetic	Poor	Good
Comments	Can be meshed for greater area (see below) Allows for extravasation of blood/serum	May use on face and fingers
Advantage	Takes well in less favourable conditions	Resists contraction, potential for growth, texture/pigment more normal
Disadvantage	Contracts significantly, abnormal pigmentation, high susceptibility to trauma	Requires well vascularized bed Must remove fat from graft before application
Uses	Large areas of skin, granulating tissue beds	Face (colour match), site where thick skin or decreased contracture is desired (e.g. finger)

- mesh graft

  Advantages
  - prevents accumulation of fluids
  - covers a larger area
  - best for contaminated recipient site

  Disadvantages
  - poor cosmesis ("alligator hide" appearance)
  - has significant contractures

Classification of methods of wound reconstruction in order of increasing complexity
- Primary closure
- Skin graft
- Local flap
- Distant flap
- Free tissue transfer

OTHER GRAFTS

Table 7. Various Tissue Grafts

Graft Type	Use	Preferred Donor Site
Bone	Repair rigid defects	Cranial, rib, iliac, fibula
Cartilage	Restore contour of ear and nose	Ear, nasal septum, costal cartilage
Tendon	Repair damaged tendon	Palmaris longus, plantaris
Nerve	Conduit for regeneration across nerve gap	Sural, forearm, cutaneous arm
Vessel	Bridge vascular gaps (i.e. free flaps)	Forearm or foot vessels for small vessels, saphenous vein for larger vessels
Dermis	Contour restoration (± fat for bulk)	Thick skin of buttock or abdomen

FLAPS
- **definition**: tissue transferred from one site to another with vascular supply (pedicle) intact (not dependent on neovascularization, unlike a graft)
- may consist of: skin, subcutaneous tissue, fascia, muscle, bone, other tissue (e.g. omentum)
- **classification**: based on blood supply to skin (random, axial) and anatomic location (local, regional, distant)
- **indications for flaps**:
  - reconstruction – replaces tissue loss due to trauma or surgical excision (i.e. after facial, breast, or lower leg tissue loss) – brings specialized tissue for reconstruction (e.g. bone, functioning muscle)
  - provides skin coverage through which surgery can be carried out later
  - soft tissue coverage (i.e. padding bony prominences)
  - provides vascular recipient bed for skin graft
  - improves blood supply to poorly vascularized bed (e.g. bone)
  - improves sensation (nerves to skin flap intact)
- **main complication**: flap loss due to vascular thrombosis, flap necrosis caused by extrinsic compression (dressing too tight) or excess tension on wound closure, hematoma, seroma, infection, fat necrosis

Random Pattern Flaps (see Figure 15)
- blood supply by dermal and subdermal plexus to skin and subdermal tissue with random vascular supply
- limited length:width ratio to ensure adequate blood supply (on face 4:1, lower extremity 2:1)
- types:
  - **rotation**: cover wounds of various sizes; common use: sacral pressure sores
  - **transposition:** useful when not enough laxity of surrounding tissue to create other types of flaps
  - **Z-plasty**: used to reorient and lengthen a scar at the expense of width (release scar contractures); common use: Dupuytren's disease
  - **advancement flaps (single/bipedicle, V-Y, Y-V)**
    - V-Y flaps: wounds with lax surrounding tissue; the pedicle is the deep tissue underlying the flap

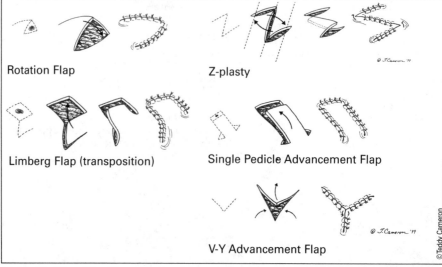

Rotation Flap

Z-plasty

Limberg Flap (transposition)

Single Pedicle Advancement Flap

V-Y Advancement Flap

© Teddy Cameron

Figure 15. Wound Care Flaps – Random Pattern

Axial Pattern Flaps (Arterialized)

- flap contains a well defined artery and vein
- allows greater length: width ratio (5-6:1)
- types:
  - **peninsular flap** – skin and vessel intact in pedicle (see Figure 16)
  - **island flap** – vessel intact, but no skin in pedicle (see Figure 17)
  - **free flap** – vascular supply anastomosed at recipient site by microsurgical techniques
- can be sub-classified according to tissue content of flap:
  - e.g. musculocutaneous/myocutaneous (Transverse Rectus Abdominal Myocutaneous (TRAM)) vs. fasciocutaneous

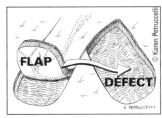

Figure 16. Peninsular Axial Pattern Flap

Free Flaps

- transplanting expendable donor tissue from one part of the body to another by isolating and dividing the dominant artery and veins to a flap and performing a microscopic anastomosis between these and the vessels in the recipient wound
- survival rates >95%
- types: muscle and skin (common), bone, nerves, tendons, jejunum, omentum
  - e.g. radial forearm, scapular, latissimus dorsi

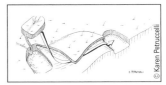

Figure 17. Island Axial Pattern Flap

Table 8. Free Flap Characteristics

Characteristic	Normal	Arterial Insufficiency	Venous Insufficiency
Colour	Pink	Pale	Purple or blue
Temperature	Warm	Cool	Warm or cool
Arterial Pulse (Doppler)	Present	Maybe present	Maybe present
Turgor	Soft, but with tissue turgor	Poor turgor	Increased (i.e. tense)

Monitor flap viability using skin colour, capillary refill (<2 sec), post-puncture bleeding, and Doppler monitoring.

Soft Tissue Infections

Erysipelas

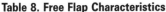

Definition
- acute skin infection that is more superficial than cellulitis

Etiology
- typically caused by Group A β-hemolytic *Streptococcus* (GABHS)

Clinical Features
- intense erythema, induration, and **sharply demarcated borders** (differentiates it from other skin infections)

Treatment
- penicillin or first generation cephalosporin (e.g. cefazolin or cephalexin)

Cellulitis

Definition
- non-suppurative infection of skin and subcutaneous tissues

Etiology
- skin flora most common organisms: *S. aureus*, β-hemolytic *Streptococcus*
- immunocompromised: Gram negative rods and fungi

Clinical Features
- source of infection
  - trauma, recent surgery
  - PVD, diabetes – cracked skin in feet/toes
  - foreign bodies (IV, orthopaedic pins)
- systemic symptoms: fever, chills, malaise
- pain, tenderness, edema, erythema with poorly defined margins, tender regional lymphadenopathy
- can lead to ascending lymphangitis (visible red streaking in skin proximal to area of cellulitis)

Table 9. Classification of Soft Tissue Infections by Depth

Erysipelas	Superficial with subcutaneous tissue involvement
Cellulitis	Full thickness with subcutaneous tissue involvement
Fasciitis	Fascia
Myositis	Muscle

Cellulitis vs. Erysipelas
Cellulitis: indistinct borders
Erysipelas: sharp borders

Investigations
- CBC, blood cultures
- culture and Gram stain wound/aspirate from wound
- plain radiographs
  - r/o bone invasion (osteomyelitis)
  - if crepitus present, may see gas in soft tissues (requires surgical correction)

Treatment
- antibiotics: first line - IV penicillin G 2 million units q6-8h + IV cloxacillin 1 g q6-8h
- outline area of erythema to monitor success of treatment

Necrotizing Fasciitis

Definition
- rapidly spreading, very painful infection of the deep fascia with necrosis of tissues. Some bacteria create gas that can be felt as crepitus and be seen on x-rays
- infection spreads rapidly along deep fascial plane and is **limb and life threatening**

Etiology
- Type I: β-hemolytic *Streptococcus*, type II: polymicrobial

Clinical Features
- **severe pain**, fever, edema, tenderness, crepitus (subcutaneous gas from anaerobes)
- infection spreads very rapidly
- patients are often very sick and toxic in appearance
- skin turns dusky blue and black (secondary to thrombosis and necrosis)
- induration, formation of bullae
- cutaneous gangrene, subcutaneous emphysema (type II)

Investigations
- generally a clinical diagnosis
- x-ray
- fascial biopsy in equivocal situations
- severely elevated CK: usually means myonecrosis
- hemostat easily passed along fascial plane

Treatment
- rigorous resuscitation
- multiple surgical debridement: remove all necrotic tissue, copious irrigation, often repeated trips to OR
- IV antibiotics: as appropriate for clinical scenario
- urgent consultation with infectious disease specialist is recommended

Special Considerations

HAND INFECTIONS

Principles
- trauma is most common cause
- 5 cardinal signs: *rubor* (red), *calor* (hot), *tumor* (swollen), *dolor* (painful) and *functio laesa* (loss of function)
- 90% caused by Gram positive organisms
- most common organisms (in order) – *S. aureus, S. viridans*, Group A *Streptococcus, S. epidermidis*, and *Bacteroides melanin*

TYPES OF INFECTIONS

Deep Palmar Space Infections
- uncommon, involve thenar or mid-palm, treated in OR

Felon
- **definition:** subcutaneous abscess in the fingertip that commonly occurs following severe paronychia or a puncture wound into the pad of digit; may be associated with osteomyelitis
- **treatment:** elevation, warm soaks, cloxacillin 500 mg PO q6h (if in early stage); I&D and PO cloxacillin if obvious abscess

Soft tissue infections: Suspect necrotizing fasciitis with rapidly spreading erythema and edema. Must **demarcate erythematous area** on admission in order to determine amount of spread.

MRSA positive cultures are now more common. Cultures must be taken. Choices of antibiotics may need to be adjusted.

Flexor Tendon Sheath Infection
(*Staph* > *Strep* > *Gram Negative Rods*)
- **definition:** acute suppurative tenosynovitis commonly caused by a penetrating injury and can lead to tendon necrosis and rupture if not treated
- **clinical features:** Kanavel's 4 cardinal signs:
    1. point tenderness along flexor tendon sheath (earliest and most important)
    2. severe pain on passive extension of DIP (second most important)
    3. fusiform swelling of entire digit
    4. flexed posture (↑ comfort)
- **treatment**
    - if early (first 24 hrs): elevation, immobilization, IV antibiotics (culture-specific or cefazolin 1 g IV q8h) and observation
    - if late (or no improvement for early treatment): OR I&D, irrigation, IV antibiotics, and resting hand splint until infection resolves

Herpetic Whitlow (HSV-1, HSV-2)
- **definition:** painful vesicle(s) around fingertip
- often found in medical/dental personnel and children
- **clinical features:** can be associated with fever, malaise and lymphadenopathy
- patient is infectious until lesion has completely healed
- **treatment:** routine culture and viral prep protection (cover), consider oral acyclovir

Paronychia (acute = *Staph;* chronic = *Candida*)
- **definition:** infection (granulation tissue) of soft tissue around fingernail (beneath eponychial fold)
- **etiology**
    - acute paronychia - a "hangnail", artificial nails, and nail biting
    - chronic paronychia - prolonged exposure to moisture
- **treatment**
    - acute paronychia - warm compresses and cephalexin 500 mg PO q6h ± drainage if abscess present
    - chronic paronychia - anti-fungals with possible debridement and marsupialization, removal of nail plate

Ulcers

Lower Limb Ulcers

Table 10. Venous vs. Arterial Ulcers vs. Diabetic Ulcers

Characteristic	Venous (70% vascular ulcers)	Arterial	Diabetic
Cause	Valvular incompetence Venous HTN	2° to small and/or large vessel disease Be aware of risk factors	Peripheral neuropathy: ↓ sensation Atherosclerosis: ↓ regional blood flow
History	Dependent edema, trauma Rapid onset ± thrombophlebitis, varicosities	Arteriosclerosis, claudication Usually >45 y.o. Slow progression	Diabetes mellitus Peripheral neuropathy
Distribution	Medial malleolus	Distal locations	Pressure point distribution
Appearance	Yellow exudates Granulation tissue	Pale/white, necrotic base ± dry eschar covering	Necrotic base
Wound margins	Irregular	Even ("punched out")	Irregular or "punched out" or deep
Depth	Superficial	Deep	Superficial/deep
Surrounding skin	Venous stasis discolouration (brown)	Thin shiny dry skin, hairless, cool Hypersensitive/ischemic	Thin dry skin ± hyperkeratotic border
Pulses	Normal distal pulses	↓ distal pulses	↓ pulses likely

Ankle-brachial index (ABI) in diabetics can be falsely normal due to incompressible arteries secondary to plaques/calcification.

Diabetic ulcers indicate mainly small vessel disease, while gangrene most likely has small and large vessel involvement.

Table 10.   Venous vs. Arterial Ulcers vs. Diabetic Ulcers (continued)

Characteristic	Venous (70% vascular ulcers)	Arterial	Diabetic
Vascular exam	ABI >0.9	ABI <0.9	ABI is inaccurately high
	Doppler; abn. venous system	Pallor on elevation, rubor on dependency	Usually assoc. with arterial disease
		Delayed venous filling	
Pain	Moderately painful	Extremely painful	Painless
	↑ with leg dependency, ↓ with elevation	↓ with dependency, ↑ with leg elevation	No claudication or rest pain
	No rest pain	and exercise (claudication)	Associated paresthesia, anesthesia
		Rest pain	
Treatment	Leg elevation, rest	Rest, no elevation, no compression	Control diabetes
	Compression at 30 mmHg (stockings	Moist wound dressing	Careful wound care
	or elastic bandages)	± topical and/or systemic abx.	Foot care
	Moist wound dressings	Modify risk factors (smoking, diet, exercise, etc.)	Orthotics
	± topical, systemic abx.	Vascular surgical consultation	Early intervention for infections
	± skin grafts	Treat underlying conditions	(topical and/or systemic abx.)
		(DM, prox. arterial occlusion, etc.)	Vascular surgical consultation

Large vessel disease may be managed
conservatively like peripheral vascular
disease (PVD) (i.e. stop smoking, lifestyle change, etc).
Arterial reconstruction may be
required.

Traumatic Ulcers
- failure of lesions to heal, usually due to compromised blood supply and unstable scar
- usually over bony prominence, ± edema, ± pigmentation changes, ± pain
- treatment: resection of ulcer, unstable scar and thin skin; reconstruction with local or distant flap

Pressure Ulcers

Common Sites
- over bony prominences; 95% on lower body

Stages of Development
1) hyperemia – disappears 1 hour after pressure removed
2) ischemia – follows 2-6 hours of pressure
3) necrosis – follows >6 hours of pressure
4) ulcer – necrotic area breaks down - N.B. skin is like tip of an iceberg

Classification
Stage I: nonblanchable erythema present >1 hr after pressure relief, skin intact
Stage II: partial-thickness skin loss
Stage III: full-thickness skin loss into subcutaneous tissue, but not through fascia
Stage IV: through fascia into muscle, bone, tendon, or joint
    ■ if an eschar is present, must fully debride before staging possible

Prevention
- good nursing care (clean dry skin, frequent repositioning), special beds or mattress (Kin Air™), proper nutrition, activity, early identification of individuals at risk (e.g. immobility, incontinence, fever and/or hypotension)

Treatment
- continue with preventative measures (up to 95% preventable)
- clean and dry wound, debridement of necrotic tissue, dressings
- topical antibiotics questionable, systemic antibiotics for complications (e.g. osteomyelitis)
- surgical intervention for definitive treatment of deep/complicated ulcers

Complications
- cellulitis, osteomyelitis, sepsis, gangrene, bacterial endocarditis

Management of Skin Lesions

- see Dermatology

Burns

Causal Conditions
- thermal (flame contact, scald)
- chemical
- radiation (UV, medical/therapeutic)
- electrical

Most Common Etiology
- children: scald burns
- adults: flame burns

Table 11. Skin Function and Burn Injury

Skin Function	Consequence of Burn Injury	Intervention Required
Thermoregulation	Prone to lose body heat	Must keep patient covered and warm
Control of fluid loss	Loss of large amounts of water and protein from the skin and other body tissues	Adequate fluid resuscitation is imperative
Mechanical barrier to bacterial invasion and immunological organ	High risk of infection	Antibiotic ointments (systemic if signs of specific infection present) Tetanus prophylaxis if necessary

Pathophysiology of Burn Wounds

- see Figure 18
- amount of tissue destruction is based on temperature, time of exposure, and specific heat of the causative agent
- **zone of hyperemia** – vasodilation from inflammation; entirely viable, cells recover within 7 days; contributes to systemic consequences seen with major burns
- **zone of stasis (edema)** – decreased perfusion; microvascular sludging and thrombosis of vessels results in progressive tissue necrosis → cellular death in 24-48 hrs without proper treatment
    - factors favoring cell survival: moist, aseptic environment, rich blood supply
    - zone where appropriate early intervention has most profound effect in minimizing injury
- **zone of coagulation (ischemia)** – no blood flow to tissue → irreversible cell damage → cellular death/necrosis

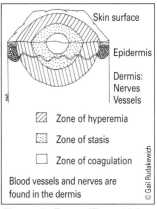

Skin surface

Epidermis

Dermis:
Nerves
Vessels

▨ Zone of hyperemia

▦ Zone of stasis

☐ Zone of coagulation

Blood vessels and nerves are found in the dermis

© Gail Rudakewich

Figure 18. Zones of Thermal Injury

Diagnosis and Prognosis

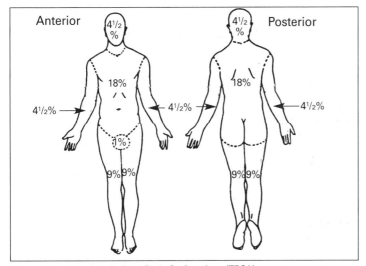

Figure 19. Rule of 9's for Total Body Surface Area (TBSA)

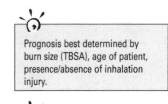

Prognosis best determined by burn size (TBSA), age of patient, presence/absence of inhalation injury.

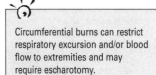

Circumferential burns can restrict respiratory excursion and/or blood flow to extremities and may require escharotomy.

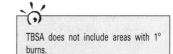

TBSA does not include areas with 1° burns.

- burn size (see Figure 19)
    - % of total body surface area (TBSA) burned – rule of 9's for 2° and 3° burns only (children <10 years old use Lund-Browder chart)
    - for patchy burns, surface area covered by patient's palm (fingers closed) represents approximately 1% of TBSA
- age: more complications if <3 or >60 years old

- depth: difficult to assess initially – history of etiologic agent and time of exposure helpful (see Table 12)
- location: face and neck, hands, feet, perineum are critical areas requiring special care of a burn unit
- inhalation injury
- associated injuries (e.g. fractures)
- comorbid factors (e.g. concurrent disability, alcoholism, seizure disorders, chronic renal failure)

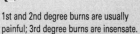

1st and 2nd degree burns are usually painful; 3rd degree burns are insensate.

Table 12. Burn Depth

Nomenclature	Traditional Nomenclature	Depth	Clinical Features
Erythema / superficial	First degree	Epidermis	Painful, sensation intact, erythema, blanchable
Superficial-partial thickness	Second degree	Into superficial dermis	Painful, sensation intact, erythema, blisters with clear fluid, blanchable, hairs follicles present
Deep-partial thickness	Second degree	Into deep (reticular) dermis	Difficult to distinguish from full thickness, ± pain, doesn't blanch, some hair follicles still attached, softer than full thickness burn
Full thickness	Third degree Fourth degree	Through epidermis and dermis Injury to underlying tissue structures (e.g. muscle, bone)	Painless (nerve endings destroyed), hard leathery eschar that is black, grey, white, or cherry red in colour, hairs don't stay attached, may see thrombosed veins

Indications for Transfer to Burn Centre

American Burn Association Criteria
- total 2° and 3° burns >10% TBSA in patients <10 or >50 years of age
- total 2° and 3° burns >20% TBSA in patients any age
- 3° burns / full thickness >5% TBSA in patients any age
- 2° or 3° burns posing a serious threat of functional or cosmetic impairment (i.e. circumferential burns, burns to face, hands, feet, genitalia, perineum, major joints)
- inhalation injury (may lead to respiratory distress)
- electrical burns, including lightning (internal injury underestimated by TBSA)
- chemical burns posing a serious threat of functional or cosmetic impairment
- burns associated with major trauma / serious illness

Acute Care of Burn Patients

Signs of CO Poisoning
- headache
- confusion
- coma
- arrhythmias

- adhere to ATLS protocol
- burn specific care
  - relieve respiratory distress – escharotomy and / or intubation (burn >40% TBSA; suggestion of inhalation or upper airway injury)
  - prevent and / or treat burn shock – 2 large bore IVs
  - identify and treat immediate life-threatening conditions (e.g. inhalation injury, CO poisoning)
  - determine BSA affected 1st, since depth is difficult to determine initially (easier to determine after 24 hrs)
- tetanus prophylaxis if needed
  - all patients with burns >10% TBSA, or deeper than superficial partial thickness, need 0.5 ml tetanus toxoid
  - also give 250 U of tetanus Ig if prior immunization is absent / unclear, or the last booster >10 yrs ago
- baseline laboratory studies (Hb, U/A, BUN, CXR, electrolytes, ECG, cross-match, ABG, carboxyhemoglobin)
- cleanse, debride, and treat the burn wound

Inhalation Injuries 101
1. Indicators of Inhalation Injury
  - injury in a closed space
  - facial burn
  - singed nasal hair/eyebrows
  - soot around nares/oral cavity
  - hoarseness
  - conjunctivitis
  - tachypnea
  - carbon particles in sputum
  - elevated blood CO levels (i.e. brighter red)
2. Suspected inhalation injury requires immediate intubation due to impending airway edema. Failure to diagnose inhalation injury can result in airway swelling and obstruction, which, if untreated, can lead to death.
3. Neither CXR or ABG can be used to rule out inhalation injury.

Respiratory Problems
- 3 major causes
  - burn eschar encircling chest
    - distress may be apparent immediately
    - perform escharotomy to relieve constriction
  - carbon monoxide (CO) poisoning
    - may present immediately or later
    - treat with 100% O_2 by facemask (decreases half-life of carboxyhemoglobin from 210 to 59 minutes) until carboxyHb <10%
  - smoke inhalation leading to pulmonary injury
    - chemical injury to alveolar basement membrane and pulmonary edema (insidious onset)

- if humidified O_2 not successful, may need to intubate and ventilate
- risk of pulmonary insufficiency (up to 48 hrs) and pulmonary edema (48-72 hrs)
- watch for secondary bronchopneumonia (3-25 days) leading to progressive pulmonary insufficiency

Burn Shock
- definition: hypovolemia due to movement of H_2O and Na in zone of stasis and generalized increased capillary permeability in all organs (occurs if >30% TBSA)
- resuscitation with **Parkland formula** to restore plasma volume and cardiac output (see Table 13)
  - 4 cc Ringer's/kg/% TBSA over first 24 hours (1/2 within first 8 hours of sustaining burn, 1/2 in next 16 hrs)
  - between 24-30 hours post-burn give 0.35-0.5 cc plasma/kg/%TBSA, then D5W at rate to maintain normal serum Na
- extra fluid administration required if:
  - burn >80% TBSA
  - 4° burns
  - associated traumatic injury
  - electrical burn
  - inhalation injury
  - delayed start of resuscitation
  - pediatric burns
- monitor resuscitation
  - urine output is best measure – maintain at >0.5 cc/kg/hr (adults) and 1.0 cc/kg/hour (children <12 years)
  - maintain a clear sensorium, HR <120/minute, mean BP >70 mmHg

Table 13. Burn Shock Resuscitation	
Hour 0-24	4 cc Ringer's/kg/% TBSA with 1/2 of total 0-8 h and 1/2 of total 8-24 h
Hour 24-30	0.35-0.5 cc plasma/kg/%TBSA
>Hour 30	D5W at rate to maintain normal serum sodium

* don't forget to add maintenance fluid to resuscitation

Burn Wound Healing

Table 14. Burn Wound Healing

Depth	Healing
First degree	No scarring. Complete healing.
Second degree (Superficial partial)	Spontaneously re-epithelialize in 7 to 14 days from retained epidermal structures ± residual skin discolouration. Hypertrophic scarring uncommon. Grafting rarely required.
Deep second degree (Deep partial)	Re-epithelialize in 14-35 days from retained epidermal structures. Hypertrophic scarring frequent. Grafting recommended to expedite healing.
Third degree (Full thickness)	Re-epithelialize from the wound edge. Grafting necessary to replace dermal integrity, limit hypertrophic scarring.

Treatment
- 3 stages:
  1) assessment – depth determined
  2) management – specific to depth of burn
  3) rehabilitation
- first degree
  - treatment aimed at comfort
    - topical salves (pain control, keep skin moist) ± aloe
    - oral NSAIDs (pain control)
- superficial second degree
  - daily dressing changes with topical antibiotics, cotton gauze, and elastic wraps or use of a temporary biological or synthetic covering to close the wound; leave blisters intact unless circulation impaired
- deep second degree and third degree
  - prevent infection (one of the most significant causes of death in burn patients)
    - most common organisms: *S. aureus*, *P. aeruginosa* and *C. albicans*
      - day 1-3: Gram positive
      - day 3-5: Gram negative (*Proteus, Klebsiella*)
    - topical antimicrobials: prevent bacterial infection (from gut flora or caregiver) and secondary sepsis (Table 15)
  - remove dead tissue
    - surgically debride necrotic tissue, excise to viable (bleeding) tissue

Table 15. Topical Antibiotic Therapy

Antibiotic	Pain with Application	Penetration	Adverse Effects
Silver nitrate (0.5% solution)	None	Minimal	May cause methemoglobinemia, stains (black), leaches sodium from wounds
Silver sulfadiazine (cream) (Sulfamylon™)	Minimal	Medium, doesn't penetrate eschar	Slowed healing, leukopenia, mild inhibition of epithelialization
Mafenide acetate (solution/cream) (Silvadene™)	Moderate	Well, penetrates eschar	Mild inhibition of epithelialization, may cause metabolic acidosis with wide application

- important to obtain early wound closure
- initial dressing should decrease bacterial proliferation and provide occlusion until surgery
- indication for skin graft: deep 2° or 3° burn > size of a quarter
- prevention of wound contractures: pressure dressings, joint splints, early physiotherapy

Other Considerations in Burn Management (see Figure 20)

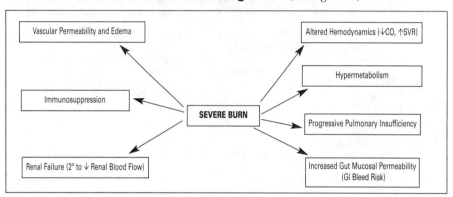

Figure 20. Systemic Effects of Severe Burns

- nutrition
  - hypermetabolism: TBSA >40% have BMR 2-2.5x predicted
  - calories, vitamin C, vitamin A, Ca, Zn, Fe
- immunosuppression and sepsis
  - must keep bacterial count <10^5 bacteria/g of tissue (monitor by tissue biopsy, blood culture may not be positive)
  - signs of sepsis: sudden onset of hyper/hypothermia, unexpected CHF or pulmonary edema, development of ARDS, ileus >48 hrs post-burn, mental status changes, azotemia, thrombocytopenia, hypofibrinogenemia, hyper/hypoglycemia (especially if burn >40% TBSA)
- gastrointestinal (GI) bleed may occur with burns >40% TBSA (usually subclinical)
  - treatment: tube feeding or NPO, antacids, H_2 blockers
- renal failure secondary to hypovolemia (rare) or nephrotoxic antibiotics
- progressive pulmonary insufficiency
  - can occur after: smoke inhalation, pneumonia, cardiac decompensation, sepsis
- wound contracture and hypertrophic scarring
  - largely preventable with timely wound closure, splinting and elastic pressure supports

Special Considerations

CHEMICAL BURNS
- major categories: acid burns, alkaline burns, phosphorous burns, chemical injection injuries
- common agents: cement, hydrofluoric acid, phenol, tar
- mechanism of injury: chemical solutions coagulate tissue protein leading to necrosis
  - acids → coagulation necrosis
  - alkalines → saponification followed by liquefaction necrosis
- severity related to: type of chemical (alkali worse than acid), temperature, volume, concentration, contact time, site affected, mechanism of chemical action, degree of tissue penetration
- burns are deeper than initially appear and may progress with time

Treatment (general)
- ABCs, monitoring
- remove contaminated clothing and brush off any dry powders before irrigation
- irrigation with water for 1-2 hrs under low pressure (>15-20 L water for significant chemical injury)
- inspect eyes, if affected: wash with saline and refer to ophthalmology
- inspect nails, hair and webspaces
- correct metabolic abnormalities and tetanus prophylaxis if necessary
- local wound care after 12 hours initial dilution: debridement, topical antibiotics
- wound closure same as for thermal burn
- beware of underestimated fluid resuscitation, renal, liver, and pulmonary damage

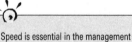

Speed is essential in the management of chemical burns as chemicals can continue to cause damage until they are removed or neutralized.

Tar: remove with repeated application of petroleum-based antibiotic ointments (e.g. Polysporin™).

Treatment (specific)
Acid burns: dilute solution of sodium bicarbonate following water irrigation.
Hydrofluoric acid: water irrigation; clip fingernails to avoid acid trapping; inactivation of fluoride ions by topical application ± subcutaneous injection and even IV administration (where exposure is copious, e.g. entire face) of IV solution of 10% calcium gluconate.

ELECTRICAL BURNS

- depth of burn depends on voltage and resistance of the tissue (injury more severe in tissues with high resistance)
- often presents as small punctate burns on skin with extensive deep tissue damage which requires debridement
- electrical burns require ongoing monitoring as latent injuries can occur
- watch for system specific damages and abnormalities:
  - abdominal: intraperitoneal damage
  - bone: fractures and dislocations especially of the spine and shoulder
  - cardiopulmonary: anoxia, ventricular fibrillation, arrhythmias
  - muscle: myoglobinuria indicates significant muscle damage —> compartment syndrome
  - neurological: seizures and spinal cord damage
  - ophthalmology: cataract formation (late complication)
  - renal: acute tubular necrosis (ATN) resulting from toxic levels of myoglobin and hemoglobin
  - vascular: vessel thrombosis —> tissue necrosis (increased Cr, K and acidity), decrease in RBC (beware of hemorrhages/delayed vessel rupture)

Tissue Resistance to Electrical Current:
nerve < vessel/blood < muscle < skin < tendon < fat < bone

Treatment

- ABC's, primary and secondary survey, treat associated injuries
- monitor: hemochromogenuria, compartment syndrome, urine output
- wound management: topical agent with good penetrating ability (silver sulfadiazine or mafenide acetate)
- debride non-viable tissue early and repeat prn (every 48 hrs) to prevent sepsis
- major amputations frequently required

FROSTBITE

- see Emergency Medicine

Hand

Table 16. Examination of the Tendons of the Hand

Tendon	Insertion	Test of Action
Flexors		
FPL (flexor pollicis longus)	Base of distal phalanx of thumb	Flex IP (interphalangeal) of thumb
FDP (flexor digitorum profundus)	Base of distal phalanx D2-5	Flex DIP (distal interphalangeal) of finger (see Figure 6)
FDS (flexor digitorum superficialis)	Base of middle phalanx	Flex PIP (proximal interphalangeal) (see Figure 7)
FCU (flexor carpi ulnaris)	Pisiform and hamate	Flex and adduct wrist
FCR (flexor carpi radialis)	Base of 2nd and 3rd metacarpals	Flex and abduct wrist
Extensors		
APL (abductor pollicis longus)	Base of thumb metacarpal	Abduct thumb at 90° to palm
EPB (extensor pollicis brevis)	Base of proximal thumb phalanx	Abduct thumb at 90° to palm
ECRL (extensor carpi radialis longus)	Base of 2nd metacarpal	Extend wrist against resistance
ECRB (extensor carpi radialis brevis)	Base of 3rd metacarpal	Extend wrist against resistance
EPL (extensor pollicis longus)	Base of distal thumb phalanx	Extend thumb in plane of palm
EDC (extensor digitorum communis)	Base of middle and distal phalanx D2-5	Extend MCP (metacarpal interphalangeal), PIP, DIP of D2 to D5
EI (extensor indicis proprius)	Base of distal and middle phalanx D2	Extend MCP, PIP, DIP of D2
EDM (extensor digiti minimi)	Base of distal and middle phalanx D5	Extend MCP, PIP, DIP of D5
ECU (extensor carpi ulnaris)	Base of 5th metacarpal	Extend and adduct wrist
Intrinsic Muscles		
APB (abductor pollicis brevis)	Base of proximal thumb phalanx	Abduct thumb perpendicular to palm
OP (opponens pollicis)	Radial side of metacarpal D1	Oppose thumb to little finger
FPB (flexor pollicis brevis)	Base of proximal phalanx thumb	Flex thumb across palm
ADP (abductor pollicis)	Base of proximal phalanx thumb	Hold paper between medial aspect of thumb and radial aspect of D2
Lumbricals	Extensor tendons	Flex MCP joint and extend IP
Palmar interossei	Extensor expansions D2-D5	Adduct D2, D4, D5 to midline
Dorsal interossei	Extensor expansions D2-D5	Abduct D2-D5 from midline
ADM (abductor digiti minimi)	Base of proximal phalanx D5	Deviate D1 ulnarly (inspect for dimpling of hypothenar skin)
ODM (opponens digiti minimi)	Ulnar side of metacarpal D5	Oppose thumb to little finger
FDM (flexor digiti minimi)	Base proximal phalanx D5	Flex little finger

High pressure injection injury is deceptively benign-looking (small pinpoint hole on finger pad) often with few clinical signs.
Intense pain and tenderness, present along the course the foreign material traveled, is present a few hours after the injury. Definitive treatment is exposure and removal of foreign material.

Approach to hand lacerations
TIN AX
Tetanus prophylaxis
Irrigate with NS
NPO
Antibiotic prophylaxis
X-rays

Never blindly clamp a bleeding vessel as nerves are often found in close association with vessels.

Arterial bleeding from a volar digital laceration may indicate nerve laceration (nerves in digits are superficial to arteries).

Compartment Syndrome:
Watch out for these signs with a closed or open injury: tense, painful extremity (worse on passive stretch), distal pulselessness (often late in process), paresthesia/paralysis, and contracture (irreversible ischemia).
Intracompartmental pressures can be measured, but a clinical diagnosis is an indication for an emergent fasciotomy. If untreated, end result is ischemic contracture of the extremity (Volkmann's).

General Management

Nerves
- direct repair for a clean injury within 14 days and without concurrent major injuries → otherwise secondary repair
- epineural repair of digital nerves with minimal tension
- post-operative: dress wound, elevate hand and immobilize
- Tinel's sign (cutaneous percussion over the repaired nerve) produces paresthesias and defines level of nerve regeneration
    - a peripheral nerve regenerates at 1 mm/day after the first 4 weeks as a result of Wallerian degeneration
    - paresthesias felt at area of percussion because re-growth of myelin (Schwann cells) is slower than axonal re-growth → percussion on exposed free-end of axon generates paresthesia

Vessels
- often associated with nerve injury (anatomical proximity)
- control bleeding with direct pressure and hand elevation
- if needed repair optimal if within 6 hours
- dress, immobilize, and splint hand with finger tips visible
- post-operatively monitor colour, capillary refill, skin turgor, fingertip temperature

Tendons
- most tendon lacerations require primary repair
- many extensors are repaired in the emergency room, flexors in the operating room within 2 weeks
- avoid excessive immobilization to minimize stiffness and facilitate rehabilitation

Amputations

Hand or Finger
- emergency management: injured patient and amputated part require attention
    - **patient**: x-rays, NPO, clean wound and irrigate with NS, dress stump with nonadherent, cover with dry sterile dressing, tetanus and antibiotic prophylaxis (cephalosporin/erythromycin)
    - **amputated part**: x-rays, gently irrigate with RL, wrap amputated part in a NS/RL soaked sterile gauze and place inside waterproof plastic bag in container of ice and water
- **indications for replantation**
    - **age**: children often better results than adults
    - **level of injury**
        - proximal, thumb and multiple digit amputations are higher priority
    - **nature of injury**: guillotine injuries have a better potential than avulsion amputations or crush injuries
- if replant contraindicated manage stump with revision amputation, or allow to heal by secondary intention, especially in children

Tendons

Common Extensor Tendon Deformities

Table 17. Extensor Tendon Deformities

Injury	Definition	Zone	Etiology/Clinical Features	Treatment
Mallet Finger	DIP flexed with loss of active extension (see Figure 22)	1	Forced flexion of the extended DIP joint leading to extensor tendon rupture at DIP joint (e.g. sudden blow to tip of the finger).	Splint DIP in extension for 6 wks followed by 2 wks of night splinting. If inadequate improvement after 6 wks, check splinting routine and recommend 4 more wks of continous splitting.
Boutonniere Deformity	PIP flexed, DIP hyperextended (see Figure 23)	3	Injury or disease affecting the extensor tendon insertion into the dorsal base of the middle phalanx. Associated with Rheumatoid Arthritis (RA) or trauma (laceration, volar dislocation, acute forceful flexion of PIP).	Splint PIP in extension and allow active DIP motion.
Swan Neck Deformity	PIP hyperextended, DIP flexed (see Figure 24)	3	Trauma (PIP volar plate injury). Associated with RA and old, untreated mallet deformity.	Splint to prevent PIP hyperextension or DIP flexion. Consider arthrodesis/arthroplasty.

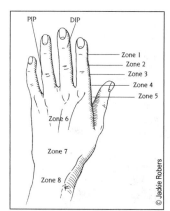

Figure 21. Zone of Extensor Tendon Injury

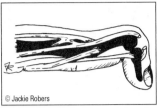

Figure 22. Mallet Finger Deformity

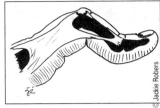

Figure 23. Boutonniere Deformity

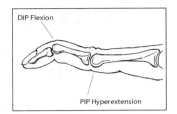

Figure 24. Swan Neck Deformity

De Quervain's Tenosynovitis (zone 7; most common cause of radial wrist pain)
- definition: inflammation in 1st dorsal wrist compartment (APL and EPB)
- clinical features
  - +ve Finkelstein's test (pain over the radial styloid induced by making fist, with thumb in palm, and ulnar deviation of wrist)
  - pain localized to the 1st extensor compartment
  - tenderness and crepitation over radial styloid may be present
  - differentiate from CMC joint arthritis (CMC joint arthritis will have a positive grind test, whereby crepitus and pain are elicited by axial pressure to the thumb)
- treatment
  - mild: NSAIDs, splinting and steroid injection into the tendon sheath (successful in over 60% of cases)
  - severe: surgical release of stenotic tendon sheaths (APL and EPB); remember there may be 2 or more sheaths

Ganglion Cyst (zone 7)
- definition
  - fluid-filled synovial lining that protrudes between carpal bones (commonly carpal) or from a tendon sheath
  - most common soft tissue tumour of hand and wrist (60% of masses)
- clinical features
  - most common around scapholunate ligament junction
  - 3 times more common in women than in men
  - more common in younger individuals
  - can be large or small – may drain internally so size may wax and wane
  - often non-tender although tenderness ↑ when cyst smaller (from ↑ pressure within smaller cyst sac)
- treatment
  - conservative treatment: watch and wait
  - aspiration (recurrence rate 65%)
  - consider operative excision of cyst and stalk (recurrence is possible)
  - steroids if painful

Common Flexor Tendon Deformities (see Figure 25)
- flexor tendon zones (important for prognosis of tendon lacerations)
- "no-man's land"
  - between distal palmar crease and mid-middle phalanx
  - zone where superficialis and profundus lie ensheathed together
  - recovery of glide very difficult after injury

Stenosing Tenosynovitis (trigger finger/thumb)
- definition: inflammation of synovium causes size discrepancy between tendon and sheath/pulley (most commonly at A-1 pulley) = locking of thumb or finger in flexion/extension
- etiology: idiopathic or associated with RA, diabetes, hypothyroidism and gout
- clinical features
  - thumb, ring and long fingers most commonly affected
  - patient complains of catching, snapping or locking of affected finger
  - tenderness to palpation/nodule at palmar aspect of MCP over A1 pulley
  - women are 4 times more likely than men to be affected
- conservative treatment
  - NSAIDs and steroid injection into the sheath; surgical release necessary if unresponsive to conservative/medical therapy
  - injections less likely to be successful in patients with DM or symptoms greater than 6 months
- surgical treatment
  - incise A-1 flexor tendon pulley to permit unrestricted, full active finger motion

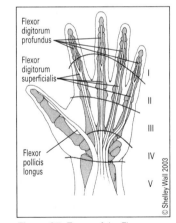

Figure 25. Zones of the Flexor Tendons

Fractures and Dislocations

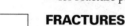

- for Fracture principles, see Orthopaedics

FRACTURES
- about 90% of hand fractures are stable in flexion (lock/prevent extension)
- **position of function** (like a hand holding a pop can) (see Figure 26)
    - wrist extension 15°
    - MCP flexion 45°
    - IP flexion (slight)
    - thumb abduction/rotation
    - **contraindications**: post repair of flexor tendons, median/ulnar nerve
- **position of safety** (see Figure 27)
    - wrist extension 45° (position most beneficial for hand function if immobilized)
    - MCP flexion 60° (maximal collateral ligament stretch)
    - PIP and DIP in full extension (maximal volar plate origin stretch)
    - thumb abduction and opposition (functional position)
- **stiffness** secondary to immobilization is the most important complication; Tx = **early motion**

Figure 26. Position of Function

Figure 27. Position of Safety

Distal Phalanx Fractures
- most commonly fractured bone in the hand
- usual mechanism is crush injury and thus accompanied by soft tissue injury
- subungual hematoma is common and must be decompressed if painful
- treatment consists of 3 weeks of digital splinting (with IP joint movement preserved)

Proximal and Middle Phalanx Fractures
- check for: rotation, scissoring (overlap of fingers on making a fist), shortening of digit
- undisplaced or minimally displaced – closed reduction (if extra-articular) buddy tape to neighbouring stable digit, elevate hand, motion in guarded fashion 10-14 days post injury
- displaced, non-reducible or not stable with closed reduction – percutaneous pins (K-wires) or ORIF, and splint

Metacarpal Fractures
- **Boxer's fracture (extra-articular)**: acute angulation of head or neck of metacarpal of little finger into palm (see Figure 28)
    - mechanism: blow on the distal-dorsal aspect of closed fist
    - loss of prominence of metacarpal head, volar displacement of head
    - check for scissoring of fingers on making a fist
    - up to 30-40° angulation may be acceptable
    - closed reduction should be considered to decrease the angle and to eliminate scissoring
    - if stable ulnar gutter splint x 3 weeks with PIP and DIP joints free
- **Bennett's fracture (intra-articular)**: fracture/dislocation of the base of the thumb metacarpal (see Figure 29)
    - unstable fracture
    - abductor pollicis longus pulls MC shaft proximally and radially causing adduction of thumb
    - treat with percutaneous pinning, thumb spica x 6 weeks
- **Rolando's fracture (intra-articular)**: T- or Y-shaped fracture of the base of the thumb metacarpal (see Figure 30)
    - treat with open reduction, internal fixation (ORIF)

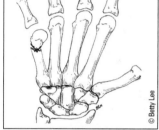

Figure 28. Boxer's Fracture

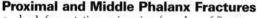

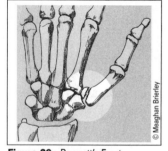

Figure 29. Bennett's Fracture

DISLOCATIONS

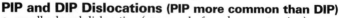

PIP and DIP Dislocations (PIP more common than DIP)
- usually dorsal dislocation (commonly from hyperextension)
- if closed dislocation: closed reduction and splinting (30° flexion for PIP and full extension for DIP) or buddy taping and early mobilization (prolonged immobilization causes stiffness)
- open injuries are treated with wound care, closed reduction and antibiotics

MCP Dislocations (relatively rare)
- dorsal dislocations much more common than volar dislocations
- dorsal dislocation of proximal phalanx on metacarpal head; most commonly index finger (hyperextension)
- two types of dorsal dislocation
    - simple (reducible with manipulation)
    - complex (volar plate blocks reduction)

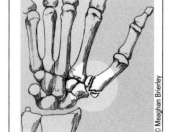

Figure 30. Rolando's Fracture

- simple dislocations are treated with reduction and 2 weeks of splinting at 60° MCP flexion
- complex dislocations are treated with open reduction + extension-blocking splint

Gamekeeper's Thumb: MCP ulnar collateral ligament (UCL) rupture
- **mechanism**: forced abduction of thumb (ski pole injury)
- **evaluation:** radially deviate joint in full extension and at 30° flexion and compare with non-injured hand. UCL rupture is presumed if injured side deviates more than 30° in full extension or more than 15° in flexion
- Stener's lesion: the UCL has bony attachments to the adductor aponeurosis and the proximal ligament can displace while the distal attachment remains deep to the aponeurosis, forming a barrier that blocks healing and leads to chronic instability; requires surgery

Dupuytren's Disease

Definition
- contraction of longitudinal palmar fascia, forming nodules (usually painless), fibrous cords and eventually flexion contractures at the MCP and interphalangeal joints (see Figure 31)
- flexor tendons not involved

Epidemiology
- genetic disorder (unusual in patients from African and Asian countries, high incidence in northern Europeans), men > women, often presents in 5th-7th decade of life, associated with but not caused by alcohol use and diabetes

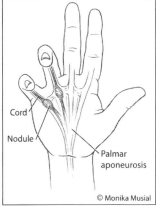

Figure 31. Dupuytren's disease

Clinical Features
- order of digit involvement (most common to least common): ring > little > long > thumb > index
- may also involve feet (Lederhosen's) and penis (Peyronie's)
- stages
  1. palmar pit or nodule – no surgery
  2. palpable band / cord with no limitation of extension of either MCP or PIP – no surgery
  3. lack of extension at MCP or PIP – surgical fasciectomy indicated
  4. irreversible periarticular joint changes / scarring – surgical treatment possible but poorer prognosis compared to stage 3

Treatment
- surgical fasciectomy is indicated when MCP joint contractures exceed 30° and when there is no PIP contracture. Fasciotomy is not curative but can provide a temporary relief
- enzymatic fasciotomy (collegenase injections) has shown promise with MCP contractures
- may recur, especially in Dupuytren's diathesis
  - early age of onset, strong family history, and involvement of sites other than palmar aspect of hand

Carpal Tunnel Syndrome (CTS)

Definition
- nerve compressed by nearby anatomic structures, often idiopathic
- can possibly be secondary to localized, repetitive mechanical trauma with additional vascular injury to the nerve

Etiology
- median nerve entrapment at wrist, usually bilateral

Epidemiology
- female:male = 4:1, **most common entrapment neuropathy**

Clinical Features
- sensory loss in nerve distribution (often discriminative touch lost first)
- classically, patient awakened at night with numb / painful hand, relieved by shaking / dangling / rubbing
- distribution: radial 3.5 digits
- decreased light touch, 2-point discrimination, especially fingertips
- job / hobby related repetitive trauma, especially forced wrist flexion
- advanced cases: wasting / weakness of abductor pollicis brevis
- ± Tinel's sign (tingling sensation on percussion of nerve)
- ± Phalen's sign (wrist flexion induces symptoms)

Accuracy of the clinical assessment for carpal tunnel syndrome –
Hand Surgery Update 1996; p.223
1. Phalen's:
   - sensitivity: 0.75   specificity: 0.47
2. Tinel's:
   - sensitivity: 0.60   specificity: 0.67
3. Carpal Tunnel Compression Test:
   - sensitivity: 0.87   specificity: 0.90

Development and Validation of Diagnostic Criteria for Carpal Tunnel Syndrome
J Hand Surg, 2006, Vol 31 No. 6 p.919

Purpose: To develop a clinical diagnostic criteria for carpal tunnel syndrome that modeled the clinical diagnostic practices of experts.
Methods: Out of 57 clinical findings associated with CTS, eight were ranked highly by a panel of expert clinicians. Using 256 case histories, a panel of experts decided whether a case did or did not have a diagnosis of CTS. This diagnosis represented the dependent variable for a logistic regression model, to which the eight clinical findings were applied. The regression model was then validated against the consensus of a second panel on the diagnosis of CTS for the case histories.
Results: The correlation between the probability of CTS predicted by the regression model and the panel of clinicians was 0.71. The following is the final list of unweighted clinical diagnostic criteria that contributed significantly to the model:
1. Numbness and tingling in median nerve distribution
2. Nocturnal numbness
3. Weakness and/or atrophy of the thenar musculature
4. Tinel's sign
5. Phalen's test
6. Loss of 2-point discrimination

Investigations
- confirm with nerve conduction velocities (NCV), EMG pre-operatively

Treatment
- avoid repetitive wrist and hand motion, wrist splints when repetitive wrist motion required
- **conservative**: night time splinting to keep wrist in neutral position
- **medical**: NSAIDs, local corticosteroids injection, oral corticosteroids
- **surgical decompression**: palmar fascia and transverse carpal ligament incised to decompress median nerve
- **indications for surgery**: numbness and tingling ± sensory loss, weakness ± muscle atrophy, unresponsive to conservative measures
- **complications**: injury to median motor branch, palmar cutaneous branch, superficial transverse vascular arch, local pain (pilar pain), scar

Rheumatoid Hand

Radiographic evolution of the rheumatoid hand:
Earliest sign: erosion of the ulnar styloid
Progression: chracterized by symmetrical joint space narrowing and erosions of the carpal bones, MCP and PIP (with DIP relatively spared)
Late stage: Swan neck and Boutonniere deformities

General Principles
- non-surgical treatments form the foundation in the management of the rheumatoid hand
- surgery only for patients whose goals (improved cosmesis or function) may be achieved

Surgical Treatment of Common Problems
- synovitis: requires tendon repair if ruptured; can lead to carpal tunnel syndrome and trigger finger
- ulnar drift: MCP arthroplasty, resection of distal ulna, soft tissue reconstruction around wrist
- thumb deformities: can be successfully treated by arthrodesis (surgical fixation of joint to promote bone fusion)

Brachial Plexus

- common causes of brachial plexus injury: complication of childbirth and trauma
- other causes of injury: compression from tumours, ectopic ribs

Common Palsies

Table 18. Named Neonatal Palsies of the Brachial Plexus

Palsy	Location of Injury	Mechanism of Injury	Features
Duchenne-Erb Palsy	Upper brachial plexus (C5-C6)	Head/shoulder distraction (e.g. motorcycle)	Waiter's tip deformity (shoulder internal rotation, elbow extension, wrist flexion)
Klumpke's Palsy	Lower brachial plexus (C7-T1)	Traction on abducted arm	May include Horner's syndrome ("claw hand")

Differential Diagnosis

- trauma (blunt, penetrating)
- thoracic outlet syndrome
  - neurogenic – associated with cervical rib; compression of C8/T1
  - vascular – pain or sensory symptoms without cervical rib; cessation of radial pulse with provocative maneuvers
- tumour
  - schwannoma – well-defined margins makes it easier for total resectio
  - neurofibromas – neurofibromatosis type I (NF-1)
  - other – e.g. Pancoast's syndrome (lung tumour)
- neuropathy (compressive, post-irradiation, viral, diabetic, idiopathic)

Investigations

- EMG
- MRI – gold standard for identifying soft tissue masses
- CT myelogram – better than MRI for identification of nerve root avulsion and identification of pseudomeningocele. Important for preoperative identication of patients likely to require neurotisation procedures (esp. for patients with blunt trauma)

Management

Table 19. Management of Brachial Plexus Injuries

	Type	Treatment
Non-penetrating Trauma	Concussive/compressive	Usually improves (unless expanding mass, e.g. hematoma)
	Traction/stretch	If no continued insult, follow for 3-4 mos for improvement
	Obstetric palsy	Surgery if no significant improvement and/or residual paresis at 6 mos of age
Penetrating Trauma	Sharp or vascular injury	Explore immediately in OR
	Blunt	Repair within 2-3 weeks

Craniofacial Injuries

- low velocity vs. high velocity injuries determine degree of damage
- fractures → bruising, swelling and tenderness → loss of function
- frequency: nasal > zygomatic > mandibular > maxillary
- management: can wait up to 10 days for swelling to decrease before ORIF are required

Approach to Facial Injuries

- see Emergency Medicine

- ATLS protocol
- wound irrigation with physiologic solution and remove foreign materials
- palpate/explore wounds for injury to underlying structures (e.g. facial nerve)
- visual assessment
- tetanus prophylaxis, antibiotics if indicated
- radiological evaluation
- conservative debridement of detached or nonviable tissue
- repair when patient's general condition allows (soft tissue injury: <8 hrs preferable, primary closure <24 hrs)

Investigations (see Table 20)
- CT:
  - axial and coronal – for fractures of upper and middle face (not good for mandible)
  - indicated for high velocity trauma, complex facial fractures, orbital floor, panface fractures, pre-op assessment
- panorex radiograph – shows entire upper and lower jaw

Table 20. Imaging of the Craniofacial Skeleton

Structure	Appropriate Imaging
Mandible	**Panoramic (panorex)*** CT
Zygomatic and orbital bones	**CT scan*** Water's view (occipitomental, A-P "from below")
Nasal bones	No x-ray required - clinical
Maxilla	CT scan – axial and **coronal***

*best imaging method

Treatment
- consultation when indicated (dentistry, ophthalmology)
- re-establish normal occlusion
- pursue normal eye function
- retore stability of face and appearance
- be alert for bleeding, CSF leak (can lead to meningitis in future), and SIADH

Patient with major facial injuries are at risk of developing upper airway obstruction (displaced blood clots, teeth or fracture fragments; swelling of pharynx and larynx; loss of support of hyomandibular complex → retroposition of tongue)

Suspect C-spine injury with any facial trauma. C-spine evaluation before radiographs are ordered.

Consider intracranial trauma; rule out skull fracture.

Signs of Basal Skull / Le Fort III Fracture
1. Battle sign (bruised mastoid process)
2. Hemotympanum
3. Raccoon eyes (periorbital bruising)
4. CSF otorrhea

Most facial bone fractures (especially orbital injuries) require ophthalmology consult.

Complications
- diplopia / enophthalmos / blindness
- cerebrospinal fluid (CSF) leak
- sinusitis
- extraocular muscle entrapment
- cosmesis
- functional abnormalities
- infection (see Table 20)

Table 21. Head and Neck Infections – Cause and Treatment

Infection	Usual Cause	Treatment
Facial cellulitis	*Staph* or *Strep*	cephalosporin
Oral cavity infection	Anaerobic Strep, Bacteroides	extended spectrum penicillin/anaerobic coverage
Acute sialadenitis – fever, pain, swelling over parotid gland	Dehydration, debilitation, diabetes, poor oral hygiene	abx, fluids
Atypical mycobacterium – enlarged lymph node	Atypical mycobacterium	special cultures, specific drugs, ± drainage

Mandibular Fractures

- often bilateral, at sites of weakness (condylar neck, angle of mandible, region of 3rd molar or canine tooth)

> Panorex is the appropriate imaging for a suspected mandibular fracture. If needed for other possible fractures, a CT can be helpful.

Etiology
- anterior force: bilateral fractures
- lateral force: ipsilateral subcondylar and contralateral angle or body fracture
- note: classified as open if fracture into tooth bearing area (alveolus)

Clinical Features
- pain, swelling, trismus
- malocclusion, asymmetry of dental arch
- damaged, loose, or lost teeth
- palpable "step" along mandible
- numbness in V_3 distribution
- intra-oral lacerations or hematoma (sublingual)
- chin deviating toward side of a fractured condyle

Classification

Table 22. Mandibular fracture classifications by anatomic region (Please refer to figure 32)

	Areas/Boundaries
Symphysis	Midline of the mandible; between the central incisors from the alveolar process through the inferior border of the mandible
Body*	From the symphysis to the distal alveolar border of the third molar
Angle	Triangular region between the anterior border of the masseter and the posterosuperior insertion of the masseter distal to the third molar)
Ramus	Part of the mandible that extends posteriosuperiorly into the condylar and coronoid processes
Condylar	Area of condylar process of mandible
Subcondylar	Area below the condylar neck (i.e. sigmoid notch) of the mandible
Coronoid Process	Area of the coronoid process of mandible

*Most common mandibular fracture type

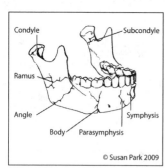

Figure 32. Mandibular Fracture

Treatment
- maxillary and mandibular arch bars wired together (intramaxillary fixation) or ORIF
- antibiotics to cover against *S. aureus* and anaerobes if fracture is open into the mouth

Complications
- malocclusion, malunion
- tooth loss, and possible sensation loss(es)
- temporomandibular joint (TMJ) ankylosis

Maxillary Fractures

Table 23. Le Fort Classification

	Le Fort I	Le Fort II	Le Fort III
Alternative Name	Guerin fracture	Pyramidal fracture	Craniofacial dysjunction
Type of fracture	Horizontal	Pyramidal	Transverse
Structures involved	Piriform aperture Maxillary sinus Pterygoid plates	Nasal bones Medial orbital wall Maxilla Pterygoid plates	Nasofrontal suture Zygomatofrontal suture Zygomatic arch Pterygoid plates
Anatomical result	Maxilla divided into 2 segments	Maxillary teeth separated from face	Detach entire midfacial skeleton from cranial base

Le Fort I Fractures   Le Fort II Fractures   Le Fort III Fractures

©Ryo Sakai 2007

Clinical Features
- dish pan / equine facies (flat or protruding facies)
- periorbital hematoma, epistaxis
- malocclusion
- mobility of maxilla: tested by trying to move maxilla while watching and palpating for mobility of nasal and zygomatic bones (may not move if fragment is impacted)

Treatment
- primary goal is restoration of occlusion and functional rehabilitation (speech, bite)
- intermaxillary fixation (IMF: wiring jaws together)
- usually also require ORIF to restore projection of the face

Complications
- malocclusion; facial deformities
- airway compromise
- areas of altered sensation

Nasal Fractures

Etiology
- lateral force → more common, good prognosis
- anterior force → can produce more serious injuries

Clinical Features
- epistaxis/hemorrhage, deviation/flattening of nose, swelling, periorbital ecchymosis, tenderness over nasal dorsum, crepitus, septal hematoma, respiratory obstruction, subconjunctival hemorrhage
- depression and splaying of nasal bones causing a saddle deformity

Treatment
- nothing
- always drain **septal hematomas** as this is a cause of septal necrosis with perforation (saddle nose deformity)
- closed reduction with Asch or Walsham forceps under anesthesia, pack nostrils with Adaptic™, nasal splint for 7 days
- best reduction immediately (<6 hrs) or when swelling subsides (5-7 days)
- rhinoplasty may be necessary later for residual deformity (30%)

Zygomatic Fractures

Suspect a fracture of the zygoma when there is a history of direct injury to the malar region with unilateral epistaxis and subconjunctival hemorrhage.

- 3 categories (please see Figure 33)
  1. fracture restricted to zygomatic arch
  2. depressed fracture of zygomatic complex (zygoma)
  3. unstable fracture of zygomatic complex (tripod fracture) – zygoma separates from maxilla, frontal, temporal bone

Clinical Features
- flattening of malar prominence (view from above)
- pain over fractures on palpation
- numbness in V_2 distribution (infraorbital and superior dental nerves)
- palpable step deformity in bony orbital rim (especially inferiorly)
- often associated with fractures of the orbital floor
- enophthalmos, diplopia, proptosis, vertical dystrophia; periorbital ecchymosis and ipsilateral subconjunctival hemorrhage (lateral to limbus); inferior displacement of eyeball (loss of alignment or entrapment of inferior rectus in fracture)
- ipsilateral epistaxis; trismus (lock jaw)

Treatment
- if undisplaced and no symptoms, then no treatment necessary
- ophthalmologic evaluation
- elevate using Gillies approach: leverage on the anterior part of the zygomatic arch via a temporal incision
- if Gillies approach fails or a comminuted fracture, then ORIF

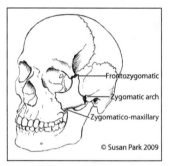

Figure 33. Zygomatic Fractures

Labels: Frontozygomatic; Zygomatic arch; Zygomatico-maxillary; © Susan Park 2009

Orbital Blow-Out Fractures

Definition
- fracture of floor of orbit with intact infraorbital rim (see Figure 34)
- may be associated with nasoethmoid fracture

Etiology
- blunt force to eyeball $\rightarrow$ sudden increase in intra-orbital pressure (e.g. baseball or fist)

Clinical Features
- **check visual fields and acuity for injury to globe**
- periorbital edema and bruising, subconjunctival hemorrhage
- ptosis, exophthalmos, exorbitism, or enophthalmos
- diplopia looking up or down (entrapment of inferior rectus), limited EOM

Investigations
- CT (coronals)
- forced duction test for entrapment – i.e. pull on inferior rectus muscle

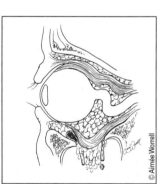

Figure 34. Blow-Out Fracture

© Aimée Worrell

Diplopia can present late in orbital blow-out fractures.

Treatment
- may require open reduction with reconstruction of orbital floor with bone graft or alloplastic material
- ophthalmologic evaluation mandatory within 24 hrs

Indications for open reduction of orbital blow-out fractures
- immediate repair if have:
  - oculocardiac reflex resulting in bradycardia and cardiovascular instability
  - early enophthalmos or hypoglobus
  - orbital tissue entrapment (e.g. inferior rectus muscle entrapment)
- repair in 2 weeks if have:
  - symptomatic diplopia affecting function
  - fracture involving >50% of orbital floor leading to enophthalmous when edema resolves
  - progressive infraorbital hypoesthesia

Superior Orbital Fissure (SOF) Syndrome
- fracture of SOF causing ptosis, proptosis, paralysis of CN III, IV, VI, and anesthesia in V_1 distribution
- requires **urgent surgical decompression**

Orbital Apex Syndrome
- fracture through optic canal with division of CN II at apex of orbit
- symptoms are the same as SOF syndrome plus blindness; treatment is the same **(urgent surgical decompression)**

Breast Surgery

Breast Reconstruction

Information for the *Breast Reconstruction* section provided courtesy of Dr. P. Neligan
- integral part breast cancer treatment
- two basic methods: implants and autologous tissue (see Table 24 below)
  - choice of method depends on: several factors: patient age, prognosis, body weight, characteristics of the chest, contralateral breast, availability of suitable donor tissue for autologous reconstruction, surgical history, radiation treatment, patient's attitude, and surgeon's experience
- timing
  - immediate vs. delayed: immediate preferred in cases with no increased risk of cancer recurrence; delayed in cases requiring radiation following mastectomy
- contralateral breast
  - may not be possible to reconstruct a breast of the same shape and size as the contralateral breast
  - contralateral reduction/mastopexy at time of reconstruction in large breasted women may be considered

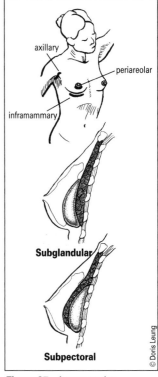

Figure 35. Augmentation Mammoplasty-incision lines and implant placement

Table 24. Common Surgical Procedures of the Breast

Procedure	Definition	Surgical Details	Other Comments
Augmentation (Breast Implants)	Increase in the size of the breast	Implantation of saline or silicone filled implants (subglandular or submuscular)	See Figure 35 for anatomic location of implants
Mastopexy	Raises nipple in ptotic breasts	3 surgical approaches with many different procedures	
Reduction Mammoplasty (Breast Reduction)	Reduction of breast for relief of physical discomfort, improvement of breast size/shape	1. Incisions: e.g. Circular around areola, vertical from areola incision to infra-mammary fold, along natural infra-mammary fold 2. Fat, breast tissue, and skin removal division between breast tissue and pectoralis muscle 3. Nipple and areola complex moved to higher position	Complications include: infection, hemorrhage, decreased nipple sensation, inability to breast feed, breast/nipple asymmetry, nipple loss (partial or complete)
Implant Reconstruction	Use of synthetic material to remodel original breast after mastectomy	1. Usually tissue expanders (placed at time of mastectomy) prior to placement of implants to facilitate breast ptosis. Not required in skin-sparing mastectomies (see further discussion of tissue expanders below.) 2. Breast implants replace expander 2 weeks after expansion complete (details in augmentation above)	Complications include: capsular contraction (foreign body reaction) unique to implants, increased risk of infection, risk of complications increased in previously irradiated breast
Autologous Reconstruction	Use of autologous tissue to remodel original breast after mastectomy	Many options: DIEP (deep inferior epigastric perforator) flap, TRAM (transverse rectus abdominus myocutaneous) flap, SIEA (superficial inferior epigastric artery) flap, SGAP (superior gluteal artery perforator) flap, latissimus dorsi flap	Considered gold standard: offers reduced long-term morbidity and natural consistency Complications: see *Grafts and Flaps* section
Nipple/Areola Reconstruction	Final stage of breast reconstruction	Usually require tattooing for areola reconstruction Local vs. distant flaps/grafts: 1. Local: fish tail flap or skate flap most common; these flaps allow simultaneous nipple and areola reconstruction 2. Distant: opposite nipple, earlobes, abdominal skin, costal cartilage	Usually performed 3 months post-reconstruction

Always check for arterial insufficiency (pale pink colour to flap, poor capillary refill and absent Dopplers) and venous congestion (bluish colour to flap and rapid capillary refill) after vessel anastamoses or flap transfer.

Breast Tissue Expanders

- types: textured vs. smooth, integrated port vs. remote port (axilla location)
- placement: sub-mammary vs. sub-pectoral
    - subpectoral preferred: lower incidence of capsular contracture, extra layer of tissue between expander and skin
- size: depends on chest size, contralateral breast, desired size
    - generally over-expanded to facilitate ptosis
- timing of expansion: 8-10 week process which begins when wound fully healed (usually 2 weeks post-op), implant re-expanded weekly or bi-weekly until complete

Aesthetic Surgery

Table 25. Aesthetic Surgical Procedures

Location	Procedure	Description
Head/Neck	Hair transplants	Aesthetic improvement of hair growth patterns using grafts of flaps.
	Otoplasty	Surgical correction of "outstanding" ears.
	Brow lift	Surgical procedure to lift low brows or to reduce deep frown lines.
Face	Rhytidectomy	Surgical procedure to reduce wrinkling and sagging of the face and neck. "Face lift".
	Blepharoplasty	Surgical procedure to shape or modify the appearance of eyelids by removing excess eyelid skin ± fat pads.
	Rhinoplasty	Intranasal surgical reconstruction of the nose.
	Genioplasty	Chin augmentation via osteotomy or synthetic implant to improve contour.
	Lip Augmentation	Procedure to create fuller lips and to reduce wrinkles around the mouth using collagen injections, fat transferred from other body parts, or implantable materials.
Skin	Chemical peel	Application of one or more exfoliating agents to the skin resulting in destruction of portions of the epidermis and/or dermis with subsequent tissue regeneration.
	Dermabrasion	Skin re-surfacing by sanding with a rapidly rotating abrasive tool. Often used to reduce scars, irregular skin surfaces and fine lines.
	Laser resurfacing	Application of laser to the skin which ultimately results in collagen reconfiguration and subsequent skin shrinking and tightening. Often used to reduce scars and wrinkles.
	Collagen Injections	Injectable collagen is used to replenish natural collagen in the skin that is lost due to aging. Often used to decrease frown lines, wrinkles and nasolabial folds
Other	Liposuction	Surgical removal of adipose tissue for contouring and not weight loss.
	Abdominoplasty	Surgical removal of abdominal pannus or tightening of abdominal muscles separated and weakened by pregnancy. "Tummy tuck".
	Calf augmentation	Surgical implantation to enhance appearance of calf muscle.

Pediatric Plastic Surgery

Craniofacial Anomalies

Table 26. Pediatric Craniofacial Anomalies

	Definition	Epidemiology	Clinical Features	Treatment
Cleft Lip	Failure of fusion of maxillary and medial nasal processes	1 in 1000 live births (1 in 800 Caucasians, ↑Asians, ↓Blacks) M:F = 2:1 Cleft of left lip/palate in boys has hereditary component	Classified as incomplete/complete & uni/bilateral 2/3 cases: unilateral, left-sided, male	Cleft lip team; Surgery (3 months): Milliard or Tennison-Randall; corrections usually required later on (esp. for nasal deformity)
Cleft Palate	Failure of fusion of lateral palatine/median palatine processes and nasal septum	Isolated Cleft Palate: 0.5 per 1000 (no racial variation) F > M	Classified as incomplete/complete & uni/bilateral Isolated (common in females) or in conjunction with cleft lip (common in males)	Special bottles for feeding Speech pathologist Surgery (6-9 months): Von Langenbeck or Furlow Z-Plasty ENT consult – often recurrent OM, requiring myringotomy tubes
Craniosynostosis	Premature fusion of 1+ cranial sutures Primary – abnormal suture, no known cause This may limit brain development in the direction perpendicular to the suture and cause compensatory growth parallel to the fused suture	1 in 2000 live newborns; M:F = 52:48 Syndromic includes: Crouzon's, Apert's Saethre-Chotzen, Carpenter's, Pfeiffer's Jackson-Weiss and Boston-type syndromes	Syndromic – assoc. with genetic mutation Secondary (to microcephaly, hyperthyroid, rickets, etc.) Dx: irregular head shape, craniofacial abnormalities, X-ray	Multidisc. team (incl neurosurg, ENT, genetics, dentistry, peds, SLP) Early surgery prevents secondary deformities ↑ICP is an indication for emergent surg ICU bed may be req'd post-surgically

Congenital Hand Anomalies

Table 27. American Society for Surgery of the Hand (ASSH) Classification of Congenital Hand Anomalies

Classification	Example	Features	Treatment
A. Failure of formation	Transverse Absence (congenital amputation)	At any level (often below elbow/wrist)	Early prosthesis
	Longitudinal Absence (phocomelia)	Absent humerus Thalidomide-assoc.	
	Radial Deficiency (radial club hand)	Radial deviation Thumb hypoplasia M>F	Physio + splinting Soft tissue release if splinting fails Distraction osteogenesis (Ilizarov) ± wedge osteotomy Tendon transfer Pollicization
	Thumb Hypoplasia	Degree ranges from small thumb with all components to complete absence	Depends on degree - may involve no treatment, webspace deepening, tendon transfer, or pollicization of index finger
	Ulnar Club Hand	Rare, compared to Radial club hand Stable wrist	Splinting & soft-tissue stretching therapies Soft-tissue release (if above fails) Correction of angulation (Ilizarov distraction)
	Cleft Hand	Autosomal dominant Often functionally normal (depending on degree)	First web space syndactyly release Osteotomy/tendon transfer of thumb (if hypoplastic)
B. Failure of differentiation/ separation	Syndactyly	Fusion of 2+digits 1/3000 live births M:F = 2:1 Classified as partial/complete Simple (skin only) vs. complex (osseous or cartilaginous bridges)	Surgical separation before 6-12 mos of age Usually good result
	Symbrachydactyly	Short fingers with short nails at fingertips	Digital separation (more difficult) Webspace deepening
	Camptodactyly	Congenital flexion contracture (usually at PIP, esp. 5th digit)	Early splinting Volar release Arthroplasty (rarely)
	Clinodactyly	Radial or ulnar deviation Often middle phalanx	None (usually) If severe, osteotomy with grafting

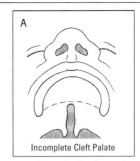

A – Defects of soft palate only

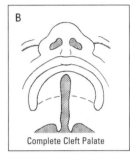

B – Defects of soft and hard palate

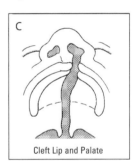

C – Defects of soft palate to alveolus, usually involving lip

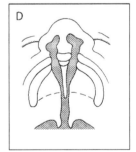

D – Complete bilateral cleft

© Adrian Yen (2006)

Figure 36. Types of Cleft Lips and Palates

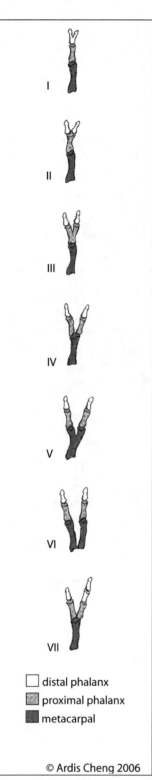

I

II

III

IV

V

VI

VII

☐ distal phalanx
▨ proximal phalanx
■ metacarpal

© Ardis Cheng 2006

Figure 37. Wassel Classification of Thumb Duplication

Table 27. American Society for Surgery of the Hand (ASSH) Classification of Congenital Hand Anomalies (continued)

Classification	Example	Features	Treatment
C. Duplication	Polydactyly	Congenital duplication of digits May be radial (↑Native Indians, ↑Asians) or central or ulnar (↑Blacks)	Amputation of least functional digit Usually >1 yr of age (when functional status can be assessed)
D. Overgrowth	Macrodactyly	Rare	None (if mild) Soft tissue/bony reduction
E. Undergrowth	Brachydactyly	Short phalanges	Removal of non-functional stumps Osteotomies/tendon transfers Distraction osteogenesis Phalangeal/free toe transfer
	Symbrachydactyly (Brachysyndactyly)	Short webbed fingers	As above + syndactyly release
F. Constriction band syndrome	AKA amniotic (annular) band syndrome	Variety of presentations	Urgent release for acute, progressive edema distal to band in newborn Other reconstruction is case-specific
G. Generalized skeletal abnormality	Achondroplasia, Marfan's, Madelung's	Variety of presentations	Treatment depends on etiology

Common Medications

Table 28. Commonly Used Medication

Drug Name (Brand Name)	Dosing Schedule	Indications/Comments
cefazolin (Ancef™)	1-2 g IV q8h	Surgical prophylaxis, flexor tenosynovitis
cloxacillin	250-500 mg PO q6h	Staph. infections – felons, skin infections
cephalexin (Keflex™)	500 mg PO q6h	Staph. infections – paronychia, skin infections
amoxicillin + clavulanate potassium (Clavulin™)	250-500 mg PO q8h	Skin infections – human bites, animal bites
clindamycin (Biaxin™ in PO form)	150-450 mg PO q6h 1.2-1.8 g/day IV divided bid or tid	Human bites with penicillin allergy (add ciprofloxacin)
ciprofloxacin (Cipro™)	250-500 mg PO bid	Human bites with penicillin allergy
acetaminophen + codeine (Tylenol #3™)	1-2 tabs PO q4-6h prn	Pain relief
acetaminophen + oxycodone (Percocet™)	1-2 tabs PO q4-6h prn	Pain relief – for patients with codeine allergy
dimenhydrinate (Gravol™)	25-50 mg PO/IV/IM q4-6h prn	Anti-emetic
lidocaine (Xylocaine®) (with or without epinephrine)	Plain: 4 mg/kg (max) With epi: 7 mg/kg (max)	Local anaesthetic ± vasoconstrictor (epinephrine)
bupivicaine (Marcaine ®)	2 mg/kg (max)	Local anaesthetic

PH | Population and Community Health

Adam Lenny and Shauna Tsuchiya, chapter editors
Justine Chan and Angela Ho, associate editors
Billie Au, EBM editor
Dr. Richard Glazier and Dr. Ian Johnson, staff editors

Historical Context of Public Health

For the LMCC exam, it is recommended that you read all of Chapter 15 in Shah CP. *Public Health and Preventative Medicine in Canada.* 5th edition. Elsevier Canada. 2003.

Definitions
- **Population Health**
  - health of the population as measured by health status indicators
  - influenced by physical, biological, social and economic factors in the environment as well as personal health behaviours and health care services
  - refers to the prevailing or desired level of health in the population of a specific country, region or subset of population

- **Public Health**
  - systematic efforts of society to protect, promote and restore the health of the public
  - refers to the practices, procedures, institutions and disciplines required to achieve the desired state of population health

- **Community Medicine**
  - the study of health and disease in the population or a specified community
  - goal: to identify and address health problems and evaluate the extent to which health services address these issues

Source: Last JM. *A Dictionary of Epidemiology*, 4th ed. Oxford University Press. 2001.

Historical perspective
Public health has evolved through three main epidemiological phases:

1. Infectious diseases
  - examples of this era include smallpox, plagues, and tuberculosis
  - most illness, such as malaria, were successfully treated in the developed world but still remain an issue in some developing countries
  - notable successes in this era of public health include the eradication of smallpox and near eradication of polio

2. Chronic diseases
  - examples of this era include heart disease and cancer
  - these diseases became the most common causes of death and disability due to:
    - changes in lifestyle such as an increase in the prevalence of smoking and sedentary lifestyle
    - reduction in infectious disease mortality resulting in increasing life span and therefore prevalence of chronic diseases
    - exposure to other factors, such as asbestos, leading to cancer
    - increasing urbanization and changes in social structure

3. Re-emerging infectious diseases
  - examples of this era include AIDS, hantavirus and drug-resistant tuberculosis
  - this new era has emerged due to:
    - encroachment on natural environments and contact with unfamiliar pathogens (e.g. HIV)
    - fast international travel facilitating the rapid spread of organisms
    - inefficient and inappropriate use of antibiotics leading to drug-resistant organisms, e.g. drug resistant TB, MRSA, VRE
    - global warming, which may possibly increase the size of regions at high-risk for transmission of vector-borne diseases such as malaria and dengue

Public Health Services in Canada

Five Core Functions for All Public Health Units
1. population health assessment
2. health surveillance
3. health promotion
4. disease and injury prevention
5. health protection

Mission: to promote and protect the health of Canadians through leadership, partnership, innovation and action in public health.

- local public health unit provides programs and activities for health protection, promotion and disease prevention at local and regional levels
- catchment-areas can have populations a hundred to two million people, covering areas of 15 to 1.5 million km^2

Legislation and Public Health in Canada

Federal
- 3 divisions of the federal government are responsible for public health:
  - Health Canada
    - provides health services to First Nations and Aboriginal peoples
    - approval of new drugs and medical devices
    - liaising with other national health organizations, e.g. WHO
  - Canadian Food Inspection Agency
    - monitoring of genetically modified foods
    - monitoring food importation
    - animal-related infections (e.g. BSE)
  - Public Health Agency of Canada
    - an agency created to strengthen public health by forming an independent body that reports to federal government via the Chief Public Health Officer
    - immigration screening, protecting Canadian borders (e.g. airport health inspection)

Provincial
- legislation is in the form of Acts and Regulations
- each province has its own *Public Health Act* or equivalent. In Ontario, it is the *Health Promotion and Protection Act*
  - designates the creation of local health units or geographic areas for the provision of public health services
  - gives powers to the Chief Medical Officer of Health to control public health hazards
  - specifies infectious diseases to be reported to public health units by physicians, laboratories and hospitals (see Appendix 1)
  - has the ability to mandate programs that address public health issues, i.e. injury prevention programs, infectious disease control programs, healthy environments and chronic disease prevention

Municipal
- delivers programs mandated by provincial legislation in accordance with local needs
- Public health is directed at the regional level in Ontario, e.g. York Region. Regional health units are responsible for the delivery of most public health services such as:
  - infectious disease control, including the follow-up of reported diseases and management of outbreaks
  - inspection of food premises including those in hospitals, nursing homes and restaurants
  - family health services including pre-conception, preschool, school-aged and adult health programs
  - tobacco control legislation enforcement
  - assessment and management of local environmental health risks
  - collection and dissemination of local health status reports
  - some public dental health services to children
- by-laws may be legislated by municipal government to facilitate issues of zoning

Medical Officer of Health
- appointed to each public health unit by the board of health, which itself is composed of individuals appointed by the municipality and the province
- full-time position that can only be held by a physician
- physicians can also be appointed as Associate Medical Officers of Health if needed
- responsibilities of the Medical Officer of Health include:
  - reporting to the board of health on matters of public health
  - supervision of community sanitation, including food premises and places of lodging
  - control of infectious and reportable diseases, including immunization
  - implementation of disease and injury prevention as well as health promotion and protection programs as needed
  - collection and analysis of epidemiological data
  - occupational and environmental health surveillance
  - implementation of family health programs, including:
    - counseling
    - family planning services
    - parenting programs, prenatal courses
    - preschool and school health services
    - disease screening programs to reduce morbidity and mortality

> > > > ◆ tobacco use prevention programs
> > > > ◆ nutrition services to schools and seniors' centres
> > • authority
> > > ▪ the Medical Officer of Health can require an individual to take or refrain from any action due to a public health hazard including an order to:
> > > > ◆ vacate a premises or close a business
> > > > ◆ update or maintain a business or home with maintenance work
> > > > ◆ receive treatment by a physician if infected
> > > > ◆ give a blood sample
> > > ▪ the Medical Officer of Health can also:
> > > > ◆ prohibit or regulate the manufacturing, storage, handling, sale or distribution of any item
> > > > ◆ order the isolation or quarantine of individuals who have or may have communicable diseases

Determinants of Health

Concepts of Health

- **Disease:** abnormal, medically defined changes in the structure or function of the human body
- **Illness:** an individual's experience or subjective perception of a lack of physical or mental well-being and consequent inability to function normally in social roles
- **Impairment:** any loss or abnormality of psychological, physiological or anatomical structure or function, i.e. a change in the individual's body
- **Disability:** any restriction or lack of ability to perform an activity within the range considered normal for a human being, i.e. changes in what the individual can or cannot do
- **Handicap:** the disadvantage for an individual arising due to impairment and disability. A handicap limits or prevents the fulfillment of an individual's normal role as determined by society and depends on age, sex, social and cultural factors. A handicap changes the individual's relationship with the physical and social environment

Determinants of Health
- four elements that interact to determine **health: human biology, environment, lifestyle and the health care organization**
- comprehensive view of the determinants of health put forward in 1974 by Marc Lalonde, Minister of Health, in a health field concept entitled *A New Perspective on the Health of Canadians* (see sidebar)
- the **Population Health Model** expands on the previous list of health determinants and can be organized into 5 categories:

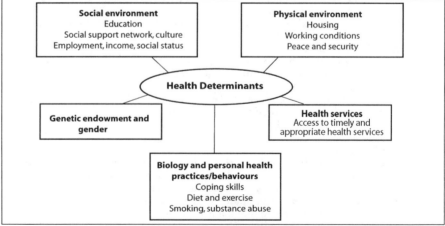

Figure 1. Population Health Model

Definitions of Health
- First multidimensional definition of health, as defined by the World Health Organization (WHO) in 1948: "A complete state of physical, mental and social well being and not merely the absence of illness"
- WHO updated the definition (socioecological definition) of health in 1986: *"The ability to identify and to realize aspirations, to satisfy needs, and to change or cope with the environment. Health is therefore a resource for everyday life, not the objective of living. Health is a positive concept emphasizing social and personal resources, as well as physical capacities."*

Determinants of Health
1. income and social status
2. social support networks
3. education and literacy
4. employment and working conditions
5. social environment
6. physical environment
7. personal health practices and coping skills
8. healthy child development
9. biology and genetic endowment
10. health services
11. gender
12. culture
Source: Public Health Agency of Canada

Vulnerable Populations

Table 1. Health Determinants of Vulnerable Populations

	Psychosocial/socioeconomic	Physical environment	Lifestyle and behaviour
Aboriginal peoples	Low income Family violence Low education status Unemployment Homelessness	Crowded housing Inefficient ventilation Environmental toxins	Smoking Substance abuse Problem gambling Poor nutrition Sedentary lifestyle High BMI High risk behaviours
Seniors	Elder abuse Lack of emotional support	Low hazard tolerance Institutionalization	Inactivity Polypharmacy Medical co-morbidities
Children in poverty	Low income Family dysfunction Lack of educational opportunities	Housing availability Unsafe housing Lack of recreational space	Poor supervision Food insecurity High risk behaviours
People with disabilities	Low income Low education status Discrimination	Institutionalization (7%) Barriers to access TraDnsportation challenges	Substance abuse Poor nutrition Inactivity Dependency for ADLs
Immigrants	Access to community services Cultural perspectives	Diseases & conditions in country of origin (e.g. smoke from wood fires, incidence of TB, etc.)	
Homeless persons	Low income Mental illness	Exposure to temperature extremes	Substance abuse Violence

Disease Prevention

Disease Prevention Strategies
- measures aimed at preventing, interrupting or slowing the progression of disease

Primary Prevention (Immunization)
- immunization programs exist in most countries to address 6 major causes of pediatric morbidity and mortality that are preventable by vaccines:
    1. measles
    2. diphtheria
    3. pertussis
    4. tetanus
    5. polio
    6. tuberculosis (not routine in Canada or the U.S.)
- additional immunization are offered in Canada depending on jurisdiction: mumps, rubella, hepatitis B, *Haemophilus influenzae* type B, varicella, HPV, conjugated pneumococcal and meningococcal vaccines (see <u>Pediatrics</u>, P5)

Secondary Prevention (Screening)
- presumptive identification of unrecognized disease or defect by the application of tests, examinations or other procedures which can be applied rapidly
- **types of screening**
    - mass screening: screening all members of a population for a disease, e.g. phenylketonuria and hypothyroidism in newborns
    - selective screening: screening of a specific subgroup of the population at risk for a disease, e.g. mammography in women >50 years old
    - multiphasic screening: the use of many measurements and investigations to look for many disease entities, e.g. periodic health exam
- **criteria for screening tests**
    - disease
        - must cause significant suffering and/or death
        - natural history must be understood
        - must have an asymptomatic stage that can be detected by a test
        - early detection and intervention result in favorable outcomes
        - incidence is not too high or too low
    - test
        - high specificity and sensitivity
        - safe, rapid, easy, relatively inexpensive
        - acceptable to providers and population

Disease Prevention Strategies
- **Primary:** before disease occurs
    - e.g. immunizations, seatbelt use, smoking cessation programs for lung cancer prevention

- **Secondary:** early detection of disease
    - e.g. mammography, routine Pap smears

- **Tertiary:** treatment and rehabilitation of existing disease
    - e.g. ACEI for hypertension

- **Passive prevention:** measures that operate without the person's active involvement
    - e.g. airbags in cars

- **Active prevention:** measures that a person must do on their own
    - e.g. put on a seatbelt

- healthcare system
  - ◆ adequate capacity for reporting, follow-up and treatment of positive screens
  - ◆ cost effective
  - ◆ sustainable program
  - ◆ clear policy guidelines

Tertiary Prevention
- treatment and rehabilitation of disease after it has been diagnosed so as to prevent progression and permanent disability (e.g. ACEI for hypertension, insulin for diabetes, etc.)

Health Promotion Strategies

Canadian Task Force on Preventive Health Care grading of health promotion actions

A: *Good evidence to recommend* the preventive health measure

B: *Fair evidence to recommend* the preventive health measure

C: *Existing evidence is conflicting* and does not allow making a recommendation for or against use of the clinical preventive action, however other factors may influence decision-making

D: *Fair evidence to recommend against* the preventive health measure

E: *Good evidence to recommend against* the preventive health measure

I: *Insufficient evidence* (in quantity and/or quality) to make a recommendation, however other factors may influence decision-making

Source: Canadian Task Force on Preventive Health Care. 2003. CMAJ 169 (3):213-214

Table 2. Disease Prevention versus Health Promotion Approach

Disease Prevention	Health Promotion
Health = absence of disease	Health = positive and multidimensional concept
Medical model (passive role)	Participatory model of health
Aimed mainly at high-risk groups in the population	Aimed at the population in its total environment
Concerns a specific pathology	Concerns a network of issues
One-shot strategy	Diverse and complementary strategies
Directive and persuasive strategies	Facilitating and enabling approaches
Directive measures enforced in target groups	Incentive measures offered to the population
Focused mostly on individuals and groups of subjects	Focus on a person's health status and environment
Preventive programs considered the affairs of professional groups from health disciplines	Non-professional organizations, civic groups, local, municipal, regional and national governments necessary for achieving the goal of health promotion

Source: Shah CP. *Public Health and Preventive Medicine in Canada.* 5th ed. Elsevier Canada. 2003.

Ottawa Charter for Health Promotion (1986)
- **health promotion:** the process of enabling people to increase control over and to improve their health
- the charter states that governments and health care providers should be involved in a **health promotion process** that includes:
  1. building healthy **public policy**
  2. creating supportive **environments**
  3. strengthening **community action**
  4. developing **personal skills**
  5. reorienting **health services**

Jakarta Declaration on Health Promotion into the 21st Century (WHO 1997)
- reiterated the commitment of health promotion
- first of the health promotion conferences to involve the private sector
- formally cited poverty as the greatest threat to health priorities for health promotion:
  - promote social responsibility for health
  - increase investments for health development
  - consolidate and expand partnerships for health
  - increase community capacity and empower the individual
  - secure an infrastructure for health promotion

Healthy Public Policy
1. **Fiscal**
   - tax and pricing policies established to impose additional costs to undertake "unhealthy" behaviours
     - ◆ e.g. taxes on tobacco and alcohol
2. **Legislative**
   - implementation of legal deterrents to individual behaviors
     - ◆ e.g. anti-smoking bylaws, seat belt legislation, bicycle helmet bylaws, legal drinking age

3. **Social**
- responsibility of improving health beyond providing traditional health services, the premise of universal health care under the *Canada Health Act*
  - e.g. providing affordable housing and ensuring adequate income
- may improve the health of the population independently of the health care system

Community Development
- process of community members identifying issues and problems affecting their community and subsequently developing the skills and capacity to implement change

Community-Based Prevention
- health promotion focused on an entire community as opposed to only high risk groups
- "community-based approaches" are population-based multifactorial initiatives that make use of communication-behavior change, community organization, and social marketing to elicit change at the community level
  - e.g. Canadian Heart Health Initiative
- numerous preventable risk factors are being addressed by multiple health promotion strategies

Health Marketing
- application of the principles of commercial marketing to promote healthy changes
- involves target group analysis and segmentation of the market for specific messages and promotion strategies
- employed by both the health care system (e.g. pamphlets providing health information about HIV) and by industry (e.g. in medication advertisements)

Behavior Change
- Health Education serves to:
  - increase knowledge and skills
  - encourage positive lifestyle changes and discourage unhealthy choices
- Health Education is an important component of eliciting behavior change, however behavior is not only dictated by knowledge, e.g. many smokers know smoking is bad for them but they still continue to smoke
- Behavior is a result of three factors:
  1. **Predisposing factors** - knowledge, attitude, beliefs, values, intentions
  2. **Enabling factors** - skills, supports
  3. **Reinforcing factors** - health care professionals and the social context of family and community
- **Health Belief Model** (1975)
  - behaviors undertaken by individuals in order to remain healthy are a function of a set of interacting beliefs
  - beliefs include an individual's perception of his or her susceptibility to a disease, the severity of the disease and the benefits and costs of health related actions
  - beliefs are modified by **socio-demographic** and **psychosocial variables**
  - individuals must believe that the action will have positive consequences
  - individuals must be in a state of readiness
  - behavior can be stimulated by cues to action, which are specific events that can encourage preventive health decisions and actions, e.g. physician recommendation, public advertising
- **Stages of Change Model**
  - provides a framework in which the Health Belief Model is applied to facilitating behavior change (see Figure 2)

Labonte Model of Community Development
- personal empowerment
- small group development
- community organization
- coalition advocacy
- political action

4 P's Influencing Health Marketing
1. **Product** = good health
2. **Price** = what a person must give up if he or she accepts the product "pursuing good health"
3. **Place** = the distribution channels used to reach the consumer (e.g. distributing pamphlets at the doctor's office)
4. **Promotion** = the way in which the product is promoted to the consumer

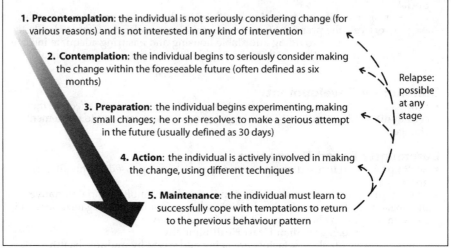

Figure 2. Stages of Change Model
Source: Prochaska JO, DeClement CC, and Norcross JC, In Search of How People Change. Applications to Addictive Behaviours. Am Psychol 47(9):1102-1114, 1992.

Risk Reduction Strategies
- **risk reduction:** lower the risk to health without eliminating it, e.g. avoid sun, exercise; eat healthy to lower risk of cancer
- **harm reduction:** tolerance of some degree of risk behavior, while aiming to minimize the adverse outcomes associated with these behaviors, e.g. needle exchange programs for intravenous drug abusers to minimize exchange of blood-borne infections

Innovation-Diffusion Theory
- theory that describes the process by which health promotion efforts spread in populations
- aims to identify the most effective methods of health promotion within a population
- **Roger's diffusion theory** illustrates the following hierarchy within populations:
    1. early adapters (community leaders)
    2. early majority
    3. late majority group
    4. late adapters
- characteristics of **innovations** that influence adaptability:
    - simple
    - workable
    - reversible
    - flexible
    - advantageous
    - cost effective
    - low risk
    - compatible with value systems

Measurements of Health and Disease in a Population

Life Expectancy
- the average number of years that an individual will live
- usually qualified by country, gender and age

Crude Death Rate
- mortality rate from all causes of death per 1,000 population

Standardized Mortality Rate
- the ratio of the observed (actual) number of deaths to the expected number of deaths for a group (e.g. age, race, gender, etc.)
- useful for comparing populations that are significantly different in some aspect (e.g. the causes of death in developing and developed world countries)

Potential Years of Life Lost (PYLL)
- the difference between the actual age of death and a standard age (e.g. 70 or 75)
- heavier weight is given to deaths that cause early mortality
- males are more likely to die at younger ages, due to unintentional injuries; therefore, PYLL is much higher for males than for females

Infant Mortality Rate (IMR)
- number of deaths among children under 1 year of age reported during a given time period divided by the number of live births reported during the same time period and expressed per 1,000 live births

Maternal Mortality Rate (MMR)
- annual number of deaths of women during pregnancy and due to puerperal causes per 100,000 live births

Proportional Mortality Ratio (PMR)
- proportion of deaths in a specified population over a given period of time attributable to a specific cause. Each cause is expressed as a percentage of all deaths, with the sum of all causes adding to 100%
- these proportions are not mortality rates, as the denominator is all deaths and not the specific population in which the deaths occurred

Disability Adjusted Life Year (DALY)
- quantitative indicator of the burden of disease that reflects the total amount of healthy life lost. Includes loss from premature mortality or loss due to a degree of disability over a specific period of time; these disabilities can be physical or mental
- two purposes:
    1. measure the burden of disease
    2. increase the budget allocative efficiency by identifying health interventions that will purchase the largest improvement in health

Quality Adjusted Life Year (QALY)
- a value from 0 to 1 assigned to a year of life adjusted for its quality. A year in perfect health is considered equal to 1 QALY. The value of a year in ill health would be discounted

For additional rate calculations, see *Outbreak of Infectious Diseases, PH18*

Epidemiology

Definitions

Population
- a collection of individuals who share a common trait

Sample
- a selection of individuals from a population or set of possible observations
- types:
    - random - all are equally likely to be selected
    - systematic - an algorithm is used to randomly select a subset
    - stratified - separate representation of more than one subgroup
    - cluster - grouped in space/time to reduce costs
    - convenience - non-random

Sample Size
- sample size contributes to the statistical precision of the estimate
- increasing the sample size decreases the probability of type I and type II error

Sampling Bias
- selection of a sample that does not truly represent the population
- sampling procedures should be chosen to prevent or minimize bias

Bias
- non-random error leading to a deviation of inferences or results from the truth
- any trend in the collection, analysis, interpretation, publication or review of data that can lead to conclusions that are systematically different from the truth

- **lead-time**: time between early diagnosis with screening and when diagnosis would have been made without screening
- **lead-time bias**: over-estimation of survival when the estimate is made from the time of actual diagnosis, instead of the time when the disease would have been diagnosed without screening
- **incidence-prevalence bias**: when prevalent cases include long-term survivors who have a better prognosis than incident cases
- **length time bias**: overestimation of the survival time due to the sampling of prevalent as opposed to incident cases. Selection of prevalent cases will favour the over-inclusion of longer-living cases rather than newly-diagnosed incident cases, some of whom may have short survival times

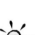

E ⟶ D

CF

Interrelation between exposure (E), disease (D) and confounding factors (CF).

Confounder
- a variable that is related to both the exposure and outcome but is not measured or is not distributed equally between groups
- distorts the apparent effect of an exposure or risk because it is not logically possible to separate the contribution of a single causal factor to an effect, e.g. smoking and alcohol with head and neck cancer

Prevalence
- total number of cases in a population over a defined period of time
- two forms of prevalence
  - **point prevalence**: attempts to measure the frequency of all disease at one specific point in time, therefore knowledge of the time of onset of disease is not required
  - **period prevalence**: measure constructed from prevalence at a point in time, plus new cases and recurrences over a defined period of time
- depends on the incidence rate and the duration of disease from onset to termination
- favours the inclusion of chronic over acute cases and therefore presents a biased picture of the disease
- prevalence studies are cross-sectional and cannot be used for causal inferences
- prevalence figures are useful for determining the extent of a disease and can aid in the rational planning of facilities and services

Incidence and Prevalence

$$\text{Incidence} = \frac{\text{number of new cases of disease in a time interval}}{\text{total population at risk}} \times [\text{per unit population (e.g. 100,000)}]$$
(measures the rate of new infections)

$$\text{Prevalence} = \frac{\text{number of existing cases of disease at a point in time}}{\text{total population}} \times [\text{per unit population (e.g. 100,000)}]$$
(measures the disease at a point in time)

Standardization
- adjustment made to the crude rate of a health-related event in a specific population when compared to a "standard" population
- standard population is one with a fixed number of persons in each age and sex group, e.g. the 1991 census data for Canada using 5 year age groups for males and females
- adjustment can be made on the basis of any characteristics of a population
- standardization prevents bias which could be made by comparing crude rates from two dissimilar populations, e.g. crude death rates between decades are not comparable as the population age distribution has changed with time

Pre-test Probability
- an estimate of the likelihood a particular patient has a given disease based on known factors

Post-test Probability
- a revision of the probability of disease after a patient has been interviewed and examined. The calculation process can be more explicit using results from epidemiologic studies, knowledge of the accuracy of tests and Bayes' theorem
- the post-test probability from clinical examination is the basis of consideration when ordering diagnostic tests or imaging studies. After each iteration the resultant post-test probability becomes the pre-test probability when considering new investigations

Intention-To-Treat
- a strategy for analyzing data in which all participants are included in the group to which they were assigned, whether or not they completed the requirements of that group. This is to limit the bias introduced by issues of compliance and to simulate real world situations in which not all patients comply

Relative Risk (RR)
- ratio of the incidence of a health outcome among the exposed population to the incidence of the health outcome in the non-exposed population

Attributable Risk (AR)

- rate of a health outcome attributable to a hypothetical risk factor for that outcome
- [incidence in exposed population] - [incidence in non-exposed]
- attributable risk assumes causation

Odds Ratio (OR)

- ratio of the odds of exposure to a hypothetical risk factor among cases to the odds of exposure among non-cases
- can be interpreted as the ratio of the odds of developing the outcome (i.e. disease) among those exposed to the hypothetical risk factor to those who are not exposed
- OR approximates RR when the prevalence of disease in the population is low

Source: Last J. M. *A Dictionary of Epidemiology*, 4th ed. Oxford University Press. 2001

		Disease	
		Present	**Absent**
Test result	**Positive**	TP	FP
	Negative	FN	TN

TP = True Positive   **TN = True Negative**   **FP = False Positive**   **FN = False Negative**

Sensitivity: proportion of people with disease who have a positive test $\dfrac{TP}{TP + FN}$

Specificity: proportion of people without disease who have a negative test $\dfrac{TN}{TN + FP}$

Likelihood ratio (LR): likelihood that a given test result would be expected in a patient with disease compared with the likelihood that that same result would be expected in a patient without disease. LR+ indicates how much to increase the probability of disease if the test is positive, while LR- indicates how much to decrease it if the test is negative

$$LR+ = \frac{Sensitivity}{1 - Specificity} = \frac{[TP/(TP + FN)]}{[FP/(TN + FP)]} \qquad LR- = \frac{1 - Sensitivity}{Specificity} = \frac{[FN/(TP + FN)]}{[TN/(TN + FP)]}$$

Positive predictive value (PPV): proportion of people with a positive test who have the disease
Negative predictive value (NPV): proportion of people with a negative test who are free of disease

$$PPV = \frac{TP}{TP + FP} \qquad NPV = \frac{TN}{TN + FN}$$

$$Pre\text{-}test\ odds = \frac{prevalence}{1 - prevalence}$$

$$Post\text{-}test\ odds = pretest\ odds \times LR \qquad Post\text{-}test\ probability = \frac{post\text{-}test\ odds}{post\text{-}test\ odds + 1}$$

$$Relative\ Risk\ (RR) = PPV/(1\text{-}NPV) = \frac{TP}{TP + FP} \div \frac{FN}{TN + FN} \qquad Attributable\ risk = PPV - (1 - NPV) = \frac{TP}{TP + FP} - \frac{FN}{TN + FN}$$

Figure 3. Clinical Epidemiology Equations

SPIN: use a **sp**ecific test to rule **in** a hypothesis. Note that specific tests have very few false positives. If you get a positive test, you can count on it being a true positive.
SNOUT: use a **sen**sitive test to rule **out** a hypothesis. Note that sensitive tests have very few false negatives. If you get a negative test, you can count on it being a true negative.

Sensitivity and specificity are characteristics of the test

LR depends on the test characteristics, not the prevalence

PPV and NPV depend on the prevalence of the disease in the population

	Disease (e.g. lung CA)		
	Present	**Absent**	**Total**
Exposure (e.g. smoking) **Present**	A	B	A + B
Absent	C	D	C + D
Total	A + C	B + D	A + B + C + D

Case-Control Study

odds ratio (OR) $= \dfrac{A}{B} \div \dfrac{C}{D} = \dfrac{A \times D}{B \times C}$

Cohort Study

$\dfrac{A}{A+B}$ = incidence rate of disease in smokers $\dfrac{C}{C+D}$ = incidence rate of disease in non-smokers

relative risk (RR) $= \dfrac{A}{A+B} \div \dfrac{C}{C+D}$ attributable risk (AR) $= \dfrac{A}{A+B} - \dfrac{C}{C+D}$

Figure 4. Results Tabulation by Study Design

Types of Study Design

Observational Studies
- ecological study
- prevalence study (cross-sectional)
- case-control (retrospective)
- cohort (prospective, incidence, longitudinal)

Experimental Studies
- non-randomized control trials (e.g. allocation by clinic or other non-random basis) can be performed when randomization is not possible
- randomized controlled trial (RCT)
  - **clinical trial**: tests a treatment or laboratory test in human subjects

Ecological Study

- **observational study of an aggregate**

Subjects
- population, rather than individuals (e.g. geographic areas such as countries or census tracts)

Methods
- hypotheses generated, often providing accurate descriptions of the average exposure or risk of disease for a population

Advantages
- quick, easy to do, makes use of readily available data

Disadvantages
- cannot be used for direct assessment of causal relationships because adequate control of all confounding variables cannot be achieved
- cannot infer about an individual in the population; this is an ecological fallacy
  - e.g. an ecological study may show that France has a higher rate of red wine consumption and a lower rate of death from cardiovascular (CVS) causes
  - one cannot conclude that red wine drinking leads to lower risk of death from CVS disease because the individuals dying from CVS disease were not investigated for their red wine drinking habits

Prevalence Study (Cross-Sectional Study)

- status of individual with respect to presence and absence of both exposure and disease assessed at one point in time

Subjects
- a population (total or sample)

Methods
- collect information from each person at one particular time (or retrospectively from one particular time)
- tabulate the numbers in groups (i.e. by presence or absence of disease and presence or absence of a factor)
- do appropiate analysis (i.e. make 2 x 2 table and compare groups)

Advantages
- allows for determination of association between variables

Disadvantages
- does not allow for assessment of temporal relationship between variables

Case-Control Study (Retrospective)

- samples a group of people who already have a particular outcome (cases) and compares them to a similar sample group without that outcome (controls)

Subjects
- two study populations are compared: cases and controls

Methods
- retrospective
- hypothesizes that cases have had significantly more exposure to the risk factors than controls
- select all the cases of a specific disease during a specific time frame
    - cases should be representative of spectrum of clinical disease under investigation
- select control(s)
    - controls should represent the general population
- to minimize risk of bias, may select more than one control group and/or match controls to cases (i.e. age, gender)
- if a presumed risk factor is present in cases significantly more frequently than in controls, then an association exists between the risk factor and the disease (expressed as an **odds ratio**, an estimate of relative risk)

Advantages
- commonly used when disease in population is rare (less than 10% of population) due to increased efficiency
- less costly and time consuming than cohort studies

Disadvantages
- may suffer from **recall bias**: people with a disease may be more prone to recalling or believing that they were exposed to a possible causal factor than those who are free of the disease
- confounding may occur
- selection bias for controls
- only one outcome can be measured

Cohort Study
(Prospective, Incidence, Longitudinal)

- subjects are sampled and as a group are classified on the basis of presence or absence of exposure to a particular risk factor

Subjects
- population separated into cohorts
    - cohort is a group of people with a common characteristic (e.g. year of birth, place of residence, occupation, exposure to a suspected cause of disease)

Methods
- subjects are followed for a specific period of time (often years) to determine development of disease in each exposure group
- start with persons who are free of disease and follow forward for a period of time

- measure exposure to a risk factor (e.g. smoking)
- define one or more outcomes
- collect information on factors from all persons at the beginning of the study
- tabulate the number of persons who develop the disease or other measured outcomes of morbidity
- provides estimates of incidence, relative risk, attributable risk

Advantages
- can show an association between a factor and an outcome/several outcomes
- generally provides stronger evidence for causation than case-control study

Disadvantages
- by itself, cannot establish causation
- confounding common as the cohort self-selects the exposure
- cost, duration of time needed to follow cohort both high

Randomized Controlled Trial (RCT)

- **subjects are randomly assigned to two or more groups, one of which is the control group, the other group(s) receive(s) an experimental intervention**

Randomized Controlled Trial (RCT)
- 'gold standard' of studies upon which the school of Evidence Based Medicine (EBM) is founded
- provides **strongest evidence for causation**
- clinical trial tests a treatment in human subjects
- *random distribution of baseline* characteristics and treatment between groups allows prospective assessment of the effects of intervention without introducing bias:
- one group receives *intervention* under study
- one group receives *placebo* or standard therapy
- all other conditions are kept the same between groups
- the outcome is measured and the groups are compared

Subjects
- individuals

Methods
- random distribution of individuals into two or more treatment groups
- one group receives placebo or standard therapy
- one or more groups receive(s) the intervention(s) under study
- the outcome is measured and the groups are compared

Advantages
- 'gold standard' of studies, upon which the school of EBM is founded
- provides the strongest evidence for causation
- with sufficient sample size and appropriate randomization, confounding variables are eliminated

Disadvantages
- some concepts are not amenable to randomization (e.g. cannot randomize subjects to poverty/wealth or to harmful exposures such as smoking)
- costly

Considerations
A. **What is the method of randomization?**
  - is it a centralized concealed process?
  - **single-blind**: subjects do not know group assignment (intervention or placebo)
  - **double-blind**: subject and observer both unaware of group assignment
  - **triple-blind**: subject, observer, and analyst unaware of group assignment

B. **Are the groups truly randomized?**
  - are the groups balanced on demographics and other potential confounders?
  - if not, was there selection bias in group assignment?

C. **Is the follow-up of sufficient duration to assess potential harm? How many subjects have been lost to follow-up?**

D. **Are the groups treated equally except for the intervention being studied?**

E. **Are the outcomes meaningful?**

Common Statistical Tests

Z-Test (known as t-test for samples of fewer than 30 points)
• designed to test the difference between two sample means for continuous data

Chi-square Test (χ^2)
• designed to test the correspondence between a theoretical frequency distribution and an observed frequency distribution of categorical data
  ▪ e.g. if one sample of 20 patients is 30% hypertensive and another comparison group of 25 patients is 60% hypertensive, a chi-squared test can be used to determine if this variation is different than might be expected due to chance alone

Analysis of Variance (ANOVA)
• similar to the Z/t-test, but compares mean values from three or more groups simultaneously considering one or more factors
• one-way ANOVA compares 2 or more groups considering one factor
• two-way ANOVA compares 2 or more groups considering two or more factors
  ▪ e.g. the blood pressure reductions in groups that have undergone some combination of two possible interventions: an education program and on-site therapy. The options are listed in Table 3

Table 3. Example of ANOVA Combinations

	Education Program	No Education Program
Onsite Therapy	+/+	+/–
No Onsite Therapy	–/+	–/–

Regression
• **linear regression**
  ▪ a technique used to describe the relationship between two continuous variables, where one variable might be used to predict or to explain changes in the other though not necessarily causal
  ▪ assumes a linear relationship between variables
  ▪ the slope of the line of best fit can be estimated
• **logistic regression**
  ▪ requires discrete outcomes, e.g. disease or disease free
  ▪ may produce an adjusted odds ratio for individual variables

Distributions

• distribution describes the probability of events
• normal (Gaussian) or non-normal (skewed, bimodal, etc.)
• characteristics of the normal distribution
  ▪ mean = median = mode
  ▪ 67% of observations fall within one standard deviation of the mean
  ▪ 95% of observations fall within two standard deviations of the mean
• measures of central tendency
  ▪ **mean**: sum of all observations divided by total number of variables
  ▪ **median**: value at the 50th percentile, this is a better reflection of the central tendency for a skewed distribution
  ▪ **mode**: most frequently observed value in a series
• measures of dispersion
  ▪ **range**: the largest value minus the smallest value
  ▪ **variance**: a measure of the spread of data
    ◆ average squared deviation of each number from the mean of a data set
  ▪ **standard deviation**: the average distance of data points from the mean (the positive square root of variance)
• given the mean and standard deviation of a normal or binomial distribution curve, a description of the entire distribution of data is obtained

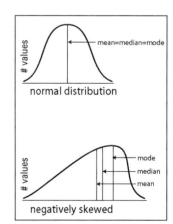

Figure 5. Distribution Curves

Critical Appraisal

Data Analysis

Statistical Hypotheses
- null (H_0)
    - no relationship exists between the two stated variables, i.e. no association between the proposed risk factor and the disease
- alternative (H_1)
    - a relationship does exists between the two stated variables

Type I Error (α Error)
- the null hypothesis is falsely rejected, i.e. declaring an effect to be present when it is not
- the probability of this error is denoted by the p-value

Type II Error (β Error)
- the null hypothesis is falsely accepted, i.e. declaring a difference/effect to be absent when it is present
    - can also be used to calculate statistical power

		Actual Situation	
		No Effect (H_0)	Effect (H_1)
Results of Statistical Analysis	No Effect	No error ($p=1-\alpha$)	Type II (β) error ($p=\beta$)
	Effect	Type I (α) error ($p=\alpha$)	No error ($p=1-\beta$)

Figure 6. Types of Error. p = probability

Power
- probability of correctly rejecting a null hypothesis when it is in fact false i.e. the probability of finding a specified difference to be statistically significant at a given p-value
- power increases with an increase in sample size
- power = $1 - \beta$, and is therefore equal to the probability of a true positive result

Statistical Significance
- the probability that the statistical association found between the variables is due to random chance alone (i.e. that there is no association)
- the preset probability is set sufficiently low that one would act on the result; frequently p=0.05
- when statistical tests result in a probability less than the preset limit the results are said to be statistically significant, i.e. p<0.05

Clinical Significance
- measure of clinical usefulness, e.g. 1 mmHg BP reduction may be statistically significant, but may not be clinically significant
- depends on factors such as cost, availability, patient compliance and side effects in addition to statistical significance

Confidence Interval (CI)
- provides a range of values within which the true population mean lies
- frequently reported as 95% CI, i.e. one can be 95% certain that the true value is within this data range
- bounded by the upper and lower confidence limits

Data
- information collected about a sample or population
- there are 3 classes of data listed with examples:
    - **discrete** - number of strokes experienced
    - **continuous** - serum cholesterol, hemoglobin, age
    - **categorical** - gender, marital status

Accuracy
- how closely a measurement approaches the true value

Reliability
- how consistent a measurement is when performed by different observers under the same conditions or by the same observer under different conditions

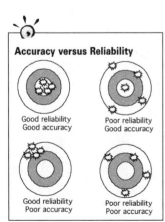

Accuracy versus Reliability

Good reliability
Good accuracy

Poor reliability
Good accuracy

Good reliability
Poor accuracy

Poor reliability
Poor accuracy

Validity
- extent to which a measurement approaches what it is designed to measure
- determined by the accuracy and reliability of a test

Effectiveness of Interventions

DEFINITIONS

Relative Risk Reduction (RRR)
- proportional reduction in rates of bad outcomes between experimental and control participants in a trial

Absolute Risk Reduction (ARR)
- absolute arithmetic difference in rates of bad outcomes between experimental and control participants in a trial
- events occur more often in control group than in experimental group

Absolute Risk Increase (ARI)
- absolute arithmetic difference in rates of bad outcomes between control and experimental participants in a trial
- events occur more often in experimental group than in control group

Number Needed to Treat (NNT)
- number of patients who need to be treated to achieve one additional favourable outcome, calculated as 1/(ARR)

Number Needed to Harm (NNH)
- number of patients who, if they received the experimental treatment, would lead to one additional patient being harmed, compared with patients who received the control treatment, calculated as 1/(ARI)

Compliance/Adherence
- degree to which a patient adheres to a treatment plan

Effectiveness, Efficacy, Efficiency
- three measurements indicating the relative value (beneficial effects vs. harmful effects) of an intervention
- **efficacy**: the extent to which a specific intervention produces a beneficial result under ideal conditions
    - ideally, based on the results of a randomized control trial (the theoretical impact)
- **effectiveness**: measures the benefit of an intervention under usual conditions of clinical care
    - considers both the efficacy of an intervention and its actual impact on the real world, taking into account access to the intervention, whether it is offered to those who can benefit from it, its proper administration, acceptance of intervention and degree of adherence to intervention
- **efficiency**: a measure of economy of an intervention with known effectiveness
    - considers the optimal use of resources (i.e. monetary, time, personnel, equipment, etc.)

Assessing Evidence

- critical appraisal is the process of systematically examining research evidence to assess validity, results and relevance before using it to inform a decision:

A. **Are the results of the study valid?**

B. **What are the results?**
    - what was the impact of the treatment effect?
    - how precise was the estimate of treatment effect?
    - what were the confidence intervals and power of the study?

C. **Will the results help me in caring for my patients?**
    - are the results clinically significant?
    - can I apply the results to my patient population?
    - were all clinically important outcomes considered?
    - are the likely treatment benefits worth the potential harm and costs?

Equations to Assess Effectiveness

CER = control group event rate
EER = experimental group event rate
RRR = (CER - EER)/CER
ARR = CER - EER
ARI = EER - CER
NNT = 1/ARR
NNH = 1/ARI

Validity
- the degree to which the outcome observed in the study can be attributed to the intervention

5 Questions About the Validity of Primary Studies
1. Were the patients *randomized*?
2. Was the *follow-up* of patients sufficiently long and complete?
3. Were all patients *analyzed in the groups* to which they were randomized?
4. Were the *groups treated equally* except for the intervention?
5. Were the patients and clinicians kept *blind* to treatment?

Other Questions to Consider
- Were the groups similar (i.e. demographics, prognostic factors) at the start of the trial?
- Were the appropriate and valid exposure and outcome measures obtained?
- Were outcome assessors aware of group allocation?
- Was contamination reported?
- Were ethical issues continuously upheld?

Causation

Criteria for causation (Sir Bradford Hill)
• general guide for causation

Other criteria to consider:
• **biological gradient:** finding a quantitative relationship between the factor and the frequency (i.e. dose response relationship)
• **consistency:** is it the same outcome with different populations or study design?
• **analogy:** do other established associations provide a model for this type of the relationship?
• **strength of association:** the frequency with which the factor is found in the disease and the frequency with which it occurs in the absence of disease
• **experimental evidence:** experiment that investigates what happens when the suspected offending agent is removed (i.e. is there improvement?)

Outbreak of Infectious Diseases

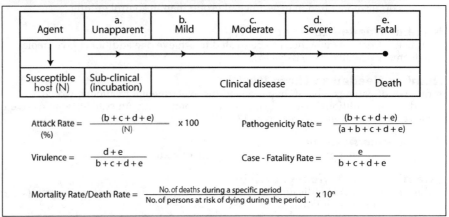

Agent	a. Unapparent	b. Mild	c. Moderate	d. Severe	e. Fatal
Susceptible host (N)	Sub-clinical (incubation)	Clinical disease			Death

$$\text{Attack Rate (\%)} = \frac{(b+c+d+e)}{(N)} \times 100 \qquad \text{Pathogenicity Rate} = \frac{(b+c+d+e)}{(a+b+c+d+e)}$$

$$\text{Virulence} = \frac{d+e}{b+c+d+e} \qquad \text{Case - Fatality Rate} = \frac{e}{b+c+d+e}$$

$$\text{Mortality Rate/Death Rate} = \frac{\text{No. of deaths during a specific period}}{\text{No. of persons at risk of dying during the period}} \times 10^{n}$$

Figure 7. Spectrum of Infectious Disease
Source: Shah CP. *Public Health and Preventative Medicine in Canada.* 5th edition. Elsevier Canada. 2003.

Definitions

Outbreak
• occurrence of new cases clearly in excess of the baseline frequency of the disease in a defined community or population over a given period of time
• synonymous with epidemic although generally considered to be an epidemic that is localized, has an acute onset or is relatively short in duration

Epidemic
• any disease, infectious or chronic, occurring at a greater frequency than usually expected in a defined community or institutional population over a given time period (i.e. excessive rate of disease)

Endemic
• constant presence of disease or infectious agent in a given geographic area or population subgroup (i.e. usual rate of disease)

Pandemic
• epidemic over a wide area, crossing international boundaries and affecting a large number of people

Attack Rate
• cumulative incidence of infection within a defined group observed during a specific period of time in an epidemic
• calculated by dividing the total number of people who develop clinical disease by the population at risk, usually expressed as a percentage (see Figure 7)

Secondary Attack Rate
- number of cases among contacts occurring within the incubation period following exposure to the primary case, in relation to the total exposed contacts
- infectiousness reflects the ease of disease transmission and is usually measured by the secondary attack rate

Pathogenicity Rate
- power of an organism to produce clinical disease in those that are affected (see Figure 7)

Virulence
- severity of the disease produced by the organism in a given host
- expressed as the ratio of the number of cases of severe and fatal infection to the total number of clinically affected (see Figure 7)

Case-Fatality Rate
- proportion of individuals contracting a disease who die as a result of that disease (see Figure 7)
- most frequently applied to a specific outbreak of acute disease in which all patients have been followed for an adequate period of time to include all attributable deaths
- must be clearly differentiated from the mortality rate

Mortality Rate/Death Rate
- estimate of the portion of the population that dies during a specified period from all causes of death (see Figure 7)

Steps to Controlling an Outbreak

1. Define the problem
- is it an outbreak?

2. Appraise existing data and institution of a surveillance system
- **case definition**: formulated from the most common symptoms or signs; definition includes the likely date of onset of illness of the first case
    - example: any person with onset of fever higher than 38.5°C and cough within past 28 days
    - laboratory confirmation of the clinical diagnosis via culture or serology is sought as soon as possible as results can define a case more precisely
- **active surveillance**: identify those who may have been exposed to the infectious agent and who fit the case definition through active efforts, including:
    - contacting emergency rooms, physicians' offices, local schools
    - obtaining records from other health units, mortality or laboratory records

3. Formulate hypotheses and implementation of initial control measures
- depends on symptoms, suspected agent, population at risk and location
- effective outbreak management includes infection control when outbreak is due to infectious agent

4. Test the hypothesis through analysis of surveillance data or special studies
- analyze raw data and generate epidemic curves (see below)

5. Draw conclusions, re-adjust hypothesis and control measures

6. Write report, make recommendations for long-term prevention and surveillance
- modify control measures to stop the outbreak
    - remove/neutralize agent (e.g. isolating residents in a facility)
    - strengthen resistance of hosts (e.g. immunization)
    - interrupt means of transmission in environment (e.g. improvements in food processing)
- communicate outbreak information to the public in an effective manner
    - provide education
    - recommend specific prevention and control strategies clearly
    - deliver a unified message, e.g. local public health department, chief officer of health

For specific examples, see "Communicable Diseases" section in: Shah CP. *Public Health and Preventive Medicine in Canada. 5th edition.* Elsevier Canada. 2003.

Steps to Controlling an Outbreak
- Surveillance
- Defining purpose
- Data collection
- Data analysis
- Interpretation
- Dissemination
- Action to prevent disease/injury

Active Surveillance
Outreach such as visits or phone calls by the public health/surveillance authority to detect unreported cases (e.g. an infection control nurse goes to the ward and reviews temperature charts to see if any patient has a nosocomial infection)

Passive Surveillance
A surveillance system where the public health/surveillance authority depends on others to submit standardized forms or other means of reporting cases (e.g. ward staff notify infection control when new cases of nosocomial infections are discovered)

Figure 8. Epidemic Curves

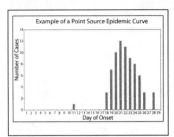

Figure 8a. Point Source Epidemic Curve

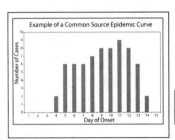

Figure 8b. Common Continuous Source Epidemic Curve

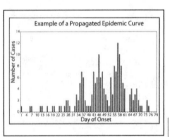

Figure 8c. Propagated Source Epidemic Curve

Epidemic Curves

Epidemic Curve
- generated from data collected in active surveillance
- usually a frequency histogram, with the number of cases plotted on the vertical axis and their dates or times of onset along the horizontal axis
- curve can indicate whether the epidemic (outbreak) has a common source or whether it is propagated

Common-Source Epidemics
- people become ill because of exposure to a single (common) source of infection
- **point source epidemic:** exposure is brief and essentially simultaneous (see Figure 8a)
- **extended source epidemic:** exposure lasts for a period of days to weeks
    - extended exposure can be continuous (no irregular peaks, see Figure 8b) or intermittent (irregularly spaced peaks)

Propagated Epidemic
- begins with only a few exposed persons but is maintained by person-to-person transmission (e.g. measles/influenza); epidemic curve shows a series of peaks (see Figure 8c)

Environmental Health

Definition
- study of conditions in the natural and human-made environment that influence human health and well-being
- environmental exposures
    - four main reservoirs: air, food, water and soil
    - three main routes: inhalation, ingestion or absorption (skin)
- usually divided into two main settings:
    - workplace: often high level exposure in healthy adults (see *Occupational Health* section, PH23)
    - non-workplace: generally low level but chronic exposure; population at risk includes extremes of age, developing fetuses, and ill or immunocompromised

Environmental Health Jurisdiction

Public Health Unit
- enforcement of water and food safety regulations (including restaurant food safety)
- sanitation
- assessment of local environmental risks
- monitoring and follow-up of reportable diseases

Municipal Government
- garbage disposal
- recycling

Provincial and Territorial Government
- water and air quality standards
- industrial emission regulation
- toxic waste disposal

Federal Government
- designating and regulating toxic substances
- regulating food products (e.g. Health Canada)
- setting policy for pollutants that can travel across provincial boundaries

International
- multilateral agreements (e.g. Kyoto Protocol, UN Convention on Climate Change)

Hazard Identification

- two major approaches
    - toxicological: examines the adverse effects of poisons on animals (including humans), has the potential to identify health hazards before humans become ill
    - epidemiological: provides information about health hazards in humans after humans have become ill

Air

Physical Contaminants
- sound waves
- ionizing radiation
    - radon is naturally produced by soil containing uranium or radium, can contaminate indoor air and is associated with a small proportion of lung cancers
    - ultraviolet radiation is increasing due to ozone layer destruction caused by chlorofluorocarbons (CFCs), and increases risk of skin cancer
    - alpha-particles are larger and damage the skin and bronchial lining (airway irritation)
    - beta-particles are smaller and cause deeper damage (alveoli)
- non-ionizing radiation
    - electromagnetic fields

Chemical Contaminants
- ground-level ozone
    - main component of smog
    - worsens asthma, irritates upper airway
    - implicated in skin cancer, cataracts and depressed immune function
    - levels increasing in Canadian cities
- carbon monoxide (fossil fuel related)
    - combustion byproduct
    - invisible, odourless gas
    - aggravates cardiac disease at low levels
    - headache, nausea, dizziness at moderate level
    - fatal at elevated concentrations
    - levels decreasing in Canadian cities
- sulphur dioxide (fossil fuel related), nitrogen oxides
    - contribute to acid rain
    - exacerbate breathing difficulties
    - levels decreasing in Canadian cities
- organic compounds
    - benzene, methylene chloride, tetrachloroethylene, among others
    - variety of health effects at high levels, e.g. benzene is a known carcinogen
    - tend to be fat soluble, easily absorbed through skin and difficult to excrete
- heavy metals
    - e.g. nickel, cadmium, chromium
    - present in industrial emissions
    - variety of health effects, upper airway disease, asthma, decreased lung function
- second hand tobacco smoke
    - respiratory problems, increase risk of lung cancer

Biological Contaminants
- particulates
    - pollen, fungal spores, aerosols
    - associated with decreased lung function, asthma, upper airway irritation
    - levels decreasing in Canadian cities
- biological agents
    - moulds thrive in moist areas; 10-15% of the population allergic
    - bacteria survive as spores and aerosols, can be distributed through ventilation systems (e.g. *Legionella*)
    - dust mites and pollens can trigger upper and lower-airway symptoms
        - dust mites are year-round and concentrate indoors
        - pollen is seasonal and outdoors

Climate Change
- anthropogenic greenhouse gas emissions (e.g. carbon dioxide, methane, etc.) leading to adverse changes in the global environment
    - increased extreme weather conditions (e.g. floods, hurricanes, heat waves)
    - increased distribution of vectors of disease (e.g. mosquitoes & malaria)
    - increased malnutrition from crop failures
    - increased diarrhoeal diseases

Water

Biological Contaminants
- mostly due to human and animal waste
- aboriginal Canadians, rural Canadians at higher risk
- bacteria: *Escherichia coli* (e.g. Walkerton, ON), *Salmonella, Pseudomonas, Shigella*
- protozoa: *Giardia*, cryptosporidium (e.g. North Battleford, SK)

Chemical/Industrial Contaminants
- chlorination by-products (e.g. chloroform can cause cancer at high levels)
- volatile organic compounds, heavy metals, pesticides and other industrial waste products can be present in groundwater
- fluoride at high levels (greater than that of municipal fluoridation) can cause skeletal fluorosis

Soil

- contamination sources: rupture of underground storage tanks, use of pesticides and herbicides, percolation of contaminated water runoffs, leaching of wastes from landfills, dust from smelting and coal burning power plants, direct discharge of industrial wastes, lead deposition, leakage of transformers
- most common chemicals: petroleum hydrocarbons, solvents, lead, pesticides, motor oil, other industrial waste products
- health effects:
    - infants and toddlers at highest risk of exposure
    - dependent on contaminant: leukemia, kidney damage, liver toxicity, neuromuscular blockade, developmental damage to the brain and nervous system, skin rash, eye irritation, headache, nausea, fatigue

Food

Table 4. Comparison of Select Biological Contaminants

	Source	Effects on human health
Salmonella	Raw eggs, poultry, meat	GI symptoms
Campylobacter	Raw poultry, raw milk	Joint pain GI symptoms
Escherichia coli	Various including meat, sprouts Primarily undercooked hamburger	Watery or bloody diarrhea Hemolytic uremic syndrome (esp. children)
Listeria monocytogenes	Unpasteurized cheeses, prepared salads, cold cuts	Listeriosis: nausea, vomiting, fever, headache, rarely meningitis or encephalitis
Clostridium botulinim	Unpasteurized honey, canned foods	Dizziness, weakness, respiratory failure GI symptoms: thirst, nausea, constipation
BSE	Beef and beef products	Creutzfeldt-Jakob Disease
Avian influenza	Poultry, usually agricultural exposure	Spectrum from mild flu-like illness to death

- other biological food contaminants include:
    - viruses
    - mould toxins (e.g. aflatoxin→liver cancer)
    - parasites (e.g. toxoplasmosis, tapeworm)
    - paralytic and shellfish poisoning (rare)
    - genetically modified organisms (GMO) - controversial

Chemical Contaminants
- many persistent organic pollutants are fat soluble so they "bio-accumulate" with increasing amount of the contaminant in organisms higher up the food chain
- drugs (antibiotics, hormones)
    - emerging field of study, organic pollutants can have hormonal effects and cause endocrine disruption
- alternate herbal medications
- food additives and preservatives
    - nitrites can be converted to carcinogenic nitrosamines; highest in cured meats
    - sulphites commonly used as preservatives; associated with sulphite allergy (hives, nausea, shock) rarely

- pesticide residues
    - older pesticides (i.e. DDT) have considerable human health effects
    - many older pesticides still being used in countries where restrictions are less strict than in Canada
    - current debate about DDT use in malaria-endemic countries, weighing risks of DDT vs. risks of malaria
- polychlorinated biphenyls (PCBs)
    - levels continue to increase in the Arctic
    - effects (severe acne, numbness, muscle spasm, bronchitis) much more likely to be seen in occupationally exposed individuals than in the general population
- dioxins and furans
    - levels highest in fish and marine mammals, also present in breast milk
    - can cause immunosuppression, liver disease, respiratory disease

Heavy Metal Toxicity

Background
- 100+ elements, 80 are metals, <30 have described toxic effects
- exposure may be acute or chronic, local or systemic
- after exposure, superabundant metals bind to proteins, changing their enzymatic activity, leading to diffuse disease manifestations

At-risk Groups
- children: hand-to-mouth, incomplete BBB
- pregnant women and developing foetus: heavy metals cross placenta, mothers release heavy metal stores at times of calcium stress e.g. pregnancy
- adults (higher threshold): occupational, developing countries, hobbies

Etiology
- iatrogenic (e.g. gold, gallium, lithium, aluminum)
- inhalation (e.g. zinc oxide, lead gasoline fumes)
- ingestion (e.g. lead paint, mercury in fish, folk remedies)
- industry (e.g. methyl mercury, Minamata disease)

Treatment
- generalized workup – symptoms are usually wide-ranging and non-specific
- chelation therapy (e.g. dimercaprol)

Occupational Health

- occupational health is the maintenance and promotion of health in the work environment
- 920 workplace fatalities (more deaths than due to HIV/AIDS) and 373,216 lost time injuries in Canada in 2001
- 5,703 fatal work injuries in the United States in 2006; rate = 3.9 per 100,000 workers
- occupational health services include physicians, nurses, engineers, ergonomists, safety officers, physicists, technicians and others
- services encompass health promotion and protection (primary prevention), disease prevention (secondary prevention) and treatment and rehabilitation (tertiary prevention)
- general bias towards reporting occupational injuries versus occupational disease, as occupational disease is harder to identify

Health Promotion and Protection

- take action in the workplace so the worker is protected from injury or illness
    - identifying workplace hazards (e.g. through material safety data sheets (MSDS))
    - assessing risk
    - reducing exposure
        - **source**: substituting a less toxic chemical
        - **path**: enclosing a source of noise in a sound-proof room
        - **worker**: personal protection equipment (e.g. reflective vests, helmets)
        - worker education (e.g. emergency protocols, material safety education)
        - rotation of workers: decrease exposure for each worker but more workers exposed

Reducing Exposure in the Workplace
Source - engineering controls
Path - administrative/work practices
Worker - personal protective equipment

Disease Prevention

- monitor workers' health to prevent the development of disease
- examples:
  - periodic examinations to facilitate pre-symptomatic diagnosis (e.g. screening for lead exposure)
  - substance abuse screening where performance impairment is suspected

Treatment and Rehabilitation

- treat injury or illness with safe return to the workplace
- may require rehabilitation, retraining, change in job duties and/or workers' compensation involvement

Legislation

- universal across Canada for corporate responsibility in the workplace: due diligence, application of WHMIS, existence of joint health and safety committees in the workplace with representatives from workers and management
- jurisdiction in Canada is provincial (90% of Canadian workers), except for 16 federally regulated industries (e.g. airports, banks, highway transport) under the *Canada Labour Code*
- Ontario's *Occupational Health and Safety Act*
  - sets out rights of workers and duties of employers, procedures for dealing with workplace hazards and law enforcement
  - workers have the right to:
    - **participate** (e.g. have representatives on joint health and safety committees)
    - **know** (e.g. be trained and have information about workplace hazards)
    - **refuse work** (e.g. workers can decline tasks they feel are overly dangerous)
    - **stop work** (e.g. 'certified' workers can halt work they feel is dangerous to other workers)
  - employers must take precautions to protect the health and safety of employees and investigate concerns
  - enforced by Ministry of Labour via inspectors
- *Health Protection and Promotion Act* (HPPA)
  - medical officer of health has right to enter and shut down workplace
  - enforced by Ministry of Health

Ontario's *Workplace Safety and Insurance Act*

- establishes Workplace Safety and Insurance Board (WSIB), an **autonomous** government agency which oversees workplace safety training and administers insurance for workers and employers (previously Workers' Compensation Board, WCB)
- WSIB decides benefits for workers, which may include reimbursement for
  - loss of earned income
  - non-economic loss (e.g. physical, functional or psychological loss extending beyond the workplace)
  - loss of retirement income
  - health care expenses (e.g. first-aid, medical treatment)
  - survivor benefits (e.g. dependents and spouses can receive benefits)
- employers pay for costs (e.g. no government funding)
- no-fault insurance (e.g. worker has no right to sue the employer) in return for guaranteed compensation for accepted claims
- negligence is not considered a factor
- physicians are required to provide the WSIB with information about a worker's health without a medical waiver once a claim is made

Assessing Occupational Health and Safety

- symptoms of disease and job-related injuries
- work description including occupational profile
- prior or current exposure to dusts, chemicals, solvents, radiation, biological agents, loud noise, mechanical or psychosocial stressors
- review of relevant workplace material safety data sheets (ask patient to provide these)
- temporal relationship between symptoms and exposure
- description of other environments (home, neighbourhood)
- hobbies
- occupation of family members

Occupational Hazards

Physical

- general trauma: fractures, lacerations
- noise/hearing loss
- temperature (heat cramps, heat exhaustion, heat stroke)
- air pressure (barotraumas, decompression sickness)
- ergonomic
  - repetitive use/overuse injuries, excessive force, awkward postures, poorly designed physical work environment
  - may cause tenosynovitis, bursitis, carpal tunnel syndrome
- radiation
  - non-ionizing: UV, infrared
  - ionizing: x-rays, gamma rays, etc.
- electricity

Chemical

- organic solvents (e.g. benzene, methyl alcohol; most toxic is carbon tetrachloride)
- mineral dusts (e.g. silica leads to silicosis and predisposition to TB, asbestos leads to diffuse fibrosis, coal leads to pneumoconiosis)
- heavy metals (e.g. nickel, cadmium, mercury, lead)
  - lead is ubiquitous and can cause severe disability
- gases (sulphur dioxide, carbon monoxide, silo filler's disease, halogen gas)
- second hand smoke – causal factor for lung cancer, lung disease, heart disease, asthma exacerbations; may be linked to miscarriage. Exposure restricted in most municipal, provincial and federal jurisdictions
- skin diseases are the major portion of compensations (e.g. contact dermatitis, occupational acne, pigmentation disorders)

Biological

- exposure to bacteria, viruses, fungi, protozoa, rickettsia
- blood should be considered a potentially toxic substance due to blood-borne infectious diseases (e.g. HIV, hepatitis B)

Psychosocial Stresses

- due to workload, responsibility, fear of job loss, geographical isolation, shift work, harassment (sexual/non-sexual)
- incurs high cost from absenteeism, poor productivity, mental illness (e.g. post-traumatic stress disorder)

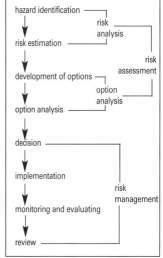

Figure 9. Risk Assessment and Management

Appendix 1. Reportable Diseases

In general, diseases are reportable to public health units if they present the threat of an outbreak (e.g. cholera, salmonella), if they present a significant threat to individuals or a subset of the population (e.g. Lassa Fever, congenital rubella, respiratory diseases in institutions), or if they are preventable with immunization (e.g. polio, diphtheria) or education and contact tracing (e.g. gonorrhoea, TB). Physicians should also report unlisted diseases that appear in clusters (e.g. severe respiratory illness later identified as SARS, C. difficile in nursing homes). The following list is based on the reportable diseases in Ontario for 2008.

Acquired Immunodeficiency Syndrome (AIDS)
Amebiasis
Anthrax

Botulism
Brucellosis

Campylobacter enteritis
Chancroid
Chickenpox (Varicella)
Chlamydia trachomatis infections
Cholera
Cryptosporidiosis
Cyclosporiasis
Cytomegalovirus infection, congenital

Diphtheria

Encephalitis, including,
   i.   Primary, viral
   ii. Post-infectious
   iii. Vaccine-related
   iv. Subacute sclerosing panencephalitis
   v. Unspecified

Food poisoning, all causes

Gastroenteritis, institutional outbreaks
Giardiasis, except asymptomatic cases
Gonorrhoea
Group A Streptococcal disease, invasive
Group B Streptococcal disease, neonatal

Haemophilus influenzae b disease, invasive
Hantavirus pulmonary syndrome
Hemorrhagic fevers, including,
   i.   Ebola virus disease
   ii. Marburg virus disease
   iii. Other viral causes
Hepatitis, viral,
   i.   Hepatitis A
   ii. Hepatitis B
   iii. Hepatitis C
   iv. Hepatitis D (Delta hepatitis)
Herpes, neonatal

Influenza

Lassa Fever
Legionellosis
Leprosy
Listeriosis
Lyme Disease

Malaria
Measles
Meningitis, acute,
   i.   Bacterial
   ii. Viral
   iii. Other
Meningococcal disease, invasive
Mumps

Ophthalmia neonatorum

Paratyphoid Fever
Pertussis (Whooping Cough)
Plague
Pneumococcal disease, invasive
Poliomyelitis, acute
Psittacosis/Ornithosis

Q Fever

Rabies
Respiratory infection outbreaks in institutions
Rubella
Rubella, congenital syndrome

Salmonellosis
Severe Acute Respiratory Syndrome (SARS)
Shigellosis
Smallpox
Syphilis

Tetanus
Transmissible Spongiform Encephalopathy, including,
   i.   Creutzfeldt-Jakob Disease, all types
   ii. Gerstmann-Sträussler-Scheinker Syndrome
   iii. Fatal Familial Insomnia
   iv. Kuru
Trichinosis
Tuberculosis
Tularemia
Typhoid Fever

Verotoxin-producing E. coli infection indicator conditions, including Hemolytic Uremic Syndrome (HUS)

West Nile Virus illness

Yellow Fever
Yersiniosis

Source: Health Protection and Promotion Act, O. Reg. 559/91, amended to O. Reg. 49/07.
For updates refer to: http://www.canlii.org/on/laws/regu/1991r.559/index.html

Appendix 2. Global Health Statistics

Region	Country	Demographics		Healthcare Resources & Spending					Mortality & Burden of Disease						
		Gross national Income per capita (PPP intl. $)	Population annual Growth rate (%)	Healthcare Resources (density per 10,000 population)			Per capita health expenditures		Life expectancy (years)		Mortality rate (per 1000 live births)		Years of life lost to (%)		
				Hospital beds	Nurses & Midwives	Physicians	(PPP intl. $)	(US$)	Total	Healthy	Infant	Under-5	Communicable diseases	Injuries	Non-communicable diseases
		2006	2006	2000-2006	1998-2006	1997-2006	2005	2005	2006	2003	2006	2006	2002	2002	2002
Sub-Saharan Africa	Congo, DR	270	3.2	11	5	1	17	5	47	37	129	205	82	11	7
	Kenya	1470	2.6	14	12	1	95	24	53	44	79	121	81	8	11
	Nigeria	1410	2.4	5	17	3	45	27	48	42	99	191	83	7	10
	Sierra Leone	610	2.8	4	5	<1.0	41	8	40	29	159	269	86	8	6
	Uganda	880	3.2	11	7	<1.0	130	22	50	43	78	134	84	8	8
Americas	Argentina	11670	1	41	8	30	1529	484	75	65	14	17	18	17	66
	Bolivia	3810	1.9	11	21	12	206	73	66	54	50	61	55	11	34
	Canada	**36280**	**0.9**	**34**	**101**	**19**	**3452**	**3463**	**81**	**72**	**5**	**6**	**6**	**15**	**80**
	Cuba		0.1	49	74	59	333	310	78	68	5	7	10	17	73
	Haiti	1070	1.6	8	1	3	71	28	61	44	60	80	84	2	15
	Jamaica	7050	0.6	17	17	9	210	170	72	65	26	32	30	4	66
	Mexico	11990	1	10	9	20	725	474	74	65	29	35	27	19	54
	U.S.A	44070	1	32	94	26	6347	6347	78	69	7	8	9	17	75
E. Mediterranean	Egypt	4940	1.8	22	34	24	279	78	68	59	29	35	32	8	61
	Pakistan	2410	1.8	12	5	8	49	15	63	53	78	97	70	8	21
	Tunisia	6490	1.1	19	29	13	477	158	72	62	19	23	18	19	63
Europe	France	32240	0.6	73	80	34	3406	3926	81	72	4	5	6	16	78
	Germany	32680	0	83	80	34	3250	3628	80	72	4	5	5	10	86
	Norway	50070	0.6	41	162	38	4331	5942	80	72	3	4	5	12	83
	Russia	12740	-0.5	97	85	43	561	277	66	58	10	13	8	28	64
	U.K.	33650	0.4	39	128	23	2598	3065	79	71	5	6	10	9	82
SE Asia	India	2460	1.5		13	6	100	36	63	53	57	76	58	13	29
	Thailand	7440	0.7		28	4	323	98	72	60	7	8	43	17	40
Western Pacific	Australia	33940	1.1	40	97	25	3001	3181	82	73	5	6	5	17	77
	China	4660	0.6	22	10	14	315	81	73	64	20	24	23	21	56
	Japan	32840	0	141	95	21	2474	2908	83	75	3	4	8	16	76

Notes

PS Psychiatry

Sivan Durbin, Katie Ker and Shail Rawal, chapter editors
Justine Chan and Angela Ho, associate editors
Billie Au, EBM editor
Dr. Jodi Lofchy, staff editor

Diagnostic Criteria reprinted with permission from the Diagnostic and Statistical Manual of Mental Disorders, Fourth Edition, Text Revision. © 2000 American Psychiatric Association.

The Psychiatric Assessment

History

Identifying Data
- name, sex, age, ethnicity, marital status, religion, occupation, education, living situation, referral source

Reliability of Patient as a Historian
- may need collateral source for history (e.g. parent, teacher) if patient unable/unwilling to cooperate

Chief Complaint
- in patient's own words
- duration, previous history of disorder or treatment

History of Present Illness
- reason for seeking help (that day), current symptoms (onset, duration and course), stressors, supports, functional status, relevant associated symptoms (pertinent positives and negatives)

Psychiatric Functional Inquiry
- mood: depressed, manic
- anxiety: worries, obsessions, compulsions, panic attacks, phobias
- psychosis: hallucinations, delusions, thought form disorders
- suicide/homicide: ideation, plan, history of attempts
- organic: EtOH/drug use or withdrawal, illness, dementia

Past Psychiatric History
- all previous psychiatric diagnoses, psychiatric contacts, treatments (pharmacological and non-pharmacological) and hospitalizations
- also include past suicide attempts, substance use/abuse, and legal problems

Past Medical/Surgical History
- all medical, surgical, neurological (e.g. head trauma, seizures), and psychosomatic illnesses
- medications, allergies

Family Psychiatric/Medical History
- family members: ages, occupations, personalities, medical or genetic illnesses and treatments, relationships with parents/siblings
- family psychiatric history: any past or current psychiatric illnesses and hospitalizations, suicide, depression, substance abuse, history of "nervous breakdown/bad nerves", forensic history, any past treatment by psychiatrist or other therapist

Past Personal History
- prenatal and perinatal history (desired pregnancy or not, maternal and fetal health, domestic violence, maternal substance use, complications of pregnancy/delivery)
- early childhood to age 3 (developmental milestones, activity/attention level, family stability, attachment figures)
- middle childhood to age 11 (school performance, peer relationships, fire-setting, stealing, incontinence)
- late childhood to adolescence (drug/EtOH, legal problems, peer and family relationships)
- adulthood (education, occupations, relationships)
- psychosexual history (paraphilias, gender roles, sexual abuse, sexual dysfunction)
- personality before current illness, recent changes in personality

Mental Status Exam (MSE)

General Appearance and Behaviour
- dress, grooming, posture, gait, physical characteristics, body habitus, apparent vs. chronological age, facial expression (e.g. sad, suspicious)
- psychomotor activity (agitation, retardation), abnormal movements or lack thereof (tremors, akathisia, tardive dyskinesia, paralysis), attention level and eye contact, attitude toward examiner (ability to interact, level of cooperation)

The MSE is analogous to the physical exam. It focuses on current signs, symptoms, affect, behaviour and cognition.

Speech
- rate (e.g. pressured, slowed), rhythm/fluency, volume, tone, articulation, quantity, spontaneity

Mood and Affect
- mood – subjective emotional state; in patient's own words
- affect – objective emotional state; described in terms of quality (euthymic, depressed, elevated, anxious), range (full, restricted, blunted, flat), stability (fixed, labile), mood congruence, appropriateness, intensity

Thought Process
- coherence – coherent, incoherent
- logic – logical, illogical
- stream
  - goal-directed
  - circumstantiality – speech that is indirect and delayed in reaching its goal; eventually comes back to the point
  - tangentiality – speech is oblique or irrelevant; does not come back to the original point
  - loosening of associations – illogical shifting between topics
  - flight of ideas – quickly skipping from one idea to another where the ideas are marginally connected; associated with mania
  - word salad – jumble of words lacking meaning or logical coherence
- perseveration – repetition of the same verbal or motor response to stimuli
- echolalia – repetition of phrases or words spoken by someone else
- thought blocking – sudden cessation of flow of thought and speech
- clang associations – speech based on sound such as rhyming or punning
- neologism – use of novel words or of existing words in a novel fashion

Thought Content
- suicidal ideation/homicidal ideation
  - low – fleeting thoughts, no formulated plan, no intent
  - intermediate – more frequent ideation, well-formulated plan, no active intent
  - high – persistent ideation and profound hopelessness/anger, well-formulated plan and active intent, believes suicide/homicide is the only helpful option available
- obsession – recurrent and persistent thought, impulse or image which is intrusive or inappropriate
  - cannot be stopped by logic or reason
  - causes marked anxiety and distress
  - common themes: contamination, orderliness, sexual, pathological doubt/worry/guilt
- pre-occupations, ruminations (reflections/thoughts at length)
- overvalued ideas – unusual/odd beliefs that are not of delusional proportions
- magical thinking – belief that thinking something will make it happen; normal in kids
- ideas of reference – similar to delusion of reference but the reality of the belief is questioned
- delusion – a fixed false belief that is out of keeping with a person's cultural or religious background and is firmly held despite incontrovertible proof to the contrary
- thought insertion/withdrawal/broadcasting, delusions of control – belief that one's thoughts/actions are controlled by some external source

Perception
- hallucination – sensory perception in the absence of external stimuli that is similar in quality to a true perception; auditory (most common), visual, gustatory, olfactory, tactile
- illusion – misperception of a real external stimulus
- depersonalization – change in self-awareness such that the person feels unreal, detached from his or her body, and/or unable to feel emotion
- derealization – feeling that the world/outer environment is unreal

Cognition
- level of consciousness
- orientation - time, place, person
- memory - immediate, recent, remote
- global evaluation of intellect - below average, average, above average
- intellectual functions - attention, concentration, calculation, abstraction (proverb interpretation, similarities test), language, communication

Mental Status Exam
"ASEPTIC"
Appearance and behaviour
Speech
Emotion (mood and affect)
Perception
Thought content and process
Insight and judgment
Cognition

Spectrum of Affect
Full > Restricted > Blunted > Flat

There is poor correlation between clinical impression of suicide risk and frequency of attempts.

Delusions
- Persecutory – belief that others are trying to cause harm
- Delusions of reference – interpreting publicly known events/celebrities as having direct reference to the patient
- Erotomania – belief that another is in love with you
- Grandiose – belief of an inflated sense of self-worth or power
- Religious – belief of receiving instructions/powers from a higher being; of being a higher being
- Somatic – belief that one has a physical disorder/defect
- Nihilistic – belief that things do not exist; a sense that everything is unreal

Cognitive Assessment
Use Folstein Mini Mental State Exam (MMSE) to assess:
- Orientation (time and place)
- Memory (immediate and delayed recall)
- Attention and Concentration
- Language (comprehension, reading, writing, repetition, naming)
- Spacial ability (intersecting pentagons)

Gross screen for cognitive dysfunction:
Total score is out of 30; <24 abnormal
20-24 mild, 10-19 moderate, <10 severe

Insight
- patient's ability to realize that he or she has a physical or mental illness and to understand its implications

Judgment
- ability to understand relationships between facts and draw conclusions that determine one's action

Axis V: Global Assessment of Functioning	
91-100	Superior functioning in a wide range of activities
81-90	Absent or minimal symptoms
71-80	If symptoms are present, they are transient and expected reactions to psychosocial stressors
61-70	Some mild symptoms or some difficulty but generally functioning well
51-60	Moderate symptoms or difficulty
41-50	Serious symptoms or difficulty
31-40	Some impairment in reality testing/ communication, impairment in several areas
21-30	Behaviour is influenced by delusions/ hallucinations or serious impairment in communication/judgment
11-20	Some danger of hurting self or others or occasionally fails to maintain minimal hygiene or gross impairment in communication
1-10	Persistent danger of severely hurting self or others or persistent inability to maintain minimal personal hygiene or serious suicidal act
0	Inadequate information

Summary of Axes

Multiaxial Assessment
Axis I – differential diagnosis of DSM-IV clinical disorders
Axis II – personality disorders, mental retardation
Axis III – general medical conditions that are potentially relevant to the understanding or management of the mental disorder
Axis IV – psychosocial and environmental issues
Axis V – global assessment of functioning (GAF, 0 to 100) incorporating effects of axes I to IV

Formulation
- a diagram outlining current issues and interrelations between an individual's biological, psychological, and social factors
- for each category: predisposing, precipitating, perpetuating, and protecting factors

Approach to Management
- consider subdividing management into 1) biological (e.g. pharmacotherapy), 2) psychological (e.g. CBT) and 3) social (e.g. support group)

Psychotic Disorders

Definition
- characterized by a significant impairment in reality testing
  - delusions or hallucinations (with/without insight into their pathological nature)
  - behaviour so disorganized that it is reasonable to infer that reality testing is disturbed

Differential Diagnosis of Psychosis

Differential Diagnosis of Psychosis - "GASPP"
General medical condition
Affective disorders
Substance induced
Psychotic disorders
Personality disorders

- primary psychotic disorders: schizophrenia, schizophreniform, brief psychotic, schizoaffective, delusional disorder
- mood disorders: depression with psychotic features, bipolar disorder (manic episode with psychotic features)
- personality disorders: schizotypal, schizoid, borderline, paranoid, obsessive-compulsive
- general medical conditions: tumour, head trauma, dementia, delirium, metabolic
- substance-induced psychosis: intoxication or withdrawal

Schizophrenia

DSM-IV-TR Diagnostic Criteria for Schizophrenia
A. characteristic symptoms (active phase): ≥2 of the following, each present for a significant portion of time during a **1-month period** (or less if successfully treated):
  - delusions
  - hallucinations
  - disorganized speech (e.g. frequent derailment or incoherence)
  - grossly disorganized or catatonic behaviour
  - negative symptoms, e.g. affective flattening, alogia (inability to speak), or avolition (inability to initiate and persist in goal-directed activities)

  Note: only 1 "A" symptom is required if delusions are bizarre or hallucinations consist of a voice keeping a running commentary on the person's behaviour or thoughts, or 2 or more voices conversing with each other
B. social/occupational dysfunction: ≥1 major areas of functioning (work, interpersonal relations, self-care) markedly below the level achieved prior to the onset of symptoms

C. continuous signs of disturbance for ≥**6 months**, including ≥**1 month** of active phase symptoms; may include prodromal or residual phases
D. schizoaffective and mood disorders excluded
E. the disturbance is not due to the direct physiological effects of a substance or a general medical condition (GMC)
F. if history of pervasive developmental disorder, additional diagnosis of schizophrenia is made only if prominent delusions or hallucinations are also present for at least 1 month

Subtypes
- paranoid
    - preoccupation with one or more delusions (typically persecutory or grandiose) or frequent auditory hallucinations
    - relative preservation of cognitive functioning and affect; onset tends to be later in life; believed to have the best prognosis
- catatonic
    - at least two of: motor immobility (catalepsy or stupor); excessive motor activity (purposeless, not influenced by external stimuli); extreme negativism (resistance to instructions/attempts to be moved) or mutism; peculiar voluntary movement (posturing, stereotyped movements, prominent mannerisms); echolalia (repeating words/phrases of another's speech) or echopraxia (imitative repetition of another's movements, gestures or posture)
- disorganized
    - disorganized speech and behaviour; flat or inappropriate affect
    - poor premorbid personality; early and insidious onset; and continuous course without significant remissions
- undifferentiated
    - symptoms from criteria A met, but does not fall into the 3 previous subtypes
- residual
    - absence of prominent delusions, hallucinations, disorganized speech, grossly disorganized or catatonic behaviour
    - continuing evidence of disturbance indicated by the presence of negative symptoms or two or more symptoms from criteria A present in attenuated form

Epidemiology
- prevalence: 0.5%-1%; M:F = 1:1
- mean age of onset: females ~27; males ~21

Etiology
- multifactorial: disorder is a result of interaction between both biological and environmental factors
    - genetic – 50% concordance in monozygotic (MZ) twins; 40% if both parents have schizophrenia; 10% of dizygotic (DZ) twins, siblings, children affected
    - neurochemistry – "dopamine hypothesis" theory: excess activity in the mesolimbic dopamine pathway may mediate the positive symptoms of psychosis (i.e. delusions, hallucinations, disorganized speech and behaviour, and agitation)
    - neuroanatomy – decreased frontal lobe function, asymmetric temporal/limbic function, decreased basal ganglia function; subtle changes in thalamus, cortex, corpus callosum, and ventricles; cytoarchitectural abnormalities
    - neuroendocrinology – abnormal growth hormone, prolactin, cortisol, and adrenocorticotropic hormone
    - neuropsychology – global defects seen in attention, language, and memory suggest lack of connectivity of neural networks
    - indirect evidence of geographical variance, winter season of birth, and prenatal viral exposure

Pathophysiology
- neurodegenerative theory
    - natural history may be rapid or gradual decline in function and ability to communicate
    - glutamate system may mediate progressive degeneration by excitotoxic mechanism which leads to production of free radicals
- neurodevelopmental theory – abnormal development of the brain from prenatal life
    - neurons fail to migrate correctly, make inappropriate connections, and break down in later life
    - inappropriate apoptosis during neurodevelopment resulting in faulty connections between neurons

Suggested Criteria for Prodromal Syndromes
- **Attenuated positive symptom syndrome:** Abnormal unusual thought content, suspiciousness, grandiosity, perceptual abnormalities, and/or organization of communication; onset or worsening in past year
- **Brief intermittent psychotic syndrome:** Frankly psychotic unusual thought content, suspiciousness, grandiosity, perceptual abnormalities, and/or organization of communication; onset in past three months
- **Genetic risk plus functional deterioration:** First-degree relative with history of any psychotic disorder or schizotypal personality disorder in patient; substantial functional decline in past year

Adapted from Sadock, B. J. and Sadock, V. A. Kaplan and Sadock's Comprehensive Textbook of Psychiatry, 8th Edition. Lippincott Williams & Wilkins, 2005.

Relationship between duration of untreated psychosis (DUP) and outcome in first-episode schizophrenia
Am J Psychiatry. 2005 Oct; 162:1785-1804
Purpose: To review the association between DUP and symptom severity at first treatment contact, and between DUP and treatment outcomes.
Study Characteristics: Critical review and meta-analysis of 43 studies with 4177 patients.
Participants: Patients with non-affective psychotic disorders at or close to first treatment.
Results: Shorter DUP was associated with greater response to antipsychotic treatment, as measured by global psychopathology, positive symptoms, negative symptoms, and functional outcomes. At the time of treatment initiation, longer DUP was associated with the severity of negative symptoms but not with the severity of positive symptoms, global psychopathology, or neurocognitive function.
Conclusions: DUP may be a potentially modifiable prognostic factor.

Supportive Evidence for Dopamine Hypothesis
- Dopamine (DA) agonists exacerbate schizophrenia
- Antipsychotic drugs act by blocking post-synaptic DA receptors
- Potency of many antipsychotic drugs correlates with D2 blockade of post-synaptic receptors
- Antipsychotic drugs are associated with an increase in the number of D2 and D4 post-synaptic receptors

Management of Schizophrenia

- pharmacological
    - acute treatment and maintenance with antipsychotics ± anticonvulsants ± anxiolytics
    - management of side effects
- psychosocial
    - psychotherapy (individual, family, group): supportive, cognitive behavioural therapy (CBT)
    - assertive community treatment (ACT)
    - social skills training, employment programs, disability benefits
    - housing (group home, boarding home, transitional home)

Good Prognostic Factors
- acute onset
- precipitating factors
- good cognitive functioning
- good premorbid functioning
- no family history
- presence of affective symptoms
- absence of structural brain abnormalities
- good response to drugs
- good support system

Prognosis

- majority of individuals display some type of prodromal phase
- course is variable – some individuals have exacerbations and remissions and others remain chronically ill; accurate prediction of the long term outcome is not possible
- early in the illness, negative symptoms may be prominent; positive symptoms appear and typically diminish with treatment; negative symptoms may become more prominent and more disabling
- over time, 1/3 improve, 1/3 remain the same, 1/3 worsen

Schizophreniform Disorder

- **diagnosis**: criteria A, D & E of schizophrenia are met; an episode of the disorder lasts at least **1 month** but **less than 6 months**
- **treatment**: similar to acute schizophrenia
- **prognosis**: better than schizophrenia; begins and ends more abruptly; good pre- and post-morbid function

Brief Psychotic Disorder

- **diagnosis**: acute psychosis (presence of 1 or more positive symptoms in criteria A1-4 of schizophrenia) lasting from **1 day to 1 month**, with eventual full return to premorbid level of functioning
- can occur after a stressful event or postpartum (see *Postpartum Mood Disorders* section, PS10)
- **treatment**: secure environment, antipsychotics, anxiolytics
- **prognosis**: good, self-limiting, should return to pre-morbid function in about 1 month

Schizoaffective Disorder

DSM-IV-TR Diagnostic Criteria for Schizoaffective Disorder

A. uninterrupted period of illness during which there is either a major depressive episode (MDE), manic episode, or a mixed episode concurrent with symptoms meeting criterion A for schizophrenia

B. in the same period, delusions or hallucinations for **at least 2 weeks** in the absence of prominent mood symptoms

C. symptoms that meet criteria for a mood episode are present for a substantial portion of total duration of active and residual periods of the illness

D. the disturbance is not due to the direct physiological effects of a substance or GMC

- **treatment**: antipsychotics, mood stabilizers, antidepressants
- **prognosis**: between that of schizophrenia and that of mood disorder

Delusional Disorder

DSM-IV-TR Diagnostic Criteria for Delusional Disorder

A. non-bizarre delusions for at least **1 month**

B. **criterion A for schizophrenia has never been met** (though patient may have tactile or olfactory hallucinations if they are related to the delusional theme)

C. functioning not markedly impaired; behaviour not obviously odd or bizarre

D. if mood episodes occur concurrently with delusions, total duration has been brief relative to duration of the delusional periods

E. the disturbance is not due to the direct physiological effects of a substance or GMC

Non-bizarre delusions involve situations that could occur in real life (e.g. being followed, poisoned, loved at a distance).

- **subtypes**: erotomanic, grandiose, jealous, persecutory, somatic, mixed, unspecified
- **treatment**: psychotherapy, antipsychotics, antidepressants
- **prognosis**: chronic, unremitting course but high level of functioning

Shared Psychotic Disorder (Folie à Deux)

- **diagnosis**: delusion that develops in an individual who is in a close relationship with another person who already has a psychotic disorder with prominent delusions; the delusion is similar in content to that of the other person
- **treatment**: separation of the two people results in the disappearance of the delusion in the healthier member; antipsychotics may play a role
- **prognosis**: good

Table 1. Differentiating Psychotic Disorders

Disorder	Psychotic symptoms	Duration	Mood symptoms
Schizophrenia	Criterion A	>6 months	None
Schizophreniform disorder	Criterion A	1-6 months	None
Schizoaffective disorder	≥2 weeks (with no mood symptoms)	>1 month	Present
Delusional disorder	Non-bizarre delusions, hallucinations	>1 month	If present, 2°
Brief psychotic disorder	≥1 positive symptoms of criterion A	<1 month	None
2° to substance intoxication/withdrawal	Criterion A	During intoxication or ≤1 month after withdrawal	Variable
2° to mood disorder	Delusions/hallucinations (mood congruent)	Unspecified	1°

Mood Disorders

Definitions
- mood disorders are defined by the presence of mood episodes
- mood episodes represent a combination of symptoms comprising a predominant mood state that is abnormal in quality or duration; e.g. major depressive, manic, mixed, hypomanic
- types of mood disorders include:
  - depressive (major depressive disorder, dysthymia)
  - bipolar (bipolar I/II disorder, cyclothymia)
  - secondary to GMC, substances, medications

Secondary Causes of Mood Disorders
- infectious: encephalitis/meningitis, hepatitis, pneumonia, TB, syphilis
- endocrine: hypothyroidism, hyperthyroidism, hypopituitarism, SIADH
- metabolic: porphyria, Wilson's disease, diabetes
- vitamin disorders: Wernicke's, beriberi, pellagra, pernicious anemia
- collagen vascular diseases: SLE, polyarteritis nodosa
- neoplastic: pancreatic cancer, carcinoid, pheochromocytoma
- cardiovascular: cardiomyopathy, CHF, MI, CVA
- neurologic: Huntington's disease, multiple sclerosis, tuberous sclerosis, degenerative (vascular, Alzheimer's)
- drugs: antihypertensives, antiparkinsonian, hormones, steroids, antituberculous, interferon, antineoplastic medications

Medical Workup of Mood Disorder
- routine screening:
  - physical examination
  - complete blood count
  - thyroid function test
  - electrolytes
  - urinalysis, urine drug screen
- addtional screening:
  - neurological consultation
  - chest x-ray
  - electrocardiogram
  - CT scan

Mood Episodes

DSM-IV-TR Criteria for Major Depressive Episode

A. ≥5 of the following symptoms have been present during the same **2-week** period and represent a change from previous functioning; at least one of the symptoms is either **1) depressed mood**, or **2) loss of interest or pleasure (anhedonia)**
   Note: Do not include symptoms that are clearly due to a general medical condition, or mood-incongruent delusions or hallucinations
   - depressed mood most of the day, nearly every day, as indicated by either subjective report or observation made by others
   - markedly diminished interest or pleasure in all, or almost all, activities most of the day, nearly every day
   - significant unintentional weight loss or gain or decrease or increase in appetite nearly every day
   - insomnia or hypersomnia nearly every day
   - psychomotor agitation or retardation nearly every day
   - fatigue or loss of energy nearly every day
   - feelings of worthlessness or excessive or inappropriate guilt (which may be delusional) nearly every day; not merely self-reproach or guilt about being sick
   - diminished ability to think or concentrate, or indecisiveness, nearly every day
   - recurrent thoughts of death (not just fear of dying), recurrent suicidal ideation without a specific plan, or a suicide attempt or a specific plan for committing suicide

B. the symptoms do not meet criteria for a Mixed Episode (see below)

C. the symptoms cause clinically significant distress or impairment in social, occupational, or other important areas of functioning

D. the symptoms are not due to the direct physiological effects of a substance or a GMC

E. the symptoms are not better accounted for by bereavement, i.e. after the loss of a loved one, the symptoms persist for longer than 2 months or are characterized by marked functional impairment, morbid preoccupation with worthlessness, suicidal ideation, psychotic symptoms, or psychomotor retardation

DSM-IV-TR Criteria for Manic Episode

A. a distinct period of abnormally and persistently elevated, expansive, or irritable mood, lasting **≥1 week** (or any duration if hospitalization is necessary)

B. during the period of mood disturbance, ≥3 of the following symptoms have persisted (4 if the mood is only irritable) and have been present to a significant degree:
   - inflated self-esteem or grandiosity
   - decreased need for sleep (e.g. feels rested after only 3 hours of sleep)
   - more talkative than usual or pressure to keep talking
   - flight of ideas or subjective experience that thoughts are racing
   - distractibility (i.e. attention too easily drawn to unimportant or irrelevant external stimuli)
   - increase in goal-directed activity (either socially, at work or school, or sexually) or psychomotor agitation
   - excessive involvement in pleasurable activities that have a high potential for painful consequences (e.g. engaging in unrestrained buying sprees, sexual indiscretions, or foolish business investments)

C. the symptoms do not meet criteria for a Mixed Episode (see below)

D. the mood disturbance is sufficiently severe to cause marked impairment in occupational functioning or in usual social activities or relationships with others, or to necessitate hospitalization to prevent harm to self or others, or there are psychotic features

E. the symptoms are not due to the direct physiological effects of a substance (e.g. drug of abuse, medication, or other treatment) or a general medical condition (e.g. hyperthyroidism). **Note:** Manic-like episodes that are clearly caused by somatic antidepressant treatment (e.g. medication, electroconvulsive therapy, light therapy) should not count toward a diagnosis of Bipolar I Disorder

Mixed Episode

- criteria met for both manic episode and major depressive episode (MDE) nearly every day for 1 week
- criteria D and E of manic episodes are met

Hypomanic Episode

- criterion A of a manic episode is met, but duration is **≥4 days**
- criterion B and E of manic episodes are met
- episode associated with an uncharacteristic decline in functioning that is observable by others
- change in function is **not severe enough** to cause marked impairment in social or occupational functioning or to necessitate hospitalization
- absence of psychotic features

Criteria for Depression (≥5):
"MSIGECAPS"

M	Depressed **M**ood
S	Increased/decreased **S**leep
I	Decreased **I**nterest
G	**G**uilt
E	Decreased **E**nergy
C	Decreased **C**oncentration
A	Increased/decreased **A**ppetite
P	**P**sychomotor agitation/retardation
S	**S**uicidal ideation

Criteria for Mania (≥3):
"GST PAID"

Grandiosity
Sleep (decreased need)
Talkative
Pleasurable activities, **P**ainful consequences
Activity
Ideas (flight of)
Distractable

An example of a mixed episode would be manic behaviour, racing thoughts with depressive or nihilistic content.

Depressive Disorders

MAJOR DEPRESSIVE DISORDER

DSM-IV-TR Diagnostic Criteria for Major Depressive Disorder (MDD), Single Episode (vs. Recurrent)
A. presence of a single Major Depressive Episode (vs. Recurrent, which requires presence of two or more Major Depressive Episodes; to be considered separate episodes, there must be an interval of at least 2 consecutive months in which criteria are not met for a MDE)
B. the Major Depressive Episode is not better accounted for by Schizoaffective Disorder and is not superimposed on Schizophrenia, Schizophreniform Disorder, Delusional Disorder, or Psychotic Disorder not otherwise specified
C. there has never been a Manic Episode, a Mixed Episode, or a Hypomanic Episode
Note: This exclusion does not apply if all of the manic-like, mixed-like, or hypomanic-like episodes are substance- or treatment-induced or are due to the direct physiological effects of a general medical condition

Features/Specifiers
- **psychotic** – with hallucinations or delusions
- **chronic** – lasting 2 years or more
- **catatonic** – at least two of: motor immobility, excessive motor activity, extreme negativism or mutism; peculiarities of voluntary movement; echolalia or echopraxia
- **melancholic** – quality of mood is distinctly depressed, mood is worse in the morning, early morning awakening, marked weight loss, excessive guilt, psychomotor retardation
- **atypical** – increased sleep, weight gain, leaden paralysis, rejection hypersensitivity
- **postpartum** (see *Postpartum Mood Disorders* section, PS10)
- **seasonal** – pattern of onset at the same time each year (most often in the fall or winter)

Epidemiology
- prevalence: male 5-12%, female 10-25% (M:F = 1:2)
- mean age of onset: ~30 years

Etiology
- biological
  - genetic: 65-75% MZ twins; 14-19% DZ twins
  - neurotransmitter dysfunction at level of synapse (decreased activity of serotonin, norepinephrine, dopamine)
  - secondary to general medical condition
- psychosocial
  - psychodynamic (e.g. low self-esteem)
  - cognitive (e.g. negative thinking)
  - environmental factors (e.g. job loss, diet (omega 3 fatty acids), bereavement, history of abuse)
  - co-morbid psychiatric diagnoses (e.g. anxiety, substance abuse, mental retardation, dementia, eating disorder)

Risk Factors
- sex: female > male
- age: onset between 25-50 years of age
- family history: depression, alcohol abuse, sociopathy
- childhood experiences: loss of parent before age 11, negative home environment (abuse, neglect)
- personality: insecure, dependent, obsessional
- recent stressors (illness, financial, legal)
- postpartum <6 months
- lack of intimate, confiding relationships or social isolation

Depression in the Elderly
- accounts for about 50% of acute psychiatric admissions in the elderly
- affects about 15% of community residents >65 years old
- high suicide risk due to social isolation, chronic medical illness
- suicide peak: males aged 80-90; females aged 50-65
- often present with somatic complaints (e.g. changes in weight, sleep, energy) or anxiety symptoms
- refer to Table 2 to compare with delirium and dementia

Treatment
- biological: antidepressants, lithium, antipsychotics, anxiolytics, electroconvulsive therapy (ECT), light therapy
- psychological
  - individual therapy: psychodynamic, interpersonal, cognitive behavioural therapy
  - family therapy
  - group therapy

Selective serotonin reuptake inhibitors (SSRIs) versus other antidepressants for depression (Cochrane Review)
Cochrane Database of Systematic Reviews 2004; Issue 3
Last substantive amendment: 15 July 1999.
This systematic review of 98 RCTs compared the efficacy of SSRIs with other kinds of antidepressants in the treatment of patients with depressive disorders.
Conclusions: There is no significant difference in the effectiveness of SSRIs versus TCAs. Consider relative patient acceptability, toxicity and cost when choosing.

Antidepressants for depression in medical illness (Cochrane Review)
Cochrane Database of Systematic Reviews 2004; Issue 3
Last substantive amendment: 22 August 2000.
This systematic review of 18 RCTs compared antidepressants to placebo or no treatment in patients with a physical disorder (e.g. cancer, MI) who have been diagnosed as depressed.
Conclusions: Antidepressants cause a significant improvement in patients with physical diseases, as compared to placebo or no treatment (NNT 4).

- social: vocational rehabilitation, social skills training
- experimental: deep brain stimulation, transcranial magnetic stimulation, vagal nerve stimulation

Prognosis
- one year after diagnosis of a MDE without treatment, 40% of individuals still have symptoms that are sufficiently severe to meet criteria for a full MDE, 20% continue to have some symptoms that no longer meet criteria for a MDE, 40% have no mood disorder

DYSTHYMIA

DSM-IV-TR Diagnostic Criteria for Dysthymic Disorder
A. depressed mood for most of the day, for more days than not, as indicated either by subjective account or observation by others, for ≥ 2 years. **Note**: In children and adolescents, mood can be irritable and duration must be at least 1 year
B. presence, while depressed, of ≥2 of the following:
  - poor appetite or overeating
  - insomnia or hypersomnia
  - low energy or fatigue
  - low self-esteem
  - poor concentration or difficulty making decisions
  - feelings of hopelessness
C. during the 2-year period (1 year for children or adolescents) of the disturbance, the person has never been without the symptoms in criteria A and B for more than 2 months at a time
D. no MDE has been present during the first 2 years of the disturbance (1 year for children and adolescents); i.e. the disturbance is not better accounted for by chronic MDD, or MDD in partial remission
E. there has never been a Manic Episode, a Mixed Episode, or a Hypomanic Episode, and criteria have never been met for Cyclothymic Disorder
F. the disturbance does not occur exclusively during the course of a chronic Psychotic Disorder, such as Schizophrenia or Delusional Disorder
G. the symptoms are not due to the direct physiological effects of a substance or a GMC
H. the symptoms cause clinically significant distress or impairment in social, occupational, or other important areas of functioning

Epidemiology
- point prevalence: 3%; life prevalence: 6%; M:F = 1:2-3

Treatment
- psychological treatment
  - principle treatment for dysthymia
  - individual, group, and family therapy
- medical treatment
  - antidepressant therapy (SSRIs/SNRIs) as an outpatient

Postpartum Mood Disorders

Postpartum "Blues"
- transient period of mild depression, mood instability, anxiety, decreased concentration, increased concern over own health and health of baby; considered to be normal emotional changes related to the puerperium
- occurs in 50-80% of mothers; begins 2-4 days postpartum, usually lasts 48 hours, can last up to 10 days
- does not require psychotropic medication
- patient at increased risk of developing postpartum depression

Postpartum Depression (PPD)
- **diagnosis**: MDE, onset within 4 weeks postpartum
- **clinical presentation**
  - typically lasts 2 to 6 months; residual symptoms can last up to 1 year
  - may present with psychosis - rare (0.2%), usually associated with mania, but can be MDE
  - severe symptoms include extreme disinterest in baby, suicidal and infanticidal ideation
- **epidemiology**: occurs in 10% of mothers, risk of recurrence 50%
- **risk factors**
  - previous history of a mood disorder (postpartum or otherwise)
  - psychosocial factors: stressful life events, unemployment, marital conflict, lack of social support, unwanted pregnancy, colicky or sick infant
- **treatment**
  - psychotherapy
  - short-term safety of maternal SSRIs for breastfeeding infants established; long-term effects unknown

Cognitive therapy vs medications in the treatment of moderate to severe depression
Arch Gen Psychiatry. 2005;62:409-416
Study: Randomized control trial.
Patients: 240 outpatients with moderate to severe MDD, aged 18-70.
Intervention: 16 weeks of paroxetine with or without augmentation with lithium carbonate or desipramine hydrochloride (n=120) versus cognitive behavioural therapy (n=60). Response up to 8 weeks was controlled by pill placebo (n=60)
Main Outcomes: The Hamilton Depression Rating scale was used to determine response to treatment.
Results: At 8 weeks, 50% (95%CI 41-59%) of patients on medication and 43% (95%CI 31-56%) of patients on CBT had responded in comparison to 25% (95%CI 16-38%) of patients on pill placebo. There was no significant difference between medication and CBT. At 16 weeks, 46% of patients on medication and 40% of patients on CBT achieved remission.
Summary: There is no difference in efficacy between CBT vs. paroxetine in the treatment of moderate to severe depression.

Health Canada advises of potential adverse effects of SSRIs and other antidepressants on newborns
August 9, 2004
Health Canada was concerned that newborns exposed to SSRIs and other antidepressants during the third trimester of pregnancy may be adversely affected, because of reports of complications at birth requiring longer hospitalization, breathing support and tube feeding. Advisory applied to: bupropion (used for depression or smoking cessation), citalopram, fluoxetine, fluvoxamine, mirtazapine, paroxetine, sertraline and venlafaxine.
Conclusions: Physicians and patients should carefully consider risks, benefits and options for both the mother and unborn baby when treating depression in pregnant women. Consider tapering in the third trimester. Women should consult their doctors before stopping these medications.

- supportive, non-directive counselling by trained home visitors
  - if depression severe, consider ECT
- **prognosis**: impact on child development – increased risk of cognitive delay, insecure attachment, behavioural disorders; treatment of mother improves outcome for child at 8 months through increased mother-child interaction

Premenstrual Dysphoric Disorder (PMDD)

DMS-IV-TR Diagnostic Criteria for Premenstrual Dysphoric Disorder

A In most menstrual cycles during the past year, **five (or more)** of the following symptoms were present for most of the time during the last week of the luteal phase, began to remit within a few days after the onset of the follicular phase, and were absent in the week post-menses, with at least one of the symptoms being one of the first four listed:
   1. markedly depressed mood, feelings of hopelessness, or self-deprecating thoughts
   2. marked anxiety, tension, feeling of being "keyed up" or "on edge"
   3. marked affective lability
   4. persistent and marked anger, irritability, or increased interpersonal conflicts
   5. decreased interest in usual activities
   6. difficulty concentrating
   7. lethargy, easily fatigued, lack of energy
   8. change in appetite - overeating or specific food cravings
   9. hypersomnia or insomnia
   10. a sense of being overwhelmed or out of control
   11. physical symptoms - breast tenderness or swelling, headaches, joint or muscle pain, sensation of bloating or weight gain
B. The disturbance markedly interferes with work, school, social activities, or relationships with others
C. The disturbance is not merely an exacerbation of the symptoms of another disorder such as Major Depressive Disorder, Panic Disorder, Dysthymic Disorder or Personality Disorder
D. Criteria A, B and C must be confirmed by prospective daily recordings and/or ratings during at least two consecutive symptomatic cycles

Treatment

- 1st line: SSRIs highly effective in treating PMDD
  - fluoxetine and sertraline most studied
  - can be used intermittently in luteal phase x 14 days
- 2nd line
  - clomipramine
  - alpraxolam (Xanax®) for anxiety symptoms
- 3rd line
  - OCP containing progesterone drospirenone (e.g. Yasmin®)
  - GnRH agonists (e.g. leuprolide)
    - if GnRH agonist completely relieves symptoms may consider definitive surgery (i.e. total abdominal hysterectomy + bilateral salpingo-oophorectomy)
- see Gynecology

Bipolar Disorders

BIPOLAR I / BIPOLAR II DISORDER

Definition

- Bipolar I Disorder
  - disorder in which **at least one manic or mixed episode** has occurred
  - commonly accompanied by at least 1 MDE but not required for diagnosis
- Bipolar II Disorder
  - disorder in which there is at least 1 MDE and at least 1 hypomanic episode
  - **no past manic or mixed episode**

Epidemiology

- prevalence: 0.6-0.9%; M:F = 1:1
- age of onset: teens to 20s

Risk Factors

- slight increase in upper socioeconomic groups
- 60-65% of bipolar patients have family history of major mood disorders

Classification

- classification of bipolar disorder involves describing the current or most recent mood episode as either manic, hypomanic, mixed or depressed

Antidepressant treatment for post-natal depression (Cochrane Review)
Cochrane Database of Systematic Reviews 2004; Issue 3
Last substantive amendment: 12 January 2001
This systematic review of trials included only one trial in which postpartum depressed women received fluoxetine or placebo.
Conclusions: Fluoxetine was significantly more effective than placebo, and as effective as a course of CBT in the short term. More trials are needed.

A randomized controlled trial of cognitive therapy for bipolar disorder: focus on long-term change
J Clin Psychiatry. 2006 Feb; 67(2):277-86
Study: Randomized, blinded clinical trial.
Patients: 52 patients with DSM-IV bipolar 1 or 2 disorder.
Intervention: Patients allocated to either a 6 month trial of cognitive therapy (CT) with emotive techniques or treatment as usual. Both groups received mood stabilizers.
Main Outcomes: Relapse rates, dysfunctional attitudes, psychosocial functioning, hopelessness, self-control, medication adherence. Patients were assessed by independent raters blinded to treatment group.
Results: At 6 months, CT patients experienced fewer depressive symptoms and fewer dysfunctional attitudes. There was a non-significant (p=.06) trend to greater time to depressive relapse. At 12 month follow up, CT patients had lower Young Mania Rating scores and improved behavioural self-control. At 18 months, CT patients reported less severity of illness.
Conclusions: CT appears to provide benefits in the 12 months succeeding completion of therapy.

- the current or most recent episode can be further classified as without psychotic features, with psychotic features, with catatonic features, with postpartum onset, with seasonal pattern, with rapid cycling (at least 4 episodes of a mood disturbance in the previous 12 months that meet criteria for a Major Depressive, Manic, Mixed, or Hypomanic Episode)

Treatment
- biological: mood stabilizers, anticonvulsants, antipsychotics, antidepressants, ECT
  Note: Treatment of bipolar depression must be done extremely cautiously, as a switch from depression to mania can result. Monotherapy with antidepressants should be avoided
- psychological: supportive and psychodynamic psychotherapy, cognitive or behavioural therapy
- social: vocational rehabilitation, leave of absence from school/work, drug and EtOH cessation, substitute decision maker for finances, sleep hygiene, social skills training, education for family members

CYCLOTHYMIA

Diagnosis
- presence of numerous periods of hypomanic and depressive symptoms (not meeting criteria for MDE) for ≥2 **years**; never without symptoms for >2 **months**
- no MDE, manic or mixed episodes; no evidence of psychosis
- symptoms are not due to the direct physiological effects of a substance or GMC
- symptoms cause clinically significant distress or impairment in social, occupational, or other important areas of functioning

Treatment
- similar to Bipolar I
- anticonvulsants ± psychotherapy

Anxiety Disorders

Definition
- anxiety is a universal human characteristic involving tension, apprehension, or even terror, which serves as an adaptive mechanism to warn about an external threat by activating the sympathetic nervous system (fight or flight)
- manifestations of anxiety can be described along a continuum of physiology, psychology, and behaviour
  - physiology – main brain structure involved is the amygdala; neurotransmitters involved include serotonin, cholecystokinin, epinephrine, norepinephrine, dopamine
  - psychology – one's perception of a given situation is distorted which causes one to believe it is threatening in some way
  - behaviour – once feeling threatened, one responds by escaping or facing the situation, thereby causing a disruption in daily functioning
- anxiety becomes pathological when
  - fear is greatly out of proportion to risk/severity of threat
  - response continues beyond existence of threat or becomes generalized to other similar/dissimilar situations
  - social or occupational functioning is impaired

Differential Diagnosis
- endocrine: hyperthyroidism, pheochromocytoma, hypoglycemia, hyperadrenalism, hyperparathyroidism
- CVS: congestive heart failure, pulmonary embolus, arrhythmia, mitral valve prolapse
- respiratory: asthma, pneumonia, hyperventilation
- metabolic: vitamin B12 deficiency, porphyria
- neurologic: neoplasm, vestibular dysfunction, encephalitis
- substance-induced: intoxication (caffeine, amphetamines, cocaine), withdrawal (benzodiazepines, alcohol)

Medical Workup of Anxiety Disorder
- routine screening: physical examination, CBC, thyroid function test, electrolytes, urinalysis, urine drug screening
- additional screening: neurological consultation, chest x-ray, electrocardiogram (ECG), CT scan

Panic Disorder

DSM-IV-TR Diagnostic Criteria for Panic Disorder without Agoraphobia

A. Both (1) and (2):
  - (1) recurrent unexpected panic attacks: a discrete period of intense fear or discomfort, in which ≥4 of the following symptoms develop abruptly and reach a **peak within 10 minutes**
    - palpitations, pounding heart, or accelerated heart rate
    - sweating
    - trembling or shaking
    - sensations of shortness of breath or smothering
    - feeling of choking
    - chest pain or discomfort
    - nausea or abdominal distress
    - feeling dizzy, unsteady, lightheaded, or faint
    - derealization (feelings of unreality) or depersonalization (being detached from oneself)
    - fear of losing control or going crazy
    - fear of dying
    - paresthesias (numbness or tingling sensations), chills or hot flushes
  - (2) at least one of the attacks has been followed by **1 month** (or more) of ≥1 of the following:
    - persistent concern about having additional attacks
    - worry about the implications of the attack or its consequences (e.g. losing control, having a heart attack, "going crazy")
    - a significant change in behavior related to the attacks
B. absence of agoraphobia
C. the panic attacks are not due to the direct physiological effects of a substance or GMC
D. the panic attacks are not better accounted for by another mental disorder, such as Social Phobia, Specific Phobia, Obsessive-Compulsive Disorder, Post-Traumatic Stress Disorder, Separation Anxiety Disorder

Epidemiology
- prevalence: 1.5-5% (one of the top five most common reasons to see a family doctor); M:F = 1:2-3
- onset: average late 20s, familial pattern

Treatment
- supportive psychotherapy, relaxation techniques (visualization, box-breathing), cognitive behavioural therapy (correct distorted thinking, desensitization/exposure therapy)
- pharmacotherapy
  - benzodiazepines (short term, low dose, regular schedule, long half-life, no prn)
  - SSRIs/SNRI (start low, go slow, aim high since anxiety patients are very sensitive)
  - other antidepressants (trazodone, Remeron™, MAOIs; avoid Wellbutrin™)

Prognosis
- 6-10 years post-treatment: 30% well, 40-50% improved, 20-30% no change or worse
- clinical course: chronic, but episodic with psychosocial stressors

Panic Disorder with Agoraphobia
- agoraphobia
  - anxiety about being in places or situations from which escape might be difficult (or embarrassing) or where help may not be available in the event of having an unexpected panic attack
  - fears commonly involve being out alone, being in a crowd, standing in a line, or travelling on a bus
- situations are avoided, endured with anxiety or panic, or require companion
- **treatment**: as per panic disorder

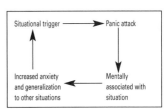

Figure 1. Panic Attack

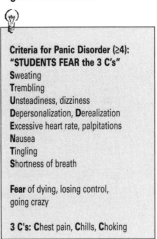

Criteria for Panic Disorder (≥4): "STUDENTS FEAR the 3 C's"
Sweating
Trembling
Unsteadiness, dizziness
Depersonalization, **D**erealization
Excessive heart rate, palpitations
Nausea
Tingling
Shortness of breath

Fear of dying, losing control, going crazy

3 C's: **C**hest pain, **C**hills, **C**hoking

Generalized Anxiety Disorder (GAD)

DSM-IV-TR Diagnostic Criteria for Generalized Anxiety Disorder

A. excessive anxiety and worry (apprehensive expectation), occurring more days than not for at least **6 months**, about a number of events or activities (such as work or school performance)
B. the person finds it difficult to control the worry
C. the anxiety and worry are associated with ≥3 of the following 6 symptoms (with at least some symptoms present for more days than not for the past **6 months**). **Note**: Only one item is required in children
  - (1) restlessness or feeling keyed up or on edge
  - (2) being easily fatigued

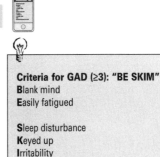

Criteria for GAD (≥3): "BE SKIM"
Blank mind
Easily fatigued

Sleep disturbance
Keyed up
Irritability
Muscle tension

(3) difficulty concentrating or mind going blank
(4) irritability
(5) muscle tension
(6) sleep disturbance (difficulty falling or staying asleep, or restless unsatisfying sleep)

D. the focus of the anxiety and worry is not confined to features of an Axis I disorder, such as panic disorder, social phobia, etc.
E. the anxiety, worry, or physical symptoms cause clinically significant distress or impairment in social, occupational, or other important areas of functioning
F. the disturbance is not due to the direct physiological effects of a substance or a GMC and does not occur exclusively during a Mood Disorder, a Psychotic Disorder, or a Pervasive Developmental Disorder

Epidemiology
* 1-year prevalence: 3-8%; M:F = 1:2; if considering only those receiving inpatient treatment, ratio is 1:1
* most commonly presents in early adulthood

Treatment
* psychotherapy, relaxation, mindfulness, and CBT
* caffeine and EtOH avoidance, sleep hygiene
* pharmacotherapy
    * benzodiazepines (short term, low dose, regular schedule, long half-life, no prn)
    * buspirone (tid dosing)
    * others: SSRIs/SNRI, TCAs, β-blockers
* combinations of above

Prognosis
* chronically anxious adults become less so with age
* depends on pre-morbid personality functioning, stability of relationships, work, and severity of environmental stress
* difficult to treat

Phobic Disorders

Specific Phobia
* definition: marked and persistent fear that is excessive or unreasonable, cued by presence or anticipation of a specific object or situation
* lifetime prevalence: 12-16%; M:F ratio variable
* types: animal/insect, environment (heights, storms), blood/injection/injury, situational (airplane, closed spaces), other (loud noise, clowns)

Social Phobia (Social Anxiety Disorder)
* definition: marked and persistent fear of social or performance situations in which person is exposed to unfamiliar people or to possible scrutiny by others; person fears he/she will act in a way that may be humiliating or embarrassing (e.g. public speaking, initiating or maintaining conversation, dating, eating in public)
* lifetime prevalence may be as high as 13-16%; M<F

Diagnostic Criteria for Phobic Disorders
* exposure to stimulus almost invariably provokes an immediate anxiety response; may present as a panic attack
* person recognizes fear as excessive or unreasonable
* situations are avoided or endured with anxiety/distress
* significant interference with daily routine, occupational/social functioning, and/or marked distress
* if person is <18 years, duration is at least 6 months

Treatment
* exposure therapy/desensitization, insight-oriented psychotherapy
* pharmacotherapy
    * β-blockers or benzodiazepines in acute situations (e.g. public speaking)
    * SSRIs, MAOIs; no TCAs
* behavioural therapy is more efficacious than medication

Prognosis
* chronic

Obsessive-Compulsive Disorder (OCD)

DSM-IV-TR Diagnostic Criteria for Obsessive-Compulsive Disorder
A. either obsessions or compulsions:
    obsessions as defined by (1), (2), (3), and (4):

      (1) recurrent and persistent thoughts, impulses, or images that are experienced, at some time during the disturbance, as intrusive and inappropriate and that cause marked anxiety or distress

      (2) the thoughts, impulses, or images are not simply excessive worries about real-life problems

      (3) the person attempts to ignore or suppress such thoughts, impulses, or images, or to neutralize them with some other thought or action

      (4) the person recognizes that the obsessional thoughts, impulses, or images are a product of his or her own mind (not externally imposed as in thought insertion)

  compulsions as defined by (1) and (2):

      (1) repetitive behaviours or mental acts that the person feels driven to perform in response to an obsession, or according to rules that must be applied rigidly

      (2) the behaviours or mental acts are aimed at preventing or reducing distress or preventing some dreaded event or situation; however, these behaviours or mental acts either are not connected in a realistic way with what they are designed to neutralize or prevent or are clearly excessive

B.   at some point during the course of the disorder, the person has recognized that the obsessions or compulsions are excessive or unreasonable (ego-dystonic)
Note: This does not apply to children

C.   the obsessions or compulsions cause marked distress, are time consuming (take **≥1 hour** a day), or significantly interfere with the person's normal routine, occupational/academic functioning, or usual social activities or relationships

D.   if another Axis I disorder is present, the content of the obsessions or compulsions is not restricted to it (e.g. preoccupation with food in the presence of an Eating Disorder)

E.   the disturbance is not due to the direct physiological effects of a substance or a GMC

Epidemiology
- lifetime prevalence: 2-3%; M=F
- rate of OCD in first-degree relatives is higher than in the general population

Treatment
- CBT – desensitization, flooding, thought stopping, implosion therapy, aversive conditioning
- pharmacotherapy
  - clomipramine, SSRIs (higher doses and longer treatment needed than for treatment of depression, i.e. up to 8-12 weeks)
  - atypical and typical antipsychotics – risperidone, haloperidol

Prognosis
- tends to be refractory and chronic

Post-Traumatic Stress Disorder (PTSD)

DSM-IV-TR Diagnostic Criteria for Post-Traumatic Stress Disorder
A.   the person has been **exposed to a traumatic event** in which both of the following were present:

      (1) the person experienced, witnessed, or was confronted with an event or events that involved actual or threatened death or serious injury, or a threat to the physical integrity of self or others

      (2) the person's response involved intense fear, helplessness, or horror. **Note**: In children, this may be expressed instead by disorganized or agitated behaviour

B.   the traumatic event is **persistently re-experienced** in ≥1 of the following ways:

      (1) recurrent and intrusive distressing recollections of the event, including images, thoughts, or perceptions. **Note**: In young children, repetitive play may occur in which themes or aspects of the trauma are expressed

      (2) recurrent distressing dreams of the event. **Note**: In children, there may be frightening dreams without recognizable content

      (3) acting or feeling as if the traumatic event were recurring (includes a sense of reliving the experience, illusions, hallucinations, and dissociative flashback episodes, including those that occur on awakening or when intoxicated) **Note**: In young children, trauma-specific reenactment may occur

      (4) intense psychological distress at exposure to internal or external cues that symbolize or resemble an aspect of the traumatic event

      (5) physiological reactivity on exposure to internal or external cues that symbolize or resemble an aspect of the traumatic event

C.   persistent **avoidance of stimuli** associated with the trauma and numbing of general responsiveness (not present before the trauma), as indicated by ≥3 of the following:

      (1) efforts to avoid thoughts, feelings, or conversations associated with the trauma

      (2) efforts to avoid activities, places, or people that arouse recollections of the trauma

      (3) inability to recall an important aspect of the trauma

      (4) markedly diminished interest or participation in significant activities

      (5) feeling of detachment or estrangement from others

(6) restricted range of affect (e.g. unable to have loving feelings)
(7) sense of a foreshortened future (e.g. does not expect to have a career, marriage, children, or a normal life span)
D. persistent **symptoms of increased arousal** (not present before the trauma), as indicated by ≥**2** of the following:
    (1) difficulty falling or staying asleep
    (2) irritability or outbursts of anger
    (3) difficulty concentrating
    (4) hypervigilance
    (5) exaggerated startle response
E. duration of the disturbance (symptoms in Criteria B, C, and D) is ≥**1 month**
F. the disturbance causes clinically significant distress or impairment in social, occupational, or other important areas of functioning

Epidemiology
• lifetime prevalence: 1-3%
• men's trauma is most commonly combat experience; women's trauma is usually physical or sexual assault

Treatment
• CBT – systematic desensitization, relaxation techniques, thought stopping
• pharmacotherapy
    ▪ SSRIs
    ▪ benzodiazepines (for acute anxiety)
    ▪ first-line adjunct – atypical antipsychotics (quetiapine, olanzapine, risperidone)
• EMDR (eye movement desensitization and reprocessing): an experimental method of reprocessing memories of distressing events by recounting them while using a form of dual attention stimulation such as eye movements, bilateral sound, or bilateral tactile stimulation

Complications
• substance abuse, relationship difficulties, depression, impaired social and occupational functioning, Axis II disorders

Adjustment Disorder

DSM-IV-TR Diagnostic Criteria for Adjustment Disorder
A. the development of emotional or behavioral symptoms in response to an identifiable stressor(s) occurring **within 3 months** of the onset of the stressor(s)
B. these symptoms or behaviours are clinically significant as evidenced by either of the following:
    (1) marked distress that is in excess of what would be expected from exposure to the stressor
    (2) significant impairment in social or occupational (academic) functioning
C. the stress-related disturbance does not meet the criteria for another specific Axis I disorder and is not merely an exacerbation of a pre-existing Axis I or Axis II disorder
D. the symptoms do not represent bereavement
E. once the stressor (or its consequences) has terminated, the symptoms do not persist for more than an additional 6 months
    ▪ specify if:
        ◆ **acute**: if the disturbance lasts less than 6 months
        ◆ **chronic**: if the disturbance lasts for 6 months or longer
    ▪ adjustment disorders are coded based on the subtype, which is selected according to the predominant symptoms

Classification
• types of stressors
    ▪ single (e.g. termination of romantic relationship)
    ▪ multiple (e.g. marked business difficulties and marital problems)
    ▪ recurrent (e.g. seasonal business crises)
    ▪ continuous (e.g. living in a crime-ridden neighbourhood)
    ▪ developmental events (e.g. going to school, leaving parental home, getting married, becoming a parent, failing to attain occupational goals, retirement)
      Note: the specific stressor is specified on Axis IV
• **subtypes**, adjustment disorder with:
    ▪ depressed mood
    ▪ anxiety
    ▪ mixed anxiety and depressed mood
    ▪ disturbance of conduct
    ▪ mixed disturbance of emotions and conduct
    ▪ unspecified

Epidemiology
- M=F

Treatment
- brief psychotherapy (group, individual), crisis intervention
- medications
  - benzodiazepines may be used for those with anxiety symptoms; short-term, low-dose, regular schedule, long half-life, no prn
  - SSRIs for both depressed and anxiety symptoms

Cognitive Disorders

Delirium

- see Neurology

DSM-IV-TR Diagnostic Criteria for Delirium due to a GMC
A. **disturbance of consciousness** (i.e. reduced clarity of awareness of the environment) with reduced ability to focus, sustain, or shift attention
B. a **change in cognition** (such as memory deficit, disorientation, language disturbance) or the development of a perceptual disturbance that is not better accounted for by a pre-existing, established, or evolving dementia
C. the disturbance develops over a short period of time (usually **hours to days**) and tends to fluctuate during the course of the day
D. there is evidence from the history, physical examination, or laboratory findings that the disturbance is caused by the direct physiological consequences of a GMC

> **Delirium - "I WATCH DEATH"**
> **I**nfectious
>
> **W**ithdrawal from drugs
> **A**cute metabolic disorder
> **T**rauma
> **C**NS pathology
> **H**ypoxia
>
> **D**eficiencies in vitamins
> **E**ndocrinopathies
> **A**cute vascular insults
> **T**oxins
> **H**eavy metals

Clinical Presentation and Assessment
- common symptoms
  - wandering attention
  - distractibility
  - disorientation (time, place, rarely person)
  - misinterpretations, illusions, hallucinations
  - speech/language disturbances (dysarthria, dysnomia, dysgraphia)
  - affective symptoms (anxiety, fear, depression, irritability, anger, euphoria, apathy)
  - shifts in psychomotor activity (groping/picking at clothes, attempts to get out of bed when unsafe, sudden movements, sluggishness, lethargy)
- Folstein exam is helpful to assess baseline of altered mental state – i.e. score will improve as symptoms resolve

Risk Factors
- hospitalization (incidence 10-40%)
- nursing home residents (incidence 60%)
- childhood (e.g. febrile illness, anticholinergic use)
- old age (especially males)
- severe illness (e.g. cancer, AIDS)
- pre-existing cognitive impairment or brain pathology
- recent anesthesia
- substance abuse

Etiology
- **I**nfectious (encephalitis, meningitis, UTI, pneumonia)
- **W**ithdrawal (alcohol, barbiturates, benzodiazepines)
- **A**cute metabolic disorder (electrolyte imbalance, hepatic or renal failure)
- **T**rauma (head injury, postoperative)
- **C**NS pathology (stroke, hemorrhage, tumour, seizure disorder, Parkinson's)
- **H**ypoxia (anemia, cardiac failure, pulmonary embolus)
- **D**eficiencies (vitamin B_{12}, folic acid, thiamine)
- **E**ndocrinopathies (thyroid, glucose, parathyroid, adrenal)
- **A**cute vascular (shock, vasculitis, hypertensive encephalopathy)
- **T**oxins: substance use, alcohol or alcohol withdrawal, sedatives or sedative withdrawal, narcotics (especially morphine), anesthetics, anticholinergics, anticonvulsants, dopaminergic agents, steroids, insulin, glyburide, antibiotics (especially quinolones), NSAIDs
- **H**eavy metals (arsenic, lead, mercury)

Investigations
- standard: CBC + diff, electrolytes, calcium, phosphate, magnesium, glucose, ESR, LFTs (AST, ALT, ALP, albumin, bilirubin), RFTs (Cr, BUN), TSH, vitamin B_{12}, folate, albumin, urine C&S, R&M
- as indicated: ECG, CXR, CT head, toxicology/heavy metal screen, VDRL, HIV, LP, LE preparation, EEG (typically abnormal: generalized slowing or fast activity), blood cultures
- indications for radiological intervention: focal neurological deficit, acute change in status, anticoagulant use, acute incontinence, gait abnormality, history of cancer

Management
- intrinsic
  - identify and treat underlying cause immediately
  - stop all non-essential medications
  - maintain nutrition, hydration, electrolyte balance and monitor vitals
- extrinsic
  - environment should be quiet and well-lit
  - optimize hearing and vision
  - room near nursing station for closer observation; constant care if patient jumping out of bed, pulling out lines
  - family member present for reassurance and re-orientation
  - calendar, clock for orientation cues
- pharmacological
  - haloperidol or risperidone (low dose)
  - lorazepam
- physical restraints if patient becomes violent

Prognosis
- up to 50% 1-year mortality rate after episode of delirium

Dementia

- see Neurology

Differential Diagnosis of Dementia
Alzheimer's dementia
Vascular dementia
Lewy-Body dementia
Fronto-temporal dementia

DSM-IV-TR Diagnostic Criteria for Dementia (Alzheimer's Type)
A. the development of multiple cognitive deficits manifested by both
  1. **memory impairment** (impaired ability to learn new information or to recall previously learned information)
  2. **≥1** of the following **cognitive disturbances**:
      (a) aphasia (language disturbance)
      (b) apraxia (impaired ability to carry out motor activities despite intact motor function)
      (c) agnosia (failure to recognize or identify objects despite intact sensory function)
      (d) disturbance in executive functioning (i.e. planning, organizing, sequencing, abstracting)
B. the cognitive deficits in Criteria A1 and A2 each cause significant impairment in social or occupational functioning and represent a significant decline from a previous level of functioning
C. the course is characterized by gradual onset and continuing cognitive decline
D. the cognitive deficits in Criteria A1 and A2 are not due to any of the following:
  1. other central nervous system conditions that cause progressive deficits in memory and cognition
  2. systemic conditions that are known to cause dementia
  3. substance-induced conditions
E. the deficits do not occur exclusively during the course of a delirium
F. the disturbance is not better accounted for by another Axis I disorder

Epidemiology
- prevalence increases with age: 10% in patients over 65 years; 25% in patients over 85 years
- prevalence is increased in people with Down syndrome and head trauma
- Alzheimer's dementia comprises >50% of cases; vascular causes comprise approximately 15% of cases (other causes of dementia – see Neurology)
- 10% of dementia cases are potentially curable (mainly vascular etiology)
- average duration of illness from onset of symptoms to death is 8-10 years

Subtypes
- with or without behavioural disturbance (e.g. wandering, agitation)
- early onset: age of onset <65 years
- late onset: age of onset >65 years

Investigations (rule out reversible causes)
- standard: as in *Delirium*
- as indicated: VDRL, HIV, SPECT, CT head in dementia
- indications for CT head, as in *Delirium* section plus: age <60, rapid onset (unexplained decline in cognition or function over 1-2 months), dementia of relatively short duration (<2 years), recent significant head trauma, unexplained neurological symptoms (new onset of severe headache/seizures)

Management
- treat medical problems and prevent others
- provide orientation cues (e.g. clock, calendar)
- provide education and support for patient and family (day programs, respite care, support groups, home care)
- consider long-term care plan (nursing home) and power of attorney/living will
- inform Ministry of Transportation about patient's inability to drive safely
- consider pharmacological therapy
    - cholinesterase inhibitors (e.g. donepezil (Aricept™)) for mild to severe disease
    - glutamatergic NMDA receptor antagonist (e.g memantine) for moderate to severe disease
    - low-dose neuroleptics (e.g. haloperidol, risperidone) and antidepressants if behavioural or emotional symptoms prominent - start low and go slow
    - reassess pharmacological therapy every 3 months

Table 2. Comparison of Dementia, Delirium and Pseudodementia of Depression

	Dementia	Delirium	Pseudodementia of Depression
Onset	Gradual/step-wise decline	Acute (hours – days)	Subacute
Duration	Months – years	Days – weeks	Variable
Natural History	Progressive Usually irreversible	Fluctuating, reversible High morbidity/ mortality in very old	Recurrent Usually reversible
Level of Consciousness	Normal	Fluctuating (over 24 hours)	Normal
Attention	Not initially affected	Decreased (wandering, easily distracted)	Difficulty concentrating
Orientation	Intact initially	Impaired (usually to time and place), fluctuates	Intact
Behaviour	Disinhibition, impairment in ADL/IADL, personality change, loss of social graces	Severe agitation/retardation	Importuning, self-harm/suicide
Psychomotor	Normal	Fluctuates between extremes	Slowing
Sleep Wake Cycle	Fragmented sleep at night	Reversed sleep wake cycle	Early morning awakening
Mood and Affect	Labile but not usually anxious	Anxious, irritable, fluctuating	Depressed, stable
Cognition	Decreased executive functioning, paucity of thought	Fluctuating preceded by mood changes	Fluctuating
Memory Loss	Recent, eventually remote	Marked recent	Recent
Language	Agnosia, aphasia, decreased comprehension, repetition, speech (echolalia, palilalia)	Dysnomia, dysgraphia, speech rambling, irrelevant, incoherent, subject changes	Not affected
Delusions	Compensatory	Nightmarish and poorly formed	Nihilistic, somatic
Hallucinations	Variable	Visual common	Less common, auditory predominates
Quality of Hallucinations	Vacuous/bland	Frightening/ bizarre	Self-deprecatory
Medical Status	Variable	Acute illness, drug toxicity	R/O systemic illness, meds

Risk of death with atypical antipsychotic drug treatment for dementia
Schneider et al. JAMA. 2005 Oct; 294(15):1934-1943
Purpose: To assess the evidence for increased mortality from atypical antipsychotic drug treatment for delusions, aggression and agitation in dementia.
Study Characteristics: Meta-analysis of 15 RCTs with 5110 patients.
Participants: Patients with Alzheimer disease or dementia.
Results: Death occurred more often among patients randomized to drugs (118 [3.5%] vs. 40 [2.3%]. The odds ratio by meta-analysis was 1.54; 95% confidence interval [CI], 1.06-2.23; P=0.02). Sensitivity analyses did not show evidence for differential risks for individual drugs or diagnosis.
Conclusions: Atypical antipsychotic drugs may be associated with a small increased risk of death compared to placebo. This risk should be considered within the context of medical need for the drugs, efficacy evidence, medical comorbidity, and the efficacy and safety of alternatives.

Substance-Related Disorders

Types of Substance Disorders
- 47% of those with substance abuse have mental health problems
- 29% of those with a mental health disorder have a substance - use disorder (concurrent disorder) - 47% of those with schizophrenia, 25% of those with an anxiety disorder

A. Substance-use disorders
1. **substance abuse**: maladaptive pattern of substance use leading to clinically significant impairment or distress, as manifested by ≥1 of the following occurring within a 12 month period:
   - recurrent use resulting in failure to fulfill major role obligation
   - recurrent use in situations in which it is physically hazardous (e.g. driving)
   - recurrent substance-related legal problems
   - continued use despite interference with social or interpersonal function
2. **substance dependence**: maladaptive pattern of substance use leading to clinically significant impairment or distress as manifested by ≥3 occurring at any time in the same 12 month period:
   - tolerance (need for increased amount to achieve intoxication or diminished effect with same amount of substance)
   - withdrawal/use to avoid withdrawal
   - taken in larger amount or over longer period than intended
   - persistent desire or unsuccessful efforts to cut down
   - excessive time to procure, use substance, or recover from its effects
   - important interests/activities given up or reduced
   - continued use despite physical/psychological problem caused/ exacerbated by substance

B. Substance-induced disorders
1. **substance intoxication**: reversible physiological and behavioural changes due to recent exposure to psychoactive substance
2. **substance withdrawal**: substance-specific syndrome that develops following cessation of or reduction in dosage of regularly used substances

---

**Substance Dependence
The 3 Cs:**
Compulsive use
Loss of **C**ontrol
Consequences of use

Alcohol

- see <u>Family Medicine</u>

History
- validated screening questionnaire:
  - **C**   ever felt the need to **C**ut down on drinking?
  - **A**   ever felt **A**nnoyed at criticism of your drinking?
  - **G**   ever feel **G**uilty about your drinking?
  - **E**   ever need a drink first thing in morning (**E**ye opener)?
    - for men, a score of ≥2 is a positive screen and for women, a score of ≥1 is a positive screen
    - if positive CAGE, then assess further to distinguish between problem drinking and alcohol dependence

General Assessment
- When was your last drink?
- Do you have to drink more to get the same effect?
- Do you get shaky or nauseous when you stop drinking?
- Have you had a withdrawal seizure?
- How much time and effort do you put into obtaining alcohol?
- Has your drinking affected your ability to work, go to school, or have relationships?
- Have you suffered any legal consequences?
- Has your drinking caused any medical problems?

A "Standard Drink"
Spirit (40%) – 1.5 oz. or 43 mL
Table Wine (12%) – 5 oz. or 142 mL
Fortified Wine (18%) – 3 oz. or 85 mL
Regular Beer (5%) – 12 oz. or 341 mL

OR

1 pint beer = 1.5 SD
1 bottle wine = 5 SD
1 "mickey" = 8 SD
"26-er" = 17 SD
"40 oz." = 27 SD

Make sure to ask about other alcohols: mouthwash, rubbing alcohol, methanol, ethylene glycol, aftershave (may be used as a cheaper alternative).

Alcohol abuse can only be diagnosed in the absence of alcohol dependence. The criteria for abuse and dependence are outlined under substance-use disorders.

Table 3. Differentiating Moderate Drinking from a Drinking Problem

Moderate Drinking	Drinking Problem
Drinking within the recommended guidelines (U.S. Department of Health and Human Services) Men: 2 or less/day Women: 1 or less/day Elderly: 1 or less/day	Drinking above the recommended guidelines, associated with: • Drinking to reduce depression or anxiety • Loss of interest in food • Lying/hiding drinking habits • Drinking alone • Injuring self or others while intoxicated • Were drunk more than three or four times last year • Increasing tolerance • Withdrawal symptoms: feeling irritable, resentful, unreasonable when not drinking • Experiencing medical, social, or financial problems caused by drinking

Alcohol Intoxication
- legal limit for impaired driving is 17 mmol/L (80 mg/dL) reached by 4 drinks/hr for men and 2-3 drinks/hr for women
- coma can occur with 60+ mmol/L (non-tolerant drinkers) and 90-120 mmol/L (tolerant drinkers)

Alcohol Withdrawal
- occurs within 12 to 48 hours after prolonged heavy drinking and can be life-threatening
- alcohol withdrawal can be described as having 4 stages, however not all stages may be experienced
    - stage 1 (onset 6-12 hours after last drink): tremor, sweating, agitation, anorexia, cramps, diarrhea, sleep disturbance
    - stage 2 (onset 1-7 days): visual, auditory, olfactory or tactile hallucinations
    - stage 3 (onset 12-72 hours and up to 7 days): seizures, usually grand mal (non-focal, brief)
    - stage 4 (onset 3-5 days): delirium tremens, confusion, delusions, hallucinations, agitation, tremors, autonomic hyperactivity (fever, tachycardia, hypertension)
- course: in young almost completely reversible; elderly often left with cognitive deficits
- mortality rate 20% if untreated

Delirium Tremens (alcohol withdrawal delirium)
Autonomic hyperactivity (diaphoresis, tachycardia, increased respiration)
Hand tremor
Insomnia
Psychomotor agitation
Anxiety
Nausea or vomiting
Grand mal seizures
Visual/tactile/auditory hallucinations
Persecutory delusions

Management of Alcohol Withdrawal
- monitor using the Clinical Institute Withdrawal Assessment for Alcohol (CIWA-A) scoring system
    - areas of assessment include
        - nausea and vomiting
        - tactile disturbances
        - tremor
        - auditory disturbances
        - agitation
        - paroxysmal sweats
        - visual disturbances
        - anxiety
        - headache, fullness in head
        - orientation and clouding of sensorium
    - all categories are scored from 0-7 (except: orientation/sensorium 0-4), maximum score of 67
        - mild <10
        - moderate 10-20
        - severe >20
- basic treatment protocol using CIWA-A scale
    - diazepam 20 mg PO q1-2h prn until CIWA-A <10 points; tapering dose not required
    - observe 1-2 h after last dose and re-assess on CIWA-A scale
    - thiamine 100 mg IM then 100 mg PO OD for 3 days
    - supportive care (hydration and nutrition)
- if history of withdrawal seizures
    - diazepam 20 mg q1h for minimum of three doses regardless of subsequent CIWA-A scores
- if history of seizure disorder or multiple withdrawal seizures despite diazepam, use anti-seizure medication (e.g. Dilantin™)
- if oral diazepam not tolerated
    - diazepam 2-5 mg IV/min – maximum 10-20 mg q1h; or lorazepam SL
- if >65 yr or severe liver disease, severe asthma, or respiratory failure are present, use short acting benzodiazepine
    - lorazepam PO/SL/IM 1-4 mg q1-2h
- if hallucinosis present
    - haloperidol 2-5 mg IM/PO q1-4h – max 5 doses/day or atypical antipsychotics (olanzapine, risperidone)
    - diazepam 20 mg x 3 doses as seizure prophylaxis (haloperidol lowers seizure threshold)
- admit to hospital if:
    - still in withdrawal after >80 mg of diazepam
    - delirium tremens, recurrent arrhythmias, or multiple seizures
    - medically ill or unsafe to discharge home

Wernicke-Korsakoff Syndrome
- alcohol-induced amnestic disorders due to thiamine deficiency
- necrotic lesions – mammillary bodies, thalamus, brain stem
- Wernicke's encephalopathy (acute and reversible): triad of nystagmus (CN VI palsy), ataxia and confusion
- Korsakoff's syndrome (chronic and only 20% reversible with treatment): anterograde amnesia and confabulations; cannot occur during an acute delirium or dementia and must persist beyond usual duration of intoxication/withdrawal
- management
    - Wernicke's: thiamine 100 mg PO OD x 1-2 weeks
    - Korsakoff's: thiamine 100 mg PO bid/tid x 3-12 months

Treatment of Alcohol Dependence

Non-pharmacological
- behaviour modification: hypnosis, relaxation training, aversion therapy, assertiveness training, operant conditioning
- supportive services: half-way houses, detoxification centres, Alcoholics Anonymous
- psychotherapy, motivational interviewing
- medications important as adjunctive treatment: SSRIs, ondansetron, topiramate

Pharmacological
- naltrexone: opioid antagonist, shown to be successful in reducing the "high" associated with alcohol, moderately effective in reducing cravings and frequency or intensity of alcohol binges
- disulfiram (Antabuse™): blocks oxidation of EtOH; with EtOH consumption, acetaldehyde accumulates to cause a toxic reaction (vomiting, tachycardia, death); if patient relapses, must wait 48 hours before restarting Antabuse™

Opioids

- types of opioids: heroin, morphine, oxycodone, Tylenol # 3 (codeine)
- major risks associated with the use of contaminated needles: increased risk of hepatitis B and C, bacterial endocarditis, HIV

Acute Intoxication
- direct effect on receptors in CNS resulting in decreased pain perception, sedation, decreased sex drive, nausea/vomiting, decreased GI motility (constipation and anorexia), and respiratory depression

Toxic Reaction
- typical syndrome includes shallow respirations, miosis, bradycardia, hypothermia, decreased level of consciousness
- treatment
  - ABCs
  - IV glucose
  - naloxone hydrochloride (Narcan™): 0.4 mg up to 2 mg IV for diagnosis
  - treatment: intubation and mechanical ventilation, ± naloxone drip, until patient alert without naloxone (up to 48+ hours with long-acting opioids)
- caution with longer half-life; may need to observe for toxic reaction for at least 24 hours

Withdrawal
- symptoms: depression, insomnia, drug-craving, myalgias, nausea, chills, autonomic instability (lacrimation, rhinorrhea, piloerection)
- onset: 6-12h, duration: 5-10 days
- complications: loss of tolerance (overdose on relapse), miscarriage, premature labour
- management: long-acting oral opioids (methadone, buprenorphine), α-adrenergic agents (e.g. clonidine)

Treatment of Chronic Abuse
- psychosocial treatment (e.g. Narcotics Anonymous); usually emphasize total abstinence
- long-term treatment may include withdrawal maintenance treatment
  - methadone relieves drug cravings and withdrawal symptoms without inducing sedation or euphoria
- naltrexone or naloxone (opioid antagonists) may also be used to extinguish drug-seeking behaviour

Cocaine

- street names: blow, C, coke, crack, flake, freebase, rock, snow
- alkaloid extracted from leaves of the coca plant; blocks presynaptic uptake of dopamine (causing euphoria), norepinephrine and epinephrine (causing vasospasm, hypertension)
- self-administered by inhalation or intravenous route

Intoxication
- elation, euphoria, pressured speech, restlessness, sympathetic stimulation (i.e. tachycardia, mydriasis, sweating)
- prolonged use may result in paranoia and psychosis

Overdose
- medical emergency: hypertension, tachycardia, tonic-clonic seizures, dyspnea, and ventricular arrhythmias
- treatment with IV diazepam to control seizures and propanolol or labetalol to manage hypertension and arrhythmias

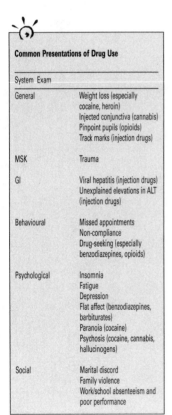

Common Presentations of Drug Use

System	Exam
General	Weight loss (especially cocaine, heroin) Injected conjunctiva (cannabis) Pinpoint pupils (opioids) Track marks (injection drugs)
MSK	Trauma
GI	Viral hepatitis (injection drugs) Unexplained elevations in ALT (injection drugs)
Behavioural	Missed appointments Non-compliance Drug-seeking (especially benzodiazepines, opioids)
Psychological	Insomnia Fatigue Depression Flat affect (benzodiazepines, barbiturates) Paranoia (cocaine) Psychosis (cocaine, cannabis, hallucinogens)
Social	Marital discord Family violence Work/school absenteeism and poor performance

Withdrawal
- initial "crash" (1-48 hrs): increased sleep, increased appetite
- withdrawal (1-10 wks): dysphoric mood plus fatigue, irritability, vivid, unpleasant dreams, insomnia or hypersomnia, psychomotor agitation or retardation
- complications: relapse, suicide (significant increase in suicide during withdrawal period)
- management: supportive management

Treatment of Chronic Abuse
- optimal treatment not established
- psychotherapy, group therapy, and behaviour modification useful in maintaining abstinence
- studies of dopamine agonists to block cravings show inconsistent results

Complications
- cardiovascular: arrhythmias, MI, CVA, ruptured AA
- neurologic: seizures
- psychiatric: psychosis, paranoia, delirium, suicidal ideation

Cannabis

- marijuana, hashish (hash) and hash oil come from cannabis sativa
- street names: weed, herb, chronic, jay, bud, blunt, bomb, doobie, hydro, sinsemilla, hash, joint, pot, grass, reefer, Mary Jane (MJ), ganja, homegrown, dope, spliff
- marijuana is the most often used illicit drug
- psychoactive substance delta-9-tetrahydrocannabinol (Δ^9-THC)
- smoking is the most common mode of self-administration
- intoxication characterized by tachycardia, conjunctival vascular engorgement, dry mouth, increased appetite, increased sense of well-being, euphoria/laughter, muscle relaxation, impaired performance on psychomotor tasks including driving
- high doses can cause depersonalization, paranoia, and anxiety
- may trigger psychosis and schizophrenia in predisposed individuals
- chronic use associated with tolerance and an apathetic, amotivational state
- cessation does not produce significant withdrawal phenomenon
- treatment of dependence includes behavioural and psychological interventions to maintain an abstinent state

Amphetamines

- types of amphetamines: amphetamine, methamphetamine, dextroamphetamine
- street names: speed, bennies, glass, crystal, crank, pep pills, uppers
- class of drugs structurally related to catecholamine neurotransmitters, includes methamphetamine (see *Club Drugs*)
- intoxication characterized by euphoria, improved concentration, sympathetic and behavioural hyperactivity
- at high doses can cause coma
- chronic use can produce a paranoid psychosis diagnostically similar to schizophrenia with agitation, paranoia, delusions and hallucinations; antipsychotics useful in treatment of stimulant psychosis
- withdrawal symptoms include dysphoria, fatigue, and restlessness

Hallucinogens

- types of hallucinogens: LSD, mescaline, psilocybin, PCP, cannabis, ecstasy, salvia (see *Club Drugs*)
- LSD is a highly potent drug; intoxication characterized by tachycardia, hypertension, mydriasis, tremor, hyperpyrexia, and a variety of perceptual and mood changes
- treatment of agitation and psychosis: support, reassurance, diminished stimulation; benzodiazepines or high potency antipsychotics seldom required
- high doses can cause depersonalization, paranoia, and anxiety
- no specific withdrawal syndrome characterized

Phencyclidine

- street names: PCP, angel dust
- widely used in veterinary medicine to immobilize large animals; mechanism of action not well understood
- taken orally, smoked, or IV
- intoxication characterized by an amnestic, euphoric, hallucinatory state; horizontal/vertical nystagmus, myoclonus, ataxia, and autonomic instability common
- effects unpredictable and often include prolonged agitated psychosis; individuals at high risk for suicide or violence towards others

Medical Uses of Marijuana:
- Anorexia-cachexia (AIDS, cancer)
- Spasticity, muscle spasms (multiple sclerosis, spinal cord injury)
- Levodopa-induced dyskinesia (Parkinson's Disease)
- Controlling tics and obsessive-compulsive behaviour (Tourette's syndrome)
- Reducing intra-ocular pressure (glaucoma)

Cannabis use and risk of psychotic or affective mental health outcomes: a systematic review
The Lancet. 2007 370:319-328
Purpose: To review the evidence for cannabis use and occurrence of psychotic or affective mental health outcomes.
Study Characteristics: A meta-analysis of 35 population-based longitudinal studies, or case-control studies nested within longitudinal designs.
Results: There was an increased risk of any psychotic outcome in individuals who had ever used cannabis (pooled adjusted odds ratio =1.41, 95% CI 1.20-1.65). Findings were consistent with a dose-response effect, with greater risk in people who used cannabis more frequently (2.09, 95% CI, 1.54-2.84). Findings for depression, suicidal thoughts and anxiety outcomes were less consistent. In both cases (psychotic and affective outcomes) a substantial confounding effect was present.
Conclusions: The findings are consistent with the view that cannabis increases risk of psychotic outcomes independent of transient intoxication effects, although evidence is less strong for affective outcomes. Although cannabis use and the development of psychosis are strongly associated, it is difficult to determine causality and it is possible that the association results from confounding factors or bias. The authors did conclude that there is sufficient evidence to warn young people that using cannabis could increase their risk of developing a psychotic illness later in life.

- at high doses, can cause coma
- treatment of toxic reaction: room with minimal stimulation; diazepam IV for muscle spasm/seizures; haloperidol to suppress psychotic behaviour

"Club Drugs"

MDMA ("Ecstasy", "X", "E")
- has properties of a hallucinogen and an amphetamine; acts on serotonergic and dopaminergic pathways
- enhances sensorium; increased feelings of well-being and empathy
- adverse effects: sweating, tachycardia, fatigue, muscle spasms (especially jaw clenching), ataxia
- severe complications (not necessarily dose-dependent): hyperthermia, arrhythmias, DIC, rhabdomyolysis, renal failure, seizures and death
- animal studies suggest long-term neurotoxicity to serotonergic system

Gamma Hydroxybutyrate (GHB, "G", "Liquid Ecstasy")
- produces biphasic dopamine response and releases opiate-like substance
- purported euphoric effects, increased aggression and impaired judgement
- adverse effects: nystagmus, ataxia, amnesia, apnea with sudden awakening and violence, bradycardia
- abrupt cessation of high doses can cause severe withdrawal with tremor, seizures and psychosis

Flunitrazepam (Rohypnol™, "Roofies", "Rope", "The Forget Pill")
- one of the most potent benzodiazepines; rapidly absorbed after oral administration
- produces sedation, psychomotor impairment and amnestic effects
- decreased sexual inhibition, CNS depression with EtOH

Date Rape Drugs:
GHB
Flunitrazepam (Rohypnol)
Ketamine

Ketamine ("Special K", "Kit-Kat")
- a general anesthetic still in use to sedate children for short procedures
- NMDA receptor antagonist
- rapid-acting; produces a "dissociative" state with profound amnesia and analgesia; also hallucinations and sympathomimetic effects
- strong potential for psychological distress or accidents due to intensity of experience and lack of bodily control
- may be packaged to look like Ecstasy
- toxicity: decreased LOC, respiratory depression, catatonia

Methamphetamine ("speed", "meth", "chalk", "ice", "crystal")
- stimulant similar to amphetamine with more pronounced effects on CNS
- may be smoked, snorted, injected, orally ingested
- initial rush begins in minutes and overall effects last 6-8 hours
- tolerance occurs quickly, users often binge and crash
- usually results in increased activity, decreased appetite, general sense of well-being
- can cause state of high agitation, rage and violent behaviour, occasionally hyperthermia and convulsions
- long-term use results in addiction, anxiety, confusion, insomnia, paranoia, auditory and tactile hallucinations (especially formication), delusions, mood disturbance, suicidal and homicidal thoughts, stroke
- illegal methamphetamine production may be contaminated with lead, and IV users may present with acute lead poisoning

Formication – tactile hallucination that insects or snakes are crawling over or under the skin

Suicide

Epidemiology
- attempted:completed = 120:1
- M:F = 3:1 for completed; 1:4 for attempts

Risk Factors
- epidemiologic factors
  - age: increases after age 14; second most common cause of death for ages 15-24; highest rates in persons >65 years
  - sex: male
  - race/ethnic background: white or native Canadians on reserves
  - marital status: widowed/divorced
  - living situation: alone; no children <18 years old in the household
  - other: stressful life events; access to firearms

- Asking patients about suicide will not give them the idea or the incentive to commit suicide.
- The best predictor of completed suicide is a history of attempted suicide.
- The most common psychiatric disorders associated with completed suicide are major depression and alcohol abuse.

- psychiatric disorders
  - mood disorders (15% lifetime risk in depression; higher in bipolar)
  - anxiety disorders (especially panic disorder)
  - schizophrenia (10-15% risk)
  - substance abuse (especially EtOH – 15% lifetime risk)
  - eating disorders (5% lifetime risk)
  - adjustment disorder
  - conduct disorder
  - personality disorders (borderline, antisocial)
- past history
  - prior suicide attempt
  - family history of suicide attempt/completion

Clinical Presentation
- symptoms associated with suicide
  - hopelessness
  - anhedonia
  - insomnia
  - severe anxiety
  - impaired concentration
  - psychomotor agitation
  - panic attacks

Pharmacotherapy and Suicide Risk
Once antidepressant therapy is initiated, patients should be followed frequently as there is a "suicide window" in which the patient may still be depressed, but now has enough energy to carry out suicide. Avoid tricyclic antidepressants (TCAs) as high lethality in overdose!

Approach
Every Patient: "Have you had any thoughts of wanting to hurt yourself?"
- Ideation – "Do you have thoughts about ending your life, committing suicide?"
- Passive – would rather not be alive but doesn't admit to idea that involves act of initiation
  - "I'd rather not wake up"
  - "I wouldn't mind if a car hit me"
- Active
  - "I think about killing myself"
- Plan – "Do you have a plan as to how you would end your life?"
- Intent – "You talk about wanting to die, but are you planning to do this?", "What has stopped you from ending your life?"
- Past attempts - Highest risk if previous attempt in past year, ask about lethality, outcome, medical intervention

Assessment of Suicidal Ideation
- Onset and frequency of thoughts - "When did this start? How often do you have these thoughts?"
- Control over suicidal ideation - "Can you stop the thoughts or call someone for help?"
- Lethality - "Do you want to end your life? Or get a 'release' from your emotional pain?"
- Access to means - "How will you get a gun?" "Which bridge do you think you would go to?"
- Time and place - "Have you picked a date and place? Is it in an isolated location?"
- Provocative factors - "What makes you feel worse (e.g. being alone)?"
- Protective factors - "What keeps you alive (e.g. friends, family, pets, faith, therapist)?"
- Final Arrangements - "Have you written a suicide note? Made a will? Given away your belongings?"
- Practised suicide or aborted attempts - "Have you put the gun to your head? Held the medications in your hand? Stood at the bridge?"
- Ambivalence - "There must be a part of you that wants to live - you came here for help"

Suicide Risk Factors:
"SAD PERSONS"
Sex (male)
Age >60 years old
Depression
Previous attempts
Ethanol abuse
Rational thinking loss (delusions, hallucinations, hopelessness)
Suicide in family
Organized plan
No spouse (no support systems)
Serious illness, intractable pain

Assessment of Suicide Attempt
- Setting – isolated vs. others present, chance of discovery
- Planned vs. impulsive attempt, triggers/stressors
- Intoxication
- Medical attention – brought in by another person vs. brought in by self to ER
- Time lag from suicide attempt to ER arrival
- Expectation of lethality, dying
- Reaction to survival: guilt/remorse vs. disappointment/self-blame

Management
- depends on the level of risk identified
- higher risk:
  - patients with a plan, access to lethal means, recent social stressors, and symptoms suggestive of a psychiatric disorder should be hospitalized immediately
  - do not leave patient alone; remove potentially dangerous objects from room
  - if patient refuses to be hospitalized, complete form for involuntary admission
- lower risk:
  - patients who are not actively suicidal, with no plan or access to lethal means
  - discuss protective factors and supports in their life, remind them of what they live for (as identified above), promote survival skills that helped them through previous suicide attempts

- make a safety plan - an agreement that they will not harm themselves, that they will try to avoid alcohol, drugs, and situations that may trigger suicidal thoughts, that they will follow up with you at a designated time, and that they will contact a health care worker, call a crisis line or go to an emergency department if they feel unsafe or if their suicidal feelings return or intensify
- depression: hospitalize if severe or if psychotic features are present; otherwise outpatient treatment with good supports and SSRIs/SNRIs
- alcohol-related: usually resolves with abstinence for a few days; if not, suspect depression
- personality disorders: crisis intervention/confrontation, may or may not hospitalize
- schizophrenia/psychosis: hospitalization
- parasuicide/self-mutilation: long-term psychotherapy with brief crisis intervention when necessary
- proper documentation of the clinical encounter and rationale for management is essential

Somatoform Disorders

General Characteristics
- physical signs and symptoms lacking a known medical basis in the presence of psychological factors that are judged to be important in the initiation, exacerbation, or maintenance of the disturbance
- cause significant distress or impairment in functioning
- symptoms are produced unconsciously
- symptoms are **not** the result of malingering or factitious disorder which are under conscious control
- primary gain: somatic symptom represents a symbolic resolution of an unconscious psychological conflict; serves to reduce anxiety and conflict; no external incentive
- secondary gain: the sick role; external benefits obtained or unpleasant duties avoided (e.g. work)

Management of Somatoform Disorders
- brief frequent visits
- limit number of physicians involved in care
- focus on psychosocial not physical symptoms
- minimize medical investigations; co-ordinate necessary investigations
- biofeedback
- psychotherapy – conflict resolution
- minimize psychotropic drugs (anxiolytics in short term only; antidepressants for depressive symptoms)
- attend to transference and countertransference

Conversion Disorder

- one or more symptoms or deficits affecting voluntary motor or sensory function that mimic a neurological or general medical condition (e.g. impaired co-ordination, local paralysis, double vision, seizures or convulsions)
- psychological factors thought to be etiologically related to the symptoms as the initiation of symptoms is preceded by conflicts or other stressors
- 11-300/100,000 in general population; focus of treatment in 1-3% of outpatient referrals to mental health clinics
- more common in rural populations and in individuals with little medical knowledge
- spontaneous remission in 95% of acute cases, 50% of chronic cases (>6 months)

Somatization Disorder

- recurring, multiple, clinically significant physical complaints which result in patient seeking treatment or having impaired functioning
- ≥8 physical symptoms that have no organic pathology including each of:
  - four pain symptoms related to at least four different sites or functions
  - two gastrointestinal symptoms, not including pain
  - one sexual symptom, not including pain
  - one pseudo-neurological symptom, not including pain (e.g. numbness, paresthesias)
- onset before age 30; extends over a period of years
- lifetime prevalence 0.2-2% among women and 0.2% among men
- cultural factors may influence sex ratio
- complications: anxiety, depression, unnecessary medications or surgery

Malingering – intentional production of false or grossly exaggerated physical or psychological symptoms, motivated by external reward (e.g. avoiding work, obtaining financial compensation or obtaining drugs)

Factitious disorder – intentional production or feigning of physical or psychological signs or symptoms in order to assume the sick role where external incentives (e.g. economic gain) are absent

- often a misdiagnosis for an insidious illness so rule out all organic illnesses (e.g. multiple sclerosis)

Pain Disorder

- pain is primary symptom and is of sufficient severity to warrant medical attention
- usually no organic pathology but when it exists reaction is excessive
- lifetime prevalence 12%
- psychiatric disorders (mood, anxiety, substance) may precede, co-occur or result from pain disorder

Elements of pain perception:
- cognition
- affect
- nociception

Hypochondriasis

- preoccupation with fear of having, or the idea that one has, a serious disease based on a misinterpretation of one or more bodily signs or symptoms
- evidence does not support diagnosis of a physical disorder
- fear of having a disease despite medical reassurance
- belief is not of delusional intensity (as in delusional disorder, somatic type) as person acknowledges unrealistic interpretation
- duration is ≥6 months; onset in 3rd-4th decade of life
- community prevalence 1.1-4.5%; prevalence in general medical practice 4-9%; higher in psychiatric settings

Body Dysmorphic Disorder

- preoccupation with imagined defect in appearance or excess concern around slight anomaly
- usually related to face
- M=F, prevalence 1-2.2% in the community; 6-15% in dermatology/cosmetic surgery clinics
- may lead to avoidance of work or social situations

Dissociative Disorders

Definition
- dissociation so severe that the usually integrated functions of consciousness and perception of self break down
- sudden or gradual onset, transient or chronic course
- symptoms cause distress or impaired functioning

Manifestations
- dissociative amnesia, dissociative fugue, dissociative identity disorder, and depersonalization disorder
- differential diagnosis: PTSD, acute stress disorder, somatization disorder, substance abuse, general medical condition (e.g. complex/partial seizures)

Table 4. Dissociative Disorders

	Amnesia	Fugue	Identity Disorder	Depersonalization Disorder
Diagnosis	Inability to recall important personal information, usually of a traumatic or stressful nature; may be localized, selective or generalized	Sudden, unexpected travel away from home or workplace with inability to recall some or all of one's past; may assume new identity	Two or more distinct personalities that take control of an individual's behaviour; amnesia regarding personal history (a.k.a. Multiple Personality Disorder)	Persistent or recurrent experiences of feeling detached from one's mental processes or body (i.e. like being in a dream)
Epidemiology	6% prevalence Increased in survivors of trauma (war, abuse)	0.2% prevalence May occur under traumatic circumstances (combat, rape, natural disasters)	1.3% prevalence, M:F=1.3:9 May have history of physical or sexual abuse	Rare disorder Approximately 50% of adults have experienced a single brief episode of depersonalization, precipitated by extreme stress
Treatment	Psychotherapy, hypnosis No proven role for barbiturates/pharmacologically-assisted interviewing	Usually spontaneous recovery Psychotherapy, hypnosis Ensure stability and safety No proven role for barbiturates/pharmacologically-assisted interviewing	Three stages: symptom stabilization, attention to trauma, reintegration Psychotherapy, hypnosis Symptom-oriented adjuvants (antidepressants, anxiolytics) No proven role for barbiturates/pharmacologically-assisted interviewing	Psychotherapy Pharmacotherapy: clonazepam, fluoxetine, clomipramine

Sleep Disorders

Criteria for Diagnosis
- causes significant distress or impairment in functioning
- not due to medications, drugs, or a GMC

Nocturnal Myoclonus

- middle-aged and elderly
- myoclonic jerks every 20-40 seconds
- bed partner complaints
- treatment: benzodiazepines (clonazepam, nitrazepam)

Narcolepsy

Symptoms of Narcolepsy: "CHAP"
Cataplexy
Hallucinations
Attacks of Sleep
Paralysis on waking

- irresistible sleep attacks (up to 30 minutes) and persistent day time drowsiness occurring daily for ≥**3 months**
- cataplexy (sudden temporary episodes of paralysis with loss of muscle tone)
- sleep paralysis
- hypnogogic (while falling asleep)/hypnopompic (while waking) hallucinations are manifestations of recurrent invasions of rapid eye movement (REM) sleep into the transition between sleep and wakefulness
- incidence 4:10,000 cases; M=F
- treatment: stimulants (methylphenidate, D-amphetamine), TCAs, SSRIs

PRIMARY INSOMNIA
- see Family Medicine

SLEEP APNEA
- see Respirology

Sexuality and Gender

Sexual Orientation

- describes the degree of a person's erotic attraction to people of the same sex (homosexual), the opposite sex (heterosexual), or both sexes (bisexual)
- individuals may fall anywhere along a continuum between exclusive homosexuality and exclusive heterosexuality
- homosexuals and bisexuals undergo a developmental process of identity formation
    - **sensitization** – sensation of being different from one's peers
    - **identity confusion** – after puberty, awareness of same-sex attraction may conflict with social expectations
    - **identity assumption** – self-definition as homosexual or bisexual, but not yet fully accepted
    - **commitment** – self-acceptance and comfort with identity; disclosure to family, social, occupational settings

Paraphilias

- **definition**: sexual arousal, fantasies, sexual urges or behaviour involving non-human objects, suffering or humiliation of oneself or one's partner, children or other non-consenting person
- **subtypes**: exhibitionism, fetishism, frotteurism, voyeurism, pedophilia, sexual masochism, sexual sadism, transvestite fetishism, not otherwise specified (NOS)
- rarely self-referred; come to medical attention through interpersonal or legal conflict
- person usually has more than one paraphilia; only 5% of paraphilia diagnoses attributed to women
- **typical presentation:**
    - begins in childhood or early adolescence; increasing in complexity and stability with age
    - chronic, decreases with advancing age
    - may increase with psychosocial stressors
- **treatment:**
    - anti-androgen drugs
    - behaviour modification
    - psychotherapy

Gender Identity Disorder

- gender identity is set at approximately 3 years of age
- **typical presentation:**
  - strong and persistent cross-gender identification
  - repeated stated desire or insistence that one is of the opposite sex
  - preference for cross-dressing, cross-gender roles in make-believe plays
  - intense desire to participate in the stereotypical games and pastimes of the opposite sex
  - strong preference for playmates of the opposite sex
  - significant distress or impairment in functioning and persistent discomfort with his or her sex or gender role
- **treatment:**
  - psychotherapy
  - hormonal therapy
  - sexual reassignment surgery

SEXUAL DYSFUNCTION
- see Gynecology and Urology

Eating Disorders

Epidemiology
- anorexia nervosa (AN) – 1% of adolescent and young adult females; onset 13-20 years old
- bulimia nervosa (BN) – 2-4% of adolescent and young adult females; onset 16-18 years old
- F:M=10:1; mortality 5-10%

Etiology
- commonly multifactorial – psychological, sociological and biological associations
- **individual:** perfectionism, lack of control in other life areas, history of sexual abuse
- **personality:** obsessive-compulsive, histrionic, borderline
- **familial:** maintenance of equilibrium in dysfunctional family
- **cultural factors:** prevalent in industrialized societies, idealization of thinness in the media
- **genetic factors:**
  - AN: 6% prevalence in siblings, with one study of twin pairs finding concordance in 9 of 12 monozygotic pairs versus concordance in 1 of 14 dizygotic pairs
  - BN: higher familial incidence of affective disorders than the general population

Risk Factors
- **physical factors:** obesity, chronic medical illness (e.g. diabetes mellitus)
- **psychological factors:** individuals who by career choice are expected to be thin, family history (mood disorders, eating disorders, substance abuse), history of sexual abuse, homosexual men, competitive athletes, concurrent associated mental illness (depression, OCD, anxiety disorder (especially panic and agoraphobia), substance abuse (BN))

Anorexia Nervosa

DSM-IV-TR Diagnostic Criteria for Anorexia Nervosa
A. refusal to maintain body weight at or above a minimally normal weight for age and height (e.g. weight loss leading to maintenance of body weight less than 85% of that expected; or failure to make expected weight gain during period of growth, leading to body weight less than 85% of that expected)
B. intense fear of gaining weight or becoming fat, even though underweight
C. disturbance in the way in which one's body weight or shape is experienced, undue influence of body weight or shape on self-evaluation, or denial of the seriousness of the current low body weight
D. in postmenarcheal females, amenorrhea, i.e. the absence of at least three consecutive menstrual cycles

Specific Type
- **restricting:** during the current episode of anorexia nervosa, the person has not regularly engaged in binge-eating or purging behaviour (i.e. self-induced vomiting or the misuse of laxatives, diuretics, or enemas)
- **binge-eating/purging:** during the current episode of anorexia nervosa, the person has regularly engaged in binge-eating or purging behavior (i.e. self-induced vomiting or the misuse of laxatives, diuretics, or enemas)

Associated Features
- deteriorating mood (irritable, anxious, extreme sensitivity, sadness)
- isolation

Athletic Triad
1. Disordered eating
2. Amenorrhea
3. Osteoporosis

- trouble concentrating due to repetitive, intrusive, irresolvable and anxiety-provoking thoughts about food and weight
- malnutrition
- poor sleep

Management
- criteria for admission vary among hospitals
- admit to hospital if: <65% of standard body weight (<85% of standard body weight for adolescents), hypovolemia requiring intravenous fluid, heart rate <40 bpm, abnormal serum chemistry or if actively suicidal
- agree on target body weight on admission and reassure this weight will not be surpassed
- psychotherapy (individual/group/family) – addressing food and body perception, coping mechanisms, health effects
- monitor for complications of AN (see Table 5)
- monitor for **refeeding syndrome**:
    - a potentially life-threatening metabolic response to refeeding in severely malnourished patients resulting in severe shifts in fluid and electrolyte levels
    - complications include hypophosphatemia, congestive heart failure, cardiac arrhythmias, delirium and death
    - prevention: slow refeeding, gradual increase in nutrition, supplemental phosphorus, close monitoring of electrolytes and cardiac status

Prognosis
- early intervention much more effective
- with treatment, 70% resume a weight of at least 85% of expected levels and about 50% resume normal menstrual function
- eating peculiarities and associated psychiatric symptoms are common and persistent
- long-term mortality – 10% to 20% of patients hospitalized will die in next 10 to 30 years (secondary to severe and chronic starvation, metabolic or cardiac catastrophies, with a significant proportion committing suicide)

Bulimia Nervosa

DSM-IV-TR Diagnostic Criteria for Bulimia Nervosa
A. recurrent episodes of binge eating, characterized by both of the following:
    (1) eating, in a discrete period of time (e.g. within any 2-hour period), an amount of food that is definitely larger than most people would eat during a similar period of time and under similar circumstances
    (2) a sense of lack of control over eating during the episode (e.g. a feeling that one cannot stop eating or control what or how much one is eating)
B. recurrent inappropriate compensatory behaviour in order to prevent weight gain, such as self-induced vomiting, misuse of laxatives, diuretics, enemas, or other medications, fasting, or excessive exercise
C. the binge eating and inappropriate compensatory behaviours both occur, on average, at least twice a week for 3 months
D. self-evaluation is unduly influenced by body shape and weight
E. the disturbance does not occur exclusively during episodes of Anorexia Nervosa

Specific Type
- **purging**: during the current episode of bulimia nervosa, the person has regularly engaged in self-induced vomiting or the misuse of laxatives, diuretics, or enemas
- **non-purging**: during the current episode of bulimia nervosa, the person has used other inappropriate compensatory behaviours, such as fasting or excessive exercise, but has not regularly engaged in self-induced vomiting or the misuse of laxatives, diuretics, or enemas

Associated Features
- fatiguability and muscle weakness due to repetitive vomiting and fluid/electrolyte imbalance
- tooth decay
- swollen appearance around angle of jaw and puffiness of eye sockets due to fluid retention
- reddened knuckles, Russell's sign (knuckle callus)
- trouble concentrating
- weight fluctuation over time

Management
- criteria for admission: significant electrolyte abnormalities
- biological
    - treatment of starvation effects
    - SSRIs
- psychological
    - develop trusting relationship with therapist to explore personal etiology and triggers

Ipecac syrup
- Was commonly used to induce vomiting in accidental poisoning or drug overdose
- Used chronically by some patients with ED to induce vomiting

- reality-oriented feedback, cognitive behavioural therapy, family therapy
- recognition of health risks
  - social
    - challenge destructive societal views of women
    - use of hospital environment to provide external patterning for normative eating behaviour

Prognosis
- few recover without recurrence
- good prognostic factors: onset before age 15, achieving a healthy weight within 2 years of treatment
- poor prognostic factors: later age of onset, previous hospitalizations, individual and familial disturbance

Table 5. Physiologic Complications of Eating Disorders

System	Starvation	Binge-purge
General	Low BP, low HR, significant orthostatic changes ± syncopal episodes, low temperature, vitamin deficiencies	Russell's sign (knuckle callus) Parotid gland enlargement Perioral skin irritation Periocular and palatal petechiae Loss of dental enamel and caries Aspiration pneumonia Metabolic alkalosis secondary to hypokalemia and loss of acid
Endocrine	Primary or secondary amenorrhea, $\downarrow T_3/T_4$	
Neurologic	Grand mal seizure ($\downarrow$Ca, Mg, PO$_4$)	
Cutaneous	Dry skin, lanugo hair, hair loss or thinning, brittle nails, yellow skin from high carotene	
GI	Constipation, GERD, delayed gastric emptying	Acute gastric dilation/rupture, pancreatitis, GERD, hematemesis secondary to Mallory-Weiss tear
CVS	Arrhythmias, CHF	Arrhythmias, cardiomyopathy (from use of ipecac), sudden cardiac death ($\downarrow$K)
MSK	Osteoporosis secondary to hypogonadism	Muscle wasting
Renal	Pre-renal failure (hypovolemia), renal calculi	Renal failure (electrolyte disturbances)
Extremities	Pedal edema ($\downarrow$ albumin)	Pedal edema ($\downarrow$ albumin)
Lab Values	Starvation: $\downarrow$RBCs, $\downarrow$WBCs, $\downarrow$LH, $\downarrow$FSH, $\downarrow$estrogen, $\downarrow$testosterone, $\uparrow$growth hormone, $\uparrow$cholesterol Dehydration: $\uparrow$BUN	Vomiting : $\downarrow$Na, $\downarrow$K, $\downarrow$Cl, $\downarrow$H, $\uparrow$amylase; hypokalemia with metabolic alkalosis Laxatives : $\downarrow$Na, $\downarrow$K, $\downarrow$Cl, $\uparrow$H; metabolic acidosis

Personality Disorders

General Diagnostic Criteria
- an enduring pattern of inner experience and behaviour that deviates markedly from the expectations of the individual's culture; manifested in two or more of: cognition, affect, interpersonal functioning, impulse control
- inflexible and pervasive across a range of situations
- causes distress or impaired functioning not necessarily for the person with the personality disorder, but for those around him/her
- pattern is stable and well established by adolescence or early adulthood
- associated with many complications, such as depression, suicide, violence, brief psychotic episodes, multiple drug use and treatment resistance
- each personality disorder is present in 1% of the population
- personality disorders are lifelong and chronic
- the mainstay of treatment is psychotherapy with the addition of pharmacotherapy to treat associated axis I disorders (i.e. depression, anxiety, substance abuse)

Table 6. Classifying and Diagnosing the Personality Disorders

NB. For each personality disorder, the most recognizable feature is indicated in *italics*

Diagnostic Cluster	Diagnosis

Cluster A "Mad"
Patients seem odd, eccentric, withdrawn

Familial association with psychotic disorders

Common defense mechanisms:
intellectualization, projection, magical thinking

Paranoid Personality Disorder
Pervasive distrust and suspiciousness of others, interpret motives as malevolent.
Blame problems on others and seem angry and hostile.

Diagnosis requires 4 of:
1. Suspicious that others are exploiting or deceiving them
2. Pre-occupied with trustworthiness of acquaintances
3. Reluctant to confide in others
4. Interpret benign remarks as threatening, demeaning
5. Holds grudges
6. Perceives attacks on character and is quick to counterattack
7. Questions fidelity of partner without justification

Schizoid Personality Disorder
Neither desires nor enjoys close relationships including being a part of a family; prefers to be alone.
Lifelong pattern of social withdrawal
Seen as eccentric and reclusive with restricted affect.

Diagnosis requires 4 of:
1. Does not enjoy or desire close relationships
2. Chooses solitary activities
3. Little to no interest in sexual activity with others
4. Takes pleasure in few (if any) activities
5. Few or no close friends
6. Indifference to praise or criticism
7. Emotionally cold, detached, or have flattened affect

Schizotypal Personality Disorder
Pattern of eccentric behaviours, peculiar thought patterns.

Diagnosis requires 5 of:
1. Ideas of reference
2. Odd beliefs, magical thinking (inconsistent with cultural norms i.e. belief in telepathy, superstitions)
3. Unusual perceptual experiences (i.e. bodily illusions)
4. Suspiciousness
5. Inappropriate or restricted affect
6. Odd, eccentric appearance or behaviour (i.e. involved in cults, strange religious practices)
7. Few close friends
8. Odd thinking, odd speech (i.e. vague, stereotyped)
9. Excessive social anxiety

Cluster B "Bad"
Patients seem dramatic, emotional, inconsistent

Familial association with mood disorders

Common defense mechanisms:
denial, acting out, regression (histrionic PD), splitting (borderline PD), projective identification, idealization/devaluation

> **Borderline Personality: "IMPULSIVE"**
> **I**mpulsive
> **M**oody
> **P**aranoid under stress
> **U**nstable self image
> **L**abile intense relationships
> **S**uicidal
> **I**nappropriate anger
> **V**ulnerable to abandonment
> **E**mptiness

Borderline Personality Disorder
Unstable moods and behaviour, feel alone in the world, problems with self image
History of repeated suicide attempts, self-harm behaviours
10% suicide rate

Diagnosis requires 5 of:
1. Frantic efforts to avoid real or imagined abandonment
2. Unstable and intense relationships
3. Unstable sense of self
4. Impulsivity in two potentially harmful ways (sexual, drugs, spending)
5. Recurrent suicidal behaviour/self-harm
6. Unstable mood/affect
7. General feelings of emptiness
8. Difficulty controlling anger
9. Transient dissociative symptoms or paranoid ideation associated with stress

Antisocial Personality Disorder
Lack of remorse for actions, manipulative and deceitful, often violate the law. May appear charming on first impression.
Pattern of disregard for others and violation of rights of others must be present before the age of 15, however, for the diagnosis of ASPD patients must be at least 18.

Diagnosis requires 3 of the following:
1. Failure to conform to social norms by committing unlawful acts
2. Deceitfulness, lying, manipulating others for personal gain
3. Impulsive, fails to plan ahead
4. Irritable, aggressive, repeated fights or assaults
5. Recklessness and disregard for personal safety, safety of others
6. Irresponsible, cannot sustain work
7. Lack of remorse for actions

Narcissistic Personality Disorder
Sense of superiority, needs constant admiration, lacks empathy, but with fragile sense of self.
Consider themselves "special" and will exploit others for personal gain.

Diagnosis requires 5 of:
1. Exaggerated sense of self-importance (grandiosity)
2. Preoccupied with fantasies of unlimited success, power, beauty, love
3. Believes he/she is "special" and should associate with other "special" people
4. Requires excessive admiration
5. Sense of entitlement
6. Takes advantage of others
7. Lacks empathy
8. Envious of others or believes that others are envious of him/her
9. Arrogant attitudes

Histrionic Personality Disorder
Attention-seeking behaviour and excessively emotional. Are dramatic, flamboyant and extroverted. Cannot form meaningful relationships.
Often sexually inappropriate.

Diagnosis requires 5 of:
1. Not comfortable unless center of attention
2. Inappropriately sexually seductive
3. Uses physical appearance to attract attention
4. Speech is impressionistic, lacks detail
5. Theatrical and exaggerated expression of emotion
6. Easily influenced by others
7. Perceives relationships as more intimate than they actually are

---

Cluster C "Sad"
Patients seem anxious, fearful

Familial association with anxiety disorder

Common defense mechanisms:
isolation, avoidance, hypochondriasis

> A key distinction between obsessive compulsive disorder (OCD) and obsessive compulsive personality disorder (OCPD) is that in OCD the symptoms are ego-dystonic (i.e. the patient realizes the obsessions are not reasonable) whereas in OCPD the symptoms are ego-syntonic (i.e. consistent with the patient's way of thinking).

Avoidant Personality Disorder
Timid and socially awkward with a pervasive sense of inadequacy and fear of criticism.
Fear of embarrassing or humiliating themselves in social situations so remain withdrawn and socially inhibited.

Diagnosis requires 4 of:
1. Avoids occupational activities that involve significant interpersonal contact for fear of criticism or rejection
2. Unwilling to get involved with people unless certain of being liked
3. Restrained in intimate relationships for fear of being shamed or ridiculed
4. Preoccupied with being rejected or criticized in social situations
5. Inhibited in new interpersonal situations due to fear of inadequacy
6. Views him or herself as inferior, socially inept or personally unappealing
7. Reluctant to engage in new activities for fear of embarassment

Dependent Personality Disorder
Pervasive and excessive need to be taken care of, excessive fear of separation, clinging and submissive behaviours.
Difficulty making everyday decisions.

Diagnosis requires 5 of:
1. Difficulty making everyday decisions without advice and reassurance from others
2. Needs others to assume responsibility for most major areas of his/her life
3. Difficulty expressing disagreement

4. Difficulty initiating projects due to lack of self-confidence
5. Goes to excessive lengths to obtain support
6. Uncomfortable or helpless when alone because of fear of being unable to take care of him/herself
7. Urgently seeks another relationship as a source of care and support when a close relationship ends
8. Unrealistically preoccupied with fears of being left to take care of him/herself

Obsessive-Compulsive Personality Disorder
Preoccupation with orderliness, perfectionism, and mental and interpersonal control.
Is inflexible, closed-off, and inefficient.

Diagnosis requires 4 of:
1. Preoccupation with details, rules, lists, order, organization, or schedules to extent that point of activity is lost
2. Perfectionism interferes with task completion
3. Excessively devoted to work to the exclusion of leisure activities and friendships
4. Inflexible about morality/ethics/values
5. Unable to discard worthless objects of no sentimental value
6. Reluctant to delegate tasks to others
7. Miserly spending style (money is hoarded for future disasters)
8. Rigid and stubborn

Child Psychiatry

The Child Psychiatric Interview

- ID
  - name, age, family situation, school grade
- chief complaint
  - onset, time course, stressors, impact on child's and family's functioning, supports
  - child's functioning and behaviour at home, at school, and with peers
  - mental status (see adult mental status exam)
- history of present illness
  - symptoms and features of most likely diagnostic area (e.g. disruptive behaviour disorders (ADHD, CD, ODD), developmental disorders, learning disorders, abuse, mood disorders, and anxiety disorders)
  - in adolescents, consider psychotic disorders, eating disorders, and substance abuse disorders
  - screen for comorbid conditions
- risk assessment
  - physical/sexual abuse, suicidality, aggression/homicidality, firesetting, risky behaviour
  - past assessments (e.g. psychiatric, psychological, educational), treatments, risk issues (past suicide attempts, past aggression), previous contact with child protection services
  - brief developmental history – pregnancy, birth, milestones, general behaviour, parents' method of discipline, school functioning, peer relationships

> **HEADSSS Interview:**
> **H**ome environment
> **E**ducation/employment
> **A**ctivities
> **D**rugs/diet
> **S**ex
> **S**afety
> **S**uicide/depression

Developmental Concepts

Table 7. Developmental Stages

Freud	Erikson	Piaget
Oral	Trust/mistrust (birth-1 year)	Sensorimotor (birth-2 years old)
Anal	Autonomy/shame, doubt (1-3 years old)	Object permanence (15 months) – Child begins to understand the concept that objects exist even when not visible
		Object constancy (18 months) – Child becomes comfortable with mother's absence by internalizing her image and the knowledge she will return
Oedipal	Initiative/guilt (4-6 years old)	Preoperational (2-7 years old)
Latency	Industry/inferiority (6-12 years old)	Concrete operations (7-11 years old)
	Identity/role confusion (adolescence)	Formal operations (11+ years)
	Erikson stages continue throughout life: Intimacy/isolation (young adult)	
	Generativity/stagnation (middle age)	
	Integrity/despair (later life)	

- **temperament**: innate psycho-physiological and behavioural characteristics of a child (e.g. emotionality, activity, and sociability); spectrum from "difficult" to "slow-to-warm-up" to "easy temperament", plotted on nine parameters:
  - activity level, adaptation, attention span and persistence, distractibility, intensity of reaction, quality of mood, response to a new stimulus, rhythmicity, threshold of responsiveness
- **parental fit**: the congruence between parenting style (authoritative, authoritarian, permissive) and child's temperament
- **attachment**: special relationship between child and primary caretaker(s); develops during first year (see Table 8); best predictor of a child's attachment style is their parent's attachment style
- **stranger anxiety** (8 months): infants cry at approach of stranger
- **separation anxiety** (10-18 months): separation from attachment figure results in distress

Attachment type can be assessed in infants 10-18 months of age using the Strange Situation test, in which the child is stressed by the caregiver being removed from the situation and the stranger staying. Attachment style is measured by the child's behaviour during the reunion with the caregiver.

Attachment problems may present as a child who is difficult to soothe, has difficulty sleeping, problems feeding, tantrums or behaviours.

Health Canada advises Canadians under the age of 18 to consult physicians if they are being treated with SSRIs, SNRIs, or mirtazapine. This request was made as a result of international reports that some of these drugs may be associated with an increased risk of suicidal ideation in patients under the age of 18. There was no increased risk of suicide completion.

Selective serotonin reuptake inhibitors in childhood depression: systematic review of published versus unpublished data
Lancet. 363(9418): 1341-5, 2004 Apr 24
Purpose: To evaluate the safety and effectiveness of SSRIs in the treatment of childhood depression, comparing published and unpublished data.
Study Characteristics: Meta-analysis of 5 double-blind RCTs published in peer-reviewed journals, 6 unpublished studies, and data reviewed in the Committee on Safety of Medicines report for SSRIs in pediatric major depressive disorder.
Participants: Patients age 5-18 years who were diagnosed with depression.
Intervention: Any SSRI.
Main Outcomes: Remission and response, mean depression level, serious adverse events, discontinuation attributable to any adverse event.
Results: Fluoxetine had a favourable risk-benefit profile, and was more likely than placebo to bring about remission by 7-8 weeks (NNTB 6, 95% CI 4-15) and lead to a clinically meaningful response (NNTB 5, 95% CI 4-13). This was supported by unpublished data. The one published trial for paroxetine and the two for sertraline have weak positive risk-benefit profiles, contradicted by unpublished data. Unpublished trials of citalopram and venlafaxine show similarly unfavourable profiles.
Conclusions: Fluoxetine has a favourable risk-benefit profile and can be used in the treatment of adolescent depression. The composite of published and unpublished data suggests other SSRIs have an unfavourable risk-benefit profile.

Table 8. Attachment Models

Parent/Caregiver	Attachment Type	Features in Child
Loving, consistently available, sensitive, and receptive	Secure	Able to use caregiver to calm self
Rejecting, unavailable psychologically, insensitive responses	Insecure (avoidant)	Not reliant on caregiver for soothing
Inconsistent, insensitive responses, role reversal	Insecure (ambivalent/resistant)	
Frightening, dissociated, sexualized, or atypical	Disorganized	

Mood Disorders

DEPRESSIVE DISORDER

Epidemiology
- pre-pubertal 1-2%; post-pubertal 4-8%; F:M = 2:1

Clinical Presentation
- see adult mood disorder (DSM-IV)
- more cognitive and fewer vegetative symptoms than adults
- physical factors: insomnia (children), hypersomnia (adults), somatic complaints, substance abuse
- psychological factors: boredom, irritability, anhedonia, discouragement, helplessness, low self-esteem, deterioration in academic performance, social withdrawal, lack of motivation
- comorbid diagnoses of anxiety, ADHD, conduct disorder, and eating disorders

Treatment
- majority never seek treatment
- individual/family psychotherapy and education, modified school program
- SSRIs, SNRIs (see side note)
- ECT (only in adolescents)
- light therapy, self-help books

Prognosis
- prolonged, up to 1-2 years
- adolescent onset predicts chronic mood disorder; 2/3 will have another depressive episode within 5 years
- complications
  - negative impact on family and peer relationships
  - school failure
  - significantly increased risk of suicide attempt (10%) or completion
  - substance abuse

BIPOLAR DISORDER

Clinical Presentation
- see adult bipolar disorder/mania (DSM-IV)
- triad: inappropriate sexual behaviour, physical violence, mood swings in 24 hours
- may look like children with ADHD
- more likely to have bipolar II or rapid-cycling, particularly if early onset
- often comorbid or pre-existing ADHD/conduct disorder
- mixed presentation more common in adolescent population than adult population
- unipolar depression may be an early sign of adult bipolar disorder
  - ~30% of psychotic depressed adolescents receive a bipolar diagnosis within 2 years of presentation
  - associated with rapid onset of depression, psychomotor retardation, mood-congruent psychosis, affective illness in family, pharmacologically-induced mania

Treatment
- mood stabilizers ± antidepressants
- benzodiazepines (careful of disinhibiting effect) ± antipsychotics

Anxiety Disorders

- prevalence: 2-15%; F:M = 2:1

Diagnosis
- school problems, recurrent physical symptoms (stomach aches, headaches) especially in mornings, social and relationship problems, social withdrawal and isolation, family conflict, irritability and mood symptoms, alcohol and drug use in adolescents

Treatment
- family and individual psychotherapy
- behaviour modification techniques, stress reduction, parental education, predictive and supportive environment, relaxation techniques
- pharmacotherapy: SSRIs (e.g. fluoxetine), benzodiazepines (e.g. clonazepam - use with caution, may have disinhibiting effect)

SEPARATION ANXIETY DISORDER

Epidemiology
- prevalence: 4% of children/teens
- on average 7.5 years old at onset, 10 years old at presentation
- common for mother to have an anxiety or depressive disorder

Differential Diagnosis
- simple or social phobia, depression, learning disorder, truancy, conduct disorder, school-related problems (e.g. bullying)

Clinical Presentation
- school refusal (75%)
- excessive and developmentally inappropriate anxiety on separation from primary caregiver with physical or emotional distress for at least two weeks
- persistent worry, refusal to sleep, clinging, nightmares, somatic symptoms
- comorbid major depression common (2/3)
- worry about something happening to parent or themselves

Prognosis
- if inadequately treated early on, may present later in a more severe form
- may develop into panic disorder with/without agoraphobia

SOCIAL ANXIETY DISORDER
- must distinguish between shy child and child with social anxiety
  - diagnosis only if anxiety interferes significantly with daily routine, social life, academic functioning, or if markedly distressed
- features: temper tantrums, freezing, clinging behaviour, mutism, excessively timid, stays on periphery, refuses to be involved in group play
- must be capable of developing social relationships
- must occur in settings with peers, not just adults
- selective mutism:
  - does not speak in front of others; no problems speaking at home
  - must rule out language or communication problems
  - severe form of social anxiety

The shy child is quiet and reluctant to participate but slowly 'warms up'.

POST-TRAUMATIC STRESS DISORDER (PTSD)
- diagnostic criteria same as adults
  - in children, one often sees repetitive play involving the event, generalized nightmares, psychosomatic symptoms, omen formation
- common examples of trauma include: sexual/physical abuse, witnessing family violence, natural disasters
- can also be associated with onset of sexual activity

OBSESSIVE-COMPULSIVE DISORDER (OCD)
- diagnostic criteria same as adults, except it is not necessary for child to recognize thoughts/actions as excessive or unreasonable
- 0.3-1% of children/adolescents; tends to begin earlier in boys than girls
  - tend to engage in rituals at home rather than in front of others
  - associated with Tourette's Disorder

PANIC DISORDER
- diagnostic criteria same as adults
- genetic/parental modeling/identification hypothesized as cause
- often parent with panic or depressive disorder

GENERALIZED ANXIETY DISORDER (GAD)
- diagnostic criteria same as adults
- often redo tasks, show dissatisfaction with their work and tend to be perfectionistic
- often require reassurance and support to take on new tasks

SPECIFIC PHOBIA
- common phobias in childhood include a fear of heights, small animals, doctors, dentists, darkness, loud noises, thunder and lightening

Childhood Schizophrenia

Epidemiology
- 1/2,000 in childhood; increases after puberty to adult rates (1%) in late adolescence
- diagnostic criteria same as in adults
- <6 years old may present in similar fashion to Autism prior to onset of core symptoms
- prognosis poor as cognitive, language, social and personality development are disrupted

Treatment
- psychotherapy, family education
- low dose antipsychotics for target behaviours (i.e. aggression, hyperactivity, impulsiveness)
- hospitalization or residential placement, if severe

Pervasive Developmental Disorders (PDD)

- include Autism, Asperger's, Childhood Disintegrative Disorder, Rett's Disorder, and PDD NOS
- M:F = 3-4:1 (except for Rett's with female predominance)

Differential Diagnosis
- mental retardation, childhood schizophrenia, social phobia, OCD, communication disorder, non-verbal learning disorder, ADHD, abuse, hearing or visual impairment, seizure disorder, motor impairment

Management
- hearing test to rule out impairment
- chromosomal analysis to rule out abnormalities (e.g. trisomy 21)
- rule out psychotic disorders, social problems, depression, anxiety, abuse

Treatment
- team-based – school, psychologist, occupational therapist, physiotherapist, speech and language therapy, audiology, pediatrics, psychiatry
- family education and support
- treat concomitant disorders such as tics, OCD, anxiety, depression, and seizure disorder
- behaviour management, school programming
- pharmacotherapy – atypical antipsychotics (for bizarre behaviours, agitation, self-mutilation, tics), SSRIs (for anxiety, depression), stimulants (for associated hyperactivity)

Prognosis
- variable, but improves with early intervention
- better if IQ >60 and able to communicate

AUTISM
- prevalence 1/1000
- abnormalities in three areas:
    - social interaction – impaired non-verbal behaviours (eye contact, facial expression, hand gestures), failure to develop appropriate peer relationships, lack of social/emotional reciprocity
    - communication – delayed or absent speech or marked impairment to initiate or sustain a conversation; stereotyped/repetitive or idiosyncratic use of language; absence of appropriate make-believe play
    - restricted and repetitive behaviours, interests, and activities – inflexible adherence to specific, non-functional routines, stereotyped hand or body movements (e.g. rocking)
- at least 6 features before 3 years old (at least 2 from social interaction and 1 from other 2 categories)

ASPERGER'S SYNDROME
- prevalence 3/1000
- no early speech and language delay, no cognitive deficits, normal to high intelligence
- impaired social interaction with ≥2 of:
    - nonverbal interactions, peer relationships, spontaneous sharing of enjoyment/activities, social/emotional reciprocity
- restricted repetitive patterns of behaviour/interests with ≥1 of:
    - restricted interest with high intensity, inflexible nonfunctional routines, repetitive mannerisms, preoccupation with parts
- causes impairment, no delay in language or cognitive development, not caused by another PDD

CHILDHOOD DISINTEGRATIVE DISORDER (CDD)
- similar to autism, but there must be a period of at least 2 years (and up to ten years) of normal development
- rule out degenerative brain disease, schizophrenia

RETT'S DISORDER
- X-linked dominant disorder, therefore predominantly in girls
- restriction of brain growth beginning in first year of life
- normal development between 6 months to 4 years, then regression (loss of purposeful hand movements, mental retardation, seizures, neurological, respiratory and motor deficits)

PDD NOS
- marked deficits in above areas, but does not meet full criteria for another PDD

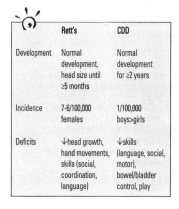

	Rett's	CDD
Development	Normal development, head size until ≥5 months	Normal development for ≥2 years
Incidence	7-6/100,000 females	1/100,000 boys>girls
Deficits	↓head growth, hand movements, skills (social, coordination, language)	↓skills (language, social, motor), bowel/bladder control, play

Attention Deficit Hyperactivity Disorder (ADHD)

- prevalence: 5-12% of school-aged children; M:F = 4:1, although girls may be under-diagnosed
    - girls tend to have inattentive/distractible symptoms; boys have impulsive/hyperactive symptoms

Etiology
- genetic – dopamine candidate genes, catecholamine/neuroanatomical hypothesis
- cognitive – MR, inhibitory control and other errors of executive function
- arousal – alterations in the sensory system filters

Diagnosis
- differential: learning disorders, hearing/visual defects, thyroid, atopic conditions, congenital problems (e.g. FAS, Fragile X), lead poisoning, history of head injury, traumatic life events (e.g. abuse)

- diagnosis (using Conner's Teacher's and Parent's ADHD Scales)
  - six or more symptoms of inattention and/or hyperactivity-impulsivity persisting for at least 6 months
  - onset before age 7
  - symptoms present in at least two settings (i.e. home, school, work)
  - interferes with academic, family, and social functioning
  - does not occur exclusively during the course of another psychiatric disorder

Table 9. Core Symptoms of ADHD (DSM-IV)

Inattention	Hyperactivity	Impulsivity
Careless mistakes	Fidgets, squirms in seat	Blurts out answers before questions completed
Cannot sustain attention in tasks or play	Leaves seat when expected to remain seated	Difficulty awaiting turn
Does not listen when spoken to directly		Interrupts/intrudes on others
Fails to complete tasks	Runs and climbs excessively	
Disorganized	Cannot play quietly	
Avoids, dislikes tasks that require sustained mental effort	On the "go", driven by a motor	
Loses things necessary for tasks or activities	Talks excessively	
Distractible		
Forgetful		

A 14-month randomized clinical trial of treatment strategies for attention-deficit/hyperactivity disorder
Arch Gen Psychiatry. 56:1073-1086, 1999
Purpose: To investigate the long-term efficacy of pharmacotherapy and behaviour therapy, as well as their combination.
Study Characteristics: Single blinded RCT with 579 children, and 14 month follow-up.
Participants: Age 7-9.9 with characteristics typical of other ADHD samples.
Intervention: 14 months of one of four interventions: 1) medication management, with methylphenidate used as a first line agent, followed by other drugs as required, and monthly follow-up; 2) intensive behavioural therapy (parent, school, and child); 3) the two combined; or 4) standard community care.
Main Outcomes: ADHD symptoms, oppositional/aggressive symptoms, social skills, internalizing symptoms (anxiety and depression), parent-child relation, and academic achievement
Results: All groups showed a reduction in symptoms over time. Medication was found to be superior to behavioural treatment for ADHD symptoms, but no other outcomes. Combined treatment and medication did not differ significantly across any domain in direct comparison. MTA medication treatments were superior to community care, despite the fact that two-thirds of community-treated subjects received medication during the study period.
Conclusions: Use of psychostimulant medications is superior to behavioural interventions or community care in treating ADHD symptoms. Combined medical and behavioural treatment is not more efficacious than medication alone in treating ADHD symptoms.

Features
- average onset 3 years old
- identification upon school entry
- rule out developmental delay, genetic syndromes, encephalopathies or toxins (alcohol, lead)
- risk of substance abuse, particularly cannabis and cocaine, depression, anxiety, academic failure, poor social skills, risk of comorbid CD and/or ODD, risk of adult ASPD
- associated with family history of ADHD, difficult temperamental characteristics

Treatment
- non-pharmacological – parent management, anger control strategies, positive reinforcement, social skills training, individual/family therapy, resource room, tutors, classroom intervention, exercise routines, extracurricular activities
- pharmacological
  - standard treatment – stimulants (methylphenidate - Ritalin®, Concerta® (long-acting), dextromethamphetamine, atamoxetine – Strattera®)
  - for comorbid symptoms – antidepressants, neuroleptics, clonidine, anticonvulsants, β-agonists

Prognosis
- 65% continue into adulthood; secondary personality disorders and compensatory anxiety disorders are identifiable
- 70-80% continue into adolescence, but hyperactive symptoms usually abate

Conduct Disorder (CD)

- prevalence: 1.5-3.4%; M:F = 4-12:1

Etiology
- parental/familial factors - parental psychopathology (e.g. ASPD, substance abuse), child rearing practices (e.g. child abuse, discipline), low SES, family violence
- child factors – difficult temperament, ODD, learning problems, neurobiology

Diagnosis
- differential: ADHD, depression, head injury, substance abuse
- diagnosis: use multiple sources (Achenbach Child Behavioural Checklist, Teacher's Report Form)
  - pattern of behaviour that violates rights of others and age-appropriate social norms with ≥3 in past 12 months and ≥1 in past 6 months:
    - aggression to people and animals (bullying, physical fights, use of weapons, forced sex)
    - destruction of property, firesetting with intent to damage
    - deceitfulness or theft (breaking and entering, car theft)
    - violation of rules (out all night before 13, runaway ≥2 times or for long periods time, often truant from school before 13)

- disturbance causes clinically significant impairment in social, academic, or occupational functioning
- if individual is 18 years or older, criteria not met for antisocial personality disorder
- diagnostic types
  - childhood onset: at least one criterion prior to age 10
    - poor prognosis: associated with ODD, aggressiveness, impulsiveness
  - adolescent onset: absence of any criteria until age 10
    - better prognosis; least aggressive, gang-related delinquency
  - mild, moderate, severe

Treatment
- early intervention necessary and more effective, long-term follow-up required
- parent management training, anger replacement training, CBT, family therapy, education/employment programs, social skills training, medications for aggressiveness or comorbid disorders
- pharmacotherapy is insufficient; mainly used for treatment of comorbid disorders

Prognosis
- poor prognostic indicators include early-age onset, high frequency and variety of behaviours, pervasiveness (i.e. in home, school, community), comorbid ADHD, early sexual activity, substance abuse
- 50% of CD children progress to adult ASPD

Oppositional Defiant Disorder (ODD)

- prevalence: 2-16%

Diagnosis
- pattern of negativistic/hostile and defiant behaviour for ≥6 months with ≥4 of:
  - loses temper, argues with adults, defies adult rules, deliberately annoys, blames others, touchy/easily annoyed, angry and resentful, spiteful or vindictive
- behaviour causes significant impairment in social, academic or occupational functioning
- behaviours do not occur exclusively during the course of a psychotic or mood disorder
- criteria not met for CD; if 18 years or older, criteria not met for ASPD
- features that typically differentiate ODD from transient developmental stage: onset <8 years, chronic duration (>6 months), frequent intrusive behaviour
- impact of ODD: poor school performance, few friends, strained parent/child relationships
- may progress to CD

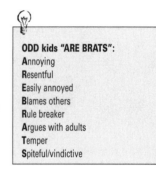

ODD kids "ARE BRATS":
Annoying
Resentful
Easily annoyed
Blames others
Rule breaker
Argues with adults
Temper
Spiteful/vindictive

Treatment
- establish generational boundaries
- parent management training and psychoeducation
- individual/family therapy
- pharmacotherapy for comorbid disorders
- school/daycare interventions to help with behaviour management

SEE PEDIATRICS:
CHILD ABUSE
CHRONIC RECURRENT ABDOMINAL PAIN
DEVELOPMENTAL DELAY
ELIMINATION DISORDERS
LEARNING DISORDERS
MENTAL RETARDATION
SLEEP DISTURBANCES
TIC DISORDERS

The role of the therapeutic alliance in psychotherapy and pharmacotherapy outcome: findings in the National Institute of Mental Health Treatment of Depression Collaborative Research Program
J Consult Clin Psychol. 1996 Jun; 64(3):532-9
Study: Randomized clinical trial.
Participants: 255 male and female adults fulfilling research criteria for major depressive episode and who completed follow-up (total of 619 sessions).
Intervention: Four treatment arms: cognitive-behavioural therapy, interpersonal therapy, imipramine plus clinical management and placebo plus clinical management.
Methods: Clinical raters scored videotapes of early, middle and late therapy session.
Outcomes: Patients' and clinicians' perspectives and depressive symptomatology.
Results: Therapeutic alliance was found to have a significant effect on outcome in all treatment arms. Patient contribution to alliance had a significant effect on outcomes, whereas therapist contribution to alliance had no significant effect.
Conclusions: Therapeutic alliance is a common factor which significantly influences outcome.

Psychotherapy

Psychodynamic Therapies

- theory: one's present outlook is shaped by one's past and unconscious psychological forces
- insight allows change in personality and behaviour
- conflict - three stages:
  - non-resolvable conflict
  - attempt to repress
  - return of conflict in disguised form (symptom or character trait)
- emphasis on early interaction with caregiver
- sources of information:
  - past and present experiences and relationships
  - relationship with therapist
    - **transference**: unconscious re-enactment of early interpersonal patterns in relationship with therapist
    - **countertransference**: therapist's transference to patient
    - **resistance**: elements in the patient which oppose treatment
- techniques:
  - free association – patient says whatever comes to mind
  - dream analysis
- stage of change important for all conflict resolutions (see Population and Community Health)

Defense Mechanisms

- defence mechanisms are unconsciously activated by the patient in response to anxiety provoking events and feelings.

Table 10. Defense Mechanisms

Level 1: Psychotic defenses
Common in psychosis; normally seen throughout childhood and in dreams
- **denial**: replacing external reality with wishful fantasy
- **distortion**: reshaping of reality to meet inner beliefs, resulting in unrealistic and overvalued ideas
- **projection**: interpreting internal impulses as though they are outside self; in psychosis seen as frank delusion about reality (i.e. persecutory delusions)

Level 2: Immature defenses
Common in personality disorders, severe depression. Normally seen throughout adolescence
- **acting out**: express unconscious wish through impulsive action, rather than inhibit it
- **blocking**: of thinking, affect, or impulse
- **hypochondriasis**: exaggeration of illness in order to avoid anxiety-provoking situations
- **introjection**: internalizing qualities of an object (i.e. victim identifying with aggressor)
- **passive-aggressive behaviour**: express aggression through passivity and masochism
- **regression**: returning to an earlier stage of development to avoid present stressors
- **somatization**: unconscious expression of psychic pain/tension as physical symptoms

Level 3: Neurotic defenses
Common in adults
- **controlling**: managing events to reduce inner conflict
- **displacement**: shifting emotional response to an object/idea resembling that which is anxiety provoking
- **externalization**: attributing personal aspects (i.e. moods, attitudes, conflicts) to external world and objects
- **inhibition**: limiting function to avoid anxiety producing internal conflicts
- **intellectualization**: using intellectual processing to avoid experiencing affect
- **isolation**: separating objects/ideas from their associated affect (which is repressed)
- **rationalization**: using rational explanations to justify behaviours that are unacceptable
- **dissociation**: temporary modification of sense of self to avoid emotional distress
- **reaction formation**: transforming an unacceptable impulse into its opposite
- **repression**: withholding or removing from consciousness an idea/feeling
- **sexualization**: bestowing sexual importance to objects

Level 4: Mature defenses
Common in emotionally healthy adults
- **altruism**: constructive service to others to experience empathy
- **anticipation**: planning for future discomfort
- **asceticism**: denying pleasurable effects of an experience (i.e. gratification from renunciation)
- **humour**: overt expression of feelings in a comic fashion
- **suppression**: postpone attention to impulse or conflict

Varieties of Psychodynamic Therapy

- **psychoanalysis** (exploratory psychotherapy)
  - original therapy developed by Freud, goal is self-revelation and insight
  - the exploration of the meaning of early experiences and how they affect emotions and patterns of behaviour presently
  - time intensive (e.g. 4-5 times/week for 3-7 years)
  - for individuals who can tolerate ambiguity in explorations of feelings and treatment

- **supportive psychotherapy**
  - goal is not insight but reduction of anxiety
  - strengthen healthy defense mechanisms to assist day-to-day functioning
  - techniques include: enhancing self-esteem, clarification, confrontation, rationalization, reframing, encouragement, rehearsal/anticipation, de-catastrophizing, allowing "ventilation" of frustrations
- **short term/brief psychotherapy**
  - resolution of particular emotional problems, or acute crisis
  - number of sessions agreed on at outset (6-20)
- **interpersonal psychotherapy**
  - short-term treatment looking at relationship patterns and teaching coping mechanisms
  - focus on personal social roles and relationships to help deal with problems in current functioning

Behaviour Therapy

- modification of internal or external events which precipitate or maintain emotional distress; useful in the treatment of anxiety disorders, substance abuse, paraphilias
- **systematic desensitization:** mastering anxiety-provoking situations by approaching them gradually and in a relaxed state that limits anxiety
- **flooding**: confronting feared stimulus for prolonged periods until it is no longer frightening
- **positive reinforcement**: strengthening behaviour and causing it to occur more frequently by rewarding it
- **negative reinforcement**: causing behaviour to occur more frequently by removing a noxious stimulus when desired behaviour occurs
- **extinction**: causing a behaviour to diminish by not rewarding it
- **punishment** (aversion therapy): causing a behaviour to diminish by applying a noxious stimulus

Cognitive Therapy

- theory: moods and feelings are influenced by one's thoughts
- psychiatric disturbances are frequently caused by habitual errors in thinking
- goal is to help patient become aware of automatic thoughts and correct assumptions with a more balanced view
- useful for depression, anxiety disorders, self-esteem problems
- use of this therapy presupposes a significant level of functioning
- patients asked to keep thought journal (often in chart form, with column headings "situation", "feeling", "thought" and "cognitive distortion") to monitor their thoughts, when/where they think these thoughts, how the thoughts make them feel and what their underlying error in thinking might be

Cognitive Behaviour Therapy

- combines cognitive and behaviour therapies to teach the patient to weaken connections between thinking patterns, habitual behaviours and mood/anxiety problems
- good for treatment of mild/moderate depression/anxiety

Other Therapies

- **group psychotherapy**
  - goals: self-understanding, acceptance, social skills
  - creates a microcosm of society
- **family therapy**
  - family system considered more influential than individual
  - structural focus
    - here and now
    - re-establish parental authority
    - strengthen normal boundaries
    - re-arrange alliances
- **hypnosis**: mixed evidence for the treatment of pain, phobias, anxiety, and smoking cessation
- **dialectical behaviour therapy**: a form of CBT originally developed for borderline patients but since found to be effective for the treatment of several other disorders; focuses on four types of skills: mindfulness, emotion regulation, interpersonal effectiveness, and distress tolerance; individual and group therapy settings
- **mindfulness-based cognitive therapy**: derived from Buddhist meditative practices; aims to help people attend to thoughts, behaviours and emotions non-judgmentally and in the moment using guided breathing exercises

Two-year randomized controlled trial and follow-up of dialectical behaviour therapy vs. therapy by experts for suicidal behaviours and borderline personality disorder
Arch Gen Psychiatry. 2006 Jul; 63(7):757-66

Objective: To determine how DBT compares with non-behavioural psychotherapy.
Study: One-year randomized controlled trial followed by one year follow-up period.
Patients: 100 women with recent suicidal and self-injurious behaviours meeting DSM criteria and matched to various demographic data.
Intervention: One year of DBT or one year of non-behavioural therapy.
Outcomes: Trimester assessments of suicidal behaviour, emergency services use, general psychological well-being.
Results: Patients receiving DBT were half as likely to attempt suicide, required less hospitalization for suicidal ideation, had lower medical risk for suicide attempts, were less likely to drop out of therapy and had fewer emergency room visits for suicidal ideation.
Conclusions: DBT is effective in reducing suicidal behaviour in patients with borderline personality disorder.

Pharmacotherapy

Antipsychotics

- "antipsychotics" and "neuroleptics" are terms used interchangeably
- **indications**: schizophrenia and other psychotic disorders, mood disorders with or without psychosis, violent behaviour, autism, Tourette's, somatoform disorders, dementia, OCD
- **onset**: immediate calming effect and decrease in agitation; thought disorder responds in 2-4 weeks
- **mechanism of action**
  - "typical" – blocks D2 receptors (dopamine); treats only positive symptoms (hallucinations, delusions)
  - "atypical" – blocks D2 and/or D1, 5-HT receptors (dopamine + serotonin); treats both positive and negative symptoms (flat affect, anhedonia, avolition)
  - specific "typical" and "atypical" antipsychotics vary in terms of binding to adrenergic, 5-HT, cholinergic and histaminergic sites leading to different side effect profiles

Rational Use of Antipsychotics

- no reason to combine antipsychotics
- choosing an antipsychotic
  - all antipsychotics are equally effective
  - atypical antipsychotics are as effective as typical antipsychotics but have better side effect profiles
  - choose a drug patient has responded to in the past or was used successfully in a family member
- route: PO; short-acting or long-acting depot IM injections
- minimum 6 months, usually for life

Table 11. Common Antipsychotic Agents

	Starting Dose	Maintenance	Maximum	Relative Potency (mg)
Typicals				
(In order of potency from high to low)				
Pimozide (Orap™)	0.5-1 mg PO bid	2-12 mg/d PO	20 mg/d PO	1
Haloperidol (Haldol™)	2-5 mg IM q4-8h 0.5-5 mg PO b/tid 0.2 mg/kg/d PO	Based on clinical effect	20 mg/d PO	2
Fluphenazine enanthate (Moditen™, Modecate™ for IM formulation)	2.5-10 mg/d PO	1-5 mg PO qhs 25 mg IM/SC q1-3 weeks	20 mg/d PO	2
Zuclopenthixol HCl (Clopixol™)	20-30 mg/d PO	20-40 mg/d PO	100 mg/d PO	4
Zuclopenthixol acetate (Acuphase™)	50-150 mg IM q48-72h		400 mg IM (q2 weeks)	
Zuclopenthixol decanoate (Cloxipol Depot™)	100 mg IM q1-4 weeks	150-300 mg IM q2 weeks	600 mg IM/week	
Trifluoperazine (Stelazine™)	2-5 mg PO bid	2-15 mg PO bid	60 mg/d PO	5
Perphenazine (Trilafon™)	8-16 mg PO b/tid	4-8 mg PO t/qid	64 mg/d PO	10
Loxapine HCl (Loxitane™)	10 mg PO tid 12.5-50 mg IM q4-6h	60-100 mg/d PO	250 mg/d PO	10
Thioridazine (Mellaril™)	25-100 mg PO tid	100-400 mg PO bid	800 mg/d PO	100
Chlorpromazine (Largactil™)	10-15 mg PO b/t/qid	400 mg/d PO	1000 mg/d PO	100
Atypicals				
Risperidone (Risperdal™, Risperdal Consta™ for IM long acting preparation)	1-2 mg OD/bid	4-8 mg/d PO 25 mg IM q2 weeks	8 mg/d PO	High potency
Olanzapine (Zyprexa™, Zydis™)	5 mg/d PO	10-20 mg/d PO	30 mg/d PO	
Ziprasidone (not yet approved in Canada)	40 mg/d IM	80-160 mg/d IM	160 mg/d IM	
Clozapine (Clozaril™)	25 mg PO bid	300-600 mg/d PO	900 mg/d PO	
Quetiapine (Seroquel™)	25 mg PO bid	400-800 mg/d PO	800 mg/d PO	
Aripiprazole (not yet approved in Canada)	10-15 mg/d PO	10-15 mg/d PO	30 mg/d PO	Low potency

Side effects of typical antipsychotics

- low potency: anticholinergic, antiadrenergic, anti-histaminic side effects
- high potency: risk of movement disorder side effects (extrapyramidal side effects) and neuroleptic malignant syndrome (allergic reaction)

Table 12. Commonly Used Atypical Antipsychotics

	Risperidone	Olanzapine	Quetiapine	Clozapine	Ziprasidone
Mechanism	Blocks 5-HT$_2$, D2 and adrenergic receptors	Blocks 5- HT$_{2,3,6}$, D1-D4, muscarinic, adrenergic ,histaminergic receptors	Blocks 5-HT$_{2A}$, D1-2, adrenergic and histaminergic receptors	Blocks 5-HT$_{2,3}$, D1-4, muscarinic, histaminergic receptors	Blocks 5-HT$_{2A}$ and moderate D2 receptor antagonism; moderately potent adrenergic and histaminergic blocker
Advantages	Low incidence of EPS at lower doses (<8mg)	Better overall efficacy compared to haloperidol Well tolerated Low incidence of EPS and TD	Associated with less weight gain compared to clozapine and olanzapine	Most effective for treatment-resistant schizophrenia Does not worsen tardive symptoms; may treat them Approximately 50% of patients benefit, especially paranoid patients and those with onset after 20 years	
Disadvantages	SE: insomnia, agitation, **EPS**, h/a, anxiety, ↑ prolactin, postural hypotension, constipation, dizziness, weight gain	SE: mild sedation, insomnia, dizziness, minimal anticholinergic, early AST and ALT elevation, restlessness **Weight gain associated with increased risk of diabetes mellitus and hyperlipidemia**	SE: h/a, sedation, dizziness, constipation **Most sedating of first line atypicals**	SE: drowsiness/sedation, hypersalivation, tachycardia, dizziness, EPS, NMA **1% agranulocytosis**	SE: sedation, nausea, constipation, dyspepsia
Comments	Quick dissolve (M-tabs), and long-acting (Consta®) formulations available	Quick dissolve formulation (Zydis™) used commonly in ER setting for better compliance IM form available		**Weekly blood counts for at least 1 month, then q2weeks** Do not use with drugs which may cause bone marrow suppression due to risk of agranulocytosis	

Note: Risk of weight gain: Clozapine/Olanzapine > Risperidone/Quetiapine > Ziprasidone.

Atypical Antipsychotics: "ROCS"
Risperidone
Olanzapine
Clozapine
Seroquel (Quetiapine)

Atypical Antipsychotics
- fewer EPS than typicals (except risperidone above 8 mg/d)
- risperidone, olanzapine, quetiapine are the "first line atypical antipsychotics"
- no significant difference in efficacy, speed of response and stability of remission between first line atypicals
- disadvantage: expensive, metabolic side effects

Long-Acting Preparations
- antipsychotics formulated in oil for deep IM injection (see Table 11)
- received on an outpatient basis
- indications: individuals with schizophrenia or other chronic psychoses who relapse because of non-adherence
- dosing: start at low dosages, and then titrate every 2 to 4 weeks to maximize safety and minimize side effects
- should be exposed to oral form prior to first injection
- side effects: risk of EPS, parkinsonism, increased risk of neuroleptic malignant syndrome

Canadian Guidelines for the Treatment of Acute Psychosis in the Emergency Setting
- haloperidol 5 mg IM +/- 2 mg IM lorazepam
- olanzapine 2.5 – 10 mg (PO, IM, quick dissolve)
- risperidone 2 mg (M-tab, liquid)

Anticholinergic Effects
Red as a beet
Hot as a hare
Dry as a bone
Blind as a bat
Mad as a hatter

Table 13. Side Effects of Antipsychotics

System	Side Effects
Anticholinergic	Dry mouth, difficulty urinating, constipation, blurred vision, toxic-confusional states
Alpha-adrenergic blockade	Orthostatic hypotension, impotence, failure to ejaculate
Dopaminergic blockade	Extrapyramidal syndromes (dystonia, akathisia, pseudo Parkinsonism, dyskinesia), galactorrhea, amenorrhea, impotence, weight gain
Anti-histamine	Sedation
Hematologic	Agranulocytosis (Clozapine)
Hypersensitivity reactions	Liver dysfunction Blood dyscrasias Skin rashes Neuroleptic Malignant Syndrome Altered temperature regulation (hypothermia or hyperthermia)
Endocrine	Metabolic syndrome (see sidebar)

Metabolic Syndrome
Atypical antipsychotics have been linked to weight gain, hyperglycemia, and lipid abnormalities and are associated with an increased risk of metabolic syndrome (a collection of clinical and laboratory abnormalities including abdominal obesity, insulin resistance, hypertension, low levels of high-density lipoprotein cholesterol, and high levels of triglycerides).

Neuroleptic Malignant Syndrome
- due to massive dopamine blockade; increased incidence with high potency and depot neuroleptics
- **risk factors:**
    - medication factors
        - sudden increase in dosage, or starting a new drug
    - patient factors
        - medical illness
        - dehydration
        - exhaustion
        - poor nutrition
        - external heat load
        - sex: male
        - age: young adults
- **clinical presentation:**
    - fever, autonomic reactivity, rigidity, mental status changes (usually occur first)
    - develops over 24-72 hours
    - labs: increased CPK, leukocytosis, myoglobinuria
- **treatment:** discontinue drug, hydration, cooling blankets, dantrolene (hydantoin derivative, used as a muscle relaxant), bromocriptine (DA agonist)
- **mortality:** 5%

Features of Neuroleptic Malignant Syndrome: "FARM"
Fever
Autonomic changes
(i.e. increased HR/BP, sweating)
Rigidity of muscles
Mental status changes
(i.e. confusion)

Extrapyramidal Symptoms (EPS)
- incidence related to increased dose and potency
- acute (early-onset; reversible) vs. tardive (late-onset; often irreversible)

Table 14. Extrapyramidal Symptoms

	Dystonia	Akathisia	Pseudoparkinsonism	Dyskinesia
Acute or tardive	Both	Both	Acute	Tardive
Risk group	Acute: Young Asian and Black males		Elderly females	Elderly females
Presentation	**Sustained abnormal posture**; torsions, twisting, contraction of muscle groups; muscle spasms **(e.g. oculogyric crisis, laryngospasm, torticollis)**	**Motor restlessness;** Crawling sensation in legs relieved by walking; very distressing, increased risk of suicide and poor adherence	**T**remor **R**igidity (cogwheeling) **A**kinesia **P**ostural instability (decreased/absent arm-swing, stooped posture, shuffling gait, difficulty pivoting)	Purposeless, constant movements, **involving facial and mouth musculature**, or less commonly, the limbs
Onset	Acute: within 5 d Tardive: >90 d	Acute: within 10 d Tardive: >90 d	Acute: within 30 d	Tardive: >90 d
Treatment	Acute: benztropine or diphenhydramine	Acute: lorazepam, propanolol or diphenhydramine; reduce or change neuroleptic to lower potency	Acute: benztropine (or benzodiazepine if side effects); reduce or change neuroleptic to lower potency	Tardive: no good treatment; may try clozapine; discontinue drug or reduce dose

Tardive Dyskinesia may include grimacing, tongue protrusion, lip smacking, and rapid eye movement.

Antiparkinsonian Agents (Anticholinergic Agents)
- do not always prescribe with neuroleptics; give only if at high risk for acute EPS or if develop acute EPS
- do not give these for tardive syndromes, because they worsen the condition
- types
    - benztropine (Cogentin™) 2 mg PO, IM or IV OD (~1-6 mg)
    - amantadine (Symmetrel™) 100 mg PO bid (100-400 mg)
    - diphenhydramine (Benadryl™) 25-50 mg PO/IM qid

Antidepressants

- onset of effect
    - neurovegetative symptoms – 1-3 weeks
    - emotional/cognitive symptoms – 2-6 weeks
- may use mild stimulant (e.g. methylphenidate) for severe neurovegetative symptoms briefly and taper down as antidepressant effect increases
- taper TCAs slowly (over weeks-months) because they can cause withdrawal reactions
- tapering of any kind of antidepressant may be required based on the half-life of the medication and the patient's individual sensitivity
- it is important to be particularly vigilant over the first 2 weeks of therapy as neurovegetative symptoms have begun to resolve but emotional and cognitive symptoms have not (patients may be particularly at risk for suicidal behaviour during this time)
- treatment of bipolar depression: monotherapy with antidepressants is not advisable as a switch from depression to mania can occur. If the patient is medication-naïve, initiate therapy with a mood stabilizer plus an SSRI or buproprion. For patients taking mood stabilizers, consider adding or switching to lithium or lamotrigine, or adding an SSRI or buproprion

Table 15. Common Antidepressants

Class	Drug	Daily Starting dose (mg)	Therapeutic dose (mg)
SSRI	fluoxetine (Prozac™)	20	20-80
	fluvoxamine (Luvox™)	50-100	150-300
	paroxetine (Paxil™)	10	20-60
	sertraline (Zoloft™)	50	50-200
	citalopram (Celexa™)	20	20-60
	escitalopram (Cipralex™)	10	10-20
SNRI	venlafaxine (Effexor™)	37.5-75	75-225
	duloxetine (Cymbalta™)	40	40-60
NDRI	bupropion (Wellbutrin™)	100	300-450
TCA (3° Amines)	amitriptyline (Elavil™)	75-100	150-300
	imipramine (Tofranil™)	75-100	150-300
TCA (2° Amines)	nortriptyline (Aventyl™)	75-100	75-150
	desipramine (Norpramin™)	100-200	150-300
MAOI	phenelzine (Nardil™)	45	60-90
	tranylcypromine (Parnate™)	30	10-60
RIMA	moclobemide (Manerix™)	300	300-600
NASSA	mirtazapine (Remeron™)	15	15-45

(SSRI=selective serotonin reuptake inhibitors; SNRI=serotonin and norepinephrine reuptake inhibitors; NDRI=norepinephrine and dopamine reuptake inhibitors; TCA=tricyclic antidepressants; MAOI= monoamine oxidase inhibitors; RIMA=reversible inhibition of MAO-A; NASSA=noradrenergic and specific serotonin antagonists)
*Please note divided dosing is often required with these medications

Treatment Strategies for Refractory Depression (see Figure 2)
- **optimization**: ensuring adequate drug doses for the individual
- **augmentation**: the addition of a medication that is not considered an antidepressant to an antidepressant regimen (i.e. thyroid hormone, lithium, atypical antipsychotics)
- **combination**: the addition of another antidepressant to an existing treatment regimen (i.e. the addition of bupropion to an SSRI or SNRI)
- **substitute**: change in the primary antidepressant (within or outside a class)
  Note: it is important to fully treat the symptoms of depression in order to decrease rates and severity of relapses

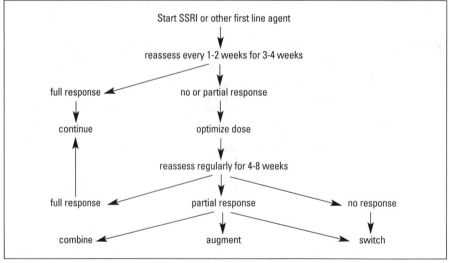

Figure 2. Treatment of Depression

Table 16. Commonly Used Antidepressants

	TCA	SSRI	MAOI	SNRI
Considerations	OCD (clomipramine) Melancholic depression	Anxiety states, OCD, eating disorders, seasonal depression, typical and atypical depression	For moderate/severe depression that does not respond to SSRI Atypical depression	Depression, anxiety disorders
Mode of Action	Block norepinephrine and serotonin reuptake	Block serotonin reuptake only	Irreversible inhibition of monoamine oxidase A and B Leads to ↑ norepinephrine and serotonin	Block norepinephrine and serotonin reuptake
Side Effects	Anticholinergic effect Noradrenergic effects: tremors, tachycardia, sweating, insomnia, erectile and ejaculation problems α 1 adrenergic: orthostatic hypotension Antihistamine: sedation, weight gain CNS: sedation, stimulation, ↓ seizure threshold CVS: ↑ HR, conduction delay	Fewer than TCA, therefore increased compliance CNS: restlessness, tremor, insomnia, headache, drowsiness GI: N/V, diarrhea, abdominal cramps, weight loss Sexual dysfunction: impotence, anorgasmia CVS: increased HR, conduction delay Serotonin syndrome, SIADH	**Hypertensive crises with tyramine rich foods (e.g. wine, cheese)** develop headache, flushes, palpitations, N/V, photophobia Dizziness, reflex tachycardia, postural hypotension, sedation, insomnia Weight gain, social dysfunction Energizing Minimal anticholinergic and antihistamine effects	Low dose side effects (Serotonergic): Insomnia Higher dose side effects (Noradrenergic): tremors, tachycardia, sweating, insomnia, dose-dependent increase in diastolic BP
Risk in Overdose	Toxic in OD **3 times therapeutic dose is lethal** *Presentation:* anticholinergic effects, CNS stimulation, then depression and seizures *ECG:* ↑ QT (duration reflects severity) *Treatment:* activated charcoal, cathartics, supportive treatment, IV diazepam for seizure, physostigmine salicylate for coma Do not give ipecac, as can cause rapid neurologic deterioration and seizures	Very safe	Toxic in OD, but wider margin of safety than TCA	Tachycardia and N/V seen in acute overdose
Drug Interactions	MAOI, SSRI EtOH	SSRIs inhibit P450 enzymes; therefore will ↑ levels of drugs metabolized by P450 system	EtOH Hypertensive crises with noradrenergic medications (e.g. TCA, decongestants, amphetamines) Serotonin syndrome with serotonergic drugs (e.g. SSRI, tryptophan, dextromethorphan)	MAOI, SSRI Does not seem to inhibit P450 system

	NDRI	RIMA	NASSA
Considerations	Depression, seasonal depression	Depression unresponsive to other therapies	Useful in patients with insomnia, agitation or depression with cachexia
Mode of Action	Block norepinephrine and dopamine reuptake	Reversible inhibitor of monoamine oxidase A Leads to ↑ norepinephrine and serotonin	Enhance central noradrenergic and serotonergic activity by inhibiting presynaptic α-2 adrenergic receptors
Side Effects	CNS: dizziness, headache, tremor, insomnia CVS: dysrhythmia, hypotension GI: dry mouth, N/V, constipation, ↑ appetite Other: agitation, anxiety, anaphylactoid reaction	CNS: dizziness, headache, tremor, insomnia CVS: dysrhythmia, hypotension GI: dry mouth, N/V, diarrhea, abdominal pain, dyspepsia GU: delayed ejaculation Other: diaphoresis	CNS: somnolence, dizziness, seizure (rare) Endocrine: ↑cholesterol, ↑ triglycerides GI: Constipation, ↑ALT
Risk in Overdose	Tremors and seizures seen in acute overdose	Risk of fatal overdose when combined with citalopram or clomipramine	Mild symptoms with overdose
Drug Interactions	MAOI Drugs that reduce seizure threshold: antipsychotics, systemic steroids, quinolone antibiotics, antimalarial drugs	MAOI, SSRI, TCA Narcotics	MAOI, SSRI, SNRI, RIMA

Serotonin Syndrome
- rare but potentially life-threatening adverse reaction to SSRIs, especially when switching from an SSRI to an MAOI
- thought to be due to over-stimulation of the serotonergic system
- symptoms include nausea, diarrhea, palpitations, chills, restlessness, confusion, and lethargy but can progress to myoclonus, hyperthermia, rigors and hypertonicity
- treatment: discontinue medication and administer emergency medical care as needed

Discontinuation Syndrome
- caused by the abrupt cessation of an antidepressant
- observed most frequently with paroxetine, fluvoxamine, and venlafaxine
- symptoms usually begin within 1-3 days, and include: anxiety, insomnia, irritability, mood lability, N/V, dizziness, headache, dystonia, tremor, chills, fatigue, lethargy and myalgia
- treatment: symptoms may last between 1-3 weeks, but can be relieved within 24 hours by restarting antidepressant therapy at the same dose the patient was taking, and initiating a slow taper over several weeks
- consider drug with longer half-life such as fluoxetine

Mood Stabilizers

- before initiating, get baseline: CBC, ECG (if patient >45 years old or cardiovascular risk), urinalysis, BUN, Cr, electrolytes, TSH
- before initiating lithium: screen for pregnancy, thyroid disease, seizure disorder, neurological, renal, cardiovascular diseases
- use lithium or valproic acid first (± an antipsychotic), may need acute coverage with benzodiazepines or antipsychotics
- use carbamazepine in non-responders and rapid cycling
- can combine lithium and carbamazepine or valproic acid safely in lithium non-responders
- olanzapine may be used as a mood stabilizer, in conjunction with other mood stabilizers
- lithium and lamotrigine have established antidepressant efficacy

Lithium Toxicity (see Table 17)
- clinical diagnosis, as toxicity can occur at therapeutic levels
- **common causes:**
  - overdose
  - sodium or fluid loss
  - concurrent medical illness
- **clinical presentation:**
  - GI: severe nausea/vomiting and diarrhea
  - cerebellar: ataxia, slurred speech, lack of coordination
  - cerebral: drowsiness, myoclonus, choreiform or Parkinsonian movements, upper motor neuron signs, seizures, delirium, coma
- **management:**
  - discontinue lithium for several doses and begin again at a lower dose when lithium level has fallen to a nontoxic range
  - serum lithium levels, BUN, lytes
  - saline infusion
  - hemodialysis if lithium >2 mmol/L, coma, shock, severe dehydration, failure to respond to treatment after 24 hours, or deterioration

Second-line/Adjuvant Mood Stabilizers
Lamotrigine (Lamictal™):
- **indications:** treatment of dysphoric mania, mixed episodes and rapid cycling BAD, bipolar type 1 depression, prevention of mania and depression
- **mechanism:** may inhibit 5-HT$_3$ receptors and potentiate DA activity
- **side effects:**
  - CNS: dizziness, headache, ataxia, nausea, somnolence, fever, anxiety
  - Skin: rash, Stevens-Johnson syndrome (0.001%)

Symptoms of Discontinuation:
"FINISH"
Flu-like symptoms
Insomnia
Nausea
Imbalance
Sensory disturbances
Hyperarousal (anxiety/agitation)

Long term lithium use can lead to a nephropathy and diabetes insipidus in some patients.

Lithium Side Effects
"LITHIVM"
Leukocytosis
Insipidus (diabetes)
Tremor, teratogenicity
Hypothyroidism
Increased weight
"V"omiting, nausea
Miscellaneous (e.g. ECG changes, acne)

Table 17. Commonly Used Mood Stabilizers

	Lithium	Lamotrigine (Lamictal™)	Divalproex (Epival™)	Carbamazepine (Tegretol™)
Indications	Maintenance therapy of bipolar disorder Treatment of acute mania Augmentation of antidepressants in MDE and OCD Schizoaffective disorder Chronic aggression and antisocial behaviour Recurrent depression	Treatment of bipolar disorder Rapid cycling bipolar disorder Mixed phase/Dysphoric mania Prevention of mania and depression	Maintenance therapy of bipolar disorder Treatment of acute mania Rapid cycling bipolar disorder Mixed phase/Dysphoric mania	Maintenance therapy of bipolar disorder Treatment of acute mania Rapid cycling bipolar disorder
Mode of Action	Unknown Therapeutic response within 7-14 days	May inhibit 5-HT$_3$ receptors May potentiate DA activity	Depresses synaptic transmission Raises seizure threshold	Depresses synaptic transmission Raises seizure threshold
Dosage	*Adult* 600-1500 mg/day *Geriatric* 150-600 mg/day Usually once/day dosing	Starting: 12.5-15mg/day Maximum: 500 mg/day Dose adjusted in patients taking other anti-convulsants	750-2500 mg/day Usually tid dosing	400-1600 mg/day Usually bid or tid dosing
Therapeutic Level	*Adult* 0.5-1.2 mmol/L (1.0-1.25 mEq/L for acute mania) *Geriatric* 0.3-0.8 mmol/L	Therapeutic plasma level not established Dosing based on therapeutic response	17-50 mmol/L	350-700 μmol/L
Monitoring	Monitor serum levels until therapeutic (always wait 12 hours after dose) Then monitor biweekly or monthly until a steady state is reached, then q2 months Monitor thyroid function q6 months, creatinine q6 months, urinalysis q1 year	Monitor for suicidality, particularly when initiating treatment	LFTs weekly x 1 month, then monthly, due to risk of liver dysfunction Watch for signs of liver dysfunction: nausea, edema, malaise	Weekly blood counts for first month, due to risk of agranulocytosis Watch for signs of blood dyscrasias: fever, rash, sore throat, easy bruising
Side Effects	*GI:* N/V, diarrhea, stomach pain *GU:* polyuria, polydipsia, GN, renal failure, nephrogenic DI *CNS:* fine tremor, lethargy, fatigue, headache *Hematologic:* reversible leukocytosis, *Other:* teratogenic (Ebstein's anomaly), weight gain, edema, psoriasis, hypothyroidism, hair thinning, muscle weakness, ECG changes	*GI:* N/V, diarrhea *CNS:* ataxia, dizziness, diplopia, headache, somnolence *Skin:* rash (should d/c drug because of risk of Stevens-Johnson syndrome *Other:* anxiety	*GI:* liver dysfunction, N/V, diarrhea *CNS:* ataxia, drowsiness, tremor, sedation, cognitive blurring *Other:* hair loss, weight gain, transient thrombocytopenia, neural tube defects when used in pregnancy	*GI:* N/V, diarrhea, hepatic toxicity (↑SGOT, ↑GSPT, ↑LDH) *CNS:* ataxia, dizziness, slurred speech, drowsiness, confusion, nystagmus, diplopia *Hematologic:* transient leukopenia (10%), agranulocytosis, aplastic anemia *Skin:* rash (5% risk; should d/c drug because of risk of Stevens-Johnson syndrome) *Other:* neural tube defects when used in pregnancy
Interactions	NSAIDs decrease clearance	↑lamotrigine levels = ↑risk of rash; OCP		OCP

*SGOT: serum glutamic-oxaloacetic transaminase, SGPT: serum glutamic-pyruric transaminase; LDH: lactate

Anxiolytics

- **indications:**
  - short term treatment of transient forms of anxiety disorders, insomnia, alcohol withdrawal (especially delirium tremens), barbiturate withdrawal, organic brain syndrome (agitation in dementia), EPS and akathisia due to antipsychotics, seizure disorders, musculoskeletal disorders
- **relative contraindications:**
  - major depression (except as an adjunct to other treatment), history of drug/alcohol abuse, pregnancy, breast feeding
- **mechanism of action:**
  - benzodiazepines: potentiate binding of GABA to its receptors; results in decreased neuronal activity
  - buspirone: partial agonist of 5-HT type IA receptors

Rational Use of Anxiolytics (see Table 18)
- anxiolytics mask or alleviate symptoms, they do not cure them

Benzodiazepines
- should be used for limited periods (weeks-months) to avoid dependence
- all benzodiazepines are sedating
- have similar efficacy, so choice depends on half-life, metabolites and route of administration, OD or bid
- taper slowly over weeks-months because they can cause withdrawal reactions
  - low dose withdrawal: tachycardia, hypertension, panic, insomnia, anxiety, impaired memory and concentration, perceptual disturbances
  - high dose withdrawal: hyperpyrexia, seizures, psychosis, death
- avoid alcohol because of potentiation of CNS depression; caution with drinking and use of machinery
- **side effects:**
  - CNS: drowsiness, cognitive impairment, reduced motor coordination, memory impairment
  - physical dependence, tolerance develops
- **withdrawal:**
  - symptoms: anxiety, insomnia, dysperceptions, autonomic hyperactivity (less common)
  - onset: 1-2 days (short-acting), 2-4 days (long-acting)
  - duration: weeks/months
  - complications: above 50 mg diazepam/day: seizures, delirium, arrhythmias, psychosis
  - management: taper with long-acting benzodiazepine
  - similar to, but less severe than alcohol withdrawal; can be fatal
  - commonly used drug in overdose
    - overdose is rarely fatal
    - in combination with alcohol, other CNS depressants, or TCAs is more dangerous and may cause death

Benzodiazepine Antagonist – Flumazenil (Anexate™)
- use for suspected benzodiazepine overdose
- specific antagonist at the benzodiazepine receptor site

Buspirone (Buspar™)
- primary use: generalized anxiety disorder (GAD)
- non-sedating and not prone to abuse; therefore, may be preferred over benzodiazepines
- does not interact with or show cross tolerance to other sedating drugs (e.g. alcohol, barbiturates, benzodiazepines)
- does not alter seizure threshold, interact with EtOH, act as a muscle relaxant
- **onset of action**: 2 weeks
- **side effects**: dizziness, drowsiness, nausea, headache, nervousness, extrapyramidal

Table 18. Common Anxiolytics

Class	Drug	Dose Range (mg/day)	T1/2 (hours)	Appropriate use
Benzodiazepines				
Long-acting	clonazepam (Rivotril™)	0.25-4	18-50	Akathisia, generalized anxiety seizure prevention, panic disorder
	diazepam (Valium™)	2-40	30-100	Generalized anxiety, seizure prevention, muscle relaxant, alcohol withdrawal
	chlordiazepoxide (Librium™)	5-300	30-100	Sleep, anxiety, alcohol withdrawal
	flurazepam (Dalmane™)	15-30	50-160	Sleep
Short-acting	alprazolam (Xanax™)	0.25-4.0	6-20	Panic disorder, high dependency rate
	lorazepam (Ativan™)	0.5-6.0	10-20	Sleep, generalized anxiety, akathisia, alcohol withdrawal, sublingual available for very rapid action
	oxazepam (Serax™)	10-120	8-12	Sleep, generalized anxiety, alcohol withdrawal
	temazepam (Restoril™)	7.5-30	8-20	Sleep
	triazolam (Halcion™)	0.125-0.5	1.5-5	Shortest $t_{1/2}$, rapid sleep, but rebound insomnia
Azapirones	buspirone (Buspar™)	20-60	2-11	Generalized anxiety
	zopiclone (Imovane™)	5-7.5	3.8-6.5	Sleep

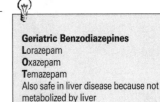

Geriatric Benzodiazepines
Lorazepam
Oxazepam
Temazepam
Also safe in liver disease because not metabolized by liver

Benzos used for Alcohol Withdrawal
Diazepam 20 mg PO/IV q1h prn
Lorazepam 10 mg PO/IV/SL for patients with liver disease, chronic lung disease, or elderly

Efficacy of ECT in Depression: A Meta-Analytic Review
J of ECT 2004; 20: 13-20
Study: Meta-analysis of randomized and non-randomized control trials.
Patients: Individuals with unipolar and bipolar depression.
Methods: MEDLINE search for relevant papers from 1966-2003.
Main Outcomes: The Hamilton Depression Rating scale was used to determine response to treatment.
Results: ECT was found to be superior to simulated ECT, placebo, TCAs, MAOIs, and anti-depressants in general.
Summary: ECT is an efficacious treatment modality, particularly in severe and treatment-resistant depression.

ECT in Society
Prior to the 1940's, ECT was performed without the use of muscle relaxants, resulting in seizures with full-scale convulsions and rare but serious complications such as vertebral and long-bone fractures. This practice may have led to negative societal perceptions of ECT, further perpetuated by barbaric depictions in popular culture.
Despite ongoing stigmatization, ECT as it is practiced today is an effective and safe option for patients struggling with mental illness.

Electroconvulsive Therapy

- induction of a grand mal seizure using an electrical pulse through the brain while the patient is under general anesthesia and a muscle relaxant
- unilateral vs. bilateral electrode placement
- **indications:**
  - depression refractory to adequate pharmacological trial
  - high suicide risk
  - medical risk in addition to depression (dehydration, electrolytes, pregnancy)
  - previous good response to ECT
  - familial response to ECT
  - elderly
  - psychotic depression
  - catatonic features
  - marked vegetative features
  - acute schizophrenia
  - mania unresponsive to meds
- **side effects:** risk of anesthesia, memory loss (may be retrograde and/or anterograde, tends to resolve by 6 to 9 months, permanent impairment controversial), headaches, myalgias
- evidence that unilateral ECT causes less memory loss than bilateral but may not be as effective
- **contraindications:** increased intracranial pressure

Experimental Therapies

Deep Brain Stimulation (DBS)
- constant electrical stimulation of neuroanatomical targets that have been identified in the biological model of depression
- areas identified include the nucleus accumbens, internal capsule and subgenual cingulate cortex
- parameters such as active electrode location, pulse width, frequency and voltage may be manipulated

Transcranial Magnetic Stimulation (TMS)
- non-invasive magnetic stimulation of superficial neurons in the frontal cortex (main target: dorsolateral prefrontal cortex) hypothesized to normalize cortical activity in depressed patients
- meta-analyses show modest acute efficacy

Legal Issues

Common Forms

Form 1: A Primer
- Based on any combination of the physician's own observations and facts communicated by others
- Box A or Box B completed
- **Box A:** Serious Harm Test
  - The Past/Present Test assesses current behaviours/threats/attempts
  - The Future Test assesses the likelihood of serious harm occurring as a result of the presenting mental disorder
- **Box B:** Patients with a known mental disorder, who are incapable of consenting to treatment (existing substitute decision-maker), have previously received treatment and improved, and are currently at risk of serious harm due to the same mental disorder

Table 19. Common Forms Under the Mental Health Act (in Ontario)

Form	Who signs	When	Expiration Date	Right of Patient to Review Board Hearing	Options Before Form Expires
Form 1: Application by physician to hospitalize a patient for psychiatric assessment against his/her will to a schedule 1 facility **(Form 42 to patient)**	Any MD	Within 7 days after examination	72 hours after hospitalization Void if not implemented within 7 days	No	Form 3 *or* Voluntary admission (Form 5) *or* Send home ± Follow-up
Form 2: Order for hospitalization and medical examination against his/her will by Justice of the Peace	Justice of the Peace	No statutory time restriction	7 days from when completed Purpose of form is complete once patient brought to hospital	No	Form 1 *or* Send home ± Follow-up
Form 3: Certificate of involuntary admission to a schedule 1 facility **(Form 30 to patient, notice to rights advisor)**	Attending MD (different than MD who completed Form 1)	Before expiration of Form 1 Any time to change status of an informal patient	14 days	Yes (within 48 hours)	Form 4 *or* Form 5
Form 4: Certificate of renewal of involuntary admission to a schedule 1 facility **(Form 30 to patient, notice to rights advisor)**	Attending MD following patient on Form 3	Prior to expiration of Form 3	First: 1 month Second: 2 months Third: 3 months (max)	Yes (within 48 hours)	Form 4 *or* Form 5
Form 5: Change to informal/voluntary status	Attending MD following patient on Form 3/4	Whenever deemed appropriate	N/A	N/A	N/A
Form 14: Consent to Disclosure of Clinical record	Patient	Whenever deemed appropriate	N/A	N/A	N/A
Form 33: Notice to patient that patient is incompetent to consent to treatment of mental disorder and/or management of property	Attending MD	Whenever deemed appropriate	N/A	N/A	N/A

*Forms available at: www.health.gov.on.ca/english/public/forms/forms_menus/mental_fm.html

Consent

- see *Ethics* in <u>Ethical, Legal and Organizational Aspects of Medicine</u>

Community Treatment Order (CTO)

- known as "Brian's Law," Ontario passed legislature regarding CTOs on December 1, 2000. Similar CTOs have been implemented in Saskatchewan (1995), Manitoba (1997) and British Columbia (1999)
- purpose: to provide a person who suffers from a serious mental disorder with a comprehensive plan of community-based treatment and supervision that is less restrictive than being detained in a psychiatric facility
- intended for those who:
    - as a result of their serious mental disorder, experience a pattern of admission to a psychiatric facility where their condition is usually stabilized
    - after being released, these patients often lack supervision and stop treatment
    - due to the destabilization of their condition, these patients usually require re-admission to hospital
- criteria for a physician to issue a CTO:
    - patient with a prior history of hospitalization
    - a community treatment plan for the person has been made
    - examination by a physician within the previous 72 hours before entering into the CTO plan
    - ability of the person subject to the CTO to comply with it
    - consultation with a rights adviser and consent of the person and the person's substitute decision maker, if any
- CTOs are valid for six months unless they are renewed or terminated at an earlier date
    - where the person fails to comply with the CTO
    - when the person or his/her substitute decision-maker withdraws consent to the community treatment plan
- CTO process is consent-based and all statutory protections governing informed consent apply
- the rights of a person subject to a CTO include:
    - the right to a review by the Consent and Capacity Board with appeal to the courts each time a CTO is issued or renewed
    - a mandatory review by the Consent and Capacity Board every second time a CTO is renewed
    - the right to request a re-examination by the issuing physician to determine if the CTO is still necessary for the person to live in the community
    - the right to review findings of incapacity to consent to treatment
    - provisions for rights advice

Duty to Inform/Warn

- see Ethical, Legal, and Organizational Aspects of Medicine

Notes

R

Respirology

Adil Bhatti, Alex Mansfield, and Jonathan Wong, chapter editors
Deepti Damaraju and Elliott Owen, associate editors
Erik Venos, EBM editor
Dr. William Geerts, Dr. John Granton and Dr. Jae Yang, staff editors

An approach to chest x-rays can be found online at http://www.torontonotes.ca, located under Resources → Essentials of Medical Imaging.
Please refer to the online Radiology Atlas for additional medical imaging resources, including x-rays and CT imaging for common respiratory conditions discussed in this chapter.

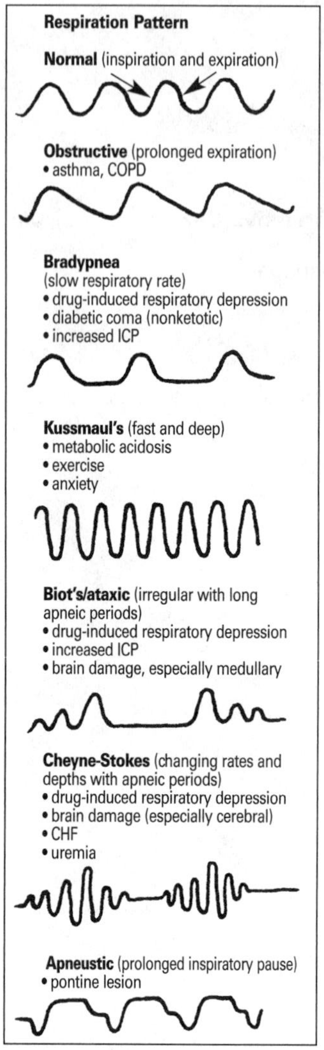

Respiration Pattern
Normal (inspiration and expiration)
Obstructive (prolonged expiration)
• asthma, COPD
Bradypnea
(slow respiratory rate)
• drug-induced respiratory depression
• diabetic coma (nonketotic)
• increased ICP
Kussmaul's (fast and deep)
• metabolic acidosis
• exercise
• anxiety
Biot's/ataxic (irregular with long apneic periods)
• drug-induced respiratory depression
• increased ICP
• brain damage, especially medullary
Cheyne-Stokes (changing rates and depths with apneic periods)
• drug-induced respiratory depression
• brain damage (especially cerebral)
• CHF
• uremia
Apneustic (prolonged inspiratory pause)
• pontine lesion

Figure 2. Respiration Patterns in Normal and Disease States

Approach to the Respiratory Patient

Basic Anatomy Review

Superior lobar bronchus
Right upper lobe
Middle lobar bronchus
Right middle lobe
Inferior lobar bronchus
Right lower lobe
Right and left main bronchi
Carina
Superior lobar bronchus
Superior division bronchus
Left upper lobe
Lingular bronchus
Inferior lobar bronchus
Left lower lobe
Lingula
B1
B2
B3
B4
B5
B6
B7
B8
B9
B10
B1+2
B7+8
© Hyun Joo Lee 2005

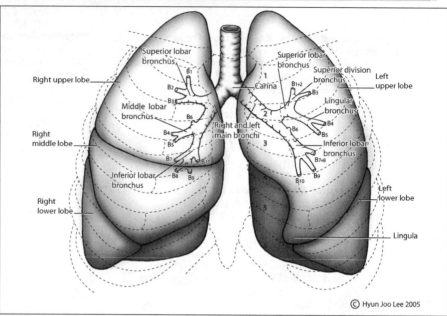

Figure 1. Lung Lobes and Bronchi

Differential Diagnoses of Common Presentations

Table 1. Differential Diagnosis of Dyspnea

- **Respiratory**
  - Airway disease (wheeze)
    - Asthma*
    - COPD exacerbation*
    - Upper airway obstruction (anaphylaxis, foreign body, etc)*
    - Mucus plugging*
  - Parenchymal lung disease (crackles)
    - ARDS*
    - Pneumonia*
    - Interstitial lung disease
  - Pulmonary vascular disease
    - PE*
    - Pulmonary HTN
    - Pulmonary vasculitis
  - Pleural disease (pleuritic chest pain)
    - Pneumothorax* tension pneumothorax*
    - Pleural effusion
- **Neuromuscular and chest wall disorders (↓ chest expansion)**
  - Polymyositis, myasthenia gravis, Guillain-Barré syndrome, Kyphoscoliosis, C-spine injury*, ALS, diaphragmatic paresis
- **Cardiovascular (worse with dependancy/exertion)**
  - Elevated pulmonary venous pressure
    - LVF with pulmonary edema*
    - Mitral stenosis
    - Decreased cardiac output
- **Hematologic**
  - Severe anemia (pallor)
- **Psychiatric**
  - Anxiety/psychosomatic*

Table 2. Differential Diagnosis of Chest Pain

Nonpleuritic
- **Pulmonary**
  - Pneumonia
  - PE
  - Neoplastic
- **Cardiac**
  - MI
  - Myocarditis/pericarditis
- **Esophageal**
  - **GERD**
  - Spasm
  - Esophagitis
  - Ulceration
  - Achalasia
  - Neoplasm
- **Mediastinal**
  - Lymphoma
  - Thymoma
- **Subdiaphragmatic**
  - **PUD**
  - Gastritis
  - Biliary colic
  - Pancreatic
- **Vascular**
  - Dissecting aortic aneurysm
- **MSK**
  - Costochondritis
  - Skin
  - Breast
  - Ribs

Pleuritic
- **Pulmonary**
  - Pneumonia
  - PE
  - Pneumothorax
  - Hemothorax
  - Bronchiectasis
  - Neoplasm
  - TB
  - Empyema
- **Cardiac**
  - Pericarditis
  - Dressler's syndrome
- **GI**
  - Pancreatitis
  - Subphrenic abscess
- **MSK**
  - Costochondritis
  - Fractured rib
  - Myositis
  - Herpes zoster

* denotes causes that should be considered for acute dyspnea

Table 3. Differential Diagnosis of Hemoptysis

Airway Disease
 Acute or chronic bronchitis
 Bronchiectasis
 Bronchogenic CA
 Bronchial carcinoid tumour
Parenchymal Disease
 Pneumonia
 TB
 Lung abscess
 Miscellaneous:
  Goodpasture's syndrome
  Idiopathic pulmonary hemosiderosis
Vascular Disease
 PE
 Elevated pulmonary venous pressure:
  LVF
  Mitral stenosis
 Vascular malformation
Miscellaneous
 Impaired coagulation
 Pulmonary endometriosis

Table 4. Differential Diagnosis of Cough

Airway Irritants
 Inhaled smoke, dusts, fumes
 Aspiration
  Gastric contents (GERD)
  Oral secretions
  Foreign body
 Postnasal drip
Airway Disease
 URTI including postnasal drip and sinusitis
 Acute or chronic bronchitis
 Bronchiectasis
 Neoplasm
 External compression by node or mass lesion
 Asthma
 COPD
Parenchymal Disease
 Pneumonia
 Lung abscess
 Interstitial lung disease
CHF
Drug-induced (e.g. ACE inhibitor)

Reprinted from *Principles of Pulmonary Medicine, 2nd edition*, SE Weinberger, Copyright (1992), with permission from Elsevier.

Table 5. Differential Diagnosis of Clubbing

Pulmonary	Gastrointestinal	Mediastinal
CF	IBD (UC, CD)	Esophageal CA
Pulmonary fibrosis	Chronic infections	Thymoma
Chronic pus in the lung	Laxative abuse	**Other**
(bronchiectasis, abscess,	Polyposis	Graves Disease
infections, etc.)	Malignant tumours	Thalassemia
Lung CA (primary or mets)	Cirrhosis	Other malignancies
Mesothelioma	HCC	Primary hypertrophic osteoarthropathy
A-V fistula	**Cardiac**	
	Cyanotic congenital heart disease	
	Infective endocarditis	

Most common causes of chronic cough in healthy-appearing patient (cough >3 months in duration)
- GERD
- Asthma
- Post-nasal drip
- Post-viral

Normal   Clubbed

$\angle ABC < 176°$ $\angle ABC > 176°$
$\angle ABD < 192°$ $\angle ABD > 192°$

IPD>DPD   DPD>IPD

© Sherry H. Lai 2006

Figure 3. Three Signs of Clubbing
1. Profile Angle (ABC >176°)
2. Hyponychial Angle (ABD >192°)
3. Phalangeal Depth Ratio (DPD:IPD >1)
Adaped from *JAMA* 2001. 286(3): 341-7.

Clubbing is not seen in COPD alone – if present, think malignancy.

Pulmonary Function Tests (PFTs)

- useful in differentiating the pattern of lung disease (obstructive vs. restrictive) (Table 6)
- assess lung volumes, flow rates, and diffusion capacity (Figures 4a and 4b)
- normal values for FEV_1 are approximately $\pm 20\%$ of the predicted values (for age, sex and height); race may affect predicted values

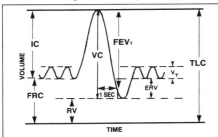

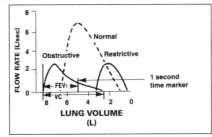

Figure 4a. Subcompartments of Lung Volumes   **Figure 4b.** Expiratory Flow Volume Curves
Reprinted from *Principles of Pulmonary Medicine, 2nd edition*, SE Weinberger, Copyright (1992), with permission from Elsevier.

Obstructive Lung Disease
- characterized by obstructed airflow, decreased flow rates (most marked during expiration), air trapping (increased RV/TLC), and hyperinflation (increased FRC, TLC)
- differential diagnosis includes asthma, chronic obstructive pulmonary disease (COPD), cystic fibrosis (CF), and bronchiectasis

Restrictive Lung Disease
- characterized by decreased lung compliance and lung volumes
- differential diagnosis includes interstitial lung disease, neuromuscular disease, chest wall disease, pleural disease, and parenchymal disease (pulmonary fibrosis)

Lung Volumes
FEV_1 – Forced Expiratory Volume in one second
MMFR – Maximal Mid-expiratory Flow Rate
FVC – Forced Vital Capacity
FEF – Forced Expiratory Flow Rate
FRC – Functional Residual Capacity
TLC – Total Lung Capacity
VC – Vital Capacity
RV – Residual Volume
Dco – Diffusion Capacity of Carbon Monoxide

Table 6. Comparison of Lung Flow and Volume Parameters in Obstructive vs. Restrictive Lung Disease

		Obstructive	Restrictive
Flow Rates	FEV_1	↓	↓ or N
	FVC	↓	↓
	FEV_1/FVC	↓	↑ or N
	FEF_{25-75}	↓	↑ or N
Lung Volumes	TLC	↑ or N	↓
	FRC	↑ or N	↓
	VC	↓ or N	↓
	RV	↑↑	↓
	RV/TLC	↑	N
Diffusion Capacity	D_{CO}	↓ or N	↓ or N

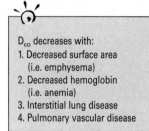

D_{CO} decreases with:
1. Decreased surface area (i.e. emphysema)
2. Decreased hemoglobin (i.e. anemia)
3. Interstitial lung disease
4. Pulmonary vascular disease

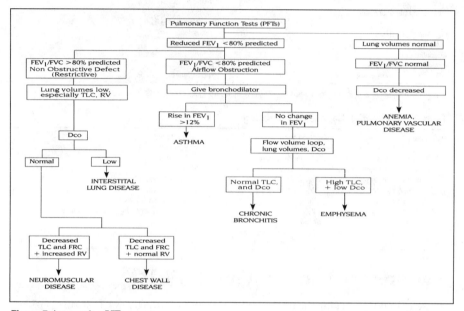

Figure 5. Interpreting PFTs

Arterial Blood Gases

- provides information on acid-base and oxygenation status
- see also Nephrology

Approach to Acid-Base Status
1. What is the pH? acidemic (pH <7.35), alkalemic (pH >7.45), or normal (pH 7.35-7.45)
2. What is the primary disturbance?
   - metabolic: change in HCO_3 and pH in same direction
   - respiratory: change in HCO_3 and pH in opposite direction
3. Has there been appropriate compensation? (Table 7)
   - metabolic compensation occurs over 2-3 days reflecting altered renal HCO_3 production/excretion
   - respiratory compensation through ventilation control of $PaCO_2$ occurs immediately
   - inadequate compensation may indicate a second acid-base disorder

Table 7. Expected Compensation for Specific Acid-Base Disorders

Disturbance	$PaCO_2$ (mmHg)	HCO_3 (mmHg)
Respiratory Acidosis		
Acute	↑10	↑1
Chronic	↑10	↑3
Respiratory Alkalosis		
Acute	↓10	↓2
Chronic	↓10	↓5
Metabolic Acidosis	↓1	↓1
Metabolic Alkalosis	↑5-7	↑10

4. If there is metabolic acidosis, what is the anion gap and osmolar gap?
  - anion gap = [Na]–([Cl]+[HCO_3]); normal = 10-15 mmol/L
  - osmolar gap = measured osmolarity – calculated osmolarity
    = measured – (2[Na] + glucose + urea); normal = 10
5. If anion gap is increased, is the change in bicarbonate the same as the change in anion gap?
  - if not, consider a mixed picture

DIFFERENTIAL DIAGNOSIS OF RESPIRATORY ACIDOSIS
characterized by increased $PaCO_2$ secondary to hypoventilation
- respiratory centre depression ($\downarrow$RR)
  - drugs (anesthesia, sedatives, narcotics)
  - trauma
  - increased ICP
  - encephalitis
  - stroke
  - central apnea
  - supplemental O_2 in chronic CO_2 retainers (i.e. COPD)
- neuromuscular disorders ($\downarrow$TV)
  - myasthenia gravis
  - Guillain-Barré syndrome
  - poliomyelitis
  - muscular dystrophies
  - ALS
  - myopathies
  - chest wall disease (obesity, kyphoscoliosis)
- airway obstruction (asthma, foreign body) ($\downarrow$FEV)
- parenchymal disease
  - COPD
  - pulmonary edema
  - pneumothorax
  - pneumonia
  - pneumoconiosis
  - acute respiratory distress syndrome (ARDS)
- mechanical hypoventilation (inadequate mechanical ventilation)

DIFFERENTIAL DIAGNOSIS OF RESPIRATORY ALKALOSIS
characterized by decreased $PaCO_2$ secondary to hyperventilation
- hypoxemia
  - pulmonary disease (pneumonia, edema, PE, interstitial fibrosis)
  - severe anemia
  - heart failure
  - high altitude
- respiratory centre stimulation
  - CNS disorders
  - hepatic failure
  - Gram-negative sepsis
  - drugs (ASA, progesterone, theophylline, catecholamines, psychotropics)
  - pregnancy
  - anxiety
  - pain
- mechanical hyperventilation (excessive mechanical ventilation)

- see <u>Nephrology</u> for differential diagnosis of metabolic acidosis and alkalosis

Calculation of A-aDO₂ Gradient (Approach to Oxygenation Status)
- calculate the oxygen gradient between the alveolus and the pulmonary capillaries
- approach includes asking 3 questions:
  1. What is the PaO_2? (normal = 95-100 mm Hg)
  2. What is the A-aDO_2 (the gradient)? (normal <15 mm Hg)
    - A-aDO_2 = PAO_2 (alveolar) – PaO_2(arterial)
      = [FiO_2 (P_{atm} – PH_2O) – $PaCO_2$/RQ] – PaO_2
        - On room air: FiO_2 = 0.21, P_{atm} = 760* mmHg, PH_2O = 47 mmHg, RQ = 0.8
        - A-aDO_2 = [150* – 1.25($PaCO_2$)] – PaO_2 (*apply at sea level)
    - the normal A-aDO_2 increases with age
  3. What is the cause of the hypoxemia? (see Figure 7)

Ventilator Failure
Think "can't breathe" vs.
"won't breathe" ($\uparrow$PaCo₂)

Won't Breathe
- respiratory centre depression
- hypothyroid
- sleep apnea

Can't Breathe
- neuromuscular disorders
- airway obstruction
- parenchymal disease

Anion Gap Metabolic Acidosis
MUDPILES
Methanol
Uremia
Diabetic ketoacidosis
Paraldehyde
Isopropyl alcohol / Iron / INH
Lactic acidosis
Ethylene glycol
Salicylates

At Sea Level
A-aDO₂ Gradient on Room Air
A-aDO₂ = {150 - 1.25 (PaCO₂)} – PaO₂

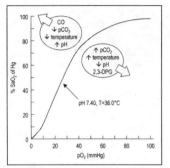

Figure 6. Oxygen-Hb dissociation curve

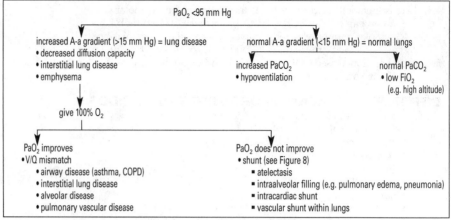

Figure 7. Approach to Hypoxemia

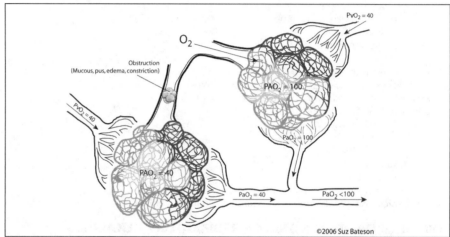

Figure 8. Pathophysiology of Shunt

Diseases of Airway Obstruction

Asthma

Definition
- chronic, generally variable inflammatory disorder of the airways resulting in episodes of reversible hyper-responsive inflammation and bronchospasm causing airflow obstruction
- paroxysmal or persistent symptoms such as dyspnea, chest tightness, wheezing, sputum production and/or cough
- associated with reversible airflow limitation and airway hyper-responsiveness to endogenous or exogenous stimuli

Epidemiology
- common (7-10% of adults), especially in children (10-15%)
- most children with asthma improve significantly in adolescence
- often family history of atopy (asthma, allergic rhinitis, eczema)
- occupational asthma

Etiology and Pathophysiology
- acute asthma: airway obstruction → V/Q mismatch → hypoxemia → ↑ ventilation → ↓ $PaCO_2$ → ↑ pH and muscle fatigue → ↓ ventilation, ↑ $PaCO_2$/↓ pH

Triggers
- URTIs, allergens (pet dander, house dusts, molds), irritants (cigarette smoke, air pollution), drugs (NSAIDs, β-blockers), preservatives (sulphites, MSG), other (emotion/anxiety, cold air, exercise, GERD)

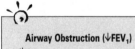

Airway Obstruction (↓FEV₁)
- asthma
- COPD (chronic bronchitis, emphysema)
- bronchiectasis
- cystic fibrosis

RED FLAG
A good predictor of a potential life-threatening attack is an excess consumption of short-acting β₂-agonists.

Signs and Symptoms
- tachypnea, wheezing, chest tightness, cough (especially nocturnal), sputum production

Table 8. Important Signs and Symptoms

Red Flags	Respiratory Distress
fatigue	nasal flaring, tracheal tug
diminished expiratory effort	inability to speak
cyanosis	accessory muscle use, intercostal indrawing
silent chest	pulsus paradoxus
decreased LOC	

Adapted with permission from *CMAJ* 1999; 161 (11 Suppl): S1-61

Table 9. Risk Factors Indicating Poor Asthma Control

Previous Non-Fatal Episodes	Ominous Signs and Symptoms
loss of consciousness during asthma attack	night time symptoms >1 night/week
frequent ER visits	silent chest
prior intubation	FEV_1 or PEF (peak expiratory flow) <60%
ICU admission	limited activities of daily living
	use of β_2 agonists >3 times/day

Adapted with permission from *CMAJ* 1999; 161 (11 Suppl): S1-61

Table 10. Criteria for determining whether asthma is well controlled

daytime symptoms <4 days/wk	No asthma-related absence from work/school
night-time symptoms, <1 night/wk	β_2 agonist use <4 times/wk
normal physical activity	FEV_1 or PEF >90% of personal best
mild, infrequent exacerbations	PEF diurnal variation <10-15%

Adapted with permission from *CMAJ* 2005; 173 (11 Suppl): S4

Investigations
- O_2 saturation
- ABGs
  - $\downarrow PaO_2$ during attack (V/Q mismatch)
  - $\downarrow PaCO_2$ in mild asthma due to hyperventilation
  - normal or $\uparrow PaCO_2$ ominous as patient is no longer able to hyperventilate (worsened airway obstruction or respiratory muscle fatigue)
- PFTs (may not be possible during severe attack, do when stable)
  - spirometry: increase in FEV_1 >12% with β_2-agonist, or >20% with 10-14 days of steroids, or >20% spontaneous variability
  - provocation testing: decrease in FEV_1 >20% with methacholine challenge

Treatment
- environmental control: avoid relevant triggers
- patient education: features of the disease, goals of treatment, self-monitoring
- pharmacological therapy:
  - symptomatic relief in acute episodes: short-acting β_2-agonist, anticholinergic bronchodilators, oral steroids, addition of a long acting β_2-agonist
  - long-term prevention of acute episodes: inhaled/oral corticosteroids, anti-allergic agent, long-acting β_2-agonist, methylxanthine, leukotriene receptor antagonists (LTRA)

Central cyanosis is not detectable until the SaO_2 is <85%.
It is more easily detected in poly-cythemia and less readily detectable in anemia.

Asthma Triad
- asthma
- ASA/NSAID sensitivity
- nasal polyps

Randomized, Placebo Controlled Trial of Effect of a Leukotriene Receptor Antagonist, Montelukast, on Tapering Inhaled Corticosteroids in Asthmatic Patients
BMJ 1999;319:87-90
Study: Double blind, randomized, placebo controlled, parallel group, multicentre study with a follow-up of 12 weeks.
Patients: 226 clinically stable patients (mean age 41 yrs, 52% female) with chronic asthma requiring moderate to high doses of corticosteroids for control.
Intervention: Patients were randomized to receive either montelukast 10 mg PO qhs or placebo while undergoing a tapering protocol in which their dose of inhaled corticosteroids was tapered, maintained, or increased (rescue) every 2 weeks based on a standardized clinical score.
Primary Outcomes: Lowest tolerated dose of inhaled corticosteroids.
Results: Patients taking montelukast were able to taper their inhaled corticosteroid dose to a significantly greater degree than those taking placebo (47% vs. 30%, P=0.046). In addition, those taking montelukast were significantly less likely to require discontinuation of the tapering protocol due to failure of increased corticosteroid dose/rescue to maintain clinical stability (16% vs. 30%, P=0.001, NNT=8).
Conclusion: Montelukast allows significantly greater reduction in the dose of inhaled corticosteroids required to maintain clinical stability in chronic asthmatics formerly requiring moderate to high doses.

Remember to step down therapy to lowest doses which control symptoms/signs of bronchoconstriction.

Guidelines for Asthma Management

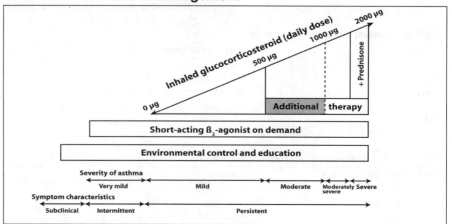

Figure 9. Guidelines for Asthma Management

Canadian Asthma Consensus Report, 1999 – Reprinted with permission from *CMAJ* Supplement to Nov. 30, 1999; 161 (11 Suppl) by permission of the publisher. © 1999 Canadian Medical Association.

Emergency Management of Asthma (see also Emergency Medicine)
1. inhaled β2-agonist first line (MDI route and spacer device recommended)
2. add anticholinergic therapy
3. ketamine and succinylcholine for rapid sequence intubation in life-threatening cases
4. SC/IV adrenaline, IV salbutamol if unresponsive
5. all patients admitted to ER for asthma exacerbations should be considered for corticosteroid therapy at discharge

Chronic Obstructive Pulmonary Disease (COPD)

Natural Progression of COPD

40s   Chronic productive cough, wheezing occasionally

50s   1st acute chest illness

60s   Dyspnea on exertion, increasing amounts of sputum production, more frequent acute exacerbations

Late Stage   Hypoxemia with cyanosis, polycythemia (↑RBCs), hypercapnia (morning headache), hypoxemia, cor pulmonale

Pulmonary Embolism in Patients with Unexplained Exacerbation of Chronic Obstructive Pulmonary Disease: Prevalence and Risk Factors
Ann Intern Med. 2006; 144:390-396.
Study: Prospective cohort study of 211 patients with COPD (all current and former smokers) who were admitted to hospital for severe exacerbation of their COPD of unknown origin.
Measurements: All patients received a spiral CT angiogram (CTA) and venous compression ultrasonography of both legs.
Results: 25% of patients met diagnostic criteria for PE (+ CTA or +U/S).
Conclusions: Prevalence of PE in patients hospitalized for COPD exacerbation of unknown origin is 25%.

Therefore, all patients presenting to hospital with COPD exacerbation without an obvious cause require a PE workup (leg dopplers or CTA- decision of which to use depends on pre-test probability of the patient).

Definition
• characterized by progressive development of irreversible airway obstruction
• 2 subtypes: usually coexist to variable degrees in most patients
• the course of COPD is characterized by a gradual decrease in FEV$_1$ over a period of time with episodes of acute exacerbations

Table 11. Clinical and Pathologic features of COPD

Chronic Bronchitis	Emphysema
Defined clinically as: Productive cough on most days for at least 3 consecutive months in 2 successive years	**Defined pathologically as:** Dilation and destruction of air spaces distal to the terminal bronchiole without obvious fibrosis
Obstruction is due to narrowing of the airway lumen by mucosal thickening and excess mucus	Decreased elastic recoil of lung parenchyma causes decreased expiratory driving pressure, airway collapse, and air trapping

	2 types:
	1) **centriacinar** (respiratory bronchioles predominantly affected)
	  • typical form seen in smokers, primarily affects upper lung zones
	2) **panacinar** (respiratory bronchioles, alveolar ducts, and alveolar sacs affected)
	  • responsible for less than 1% of emphysema cases, (α-1-antitrypsin deficiency), primarily affects lower lobes

Risk Factors
• smoking is the most important risk factor (likelihood ratio of 8.3)
• other risk factors include:
  ▪ environmental factors: air pollution, occupational exposure
  ▪ treatable factors: increased BMI, α1-antitrypsin deficiency, bronchial hyperactivity
  ▪ demographic factors: age, family history, male sex, history of childhood respiratory infections, and low socioeconomic status

Signs and Symptoms

Table 12. Clinical Presentation and Investigations for Chronic Bronchitis and Emphysema

	Symptoms	Signs	Investigations
Bronchitis (Blue Bloater)	• chronic productive cough • purulent sputum • hemoptysis • mild dyspnea initially	• cyanotic ($2°$ to hypoxemia and hypercapnia) • peripheral edema from RVF (cor pulmonale) • crackles, wheezes • prolonged expiration if obstructive • frequently obese	**PFT:** • ↓ FEV_1, ↓ FEV_1/FVC • N TLC, ↑ or N D_{CO} **CXR:** • AP diameter normal • ↑ bronchovascular markings • enlarged heart with cor pulmonale
Emphysema (Pink Puffer)	• dyspnea (± exertion) • minimal cough • tachypnea • decreased exercise tolerance	• pink skin • pursed-lip breathing • accessory muscle use • cachectic appearance due to anorexia + increased work of breathing • hyperinflation/barrel chest, hyperresonant percussion • decreased breath sounds • decreased diaphragmatic excursion	**PFT:** • ↓ FEV_1, ↓ FEV_1/FVC • ↑ lung volume • ↓ D_{CO} **CXR:** • ↑ AP diameter • flat hemidiaphragm (on lateral CXR) • ↓ heart shadow • ↑ retrosternal space • bullae • ↓ peripheral vascular markings

Treatment of Stable COPD
- prolong survival
    - smoking cessation: nicotine replacement, bupropion (Zyban™)
    - vaccination: influenza prophylaxis, pneumovax
    - home oxygen: to prevent cor pulmonale and decrease mortality if used >15 hrs/day → indications: PaO_2 ≤55 mmHg; O_2 saturation ≤89% consistently
- symptomatic relief
    - bronchodilators: mainstay of current drug therapy, used in combination
        - anticholinergics (e.g. ipratropium bromide, tiotropium bromide)
            - more effective than β_2-agonists with fewer side effects
            - slower onset of action; take daily rather than on prn basis
        - short acting β_2-agonists (e.g. salbutamol, terbutaline)
            - rapid onset of action
            - significant side effects at high doses (e.g. hypokalemia)
        - long acting β_2-agonists (e.g. salmeterol, formoterol) – may delay hospitalization
        - theophylline – increases collateral ventilation, mucociliary clearance, and may reduce airway inflammation; used as 4th line
            - side effects include: nervous tremor, nausea/vomiting/diarrhea, tachycardia, arrhythmias, sleep changes, headache, gastric acid, toxicity
    - corticosteroids
        - chronic treatment of COPD with systemic glucocorticoids should be avoided
        - COPD airways are usually inflamed, but *not* generally responsive to steroids
        - inhaled steroids used in spirometric responsive symptomatic patients. Trial of 6 wks to 3 months. If FEV_1 improves 20%, inhaled steroids can be used in the long term. However, long term benefits have yet to be determined. Consider use in patients with FEV_1 ≤35% (GOLD guidelines)
    - surgical treatment
        - lung reduction surgery: bullectomy of emphysematous parts of lung to improve ventilatory function, associated with higher mortality in certain risk groups (FEV_1 <20%)
        - lung transplant
- others
    - patient education, eliminate respiratory irritants/allergens (occupational/environmental), exercise rehabilitation to improve physical endurance

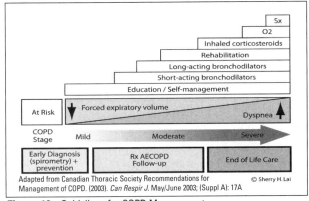

Adapted from Canadian Thoracic Society Recommendations for Management of COPD. (2003). *Can Respir J.* May/June 2003; (Suppl A): 17A   © Sherry H. Lai

Figure 10. Guidelines for COPD Management

Effects of Smoking Intervention and the Use of an Inhaled Anticholinergic Bronchodilator on the Rate of Decline of FEV_1
JAMA 1994;272:1497-1505
Study: Randomized, double-blind, placebo-controlled, multicentre trial with follow-up of 5 years.
Patients: 73,684 otherwise healthy smokers between the ages of 35 and 60 years were screened with spirometry for evidence of mild to moderate airway obstruction (defined as FEV_1/FVC <70%, and FEV_1 of 55-90% of predicted normal). 12,670 (17%) patients met these criteria and were therefore thought to be at high risk for, or indeed be in the early stages of COPD. Application of exclusion criteria yielded a final study population of 5,887 (8%) smokers with evidence of mild to moderate airway obstruction (mean age 48 yrs, 63% male).
Intervention: Patients were randomized to receive one of usual care (UC), smoking intervention and inhaled Atrovent (SIA), or smoking intervention and inhaled placebo (SIP) for 5 years.
Primary Outcomes: Decline in FEV_1 over a 5 year period.
Results: Patients in the smoking intervention groups had significantly smaller declines in FEV_1 than those receiving usual care. FEV_1 results were most striking at 1 year with a mean *decrease* of 34.3 mL in the UC group and mean *increases* of 11.2 and 38.8 mL in the SIP and SIA groups, respectively (P<0.005). Between 1 year and 5 years, FEV_1 declined at similar rates in all three groups (52.3-56.2 mL/yr). However, subgroup analysis revealed that quitters in the SIP group who remained abstinent throughout the study's 5 year follow-up experienced a cumulative decline in FEV_1 of only 72 mL in the same period, compared with a cumulative decline of 301 mL in those who continued to smoke. The small benefit associated with Atrovent was reversible with discontinuation, and therefore did not impact the long-term decline in FEV_1.
Conclusion: Spirometry is an effective screening method for the detection of early COPD. Smoking intervention programs can significantly reduce the decline in FEV_1 in this population. Atrovent did not impact the long-term decline in FEV_1.

COPD - *JAMA* 2000; 283:1853-57

Finding	Likelihood Ratio (+)
Smoking >40 pk years	8.3
Self reported Hx of obstructive lung disease	7.3
Maximum laryngeal Height of <4 cm	2.8
Age at least 45 years	1.3

Patients having 4 findings had an LR+ of 220. Those with none had LR- of 0.13.

Early Use of Non-invasive Ventilation for Acute Exacerbations of COPD on General Respiratory Wards – A Multicentre Randomized Controlled Trial
Lancet 2000;355: 1931-5
Study: Prospective, randomized, controlled, multicentre trial.
Patients: 236 adult patients (mean age 69 yrs, 50% female) admitted to hospital for an acute exacerbation of COPD, who were also tachypneic (RR>23) and acidemic (pH 7.25-7.35) with a high P_aCO_2 (>45mmHg).
Intervention: Patients were randomized to receive either standard treatment (oxygen, salbutamol, ipratropium, corticosteroids, antibiotics) or standard treatment with the addition of non-invasive ventilation (NIV, bilevel assist-mode).
Primary Outcomes: Need for endotracheal intubation as defined by objective criteria.
Results: Fewer patients in the NIV group required endotracheal intubation compared with those in the standard treatment group (15.3% vs. 27.1%, p<0.02, NNT=9). In addition, in hospital mortality was reduced in the NIV group relative to the standard treatment group (10.2% vs. 20.3%, p=0.05, NNT=10). NIV also led to faster improvement in pH in the first hour, greater reduction in respiratory rate at 4 hours, and reduced duration of the subjective experience of breathlessness.
Conclusion: Early NIV reduces mortality and the need for endotracheal intubation in tachypneic and mildly to moderately acidemic patients admitted to hospital for an acute exacerbation of COPD.

Oral Prednisone for COPD Exacerbation
NEJM 2003; 348:2618-25
Study: Randomized, double-blind, placebo-controlled trial with 30 day follow-up
Patients: 147 patients (mean age 69y, 97% male, 97% white) with COPD, presenting to the ER with at least 2 of the following: recent increase in breathlessness, sputum volume, or sputum purulence. Inclusion criteria also included a smoking history of ≥15 pack-years, and irreversible airflow obstruction in the ER (FEV$_1$/FVC ≤0.70). Exclusions included patients with asthma or atopy, recent oral or IV steroid use, chest x-ray consistent with pneumonia or CHF, and those requiring admission to hospital.
Intervention: All patients received 10 days of broad-spectrum antibiotics, plus inhaled albuterol and ipratropium bromide for 30 days. Patients were randomized to receive 40 mg prednisone x 10 days, or placebo.
Main Outcomes: Relapse defined as unscheduled visit to a physician or return to ER for worsening SOB within 30 days.
Results: Oral prednisone significantly reduced the rate of relapse at 30 days (27% vs. 43%, p=0.05). Prednisone prolonged the time to relapse (p=0.04). Increased appetite, weight gain, and insomnia were more prevalent in the prednisone group.
Conclusion: In COPD patients discharged from the ER with COPD exacerbation, a 10-day course of oral prednisone offers a small advantage over placebo in preventing relapse.

Influenza vaccination in COPD
Chest 2004; 125(6):2011-20
Study: Single centre, randomized, double-blinded, placebo-controlled trial.
Patients: 125 patients with COPD, stratified by FEV$_1$ into mild, moderate and severe COPD.
Intervention: Influenza vaccination.
Main Outcomes: Number of episodes and severity of acute respiratory illness, influenza-related and total.
Results: Influenza vaccinated patients experienced 6.8 influenza-related acute respiratory illnesses per 100 patient-years while those in the placebo group experienced 28.1 influenza-related acute respiratory illnesses per 100 patient-years (RR 0.24, p=0.005). This reduction held for all subgroups of FEV$_1$ level. No effect was seen on the total number of acute respiratory illnesses.
Conclusion: Influenza vaccination is effective in reducing the number of influenza-related illnesses in COPD patients, but not in other acute respiratory illness.

Prognosis in COPD
- chronic hypoxemia
- pulmonary hypertension from vasoconstriction
- cor pulmonale

Acute Exacerbations of COPD
- definition
    - episode of increased dyspnea, coughing, increase in sputum volume or purulence
- etiology: viral URTI's, bacteria, air pollution, CHF, PE, MI must be considered
- management
    1. assess ABCs, consider assisted ventilation if decreasing LOC or poor ABGs
    2. supplemental O_2 (controlled FiO_2): target 88-92% O_2 sats for CO_2 retainers
    3. bronchodilators by nebulizer
        - short acting β_2-agonists used concurrently with anticholinergics
        - salbutamol and ipratropium bromide via nebulizers x 3 back-to-back
    4. systemic corticosteroids : IV solumedrol, hydrocortisone, methylprednisolone
    5. antibiotics: often used to treat precipitating infection
        - indications (2 out of 3) ↑ SOB, ↑ sputum, or ↑ sputum purulence (change in colour)
    6. post exacerbation:
        - rehab with general conditioning to improve exercise tolerance

- ICU admission
    - for life threatening exacerbations:
        - ventilatory support:
            1. non-invasive: NIPPV, CPAP, BiPAP
            2. conventional mechanical ventilation

Prognosis in COPD
- complications
    - secondary polycythemia due to hypoxemia
    - pulmonary hypertension due to reactive vasoconstriction 2o to hypoxemia
    - cor pulmonale from chronic pulmonary HTN
    - pneumothorax due to formation of bullae in emphysema
- prognostic factors
    - severity of airflow limitation (FEV$_1$) is the single best predictor
    - development of complicating factors such as hypoxemia or cor pulmonale
- 5-year survival
    - FEV$_1$ <1 L = 50%
    - FEV$_1$ <0.75 L = 33%
- BODE index for risk of death in COPD
    - 10 point index consisting of four factors:
        - body mass index (BMI): <21 (+1 point)
        - obstruction (FEV1): 50-64% (+1), 36-49% (+2), <35% (+3)
        - dyspnea (MMRC scale): walks slower than people of same age on level surface, stops occasionally (+1), stops at 100 yards or a few minutes on the level (+2), too breathless to leave house or breathless when dressing/undressing (+3)
        - exercise capacity (6 minute walk distance): 250-349 m (+1), 150-249 m (+2), <149 m (+3)
    - greater score indicates higher probability that the patient will die from COPD; score can also be used to predict hospitalization

Bronchiectasis

Definition
- an irreversible dilatation of airways due to inflammatory destruction of airway walls resulting from persistently infected mucus
- usually affects medium to small sized airways
- once bronchiectasis is established *P. aeruginosa* is the most common pathogen

Table 13. Etiology and Pathophysiology of Bronchiectasis

Obstruction	Post-infection (results in dilatation of bronchial walls)	Impaired defenses (leads to interference of drainage, chronic infections, and inflammation)
tumours	pneumonia	hypogammaglobulinemia
foreign bodies	TB	CF
thick mucus	measles	defective leukocyte function
	pertussis	ciliary dysfunction (Kartagener's syndrome:
	allergic bronchopulmonary aspergillosis	bronchiectasis, sinusitis, situs inversus)
	MAC (mycobacteria avium complex)	

Signs and Symptoms
- chronic cough, purulent sputum (but 10-20% have a dry cough), hemoptysis (can be massive), recurrent pneumonia, local crackles (inspiratory and expiratory), wheezes
- clubbing
- often difficult to differentiate from chronic bronchitis

Investigations
- PFTs: often demonstrate obstructive pattern but may be normal
- CXR

- - nonspecific: increased markings, linear atelectasis, loss of volume in affected areas
  - specific: "tram tracking" – parallel narrow lines radiating from hilum, cystic spaces, honeycomb like structures
- bronchoscopy: used for examination of proximal airways to investigate obstructive lesions or hemoptysis
- high-resolution thoracic CT (diagnostic, gold standard):
  - 87-97% sensitivity, 93-100% specificity
  - "signet ring" : dilated bronchi with thickened walls where diameter bronchus > diameter of accompanying artery

Treatment
- vaccination: influenza and Pneumovax™
- antibiotics (oral, IV, inhaled) – routinely used for mild exacerbations, driven by sputum sensitivity; macrolides may also have an anti-inflammatory effect
- inhaled corticosteroids – decrease inflammation and improve FEV_1
- oral corticosteroids for acute, major exacerbations
- chest physiotherapy, breathing exercises, physical exercise
- pulmonary resection: in severe cases where medical therapy fails

Cystic Fibrosis (CF)

- see also Pediatrics
- chloride transport dysfunction: thick secretions from exocrine glands (lung, pancreas, skin, gonads) and blockage of secretory ducts
- results in severe lung disease, pancreatic insufficiency and azospermia
- presents in childhood with recurrent lung infections that become persistent and chronic
- chronic lung infections
  - *S. aureus*: early
  - *P. aeruginosa*: most common
  - *B. cepacia*: worse prognosis but less common
  - *Aspergillus fumigatus*

Investigations
- sweat chloride test
  - increased concentrations of sodium chloride and potassium (chloride >60 mmol/L is diagnostic in children)
  - heterozygotes have normal sweat tests (and no symptoms)
- PFTs
  - characteristic of obstructive airway disease
  - early: only small airways will be affected
  - later: characteristics of obstructive disease with airflow limitation, hyperinflation, gas trapping, decreased D_{co} (very late)
- ABGs
  - hypoxemia, hypercapnia later in disease with eventual respiratory failure and cor pulmonale
- CXR
  - hyperinflation, increased pulmonary markings, bronchiectasis

Treatment
- chest physiotherapy and postural drainage
- bronchodilators (salbutamol ± ipratropium bromide)
- inhaled mucolytic (reduces mucus viscosity)
- antibiotics (e.g. ciprofloxacin)
- lung transplant

Prognosis
- depends on: infections, FEV1, acute pulmonary exacerbations, lung transplant vs non-lung transplant

Interstitial Lung Disease

Pathophysiology
- inflammatory process in the alveolar walls → thickening and possible destruction of pulmonary vessels, and fibrosis of interstitium leading to:
  - decreased lung compliance (↑ or normal FEV_1/FVC)
  - decreased lung volumes (↓TLC, ↓VC, ↓RV)
  - impaired diffusion
  - hypoxemia without hypercarbia (V/Q mismatch) due to vasoconstriction and fibrosis
  - pulmonary HTN and subsequent cor pulmonale secondary to hypoxemia and blood vessel destruction

---

ILD's to be covered in detail
- idiopathic pulmonary fibrosis
- sarcoidosis
- Langerhans-Cell histiocytosis
- PIE syndrome
- BOOP
- hypersensitivity pneumonitis
- pneumoconiosis
- drug/radiation induced ILD

Table 14. Causes of Interstitial Lung Disease by Lung Field

Upper Lung Disease	Lower Lung Disease
Farmer's lung	**B**ronchiolitis obliterans with organizing pneumonia (BOOP)
Ankylosing spondylitis	**A**sbestosis
Sarcoidosis	**D**rugs (nitrofurantoin, hydralazine, INH, amiodarone, many chemo drugs)
Silicosis	**R**heumatologic disease
TB (miliary)	**A**spiration
Eosinophilic granuloma (histiocytosis)	**S**cleroderma
Neurofibromatosis	**H**amman Rich (interstitial pulmonary fibrosis)

In Interstitial Lung Disease think

FASSTEN and **BAD RASH**
(see Table 14)

Etiology
- >100 known disorders can cause interstitial lung disease
- 65% due to unknown agents or cause
- divided into 2 major categories: unknown etiology and known etiology

Table 15. Interstitial Lung Diseases

UNKNOWN ETIOLOGY		
idiopathic pulmonary fibrosis	bronchiolitis obliterans with organizing pneumonia (BOOP)	
sarcoidosis	lymphocytic interstitial pneumonia	
Langerhans-cell histiocytosis (histiocytosis X)	lymphangioleiomyomatosis	
pulmonary infiltrates with eosinophilia (PIE Syndrome)		

KNOWN ETIOLOGY		
ILD Associated With Systemic Rheumatic Disorders scleroderma rheumatoid arthritis SLE polymyositis/dermatomyositis mixed connective tissue disease	**ILD Associated With Drugs or Treatments** antibiotics (nitrofurantoin) anti-inflammatory agents cardiovascular drugs (amiodarone) antineoplastic agents (chemotherapy agents) illicit drugs radiation	**Alveolar Filling Disorders** chronic eosinophilic pneumonia Goodpasture's syndrome diffuse alveolar hemorrhage pulmoary alveolar proteinosis

Environment/Occupation Associated ILD
Organic dusts (hypersensitivity pneumonitis)
  farmer's lung
  air conditioner/humidifier lung
  bird breeder's lung
Inorganic dusts (pneumoconiosis)
  silicosis
  asbestosis
  coal workers' pneumoconiosis
  berylliosis
  gases/fumes/vapours
	ILD Associated With Pulmonary Vasculitis
	Wegener's granulomatosis
	Churg-Strauss syndrome
	hypersensitivity vasculitis
	necrotizing sarcoid granulomatosis
	idiopathic pulmonary hemosiderosis
	pulmonary alveolar proteinosis
		Miscellaneous
		infections (viral pneumonia, PCP, fungal, mycobacterial)
		lipoid pneumonia (oil aspiration)
		lymphangitic carcinomatosis
		lymphoma
		chronic uremia (perihilar edema, periphery)
		chronic gastric aspiration

	Inherited Disorders familial idiopathic pulmonary fibrosis neurofibromatosis tuberous sclerosis Gaucher's disease	

Signs and Symptoms
- SOB, especially on exertion
- dry crackles
- dry cough
- cyanosis
- clubbing (only in IPF and asbestosis)
- features of cor pulmonale
- note that signs and symptoms vary with underlying disease process

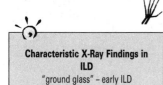

The CXR can be normal in up to 15% of patients with interstitial lung disease.

Characteristic X-Ray Findings in ILD
"ground glass" – early ILD
"honey combing" – late ILD

Investigations
- CXR/high resolution CT
  - decreased lung volumes, reticular, nodular, or reticulonodular pattern (nodular <3 mm), Kerley B lines, hilar/mediastinal adenopathy
  - diffuse ground-glass appearance early in disease progresses to honey-combing late in disease
  - DDx: pulmonary fibrosis, interstitial pulmonary edema (CHF), PCP, TB (miliary), sarcoidosis, pneumoconiosis, lymphangitic carcinomatosis
  - DDx of cystic lesions: end-stage emphysema, PCP, histiocytosis X, lymphangiomyomatosis
- PFTs
  - restrictive pattern: decreased lung volumes (VC and TLC) and compliance
  - normal or ↑FEV_1/FVC (>70-80%), i.e. flow rates are actually normal or supernormal when corrected for absolute lung volume
  - D_{CO} decreased due to less surface area for gas exchange ± pulmonary vascular disease
- ABGs
  - initially may be normal
  - with progression of disease, hypoxemia and decreased $PaCO_2$ may be present
- Other
  - bronchoscopy, bronchoalveolar lavage, lung biopsy
  - c-ANCA (Wegner's), anti-GBM (Goodpasture's), ESR, ANA (lupus), RF (RA), serum-precipitating antibodies to inhaled organic antigens (hypersensitivity pneumonitis)

Unknown Etiologic Agents

Idiopathic Pulmonary Fibrosis

Definition
- a diagnosis of exclusion
- also known as cryptogenic fibrosing alveolitis or usual interstitial pneumonitis (UIP)
- DDx:
    - nonspecific interstitial pneumonitis (NSIP)
    - desquamative interstitial pneumonitis (DIP)
    - lymphocytic interstitial pneumonitis (LIP) (usually 2° to lymphoma)
- no geographic, gender, racial, or seasonal predilections noted

Signs and Symptoms
- commonly presents between ages 40-75; males > females
- most patients present with insidious onset of SOB on exertion and nonproductive cough
- constitutional symptoms present in some patients:
    - fever, fatigue, anorexia, weight loss, myalgia, and arthralgia
- additional clinical features:
    - late inspiratory fine ("Velcro") crackles at the lung bases, clubbing

> **IPF Prevalence**
> Age 35-44 : 2-7 per 10^5
> Age >75 : 175 per 10^5

Investigations
- lab tests (nonspecific)
    - ESR increased
    - ANA and RF positive in 10%
- CXR
    - lower lung: reticulonodular or reticular pattern (starts in periphery)
    - generally bilateral and relatively symmetric
    - no pleural or hilar involvement
    - multiple cystic or honeycombed areas (0.5-1 cm) seen late in disease (indicate poor prognosis)
- CT (high resolution)
    - ground glass appearance
    - diffuse ↑ interstitial markings
    - honey-combing late in disease
- biopsy
    - required to establish the diagnosis of idiopathic pulmonary fibrosis
    - to exclude granulomas (found in sarcoidosis and hypersensitivity pneumonitis)

Treatment
- supportive: oxygen therapy if hypoxemic
- steroids ± immunosuppressants (e.g. cytotoxic agents), no benefit from interferon gamma 1b therapy
- favourable clinical response occurs in only 10-20% of patients
- mean survival of 5-7 years after diagnosis
- lung transplantation may be considered for patients unresponsive to medical therapy with end-stage disease

Sarcoidosis

Definition
- non-infectious granulomatous multi-system disease of unknown cause with lung involvement in 90%
- characterized pathologically by noncaseating granulomas
- proposed triggers include infectious, allergic, and environmental exposures (neither genetic nor specific triggers have been established)

Epidemiology
- typically affects young and middle-aged black women but other groups also affected

Signs and Symptoms
- 2/3 are asymptomatic and 1/3 may have cough, dyspnea, fever, arthralgia, malaise, erythema nodosum, chest pain
- chest exam usually normal
- common extrapulmonary manifestations
    - cardiac (arrhythmias, sudden death)
    - eye involvement (anterior uveitis)
    - skin involvement (skin papules, erythema nodosum, lupus pernio)
    - peripheral lymphadenopathy
    - arthralgia
    - hepatomegaly
- less common extra-pulmonary manifestations involve bone, CNS and kidney
- two acute sarcoid syndromes
    - Lofgren's syndrome: fever, erythema nodosum, bilateral hilar lymphadenopathy, arthralgias

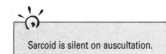

> Sarcoid is silent on auscultation.

- Heerfordt-Waldenstrom syndrome: fever, parotid enlargement, anterior uveitis, facial nerve palsy

Investigations
- leukopenia, eosinophilia
- hypercalcemia, hypercalciuria (hypercalciuria more common)
- increased ESR
- hypergammaglobulinemia, RF positive
- elevated serum ACE (non-specific)
- CXR: predominantly nodular opacities especially in upper lung zones ± hilar adenopathy
- ABG (normal, or hypoxemia and hypocapnia)
- PFTs (normal, obstructive pattern, restrictive pattern with normal flow rates and $\downarrow D_{co}$)
- ECG (to rule out arrhythmias)
- slit-lamp eye exam (to rule out uveitis)

Diagnosis
- biopsy
  - transbronchial or mediastinoscopic biopsy of lymph node for granulomas
  - in ~75% of cases, transbronchial biopsy shows granulomas in the parenchyma even if the CXR is normal

Staging
- radiographic, based on CXR
  - Stage 0:   normal radiograph
  - Stage I: bilateral hilar lymphadenopathy ± right paratracheal lymphodenopathy
  - Stage II: bilateral hilar lymphadenopathy and diffuse interstitial disease
  - Stage III: interstitial disease only (reticulonodular pattern or nodular pattern)
  - Stage IV: pulmonary fibrosis (honeycombing)

Treatment
- 85% of stage I resolve spontaneously
- 50% of stage II resolve spontaneously
- steroids for respiratory symptoms, PFT abnormalities, hypercalcemia, or involvement of eye, CNS, kidney, or heart (not for abnormal CXR alone)
- chloroquine, other immunosuppressants

Prognosis
- approximately 10% mortality secondary to progressive fibrosis of lung parenchyma

Langerhans-Cell Histiocytosis

- also called pulmonary eosinophilic granuloma, Langerhans-cell granulomatosis
- represents the pulmonary form of Histiocytosis X
- characterized by clonal proliferation of dendritic cells (Langerhans' cells)
- cells have X-bodies on EM
- epidemiology: typically affects young-middle aged smokers
- signs/symptoms: cough, tachypnea, cyanosis, inspiratory crackles, pleural effusions, chest pain, or pneumothorax
- investigations: CXR: primarily in upper lung zones
  - cystic, nodular and/or reticulonodular changes that progress to honeycombing
- course: may stabilize in some patients or may be progressive
- treatment:
  - smoking cessation
  - acute multisystem disease: methylprednisolone + either vinblastine or etoposide
  - chronic multisystem disease: cyclosporin + antithymocyte globulin + prednisolone or bone marrow transplantation

Pulmonary Infiltrates with Eosinophilia (PIE Syndrome)

Think of parasites if positive travel history.

- a broad group of disorders
  - known etiology
    - allergic bronchopulmonary aspergillosis (and other mycoses)
    - parasitic infestations (filariasis, ascariasis, tropical eosinophilia etc.)
    - drug reactions: antibiotics (penicillin, sulfonamides, tetracyclines, INH), anti-inflammatory (ASA, MTX), imipramine
    - eosinophilic myalgia syndrome
  - unknown etiology
    - idiopathic Löffler's syndrome
    - acute eosinophilic pneumonia
    - chronic eosinophilic pneumonia
    - Churg-Strauss Syndrome
    - hyper-eosinophilic syndrome

Löffler's Syndrome
- transient and migrating peripheral lung infiltrates and eosinophilia
- asymptomatic to mildly symptomatic (fever and cough) without auscultatory findings

- CXR usually resolves spontaneously within two to six weeks or upon treatment of the underlying cause (e.g. parasite, drug) if known

Chronic Eosinophilic Pneumonia
- infiltrates of eosinophils and macrophages in the interstitium and alveolar spaces
- commonly presents as fever, night sweats, cough ± hemoptysis in a middle-aged woman (similar presentation to TB)
- 2/3 of cases have a very high eosinophil count (>25 x 10⁹) and a very high ESR (100 mm/hour)
- diagnosis
  - clinical, based on history, eosinophilia, and typical CXR
  - confirmed by rapid radiological and clinical response to corticosteroids

The CXR in chronic eosinophiic pneumonia shows a peripheral alveolar infiltrate referred to as the "photographic negative of pulmonary edema" (pattern is often migratory).

Allergic Bronchopulmonary Aspergillosis (ABPA)
- airway colonization with *Aspergillus* causes an inflammatory reaction (not infection) which can lead to proximal bronchiectasis
- classic presentation: asthmatic with an exacerbation of symptoms, low grade fever, migratory infiltrates on CXR, and expectoration of golden brown mucus plugs (loaded with *Aspergillus mycelia*)
- diagnosis
  - positive culture
  - presence of serum precipitants of *A. fumigatus* (70% of patients)
  - elevation of specific IgE (>1,000 ng/mL)
  - positive skin test (immediate and/or delayed)
- treatment consists of blunting the immune response to the organism with corticosteroids, eradication of *Aspergillus* may hasten resolution
- commonly leads to remission but may recur as corticosteroid treatment is tapered

Tropical Eosinophilia
- cough, wheeze and fever (especially at night) in someone who has recently visited the tropics
- positive filarial complement fixation test
- CXR: diffuse bilateral micronodules

Churg-Strauss Syndrome (see *Pulmonary Vasculitis*, R21)

Associated With Collagen Vascular Disease (see *Pulmonary Vasculitis*, R21)

Bronchiolitis Obliterans With Organizing Pneumonia (BOOP)

- acute inflammation of bronchioles with granulation tissue and mononuclear cell infiltrate plugs
- idiopathic but may follow toxic fume inhalation/viral infection in children; associated with connective tissue diseases, and hypersensitivity pneumonitis
- presents over weeks to months with systemic and respiratory symptoms, may have URTI 2-4 months prior to SOB
- crackles on chest exam
- CXR, CT: bilateral ground glass densities; also miliary nodules and symmetric lower lobe interstitial infiltrates
- biopsy often required to distinguish BOOP from other ILDs
- treatment: corticosteroids (responds faster and more frequently than idiopathic pulmonary fibrosis)
  - often improves within days
  - continue high dose for 2-3 months; taper slowly

Known Etiologic Agents

Hypersensitivity Pneumonitis

- also known as extrinsic allergic alveolitis
- immunolgically induced inflammation of lung parenchyma (acute, subacute, and chronic forms)
- caused by intense/repeated inhalation and sensitization to certain organic agents
- lymphocytic granulomas present, airway centered

- exposure usually related to occupation or hobby
  - Farmer's Lung (*Thermophilic actinomycetes*)
  - Bird Breeder's/Bird Fancier's Lung (*Chlamydia psittaci* in bird droppings)
  - Humidifier Lung (*Aureobasidium pullulans*)
  - Sauna Taker's Lung (*Aureobasidium spp*)

Signs and Symptoms
- acute presentation: (4-6 hours after exposure)
  - dyspnea, cough, fever, chills, malaise (lasting 18-24 hrs)
  - PFTs: modestly and transiently restrictive
  - CXR: diffuse infiltrates
  - type III (immune complex) reaction
- subacute presentation: more insidious onset than acute presentation
- chronic presentation
  - insidious onset
  - dyspnea, cough, malaise, anorexia, weight loss
  - PFTs: progressively restrictive
  - CXR: predominantly upper lobe, nodular/reticulonodular pattern
  - type IV (cell mediated, delayed hypersensitivity) reaction (see Rheumatology)
- in both acute and chronic reaction, serum precipitins detectable (neither sensitive nor specific)

Treatment
- goal is to prevent chronic fibrotic changes
- early diagnosis: avoidance of further exposure is critical as chronic changes are irreversible
- systemic corticosteroids can relieve symptoms in acute phase
- steroids for persistent disease

Pneumoconioses

- reaction to inhaled inorganic dusts 0.5-5 mm in size
- no effective treatment, therefore key is exposure prevention through the use of protective equipment

Asbestosis
- population at risk: insulation, shipyard, construction, brake linings, pipe fitters, plumbers
- slowly progressive diffuse interstitial fibrosis from dose-related inhalation of asbestos
- etiology: usually >10-20 yrs of exposure; may develop with shorter but heavier exposure; typically prolonged interval (20-30 yrs) between exposure and clinical manifestations of disease
- signs and symptoms
  - insidious onset
  - SOB on exertion usually first symptom with increased dyspnea as disease progresses
  - cough: paroxysmal, non-productive
  - fine end-respiratory crackles (increased at bases)
  - clubbing (much more likely in asbestosis than silicosis or coal workers' pneumoconioses), edema, jugular venous distention
- investigations: CXR
  - rounded atelectasis
  - lower > upper lobe
  - early: fibrosis with linear streaking
  - later: cysts and honeycombing
  - asbestos exposure can also cause pleural and diaphragmatic plaques (± calcification) or pleural effusion
- microscopic examination reveals ferruginous bodies: yellow-brown rod-shaped structures which represent asbestos fibres coated in macrophages
- complications: increases risk of bronchogenic CA and malignant mesothelioma
  - risk dramatically increased for smokers
- treatment:
  - removal from exposure
  - smoking cessation, proper nutrition, exercise
  - home oxygen PRN
  - treatment of respiratory infections, annual influenza and pneumococcal vaccinations

CXR Fibrotic Patterns
Asbestosis: lower > upper lobes
Silicosis: upper > lower lobes
Coal: upper > lower lobes

Remember to involve occupational health at place of work for data collection and treatment plan. Also counsel re: worker's insurance as per jurisdiction (eg. WSIB in Ontario).

Silicosis
- at risk population: sandblasters, rock miners, stone cutters, quarry and highway workers
- etiology: generally requires >20 years exposure; may develop with much shorter but heavier exposure
- signs & symptoms: dyspnea, cough and wheezing
- investigations: CXR
  - upper > lower lobe
  - early: nodular disease (simple pneumoconiosis)
  - late: nodules coalesce into masses (progressive massive fibrosis)
- when nodules become larger and coalesce into masses, disease has changed from simple silicosis to complicated silicosis (progressive massive fibrosis)
- possible hilar lymph node enlargement (frequent calcification) and egg shell calcifications
- complications: mycobacterial infection (i.e. TB)
- treatment: prevention, removal from exposure, treat associated TB if present, supportive measures (oxygen, bronchodilators), lung transplant

Coal Worker's Pneumoconiosis (CWP)
- at risk population: coal workers, graphite workers
- etiology: coal and silica, coal is less fibrogenic than silica
- pathologic hallmark is coal macule:
  - coal dust surrounded by minimal tissue reaction and focal emphysema
  - found around respiratory bronchioles
- simple CWP
  - no signs or symptoms
  - CXR: multiple nodular opacities, mostly upper lobe
  - respiratory function well preserved
- complicated CWP (also known as progressive massive fibrosis)
  - dyspnea
  - CXR: opacities larger and coalesce
- course: few patients progress to complicated CWP
- Caplan's syndrome: rheumatoid arthritis and CWP present as larger nodules
- treatment: minimize future exposure, cardiopulmonary rehabilitation, follow periodically

ILD Associated with Drugs or Treatments

Drug-Induced
- antineoplastic agents: bleomycin, mitomycin, busulfan, cyclophosphamide, methotrexate, chlorambucil, BCNU (carmustine)
- antibiotics: nitrofurantoin, penicillin, sulfonamide
- cardiovascular drugs: amiodarone, tocainide
- anti-inflammatory agents
- gold salts
- illicit drugs

Radiation-Induced
- early pneumonitis: approximately 6 weeks post-exposure
- late fibrosis: 6-12 months post-exposure
- infiltration conforms to the shape and field of the irradiation

Pulmonary Vascular Disease

Pulmonary Hypertension

- mean pulmonary arterial pressure >25 mmHg at rest and >30 mmHg with exercise, or a systolic pulmonary artery pressure of >40 mmHg at rest
- in the past, pulmonary hypertension was classified as primary or secondary pulmonary hypertension, but this classification was modified to a more clinically useful, treatment based classification (Table 16)

Table 16. Diagnostic Classification of Pulmonary Hypertension (WHO 1998)

Classification	Causes

• pulmonary arterial hypertension	primary pulmonary hypertension - sporadic vs. familial
	related to:
	    collagen vascular disease (scleroderma, SLE, RA)
	    congenital systemic-to-pulmonary shunts (Eisenmenger syndrome)
	    portopulmonary hypertension
	    HIV infection
	    drugs and toxins (e.g. anorexigens)

• pulmonary venous hypertension	left sided atrial or ventricular heart disease (e.g. LV dysfunction) left sided valvular heart disease (e.g. aortic stenosis, mitral stenosis) pulmonary veno-occlusive disease extrinsic compression of central pulmonary veins (tumour, adenopathy, fibrosing mediastinitis)
• associated with disorders of the respiratory system and/or hypoxemia	parenchymal lung disease (COPD, interstitial fibrosis, cystic fibrosis) chronic alveolar hypoxia (chronic high altitude, alveolar hypoventilation disorders, sleep disordered breathing)
• due to chronic thrombotic and/or embolic disease	thromboembolic obstruction of proximal pulmonary arteries obstruction of distal pulmonary arteries – PE (thrombus, foreign material, tumour, schistosomiasis, in situ thrombosis, sickle cell disease)
• due to disorders directly affecting the pulmonary vasculature	inflammatory (sarcoidosis, schistosomiasis) pulmonary capillary hemangiomatosis

Mechanisms of Pulmonary Hypertension
• the approach is simplified, as some causes could fall under more than one mechanism:
  ▪ hypoxic vasoconstriction
    ◆ chronic hypoxia causes pulmonary vasoconstriction by a variety of actions on the pulmonary artery endothelium and smooth muscle cells, such as: down regulation of endothelial nitric oxide synthase and alteration of voltage gated potassium channels leading to vasoconstriction
    ◆ causes: COPD, chronic alveolar hypoxia
  ▪ decreased area of pulmonary vascular bed
    ◆ a decrease in the area of the pulmonary vascular bed causes rise in resting pulmonary arterial pressure
    ◆ causes: collagen vascular disease, HIV infection, drugs and toxins, thrombotic or embolic disease, inflammatory, pulmonary capillary hemangiomatosis, interstitial fibrosis, cystic fibrosis
  ▪ volume and pressure overload
    ◆ significant hypertension only occurs with excessive volume overload, since pulmonary artery pressure will not rise in otherwise normal lung until pulmonary blood flow exceeds 2.5 times the basal rate
    ◆ causes: congenital systemic to pulmonary shunts (e.g. VSD, ASD, PDA), portopulmonary hypertension, left-sided heart conditions, pulmonary veno-occlusive disease, extrinsic compression of central pulmonary veins

PULMONARY ARTERIAL HYPERTENSION (AKA PRIMARY PULMONARY HYPERTENSION (PPH))

Definition
• the diagnostic criteria used in the National Institutes of Health (NIH) registry include a mean pulmonary-artery pressure of more than 25 mmHg at rest, or more than 30 mmHg with exercise. A diagnosis of idiopathic pulmonary hypertension is made in the absence of a demonstrable cause; also excluding left-sided cardiac valvular disease, myocardial disease, congenital heart disease, and any clinically significant parenchymal lung disease, systemic connective-tissue, or chronic thromboembolic disease

Epidemiology
• disease of young women (20-40 years); mean age of diagnosis is 36 yrs
• most cases are sporadic; familial predisposition in 10% of cases

Signs and Symptoms
• exertional dyspnea, fatigue, syncope, exertional chest pain, Raynaud's syndrome (see Table 17)

Prognosis
• 2-3 year mean survival from time of diagnosis
• may be associated with the use of anorexic drugs (e.g. aminorex, fenfluramine), also amphetamines and cocaine
• survival decreases to approximately 1 year if severe pulmonary HTN or right-heart failure

---

Guildelines for Vasodilator Response

1. Evidence for the use of CCBs after a positive vasodilator challenge is limited to patients with IPAH.

2. The precise definition about what constitutes a "positive" result is controversial. The latest consensus according to the European Society of Cardiology was that a positive result constitutes a fall of mean PAP pressure of 10 mmHg to less than or equal to 40 WITHOUT a change in cardiac output.

3. Best agents to use: NO or epoprostenol (prostacyclin) analogue (best safety profile).

4. Those who have a "significant" response (as determined by the criteria in #2) should be treated cautiously with a CCB (nifedipine, diltiazem, amlodipine are good choices, NOT verapamil). Evidence suggests these patients will have improved survivals.

Reference: Badesch et al. Medical Therapy For Pulmonary Arterial Hypertension. ACCP Evidence-Based Clinical Practice Guidelines. CHEST 126, supplement, July, 2004.

Table 17. Signs and Symptoms of Pulmonary Hypertension

Symptoms	Signs
dyspnea	loud, palpable P2
fatigue	RV heave
substernal chest pain	right sided S4 (due to RVH)
syncope	systolic murmur (TR)
symptoms of underlying disease	if RV failure: right sided S3, increased JVP, positive HJR, peripheral edema, TR

Investigations
- CXR: enlarged central pulmonary arteries, cardiac changes due to RV enlargement (filling of retrosternal air space)
- ECG
  - RVH/right-sided strain and RA enlargement, rightward axis deviation
  - R/S ratio >1 in V_1
  - increased P wave amplitude in lead II
  - incomplete or complete R bundle branch block
- 2-D echo doppler assessment of RVSP
- cardiac catheterization: direct measurement of pulmonary artery pressures
- PFTs to rule out lung disease
- spiral CT to assess lung parenchyma and possible PE
- V/Q scan ± pulmonary angiogram to rule out thromboembolic disease
- serology: ANA positive in 30% of patients wih primary pulmonary hypertension

Treatment
- **Primary Pulmonary Hypertension**
  - anticoagulation in patients at increased risk for intrapulmonary thrombosis and thromboembolism (anticoagulation of choice is warfarin, target INR approximately 2.0)
  - vasodilators: oral (nitric oxide), parenteral (epoprostenol, treprostanil)
  - calcium channel blockers: nifedipine, diltiazem, NOT verapamil
  - lung transplantation
- **Other Causes of Pulmonary Hypertension**
  - continuous oxygen therapy for patients who are hypoxic
  - treat underlying condition before irreversible damage occurs
  - phlebotomy for polycythemia (rarely required)
  - treatment of exacerbating factors: smoking, infection, sleep apnea
  - epoprostenol – beneficial in cardiomyopathy, and NYHA class III-IV symptoms
  - endothelin receptor antagonists (bosentan, sitaxentan)
  - phosphodiesterase inhibitors (sildenafil)

Pulmonary Embolism (PE)

Definition
- lodging of a blood clot in the pulmonary arterial tree with subsequent increase in pulmonary vascular resistance and possible obstruction of blood supply to the lung parenchyma

Etiology and Pathophysiology
- one of the most common causes of preventable death in the hospital
- proximal leg thrombi (popliteal, femoral or iliac veins) are the source of most clinically recognized pulmonary emboli
- thrombi often start in calf, but must propagate into proximal veins to create a sufficiently large thrombus for a clinically significant PE
- fewer than 30% of patients have clinical evidence of DVT (i.e. leg swelling, pain or tenderness)
- always suspect PE if patient suddenly collapses 1-2 weeks after surgery

Risk Factors (Virchow's Triad)
- stasis
  - immobilization: paralysis, stroke, bed rest, prolonged sitting during travel, immobilization of an extremity after fracture
  - obesity, CHF
  - chronic venous insufficiency
- **endothelial cell damage**
  - post-operative injury, trauma
- **hypercoagulable states**
  - underlying CA (particularly adenocarcinoma)
  - cancer treatment (chemotherapy, hormonal)
  - exogenous estrogen administration (OCP, HRT)
  - pregnancy, post-partum
  - prior history of DVT/PE, family history
  - nephrotic syndrome
  - coagulopathies: Factor V Leiden, Prothrombin 20210A variant, inherited deficiencies of antithrombin/protein C/protein S, antiphospholipid antibody, hyperhomocysteinemia, ↑ Factor VIII levels, and myeloproliferative diseases
- increasing age

Virchow's Triad
- venous stasis
- endothelial cell damage
- hypercoagulable states

Clinical Prediction Rule for Pulmonary Embolism
Thrombosis and Hemostasis 2000; 83(3):416-20.

Risk Factors	Points
Clinical signs of DVT	3.0
No more likely alternative diagnosis (using H&P, CXR, ECG)	3.0
Immobilization or surgery in the previous 4 weeks	1.5
Previous PE/DVT	1.5
Heart rate >100 beats/min	1.5
Hemoptysis	1.0
Malignancy	1.0

Clinical probability	
Low	3%
Intermediate	28%
High	78%

Simplified wells: >4 likely; ≤4 unlikely for PE
JAMA 2006

Evaluation of a Suspected Pulmonary Embolism

Low clinical probability of embolism:

D-dimer (+ve) → **CT scan (+ve)** → ruled in
(–ve) ↓   (–ve) ↓
ruled out   ruled out

Intermediate or high probability:

CT scan (–ve) → ruled out
(+ve) ↓
ruled in

Notes:
- use D-dimers only if low clinical probability, otherwise, go straight to spiral CT
- if using V/Q scans (CT contrast allergy or renal failure):
  - negative V/Q scan rules out the diagnosis
  - high probability V/Q scan only rules in the diagnosis if have high clinical suspicion
  - inconclusive V/Q scan requires ultrasound, or spiral CT

Symptoms and Signs (neither sensitive nor specific)
- **symptoms**: dyspnea, pleuritic chest pain, hemoptysis, presyncope/syncope
  - leg symptoms (swelling, pain) occur in <30% of cases
- **signs**: may include tachypnea, tachycardia, SaO_2 <92%, pleural rub, hypotension, fever
- in severe hemodynamic compromise: elevated JVP, hypotension, shock, cardiac arrest

Investigations (if highly suspicious, go straight to spiral CT)
- D-dimer (products of thrombotic/fibrinolytic process)
  - ELISA better than latex agglutination
  - D-dimer results alone do not rule in or out DVT/PE
  - consider only in out-patients with low pretest probability
  - need to use in conjunction with leg Dopplers
- ABG
  - of NO diagnostic use in PE (insensitive and nonspecific)
  - respiratory alkalosis (due to hyperventilation)
- ECG
  - findings not sensitive or specific
  - sinus tachycardia most common; may see non-specific ST segment and T wave changes
  - RV strain, RAD, RBBB, S1-Q3-T3 with massive embolization
- CXR
  - frequently normal; no specific features
  - atelectasis (subsegmental), elevation of a hemidiaphragm
  - pleural effusion – usually small
  - Hampton's hump – cone-shaped area of peripheral opacification representing infarction
  - Westermark's sign – dilated proximal pulmonary artery with distal oligemia/decreased vascular markings (difficult to assess without prior films)
  - dilatation of proximal PA – rare
- echo
  - of little diagnostic value
  - ↑RVSP, RV hypokinesis, seen in massive PE
- V/Q scan (very sensitive but low specificity)
  - order scan if
    - CXR normal, no COPD
    - contraindication to CT (contrast allergy, renal dysfunction)
  - avoid V/Q scan if
    - CXR abnormal or COPD
    - inpatient
    - suspect massive PE
  - results
    - normal – excludes the diagnosis of PE
    - high probability – most likely means PE present, unless pre-test probability is low
    - 60% of V/Q signs are nondiagnostic
- spiral CT scan with contrast is both sensitive and specific for PE
  - diagnosis and management uncertain for small filling defects
  - spiral CT may identify the alternative diagnosis if PE is not present
  - CT scanning of the proximal leg and pelvic veins is often done at the same time and may be helpful
- venous duplex ultrasound or doppler
  - with leg symptoms
    - positive test can rule in a proximal DVT
    - negative test can rule out a proximal DVT
  - without leg symptoms
    - positive test rules in proximal DVT
    - negative test does not rule out a DVT – patient may have a non-occlusive or calf DVT

Treatment
- admit if unstable or very high bleeding risk
- oxygen: provide supplemental O_2 if hypoxemic or short of breath
- pain relief: analgesics if chest pain – a narcotic or NSAID
- acute anticoagulation: therapeutic-dose SC LMWH or IV heparin – start ASAP
  - anticoagulation stops clot propagation, prevents new clots and allows endogenous fibrinolytic system to dissolve existing thromboemboli over months
  - get baseline CBC, INR, aPTT ± renal function ± liver function
  - for SC LMWH: dalteparin 200 U/kg once daily or enoxaparin 1 mg/kg bid – no lab monitoring – avoid or reduce dose in renal dysfunction
  - for IV heparin: bolus of 75 U/kg (usually 5,000 U) followed by infusion starting at 20 U/kg/hr – aim for aPTT 2-3 times control

> Classic ECG finding of PE is S1-Q3-T3 (inverted T_3), but most commonly see only sinus tachycardia.

Excluding Pulmonary Embolism at Bedside
Ann Intern Med 2001;135:98-107.
Study: Multicentre, prospective cohort study.
Patients: 930 patients with suspected PE at emergency departments at 4 tertiary care hospitals in Canada.
Intervention: A Wells score was used to determine patient's pretest probability (PTP) of pulmonary embolism and then a D-dimer test was performed. Patients with low PTP and a negative D-dimer test had no further testing and the diagnosis of pulmonary embolism was excluded. All other patients had V/Q scanning, and if non-diagnostic, had bilateral deep venous ultrasonography. Further serial ultrasonography and angiography were done depending on the patients PTP and lung-scanning results.
Main outcomes: Diagnosis of pulmonary embolism and the development of thromboembolic events at 3 months follow-up.
Results: One of 759 patients in whom PE was initially ruled out developed a thromboembolic event during follow-up (0.1% [CI 0.0%-0.7%]). One of the 437 patients with negative D-dimers and low clinical PTP developed PE during follow up (NPV 99.5%, CI 99.1-100%).
Conclusion: Managing patients with suspected pulmonary embolism on the basis of PTP and D-dimer results is safe and decreases the need for diagnostic imaging.

- long term anticoagulation: warfarin – start the same day as LMWH/heparin – over lap warfarin with LMWH/heparin for at least 5 days and until INR in target range of 2-3 for at least 2 days
    - LMWH instead of warfarin for pregnancy, active cancer, high bleeding risk
- IV thrombolytic therapy: if patient has massive PE (hypotension or clinical right heart failure) and no contraindications – hastens resolution of PE but may not improve survival or long-term outcome and doubles risk of major bleeding
- interventional thrombolytic therapy: massive PE is preferentially treated with catheter-directed thrombolysis by an interventional radiologist – works better than IV thrombolytic therapy and fewer contraindications
- IVC filter: only if recent proximal DVT + absolute contraindication to anticoagulation
- duration of long-term anticoagulation: individualized, however generally:
    - if reversible cause for PE (surgery, injury, pregnancy, etc.): 3-6 months
    - if PE unprovoked: 6 mos to indefinite
    - if ongoing major risk factor (active cancer, antiphospholipid antibody, etc.): indefinite

Thromboprophylaxis
- mandatory for most hospital patients: reduces DVT, PE, all-cause mortality, cost-effective
- start ASAP
- continue at least until discharge or at least 10 days if major ortho surgery

Table 18. VTE Risk Categories and Prophylaxis

Risk Group	Prophylaxis Options
Low thrombosis risk: • medical patients – fully mobile • surgery – <30 minutes, fully mobile	• no specific prophylaxis • frequent ambulation
Moderate thrombosis risk: • most general, gynecologic, urologic surgery • sick medical patients	• LMWH • low dose heparin
High thrombosis risk: • arthoplasty, hip fracture surgery • major trauma, spinal cord injury	• LMWH • fondaparinux • warfarin (INR 2-3)
High bleeding risk: • neurosurgery, intracranial bleed • active bleeding	• TED stockings, pneumatic compression devices • LMWH or low dose heparin when bleeding risk decreases

Multidetector computed tomography for acute pulmonary embolism (PIOPED II Trial)
N Engl J Med. 2006 Jun 1;354(22):2317-27.
Study: Multicentre, prospective study investigating accuracy of computed tomography angiography (CTA) alone and combined with venous phase imaging (CTA-CTV).
Patients: 824 patients of several thousand eligible for study received reference diagnosis to confirm absence or presence of PE (V/Q scan, venous compression U/S of lower extremities, and pulmonary digital-subtraction angiography (DSA) if necessary). To confirm absence, patients in whom PE was excluded were telephoned 3-6 months after enrollment. Any deaths were reviewed by an outcome committee. All patients enrolled also underwent clinical assessment of PE (including a Well's score) prior to imaging.
Outcomes: Diagnosis of pulmonary embolism.
Results: 773 of 824 patients had adequate CTAs for interpretation. PE was diagnosed in 192 of the 824 patients. Sensitivity was 83% (150 of 181 patients, 95% CI, 0.76-0.92) and specificity was 96% (567 of 592 patients, 95% CI, 0.93-0.97). However, the predictive value of CTA-CTV varied when clinical pre-test probability was taken into account. PPV of CTA for high, intermediate and low clinical probability were 96% (95% CI, 0.78-0.99), 92% (95% CI, 0.84-0.96), and 58% (95% CI, 0.40-0.73) respectively. NPV of CTA for high, intermediate and low clinical probability were 60% (95% CI, 0.32-0.83), 89% (95% CI, 0.82-0.93), and 96% (95% CI, 0.92-0.98) respectively.
Conclusion: CTA is effective for diagnosing or excluding PE in accordance with assessment of clinical pretest probability. When clinical probability is inconsistent with imaging results, further investigations are required to rule out PE.

Pulmonary Vasculitis

Wegener's Granulomatosis
- see Rheumatology
- definition: systemic vasculitis of the medium and small arteries with many extravascular manifestations
- triad: necrotizing granulomatous lesions of the upper and lower respiratory tract, focal necrotizing lesions of arteries and veins, and focal glomerulonephritis
- characteristically has pulmonary, renal, and ENT signs and symptoms
- signs and symptoms: persistent rhinorrhea, purulent/bloody nasal discharge, oral and/or nasal ulcers, polyarthralgias, myalgias, sinus pain, cough, dyspnea, hemoptysis, pleuritic pain, constitutional symptoms (fever, anorexia, weight loss, night sweats, malaise)
- investigations
    - CXR: nodules (solitary or multiple, 1-10 cm, cavities), alveolar opacities
    - definite diagnosis by positive c-ANCA, renal or lung biopsy
- treatment: corticosteroids and cyclophosphamide
- prognosis: excellent with treatment (complete and long term remission in >90% of patients)

Churg-Strauss Syndrome (Allergic Granulomatosis and Angiitis)
- definition: a multisystem disorder characterized by allergic rhinitis, asthma, and prominent peripheral eosinophilia (no renal symptoms)
- epidemiology: approximately 10% of patients with major vasculitis, mean age at diagnosis is 50 years old
- signs and symptoms: asthma is a cardinal feature (prodromal phase), constitutional symptoms of malaise, fever, weight loss, and a life-threatening systemic vasculitis involving the lungs, pericardium and heart, kidneys, skin, and PNS (mononeuritis multiplex is the 2nd most common clinical manifestation)
- investigations: no specific investigations, peripheral eosinophilia is the most common finding
- treatment: corticosteroids and cyclophosphamide typically effective

Goodpasture's Syndrome
- definition: a disorder characterized by diffuse alveolar hemorrhage and glomerulonephritis caused by anti-GBM antibodies which cross-react with basement membranes of the lung and the kidney
- signs and symptoms: hemoptysis, anemia
- risk factors: onset of disease may follow an influenza infection, increased risk in smokers
- investigations
  - CXR: may be normal but alveolar infiltrates may be seen if hemorrhage is profuse
  - ELISA test with anti-GBM antibodies
  - Renal biopsy/indirect immunofluorescence: looking for anti-GBM antibodies in renal tissue
- treatment (may be fatal if left untreated)
  - acutely: corticosteroids, plasmapheresis to remove anti-GBM antibodies
  - immunosuppressive therapy (corticosteroids, cyclophosphamide) to decrease anti-GBM antibody production
  - severe/unresponsive cases: bilateral nephrectomy

> Scleroderma is the most common collagen vascular disease to affect the lung.

Systemic Lupus Erythematosus (SLE)
- see Rheumatology

Rheumatoid Arthritis (RA)
- see Rheumatology

Scleroderma
- see Rheumatology

Diseases of the Mediastinum and Pleura

Mediastinal Masses

Definition
- mediastinum structures that are bound by the thoracic inlet, diaphragm, sternum, vertebral bodies and the pleura
- can be broken down into 3 compartments: anterior upper, middle and posterior

Etiology and Pathophysiology
- diagnosis is made by location and patient's age
- **anterior compartment** (sternum to anterior border of pericardium) – more likely to be malignant
  - "Tive Ts" (see sidebar), lymphoma, lipoma, pericardial cyst
- **middle compartment** (anterior to posterior pericardium)
  - pericardial cyst, bronchogenic cyst/tumour, lymphoma, lymph node enlargement, aortic aneurysm
- **posterior compartment** (posterior pericardium to vertebral column)
  - neurogenic tumours, meningocele, enteric cysts, lymphomas, diaphragmatic hernias, esophageal tumour, aortic aneurysm

> **Anterior Compartment: 5T's**
> **T**hymoma
> **T**hyroid enlargement (goiter)
> **T**eratoma
> **T**horacic aortic aneurysm
> **T**umours
> (lymphoma, parathyroid, esophageal, angiomatous)

Signs and Symptoms
- 50% asymptomatic (most of these are benign); when symptomatic, 50% are malignant
- chest pain, cough, dyspnea, recurrent respiratory infections
- hoarseness, dysphagia, Horner's syndrome, facial/upper extremity edema (SVC compression)
- paraneoplastic syndromes (e.g. myasthenia gravis (thymomas))

Investigations
- CXR (compare to previous)
- CT with contrast (provides information regarding anatomic location, density, relation to mediastinal vascular structures)
- MRI – specifically indicated in the evaluation of neurogenic tumours
- ultrasound (best for assessment of structures in close proximity to the heart and pericardium)
- radionuclide scanning – ^{131}I (for thyroid), Gallium (for lymphoma)
- biochemical studies – thyroid function, serum calcium, phosphate, parathyroid hormones, AFP, β-hCG
- biopsy (mediastinoscopy, percutaneous needle aspiration)

Management
- depends on the diagnosis
- decide if the lesion should be excised (most isolated benign masses should be removed)
- needle aspiration of suspected benign cystic lesion
- resection via minimally invasive video assisted procedures (bronchogenic cysts, localized neurogenic tumours)
- exploration via sternotomy or thoracotomy
- diagnostic biopsy rather than major operation if mass is likely to be a lymphoma, germ cell tumour, or unresectable invasive malignancy
- ± post-op radiotherapy / chemotherapy if malignant

Mediastinitis

- most common causes of mediastinitis are postoperative complications of cardiovascular or other thoracic surgical procedures

Acute
- etiology
  - complication of endoscopy (e.g. esophageal perforation providing entry point for infection)
  - esophageal or cardiac surgery
  - tumour necrosis
- signs and symptoms
  - fever, substernal pain
  - pneumomediastinum, mediastinal compression
  - Hamman's sign (auscultatory "crunch" during cardiac systole)
- treatment
  - antibiotics, drainage, ± surgical closure of perforation

Chronic
- usually a granulomatous process (e.g. histoplasmosis, TB, sarcoidosis, syphilis)

Pleural Effusions

Definition
- a pleural effusion is present when there is an excess amount of fluid in the pleural space (normally, up to 25 ml of pleural fluid is present in pleural space)

Etiology
- disruption of normal equilibrium between pleural fluid formation/entry and pleural fluid absorption/exit
- pleural effusions are classified as transudative or exudative – distinguish clinically using Light's Criteria (Table 19)

Table 19. Laboratory Values in Transudative and Exudative Pleural Effusion ("Light's Criteria")

	Transudate	Exudate
Protein – pleural/serum	<0.5	>0.5
LDH – pleural/serum	<0.6	>0.6
Pleural LDH	<2/3 upper limit of N serum LDH	>2/3 upper limit of N serum LDH

Light RW, Macgregor MI, Luchsinger PC et al. Ann Intern Med 1979; 77(4):507-513

Transudative Pleural Effusions
- pathophysiology: alteration of systemic factors that affect the formation and absorption of pleural fluid (i.e. increased capillary hydrostatic pressure, decreased plasma oncotic pressure)
- etiology
  - congestive heart failure
  - cirrhosis
  - nephrotic syndrome
  - pulmonary embolism (may cause transudative or exudative effusion)
  - peritoneal dialysis, hypothyroidism, CF, urinothorax

Exudative Pleural Effusions
- pathophysiology: increased permeability of pleural capillaries or lymphatic dysfunction

Light's Criteria: Sensitivity and Specificity
Comparative analysis of the biochemical parameters used to distinguish between pleural transudates and exudates. Chest. 1995 Jun;107(6):1604-9.

Study: Pleural fluid and medical records for 500 patients were analyzed and the diagnostic accuracy's of the Light's Criteria was assessed. The Light's criteria was compared to other biochemical methods.
Results: Sensitivity: 98%, Specificity: 83%, for identifying exudative pleural effusions.

Comparative analysis of Light's criteria and other biochemical parameters for distinguishing transudates from exudates. Respirology Medicine. 92(5) 1998: 762-765.

Study: Pleural fluid and medical records for 241 patients were assessed and the accuracy of the Light's Criteria for detecting exudative pleural effusions was analyzed. The results were compared to other potential methods for distinguishing between exudative and transudative pleural effusions.
Results: Sensitivity: 97%, Specificity: 71% for identifying exudative pleural effusions.

Note: to determine if transudate or exudate, use fluid from thoracentesis and blood sample (taken at same time); all criteria for transudate must be fulfilled. Even if 1 criteria for exudates is met – it is an exudate (see Table 19).

Transudative effusions are usually bilateral, not unilateral

Exudative effusions can be bilateral or unilateral

- etiology
    - infectious
        - parapneumonic effusion (associated with bacterial pneumonia, lung abscess)
        - empyema (bacterial, fungal, TB), TB pleuritis, viral infection
    - malignancy
        - lung carcinoma (35%)
        - lymphoma (10%)
        - metastases: breast (25%), ovary, kidney
        - mesothelioma
    - vascular/cardiac
        - collagen vascular diseases: RA, SLE
        - pulmonary embolism, after coronary artery bypass surgery
    - intra-abdominal
        - subphrenic abscess
        - esophageal perforation (elevated pleural fluid amylase)
        - pancreatic disease (elevated pleural fluid amylase)
        - Meigs' syndrome (ascites and hydrothorax associated with an ovarian fibroma or other pelvic tumour)
    - trauma
        - chylothorax: occurs when the thoracic duct is disrupted and chyle accumulates in the pleural space, due to trauma, tumours
        - hemothorax: due to rupture of a blood vessel, commonly by trauma or tumours
    - other
        - pneumothorax (spontaneous, traumatic, tension)
        - pleural thickening (chronic infection, neoplasm, inflammatory)

Signs and Symptoms
- dyspnea: varies with size of effusion and underlying lung function
- pleuritic chest pain
- often asymptomatic
- inspection: trachea deviates away from effusion, ipsilateral decreased expansion
- percussion: decreased tactile fremitus, dullness
- auscultation: decreased breath sounds, bronchial breathing and egophony at upper level, pleural friction rub

Investigations
- CXR
    - must have >250 ml of pleural fluid for visualization
    - lateral: small effusion leads to blunting of posterior costophrenic angle
    - PA: blunting of lateral costophrenic angle
    - dense opacification of lung fields with concave meniscus
    - decubitus: fluid will shift unless it is loculated
    - supine: fluid will appear as general haziness
- thoracentesis: indicated if pleural effusion is a new finding
    - risk of re-expansion pulmonary edema if 2 L of fluid is removed
    - inspect for colour, character, and odour of fluid
    - analyze fluid (see Table 19, 20)

Table 20. Analysis of Pleural Effusion

Measure	Purpose
Protein, LDH	transudate vs. exudate (see Table 19)
Gram stain, Ziehl-Nielsen stain (TB), culture	looking for specific organisms
Cell count differential	neutrophils vs. lymphocytes (lymphocytic TB, lymphoma)
Cytology	malignancy, infection
Glucose (low)	RA, TB, empyema, malignancy, esophageal rupture
Rheumatoid factor, ANA, complement	collagen vascular disease
Amylase	pancreatitis, esophageal perforation, malignancy
pH	empyema <7.2, TB and mesothelioma <7.3
Blood	mostly traumatic, malignancy, PE with infusion, TB
Triglycerides	chylothorax from thoracic duct leakage, mostly due to trauma, lung CA, or lymphoma

- pleural biopsy: indicated if suspect TB, mesothelioma, or other malignancy (and if cytology negative)
- ± U/S: detects small effusions and can guide thoracentesis
- treatment depends on cause, ± drainage if symptomatic
- CT can be helpful in differentiating parenchymal from pleural abnormalities

Treatment
- thoracentesis
- treat underlying cause

Appearance of Pleural Fluid
Bloody - trauma, malignancy
White - chylothorax, empyema
Black - aspergillosis, amoebic liver abscess
Yellow-green - rheumatoid pleurisy
Viscous - malignant mesothelioma
Ammonia odour - urinothorax
Food particles - esophageal rupture

Role of CT in Pleural Effusion
- for further assessment of pleural thickening identified on CXR
- helps to distinguish benign from malignant effusion and transudative from exudative effusion
- does not help to distinguish empyema from parapneumonic effusion
- does not predict the severity of infection and need of surgical intervention

Features of Malignant Effusion
- multiple pleural nodules
- nodular pleural thickening

Features of Exudative Effusion
- loculation
- pleural thickening
- pleural nodules
- extrapleural fat of increased density

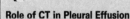

Complicated Effusion

- persistent bacteria in the pleural space, but fluid is non-purulent
- neutrophils, pleural fluid acidosis, and high LDH
- often no bacteria grown, since rapidly cleared from pleural space
- fibrin layer leading to loculation of pleural fluid
- treatment: antibiotics and drainage, treat as an empyema

Simple Effusion
pH >7.2, LDH <1/2 serum, glucose >2.2.
Complicated Effusion
pH <7.2, LDH >1/2 serum, glucose <2.2,
positive gram stain. Needs drainage.

Empyema

Definition
- pus in pleural space *or* an effusion with organisms seen on a gram stain or culture (i.e. pleural fluid is grossly purulent)
- positive culture is not required for diagnosis

Etiology
- contiguous spread from lung infection (most commonly anaerobes), or infection through chest wall (e.g. trauma, surgery)

Signs and Symptoms
- fever, pleuritic chest pain

Investigations
- CT chest
- thoracentesis
- PMNs (lymphocytes in TB), ± visible organisms on Gram stain

Treatment
- antibiotic therapy for at least 4-6 weeks (rarely effective alone)
- complete pleural drainage with chest tube
- if loculated, more difficult to drain – may require surgical drainage

When possible, organism-directed
therapy, guided by culture sensitivities or local patterns of drug
resistance should be utilized.

Pneumothorax

Definition
- presence of air in the pleural space

Pathophysiology
- positive intrapleural pressure reduces lung inflation

Etiology
- traumatic – penetrating or non-penetrating chest injuries
- iatrogenic (CVP line, thoracentesis, mechanical ventilation and ↑ alveolar pressure)
- spontaneous (no history of trauma)
  - primary (no underlying lung disease)
    - spontaneous rupture of apical subpleural bleb of lung into pleural space
    - predominantly healthy young tall males
  - secondary (underlying lung disease)
    - rupture of subpleural bleb which migrates along bronchioalveolar sheath to the mediastinum then to the intrapleural space
    - necrosis of lung tissue adjacent to pleural surface (e.g. pneumonia, abscess, PCP, lung CA, emphysema)

**Need to rule out life-threaten-
ing tension pneumothorax**

If pneumothorax with:
- severe respiratory distress
- tracheal deviation to contralateral side
- distended neck veins
- hypotension

**Do not perform CXR.
Needs immediate treatment.**
See <u>Emergency Medicine</u>, ER12

Signs and Symptoms
- can be asymptomatic
- acute-onset pleuritic chest pain
- acute-onset dyspnea
- tracheal deviation (contralateral deviation in tension pneumothorax, ipsilateral deviation in non-tension pneumothorax)
- ipsilateral diminished expansion
- decreased tactile/vocal fremitus
- hyperresonant percussion note
- ipsilateral diminished breath sounds

Investigations
- CXR
  - small: separation of visceral and parietal pleura seen as fine crescentic line parallel to chest wall at apex
  - large: increased density and decreased volume of lung on side of pneumothorax
  - see <u>Diagnostic Medical Imaging</u>

Treatment
- small pneumothoraces (<20% with no signs of respiratory/circulatory collapse) resolve spontaneously; can use 100% oxygen
- small intercostal tube with Heimlich valve for most spontaneous pneumothoraces
- large pneumothoraces or those complicating underlying lung disease require placement of a chest tube connected to underwater seal ± suction
- for repeated episodes: pleurodesis with sclerosing agent or partial pneumonectomy/bleb resection
- treat underlying cause (e.g. antibiotic for PCP)

Asbestos-Related Pleural Disease and Mesothelioma

Etiology and Pathophysiology
- exudative pleural effusion
- pleural thickening or calcification, pleural plaque (Hyalinosis Simplex)
- mesothelioma
  - primary malignancy of the pleura
  - decades after asbestos exposure (even light exposure)
  - smoking is not a risk factor (but greatly increases risk of other asbestos induced cancers)

Signs and Symptoms
- persistent chest pain, dyspnea, cough, bloody pleural effusion, weight loss, clubbing

Investigations
- biopsy (pleuroscopic or open)

Treatment
- resection (requires careful patient selection); however, rarely successful (average survival <1 year)

Respiratory Failure

Etiology and Pathophysiology
- due to impairment of gas exchange between ambient air and circulating blood
- hypoxemic (PaO_2 <60 mm Hg), or hypercapnic ($PaCO_2$ >40 mm Hg)
- acute vs. chronic (compensatory mechanisms activated)
- airway obstruction: COPD, bronchiectasis, CF, asthma, bronchiolitis, upper airway obstruction
- abnormal parenchyma: pneumonia, pulmonary edema, pulmonary fibrosis, acute respiratory distress syndrome (ARDS), pleural effusion
- hypoventilation without bronchopulmonary disease: CNS disorder (drugs, increased ICP, spinal cord lesion, sepsis), neuromuscular (myasthenia gravis, Guillain-Barré, muscular dystrophies), chest wall (kyphoscoliosis, obesity)

Signs and Symptoms
- signs of underlying disease
- hypoxemia: restlessness, confusion, cyanosis, coma, cor pulmonale
- hypercapnia: headache, dyspnea, drowsiness, asterixis, warm periphery, plethora, increased ICP (secondary to vasodilatation)

Investigations
- serial ABGs

Hypoxemic Respiratory Failure

- PaO_2 decreased, $PaCO_2$ normal or decreased

Pathophysiology
- low inspired FiO_2 (e.g. high altitude)
- normal FiO_2
  - diffusion impairment: interstitial lung disease
  - V/Q mismatch: airway disease (asthma, COPD), alveolar disease (pneumonia, edema), vascular disease (PE)
  - shunts: alveolar collapse, intra-alveolar filling (pneumonia, edema), intracardiac (R to L), intrapulmonary (AVM)
  - diffusion/ventilation imbalance: anemia, low cardiac output, hypermetabolism

Causes of Hypoxemia
1. Low FiO_2
2. Hypoventilation
3. Shunting
4. Low mixed venous O_2 content
5. V/Q Mismatch

Treatment

- reverse the underlying pathology
- maintain oxygenation
- enrichment of FiO_2: remember that if shunting is the problem, supplemental O_2 is not nearly as effective
- positive pressure: use of PEEP and CPAP will recruit alveoli and redistribute lung fluid
- ± hemodynamic support: fluids, vasopressors, inotropes, reduction of O_2 requirements

Table 21. Approach to Hypoxemia*

Type of Hypoxemia	Settings	PaCO₂	A-aDO₂*	Oxygen Therapy	Ventilation, BiPAP & PEEP	Improved Cardiac Output
1. Low FiO₂	Postop, high altitude	Normal, Low	Normal	Improves	No change	No change
2. Hypoventilation	Drug OD	High	Normal	Improves	Improves with ventilation	No change
3a. Shunt	ARDS, Pneumonia	Low, Normal	Increased	No change	Improves (except if one-sided)	Improves
3b. Shunt (Right to Left)	Pulmonary HTN	Normal, Low	Increased	No change	Worsens	Worsens
4. Low mixed venous O₂ content	Shock	Low	Increased	No change	Worsens	Improves
5. V/Q Mismatch	COPD	High, Normal	Increased	Improves with small amounts	Often Improves	Improves

* with permission from Dr. Ian Fraser

Hypercapnic Respiratory Failure

- $PaCO_2$ increased, PaO_2 decreased

Pathophysiology

- increased CO_2 production: fever, sepsis, seizure, acidosis, carbohydrate load
- alveolar hypoventilation: COPD, asthma, CF, chest wall disorder, rapid shallow breathing
- hypoventilation
  - central: brainstem stroke, hypothyroidism, severe metabolic alkalosis, drugs (opiates, benzodiazepines)
  - neuromuscular: myasthenia gravis, Guillain-Barré, phrenic nerve injury, muscular dystrophy, polymyositis, kyphoscoliosis
  - muscle fatigue

Treatment

- reverse the underlying pathology
- if $PaCO_2$ >50 mmHg and pH is acidemic consider noninvasive or mechanical ventilation
- correct exacerbating factors
  - NTT/ETT suction: clearance of secretions
  - bronchodilators: reduction of airway resistance
  - antibiotics: treatment of co-morbid infections
- maintain oxygenation (see above)
- increased carbohydrate feeding can increase $PaCO_2$ in those with mechanical or limited alveolar ventilation; high lipids decrease $PaCO_2$

Causes of Hypercarbia
1. High Inspired CO₂
2. Low Total Ventilation
3. High Deadspace Ventilation
4. High CO₂ Production

In chronic hypercapnia, supplemental O₂ may decrease the hypoxic drive to breathe, *but do not* deny oxygen if the patient is hypoxic

In COPD patients with chronic hypercapnia ("CO₂ retainers") provide supplemental oxygen to achieve target O₂ saturation from 88-92%.

Acute Respiratory Distress Syndrome (ARDS)

- clinical syndrome characterized by severe respiratory distress, hypoxemia, and noncardiogenic pulmonary edema
- American-European Consensus Conference (1994) criteria for ARDS:
  1. acute onset
  2. bilateral infiltrates on CXR
  3. PCWP <18 or no evidence of increased left atrial pressure
  4. PaO_2/FiO_2 ≤200

Etiology

- may result from direct or indirect lung injury:
  - airway: aspiration (gastric contents, drowning), pneumonia, gas inhalation (oxygen toxicity, nitrogen dioxide, smoke)
  - circulation: sepsis, shock, trauma, pancreatitis, DIC, blood transfusion, embolism (fat, amniotic fluid), drug overdose (narcotics, sedatives, TCAs)
  - neurogenic: head trauma, intracranial hemorrhage

Pathophysiology

- disruption of alveolar capillary membranes → leaky capillaries → interstitial and alveolar pulmonary edema → reduced compliance, V/Q mismatch, shunt, hypoxemia, pulmonary HTN

Signs and Symptoms

- four phases of clinical presentation:
  1. beginning several hours after injury and lasting a few hours to days: hyperventilation, cyanosis on room air, respiratory alkalosis, normal CXR
  2. tachypnea (>20/min), respiratory distress, marked hypoxemia, alkalosis, interstitial pulmonary edema on CXR
  3. hypoxemic respiratory failure
  4. cardiac arrest

Treatment

- treat underlying disorder (e.g. antibiotics if infection present)
- mechanical ventilation using low tidal volumes (≤6 ml/kg) to prevent barotrauma and use minimal amount of PEEP (positive end-expiratory pressure) necessary to keep airways open and allow the use of lower levels of oxygen
  - may consider using prone ventilation and/or inhaled nitric oxide if conventional treatment is failing
- inotropic therapy (e.g. dopamine, vasopressin) if cardiac output inadequate
- pulmonary-arterial catheter is useful for monitoring hemodynamics
- mortality: 30-40%, usually due to non-pulmonary complications
- many survivors of ARDS have some pulmonary symptoms, such as cough, dyspnea, and sputum production, which tend to improve over time
- mild abnormalities of oxygenation, diffusion capacity, and lung mechanics may persist in some people

Mechanical Ventilation

- see Anesthesia
- artificial means of supporting ventilation and oxygenation
- mechanically ventilated patients may require some sedation and/or analgesia
- general indications
  - hypoxemic respiratory failure
  - hypercapnic respiratory failure
- specific indicators for mechanical ventilation
  - acute ventilation failure/acute respiratory acidosis
  - refractory hypoxemia
  - reduced level of consciousness
  - facilitation of surgical procedures
- ventilator strategies
  - the target tidal volume, respiratory rate, PEEP and ratio of inspiratory to expiratory time are all determined based on the underlying reason for mechanical ventilation
  - hypoxemic respiratory failure: ventilator provides supplemental oxygen and helps improve V/Q mismatch and decreases intrapulmonary shunt
  - hypercapnic respiratory failure: ventilator provides alveolar ventilation; may decrease the work of breathing, allowing respiratory muscles to rest
- ventilatory modes
  - assist-control ventilation (ACV) (**often initial mode of ventilation**)
    - every breath is delivered with a pre-set tidal volume
    - inspiration may be triggered by patient effort, or if no effort is detected within a specified amount of time the ventilator will initiate the breath
  - synchronous intermittent mandatory ventilation (SIMV)
    - ventilator provides breaths at fixed rate and tidal volume
    - patient can breathe spontaneously between ventilator breaths without triggering the ventilator
  - pressure support ventilation (PSV)
    - patient initiates all breaths and the vent supports each breath with a pre-set inspiratory pressure
    - useful for weaning off vent
  - pressure control ventilation (PCV)
    - a minimum frequency is set and patient may trigger additional breaths above the vent
    - all breaths delivered at a preset constant inspiratory pressure
  - noninvasive ventilation (NIV)
    - achieved without intubation by using a nasal mask with:
      - BiPAP (bilevel positive airway pressure): a wave of increased pressure on inspiration and lower constant pressure on expiration
      - CPAP (continuous positive airway pressure): constant pressure
- complications of mechanical ventilation
  - barotrauma

Tracheostomy
- tracheostomy should be considered in patients who require ventilator support for extended periods of time
- shown to improve patient comfort and give patients a better ability to participate in rehabilitation activities

Positive End Expiratory Pressure (PEEP)
- positive pressure applied at the end of ventilation which opens up collapsed alveoli decreasing V/Q mismatch
- used with all invasive modes of ventilation

Monitoring Ventilatory Therapy
Pulse oximetry, end-tidal CO_2 concentration
Regular arterial blood gases
Assess tolerance to ventilation regularly

Management of pneumothorax in patients on mechanical ventilation → chest tube.

- pneumothorax, tension pneumothorax, pneumomediastinum, subcutaneous emphysema, ventilator-induced lung injury (from the use of high tidal volumes – can resemble ARDS)
  - ventilator associated pneumonia (nosocomial pneumonia)
    - patients intubated 72 hours are at high risk of acquiring pneumonia
    - common organisms include enteric gram negative rods, anaerobes, *S. aureus*
  - tracheal stenosis
  - laryngeal dysfunction
  - hypotension ($\downarrow$CO)
    - increased intrathoracic pressure with decreased venous return that usually responds to intravascular volume repletion
  - stress ulcers
    - may be prevented with H2 blocker prophylaxis

Neoplasms

Approach to the Solitary Pulmonary Nodule

- also see <u>Diagnostic Medical Imaging</u>

Definition
- a round or oval, sharply circumscribed radiographic lesion up to 3-4 cm which may or may not contain calcium and is surrounded by normal lung

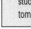

Pulmonary neoplasms may present as a solitary pulmonary nodule identified incidentally on a radiographic study (~ 10% of cases) or as a symptomatic disease (mostly).

Table 22. Differential Diagnosis for Benign vs. Malignant Solitary Nodule

Benign (70%)	Malignant (30%)
infectious granuloma (histoplasmosis, coccidiomycosis, TB, atypical mycobacteria)	**bronchogenic carcinoma**
other infections (bacterial abscess, PCP, aspergilloma)	adenocarcinoma
benign neoplasms (hamartoma, lipoma, fibroma)	squamous cell carcinoma
vascular (AV malformation, pulmonary varix)	large cell carcinoma
developmental (bronchogenic cyst)	small cell carcinoma
inflammatory (Wegener's Granulomatosis, rheumatoid nodule, sarcoidosis)	**metastatic lesions**
other (hematoma, infarct, pseudotumour, rounded atelectasis, lymph nodes, amyloidoma)	breast
	head and neck
	melanoma
	colon
	kidney
	sarcoma
	germ cell tumours
	pulmonary carcinoid

Investigations (see Figure 11)
- CXR: always compare with previous CXR (see Table 23)
- CT thorax
- sputum cytology: usually poor yield
- biopsy (bronchoscopic or percutaneous) or excision (thoracoscopy or thoracotomy): if clinical and radiographic features do not help distinguish between benign or malignant lesion
- watchful waiting: repeat CXR at 3, 6, 12 months

Terminology
"nodule" <3 cm
"mass" >3 cm

Table 23. CXR Characteristics of Benign vs. Malignant Solitary Nodule

Parameters	Benign	Malignant
Size	<3 cm, round, regular	>3 cm, irregular, spiculated
Margins	Smooth margin	Ill-defined or notched margin
Features	Calcified pattern: central, "popcorn" pattern if hamartoma, usually no cavitation; if cavitated, wall is smooth and thin, no other lung pathology	Usually not calcified; if calcified, pattern is eccentric, no satellite lesions, cavitation with thick wall, may have pleural effusions, lymphadenopathy
Doubling Time	Doubles in <1 month or >2 years	Doubles in >1 month or <2 years

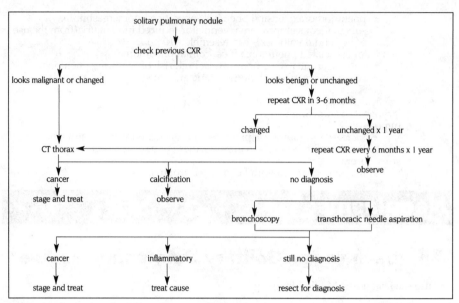

Figure 11. Evaluation of a Solitary Pulmonary Nodule

Benign Lung Tumours

Epidemiology
- less than 5% of all primary lung neoplasms
- bronchial adenomas and hamartomas comprise 90% of the benign neoplasms of the lung
- uncommon benign neoplasms of the lung include fibromas, lipomas, leiomyomas, hemangiomas, papillomas, chondromas, teratoma and endometriosis

Signs and Symptoms
- cough, hemoptysis, recurrent pneumonia, wheezing, atelectasis
- can present without symptoms or signs as a solitary pulmonary nodule (see previous section)

Classification
- bronchial adenomas
  - slow-growing, benign endobronchial tumours that rarely metastasize
  - may be carcinoids (90%), adenocystic tumours, or mucoepidermoid
  - symptoms
    - systemic symptoms usually absent
    - patients may complain of chronic cough, wheezing or give a history of recurrent pneumonia
    - hemoptysis may be present

- bronchial carcinoids
  - atypical subtype of adenoma with a high metastatic rate
  - often in young adults; smoking not a risk factor
  - clinical presentation: follows a slow course, metastasizes late, can cause symptoms of carcinoid syndrome (flushing, diarrhea, cardiac valvular lesions, wheezing)
  - may cause paraneoplastic syndromes (see Table 25)
  - treatment and prognosis: amenable to resection; 5-year survival is 95%

- hamartomas
  - composed of tissues normally present in lung (fat, epithelium, fibrous tissue and cartilage), but they exhibit disorganized growth
  - peak incidence at age 60, more common in men, 10% of benign lung lesions, 2nd to infectious granuloma (80%)
  - usually peripheral, clinically silent, and benign in behaviour
  - CXR: clustered "popcorn" pattern of calcification is pathognomonic for hamartoma

Malignant Lung Tumours

Pathological Classification
- bronchogenic cancer (90% of primary lung cancers) (for characteristics, see Table 24)
  - classified into small cell lung cancer (SCLC) and non-SCLC (NSCLC i.e. adenocarcinoma, squamous cell, large cell), bronchioalvelolar cancer (BAC)
  - incidence of adenocarcinoma is increasing
- lymphoma
- secondary metastases: breast, colon, prostate, kidney, thyroid, stomach, cervix, rectum, testes, bone, melanoma

Malignant lung tumours are the most common cause of cancer mortality throughout the world in both men and women.

Table 24. Characteristics of Bronchogenic Cancer

Cell Type	Incidence	Correlation with smoking	Location	Histology	Metastasis
Adenocarcinoma	M~35% F~40%	weak	peripheral	glandular, mucin producing	early, distant
Squamous cell cancer (SCC)	30%	strong	central	keratin, intercellular bridges	slow, local invasion, may cavitate
SCLC	25%	strong	central	oat cell, neuroendocrine	disseminated at presentation origin in endobronchial cells
Large cell cancer	10-15%	strong	peripheral	anaplastic, undifferentiated	early, distant

Adenocarcinoma has a worse prognosis than squamous cell.

Epidemiology
- most common cancer in men and women
- most common cause of cancer death in men and women
- 18% of all cancer related deaths

Risk Factors
- cigarette smoking: 85% of lung cancer related to smoking
- asbestos 5x ↑risk, asbestos + smoker 80-90x ↑risk
- radiation: radon, uranium (especially if smoker)
- arsenic, chromium, nickel
- genetic damage
- parenchymal scarring: granulomatous disease, fibrosis, scleroderma
- passive exposure to cigarette smoke
- air pollution: exact role is uncertain
- HIV

Signs and Symptoms
- cough (75%); beware of chronic cough that changes in character
- dyspnea (60%)
- chest pain (45%)
- hemoptysis (35%)
- other pain (25%)
- clubbing (21%)
- constitutional signs: anorexia, weight loss, fever, anemia

Presentation by Location of Tumour Extension
- lung, hilum, mediastinum, pleura: pleural effusion, atelectasis, wheezing
- pericardium: pericarditis, pericardial tamponade
- esophageal compression: dysphagia
- phrenic nerve: paralyzed diaphragm
- recurrent laryngeal nerve: hoarseness
- superior vena cava syndrome: obstruction of SVC causing neck and facial swelling, as well as dyspnea and cough
  - other symptoms associated with SVC compression: hoarseness, tongue swelling, epistaxis, and hemoptysis
  - physical findings include dilated neck veins, increased number of collateral veins covering the anterior chest wall, cyanosis, edema of the face, arms, and chest, Pemberton's sign
  - milder symptoms if obstruction is above the azygos vein
- lung apex (Pancoast tumour): Horner's syndrome, brachial plexus palsy, most commonly C8 and T1 nerve roots
- rib and vertebrae: erosion
- distant metastasis to brain, bone, liver, adrenals
- paraneoplastic syndromes (see Table 25)
  - a group of disorders associated with malignant disease, not related to the physical effects of the tumour itself
  - most often associated with SCLC

Horner has a MAP of the Coast
A Pan**coast** tumour compresses the cervical sympathetic plexus causing a **Horner's** syndrome
Miosis
Anhydrosis
Ptosis

Table 25. Paraneoplastic Syndromes

System	Clinical Presentation	Associated Malignancy
Skeletal	clubbing	NSCLC
Dermatologic	acanthosis nigricans	bronchogenic cancer
	dermatomyositis	bronchogenic cancer
Endocrine	hypercalcemia (osteolysis or PTHRP)	squamous cell cancer
	hypophosphatemia	squamous cell cancer
	hypoglycemia	sarcoma
	Cushing's syndrome (ACTH)	SCLC
	somatostatinoma syndrome	bronchial carcinoid
	SIADH	SCLC
Neuromyopathic	Lambert-Eaton syndrome	SCLC
	polymyositis	
	subacute cerebellar degeneration	
	spinocerebellar degeneration	
	peripheral neuropathy	
Vascular/Hematologic	nonbacterial endocarditis	bronchogenic cancer
	Trousseau's syndrome (migratory thrombophlebitis)	NSCLC
	DIC	
Renal	nephrotic syndrome	

Investigations
- initial diagnosis
    - imaging: CXR, CT chest + upper abdomen, PET scan, bone scan
    - cytology: sputum
    - biopsy: bronchoscopy, percutaneous, mediastinoscopy
- staging work-up
    - blood work: LFTs, calcium, ALP
    - imaging: CXR, CT thorax and abdomen, bone scan, neuroimaging
    - invasive: bronchoscopy, mediastinoscopy, mediastinotomy, thoracotomy

Staging/Treatment

Table 26. SCLC vs NSCLC

	Stage	Definition	Treatment	Median Survival
SCLC	limited stage	confined to single radiation port (one hemithorax and regional lymph nodes)	radiation ± chemo ± prophylactic to brain	1-2 years
	extensive stage	extension beyond a single radiation port	chemotherapy	6 months

	Stage (TNM ISS)		Treatment	5 Year Survival
NSCLC	I	no invasion beyond lung and nodes negative	surgery	~50%
	II	no invasion beyond lung and ipsilateral hilar nodes positive	surgery + radiation	30%
	IIIA	direct extension to chest wall, pleura, pericardium or ipsilateral mediastinal nodes positive	chemotherapy + radiation followed by surgery	15%
	IIIB	advanced local involvement (malignant effusion, major structures), or contralateral nodes positive	radiation + chemo + surgery	5%
	IV	distant metastasis	palliative	<2%

Therapy for Bronchogenic Cancer
- chemotherapy (no role for chemo alone, only in combination with other treatments)
    - cisplatin and etoposide
    - paclitaxel, vinorelbine, and gemcitabine are new NSCLC therapies
    - new biologics, e.g. epidermal growth factor inhibitor (Gefitinib)
    - complications:
        + acute: tumour lysis syndrome, infection, bleeding, myelosuppression, hemorrhagic cystitis (cyclophosphamide), cardiotoxicity (doxorubicin), renal toxicity (cisplatin), peripheral neuropathy (vincristine)
        + chronic: neurologic damage, leukemia, second primary neoplasms
- radiotherapy
- surgery
    - only chance for cure is resection when tumour is still localized
    - contraindications:
        + any evidence of local extension or metastases
            - patients with surgically resectable disease must undergo mediastinal node sampling since CT thorax is not accurate in 20-40% of cases
        + poor pulmonary status (i.e. unable to tolerate resection of lung)
    - perioperative mortality
        + 6% if pneumonectomy
        + 3% if lobectomy
        + 1% if segmentectomy
- palliative care for end-stage disease

Prognosis of Bronchogenic Cancer
- 5 year survival rates for different subtypes
  - squamous 25%
  - adenocarcinoma 12%
  - large cell carcinoma 13%
  - SCLC 1%
    - SCLC has the poorest prognosis
    - greatest tendency to metastasize
    - 70% present with extensive disseminated disease at initial diagnosis
    - limited-stage: 15-20% cure rate
    - extensive-stage treated: median survival of 6 months, but can live up to two years with a rare cure (1%); untreated median survival is 2-3 months
  - NSCLC
    - see Table 26

BRONCHOALVEOLAR CARCINOMA
- a type of adenocarcinoma that grows along the alveolar wall in the periphery
- may arise at sites of previous lung scarring (a scar cancer)
- clinical presentation: similar to bronchogenic cancer; late metastasis
- treatment and prognosis: solitary lesions are resectable with a 60% 5-year survival rate; overall survival rate is 25%

Sleep-Related Breathing Disorders

- normal changes during sleep: tidal volume decreases, arterial CO_2 increases (due to decreased minute ventilation), pharyngeal dilator muscles relax causing increased upper airway resistance
- sleep-related breathing disorders: a group of disorders characterized by decreased air-flow occurring only in sleep or worsening in sleep
- affects 9% of men, 4% of women
- sleep apnea (see below)
- hypoventilation syndromes
  - primary alveolar hypoventilation: idiopathic
  - obesity-hypoventilation syndrome (Pickwickian syndrome)
  - respiratory neuromuscular disorders

Sleep Apnea

Definition
- the cessation of airflow during sleep
- quantitatively measured by the Apnea/Hypopnea Index (AHI) = # of apneic and hypopneic events per hour of sleep
- sleep apnea generally accepted to be present if AHI >15

Classification
- obstructive (OSA)
  - caused by transient, episodic obstruction of the upper airway
  - absent or reduced airflow despite persistent respiratory effort
- central (CSA)
  - caused by transient, episodic withdrawal of CNS drive to breathe
  - no airflow because no respiratory effort
  - Cheyne-Stokes Respiration (CSR): a form of CSA in which central apneas alternate with hyperpneas to produce a crescendo-decrescendo pattern of tidal volume; seen in severe LV dysfunction (see pattern R2)
- mixed (MSA)
  - features of both OSA and CSA
  - loss of hypoxic and hypercapnic drives to breathe secondary to "resuscitative breathing": overcompensatory hyperventilation upon awakening from OSA induced hypoxia

Risk Factors
- for OSA: obesity, upper airway abnormality, neuromuscular disease, hypothyroidism, alcohol/sedative use, nasal congestion, sleep deprivation
- for CSA: LV failure, brain-stem lesions, encephalitis, encephalopathy, myxedema, high altitude

Signs and Symptoms
- obtain history from spouse/partner
- secondary to repeated arousals and fragmentation of sleep: daytime somnolence, personality and cognitive changes, snoring

Apneic – no breathing for ≥10 seconds

Hypopneic – >50% reduction in ventilation for ≥10 seconds

Continuous positive airways pressure for obstructive sleep apnea
The Cochrane Database of Systematic Reviews 2008, Issue 2.
Study: Pooled analysis of 36 RCTs (1718 people) comparing nocturnal CPAP with an inactive control or oral appliances in adults with obstructive sleep apnea.
Conclusions: The use of CPAP showed significant improvements in objective and subjective measures including cognitive function, sleepiness, measures of quality of life, and a lower average systolic and diastolic blood pressure. People who responded equally well to CPAP and oral appliances expressed a strong preference for oral appliances; however, participants on OA were more likely to withdraw from therapy.

- secondary to hypoxemia and hypercapnia: morning headache, polycythemia, pulmonary/systemic HTN, cor pulmonale/CHF, nocturnal angina, arrhythmias
- OSA typically presents in a middle-aged obese male snorer
- CSA can be due to neurological disease

Investigations
- sleep study (polysomnography)
    - evaluates sleep stages, airflow, ribcage movement, ECG, O_2 saturation, limb movements
    - indications:
        - excessive daytime sleepiness
        - unexplained pulmonary HTN or polycythemia
        - daytime hypercapnia
        - titration of optimal nasal CPAP
        - assessment of objective response to other interventions

Treatment
- modifiable factors: weight loss, decreased alcohol/sedatives, nasal decongestion, treatment of underlying medical conditions
- OSA or MSA: nasal CPAP, postural therapy (i.e. no supine sleeping), dental appliance, uvulopalatopharyngoplasty, tonsillectomy
- CSA or hypoventilation syndromes: nasal BiPAP/CPAP, respiratory stimulants (e.g. progesterone) in select cases
- tracheostomy rarely required and should be used as last resort

Complications
- depression, weight gain, decreased QOL, workplace and vehicular accidents, cardiac complications (OSA is independent risk-factor for HTN), reduced work/social function

CPAP has been shown to reduce cardiovascular risk and cardiovascular related deaths in patients with obstructive sleep apnea.

Introduction to Intensive Care

- goal of the intensive care unit (ICU) is to provide stabilization in the setting of an acutely or severely ill patient
- insults that result in hemodynamic, respiratory or cardiac instability, or widespread infection warrant ICU admission
- ICUs are intended to reverse the abnormal physiology, contain the underlying problem and create a favourable environment for recovery until the patient is stable enough to be transferred
- features unique to ICU are:
    - high nurse to patient ratio
    - extensive invasive cardiopulmonary and other system support monitoring

ICU Basics

Lines and Catheters
- arterial lines
    - used to monitor beat-to-beat blood pressure variations, obtain blood for routine ABGs, administer high flow medications, can use to monitor cardiac compliance (common sites are femoral or radial lines)
- central venous catheter (central line)
    - used to administer IV fluids, monitor central venous pressure, insert pulmonary artery catheters, give parenteral nutrition, give agents which are too irritating to be given via a peripheral line, when peripheral access is not possible
    - common sites include: internal jugular vein, subclavian vein, femoral vein
- pulmonary arterial catheter
    - uses a balloon "sail" to guide the catheter from a major vein to the right heart
    - "wedged" in the pulmonary artery temporarily to take a variety of measurements
    - indications:
        - diagnosis of shock states
        - differentiation of high- versus low-pressure pulmonary edema
        - diagnosis of primary pulmonary hypertension (PPH)
        - assessment of response to treatment in patients with PPH
        - diagnosis of valvular disease, intracardiac shunts, cardiac tamponade, and pulmonary embolism (PE)
        - monitoring and management of complicated MI
        - assessing hemodynamic response to therapies

A catheter "wedged" in the distal pulmonary artery measures pressure transmitted from the pulmonary venous system. This is known as the pulmonary capillary wedge pressure (PCWP). The PCWP reflects left atrial pressure (as long as there is no pulmonary venous disease) and LV diastolic pressure (as long as there is no mitral valve disease).
Source: Cecil Essentials of Medicine, 6th Edition.

- management of multiorgan system failure and/or severe burns
- management of hemodynamic instability after cardiac surgery
  - absolute contraindications:
    - tricuspid or pulmonary valve mechanical prosthesis
    - right heart mass (thrombus and/or tumour)
    - tricuspid or pulmonary valve endocarditis

Table 27. Useful Equations and Cardiopulmonary Parameters

Body Surface Area (BSA) = [Ht (cm) + Wt (kg) – 60]/100

PCWP (Pulmonary Capillary Wedge Pressure) = LVEDP (Left Ventricular End Diastolic Pressure)

Cardiac Index (CI) = Cardiac Output/BSA

Stroke Volume Index (SVI) = CI/Heart Rate

RV Ejection Fraction = SV/RVEDV

Systemic vascular resistance index (SVRI) = [(MAP – right atrial pressure (RAP)) + 80]/CI

O_2 Index = (MAP * FiO_2)/pO_2

P:F ratio = PaO_2/FiO_2

ICU Approach to Management

- the initial assessment of the critically ill patient focuses on life-threatening processes that require immediate diagnostic and/or therapeutic intervention
- management is based on the understanding of the pathophysiology of the disease process taking into consideration organ-system dependence

Organ Failure

- Respiratory Failure (see *Respiratory Failure* section)
- Coagulopathy
  - see Hematology for disorders of 1° and 2° hemostasis
  - coagulopathies commonly occur in acutely and severely ill patients
  - monitor for:
    - thrombocytopenia
    - INR, PTT elevations
    - DIC (increase in fibrin degradation products and reduction in fibrinogen)
- Liver Failure (see Gastroenterology)
  - manifested by rise in transaminases, bilirubin, and INR
- Renal Failure (see Nephrology)
  - the kidney is the major organ responsible for the maintenance of fluid and electrolyte homeostasis
  - damage sustained by hypovolemia, nephrotoxins disrupts this balance
  - patients typically develop acute tubular necrosis (ATN)
    goal of treatment: correct volume and electrolyte status, eliminate toxins
  - common treatment modalities: diuretics, dialysis (early aggressive daily dialysis is key)

Shock

- inadequate tissue perfusion potentially resulting in end organ injury
  - classifications of shock include:
    - hypovolemic: hemorrhagic, dehydration, vomiting, diarrhea, interstitial fluid redistribution
    - cardiogenic: myopathic (myocardial ischemia ± infarction), mechanical, arrhythmic, pharmacologic
    - obstructive: massive PE (saddle embolus), pericardial tamponade, constrictive pericarditis, increased intrathoracic pressure (e.g. tension pneumothorax)
    - distributive: sepsis, anaphylactic reaction, neurogenic, endocrinologic, toxic

Intensive Insulin Therapy in Critically Ill Patients
NEJM. 2001; 345:1359-67
Study: Prospective, randomized controlled clinical outcome study.
Patients: 1548 Patients admitted to the ICU
Intervention: At admission, patients were randomly assigned to either intensive insulin therapy or conventional therapy. Those in the intensive group had an infusion started if BG exceeded 61 mmol/L, and maintained to keep BG between 4.4 to 6.1 mmol/L.
Those in the conventional group were started on insulin only if BG exceeded 11.9, and the infusion was adjusted for a target between 10.0 and 11.1 mmol/L.
Primary Outcome: Death from any cause during ICU stay.
Results: 35 patients (4.6%) died in the intensive group in the ICU, versus 63 patients (8.0%) in the conventional group. This represents a 32% mortality reduction (p=0.04). Intensive insulin therapy also reduced overall in-hospital mortality, lowered deaths due to sepsis, multi-organ failure. Most of the mortality benefit was seen in long stay patients (>5 days).
Conclusion: Intensive insulin therapy in the ICU reduces mortality by 32%, and improves in-hospital mortality and morbidity.

Shock: Clinical Correlation
Hypovolemic: patients have cool extremities due to peripheral vasoconstriction.
Cardiogenic: patients usually have signs of left-sided heart failure.
Obstructive: varied presentation.
Distributive: patients have warm extremities due to peripheral vasodilation.

Table 28. Changes Seen in Different Classes of Shock

	Hypovolemic	Cardiogenic	Obstructive	Distributive
HR	↑	↑, N, or ↓	↑	↑
BP	↓	↓	↓	↓
JVP	↓	↑	↑	↓
Extremities	Cold	Cold	N or Cold	Warm
Other	look for visible hemorrhage or signs of dehydration	bilateral crackles on chest exam	depending on cause may see pulsus paradoxus, Kussmaul's sign, or tracheal deviation	look for obvious signs of infection or anaphylaxis

- treatment should be directed at underlying etiology once it becomes clear
- treatment goal is to return critical organ perfusion to normal (e.g. normalize BP)
- common treatment modalities include:
  - fluid resuscitation
  - inotropes, vasopressors (e.g. norepinephrine, dobutamine), vasopressin
  - revascularization or thrombolytics for ischemic events

Infection/Sepsis

Effect of treatment with low doses of hydrocortisone (HC) and fludrocortisone (FC) on mortality in patients with septic shock.
JAMA 2002:288:862-71.
Study: Placebo-controlled, randomized, double-blind outcome study.
Patients: 300 adult patients admitted to ICU with septic shock.
Intervention: Patients were randomly assigned to receive either HC (50 mg q6h) and FC (50 mg q24h) or placebo for 7 days.
Primary Outcome: 28-day survival in patients with relative adrenal insufficiency (nonresponders to corticotropin stimulation test).
Results: Of the 229 nonresponders, 53% of patients died in the steroid group versus 63% in the placebo group. This corresponds to a 15.9% relative risk reduction (P=0.02). There was no significant difference between groups in the responders.
Conclusion: Corticosteroid therapy in the ICU reduces mortality without increasing adverse events.

Corticosteroids for treating severe sepsis and septic shock.
Cochrane Database of Systematic Reviews 2004, Issue 1.
Study: Meta-analysis of 15 randomized and quasi randomized control trials examining the efficacy of corticosteroids on death at one month in patients with severe sepsis and septic shock.
Results: Overall, there was no difference in 28-day all cause mortality. However, a subgroup of five trials that used long-term low dose corticosteroids (200-300 mg IV) showed a significant benefit in 28 day mortality (RR=0.80 95% CI 0.67-0.95). Data from this subgroup also showed a significant reduction of in-hospital mortality and increased shock reversal by day seven.
Conclusions: The lack of an overall benefit to corticosteroids in sepsis was attributed to significant study heterogeneity. Low dose and long-term corticosteroids appear to have significant benefit for patients with sepsis. However, further research is needed to identify patients with sepsis who have adrenal insufficiency. Moreover, the optimal time to start treatment and the optimal dose require further trials.

- the leading cause of death in noncoronary ICU settings is multi-organ failure due to sepsis
- treating sepsis is one of the biggest challenges faced by ICU staff as the underlying pathophysiology of this condition is not fully understood
- the predominant theory is that sepsis is attributable to uncontrollable immune system activation
- formal definitions for sepsis-related terms are as follows:
  - infection: pathologic process caused by the invasion of normally sterile tissue or fluid by pathogenic or potentially pathogenic microorganisms
  - bacteremia: the presence of viable bacteria in the blood
  - Systemic Inflammatory Response Syndrome (SIRS): clinical insults, including both infectious and noninfectious moieties that result in a generalized inflammatory reaction manifested by one or more of the following:
    - body temperature >38°C or <36°C
    - heart rate >90/min
    - respiratory rate >20/min or $PaCO_2$ <32 mmHg
    - WBC >12,000 cells/mL or <4,000 cells/mL
  - sepsis: the clinical syndrome defined by the presence of both infection and a systemic inflammatory response and is classified by severity (see Table 29):
    - severe sepsis: sepsis associated with organ dysfunction, hypoperfusion or hypotension
    - septic shock: sepsis with arterial hypotension despite adequate fluid resuscitation
    - multiorgan dysfunction syndrome: sepsis in the presence of altered organ function such that homeostasis cannot be maintained without intervention

Table 29. Diagnostic criteria for sepsis requires documented or suspected infection and some of the following:

General Variables	Organ dysfunction variables
Fever (>38°C) or Hypothermia (<36°C)	Arterial hypoxemia (PaO_2/FiO_2 <300)
Heart rate >90/min	Acute oliguria (urine output <0.5 mL/kg /hr)
sBP <90 mmHg, MAP <70, or an sBP decrease >40 mm Hg	Creatinine increase >0.5 mg/dL
Tachypnea	Coagulation abnormalities (INR >1.5 or aPTT >60 secs)
Altered mental status	Ileus (absent bowel sounds)
Positive fluid balance (>20 mL/kg over 24 hrs)	Thrombocytopenia (platelet count <100,000/L)
Hyperglycemia (BG >7.7 mmol/L) in the absence of diabetes	Hyperbilirubinemia (plasma total bilirubin >4 mg/dL or 70 mmol/L)
Leukocytosis (WBC >12,000/L)	
Leukopenia (WBC <4,000/L)	**Tissue perfusion variables**
Normal WBC count with >10% immature forms	Hyperlactatemia (>1 mmol/L)
Plasma C-reactive protein >2 SD above the normal value	Decreased capillary refill or mottling

Table adapted with permission from Levy MM, Fink MP, Marshall JC, Abraham E, Angus D, Cook D, Cohen J, Opal SM, Vincent J-L, Ramsay G. 2001 SCCM/ESICM/ACCP/ATS/SIS International Sepsis Definitions Conference. Critical Care Medicine. 2003;31(4):1250-6

Basic Principles for the Management of Sepsis
- identify the cause and source of infection: blood, sputum, urine gram stain and culture and sensitivity
- initiate empiric antibiotic therapy
- monitor, restore and maintain hemodynamic function
    - early goal-directed therapy that involves adjustments of cardiac preload, afterload and contractility to balance oxygen delivery with demand provides significant outcome benefits
        - early goal-directed therapy should be started immediately and completed within 6 hours of recognition of severe sepsis/septic shock

Early Goal Directed Therapy
- for initiation of therapy patient should meet SIRS criteria and sBP ≤90 mmHg or lactate ≥4 mmol/L. Therapy should be initiated ASAP after presentation and for ≥6 hours
    1. supplemental oxygen ± intubation and mechanical ventilation
    2. central venous and arterial catheterization
    3. if CVP ≤8 mmHg then crystalloid/colloid fluid IV to maintain CVP 8-12 mmHg
    4. MAP maintained 65-90 mmHg with the use of vasoactive agents
    5. if central venous oxygen saturation (ScvO$_2$) <70% then
        - transfusion of red cells until Hct ≥30%
        - if ScvO$_2$ <70% after transfusion then use inotropic agents
- supportive oxygenation and ventilation using lung-protective regimen
- early nutritional support: enteral route is used to preserve function of intestinal mucosal barrier
- control hyperglycemia with insulin to decrease infectious complications
- physiologic dose corticosteroid replacement therapy in patients with relative adrenal insufficiency (nonresponders to corticotropin stimulation test)
    - consider in mechanically ventilated septic shock patients with organ dysfunction requiring vasopressors, despite early goal-directed therapy and appropriate antibiotic therapy
- recombinant activated protein C (drotrecogin alfa) may be considered in patients with severe sepsis or septic shock with an APACHE II score ≥25 despite early goal-directed therapy and appropriate antibiotic therapy
- DVT/PE prophylaxis
- advanced care planning, including the communication of likely outcomes and realistic goals of treatment with patients and families

Early goal-directed therapy in the treatment of severe sepsis and septic shock.
N.Engl J Med.2001;345(19):1368-77
Study: RCT of patients with severe sepsis or septic shock who arrived at an emergency department were randomized to receive early-goal directed therapy or standard therapy in the emergency department.
Intervention: Early-goal directed therapy consisted of specific treatment goals in the initial six hours of treatment. Specific goals were as follows:
CVP: 8-12 mmHg (Rx'd with either crystalloid or colloids)
MAP: >65 mmHg and <90 mmHg (Rx'd vasopressors or vasodilators)
SvcO2: >70% (Rx'd with transfusion of pRBCs until hemotacrit >30, then inotropic agents).
Standard therapy in the emergency department consisted of ensuring MAP >65, CVP between 8-12 mmHg, and urine output >0.5 mg/kg/hr.
Results: The in-hospital mortality for patients assigned to early-goal directed therapy was 30.5% compared to 46.5% in the standard medical care group (p= 0.009). Patients in the early-goal directed therapy group had improved APACHE II scores, higher central venous oxygen saturation, lower lactate concentrations, higher pH, and a lower base deficit.
Conclusions: Early-goal directed therapy provides significant benefits to patients presenting to hospital with severe sepsis or septic shock. These patients had improved mortality and improved physiologic function as measured between 7 and 72 hours.

Human recombinant activated protein C (APC) for severe sepsis.
Cochrane Database of Systematic Reviews 2007, Issue 3.
Study: Meta-Analysis of 4 RCTs comprising 4911 participants. Both children and adults were included (neonates were excluded).
Results: Pooled data did not show a 28-day mortality benefit for adult or pediatric patients with severe sepsis (Adults: RR: 0.92 95% CI: 0.72-1.18, Children: RR: 0.98 95% CI 0.66-1.46). It is unclear whether patients with APACHE II scores > 25 will benefit from APC. Studies that addressed this question had multiple methodological problems. There is very weak evidence that patients at high risk of death (positive blood culture) will benefit from APC. There was a significant increased risk of bleeding associated with APC.
Conclusions: Authors conclude that evidence does not show a benefit for patients with APACHE II scores less than 25 or pediatric patients. For patients at high risk of death or APACHE II scores >25, further RCTs conducted by non-profit agencies are required. Cost-analysis is also required if APC is to obtain widespread use.

Efficacy and safety of recombinant human activated protein C for severe sepsis.
N Engl J Med. 2001;344(10):699-709.
Study: Placebo-controlled, randomized, double-blind outcome study.
Patients: 1690 patients with systemic inflammation and organ failure due to acute infection were enrolled.
Intervention: Patients were randomly assigned to receive intravenous infusion of either drotrecogin alfa activated (24 mg/kg/hr) or placebo for 96 hours.
Primary Outcome: 28-day survival.
Results: The mortality rate was 24.7% in the drotrecogin alfa activated group and 30.8% in the placebo group which is associated with a 19.4% relative risk reduction (P=0.05).
Conclusion: Treatment with drotrecogin alfa significantly reduced mortality in patients with severe sepsis but with an increased risk of bleeding.

Common Medications

Table 30. Common Medications for Respiratory Diseases

	Drug	Adult dose	Indications	Side effects
BETA-2 AGONISTS				
Short-acting	salbutamol/albuterol (Ventolin®) (light blue/navy), terbutaline (Bricanyl®)	1-2 puffs q4-6h prn	Bronchodilator in acute reversible airway obstruction	CV (angina, flushing, palpitations, tachycardia, can precipitate Afib), CNS (dizziness, headache, insomnia, anxiety), GI (diarrhea, nausea, vomiting), rash, hypokalemia, paroxysmal bronchospasm
Long-acting	salmeterol (Serevent®), formoterol (Oxeze®)	1-2 puffs bid	Maintenance treatment (prevention of bronchospasm) in chronic obstructive lung disease, asthma	
Long-acting beta-2 agonist and inhaled corticosteroid	fluticasone and salmeterol (Advair®) (purple discus) Budesonde and formoterol (Symbicort®) (red puffer)	1 puff bid	COPD and asthma	Common: CNS, headache, dizziness, Resp: URTI, GI (N/V, diarrhea, pain/discomfort, oral candidiasis)
ANTICHOLINERGICS				
	ipratropium bromide (Atrovent®) (clear/green), tiotropium bromide (Spiriva®)	2-3 puffs qid 1 puff qam	Bronchodilator used in COPD, bronchitis and emphysema	Palpitations, anxiety, dizziness, fatigue, headache, nausea, dry mucous membranes, increased toxicity in combination with other anticholinergic drugs
CORTICOSTEROIDS				
Inhaled	fluticasone (Flovent®) (orange/peach)	2-4 puffs bid	Maintenance treatment of asthma	Headache, fever, n/v, MSK pain, URTI, throat irritation, growth velocity reduction in children/adolescents, HPA axis suppression
	budesonide (Pulmicort®) ciclesonide (Alvesco®)	2 puffs bid 1-4 puffs OD		
	beclomethasone (QVAR®, Vanceril®)	1-4 puffs bid (40 µg), 1-2 puffs bid (80 µg)		
Systemic	prednisone (Apo-prednisone®, Deltasone®)	2 mg/kg/day PO (max 60 mg/day)	Acute exacerbation of COPD; severe, persistent asthma, PCP	Endocrine (hirsutism, DM/glucose intolerance, Cushing's syndrome, HPA axis suppression), GI (increased appetite, indigestion), ocular (cataracts, glaucoma), edema, AVN, osteoporosis, headache, psych (anxiety, insomnia), easy bruising
	methylprednisolone (Depo-Medrol®, Solu-Medrol®)	2 mg/kg sodium succinate IV then 0.5-1 mg/kg q6h for 5 days		
ADJUNCT AGENTS	theophylline (Elixophyllin®, Theo-Dur®)	5-13 mg/kg/day PO in divided doses, max 900 mg/day	Treatment of symptoms of reversible airway obstruction due to COPD	GI upset, diarrhea, n/v, anxiety, headache, insomnia, muscle cramp, tremor, tachycardia, PVCs, arrhythmias, Toxicity: persistent, repetitive vomiting, seizures
LEUKOTRIENE ANTAGONISTS				
	montelukast (Singular®)	10 mg PO qhs	Prophylaxis and chronic treatment of asthma	Headache, dizziness, fatigue, fever, rash, dyspepsia, cough, flu-like symptoms
	zileuton (Zyflo®)	600 mg PO qid not available in Canada		Headache, hepatotoxic (ALT elevation), potentiates warfarin and theophylline, chest pain, anxiety, myalgia, arthralgia
ANTIBIOTICS – COMMUNITY ACQUIRED PNEUMONIA				
Macrolide	erythromycin	25-50 mg bid x 7-10 d	Alternate to doxycycline or fluoroquinolone	GI (abdominal pain, diarrhea, n/v), headache, prolonged QT, ventricular arrhythmias, hepatic impairment
	azithromycin	500 mg PO OD x 7-10 d		GI (diarrhea, n/v, abd pain), renal failure, deafness
	clarithromycin	250 mg PO bid x 7-10 days		Headache, rash, GI (diarrhea, n/v, abnormal taste, heartburn, abdo pain), increased BUN
Doxycycline		100 mg PO bid x 7-10 d	Alternate to macrolide or fluoroquinolone	Photosensitivity, rash, urticaria, anaphylaxis, diarrhea, enterocolitis, tooth discoloration in children
Fluoroquinolone	levofloxacin (Levaquin®)	500 mg PO OD x 7-10d	Alternate to macrolide or doxycycline	CNS (dizziness, fever, h/a), GI (n/v, diarrhea, constipation), prolonged QT
	moxifloxacin (Avelox®)	400 mg PO OD x 5 d		
ANTIBIOTICS – HOSPITAL ACQUIRED PNEUMONIA				
3rd gen Cephalosporin	ceftriaxone (Rocephin®)	1-2 g IV bid x 7-10 d	Combine with fluoroquinolone	Rash, diarrhea, eosinophilia, thrombocytosis, leukopenia, elevated transaminases
Fluoroquinolone	levofloxacin moxifloxacin	see above	Combine with 3rd gen cephalosporin	See above
Piperacillin (Pipracil®)		3-4g IV q 4-6h x 7-10 d	Suspect Pseudomonas	CNS (confusion, convulsions, drowsiness), rash, Hematologic (abnormal platelet aggregation, prolonged PT, positive Coombs)
Vancomycin (Vancocin®)		1g IV bid x 7-10 d	Suspect MRSA	CNS (chills, drug fever), hematologic (eosinophilia), rash interstitial nephritis, renal failure, ototoxicity
Macrolide	azithromycin	500 mg PO OD x 7-10 d	Suspect Legionella	See above
	clarithromycin	250 mg PO bid x 7-10 d		See above
ICU MEDICATIONS				
Pressors/Inotropes	Norepinephrine (Levophed©)	1-40 µg/min	Acute hypotension	Angina, bradycardia, dyspnea, hyper/hypotension, arrhythmias
	Phenylephrine	10-300 µg/min	Severe hypotension	See above
	Dobutamine	2-20 µg/kg/min	Inotropic support	See above
Sedatives/Analgesia	Fentanyl (opioid class)	50-100 µg then 50-unlimited µg/hr	Sedation and/or analgesia	Bradycardia, respiratory depression, drowsiness, hypotension
	Propofol (anesthetic)	1-3 mg/kg then 0.3-5 mg/kg/hr	Sedation and/or analgesia	Apnea, bradycardia, hypotension (good for ventilator sedation)

See Infectious Diseases for the management of pulmonary tuberculosis

RH Rheumatology

Neesha Merchant, Laura Waltman and Adina Weinerman, chapter editors
Deepti Damaraju and Elliott Owen, associate editors
Erik Venos, EBM editor
Dr. Dana Jerome and Dr. Heather McDonald-Blumer, staff editors

Basic Anatomy Review

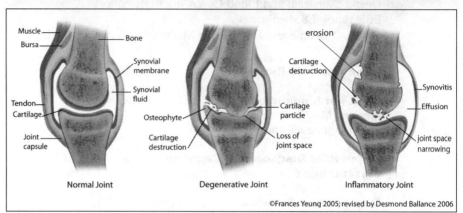

©Frances Yeung 2005; revised by Desmond Ballance 2006

Figure 1. Structure of normal, degenerative and inflammatory joint

Basics of Immunology

Immune Mechanisms of Disease

> **Terminology in Rheumatology**
>
> **arthritis** = inflammation of the joint
>
> **arthralgia** = perception of joint pain without clinical findings to support evidence of arthritis
>
> **"active joint"** = swelling, joint tenderness or stress tenderness

- fundamental principles of pathogenesis of autoimmune diseases
    - disease results from a failure to discriminate between self and non-self
    - activated immune system against self → cell damage/destruction → altered cell function
    - autoreactive T cell is a common effector of many of these diseases
    - certain human leukocyte antigen (HLA) haplotypes are associated with increased susceptibility to disease (see Table 2)
- mechanisms of immunologically mediated disorders (4 types of immune reactions):
    - i. **anaphylactic (type I)**
        - ◆ formation of IgE → release of mediators from basophils/mast cells → diffuse inflammation
        - ◆ e.g. asthma, allergic rhinitis, anaphylaxis
    - ii. **cytotoxic (type II)**
        - ◆ formation of antibody (Ab) → deposit and bind to antigen (Ag) on cell surface → phagocytosis or lysis of target cell
        - ◆ e.g. autoimmune hemolytic anemia, Goodpasture's syndrome, Graves' disease, pernicious anemia
    - iii. **immune complex (type III)**
        - ◆ formation of Ag-Ab complexes form → activate complement → attracts inflammatory cells and release of cytokines
        - ◆ e.g. SLE, PAN, post-streptococcal glomerulonephritis
    - iv. **cell-mediated/delayed hypersensitivity (type IV)**
        - ◆ release of cytokines by sensitized T cells and T-cell mediated cytotoxicity
        - ◆ e.g. contact dermatitis

Immunogenetics and Disease

- cell surface molecules called HLA play a role in mediating immune reactions
- major histocompatibility complex (MHC) are the genes on the short arm of chromosome 6 that encode HLA molecules
- discrete domains of hypervariability within MHC molecules appear to represent "susceptibility determinants"
- there are three classes of MHC (see Table 1)

Table 1. Classes of Major Histocompatibility Complexes (MHCs)

MHC Class	Types	Location	Function
I	HLA-A, -B, -C	All cells	Recognized by CD8+ (cytotoxic) T lymphocytes
II	HLA-DP, -DQ, -DR	Antigen presenting cells (mononuclear phagocytes, B cells, others)	Recognized by CD4+ (helper) T lymphocytes
III	Complement components	In plasma	Chemotaxis, opsonization, lysis of bacteria and cells

Table 2. HLA-Associated Rheumatic Disease

HLA Type	Associated Conditions	Comments
B27	Ankylosing spondylitis (AS) Reactive arthritis IBD arthropathy (spine)	In AS, relative risk = 70-90 In reactive arthritis, relative risk = 40
DR4, DR1	Rheumatoid arthritis	93% of patients
DR3	Sjögren's syndrome SLE	DR3 associated with many non-rheumatic conditions (Celiac disease, Type 1 DM, Graves' disease, Chronic active hepatitis)

Differential Diagnoses of Common Presentations

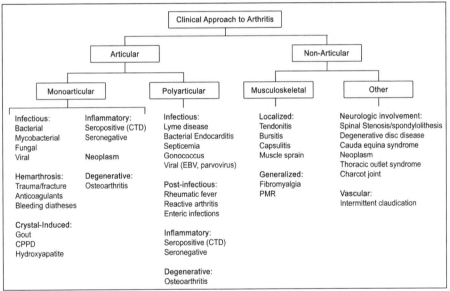

Figure 2. Approach to Joint Pain

**Joint Pain Causes
SOFTER TISSUE**

Sepsis
OA
Fracture
Tendon/muscle
Epiphyseal
Referred

Tumour
Ischemia
Seropositive arthritides
Seronegative arthritides
Urate (gout)/other crystal
Extra-articular rheumatism (polymyalgia/fibromyalgia)

Patterns of Joint Involvement
- symmetrical vs. asymmetrical
- small vs. large
- mono vs. oligo vs. polyarticular
- axial vs. peripheral

Table 3. Differential Diagnosis of Joint Pain: Patterns of Joint Involvement

Symmetrical	Asymmetrical

Large Joint Polyarthritis
• Ankylosing spondylitis
• Rheumatoid arthritis
• Polymyalgia rheumatica
• Osteoarthritis
	Oligoarthritis
	• Seronegative disorders
	  ▪ Psoriatic arthritis
	  ▪ Reactive arthritis
	• Infectious arthritis
	• Crystal-induced arthritis

Small Joint Polyarthritis • Seropositive disorders (RF+, ANA+) • Psoriatic arthritis	• Psoriatic arthritis • Tophaceous gout

---

Septic Arthritis is a Medical Emergency! Consider empiric antibiotic treatment until septic arthritis is excluded by history, physical exam and synovial fluid analysis. (see Infectious Diseases, ID22)

Table 4. Seropositive vs. Seronegative Rheumatic Diseases

	Seropositive	Seronegative
Demographics	F>M	M>F
Peripheral Arthritis	Symmetrical Small and large joints DIP less involved	Usually larger joints, lower extremities (Psoriatic arthritis may be the exception) Dactylitis Enthesitis DIP in Psoriatic arthritis
Pelvic/Axial Disease	No (except for C-spine)	Yes
Enthesitis	No	Yes
Extra-Articular	Nodules Vasculitis Sicca Raynaud's phenomenon	Iritis (= Anterior Uveitis) Oral ulcers GI GU Dermatological features

Extra-Articular Features
- consider skin and appendages, eyes, lungs, cardiac, pulmonary, GI, GU, neurologic, psychiatric

Degenerative Arthritis: Osteoarthritis (OA)

Definition
- primary (idiopathic)
  - most common, of unknown etiology
- secondary
  - post-traumatic or mechanical
  - post-inflammatory (e.g. RA) or post-infectious
  - heritable skeletal disorders (e.g. scoliosis)
  - endocrine disorders (e.g. acromegaly, hyperparathyroidism, hypothyroidism)
  - metabolic disorders (e.g. gout, pseudogout, hemochromatosis, Wilson's disease, ochronosis)
  - neuropathic (also known as Charcot joints)
    - atypical joint trauma due to loss of proprioceptive senses (e.g. diabetes, syphilis)
  - avascular necrosis (e.g. fracture, steroids, alcohol, gout, sickle cell)
  - other (e.g. congenital malformation)

Etiology and Pathophysiology
- abnormal physical forces lead to altered joint function and damage
- primary event is deterioration of articular cartilage due to local biomechanical factors and release of proteolytic and collagenolytic enzymes
  - OA develops when cartilage catabolism > synthesis
  - loss of proteoglycans and water exposes underlying bone
- abnormal local bone metabolism further damages joint
- synovitis is secondary to cartilage damage therefore may see small effusions in OA

Epidemiology
- most common arthropathy (12% of age 25-74)
- increased prevalence with increasing age (35% of 30-year olds, 85% of 80-year olds)

Risk Factors
- genetic predisposition, advanced age, obesity (for knee OA), female, trauma

Signs and Symptoms
- signs and symptoms localized to affected joints (not a systemic disease)
- pain is often insidious, gradually progressive, with intermittent flare-ups and remissions

Table 5. Signs and Symptoms of OA

Symptoms	Signs
joint pain with motion; relieved with rest	joint line tenderness; stress pain
short duration of stiffness (<1/2 hr) after immobility	bony enlargement at affected joints
joint instability/buckling	malalignment/deformity (angulation)
joint locking due to "joint mouse" (bone or cartilage fragment)	limited ROM
loss of function or other internal derangements (e.g. meniscal tear)	crepitus on passive ROM
	inflammation (mild if present)
	periarticular muscle atrophy

Joint Involvement
- asymmetric joint involvement
- any joint can be affected especially knee, hip, hand, spine (see Figure 3)

Glucosamine therapy for treating osteoarthritis
(Towheed TE, Maxwell K, Anastassiades TP, et al. *Cochrane Database of Systemic Reviews* 2005, Issue 2. Art. No.: CD002946. DOI: 10,1002/14651858. CD002946. pub2)
Study: Meta-analysis of 20 RCTs (n=2750) examining the efficacy of glucosamine on OA.
Results: Overall analysis of 15 RCTs favoured glucosamine over placebo for total reduction in pain (measured by a variety of methods). Significant differences between glucosamine and placebo were also observed when compared to Levesque Index scores. Only the glucosamine containing Rotta preparation was found to be significant. No significant differences in WOMAC (in pain, stiffness and function subscales) were found between glucosamine and placebo when only studies with adequate allocation concealment were included. There was evidence to suggest that glucosamine may slow the radiologic progression of OA at 3 years. Glucosamine had an excellent safety profile.
Conclusion: Glucosamine appears helpful for pain when all studies (low quality and older studies) are included. However, when only the higher quality studies are included, there is no longer a difference between glucosamine and placebo. Glucosamine was very well tolerated with low toxicity. Rotta preparation of glucosamine may be of some benefit.

Meta-analysis: Chondroitin for osteoarthritis of the knee and hip
(Annals of Internal Medicine, 17 April, 2007. Volume 146(8):580-590)
Study: Meta-analysis of 20 RCTs (n=3846) examining the efficacy of chondroitin on OA.
Results: The analysis of this review was hampered by significant trial heterogeneity. Trials with poor methodology (small numbers, inadequate randomization concealment, no intention to treat analysis) showed larger effect sizes in favour of glucosamine than more recent trials. When the authors analyzed only the newer and more robust trials, an effect size of -0.3 (CI 95%: -0.13 to 0.07) was generated.
Conclusion: There is high quality evidence to suggest there is no difference between chondroitin and placebo. Chondroitin should be disregarded from routine use in clinical practice.

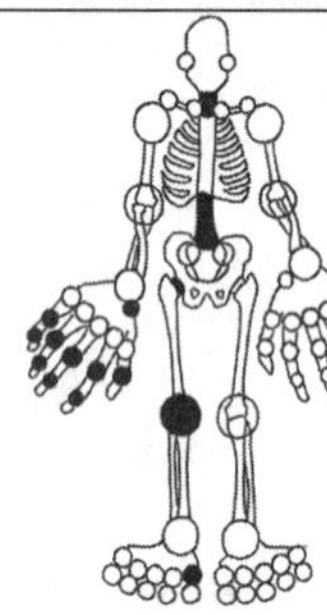

- hand (DIP, PIP, 1st CMC)
- hip
- knee
- 1st MTP
- L-spine (L4-L5, L5-S1)
- C-spine
- uncommon: ankle, shoulder, elbow, MCP, rest of wrist

© Linda Colati

Figure 3. Common sites of involvement in OA

- hand
  - DIP (Heberden's nodes = osteophytes → enlargement of joints)
  - PIP (Bouchard's nodes) (see Figure 4)
  - CMC (usually thumb squaring)
  - MCP is usually spared (except the 1st MCP)
- hip
  - dull or sharp pain in trochanter, groin, anterior thigh, or knee
  - internal rotation and abduction are lost first
- knee
  - narrowing of one compartment of the knee is the rule, medial > lateral
  - standing x-rays must be done (not supine)
- foot
  - common in first MTP
- lumbar spine
  - very common especially L4-L5, L5-S1
  - degeneration of intervertebral discs and facet joint degeneration
  - reactive bone growth can contribute to neurological impingement (e.g. sciatica, neurogenic claudication) or listhesis (slippage)
- cervical spine
  - commonly presents with neck pain, especially in lower cervical area

Investigations
- blood work
  - normal CBC and ESR
  - negative RF and ANA
- synovial fluid → non-inflammatory (see Table 18, RH24)
- radiology (4 hallmark findings, see sidebar)

Treatment
- presently no treatment alters the natural history of OA
- non-pharmacological therapy
  - weight loss (minimum 5-10 lbs. loss)
  - rest/low-impact exercise
  - physiotherapy with heat/cold, exercise programs
  - occupational therapy → aids, splints, cane, walker, bracing
- medical therapy
  - NSAIDs, acetaminophen (see *Common Medications*, RH27)
  - hyaluronic joint injections (Hyalgan™, Synvise™, etc.)
  - nutraceuticals: glucosamine ± chondroitin
- surgical treatment
  - joint debridement, osteotomy, total and/or partial joint replacement, fusion

Seropositive Rheumatic Diseases: Connective Tissue Disorders

Table 6. Features of Seropositive Arthropathies

	Rheumatoid Arthritis	Systemic Lupus Erythematosus	Scleroderma	Dermatomyositis
Clinical Features				
History	Symmetrical Polyarthritis (small joint involvement) AM stiffness (>1 hr)	Multisystemic disease - rash, photosensitivity, Raynaud's, alopecia, cardiac and pulmonary serositis, CNS symptoms, glomerulonephritis	Raynaud's, stiffness of fingers, skin tightness, heartburn/dysphagia pulmonary hypertension, renal dysfunction	Heliotrope rash (eyelids), Gottron's papules, macular erythema and poikiloderma (shoulders, neck and chest), proximal muscle weakness ± pain
Physical Examination	Effused joints Tenosynovitis Nodules Bone-on-bone crepitus Joint deformities	Confirm historical findings (rash, serositis, etc) ± effused (typically small) joints (can be minimal, look for soft tissue swelling)	Skin tightness on dorsum of hand, facial skin tightening, telangiectasia, calcinosis, non-effused joint	Rash, proximal muscle weakness
Laboratory				
Non-specific	Increased ESR in 50-60% Increased platelets Decreased Hb Decreased WBC (Felty's)	Increased ESR Decreased platelets (autoimmune) Decreased Hb (autoimmune) Decreased WBC (leukopenia, lymphopenia)	Increased ESR Increased platelets Decreased Hb Normal WBC	Possible increased ESR Normal platelets Decreased Hb Normal WBC
Specific	RF +ve in ~80%	ANA +ve in 98% Anti-SM +ve in 30% Anti-dsDNA +ve in 50-70% Decreased C3, C4, total hemolytic complement False positive VDRL (in lupus subtypes) Increased PTT (in lupus subtypes; e.g. antiphospholipid Ab)	ANA +ve in >90% Anti-topoisomerase 1 (diffuse) Anti-centromere (usually in CREST, see RH11)	CPK elevated in 80% ANA +ve in 33% anti-Jo-1, anti-Mi-2 Muscle biopsy - key for diagnosis EMG MRI
Synovial Fluid	Inflammation Leukocytosis (>10,000)	Mild inflammation with +ve ANA	Not specific	Not specific
Radiographs	Demineralization Symmetric/concentric joint space narrowing Marginal erosions Absence of bone repair	Nondestructive/nonerosive ± osteopenia ± soft tissue swelling	± pulmonary fibrosis ± esophageal dysmotility ± calcinosis	± esophageal dysmotility ± interstitial lung disease ± calcifications

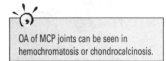

OA of MCP joints can be seen in hemochromatosis or chondrocalcinosis.

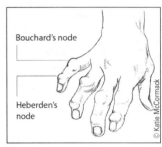

Bouchard's node

Heberden's node

© Katie McCormack

Figure 4. Bouchard's and Heberden's nodes

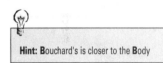

Hint: Bouchard's is closer to the **B**ody

The Radiographic Hallmarks of OA
1. joint space narrowing
2. subchondral sclerosis
3. subchondral cyst formation
4. osteophytes

Arthroscopic debridement for knee osteoarthritis.
Cochrane Database Syst Rev. 2008;(1):CD005118.
Purpose: To identify the effectiveness of AD in knee OA on pain and function.
Study Selection: Randomised controlled trials (RCT) or controlled clinical trials (CCT) assessing effectiveness of AD compared to another surgical procedure, including sham or placebo surgery and other non-surgical interventions, in patients with a diagnosis of primary or secondary OA of the knees, who did not have other joint involvement or conditions requiring long term use of non-steroidal anti-inflammatory drugs (NSAIDs). The main outcomes were pain relief and improved function of the knee.
Results: Three RCTs were included with a total of 271 patients. They had different comparison groups and a moderate risk of bias. One study compared AD with lavage and with sham surgery. Compared to lavage the study found no significant difference. Compared to sham surgery placebo, the study found worse outcomes for AD at two weeks (WMD for pain 8.7, 95% CI 1.7 to 15.8, and function 7.7, 95% CI 1.1 to 14.3; NNTH=5) and no significant difference at two years. The second trial, at higher risk of bias, compared AD and arthroscopic washout, and found that AD significantly reduced knee pain compared to washout at five years (RR 5.5, 95% CI 1.7 to 15.5; NNTB=3). The third trial, also at higher risk of bias, compared AD to closed-needle lavage, and found no significant difference.
Conclusion: There is 'gold' level evidence that AD has no benefit for undiscriminated OA (mechanical or inflammatory causes).

Common Presentation
- Morning stiffness >30 min, improves with use
- Symmetric joint involvement
- Initially involves small joints of hands and feet
- Constitutional symptoms

Criteria are 91-94% sensitive and 89% specific for RA.

Rheumatoid Arthritis (RA)

Definition
- chronic, symmetric, erosive synovitis of peripheral joints (i.e. wrists, MCP joints, and MTP joints)
- characterized by a number of extra-articular features

Table 7. Diagnostic Criteria: RA diagnosed if 4 or more of the following 7 criteria present (American Rheumatism Association, 1987)

Criteria	Definition
1. Morning stiffness	Joint stiffness >1 hour for >6 weeks
2. Arthritis of three or more joint areas	At least 3 active joints for >6 weeks; commonly involved joints are PIP, MCP, wrist, elbow, knee, ankle, MTP
3. Arthritis of hand joints	At least one active joint in wrist, MCP or PIP for >6 weeks
4. Symmetric arthritis	Bilateral involvement of PIP, MCP, or MTP for >6 weeks
5. Rheumatoid nodules	Subcutaneous nodules over bony prominences, extensor surfaces or in juxta-articular regions
6. Serum RF	Found in 60-80% of RA patients
7. Radiographic changes	Erosions or periarticular osteopenia, likely to see earliest changes at ulnar styloid, 2nd and 3rd MCP and PIP joints

Etiology and Pathophysiology
- autoimmune disorder, unknown etiology
- hallmark of RA is hypertrophy of the synovial membrane
  - outgrowth of activated rheumatoid synovium (pannus) into and over the articular surface results in destruction of articular cartilage and subchondral bone
- two theories attempt to explain chronic remissions and exacerbations seen in RA
  - **sequestered Ag**
    - during inflammation, immune complexes (ICs) are deposited at cartilage-bone junction, which is an avascular area → ICs remain free of reticulo-endothelial system but are released as further cartilage breaks down → triggers cascade
  - **molecular mimicry**
    - cartilage damage → altered configuration of cartilage resembles offending agent → triggers cascade

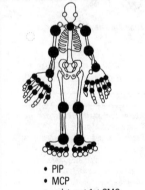

- PIP
- MCP
- wrist, not 1st CMC
- elbow
- shoulder
- knee
- ankle
- MTP
- C-spine

© Linda Colati

Figure 5. Common sites of joint involvement in RA

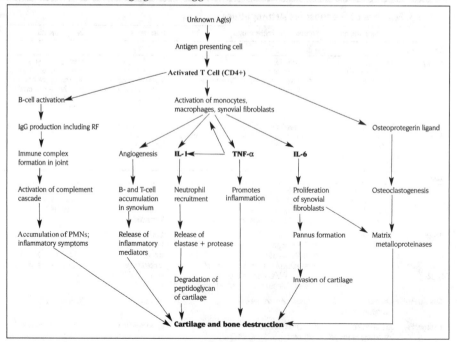

Figure 6. Proposed Pathogenesis of RA

Epidemiology
- incidence 0.6-2.9 per 1,000 population/yr, prevalence 1% of adult population
- F:M = 3:1; age of onset 20-40 yrs
- genetic predisposition: HLA-DR4/DR1 association (93% of patients have either HLA type)

Signs and Symptoms
- variable course of exacerbations and remissions
- morning stiffness >1 hr, improves with use, aggravated by rest
- symmetric joint involvement (see Figure 5)
- signs of disease activity: synovitis (assessed by tender and swollen joint count), elevated serum markers of inflammation such as ESR or CRP, decreased grip strength, increased pain
- signs of mechanical joint damage: loss of motion, instability, deformity, crepitus
- constitutional symptoms: profound fatigue; rarely myalgia or weight loss
- extra-articular features (see Figure 7) and radiographic damage
- limitation of function and decrease in global functional status

Extra-Articular Features (EAF)
- classified in terms of the underlying process: either vasculitis or a lymphocytic infiltrate

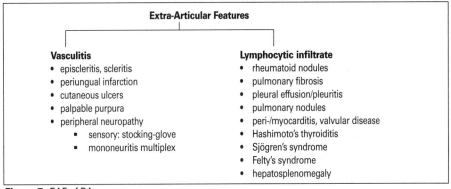

Extra-Articular Features

Vasculitis
- episcleritis, scleritis
- periungual infarction
- cutaneous ulcers
- palpable purpura
- peripheral neuropathy
  - sensory: stocking-glove
  - mononeuritis multiplex

Lymphocytic infiltrate
- rheumatoid nodules
- pulmonary fibrosis
- pleural effusion/pleuritis
- pulmonary nodules
- peri-/myocarditis, valvular disease
- Hashimoto's thyroiditis
- Sjögren's syndrome
- Felty's syndrome
- hepatosplenomegaly

Figure 7. EAF of RA

Investigations
- RF positive in 80% of patients
  - non-specific, also seen in other rheumatic diseases (e.g. SLE, Sjögren's), chronic inflammation (e.g. SBE, hepatitis, TB) and 5% of healthy population
- anti-CCP (cyclic citrullinated peptide): sensitivity (~80%)
- increased disease activity is associated with decrease Hb (anemia of chronic disease), increased platelets, elevated ESR, CRP, and RF

Classification of Global Functional Status in RA
(American College of Rheumatology, 1991)
- **Class I**: able to perform usual ADLs (self-care, vocational, avocational)
- **Class II**: able to perform self-care and vocational activities, restriction of avocational activities
- **Class III**: able to perform self-care, restriction of vocational and avocational activities
- **Class IV**: limited in ability to perform self-care, vocational, avocational activities

Complications of Chronic Synovitis
- joint deformities (see Figure 8)
  - swan neck deformity, boutonnière deformity
  - ulnar deviation of MCP; radial deviation of wrist joint
  - hammer toe, mallet toe, claw toe
  - flexion contractures
- atlanto-axial and subaxial subluxation
  - C-spine instability
  - neurological impingement (long tract signs)
  - difficult intubation
- limited shoulder mobility, spontaneous tears of the rotator cuff leading to chronic spasm
- tenosynovitis → may cause rupture of tendons
- Carpal Tunnel Syndrome
- ruptured Baker's cyst (outpouching of synovium behind the knee); presentation similar to acute DVT
- decreased functional capacity and early mortality

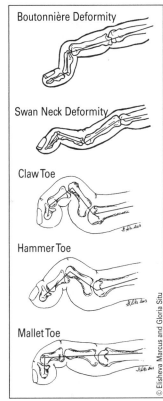

Boutonnière Deformity

Swan Neck Deformity

Claw Toe

Hammer Toe

Mallet Toe

© Elisheva Marcus and Gloria Situ

Figure 8. Joint deformities

Poor prognostic features of RA include young age of onset, high RF titer, elevated ESR, activity of >20 joints, and presence of EAF.

Common Syndromes in RA
1. Sjögren's syndrome (sicca complex – dry eyes and mouth)
2. Caplan's syndrome (multiple pulmonary nodules and pneumoconiosis)
3. Felty's syndrome (arthritis, splenomegaly, neutropenia)

Comparison of Treatment Strategies in Early Rheumatoid Arthritis
(*Ann Intern Med* 20 March 2007:146(6))
Study: RCT of 508 patients comparing 4 different treatment strategies for early rheumatoid arthritis.
Intervention:
Group 1: Sequential Monotherapy with traditional DMARDs
Group 2: Step-Up Combination Therapy
Group 3: Initial Combination Therapy with prednisone (high dose)
Group 4: Initial Combination Therapy with infliximab
Results: Patients in groups 3 and 4 responded faster and had significantly greater overall change in physical function scores after the first year of treatment. By end of the second year, groups 1 and 2 had achieved a similar response to groups 3 and 4. Groups 3 and 4 also showed significantly less radiologic progression of their disease over 2 years than groups 1 and 2. There were no significant differences in toxicity levels between the 4 groups.
Conclusions: Initial combination therapy with prednisone or infliximab results in faster response rates. Whether faster initial response rates leads to better long-term disease outcomes is not yet studied.

Only DMARDs (not analgesics or NSAIDs) alter the course of RA!

The safety of infliximab, combined with background treatments, among patients with rheumatoid arthritis and various comorbidities (START)
(*Arthritis Rheum* 2006;54:1075-86)
Study: Randomized, placebo-controlled multicentre trial.
Patients: 1084 patients (mean age 52 yrs, 80% female) with active moderate to severe rheumatoid arthritis despite treatment with methotrexate.
Intervention: Patients were randomized to receive infusions of placebo, infliximab dosed at 3 mg/kg, or infliximab dosed at 10 mg/kg at 0, 2, 6, and 14 weeks, in addition to methotrexate.
Primary Outcome: Incidence of serious infection within 22 weeks of randomization.
Results: Compared with the placebo group, the relative risk of developing serious infection was 1.0 (95%CI 0.3-3.1, P=0.995) in patients receiving infliximab at 3 mg/kg and 3.1 (95%CI 1.2-7.9, P=0.013) in patients receiving infliximab at 10 mg/kg. In addition, 31% of patients receiving infliximab at 3 mg/kg and 32% of patients receiving infliximab at 10 mg/kg were able to achieve remission at 22 weeks compared with only 14% of those receiving placebo (P<0.001, NNT=6).
Conclusions: Therapy with infliximab 3 mg/kg does not significantly increase the risk of serious infection in patients with active moderate to severe rheumatoid arthritis already receiving methotrexate. However, therapy with infliximab 10 mg/kg does significantly increase the risk of serious infection in this population.

Treatment
- goals of therapy
    - control disease activity
    - relieve pain and stiffness
    - maintain function and lifestyle
    - prevent or control joint damage
    - key is early diagnosis and early intervention with disease modifying anti-rheumatic drugs (DMARDs)

A) Education, occupational therapy, physiotherapy, vocational counselling
- therapeutic exercise program (isometrics and active ROM exercise during flares, aquatic/aerobic/strengthening exercise between flares), assistive devices and patient education
- patients may need job modification, time off work or change in occupation
- The Arthritis Society (Canada) and Arthritis Foundation (U.S.) provide resources and programs

B) Medical
- NSAIDs, DMARDs, and corticosteroids are the mainstay of pharmacological therapy

1. Reduction of Inflammation and Pain
- NSAIDS
    - individualize according to efficacy and tolerability
    - contraindicated or cautioned in some patients
- analgesics
    - add acetaminophen ± opioid prn for synergistic pain control
- corticosteroids
    - local
        - intra-articular injections to control symptoms in a specific joint
        - eye drops for eye involvement
    - systemic (prednisone)
        - low dose (5-10 mg/day) useful for (a) short term to improve symptoms if NSAIDs ineffective, (b) to bridge gap until DMARD takes effect or (c) for refractory disease
        - moderate to high dose (20-60+ mg/day) for cardiopulmonary disease
        - high dose (1 mg/kg/day) for vasculitis
        - do baseline DEXA bone density scan and start bisphosphonate, calcium, and vitamin D therapy if using corticosteroids >3 months at >7.5 mg/day
    - side effects: osteoporosis, avascular necrosis (AVN), hypertension, cataracts, glaucoma, peptic ulcer disease (PUD), susceptibility to infection, hypokalemia, hyperglycemia, hyperlipidemia, weight gain, acne
    - cautions/contraindications: active infection, osteoporosis, hypertension, gastric ulcer, diabetes, TB

2. Disease Modifying Antirheumatic Drugs (DMARDs)
- combination DMARDs are the standard of care
- start DMARDs within 3 months of diagnosis to decrease disease progression, symptoms and signs
- DMARDs reduce or prevent joint damage, and are associated with better long-term disability index
- delayed onset of action (may take 8-12 weeks)
- many DMARDs have potential toxicities that require periodic monitoring
- if repetitive flares, progressive joint damage, or ongoing disease activity after 3 months of maximal therapy → change or add other DMARDs
- **mild and early stages:**
    - hydroxychloroquine or sulfasalazine monotherapy preferred
- **moderate to severe disease** (especially if unfavourable prognostic factors):
    - methotrexate is the gold standard
    - single regimen with methotrexate or leflunomide (Arava™)
    - combination therapy: methotrexate + sulfasalazine + hydroxychloroquine; methotrexate + cyclosporine; methotrexate + leflunomide
- biologics: indicated if persistent disease activity (see *Common Medications*, RH27)
    - commonly used after failure of other DMARDs; however, evidence suggests benefit from use in early RA as well

C) Surgical Therapy
- synovectomy: debridement and/or removal of inflamed synovium from individual joints (surgical or radioactive)
- joint replacement (hip, shoulder, knee)
- joint fusion (wrist, thumb, ankle, C-spine)
- reconstruction (tendon repair)
- surgery indicated for structural joint damage

Systemic Lupus Erythematosus (SLE)

Definition
- chronic inflammatory multisystem disease of unknown etiology, characterized by production of autoantibodies and diverse clinical manifestations

Table 8. Diagnostic Criteria of SLE: 4 or more of 11 must be present serially or simultaneously (American College of Rheumatology, 1997 update)

Criteria	Description
Clinical	
Malar rash	Classic "butterfly rash", sparing of nasolabial folds, no scarring
Discoid rash	May cause scarring due to invasion of basement membrane
Photosensitivity	Skin rash in reaction to sunlight
Oral/nasal ulcers	Usually painless
Arthritis	Symmetric, involving ≥2 small or large peripheral joints, non-erosive
Serositis	Pleuritis or pericarditis
Neurologic disorder	Seizures or psychosis
Laboratory	
Renal disorder	Proteinuria (>0.5 g/day or 3+)
	Cellular casts (RBC, Hb, granular, tubular, mixed)
Hematologic disorder	Hemolytic anemia, leukopenia, lymphopenia, thromboctyopenia
Immunologic disorder	Anti-dsDNA Ab, anti-Sm Ab
	Antiphospholipid antibodies based on the finding of serum anticardiolipin Ab, lupus anticoagulant, or false positive VDRL
Antinuclear antibody (ANA)	Most sensitive test (98%)

Note: "4, 7, 11" rule → 4 out of 11 criteria (4 lab, 7 clinical) for diagnosis

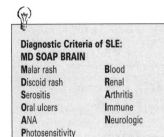

Diagnostic Criteria of SLE:
MD SOAP BRAIN

Malar rash	**B**lood
Discoid rash	**R**enal
Serositis	**A**rthritis
Oral ulcers	**I**mmune
ANA	**N**eurologic
Photosensitivity	

Radiographically, unlike RA, the arthritis of SLE is non-erosive.

Suspect SLE in a patient who has involvement of 2 or more organ systems.

Pathophysiology
- disorder characterized by autoantibodies causing multi-organ inflammation
- peripheral polyarthritis with symmetric involvement of small and large joints

Proposed Etiology
- multifactorial etiology (see Figure 9)
- **genetics**
  - common association with HLA-B8/-DR3; ~10% have positive family history
- **estrogen**
  - prepubertal and postmenopausal women have similar incidence to men
  - men with SLE have higher concentration of estrogenic metabolites
- **infection**
  - viral (nonspecific stimulant of immune response)
- **drugs**
  - anticonvulsants (phenytoin)
  - antihypertensives (hydralazine)
  - antiarrhythmics (procainamide)
  - isoniazid (INH)
  - anti-histone antibodies are commonly seen in drug-induced lupus
  - oral contraceptive pills associated with exacerbation

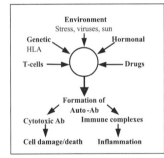

Figure 9. Multifactorial etiology of SLE

Epidemiology
- prevalence: 0.05% overall
- F:M = 10:1; age of onset in reproductive years, 13-40
- more common and severe in African-Americans and Asians
- bimodal mortality pattern
  - early (within 2 years)
    - active SLE, active nephritis, infection secondary to steroid use
  - late (>10 years)
    - inactive SLE, inactive nephritis, atherosclerosis secondary to long-term steroids and partially due to chronic inflammation

Signs and Symptoms
- characterized by periods of exacerbation and remission
- **systemic**
  - fever, malaise, fatigue, lymphadenopathy, weight loss
- **vascular**
  - Raynaud's phenomenon (see sidebar), thrombosis, vasculitis, livedo reticularis (mottled discolouration of skin due to narrowing of blood vessels, characteristic lacy or net-like appearance)

Raynaud's Phenomenon
Vasospastic disorder characteristically causing discolouration of fingers and toes (white→blue→red).
Classic triggers: cold and emotional stress.

Drug-Induced SLE
Drug-induced SLE often presents atypically with systemic features and serositis; usually associated with anti-histone antibodies.

Consider septic arthritis and avascular necrosis in patients with SLE and joint pain.

- **dermatologic**
    - maculopapular rash, photosensitivity, panniculitis (inflammation of subcutaneous fat and muscle tissue), alopecia (hair loss), urticaria, purpura, oral, nasal, genital ulcers
- **ophthalmic**
    - conjunctivitis, episcleritis, keratoconjunctivitis, cytoid bodies (cotton wool exudates on fundoscopy = infarction of nerve cell layer of retina)
- **gastrointestinal**
    - pancreatitis, lupus enteropathy, hepatitis, hepatomegaly
- **pulmonary**
    - interstitial lung disease, pulmonary hypertension, PE, alveolar hemorrhage, pleuritis
- **musculoskeletal**
    - arthralgias, arthritis, avascular necrosis, myositis
- **neurologic**
    - depression, personality disorder, cerebritis, transverse myelitis, seizures, headache, peripheral neuropathy

Investigations
- serologic hallmark is high titer ANA detected by immunofluorescence
- ANA has high sensitivity (98%) and therefore is a useful screening test, but poor specificity
- anti-dsDNA Ab (detected by Crithidia test, Farr radioimmunoassay) and anti-Sm Ab are specific for SLE (95-99%)
- a drop in anti-dsDNA titer and normalization of serum complement (C3, C4) are useful to monitor response to treatment in patients who are clinically and serologically concordant
- lupus anticoagulant may cause increased risk of arterial and venous clotting and increased PTT

Treatment
- principles of therapy:
    - treat early and avoid long term steriod use if possible
    - if high doses of steroids necessary for long-term control add steroid sparing agents and taper when possible
    - treatment is tailored to organ system involved and severity of disease
    - all medications used to treat SLE require periodic monitoring for potential toxicities
- dermatologic
    - preventative: use sunscreen, avoid UV light and estrogens
    - topical steroids for rash, antimalarials
- musculoskeletal
    - bisphosphonates, calcium, vitamin D to combat osteoporosis
    - antimalarials (hydrochloroquine if no serious internal organ involvement → improves long term control and prevents flares)
    - NSAIDs ± gastroprotective agent for arthritis (also beneficial for pleuritis and pericarditis)
- organ threatening disease
    - systemic steroids to minimize end organ damage secondary to inflammation high-dose oral prednisone/IV methylprednisone in severe disease
    - steroid sparing agents: azathioprine, methotrexate, mycophenolate
    - IV cyclophosphamide for serious organ involvement (e.g. cerebritis or SLE nephritis)

Antiphospholipid Antibody Syndrome (APS)

Definition
- multisystem vasculopathy manifested by recurrent thromboembolic events, spontaneous abortions and thrombocytopenia
- circulating antiphospholipid autoAbs (anticardiolipin Ab and lupus anticoagulant) interfere with coagulation cascade
- primary vs. secondary
    - secondary APS develops in SLE, other connective tissue diseases, malignancy, drugs (hydralazine, procainamide, phenytoin, interferon, quinidine), infections (HIV, TB, hepatitis C, infectious mononucleosis)
- catastrophic APS
    - fatal condition with sepsis, ARDS (acute respiratory distress syndrome), MODS (multi-organ dysfunction syndrome), TTP (thrombotic thrombocytopenic purpura)

Signs and Symptoms
- primary manifestation is venous or arterial thrombosis
    - venous thrombosis → DVT, PE, renal and retinal vein thrombosis
    - arterial thrombosis → stroke/TIA, multi-infarct dementia, MI, valvular incompetence, limb ischemia

A systematic review of secondary thromboprophylaxis in patients with antiphospholipid antibodies.
Arthritis Rheum. 2007;57:1487-95.
Purpose: To systematically review the efficacy and safety data of different therapeutic approaches in patients with antiphospholipid antibodies (aPL) and thrombosis.
Study Selection: Randomized controlled trials, prospective and retrospective cohort studies, and subgroup analysis (n > 15) that focused on the secondary thromboprophylaxis in patients with aPL were selected.
Results: Sixteen studies were selected. Patients with venous events and a single test for aPL showed a low recurrence rate while receiving oral anticoagulation at a target international normalized ratio (INR) of 2.0-3.0. Patients with stroke and a single positive aPL test had no increased risk compared with those without aPL. Recurrence rates in patients with definite antiphospholipid syndrome (APS) and previous venous thromboembolism were lower than in patients with arterial and/or recurrent events, both with and without therapy. Only 3.8% of recurrent events occurred at an actual INR >3.0. Mortality due to recurrent thrombosis was higher than mortality due to bleeding (18 patients versus 1 patient reported).
Conclusion: For patients with definite APS, the authors recommend prolonged warfarin therapy at a target INR of 2.0-3.0 in APS patients with first venous events and >3.0 for those with recurrent and/or arterial events. For patients with venous thromboembolism or stroke and a single positive aPL test, the authors recommend further testing to determine if they have a persisting antibody. If they do not, the same therapy as for the general population should be used (warfarin at a target INR of 2.0-3.0 and low-dose aspirin, respectively).

- recurrent spontaneous abortions including first and second trimester fetal loss, premature birth at <34 wks gestational age
- hematologic abnormalities
  - thrombocytopenia, hemolytic anemia, neutropenia
- skin
  - livedo reticularis, purpura, leg ulcers, and gangrene

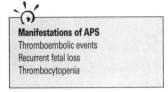

Manifestations of APS
Thromboembolic events
Recurrent fetal loss
Thrombocytopenia

Investigations
- serology
  - diagnosis: lupus anticoagulant, or anticardiolipin (IgG or IgM) antibody positive on 2 occasions, at least 12 weeks apart

Treatment
- thrombosis
  - lifelong anticoagulation with warfarin → target INR 2.5-3.5
- recurrent fetal loss
  - aspirin, heparin, ± steroids
- catastrophic APS
  - high-dose steroids, anticoagulation, cyclophosphamide, plasmapheresis

Scleroderma/Progressive Systemic Sclerosis (PSS)

Definition
- a non-inflammatory disorder characterized by widespread small vessel vasculopathy and fibrosis, which occurs in the setting of immune system activation and autoimmunity

Diagnosis
- diagnostic criteria: 1 major or ≥2 minor criteria
  - major criterion: proximal scleroderma
  - minor criteria: sclerodactyly, digital pitting scars or loss of substance from finger pads, bibasilar pulmonary fibrosis
- serology
  - anti-topoisomerase 1: specific but not sensitive for systemic sclerosis
  - anti-centromere favours diagnosis of CREST variant (limited systemic sclerosis)

Etiology and Pathophysiology
- idiopathic vasculopathy (not vasculitis) leading to atrophy and fibrosis of tissues
  - intimal proliferation and media mucinous degeneration → progressive obliteration of vessel lumen → fibrotic tissue
  - resembles malignant hypertension

Epidemiology
- F:M = 3-4:1, peaking in 5th and 6th decades
- associated with HLA-DR1
- associated environmental exposure (silica, epoxy resins, toxic oil, aromatic hydrocarbons, polyvinyl chloride)

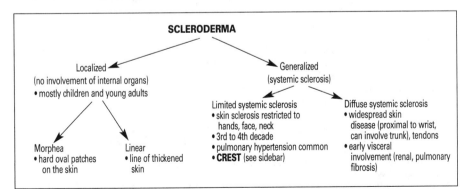

Figure 10. Forms of Scleroderma

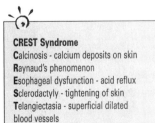

CREST Syndrome
Calcinosis - calcium deposits on skin
Raynaud's phenomenon
Esophageal dysfunction - acid reflux
Sclerodactyly - tightening of skin
Telangiectasia - superficial dilated blood vessels

Signs and Symptoms

Table 9. Clinical Manifestations of Scleroderma

System	Features
Dermatologic	Initial phase characterized by painless non-pitting edema Progressive bilateral swelling of fingers, hands and feet leading to skin tightening Characteristic face: mask-like facies with tight lip, beak nose, radial perioral furrows Atrophy, ulcerations, hypo/hyperpigmentation, telangiectasias, calcinosis, periungual erythema, pruritus
Vascular	Episodes (minutes to hours) of well-demarcated blanching and/or cyanosis of digits followed by erythema (Raynaud's phenomenon), tingling and pain Due to vasospasm following cold exposure or emotional stress If severe, can result in infarction of tissue at fingertips → digital pitting scars, frank gangrene or autoamputation of the fingers or toes
Gastrointestinal (~90%)	GI tract becomes a rigid tube leading to decreased motility Distal esophageal hypomotility → dysphagia Loss of lower esophageal sphincter function → GERD, ulcerations, strictures Small bowel hypomotility → bacterial overgrowth, diarrhea, bloating, cramps, malabsorption, weight loss Large bowel hypomotility → pathognomonic radiographic finding on barium study is large bowel wide mouth diverticuli
Renal	Mild proteinuria, creatinine elevation and/or hypertension are common "Scleroderma renal crisis" (10-15%) may lead to malignant arterial hypertension, oliguria and microangiopathic hemolytic anemia
Pulmonary	Interstitial fibrosis, pulmonary HTN, pleurisy, and pleural effusions
Cardiac	Left ventricular dysfunction, pericarditis, pericardial effusion, arrhythmias
Musculoskeletal	Polyarthralgias → polyarthritis affecting both small and large joints Subcutaneous calcifications (calcinosis) "Resorption of distal tufts" (radiological finding) Proximal weakness 2° to disuse, atrophy, low grade myopathy
Endocrine	Hypothyroidism common

Scleroderma is the most common cause of secondary Raynaud's phenomenon.

Treatment
- treatment is tailored to organ system involved
- dermatologic
    - good skin hygiene
    - low dose prednisone, methotrexate (limited evidence)
- vacular (Raynaud's)
    - patient education on cold avoidance
    - vasodilators (CCBs, local nitroglycerine cream, systemic PGE_2 inhibitors)
- gastrointestinal
    - gastroesophageal reflux disease (GERD): PPIs are first line, then H_2-receptor agonists
    - small bowel bacterial overgrowth: broad spectrum antibiotics (tetracycline, metronidazole)
- renal disease: ACE inhibitors
- cardiac
    - pericarditis: systemic steroids
    - pulmonary hypertension: bosetan (Tracleer™), epoprostenol (Flolan™), sildenafil (Viagra™)
- musculoskeletal
    - myositis: systemic steroids

Idiopathic Inflammatory Myopathy

- autoimmune diseases characterized by proximal limb and neck weakness, may be associated with muscle pain
- autoantibodies: ANA, anti-Jo-1 (DM), anti-Mi-2, other myositis-specific antibodies
- classification
    - adult polymyositis (PM)/dermatomyositis (DM)
    - juvenile DM (usually with vasculitis)
    - PM/DM associated with malignancy
    - PM/DM associated with connective tissue disease
    - inclusion body myositis (IBM)

POLYMYOSITIS (PM)/DERMATOMYOSITIS (DM)

Definition
- idiopathic inflammatory myopathy: a number of conditions in which muscle becomes damaged by a non-suppurative lymphocytic inflammatory process
- PM: inflammation of muscles, DM: inflammation of muscles and skin

Diagnosis
- definite PM/DM if 4 criteria fulfilled
- probable if fulfill 3 criteria
- possible if fulfill 2 criteria

Table 10. Diagnostic criteria for PM/DM

Criteria	Description
1. Progressive symmetric proximal muscle weakness	Typical involvement of shoulders and hips
2. Elevated muscle enzymes	Increased CK, aldolase, LDH, AST, ALT
3. EMG changes	Short polyphasic motor units, high frequency repetitive discharge, insertional irritability
4. Muscle biopsy	Segmental fibre necrosis, basophilic regeneration, perivascular inflammation and atrophy
5. Typical rash of dermatomyositis	Required for diagnosis of DM

Etiology and Pathophysiology
- PM is CD8 cell-mediated muscle necrosis, found in adults
- DM is B-cell and CD4 immune complex-mediated perifasicular vasculitis

Signs and Symptoms
- progressive symmetrical proximal muscle weakness (shoulder and hip) developing over weeks to months
- early symptom is difficulty lifting head off pillow
- **dermatological**
  - DM has characteristic dermatological features, found in children and adults, F>M
    - Gottron's papules
      - pink-violaceous, flat-topped papules overlying the dorsal surface of the interphalangeal joints
    - Gottron's sign
      - erythematous smooth or scaly patches over the dorsal IP, MCP, elbows, knees, or medial malleoli
    - heliotrope (purple) rash over the eyelids; usually with edema
    - "shawl sign"
      - erythematous rash over neck, upper chest, and shoulders
- **cardiac**
  - dysrhythmias, congestive heart failure, conduction defect, ventricular hypertrophy, pericarditis
- **gastrointestinal**
  - oropharyngeal and lower esophageal dysphagia, reflux
- **pulmonary**
  - weakness of respiratory muscles, interstitial lung disease, aspiration pneumonia

Treatment
- physical therapy and occupational therapy
- medical
  - high dose corticosteroid (1-2 mg/kg/day) and slow taper
  - immunosuppressive agents (azathioprine, methotrexate, cyclophosphamide, cyclosporine)
  - intravenous immunoglobulin for DM
- malignancy surveillance
  - detailed history and physical (breast, pelvic and rectal exam)
  - CXR, abdominal and pelvic ultrasound, stool occult blood, Pap test, mammogram ± CT scan (thoracic, abdominal, pelvic)

Prognosis
- **PM/DM Associated with Malignancy**
  - increased risk of malignancy: age >50, DM>PM, normal CK, refractory disease
  - 2.4-6.5 fold increased risk of underlying malignancy usually in internal organs

Signs of DM
Gottron's papules and Gottron's sign are pathognomonic of DM (occur in 70% of patients).

- **Inclusion Body Myositis**
  - age >50, M>F, slowly progressive, vacuoles in cells on biopsy
  - suspect when patient unresponsive to treatment
  - distal as well as proximal muscle weakness
  - muscle biopsy positive for inclusion bodies

Sjögren's Syndrome

Definition
- autoimmune condition characterized by dry eyes (keratoconjunctivitis sicca) and dry mouth (xerostomia), caused by lymphocytic infiltration of salivary and lacrimal glands
- primary and secondary form (i.e. associated with RA, SLE, DM, and HIV)
- incidence estimated at 4/100,000 people
- 90% of cases are among females
- mean age of diagnosis is 40-60 yrs

Classic Triad
(identifies 93% of Sjögren's patients)
- Dry eyes
- Dry mouth (dysphagia, xerostomia)
- Arthritis (small joint, asymmetrical, nonerosive)

Diagnosis
- Symptoms of dry eyes
- Signs of dry eye – Schirmer test (to assess tear flow) or slit lamp exam with Rose Bengal stain
- Autoantibodies anti-Ro, anti-La, ANA, RF
- Symptoms of dry mouth
- Signs of dry mouth - Sialography
- Salivary gland biopsy: gold standard

Note: Need 4 of the above criteria, one of which must be either autoantibodies or salivary gland biopsy (sensitivity 95% - European Community Criteria)

Etiology and Pathophysiology
- may evolve into systemic disorder and may lead to diminished exocrine gland activity in respiratory tract and skin

Signs and Symptoms
- systemic manifestations:
  - arthralgias, arthritis, subclinical diffuse interstitial lung disease, renal disease, palpable purpura, systemic vasculitis
- results in "sicca complex": dry eyes (keratoconjunctivitis sicca), dry mouth (xerostomia)

Complications
- xerotrachea resulting in chronic dry cough
- Staphylococcus blepharitis: most common complication
- autoimmune thyroid dysfunction in 45% of patients
- vascular involvement leads to peripheral neuropathy (most common systemic complication)
- glomerulonephritis
- lymphoma

Table 11. Signs and Symptoms of Sicca

Location	Manifestation
Ocular	Burning/dry/painful eye relieved by tears
	Foreign body sensation (worse in evening)
	Blepharitis
Oral	Dry mouth – difficulty swallowing food without drinking
	Rapidly progressive caries (secondary to decreased saliva volume and its antibacterial factors)
	Erythema of hard palate and oral mucosa
	Oral candidiasis, angular cheilitis (inflammation and fissuring at the commissures of the mouth)

Treatment
- good dental hygiene
- artificial tears or surgical punctal occlusion for xerophthalmia
- adequate hydration for xerostomia
- topical nystatin or clotrimazole x 4-6 weeks for oral candidiasis
- hydroxychloroquine, corticosteroids, immunosuppressive agents for severe systemic involvement
- agents that stimulate salivary flow (e.g. pilocarpine)

Patients with Sjögren's syndrome are at higher risk of non-Hodgkin's lymphoma.

Mixed Connective Tissue Disease (MCTD)/ Overlap Syndrome

- syndrome with features of 2 different CTD are present (e.g. SLE, PSS, PM) with presence of anti-RNP Ab (see Table 13, RH18)
- common symptoms: Raynaud's phenomenon, swollen fingers
- prognosis
  - 50-60% will evolve into SLE
  - 40% will evolve into scleroderma
  - only 10% will remain as MCTD for the rest of their lives

Vasculitides

VASCULITIS
- inflammation and subsequent necrosis of blood vessels with resulting tissue ischemia or infarction
- any organ system can be involved
- keys to diagnosis
  - clinical suspicion: suspect in cases of unexplained multiple organ ischemia or systemic illness with no evidence of malignancy or infection
  - labs non-specific: anemia, increased WBC and ESR, abnormal urinalysis
  - biopsy if tissue accessible
  - angiography if tissue inaccessible
- treatment generally entails corticosteroids and/or immunosuppressives

> **c-ANCA =** circulating anti-neutrophil cytoplasmic antibody
> **p-ANCA =** perinuclear anti-neutrophil cytoplasmic antibody

Table 12. Classification of Vasculitis and Characteristic Features

Classification	Characteristic Features
Small vessel	
• **Non-ANCA-associated**	Immune complex mediated (most common mechanism)
Predominantly cutaneous vasculitis	Also known as hypersensitivity/leukocytoclastic vasculitis
Henoch-Schönlein purpura (see <u>Pediatrics</u>, P94)	Vascular deposition of IgA causing systemic vasculitis (skin, GI, renal), seen most frequently in childhood, usually self-limiting condition
Essential cryoglobulinemic vasculitis	
• **ANCA-associated**	
Wegener's granulomatosis (c-ANCA > p-ANCA)	Granulomatous inflammation of vessels of respiratory tract and kidneys, most common in middle age, most present initially with symptoms of URTI
Churg-Strauss syndrome (50% ANCA positive)	Granulomatous inflammation of vessels with hypereosinophilia and eosinophilic tissue infiltration, sometimes associated with p-ANCA or c-ANCA Other manifestations include coronary arteritis, myocarditis and neuropathy
Microscopic polyangiitis (70% ANCA positive, usually p-ANCA)	Pauci-immune necrotizing vasculitis, affecting kidneys (necrotizing glomerulonephritis), lungs (capillaritis and alveolar hemorrhage), skin
Medium-sized vessel	
Polyarteritis nodosa	Any age (average 40-50's), unknown etiology in most cases Segmental non-granulomatous necrotizing inflammation
Kawasaki's (see <u>Pediatrics</u>, P94)	T lymphocyte response and granuloma formation
Large vessel	T lymphocyte response and granuloma formation
Giant cell arteritis (GCA)/Temporal Arteritis	Over 50 years of age, F>M, inflammation predominantly of the aorta and arteries originating from it
Takayasu's arteritis	"Pulseless disease", increased ESR, fever, night sweats, chronic inflammation, most often the aorta and its branches, usually young adults of Asian descent, F>M
Other Vasculitides	
Buerger's disease	Also known as thromboangiitis obliterans, inflammation secondary to pathological clotting, affects small and medium-sized vessels of distal extremities, most important etiologic factor is cigarette smoking, most common in Asian males, may lead to distal claudication and gangrene
Behcet's disease	Pathology: leukoclastic vasculitis, multisystem disorder presenting with ocular involvement, recurrent oral and genital ulceration, venous thrombosis, skin and joint involvement
Vasculitis mimicry	Cholesterol emboli, atrial myxoma

> **Churg-Strauss Triad**
> - Allergic rhinitis and asthma
> - Eosinophilic infiltrative disease resembling pneumonia
> - Systemic vasculitis

Predominantly Cutaneous Vasculitis

SMALL VESSEL NON-ANCA ASSOCIATED VASCULITIS
- subdivided into
  - drug-induced vasculitis
  - serum sickness reaction
  - vasculitis associated with other underlying primary diseases

Etiology and Pathophysiology
- cutaneous vasculitis following:
  - drug exposure (allopurinol, gold, sulfonamides, penicillin, phenytoin)
  - viral or bacterial infection
  - idiopathic causes
- small vessels involved (post-capillary vessels most frequently)
- usually causes a leukocytoclastic vasculitis = debris from neutrophils around vessels
- sometimes due to cryoglobulins which precipitate in cold temperatures

Signs and Symptoms
- palpable purpura ± vesicles and ulceration, urticaria, macules, papules, bullae, subcutaneous nodules

Investigations
- vascular involvement (both arteriole and venule) established by skin biopsy

Treatment
- stop possible offending drug
- usually self-limiting
- corticosteroids ± immunosuppressive agents

Wegener's Granulomatosis

SMALL VESSEL ANCA-ASSOCIATED VASCULITIS

Definition
- granulomatous inflammation of vessels that may affect the upper airways (rhinitis, sinusitis), lungs (pulmonary nodules, infiltrates), and kidneys (glomerulonephritis, renal failure)
- highly associated with cytoplasmic anti-neutrophil cytoplasmic antibody (c-ANCA)
- incidence 5 per 100,000; more common in Northern latitudes

Classic Features:
- necrotizing granulomatous vasculitis of lower and upper respiratory tract
- focal segmental glomerulonephritis

Diagnosis
- diagnosis with 2 of 4 criteria (American College of Rheumatology, 1990)
  1. nasal or oral inflammation, ulcers, epistaxis
  2. abnormal findings on CXR, including nodules, cavitations
  3. urinary sediment (protein, RBC casts)
  4. biopsy of involved tissue: lungs show granulomas, and kidneys show necrotizing segmental glomerulonephritis

Etiology and Pathophysiology
- transformation from inflammatory prodrome (serous otitis media and sinusitis) to full-blown vasculitic syndrome

Signs and Symptoms
- systemic
  - malaise, fever, weakness, weight loss
- ENT
  - sinusitis or rhinitis, nasal crusting, nasoseptal perforation, saddle nose deformity, extension into the orbit with proptosis, hearing loss
- pulmonary
  - cough, hemoptysis
- other
  - joint, skin, eye complaints, vasculitic neuropathy

Investigations
- routine investigations
  - bloodwork: decreased Hb (normal MCV), increased WBC, increased Cr, increased ESR
  - urinalysis: proteinuria, hematuria
  - CXR: pneumonitis, lung nodules, infiltrations, cavitary lesions
- other tests include
  - specific: ANCA (c-ANCA > p-ANCA)
  - biopsy: renal (segmental necrotizing glomerulonephritis), lung (trachcobronchial erosion)
- possible decline in c-ANCA and ESR used to monitor response to treatment in some patients

Treatment
- prednisone 1 mg/kg for 3-6 months ± cyclophosphamide 2 mg/kg/day PO for 3-6 months followed by high dose methotrexate (20-25 mg PO/SC weekly) or azathioprine (2 mg/kg PO OD)
- consider biologic agents (infliximab, rituximab, IVIg) and plasmapheresis in systemic disease resistant to corticosteroids plus cyclophosphamide

Polyarteritis Nodosa (PAN)

MEDIUM VESSEL VASCULITIS

Definition
- pauci-immune necrotizing vasculitis of medium to small vessles, without associated glomerulonephritis or pulmonary capillaritis (as seen in microscopic polyangiitis)
- incidence 0.7 per 100,000; affects inviduals between 40-60 yrs; M:F = 2:1

Etiology and Pathophysiology
- focal panmural necrotizing inflammatory lesions in small and medium-sized arteries
- thrombosis, aneurysm or dilatation at lesion site may occur
- healed lesions show proliferation of fibrous tissue and endothelial cells that may lead to luminal occlusion

There is an association between hepatitis B surface antigen (HBsAg) positivity and PAN.

Diagnosis
- diagnosis with >3 of 10 criteria (American Collegue of Rheumatology, 1990)
  - weight loss >4 kg
  - myalgias, weakness or leg tenderness
  - livedo reticularis (mottled reticular pattern over skin)
  - neuropathy
  - testicular pain or tenderness
  - diastolic BP >90 mmHg
  - elevated Cr or BUN
  - hepatitis B positive
  - arteriographic abnormality (commonly aneurysms)
  - biopsy of artery showing presence of granulocytes or macronuclear leukocytes in the artery wall

Consider PAN in a non-diabetic patient with mononeuritis multiplex.

Treatment
- prednisone 1 mg/kg/day ± cyclophosphamide 2 mg/kg/day PO
- ± anti-viral therapy to enhance clearance of HBV

Giant Cell Arteritis (GCA)/Temporal Arteritis

LARGE VESSEL VASCULITIS

Signs and Symptoms
- temporal headaches ± scalp tenderness due to inflammation of involved portion of the temporal or occipital arteries
- sudden, painless loss of vision and/or diplopia due to narrowing of the ophthalmic or posterior ciliary arteries
- tongue and jaw claudication (pain in muscles of mastication on chewing)
- polymyalgia rheumatica (proximal myalgia, constitutional symptoms, elevated ESR) occurs in 30% of patients
- aortic arch syndrome (involvement of subclavian and brachial branches of aorta result in pulseless disease), aortic aneurysm ± rupture

Medical Emergency
Untreated, GCA can lead to permanent blindness in 20-25%!

Investigations
- diagnosis made by clinical suspicion, increased ESR, increased CRP, temporal artery biopsy within 14 days of starting steroids, angiography

Treatment
- if suspect GCA, immediately start high dose prednisone 1 mg/kg in divided doses tapering prednisone as symptoms resolve; highly effective in treatment and in prevention of blindness and other vascular complications
- ASA 325 mg tid

GCA CRITERIA
- age >50
- new headache
- temporal artery tenderness or decreased pulse
- ESR over 50
- abnormal artery biopsy
Presence of 3 or more criteria yields sensitivity of 94%, specificity of 91%.

Investigations

Bloodwork, Urinalysis, Synovial fluid analysis
- general: CBC, BUN, creatinine
- acute phase reactants: complement (C3 and C4), fibrinogen, CRP, ferritin, albumin
- ESR increases with the increase of acute phase reactants, and chronically, with increase in gamma globulins
- C3, C4 often decrease in active SLE
- urinalysis to detect disease complications (proteinuria, active sediment)
- serology: autoantibodies (Table 13, RH18)
- synovial fluid analysis (Table 18, RH24)
- radiology (plain film, CT, MRI, ultrasound, bone densitometry, angiography, bone scan)

Differential Diagnosis of Elevated ESR
Rheumatoid arthritis, PMR, GCA, hypoalbuminemia, anemia, multiple myeloma, bacterial infections, malignancy. ESR (and CRP) is insensitive for PM/DM, AS, PSS, SLE, viral infections.

Table 13. Autoantibodies and Their Prevalence in Rheumatic Diseases

Autoantibody	Disease	Normal	Comments
RF	RA 80% Sjögren's 50% SLE 20%	<5%	Autoantibodies (IgM > IgG > IgA) directed against Fc domain of IgG 10-20% over age 65 Present in most seropositive diseases Levels correlate with disease severity in RA Non-specific; may be present in IE, tuberculosis, hep C infections, silicosis, sarcoidosis
Anti-CCP	RA 80%		
ANA	SLE 98% MCTD 95% Sjögren's 70-90% CREST 80%	<5% other CTDs	Antibodies against nuclear components (DNA, RNA, histones, centromere) 1:40 dilution found in 5-30% of the normal population Sensitive but not specific for SLE 4 patterns: 1) Rim pattern in SLE 2) Homogenous (diffuse) pattern in SLE, RA, drug-induced lupus 3) Speckled pattern in SLE, PSS, RA, MCTD, Sjögren's, scleroderma 4) Nucleolar pattern in scleroderma
Anti-dsDNA	SLE 50-70%	0%	Specific for SLE Levels correlate with disease activity
Anti-Sm	SLE <30%	0%	Specific but not sensitive for SLE
Anti-Ro (SSA)	Sjögren's 40-95%	0.5%	Subacute cutaneous SLE and mothers of babies with neonatal lupus SLE 25%
Anti-La (SSB)	Sjögren's 40% SLE 10%	0%	Usually occurs with anti-Ro
Antiphospholipid antibodies (LAC, ACLA)	APS SLE 31-40%	<5%	By definition present in APS Only small subset of SLE patients develop clinical syndrome of APS If positive will get a false positive VDRL test
Anti-histone	Drug-induced SLE >90% Idiopathic SLE >50%	0% 0%	
Anti-RNP	MCTD	0%	By definition present in MCTD; present in many other CTD
Anti-centromere Anti-topoisomerase I (formerly Scl-70)	CREST >80% PSS 26-76%	0% 0%	Specific for CREST variant of PSS
c-ANCA	Active Wegener's >90%	0%	Specific and sensitive
p-ANCA	Wegener's 10%, other vasculitis	0%	Nonspecific and poor sensitivity (found in ulcerative colitis, polyarteritis nodosa, microscopic polyangiitis, Churg-Strauss, rapidly progressive glomerulonephritis)
Anti-Mi-2	Dermatomyositis 15-20%		Specific but not sensitive
Antibodies against RBCs, WBCs, or platelets	SLE		Perform direct Coomb's test Test hemoglobin, reticulocyte, leukocyte and platelet count, antiplatelet Abs

Seronegative Rheumatic Diseases

Table 14. A Comparison of the Spondyloarthropathies

Feature	AS	PsA	ReA	IBD
M:F	5:1	1:1	8:1	1:1
Age onset	20's	35-45	20's	any
Peripheral arthritis	25%	96%	90%	Common
Distribution	Axial, LE	Any	LE	LE
Sacroiliitis	100%	40%	80%	20%
Dactylitis	Uncommon	35%	Common	Uncommon
Enthesitis	Common	Common	Common	Less Common
Skin lesions	Rare	100%	Common	Occasional
	Nil specific	Psoriasis	Keratoderma	Pyoderma, Erythema Nodosum
Uveitis	30%	Occasional	20%	Rare
Urethritis	Rare	Occasional	Common	Rare
Aortic Regurgitation	Occasional	Rare	Occasional	Occasional
HLA-B27	90%	40%	80%	30%

Ankylosing Spondylitis (AS)

Definition
- inflammatory arthritis involving the sacroiliac joints and vertebrae (see Figure 11)
- prototype of the spondyloarthropathies

Etiology and Pathophysiology
- enthesitis (inflammation of tendon or ligament at site of attachment to bone)
- inflammation leads to osteopenia, then erosion, then ossification

Epidemiology
- prevalence 0.2% of general population
- M:F = 5:1; females have milder disease
- 95% of patients have HLA-B27 (9% HLA-B27 positive in general population)

Signs and Symptoms
- axial
  - mid and lower back stiffness, prolonged morning stiffness, pain during the second half of the night, persistent buttock pain, painful sacroiliac joint (Faber's test) (see Table 15)
  - spinal restriction (decreased ROM): lumbar (decreased Schöber), thoracic (decreased chest wall expansion, normal >5 cm at T4), cervical (global decrease, often extension first)
  - postural changes: decreased lumbar lordosis, increase thoracic kyphosis, increase cervical flexion; net result is an increase in occiput to wall distance
- peripheral
  - asymmetrical large joint peripheral arthritis, most often involving lower limb
- extra-articular manifestations
  - ophthalmic: acute anterior uveitis (25-30% patients)
  - cardiac: aortitis, aortic regurgitation, pericarditis, conduction disturbances, heart failure (rare)
  - renal: amyloidosis and IgA nephropathy
  - respiratory: apical fibrosis (rare)
  - neurologic: cauda equina syndrome (rare)

Investigations
- x-ray of SI joint: "pseudowidening" of joint due to erosion with joint sclerosis → bony fusion (late), symmetric sacroiliitis
- x-ray of spine: appearance of "squaring of edges" from erosion and sclerosis on corners of vertebral bodies leading to ossification of outer fibres of annulus fibrosis (bridging syndesmophytes), this produces a "bamboo spine" radiographically

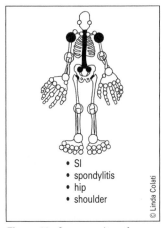

Figure 11. Common sites of involvement of AS

- SI
- spondylitis
- hip
- shoulder

© Linda Colati

Extra-articular Manifestations of Ankylosing Spondylitis (6 As):
Atlanto-axial subluxation
Anterior uveitis
Apical lung fibrosis
Aortic incompetence
Amyloidosis (kidneys)
Autoimmune bowel disease (UC)

Consider AS in the differential for causes of aortic regurgitation.

Table 15. Types of Back Pain

Parameter	Mechanical	Inflammatory
Past History	±	++
Family History	–	+
Onset	Acute	Insidious
Age (years)	15-90	<40
Sleep Disturbance	±	++
Morning Stiffness	<30 minutes	>1 hour
Involvement of Other Systems	–	+
Exercise	Worse	Better
Rest	Better	Worse
Radiation of Pain	Anatomic (L5-S1)	Diffuse (thoracic, buttock)
Sensory Symptoms	+	–
Motor Symptoms	+	–

Treatment
- conservative/non-pharmacologic
  - heat
  - prevent fusion in poor posture and disability by: exercise (e.g. swimming), postural and deep breathing exercises, outpatient PT, smoking cessation

- **medical**
  - NSAIDs
  - DMARDs for peripheral arthritis (sulfasalazine, methotrexate)
  - Biologics for axial involvement
  - manage extra-articular manifestations
- **surgical**
  - hip replacement, vertebral osteotomy for marked deformity

Prognosis
- spontaneous remissions and relapses are common and can occur at any age
- function may be excellent despite spinal deformity
- favorable prognosis if female and age of onset >40
- early onset with hip disease may lead to severe disability; may require arthroplasty

Reactive Arthritis

Definition
- a generic term for a sterile arthritis following an infection (e.g. rheumatic fever, post viral arthritis etc.)
- when capitalized i.e. Reactive Arthritis (ReA), it refers to one of the seronegative spondyloarthropathies in which patients have a peripheral arthritis (of greater than 1 month duration) accompanied by one or more extra-articular manifestations, that appears shortly after certain infections of the GI or GU tracts

Etiology
- onset following an infectious episode either involving the GI or GU tract
  - GI: *Shigella, Salmonella, Campylobacter, Yersinia* species
  - GU: *Chlamydia* (isolated in 16-44% of ReA cases), *Mycoplasma* species
- acute pattern of clinical course
  - 1-4 weeks post-infection
  - lasts weeks to years with 1/3 chronic
  - often recurring
  - spinal involvement persists

Epidemiology
- in HLA-B27 patients, axial > peripheral involvement
- M>F

Signs and Symptoms
- **musculoskeletal**
  - peripheral arthritis, asymmetric pattern, spondylitis (thick and skipped syndesmophytes), Achilles tendinitis, plantar fasciitis, dactylitis ("sausage digits")
- **ophthalmic**
  - iritis (anterior uveitis), conjunctivitis
- **dermatologic**
  - keratoderma blenorrhagicum (hyperkeratotic skin lesions on palms and soles) and balanitis circinata (small, shallow, painless ulcers of glans penis and urethral meatus) are diagnostic
- **gastrointestinal**
  - oral ulcers, diarrhea
- **urethritis and cervicitis**
  - sterile cultures; presence not related to site of initiating infection

Investigations
- diagnosis is clinical plus laboratory
- lab findings: normocytic, normochromic anemia and leukocytosis
- cultures are sterile
- HLA-B27 positive

Treatment
- appropriate antibiotics if non-articular infection is present
- NSAIDs, physical therapy, home exercise
- local therapy
  - joint protection
  - intra-articular steroid injection
  - topical steroid for ocular involvement
- systemic therapy
  - corticosteroids, sulfasalazine, methotrexate (for peripheral joint involvement only)
  - TNF inhibitors for spinal inflammation

The triad of arthritis, conjunctivitis, and urethritis is 99% specific (but 51% sensitive) for ReA.

Look for genetic predisposition (HLA-B27) and infection.

Psoriatic Arthritis

Etiology and Pathophysiology
- unclear but many genetic, immunologic and some environmental factors involved (e.g. psoriatic plaque flora, particularly Group A *Streptococcus*, and trauma)

Epidemiology
- psoriasis affects 1% of population
- arthropathy in 10% of patients with psoriasis
- 15-20% of patients will develop joint disease before skin lesions appear

Signs and Symptoms
- **dermatolgic**
  - well-demarcated erythematous plaques with silvery scale
  - nail involvement includes pitting, transverse or longitudinal ridging, discolouration, subungual hyperkeratosis, onycholysis, and oil drops
- **musculoskeletal**
  - 5 general patterns
    - asymmetric oligoarthritis (most common – 70%)
    - arthritis of DIP joints with nail changes
    - destructive (mutilans) arthritis (5%)
    - symmetric polyarthritis (similar to RA)
    - sacroiliitis and spondylitis (usually older, male patients)
- **ophthalmic**
  - conjunctivitis, iritis (uveitis)
- **cardiac and respiratory** (late findings)
  - aortic insufficiency
  - apical lung fibrosis
- **neurologic**
  - cauda equina syndrome
- **radiologic**
  - floating syndesmophytes
  - pencil and cup appearance at IP joints
  - osteolysis, periostitis

Treatment
- treat skin disease (e.g. steroid cream, salicylic and/or retinoic acid, tar, UV light)
- NSAIDs or intra-articular steroids
- DMARDs, biologic therapies to minimize erosive disease (use early if peripheral joint involvement)
- spinal disease → biologic therapies

Check "hidden" areas for psoriatic lesions (ears, hair line, umbilicus, anal cleft, nails).

Risks and benefits of tumour necrosis factor-alpha inhibitors in the management of psoriatic arthritis: systematic review and metaanalysis of randomized controlled trials.
J Rheumatol. 2008;35:883-90.
Purpose: To evaluate the efficacy and safety of tumour necrosis factor-alpha (TNF-alpha) inhibitors in the management of psoriatic arthritis (PsA).
Study Selection: Randomized controlled trials (RCT) of adalimumab, etanercept, and infliximab used in patients with PsA.
Results: Six RCT met the inclusion criteria, including 982 patients. All 3 TNF-alpha inhibitors were significantly more effective than placebo on the basis of Psoriatic Arthritis Response Criteria (PsARC) and American College of Rheumatology response criteria ACR20, ACR50, and ACR70 ratings. There were no significant differences between TNF-alpha inhibitors and placebo in the proportions of patients who withdrew for any reason (RR 0.48, 95% CI 0.20-1.18), or withdrawal due to adverse events (RR 2.14, 95% CI 0.73-6.27), serious adverse events (RR 0.98, 95% CI 0.55-1.77), or upper respiratory tract infections (RR 0.91, 95% CI 0.65-1.28). Pooled rates for injection site reactions were significantly higher for adalimumab and etanercept than for placebo (RR 2.48, 95% CI 1.16-5.29), but there was no significant difference in the proportion of patients experiencing infusion reactions with infliximab (RR 1.03, 95% CI 0.48-2.20) compared to placebo. Indirect analysis did not demonstrate any significant differences between the TNF-alpha inhibitors.
Conclusions: TNF-alpha inhibitors are effective treatments for PsA with no important added risks associated with their short-term use. There is still a need for longterm risk-benefit assessment of using these drugs for the management of PsA.

Inflammatory Bowel Disease (IBD)

- see Gastroenterology
- manifestations of ulcerative colitis and Crohn's disease include peripheral arthritis (large joint, asymmetrical), spondylitis, and hypertrophic osteoarthropathy
- arthralgia, myalgia, osteoporosis and aseptic necrosis of bone 2° to steroid treatment of bowel inflammation
- NSAIDs should be used cautiously as they may exacerbate bowel disease

Both ankylosing spondylitis and IBD-arthritis feature symmetric sacroiliitis.

Table 16. Comparing Features of Spondylitis vs. Peripheral Arthritis in IBD

Parameter	Spondylitis	Peripheral Arthritis
HLA-B27 association	yes	no
gender	M>F	M=F
onset before IBD	yes	no
parallels IBD course	no	yes
type of IBD	UC = Crohn's	Crohn's

Undifferentiated Spondyloarthropathy

- does not meet criteria for any of the well defined spondyloarthropathies
- generally good prognosis and responds well to NSAIDs

Crystal-Induced Arthropathies

Table 17. Gout vs. Pseudogout

Parameter	Gout	Pseudogout
Gender	M>F	M=F
Age	Middle-aged males Post-menopausal females	Older
Onset of disease	Acute	Acute/insidious
Crystal type	Negative birefringence, (yellow when parallel), needle-shaped	Positive birefringence, (blue when parallel), rhomboid-shaped
Distribution	First MTP, foot	Knee, wrist, polyarticular
Radiology	"Holes in bones"	Chondrocalcinosis OA (knee, wrist, 2nd and 3rd MCP)
Treatment	Indomethacin, colchicine, allopurinol	NSAIDs

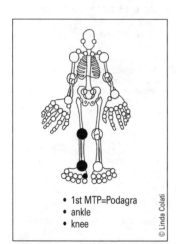

- 1st MTP=Podagra
- ankle
- knee

© Linda Colati

Figure 12. Common sites of involvement in gout (asymmetric joint involvement)

An acute gout attack may mimic cellulitis. However, joint mobility is preserved in cellulitis.

Sudden changes in uric acid concentration are more important than absolute values. Therefore, changes in pH, temperature or initiation of antihyperuricemics may precipitate an acute gouty attack.

Precipitants of Gout

Drugs are FACT:
Furosemide
Aspirin/**A**lcohol
Cytotoxic drugs
Thiazide diuretics

Foods are SALTS:
Shellfish
Anchovies
Liver and Kidney
Turkey
Sardines

Gout

Definition
- derangement in purine metabolism resulting in hyperuricemia, monosodium urate crystal deposits in tissues (tophi), synovium (microtophi)

Etiology and Pathogenesis
- sources of uric acid: diet and endogenous
- synthesis
  - hypoxanthine → xanthine → uric acid
  - both steps catalyzed by xanthine oxidase

Hyperuricemia
- **primary or genetic**
  - mostly due to idiopathic renal underexcretion (90%)
  - also idiopathic overproduction or abnormal enzyme production/function
- **secondary**
  - dietary excess
  - underexcretion (>90%) – renal failure, drugs, systemic conditions
  - overproduction (<10%) – increased nucleic acid turnover states
- majority of people with hyperuricemia do not have gout, and normal or low uric acid levels do not rule out gout
- common precipitants: EtOH, dietary excess, dehydration (e.g. thiazide and loop diuretics), trauma, illness, surgery
- other associated conditions: hypertension, obesity, diabetes, starvation

Epidemiology
- most common in males >45 years old
- extremely rare in premenopausal female

Signs and Symptoms
- recurrent episodes of acute arthritis
- **acute gouty arthritis**
  - painful, usually involving lower extremities (see Figure 12)
  - joint mobility may be limited
  - attack will subside on its own within several days to weeks and may or may not recur
- **tophi**
  - urate deposits in cartilage, tendons, bursae, soft tissues, and synovial membranes
  - common sites: first MTP, ear helix, olecranon bursae, tendon insertions (common in Achilles tendon)
- **kidney**
  - gouty nephropathy
  - uric acid calculi

Investigations
- joint aspirate: >90% of joint aspirates show crystals of monosodium urate (see Table 18, RH24) (negatively birefringent)
- differential diagnosis includes pseudogout, trauma, sepsis, OA

Treatment

A) acute gout
- NSAIDs: high dose, then taper as symptoms improve
- corticosteroids: intra-articular, oral or intra-muscular (if renal, cardiovascular or GI disease and/or if NSAIDs contraindicated or fail)
- colchicine within first 24 hours but effectiveness limited by narrow therapeutic range
- allopurinol can worsen an acute attack (**therefore do not start during acute flare**)

B) chronic gout
- not the same as treatment of acute gout
- **conservative**
  - avoid foods with high purine content (e.g. visceral meats, sardines, shellfish, beans, peas), avoid drugs with hyperuricemic effects (e.g. pyrazinamide, ethambutol, thiazide, alcohol)
- **medical**
  - antihyperuricemic drugs: decrease uric acid production (allopurinol and febuxostat inhibit xanthine oxidase)
  - uricosuric drugs (probenecid, sulfinpyrazone): use if failure on or intolerant to allopurinol; do not use in renal failure
- prophylaxis prior to starting antihyperuricemic drugs (colchicine/low-dose NSAID)
- in renal disease secondary to hyperuricemia, use low-dose allopurinol and monitor creatinine

Pseudogout (Chondrocalcinosis)

Etiology and Pathophysiology
- acute inflammatory arthritis due to phagocytosis of IgG-coated calcium pyrophosphate dihydrate (CPPD) crystals by neutrophils and subsequent release of inflammatory mediators within joint space

Epidemiology
- more frequently polyarticular, slower in onset in comparison to gout, lasts up to 3 weeks but is self-limited
- risk factors: old age, advanced OA, neuropathic joints
- other associated conditions: hyperparathyroidism, hypothyroidism, hypomagnesemia, hypophosphatasia (low ALP), diabetes, hemochromatosis

Signs and Symptoms
- affects knees, wrist, MCPs, hips, shoulders, elbows, ankles, big toe (see Figure 13)
- may present as chronic arthritis with acute exacerbations
- 5% will mimic rheumatoid arthritis (symmetrical polyarticular pattern with morning stiffness and constitutional symptoms)
- may be triggered by dehydration, acute illness, surgery, trauma
- 50% of the patients will develop degenerative joint changes

Investigations
- must aspirate joint to rule out septic arthritis, gout
- crystals of CPPD: present in 60% of patients and often only a few crystals
- x-rays show chondrocalcinosis: radiodensities in fibrocartilaginous structures (e.g. knee menisci) or linear radiodensities in hyaline articular cartilage
- chondrocalcinosis seen in 75% of pseudogout
- differential diagnosis includes gout, trauma, sepsis, RA

Treatment
- joint aspiration, rest, and protection
- NSAIDs – also used for maintenance therapy
- prophylactic colchicine PO (controversial)
- intra-articular or oral steroids to relieve inflammation

Synovial Fluid Analysis

- synovial fluid is an ultrafiltrate of plasma plus hyaluronate; it lubricates joint surfaces and nourishes articular cartilage

Three Most Important Tests of Synovial Fluid (The Three Cs)
1. Cell count and differential
2. Culture and Gram stain (bacteria, mycobacteria, fungi)
3. Crystal examination (microscopy with polarized light)
   - gout (monosodium urate) → needle-shaped, negatively birefringent (yellow)
   - pseudogout (calcium pyrophosphate dihydrate) → rhomboid-shaped, positively birefringent (blue)
- protein, LDH, glucose less helpful

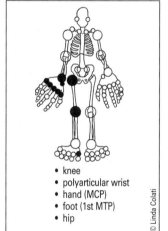

- knee
- polyarticular wrist
- hand (MCP)
- foot (1st MTP)
- hip

© Linda Colati

Figure 13. Common sites of involvement in CPPD

Differential Diagnosis of Acute Monoarthritis
- septic arthritis (see Infectious Diseases, ID22)
- gout
- pseudogout
- trauma
- hemarthrosis
- osteonecrosis
- osteoarthritis
- tumour
- systemic inflammatory disease
- polyarthritis presenting with monoarticular symptoms

Table 18. Synovial Fluid Analysis

Parameter	Normal	Non-Inflammatory	Inflammatory	Infectious	Hemorrhagic
Colour	Clear	Clear	Opaque	Opaque	Sanguinous
Viscosity	High (due to hyaluronate)	High	Low	Low	Variable
WBC/mm³	<200	<2,000	>2,000	>50,000	Variable
% PMN	<25%	<25%	>25%	>50%	Variable
Examples		Trauma Osteoarthritis Neuropathy Hypertrophic - arthropathy	Seropositives Seronegatives Crystal arthropathies	Septic arthritis	Trauma Hemophilia CPPD

Non-Articular Rheumatism

- disorders that primarily affect soft tissues or periarticular structures
- includes bursitis, tendinitis, tenosynovitis, fibromyalgia and polymyalgia rheumatica

Polymyalgia Rheumatica (PMR)

Definition
- characterized by profound pain and stiffness of the proximal extremities (girdle area)
- closely related to giant cell arteritis (15% of patients with PMR develop GCA)
- no weakness

Diagnosis
- age >50 years
- more than two affected muscle groups
- at least a one month duration
- increased ESR
- rapid and lasting response to corticosteroids
- must rule out infection, RA, SLE, PAN, polymyositis, malignancy, and giant cell arteritis

Epidemiology
- incidence 50 per 100,000 per year in those over age 50
- age of onset typically >50, F:M = 2:1

Signs and Symptoms
- constitutional symptoms prominent (fever, weight loss, malaise)
- morning stiffness of symmetrical proximal muscles (neck, shoulder and hip girdles, thighs)
- physical examination reveals tender muscles but no weakness or atrophy

Investigations
- bloodwork often shows anemia, elevated platelets, ESR and CRP; normal CK

Treatment
- goal of therapy: symptom relief
- start with steroid dose of 15-20 mg PO daily
- taper slowly over 2-year period monitoring ESR and symptoms closely
- treat relapses aggressively (50% relapse rate)

PMR Criteria
1. Age over 50
2. Bilateral aching/morning stiffness >1 month
3. ESR over 40 mm/hr
4. Prompt response to low-dose corticosteroids

Prednisone plus methotrexate for polymyalgia rheumatica: a randomized, double-blind, placebo-controlled trial
Ann Intern Med. 2004;141:493-500.
Study: Multicenter randomized, double-blind, placebo-controlled trial.
Patients: Patients with newly diagnosed polymyalgia rheumatica.
Intervention: Prednisone dosage (25 mg/d) was tapered to 0 mg/d within 24 weeks and was adjusted if flare-ups occurred. Oral methotrexate (10 mg) or placebo, with folinic acid supplementation (7.5 mg), was given weekly for 48 weeks.
Primary Outcome: The proportion of patients no longer taking prednisone, the number of flare-ups, and the cumulative prednisone dose after 76 weeks.
Results: Twenty-eight of 32 patients in the methotrexate group and 16 of 30 patients in the placebo group were no longer taking prednisone at 76 weeks (P = 0.003). The risk difference was 34 percentage points (95% CI, 11 to 53 percentage points). Similar results were obtained after adjustment for C-reactive protein level and duration of symptoms in a multivariate model. Fifteen of 32 patients in the methotrexate group and 22 of 30 patients in the placebo group had at least 1 flare-up by the end of follow-up (P = 0.04). The median prednisone dose was 2.1 g in the methotrexate group and 2.97 g in the placebo group (P = 0.03). The rate and severity of adverse events were similar.
Limitations: Follow-up was short, and a high dose of folinic acid and a relatively high starting dosage of prednisone were used. Ten of 72 patients (14%) discontinued treatment or were lost to follow-up.
Conclusions: Prednisone plus methotrexate is associated with shorter prednisone treatment and steroid sparing. It may be useful in patients at high risk for steroid-related toxicity.

Fibromyalgia

Definition
- chronic, widespread pain with characteristic tender points

Diagnosis
- history of widespread pain for at least 3 months in four quadrants of body
- pain in 11 of 18 tender points with approximate force of 4 kg by digital palpation
- must rule out numerous other causes (e.g. polymyositis, polymyalgia rheumatica, thyroid disorders, sleep apnea), although presence of second clinical disorder does not exclude the diagnosis of fibromyalgia

Epidemiology
- F:M = 3:1
- primarily ages 25 to 45, some adolescents
- prevalence of 2-5% in general population, higher in rheumatology patients
- overlaps with chronic fatigue syndrome and myofascial pain syndrome
- strong association with psychiatric illness

Investigations
- laboratory investigations typically normal unless underlying illness present
- workup includes: TSH, ESR, laboratory sleep assessment

Signs and Symptoms
- widespread aching, stiffness and reproducible tender points (see Figure 14)
- fatigue
- sleep disturbance: non-restorative sleep, difficulty falling asleep, and frequent wakening
- symptoms aggravated by physical activity, poor sleep, emotional stress
- patient feels that joints are diffusely swollen although joint examination is normal
- neurologic symptoms of hyperalgesia, paresthesias
- associated with irritable bowel or bladder syndrome, migraines, tension headaches, obesity, depression, and anxiety

Treatment
- conservative
  - education – disease is benign, non-deforming and does not progress
  - exercise program (walking, aquatic exercises)
  - support back and neck: neck support while sleeping, abdominal muscle strengthening exercises
  - stress reduction; psychiatric treatment when necessary
  - biofeedback, meditation, acupuncture, physiotherapy may be helpful
- medical
  - low dose tricyclic antidepressant (e.g. amitriptyline)
    - for sleep restoration
    - select those with lower anticholinergic side effects
  - analgesics or NSAIDs may be beneficial for pain that interferes with sleep
  - pregabalin (Lyrica™) has shown some benefit

A 14-week, Randomized, Double-Blinded, Placebo-Controlled Monotherapy Trial of Pregabalin in Patients With Fibromyalgia
J Pain. 2008 Jun 2.
Study: Multicentre, randomized, double-blinded, placebo-controlled trial.
Patients: Patients (n=750) meeting American College of Rheumatology criteria for fibromyalgia and who had a pain score of at least 40 mm on the 100-mm pain visual analog scale (VAS).
Intervention: Patients were randomly assigned to placebo or pregabalin (300 mg/d, 450 mg/d, or 600 mg/d) given twice daily in equally divided doses for 12 weeks.
Primary Outcome: Change in the mean pain score derived from the subject's daily pain diary as measured at the patient's baseline to the end point of the study.
Results: Patients in 2 pregabalin treatment groups (450 and 600 mg/d pregabalin) showed a statistically significant improvement in the end point mean pain score compared with placebo-treated subjects (mean difference, -0.50; P = .0147 [450 mg/d] and -0.45, P = .0287 [600 mg/d]). The =30% responder rate was 30% (56/184) in the placebo arm and 42% (76/183) in the 300 mg/d, 50% (94/190) in the 450 mg/d, and 48% (88/188) in the 600 mg/d pregabalin arms (P = .0172, P = .0002, P = .0006, respectively), whereas the =50% responder rate was 15% (28/184) for placebo, 24% (44/183) for 300 mg/d, 27% (52/190) for 450 mg/d, and 30% (57/188) for 600 mg/d (P = .0372, P = .0038, P = .0010, respectively). The number needed to treat (NNT) for the =30% response rate was 9.01 for 300 mg/d, 5.25 for 450 mg/d, and 5.73 for 600 mg/d. The NNT for the =50% responder rate was 11.33 for 300 mg/d, 8.23 for 450 mg/d, and 6.62 for 600 mg/d. Discontinuations due to adverse events were 12%, 16%, 22%, and 26% in placebo and pregabalin 300, 450, and 600 mg/d groups, respectively. The 450 and 600 mg/d groups were significantly different from placebo (P = .0001).
Conclusions: Pregabalin at 300 mg/d, 450 mg/d, and 600 mg/d showed statistically significant response rates as compared to placebo although discontinuation rates for the 450 mg/d and 600 mg/d regimens were significantly higher as compared to placebo.

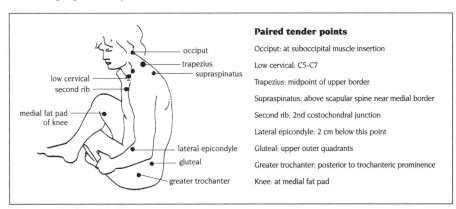

Paired tender points

Occiput: at suboccipital muscle insertion

Low cervical: C5-C7

Trapezius: midpoint of upper border

Supraspinatus: above scapular spine near medial border

Second rib: 2nd costochondral junction

Lateral epicondyle: 2 cm below this point

Gluteal: upper outer quadrants

Greater trochanter: posterior to trochanteric prominence

Knee: at medial fat pad

Figure 14. Tender Point Sites

Summary of Arthritic Diseases

Table 19. Classification of Arthritis and Characteristic Features

Classification	Characteristic Features
Degenerative	
Osteoarthritis (OA)	Insidious onset
	Older age (>50 years old)
	Negative serology
Seropositive rheumatic diseases	
1. *Connective Tissue Disease*	Serologic markers helpful
Rheumatoid Arthritis (RA)	Constitutional symptoms
Systemic lupus erythematosus (SLE)	Skin nodules, ulcers, rash
Antiphospholipid antibody syndrome (APS)	Raynaud's phenomenon
Scleroderma/progressive systemic sclerosis (PSS)	Vascular involvement
Polymyositis (PM)/dermatomyositis (DM)	Renal involvement
Mixed connective tissue disease (MCTD)	Neurological involvement
Sjögren's syndrome	Sicca syndrome
2. *Vasculitides*	see Table 12
Polyarteritis nodosa (PAN)	Medium vessel disease
Microscopic polyangiitis	Small vessel disease, ANCA associated
Wegener's granulomatosis	Small vessel disease, ANCA associated
Predominantly cutaneous vasculitis	Small vessel disease, non-ANCA associated
Giant cell arteritis (GCA)	Large vessel disease
Seronegative rheumatic diseases	Axial skeleton involvement
Ankylosing spondylitis (AS)	Anterior uveitis, conjunctivitis, urethritis
Reactive arthritis	Enthesitis, sacroiliitis, dactylitis, urethritis
Psoriatic arthritis	Psoriasis, keratoderma, E. nodosum
Inflammatory bowel disease (IBD)	Family history and HLA-B27 association
Crystal-induced	Remitting, recurring pattern
Gout (monosodium urate)	Mono or oligoarthritis
Pseudogout (calcium pyrophosphate dihydrate)	Tophi
Hydroxyapatite deposition disease	Renal involvement
Septic/infectious	Acute monoarthritis or migratory polyarthritis
	Constitutional symptoms
Non-Articular	
Localized (bursitis, capsulitis, tendinitis, myositis)	Periarticular structures affected
Generalized (fibromyalgia, polymyalgia rheumatica)	Trigger points

Common Medications

Table 20. Common Medications for Osteoarthritis

Class	Generic Drug Name	Trade Name	Dosing	Indications	Contraindications	Adverse Effects
	acetaminophen	Tylenol™	500 mg tid	1st line		Hepatotoxicity Overdose >10 g Potentiates warfarin
NSAIDs	ECASA ibuprofen diclofenac diclofenac/misoprostol naproxen meloxicam	 Advil,™ Motrin™ Voltaren™ Arthrotec™ Naprosyn™, Aleve™ Mobicox™	325-975 mg qid 200-600 mg tid 25-50 mg tid 50-75/200 mg tid 125-500 mg bid 7.5-15 mg OD	2nd line	GI bleed Renal impairment Allergy to ASA, NSAIDs Pregnancy (T3)	Nausea, tinnitus, vertigo, rash, dyspepsia, GI bleed, PUD, hepatitis, renal failure, HTN, nephrotic syndrome
COX-2 Inhibitors	celecoxib	Celebrex™	200 mg OD	High risk for GI bleed: age >65 hx of GI bleed, PUD	Renal impairment Sulfa allergy (celecoxib) Cardiovascular disease	Delayed ulcer healing Renal/hepatic impairment Rash

Other treatments	Comments
Combination analgesics (acetaminophen + codeine)	Enhanced short term effect compared to acetaminophen alone More adverse effects: sedation, constipation, nausea, GI upset
Intra-articular corticosteroid injection	Short-term (weeks-months) decrease in pain and improvement in function Do not inject >3-4 times/year in the same joint
Intra-articular hyaluronan q6months	Modest decrease in pain Used for mild-moderate OA of the knees Precaution with chicken/egg allergy
Topical NSAIDs	1.5% wt/wt topical diclofenac (Pennsaid) May use for patients who fail acetaminophen treatment and who wish to avoid systemic therapy
Capsaicin cream	Mild decrease in pain
Glucosamine sulfate/chondroitin	Limited clinical studies No regulation by Health Canada

Table 21. DMARDs Used in the Treatment of Rheumatoid Arthritis

Genetic Drug Name	Trade Name	Dosing	Contraindications	Adverse Effects
COMMONLY USED				
hydroxychloroquine $	Plaquenil™	400 mg OD initially 200-400 mg OD maintenance	Retinal disease, G6PD deficiency	GI symptoms, macular damage, neuromyopathy, skin rash
sulfasalazine $	Salazopyrim™ Azulfidine™ (US)	1000 mg bid-tid	Sulfa/ASA allergy, kidney disease, G6PD deficiency	GI symptoms, headache, leukopenia, rash
methotrexate $	Rheumatrex™ Folex/Mexate™	qweekly 7.5-25 mg PO/IM/SC	Bone marrow suppression, liver disease, significant lung disease, immunodeficiency, pregnancy, EtOH abuse	Urticaria, GI symptoms, tubular necrosis, myelosuppression, cirrhosis, pneumonitis, oral ulcers
leflunomide $$	Arava™	10-20 mg PO OD	Liver disease	Alopecia, GI symptoms, pulmonary infiltrates, liver dysfunction
NOT COMMONLY USED				
cyclosporine $$	Neoral™		Kidney/liver disease, infection, hypertension	Bleeding, hypertension, decreased renal function, hair growth, tremors
gold (oral) $			IBD, kidney/liver disease	Diarrhea, rash, stomatitis
gold (injectable) $	Solganal™ Myocrysine™	weekly or monthly injections	IBD, kidney/liver disease	Rash, mouth soreness/ulcers, proteinuria, marrow suppression
azathioprine $	Imuran™		Kidney/liver disease	Pancytopenia, biliary stasis, rash, hair loss, vomiting, diarrhea
cyclophosphamide $	Cytoxan™		Kidney/liver disease	Cardiotoxicity, GI symptoms, hemorrhagic cystitis, nephrotoxicity, bone marrow suppression, sterility
penicillamine $			Penicillin allergy hematologic/kidney disease	Rash, loss of taste/appetite, GI symptoms, nephritic syndrome
NEWER DMARDs (Biologics)			**MECHANISM OF ACTION**	
etanercept $$$	Enbrel™	25 mg biweekly or 50 mg weekly SC injections	Fusion protein of TNF receptor and Fc portion of IgG Decreases number of active joints by 50% from baseline after 6 months	
infliximab $$$	Remicade™	3-5 mg/kg IV q 8 weeks	Chimeric mouse/human monoclonal Ab against TNFα Rapidly reduces number of swollen joints	
anakinra $$$	Kineret™	100 mg SC OD	Interleukin-1 receptor antagonist Reduce joint activity and x-ray progression	
adalimumab $$$	Humira™	40 mg SC q 2 weeks	Monoclonal anti-TNFα antibody	
abatacept $$$	Orencia™	IV infusion	Costimulation modulator of T cell activation	
rituximab $$$	Rituxan™	2 IV infusions, 2 weeks apart	Causes B cell depletion, binds to CD20	

Notes

U

Urology

CB Allard, Nashwah Taha, and Melinda Wu, chapter editors
Sami Chadi and Biniam Kidane, associate editors
Emily Partridge, EBM editor
Dr. Walid Farhat and Dr. Sender Herschorn, staff editors

Basic Anatomy Review

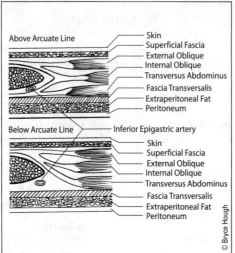

Figure 1. Midline Cross-Section of Abdominal Wall

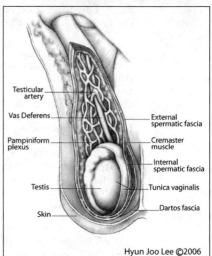

Figure 2. Anatomy of Scrotum

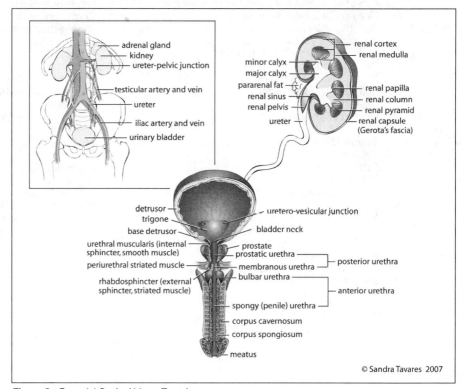

Figure 3. Essential Genito-Urinary Tract Anatomy

Common Presenting Problems

Hematuria

Classification (see Nephrology)

Table 1. Etiology of Hematuria by Age Group

Age (years)	Etiology (in order of decreasing frequency)	
0-20	Glomerulonephritis, UTI, congenital anomalies	
20-40	UTI, stones, bladder tumour	
40-60	Male: bladder tumour, stones, UTI	Female: UTI, stones, bladder tumour
>60	Male: BPH, bladder tumour, UTI	Female: bladder tumour, UTI

Etiology
- pseudohematuria (factitious hematuria)
    - menses, endometriosis
    - dyes (beets, rhodamine B in drinks, candy and juices)
    - hemoglobin (hemolytic anemia)
    - myoglobin (rhabdomyolysis)
    - drugs (rifampin, phenazopyridine, pyridium, phenytoin)
    - porphyria
    - laxatives (phenolphthalein)
- based on source of bleeding
    - pre-renal
        - anticoagulants
        - coagulation defects
        - sickle cell disease
        - leukemia
        - thromboembolism
        - adjacent inflammation (neoplasms, diverticulitis, appendicitis, PID)
    - renal
        - stone, renal cell carcinoma, transitional cell carcinoma, trauma, pyelonephritis, Wilm's tumour, glomerulonephritis, tuberculosis, interstitial nephritis, infarct, polycystic kidneys, arteriovenous malformation, exercise
    - ureter: stone, tumour
    - bladder: cystitis, tumour, stone, polyps, foreign body
    - urethra: urethritis, stone, tumour, urethral stricture

> Common urologic causes of hematuria can be grossly classified as **T**umour, **I**nfection, **T**rauma or **S**tones

History
- in addition to a full history, inquire about timing of macroscopic hematuria in urinary stream:
    - initial: anterior urethra
    - terminal: bladder neck and prostatic urethra
    - total: bladder and/or above

Investigations
- gross hematuria and symptomatic hematuria require full workup:
    - CBC (rule out anemia, leukocytosis)
    - chemistry: electrolytes, creatinine, BUN
    - urine studies
        - urinalysis (casts, crystals, cells)
        - culture and sensitivity
        - cytology
    - imaging
        - CT/IVP to investigate upper tracts (ultrasound alone is not sufficient)
        - cystoscopy to investigate lower tracts (possible retrograde pyelogram)
- microscopic hematuria defined as three or more red blood cells per high-power field
    - see Figure 4

Acute Management of Severe Bladder Hemorrhage
- secondary to advanced bladder cancer or hemorrhagic cystitis
- manual irrigation via catheter with normal saline to remove clots
- start continuous bladder irrigation (CBI) using large (22-26 Fr) 3-way Foley if bleeding is minimal to help prevent clot formation

- cystoscopy if bleeding quite active
    - identify resectable tumours
    - coagulate obvious sites of bleeding
- refractory bleeding
    - continuous intravesical irrigation with 1% alum (aluminum potassium sulfate) solution as needed
    - intravesical instillation of 1% silver nitrate solution
    - intravesical instillation of 1-4% formalin (need general anesthesia)
    - embolization or ligation of iliac arteries
    - cystectomy and diversion rarely

Gross painless hematuria is bladder cancer until proven otherwise.

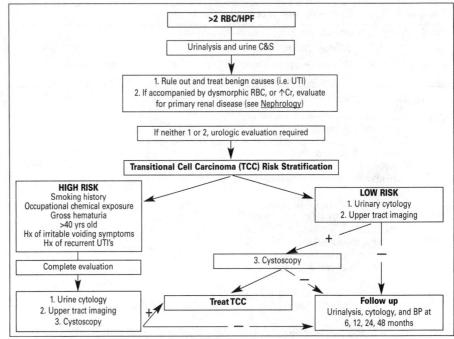

Figure 4. Workup of asymptomatic microscopic hematuria based on AUA Guidelines

Scrotal Complaints

- also see *Scrotal Mass*, U28

Painless	Painful
hydrocele	epididymitis
spermatocele	orchitis
varicocele	torsion
tumour	tumour (hemorrhagic)
indirect inguinal hernia	hematocele
idiopathic scrotal swelling	hernia (strangulated)
testicular abscess	testicular abscess
	granulomatous orchitis

Urinary Retention

- see *Failure to Void*, U7

Dysuria

Differential Diagnosis
- inflammation/infection
    - urethritis, trigonitis, cystitis, interstitial cystitis, prostatitis, pyelonephritis, vulvovaginitis, vestibulitis, Reiter's syndrome (arthritis, uveitis, urethritis)
- obstruction
    - abscess, stricture, stone, tumour, BPH, foreign body

- bladder carcinoma in situ
- atrophic vaginitis

Approach
- focused history and physical to determine cause (fever, discharge, CVA tenderness, conjunctivitis, back/joint pain)
- urine dip, C&S, R&M
- any discharge (urethral, vaginal, cervical) should be sent for gonococcus/chlamydia testing; wet mount if vaginal discharge
- may start empiric antibiotic treatment
- +/- imaging of urinary tract (tumour, stones)
- cystitis
- urethritis
- prostatitis
- interstitial cystitis
- pyelonephritis
- atrophic vaginitis
- vulvo-vaginitis
- urethral stone
- Urethral stricture
- bladder cancer (CIS)
- vaginal/urethral trauma
- foreign body
- spondyloarthropathy (e.g. Reiters syndrome)

Voiding Dysfunction

- two phases of lower urinary tract function
  - bladder filling and urine storage
    - accommodation and compliance
    - a closed outlet despite increasing intra-abdominal pressure
    - no involuntary contraction
  - bladder emptying
    - coordinated detrusor contraction
    - synchronous relaxation of outlet sphincters
    - no anatomic obstruction
- voiding dysfunction can therefore be classified as:
  - failure to store – due to bladder or outlet
  - failure to void – due to bladder or outlet
- 3 types of symptoms: storage, voiding, post-void

> **Causes of Acute and Reversible Urinary Incontinence (DRIP):**
> **D**elerium
> **R**estricted mobility/**R**etention
> **I**nflammation/**I**nfection
> **P**harmaceuticals/**P**olyuria

Failure to Store: Urinary Incontinence

Definition
- the involuntary leakage of urine

Etiology
- bladder problem
  - detrusor overactivity
    - CNS lesion, inflammation/infection (cystitis, stone, tumour), bladder neck obstruction (tumour, stone)
  - decreased compliance of bladder wall
    - CNS lesion, fibrosis
- sphincter/urethra problem
  - urethral hypermobility
    - due to weakened pelvic floor allows bladder neck and urethra to descend with increased intra-abdominal pressure
    - urethra is pulled open by greater motion of posterior wall of outlet relative to anterior wall
    - associated with childbirth, pelvic surgery, aging, levator muscle weakness
  - intrinsic sphincter deficiency (ISD)
    - pelvic surgery, neurologic problem, aging and hypoestrogen state
  - ISD and urethral hypermobility can co-exist

Epidemiology
- more frequent in the elderly, affecting 5-15% of those living in the community and 50% of nursing home residents
- F:M = 2:1

Surgical Treatment of Female Urinary Stress Incontinence
(Leach GE, Dmochowski RR, et al. J. Urol 1997; 158(3);875-880)

Study: Meta analysis incorporating 282 papers on the surgical management of USI.
Intervention: Probability estimates for the 4 major procedure categories of retropubic suspensions, transvaginal suspensions, anterior repairs and pubovaginal sling procedures were compared.
Main outcome: Objective or subjective definition of cure/dry over 3 discrete time frames (<23, 24-47, >48 months).
Results: Surgery is effective primary management of USI. Retropubic suspensions and slings are the most efficacious procedures for long-term success, but have slightly increased complication rate. Anterior repairs are the least likely of the 4 major procedure categories to be efficacious in the long term. Transvaginal suspensions have less likelihood of morbidity and/or earlier return to work.

Failure to Store
Lower Urinary Tract Symptoms (LUTS)
(irritative)
• **F**requency
• **U**rgency
• **N**octuria
• **D**ysuria

Think
Frequent **U**rgent **N**ighttime **D**iscomfort

Types of Urinary Incontinence
- stress incontinence: involuntary leaking with sudden increases in intra-abdominal pressure
  - due to urethra/sphincter problem
  - diagnose by stress test (Valsalva or cough with full bladder)
  - degrees: mild – sneezing, coughing; moderate – leaks when walking; severe – leaks when standing up
- urge incontinence: involuntaty leaking preceded by strong, sudden urge to void
  - due to bladder problem
  - diagnosis by urodynamics: uninhibited contractions (detrusor overactivity), small bladder capacity if irritable bladder
- mixed incontinence: urinary leakage associated with urgency and also with increased intrabdominal pressure
  - due to a combination of bladder and sphincter problems
  - diagnosis by stress test and urodynamics
- overflow incontinence: involuntary leakage when intravesical pressure exceeds urethral pressure
  - due to obstruction (e.g. BPH, stricture), hypotonic bladder (e.g. autonomic neuropathy from diabetes, multiple sclerosis, anticholinergic meds)
  - diagnosis by urodynamics: large bladder capacity
- total incontinence: continuous leakage of urine without warning
  - due to loss of sphincteric or bladder storage function (previous surgery, nerve damage, cancerous infiltration)
- continuous incontinence: continuous leakage of urine without warning
  - sphincter bypassed by abnormal connection between urinary tract and skin (bladder exstrophy, epispadias, vesico-vaginal fistulae, ectopic ureteral orifices)
- functional incontinence: urinary loss caused by inability to reach toilet in time
  - physical immobility, confusion

Investigations
- voiding diary
- physical exam: genito-urinary (GU), digital rectal exam (DRE), neurologic
- labs: urinalysis, urine C&S, renal function
- other investigations:
  - post-void residuals (catheterization or bladder scan)
  - U/S

Specialized Tests
- cystoscopy
- voiding cystourethrogram (VCUG)
- urodynamic studies – uroflowmetry, cystometrogram, video fluoroscopy

Treatment
- goals
  - improvement or cure
  - improvement in quality of life
  - low pressure system with minimal tubes and devices (for neurogenic bladders)
- stress
  - Kegel exercises to improve pelvic floor muscle tone
  - topical estrogen cream
  - injectable agents to proximal urethra
  - surgery – reinforce bladder neck or urethra with cystourethropexy or slings to prevent urethral descent or kink hyper-mobile urethra
- urge
  - antispasmodics (oxybutynin (Ditropan™))
  - anticholinergics (tolterodine (Detrol™), oxybutynin (Ditropan™), trospium (Trosec™), solifenacin (Vesicare™), darifenacin (Enablex™))
  - tricyclic antidepressants (imipramine)
  - neuromodulation (e.g. sacral nerve stimulation)
- retention-associated
  - catheterization to prevent bladder or kidney damage
  - further treatment directed at underlying cause of urinary retention
- total
  - usually surgical correction of underlying etiology or urinary diversion
- other treatments
  - pads, timed voiding, double voiding, condom catheter, penile clamp, artifical sphincter

Failure to Void: Urinary Retention

Etiology
- outflow obstruction
    - prostate – BPH, prostate cancer, prostatitis
    - urethra – stricture, carbuncle, traumatic disruption
    - calculus/clot/foreign body at bladder neck or urethra
- loss of bladder innervation
    - spinal cord – injury, disc herniation, multiple sclerosis
    - stroke
    - DM
    - post-pelvic surgery
- pharmacologic
    - anticholinergics
    - narcotics
    - antihypertensives (ganglionic blockers, methyldopa)
    - over the counter cold medications containing ephedrine or pseudoephedrine (e.g. Sudafed™)
    - antihistamines (e.g. Benadryl™, Nytol™, Sominex™)
    - psychosomatic substances (e.g. ecstasy)

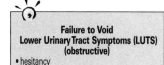

Failure to Void
Lower Urinary Tract Symptoms (LUTS)
(obstructive)
- hesitancy
- straining
- intermittency
- decreased force or calibre of stream
- prolonged voiding
- post-void dribble
- incomplete emptying

Clinical Features
- palpable and/or percussable bladder (suprapubic)
- possible purulent/bloody meatal discharge
- DRE – size of prostate, anal sphincter tone
- neurological – deep tendon reflexes, "anal wink", normal sensation

Investigations
- CBC, electrolytes, Cr, BUN, urine R&M, C&S, ultrasound, cystoscopy, urodynamic studies, bladder scan

Treatment (use least invasive technique possible)
- catheterization or suprapubic cystotomy
    - contraindicated in trauma patient unless urethral disruption has been ruled out
    - acute retention: immediate catheterization to relieve retention, leave Foley in to drain bladder, follow up to determine cause
    - chronic retentions: intermittent catheterization by patient is commonly used; definitive treatment depends on etiology
- post-operative patients
    - encourage ambulation
    - cholinergics to cause bladder contraction (occasionally)
    - α-blockers to relax bladder neck
    - may need catheterization
    - definitive treatment will depend on etiology

Benign Prostatic Hyperplasia (BPH)

Definition
- hyperplasia of stroma and epithelium in periurethral area of prostate (transition zone) – see Figure 5
- tone of prostatic smooth muscle cells plays a role in addition to hyperplasia

Etiology
- etiology unknown
    - androgen dihydrotestosterone (DHT) required (converted from testosterone by 5-α reductase)
    - possible role of impaired apoptosis, estrogens, other growth factors

Epidemiology
- age-related, extremely common (50% of 50 year olds, 80% of 80 year olds)
- 25% of men will require treatment

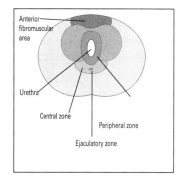

Figure 5. Cross-Section of Prostate

Clinical Features
- result from outlet obstruction and compensatory changes in detrusor function
- voiding symptoms (obstructive)
    - obstructive LUTS and UUTS (hesitancy, straining, weak/interrupted stream, incomplete bladder emptying)

Prostate size does not correlate well with symptoms in BPH.

Absolute Indications for Surgery
- refractory urinary retention
- renal insufficiency
- intolerance/failure of medical therapy

The Long-Term Effect of Doxazosin, Finasteride, and Combination Therapy on the Clinical Progression of Benign Prostatic Hyperplasia (Medical Therapy of Prostatic Symptoms (MTOPS) Trial)
(NEJM 2003; 349: 2387-2398)
Study: Randomized, double-blinded, controlled trial with mean follow-up 4.5 years.
Patients: 3047 patients with symptomatic BPH (AUA symptom score 8 to 35) were randomly assigned to placebo (n=737), doxazosin (n=756), finasteride (n=768), or combination therapy (n=786). Mean age 62.6.
Intervention: Conservative treatment vs. doxazosin vs. finasteride vs. combination therapy.
Main Outcomes: Clinical progression defined as: first occurrence of an increase over base line of at least four points in the AUA symptom score, acute urinary retention, renal insufficiency, recurrent urinary tract infection, or urinary incontinence.
Results: The 6-yr absolute reduction in cumulative incidence of clinical progression of symptomatic BPH compared to placebo for doxazosin was 39% (P<0.001), finasteride was 34% (P=0.002), and combination therapy was 66% (P<0.001). Combination therapy was more effective than either doxazosin (P<0.001) or finasteride (P<0.001) alone. There was no significant difference between doxazosin and finasteride alone.
Conclusion: Long-term combination therapy with doxazosin and finasteride reduced the risk of overall clinical progression of benign prostatic hyperplasia significantly more than did treatment with either drug alone.

- - decreased flow rates on uroflowmetry
  - due to outflow obstruction and impaired detrusor contractility
- storage symptoms (irritative)
  - urgency, frequency, nocturia, urgency incontinence
  - due to detrusor overactivity and decreased compliance
- prostate is smooth, rubbery and symmetrically enlarged on DRE
- complications
  - retention
  - incontinence
  - hydronephrosis and renal compromise
  - infection
  - gross hematuria
  - bladder stones

Investigations
- history
  - may include self-administered questionnaires (AUA symptom score) developed to follow disease progression and response to therapy
  - assess symptoms and effect on quality of life
- DRE
- urinalysis to exclude UTI
- creatinine to assess renal function +/- renal ultrasound to assess for hydronephrosis
- prostate-specific antigen (PSA) to rule out malignancy (if life expectancy >10 years)
- uroflowmetry to measure flow rate (optional)
- bladder ultrasound to determine post-void residual urine (optional)
- cystoscopy prior to potential surgical management

Treatment
- conservative for those with mild symptoms
  - watchful waiting – 50% of patients improve spontaneously
  - includes lifestyle changes (e.g. evening fluid restriction, planned voiding)
- medical treatment
  - α-adrenergic antagonists – reduce stromal smooth muscle tone (e.g. terazosin (Hytrin™), doxazosin (Cardura™), tamsulosin (Flomax™), alfuzosin (Xatral™))
  - 5-α reductase inhibitor (e.g. finasteride (Proscar™), dutasteride (Avodart™)) – blocks conversion of testosterone to DHT; acts on the epithelial component of the prostate
  - combination shown to be synergistic (see sidebox)
- transurethral resection of prostate (TURP)
  - see *Selected Urological Procedures* section, U41
- open prostatectomy
  - for large prostates or associated problems (e.g. bladder stones)
  - suprapubic (transvesically to deal with bladder pathology)
  - retropubic (through the prostatic capsule)
- minimally invasive therapy
  - prostatic stents, microwave therapy, laser ablation, cryotherapy, high intensity focused ultrasound (HIFU) and transurethral needle ablation (TUNA)

Urethral Stricture

- decrease in urethral calibre due to scar formation in urethra may also involve corpus spongiosum
- more common in males

Etiology
- congenital – failure of normal canalization
  - may cause hydronephrosis
- trauma
  - instrumentation (most common, at fossa navicularis)
  - external trauma (e.g. burns, removal of inflated Foley catheter)
- infection
  - long-term indwelling catheter
  - balanitis xerotica obliterans – causes meatal stenosis (common with past history of gonorrhea)

Clinical Features
- voiding symptoms (obstructive symptoms)
- urinary retention
- related infections: recurrent UTI, secondary prostatitis/epididymitis

Investigations
- laboratory findings
  - flow rates <10 ml/s (normal ~20 ml/s)
  - urine culture usually negative, but may show pyuria
- radiologic findings
  - retrograde urethrogram, voiding cystourethrogram (VCUG) will demonstrate location
- urethroscopy

Treatment
- urethral dilatation
  - temporarily increases lumen size by breaking up scar tissue
  - healing will often reform scar tissue and recreate stricture
- visual internal urethrotomy (VIU)
  - endoscopically incise stricture without skin incision
  - cure rate 50-80% with single treatment, <50% with repeated courses
- open surgical reconstruction
  - complete stricture excision for all, then (dependent on location and size of stricture):
    - membranous urethra – end-to-end anastomosis
    - bulbar urethra <2 cm – end-to-end anastomosis
    - bulbar urethra >2 cm or penile urethra – 1) vascularized flap of local genital skin or 2) free graft (penile shaft skin or buccal mucosa) – preferred

Neurogenic Bladder

Definition
- a malfunctioning urinary bladder due to a deficiency in some aspect of its innervation

Neurophysiology

Table 2. Efferent Sympathetic, Parasympathetic, and Somatic Nerve Supply

Nerve Fibres	Segment	Neurotransmitter	Target	Key Receptors
Sympathetic	T10-L2	Noradrenaline	Trigone, internal sphincter, proximal urethra	Adrenergic (α1)
Somatic	S2-S3	Acetylcholine	External sphincter	Nicotinic
Parasympathetic	S2-S4	Acetylcholine	Detrusor	Muscarinic (M2, M3)

> **4Cs of Bladder**
> **C**apacity (350-500 cc; Peds: (Age + 2) x 30)
> **C**ompliance (minimal DPressure/DVolume)
> **C**ontractility (voluntary and sustained)
> **C**ooperation of bladder and sphincter

- receptors in the bladder wall and mucosa relay information to pontine micturition centre (PMC) and activate micturition reflex
- the PMC, receiving inhibitory voluntary cortical input, sends excitatory/inhibitory signals to regulate micturition reflex:
  - micturition: stimulation of sacral parasympathetic neurons (bladder contraction); inhibition of sympathetic (IS relaxation) and sacral somatic neurons (ES relaxation)
  - urine storage: inhibition of sacral parasympathetic neurons (bladder relaxation) aided by sympathetic activation (bladder relaxation, IS contraction); stimulation of sacral somatic neurons (ES contraction)
- voluntary action of external sphincter (pudendal n. S2-S3) can inhibit urge to urinate
- cerebellum, basal ganglia, thalamus, and hypothalamus all have input at PMC

> Nerve roots in micturition:
> **"S2-3-4 keeps the urine off the floor."**

Classification of Neurologic Voiding Dysfunction
- lesion above PMC (e.g. stroke, tumour, multiple sclerosis (MS): neurogenic detrusor overactivity (detrusor hyperreflexia)
  - loss of voluntary inhibition of voiding
  - intact pathway inferior to PMC maintains coordination of voiding episodes
- lesion of spinal cord (e.g. MS, arteriovenous malformation (AVM)): detrusor-sphincter dyssynergia (DSD)
  - loss of coordination between detrusor and sphincter (i.e. detrusor contracts on closed sphincter and vice versa)
  - component of detrusor overactivity as well

- lesion of sacral cord or peripheral efferents (e.g. trauma, diabetes, disc herniation): detrusor atony/areflexia
  - flaccid bladder which fails to contract
  - may progress to poorly compliant bladder with high pressures
- peripheral autonomic neuropathy: deficient bladder sensation → increasing residual urine → decompensation (e.g. DM, neurosyphilis, herpes zoster)
- muscular lesion: can involve detrusor, smooth/striated sphincter

"Spinal shock" early phase following cord injury manifests as atonic bladder.

Neuro-Urologic Evaluation
- history and physical exam (urologic and general neurologic)
- urinalysis, renal profile
- imaging: intravenous pyelogram (IVP), U/S to rule out hydronephrosis and stones
- cystoscopy
- urodynamic studies
  - uroflowmetry – assess flow rate, pattern
  - filling cystometrogram (CMG) – assess capacity, compliance, detrusor overactivity
  - voiding cystometrogram – pressure-flow study, assess bladder contractility and extent of bladder outflow obstruction
  - EMG – helps ascertain presence of coordinated or uncoordinated voiding, allows accurate diagnosis of DSD
  - video study – x-ray contrast to visualize bladder/bladder neck/urethra during CMG

Treatment
- goals of treatment
  - maintenance of low pressure storage and emptying system with minimum of tubes and collecting devices is necessary to:
    - prevent renal failure
    - prevent infections
    - prevent incontinence or achieve social continence
- treatment options: depends on status of bladder and urethra
  - bladder hyperactivity → medications to relax bladder (see *Incontinence*, U5); botulinum toxin injections into bladder wall; occasionally augmentation cystoplasty
  - flaccid bladder → clean intermittent catheterization (CIC)

Autonomic Dysreflexia
- exaggerated sympathetic nervous system response to visceral stimulation below the lesion in spinal cord injury patients
  - lesion is usually above T6/T7
  - stimulation includes instrumentation, distention or stimulation of bladder, urethra, rectum (fecal impaction)
- hypertension, headache, reflex bradycardia, sweating, anxiety, piloerection
- vasoconstriction below lesion, vasodilation above lesion
- treatment: remove noxious stimulus (e.g. insert catheter), parenteral ganglionic or α-blockers or chlorpromazine, nifedipine (prophylaxis during cystoscopy)

Post Obstructive Diuresis (POD)

Definition
- polyuria resulting from relief of severe chronic obstruction
  - may occur after catheterization for bladder outflow obstruction (e.g. BPH), release from bilateral ureteral obstruction, or obstruction of a solitary kidney
- increased urine output out of proportion to fluid intake
- after relief of obstruction, >3 L over 24 hrs or more than 200 cc/hr over each of two consecutive hours is diagnostic of polyuria found with POD

Pathophysiology
- ranges in severity from a physiologic process to a pathologic sodium-wasting nephropathy
  - physiologic diuresis occurs secondary to excretion of retained urea, sodium, and water (high osmotic load) after relief of obstruction
    - self-limiting, usually resolves in 48 hrs with PO fluids but sometimes can continue even after having reached euvolemic status (i.e. pathologic POD)
  - pathologic POD occurs secondary to an impaired concentrating ability of the renal tubules due to:
    - defective generation of a medullary solute gradient secondary to a decreased reabsorption of sodium chloride in the thick ascending limb and urea in the collecting tubule

    ◆ an inability to maintain the solute gradient secondary to an increased medullary blood flow (solute washout)
    ◆ an impaired medullary gradient secondary to an increased flow and solute concentration in the distal nephron

Management
- admit patient and closely monitor hemodynamic status and electrolytes
- make sure total fluid intake is less than urine output (U/O) as this could exacerbate diuresis
- monitor U/O q2h and replace with IV 1/2 NS 0.5 cc per 1 cc U/O (can maintain on PO fluids if physiologic POD)
- avoid glucose-containing fluid replacement as it can add an iatrogenic cause of continuing diuresis
- check Na and K q6-12h and replace prn
- follow creatinine and BUN to normal

Infectious and Inflammatory Diseases

Urinary Tract Infections (UTI)

Definition
- greater than 100,000 bacteria/ml – midstream urine
  - if symptomatic, 100 bacteria/ml may be significant

Classification
- first infection = first documented UTI
- unresolved bacteriuria = urinary tract is not sterilized during therapy (most commonly due to resistant organisms or noncompliance)
- recurrent UTI
  - bacterial persistence = urine cultures become sterile during therapy but resultant reinfection of the urine by the same organisms
  - reinfection = new infections with new pathogens (80% of recurrent UTI)

Source
- ascending (most common) – GI organisms
- hematogenous (TB, perinephric abscess)
- lymphatic
- direct (inflammatory bowel disease, diverticulitis)

Risk Factors
- stasis and obstruction
  - residual urine in poorly flushing system e.g. posterior urethral valves, reflux, drugs (anticholinergics, BPH, urethral stricture)
- foreign body
  - introduce pathogen or act as nidus of infection
  - e.g. catheter, stone, instrumentation
- decreased resistance to organisms
  - diabetes, malignancy, immunosuppression
- other factors
  - trauma, anatomic variance (congenital), female (short urethra)

Clinical Features
- storage symptoms (hesitancy, post-void dribbling, double void)
- voiding symptoms (frequency, urgency, dysuria)
- pain, tenderness (costovertebral angle (CVA), abdominal, rectal)
- hematuria
- constitutional symptoms (fever, chills, malaise, nausea, vomiting)
- sepsis/shock

Organisms
- routine cultures (see box)
- non-routine cultures
  - tuberculosis (TB)
  - *Chlamydia trachomatis*

Common Pathogens in Cystitis
"KEEPS"
- *Klebsiella* sp.
- *E. coli* (90%), other Gram negatives
- Enterococci
- *Proteus mirabilis*, *Pseudomonas*
- *S. saprophyticus*, *S. fecalis*

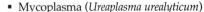

- Mycoplasma (*Ureaplasma urealyticum*)
- fungi (*Candida*)

Indications for Investigations
- persistence of pyuria/symptoms after adequate therapy
- severe infection with an increase in creatinine
- hematuria
- recurrent/persistent infections
- male
- child

Investigations
- midstream urine R&M, C&S
- hematuria workup – urine cytology, ultrasound, cystoscopy
- spiral CT (if indicated)
- *VCUG* (to visualize tract) if recurrent and/or hydronephrosis

Treatment
- confirm diagnosis
- identify organism and treat (TMP/SMX, fluoroquinolones, nitrofurantoin)
  - for mild infections 3 day course is sufficient (for treatment details see *Common Medications* section, U44)
- establish predisposing cause (if any) and correct
- consider long term, low dose prophylaxis in recurrent UTI
- if febrile, consider admission with IV therapy and rule out obstruction

Recurrent/Chronic Cystitis

- incidence of bacteriuria in females
  - pre-teens: 1%; late teens: 4%; 30-50 years: 6%
- assess predisposing factors as described above
- possible relation to intercourse (postcoital antibiotics), perineal colonization
- investigations may include cystoscopy, ultrasound, CT
- antibiotic prophylaxis if greater than three or four episodes per year in females

Etiology
- unknown
  - theories: increased epithelial permeability, autoimmune, neurogenic
  - associations: severe allergies, irritable bowel syndrome (IBS), fibromyalgia

Treatment
- daily low-dose prophylaxis (nitrofurantoin, TMP/SMX)
- lifestyle changes (limit caffeine intake, increase fluid/water intake, smoking cessation)
- daily cranberry juice
- no treatment for asymptomatic UTI except in pregnant women ± urinary tract instrumentation

Interstitial Cystitis (Painful Bladder Syndrome)

Definition
- chronic urgency, frequency ± pain without other reasonable causation

Etiology
- unknown
  - theories: increased epithelial permeability, autoimmune, neurogenic, defective glycosaminoglycan (GAG) layer overlying mucosa
  - associations: severe allergies, irritable bowel syndrome (IBS), fibromyalgia

Epidemiology
- prevalence: ~20/100,000
- 90% of cases are in females
- mean age at onset is 40 years

Classification
- non-ulcerative (more common) – younger to middle-aged
- ulcerative – middle-aged to older

Various Causes of Dysuria

Infectious: pyelonephritis, cystitis, urethritis, prostattis, epididymitis, orchitis, cervicitis, vulvovaginitis, perineal inflammation/infection, TB

Neoplasm: renal cell tumour, cancer of the bladder, prostate, penis, vagina/vulva, BPH

Calculi: bladder stone, ureteral stone, kidney stone

Inflammatory: seronegative arthropathies, drug side effects, autoimmune disorders, chronic pelvic pain syndrome (CPPS), intersitial cystitis (Painfull Bladder Syndrome)

Hormonal: endometriosis, hypoestrogenism

Trauma: catheter insertion, honeymoon cystitis

Psychogenic: somatization disorder, MDD, stress/anxiety disorder

Other: contact sensitivity

Cranberries for preventing urinary tract infections
Jepson RG and Craig JC. 2008 Cochrane Database Syst Rev Jan 23(1):CD001321

Background: Cranberries are often empirically used for the prevention and treatment of urinary tract infections (UTIs), but few studies have investigated their efficacy.
Results: Ten randomized studies (n = 1049) were included in this meta-analysis. The use of cranberry juice and/or tablets was associated with a significant reduction in the incidence of UTIs at 12 months (RR 0.65, 95% CI 0.46 to 0.90) compared with placebo/control. Greater efficacy was observed for cranberry products in women with recurrent UTIs as compared to study outcomes for elderly men and women or for patients requiring intermittent catheterization.
Conclusion: There is some evidence that among female patients with recurrent UTIs, cranberry juice may decrease the number of symptomatic UTIs over a 12 month period. Further studies are necessary to determine the effectiveness of cranberry products for other patient populations, as well as to determine the optimal dose, route of administration and duration of this treatment regime.

Diagnosis (not usually adhered to)
- required criteria
  - glomerulations (submucosal petechiae) or Hunner's ulcers on cystoscopic examination
  - pain associated with the bladder or urinary urgency
  - negative urinalysis, C&S

Differential Diagnosis
- UTI, vaginitis, bladder tumour
- radiation/chemical cystitis
- eosinophilic/TB cystitis
- bladder calculi

Treatment
- pentosan polysulfate (Elmiron™)
- amitriptyline
- bladder hydrodistention (also diagnostic) under general anesthesia
- intravesical dimethylsulfoxide (DMSO) or Cystistat™
- surgery (augmentation cystoplasty and urinary diversion ± cystectomy)

Pyelonephritis

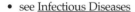

- see <u>Infectious Diseases</u>

Prostatitis/Prostatodynia

- most common urologic diagnosis in men <50 years
- incidence 10-30%

TYPE I: ACUTE BACTERIAL PROSTATITIS

Etiology
- KEEPS (see U11 sidebar): 80% *E. coli*
- ascending urethral infection and reflux into prostatic ducts
- often associated with outlet obstruction (BPH), recent cystoscopy, post prostatic biopsy
- invasion of rectal bacteria
- most infections occur in the peripheral zone (see Figure 5)

Clinical Features
- acute onset fever, chills, malaise
- rectal, low back and perineal pain
- irritative LUTS
- hematuria

Investigations
- rectal exam
  - enlarged, tender, warm prostate
- urine C&S: 4 specimens:
  - VB1: initial (urethra)
  - VB2: midstream (bladder)
  - EPS (expressed prostatic secretions): (prostate) not usually performed, as prostatic massage may cause extreme tenderness and increased risk of inducing sepsis, abscess or epididymo-orchitis
  - VB3: post-massage/DRE (prostate)
- urine R&M
- blood CBC, C&S

Treatment
- supportive measures (antipyretics, analgesics, stool softeners)
- PO antibiotics (Cipro™, Septra™)
  - treat for 4-6 wks to prevent complications
- admission criteria: sepsis, urinary retention, immunodeficiency
- IV antibiotics (ampicillin and gentamicin); mid-stream urine C&S at 1 and 3 months post antibiotic therapy to prevent chronic prostatitis
- avoid catheterization due to risk of bacteremia and systemic infection
  - small drainage catheter may be inserted if obstruction suspected

TYPE II: CHRONIC BACTERIAL PROSTATITIS

Clinical Features
- recurrent exacerbations of acute prostatitis signs and symptoms
- recurrent UTI with same organism
- frequently asymptomatic with normal prostate on DRE

Investigations
- urine C&S 4 specimens
  - colony counts in (EPS) and VB3 should exceed those of initial and midstream by 10 times

Treatment
- long course of antibiotics (3-4 months)
- fluoroquinolones, TMP/SMX or doxycycline; addition of an α-blocker may reduce symptoms

TYPE III: CHRONIC PELVIC PAIN SYNDROME
- aka chronic abacterial prostatitis
- most common and most poorly understood prostatic syndrome

Inflammatory Subtype
- pathogenesis: intraprostatic reflux of urine ± urethral hypertonia
- specific etiological agents unknown, but current proposed theories include:
  - *Mycoplasma hominis*, *Ureaplasma urealyticum*, *Trichomonas vaginalis*, *Chlamydia trachomatis*, viruses, anaerobic bacteria, coagulase-negative staphylococci, proinflammatory cytokines, autoimmune mechanisms, chemical irritation

Noninflammatory Subtype
- pathogenesis: increase tension in bladder neck muscles ± prostatic urethra ± pelvic floor tension myalgia ± psychological factors
- clinical features: pelvic pain, irritative LUTS, ejaculatory pain, postejaculatory pain DRE exam variable
- treatment
  - trial of antibiotic therapy (fluoroquinolone or doxycycline if *Chlamydia trachomatis* is suspected)
  - α–blocker to relieve sphincter spasms and symptoms
  - NSAIDs and supportive measures for symptomatic relief
  - smaller studies suggest benefit of transurethral microwave thermotherapy (TUMT), querceti, rofecoxib

Epididymitis and Orchitis

Etiology
- infection
  - <35 years – gonorrhea or *Chlamydia trachomatis* (sexually transmitted infections (STIs))
  - >35 years + homosexual males of any age – GI organisms (esp. *E.coli*)
- mumps infection may involve orchitis after parotiditis
- other rare causes
  - TB
  - syphilis
  - granulomatous (autoimmune) in elderly men
  - amiodarone (non-infectious cause, involves only head of epididymis)

If unsure between epididymitis and torsion: go to OR

Remember torsion >24 hrs is a poor prognosis

Risk Factors
- UTI, unprotected sexual contact
- instrumentation/catheter
- reflux
- increased pressure in prostatic urethra (straining, voiding, heavy lifting) may cause reflux of urine along vas deferens → sterile epididymitis

Clinical Features
- sudden onset scrotal pain and swelling ± radiation along cord to flank
- scrotal erythema and tenderness
- fever, prostration
- irritative voiding symptoms, purulent discharge
- reactive hydrocele

Investigations
- urinalysis (pyuria), urine C&S
- ± urethral discharge: Gram stain for Gram-negative cocci or rods
- if diagnosis clinically uncertain, must do:
  - colour-flow Doppler ultrasound
  - nuclear medicine scan
  - examination under anesthesia (EUA)

Prehn's sign: pain may be relieved with elevation of testicles in epididymitis but not in testicular torsion. Poor sensitivity especially in children.

Treatment
- antibiotics
  - *N. gonorrheae* or *C. trachomatis* – ceftriaxone 250 mg IM once followed by azithromycin 1 g single dose or doxycycline 100 mg bid x 10 days
  - coliforms – broad spectrum antibiotics (Septra™, Cipro™) x 2 weeks
- scrotal support, ice, analgesia

Complications
- if severe, testicular atrophy
- 30% have persistent infertility problems
- note: epididymitis is much more common than orchitis

Urethritis

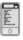

- women: vaginitis accounts for 1/3; remaining 2/3 due to gonorrhea or chlamydial infection
- men: gonococcal vs. non-gonococcal urethritis
- gonococcal
  - causative organism = *Neisseria gonorrheae*
  - diagnosis – history of sexual contact, yellow purulent discharge, irritative LUTS
  - positive Gram stain and/or culture from urethral specimen (Gram negative diplococci)
  - treatment – ceftriaxone 250 mg IM once + doxycycline 100 mg PO bid x 7 days to cover for *Chlamydia trachomatis* (can substitute ofloxacin 400 mg or ciprofloxacin 500 mg for ceftriaxone)
- non-gonococcal
  - causative organism = usually *Chlamydia trachomatis*
  - diagnosis – history of sexual contact, mucoid whitish purulent discharge, ± irritative LUTS
  - Gram stain demonstrates >4 PMN/oil immersion field, no evidence of *N. gonorrheae*
  - treatment – doxycycline 100 mg PO bid x 7 days (can use erythromycin 500 mg qid or tetracycline 500 mg qid for same duration or azithromycin 1 g single dose)

Reiter's Syndrome
Urethritis, Uveitis and Arthritis
(can't pee, can't see, can't climb a tree)

Urethral Syndrome

- dysuria in females with consistently sterile urine cultures or low bacterial counts
- some have bacterial urethrocystitis (*C. trachomatis* or other organisms) and require antimicrobial treatment
- treat: tetracycline or erythromycin
- rule out vaginitis, cancer, interstitial cystitis, psychological etiologies

Stone Disease

Incidence
- 10% of population
- male:female = 2:1
  - 50% chance of recurrence by 5 years (60-80% lifetime)
  - peak incidence 30-50 years of age

Clinical Features
- urinary obstruction → upstream distention → pain
  - flank pain from renal capsular distention (non-colicky)
  - severe waxing and waning pain radiating from flank to groin, testis, or tip of penis due to stretching of collecting system or ureter (ureteral colic)
- writhing, never comfortable, nausea, vomiting, hematuria (90% microscopic), diaphoresis, tachycardia, tachypnea

- occasionally symptoms of trigonal irritation (frequency, urgency)
- fever, chills, rigors in secondary pyelonephritis
- irritative and/or obstructive LUTS, terminal hematuria, suprapubic pain in bladder stones

Differential Diagnosis of Renal Colic
- acute ureteral obstruction (other causes)
  - UPJ obstruction
  - sloughed papillae
  - clot colic from gross hematuria
- acute abdominal crisis – biliary, bowel, pancreas, abdominal aortic aneurysm (AAA)
- gynecological – ectopic pregnancy, torsion/rupture of ovarian cyst
- pyelonephritis (fever, chills, pyuria)
- radiculitis (L1) – herpes zoster, nerve root compression

Location of Stones
- calyx
  - may cause flank discomfort, recurrent infection or persistent hematuria
  - may remain asymptomatic for years and not require treatment
- pelvis
  - tend to cause obstruction at UPJ
  - staghorn calculi (renal pelvis and one or more calyces)
  - often associated with infection that will not resolve until stone is cleared
- ureter
  - <5 mm diameter will pass spontaneously in 75% of patients

Stone Pathogenesis
- supersaturation of stone constituents (at appropriate temperature and pH)
- stasis, low flow and low volume of urine
- crystal formation and stone nidus
- loss of inhibitory factors
  - citrate (forms soluble complex with calcium)
  - magnesium (forms soluble complex with oxalate)
  - pyrophosphate
  - Tamm-Horsfall glycoprotein

> The four narrowest passage points for upper tract stones are: UPJ, pelvic brim, under vas deferens/broad ligament, UVJ.

Investigations
- screening labs
  - CBC → elevated WBC in presence of fever suggests infection
  - electrolytes, Cr, BUN → to assess renal function
  - urinalysis: R&M (WBCs, RBCs, crystals), C&S
- imaging
  - kidneys, ureters, bladders (KUB) x-ray
    - to differentiate opaque from non-opaque stones (e.g. uric acid, indinavir)
    - 90% of stones are radiopaque
  - spiral CT
    - no contrast; good to distinguish radiolucent stone from soft tissue filling defect
    - uric acid stones visible on CT
    - does not differentiate radiopaque from non-opaque stones
  - abdominal ultrasound
    - may demonstrate stone (difficult in ureter)
    - may demonstrate hydronephrosis
  - IVP (not usually done any more)
    - anatomy of urine collecting system
    - degree of obstruction
    - extravasation if present
    - renal tubular ectasia (medullary sponge kidney)
    - uric acid stones → filling defect on retrograde pyelography occasionally required to delineate upper tract anatomy and localize small calculi
- cystoscopy for suspected bladder stone
- strain all urine → stone analysis
- metabolic studies for recurrent stone formers
  - serum electrolytes, Ca, PO$_4$, uric acid, creatinine and urea
  - PTH if hypercalcemic
  - 24 hour urine x 2 for creatinine, Ca, PO$_4$, uric acid, Mg, oxalate, citrate

> Indinavir (Crixivan™) is a protease inhibitor used in the treatment of HIV.

> Indinavir stones are the only stones that are radiolucent on spiral CT as well as on plain film.

Treatment – Acute
- medical
  - analgesic (Tylenol #3™, Demerol™, morphine) ± antiemetic
  - NSAIDs help lower intra-ureteral pressure
  - alpha-blockers: increase rate of spontaneous passage in distal ureteral stones
  - ± antibiotics for UTI
  - IV fluids if vomiting (note: IV fluids do NOT promote stone passage)

- indications for admission to hospital
    - intractable pain
    - fever (suggests infection)
    - single kidney with ureteral obstruction/bilateral obstructing stones
    - intractable vomiting
    - compromised renal function
- interventional: if obstruction endangers patient (i.e. sepsis, renal failure)
    - ureteric stent (via cystoscopy)
    - percutaneous nephrostomy (image-guided)

Treatment – Elective
- medical
    - conservative if stone <5 mm and no complications
    - fluids to increase urine volume to >2 L/day (3-4 L if cystine)
    - specific to stone type
        - calcium – cellulose phosphate, orthophosphate for absorptive causes
        - calcium oxalate – thiazides, ± potassium citrate, ± allopurinol, calcium
        - uric acid – alkalinize urine (bicarbonate, potassium citrate) ± allopurinol
        - struvite – antibiotics (stone must be removed to treat infection)
        - cystine – alkalinize urine, penicillamine/α-MPG (complex cystine), captopril
    - alkalinization of urine (bicarbonate, potassium citrate)
    - patient must receive one month of therapy before being considered to have failed
- interventional
    - kidney
        - stent if stone is 1.5-2.5 cm
        - extracorporeal shockwave lithotripsy (ESWL) if stone <2.5 cm (unless cystine stone)
        - percutaneous nephrolithotomy (extraction or fragmentation) if:
            – stone >2.5 cm
            – staghorn
            – UPJ obstruction
            – calyceal diverticulum
            – cystine stones (poorly fragmented with ESWL)
            – percutaneous nephrolithotomy and ESWL or rarely open nephrolithotomy for extensively branched staghorn
    - ureter
        - ESWL is the primary modality of treatment
        - ureteroscopy (extraction or fragmentation) if:
            – failed ESWL
            – ureteric stricture
            – reasonable alternative for distal 1/3 of ureter
        - open ureterolithotomy (very rare)
    - bladder
        - transurethral cystolitholapaxy
        - remove outflow obstruction (TURP or stricture dilatation)

Prevention
- dietary modification
    - increase fluid intake to >2L/day
    - reduce animal protein intake
    - increase potassium intake
    - limit oxalate, sodium, sucrose, and fructose intake
    - avoid high-dose vitamin C supplements
- medications
    - thiazide diuretics for hypercalciuria
    - allopurinol for hyperuricosuria
    - potassium citrate for hypocitraturia

Calcium Stones (75-85%)

- 75-85% of all stones
- calcium oxalate most common, followed by calcium phosphate and mixtures of the two

ETIOLOGY
Hypercalciuria
- increased intestinal absorption
    - increased ingestion (calcium, vitamin D)
    - renal phosphate leak – decreased PO_4 leads to increased $1,25(OH)_2$ vitamin D
    - idiopathic

Efficacy of α-Blockers for the Treatment of Ureteral Stones
(J. Urol 2007; 1779: 983-987)
Study: Meta-analysis of prospective randomized trials comparing α-blockers to conservative therapy.
Data Sources: MEDLINE (January 1966 to October 2005), the Cochrane Central Search library, EMBASE (1980 to 2005), and the electronic database of abstracts presented at the Annual Meeting of the American Urological Association (2002 to 2005) were searched for literature published in English between their respective dates.
Patients: 11 studies met selection criteria (n=911). Treatment ranged from 8 days to 6 weeks.
Main Outcome: Incidence of distal ureteral stone expulsion.
Results: Administration of an α-blocker with conservative treatment increased incidence of stone expulsion over conservative treatment alone by 44% (95% CI 1.31-1.59, p<0.001).
Conclusion: α-blocker therapy is associated with significantly increased rates of distal ureteral stone expulsion.

Although hypercalciuria is a risk factor for stone formation, decreasing dietary calcium is NOT recommended to prevent stone formation. Low dietary calcium leads to increased oxalate absorption and higher urine levels of calcium oxalate.

- resorption of calcium from bone
  - hyperparathyroidism (see <u>Endocrinology</u>)
    - primary – parathyroid adenoma
    - secondary – renal leak of calcium
  - immobilization
  - malignancy (metastatic disease, multiple myeloma)
  - steroids (exogenous or endogenous)
- other: including sarcoidosis, medullary sponge kidney, distal renal tubular acidosis (RTA)

Hyperuricosuria (25% of patients with Ca stones)
- uric acid crystals can act as a nidus for calcium stone formation, independent of uric acid stone formation
- acid urine (pH <5.8), dehydration

Hyperoxaluria (<5% of patients)
- large effect on stone formation with small changes in urinary concentration
- increased intestinal absorption (majority)
  - patients with small bowel resection, inflammatory bowel disease (IBD) or other malabsorptive states
  - increased intestinal fat binds dietary calcium, which is then unavailable to bind oxalate as usual. Therefore increased oxalate absorption in large bowel (unabsorbed bile salts may aid in this) and increased urinary excretion
- endogenous overproduction
  - end product of abnormal metabolism of glycine, ascorbic acid, hydroxyproline and serine
- increased ingested oxalate
  - tea, coffee, beer, green leafy vegetables, chocolate, ethylene glycol poisoning

Hypocitraturia (12% of patients)
- citrate normally complexes with calcium and inhibits stone formation
- decreased urinary citrate in systemic acidosis (including distal renal tubular acidosis (RTA)), hypokalemia (thiazides, chronic diarrhea), high animal protein diet, idiopathic

Other
- hypomagnesemia – associated with hyperoxaluria and hypocitraturia
- high dietary sodium – increased calcium excretion, decreased urinary citrate
- decreased urinary proteins – Tamm-Horsfall glycoprotein, uropontin

Struvite Stones (5-10%)

- magnesium ammonium phosphate (MAP)
- alkaline urinary pH due to infection with urea-splitting organisms – precipitates MAP
  - *Proteus, Pseudomonas, Providencia, Klebsiella, Mycoplasma, Serratia, S. aureus*
  - NOT *E. coli*
  - perpetuate UTI because stone itself harbours organism, therefore must remove stone to cure infection
  - stone and all foreign bodies must be cleared to avoid recurrence
  - associated with staghorn calculi

Uric Acid Stones (5-10%)

- precipitate in low volume, acidic urine with a high uric acid concentration
- hyperuricosuria alone
  - low urinary pH, low urine volume (e.g. GI water loss)
  - drugs (ASA, thiazides)
  - diet (purine rich – red meats)
- hyperuricosuria with hyperuricemia
- gout
- high cell turnover (leukemias, neoplasms) or death (cytotoxic drugs)

Uric Acid Stones are radiolucent on plain x-ray (KUB).

Cystine Stones

- autosomal recessive defect in small bowel mucosal absorption and renal tubular absorption of dibasic amino acids
  - results in "COLA" in urine – cystine, ornithine, lysine, arginine
- aggressive stone disease seen in children and young adults
  - recurrent stone formation, family history
  - often staghorn calculi
- aggregation in acidic urine
- diagnosed via positive urine sodium nitroprusside test, urine chromatography for cystine

Cystine stones are radio-opaque on plain x-ray (KUB).

Urological Neoplasms

Approach to Renal Mass

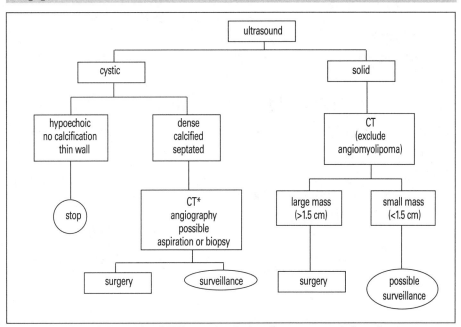

Figure 6. Workup of a Renal Mass (*MRI occassionally done if contrast contraindicated)

Benign Renal Neoplasms

RENAL CYSTS
- simple cysts
  - very common – up to 50% at age 50
  - usually incidental finding on abdominal imaging
  - Bosniak classification system depends on whether cyst is simple or complex to assess risk of malignancy based on wall, septations, calcifications and internal echoes
- polycystic kidney disease
  - autosomal recessive – massive kidneys with early renal failure in children, hepatic disease associated
  - autosomal dominant – progressive bilateral disease leading to hypertension and renal failure
    - associated with hepatic cysts and cerebral aneurysms
- medullary sponge kidney
  - dilatations of the collecting ducts
  - usually benign course, but predispose to calcium phosphate stones
- von Hippel-Lindau disease
  - renal cysts, cerebellar and retinal hemangioblastomas, pancreatic and epididymal cysts
  - 30-40% incidence of renal cell carcinoma

ANGIOMYOLIPOMA (RENAL HAMARTOMA)
- rare benign tumour (less than 0.5% of all renal tumours)
- characterized by 3 major histologic components: blood vessels, smooth muscle and fat cells
- usually asymptomatic, rarely spontaneously ruptures (especially in pregnant females)
- found in approximately 45-80% of patients with tuberous sclerosis (Bourneville's disease) which is characterized by:
  - epilepsy and mental retardation
  - sebaceous adenomas
  - hamartomas of brain and kidney
- diagnosis by CT → fat (negative density on CT) observed in kidneys is pathognomonic; echogenic on US

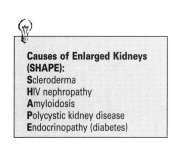

Causes of Enlarged Kidneys (SHAPE):
Scleroderma
HIV nephropathy
Amyloidosis
Polycystic kidney disease
Endocrinopathy (diabetes)

RENAL ONCOCYTOMA
- neoplasm of intercalated cells of collecting duct
- 80% are asymptomatic, found incidentally
- 20% hematuria, palpable mass or flank/abdominal pain
- difficult to distinguish from renal adenocarcinoma on imaging

RENAL ADENOMA
- cortical tumours historically thought to be benign since found incidentally at autopsy or nephrectomy
- 10 - 20% of population
- classification is controversial as pathologic diagnosis difficult and many believe this tumour has malignant potential

Malignant Renal Neoplasms

RENAL ADENOCARCINOMA (Renal Cell Carcinoma (RCC), hypernephroma)

Etiology
- cause is unknown
- originates from proximal convoluted tubule epithelial cell
- risk factors: smoking (results in 2x increased relative risk), cadmium exposure, employment in leather industry
- familial incidence seen with von Hippel-Lindau syndrome

Epidemiology
- eighth most common malignancy (accounts for 3% of all newly diagnosed cancers)
- 85% of primary malignant tumours in kidney
- male:female = 3:1
- peak incidence at 50-60 years of age

Pathology
- histological subtypes: clear, granular, and spindle cell types

Tumour may invade renal vein and inferior vena cava lumen (ascites, hepatic dysfunction, right atrial tumour, and pulmonary emboli).

Clinical Features
- usually asymptomatic – frequently diagnosed incidentally with U/S and CT
- poor prognostic indicators: weight loss, weakness, anemia, bone pain
- local effects: classic "too late triad" found in 10-15%
  - gross hematuria 50%
  - flank pain <50%
  - palpable mass <30%
- was called the "internist's tumour" because of paraneoplastic symptomatology, now called the "radiologist's tumour" because of incidental diagnosis
- systemic effects: paraneoplastic syndromes (10-40% of patients)
  - hematopoietic disturbances: anemia, polycythemia, raised ESR
  - endocrinopathies: hypercalcemia (increased vitamin D hydroxylation), erythrocytosis (increased erythropoietin), hypertension (increased renin), production of other hormones (prolactin, gonadotropins, TSH, insulin and cortisol)
  - hepatic cell dysfunction, "Stauffer's syndrome": abnormal liver function tests, decreased WBC count, fever, areas of hepatic necrosis; no evidence of metastases; reversible following removal of primary tumour
  - hemodynamic alterations: systolic hypertension (due to AV shunting), peripheral edema (due to caval obstruction)
- metastases: seen in 15% of new cases
  - bone, brain, lung, liver most common sites

Investigations
- routine labs for paraneoplastic syndromes (CBC, ESR, LFTs)
- urinalysis (60-75% have hematuria)
- renal ultrasound (solid vs. cystic lesion)
- CT scan (to distinguish solid vs. cystic lesion and to determine extent and operability)
- IVP (mass lesion): no longer routinely done
- angiography: no longer routinely done

Methods of Spread
- direct, venous, lymphatic

Staging
- involves CT, chest x-ray, liver enzymes and functions, bone scan

Table 3. TNM Classification

T	N	M
T1: tumour <7 cm, confined to renal parenchyma	N0: no regional nodes	M0: no evidence of metastasis
T1a: <4 cm	N1: metastasis to a single node, <2 cm	M1: presence of distant metastasis
T1b: 4-7 cm	N2: metastasis to a single node between	
T2: tumour >7 cm, confined to renal parenchyma	2 and 5 cm or multiple nodes <2 cm	
T3: tumour extends into major veins or adrenal,	N3: node >5 cm	
but not beyond Gerota's fascia		
T3a: into adrenal or sinus fat		
T3b: into renal vein or infradiaphragmatic IVC		
T3c: into supradiaphragmatic IVC		
T4: tumour extends beyond Gerota's fascia		

Treatment
- surgical
  - radical nephrectomy: en bloc removal of kidney, tumour, ipsilateral adrenal gland (in upper pole tumours) and intact Gerota's capsule and paraaortic lymphadenectomy
  - partial nephrectomy: <4 cm tumour or solitary kidney/bilateral tumours
  - surgical removal of solitary metastasis may be considered
- radiation for palliation – painful bony lesions
- chemotherapy: NOT effective
- immunotherapy: occasionally for metastatic disease (interferon-α, interleukin-2)
- recent: anti-angiogenesis (anti-VEGF and anti-TYR kinase; sutinib (Sorafenib™)) and anti-IL2 monoclonal antibodies (Baclizumab™) and Sunitinib (Sutent™)

Prognosis
- stage at diagnosis is the most important predictor of survival
  - T1 – 5-year survival is 90-100%
  - T2-T3 – 5-year survival is approximately 60%
  - 5-year survival of patients presenting with metastasis is 0-20%

Carcinoma of the Renal Pelvis and Ureter

Epidemiology
- rare, accounts for 4% of all urothelial cancers
- frequently multifocal, 2-5% are bilateral
- male:female = 3:1
- relative incidence – bladder:pelvis:ureter = 100:10:1

Pathology
- papillary transitional cell carcinoma (TCC); 85% (others include squamous cell, adenocarcinoma)
- TCC of kidney and ureter are histologically similar to bladder TCC

Risk Factors
- smoking
- chemical exposure (industrial dyes and solvents)
- analgesic abuse (acetaminophen, ASA, and phenacetin)
- Balkan nephropathy (chronic interstitial nephropathy in countries such as Serbia, Montenegro, Romania, Bulgaria)

Clinical Features
- gross painless hematuria (70-90% of patients)
- microscopic hematuria
- flank pain
- dysuria
- flank mass caused by tumour or associated hydronephrosis (10-20% of patients)

Investigations
- cystoscopy and retrograde; CT scan, radiolucent filling defect on IVP
- differential diagnosis of filling defect
  - transitional cell carcinoma (differentiate via cytology and CT scan)
  - uric acid stone (differentiate via cytology and CT scan)
  - blood clot
  - pyelitis cystica
  - papillary necrosis
  - fungus ball
  - gas bubble from gas producing organisms

Treatment
- radical ureteronephrectomy with cuff of bladder
- distal ureterectomy for distal ureteral tumours
- overall 5-year survival following ureteronephrectomy is 84% (depends on differentiation and depth of penetration)

Bladder Carcinoma

Etiology
- unknown, but exposure to environmental and occupational carcinogens plays a role
- risk factors
  - smoking (main factor – implicated in 60% of new cases)
  - chemicals: naphthylamines, benzidine, tryptophan, phenacetin metabolites
  - cyclophosphamide
  - prior history of radiation treatment to the pelvis
  - *Schistosoma hematobium* infection (associated with SCC)
  - chronic irritation (cystitis, chronic catheterization, bladder stones), (associated with SCC)

Epidemiology
- 2nd most common urological malignancy
- male:female = 3:1, white:black = 4:1
- mean age at diagnosis is 65 years

Pathology
- classification
  - transitional cell carcinoma (TCC) >90%
  - squamous cell carcinoma (SCC) 5-7%
  - adenocarcinoma 1%
  - others <1%
- stages of transitional cell carcinoma at diagnosis
  - superficial papillary (75%) → >80% overall survival
    - 15% of these will progress to invasive TCC
    - the majority of these patients will have recurrence
  - invasive (25%) → 50-60% 5-year survival
    - 85% have no prior history of superficial TCC (i.e. de novo)
    - 15% have occult metastases at diagnosis – lymph nodes, lung, peritoneum, liver
- carcinoma in situ → flat, non-papillary erythematous lesion characterized by dysplasia confined to urothelium
  - more aggressive, poorer prognosis
  - usually multifocal
  - may progress to invasive TCC

The "field defect" theory helps to explain why TCC has multiple lesions and has a high recurrence rate. The entire urothelium (pelvis to bladder) is bathed in carcinogens.

Clinical Features
- hematuria (key symptom: 85-90% at the time of diagnosis)
- pain (50%)
- clot retention (17%)
- asymptomatic (20%)
- storage urinary symptoms – consider carcinoma in situ
- palpable mass on bimanual exam → likely muscle invasion
- obstruction of ureters → hydronephrosis and uremia (nausea, vomiting and diarrhea)
- metastases
  - hepatomegaly, lymphadenopathy, bone lesions
  - lower extremity lymphedema if local advancement or lymphatic spread

Investigations
- urinalysis, urine C&S, urine cytology (sensitivity increases as grade/stage increases)
- ultrasound
- CT scan with contrast; intravenous pyelogram (IVP) → filling defect
- cystoscopy with bladder washings (gold standard)
- biopsy to establish diagnosis and to determine depth of penetration (although cold punch biopsy can be transurethral, resection is standard)
- new advances with specific bladder tumour markers (NMP-22, BTA, Immunocyt, FDP)

Grading
- Grade 1: well-differentiated (10% invasive)
- Grade 2: moderately differentiated (50% invasive)
- Grade 3: poorly differentiated (80% invasive)

Staging
- for invasive disease: CT or MRI, chest x-ray, liver function tests (metastatic work-up)

Table 4. TNM Classification (see Figure 7)

T	N	M
Ta: noninvasive papillary carcinoma	N status: as for renal cell carcinoma	M status: as for renal cell carcinoma
Tis: carcinoma in situ (CIS); flat tumour		
T1: tumour invades submucosa/lamina propria		
T2a: tumour invades superficial muscle		
T2b: tumour invades deep muscle		
T3: tumour invades perivesical fat		
T4a: adjacent organ involvement; prostate, uterus or vagina		
T4b: adjacent organ involvement; pelvic wall or abdominal wall		

Treatment
- superficial disease (Tis, Ta, T1)
  - transurethral resection of bladder tumour (TURBT) ± single dose or maintenance intravesical chemo-/immuno-therapy (e.g. BCG, mitomycin C) to decrease recurrence rate
  - high grade disease - TURBT + maintenance BCG OR cystectomy in select patients
- invasive disease (T2a, T2b, T3)
  - radical cystectomy + pelvic lymphadenectomy with urinary diversion or irradiation for small tumours
- advanced/metastatic disease (T4a, T4b, N+, M+)
  - initial combination systemic chemotherapy ± irradiation ± surgery

Prognosis
- depends on stage, grade, size, number of lesions, recurrence and presence of CIS
  - stage T1 – 90% at 5 years
  - stage T2 – 55%
  - stage T3 – 20%
  - stage T4/N+/M+ – <5%

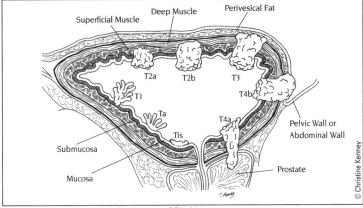

Figure 7. Transitional Cell Carcinoma of Bladder

Prostatic Carcinoma (CaP)

Etiology
- not known
- risk factors
  - urban blacks have increased incidence
  - family history
    - 1st degree relative = 2x risk
    - 1st and 2nd degree relatives = 9x risk
  - high dietary fat increases risk by 2x
  - cigarette smoking

Epidemiology
- most prevalent cancer in males
- third leading cause of male cancer deaths (following lung and colon)
- lifetime risk of a 50 y.o. man for CaP is 50%, and risk of death is 3%
- 75% diagnosed between ages of 60 and 85 and mean diagnosis at 72 years of age

Differential Diagnosis of a Prostatic Nodule
- prostate cancer (30%)
- benign prostatic hyperplasia
- prostatitis
- prostatic infarct
- prostatic calculus
- tuberculous prostatitis

Pathology
- adenocarcinoma
  - >95%
  - often multifocal
- transitional cell carcinoma (4.5%)
  - associated with TCC of bladder
  - not hormone-responsive
- endometrial (rare)
  - carcinoma of the utricle

Anatomy (see Figure 5)
- 60-70% of nodules arise in the peripheral zone
- 10-20% arise in the transition zone
- 5-10% arise in the central zone

Clinical Features
- usually asymptomatic
- most commonly detected by DRE, elevated PSA, or as an incidental finding on transurethral resection of the prostate (TURP)
  - DRE: hard irregular nodule or diffuse dense induration involving one or both lobes
  - PSA: see *Prostate Specific Antigen* section, U25
- locally advanced disease
  - storage and voiding LUTS (uncommon without spread)
  - suspect with LUTS, incontinence ± back pain
- metastatic disease
  - bony metastasis to axial skeleton is very common (osteoblastic)
  - visceral metastasis is less common with liver, lung and adrenal metastases occurring most frequently
  - leg pain and edema with nodal metastasis obstructing lymphatic and venous drainage

Methods of Spread
- local invasion
- lymphatic spread to regional nodes
  - obturator > iliac > presacral/para-aortic
- hematogenous dissemination occurs early

Investigations
- DRE
- PSA elevated in the majority of patients with CaP
- transrectal ultrasound (TRUS) → size and local staging
- TRUS-guided needle biopsy
- bone scan may be omitted in untreated CaP with PSA <10 ng/ml
- CT scanning to assess metastases

The Prostate Cancer Prevention Trial (PCPT)
(NEJM 2003;349:215-224)
Study: A randomized, double-blind, placebo-controlled study designed to determine whether treatment with finasteride could reduce the prevalence of prostate CA during a 7-year period.
Patients: 18,882 men with elevated risk of prostate CA (55 years of age or older, African-American, or a 1st degree relative having prostate CA) with a normal DRE and a PSA level of ≤3 ng/mL were enrolled. 92% white.
Intervention: Finasteride (5 mg/day) vs. placebo
Main outcome: Prevalence of prostate CA during a 7-year period.
Results: Study was closed early as objectives were met. There was a 25% relative reduction (P<0.001) in prevalence of prostate CA in the finasteride group [18% incidence] compared to placebo group [24% incidence], but an increase in the proportion of high-grade tumours (Gleason score 8-10) among those diagnosed with cancer (12% for finasteride, 5% for placebo). The majority of tumours in both groups (98%) were clinically localized disease (T1 or T2). The finasteride group also had a significantly higher incidence of sexual side effects, but fewer urinary symptoms than the placebo group.
Conclusions: Men over 55 who took finasteride for 7 years were 25% less likely to develop prostate CA compared to the placebo group, however the cancers in the finasteride group were of a higher grade.

Table 5. Staging (TNM 2002)

T	N	M
T1: clinically undetectable tumour, normal DRE and TRUS	**N:** spread to regional lymph nodes	**M:** distant metastasis
T1a: tumour incidental histologic finding in ≤5% of tissue resected		**M1a:** nonregional lymph nodes
T1b: tumour incidental histologic finding in >5% of tissue resected		**M1b:** bone(s)
T1c: tumour identified by needle biopsy (because of elevated PSA level); tumours found in 1 or both lobes by needle biopsy but not palpable or reliably visible by imaging		**M1c:** other site(s) with or without bone disease
T2: palpable, confined to prostate		
T2a: tumour involving less than half a lobe		
T2b: tumour involving less than or equal to 1 lobe		
T2c: tumour involving both lobes		
T3: tumour extends through prostate capsule		
T3a: extracapsular extension (unilateral or bilateral)		
T3b: tumour invading seminal vesicle(s)		
T4: tumour invades adjacent structures (besides seminal vesicles)		

Grading
- tumour grade (Gleason score out of 10) is also important
  - aggregate score of two most prominent histological patterns
    - ♦ 1-4 = well differentiated
    - ♦ 5-6 = moderately differentiated
    - ♦ 8-10 = poorly differentiated

Treatment
- T1 (small well-differentiated CaP are associated with slow growth rate)
  - if young consider radical prostatectomy, brachytherapy or radiation
  - follow in older population (cancer death rate up to 10%)
- T2
  - radical prostatectomy or radiation (70-85% survival at 10 years) or brachytherapy
- T3, T4
  - staging lymphadenectomy and radiation or hormonal treatment
- N >0 or M >0 (see *Common Medications* section, U44)
  - requires hormonal therapy / palliative radiotherapy to metastases
  - bilateral orchiectomy – removes 90% of testosterone
  - LHRH agonists (e.g. leuprolide (Lupron™ or Eligard™), goserelin (Zoladex™))
  - estrogens (e.g. diethylstilbestrol (DES))
  - antiandrogens
    - ♦ greater androgen blockade can be achieved by combining an antiandrogen with LHRH agonist or orchiectomy
    - ♦ local irradiation of painful secondaries or half-body irradiation
  - chemotherapy regimens that include docetaxel may improve survival in advanced prostate cancer that is no longer responsive to hormone therapy

Prognosis
- stage T1-T2: excellent, comparable with normal life expectancy
- stage T3-T4: 40-70% survival at 10 years
- stage N+ and/or M+: 40% survival at 5 years
- prognostic factors: tumour stage, tumour grade, PSA value

Prostate Specific Antigen (PSA)

- enzyme produced by epithelial cells of prostate gland to liquify the ejaculate
- leaks into circulation and is present at <4 ng/mL
- measured total serum PSA is a combination of free (unbound) PSA (15%) and complexed PSA (85%)

Screening & Investigation for Prostate Cancer: PSA, DRE, and TRUS
Ontario Ministry of Health and Long-Term Care – Ontario PSA Clinical Guidelines, 2000
- PSA may be elevated in prostate cancer and many other conditions (see sidebar); it is not specific to prostate cancer
- currently no evidence that PSA screening decreases mortality
- routine screening not currently recommended; patients should make informed decisions about whether to undergo PSA test and/or DRE

Strategies to Increase Specificity of PSA Test
- age-related cutoff values

Table 6. Normal PSA Value by Age Group

Age Range (years)	Serum PSA Concentration (g/L)
40-49	<2.5
50-59	<3.5
60-69	<4.5
70-79	<6.5

Oesterling JE et al. *JAMA.* 1993 Aug. 18; 270(7): 860-4.

- free-to-total PSA ratio
  - complexed PSA increases in prostate cancer, decreasing the percentage of the free fraction
  - <10% free PSA suggestive of cancer, >20% free suggests benign cause
- PSA velocity
  - change of >0.75 ng/mL/year associated with increased risk of cancer

In PSA testing, think "**free and easy**": increased free/total ratio suggests benign cause of high PSA.

- PSA density
  - PSA divided by prostate volume as found on TRUS
  - >0.15 ng/mL/g associated with increased risk of cancer

Testicular Tumours

Etiology
- not entirely known
- congenital: cryptorchidism (10%)
- acquired: trauma, atrophy, sex hormones

Epidemiology
- rare, but common in young adults (17-37 years of age)
- high cure rate
- any solid testicular mass in young patient – must rule out malignancy
- slightly more common in right testis (corresponds with slightly higher incidence of right-sided cryptorchidism)
- 2-3% bilateral (simultaneously or successively)

Pathology
- primary
  - 1% of all malignancies in males
  - most common solid malignancy in males aged 15-34 years
  - undescended testicle has increased risk (10-40x) of malignancy
  - 95% are germ cell tumours (all are malignant)
    - seminoma (35%) → classic, anaplastic, spermatocytic
    - nonseminomatous germ cell tumours (NSGCT) → embryonal cell carcinoma (20%), teratoma (5%), choriocarcinoma (<1%), yolk sac (<<1%), mixed cell type (40%)
  - 5% are non-germ cell tumours (usually benign) → Leydig (testosterone, precocious puberty), Sertoli (gynecomastia, decreased libido)
- secondary
  - male >50 years of age
  - usually a lymphoma
  - metastases (e.g. lung, prostate, GI)

Surgical descent (orchiopexy) of undescended testis does not reduce the risk of malignancy (10-40x). It can reduce the risk of infertility and make follow-up easier.

Clinical Features
- painless testicular enlargement (painful if intratesticular hemorrhage or infarction)
- firm, non-tender mass
- dull, heavy ache in lower abdomen, anal area or scrotum
- associated hydrocele in 10%
- coincidental trauma in 10%
- infertility (rarely presenting complaint)
- gynecomastia due to secretory tumour effects
- metastatic disease related back pain
- supraclavicular and inguinal nodes
- abdominal mass (retroperitoneal lymph node metastases)

Methods of Spread
- local spread follows lymphatics
  - right → medial, paracaval, anterior and lateral nodes
  - left → left lateral and anterior paraaortic nodes
  - "cross-over" metastases from right to left are fairly common, but they have not been reported from left to right
- hematogenous most commonly to lung, liver, bones and kidney

Investigations
- diagnosis is established by radical inguinal orchidectomy
- tumour markers
  - β-hCG and AFP are positive in 85% of non-seminomatous tumours
  - pre-orchidectomy elevated marker levels return to normal post-operatively if no secondaries
  - β-hCG positive in 7% of seminomas, AFP never elevated with seminoma
- testicular ultrasound (hypoechoic area within tunica albuginea = high suspicion of testicular cancer)
- evidence of testicular microlithiasis is not a risk factor for testicular cancer
- needle aspiration contraindicated

Testes and scrotum have different lymphatic drainage, therefore trans-scrotal approach for biopsy or orchiectomy should be avoided.

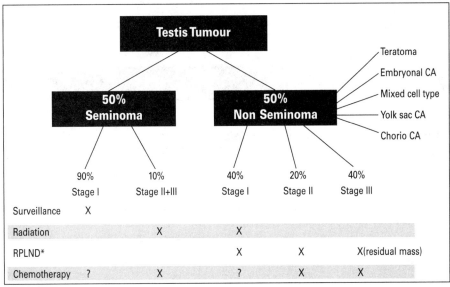

Staging
- clinical – CXR (lung metastases), markers for staging (β-hCG, AFP, LDH), CT abdomen/pelvis (retroperitoneal nodes enlarged)
  - **Stage I**: disease limited to testis, epididymis or spermatic cord
  - **Stage II**: disease limited to the retroperitoneal nodes
  - **Stage III**: disease metastatic to supradiaphragmatic nodal or visceral sites
- pathologic (at orchiectomy)
  - **T1**: tumour confined to testis and epididymis, no vascular/lymphatic invasion
  - **T2**: tumour extends beyond tunica albuginea or vascular/lymphatic invasion
  - **T3**: tumour involves spermatic cord
  - **T4**: tumour invades scrotum
  - **T4a**: tumour invades spermatic cord
  - **T4b**: tumour invades scrotal wall

Figure 8. Testicular Cancer   *RPLND = retroperitoneal lymph node dissection   Courtesy of Dr. MAS Jewett

Prognosis
- 99% cured with stage I, stage II
- 70-80% complete remission with advanced disease

Penile Tumours

- rare (<1% of cancer in males in U.S.), most common in 6th decade

Benign
- cyst, hemangioma, nevus, papilloma

Pre-malignant
- balanitis xerotica obliterans, leukoplakia, Buschke-Lowenstein tumour (large condyloma)

Pre-invasive Cancer
- carcinoma in situ (CIS)
  - Bowen's disease → crusted, red plaques on the shaft
  - erythroplasia of Queyrat → velvet red, ulcerated plaques on the glans
  - treatment options: local excision, laser, radiation, topical 5-fluorouracil

Malignant
- risk factors:
  - chronic inflammatory disease
  - STI
  - phimosis
  - uncircumcised penis
- 2% of all urogenital cancers
- squamous cell (>95%), basal cell, Paget's disease, melanoma
- definitive diagnosis requires full thickness biopsy of lesion

Table 7. TNM Staging

T	N	M
Tx: primary tumour cannot be assessed	**N1**: metastasis in a single superficial, inguinal lymph node	**M**: presence (+) or absence (0) of distant metastasis (lung, liver, bone, brain)
T0: no evidence of primary tumour	**N2**: metastasis in multiple or bilateral superficial lymph nodes	
Tis: CIS		
Ta: non-invasive carcinoma	**N3**: metastasis in deep inguinal or pelvic lymph node(s) unilateral or bilateral	
T1: tumour invades subepithelial connective tissue (Buck's and Dartos fascia)		
T2: tumour invades corpus spongiosum or cavernosum (through tunica albuginea)		
T3: tumour invades urethra or prostate		
T4: tumour invades other adjacent structures		

- lymphatic spread (superficial/deep inguinal nodes → iliac nodes) >> hematogenous

Treatment
- wide surgical excision with tumour-free margins (dependent on extent and area of penile involvement) ± lymphadenectomy

Scrotal Mass

- also see *Common Presenting Problems*, U4

Table 8. Differentiating between Scrotal Masses

Condition	Pain	Palpation	Additional Findings
torsion	+	diffuse tenderness	negative cremaster reflex, negative Prehn's sign, EMERGENCY!
epididymitis	+	epididymal tenderness	positive cremaster reflex, positive Prehn's sign
orchitis	+	diffuse tenderness	positive cremaster reflex, positive Prehn's sign
hematocele	+	diffuse tenderness	no transillumination
hydrocele	-	testis not separable from hydrocele, cord palpable	transilluminates
spermatocele	-	testis separable from spermatocele, cord palpable	transilluminates
varicocele	-	Bag of worms	no transillumination
indirect inguinal hernia	- (+ if strangulated)	testis seperable from hernia, cord not palpable, cough impulse may transmit, may be reducible	no transillumination
tumour	- (+ if hemorrhagic)	hard lump/nodule	
idiopathic	-		

Torsion

TESTICULAR TORSION (SPERMATIC CORD TORSION)
- UROLOGICAL EMERGENCY

Etiology
- testis rotates medially causing strangulation of the blood supply (varies between 180°-720°)
    - ultimately leads to necrosis of entire gonad if untreated within 5-6 hours
- any age, but most common in adolescence due to pubertal increase in testicular volume
- acute scrotal swelling in children indicates torsion until proven otherwise

Incidence
- ~1/4000 males <25 years
- left testis more frequently involved

Predisposing Factors
- cryptorchid testis
- trauma (although 50% occur during sleep)
- "bell clapper" congenital deformity
    - narrow attachment of spermatic cord on to testis/epididymis → testis falls forward and is free to rotate within tunica vaginalis
- anomalous development of tunica vaginalis or spermatic cord

Clinical Features
- acute onset of severe scrotal pain, swelling ± nausea/vomiting
- retracted and transverse testicle (horizontal lie)
- absent cremasteric reflex
- no pain relief with testicle elevation (negative Prehn's sign)
- epididymis may be palpated anteriorly in the early stages

Diagnosis
- ultrasound with colour-flow Doppler probe over testicular artery (if torsion, no blood flow)
- decrease uptake on 99m Tc-pertechnetate scintillation scan ("doughnut" sign)
- examination under anesthesia and surgical exploration

Acute scrotal swelling/pain in young boys is torsion until proven otherwise.

Treatment
- emergency detorsion (rotate outward, like opening a book) + elective bilateral orchiopexy (fixation)
- failure of manual detorsion requires surgical detorsion and bilateral orchiopexy
- <12 hours – good prognosis
- 12-24 hours – uncertain prognosis, testicular atrophy
- >24 hours – poor prognosis, orchiectomy is advised

TORSION OF TESTICULAR APPENDIX
- twisting of testicular/epididymal vestigial appendix
- often <16 years of age

Signs and Symptoms
- clinically similar to testicular torsion
- "blue dot sign" – blue infarcted appendage seen through scrotal skin (can usually be palpated as small, tender lump)
- point tenderness over the superior-posterior portion of testicle

Treatment
- analgesia – most will subside over 5-7 days
- surgical exploration and excision if diagnosis uncertain or refractory pain

Hematocele

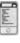

- trauma with bleed into tunica vaginalis
- ultrasound helpful to exclude fracture of testis which requires surgical repair
- treatment: ice packs, analgesics, surgical repair

Hydrocele

Definition
- collection of fluid within the tunica vaginalis
- most often seen surrounding the testis, may occur within the spermatic cord

Etiology
- usually idiopathic
- found in 5-10% of testicular tumours
- associated with trauma, orchitis, epididymitis

Classification
- communicating hydrocele: patent processus vaginalis, changes size during day (pediatrics)
- non-communicating hydrocele: processus vaginalis is not patent, does not change size during day (mainly in adults)

Investigations
- usually a non-tender cystic intrascrotal mass which transilluminates
- ultrasound (definitive), especially if <40 years of age (rule out tumour)

Treatment
- nothing if tolerated and no complications
- needle drainage ± instillation of a sclerosing agent to prevent recurrence
- surgical

Complications
- hemorrhage into hydrocele sac following trauma
- may prevent palpation of testicular mass
- compression of testicular blood supply

Spermatocele/Epididymal Cyst

Definition
- sperm filled epididymal retention cyst in the efferent ductules
- located at superior pole of testicle

Diagnosis
- may be entirely asymptomatic and often incidentally found
- round, firm, and cystic with distinct borders
- aspirate contains sperm
- transilluminates

Treatment
- usually no treatment
- needle aspiration should be avoided because it can lead to infection, spillage of irritating sperm within the scrotum and reaccumulation of spermatocele
- excise only if symptomatic

Hernia

- see General Surgery

Varicocele

In an isolated right-sided varicocele, beware of a right retroperitoneal mass.

Indications for treatment of varicocele
- impaired sperm quality or quantity
- pain or dull ache affecting quality of life
- affected testis fails to grow in adolescents
- cosmetic indications (esp. in adolescents)

Etiology
- dilated veins in the pampiniform plexus; incompetent valves in testicular veins
- 90% on left side
    - left testicular vein is longer and joins the left renal vein (extra resistance; right side empties into the vena cava)
- rarely from retroperitoneal mass
- 10% incidence in young men
- 30% of men with infertility have it (associated with testicular atrophy)

Clinical Features
- usually asymptomatic, but may be painful
- heavy sensation after walking or standing
- upright – mass of dilated, tortuous veins ("bag of worms")
- supine – venous distention abates
- pulsates with Valsalva or cough

Treatment
- surgical ligation of testicular vein above inguinal ligament
- percutaneous vein occlusion – balloon catheter, sclerosing agents
- in the presence of oligospermia, surgically correcting the varicocele may improve sperm count and motility in 50-75% of patients

Penile Complaints

Peyronie's Disease

Definition
- fibrous thickening of the penile shaft resulting in painful erections and/or penile curvature

Etiology
- can be associated with vitamin E deficiency, β-blockade, elevated serotonin levels, Dupuytren's contractures, and with HLA-B27
- inflammatory process involving the tunica albuginea secondary to penile trauma
    - results in fibrotic plaque formation that fails to stretch with erection
- commonly on dorsal surface resulting in upward curvature of erect penis due to scar tissue – may occur at any site
- chordee = ventral bend
    - in children, associated with hypospadias due to congenital shortening of ventral skin (not Peyronie's disease). See: *Congenital Abnomalities* section, U37

Clinical Features
- penis curvature ± painful erection, poor erection distal to plaque

Treatment
- depends on pain and interference with intercourse
- watchful waiting (spontaneous resolution in up to 50%)
- vitamin E, potassium paraaminobenzoate (potaba) – limited efficacy
- intralesional verapamil
- surgical excision of plaque, prosthesis for erectile dysfunction
  - wait 1 year to allow for spontaneous resolution or failure of medical treatment prior to initiation of surgical treatment

Priapism

Definition
- UROLOGICAL EMERGENCY
- tumescence (swelling) of corpora cavernosa (often painful) with flaccid glans penis (no corpora spongiosum involvement) lasting >4 hours without sexual desire

Etiology
- high-flow (unregulated arterial flow – high pO_2) vs. low-flow (ischemic venous blockage – low pO_2)
- primary – 60% idiopathic
- secondary
  - thromboembolic – including sickle cell, thalassemia, total parenteral nutrition (TPN), dialysis
  - neoplastic – pelvic tumours (prostate, bladder), leukemia, melanoma, RCC
  - neurogenic – spinal cord injury, autonomic neuropathy
  - traumatic (genital, perineal) – usually high flow and less rigid due to venous competency
  - iatrogenic (e.g. intracorporal drug injection (papaverine, phentolamine, PGE_1 = triple mix for erectile dysfunction), chlorpromazine, trazodone, hydralazine, guanethidine, prazosin, heparin, omeprazole)
  - recreational drugs – cocaine, marijuana, EtOH

Treatment
- high flow – observation vs. arterial embolization
- low flow
  - needle aspiration of blood
  - phenylephrine injection into the corpora cavernosa q10-15min
  - shunt creation between cavernosum and spongiosum
  - STAT leukophoresis if leukemia
  - treat sickle cell anemia crisis

Complications
- erectile dysfunction due to corporal fibrosis if treatment delayed (50%)
  - significantly increased risk if treatment delayed >24-48 hours

Phimosis

Definition
- inability to retract foreskin over glans penis
- may be caused by balanitis (infection of glans), often due to poor hygeine
- normal congenital adhesions separate naturally by 1-2 years of age

Treatment
- circumcision, dorsal slit, proper hygiene (trial of topical corticosteroids in children)

Complications
- balanoposthitis (inflammation of prepuce), paraphimosis, penile cancer

Paraphimosis

Definition
- UROLOGICAL EMERGENCY
- foreskin caught behind glans leading to edema; unable to reduce foreskin

Treatment
- squeeze edema out of the glans with manual pressure (analgesia required)
- pull on foreskin with fingers while pushing on glans with thumbs
  - if fails, do dorsal slit or circumcision
- elective circumcision for definitive treatment (paraphimosis tends to recur)

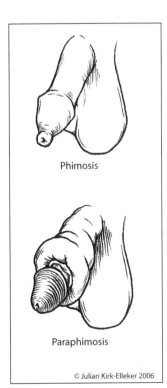

Phimosis

Paraphimosis

© Julian Kirk-Elleker 2006

Figure 9. Paraphimosis vs Phimosis

Complications
• infection, glans ischemia, gangrene

Erectile Dysfunction (ED)

Definition
• consistent (>3 months duration) or recurrent inability to obtain or maintain an adequate erection for sexual performance

Physiology
• erection involves the coordination of psychologic, neurologic, hemodynamic, mechanical and endocrine components
• erection (= POINT)
  ▪ release of nitric oxide (NO) by activated parasympathetics increased cGMP levels within corpora cavernosa: 1) arteriolar dilatation and 2) relaxation of the sinusoidal smooth muscle → increased arterial inflow and compression of penile venous drainage (decreased venous outflow)
• emission (= SHOOT)
  ▪ sensory afferents from glans
  ▪ secretions from prostate, seminal vesicles, and ejaculatory ducts enter prostatic urethra (sympathetics)
• ejaculation (= SHOOT)
  ▪ bladder neck closure (sympathetic)
  ▪ spasmodic contraction of bulbo-cavernosus and pelvic floor musculature (somatic)

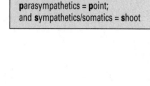

Erections POINT AND SHOOT:
parasympathetics = **p**oint;
and **s**ympathetics/somatics = **s**hoot

Classification
• psychogenic (10%)
  ▪ EtOH, tension, and/or premature ejaculation often involved
  ▪ performance anxiety
  ▪ depression, post-traumatic stress disorder (PTSD)
  ▪ widower syndrome
  ▪ sensate focus
  ▪ typically:
    ◆ younger age
    ◆ intermittent difficulty
    ◆ no risk factors for organic disease
    ◆ nocturnal penile tumescence present
    ◆ often able to achieve erection using self-stimulation
• organic (90%)
  ▪ endocrine: diabetes, gonadal or pituitary dysfunction
  ▪ vasculogenic: arterial insufficiency (many causes, including diabetes), atherosclerosis
  ▪ neurogenic: diabetes, multiple sclerosis, spinal cord injury, Alzheimer's, Guillain-Barré, stroke
  ▪ respiratory: COPD, sleep apnea
  ▪ iatrogenic: drugs (antihypertensives, sedatives, psychotropics, antinuclear agents such as cimetidine and finasteride), radiation, pelvic surgery (radical prostatectomy)
  ▪ penile: post-priapism, Peyronie's, epispadias surgery
  ▪ organ failure: liver, renal
  ▪ nutritional: malnutrition, zinc deficiency
  ▪ typically:
    ◆ older age (>50 years old)
    ◆ constant difficulty, including self-stimulation
    ◆ risk factors present (atherosclerosis, hypertension, diabetes)
• mixed (common)

Testosterone deficiency is an uncommon cause of ED.

Diagnosis
• complete history (sexual, medical, and psychosocial)
• self-administered questionnaires (International Index of Erectile Function, Sexual Health Inventory for Men Questionnaire, ED Intensity Scale, ED Impact Scale)
• focused physical exam, including vascular and neurologic examinations
• lab investigations
  ▪ risk factor evaluation: fasting blood glucose or HbA1c, cholesterol profile
  ▪ other: TSH, CBC, urinalysis
  ▪ hypothalamic-pituitary-gonadal axis evaluation: testosterone (free and total), prolactin, LH, FSH
• usually unnecessary to do further testing except in certain situations
• specialized testing
  ▪ non-invasive

- ◆ nocturnal penile tumescence monitor
  - ▪ invasive (rarely done)
    - ◆ intracavernous injection of papaverine or PGE₁ – rule out significant arterial or venous impairment
    - ◆ Doppler studies pre- and post-papaverine injection – cavernosal anatomy and arterial flow evaluation (penile-brachial index <0.6 suggestive of vascular cause)
    - ◆ angiography of pudendal artery post papaverine injection – post-traumatic ED evaluation only for possible vascular reconstruction
    - ◆ dynamic cavernosometry and cavernosography – to evaluate leakage from penile veins

Treatment
- must fully inform patient/partner of options, benefits and complications
- non-invasive
  - ▪ lifestyle changes (alcohol, smoking), psychological (sexual counseling and education)
- minimally invasive
  - ▪ oral medication (see *Common Medications* section, U44)
    - ◆ sildenafil (Viagra™), tadalafil (Cialis™), vardenafil (Levitra™): inhibits phosphodiesterase type 5
    - ◆ yohimbine: α-blocker that is best for psychogenic ED
    - ◆ trazodone: serotonin antagonist and reuptake inhibitor
  - ▪ vacuum devices: draw blood into penis via negative pressure, then put ring at base of penis once erect
  - ▪ MUSE: Male Urethral Suppository for Erection – vasoactive substance (PGE₁) capsule into urethra
- invasive
  - ▪ intracorporal vasodilator injection/self-injection
    - ◆ triple therapy (papaverine, phentolamine, PGE₁) or PGE₁ alone
    - ◆ complications include priapism (overdose), thickening of tunica albuginea at site of repeated injections (Peyronie's plaque) and hematoma
  - ▪ implants (last resort): malleable or inflatable
  - ▪ vascular surgery: microvascular arterial bypass and venous ligation (investigational)

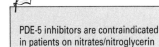

PDE-5 inhibitors are contraindicated in patients on nitrates/nitroglycerin

Premature Ejaculation

Definition
- occurrence of ejaculation prior to when one or both of partners desire it
- primary premature ejaculation
  - ▪ never experienced sexual activity without the presence of premature ejaculation
- secondary premature ejaculation
  - ▪ the individual once had acceptable ejaculatory control, but now experiences premature ejaculation, not associated with a general medical condition

Epidemiology
- 30-70% prevalence
- most common sexual dysfunction reported in men 18-30 years old, associated with secondary impotence in men aged 45-65

Investigations
- indicated by history and physical
- testosterone levels if in conjunction with impotence

Treatment
- must rule out and treat any associated general medical conditions (i.e. fear of angina)
- often thought to be due to psychological factors; identify and address specific stressors
- referral to psychiatry, couples counseling or sex therapy
- SSRI have been found to be effective in some cases

Trauma

- see also Emergency Medicine

Renal Trauma

Etiology
- blunt (80%, motor vehicle collision (MVC), assaults, falls) vs. penetrating (20%, stab and gunshots)

History
- mechanism of injury

Physical Exam
- ABCs, renal vascular injury → shock mandating resuscitation
  - upper abdominal/flank tenderness, flank contusions, lower rib/vertebral transverse process fracture suggests blunt trauma

Investigations
- urinalysis: hematuria – requires workup but degree does not correlate with the severity of injury
- imaging: CT (contrast) if patient stable – look for renal laceration, urinary extravasation, retroperitoneal hematoma, and associated intra-abdominal organ injury

Classification According to Severity
- minor: contusions and superficial lacerations/hematomas – 90% of all blunt traumas, surgical exploration seldom necessary
- major: laceration that extends into medulla and collecting system, major renal vascular injury, shattered kidney

Management
- microscopic hematuria + isolated well-staged minor injuries do not need hospitalization
- gross hematuria + contusion/minor lacerations: hospitalize, bedrest, repeat CT if bleeding persists

Surgical Management
- absolute indications: hemorrhage and hemodynamic instability
- relative indications:
  - nonviable tissue and major laceration
  - urinary extravasation
  - vascular injury
  - laparotomy for associated injury

Outcome
- follow-up with ultrasound or CT before discharge, and at 6 weeks
- hypertension in 5% of renal trauma

Bladder Trauma

- blunt (MVC, falls, and crush injury) vs. penetrating trauma to lower abdomen, pelvis, or perineum
- blunt is associated with pelvic fracture in 97% of cases

Clinical Features
- abdominal tenderness, distention, and unable to void
- may be peritoneal signs or symptoms
- associated injuries including pelvic and long bone fractures are common
- hemodynamic instability due to extensive blood loss in the pelvis

Investigations
- gross hematuria in 90%
- imaging
- cystogram and post-drainage film for extravasation

Classification
- contusions: no urinary extravasation, damage to mucosa or muscularis
- intraperitoneal ruptures: often involve the bladder dome
- extraperitoneal ruptures: involve anterior or lateral bladder wall in full bladder

Treatment
- penetrating trauma: surgical exploration
- contusion: urethral catheter until hematuria completely resolves

- extraperitoneal bladder perforations can be managed non-operatively with Foley catheter if associated injuries do not require a laparotomy and the urine is sterile at time of the injury; others will need surgical management
- intraperitoneal rupture may require surgical repair and a suprapubic catheter

Complications
- mortality is around 20%, and is usually due to associated injuries rather than bladder rupture
- complications of bladder injury itself are rare

Urethral Injuries

Etiology
- posterior urethra: common site of injury is junction of membranous and prostatic urethra due to blunt trauma, MVCs, pelvic fracture
    - shearing force on fixed membranous and mobile prostatic urethra
- anterior urethra: straddle injury can crush bulbar urethra against pubic rami
- other causes: iatrogenic (instrumentation, prosthesis insertion), penile fracture, masturbation with urethral manipulation
- always look for associated bladder rupture

Clinical Features
- signs and symptoms
    - blood at urethral meatus
    - high riding prostate on digital exam
    - sensation of voiding without urine output
    - swelling and butterfly perineal hematoma

Investigations
- do not perform cystoscopy or catheterization before retrograde urethrography if urethral trauma suspected
- retrograde urethrography – demonstrates extravasation and location of injury

Treatment
- simple contusions – no treatment
- partial urethral disruption
    - very gentle attempt at catheterization by urology staff or urology resident
    - with no resistance to catheterization – Foley x2-3 weeks
    - with resistance to catheterization – suprapubic cystostomy or urethral catheter alignment in OR
- periodic flow rates/urethrograms to evaluate for stricture formation
- complete disruption
    - immediate repair if patient stable, delayed repair if unstable (suprapubic tube in interim)

Infertility

Definition
- failure to conceive after one year of unprotected, properly timed intercourse
- incidence
    - 15% of all couples – investigate both partners
    - 1/3 female, 1/3 male, 1/3 combined problem
- primary (has never conceived before) vs. secondary (has conceived before)

Female Factors

- see Gynecology

Male Factors

Male Reproduction
- hypothalamic-pituitary-testicular axis (HPTA): GnRH from hypothalamus acts on anterior pituitary stimulating release of LH and FSH
    - LH acts on Leydig (interstitial) cells → testosterone synthesis/secretion

- FSH acts on Sertoli cells → structural and metabolic support to developing spermatogenic cells
- FSH and testosterone support germ cells (responsible for spermatogenesis)
- sperm route: epididymis → vas deferens → ejaculatory ducts → prostatic urethra

Etiology
- hormonal (see Endocrinology)
  - hypothalamic-pituitary-testicular axis (2-3%)
- testicular
  - varicocele (30% infertile males) (increased temperature)
  - tumour
  - congenital (Klinefelter's triad: small, firm testes, gynecomastia and azoospermia)
  - cryptorchidism
  - post infectious (epididymo-orchitis, STIs, mumps)
  - torsion not corrected within 6hrs
- iatrogenic
  - radiation, antineoplastic and antiandrogen drugs can interfere with sperm transport and production
- lifestyle
  - drugs (marijuana, cocaine, tobacco, EtOH, prescription)
  - increased testicular temperature (sauna, hot baths, tight pants or underwear)
- surgical complications
  - testes (vasectomy, hydrocelectomy)
  - inguinal (inadvertant ligation of vas deferens in hernia repair)
  - bladder/prostate (damage to bladder neck causing retrograde ejaculation, damage to ejaculatory ducts)
- abdomen (damage to sympathetic nerves causing retrograde ejaculation)
- transport
  - cystic fibrosis (typical – obstructive azoospermia; atypical – congenital absence of the vas deferens, bilateral ejaculatory duct obstruction, epididymal obstructions)
  - Kartagener's syndrome
  - congenital absence of vas deferens, obstruction of vas deferens
- chronic disease: liver, renal

History
- medical history (past illness, diabetes, trauma, CF, genetic syndromes)
- surgical history (orchidopexy, cryptorchidism, prostate)
- fertility history (pubertal onset, previous pregnancies, duration of infertility, treatments)
- sexual history (erection/ejaculation, timing, frequency, STIs)
- family history
- medications (e.g. nitrofurantoin, cimetidine, sulfasalazine, spironolactone, alpha blockers)
- social history (ethanol, tobacco, cocaine, anabolic steroids)
- occupational exposures

Investigations
- semen analysis (SA) – at least 2 specimens
- hormonal evaluation – indicated with abnormal semen analysis (rare to be abnormal with normal SA)
  - testosterone for evaluation of HPA
  - FSH measures state of sperm production
  - serum LH and prolactin are measured if testosterone or FSH are abnormal
- genetic evaluation
  - chromosomal studies (Klinefelter's Syndrome – XXY)
  - genetic studies (Y-chromosome microdeletion, CF gene mutation)
- immunologic studies (antisperm antibodies in ejaculate and blood)
- testicular biopsy
- scrotal U/S (varicocele, testicular size)
- vasography (assess patency of vas deferens)

Treatment
- lifestyle
  - regular exercise, healthy diet
  - eliminate lifestyle habits described above
- medical
  - endocrine therapy (see Endocrinology)
  - treat retrograde ejaculation

WHO Guidelines
Normal Semen Values
- volume: 2-5 ml
- concentration: >20 million sperm/ml
- morphology: 30% normal forms
- motility: >50% adequate forward progression
- liquefaction: complete in 20 minutes
- pH: 7.2-7.8
- WBC: <10 per high power field or <10^6 WBC/mL semen

- ▪ discontinue anti-sympathomimetic agents, may start α-adrenergic stimulation (phenylpropanolamine, pseudoephedrine, or ephedrine)
  - ▪ treat underlying infections
- • surgical
  - ▪ varicocelectomy (if indicated)
  - ▪ vasovasostomy (vasectomy reversal)
  - ▪ epididymovasostomy
  - ▪ transurethral resection of blocked ejaculatory ducts
- • assisted reproductive technologies (ART) – refer to infertility specialist
  - ▪ sperm washing + intrauterine insemination (IUI)
  - ▪ in vitro fertilization (IVF)
  - ▪ intracytoplasmic sperm injection (ICSI)

Pediatric Urology

Congenital Abnormalities

- • not uncommon; 1/200 have congenital abnormalities of the GU tract
- • UTI is the most common presentation postnatally
- • hydronephrosis is the most common finding antenatally

HYPOSPADIAS

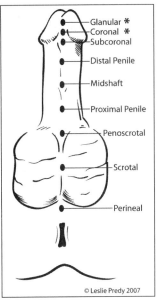

Figure 10. Classification of Hypospadias (*account for 75%)

- • very common; 1/300 live male births
- • multifactorial genetic mode of inheritance
- • white >> black
- • a condition in which the urethral meatus opens on the ventral side of the penis, proximal to the glans penis
- • may be associated with chordee, intersex states, undescended testicles or inguinal hernia
- • depending on the severity, there may be difficulty directing the urinary stream or even infertility (long-term)
- • treatment is surgical correction – optimal repair before 2 years old
- • circumcision should be deferred because the foreskin may be utilized in the correction

EPISPADIAS-EXSTROPHY COMPLEX

- • rare: incidence 1/30,000, 3:1 male to female predominance
- • epispadias-exstrophy complex: a spectrum of defects and the variant depends on the timing of the rupture of the cloacal membrane
  - ▪ bladder exstrophy (congenital absence of a portion of lower abdominal and anterior vesical wall, with eversion of bladder)
    - ◆ several variants
  - ▪ cloacal exstrophy (vesicointestinal fissure)
    - ◆ most severe
    - ◆ exposed bladder, bowel and colon with imperforate anus
    - ◆ associated with spina bifida in >50%
  - ▪ epispadias
    - ◆ least severe
    - ◆ urethra opens on dorsal penis
- • high morbidity → incontinence and infertility

Etiology

- • represents failure of closure of the cloacal membrane, resulting in the bladder and urethra opening directly through the abdominal wall

Treatment

- • surgical correction at birth, later corrections for incontinence, increasing bladder capacity and vesicoureteral reflux may be needed

ANTENATAL HYDRONEPHROSIS

- • 1 in 500 fetal U/S – detectable on U/S as early as first trimester
- • most common urological consultation in perinatal period
- • can be unilateral or bilateral
- • important to examine the rest of the GU system for anomalies

- differential diagnosis:
  - UPJ or UVJ obstruction
  - multi-cystic kidney
  - reflux
  - posterior urethral valves
  - duplication anomalies
- the majority of antenatal hydronephroses resolve during pregnancy or within the first year of life
- antenatal in utero intervention rarely indicated unless posterior urethral valves

POSTERIOR URETHRAL VALVES (PUV)
- the most common obstructive urethral lesion in male infants
- abnormal mucosal folds at the distal prostatic urethra causing varying degrees of obstruction
- most commonly recognized on prenatal ultrasound examination → bilateral hydronephrosis, thickened bladder, oligohydramnios

Clinical Presentation – depends on age and severity
- antenatal: bilateral hydronephrosis, distended bladder, oligohydramnios
- neonatal (recognized at birth): palpable abdominal mass (distended bladder, hydronephrosis), ascites (transudation of retroperitoneal urine), respiratory distress (pulmonary hypoplasia resulting from oligohydramnios) and features of oligohydramnios
- neonatal (not recognized at birth): within weeks present with urosepsis, dehydration, electrolyte abnormalities, failure to thrive
- toddlers: presents with urinary infections or voiding dysfunction
- school-aged boys: voiding dysfunction → urinary incontinence

Associated Findings
- oligohydramnios – due to low intrauterine production of urine
- renal dysplasia – due to high pressure reflux
- pulmonary hypoplasia secondary to oligohydramnios

Diagnosis
- VCUG → dilated and elongated posterior urethra, reflux

Treatment
- immediate catheterization to relieve obstruction, followed by cystoscopic resection of PUV

UPJ OBSTRUCTION
- the most common congenital defect of the ureter (but can be secondary to tumour, stone, etc.)
- twice as common in males than females
- 40% bilateral
- unclear etiology: adynamic segment of ureter, stenosis, strictures, aberrant blood vessels → extrinsic compression

Clinical Presentation
- symptoms depend on severity and age at diagnosis (mostly asymptomatic finding on antenatal U/S)
  - infants: abdominal mass, urinary infection
  - children: pain, vomiting, failure to thrive
  - some cases are diagnosed after puberty and into adulthood

Diagnosis
- antenatal U/S most commonly, Doppler U/S, IVP, and renal scan ± furosemide

Treatment
- surgical correction (pyeloplasty), consider nephrectomy if <10% renal function

Prognosis
- good since usually unilateral disease

VESICOURETERAL REFLUX (VUR)
- common condition wherein urine passes retrograde from the bladder through the UVJ into the ureter

- incidence ranges from 1-18.5% in normal children
- present in up to 70% of children with UTI
- 85% of VUR occurs in females but a male presenting with UTI has a higher likelihood of having VUR
- common cause of antenatal hydronephrosis
- 30-50% of children with reflux will have renal scarring
- common causes: trigonal weakness, lateral insertion of the ureters, short submucosal segment (all part of "primary reflux")
- many other causes including secondary reflux, subvesical obstruction, iatrogenic, secondary to ureteric abnormalities (e.g. ureterocele, ectopic ureter, or duplication), and secondary to cystitis

Presentation
- UTI, urosepsis
- pyelonephritis
- pain on voiding
- symptoms of renal failure (uremia, hypertension)
- diagnosis and staging is done using VCUG ± U/S

Grading (based on cystogram)
- grade I: ureters only fill
- grade II: ureters and pelvis fill
- grade III: ureters and pelvis fill with some dilatation
- grade IV: ureters, pelvis and calyces fill with significant dilatation
- grade V: ureters, pelvis and calyces fill with major dilatation and tortuosity

Complications
- pyelonephritis
- hydroureteronephrosis

Treatment
- many children "outgrow" reflux (60% of primary reflux)
- annual renal U/S and VCUG/RNC to monitor; renal scan if suspect new renal scar (episode of pyelonephritis)
- treatment choice is dependent on the grade
  - medical (grade I-III) – goal is to keep urine free of infection to prevent renal damage while waiting for child to "outgrow" their reflux
  - long term antibiotic prophylaxis at half the treatment dose for half the treatment time (TMP/SMX, amoxicillin, or nitrofurantoin)
  - surgical (ureteroneocystostomy ± ureteroplasty) or subureteral injection of Deflux™ or Macroplastique™
    - indications:
      - failure of medical management
      - new renal scars
      - breakthrough infections
      - high grade reflux (grade IV or V)
- prognosis depends on degree of damage done at the time of diagnosis

Interventions for primary vesicoureteric reflux
Hodson EM, Wheeler DM, Vimalchandra D, Smith GH, and Craig JC. 2007 Cochrane Database Syst Rev Jul 18(3):CD001532

Background: Vesicoureteric reflux (VUR) is a clinical condition resulting in the retrograde passage of urine through the ureter. Permanent renal parenchymal damage may occur due to recurrent urinary tract infections. Management has emphasized prevention of UTIs by antibiotic prophylaxis and/or surgical correction of reflux, but no clear consensus has been reached regarding best treatment practices.
Results: Eleven studies (n = 1148) were included in this meta-analysis. Risk of UTI by 2, 5 and 10 years was not significantly different between patients treated with antibiotics compared to surgical intervention (2 years RR 1.07, 95% CI 0.32 to 2.09; 5 years RR 0.99, 95% CI 0.79 to 1.26; 10 years RR 1.06, 95% CI 0.78 to 1.44). Combined surgical and antibiotic treatment resulted in a 50% reduction in rates of febrile UTIs by 10 years (RR 0.54, 95% CI 0.55 to 0.92), but no reduction in rates of new or progressive renal damage by 10 years (RR 1.03, 95% CI 0.53 to 2.00). Two studies failed to demonstrate significant differences in risk for symptomatic UTIs (RR 0.75, 95% CI 0.15 to 3.84) or renal parenchymal damage (RR 1.70, 95% CI 0.36 to 8.07) between antibiotic prophylaxis and no treatment.
Conclusions: It remains unclear whether the treatment of children with VUR by antibiotics or surgical intervention yields clinically significant benefit. There is a small but demonstrable additional benefit of surgery combined with antibiotics in reducing the incidence of symptomatic UTIs, but no clear impact on renal parenchymal damage. Further studies may be required to determine optimal clinical management of these patients.

Nephroblastoma (Wilm's Tumour)

- arises from abnormal proliferation of metanephric blastema
- 5% of all childhood cancers, 5% bilateral
- average age of incidence is 3 years
- 1/3 hereditary (autosomal dominant) and 2/3 sporadic
  - familial form associated with other congenital abnormalities and gene defects

Clinical Features
- abdominal mass: large, firm, unilateral (most common presentation – 80%)
- hypertension (60%)
- flank tenderness
- microscopic hematuria
- nausea/vomiting

Treatment
- always investigate contralateral kidney
- treatment of choice is radical nephrectomy ± radiation ± chemotherapy

Prognosis
- generally good; overall 5-year survival about 80%
- metastatic disease may respond well

Cryptorchidism/Ectopic Testes

- cryptorchidism refers to testes located somewhere along the normal path of descent (prepubic > external inguinal ring > inguinal canal > abdominal)
- ectopic testis (testis found outside its normal path of descent) is rare
- incidence
  - 2.7% of full term newborns
  - 0.7%-0.8% at 1 year old
- consider
  - retractile testes
  - atrophic testes
  - intersex states

Treatment
- undescended testes should be brought down to monitor for malignancy and preserve fertility (better in less than 1 year of age)
- hormonal therapy (hCG or LH may facilitate their descent)
- surgical descent (orchiopexy)

Prognosis
- untreated bilateral cryptorchidism ~100% infertility
- treated bilateral: 60-70% fertility rate
- treated/untreated unilateral: fertility is still less than the general population
- risk of malignancy is 10-40x increased in undescended testes; this risk does not decrease with surgical descent, but monitoring is made easier
- increased risk of testicular torsion (always perform bilateral orchiopexy for prevention if doing orchiopexy for torsion)

Normal Testicular Development
and Descent in utero

2nd Month – Testicle begins to form

4th Month – Begins to take on its normal appearance and migrates from its origin at the kidney to the internal inguinal ring

7th Month – The testis, surrounded its peritoneal covering, begins to descend through the internal ring, inguinal canal and external ring to terminate in the scrotum

Ambiguous Genitalia

Definition and Classification
- genitalia that do not have a normal appearance based on the chromosomal sex of the child due to the undermasculinization of genetic males or the virilization of genetic females
- considered a social emergency
- 4 major categories
  - male pseudohermaphroditism (all 46 XY, testis only)
    - defect in testicular synthesis of androgens
    - androgen resistance in target tissues
    - palpable gonad
  - female pseudohermaphroditism (all 46 XX, ovary only)
    - most due to congenital adrenal hyperplasia (21-hydroxylase deficiency most common enzymatic defect) → shunt in steroid biosynthetic pathway leading to excess androgens
  - true hermaphroditism (46 XX most common karyotype, ovary plus testis)
  - mixed gonadal dysgenesis (46 XY / 45 XO most common karyotype)
    - presence of Y chromosome → partial testis determination to varying degrees

Diagnosis and Treatment
- thorough maternal and family history needed
- other forms of abnormal sexual development
- maternal medication or drug use in pregnancy → maternal hyperandrogenemia
- parental consanguinity
- physical exam: palpable gonad (= chromosomal male), hyperpigmentation, evidence of dehydration, hypertension, stretched phallus length, position of urethral meatus
- chromosomal evaluation – sex karyotype
- laboratory tests
  - plasma 17-OH-progesterone (after 36 hours of life) → increased in 21-hydroxylase deficiency
  - plasma 11-deoxycortisol → increased in 11-β-hydroxylase deficiency
  - basal adrenal steroid levels

- - serum testosterone and DHT pre- and post-hCG stimulation (2,000 IU/day for 4 days)
  - serum electrolytes
- ultrasound of adrenals, gonads, uterus, and fallopian tubes
- endoscopy and genitography of urogenital sinus
- sex assignment (with extensive family consultation)
  - must consider capacity for sexually functioning genitalia in adulthood and psychologic impact
- reconstruction of external genitalia – between 6-12 months
- long term psychological guidance and support for both patient and family

Circumcision

Definition
- removal of some or all of the foreskin from the penis

Epidemiology
- 30% worldwide
- frequency varies depending on geographic location, religious affiliation, socioeconomic classification

Medical Indications
- phimosis
- definitive treatment of paraphimosis

Contraindications
- unstable or sick infant
- congenital genital anomalies (hypospadias)
- family history of bleeding disorders warrants laboratory investigation prior to circumcision

Complications
- bleeding
- infection
- phimosis, skin bridges
- fistula
- glans injury
- penile sensation deficits

Enuresis

- see Pediatrics

Selected Urological Procedures

Bladder Catheterization

- catheter size measured by the French (Fr) scale - circumference in mm
- each 1 mm increase in diameter = approximately 3 Fr increase (standard size 16 - 18 Fr)

Continuous Catheterization
- indications
  - accurate monitoring of urine output
  - relief of urinary retention due to medication, neurogenic bladder or intravesical obstruction
  - temporary therapy for urinary incontinence
  - perineal wounds
  - clot removal (24-28 Fr) continuous bladder irrigation
  - post-operative

Intermittent Catheterization
- indications
  - post-void residual volume measurement
  - to obtain sterile diagnostic specimens for urinalysis/cultures
  - management of neurogenic bladder or chronic urinary retention

Causes of Difficult Catheterizations and Treatment
- patient discomfort - use sufficient lubrication (± xylocaine)
- collapsing catheter - lubrication as above ± firmer catheter (silastic catheter)
- meatal/urethral stricture - dilate with progressively larger catheters/balloon catheter
- BPH - use coudé catheter as angled tip can help navigate around prostate
- urethral disruption/obstruction - filiform catheter or suprapubic catheterization
- anxious patient - anxiolytic medication

Complications of Catheterization
- infection - UTI
- meatal/urethral trauma

Contraindications
- presence of urethral trauma: blood at the meatus of the urethra, scrotal hematoma, pelvic fracture, or high riding prostate

Cystoscopy

Objective
- endoscopic inspection of the lower urinary tract (urethra, prostate, bladder neck, walls and dome, and ureteral orifices) using irrigation, illumination, and optics
- scopes can be flexible or rigid

Indications
- hematuria
- LUTS (irritative or obstructive)
- urethral and bladder neck strictures
- stones
- bladder tumour surveillance
- evaluation of upper tracts with retrograde pyelography (ureteral stents, catheters)

Complications
- during procedure
    - infection, bleeding, anesthetic-related
    - perforation (rare)
- post-procedure (short-term)
    - epididymo-orchitis (rare)
    - urinary retention
- post-procedure (long-term)
    - stricture

Radical Prostatectomy

Objective
- the removal of the entire prostate and prostatic capsule via a lower midline abdominal incision or laparoscopically
    - internal iliac and obturator vessel lymph nodes are also dissected and sent for pathology (dependent on clinical stage, grade, PSA)
    - seminal vesicle vessels are also ligated

Indications
- treatment for localized prostate cancer

Complications
- immediate (intraoperative)
    - blood loss
    - rectal injury
    - ureteral injury (extremely rare)
- perioperative
    - lymphocele formation
- late
    - moderate to severe urinary incontinence (3-10%)
    - mild urinary incontinence (20%)
    - erectile dysfunction (~50%, depending on whether one, both, or neither of the neurovascular bundles are involved in extracapsular extension of tumour)

Radical Prostatectomy versus Watchful Waiting in Early Prostate Cancer (NEJM 2005;352:1977-1984.)

Study: Randomized, blinded, controlled trial with median follow-up of 8.2 years.
Patients: 695 patients with early prostate CA (tumour stage of T1b, T1c, or T2 and PSA < 50 ng/mm) randomly assigned to radical prostatectomy (n=347) or watchful waiting (n=348). Mean age 64.7.
Intervention: Radical prostatectomy vs. watchful waiting.
Main outcome: Death due to prostate CA was the primary outcome. Secondary outcomes included death from any cause, metastasis, and local progression.
Results: Overall, 83 men in the surgery group and 106 men in the watchful-waiting group died (P=0.04). 30 (8.6%) of the surgery group and 50 (14.4%) of the watchful-waiting group died due to prostate cancer.
The 10-yr absolute reduction in cumulative incidence of prostate CA-specific and overall mortality between surgery and watchful-waiting groups was 5.3% (RR= 0.56, P=0.01) and 5.0% (RR=0.74, P=0.04) respectively. The 10-yr absolute difference in cumulative incidence for distant metastasis and for local progression were 10.2% (RR=0.60, P=0.004) and 25.1% (RR=0.33, P<0.001), respectively.
Conclusion: Radical prostatectomy resulted in lower disease-specific and overall mortality (absolute risk reductions were small), and a significantly reduced risk of metastasis and local tumour progression compared to watchful-waiting.

Transurethral Resection of the Prostate (TURP)

Objective
- to partially resect the periurethral area of the prostate (transition zone) to decrease symptoms of urinary tract obstruction
- accomplished via a cystoscopic approach using an electrocautery loop, irrigation, and illumination

Indications
- obstructive uropathy (large bladder diverticula, renal insufficiency)
- refractory urinary retention
- recurrent UTIs
- recurrent gross hematuria
- bladder stones
- intolerance/failure of medical therapy

Complications
- acute
  - intra- or extraperitoneal rupture of the bladder
  - rectal perforation
  - incontinence
  - incision of the ureteral orifice (with subsequent reflux or ureteral stricture)
  - hemorrhage
  - epididymitis
  - sepsis
  - transurethral resection syndrome (also called "post-TURP syndrome")
    - caused by absorption of a large volume of the hypotonic irrigation solution used, usually through perforated venous sinusoids, leading to a hypervolemic hyponatremic state
    - characterized by dilutional hyponatremia, confusion, nausea, vomiting, hypertension, bradycardia, visual disturbances, CHF, and pulmonary edema
    - treat with diuresis and (if severe) hypertonic saline administration
- chronic
  - retrograde ejaculation (>75%)
  - erectile dysfunction (5-10% risk increases with increasing use of cautery)
  - incontinence (<1%)
  - urethral stricture
  - bladder neck contracture

ESWL - Extracorporeal Shock Wave Lithotripsy

Objective
- to treat renal calculi, proximal calculi, and midureteral calculi which cannot pass through the urinary tract naturally
- shockwaves are generated and focused onto stone → causing fragmentation, allowing stone fragments to pass spontaneously and less painfully

Indications
- potential first-line therapy for renal and ureteral calculi less than 2 cm in size
- individuals with calculi in solitary kidneys who are at greater risk for injury and anuria if stones are treated with observation and spontaneous passage
- individuals with hypertension, diabetes or renal insufficiency

Contraindications
- acute urinary tract infection or urosepsis
- bleeding disorder or coagulopathy
- pregnancy
- obstruction distal to stone

Complications
- bacteriuria
- bacteremia
- post-procedure hematuria
- ureteric obstruction (by stone fragments)

Common Medications

Table 9. Antibiotics

Drug	Indications	Duration of Treatment	Limitiations to Use
TMP/SMX	Simple uncomplicated cystitis Recurrent cystitis Pyelonephritis Prostatitis Epididymitis/orchitis (Gram neg organism)	3 days Long term as prophylaxis 14 days 4-6 weeks 2 weeks	Stevens-Johnson syndrome ?Safety in last 2 weeks of pregnancy Resistance = 20% in the community
nitrofurantoin	Simple uncomplicated cystitis Recurrent cystitis	7 days	Contraindicated in renal failure Pulmonary toxicity
ciprofloxacin	Cystitis Pyelonephritis	3 days 7-14 days	?Safety in pregnancy
gentamicin	Severely ill patients with pyelonephritis, prostatitis		Only IV Nephrotoxic Ototoxic

Table 10. Erectile Dysfunction Medications

Drug	Class	Mechanism	Indication	Adverse Effects
sildenafil (Viagra™) tadalafil (Cialis™) vardenafil (Levitra™)	Phosphodiesterase 5 inhibitor	Selective inhibition of PDE5 (enzyme which degrades cGMP) Leads to sinusoidal smooth muscle relaxation and erection	ED when some erection present	Severe hypotension Contraindicated if Hx of priapism, or in conditions predisposing to priapism (leukemia, myelofibrosis, polycythemia, sickle cell disease) Contraindicated with nitrates
alprostadil (MUSE: Male Urethral Suppository for Erection)	Prostaglandin E_1	Activation of cAMP, relaxing sinusoidal smooth muscle Local release (capsule inserted into urethra)	ED	Penile pain Presyncope
alprostadil (intracavernosal injection) triple therapy also used: papaverine, phentolamine, PGE₁	See above	See above	ED	Thickening of tunica albuginea at site of repeated injections (Peyronie's plaque) Painful erection Hematoma Contraindicated if Hx of priapism, or in conditions predisposing to priapism

Table 11. Benign Prostatic Hyperplasia Medications

Drug	Class	Mechanism	Indication	Adverse Effects
terazosin (Hytrin™) doxazosin (Cardura™) tamsulosin (Flomax™) alfuzosin (Xatral™)	Alpha 1 blockers Alpha 1a selective Alpha 1a selective	Alpha-adrenergic antagonists reduce stromal smooth muscle tone Reduce dynamic component of bladder outlet obstruction	BPH	Presyncope Retrograde ejaculation Headache Asthenia Nasal congestion
finasteride (Proscar™) dutasteride (Avodart™)	5 alpha-reductase inhibitor	Blocks conversion of testosterone to DHT Reduces static component of bladder outlet obstruction Reduces prostatic volume	BPH	Sexual dysfunction PSA decreases

Note: All alpha-blockers developed for BPH have similar efficacy, however, alpha-1 selective agents have an improved side effect profile.

Table 12. Prostatic Carcinoma Medications

Drug	Class	Mechanism	Indication	Adverse Effects
leuprolide (Lupron™, Eligard™), goserelin (Zoladex™)	LHRH antagonists	Initially stimulates LH, increasing testosterone and causing "flare" (clinically: increased bone pain), later causes low testosterone	CaP (N>0, M>0)	Hot flashes Headache Decreased libido
*diethylstilbestrol (DES)	Estrogens	Inhibit LH and cytotoxic effect on tumour cells	As above	Increased risk of cardiovascular events
*cyproterone acetate	Steroidal antiandrogen	Competes with DHT for intracellular receptors: 1. prevent flare produced by LHRH agonist 2. use for complete androgen blockade 3. may preserve potency	As above	
flutamide (Eulexin™) bicalutamide (Casodex™)	Non-steroidal antiandrogen	As above	As above	Hepatotoxic: AST/ALT monitoring
*ketoconazole, spironolactone	Steroidogenesis inhibitors	Blocks multiple enzymes in steroid pathway, including adrenal androgens	As above	GI symptoms Hyperkalemia Gynecomastia

*Very rarely used

Table 13. Continence Agents

Drug	Class	Mechanism	Indication	Adverse Effects
oxybutynin (Ditropan™)	Antispasmotic	Inhibits action of ACh on smooth muscle Decreases frequency of uninhibited detrusor contraction Diminishes initial urge to void	Urge incontinence + urgency + frequency	Dry mouth Blurred vision Constipation Supraventricular tachycardia
oxybutynin (Ditropan™) tolterodine (Detrol™) trospium (Trosec™) solifenacin (Vesicare™) darifenacin (Enablex™)	Anticholinergic	Muscarinic receptor antagonist Selective for bladder Increases bladder volume Decreases detrusor pressure	Urge incontinence + urgency + frequency	As above
imipramine	Tricyclic antidepressant	Sympathomimetic effects: urinary sphincter Contraction Anticholinergic effects: detrusor relaxation	Stress and urge incontinence	As above Weight gain Orthostatic hypotension Prolonged PR interval

Note: All anti-cholinergics are equally effective and long acting formulations (Detrol LA™ and Ditropan XL™) are better tolerated. Newer muscarinic M3 receptor specific agents (solifenacin, darifenacin) are equally efficacious as older drugs, however, RCTs based on head-to-head comparison to long acting formulations are lacking.

Notes

Common Unit Conversions

To convert from the conventional unit to the SI unit, **multiply** by conversion factor
To convert from the SI unit to the conventional unit, **divide** by conversion factor

	Conventional Unit	Conversion Factor	SI Unit
ACTH	pg/mL	0.22	pmol/L
Albumin	g/dL	10	g/L
Bilirubin	mg/dL	17.1	μmol/L
Calcium	mg/dL	0.25	mmol/L
Cholesterol	mg/dL	0.0259	mmol/L
Cortisol	μg/dL	27.59	nmol.L
Creatinine	mg/dL	88.4	μmol/L
Creatinine clearance	mL/mon	0.0167	mL/s
Ethanol	mg/dL	0.217	mmol/L
Ferritin	ng/mL	2.247	pmol/L
Glucose	mg/dL	0.0555	mmol/L
HbA1C	%	0.01	proportion of 1.0
Hemaglobin	g/dL	10	g/L
HDL cholesterol	mg/dL	0.0259	mmol/L
Iron, total	μg/dL	0.179	μmol/L
Lactate (lactic acid)	mg/dL	0.111	mmol/L
LDL cholesterol	mg/dL	0.0259	mmol/L
Leukocytes	x 10^3 cells/mm^3	1	x 10^9 cells/L
Magnesium	mg/dL	0.411	mmol/L
MCV	$μm^3$	1	fL
Platelets	x 10^3 cells/mm^3	1	x 10^9 cells/L
Reticulocytes	% of RBCs	0.01	proportion of 1.0
Salicylate	mg/L	0.00724	mmol/L
Testosterone	ng/dL	0.0347	nmol/L
Thyroxine (T4)	ng/dL	12.87	pmol/L
Total Iron Binding Capacity	μg/dL	0.179	μmol/L
Triiodothyronine (T3)	pg/dL	0.0154	pmol/L
Triglycerides	mg/dL	0.0113	mmol/L
Urea nitrogen	mg/dL	0.357	mmol/L
Uric acid	mg/dL	59.48	μmol/L

Celsius → Fahrenheit	F = (C x 1.8) +32
Fahrenheit → Celsius	C = (F – 32) x 0.5555
Kilograms → Pounds	1 kg = 2.2 lbs
Pounds → Ounces	1 lb = 16 oz
Ounces → Grams	1 oz = 28.3 g
Inches → Centimetres	1 in = 2.54 cm

Commonly Measured Laboratory Values

Test	Conventional Units	SI Units
Arterial Blood Gases		
pH	7.35-7.45	7.35-7.45
P_{CO2}	35-45 mm Hg	4.7-6.0 kPa
P_{O2}	80-105 mm Hg	10.6-14 kPa
Serum Electrolytes		
Bicarbonate	22-28 mEq/L	22-28 mmol/L
Calcium	8.4-10.2 mg/dL	2.1-2.5 mmol/L
Chloride	95-106 mEq/L	95-106 mmol/L
Magnesium	1.3-2.1 mEq/L	0.65-1.05 mmol/L
Phosphate	2.7-4.5 mg/dL	0.87-1.45 mmol/L
Potassium	3.5-5.0 mEq/L	3.5-5.0 mmol/L
Sodium	136-145 mEq/L	136-145 mmol/L
Serum Nonelectrolytes		
Albumin	3.5-5.0 g/dL	35-50 g/L
ALP	35-100 U/L	35-100 U/L
ALT	8-20 U/L	8-20 U/L
Amylase	25-125 U/L	25-125 U/L
AST	8-20 U/L	8-20 U/L
Bilirubin (direct)	0-0.3 mg/dL	0-5 µmol/L
Bilirubin (total)	0.1-1.0 mg/dL	2-17 µmol/L
BUN	7-18 mg/dL	1.2-3.0 mmol/L
Cholesterol	<200 mg/dL	< 5.2 mmol/L
Creatinine (female)	10-70 U/L	10-70 U/L
Creatinine (male)	25-90 U/L	25-90 U/L
Creatine Kinase – MB fraction	0-12 U/L	0-12 U/L
Ferritin (female)	12-150 ng/mL	12-150 µg/L
Ferritin (male)	15-200 ng/mL	15-200 µg/L
Glucose (fasting)	70-110 mg/dL	3.8-6.1 mmol/L
HbA1C	<6%	<0.06
LDH	100-250 U/L	100-250 U/L
Osmolality	275-300 mOsm/kg	275-300 mOsm/kg
Serum Hormones		
ACTH (0800h)	<60 pg/mL	<13.2 pmol/L
Cortisol (0800h)	5-23 µg/dL	138-635 nmol/L
Prolactin	<20 ng/mL	< 20 ng/mL
Testosterone (male,free)	9-30 ng/dL	0.31-1 pmol/L
Thyroxine (T4)	5-12 (g/dL	64-155 nmol/L
Triiodothyronine (T3)	115-190 ng/dL	1.8-2.9 nmol/L
TSH	0.5-5 µU/mL	0.5-5 µU/mL
Hematologic Values		
ESR (female)	0-20 mm/h	0-20 mm/h
ESR (male)	0-15 mm/h	0-15 mm/h
Hemoglobin (female)	12.3-15.7 g/dL	123-157 g/L
Hemoglobin (male)	13.5-17.5 g/dL	140-174 g/L
Hematocrit (female)	36-46%	36-46%
Hematocrit (male)	41-53%	41-53%
INR	1.0-1.1	1.0-1.1
Leukocytes	4.5-11 x 10^3 cells/mm³	4.5-11 x 10^9 cells/L
MCV	88-100 µm³	88-100 fL
Platelets	150-400 x 10^3/mm³	150-400 x 10^9/L
PT	11-15 s	11-15 s
PTT	25-35 s	25-35 s
Reticulocytes	0.5-1.5% of RBC	20-84 x 10^9/L

μmol	micromoles
μE3	unconjugated estriol
1,25(OH)$_2$-vit D	1,25-dihydroxy-vitamin D
111-ln DTPA	111-in diethylene triamine penta acetic acid
17-KS	17-ketosteroids
17-OH prog	17-hydroxyprogesterone
18FDG	18-fluorodeoxyglucose
2-PAM	pralidoxime
5-ASA	5-aminosalicylic acid
5-HT	serotonin

A

AFib	atrial fibrillation
A/E	air entry
AA	Alcoholics Anonymous
A-a	alveolar arterial
AAA	abdominal aortic aneurysm
AaDO$_2$	arterial-alveolar oxygen diffusion gradient
AAN	American Academy of Neurology
AAT	activity as tolerated
Ab	antibody
ABCs	airway, breathing, and circulation
ABG	arterial blood gases
ABI	ankle-brachial index
ABL	acceptable blood loss
ABP	arterial blood pressure
ABPA	allergic bronchopulmonary aspergillosis
ABR	auditory brainstem response
ABVD	adriamycin, bleomycin, vincristine, decarbazine
Abx	antibiotics
ac	before meals
AC	acromioclavicular
AC	abdominal circumference
AC	activated charcoal
AC	air conduction
AC	anterior chamber
ACA	anterior cerebral artery
ACAS	asymptomatic cartic atherosclerosis study
ACC	American College of Cardiology
ACD	allergic contact dermatitis
ACE	angiotensin converting enzyme
ACEI	angiotensin converting enzyme inhibitors
ACh	acetylcholine
AChE	acetylcholinesterase
ACI	autologous chondrocyte implantation
ACG	angle closure glaucoma
ACL	anterior cruciate ligament
ACLA	anticardiolipin antibody
ACLS	advanced cardiac life support
ACR	active core rewarming
ACR	albumin to creatinine ratio
ACS	acute coronary syndrome
ACST	asymptomatic carotid surgery trial
ACT	activated clotting time
ACT-D	actinomycin D
ACTH	adrenocorticotropic hormone
ACV	assist-control ventilation
AD	Alzheimer's disease
AD	atopic dermatitis
AD	autosomal dominant
AD	right ear
ADC	apparent diffusion coefficient
ADH	antidiuretic hormone
ADHD	attention-deficit/hyperactivity disorder
ADL	activities of daily living
ADM	abductor digiti minimi
ADMD	attention deficit hyperactive disorder
ADME	absorption, distribution, metabolism and elimination
ADP	abductor pollicis
ADP	adenosine diphosphate
ADR	adverse drug reaction
ADRs	adverse drug reactions
AE	adverse event
AER	active external rewarming

AF	amniotic fluid
AFB	acid-fast bacillus
Afib	atrial fibrillation
AFLP	acute fatty liver of pregnancy
AFP	alpha-fetoprotein
AFV	amniotic fluid volume
AG	anion gap
Ag	antigen
AGA	appropriate for gestational age
AGE	advanced glycosylated end-products
AGUS	atypical glandular cells of undetermined significance
AHA	American Heart Association
AHI	apnea hypopnea index
AHTR	acute hemolytic transfusion reactions
AICA	anterior internal carotid artery
AICA	anterior inferior cerebellar artery
AIDP	acute inflammatory demyelinating polyneuropathy
AIDS	acquired immune deficiency syndrome
AIHA	autoimmune hemolytic anemia
AII	angiotensin II
AIN	acute interstitial nephritis
AIN	allergic interstitial nephritis
AIN	anterior interosseous nerve
AION	acute ischemic optic neuropathy
AION	anterior ischemic optic neuropathy
AIS	androgen insensitivity syndrome
AJR	abdominal jugular reflex
AK	actinic keratosis
AKI	acute kidney injury
ALL	acute lymphoblastic leukemia
ALND	axillary lymph node dissection
ALP	alkaline phosphatase
ALS	amyotrophic lateral sclerosis
ALT	alanine aminotransferase
AM	morning
AMA	anti-mitochondrial antibodies
AMAN	acute motor axonal neuropathy
AMI	acute myocardial infarction
AMI	acute myocardial ischemia
AML	acute myeloid leukemia
AMM	agnogenic myeloid metaplasia
AMP	adenosine monophosphate
AMSAN	acute motor-sensory axonal neuropathy
AN	acoustic neuroma
AN	anorexia nervosa
ANA	antinuclear antibody
ANC	absolute neutrophil count
ANCA	anti-neutrophil cytoplasmic antibody
ANOVA	analysis of variance
ANS	autonomic nervous system
Anti-GBM	anti-glomerular basement membrane
Anti-LKM	anti-liver kidney microsome
Anti-Sm	anti-Smith antibodies
AO	aortic root
AOM	acute otitis media
AoV	aortic valve
AP	anterior-posterior
APB	atrial premature beat
APB	abductor pollicis brevis
APC	activated protein C
APCKD	adult polycystic kidney disease
APH	antepartum hemorrhage
APL	abductor pollicis longus
APLA	anti phospholipid antibody
APLAS	anti phospholipid antibody syndrome
APML	acute promyelocytic myeloid leukemia
APO	apolipoprotein
ApoA	apolipoprotein A-1
ApoB	apolipoprotein B
APR	abdominal perineal resection
APS	antiphospholipid antibody syndrome
APTT	activated partial thromboplastin time
APUD	amine precursor uptake and decarboxylation
AR	aortic regurgitation
AR	attributable risk
AR	autosomal recessive
ARB	angiotensin II receptor blocker
ARBC	anti-ribonuclear protein complex

ARDS	acute respiratory distress syndrome
ARF	acute renal failure
ARI	absolute risk increase
ARMD	age-related macular degeneration
ARR	absolute risk reduction
ART	advanced reproductive technologies
ART	assisted reproductive technologies
ARV	anti-retroviral
AS	aortic stenosis
AS	ankylosing spondylitis
AS	left ear
ASA	above sternal angle
ASA	acetylsalicylic acid
ASA	American Society of Anesthesiology
ASC-H	atypical squamous cells, cannot exclude HSIL
ASCUS	atypical squamous cells of undetermined significance
ASD	atrial septal defect
ASIL	anal squamous intraepithelial lesion
ASIS	anterior superior iliac spine
ASO	anti-streptolysin O
ASOT	anti-streptolysin O titers
ASPD	antisocial personality disorder
AST	aspartate transaminase
AST	aspartate amino-transferase
AT II	angiotensin
ATLS	advanced trauma life support
ATN	acute tubular necrosis
ATP	adenosine triphosphate
ATRA	all-trans-retinoic acid
AU	each ear
AUB	abnormal uterine bleeding
AV	atrioventricular
AV	arteriovenous
AVA	aortic valve area
AVF	arterio-venous fistula
AVM	arteriovenous malformation
AVN	avascular necrosis
AVNRT	atrioventricular nodal reentrant tachycardia
AVPU	alert, verbal, pain, unresponsive
AVRT	atrioventricular reentrant tachycardia
AXR	abdominal x-ray
AZT	azidothymidine

B

B12	vitamin B12
BAC	bronchioalvelolar cancer
BAD	bipolar affective disorder
BAEP	brainstem auditory evoked potentials
BAL	bronchoalveolar lavage
BBB	bundle branch block
BBB	blood-brain barrier
BC	bone conduction
BCC	basal cell carcinoma
BCG	bacille Calmette-Guérin
BCP	birth control pill
BCS	breast conserving surgery
BE	barium enema
BE	Barrett's esophagus
BG	blood glucose
β-hCG	beta-human chorionic gonadotropin
BHL	bilateral hilar lymphadenopathy
bid	two times a day
BiPAP	bilevel positive airway pressure
BK	below knee
BM	basement membrane
BM	bowel movement
BMD	Becker muscular dystrophy
BMD	bone mineral density
BMI	body mass index
BMR	basal metabolic rate
BMT	bone marrow transplant
BN	bulimia nervosa
BNP	brain namuretic peptide
BOOP	bronchiolitis obliterans with organizing pneumonia
BP	blood pressure

BP	bullous pemphius
BPD	biparietal diameter
BPD	bronchopulmonary dysplasia
BPD	borderline personality disorder
BPH	benign prostatic hyperplasia
BPH	benign prostatic hypertrophy
BPP	biophysical profile
BPPV	benign paroxysmal positional vertigo
BPV	benign positional vertigo
BRAO	branch retinal artery occulsion
BRBPR	bright red blood per rectum
BRVO	branch retinal vein occlusion
BS	blood sugar
BSA	body surface area
BSE	bovine spongiform encephalopathy
BSO	bilateral salpingo-oophorectomy
BSS	balanced salt solution
BT	bleeding time
BTE	behind the ear
BUN	blood urea nitrogen
BUT	break-up time
BV	bacterial vaginosis
BW	body weight
BZ	benzodiazepine

C

C&S	culture and sensitivity
C/S	Caesarean section
C/T	cardiothoracic ratio
CA	coracoacromial ligament
Ca	calcium
CA	cancer
CA-125	cancer antigen 125
CABG	coronary artery bypass graft
CAD	coronary artery disease
CAH	congenital adrenal hyperplasia
Cal/d	calories/day
CAM	complementary alternative medicine
cAMP	cyclic adenosine monophosphate
c-ANCA	cytoplasmic antineutrophil cytoplasmic antibody
CaO2	combined arterial O2
CaO2	arterial O2 content
CAP	Canada Assistance Plan
CAP	community acquired pneumonia
CAP	prostatic carcinoma
CAS	Children's Aid Society
CAVHD	continuous arterial-venous hemodialysis
CBC	complete blood count
CBD	common bile duct
CBF	cerebral blood flow
CBGD	cortical basal ganglionic degeneration
CBT	cognitive behavioural therapy
cc	with meals
C-C	carotid-cavernous
CC	coracoclavicular ligament
CC	chief complaint
CCB	calcium channel blocker
CCB	Consent and Capacity Board
CCHD	congenital cyanotic heart disease
CCK	cholecystokinin
CCP	chronic pelvic pain
CCS	Canadian Cardiovascular Society
CCT	central corneal thickness
CCU	coronary care unit
CD	conduct disorder
CD	Crohn's disease
CDC	Center for Disease Control
CDD	childhood disintegrative disorder
CDH	congenital dislocation of the hip
CDH	congenital dysplasia of the hip
CEA	carcinoembryonic antigen
CEE	conjugated equine estrogen
CER	control group event rate
CF	counting fingers
CF	cystic fibrosis
CFCs	chlorofluorocarbons
CFPC	College of Family Physicians of Canada

CFS	chronic fatigue syndrome
CFTR	cystic fibrosis transmembrane conductama regulator
CFU	colony forming units
CGL	chronic granulocytic leukemia
CGMP	cyclic guanine monophosphate
CHA	Canada Health Act
CHD	congenital heart disease
CHF	congestive heart failure
CHL	conductive hearing loss
CHO	carbohydrate
C/I	contraindications
CI	cardiac index
CI	confidence interval
CIC	clean intermittent catheterization
CIDP	chronic inflammatory demyelinating polyneuropathy
CIN	cervical intraepithelial neoplasia
CIS	carcinoma in situ
CJD	Creutzfeldt-Jakob disease
CK	creatine kinase
CKD	chronic kidney disease
CK-MB	creatine kinase-MB
CI	cardiac index
CI	cervical incompetence
CI	chloride
CI	confidence interval
CIWA	Clinical Institute Withdrawal Assessment
CL	clearance
CL	corpus luteum
CLL	chronic lymphocytic leukemia
CM	cardiomyopathy
CMA	Canadian Medical Association
CMC	carpo-metacarpal joint
CME	continuing medical education
CMF	cyclophosphamide, methotrexate and 5-fluorouracil
CMG	cystometrogram
CML	chronic myeloid leukemia
CMPA	Canadian Medical Protective Association
CMT	Charcot Marie Tooth Disease
CMV	cytomegalovirus
CN	cranial nerve
CN	cyanide
CNH	central neurogenic hyperventilation
CNS	central nervous system
CO	carbon monoxide
CO	cardiac output
CO2	carbon dioxide
COMT	catechol-O-methyl transferase
COPD	chronic obstructive pulmonary disease
COX	cyclo oxygenase
COX-2	cyclo oxygenase-2
CP	cerebral palsy
CP	chest pain
CPA	cerebellar pontine angle
CPAP	continuous positive airway pressure
CPB	cardiopulmonary bypass
CPD	cephalopelvic disproportion
CPK	creatine phosphokinase
CPM	central pontine myelinolysis
CPM	continous passive motion
CPOE	chest pain on exertion
CPP	cerebral perfusion pressure
CPP	chronic pelvic pain
CPPD	calcium pyrophosphate dihydrate
CPR	cardiopulmonary resuscitation
CPSO	College of Physicians & Surgeons of Ontario
Cr	creatinine
CRAO	central retinal artery occlusion
CRC	colorectal cancer
CrCl	creatinine clearance
CRF	cardiac risk factor
CRF	chronic renal failure
CRH	corticotropin releasing hormone
CROS	contralateral routing of signals
CRP	C-reactive protein
CRPS	complex regional pain syndrome
CRVO	central retinal vein occlusion
CS	completed stroke
CSA	central sleep apnea
CSF	cerebrospinal fluid
CSM	central steady and maintained
C-spine	cervical spine

CSR	Cheyne-Stokes respiration
CT	cognitive therapy
CT	computed tomography
CTA	CT angiogram
CTD	connective tissue disease
CTEV	congenital talipes equinovarus
CTG	cardiotocography (fetal)
CTLA-4	cytotoxic T-lymphocyte associated protein 4
CTO	community treatment order
CTS	carpal tunnel syndrome
CUP	central venous pressure
CV	cardiovascular
CVA	cerebrovascular accident
CVA	costovertebral angle
CVD	cardiovascular disease
CVD	cerebrovascular disease
CVD	collagen vascular disease
CVP	central venous pressure
CVS	chorionic villus sampling
CVS	cardiovascular system
CVVHD	continuous venous venous hemodialysis
CWP	coal worker's pneumoconiosis
CXR	chest x-ray
CYP	cytochrome p-450

D

D	diopter
D&C	dilatation and curettage
D/T	due to
D5W	5% dextrose in water
DA	dopamine
DALY	disability adjusted life year
DASH	dietary approaches to stop hypertension
dB	decibel
dBP	diastolic blood pressure
D&C	dilatation and curettage
D/C	discontinue
DC	direct current
DCIS	ductal carcinoma in situ
DCM	dilated cardiomyopathy
Dco	diffusing capacity of carbon monoxide
DCR	dacryocystorhinostomy
DCT	distal convoluted tubule
DDAVP	1-desamino-8-d-arginine vasopressin
DDH	developmental dysplasia of hip
DDT	dichloradiphenyl trichloroethane
DDx	differential diagnosis
DES	diethylstilbestrol
DES	diffuse esophageal spasm
DES	drug eluting stent
DEXA	dual-energy x-ray absorptiometry
DF	dissociative fugue
DFA	direct fluorescent antibody
DH	dermatitis herpetiformis
DHE	dihydroergotamine
DHEA	dihydroepiandrosterone
DHEAS	dihydroepiandrosterone sulfate
DHP	dihydropyridine
DHP-CCB	dihydropyridine calcium channel blocker
DHT	dihydrotestosterone
DI	diabetes insipidus
DIC	disseminated intravascular coagulation
DID	dissociative identity disorder
DIEP	deep inferior epigastric perforator
DIP	distal interphalangeal joint
DKA	diabetic ketoacidosis
DM	dermatomyositis
DM	diabetes mellitus
DM1	type 1 diabetes
DM2	type 2 diabetes
DMARD	disease modifying anti-rheumatic drugs
DMC	dilated cardiomyopathy
DMD	Duchenne muscular dystrophy
DMSA	dimercaptosuccinic acid
DMSO	dimethylsulfamethoxazole
DMT	disease-modifying therapy

DMY	dermatomyositis
DNA	deoxyribonucleic acid
DNCB	dinitrochlorobenzene
DNET	dsyembryoplastic neuroepheral tumour
DNR	do not resuscitate
DNSI	deep neck space infections
DPD	distalphalangeal depth
DPG	diphosphoglycerate
DPL	diagnostic peritoneal lavage
DR	diabetic retinopathy
DRD	dopamine responsive dystonia
DRE	digital rectal exam
DRUJ	distal radioulnar joint
DS	double strength
DS	Down syndrome
DSA	digital subtraction angiography
DSD	detrusor-sphincter dyssynergia
DSM	Diagnostic and Statistical Manual of Mental Disorders
DST	dexamethasone suppression test
DT	delirium tremens
DTaP	diphtheria, tetanus, pertussis
DTPA	diethylene triaminepentacetic acid
DTR	deep tendon reflexes
DU	duodenal ulcer
DUB	dysfunctional uterine bleeding
DVT	deep vein thrombosis
DWI	diffusion-weighted image
Dx	diagnosis
DXM	dexamethasone
DZ	dizygotic

E

E	estrogen
EAF	extra-articular features
EBM	evidence based medicine
EBV	Epstein-Barr virus
EBV	estimated blood volume
EBW	estimated birth weight
EC	emergency contraception
EC50	effective concentration of a drug
ECASA	enteric coated aspirin
ECC	endocervical curettage
ECD	endocardial cushion defect
ECDR	extracorporeal drug removal
ECF	extracellular fluid
ECFV	extracellular fluid volume
ECFV	effective circulating fluid volume
ECG	electrocardiogram
ECHO	echocardiogram
ECM	erythema chronicum migrans
ECMO	extracorporeal membrane oxygenation
ECRB	extensor carpi radialis brevis
ECRL	extensor carpi radialis longus
ECT	electroconvulsive therapy
ECU	extensor carpi ulnaris
ED	electrodessication
ED	emergency department
ED	erectile dysfunction
ED50	effective dose - 50%
ED+C	electrodesiccation and curettage
EDC	estimated date of confinement
EDC	extensor digitorum communis
EDD	electron dense deposits
EDM	extensor digiti minimi
EDS	electrodiagnostic studies
EEG	electroencephalogram
EER	experimental group event rate
EF	ejection fraction
EFW	estimated fetal weight
e.g.	example
EGD	esophageal gastroduodenoscopy
EHEC	enterohemorrhagic E. coli
EHL	extensor hallucis longus
EIA	enzyme immunoassay
EIC	extensive in-situ component
EIEC	entero invasive E. coli
EIP	extensor indicis proprius
ELISA	enzyme-linked immunosorbent assay
EM	electron microscopy
EM	erytherma multiforme
EMA	anti-endomysial antibody

EMA	emergency medical attendant
EMA-CO	etoposide, MTX, ACT-D, cyclophosphamide, vincristine
Emax	maximal response that a drug can elicit
EMD	electromechanical dissociation
EMG	electromyography
EMLA	eutectic mixture of local anesthetic
EMS	esophageal motility study
ENG	electronystagmogram
ENT	ear, nose, throat
EOM	extraocular movement
EOM	extraocular muscle
EPB	extensor pollicis brevis
EPC	emergency postcoital contraception
EPF	Established Programs Financing
EPL	extensor pollicis longus
EPO	erythropoietin
EPS	electrophysiological studies
EPS	expressed prostatic secretions
EPS	extrapyramidal side effects
ER	emergency room
ER	estrogen receptor
ERCP	endoscopic retrograde cholangio-pancreatography
ERV	expiratory reserve volume
ESR	erythrocyte sedimentation rate
ESRD	end-stage renal disease
ESWL	extracorporeal shockwave lithotripsy
ET	essential thrombocythemia
ETCO2	end-tidal carbon dioxide
ETEC	enterotoxigenic E. coli
EtOH	ethanol/alcohol
ETT	endotracheal tube
EUA	examination under anesthesia
EVL	endoscopic variceal ligation
EVLT	endovenous laser therapy

F

F	female
F/U	follow-up
FA	folinic acid
FA	fluorescein angiography
FAB	fragment antigen binding
FAB	French-American-British
FAE	fetal alcohol effects
FAP	familial adenomatous polyposis
FAS	fetal alcohol syndrome
FASD	fetal alcohol spectrum disorder
FAST	focused abdominal sonogram for trauma
FB	foreign body
FBG	fasting blood glucose
FBS	fasting blood sugar
FCR	flexor carpi radialis
FCU	flexor carpi ulnaris
FDM	flexor digiti minimi
FDP	flexor digitorum profundus
FDPs	fibrinogen degradation products
FDS	flexor digitorum superficialis
FEF	forced expiratory flow rate
FEF25-75	forced expiratory flow at 25-75% of maximum flow rate
FE$_{NA}$	fractional excretion of sodium
FEP	free erythrocyte protoporphyrin
FESS	functional endoscopic sinus surgery
FET	forced expired time
FEV$_1$	forced expiratory volume in 1 second
FF	filtration fraction
FFA	free fatty acid
FFP	fresh frozen plasma
FHR	fetal heart rate
FHx	family history
FIGO	International Federation of Gynecology and Obstetrics
FiO2	fraction of oxygen in inspired air
FISH	fluorescence in situ hybridization
FL	femur length
FLAIR	fluid-attenuated inversion recover
FN	false negative
FNA	fine needle aspiration
FNHTR	febrile nonhemolytic transfusion reactions
FOBT	fecal occult blood test

FOOSH	fall on outstretched hand
FP	false positive
FPB	flexor pollicis brevis
FPG	fasting plasma glucose
FPL	flexor pollicis longus
FRC	functional residual capacity
FRCPC	Fellow of the Royal College of Physicians of Canada
FRCSC	Fellow of the Royal College of Surgeons of Canada
FSGS	focal segmental glomerular sclerosis
FSH	follicular stimulating hormone
FT4I	free thyroxine index
FTA-ABS	fluorescent treponemal antibody-absorption
FTS	first trimester screen
FTSG	full thickness skin graft
FTT	failure to thrive
FU	fluorouracil
FUO	fever of unknown origin
FVC	forced vital capacity

G

g	gram(s)
G/U	genitourinary
G6PD	glucose-6-phosphate dehydrogenase
GA	general anesthetic
GA	gestational age
GABA	gamma aminobutyric acid
GABHS	group A β-hemolytic streptococcus
GAD	generalized anxiety disorder
GAF	global assessment of functioning
GAS	Group A β-hemolytic streptococcus
GAT	goldmann applanation tonometry
GB	gallbladder
GBM	glioblastoma multiforme
GBM	glomerular basement membrane
GBS	group B streptococcus
GBS	Guillain-Barré syndrome
GC	Neisseria gonorrhea/ gonococcus
GCA	giant cell arteritis
GCS	Glasgow coma scale
G-CSF	granulocyte - colony stimulating factor
GCT	glucose challenge test
GDM	gestational diabetes mellitus
GDP	gross domestic product
GE	gastroesophageal
GERD	gastroesophageal reflux disease
GFR	glomerular filtration rate
GGT	gamma-glutamyltranspeptidase
GH	growth hormone
GHB	gamma hydroxybutyrate
GHRH	growth hormone-releasing hormone
GI	gastrointestinal
GIFT	gamete intra fallopian transfer
GIT	gamete-immediate transfer
GTN	gestational trophoblastic neoplasia
GIST	gastrointestinal stromal tumour
GM	germinal matrix
GMC	general medical condition
GM-CSF	granulocyte macrophage - colony stimulating factor
GMN	glomerulonephritis
GMO	genetically modified organism
GN	glomerulonephritis
GN	Gram negative
GNB	Gram negative bacilli
GNG	gluconeogenesis
GNP	gross national product
GnRH	gonadotropin-releasing hormone
GPC	giant papillary conjunctivitis
GPe	globus pallidus pars externa
GPi	globus pallidus pars interna
GSW	gunshot wound
GT	glucose tolerance
GTN	gestational trophoblastic neoplasia
GTPAL	gravidity, term infants, parity, abortions, living children
gtt	drops
GU	genito-urinary
GVHD	graft versus host disease

H

h	hour
H	hydrogen
H/A	headache
HA	hemagglutinin
HA	hemolytic anemia
HAART	highly active antiretroviral treatment
HAV	hepatitis A virus
Hb	hemoglobin
HbA1C	glycosylated hemoglobin
HBIg	hepatitis B immune globulin
HBsAg	hepatitis B surface antigen
HBV	hepatitis B virus
HC	head circumference
HCC	hepatocellular carcinoma
HCCA	Health Care Consent Act
hCG	human chorionic gonadotropin
HCl	hydrochloric acid
HCM	hypertrophic cardiomyopathy
HCO3	bicarbonate
HCP	hydrocephalus
Hct	hematocrit
HCTZ	hydrochlorothiazide
HCV	hepatitis C virus
HD	heart disease
HD	Huntington's disease
HDL	high density lipoprotein
HDV	hepatitis D virus
HE	hypaque enema
HELLP	hemolysis, elevated liver enzymes, low platelets
HF	heart failure
HHT	hereditary hemorrhagic telangiectasia
HHV	human herpes virus
HI	head injury
Hib	Haemophilus influenzae b
HIDA scan	hepatobiliary iminodiacetic acid scan
HIDS	Hospital Insurance and Diagnostic Services Act
HIE	hypoxic ischemic encephalopathy
HIFU	high intensity focused ultrasound
HIT	heparin induced thrombocytopenia
HIV	human immunodeficiency virus
HJR	hepatojugular reflex
HL	hearing loss
HLA	human leukocyte antigen
HLHS	hypoplastic left heart syndrome
HM	hand motion
HMD	hyaline membrane disease
HMG-CoA	hydroxymethylglutamyl coenzyme A
HMO	Health Maintenance Organization
HMPAO	hexamethylpropene aminooxime
HMSN	hereditary motor-sensory neuropathy
HNPCC	heroditary non-polyposis colorectal cancer
HO	heterotopic ossification
HOCM	hypertrophic obstructive cardiomyopathy
HONK	hyperglycemic hyperosmolar non-ketotic coma
HP	hydrostatic pressure
HPA	hypothalamic pituitary adrenal
HPD	histrionic personality disorder
HPF	high power field
HPI	history of present illness
HPL	human placenta lactogen
HPO	high frequency oscillation
HPS	hepatopulmonary syndrome
HPV	human papilloma virus
HR	heart rate
HRCT	high resolution CT scan
HRT	hormone replacement therapy
HSG	hysterosalpingography
HSIL	high grade squamous intraepithelial lesion
HSP	Henoch-Schönlein Purpura
HSV	herpes simplex virus
HT	height
HTLV	human T-cell leukemia/lymphoma virus
HTN	hypertension
HUS	hemolytic uremic syndrome
HVA	homovanillic acid
Hx	history
HZ	herpes zoster
HZV	herpes zoster virus

I

I	iodide
I&D	incision and drainage
I&D	irrigation and debridement
IA	intra-arterial
IABP	intra-aortic balloon pump
IADL	instrumental activities of daily living
IBD	inflammatory bowel disease
IBM	inclusion body myositis
IBM	intermenstrual bleeding
IBS	irritable bowel syndrome
IBW	ideal body weight
IC	ileocecal
IC	immune complex
IC	inspiratory capacity
ICD	implantable cardioverter defibrillator
ICD	irritant contact dermatitis
ICF	intracellular fluid
ICH	intracerebral hemorrhage
ICH	intracranial hemorrhage
ICP	intracranial pressure
ICSI	intracytoplasmic sperm injection
ICU	intensive care unit
ID	identifying data
ID	internal diameter
IDL	intermediate density lipoprotein
IDM	infant of diabetic mother
IE	infective endocarditis
IEM	inborn errors of metabolism
IF	immunofluorescence
IF	internal fixation
IF	intrinsic factor
IFA	immunofluorescence assay
IFG	impaired fasting glucose
Ig	immunoglobulin
IgA	immunoglobulin A
IGF-1	insulin-like growth factor
IgG	immunoglobulin G
IgM	immunoglobulin M
IGT	impaired glucose tolerance
IHD	ischemic heart disease
IL	interleukins
IL-1	interleukin-1
IL-6	interleukin-6
ILD	interstitial lung disease
ILR	implantable loop recorder
IM	intramedullary
IM	intramuscular
IMA	inferior mesenteric artery
IMB	intermenstrual bleeding
IMF	idiopathic myelofibrosis
IMF	intermaxillary fixation
IMR	infant mortality rate
IMV	intermittent mandatory ventilation
INF	interferon
INF-α	interferon-α
INH	isoniazid
INO	internuclear ophthalmoplegia
INR	international normalized ratio
IO	intraosseous
IOC	intra-operative cholangiography
IOL	induction of labour
IOL	intraocular lens
IOP	intraocular pressure
IP	interphalangeal
IP	intraperitoneal
IPAA	ileal pouch-anal anastomosis
IPAH	idiopathic pulmonary arterial hypertension
IPD	interphalangeal depth
IPF	idiopathic pulmonary fibrosis
IPMN	intraductal papillary mucinous neoplasm
IPS	integrated prenatal screen
IPV	injected polio vaccine
IQ	intelligence quotient
IR	immediate release
IRMA	intra retinal microvascular abnormalities
ISA	intrinsic sympathomimetic action
ISD	intrinsic sphincter deficiency
ITE	in the ear
ITP	immune thrombocytopenic purpura
IU	international units
IUD	intrauterine death
IUD	intrauterine device
IUFD	intrauterine fetal demise
IUGR	intrauterine growth restriction
IUI	intrauterine insemination
IV	intra venous
IVC	inferior vena cava
IVDU	intravenous drug use
IVF	in-vitro fertilization
IVH	intraventricular hemorrhage
IVIG	intravenous immunoglobulin
IVM	in-vitro maturation
IVP	intravenous pyelogram
IVU	intravenous urography

J

J	jaeger
JA	juvenile arthritis
JC	Jakob-Creutzfeldt
JGA	juxtaglomerular apparatus
JIA	juvenile idiopathic arthritis
JNA	juvenile nasopharyngeal angiofibroma
JRA	juvenile rheumatoid arthritis
JVP	jugular venous pulsation

K

K	potassium
KCl	postassium chloride
kg	kilogram
KOH	potassium hydroxide
KRP	Kolmer Reiter Protein
KS	Kaposi's sarcoma
KUB	kidney, ureter, bladder

L

L	litre
L	live births
L/S	lecithin/sphingomyelin
LA	left atrium
LA	local anesthetic
LA	long-acting
LAC	lupus anticoagulant
LAD	left anterior descending
LAD	left axis deviation
LAD	lymphadenopathy
LAE	left atrial enlargement
LAFB	left anterior fascicular block
LAP	left atrial pressure
LAP	leukocyte alkaline phosphatase
LAR	lower abdominal resection
LAR	lower anterior resection
LASIK	laser-assisted in-situ keratomileusis
LBB	left bundle branch
LBBB	left bundle branch block
LBD	Lewy body disease
LBO	large bowel obstruction
LPB	lower back pain
LBW	low birth weight
LCA	left circumflex artery
LCA	left coronary
LCAT	lecithin-cholesterol acyltransferase
LCCN	light chain cast nephropathy
LCD	liquor carbonis detergens
LCDC	Laboratory Center for Disease Control
LCIS	lobular carcinoma in situ
LCL	lateral collateral ligament
LCx	left circumflex artery
LD	loading dose
LD50	lethal dose - 50%
L-dopa	levodopa
LDH	lactate dehydrogenase
LDL	low density lipoprotein
LE	lower extremities
LEEP	loop electrosurgical excision procedure
LEMS	Lambert-Eaton myasthenic syndrome
LES	lower esophageal sphincter
LFT	liver function test
LGA	large for gestational age
LGI	lower gastrointestinal
LH	luteinizing hormone

LHF	left heart failure
LHRH	luteinizing hormone releasing hormone
Li	lithium
LICS	left intercostal space
LIMA	left internal mammary artery
LITA	left internal thoracic artery
LKM	liver kidney microsome
LLD	left lateral decubitus
LLDP	left lateral decubitus position
LLL	left lower lobe
LLQ	left lower quadrant
LLSB	left lower sternal border
LM	light microscope
LMA	laryngeal mask airway
LMCC	Licentiate of the MCC
LMN	lower motor nerve
LMN	lower motor neuron
LMNL	lower motor neuron lesion
LMP	last menstrual period
LMW	low molecular weight
LMWH	low molecular weight heparin
LN	lymph node
LNMP	last normal menstrual period
LOC	level of conciousness
LP	light perception
LP	lumbar puncture
LPFB	left posterior fascicular block
LPL	lipoprotein lipase
LPS	lipopolysaccharide
LR	likelihood ratio
LRA	leukotriene receptor antagonist
LRTI	lower respiratory tract infection
LSB	left sternal border
LSC	lichen simplex chronicus
LSD	lysergic acid diethylamide
LSIL	low grade squamous intraepithelial lesion
L-T4	L-thyroxine, levothyroxine
LTP	laryngotracheoplasty
LTRA	leukotriene receptor antagonist
LUD	left uterine displacement
LUL	left upper lobe
LUQ	left upper quadrant
LUTS	lower urinary tract symptoms
LV	left ventricle
LVAD	left ventricular assist device
LVED	left ventricular end diastolic
LVEDP	left ventricular end diastolic pressure
LVEF	left ventricular ejection fraction
LVES	left ventricular end systolic
LVF	left ventricular failure
LVF	left ventricular function
LVFP	left ventricle filling pressure
LVH	left ventricular hypertrophy
LVI	lymphovascular space invasion
LVOT	left ventricular outflow tract
LVP	left ventricular pressure

M

M	male
M	Muscarinic
MABP	mean arterial blood pressure
MAC	minimum alveolar concentration
MAC	Mycobacterium avium complex
MAHA	microangiopathic hemolytic anemia
MAI	mycobacterium avium-intracellulare
MALT	mucosal associated lymphomatous tissue lymphoma
MAO	monoamine oxidase
MAOI	monoamine oxidase inhibitor
MAOIs	monoamine oxidase inhibitors
MAP	magnesium ammonium phosphate
MAP	mean arterial pressure
MAS	meconium aspiration syndrome
MAST	military anti-shock trousers
MAT	multifocal atrial tachycardia
MC	metacarpal
MCA	middle cerebral artery
MCC	Medical Council of Canada
MCCQE	Medical Council of Canada qualifying exam
MCD	minimal change diesease

MCH	mean corpuscular hemoglobin
MCHC	mean corpuscular hemoglobin concentration
MCI	mild cognitive impairment
MCL	medial collateral ligament
MCN	mucinous cystic neoplasm
MCP	metacarpal phalangeal joint
MCT	medium chain triglycerides
MCTD	mixed connective tissue disease
MCV	mean corpuscular volume
MCV	molluscum contagiosum virus
MD	maintenance dose
MD	muscular dystrophy
MDAC	multidose activated charcoal
MDCT	miltidetector computed tomography
MDD	major depressive disorder
MDE	major depressive episode
MDI	metered dose inhaler
MDI	multiple daily injections
MDMA	3,4-methlenedioxy-methamphetamine (ecstacy)
MDR	multi-drug resistance
MDS	myelodysplastic syndrome
MEA	microwave endometrial ablation
MEE	middle ear effusion
MEI	middle ear inflammation
MELAS	mitochondrial myopathy, encephalopathy, lactic-acidosis and stroke like episodes
MELD	model for end stage liver disease
MEN	multiple endocrine neoplasia
MF	mycosis fungoides
mg	milligram
Mg	magnesium
MG	myasthenia gravis
MGUS	monoclonal gammopathy of unknown significance
MH	malignant hyperthermia
MHA	Mental Health Act
MHA-TP	microhemoglutination test for Ab to T. pallidium
MHC	major histocompatibility complex
MI	myocardial infarction
MIBG	meta-iodo-benzoguanide
MIDD	monoclonal 1g depostion disease
min	minutes
MLF	medial longitudinal fasciculus
MM	malignant melanoma
MM	millimeters
MM	multiple myeloma
MMF	mycophenolate mofetil
MMFR	maximal mid-expiratory flow rate
MMFR	mid maximal flow rate
MMI	methimazole
MMLE	mini-mental status exam
MMR	maternal mortality rate
MMR	measles/mumps/rubella
MMSE	mini mental status examination
MOA	mechanism of action
MOCA	Montreal cognitive assessment
MODS	multiple organ dysfunction syndrome
MODY	maturity-onset diabetes of the young
MOSF	multi-organ system failure
MP	mercaptopurine
MPA	medroxyprogesterone acetate
MPGN	membranous proliferative glomerulonephritis
MPI	myocardial perfusion imaging
MPTP	methylpheyl tetra hydropindine
MPV	mean platelet volume
MR	mitral regurgitation
MR	magnetic resonance
MR	mental retardation
MR	mitral regurgitation
MRA	magnetic resonance angiogram
MRC	Medical Research Council
MRCP	magnetic resonance cholangiopancreatography
MRI	magnetic resonance imaging
MRM	modified radical mastectomy
MRSA	methicillin-resistant S. aureus
MS	mitral stenosis
MS	multiple sclerosis
MSA	mixed sleep apnea

MSA	multiple system atrophy
MSAFP	maternal serum alphafetoprotein
MSDS	material safety data sheets
MSE	mental status examination
MSG	monsodium glutamate
MSH	melanocyte-stimulating hormone
MSK	musculoskeletal
MSM	men who have sex with men
MSS	maternal serum screen
MSSA	methicillin sensitive S. aureus
MSU	mid-stream urine
MT	metatarsal
MTC	medullary thyroid cancer
MTP	metatarso phalangeal joint
MTX	methotrexate
MTX-FA	methotrexate-folinic acid
MUA	manipulation under anesthesia
MUGA	multiple gated acquisition scan
MUSE	male urethral suppository for erection
MV	mitral valve
MVA	mitral valve area
MVA	motor vehicle accident
MVC	motor vehicle collision
MVO$_2$	myocardial O$_2$ consumption
MVP	mitral valve prolapse
MW	molecular weight
MZ	monozygotic

N

N	normal
Na	sodium
N/A	not applicable
N2O	nitrous oxide
NA	neuraminidase
NA	noradrenaline
NAC	n-acetyl
NAFLD	non-alcoholic fatty liver disease
NASH	nonalcoholic steatohepatitis
NASSA	noradrenergic and specific serotonin antagonists
NATP	neonatal alloimmune thrombocytopenia purpura
NBUVB	narrow band ultraviolet B
NBUVC	narrow band untraviolet C
NC	neurogenic claudication
NCEP	National Cholesterol Education Program
NCN	neocellular nevus
NCS	nerve conduction studies
NCV	nerve conduction velocity
NDRI	norepinephrine and dopamine reuptake inhibitors
NE	norepinephrine
NEC	necrotizing enterocolitis
NERD	non-erosive reflux disease
NF	neurofibromatosis
NF-1	neurofibromatosis type 1
NF-2	neurofibromatosis type 2
NG	nasogastric
NG-tube	nasogastric tube
NHL	non-Hodgkin's lymphoma
NICU	neonatal intensive care unit
NIPPV	noninvasive positive pressure ventilation
NIV	noninvasive ventilation
NK	natural killer
NLD	nasolacrimal duct
NLE	neonatal lupus erythematosus
NLP	no light perception
NMDA	N-methyl-D-aspartic acid
NMJ	neuromuscular junction
NMR	neonatal mortality rate
NMS	neuroleptic malignant syndrome
NMSC	nonmelanoma skin cancers
NNH	number needed to harm
NNT	number needed to treat
NO	nitric oxide
NOS	not otherwise specified
NP	nasopharyngeal
NPC	nasopharyngeal carcinoma
NPH	normal pressure hydrocephalus
NPO	nothing by mouth, nil per os
NPV	negative predictive value

NREM	non-REM
NRFHR	non-reassuring fetal heart rate
NRT	nicotine replacement therapy
NS	nasogastric tube
NS	nephrotic syndrome
NS	normal saline
NSAIDs	nonsteroidal anti-inflammatory drugs
NSCLC	non-small cell lung cancer
NSR	normal sinus rhythm
NST	non-stress test
NSTEMI	non ST elevation myocardial infarction
NT	nuchal translucency
NTD	neural tube defects
NTG	nitroglycerin
NTT	nasotracheal tube
NTUS	nuchal translucency ultrasound
N/V	nausea and vomiting
N/V/D	nausea/vomiting and diarrhea
NVI	neurovascular intact
NVS	neurovascular status
NWB	non-weightbearing
NYD	not yet diagnosed
NYHA	New York Heart Association

O

O&P	ova and parasites
O/E	on examination
O2	oxygen saturation
OA	occiput anterior
OA	osteoarthritis
OAF	osteoclast activating factor
OCD	obsessive compulsive disorder
OCP	oral contraceptive pill
OCPD	obsessive-compulsive personality disorder
OD	oculus dexter
OD	once a day
OD	overdose
OD	right eye
ODB	Ontario Drug Benefit
ODD	oppositional defiant disorder
ODM	opponens digiti minimi
OE	otitis externa
OECD	Organization for Economic Co-operation and Development
OGCT	oral glucose challenge test
OGD	oesophagogastro-duodenoscopy
OGTT	oral glucose tolerance test
OHA	oral hypoglycemic agent
OHIP	Ontario Health Insurance Plan
OHL	oral hairy leukoplakia
OM	otitis media
OME	otitis media with effusion
ONTD	open neural tube defect
OP	occiput posterior
OC	oncotic pressure
OP	opponens pollicis
OPC	oral contraceptive pill
OPCA	olivopontocerebellar atrophy
OPCAB	off pump coronary artery bypass
OPLL	ossification of posterior longitudinal ligament
OPV	oral polio vaccine
OR	odds ratio
OR	operating room
ORIF	open reduction internal fixation
OS	oculus sinister; left eye
OSA	obstructive sleep apnea
OT	occiput transverse
OT	occupational therapy
OTC	over the counter
OU	oculus uterque
OU	each eye

P

P	progesterone
P	psoralens
P/E	physical exam
PA	posteroanterior
PA	pulmonary artery
PAB	premature atrial beat

PABA	para-aminobenzoic acid
PAC	premature atrial contraction
PaCO2	arterial partial pressure of carbon dioxide
PACs	premature atrial contractions
PACG	primary angle closure glaucoma
PACU	post-anesthetic care unit
PAD	phlegmasia alba dolens
PAG	plasma anion gap
PAHO	Pan American Health Organization
PAI-I	plasminogen activator inhibitor
PAN	polyarteritis nodosa
p-ANCA	perinuclear anti-neutrophil cytoplasmic antibody
PaO2	arterial oxygen pressure
PAO2	partial pressure of oxygen in alveolar gas
PAP	Papanicolaou
PAP	pulmonary arterial pressure
PAPP-a	pregnancy-associated plasma protein
PAS	periodic acid-schiff reaction
PAS	peripheral anterior synechiae
PASP	pulmonary artery systolic pressure
PAT	paroxysmal atrial tachycardia
Patm	atmospheric pressure
PB	protein bound
PBC	primary biliary cirrhosis
PBD	percutaneous biliary drainage
pc	after meals
PC	peak concentration
PCA	patient controlled analgesia
PCA	posterior cerebral artery
PCB	polychlorinated biphenyls
PCD	phlegmasia cerulea dolens
PCI	percutaneous coronary intervention
PCKD	polycystic kidney disease
PCL	posterior cruciate ligament
PCNSL	primary central nervous system lymphoma
PCO	posterior capsular opacification
PCO2	partial pressure of carbon dioxide
PCOD	polycystic ovarian disease
PCOS	polycystic ovarian syndrome
PCP	pneumocystis carinii pneumonia
PCP	phenylclidine
PCR	polymerase chain reaction
PCT	porphyria cutanea tarda
PCT	proximal convoluted tubule
PCV	pressure control ventilation
PCWP	pulmonary capillary wedge pressure
PD	Parkinson's disease
PD	personality disorder
PD	posterior descending (artery)
PDA	parent ductus arteriosus
PDD	pervasive developmental disorder
PDE	phosphodiesterase
PDPHA	postdural puncture headache
PDR	proliferative diabetic retinopathy
PE	pulmonary embolism
PEEP	positive end expiratory pressure
PEF	peak expiratory flow
PEI	Prince Edward Island
PER	passive external rewarming
PERLA	pupils equal and reactive to light and accomodation
PET	positron emission tomography scan
PET	preeclampsia
PF	patellofemoral joint
PF	plain films
PFO	patent foramen ovale
PFT	pulmonary function tests
PG	plasma glucose
PG	prostaglandin
PGE1	prostaglandin E1
PGE2	prostaglandin E2
PH2O	partial pressure of water
PHE	periodic health examination
PHH	posthemorrhagic hydrocephalus
PHIPA	Ontario Personal Health Information Protection Act
PHPV	persistent hyperplastic primary vitreous
PICA	posterior inferior cerebral artery
PICC	peripherally inserted central catheter
PID	pelvic inflammatory disease
PIE	pulmonary infiltration with eosinophilia

PIH	pregnancy-induced hypertension
PIN	posterior interosseous nerve
PIP	proximal interphalangeal joint
PIPEDA	Personal Information Protection and Electronic Documents Act
PIV	posterior interventricular artery
PK	pyruvate kinase
PKU	phenylketonuria
PL	palmaris longus
PLT	platelets
PM	evening
PM	polymyositis
PMC	pontine micturition center
PMDD	premenstrual dysphoric disorder
PMH	past medical history
PMI	point of maximal impulse
PML	progressive multifocal leukoencephalopathy
PMN	polymorphonuclear neutrophils
PMNs	polymorphonuclear cells
PMR	proportional mortality rate
PMS	premenstrual syndrome
PMY	polymyositis
PND	paroxysmal nocturnal dyspnea
PND	post nasal drip
PNET	primitive neuroectodermal tumour
PNH	paroxysmal nocturnal hemoglobinuria
PNS	parasympathetic nervous system
PNS	peripheral nervous system
PO	per os, oral, by mouth
pO2	partial pressure of oxygen
PO4	phosphate
POAG	primary open angle glaucoma
POD	post-operative day
POD	post obstructive diuresis
POMC	pro-opiomelanocortin
PONV	post-operative nausea and vomiting
PPD	post-partum depression
PPD	purified protein derivative
PPH	postpartum hemorrhage
PPH	primary pulmonary hypertension
PPHN	persistent pulmonary hypertension of the newborn
PPI	proton pump inhibitor
PPRF	paramedian pontine reticular formation
PPROM	preterm premature rupture of membranes
PPS	progressive systemic sclerosis
PPV	positive predictive value
PPV	positive pressure ventilation
PR	per rectum
PR	progesterone receptor
PR	pulmonary regurgitation
PRBCs	packed red blood cells
PRK	photorefractive keratectomy
PRL	prolactin
PRN	pro re nata, as needed
PROM	premature rupture of membranes
PRSA	penicillin-resistant S. aureus
PRSP	penicillin-resistant Streptococcus pneumoniae
PRUJ	proximal radio ulnar joint
PRV	polycythemia rubra vera
PS	pulmonary stenosis
PSA	progressive supranuclear palsy
PSA	prostate specific antigen
PsA	psoriatic arthritis
PSC	primary sclerosing cholangitis
PSD	Parkinson plus syndrome
PSGN	poststreptococcal glomerulonephritis
PSIS	posterior superior iliac spine
PSP	progressive supranuclear palsy
PSS	progressive systemic sclerosis
PSSA	penicillin sensitive S. aureus
PSV	pressure support ventilation
PSVT	paroxysmal supraventricular tachyarrythmia
PT	physiotherapy
PT	prothrombin time
PTA	percutaneous transluminal angioplasty
PTA	pure tone audiometry
PTC	percutaneous transhepatic cholangiography
PTCA	percutaneous transluminal coronary angioplasty

PTCI	percutaneous transluminal coronary interventional
PTFE	polytetra fluroethylene
PTH	parathyroid hormone
PTHrP	PTH-related peptides
PTL	preterm labor
PTSD	post-traumatic stress disorder
PTT	partial thromblastin time
PTU	propylthiouracil
PUD	peptic ulcer disease
PUV	posterior urethral valve
PUVA	psoralens and long wave ultraviolet radiaton
PV	pulmonary valve
PVB	premature ventricular beat
PVCs	premature ventricular contractions
PVD	peripheral vascular disease
PVD	posterior vitreous detachment
PVR	peripheral venous return
PVR	pulmonary vascular resistance
PYLL	potential years of life lost

Q

q	each, every
Q	perfusion
QALY	quality adjusted life year
QD	once a day
qhs	every night, at bedtime
QID	four times a day
QOL	quality of life
QST	quantitative sensory testing

R

R&M	routine and microscopy
R/O	rule out
RA	rheumatoid arthritis
RA	right atrium
RAD	right axis deviation
RAE	right atrial enlargement
RAIU	radioactive iodine uptake
RAP	recurrent abdominal pain
RAP	right atrial pressure
RAPD	relative afferent pupillary defect
RAS	renal artery stenosis
RAS	reticular activating system
RBB	right bundle branch
RBBB	right bundle branch block
RBC	red blood cell
RBF	renal blood flow
RCA	right coronary artery
RCC	renal cell carcinoma
RCM	restrictive cardiomyopathy
RCPSC	Royal College of Physicians/Surgeons of Canada
RCT	randomized controlled trial
RD	retinal detachment
RDS	respiratory distress syndrome
RDT	rapid antigen detection test
RDW	red blood cell distribution width
ReA	reactive arthritis
REM	rapid eye movement
RES	reticuloendothelial system
RIND	reversible ischemic neurological deficit
RF	radiofrequency
RF	rheumatoid factor
RF	risk factor
RFT	renal function tests
Rh	Rhesus
RHF	right heart failure
RIA	radio-immune assay
RICS	right intercostal space
RIMA	reversible inhibitor of MAO-A
RIMA	right internal mammary artery
RIND	reversible ischemic neurological deficit
RITA	right internal thoracic artery
RL	Ringer's lactate
RLL	right lower lobe
RLQ	right lower quadrant
RLSB	right lateral sternal border

RML	right middle lobe
RNA	radionucleotide angiography
RNA	ritonucleic acid
RNAO	Registered Nurses' Association of Ontario
RNC	radionuclide cystography
RNI	recommended nutrient intake
ROM	range of motion
ROM	rupture of membranes
ROP	retinopathy of prematurity
RP	retinitis pigmentosa
RPE	retinal pigment epithelium
RPF	renal plasma flow
RPGN	rapidly progressive glomerulonephritis
RPR	rapid plasma reagin
RPS	rapid primary survey
RQ	respiratory quotient
RR	relative risk
RR	respiratory rate
RRR	relative risk reduction
RRT	renal replacement therapy
RSD	reflex sympathetic dystrophy
RSI	rapid sequence induction
RSV	respiratory syncytial virus
RT	radiation therapy
rT3	reverse triiodothyronine
RTA	renal tubular acidosis
RTI	respiratory tract infection
rt-PA	recombinant tissue plasminogen activator
RUL	right upper lobe
RUQ	right upper quadrant
RV	residual volume
RV	right ventricle
RVAD	right ventricular assist device
RVEDP	right ventricular end-diastolic pressure
RVF	right ventricular failure
RVH	right ventricular hypertrophy
RVOT	right ventricular outflow tract
RVOTO	right ventricular outflow tract obstruction
RVP	right ventricular pressure
RVSP	right ventricular strain pattern
RVSP	right ventricular systolic pressure
Rx	treatment

S

S&S	signs and symptoms
S/E	side effects
SA	sinoatrial
SA	sinus arrhythmia
SA	spontaneous abortion
SACD	subacute combined degeneration
SAH	subarachnoid hemorrhage
SaO2	hemoglobin oxygen percent saturation
SARS	severe acute respiratory syndrome
SBE	spontaneous bacterial endocarditis
SBO	small bowel obstruction
SBP	spontaneous bacterial peritonitis
sBP	systolic blood pressure
SC	sternoclavicular
SC	subcutaneous
SCA	spinocerebellar ataxia
SCA	superior cerebellar artery
SCC	squamous cell carcinoma
SCD	sickle cell disease
SCD	sudden cardiac death
SCFA	short chain fatty acids
SCFE	slipped capital femoral epiphysis
SCh	succinylcholine
SCI	spinal cord injury
SCID	severe combined immunodeficiency
SCIWARA	spinal cord injury without radiologic abnormality
SCLC	small cell lung cancer
SCM	sternocleidomastoid
SCr	serum creatinine
ScvO2	central venous oxygen saturation
SD	standard deviation
SDAC	single dose activated charcoal
SDM	substitute decision maker
SDRI	selective dopamine re-uptake inhibitor

SDS	Shy-Drager syndrome
Seb. K	seborrheic keratosis
SEM	systolic ejection murmur
SERM	selective estrogen receptor modulator
SERMs	selective estrogen receptor modifiers
SES	sick euthyroid syndrome
SES	social economic status
SF	synovial fluid
SFH	symphysis fundal height
SG	specific gravity
SGA	small for gestational age
SH	sex hormones
SHBG	sex hormone binding globulin
SHG	sonohysterography
SI	sacroiliac
SIADH	syndrome of inappropriate antidiuretic hormone
SIDS	sudden infant death syndrome
SIL	squamous intraepithelial lesion
SIMV	synchronous intermittent mandatory ventilation
SIRS	systemic inflammatory response syndrome
SJS	Stevens-Johnson Syndrome
SL	sublingual
SLE	systemic lupus erythematosis
SLP	speech language pathologist
SLR	straight leg raise
SMA	smooth muscle antibody
SMA	superior mesenteric artery
SMV	superior mesenteric vein
SMX	sulfamethoxazole
SNB	sentinel node biopsy
SND	striatonigral degeneration
SNHL	sensorineural hearing loss
SNpc	substantia nigra pars compacta
SNRI	serotonin and norepinephrine reuptake inhibitors
SNS	striatonigral degeneration
SNS	sympathetic nervous system
SOB	shortness of breath
SOBOE	shortness of breath on exertion
SOF	superior orbital fissure
SOGC	Society of Obstetricians and Gynecologists of Canada
SPAK	spreading pigmented actinic keratosis
SPECT	single photon emission computed tomography
SPEP	serum protein electrophoresis
SPF	sun protection factor
SPK	superficial punctate keratitis
SR	sinus rhythm
SRS	stereotactic radiosurgery
SRT	speech reception threshold
SSA	Sjögren's syndrome A
SSB	Sjögren's syndrome B
SSPE	subacute sclerosing panencephalitis
SSRI	selective serotonin reuptake inhibitor
SSS	sick sinus syndrome
SSSS	staphylococcal scalded skin syndrome
STAR	sore throat, arthritis, rash
STDs	sexually transmitted diseases
STEMI	ST elevation myocardial infarction
STfR	soluble transferrin receptor
STIs	sexually transmitted infections
STN	subthalamic nucleus
STP	sodium thiopental
STS	Stevens-Johnson Syndrome
STSG	split thickness skin graft
STSH	sensitive thyroid-stimulating hormone
SV	stroke volume
SVI	stroke volume index
SVC	superior vena cava
SVG	saphenous vein graft
SVR	systemic vascular resistance
SVRI	systemic vascular resistance index
SVT	supraventricular tachycardia
SWU	septic work-up

T

T1	first trimester
T2	second trimester
T3	trird trimester
t1/2	half-life
T3	triiodothyronine
T3RU	T3 resin uptake
T4	thyroxine
TA	therapeutic abortion
TAA	thoracic aortic aneurysm
TACE	transcateter arterial chemoembolization
TAH	total abdominal hysterectomy
TAH/BSO	total abdominal hysterectomy+bilateral salpingo-oophorectomy
TB	tuberculosis
TBB	transbronchial biopsy
TBG	thyroid binding globulin
TBSA	total body surface area
TBUT	tear break up time
TBW	total body water
TC	total cholesterol
TC	transcobalamin
Tc99m MIBI	technetium-99m methoxyisobatyl-isonitrile
TCA	trichloroacetic acid
TCA	tricyclic antidepressant
TCC	transitional cell carcinoma
TCF	tracheoesophogeal fistula
TCM	traditional chinese medicine
TD50	toxic dose - 50%
TDEE	total daily energy expenditure
TDM	therapeutic drug monitoring
TdP	tetanus, diphtheria, polio
TE	tracheoesophageal
TED	thromboembolic disease
TEE	transesophageal echocardiography
TEF	tracheoesophageal fistula
TEN	total enteral nutrition
TEN	toxic epidermal necrolysis
TENS	transcutaneous electrical neuro stimulation
TET	tubal embryo transfer
TFCC	triangular fibrocartilage complex
TG	triglyceride
TGA	transposition of the great arteries
THA	total hip arthroplasty
TI	therapeutic index
TIA	transient ischemic attack
TIBC	total iron binding capacity
tid	three times a day
TIG	tetanus immune globulin
TIN	tubuloInterstitial nephritis
TIPS	transjugular intrahepatic portasystemic shunt
TIVA	total intravenous anesthesia
TKA	total knee arthroplasty
TKVO	to keep vein open
TLC	total lung capacity
TLE	temporal lobe epilepsy
TM	tympanic membrane
TMB	transient monocular blindness
TMJ	temporomandibular joint
TMP	trimethoprim
TMP/SMX	trimethoprim-sulfamethoxazole
Tn	troponin
TN	true negative
TNF	tumour necrosis factor
TNFα	tumour necrosis factor alpha
TNM	tumour/node/metastasis staging
TOF	tetralogy of Fallot
TOF	train of four
TORCHS	toxoplasmosis, rubella; cytomegalovirus, hepatitis
TOT	tension-free obturator tape
t-PA	tissue plasminogen activator
TP	true positive
TP	tympanic membrane
TPE	tropical pulmonary eosinophilia
TPI	treponemal pallidum immobilization
TPN	total parenteral nutrition
TPO	thyroid peroxidase
TPR	total peripheral resistance
TR	tricuspid regurgitation

TRALI	transfusion related acute lung injury
TRAM	transverse rectus abdominus myocutaneous
TRH	thyrotropin releasing hormone
TRUS	transrectal ultrasound
TS	tricuspid stenosis
TSAb	thyroid stimulating antibodies
TSH	thyroid stimulating hormone
TSI	thyroid stimulating immunoglobulin
tsp	teaspoon
T-spine	thoracic spine
TSS	toxic shock syndrome
TT	thrombin time
TTB	transthoracic biopsy
TTE	transthoracic echocardiography
TTG	tissue transglutaminase
TTKG	transtubular potassium gradient
TTN	transient tachypnea of the newborn
TTP	thrombotic thrombocytopenic purpura
TUIP	transurethral incision of the prostate
TUMT	transurethral microwave therapy
TUNA	transurethral needle ablation
TURBT	transurethral resection of bladder tumour
TURP	transurethral resection of the prostate
TV	tricuspid valve
TVOT	tension-free vaginal obturator tape
TVT	tension-free vaginal tape
TVUS	trans-vaginal ultrasound
TXA2	thromboxane 2
TZ	transformation zone
TZD	thiazolidinedione

U

U	unit
U/A	urinalysis
ud	as directed
U/O	urine output
U/S	ultrasound
UA	unstable angina
UAE	uterine artery embolization
UC	ulcerative colitis
UCL	ulnar collateral ligament
UE	upper extremity
UES	upper esophageal sphincter
UFH	unfractionated heparin
UGI	upper gastrointestinal
UGIB	upper gastrointestinal (GI) bleed
UIP	usual interstitial pneumonitis
ULSB	upper left sternal border
UMN	upper motor nerve
UMN	upper motor neuron
UMNL	upper motor neuron lesion
ung	ointment
Uosm	urine osmolality
UPEP	urine protein electrophoresis
UPJ	ureteropelvic junction
UPPP	uvolopalatopharyngoplasty
UPV	UV protection factor
URI	upper respiratory infection
URTI	upper respiratory tract infection
UTI	urinary tract infection
UUTS	upper urinary tract symptoms
UV	ultraviolet
UVA	ultraviolet radiation
UVA	ultraviolet wavelength A
UVB	ultraviolet wavelength B
UVC	ultraviolet wavelength C
UVJ	ureterovesical junction
UVR	ultraviolet radiation

V

V fib	ventricular fibrillation
V	ventilation
VA	ventriculo-artial
VA	visual acuity
Vd	volume of distribution
VAC	vacuum assisted closure
VADs	ventricular assist devices
VAIN	vaginal intraepithelial neoplasia
VBAC	vaginal birth after cesarean
VBI	vertebrobasilar insufficiency
VC	vital capacity
VCUG	voiding cystourethrogram
VDRL	venereal disease research laboratory
VFib	ventricular fibrillation
VF	visual field
VHL	von Hippel Lindau syndrome
VIN	vulvar intraepithelial neoplasia
VIP	vasoactive intestinal peptide
Vit. A	vitamin A
VIU	visual internal urethrotomy
VLDL	very low density lipoprotein
VMA	vanillyl mandellic acid
VOR	vestibulo-ocular reflex
VP	vasopressin
VP	ventriculoperitoneal
VPB	ventricular premature beat
VPI	velopharyngeal insufficiency
VPL	ventral posterolateral
VPL	ventral posteromedial
V/Q	ventilation-to-perfusion
VRE	vancomycin-resistant Enterococci
VSD	ventricular septal defect
VSR	vital signs routine
VT	ventricular tachycardia
VT	tidal volume
VTE	venous thromboembolism
VUR	vesicoureteral reflux
vWD	von Willebrand's disease
vWF	von Willebrand's factor
VZIG	Varicella-Zoster immunoglobulin
VZV	Varicella-Zoster virus

W

WBC	white blood cell
WBRT	whole brain radiation therapy
WC	waist circumference
WCB	Workers' Compensation Board
WHI	Women's Health Initiative
WHI	Women's Health Institute
WHMIS	Workplace Hazardous Materials Information System
WHO	World Health Organization
WPW	Wolff-Parkinson-White
WSIB	Workplace Safety and Insurance Board
WT	weight

X

XRT	radiation therapy

Z

ZE	Zollinger-Ellison
ZIFT	zygote intrafallopian transfer
ZIFT	zygote-transfer
ZN	Ziehl-Neelsen
ZPP	zinc protoporphyrin

Index

M

T

References

ANESTHESIA AND PERIOPERATIVE MEDICINE

Barash PG, Cullen BF, Stoelting RK (2001). (4th ed.). Clinical Anesthesia. Lippincott, Philadelphia, USA.

Blanc VF, Tremblay NA. The complications of tracheal intubation: a new classification with review of the literature. Anesth Analg 1974; 53: 202.

Chih HN (ed.) (1998). Anaesthesia A Practical Handbook. Singapore General Hospital, Oxford University Press Singapore.

Collins, VJ (1996). Physiologic and Pharmacologic Bases of Anesthesia. Williams & Wilkins, Pennsylvania, USA.

Craft TM, Upton PM (2001) (3rd ed.) Key Topics In Anesthesia, Clinical Aspects. BIOS Scientific Publishers Ltd., UK

Duke J (2000). Anesthesia Secrets, 2nd ed. Hanley and Beltus Inc.

Eagle KA et al. ACC/AHA Guideline update for perioperative cardiovascular evaluation for noncardiac surgery - executive summary. Circulation. 105: 1257-1267, 2002.

Ezekiel MR (2002-2003). Handbook of Anesthesiology. Current Clinical Strategies Publishing.

Frank SM, Fleisher LA, Breslow MJ et al: Perioperative maintenance of normothermia reduces the incidence of morbid cardiac events: A randomized clinical trial. JAMA 227:1127-1134, 1997.

Guidelines to the Practice of Anesthesia Revised 2005 Supplement to the Canadian Journal of Anesthesia Vol 52, No 9, November 2005.

Hebert PC et al. NEJM 1999; 340: 409-417.

Henderson JJ, Popat MT, Latto IP, Pearce AC. Difficult Airway Society Guidelines for management of the unanticipated difficult intubation. Anaesthesia. 59: 675-694, 2004.

Hurford WE (2002). Clinical Anesthesia Procedures of the Massachusetts General Hospital , Sixth Edition. Lippincott Williams and Wilkins.

Kalant H, Roschlau WH (1998). Principles of Medical Pharmacology. Oxford University Press, New York, USA.

Lawrence PF (1997). Anesthesiology, Surgical Specialties. Lippencott Pub.

Lette J et al. Ann Surg 1992; 216:192-204.

Mangano DT et al. JAMA 1992; 268: 233-240.

Mangano DT et al. NEJM 1996; 335:1713-1720.

Miller RD (2000). Anesthesia, 5th ed. Churchill Livingstone, Inc.

Morgan GE Jr (2002). Clinical Anesthesiology, 3rd ed. McGraw-Hill Companies, Inc.

Palda V et al. Ann Intern Med 1997; 127:313-328.

Poldermans D et al. NEJM 1999; 341:1789-1794.

Posner K et al. Anesth Analg 1999; 89:553.

Rao T, Jacobs "KH, EI-Etr AA. Reinfarction following anaesthesia in patients with myocardial infarction. Anaesthesiology. 59: 499-505, 1983.

Roberts JR, Spadafora M, Cone DC. Proper depth placement of oral endotracheal tubes in adults prior to radiographic confirmation.

Rogers A et. al. Acad Emerg Med. 1995 Jan;2(1):20-4. BMJ 2000; 321:1-12.

Salpeter S et al. Cochrane Database of Systematic Reviews 2003; Issue 3.

Sessler DI: Temperature monitoring. Complications and treatment of mild hypothermia. Anesthesiology 95:531-543, 2001.

Sullivan P (1999). Anesthesia for Medical Students. Doculink International, Ottawa, Canada.

www.mhaus.org accessed September 23, 2007.

Zwillich CW, Pierson DJ, Creagh CE. Complication of assisted ventilation. Am J Med 1974; 57: 161-9.

CARDIOLOGY AND CARDIOVASCULAR SURGERY

Ischemic Heart Disease

Cannon CP., et al. Intensive versus moderate lipid lowering with statins after acute coronary syndromes. NEJM 2004;350(15):1495-504.

Lindahl, B., et al. Markers of Myocardial Damage and Inflammation in Relation to Long-Term Mortality in Unstable Coronary Artery Disease. New England Journal of Medicine. 2000; 343:1139-1147.

Pitt B., et al. Eplerenone, a selective aldosterone blocker, in patients with left ventricular dysfunction after myocardial infarction. NEJM 2003; 348(14):1309-21.

Rauch, U., et al. Thrombus Formation on the Atherosclerotic Plaques: Pathogenesis and Clinical Consequences. Annals of Internal Medicine. 2001; 134: 224-238.

The Arterial Revascularization Therapies Study Group. Comparison of Coronary-Artery Bypass Surgery and Stenting for the Treatment of Multivessel Disease. New England Journal of Medicine. 2001; 344:1117-1124.

Turpie, A. G. G. and Antman, E. M. Low-Molecular-Weight Heparins in the Treatment of Acute Coronary Syndromes. Archives of Internal Medicine. 2001; 161: 1484-1490.

Yeghiazarians, Y., Braunstein, J. B., Askari, A., and Stone, P. H. Review Article: Unstable Angina Pectoris. New England Journal of Medicine. 2000; 342:101-114.

Nuclear Cardiology

Lee TH and Boucher CA. Noninvasive tests in patients with stable coronary artery disease (Review). N Engl J Med 2000;344:1840-5.

Cardiomyopathies

Feldman AM and McNamara D. Myocarditis (Review). N Engl J Med 2000; 343:1388-98.

Guidelines

ACC/AHA guidelines for percutaneous coronary intervention. Circulation. 2001;103:3019–3041.

ACC/AHA 2002 guideline update for the management of patients with unstable angina and non-ST-segment elevation myocardial infarction. (Available at: http://www.acc.org)

ACC/AHA Guideline update for the Diagnosis and Management of Chronic Heart Failure in the Adult. Circulation 2005; 112:e154.

ACC/AHA guidelines for the management of patients with ST-elevation myocardial infarction: a report of the American College of Cardiology/American Heart Association Task Force on Practice Guidelines (Committee to Revise the 1999 Guidelines for the Management of Patients with Acute Myocardial Infarction). Circulation 2004; 110(9):e82-292.

Antman EM et al. ACC/AHA Guidelines for the Management of Patients with ST-elevation Myocardial Infarction - summary: A Report of the American College of Cardiology. American Heart Association Task Force on Practice Guidelines. Circulation. 2004; 110-588.

CCS. 2001 Canadian cardiovascular society consensus guideline update for the management and prevention of heart failure. Canadian Journal of Cardiology. 2001;17(suppE):5-24.

Aurigemma, GP et al. Clinical Practice, Diastolic Heart Failure. NEJM 2004; 351:1097.

www.acc.org – The American College of Cardiology (clinical guidelines, etc).

www.ccs.ca – Canadian Cardiovascular Society 2005 Consensus Conference Peripheral Aterial Disease (Draft).

www.theheart.org – Cardiology Online (requires registration).

www.heartvalverepair.net – Heart Valve Repair Online.

Beard JD. Chronic lower limb ischemia. BMJ. 2000;320:854-857.

Fuchs JA. Atherogenesis and the Medical Management of Atherosclerosis. In Vascular Surgery 4th edition, Robert B. Rutherford Ed. 1995. WB. Saunders Co., Toronto. pp 222-234.

Harrington RA et al. Antithrombotic Therapy for Coronary Artery Disease: the Seventh ACCP Conference on Antithrombotic and Thrombolytic Therapy. Chest. 2004; 126 (3 suppl):513s-584s.

May J, White GH, and Harris JP. The complications and downside of endovascular therapies. Adv Surg 35: 153-72, 2001.

Schmieder FA and Comerota AJ. Intermittent claudication: magnitude of the problem, patient evaluation, and therapeutic strategies. Am J Card 87 (Suppl): 3D-13D, 2001.

Way LW, Doherty GM, editors. Current Surgical Diagnosis and Treatment, 11th edition. Lange Medical Books/McGraw-Hill. 2004.

Yang SC, Cameron DE, editors. Current therapy in thoracic and cardiovascular medicine. McGraw-Hill Inc, 2004.

Ambulatory ECG

Peter J. Zimetbaum, MD, and Mark E. Josephson, MD,

Zimerbaum, P., Josephson, M. The Evolving Role of Ambulatory Arrhythmia Monitoring in General Clinical Practie. Annals of Internal Medicine. 130 (10). 1999.

Kadish AH, Buxton AE, Kennedy HL. ACC/AHA clinical competence statement on electrocardiography and ambulatory electrocardiography: a report of the ACC/AHA/ACP-ASIM task force on clinical competence. Circulation. 104:3169 –3178. 2001.

Krahn, A., Klein, G., Skanes, A., Yee, R. Insertable Loop Recorder Use for Detection of Intermittent Arrhythmias. Pacing and Clinical Electrophysiology. 27 (5). 2004.

Stress Testing
Allison, T., Bardsley, W., Behrenbeck, T., Christian, T., Clements, I., Edwards, B., Gibbons, R., Miller, T., Oh, J., Pellikka, P., Roger, V., Squires, R., Weissler, A. 1996 Mayo Foundation for Medical Education and Research. 71(1): 43-52. 1996.
GIBBONS ET AL. Exercise Testing Guidelines. JACC. 30 (1):260-315. 1997.

Echocardiography
Picano, E. Stress Echocardiography: A historical perspective. Am J Med. 114:126–130. 2003.
Heatlie, G., Giles, M. Echocardiography and the general physician. Postgrad Med. J. 80;84-88. 2004.
Cheitlin, M. ACC/AHA/ASE 2003 Guideline Update for the Clinical Application of Echocardiograohy: Summary Article. Journal of the American Society of Echocardiography. 16 (10). 2003.
Gowda, R., Khan, I., Sacchi, T., Patel, R. History of the evolution of echocardiography. International Journal of Cardiology. 97 (1): 1-6. 2004.

Nuclear Cardiology
Sabharwal, N. Lahiri, A. Role of myocardial perfusion imaging for risk stratification in suspected or known coronary artery disease. Heart. 89:1291-1297. 2003.
Beller, G., Zaret, B. Contributions of Nuclear Cardiology to Diagnosis and Prognosis of Patients with Coronary Artery Disease. Circulation. 2000.

MR
Danias, P., Roussakis, A. Ioannidis J. Cardiac imaging Diagnostic performance of coronary magnetic resonance angiography as compared against conventional x-ray angiography A meta-analysis Journal of the American College of Cardiology 44(2): 1867-1876. 2004.

CT
Schoepf, J., Becker, C., Ohnesorge, B., Yucel, K. CT of Coronary Artery
Disease. Radiology . 232:18–37. 2004.
Somberg, J. Arrhythmia Therapy. Lippincott Williams & Wilkins, Inc. 9(6): 537-542. 2002.

Cath/EPS
Hayes, D., Furman, S. Cardiac Pacing: How it Started, Where We Are, Where We Are Going. Journal of Cardiovascular Electrophysiology. 15 (5) 2004.
Zipes et al. ACC/AHA Task Force Report Guidelines for Clinical Intracardiac Electrophysiological and Catheter Ablation Procedures. JACC. 26 (2): 555-573. 1995.
Wellens, J. Cardiac Arrhythmias: the quest for a cure. Journal of the American College of Cardiology. 44 (6): 1155-1163. 2004.
Conti, J. ACC 2005 Annual Session Highlight. Cardiac Arrhythmias. Journal of the American College of Cardiology. 45 (11):B30-B32. 2005.
Keane, D. New Catheter Ablation Techniques for the Treatment of Cardiac Arrhythmias. Cardiac Electrophysiology Review. 6:341-348. 2002.
Skanes, A., Klein, G., Krahn, A. Yee, R. Cryoablation: Potentials and Pitfalls. J Cardiovasc Electrophysiol. 15:528-534. 2004.
Packer, D. Evolution og Mapping and Anatomic Imaging of Cardiac Arrhythmias. Journal of Cardiovascular Electrophysiology. 15 (7). 2004.
Zipes, D. The year in electrophysiology. Journal of the American College of Cardiology. 43 (7):1306-1324. 2004.
Ryan TJ, Faxon DP, Gunnar RM, et al. Guidelines for percutaneous

Percutaneous Angiography/PCI
transluminal coronary angioplasty: a report of the American College of Cardiology/Am Heart Association Task Force on Assessment of Diagnostic and Therapeutic Cardiovascular Procedures Subcommittee on Percutaneous Transluminal Coronary angioplasty). J Am Coll Cardiol.12:529–545. 1988.
O'Neil W., Dixon, S., Grines, C. The year in interventional cardiology. Journal of the American College of Cardiology. 45 (7):1117-1134. 2005.
Bashore et al. ACC/SCA&I expert concensus document. American College of Cardiology/Society for Cardiac Angiography and Interventions Clinical Expert Consensus Document on Cardiac Catheterization Laboratory Standards. Journal of the American College of Cardiology. 37 (8):2170-2214. 2001.
Baim, D. New devices for percutaneous coronary intervention are rapidly making bypass surgery obsolete. Lippincott Williams & Wilkins, Inc.19(6): 593-597. 2004.

Cardiovascular Surgery
www.acc.org – The American College of Cardiology (clinical guidelines, etc)
www.theheart.org – Cardiology Online (requires registration)
www.heartvalverepair.net – Heart Valve Repair Online
Alexander P and Giangola G. Deep venous thrombosis and pulmonary embolism: Diagnosis, prophylaxis, and treatment. Ann Vasc Surg 13: 318-27, 1999.
Beard JD. Chronic lower limb ischemia. BMJ. 2000;320:854-857.
Bojar RM. Manual of perioperative care in cardiac surgery, 3rd edition. Massachusetts: Blackwell Science Inc., 1999.
Cheng DCH, David TE eds. Perioperative care in cardiac anesthesia and surgery. Austin: Landes Bioscience, 1999.
Coulam CH and Rubin GD. Acute aortic abnormalities. Semin Roentgenol 36: 148-64, 2001.
Crawford ES and Crawford JL. Thoracoabdominal Aortic Aneurysm. In: Vascular surgery: Principles and Practice 2nd edition, Veith FJ, Hobson RW, Williams RA, and Wilson SE Eds 1994. McGraw-Hill Inc, Toronto.
Fuchs JA. Atherogenesis and the Medical Management of Atherosclerosis. In Vascular Surgery 4th edition, Robert B. Rutherford Ed. 1995. WB Saunders Co., Toronto. pp 222-234.
Freischlag JA. Abdominal Aortic Aneurysms. In: Vascular surgery: Principles and Practice 2nd edition, Veith FJ, Hobson RW, Williams RA, and Wilson SE Eds 1994. McGraw-Hill Inc, Toronto.
Hallett JW Jr. Abdominal aortic aneurysm: natural history and treatment. Heart Dis Stroke 1: 303-8, 1992.
Hallett JW Jr. Management of abdominal aortic aneurysms. Mayo Clin Proc 75: 395-9, 2000.
Harlan BJ, Starr A, Harwin FM. Illustrated handbook of cardiac surgery. New York: Springer-Verlag Inc., 1996.
May J, White GH, and Harris JP. The complications and downside of endovascular therapies. Adv Surg 35: 153-72, 2001.
Pitt MPI and Bonser RS. The natural history of thoracic aortic aneurysm disease: An overview. J Card Surg 12(Suppl): 270-8, 1997.
Powell JT and Brown LC. The natural history of abdominal aortic aneurysms and their risk of rupture. Adv Surg 35: 173-85, 2001.
Rosen CL and Tracy JA. The diagnosis of lower extremity deep venous thrombosis. Em Med Clin N Am 19: 895-912, 2001.
Schmieder FA and Comerota AJ. Intermittent claudication: magnitude of the problem, patient evaluation, and therapeutic strategies. Am J Card 87 (Suppl): 3D-13D, 2001.
Verma S, Szmitko PE, et al. Clinician Update: Should radial arteries be used routinely for coronary artery bypass grafting? Circulation. 2004;110:e40-e46.
Way LW, Doherty GM, editors. Current Surgical Diagnosis and Treatment, 11th edition. Lange Medical Books/McGraw-Hill. 2004.
Yang SC, Cameron DE, editors. Current therapy in thoracic and cardiovascular medicine. McGraw-Hill Inc, 2004.

CLINICAL PHARMACOLOGY

Baker GR, Norton PG, Flintoft V et al. The Canadian Adverse Events Study: the incidence of adverse events among hospital patients in Canada. CMAJ 2004; 170:1678-86.
Canadian Adverse Drug Reaction Monitoring Program (CADRMP) Adverse Reaction Database http://www.hc-sc.gc.ca/dhp-mps/medeff/databasdon/index_e.html
Hardman JG and Limbird LR (eds) (1996). Goodman and Gilman's the Pharmacological Basis of Therapeutics (9th ed). McGraw-Hill, New York.
Hardy B, Bedard M (2002). Serum Drug Concentration Monitoring. In: Compendium of Pharmaceuticals and Specialties 2002. Repchinsky C (ed.). Canadian Pharmacists Association, Ottawa.
Kalant H and Roschlau W (eds) (1999). Principles of Medical Pharmacology (6th ed.). Oxford University Press, New York.
Katzung BG (ed) (2001). Basic and Clinical Pharmacology (8th ed.). McGraw-Hill Companies, New York.
Rang H, Dale M, Ritter J (eds) (1999). Pharmacology (4th ed.). Churchill Livingstone, Edinburgh.
Lewis, T. (2004) Using the NO TEARS tool for medication review. BMJ. 329(7463):434.

DERMATOLOGY

Textbooks
Bolognia JL, Jorizzo JL, Rapini RP, editors. Textbook of Dermatology. Vol. 1 and 2. Toronto: Mosby, 2003.
Fitzpatrick JE and Aeling JL. Dermatology Secrets. 2nd ed. Philadelphia: Hanley & Belfus, 2001.
Johnson RA, Suurmond D, Wolff K, editors. Color atlas and synopsis of clinical dermatology. 5th ed. New York: McGraw Hill, 2005.
Kraft J, Ng C, Bertucci V. University of Toronto Pharmacology Handbook: Dermatology Chapter. Toronto: publication pending.
Lebwohl MG, Heymann WR, Berth-Jones J, Coulson I, editors. Treatment of skin disease: Comprehensive therapeutic strategies. 2nd ed. Philadelphia: Mosby, 2006.
Paller AS, Mancini AJ. Hurwitz clinical pediatric dermatology: A textbook of skin disorders of childhood and adolescence. 3rd ed. China: Elsevier, 2006.

Articles
Cribier B et al. Erythema nodosum and associated diseases. Int J Dermatol. 1998;637-667.
Cummings SR et al. Approaches to the prevention and control of skin cancer. Cancer Metastatis Rev. 1997;16:309.
DeShazo RD et al. Allergic reactions to drugs and biologic agents. JAMA. 1997;278:1895.
Ellis C, et al. ICCAD II Faculty. International Consensus Conference on Atopic Dermatitis II (ICCAD II): Clinical update and current treatment strategies. Br J Dermatol. 2003; 148 (suppl 63):3-10.
Faergemann J, Baron R. Epidemiology, clinical presentation, and diagnosis of onychomycosis. Br J Dermatol. 2003; 149 (suppl 65):1-4.
Friedmann PS. Assessment of urticaria and angio-edema. Clin Exper Allergy. 1999;29 (suppl 3):109.
Gordon ML et al. Care of the skin at midlife: Diagnosis of pigmented lesions. Geriatrics. 1997;52:56-67.
Krafchik, BR. Treatment of atopic dermatitis. J Cut Med Surg 3. 1999; 3(suppl 2):16-23.
Mastrolorenzo A, Urbano FG, Salimbeni L, et al. Atypical molluscum contagiosum in an HIV-infected patient. Int J Dermatol. 1998; 27:378-380.
Price VH. Treatment of hair loss. NEJM. 1999;341:964.
Roujeau JC. Stevens-Johnson syndrome and toxic epidermal necrolysis are severe variants of the same disease which differs from erythema multiforme. J Dermatol. 1997;274-276.
Walsh SRA and Shear NH. Psoriasis and the new biologic agents: Interrupting a T-AP dance. CMAJ. 2004;170(13):1933-1941.
Whited JD et al. Does this patient have a mole or a melanoma? JAMA. 1998;279-676.
Wilkin J, Dahl M, Detmar M, Drake L, Feinstein A, Odom R, Powell F. Standard classification of rosacea: Report of the National Rosacea Society Expert Committee on the Classification and Staging of Rosacea. J Amer Acad Dermatol. 2002;46(4):584-587.

Other Sources
Canadian Dermatology Association 82nd Annual Conference. June 29-July 4, 2007. Toronto, Ontario, Canada.
Pope E. Pediatric Exanthems. Lecture presentation to 2006-2007 University of Toronto Year 3 Medical Students.

DIAGNOSTIC MEDICAL IMAGING

Gay S, Woodcock Jr RJ (2000). Radiology Recall. Baltimore: Lippincott Williams & Wilkins.
Brant WE, Helms CA (1999). Fundamentals of diagnostic radiology. Philadelphia. Lippincott Williams and Wilkins.
Chen MYM, Pope, TL, Ott DJ. (2004) Basic Radiology. New York. Lange Medical Books/McGraw Hill.
Daffner RH (1993). Clinical radiology: the essentials. Baltimore: Williams & Wilkins.
Erkonen WE, Smith WL. (2005). Radiology 101. Philadelphia: Lippincott Williams & Wilkins.
Fleckenstein P, Tranun-Jensen J (2001). Anatomy in Diagnostic Imaging. 2nd ed. Copenhagen: Blackwell Publishing.
Goodman LR (2007). Felson's Principles of Chest Roentgenology: A Programmed Text. 3rd ed. Philadelphia: Saunders.
Joffe SA, Servaes S, Okon S, Horowitz M. Multi-detector row CT urography in the evaluation of hematuria. Radiographics. 2003, 23(6):1441-55.
Juhl JH, Crummy AB, Kuhlman JE (1998). Paul and Juhl's Essentials of Radiologic Imaging. Phildelphia: Lippincott-Raven.
Katz DS, Math KR, Groskin SA (1998). Radiology secrets. Philadelphia: Hanley and Belfus.
Novelline RA (2004). Squire's Fundamentals of Radiology. 6th ed. Cambridge:Harvard.
Ouellette H, Tetreault P. (2002). Clinical Radiology made ridiculously simple. Miami: MedMaster.
Sam PM, Curtin HD (1996). Head and neck imaging. 3rd ed.. St. Louis: Mosby.
Weissleder R, Rieumont MJ, Wittenberg J. (1997) Primer of Diagnostic Imaging, 2nd ed. Philadelphia: Mosby.

EMERGENCY MEDICINE

Books
Clinical Anesthesia 4th ed. Barash PG, Cullen BF, Stoelting RK. Philadelphia: Lippincott, 2001.
Cecil's Essentials of Medicine 7th ed. Andreoli TE, Carpenter CJ, Griggs RC, Benjamin IJ. Saunders, 2007.
Physiologic and Pharmacologic Bases of Anesthesia. Collins VJ. Pennsylvania: Williams & Wilkins, 1996.
Practical Guide to the Care of the Medical Patient, 5th ed. Ferri F (ed). Mosby, 2001.
Principles of Medical Pharmacology. Kalant H, Roschlau WH New York: Oxford University Press, 1998.
Emergency Medicine On Call. Keim, Setal. McGraw Hill. 2004.
Rosen's Emergency Medicine: Concepts and Clinical Practice, 5th ed. Marx (ed). Mosby 2002.
Clinical procedures in emergency medicine. 3rd ed. Roberts JR and Hedges JR (ed). WB Saunders Co, 1998.
Emergency medicine: A comprehensive study guide, 5th ed. Tintinalli JE and Kelen GE (ed). McGraw-Hill Professional Publishing, 1999.
Emergency Medicine Recall. Woods, WA et al (ed). Lippincott Williams and Wilkins, 2000.

Journal Articles
Varon J, Marik P. The Diagnosis and management of hypertensive crises. Chest. 2000;118(1):214-27.
Vidt DG. Emergency room management of hypertensive urgencies and emergencies. J Clin Hypertens, 2001;3(3):158-64.
Wells PS, Anderson DR, Rodger M, et al. Derivation of a simple clinical model to categorize patients probability of pulmonary embolism: increasing the models utility with the simpliRED d-dimer. Thromb Haemost. 2000;83: 416-20.
Wells PS, Anderson DR, Rodger M, et al. Excluding pulmonary embolism at the beside without diagnostic imaging: Management of patients with suspected pulmonary embolism presenting to the emergency department by using a simple clinical model. Ann Int Med. 2000;135: 98-107.
Epstein M. Diagnosis and management of hypertensive emergencies. Clin Cornerstone. 1999; 2(1):41-54.
Elliott WJ. Hypertensive emergencies. Crit Care Clin. 2001; 17(2):435-51.
Dargan P, Wallace C, Jones AL. An evidence based flowchart to guide the management of acute salicylate (aspirin) overdose. Emerg Med J. 2002;19;206-209.
Munro P. Management of eclampsia in the accident and emergency department. Emerg. Med. J. 2000;17;7-11.
Frampton A. Reporting of gunshot wounds by doctors in emergency departments: A duty or a right? Some legal and ethical issues surrounding breaking patient confidentiality. Emerg. Med. J. 2005;22;84-86
Warden C et al. Evaluation and management of febrile seizures in the out-of-hospital and emergency department settings. Ann Emerg Med. 2003;41;215-222
American college of emergency physicians: clinical policy for the initial approach to patients presenting with altered mental status. Ann Emerg Med Feb 1999;33: 251 – 280
Chu, P. Blunt Abdominal Trauma: current concepts. Current Orthopedics 2003;17, 254-259.

ENDOCRINOLOGY

Agus AZ Etiology of hypercalcemia. 2002 Uptodate online version 10.2. www.uptodate.com

Agus AZ. Overview of metabolic bone disease. 2002 Uptodate online version 10.2. www.uptodate.com

American Diabetes Association. (2002). Management of dyslipidemia in adults with diabetes (Position Statement). Diabetes Care 25(S1): S74-77.

Arnold A. Classification and pathogenesis of the multiple endocrine neoplasila syndromes. 2002 Uptodate online version 10.2. www.uptodate.com

Blood glucose control in type 2 DM-UK PDS33 on page E5 reprinted from the Lancet, 352, United Kingdom Prospective Diabetes Study (UKPDS) Group. Intensive blood-glucose control with sulfonylureas or insulin compared with conventional treatment and risk of complications in patients with type 2 diabetes (UKPDS 33). 837-53, 1998. With permission from Elsevier.

Braunwald E, Fauci A, Kasper D, Hauser S, Longo D, Jameson. J, Eds. New York. p. 2109-2135.

Burman KD. Overview of thyroiditis. 2002 Uptodate online version 10.2. www.uptodate.com

Canadian Diabetes Association Clinical Practice Guidelines. Expert Committee. Canadian Diabetes Association 2003. Clinical practice guidelines for the prevention and management of diabetes in Canada. Can J Diabetes. 2003; 27(suppl2).

Canadian Journal of Diabetes. Dec 2003; 27 (S2)

Canadian Task Force on Preventive Health Care. CMAJ. May 25, 2004: 170 (11).

Cheng A et al. Oral antihyperglycemic therapy for type 2 diabetes mellitus. CMAJ. 18 January 2005; 172(2): 213-226.

Cheung, A et al. Prevention of osteoporosis and osteoporotic fractures in post-menopausal womem: recommendation statement from the Canadian Diabetes Association 2003 Clinical Practice Guidelines for the Prevention and Management of Diabetes in Canada.

Cheung, A et al. Prevention of osteoporosis and osteoporotic fractures in post-menopausal women: recommendation statement from the Canadian Task Force on Preventive Health Care. CMAJ. May 25, 2004: 170 (11).

Dayan CM. (2001). Interpretation of thyroid function tests. Lancet 357: 619-624.

Fodor JG et al. 2000). Recommendations for the management and treatment of dyslipidemia. CMAJ 162(10): 1441-1447.

Genest J et al. Recommendations of the management of dyslipidemia and the prevention of cardiovascular disease: 2003 update. CMAJ Oct 28, 203: 169 (9)

Greenspan FS. Garber DG. 2001. Basic and clinical endocrinology. New York: Lange Medical Books/ McGraw Hill. p. 100-163, 201-272, 623-761.

Hirsch IB et al. (1995). Inpatient management of adults with diabetes. Diabetes Care 18(6): 870-878.

Kitabachi AE et al. (2001). Management of hyperglycemic crises in patients with diabetes. Diabetes Care 24 (1): 131-152.

Kronenberg HM, Larsen PR et al. Williams Textbook of Endocrinology. 9th edition. 1998. W.B. Saunders Company

Metlzer S et al. (1998). Clinical practice guidelines for the management of diabetes in Canada. CMAJ 159 (8 suppl).

NIH Consensus Conference. (2001). Osteoporosis prevention, diagnosis, and therapy. JAMA 285:785-795.

Orth DN. Evaluation of the response to ACTH in adrenal insufficiency. 2002 Uptodate online version 10.2. www.uptodate.com

Physician's guide to prevention and treatment of osteoporosis. National Osteoporosis Foundation, 2003.

Powers AC. (2001). Diabetes Mellitus. In Harrisons's Principles of Internal Medicine.

Rosen HN and Rosenblatt M. Overview of the management of osteoporosis in women. 2002 Uptodate online version 10.2. www.uptodate.com

Ross DS. Disorders that cause hypothyroidism. 2002 Uptodate online version 10.2. www.uptodate.com

Ryan EA. (1998). Pregnancy in diabetes. Med Clin of N Amer 82(2): 823-845.

Simvastatin to lower CAD risk – The Heart Protection Study on page E15 reprinted from Lancet, 360, Heart Protection Study Collaborative Group, Heart Protection Study of Cholesterol lowering with Simvastatin in 20,536 high risk individuals: a randomized placebo-controlled trial. 7-22, 2002, with permission from Elsevier.

Statins and CHD in Dyslipidemia – 45 Trial on page E15 reprinted from the Lancet, 344. Randomized trial of cholesterol lowering in 4,444 patients with coronary heart disease: The Scandinavian Simvastatin Survival Study (45):1283-89, 1994, with permission from Elsevier.

Tsui E et al. (2001). Intensive insulin therapy with insulin lispro. Diabetes Care 24(10): 1722-1727.

Young WF and Kaplan NM. Diagnosis and treatment of pheochromocytoma in adults. 2002 Uptodate online version 10.2. www.uptodate.com.

ETHICAL, LEGAL AND ORGANIZATIONAL ASPECTS

Baile WF, Buckman R, Lenzi R, et al. (2000). SPIKES - A six-step protocol for delivering bad news: application to the patient with cancer. Oncologist. 5(4): 302-11.

Baker GR, Norton PG, Flintoft V, Blais R, Brown A, Cox J, Etchells E, Ghali WA, Hebert P, Majumdar SR, O'Beirne M, Palacios-Derflingher L, Reid RJ, Sheps S, Tamblyn R. The Canadian Adverse Events Study: the incidence of adverse events among hospital patients in Canada. CMAJ 2004;170(11):1678-86.

Canadian Institute for Health Information www.cihi.ca

Canadian Medical Association Journal "Bioethics for Clinicians" Series.

Canadian Medical Association www.cma.ca

Canadian Public Health Association and WHO. Ottawa Charter for Health Promotion. Ottawa: Health and Welfare Canada, 1986.

CMA Code of Ethics, Canadian Medical Association www.cma.ca

Centers for Medicare and Medicaid Services www.cms.hhs.gov

College of Physicians and Surgeons of Ontario www.cpso.on.ca

CPSO Policy Statements, College of Physicians and Surgeons of Ontario www.cpso.on.ca/policies/mandatory.htm

Devereaux P.I, Choi PT, Lacchetti C, Weaver B, Schunemann HJ, Haines T, Lavis JN, Grant BJ, Haslam DR, Bhandari M, Sullivan T, Cook DJ, Walter SD, Meade M, Khan H, Bhatnagar N, Guyatt GH. A systematic review and meta-analysis of studies comparing mortality rates of private for-profit and private not-for-profit hospitals. CMAJ 2002;166(11):1399-406.

Devereaux PJ, Heels-Ansdell D, Lacchetti C, Haines T, Burns KE, Cook DJ, Ravindran N, Walter SD, McDonald H, Stone SB, Patel R, Bhandari M, Schunemann HJ, Choi PT, Bayoumi AM, Lavis JN, Sullivan T, Stoddart G, Guyatt GH. Payments for care at private for-profit and private not-for-profit hospitals: a systematic review and meta-analysis. CMAJ 2004;170(12):1817-24.

Etchells E, Sharpe G, Elliott C and Singer PA. Bioethics for clinicians: 3. Capacity. CMAJ 1996,155(6):657-661.

Ferris LE, Barkun H, Carlisle J, Hoffman B, Katz C, and Silverman M. Defining the physician's duty to warn: consensus statement of Ontario's Medical Expert Panel on Duty to Inform. CMAJ 1998;158:1473-1479.

Fisher ES, Wennberg DE, Stukel TA, Gottlieb DJ, Lucas FL, Pinder EL. The implications of regional variations in Medicare spending. Part 1: the content, quality, and accessibility of care. Ann Intern Med 2003;138:273-87.

Fisher ES, Wennberg DE, Stukel TA, Gottlieb DJ, Lucas FL, Pinder EL. The implications of regional variations in Medicare spending. Part 2: health outcomes and satisfaction with care. Ann Intern Med 2003;138:288-98.

Government of Canada: Interagency Advisory Panel on Research Ethics www.pre.ethics.gc.ca/english/index.cfm

Health Care Consent Act, 1996. S.O. 1996, c. 2, Sched. A.

Health Protection and Promotion Act, R.S.O. 1990., c.H.7; O. Re.g. 559/91, amended to O. Re.g. 96/03.

Hebert P. Doing Right: A Practical Guide to Ethics for Physicians and Medical Trainees, Toronto, Oxford University Press; 1996.

Hebert PC, Hoffmaster B, Glass KC, Singer PA. Bioethics for clinicians: 7. Truth telling. CMAJ 1997;156:225-8.

Institute of Medicine. Care Without Coverage: Too Little, Too Late. Washington D.C., The National Academies Press; 2002. Online (www.iom.edu)

Kirby, M. The Kirby Commission: The Health of Canadians – The Federal Role. 2002. Online at the Senate Canada website: http://www.parl.gc.ca/37/2/parlbus/commmbus/senate/Com-e/soci-e/rep-e/repoct02vol6-e.htm

Lewis S, Donaldson C, Mitton C, Currie G. The future of health care in Canada. BMJ 2001;323:926-9.

Medical Council of Canada. Objectives of the considerations of the legal, ethical and organizational aspects of the practice of medicine. 1999. Online at the Medical Council of Canada website (www.mcc.ca)

National Center for Health Statistics, Center for Disease Control and Prevention website (www.cdc.gov/nchs)

Naylor CD. Health care in Canada: incrementalism under fiscal duress. Health Affairs 1999;18:9-26.

OECD. Health Data, 2008. www.oecd.org

Ontario Medical Association www.oma.org

Ontario's Office of the Chief Coroner www.mpss.jus.gov.on.ca

Physician Privacy Toolkit (2004), Ontario Medical Association www.oma.org/phealth/privacymain.htm

Romanow, R. The Romanow Report: Royal Commission on the Future of Health Care in Canada. 2002. Online at the Senate Canada website: http://www.hc-sc.gc.ca/hcs-sss/alt_formats/hpb-dgps/pdf/hhr/romanow-eng.pdf

Shah CP. Public health and preventive medicine in Canada. 5th ed. Toronto: Elsevier Canada; 2003. p 357-360, 426. Reprinted by permission of Elsevier Canada, 2006.
WHO. World Health Report 2005. http://www.who.int/whr/en
Woolhandler S, Campbell T, Himmelstein DU. Costs of Health Care Administration in the United States and Canada. N Engl J Med 2003; 349:768-75.

FAMILY MEDICINE

Abuse
Fogarty CT, Burge S, McCord E. Communicating with patients about intimate partner violence: screening and interviewing approaches. Fam Med 2002; 34(5): 369-75.
National Center on Elder Abuse at the American Public Human Services Association. National Elder Abuse Incidence Study:
http://www.aoa.gov/eldfam/Elder_Rights/Elder_Abuse/AbuseReport_Full.pdf
Wathen CN, MacMillan HL. Interventions for violence against women. JAMA 2003;289(5):589-99.

Diabetes
Canadian Diabetes Association Clinical Practice Guidelines Expert Committee. 2003 Guidelines for the Prevention and Management of Diabetes in Canada. Can J Diabetes 2003;27(Suppl 2).
Nield L et al. Dietary advice for treatment of type 2 diabetes mellitus in adults. Cochrane Database of Systematic Reviews 2007; Issue 3.
Norris SL et al. Long-term non-pharmacological weight loss interventions for adults with pre-diabetes. Cochrane Database of Systematic Reviews 2006; Issue 3.
Saenz A et al. Metformin monotherapy for type 2 diabetes mellitus. Cochrane Database of Systematic Reviews 2005; issue 3.

Diet and Obesity
Calle E, Thun MJ, Petrelli JM, et al. Body-mass index and mortality in a prospective cohort of US adults. N Eng J Med 1999;341(15):1097-1105.
Canada's Food Guide to Healthy Eating. Health Canada. Last updated 2007.
2006 Canadian clinical practice guidelines on the management and prevention of obesity in adults and children [summary]. CMAJ 10-Apr-07; 176(8): S1-S13.
Classification of Overweight and Obesity by BMI, Waist Circumference, and Associated Disease Risks, National Institute of Health, National Heart Lung and Blood Institute, Obesity Education Initiative. http://www.nhlbi.nih.gov/health/public/heart/obesity/lose_wt/bmi_dis.htm.
Dansinger ML et al. 2005. Comparison of the Atkins, Ornish, Weight Watchers, and Zone diets for weight loss and heart disease risk reduction. JAMA, Jan 2005 vol 293(1): 43-53.
Health Canada. Canada's Food Guide to Healthy Eating. Last updated 2005-06-07. http://www.hc-sc.gc.ca/fn-an/food-guide-aliment/fg-rainbow-arc_en_cie_ga_e.html.
Health Canada. Canada's Physical Activity Guide to Healthy Active Living. http://www.hc-sc.gc.ca/hppb/paguide/main.html.
Krauss RM, et al. 2000. AHA Dietary Guidelines. Revision 2000: A statement for healthcare professionals from the nutrition committee of the American Heart Association. Stroke: 31: 2751-66.

Dyslipidemia, Hypertension and Heart Disease
Evidence-Based Recommendations Task Force of the Canadian Hypertension Education Program. 2006 Canadian Recommendations for the Management of Hypertension.
Genest J, Frohlich J, Fodor G. Recommendations for the management of dyslipidemia and the prevention of cardiovascular disease: summary of the 2003 update. CMAJ 2003;169(9):921-924.
McPherson R et al. Canadian Cardiovascular Society position statement – Recommendations for the diagnosis and treatment of dyslipidemia and prevention of cardiovascular disease. Can J Cardiol 2006; 22(11):913-927.
Ontario Drug Therapy Guidelines for Stable Ischemic Heart Disease in Primary Care (2000). Ontario Program for Optimal Therapeutics. Toronto: Queen's Printer of Ontario, pp. 10.
Recommendations for the management of dyslipidemia and the prevention of cardiovascular disease: Summary of the 2003 update. Reprinted from CMAJ 28 October 2003; 169(1): 921-924

Smoking
Health Canada. Canadian Tobacco Use Monitoring Survey (CTUMS). Annual Results 2001. http://www.hc-sc.gc.ca/hecs-sesc/tobacco/research/ctums/2001/summary.html.
Hughes JR et al. Antidepressants for smoking cessation. Cochrane Database of Systematic Reviews 2007; Issue1.
Lancaster T et al. Physician advice for smoking cessation. Cochrane Database of Systematic Reviews 2004; Issue 4.
Shroeder SA. What to do with a patient who smoked. JAMA 2005; 294(4): 482-7.
Silagy C et al. Nicotine replacement therapy for smoking cessation. Cochrane Database of Systematic Reviews 2004; Issue 3.

Other
Bagai A, et al. Does this patient have hearing impairment? JAMA 2006;295:416-428.
Beck E, Sieber WJ, Trejo R. Management of cluster headaches. Am Fam Physician 2005; 71(4): 717-24.
Brown JP, Josse RG. 2002 clinical practice guidelines for the diagnosis and management of osteoporosis in Canada. CMAJ 2002;167:S1-S34.
Burge SK, Schneider FD. Alcohol-related problems: recognition and intervention. Am Fam Phys 1999;59(2):361-70, 372.
Canadian Task Force on Preventive Health Care. The Canadian Guide to Clinical Preventive Health Care. Ottawa: Minister of Supply and Services Canada and http://www.ctfphc.org.
Centor RM et al. (1981). The diagnosis of strep throat in adults in the emergency room. Med Decis Making. 1: 239-46.
Cheung AM, Feig DS, Kapral M, et al. Prevention of osteoporosis and osteoporotic fractures in post-menopausal women: Recommendation statement from the Canadian Task Force on Preventative Health Care. CMAJ 2004;170(11):1665-7.
Comuz J, Guessous I, Farrat B. Fatigue: a practical approach to diagnosis in primary care. CMAJ 2006; 174(6): 765-7.
Ebell MH. Treating adult women with suspected UTI. Am Fam Physician 2006; 73(2): 293-6.
Evans M. Mosby's Family Practice Sourcebook: An Evidence Based Approach to Care, 4th ed., Elsevier Canada, 2006
Evans M, Bradwejn J, Dunn L (Eds). Guidelines for the Treatment of Anxiety Disorders in Primary Care. Toronto: Queen's Printer of Ontario. 2002: 41.
Health Canada. Natural Health Products Directorate 2004. http:// www.hc-sc.gc.ca/hpfb-dgpsa/nhpd-dpsn/.
Holbrook AM (Chair) for Ontario Musculoskeletal Therapy Review Panel. Ontario Treatment Guidelines for Osteoarthritis, Rheumatoid Arthritis, and Acute, Musculoskeletal Injury. Toronto; Queen's Printer of Ontario, 2000:13-24.
Hueston WJ, Mainous AG. Acute bronchitis. Am Fam Phys 1998;57:1270-9.
Hunt P (2001). Motivating Change. Nursing Standard, 16(2): 45-52, 54-55.
Low DE, Desrosiers M, McSherry J et al. A practical guide for the diagnosis and treatment of acute sinusitis. CMAJ 1997;156:1S.
Mclsaac WJ, White D, Tannenbaum D, Low DE (1998). A clinical score to reduce unnecessary antibiotic use in patients with sore throat. CMAJ. 158(1):75-83.
Mosby's Family Practice Sourcebook: An Evidence Based Approach to Care, edited by Dr M. Evans, 4th ed., Elsevier Canada, 2006: 343-345.
Walsh PC et al. Campbell's Urology. 8th ed. Philadelphia: WB Saunders Co, 1998
Zink T, Chaffin J. Herbal "health" products: What family physicians need to know, American Family Physician. 1998. 58(5):1133-1140.

GASTROENTEROLOGY

Atlas
Kandel, G., Division of Gastroenterology, SMH.
Olscamp, G., Division of Gastroenterology.
Saibil, F., Division of Gastroenterology, SWCHSC.
Haber, G., Division of Gastroenterology, Lennox Hall Hospital, New York.

Esophageal and Gastric Disease
Devault, K.R., Castell, D.O.: Guidelines for the diagnoses and treatment of gastroesophageal reflux disease. Arch Intern Med. 115:2165-2173, 1995.
DiPalma JA. Management of severe gastroesophageal reflux disease. Journal of Clinical Gastroenterology. 32(1): 19 –26, 2001.
Wilcox, C.M., Karowe, M.W.: Esophageal infections: etiology, diagnosis, and management. Gastroenterology. 2:188, 1994.

Stomach and Duodenum
American Gastroenterological Association Position statement: Evaluation of dyspepsia. Gastroenterology. 114:579-581, 1998.
Howden, C.W., Hunt,R.H.: Guidelines for the management of Helicobacter Pylori infection. Am J Gastroenterology. 93:2330-2338, 1998.
Hunt RH, Fallone CA, Thomson ABR. (1999). Canadian Helicobacter pylori consensus conference update: infection in adults. J. Gastroenterol, 13: 213-6.
Laine, L., Peterson W.L.: Bleeding peptic ulcer. NEJM. 331:717-727, 1994.
Lanza, F.L.: A guideline fo the treatment and prevention fo NSAID-induced ulcer. Am J Gastroenterology. 93:2037-2046, 1998.
Peek, R.M., Blaser M.J.: Pathophysiology of Helicobacter Pylori-induced gastritis and peptic ulcer disease. Am J Med. 102:200-207, 1997.
Salcedo JA, Al-Kawas F. (1998). Treatment of Helicobacter pylori infection. Arch Intern Med, 158: 842-51.
Schmid CH, Whiting G, Cory D et al. (1999). Omeprazole plus antibiotics in the eradication of Helicobacter pylori infection: a meta-regression analysis of randomized controlled trials. Am J Ther, 6(1): 25-36.
Soll AH. Practice Parameters: committee of the American College of Gastroenterology: Medical treatment of peptic ulcer disease. I. 275: 622, 1996.
Thijs JC, van Zwet AA, Thijs WJ, et al. (1996). Diagnostic tests for Helicobacter pylori: A prospective evaluation of their accuracy, without selecting a single test as the gold standard. Am J Gastroenterology, 91(10): 2125-29.

Small and Large Bowel
Aranda-Michel, J., Giannella, R. Acute Diarrhea: A Practical Review. American Journal of Medicine. 10(6): 670:676, 1999.
Colorectal cancer screening: Recommendation statement from the Canadian Task Force on Preventative Health Care. CMAJ. 165(2): 206-8, 2001.
Donowitz M., Kokke FT., Saidi R. Evaluation of Patients with Chronic Diarrhea. NEJM. 332 (11): 725:729, 1995.
Drossma DA. The Functional Gastrointestinal disorders and the Rome III process. Gastroenterology. 130:1377-1390, 2006.
Forrest JA, Finlayson ND, Shearman DJ. Endoscopy in Gastrointestinal Bleeding. Lancet. 1974(17):394-397.
Ghosh, S., Shand A. Ulcerative Colitis. BMJ. 320 (7242) 1119-1123, 2000.
Hanauer SB. Drug therapy: Inflammatory Bowel Disease. NEJM. 334(13): 841-848, 1996.
Horwitz, BJ., Fisher RS. Current Concepts: The Irritable Bowel Syndrome. NEJM. 344(24): 1846-1850, 2001.
Jennings, JSR., Howdle, PD. Celiac Disease. Current Opinion in Gastroenterology. 17(2): 118:126, 2001.

Liver and Biliary Tract
Angulo P. Primary biliary cirrhosis and primary sclerosing cholangitis. Clinics in Liver Disease. 3(3): 529-70, 1999.
Bockus Gastroenterology. Volume 4 Haubrich, W.S., Schaffner, F, Berk, J.E. 5th Edition W.B. Saunders Company. Chapter 74. Pregnancy-Related Hepatic and Gastointestinal Disorders. Pages: 1448-1458
Cecil Essentials of Medicine. 5th edition. Andreoli, T., Carpenter, C., Griggs, R. and Loscalzo, J. eds. W.B. Saunders Company, Philadelphia, 2001.
Custis K. Common biliary tract disorders. Clin Fam Pract. 2(1): 141-154, 2000.
Diehl AM. Alcoholic liver disease. Clinics in Liver Disease. 2(1): 103-118, 1998.
Gastrointestinal and Liver Disease. Pathophysiology/Diagnosis/Management. Volume 2 Feldman, M., Friedman, L.S. and Sleisenger, M.H. 7th Edition Malik AH. Acute and chronic viral hepatitis. Clin Fam Pract. 2(1): 35-57, 2000.
Reynolds, T. Ascites. Clinics in Liver Disease. 4(1): 151-168, 2000.
Sandowski SA. Cirrhosis. Clin Fam Pract. 2(1): 59-77, Mar 2000.
Saunders. Chapter 184: Pregnancy and the Gastrointestinal Tract. Pages 3446-3452.
Sherman, M. Chronic viral hepatitis and chronic liver disease. The Canadian Journal of Diagnosis. 18(6):81-90, 2001.
Sternlieb I. Wilson's disease. Clinics in Liver Disease. 4(1): 229-239, 2000.
Williams, Simmel. Does this patient have ascites? JAMA. May 20, 1992. Vol 287, No 19.
Yapp TR. Hemochromatosis. Clinics in Liver Disease. 4(1): 211-228, 2000.
Yu AS. Management of ascites. Clinics in Liver Disease. 5(2): 541, 2001.

Pancreas
Beckinham IJ, Borman PC. Acute Pancreatitis. BMJ. 322: 595-598. 2001
Beckinham IJ, Borman PC. Chronic Pancreatitis. BMJ. 322: 595-598. 2001
Steer, M.L. Chronic pancreatitis. NEJM. 332:1482-1490, 1995.
Sternby B et al. What is the best biochemical test to diagnose acute pancreatitis? A prospective clinical study. Mayo Clin Proc. 71: 1138, 1996.
Whytcomb DC. Acute pancreatitis. NEJM. 2142-2150, 2006.

Rational Clinical Examination
Grover SA, Barkun AN, Sackett DL. Does this patient have splenomegaly? JAMA. 270(18): 2218-21, 1993.
Kitchens JM. Does this patient have an alcohol problem? JAMA. 272(22): 1782-1787, 1994.
Naylor CD. Physical exam of the liver. JAMA. 271 (23): 1859:1865, 1994.
Williams JW, Simel DL. Does this patient have ascites? How to divine fluid in the abdomen. JAMA. 267 (19): 2645-48, 1992.
Haber, Greg, MD, FRCP. Division of Gastroenterology. SMH.
Kandel, Gabor,, MD, FRCP. Division of Gastroenterology. SMH.
Oslcamp, G., MD, FRCP. Division of Gastroenterology.
Saibil, Fred, MD, FRCP. Division of Gastroenterology. SWCHSC.
Williams, Simmel. Does this patient have ascites? JAMA. May 20, 1992. Vol 287, No 19.

GENERAL SURGERY

Andreoli TE et al. Cecil Essentials of Medicine. Fifth Edition. W.B. Saunders Co, Philadelphia 2001
Bateson MC. Gallbladder disease. BMJ. 318:1745-8. 1999.
Bazarah BM, Peltekian KM, McAlister VC et al. Utility of MELD and Child-Turcotte-Pugh Scores and the Canadian Waitlisting Algorithm in predicting short-term survival after liver transplant. Clin Invest Med 27(4): 162. 2004
Bland KI et al. The Practice of General Surgery. First Edition. W.B. Saunders Co, Toronto. 2002.
Canadian Task Force on Preventive Health Care. Colorectal cancer screening. CMAJ. 165(2):206-208. 2001
Preoperative antibiotic prophylaxis. CDC website: www.cdc.gov/ncidod/hip/SSI/SSI.pdf
Chandler C et al. Prospective evaluation of early versus delayed laparoscopic cholecystectomy for treatment of acute cholecystitis. Am J Surg. 66(9): 896-900. 2000.
Classen DC et al.; The timing of prophylactic administration of antibiotics and the risk of surgical-wound infection. NEJM. 326(5):281-6. 1992.
De Groen PC et al. Biliary tract cancers. NEJM. 341(18):1368-1378. 1999.
Doherty GM. Current Surgical Diagnosis and Treatment, 12th ed. McGraw-Hill, New York, 2006.
Edell SL and Eisen MD. Current imaging modalities for the diagnosis of breast cancer. Delaware Med J. 71:377-82. 1999
Ferzoco LB et al. Acute diverticulitis. NEJM. 338(21):1521-26. 1998.
Goldhirsh A et al. Meeting Highlights: International Consensus Panel on the Treatment of Primary Breast Cancer. J Clin Oncol, 19(18):3817-27, 2001.
Graham DJ and McHenry CR. The adrenal incidentaloma: guidelines for evaluation and recommendations for management. Surg Onc Clin North Am.7(4):749. 1998.
Harken AH and Moore EE. Abernathy's Surgical Secrets. Hanley and Belfus, Inc. Philadelphia, 2000
Hartmann LC et al. Efficacy of bilateral prophylactic mastectomy in women with a family history of breast cancer. NEJM. 340(2): 77-84. 1999.
Hong Z, Wu J, Smart G, Kaita K, Wen SW, Paton S, Dawood M. Survival analysis of liver transplant patients in Canada 1997-2002. Transplant Proc. 38(9):2951-6. 2006.
Hortobagyi GN. Treatment of breast cancer. NEJM. 339(14):974-984. 1998
Ivanovich JL et al. A practical approach to familial and hereditary colorectal cancer. Am J Med. 107(1):68-77. 1999.
Janne PA et al. Chemoprevention of colorectal cancer. NEJM. 342(26):1960-1968. 2000.
Johnson CD. Upper abdominal pain: Gallbladder. BMJ. 323:1170-3. 2001.
Kanwal F, Dulai GS, Spiegel BMR et al. A comparison of liver transplantation outcomes in the pre- vs. post-MELD eras. Aliment Pharmacol Ther. 21: 169-177. 2005.
Kasper, Dennis L. Harrison's Principles of Internal Medicine. 16th ed. 2005.
Kehlet H et al. Review of postoperative ileus. Am J Surg. 182(Suppl):3S-10S. 2001.
King JE et al. Care of patients and their families with familial adenomatous polyposis. Mayo Clin Proc. 75(1):57-67. 2000
Kosters JP, Gotzsche PC. Regular self-examination or physical examination for early detection of breast cancer. Cochrane Library. 2, 2002.
Latif A. Gastric Cancer Update on Diagnosis, Staging and Therapy. Postgraduate Medicine. 1997:102(4):231-6.
Lawrence PF. Essentials of General Surgery. Lippincott Williams & Wilkins, Philadelphia, 2000.
Levine CD. Toxic megacolon: diagnosis and treatment challenges. AACN Clinical Issues. 10(4):492-99. 1999
Li CI, Anderson BO, Daling JR, Moe RE. Trends in Incidence Rates of Invasive Lobular and Ductal Breast Carcinoma. JAMA. 289(11): 1421-24. 2003.
Madan AK et al. How early is early laparoscopic treatment of acute cholecystitis? Am J Surg. 183:232-236. 2002
Mandel JS, Bond JH, Church TR, et al.. Reducing Mortality from Colorectal Cancer by Screening for Fecal Occult Blood. Minnesota Colon Cancer Control Study. NEJM, 328(19):1365-71. 1993.
Mandel JS, Church TR, Bond JH, et al.. The Effect of Fecal Occult Blood Screening on the Incidence of Colorectal Cancer. NEJM, 343:1603-7). 2000
Martin RF, Rossi RL. The Acute Abdomen: An Overview and Algorithms. Surg Clin North Am. 1997:77(6):1227-43.
McDonnell SK. Efficacy of contralateral prophylactic mastectomy in women with a personal and family history of breast cancer. J Clin Oncol. 19(19):38-43, 2001.
Olivotto I, Levine M. Clinical practice guidelines for the care and treatment of breast cancer: The management of ductal carcinoma in situ (summary of the 2001 update). CMAJ 165(7):912-913, 2001.
Olsen O, Gøtzsche PC. Screening for breast cancer with mammography (Cochrane review) In: the Cochrane Library, Issue 3, 2003. Oxford: Update Software.
Paulsan, EK et al. Suspected appendicitis. NEMJ. 348(3): 236-42. 2003 Jan 16.
Paulson EK, Kalady MF, Pappas TN. Suspected Appendicitis. NEJM. 2003. Jan 16; 348(3):236-42.
Polk H, Christmas B. Prophylactic antibiotics in surgery and surgical wound infections. Am Surgeon, 66(2): 105-111. 2000
Ransohoff DF and Sandler RS. Screening for colorectal cancer. NEJM. 346(1):40-44. 2002
Ringash J. Preventive health care, 2001 update: screening mammography among women aged 40-49 years at average risk of breast cancer. CMAJ. 164(4):469-76, 2001.
Ross NS and Aron DC. Hormonal evaluation of the patient with an incidentally discovered adrenal mass. NEJM. 323:1401. 1990.
Roy MA. Inflammatory bowel disease. Surg Clin North Am. 77(6):1419-1431. 1997
Rubin BP, Heinrich MC, Corless CL. Gastrointestinal Stromal Tumour. Lancet. 2007. May 19; 369(9574):1731-41.
Rustgi AK. Hereditary gastrointestinal polyposis and nonpolyposis syndromes. NEJM. 331(25):1694-1702. 1994.
Saini S. Imaging of the hepatobiliary tract. NEJM. 336(26):1889-1894. 1997.
Sheth SG and LaMont JT. Toxic megacolon. Lancet. 351: 509-513. 1998.
Styblo TM, Wood WC. The management of ductal and lobular breast cancer. Surgical Oncology. 8(2): 67-75. 1999.
The University of Cincinnati Residents. The Mont Reid Surgical Handbook. Mosby Inc., St. Louis, 1997.
Waki, K. UNOS Liver Registry: ten year survivals. HYPERLINK "javascript:AL_get(this,%20'jour',%20'Clin%20Transpl.');" Clin Transpl. 2006:29-39.
Way, LW. Current Surgical Diagnosis and Treatment. 11th ed. 2003.

GERIATRIC MEDICINE

Health Status
Heron M. Deaths: Leading Causes for 2004. Health E-Stats. Released Nov 20, 2007.
Hoyert DL, Heron M, Murphy SL, Kung HC. Deaths: final data for 2003. Health E-stats. Released January 19, 2006.
Statistics Canada. The leading causes of death at different ages, Canada. Ottawa: 2000.

Physiology and Pathology of Aging
Braunwald, E. Fauci, AS. Hauser, SL. Longo, DL. Jameson, JL. (Eds). Harrison's Priniciples of Internal Medicine. New York: McGraw-Hill, 2004.

Elder Abuse
Health Canada. The Canadian Guide to Clinical Perventative Health Care. Ottawa: Canadian Task Force on Preventative Health Care. 2002
Kergoat, MJ. (2000) Preventative Health Care in the Elderly. The Canadian Journal of CME. August 2000.
Lachs MS, Pillemer K (1995). Abuse and neglect of elderly persons. N Engl J Med, 332(7):437-443.
Lachs M, Pillemer K. (2004). Elder Abuse. Lancet. 1192-1263.
Periodic health examination, 1994 update: 4. secondary prevention of elder abuse and mistreatment. CMAJ, 151(10):1413-1420.
Schmorler KE (ed). UpToDate. Sokol HN. 2008.
Sillman JS. Elder abuse. UpToDate.

Failure to Thrive
Robertson RG, Montagnini M. (2004). "Geriatric failure to thrive." Am Fam Phys 70(2): 343-348.
Sarkersian CA, Laches MS (1996). Failure to thrive in older adults. Ann Intern Med. 124: 1072-1078.
Verdery RB. (1997) "Clinical evaluation of failure to thrive in older people." Clin Geriatr Med 13:769-78.

Falls
Close J, Ellis M, Hooper R, Glucksman E, Jackson S, Swift C. (1999). Prevention of falls in the elderly trial (PROFET): a randomized controlled trial. Lancet. 353(9147): 93-7.
Fuller, George (2001) "Falls in the elderly." Am Fam Phys 61(7): 2159-2172.

Ganz, DA, Bao Y, Shekelle PE, Rubenstein LZ. (2007). Will my patient fall? JAMA. 297: 77-86.
Gillespie LD, Gillespie WJ, Robertson MC, et al. Interventions for preventing falls in elderly people (Cochrane Review). In: The Cochrane Library, Issue 2, 2002.
Gillespie LD, Gillespie WJ, Robertson MC, Lamb SE, Cumming RG, Rowe BH. Interventions for preventing falls in elderly people. The Cochrane Database of Systematic Reviews 2003, Issue 4.
Goldlist B, Turpic I, Borins M. (1997) Essential Geriatrics: Managing 6 conditions: Patient Care Canada. 8(9): 61-74.
Hartikainen S, Lönnroos E, Louhivuori K (2007). Medication as a risk factor for falls: critical systematic review. J Gerontol A Biol Sci. 62(10): 1172-81.
Kiel, DP. Overview of falls in the elderly. UpToDate. Rose, BD (Ed). UpToDate. Wellesly, MA. 2005.
Tinetti ME, Baker DI, McAvay G, et al. (1994). A multifactorial intervention to reduce the risk of falling among elderly people living in the community. N Engl J Med, 331(13):821-827.

Gait Disorders
Sudarsky L (1990). Geriatrics: gait disorders in the elderly. N Engl J Med. 322(20):1441-1446.

Hazards of Hospitalization
Creditor MC (1993). Hazards of Hospitalization of the Elderly. Ann Intern Med. 118(3): 219-223.
Inouye AK, Bogardus ST, Charpentier PA, et al. (1999). A multi-component intervention to prevent delirium in hospitalized older patients. N Engl J Med, 340(9):669-676.
Sager MA, Franke T, Inouye SK, et al. (1996). Functional outcomes of acute medical illness and hospitalization in older persons. Arch Internal Med, 156(6):645-52.

Hypertension
ALLHAT officers and coordinators for the ALLHAT collaborative research group. The antihypertensive and lipid-lowering treatment to prevent heart attack trial. Major outcomes in high-risk hypertensive patients randomized to angiotensin-converting enzyme inhibitor or calcium channel blocker vs diuretic: The Antihypertensive and Lipid-Lowering Treatment to Prevent Heart Attack Trial (ALLHAT). JAMA. 2002 Dec 18;288(23):2981-97.
Appel, LJ. Espeland, MA. Easter, L. Wilson, AC. Folmar, S. Lacy, CR. (2001) Effects of reduced sodium intake on hypertension control in older individuals: results from the Trial of Nonpharmacologic Interventions in the Elderly (TONE). Arch Intern Med. 2001 Mar 12;161(5):685-93.
Beckett NS et al. (2008). Treatment of hypertension in patients 80 years of age or older. N Engl J Med. 358(18):1887-98.
Folmar KC, S. Cutler, JA. (1998). Sodium reduction and weight loss in the treatment of hypertension in older persons: a randomized controlled trial of nonpharmacologic interventions in the elderly (TONE). JAMA. 1998 Mar 18;279(11):839-46.
Heyneman A, Beele H, Vanderwee K, Defloor T. (2008). A systematic review of the use of hydrocolloids in the treatment of pressure ulcers. J Clin Nurs. 17(9):1164-73.
Kannel, WB. (1996) Blood pressure as a cardiovascular risk factor: prevention and treatment. JAMA. 1996 May 22-29;275(20):1571-6.
Kaplan, NM. Rose, BD. Treatment of hypertension in the elderly. UpToDate. Rose, BD (Ed). UpToDate. Wellesly, MA. 2005.
Mulrow C, Lau J, Cornell J, Brand M. Pharmacotherapy for hypertension in the elderly (Cochrane Review). In: The Cochrane Library, Issue 2, 2002.
Staessen JA et al. (1998). Calcium channel blockade and cardiovascular prognosis in the European trial on isolated hypertension. Hypertension. 32(3): 410-6.
Whelton, PK. Appel, LJ. Espeland, MA. Applegate, WB. Ettinger, WH Jr. Kostis, JB. Kumanyika, S. Lacy, CR. Johnson,
Canadian Hypertension Recommendations Working Group (2002). The 2001 Canadian hypertension recommendations. Perspectives in Cardiology. 38-46.

Immunizations
Rivetti D et al. (2006). Vaccines for preventing influenza in the elderly. Cochrane Database Syst Rev. 19;3:CD004876

Malnutrition
Halsted, CH. Malnutrition and nutritional assessment. Pp. 411-415. Harrison's Principles of Internal Medicine. 16th edition. Kasper, DL.

Pressure Ulcers
Berlowitz, D. Pressure ulcers: staging; epidemiology; pathogenesis; clinical manifestations. UpToDate. Rose, BD (Ed). UpToDate. Wellesly, MA. 2005.

Driving Competency
AMA. Physicians Guide to Assessing and Counseling Older Drivers. National Highway Traffic Safety Administration. 2006.
CMA. Determining Medical Fitness to Drive: A Guide for Physicians. Ottawa. 2006.
Grabowski DC, Campbell CM, Morrisey MA (2004). Elderly Licensure Laws and Motor Vehicle Fatalities. JAMA. 291(3): 2840-2846.
Hogan DB. (2007). Systematic review of driving risk and the efficacy of compensatory strategies in persons with dementia. J Am Geriatr Soc. 55:878-84.

Palliative and End of Life Care
AGS Panel on Persistent Pain in Older Persons (2002). The management of persistent pain in older persons. J Am Geriatr Soc. 50(6): Supplement.
Knowles, S. (1993). Symptom management in palliative care. On Continuing Practice. 20(1): 20-25.

Geriatric Pharmacology
Beers MH (1997). Explicit criteria for determining potentially inappropriate medication use by the elderly. Arch Intern Med, 157:1531-1536.
Carlson JE (1996). Perils of polypharmacy: 10 steps to prudent prescribing. Geriatrics, 51(7):26-35.
Fick DM, Cooper JW, Wade WE, Waller JL, Maclean R, Beers MH (2003). Updating the Beers Criteria for potentially inappropriate medication use in older adults. Arch Intern Med, 163: 2716-2724.
Fordyce, M. Geriatric Pearls. Philadelphia: FA Davis Company, 1999.
Lewis, T. (2004) Using the NO TEARS tool for medication review. BMJ. 329(7463):434

GYNECOLOGY

Books/Manuals

American Psychiatric Association. Diagnostic and Statistical Manual of Mental Disorders-Fourth Edition, Text Revision. Washington, DC. American Psychiatric Publishing Inc., 2000.
Dickey R. Managing Contraceptive Pill Patients 9th edition. EMIS Inc. Medical Publishers., USA 1998.
Cunningham FG, McDonald PC, and Gant NF (eds.), Williams Obstetrics, 14th ed, Appleton and Lange, 1993.
Hacker NF and Moore JG (eds), Essentials of Obstetrics and Gynecology. 2nd ed. N.F. Hacker and J.G. Moore (eds). W.B. Saunders Co., 1992.

Guidelines

ACOG Practice Bulletin – Clinical Management Guidelines for Obstetrician-Gynecologists. Premenstrual Syndrome. Number 15, April 2000.
Centers for Disease Control and Prevention. 2002 STD Treatment Guidelines: New Recommendations. http://www.cdc.gov/std/treatment/2002TreatmentSlides/2002STDTreatGuide
Davis V and Dunn S. Emergency Postcoital Contraception. SOGC Clinical Practice Guidelines. No. 82 July 2000.
National guideline for the treatment of bacterial vaginosis. Clinical Effectiveness Group (Association of Genitourinary Medicine and the Medical Society for the Study of Venereal Diseases). Sex Transm Infect. 1999; 75 Suppl 1: S1 6-8.
Ontario Cervical Screening Practice Guidelines. June 2005. http://www.cancercare.on.ca/index – cervical screening.htm
Paley PJ. Screening for the major malignancies affecting women: current guidelines. Am J Obstet Gynecol 2001;184(5): 1021-30.
SOGC News Release. New recommendations from national ob/gyn society address Depo-Provera, bone loss. May 2006. http://www.sogc.org/media/pdf/advisories/dmpa-may2006_e.pdf.

Journal Articles

Anderson, GL, Limacher, M, et al. (WHI Steering Committee). Effects of Conjugated Equine Estrogen in Postmenopausal Women with Hysterectomy – The Women's Health Initiative Randomized Controlled Trial. JAMA 2004; 291(14): 1701-1712.
Canadian Consensus Conference on Menopause, 2006 Update. JOGC 2006;171.
Davey E, Barratt A, Irwig L et al. Effect of study design and quality of unsatisfactory rates, cytology classifications, and accuracy in liquid-based versus conventional cervical cytology: a system-

atic review. Lancet 2006; 367: 122-32.

Espeland, MA, Rapp SR, Shumaker SA, et al. Conjugated Equine Estrogens and Global Cognitive Function in Postmenopausal Women – Women's Health Initiative Memory Study. JAMA 2004; 291(24): 2959-2968.

Hulley S, Grady D, Bush T, et al. Randomized trial of estrogen plus progestin for secondary prevention of coronary heart disease in postmenopausal women. JAMA 1998;280:605-613.

Lipscomb GH, McCord ML, Stovall TG et al. Predictors of success of methotrexate treatment in women with tubal ectopic pregnancies. NEJM 2001; 341: 1974-1978.

Luciano AA, Solima RG. Ectopic Pregnancy: From Surgical Emergency to Medical Management. Ann NY Acad Sci 2001; 943: 235-254.

Manson JE, Martin KA. Postmenopausal hormone replacement therapy. NEJM 2001;345(1):34-40.

Marchbanks PA, Aneger JF, Coulman CB, et al. Risk factors for ectopic pregnancy: a population based study. JAMA 1998; 259: 1823-1827.

Martin JL, Williams KS, Abrams KR, et al. Systematic review and evaluation of methods of assessing urinary incontinence. Health Technol Assess 2006;10(6):1-132, iii-iv.

Rambout L, Hopkins L, Fung Kee Fung M, et al. Prophylactic vaccination against human papillomavirus infection in women: a systematic review of randomized controlled trials. CMAJ 2007;177.

Ratner S and Ofri D. Menopause and hormone replacement therapy. West J Med 2001;175:32-34.

Shapter AP. Gestational trophoblastic disease. Obs Gynecol Clin North Am 2001; 28(4): 805-17.

Shumaker SA, Legault C, Kuller L, et al. Conjugated Equine Estrogens and Incidence of Probable Dementia and Mild Cognitive Impairment in Postmenopausal Women – Women's Health Initiative Memory Study. JAMA 2004; 291(24): 2947-2958.

Wooltorton, E. The Evra (ethanyl estradiol/norelgestromin) Contraceptive patch: estrogen exposure concerns. CMAJ 2006; 174(2): 164-165.

Wooltorton E. Medroxyprogesterone acetate (Depo-Provera) and bone mineral density loss. JAMA 2005; 172 (6): 746.

Women's Health Coordinating Council. Clinician Information Sheet: HPV Vaccine for Cervical Cancer Prevention. Massachusetts General Hospital. August 21, 2006.

Websites

Management of Uterine Fibroids. Summary, Evidence Report/Technology Assessment: Number 34. AHRQ Publication No. 01-E051, January 2001.

Agency for Healthcare Research and Quality, Rockville, MD. http://www.ahrq.gov/clinic/utersumm.htm

Sexuality and U. Society of Obstetricians and Gynaecologists of Canada. http://www.sexualityandu.ca

Women's Health Matters. Sexual Health Centre: Birth Control. http://www.womenshealthmatters.ca/centres/sex/birthcontrol/mirena.html

HEMATOLOGY

Armitage JO. Treatment of Non-Hodgkin's lymphoma. NEJM. 1993;328:1023-1030.

Bataiile R, Harousseua J. Multiple myeloma. NEJM. 1997;336:1657-64.

Bates SM and Ginsberg JS. Treatment of deep-vein thrombosis. NEJM, 2004;351:268-277.

Bazemore AW, Smucker DR. Lymphadenopathy and Malignancy. American Family Physician. 2002:66;2103-2110.

Bottomley SS. Causes of the hereditary and acquired sideroblastic anemias. In: UpToDate, Rose, BD (Ed). UpToDate, Waltham, MA 2006.

Callum JL, Pinkerton PH. Bloody Easy: Blood Transfusions, Blood Alternatives and Transfusion Reactions. Sunnybrook and Women's College Health Sciences Centre: Toronto, 2003.

Canadian Pediatric Society. Transfusion and risk of infection in Canada: Update 2006. Pediatrics and Child Health. 2005;11(3):158-162.

Castellone DD. Evaluation of Bleeding Disorders. In Saunders Manual of Clinical Laboratory Science. Craig Lehman ED. WB Saunders CO, Philadelphia, PA, 1998.

Christiansen SC, et al. Thrombophilia, Clinical Factors, and Recurrent Thrombotic Events. JAMA. 2005; 293 (18):2353-2361.

Cines DB and Blanchette VS. Immune Thrombocytopenic Purpura. NEJM. 2002;346:995-1008.

Coates TD and Baehner RL. Causes of neutrophilia. In: UpToDate, Rose, BD (Ed), UpToDate, Waltham, MA 2006.

Cohen K, Scadden D.T. Non-Hodgkin's lymphoma: pathogenesis, clinical presentation, and treatment. Cancer Treat Res. 2001;104:201-203.

Decousus et al. A clinical trial of vena caval filters in the prevention of pulmonary embolism in patients with proximal deep-vein thrombosis. NEJM. 1998; 338: 409-415.

Driscoll MC. Sickle Cell Disease. Pediatrics in Review. 28:7 259 - 286

Geerts WH, Pineo GF, Heit JA, et al. Prevention of venous thromboembolism. Seventh ACCP conference on antithrombotic and thrombolytic therapy. Chest. 2004; 126L 3385-4005.

George JN. Treatment and prognosis of idiopathic thrombocytopenic purpura. In: UpToDate, Rose, BD (Ed), UpToDate, Waltham, MA 2005.

Goldman J. ABC of clinical haematology: Chronic myeloid leukaemia. BMJ. 1997; 314:657.

Habermann TM, Steensma DP. Lymphadenopathy. Mayo Clinic Proc, 2000: 75(7);723-732.

Hasenclever D, Diehl V, et al. A prognostic score for advanced Hodgkin's disease. International Prognostic Factors Project on Advanced Hodgkin's Disease. NEJM. 1998; 339:1506-14.

Health Canada. Effects of Lead on Human Health. http://www.hc-sc.gc.ca/hl-vs/iyh-vsv/environ/lead-plomb-eng.php

Heaney M.L., Golde D.W. Myelodysplasia. NEJM. 1999; 340:1649-60.

http://cancernet.nci.nih.gov

Kovacs MJ et al. Comparison of 10-mg and 5-mg warfarin initiation monograms together with low-molecular-weight heparin for out patient treatment of acute venous thromboembolism. Ann Intern Med, 2003; 138: 714-719.

Kyle RA and Rajkumar SV. Chemotherapy in multiple myeloma. In: UpToDate, Rose, BD (Ed), UpToDate, Waltham, MA 2006.

Kyle RA and Rajkumar SV. Clinical manifestations and diagnosis of Waldenstrom's macroglobulinemia. In: UpToDate, Rose, BD (Ed), UpToDate, Waltham, MA 2006.

Landaw, SA. Approach to the adult patient with thrombocytopenia. In: Up To Date, Rose, BD (Ed), Up To date, Waltham, MA 2005.

Leonardi-Bee J, Bath PM, Bousser MG, et al. Review: Dipyridamole given with or without aspirin reduces recurrent stroke. In ACP Journal Club. July/Aug 2005; 143 (1):10.

Liesner RJ and Machin SJ. ABC of clinical haematology: Platelet disorders. BMJ. 1997;314:809.

Liesner RJ and Goldstone AH. ABC of clinical haematology: The acute leukaemias. BMJ. 1997;314:733.

Lowenberg B. Downing JR, Burnett A. Acute myeloid leukemia. 1999. NEJM. 341:1051-62.

Mackie IJ, and Bull HA. Normal haemostasis and it regulation. Blood Rev. 1989;3:237.

Markovic M, et al. Usefulness of soluble transferrin receptor and ferritin in irron deficiency and chronic disease. Scan J Clin Lab Invest. 2005; 65:571-576.

Mead GM. ABC of clinical haematology: Malignant lymphomas and chronic lymphocytic leukaemia. BMJ. 1997;314:1103.

Messinezy M and Pearson TC. ABC of clinical haematology: Polycythaemia, primary (essential) thrombocythaemia and myelofibrosis. BMJ. 1997; 314: 587.

Mechanisms of severe transfusion reactions. Transfus Clin Biol. 2001;8:278-81.

Pangalis GA, Vassilakopoulos TP, Boussiotis VA, Fessas P. Semin Oncol 1993; 20:570

Pillot G, Chantler M, Magiera H, et al [Eds]. The Washington Manual Hematology and Oncology Subspecialty Consult. Lipincott Williams and Wilkins, Philadelphia PA, 2004.

Pui C., Evans W.E. Acute lymphoblastic leukemia. NEJM. 1998;339:605-15.

Rozman C., Montserrat E. Chronic lymphocytic leukemia. NEJM. 1995;333:1052-57.

Sabatine MS (Ed). Hematology-Oncology. In Pocket Medicine, 2nd edition: The Massachusetts General Hospital Handbook of Internal Medicine. Lippincott Williams and Wilkins: Philadelphia PA, 2004.

Satake N and Sakamoto K. Acute Lymphoblastic Leukemia. E-medicine 2006 accessed at: http://www.emedicine.com/ped/topic2587.html

Sawyers C. Chronic myeloid leukemia. NEJM. 1999;340:1330-40.

Streiff MB, Smith B, Spivak JL. "The diagnosis and management of polycythemia vera in the era since the Polycythemia Vera Study Group: a survey of American Society of Hematology members' practice patterns". Blood 99 (4): 1144–9.

Tefferi A. Approach to the patient with thrombocytosis. In: UpToDate, Rose, BD (Ed), UpToDate, Waltham, MA 2005.

The Merck Manual; Section 11, Chapter 133: platelet disorders.

Thomas RH. Hypercoagulability syndromes. Arch Intern Med. 2001;161:2433-2439.

U.S. Consumer Product Safety Commission. Ban of Lead-Containing Paint and Certain Consumer Products Bearing Lead-Containing Paint. http://www.cpsc.gov/BUSINFO/regsumleadpaint.pdf

Valentine KA and Hull RD. Clinical use of warfarin. In: UpToDate, Ros,e BD (Ed), UpToDate, Waltham, MA 2006.

Valentine KA and Hull RD. Clinical use of heparin and low molecular weight heparin. UpToDate, Rose BD (Ed), UpToDate, Waltham MA 2006.

Wells PS, et al. Evaluation of D-dimer in the diagnosis of suspected deep-vein thrombosis. NEJM 2003;349:1227-1235.

Wilson SE, Watson HG, Crowther MA. Low-dose oral vitamin K therapy for the management of asymptomatic patients with elevated international normalized ratios: a brief review. CMAJ. 2004;170:821-4.

INFECTIOUS DISEASES

Principles of Microbiology

Andreoli TE. Cecil Essentials of Medicine. 6th edition. W.B. Saunders Company; 2003.
Hawley, LB. High Yield Microbiology and Infectious Diseases. Lippincott Williams & Wilkins; 2000.
Mandell, GL. Mandell, Douglas, and Bennett's Principles and Practice of Infectious Disease. 6th Edition. Churchill Livingstone 2005.
Levinson, Warren and Ernest Jawetz. Medical Microbiology & Immunology: Examination and Board Review. 7th Edition. McGraw Hill 2003.
McGraw Hill. Harrison's Online. Website: HYPERLINK "http://www.harrisonsonline.com" http://www.harrisonsonline.com
Schaechter M, Engleberg N, Eisenstein B, Medoff G. Mechanisms of Microbial Disease. Lippincott Williams & Wilkins; 1998.

Neurological Infections

Peterson LR, et al. West Nile Virus. JAMA. 2003. 290(4): 524-527.
Roberts L. Mosquitos and Disease. Science. 2002. 298(5591): 82-3.

Respiratory Infections

Mandell LA, Wunderink RG, Anzueto A, et al. Infectious Diseases Society of America / American Thoracic Society Consensus Guidelines on the Management of Community-Acquired Pneumonia in Adults. CID 2007, 44(Suppl 2): S27-S72.

Cardiac Infections

Wilson W et a.l. Prevention of Infective Endocarditis. Guidelines from the American Heart Association. Circulation 2007 Apr 19; [Epub ahead of print].

Gastrointestinal Infections

American Academy of Pediatrics. Pickering LK, Baker CJ, Long SS, McMillan JA, eds. Red Book: 2006 Report of the Committee on Infectious Diseases. 27th ed. Elk Grove Village, IL: American Academy of Pediatrics; 2006.

Bone and Joint Infections

Hellman, D.B., and Imboden, J.B. Arthritis and Musculoskeletal disorders. In: Current Medical Diagnosis & Treatment. 2008. Edited by McPhee, S.J., Papadakis, M.A., and Tierney, L.M. The McGraw-Hill Companies, Inc.
Gilbert, DN, Moellering, RC, Eliopoulos, GM, and Sande, MA. The Sandford Guide to Antimicrobial Therapy 2008, 38th ed.
Margaretten ME, Kohlwes J, Moore D, and Bent S. Does this adult patient have septic arthritis? JAMA. 2007;297:1478-1488.

Systemic Infections

Alejandria MM, Lansang MA, Dans LF, Mantaring JBV. Intravenous immunoglobulin for treating sepsis and septic shock (Cochrane Review). In: The Cochrane Library, Issue 2, 2002. Oxford: Update Software.
American College of Chest Physicians/Society of Critical Care Medicine Consensus Conference: definitions for sepsis and organ failure and guidelines for the use of innovative therapies in sepsis. SO - Crit Care Med 1992 Jun;20(6):864-74.
Bernard GR, Vincent JL, LaTerre PF, LaRosa SP, Dhainaut JF, Lopez-Rodriguez A, et al. Efficacy and safety of recombinant human activated protein C for severe sepsis. N Eng J Med 2001;344:699-709.
Fourrier F, Chopin C, Gouemand J, et al. Septic shock, multiple organ failure, and disseminated intravascular coagulation: compared patterns of antithrombin III, protein C and protein S deficiencies. Chest 1992;101:816-23.
Smieja MJ, Marchetti CA, Cook DJ, Smaill FM (2002). Isoniazid for preventing tuberculosis in non-HIV infected persons (Cochrane Review). In: The Cochrane Library, Issue 2. Oxford: Update Software.
Steere AC. Lyme disease. New England Journal of Medicine. 2001. July 12; 345(2):115-25.
Targeted Tuberculin Testing and Treatment of Latent Tuberculosis Infection Am J Respir Crit Care Med, Vol 161 pp.S221-S247, 2000
Tuberculosis: selected series. Mechanisms of microbial disease. CMAJ. 1999. 160.

HIV and AIDS

2006 Guidelines for the Use of Antiretroviral Agents in HIV-1-Infected Adults and Adolescents. Available at: HYPERLINK "http://aidsinfo.nih.gov/ContentFiles/AdultandAdolescentsGL.pdf" http://aidsinfo.nih.gov/ContentFiles/AdultandAdolescentsGL.pdf
Guidelines for Preventing Opportunistic Infections Among HIV-Infected Persons – 2002. Recommendations of the U.S. Public Health Service and the Infectious Diseases Society of America. Available at: HYPERLINK "http://aidsinfo.nih.gov/ContentFiles/OlpreventionGL.pdf" http://aidsinfo.nih.gov/ContentFiles/OlpreventionGL.pdf
Hammer SM, Saag MS, Schecheter et al. Treatment for adult HIV Infection: 2006 recommendations of the International AIDS Society - USA Panel. JAMA 2006: 296(7): 827-43.
Moylett EH and Shearer WT. HIV: clinical manifestations. J Allergy Clin Immunol 2002:110;3-16.
Public Health Agency of Canada. HIV and AIDS in Canada. Selected Surveillance Tables to June 30, 2007. Surveillance and Risk Assessment Division, Centre for Infectious Disease Prevention and Control, Public Health Agency of Canada, 2007. (HYPERLINK "http://www.phac-aspc.gc.ca/aids-sida/publication/index.html" \l "surveillance" http://www.phac-aspc.gc.ca/aids-sida/publication/index.html#surveillance)
WHO. WHO AIDS Epidemic Update 2007. HYPERLINK "http://data.unaids.org/pub/EPISlides/2007/2007_epiupdate_en.pdf" http://data.unaids.org/pub/EPISlides/2007/2007_epiupdate_en.pdf
Wilkinson D (2002). Drugs for preventing tuberculosis in HIV infected persons (Cochrane Review). In: The Cochrane Library, Issue 2. Oxford: Update Software.

Parasitic Infections

Center for Disease Control & Prevention. DPDX: Identification and Diagnosis of Parasites of Public Health Concern.
Website: HYPERLINK "http://www.dpd.cdc.gov/dpdx/Default.htm" http://www.dpd.cdc.gov/dpdx/Default.htm

Infections in the Immunocompromised Host

Hughes, Armstrong, Bodey, Bou, Brown, Caladra et al. 2002. Guidelines for the Use of Antimicrobial Agents in Neutropenic Patients with Cancer. CID 2002: 34: 731-757.

Fever of Unknown Origin

Kncokaert DC, et a.l. Fever of Unknown Origin in adults: 40 years on. Journal of Internal Medicine. 2003. 253: 263-275.
Spira AM. Assessment of traveller's who return home ill. Lancet. 2003; 361(9367): 1459-69.

MRSA

American Academy of Pediatrics. Staphylococcal Infections. In: Pickering LK, Baker CJ, Long SS, McMillan JA, eds. Red Book: 2006 Report of the Committee on Infectious Diseases. 27th ed. Elk Grove Village, IL: American Academy of Pediatrics; 2006.
Simor AE, Ofner-Agostini M, Gravel D, Varia M, Paton S, McGeer A, Bryce E, Loeb M, Mulvey M, Canadian Nosocomial Infection Surveillance Program (CNISP). Surveillance for Methicillin-Resistant Staphylococcus aureus in Canadian Hospitals – A Report Update from the Canadian Nosocomial Infection Surveillance Program. CCDR 2005; 31(3):1-7.
Simor AE, Phillips E, McGeer A, Konvalinka A, Loeb M, Devlin HR, Kiss A. Randomized controlled trial of chlorhexidine gluconate for washing, intranasal mupirocin, and rifampin and doxycycline versus no treatment for the eradication of methicillin-resistant Staphylococcus aureus colonization. Clin Infect Dis. 2007 Jan 15;44(2):178-85.

Antimicrobials

e-CPS. Canadian Pharmacists Association. 2008. Available: HYPERLINK "http://e-cps.pharmacists.ca" http://e-cps.pharmacists.ca
MD consult drugs online website: HYPERLINK "http://home.mdconsult.com/das/drugs/" http://home.mdconsult.com/das/drugs/
Schlossberg, D, Ed. Current Therapy of Infectious Disease. 2nd Edition. Mosby Inc, St Louis, Missouri, 2001.

NEPHROLOGY

Adler SG, Salant DJ. Amer J Kid Dis. (2003). Vol. 42: 395-418.

Andreoli TE et al. Cecil's Eesentials of medicine 6th ed. (2004). Saunder Publishing, Philadelphia.

Androgue HJ, Madias NM. Hyponatremia. 1998. NEMJ, 342:21 1581-1589.

Androgue HJ, Madias NM. Management of life threatening acid-base disorders part I. N Engl J Med, Vol. 338 (1): 26-33.

Androgue HJ, Madias NM. Management of life threatening acid-base disorders part II. N Engl J Med, Vol. 338 (2): 107-11.

Androgue HJ, Madias NM. Management of life threatening acid-base disorders part I. N Engl J Med, Vol. 338 (1): 26-33.

Androgue HJ, Madias NE. Hyponatremia. (2000). N Engl J Med, Vol. 342 (20): 1493-1499.

Androgue HJ, Madias NE. Hyponatremia. (2000). N Engl J Med, Vol. 342 (21): 1581-1588.

Barnett AH, Bain SC, Bouter P, Karlberg B, Madsbad S, Jervell J, et at. (2004). Angiotensin-Receptor Blockade versus Converting-Enzyme Inhibition in Type 2 Diabetes and Nephropathy, N Engl J Med, Vol. 351(1); 1952-61

Brenner BM, Cooper ME. de Zeeuw D, Keane WF, Mitch WE, et al. (2001). Effects of Losartan on Renal Cardiovascular Outcomes in Patients with Type 2 Diabetes and Nephropathy, N Engl J Med, Vol. 345(12);861-869.

Churchill, DN, Blacke, PG, Jindal KK, Toffelmire EB, Goldstein MB. Clinical practice guidelines for initiation of dialysis. Canadian Society of Nephrology. J Am Soc Nephrol 1999; 10 (Suppl 13): S238-91.

Clinical Practice Guidelines for the Management of Diabetes in Canada. CMAJ, 159(8):973-978.

Donadio JV, Grande JP. (2002). Medical progress: IgA nephropathy. N Eng J Med, Vol. 347: 738-748.

Gabow PA (1993). Autosomal dominant polycystic kidney disease. N Engl J Med, 329(5):332-342.

Greenberg, Arthur. Primer on Kidney Diseases, 3rd ed. San Diego: Academic Press, 2001.

Hakim R, Lazarus M (1995). Initiation of Dialysis. J Am Soc Nephrol, Vol. 6:1319-28.

Halperin ML, Goldstein MB, Kersey R, eds (1998). Fluid, electrolyte, and acid-base physiology: a problem-based approach, 3ed. Harcourt Brace & Co.: New York.

Halperin H, Kamel K. (1998). Potassium. The Lancet. Vol 352: 135-40.

Harris SB, Meltzer SJ, Zinman B (1998). New guidelines for the management of diabetes: a physician's guide. Steering Committee for the Revision of the Hemphill RR et al. Review of acute renal failure. http://www.embbs/com/cr/rf/rf.html.

Hudson BG, Tryggvason K, Sundaramoorthy M, Neilson EG. (2003). N Engl J Med, Vol. 348: 2543-2556.

Johnson RJ, Feehally J, eds (1999). Comprehensive clinical nephrology. Mosby: New York.

K/DOQI clinical practice guidelines for chronic kidney disease: evaluation, classification, and stratification: 2000 executive update.http://www. kidney.org/professionals/dogi/kdogi/toc.htm

Keane WF, Garabed E. (1999). Proteinuria, albuminuria, risk, assessment, detection, elimination (PARADE): a position paper of the National Kidney Foundation. Amer J Kid Dis. Vol 33(5): 1004-1010.

Lewis EJ, Hunsicker LG, Bain RP, Rohde RD (1993). The Effects of Angiotensin-Converting Enzyme Inhibition on Diabetic Nephropathy, N Engl J Med, Vol.329(20);1456-62.

McFarlane P, Tobe S, Houlden R, Harris S. (2003). Nephropathy: Canadian Diabetes Association clinical practice guidelines expert committee. http://www.diabetes.ca/cpg2003/downloads/nephropathy.pdf.S66-S71.

Myers, Allen. Medicine 4th ed. Baltimore: Lipincott Williams & Wilkins, 2001.

ONTARGET Investigators. Telmisartan, ramipril, or both in patients at high risk for vascular events. 2008. N Engl J Med. 358:1547-59.

Sabatine M. (2004). Pocket Medicine: The Massachusetts General Hospital Handbook of Internal Medicine. 2nd ed. Chapter 4, 1-20. New York. Lippincott Williams & Wilkins.

Schiffl H, Lang SM, Fischer R (2002). Daily Hemodialysis and the Outcome of Acute Renal Failure, N Engl J Med, Vol. 346(5);305-10.

Schreiber M. Seminars for year 3 clinical clerks on medicine: hyponatremia and hypernatremia. October 29, 2002.

Smith, Kinsey. Renal Disease: A Conceptual Approach. New York: Churchill Livingstone, 1987.

Thadhani R, Pascual M, Bonventre JV (1996). Acute renal failure. N Engl J Med, 334(22):1448-1460.

NEUROLOGY

Brain Death

Wijdicks EF. The Diagnosis of Brain Death. NEJM 2001; 344(16): 1215-21.

Coma

Bhidayasiri R, Waters MF, Giza CC (2005). Neurological differential diagnosis: a prioritized approach. Massachusettes: Blackwell Publishing, Inc., pp.71-2.

Kasper DL, Braunwald E, Fauci AS, Hauser SL, Longo DL, Jameson JL, eds (2005). Harrison's principles of internal medicine, 16th edition. Toronto: McGraw-Hill Companies, Inc, pp. 1629-30.

Common Presenting Complaints

Bhidayasiri R, Waters MF, Giza CC (2005). Neurological differential diagnosis: a prioritized approach. Massachusettes: Blackwell Publishing, Inc, pp. 12-13, 305-14.

Headache

Headache Classification Subcommittee of the International Headache Society. The International Classification of Headache Disorders, 2nd edition. Cepahalagia. 2004; 24(S1):9-160. http://www.ihs-classification.org.

Multiple Sclerosis

Ambati BK, Smith WT, Azer-Bentsianov MT (2001). Residents manual of medicine. Hamilton: BC Decker, pp. 211-13.

Carpenter CCJ, Griggs RC, Loscalzo J, eds (2001). Cecil Essentials of medicine, 5th edition. Philadelphia: WB Saunders Co, pp. 973-6.

Ferri FF (2001). Practical guide to the care of the medical patient. St. Louis: Mobsy Inc, pp. 654-656.

Noseworthy JH, Lucchinetti C, Rodriguez M, Weinshenker BG. Multiple sclerosis. NEJM 2000; 343(13): 938-52.

Olek MJ, ed (2005). Multiple sclerosis: etiology, diagnosis, and new treatment strategies. New Jersey: Humana Press Inc, pp. 36-40, 57, 131, 222-23.

Samuels MA, Feske SK, eds (2003). Office practice of neurology, 2nd edition. Philadelphia: Elsevier Science, pp. 410-11.

Polman CH, Reingold SC, Edan G, Filippi M, Hartung HP, Kappos I, et al. Diagnostic criteria for multiple sclerosis: 2005 revisions to the "McDonald Criteria". Ann Neurol 2005 Dec;58(6):840-6.

Persistent Vegetative State

Kasper DL, Braunwald E, Fauci AS, Hauser SL, Longo DL, Jameson JL, eds (2005). Harrison's principles of internal medicine, 16th edition. Toronto: McGraw-Hill Companies, Inc, pp. 1625.

Seizures and Epilepsy

Ambati BK, Smith WT, Azer-Bentsianov MT (2001). Residents manual of medicine. Hamilton: BC Decker, pp. 203-205.

Ferri FF (2001). Practical guide to the care of the medical patient. St. Louis: Mobsy Inc, pp. 617-9.

Carpenter CCJ, Griggs RC, Loscalzo J, eds (2001). Cecil Essentials of medicine, 5th edition. Philadelphia: WB Saunders Co, pp. 956-64.

Epilepsy

Griggs RC Cecil Essentials of Medicine 7th Edition Andreoli, Carpenter, Griggs, Benjamin.   Saunders Elsevier pp 1120-8.

Status Epilepticus

Lowenstein DH, Alldredge BK. Status epilepticus. NEJM 1998;338(14):970-6.

Spinal Cord Syndrome

Wagner R, Jagoda A. Neurologic Emergencies: Spinal cord syndromes. Emerg Med Clinic North America 1997; 15(3): 699-711.

Stroke

Lindsay K, Bone I., 2003 Neurology and Neurosurgery Illustrated. Philadelphia: Churchill Livingstone p. 244.
Frontera W, Silver J. (2002) Essentials of Physical Medicine and Rehabilitation. Philadelphia: Hanley and Belfus Inc., p. 778-782.
Organized Inpatient (stroke unit) care for stroke (Stroke Unit Trialists' Collaboration). The Cochrane Database of Systematic Reviews 2001; Issue 3.
Johnston SC, Rothwell PM, Nguyen-Huynh MN, Giles MF, Elkins JS, Bernstein AL, et al. Validation and refinement of scores to predict very early stroke risk after transient ischaemic attack. Lancet 2007;369:283-92.

Neuropathic Pain

Marcus, D. (2005). Chronic Pain – A Primary Guide to Practical Management. New Jersey: Humana Press. p. 111-28.

Wilson's Disease

Aminoff MJ, Greenberg DA, Simon RP. Lange: Clinical Neurology, 6th edition. Toronto: McGraw-Hill Companies, Inc. pp. 254-56.

Disorders of the Motor System

Marshall FJ. Cecil Essentials of Medicine 7th Edition Andreoli, Carpenter, Griggs, Benjamin. Saunders Elsevier pp 1090-100.

Dementia

Patterson C, Feightner JW, Garcia A, Hsiung GY, MacKnight C, Sadovnick AD. Diagnosis and treatment of dementia: 1. Risk assessment and primary prevention of Alzheimer disease. CMAJ. 2008 Feb 26;178(5):548-56.Review.
Feldman HH, Jacova C, Robillard A, Garcia A, Chow T, Borrie M, et al. Diagnosis and treatment of dementia: 2. Diagnosis. CMAJ. 2008 March 25; 178(7):825-36. Review.

Predicting and Preventing Post-herpetic Neuralgia: Are current risk factors useful in clinical practice?

Coen PG, Scott F, Leedham-Green M et al. European Journal of Pain 2006;10:695-700.
Chapter 24 Neurologic Disorders
Yamada KA, Awadalla S. The Washington Manual of Medical Therapeutics, 31st Edition. Lippincot Williams and Wilkins pp 531-534.

NEUROSURGERY

Ahn NU, Ahn UM, Nallamshetty L, et al. Cauda equina syndrome in ankylosing spondylitis (the CES-AS syndrome): meta-analysis of outcomes after medical and surgical treatments. Journal of Spinal Disorders 2001;14:427-33.
Aids to the examination of the peripheral nervous system. London, UK: Balliere Tindall, 1986.
Al-Shahi R, Warlow CP. Interventions for treating brain arteriovenous malformations in adults. The Cochrane Library 2004;Volume 2.
Barker FG 2nd, Ogilvy CS. Efficacy of prophylactic nimodipine for delayed ischemic deficit after subarachnoid hemorrhage: a metaanalysis. Journal of Neurosurgery 1996;84:405-14.
Barnett H, Taylor W, Eliasziw M, et al. Benefit of carotid endarterectomy in patients with symptomatic moderate or severe stenosis. NEJM 1998;339:1415-25.
Bracken MB, Shepard MJ, Holford TR, et al. Methylprednisolone or tirilazad mesylate administration after acute spinal cord injury: 1-year follow up. Results of the third National Acute Spinal Cord Injury randomized controlled trial. Journal of Neurosurgery 1998;89:699-706.
Crossman AR, Neary D. Neuroanatomy: an illustrated colour text. Toronto, ON: Churchill Livingston, 1998.
Edlow J, Caplan L. Avoiding pitfalls in the diagnosis of subarachnoid hemorrhage. NEJM. 2000;342(1):29-36.
Executive Committee for the Asymptomatic Carotid Atherosclerosis Study (ACAS).
Endarterectomy for asymptomatic carotid artery stenosis. JAMA 1995;273:1421-28.
Fitzgerald MJT. Neuroanatomy: basic and clinical (3rd edition). Philadelphia: WB Saunders, 1997.
Goetz CG, Pappert EJ. Textbook of clinical neurology (1st edition). Toronto, ON: WB Saunders, 1999.
Greenberg MS. Handbook of neurosurgery (5th edition). New York: Thieme, 2001.
Guy M. McKhann, Guy Mckhann II, Neil Kitchen. Clinical Neurology and Neurosurgery. Theme Medical Publishers. 2003
Kun, LE. Brain Tumours: Challenges and Directions. Pediatric Clinics of North America. 1997; Vol 44(4):907-17.
Lindsay KW, Bone I. Neurology and neurosurgery illustrated. New York: Churchill Livingstone, 2004.
MRC Asymptomatic Carotid Surgery Trial (ACST) Collaborative Group. Prevention of disabling and fatal strokes by successful carotid endarterectomy in patients without recent neurological symptoms: randomised controlled trial. Lancet 2004;363:1491-502.
Nieuwenhuys R, Voogd J, van Huijzen C. The human central nervous system (3rd edition). New York: Springer-Verlag, 1988.
Nursing 2004 Drug Handbook (24th edition). New York, NY: Springhouse Lippincott Williams & Wilkins, 2004.
Ogilvy CS, Stieg PE, Awad I., et al. Recommendations for the management of intracranial arteriovenous malformations. Circulation 2001;103:2644-57.
Porter PJ, Willinsky RA, Harper W, et al. Cerebral cavernous malformations: natural history and prognosis after clinical deterioration with or without hemorrhage. Journal of Neurosurgery 1997;87:190-7.
Saal JS, Saal JA, Yurth EF. Nonoperative management of herniated cervical intervertebral disc with radiculopathy. Spine. 21(16):1877-83, 1996.
Shapiro S. Medical realities of cauda equina syndrome secondary to lumbar disc herniation. Spine. 25(3):348-51; discussion 352, 2000.
Shemie S, Doig C, Dickens B, et al. Severe brain injury to neurological determination of Death: Canadian forum recommendations. CMAJ 2006; 174(6): S1-30.
Short DJ, El Masry WS, Jones PW. High dose methylprednisolone in the management of acute spinal cord injury - a systematic review from a clinical perspective. Spinal Cord 2000;38:273-86.
Spetzler RF, Martin NA. A proposed grading system for arteriovenous malformations. Journal of Neurosurgery 1986;65:476-83.
The North American Symptomatic Carotid Endarterectomy Trial (NASCET). Beneficial effects of carotid endarterectomy in symptomatic patients with high-grade carotid stenosis. NEJM 1991;325:445-53.

OBSTETRICS

American College of Obstetricians and Gynecologists www.acog.org
The Society of Obstetricians and Gynaecologists of Canada www.sogc.org
ABC of labour care: Care of the newborn in the delivery room. BMJ 1999; 318: 1403-1406.
ABC of labour care: Obstetric emergencies. BMJ 1999; 318: 1342-1345.
ABC of labour care: Operative delivery. BMJ 1999; 318: 1260-1264.
ABC of labour care: Induction. BMJ 1999; 318: 995-998.
ABC of labour care: Labour in special circumstances. BMJ 1999; 318: 1124-1127.
ABC of labour care: Physiology and management of normal labour. BMJ 1999; 318: 793-796.
ABC of labour care: Place of birth. BMJ 1999; 318: 721-723.
ABC of labour care: Preterm labour and premature rupture of membranes. BMJ 1999; 318: 1059-1062.
ABC of labour care: Relief of pain. BMJ 1999; 318: 927-930.
ABC of labour care: Unusual presentations and positions and multiple pregnancy. BMJ 1999; 318: 1192-1194.
Alfirevic Z. (2002). Oral misoprostol for induction of labour (Cochrane Review). The Cochrane Library, Issue 2.
Antenatal Corticosteroid Therapy for Fetal Maturation. SOGC Clinical Practice Guidelines Policy Statement, December 1995: 53.
Baskett, T. Essential Management of Obstetric Emergencies. 3rd ed. Clinical Press, Bristol, 1999.
Bastian LA, Piscitelli JT. Is this patient pregnant? Can you reliably rule in or rule out early pregnancy by clinical examination? JAMA. 1997 Aug 20; 278(7): 586-91. Review
Berghella V, et al. (2004). Cerclage for prevention of preterm birth in women with a short cervix found on transvaginal examination: A randomized trial. Amer J Obs Gyn. 191:1311-7.
Boucher, M. Mode of Delivery for Pregnant Women infected by the Human Immunodeficiency Virus. SOGC Clinical Practice Guidelines. April 2001: 101.
Boucher, M. and Gruslin, A. The Reproductive Care of Women living with Hepatitis C Infection. SOGC Clinical Practice Guidelines. October 2000: 96.
Bricker L, Luckas M. (2002). Amniotomy alone for induction of labour (Cochrane Review). The Cochrane Library, Issue 2.
Chyu JK, Strassner HT. Prostaglandin E2 for cervical ripening: a randomized comparison of cervidil vs. prepidil. AMJ Obstet Gynecol 1997. 177: 606-11.
Crane, J. (2001). Induction of labour at term. SOGC Clinical Practice Guideline, 107:1-12.

Fetal health Surveillance in Labour - Parts 1 and 2. SOGC Clinical Practical Guideline. January 1996, 45.
Guidelines for exercise in pregnancy. SOGC Clinical Practical Guidelines. Committee Opinion. June 2003.
Guidelines for the Management of Nausea and Vomiting in Pregnancy. SOGC Clinical Practice Guidelines Committee Opinion. November 1995: 12.
Guise JM, Berlin M, McDonagh M, Osterweil P, Chan B, Helfand M. Safety of vaginal birth after caesarean: a systematic review. Obstet Gynec. 2004 Mar; 103(3):420-9.
Hannah, M. Post-term Pregnancy. SOGC Clinical Practice Guidelines Committee Opinion. March 1997: 15.
Healthy Beginnings: Guidelines for Care during Pregnancy and Childbirth. SOGC Clinical Practice Guidelines Policy Statement. December 1998: 71.
Hennessey MH, Rayburn WF, Stewart JD, Likes EC. Pre-eclampsia and induction of labour: a randomized comparision of prostaglandin E2 as an intracervical gel, with oxytocin immediately, or as a sustained - release vaginal insert. AMJ Obstet Gynecol. 1998. 179(5): 1204-9.
Howarth GR, Botha DJ. (2002). Amniotomy plus intravenous oxytocin for induction of labour (Cochrane Review). The Cochrane Library, Issue 2.
Kelly AJ, Tan B. (2002). Intravenous oxytocin alone for cervical ripening and induction of labour (Cochrane Review). The Cochrane Library, Issue 2.
Kent, N. Prevention and Treatment of Venous Thromboembolism (VTE) in Obstetrics. SOGC Clinical Practice Guidelines. September 2000: 95.
Ling, F. and Duff, P. Obstetrics and Gynecology, Principles for practice. USA: McGraw-Hill Companies, 2002.
Luckas M, Bricker L. (2000). Intravenous prostaglandin for induction of labour (Cochrane Review). The Cochrane Library, Issue 2.
Meltwer, S., Leiter, L., Daneman, D., Gerstein, HC., Lau, D., Ludwig S., Yale, JF., Zinman, B., Lillie, D. 1998 Clinical Practice Guidelines for the Management of Diabetes in Canada. CMAJ. 1998, 159 (B suppl): S1-29.
Midmer D, Biringer A, Carroll JC, Reid AJ, Wilson L, Stewart D, Tate M, Chalmers B. A Reference Guide for Providers: The ALPHA Form - Antenatal Psychosocial Health Assessment Form, 2nd Edition. Toronto: University of Toronto, Faculty of Medicine, Department of Family and Community Medicine, 1996.
Ministry of Health and Long Term Care and Canadian Medical Association. Antenatal Record 1. Ontario.
Ministry of Health and Long Term Care and Canadian Medical Association. Antenatal Record 2. Ontario.
Money, D and Dobson, S. The prevention of early-onset group B streptococcal disease. SOGC Clinical Practice Guidelines. September 2004.
Mount Sinai Hospital. First Trimester Combined Screening Program. 2001.
North York General Hospital Genetics Program. Integrated Prenatal Screening. 1999.
Ottinyer WS, Menara MK, Brost BC. A randomized control trial of prostaglandin E2 intracervical gel and a slow release vaginal for preinduction cervical ripening. AMJ Obstet Gynecol. 1998. 179(2): 349-53.
Schuurmans, N., MacKinnon, C., Lane C., Etches, D. Prevention and Management of Postpartum Hemorrhage. SOGC Clinical Practice Guidelines. April 2000: 88.
SOGC. Fetal Health Surveillance: Antepartum and Intrapartum Consensus Guideline, Sept. 2007.
Statistics Canada. 2005. Induced Abortion Statistics, 82-223-XWE, page 16 of 32.
Stewart JD, Rayburn WF, Farmer KC, Ciles EM, Schipaul AH Jr., Stanley JR. Effectiveness of prostaglandin E2 intracervical gel (prepidil) with immediate oxytocin vs. vaginal insert (cervidil) for induction of labour. AMJ Obstet Gynecol 1998. 179: 1175-80.
Van den Hof, M. and Crane, J. Ultrasound Cervical Assessment in Predicting Preterm Birth. SOGC Clinical Practice Guidelines. May 2001: 102.

OPHTHALMOLOGY

Books
Bradford C. Basic Ophthalmology for Medical Students and Primary Care Residents. 7th ed. San Francisco: American Academy of Ophthalmology, 1999.
Wilson FM. Practical Ophthalmology: A Manual for Beginning Residents. 4th ed. American Academy of Ophthalmology, 2005.
Friedman N, Pineda R, Kaiser P. The Massachusetts Eye and Ear Infirmary Illustrated Manual of Ophthalmology. Toronto: W.B. Saunders Company, 1998.
Kanski JJ. Clinical Ophthalmology: A Systematic Approach. 6th ed. Oxford: Butterworth-Heinemann, 2007.
Stein R, Stein H. Management of Ocular Emergencies. 4th ed. Montreal: Mediconcept, 2006.

Guidelines
Hux J, et al. Diabetes in Ontario: an ICES Practice Atlas. Toronto: Institute for Clinical Evaluative Sciences, 2003.
The committee for the classification of retinopathy of prematurity. An international classification of retinopathy of prematurity. Arch Ophthalmology. 1984; 102: 1130-34.

Images
Red Atlas. www.redatlas.org
Atlas of Ophthalmology www.atlasophthalmology.com/atlas/frontpage.jsf

Lectures/Cases
University of Michigan Kellogg Eye Centre www.kellogg.umich.edu/theeyeshaveit/index.html

ORTHOPAEDICS

Textbooks
Adams JC, Hamblen DL. Outline of fractures: including joint injuries. 11th ed. Toronto (ON): Churchill Livingstone, 1999.
Blackbourne LH. Surgical recall. 3rd ed. LH Blackbourne. Philadelphia (PA): Lippincott Williams & Wilkins, 2002.
Brinker MR. Review of orthopaedic trauma. Toronto (ON): W.B. Saunders Company, 2001.
Brinker M, Miller M. Fundamentals of orthopaedics. Philadelphia (PA): W.B. Saunders, 1999.
Dee R, Hurst LC, Gruber MA, Kottmeier SA, editors. Principles of orthopaedic practice. 2nd Toronto (ON): McGraw-Hill, 1997.
Kao LD. Pre-test surgery. Toronto (ON): McGraw-Hill, 2002
Ochiai DH. The orthopaedic intern pocket survival guide. McLean (VA): International Medical Publishing, 2007.
Rockwood CA Jr, Greene DP, Bucholz RU, Heckman JD, editors. Rockwood and Green's fractures in adults. 4th ed. Philadelphia (PA): Lippincott Raven, 1996.
Skinner HB. Current diagnosis and treatment in orthopaedics. 4th ed. New York (NY): McGraw-Hill, 2006.
Solomon L, Warwick DJ, Nayagam, S. Apley's system of orthopaedics and fractures. 8th ed. New York (NY): Hodder Arnold, 2001.
Thompson JC. Netter's concise altas of orthopaedic Anatomy. [USA]: Elsivier, 2001.

Journal Articles
Adkins SB. Hip pain in athletes. Am Fam Physician. 2000;61(7):2109-2118.
Armagan OE, Shereff MJ. Injuries of the toes and metatarsals. Orthop Clin North Am. 2001;32(1):1-10.
Barei DP, Bellabarba C, Sangeorzan BJ, Benirschke SK. Fractures of the calcaneus. Orthop Clin North Am. 2001;33(1):263-285.
Barrett SL. Plantar fasciitis and other causes of heel pain. Am Fam Physician. 1999;59(8):2200-2206.
Brand DA, Frazier WH, Kohlhepp WC, et al. A protocol for selecting patients with injured extremities who need x-rays. N Engl J Med. 1982;306:833-339.
Carek PJ. Diagnosis and management of osteomyelitis. Am Fam Physician. 2001;63(12): 2413-2420.
Donatto KC. Ankle fractures and syndesmosis injuries. Orthop Clin North Am. 2001;32(1):79-90.
Fernandez M. Discitis and vertebral osteomyelitis in children: an 18-year review. Pediatrics. 105(6): 1299-1304.
Fortin PT. Talus fractures: evaluation and treatment. J Am Acad Orthop Surg. 2001;9(2): 114-127.
French B, Tornetta III P. High energy tibial shaft fractures. Orthop Clin North Am. 2002;33(1):211-230.
Gustilo RB, Mendoza RM, Williams DN. Problems in the management of type III (severe) open fractures: a new classification of type III open fractures. J Trauma. 1984;24:742–746.
Geerts WH, Heit JA, Clagett, GP et al. Prevention of venous thromboembolism. Chest. 2001;119(1 Suppl): 132S-175S.
Harty MP. Imaging of pediatric foot disorders. Radiol Clin North Am. 2001;39(4):733-748.

Irrgang JJ. Rehabilitation of multiple ligament injured knee. Clin Sports Med. 2000;19(3): 545-571.

Lawrence LL. The limping child. Emerg Med Clin North Am. 1998;169(4):911-929.

Luime JJ, Verhagen AP, Miedema HS, Kuiper JI, Burdorf A, Verhaar JAN, Koes BW. An Evaluation of the Apprehension, Relocation, and Surprise Tests for Anterior Shoulder Instability. The American Journal of Sports Medicine. 2004;32:301-307.

Mazzone MF. Common conditions of the Achilles tendon. Am Fam Physician. 2000;65(9):1805-1810.

Steele PM, Bush-Joseph C, Bach Jr B. Management of acute fractures around the knee, ankle, and foot. Clin Fam Pract. 2000;2(3):661-705.

Miller SL. Malignant and benign bone tumours. Radiol Clin North Am. 2000;39(4): 673-699.

Oudjhane K. Imaging of osteomyelitis in children. Radiol Clin North Am. 2001;39(2): 251-266.

Patel DR. Sports injuries in adolescents. Med Clin North Am. 2000;84(4):983-1007.

Roberts DM, Stallard TC. Emergency department evaluation and treatment of knee and leg injuries. Emerg Med Clin North Am. 2000;18(1):67-84.

Russell GV Jr. Complicated femoral shaft fractures. Orthop Clin North Am. 2002;33(1): 127-142.

Solomon DH, Simel DL, Bates DW, Katz JN, Schaffer JL. The rational clinical examination. Does this patient have a torn meniscus or ligament of the knee? Value of the physical examination. JAMA. 2001;286(13):1610-20.

St Pierre P. Posterior cruciate ligament injuries. Clin Sports Med. 1999;18(1): 199-221.

Steele PM, Bush-Joseph C, Bach Jr B. Management of acute fractures around the knee, ankle, and foot. Clin Fam Pract. 2000;2(3):661-705.

Stewart DG, Kay RM, Skaggs DL. Open fractures in children. Principles of evalution nd management. JBJS Am. 2005;87: 2784-2798.

Swenson TM. The dislocated knee: physical diagnosis of the multiple-ligament-injured knee. Clin Sports Med. 2000;19(3):415-423.

Zollinger PE, Tuinebreijer WE, Kreis RW, Breederveld RS. Effect of vitamin C on frequency of reflex sympathetic dystrophy in wrist fractures: a randomized trial. Lancet. 1999;354(9195): 2025-2028.

OTOLARYNGOLOGY - HEAD AND NECK SURGERY

Textbooks

Bailey BJ. Head and Neck Surgery-Otolaryngology. 2nd ed. Philadelphia. Lippincott Williams and Wilkins. 1998.

Becker W, Naumann HH, Pfaltz CR. Ear, Nose, and Throat Diseases. 2nd ed. New York. Theme Medical Publishers. 1994.

Dhillon RS, East CA. Ear, Nose, and Throat, and Head and Neck Surgery: an illustrated colour text. 2nd ed. New York. Churchill & Livingston. 1999. 122p.

Jafek BW, Murrow BW. ENT Secrets. 2nd ed. Philadelphia. Hanley & Belfus. 2001: 608 p.

Lee KJ (ed), Essential Otolaryngology: Head and Neck Surgery. 8th ed. McGraw-Hill. New York. 2003: 1136 p.

Lucente FE and Har-El G. (eds). Essentials of Otolaryngology. 4th ed. Philadelphia. Lippincott Williams and Wilkins. 1999. 488 p.

Layland MK (ed). Washington manual otolaryngology survival guide. Philadelphia. Lippincott Williams and Wilkins. 2003. 187p.

Journal Articles

Berman S, Current Concepts: Otitis Media in Children. NEJM. 1995; 332(23): 1560-1565.

Forastiere A, Koch W, Trotti A, Sidransky D. Head and Neck Cancer. Review Article. NEJM. 2001; 345(26): 1890-1900.

Furman JM, Cass SP. Benign Paroxysmal Positional Vertigo. NEJM. 1999; 341(21):1590-1596.

Hilton M, Pinder D. The Epley (canalith repositioning) manoeuvre for benign paroxysmal positional vertigo. Cochrane Ear, Nose, and Throat Disorders Group. Cochrane Database of Systematic Reviews. 2004; Issue 4.

Jackson CG, von Doersten PG. The Facial Nerve: Current Trends in Diagnosis, Treatment, and Rehabilitation. Otolaryngology for the Internist. 1999; 83(1): 179-195.

Javer AR, Mechor B. Allergic Fungal Rhinosinusitis: A Review of Management Strategies. Allergy and Asthma.

Javer AR. Appropriate Pharmacotherapy for Acute Rhinosinusitis: Are We Overprescribing Antibiotics? Allergy and Asthma.

Low DE, Desrosers M, McSherry J, et al. A practical guide for the diagnosis and treatment of acute sinusitis. CMAJ. 1997; 156(suppl 6): S1-14.

MacCallum PL et al. Comparison of open, percutaneous and translaryngeal tracheostomies. Otolaryngology Head Neck Surgery. 2000. 122: 686-690.

Mclsaac WJ, Coyte PC. Croxford R, Asche CV, Freidberg J, Feldman W. Otolaryngologists' perceptions of the indications for typanostomy tube insertion in children. CMAJ. 2000;162(9): 1285-1288.

Srafford ND, Wilde A. Parotid Cancer. Review. Surgical Oncology. 1997; 6(4). 209-213.

Useful Websites

http://www.utoronto.ca/otolaryngology/
http://www.utmb.edu/otoref/Grnds/GrndsIndex.html
http://icarus.med.utoronto.ca/otolaryngology/OTL300/
http://icarus.med.utoronto.ca/carr/manual/sprays.html

PEDIATRICS

Cardiology

Smythe J. Does every childhood heart murmur need an echocardiogram? The Canadian Journal of Pediatrics. Volume 2 – Number 4.

Task Force on Blood Pressure Control in Children: Report of the Second Task Force on Blood Pressure Control in Children - 1987. Task Force on Blood Pressure Control in Children. National Heart, Lung, and Blood Institute, Bethesda, Maryland. Pediatrics. 1987 Jan; 79(1):1-25.

Endocrinology

American Diabetes Association. Type 2 Diabetes in Children and Adolescents. Pediatrics. 2000; 105(3): 671-681.

Lenhard MJ, Reeves GD. Continuous subcutaneous insulin infusion: a comprehensive review of insulin pump therapy. Archives of Internal Medicine. 2001;161(19):2293-3000.

Muir, A., et al. Precocious Puberty. Pediatrics in Review. 2006;27(10): 373-380.

Styne DM, Glaser NS. Endocrinology. Nelson's Essentials of Pediatrics. 4th Edition. W.B. Saunders co. pp 711-766, 2002.

Gastroenterology

Kirshner BS, Black DD. The Gastrointestinal Tract. In Nelson's Essentials of Pediatrics. 3rd Edition. pp. 419-458, 1998.

Nutrition for Healthy Infants - Statement of the Joint Working Group: Canadian Pediatric Society, Dieticians of Canada, Health Canada.

Scott, RB. Recurent abdominal pain during childhood. Canadian Family Physician. 1994;40:539-547.

General Topics

Albright EK. Current Clinical Strategies. Pediatric History and Physical Examination. 4th Edition. Current Clinical Strategies Publishing 2003.

McGahren E, Wilson W. Pediatrics Recall. Williams and Wilkins. 1997.

Objectives for the Qualifying Examination. Medical Council of Canada. Third Edition, 2004.

 Scruggs K, Johnson MT. Pediatrics 5-minute reviews. Current Clinical Strategies Publishing. 2001-2002.

Genetic Disorders and Developmental Disorders

Amato RSS. Human Genetics and Dysmorphology. Nelson's Essentials of Pediatrics. 3rd Edition. W.B. Saunders co. pp 129-146, 2002.

Biggar W. Duchenne Muscular Dystrophy. Pediatrics in Review. 2006;27(3):83-88.

Chudley, AE et al. Fetal alcohol spectrum disorder: Canadian guidelines for diagnosis. CMAJ. 172 (5 supplement): S1 – S21.

Nicholson JF. Inborn errors of metabolism. Nelson's Essentials of Pediatrics. 4th Edition. W.B. Saunders co. pp 153-178, 2002.

Hematology
Corrigan J, Boineau F. Hemolytic-Uremic Syndrome. Pediatrics in Review. 2001 Nov; 22(11).
Pearce JM, Sills RH. Childhood Leukemia. Pediatrics in Review. 2005; 26(3):96-102.
Segel GB. Anemia. Pediatrics in Review. 1988 Sep; 10(3).
Silverstein J. et al. Care of Children and Adolescents with Type 1 Diabetes: A Statement of the American Diabetes Association. Diabetes Care. 2005; 28(1):186-208.

Infectious Disease and Immunizations
Black S, Shinefield H, Fireman B, et al. Efficacy, safety and immungenicity of heptavalent pneumococcal conjugate vaccine in children. Pediatric Infectious Disease Journal. 2000;19(3):187-195.
Canada Communicable Disease Report. Statement on recommended use of varicella virus vaccine. An Advisory Committee Statement (ACS) National Advisory Committee on Immunization. 1999; Volume 25. ACS-1.
Canada Communicable Disease Report. Statement on recommended use of meningococcal vaccines. An Advisory Committee Statement National Advisory Committee on Immunization. 2001; Volume 27. ACS-6.
Canada Communicable Disease Report. Statement on recommended use of pneumococcal conjugate vaccine. An Advisory Centers for Disease Control and Prevention. Managing acute gastroenteritis among children. 2003; 52 (No.RR-16)
Advisory Committee Statement National Advisory Committee on Immunization. Volume 28. ACS-2.
National Advisory Committee on Immunization. Recommended Immunization Schedule for Infants, Children, and Youth (updated March 2005). Canadian Immunization Guide - 6th Edition.
Routine immunization schedule. Canadian Pediatric Society. May 2004.
Treatment of acute otitis media in an era of increasing microbial resistance. Pediatric Infectious Diseases Journal. 1998; 17:576-579.
Wubbel L, McCracken D, McCracken GH. Management of Bacterial Meningitis. Pediatrics in Review. 1998 Mar; 19(3).

Neonatology
Gomella TL, Cunningham MD, Eyal FG, Zenk KE. Assessment of gestational age. Neonatology: Management, Procedures, On-call Problems, Diseases and Drugs. 5th edition. McGraw-Hill Companies. pp 21-28, 491-6, 559-62, 2004.
Niermeyer S. et al. International Guidelines for Neonatal Resuscitation: An excerpt from the Guidelines 2000 for Cardiopulmonary Resuscitation and Emergency Cardiovascular Care: International Consensus on Science. Contributors and Reviews for the Neonatal Resuscitation. Guidelines. Pediatrics. 2000; 106(3):E29.

Nephrology
Hogg RJ, Portman RJ, Milliner D, Lemley KV, Eddy A, Ingelfinger J. Evaluation and management of proteinuria and nephrotic syndrome in children: Recommendations from a pediatric nephrology panel established at the National Kidney Foundation Conference on proteinuria, albuminuria, risk, assessment, detection and elimination (PARADE). Pediatrics. June; 105(6):1242-1249.
Michael RS. Toilet training. Pediatrics in Review. 1999; 20(7).

Neurology
Bergman I, Painter MJ. Neurology. Nelson's Essentials of Pediatrics. 4th Edition. W.B. Saunders co. pp 767-820, 2002.
Hirtz D, Ashwal S, Berg A, et al. Practice parameter: Evaluation a first nonfebrile seizure in children. Report of the quality standards subcommittee of the American Epilepsy Academy of Neurology. The Child Neurology Society and The American Epilepsy Society. Neurology. 2000 Sep 12; 55(5):616-23.
Lewis DW, Ashawal S, Dahl G, et al. The Quality Standards Subcommittee of the America Academy of Neurology. The Practice Committee of the Child Neurology Society. Practice parameter: Evaluation of children and adolescents with recurrent headaches. Report of the Quality Standards Subcommittee of the American Academy of Neurology and the Practice Committee of the Child Neurology Society. Guideline. Neurology. 2002 Aug 27; 59(4):490-498.
Lewis, D et al. Practice Parameter: Pharmacological treatment of migraine headache in Children and adolescents. American Academy of Neurology. Neurology. 2004; 63:2215-2224.

Pharmacology
Hospital for Sick Children. Formulary of Infant and Enteral Formulas. February 2006.
Kowalczyk A (Ed.). The 2004-2005 Formulary –The Hospital for Sick Children. Toronto: The Graphic Centre, HSC.

Respirology
Garrison MM, Christakis DA, Harvey E, Cummings P, Davis RL. Systemic corticosteroids in infant bronchiolitis: a meta-analysis. Pediatrics. 2000;105:e44.

Rheumatology
Olson JC. Rheumatic Diseases of Childhood. Nelson's Essentials of Pediatrics. Third Edition. W.B. Saunders co. pp299-314, 1998.
Schneider R. Pinpointing the cause of limb pain in children. Pediatrics. 1993:576-583.

Web-based Resources
http://www.medscape.com/home/topics/pediatrics
http://www.uptodate.com
http://www.icondata.com/health/pedbase
http://www.cda-adc.ca

PLASTIC SURGERY

General Plastic Surgery Concepts
Brown DL, Borschel GH. Michigan manual of plastic surgery. Philadelphia: Saunders, 2004.
Daver BM, Antia NH, Furnas DW. Handbook of plastic surgery for the general surgeon second edition. New Delhi: Oxford University Press, 1995.
Georgiade GS, Riefkohl R, Levin LS. Georgiade plastic, maxillofacial and reconstructive surgery third edition. Baltimore: Williams and Wilkins, 1997.
Hunt TK. Wound Healing. In: Doherty GM, Way LW, eds. Current surgical diagnosis & treatment twelfth edition. Norwalk, CT: McGraw-Hill, 2006.
Noble J. Textbook of primary care medicine third edition. St. Louis: Mosby Inc, 2001.
Plastic Surgery Educational Foundation. Plastic and reconstructive surgery essentials for students. Arlington Heights, IL: Plastic Surgery Educational Foundation, 2007.
http://www.plasticsurgery.org/medical_professionals/publications/Essentials-for-Students.cfm.
Richards AM. Key notes in plastic surgery. Great Britain: Blackwell Science Ltd, 2002.
Sermer NB. Practical plastic surgery for non-surgeons. Philadelphia: Hanley & Belfus Inc, 2001.
Smith DJ, Brown AS, Cruse CW et al. Plastic and reconstructive surgery. Chicago: Plastic Surgery Educational Foundation, 1987.
Stone C. Plastic surgery: facts. London: Greenwich Medical Media Ltd, 2001
Townsend CM. Sabiston textbook of surgery – the biological basis of modern surgical practice sixteenth edition. Philadelphia: W.B. Saunders Company, 2001.
Vasconez HC, Ferguson REH, Vasconez LO. Plastic & reconstructive surgery. In: Doherty GM, Way LW, eds. Current surgical diagnosis & treatment twelfth edition. Norwalk, CT: McGraw-Hill, 2006.
Weinzweig J. Plastic surgery secrets. Philadelphia: Hanley and Belfus Inc, 1999.

Hand
American Society for Surgery of the Hand. The hand: examination and diagnosis third edition. Philadelphia: Churchill-Livingston, 1990.
Beredjiklian PK, Bozenika DJ. Review of hand surgery. Philadelphia: Saunders, 2004.
Graham B, Regehr G, Naglie G, Wright J. Development and validation of diagnostic criteria for carpal tunnel syndrome. J Hand Surg 2006; 31(6): 919.e1 - 919.e7.

POPULATION AND COMMUNITY HEALTH

Journals
Bradford-Hill A – "The Environment and Disease: Association or Causation?" Proc. Royal Soc. Med. 1966;58: 295.
Kass NE. An ethics framework for public health. Am J Public Health 2001;91:1776-1782.

Government Resources
Hamilton N, and T. Bhatti. Integrated model of population health and health promotion. Ottawa: Health promotion and programs branch; 1996.
Canadian Public Health Association and WHO. Ottawa Charter for Health Promotion. Ottawa:
Health and Welfare Canada, 1986.
Health Canada. Health and environment: partners for life. Ottawa: Minister of Public Works and Government Services Canada; 1997.
Health Protection and Promotion Act, R.S.O. 1990, c. H.7.
Health Protection and Promotion Act, R.S.O. 1990., c.H.7; O. Reg. 559/91, amended to O. Reg. 49/07.

Textbooks
Hennekens, C. Buring J. Epidemiology in medicine. Philidelphia: Lippincott, Williams & Wilkins, 1987.
Hully SB and Cummings SR. Designing clinical research: an epidemiologic approach. Baltimore: Williams & Wilkins, 1988.
Kelsey JL et al. Methods in Observational Epidemiology, Second Edition. Oxford University Press, 1996.
Last JM. A Dictionary of Epidemiology. 4th e.d. Oxford University Press, 2001.
Sackett DL, Strauss SE, Richardson WS, Rosenberg W and Haynes RB. Evidence-Based Medicine: How to practice and teach EBM. 2nd ed. Toronto: Churchill, Livingstone, 2002.
Shah CP. Public health and preventive medicine in Canada. 4th ed. Toronto: University of Toronto Press, 1998.
Shah CP. Public health and preventive medicine in Canada. 5th ed. Toronto: Elsevier Canada, 2003.

Websites
Association of Workers' Compensation Boards of Canada www.awcbc.org
Bureau of Labour Statistics www.bls.gov
Canada's National Occupational Health and Safety www.canoshweb.org
Canadian Centre for Occupational Health and Safety www.ccohs.ca
Canadian Food Inspection Agency www.inspection/gc.ca/english/agen/agene.shtml
Canadian Institute for Health Information www.cihi.ca
Canadian Medical Association www.cma.ca
Canadian Public Health Association www.cpha.ca
Canadian Society for International Health www.csih.org
Canadian Task Force on Preventative Health Care www.ctfphc.org
Center for Disease Control and Prevention www.cdc.gov
Health Canada www.hc-sc.gc.ca
Institute for Population and Public Health, Canadian Institutes for Health Research www.cihr-irsc.gc.ca/e/13970.html
Intergovernmental Panel on Climate Change www.ipcc.ch
Medical Council of Canada www.mcc.ca
MedTerms www.medterms.com
National Advisory Committee on Immunization www.phac-aspc.gc.ca/naci-ccni/
Ontario Ministry of Labour Occupational Health and Safety www.gov.on.ca/LAB/ohs
Pan-American Health Organization www.paho.org
Public Health Agency of Canada www.phac-aspc.gc.ca/about_apropos/index/html.
WHO, World Health Report 2006 www.who.int/whr/2006/en/index.html
Workplace Safety and Insurance Board www.wsib.on.ca
World Bank www.worldbank.org

Evidence-Based Medicine Resources
Up-to-Date www.uptodate.com
Clinical Evidence www.clinicalevidence.com
Pier (ACP) pier.acponline.org
OVID EBM Reviews gateway.ovid.com/ovidweb.cgi
PubMed - Clinical Queries www.pubmed.com
BMJ Updates bmjupdates.mcmaster.ca
Users' Guide Series www.cche.net/usersguides/main.asp

PSYCHIATRY

American Psychiatric Association. Diagnostic and Statistical Manual of Mental Disorders-Frouth Edition, Text Revision. Washington, DC, American Psychiatric Publishing Inc., 2000.
Ball JR, Mitchell PB, Corry JC, Skilecorn A, Smith M, Malhi GS. A randomized controlled trial of cognitive therapy for bipolar disorder: focus on long-term change. J Clin Psychiatry. 67(2): 277-86, 2006.
Clinical Practice Guidelines: Treatment of Schizophrenia in Can J Psychiatry vol 50, suppl 1 Nov 2005, p19-28.
Conley RR, Kelly DL. Pharmacologic Treatment of Schizophrenia. First Edition. Professional Communications Inc., U.S.A., 2000.
DeRubeis RJ et al. Cognitive therapy vs. medications in the treatment of moderate to severe depression. Arch Gen Psychiatry. 62(4): 409-16, 2005.
Ditto KE. SSRI discontinuation syndrome. Awareness as an approach to prevention. Postgrad Med. 2003 Aug;114(2):79-84.
Folstein MF, Folstein SE and McHugh PR (1975). Mini-Mental State: A practical method for grading the state of patients for the cllinician. Journal of Psychiatric Research. 12: 189-198.
Gliatto MF, Rai AK. "Evaluation and Treatment of Patients With Suicidal Intention." American Family Physician, Volume 59, Number 6, 1999 pp. 1500-14.
Hembree EA, Foa, EB. "Posttraumatic Stress Disorder: Psychological Factors and Psychosocial Interventions." Journal of Clinical Psychiatry, Volume 61, Supplement 7, 2000, pp. 33-9.
Herrmann N. "Recommendations for the Management of Behavioural and Psychological Symptoms of Dementia." Canadian Journal of Neurological Sciences, Volume 28, Supplement 1, 2001, pp. S96-107.
Kahan, M, Wilson, L. Managing Alcohol, Tobacco and other Drug Problems: A pocket guide for physicians and nurses. Toronto, ON. Centre for Addiction and Mental Health. 2002.
Kapur S, Zipursky RB, Remington G. "Clinical and Theoretical Implications of 5-HT2 and D2 Receptor Occupancy of Clozapine, Risperidone, and Olanzapine in Schizophrenia." American Journal of Psychiatry, Volume 156, Number 2, 1999, pp. 286-93.
Koch, T. "A Tour of the Psychotropics." 4th ed. Mental Health Service-St-Michael's Hospital. Toronto, Canada.
Krupnick JL et al. The role of the therapeutic alliance in psychotherapy and pharmacotherapy outcome: findings in the National Institute of Mental Health Treatment of Depression Collaborative Research Program. J Consult Clin Psychol. 64(3): 532-9, 1996.
Lineham MM et al. Two-year randomized controlled trial and follow-up of dialectical behaviour therapy vs. therapy by experts for suicidal behaviours and boderline personality disorder. Arch Gen Psychiatry. 63(7): 757-66, 2006.
Long. P. www.mentalhealth.com. 2003.
Lopez M, Torpac MG. "The Texas Children's Medication Algorithm Project: Report of the Texas Consensus Conference Panel on Medication Treatment of Childhood Attention-Deficit/Hyperactivity Disorder. Part I." American Academy of Child and Adolescent Psychiatry, Volume 39, Number 7, 2000, pp. 908-19.
National Institute on Drug Abuse Research Report Series, Methamphetamine Abuse and Addiction, NIH Publication Number 02-4210 reprinted January 2002.
Noble. Textbook of Primary Care Medicine, p.466, 470. 3rd edition.

Patterson CJ, Gauthier S, Bergman H, Cohen C, Freightner JW, Feldman H, Hogan D. "Canadian Consensus Conference on Dementia: A Physician's Guide to Using the Recommendations." CMAJ, Volume 160, Number 12, 1999, pp. 1738-42.

Pliszka SR, Greenhill LL, Crismon ML, Sedillo A, Carlson C, Conners CK, McCracken JT, Swanson JM, Hughes CW, Llana ME.

Rees L, Lipsedge M, Ball C, ed. (1997). Textbook of Psychiatry. London: Oxford University Press, P. 109.

Stahl SM. Psychopharmacology of Antidepressants. London: Martin Dunitz, 1998.

Stahl SM. Psychopharmacology of Antipsychotics. London: Martin Dunitz, 1999.

Szewczyk M. "Women's Health: Depression and Related Disorders." Primary Care, Volume 24, Number 1, 1997, pp. 83-101.

Tasman. Psychiatry 1st ed. 1997. p.1208.

Troiden, 1989, Journal of Homosexuality. 17: 253-267.

Warneke L. "Breaking the urges of obsessive-compulsive disorder." Canadian Journal of Diagnosis, December 1996, h. page.

Weller EB, Weller RA, Fristad MA. "Bipolar Disorder in Children: Misdiagnosis, Underdiagnosis, and Future Directions." Journal of the American Academy of Child and Adolescent Psychiatry, Volume 34, Number 6, 1995, pp. 709-714.

Zimmerman, M. Interview Guide for Evaluating DSM-IV Psychiatric Disorders and the Mental Status Examination. East Greenwich, RI. Psych Products Press. 1994.

RESPIROLOGY

Andreoli, TE. Cecil Essentials of Medicine, sixth ed. WB Saunders Company. Philadelphia: 2004.

Bach PB, Brown C, Gelfand SE. Management of Acute Exacerbations of Chronic Obstructive Pulmonary Disease: A summary and Appraisal of Published Evidence. Annals of Internal Medicine 2001;134:600-620.

Augustino P, Ouriel K. Invasive approaches to treatment of venous thromboembolism. Circulation 2004;110(suppl 1): 1-27-1-34.

Balk RA. Optimum treatment of severe sepsis and septic shock: evidence in support of the recommendations. Disease-A-Month. 2004;50(4):168-213.

Bartlett JG, Dowell SF, Mandell LA et al. Practice Guidelines for the Management of Community-Acquired Pneumonia in Adults. Clin Infect Dis 2000;31:347-82.

Bass JB Jr, Farer LS, Hopewell PC, O'Brien R, Jacobs RF, Ruben F, Snider DE Jr, Thornton G. Treatment of tuberculosis and tuberculosis infection in adults and children. American Thoracic Society and The Centers for Disease Control and Prevention. Am J Respir Crit Care Med. 1994 May; 149(5):1359-74.

Baumann MH. Treatment of spontaneous pneumothorax. Curr Opin Pulm Med. 2000 Jul;6(4):275-80. Review.

Boulet LP, Becker A, Berube D, Beveridge R, Ernst P. Canadian Asthma Consensus Report, 1999. CMAJ 1999;161 (11 Suppl):S1-61.

Buller HR, Agnelli G, Hull RD, et al. Antithrombotic therapy for venous thromboembolic disease. Chest 2004;126:401S-428S.

Chunilal SD, Eikelboom JW, Attia J, et al. Dose this patient have pulmonary embolism? JAMA 2003;290:2849-2858.

Crapo JD, Glassroth JL, Karlinsky JB, Talmadge EK. Baum's Textbook of Pulmonary Diseases, seventh ed. Lippincott Williams & Wilkins. USA: 2003.

Dellinger RP, Carlet JM, Masur H, Gerlach H, Calandra T, Cohen J, Gea-Banacloche J, Keh D, Marshall JC, Parker MM, Ramsay G, Zimmerman JL, Vincent J-L, Levy MM. Surviving Sepsis Campaign guidelines for management of severe sepsis and septic shock. Critical Care Medicine 2004; 32(3):536-55.

Ferguson GT, Cherniack RM. Management of Chronic Obstructive Pulmonary Disease. N Engl J Med 1993; 328:1017.

Ferri, Fred F. Ferri's Clinical Advisor. Mosby/Elsevier Health Sciences: 2002.

Ferri, Fred F. Practical Guide to the Care of the Medical Patient, fifth ed. Mosby/Elsevier Sciences. St.Louis: 2001.

File TM. The epidemiology of respiratory tract infections. Semin Respir Infect 2000 Sep;15(3):184-94. Review.

Fine MJ, Auble TE, Yealy DM, Hanusa BH, Weissfeld LA, Singer DE, Coley CM, Marrie TJ, Kapoor WN. A prediction rule to identify low-risk patients with community-acquired pneumonia. N Engl J Med. 1997 Jan 23;336(4):243-50.

Gaine S. Pulmonary Hypertension. JAMA Dec 27, 2000. 284(25): 3160-3168.

Garcia D, Ageno W, Libby E. Update on the diagnosis and management of pulmonary embolism. Brit J Haematol 2005;131:301-312.

Geerts WH, Pineo GF, Heit JA, et al. Prevention of venous thromboembolism. Chest 2004;126:338S-400S.

Gorecka et al. Effect of long term oxygen therapy on survival in patients with chronic obstructive pulmonary disease with moderate hypoxaemia. Thorax 1997; 52(8):674-679.

Gotfried M, Freeman C. An update on community-acquired pneumonia in adults. Compr Ther 2000 Winter;26(4):283-93. Review.

Green DS, San Pedro GS. Empiric therapy of community-acquired pneumonia. Semin Respir Infect. 2000 Sep;15(3):227-33. Review.

Health Canada: Population and Public Health Branch. Management of Severe Acute Respiratory Syndrome (SARS) in Adults: Interim Guidance for Health Care Providers. Ottawa: 2003 July 2. Available: http://www.hc-sc.gc.ca/pphb-dgspsp/sars-sras/pdf/sars-clin-guide-20030703_e.pdf (accessed 2003 Oct 26).

Health Canada: Population and Public Health Branch. Recommended Laboratory Investigation of Severe Acute Respiratory. Ottawa: 2003 March 20. Available: http://www.hc-sc.gc.ca/pphb-dgspsp/sars-sras/sarslabrec_e.html (accessed 2003 Oct 26).

Health Canada: Population and Public Health Branch. Early Detection of Severe or Emerging Respiratory Infections through Severe Respiratory Illness (SRI) surveillance. Ottawa: 2004 Feb 4. Available: http://www.hc-sc.gc.ca/pphb-dgspsp/sars-sras/sri.html (accessed 2004 August 5).

Health Canada: Population and Public Health Branch. Outbreak Period. Otawa: 2003 Nov 4. Available: http://www.hc-sc.gc.ca/pphb-dgspsp/sars-sras/sarscasedef_e.html (accessed 2004 August 5).

Hershfield E. Tuberculosis: 9. Treatment. CMAJ 1999;161(4):405-11.

Holleman D, Simel D. Does the clinical examination predict airflow limitation? JAMA 1995; 273:313-319.

Hotchkiss RS and Karl IE. The pathophysiology and treatment of sepsis. N Engl J Med. 2003;348(2):138-150.

Lexi-Comp Inc. (Lexi-Drugs (Comp + SpecialitiesTM) Lexi-Comp Inc; Oct.12/2002 version

Light RW, Macgregor MI, Luchsinger PC, et al. Pleural effusions: the diagnostic separation of transudates and exudates. Ann Intern Med. 1972;77(4): 507-13.

Light RW. The management of parapneumonic effusions and empyema. Curr Opin Pulm Med. 1998 Jul;4(4):227-9. Review.

Light RW. Useful tests on the pleural fluid in the management of patients with pleural effusions. Curr Opin Pulm Med. 1999 Jul;5(4):245-9. Review.

Kasper DL, Braunwald E, Fauci AS, Hauser SL, Longo DL, Jameson JL, Isselbacher KJ. Eds. Harrison's Principles of Internal Medicine, sixteenth ed. McGraw-Hill Professional. USA: 2004.

Long R, Njoo H, Hershfield E. Tuberculosis: 3. Epidemiology of the disease in Canada. CMAJ 1999;160(8):1185-90.

Mansharamani NG, Koziel H. Chronic lung sepsis: lung abscess, bronchiectasis, and empyema. Current Opinion in Pulmonary Medicine 2003, 9:181-185.

McLoud TC, Swenson SJ. Lung carcinoma. Clin Chest Med. 1999 Dec;20(4):697-713, vii. Review.

McPhee SJ, Papadakis MA, Tierney LM. Current Medical Diagnosis and Treatment 2007, forty-seventh ed. McGraw-Hill Professional. USA: 2006.

Nguyen HB, Rivers EP, Abrahamian FM, Moran GJ, Abraham E, Trzeciak S, Huang DT, Osborn T, Stevens D. Severe sepsis and septic shock: Review of the literature and emergency department management guidelines. Ann Emerg Med. 2006. July; 48(1): 28-54.

O'Donnell DE, Aaron S, Bourbeau J et al. Canadian thoracic society recommendations for management of chronic obstructive pulmonary disease. Can Respir J. 2003; May-June;11(1) Suppl A: 17A.

Ost D, Fein A. Evaluation and management of the solitary pulmonary nodule. Am J Respir Crit Care Med. 2000 Sep;162(3 Pt 1):782-7. Review.

Ost D, Fein AM and Feinsilver SH. The solitary pulmonary nodule. NEJM. 2003 348: 2535-2542.

Parfrey H, Chilvers ER. Pleural disease—diagnosis and management. Practitioner. 1999 May;243(1598):412, 415-21. Review.

Pauwels RA, Buist AS, Calverly PM. Global Startegy for the Diagnosis, Management, and Prevention of Chronic Obstructive Pulmonary Disease. NHLBI/WHO Global Intiative for Chronic Obstructive Lung Disease (GOLD) Workshop Summary. Americal Journal of Respiratory and Critical Care Medicine. 2001;163:1256-1276.

Peiris JSM, Kwok DP, Osterhaus, ADME, Stohr K. The Severe Acute Respiratory Syndrom. NEJM. 2003 Dec:349(25):2431-41.

Reimer LG. Community-acquired bacterial pneumonias. Semin Respir Infect. 2000 Jun;15(2):95-100. Review.

Rivers E, Nguyen B, Havstad S, et al. Early goal-directed therapy in the treatment of severe sepsis and septic shock. N Engl J Med. 2001; 345(19): 1368-1377.

Sabatine MS. 2004. Pocket Medicine: The Massachusetts General Hospital Handbook of Internal Medicine. Philadelphia: Lippincott Williams and Wilkins. pp. 6-1 & 5-2.

Scharschmidt, Bruce F. Pocket Medicine: Internal Medicine Pulmonary Medicine. PocketMedicine.com: 2002.

Stein, PD, Saltzman, HA, Weg, JG. Clinical characteristics of patients with acute pulmonary embolism. Am J Cardiol 1991; 68:1723.

Stein PD, Fowler SE, Goodman LR, et al. Multidetector computed tomography for acute pulmonary embolism. NEJM 2006;354:2317-2327.

Tarascon Inc. 2004. Tarascon Pocket PharmacopoeiaTM 2004 edition. Lompoc: Tarascon Publishing.

Thrombosis Interest Group of Canada. Clinical Guides. 27 brief, evidence-based guides on thrombosis for general practitioners, downloadable to a pda. Available: www.tigc.org.

US Centers for Disease Control and Prevention (CDC). Severe acute respiratory syndrome (SARS): Information for Clinicians. Atlanta: The CDC; 2003 Oct 14. Available: http://www.cdc.gov/ncidod/sars/clinicians.htm (accessed 2003 Oct 26).

RHEUMATOLOGY

Crystal Induced Arthropathy
Cibere J. 4. Acute monoarthritis. CMAJ 2000;162(11):1577-83.

Degenerative Arthritis (DA)
ACR. Guidelines for the Medical Management of Osteoarthritis of the Hip — 11/95.
ACR. Guidelines for the Medical Management of Osteoarthritis of the Knee — 11/95.
Brady OH, Masri BA, Garbuz DS, Duncan CP. 10. Joint replacement of the hip and knee - when to refer and what to expect. CMAJ 2000;163(10):1285-91.
Wade, J.P. 15. Osteoporosis. CMAJ 2001;165(1):45-50.

General
Bookman AM. Clinical Evaluation of Arthritis. University of Toronto Foundations of Medical Practice Lecture. 2006.
Brater DC, Harris C, Redfern JS, Gertz BJ. Renal effects of COX-2-selective inhibitors. Amer J Nephrology 2001;21(1):1-15.
CMAJ Clinical Basics Rheumatology Series.
Clark BM 9. Physical & occupational therapy in the management of arthritis. CMAJ 2000;163(8):999-1005.
Ensworth S. 1. Is it arthritis? CMAJ 2000;162(7):1011-6.
Huang SHK. 7. Basics of therapy. CMAJ 2000;163(4):417-23
Klippel JH, Weyand CM, and Wortmann RL. Primer on Rheumatic Diseases, 11th ed. Arthritis Foundation, 1997.
Klinkhoff A. 5. Diagnosis and management of inflammatory polyarthritis. CMAJ 2000;162(13):1833-38.
Lacaille D. 8. Advanced therapy. CMAJ 2000;163(6):721-8.
Musculoskeletal Injury; (OPOT). Queen's Printer of Ontario, June 2000. www.opot.org
Ontario Musculoskeletal Therapeutics Review Panel. Ontario Treatment Guidelines for Osteoarthritis, Rheumatoid Arthritis, and Acute Price GE. 6. Localized therapy. CMAJ 2000;163(2):176-83.
Puttick MPE. 11. Evaluation of the patient with pain all over. CMAJ 2001;164(2):223-27.
Reid G, Esdaile JM. 3. Getting the most out of radiology. CMAJ 2000;162(9):1318-25.
Shojania K. 2. What laboratory tests are needed? CMAJ 2000;162(8):1157-63.
Taunton JE, Wilkinson M. 14. Diagnosis and management of anterior knee pain. CMAJ 2001;164(11):1595-601.
Tsang I. 12. Pain in the neck. CMAJ 2001;164(8):1182-7.
Wing PC. 13. Minimizing disability in patients with low-back pain. CMAJ 2001;164(19):1459-68.

Seropositive Rheumatic Disease
ACR Subcommittee on Rheumatoid Arthritis Guidelines, 2002. Guidelines for the Management of Rheumatoid Arthritis: 2002 Update.
Arthritis & Rheumatism 46(2):328-346.
ACR. Guidelines for Referral and Management of Systemic Lupus Erythematosus in Adults - 9/99.
Bathon JM, Martin RW, Fleischmann RM, et al. A comparison of etanercept and methotrexate in patients with early rheumatoid arthritis. N Engl J Med 2000;343:1586-93.
Bombardier C, Laine L, Reicin A, et al. Comparison of upper gastrointestinal toxicity of rofecoxib and naproxen in patients with rheumatoid arthritis. The VIGOR Study Group. N Engl J Med 2000;343:1520-28.
Kremer, JM. Rational use of new and existing disease-modifying agents in rheumatoid arthritis. Ann Intern Med 2001:134: 695-706.
Smetana, GW and Shmerling RH. Does this patient have temporal arteritis? JAMA 2002; 287:92-101.

UROLOGY

General Information
American Urological Association. http://www.auanet.org/guidelines/
American Association of Family Physicians. http://www.aafp.org/afp/20020415/1589.html
Ferri F. Practical Guide to the care of the medical patient (6th ed.) 2006. St. Louis: Mosby.
Goldman L, Ausiello D. Cecil Textbook of Medicine (22nd ed.) 2004. Philadelphia: Saunders (Elsevier).
Macfarlane MT. House Officer Series: Urology. (3rd ed.) 2001. Philadelphia: Lippincott Williams & Wilkins.
Tanagho EA, McAninch JW. Smith's General Urology. (16th ed.) 2004. McGraw-Hill Companies, Inc.
Urology Channel. http://www.urologychannel.com
Wein AJ, Kavoussi LR, Novick AC, Partin AW and C Peters CA. Campbell's Urology. (9th ed.) 2006. Philadelphia: WB Saunders Co.

Common Presenting Problems
Cohen RA and Brown RS. Microscopic hematuria. New England Journal of Medicine. 2003;348:2330-2338
Morton AR, Iliescu EA and Wilson JWL. Nephrology: 1. Investigation and treatment of recurrent kidney stones. CMAJ 166(2):213-218, Jan 2002
Teichman JMH. Acute renal colic from ureteral calculus. New England Journal of Medicine. 2004;350:684-693

Urological Emergencies
Galejs LE. Diagnosis and treatment of the acute scrotum. American Family Physician. 1999;59(4):817-24

Medications
Common Medications: Gray J (Editor). Therapeutic Choices (4th ed). Canadian Pharmacists Association, Ottawa, 2003.
Micromedex health care series. www.micromedex.com